Principles and Practice of Orthopaedic Sports Medicine

Principles and Practice of Orthopaedic Sports Medicine

Editors

WILLIAM E. GARRETT, JR., MD, PhD
Frank C. Wilson Professor and Chairman
Department of Orthopaedics
University of North Carolina School of Medicine
Chapel Hill, North Carolina

KEVIN P. SPEER, MD
Cary Orthopedic and Sports Medicine Specialists
Cary, North Carolina

DONALD T. KIRKENDALL, PhD
Clinical Assistant Professor
Department of Orthopaedics
University of North Carolina School of Medicine
Chapel Hill, North Carolina

Medical Illustrations by
Marsha Dohrmann Kitkowski

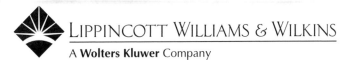

LIPPINCOTT WILLIAMS & WILKINS
A **Wolters Kluwer** Company
Philadelphia · Baltimore · New York · London
Buenos Aires · Hong Kong · Sydney · Tokyo

Acquisitions Editor: James Merritt
Developmental Editors: Sonya L. Seigafuse and Tanya Lazar
Production Editor: Steven P. Martin
Manufacturing Manager: Benjamin Rivera
Cover Designer: Catherine Lau Hunt
Compositor: The PRD Group, Inc.
Printer: Edwards Bros.

© 2000 by LIPPINCOTT WILLIAMS & WILKINS
530 Walnut Street
Philadelphia, PA 19106 USA
LWW.com

Printed in the USA

Library of Congress Cataloging-in-Publication Data

Principles and practice of orthopaedic sports medicine/editors, William E. Garrett, Jr.,
Kevin P. Speer, Donald T. Kirkendall; medical illustrations by Marsha Dohrmann Kitkowski,
    p.; cm.
  Includes bibliographical references.
  ISBN 0-7817-2578-X (casebound)
  1. Sports injuries. 2. Orthopedics. I. Garrett, William E. II. Speer, Kevin P. III.
Kirkendall, Donald T.
    [DNLM: 1. Sports Medicine. 2. Orthopedics. QT 260 P9565 2000]
RD97 .P77 2000
    617.1′027—dc21   00-027377

---

10 9 8 7 6 5 4 3 2 1

To my family: Both the family at home who makes work meaningful
And to the extended family at the office, laboratory, clinic,
And operating theater who makes work productive and fun.

WEG, Jr.

To the four women who make everything in my life possible:
Marcy, Kira, Casey, and my mother Willie.

KPS

To Mac and Louise for every opportunity,
Fritz for the direction,
Sara, Trevor, and Katy for the reason.

DTK

Contents

Contributing Authors xi

Preface xix

Part One: Basic Science for the Clinician

1. Skeletal Muscle Anatomy and Physiology 3
   Richard L. Lieber

2. Basic Science of Tendons 21
   Pekka Kannus, Laszlo Jozsa, and Markku Järvinen

3. Biomechanics of Ligaments: Healing and Reconstruction 39
   *Savio L.-Y. Woo, C. Benjamin Ma, Eric K. Wong, and
   A. Kihiro Kanamori*

4. Structure and Function of Articular Cartilage 53
   Farshid Guilak and Lori A. Setton

5. Bone Adaptation to Exercise in the Basic Science of Sports Medicine 75
   *Bert R. Mandelbaum, Luc Teurlings, and
   Joseph A. Buckwalter*

6. Acute and Chronic Compartment Syndrome 87
   Robert A. Pedowitz and Alan R. Hargens

7. Impact of Magnetic Resonance Imaging in Sports Medicine 99
   Charles E. Spritzer

8. Statistical Practices in Sports Medicine 121
   Mary Lou V. H. Greenfield

Part Two: Torso and Axial Skeleton

9. Intracranial and Cervical Spine Injuries 153
   Joseph S. Torg and Thomas A. Gennarelli

10. Brachial Plexus/Stingus 183
    Eliot Hershman and Jeffrey Berg

11. Low Back and Lumbar Spine Injuries in the Athlete 203
    William J. Richardson and Christopher G. Furey

12. Pelvis, Abdominal Wall and Adductors 215
    Scott A. Lynch and Per A.F.H. Renström

13. Athletic Pubalgia and Groin Pain 223
William C. Meyers, Rocco Ricciardi, Brian D. Busconi,
Bert R. Mandelbaum, and Richard J. Waite

Part Three: Upper Extremity

14. Hand Fractures 233
Robert J. Heaps and L. Scott Levin

15. Soft Tissue Injuries of the Hand 243
Richard S. Moore, Jr., Melissa Evans Talley, and
James R. Urbaniak

16. Fractures of the Carpal Bones 257
Andrew E. Caputo and Richard D. Goldner

17. Injuries to the Soft Tissues of the Wrist 273
James A. Nunley and Thomas Goetz

18. Tendiopathies about the Elbow 289
Jeffrey E. Budoff and Robert P. Nirschl

19. Elbow Injuries 307
Laura A. Timmerman

20. Anatomy of the Shoulder 329
Jeffrey R. Dugas, Bryan T. Kelly, and Stephen J. O'Brien

21. Biomechanics of the Shoulder 367
Louis J. Soslowsky, James E. Carpenter, and John E. Kuhn

22. Anterior Shoulder Instability 399
Daniel J. Stechschulte, Jr. and Russell F. Warren

23. Posterior Shoulder Instability 413
James P. Bradley and James E. Tibone

24. Labral Injuries in Contact Sports 431
Anthony J. Delfico and Kevin P. Speer

25. Labral Tears in Throwing Sports 457
James R. Andrews, John H. (Rus) Fairbanks, Kevin E. Wilk,
Glenn S. Fleisig, and Martin L. Schwartz

26. Rotator Cuff Injuries 479
Guido Marra and Evan L. Flatow

27. Scapular Disorders 497
W. Ben Kibler

28. Acromioclavicular Injuries 511
Carl J. Basamania

29. Clavicular and Sternoclavicular Injuries 535
William N. Levine and Claude T. Moorman, III

30. Nerve Injuries in the Upper Extremity 543
Scott Lintner

31. The Concept of Overhead Athletic Injuries 551
Marilyn M. Pink and Frank W. Jobe

Part Four: Lower Extremity

32. Hip Injuries in Sports: Evaluation and Treatment of the Painful Hip 571
Thomas Parker Vail and Diane Beal Covington

33. Injuries to the Thigh and Groin 583
Rolf H. Langeland and Robert J. Carangelo

34. The Physical Examination of the Knee 613
John A. Feagin, Jr.

35. Anatomy and Biomechanics of the Knee 623
Bruce D. Beynnon

36. Knee Meniscus 645
Julie A. Dodds, Douglas P. Dietzel, and Steven P. Arnoczky

37. Medial and Posteromedial Ligament Injuries of the Knee 663
C. Christopher Stroud and Bruce Reider

38. Posterolateral Injuries of the Knee 675
Michael J. Maynard

39. Diagnosis and Treatment of Knee Tendon Injury 687
Scott A. Rodeo and Kazutaka Izawa

40. Acute and Chronic Injuries to the Patellofemoral Joint 709
Nader Q. Kasim and John P. Fulkerson

41. Treatment of Anterior Cruciate Ligament Injuries 743
Donald Shelbourne and Douglas A. Foulk

42. Posterior Cruciate Ligament 763
Leslie J. Bisson and William G. Clancy, Jr

43. Articular Cartilage 787
Andrew S. Levy and David H. Goltz

44. Acute Multi-ligament Injuries of the Knee 805
Laurence Higgins and Christopher D. Harner

45. Ankle Impingement Syndromes 819
*Thomas P. Knapp, William M. Hayes, and
Bert R. Mandelbaum*

46. Surgical Complications of the Knee 825
Herb O. Boté and Lonnie E. Paulos

47. The Degenerative Knee 845
Garron G. Weiker and James DeVellis

48. Anterior Cruciate Ligament Functional Bracing 863
Edward M. Wojtys

49. The Leg 869
Barry P. Boden

50. Athletic Injuries of the Midfoot and Hindfoot 893
Michael W. Bowman

51. Forefoot Injuries in the Athlete 945
James A. Nunley and Penny Jo Lawlin

52. Toe Injuries and Related Conditions 965
Lamar L. Fleming

53. The Foot and Ankle Tendons 979
Roger A. Mann, Mark M. Casillas, and Michael J. Coughlin

54. The Concepts of Running Injuries 1011
Stanley L. James

Index 1027

Contributing Authors

James R. Andrews, MD
Clinical Professor of Orthopaedic Surgery
University of Alabama at Birmingham
Birmingham, Alabama 35205

Steven P. Arnoczky, DVM
Director
Laboratory for Comparative Orthopaedic
* Research*
Wade O. Brinker Endowed Professor of
* Surgery*
College of Veterinary Medicine
Professor of Surgery (Orthopaedic)
College of Osteopathic Medicine
Michigan State University
East Lansing, Michigan 48824

Carl J. Basamania, MD, FACS
Assistant Professor of Surgery
Division of Orthopedic Surgery
Duke University Medical Center
Durhama, North Carolina 27705

Jeffrey Berg
Lennox Hill Hospital
1307 East 77th Street
New York, New York 10021

Bruce D. Beynnon, PhD
Associate Professor
Director Of Research
Department Of Orthopaedics & Rehabilitation
McClure Musculoskeletal Research Center
University of Vermont
438A Stafford Hall
Burlington, Vermont 05405-0084

Leslie J. Bisson, MD
Attending Surgeon
Orthopaedics
Kalinda Hospital System
Buffalo, New York
Northtowns Orthopaedics, P.C.
8750 Transit Road
East Amherst, New York 14051

Barry P. Boden, MD
Adjunct Assistant Professor
Department of Surgery
The Uniformed Services University of the
* Health Sciences*
2101 Medical Park Drive No.305
Silver Spring, Maryland 20902
The Orthopaedic Center
9711 Medical Center Drive No.201
Rockville, Maryland 20850

Herb O. Boté, MD
Stephens Memorial Hospital
181 Main Street
Norway, Maine 04268

Michael W. Bowman, MD, FACS
Clinical Assistant Professor
University Of Orthopaedics
University Of Pittsburgh
5820 Center Avenue
Pittsburgh, Pennsylvania 15206

James P. Bradley, MD
Clinical Associate Professor
University of Pittsburgh
Department of Orthopaedic Surgery
Team Physician
Pittsburgh Steelers Football Club
Director
Pittsburgh Center For Sports Medicine
UPMC Shadyside Hospital
5230 Center Avenue
Pittsburgh, Pennsylvania 15232

Joseph A. Buckwalter, MD
University of Iowa Hospital
Department of Orthopaedics
200 Hawkins Drive
Iowa, City, Iowa 52242

Jeffrey E. Budoff, MD
Assistant Professor
Department Of Orthopaedic Surgery
Baylor College Of Medicine
6550 Fannin Road #2525
Houston, Texas 77030

Brian D. Busconi, MD
Assistant Professor
University of Massachusetts Medical Center
Department of Orthopaedics
55 Lake Avenue North
Worcester, Massachusetts 01655

Andrew E. Caputo, MD
Assistant Clinical Professor
Department of Orthopaedic Surgery
University of Connecticut Health Center
10 Talcott Notch
Farmington, Connecticut 06032
Co-Director
Hand Surgery Service
Hartford Hospital & Connecticut Children's
* Medical Center*
Hartford, Connecticut 06106

Robert J. Carangelo, MD
Associate Clinical Professor
Department Of Orthopaedic Surgery
University of Connecticut
10 Talcott Notch
Farmington, Connecticut 06034
Attending Surgeon
Department of Orthopaedics
New Britain General Hospital
40 Hart Street, Bldg. 4
New Britain, Connecticut 06052

James E. Carpenter, MD
Associate Professor of Orthopaedic Surgery
Department Of Surgery
University Of Michigan
Associate Medical Director
MedSport
University of Michigan
24 Frank Lloyd Wright Drive
Ann Arbor, Michigan 48106-0363

Mark M. Casillas, MD
Orthopaedic Surgeon
Orthopaedic Surgery Associates
San Antonio, Texas 78205

William G. Clancy, Jr., MD
Clinical Professor of Orthopaedic Surgery
University of Alabama at Birmingham
Birmingham, Alabama 35205

Mark Clatworthy, MD
Fellow, Sports Medicine
University of Pittsburgh
Pittsburgh, Pennsylvania 15232

Michael J. Coughlin, MD
Staff Orthopaedic Surgeon
St. Alphonsus Regional Medical Center
Boise, Idaho 83706

Diane Beal Covington, PA-C, ATC
Senior Physician Assistant
Division of Orthopaedic Surgery
Department Of Surgery
Box 3332
Duke University Medical Center
Durham, North Carolina 27710

Anthony J. Delfico, MD
Duke University Medical Center
Division of Orthopaedic Surgery
Section of Sports Medicine & Shoulder
* Surgery*
Durham, North Carolina 27710

James DeVellis, MD
Department of Orthopaedic Surgery
A-41
Cleveland Clinic Foundation
9500 Euclid Avenue
Cleveland, Ohio 44195

Douglas P. Dietzel, DO, ATC
Assistant Professor
Department of Osteopathic Surgical Specialties
College of Osteopathic Medicine
Michigan State University
East Lansing, Michigan 48824
Orthopaedic Surgeon
Ingham Regional Medical Center
Lansing, Michigan 48910

Julie A. Dodds, MD
Associate Professor
College of Human Medicine
Orthopaedic Consultant
Department of Intercollegiate Athletics
Michigan State University
East Lansing, Michigan 48823

Jeffrey R. Dugas, MD
Othopaedic Sports Medicine Fellow
American Sports Medicine Institute
1313 13th St, South
Birmingham, Alabama 35205

John H. (Rus) Fairbanks, MD
Clinical Professor of Orthopaedic Surgery
University of Alabama at Birmingham
Birmingham, Alabama 35205

John A. Feagin, Jr., MD
Professor Of Surgery
Department Of Surgery
Duke University Medical Center
Box 3698-DUMC
Durham, North Carolina 27709

Evan L. Flatow, MD
Professor
Department of Orthopaedics
Mount Sinai Medical School
5 East 98th Street
Box 1188
New York, New York 10029

Glenn S. Fleisig, PhD
Clinical Professor of Orthopaedic Surgery
University of Alabama at Birmingham
Birmingham, Alabama 35205

Lamar L. Fleming
Professor
Department Of Orthopaedics
Emory University
69 Butler Street SE, Room 402
Atlanta, Georgia 30302

Douglas A. Foulk, MD
Department of Orthopaedics
University of Colorado Health Science Center
5250 Leetsdale
Denver, Colorado 80222

John P. Fulkerson, MD
Associate Professor
Department Of Orthopaedic Surgery
University Of Connecticut Medical School
270 Farmington Ave., Suite 364
Farmington, Connecticut 06032

Christopher G. Furey, MD
Division of Orthopedic Sugery
Duke University Medical Center
Durham, North Carolina 27710

Thomas A. Gennarelli, MD
Professor and Chairman
Department of Neurosurgery
Medical College of Wisconsin
8701 Watertown Plank Road
Milwaukee, Wisconsin 53226

Thomas Goetz, MD
Orthopaedic Surgery
Duke University Medical Center
Box 2923 DUMC
Durham, North Carolina 27710

Richard D. Goldner, MD
Associate Professor
Division of Orthopaedic Surgery
Duke Medical Center
Durham, North Carolina 27710

David H. Goltz, MD
Department of Orthopaedic Surgery
New Jersey Medical School
Newark, New Jersey

Mary Lou V.H. Greenfield, MPH, MS
Senior Research Associate
The University of Michigan
Department of Anesthesiology
Clinical Research Offices
1G323 University Hospital
1500 East Medical Center Drive
Ann Arbor, Michigan 48109-0048

Farshid Guilak, PhD
Director of Orthopaedic Research
Department Of Surgery
Duke University Medical Center
375 Medical Sciences Research Building
Box 3093
Durham, North Carolina 27710

Alan R. Hargens, PhD
University of California, San Diego
Department of Orthopaedics
350 Dickinson Street
San Diego, California 92103-8894

Christopher D. Harner, MD
Professor
Chief, Division of Sports Medicine
Department of Orthopaedic Surgery
University of Pittsburgh
4601 Baum Boulevard.
Pittsburgh, Pennsylvania 15213

William M. Hayes, MD
Department of Orthopaedics
UTMB/Conroe Family Practice Residency
  Program
701 East Davis
Suite C
Conroe, Texas 77301
Orthopaedic and Sports Medicine
Tomball Regional Hospital
605 Holderrieth
Tomball, Texas 77375

Robert J. Heaps, MD
Attending Surgeon
The Orthopaedic Center
505 West Hollis Street
Nashua, New Hampshire 03062

Elliott B. Hershman, MD
Executive Associate Director
Department Of Orthopaedic Surgery
Lenox Hill Hospital
130 East 77th Street
New York, New York 10021

Laurence D. Higgins, MD
Assistant Professor
Department of Surgery
Division of Orthopaedics
Duke University Medical Center
Box 3615
Durham, North Carolina 27710

Kazutaka Izawa, MD
Attending Orthopaedic Surgeon
Department Of Orthopaedic Surgery
Toneyama National Hospital
511 Toneyama, Toyemaka City
Osaka, 560-8552, Japan

Stan L. James, MD
Courtesy Professor
Department Of Exercise And Movement
Science
University Of Oregon
Eugene, Oregon 97403
1200 Hillard Street, No. 600
Eugene, Oregon 97401

Frank W. Jobe, MD
Clinical Professor
University Of Southern California
School Of Medicine
Los Angeles, California 90045

Markku Järvinen, MD, PhD
Professor
Medical School and Department of Surgery
Tampere Medical School and University
Hospital
PO Box 617
FIndiana-33501, Tampere, Finland

Laszlo Jozsa, MD, PhD
Chief Physician
Department of Morphology
National Institute of Traumatology
PO Box 21
H-1430 Budapest, Hungary

Pekka Kannus, MD, PhD
Chief Physician And Head
Accident & Trauma Research Center and
Tampere Research
Center of Sports Medicine, UKK Institute
PO Box 30
FIN - 33501 Tampere, Finland

Kihiro Kanamori
Research Fellow
Department Of Orthopaedic Surgery
University Of Pittsburgh
E1641 Biomedical Science Tower
PO Box 71199
Pittsburgh, Pennsylvania 15213

Nader Q. Kasim, MD
Orthopaedic Surgeon
Department of Orthopaedic Surgery
JFK Medical Center
65 James Street
Edison, New Jersey

Bryan T. Kelly, MD
Department of Orthopaedic Surgery
The Hospital for Special Surgery
535 E. 70th Street
New York, New York 10021

Benjamin W. Kibler, MD
Medical Director
Lexington Sports Medicine Center
1221 S. Broadway
Lexington, Kentucky 40504

Thomas P. Knapp, MD
Clinical Instructor
Department of Orthopaedic Surgery
University of Southern California
1301 21st Street, Suite 150
Associate Chair
Department of Orthopaedic Surgery
Saint John's Health Center
1328 22nd Street
Santa Monica, California 90404

Virginia B. Kraus, MD, PhD
Assistant Professor
Division of Rheumatology, Allergy and
Clinical Immunology
Department of Medicine
Duke University Medical Center
Durham, North Carolina 27710

John E. Kuhn, MD
Assistant Professor of Orthopaedic Surgery
MedSport
University of Michigan Shoulder Group
24 Frank Lloyd Wright Dr.
Ann Arbor, Michigan 48106

Rolf H. Langeland, MD
Orthopaedic Surgeon
Orthopaedic Specialty Group
75 Kings Highway Cutoff
Fairfield, Connecticut 06430
Department of Surgery
Bridgeport Hospital
Mill Hill Avenue
Bridgeport, Connecticut 06610

L. Scott Levin, MD
Associate Professor
Orthopaedic & Plastic Surgery
Chief
Division of Plastic Surgery
Duke University Medical Center
134 Baker House, Box 3945
Durham, North Carolina 27710

William N. Levine, MD
Director, Sports Medicine
Assistant Professor Orthopaedic Surgery
Columbia-Presbyterian Medical Center
622 West 168th Street, PH-1117
New York, New York 10032

Andrew S. Levy, MD
Overlook Hospital
Medical Arts Center Building
33 Overlook Road, Suite 409
Summit, New Jersey 07902

Richard L. Lieber, PhD
Professor of Orthopaedics and Bioengineering
Biomedical Sciences Graduate Group
Departments of Orthopaedics and
  Bioengineering
University of California San Diego School of
  Medicine
VA Medical Center
9500 Gilman Drive
La Jolla, California 92093-9151

Scott A. Lintner, MD
Orthopaedics Indianapolis
8450 Northwest Boulevard
Medical Director-Sports Medincine
Orthopaedic Surgery
Street Vincent Hospital
Indianapolis, Indiana 46278

Scott A. Lynch, MD
Assistant Professor
Department of Orthopaedics and
  Rehabilitation
College of Medicine
Penn State University
P.O. Box 850, H089
Hershey, Pennsylvania 17033
Hershey Medical Center
P.O. Box 850, H089
Hershey, Pennsylvania 17033

C. Benjamin Ma, MD
Musculoskeletal Research Center
Department Of Orthopaedic Surgery
Kaufmann Building
3471 5th Avenue 101
Pittsburgh, Pennsylvania 15213

Bert R. Mandelbaum, MD
Fellowship Director
Santa Monica Orthopaedic and Sports
  Medicine Group
1301 20th Street
Suite 150
Santa Monica, California 90404

Roger Mann, MD
Director
Foot and Ankle Fellowship
Oakland, California 94609

Guido Marra, MD
Instructor
Department of Orthopaedic Surgery
Loyola University Medical Center
2160 South First Avenue
Maywood, Illinois 60153

Michael J. Maynard, MD
The Hospital for Special Surgery
535 E. 70th Street
Department of Orthopaedic Surgery
New York, New York 10021

William C. Meyers, MD
Professor & Chairman
University of Massachusetts Medical School
Department of Surgery
55 Lake Avenue North
Worcester, Massachusetts 01655

Richard S. Moore, Jr., MD
Assistant Professor of Surgery
Division of Orthopaedic Surgery
Duke University Medical Center
Box 3384
Trent Drive
Durham, North Carolina 27710

Claude T. Moorman, III, MD
Assistant Professor of Surgery
University of Maryland School of Medicine
Director of Sports Medicine
University of Maryland Medical Center
2200 Kernan Drive
Baltimore, Maryland 21207

Robert P. Nirschl, MD
Associate Clinical Professor
Department of Orthopaedic Surgery
Georgetown University
1715 N. George Mason Drive #504
Director of Orthopaedic Sports Medicine
Nirschl Clinic
Arlington Hospital
1715 N. George Mason Drive
Arlington, Virginia 22205

James A. Nunley, MD
Professor and Vice-Chairman
Department Of Orthopaedic Surgery
Duke University Medical School
Box 2923
Durham, North Carolina 27710

Stephen J. O'Brien, MD
Associate Professor
Department of Orthopaedic Surgery
The Hospital for Special Surgery
535 E. 70th Street
New York, New York 10021

Lonnie E. Paulos, MD
The Orthopedic Specialty Hospital
5848 South 300 East
Salt Lake City, Utah 84107

Robert A. Pedowitz, MD, PhD
Associate Professor of Clinical Orthopaedics
Department Of Orthopaedics
University Of California, San Diego
200 West Arbor Dr., Dept. 8894
San Diego, California 92103-8894

Marilyn M. Pink, PhD, PT
Director, Biomechanics Laboratory
Centinela Hospital Medical Center
555 E. Hardy Street
Inglewood, California 90301

Bruce Reider, MD
Professor
Department of Orthopaedic Surgery
University Of Chicago
5841 S. Maryland Ave.
Box 421
Chicago, Illinios 60637

Per A. F. H. Renström, MD, PhD
Professor
Section of Sports Medicine
Department of Orthopedics
Karolinska Hospital
S-17176 Stockholm, Sweden

Rocco Ricciardi, MD
Surgical Research Fellow
University of Massachusetts Medical School
Department of Surgery
55 Lake Avenue North
Worcester, Massachusetts 01655

William J. Richardson, MD
Division of Orthopedic Surgery
Duke University Medical Center
Box 3077
Durham, North Carolina 27710

Scott A. Rodeo, MD
Department of Orthopaedic Surgery
The Hospital for Special Surgery
535 East 70th Street
New York, New York 10021

Martin L. Schwartz, PhD
Clinical Professor of Orthopaedic Surgery
University of Alabama at Birmingham
Birmingham, Alabama 35205

Lori A. Setton, PhD
Department of Biomedical Engineering
Duke University
Durham, North Carolina 27710

K. Donald Shelbourne, MD
Associate Professor
Department of Orthopaedics
Indiana University
School of Medicine
Orthopaedic Surgeon
Methodist Sports Medicine Center
1815 N. Capitol Ave.
Suite 530
Indianapolis, Indiana 46202

Louis J. Soslowsky, PhD
Associate Professor of Orthopaedic Surgery
* and Bioengineering*
Director of Orthopaedic Research
Mckay Orthopaedic Research Laboratory
University of Pennsylvania
424 Stemmler Hall
Philadelphia, Pennsylvania 19104-6081

Kevin P. Speer, MD, FACSM
Cary Orthopedic and Sports Medicine
* Specialists*
101 SW Cary Parkway, Suite 100
Cary, North Carolina 27511

Charles E. Spritzer, MD
Associate Professor of Radiology
Department of Radiology
Duke University Medical Center
Box 3808
Durham, North Carolina 27710

Daniel J. Stechschulte, Jr., MD, PhD
Assistant Clinical Professor of Surgery
* (Orthopaedics)*
Department of Surgery
University of Kansas Medical Center
3901 Rainbow Boulevard
Kansas City, Kansas 66160
Attending Orthopaedic Surgeon
Kansas City Orthopaedic Institute
10400 Mohawk Lane,
Leawood, Kansas 66206

C. Christopher Stroud, MD
Attending Physician
Department of Orthopaedic Surgery
Union Memorial Hospital
3333 N. Calvert Street, Suite 400
Baltimore, Maryland 21218

Melissa Evans Talley, OTR/L
Hand Therapist
Department of Physical and Occupational
* Therapy*
Duke University Medical Center
Durham, North Carolina 27710

Luc Teurlings, MD
Orthopaedic Surgeon
Department of Orthopaedics
Diagnostic Clinic
3131 N. McMullen Booth Road
Clearwater, FL 33761

James E. Tibone, MD
Clinical Professor
Department of Orthopaedics
University of Southern California
1510 San Pablo No. 322
Los Angeles, California 90033
Associate
Kerlan Jobe Orthopaedic Clinic
6801 Park Terrace
Los Angeles, California 90045

Laura A. Timmerman, MD
Team Physician
Department of Health Services
University of California, Berkeley
Orthopaedic Surgeon Private Practice,
Walnut Creek, California 94598
112 La Casa Via
Suite 125
Walnut Creek, California 94598

Joseph S. Torg, MD
Professor and Interim Chairman
Department of Orthopedic Surgery
MCP Hahnemann University & Hospital
* School of Medicine*
245 N. 15th Street, Mail Stop 420
Broad & Vine Street
Philadelphia, Pennsylvania 19102

James R. Urbaniak, MD
Professor and Chief
Division of Orthopaedic Surgery
Duke University Medical Center
Durham, North Carolina 27710

Thomas Parker Vail, MD
Division of Orthopaedic Surgery
Box 3332
Duke University Medical Center
Durham, North Carolina 27710

Richard J. Waite, MD
Associate Professor
Department of Radiology
University of Massachusetts Medical Center
Department of Surgery
55 Lake Avenue North
Worcester, Massachusetts 01655

Russell F. Warren, MD
The Sports Medicine/Shoulder Service
The Hospital for Special Surgery
Affiliated with the New York Hospital -
  Cornell University Medical College
535 East 70th Street
New York, New York 10021

Garron G. Weiker, MD
Orthopaedic Surgeon
Department of Orthopaedic Surgery
Desk A-41
Cleveland Clinic Foundation
9500 Euclid Avenue
Cleveland, Ohio 44195

Kevin Wilk, PT
Director, Rehabilitative Research
American Sports Medicine Institute
Birmingham, Alabama 35205

Edward M. Wojtys, MD
MedSport
24 Frank Lloyd Wright Drive
PO Box 363
Ann Arbor, Michigan 48106-0363

Eric K. Wong
Kaufmann Building
3471 5th Avenue 101
Pittsburgh, Pennsylvania 15213

Savio L. Y. Woo, PhD, DSc
Ferguson Professor
Department of Orthopaedic Surgery
University of Pittsburgh
Kaufmann Building
3471 5th Avenue 101
Pittsburgh, Pennsylvania 15213

Preface

Principles and Practice of Orthopaedic Sports Medicine is the orthopaedic component of a three-volume series on sports medicine. Although the subject matter is complex and the audience is diverse, including exercise physiologists, biomechanists, and sports medicine physicians, we hope that the text will serve as the definitive reference for all serious students of sports medicine.

Perhaps the simplest component of sports medicine is the study of "performance" as applied to exercise of athletic participation. All of the basic science of sports medicine builds from its very component. For exercise physiologists, the study of sports medicine has led to investigations of the responses to exercise and the adaptations to training of those individuals with acute or chronic disease, normal or untrained persons, and competitive athletes. Biomechanists have defined the mechanics of both the specific skills required in each sport and the injuries that can occur in that sport. They have also described cellular and tissue biomechanics.

This volume focuses on the diagnosis, evaluation, and treatment of the musculoskeletal aspects of sports medicine. Our goal is to present musculoskeletal injury in a broad continuum. This book emphasizes diagnosis, evaluation, and conservative care for these injuries. Surgical treatment is also discussed where appropriate in the management of each condition. The material is organized according to anatomic parts that support the differential approaches that clinicians use when evaluating an injury. In addition, aspects of injury within the most common sports are presented because of the uniqueness of the demands and challenges within that sport. Each author has a great deal of experience regarding the subject matter in their assigned chapter, so as to reflect not only a literature consensus on approaches and strategies for treating a musculoskeletal injury, but the benefit of enhanced experience and expertise. When it comes to the care of musculoskeletal injuries in athletes and athletic individuals, there is no substitute for experience.

We hope that *Principles and Practice of Orthopaedic Sports Medicine* will be useful not only to the basic scientists involved in the study of sports medicine, but to all other experts in the discipline, because the understanding of these topics will form the basis of future developments in sports medicine. In the other volumes we cover exercise and sport science and primary care aspects of sports medicine.

All of us involved in this project are indebted to the staff at Lippincott Williams & Wilkins: Darlene Cook and Fran Klass, who helped us get this project under way and Danette Knopp, Tanya Lazar, Sonya Seigafuse, and Steven Martin, whose continued patience throughout this project must be commended. The guidance of Lottie Applewhite, the author's editor, and the efforts of Marsha Dohrmann Kitkowski, medical illustrator, cannot be overstated. Without the help of these people, we would still be way over our heads and struggling to complete our work.

William E. Garrett, Jr., MD, PhD
Kevin P. Speer, MD
Donald T. Kirkendall, PhD

PART I

Basic Science for the Clinician

Principles and Practice of Orthopaedic Sports Medicine,
edited by William E. Garrett, Jr., Kevin P. Speer, and Donald T. Kirkendall.
Lippincott Williams & Wilkins, Philadelphia © 2000.

CHAPTER 1

Skeletal Muscle Anatomy and Physiology

Richard L. Lieber

Skeletal muscle represents a classic example of a structure–function relationship. At both the macro- and microscopic levels, skeletal muscle is exquisitely tailored for force generation and movement. This chapter reviews basic muscle structure and the physiologic properties of skeletal muscle that are relevant to the field of sports medicine. First, the structure of the skeletal muscle cell is reviewed. The manner in which cells are organized into muscle tissue is then explained in the context of muscle architecture. Next, the specialization of cells into fiber types is presented along with the functional implications of such specialization. Finally, the physiologic processes involved in muscle contraction and, somewhat, in normal movement are presented. It will be seen that skeletal muscle is an extremely well-studied tissue and that an understanding of muscle physiology is requisite for understanding the basis of exercise programs, muscle injury, surgical repair of skeletal muscle, and possible applications of gene therapy to repair of injured muscle tissue.

SKELETAL MUSCLE CELL STRUCTURE

Skeletal muscle fibers are cells that in many ways are like any other bodily cell. However, because muscle cell function is highly specialized to produce force and movement, the cellular components are also highly specialized (Fig. 1.1).

Muscle Fiber Diameter and Length

Muscle cells (fibers) are cylindrical, with a diameter ranging from about 10 to about 100 μm—less than the diameter of a human hair. Muscle fiber diameter is of

R. L. Lieber: Departments of Orthopaedics and Bioengineering, University of California, San Diego, La Jolla, California 92093-9151.

profound importance for at least two reasons. First, a muscle fiber's diameter determines its maximum isometric strength, and second, when fiber diameter changes in mature muscle, this suggests that the level of muscle use has changed. Increased muscle fiber diameter represents the response to increased loading and represents cellular hypertrophy (increased cell diameter with no change in cell number). This is the primary response of skeletal muscle to strength training. There is evidence, especially in chicken muscle, that muscle fiber number can increase (1), but this cannot, in general, account for much of muscle's strength gain after strength training. Decreased muscle fiber diameter represents the response to decreased use, such as is observed after muscle immobilization, space flight, or prolonged bedrest. Muscle fiber size is highly regulated so that muscle will attempt to maintain appropriate strength to support the loads imposed upon it.

In addition to muscle cell diameter, muscle cell length is also highly variable, depending on muscle architecture (see below). Fiber length has the greatest influence on fiber contraction velocity compared with any other single structural feature within the cell.

Muscle Connective Tissue Matrix

A meshlike sheath of collagenous tissue, called the endomysium, surrounds each muscle fiber. The endomysium may play some role in the passive mechanical properties of the cell, but this has not been definitively determined. Bundles of fibers, each surrounded by endomysial tissue, are organized into muscle fascicles, each surrounded by a more stout perimysial tissue (Fig. 1.2). Finally, bundles of fascicles are organized into muscles, surrounded by epimysial connective tissue. Recent studies suggest that muscle fibers are intimately associated with this complex connective tissue matrix and that muscle fibers themselves do not simply extend from one tendon plate to the other (2–5). This organization im-

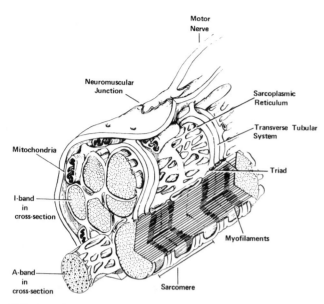

FIG. 1.1. Skeletal muscle cell. The cell is specialized for force production but, like other cells, contains nuclei, mitochondria, cytoskeletal components, and metabolic enzymes.

plies that the connective tissue matrix may play a central role in muscle fiber-to-tendon tension transmission and not merely a supportive one.

Muscle Contractile Protein Hierarchy

Perhaps the most distinctive feature of the muscle cell is the ordered array of contractile filaments that are arranged throughout the cell (Fig. 1.3). There is a well-defined hierarchy of filament organization that proceeds from a large scale (on the order of microns) to a small scale (on the order of angstroms). The largest functional unit of contractile filaments is the myofibril. A myofibril is simply a string of sarcomeres arranged in series. Myofibrillar diameter is about 1 μm, indicating that thousands of myofibrils can be packed into a single muscle fiber. Myofibrils are arranged in parallel to make up the muscle fiber. However, their arrangement might not simply be like a bundle of spaghetti; there is some evidence that myofibrils within the fiber are arranged similar to the weave in a rope (6).

Myofibrils are subdivided into their component units known as sarcomeres (Fig. 1.3), the functional unit of muscle contraction. A myofibril is therefore hundreds or thousands of sarcomeres arranged in series. The total number of sarcomeres within a fiber depends on muscle fiber length and diameter. Because of the series arrangement of sarcomeres within a myofibril, the total distance of myofibrillar shortening is equal to the sum of the individual shortening distances of the individual sarcomeres. This is why a whole muscle may shorten several

centimeters even though each sarcomere can only shorten about 1 μm.

Sarcomeres are composed of contractile filaments. Two major sets of contractile filaments exist within the sarcomere, and these thick and thin filaments represent large polymers of the proteins myosin and actin, respectively. The myosin-containing filaments (thick filaments) and the actin-containing filaments (thin filaments) interdigitate to form a hexagonal lattice (Fig. 1.4). It is the active interdigitation of these microscopic filaments that produces muscle shortening. It is also this interdigitated pattern that gives the muscle its striated or striped appearance that is observable microscopically.

Various regions of the sarcomere are named so that reference can be made to them (Fig. 1.4). For example, the sarcomere region containing the myosin filaments is known as the A band (A stands for "anisotropic," which is an optical term describing what this band does to incoming light). The region containing the actin filament is known as the I band (I stands for "isotropic"). The region of the A band where there is no actin–myosin overlap is called the H zone (H stands for *helle*, which is German for "light"). The dark narrow line that bisects the I band is the Z band (Z stands for *zwitter*, which is German for "between"). Finally, the relatively dense structures noted in the center of the A band are

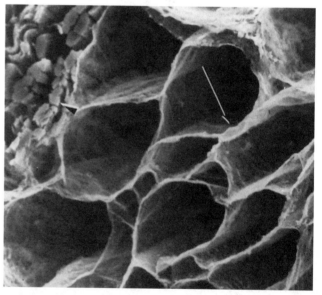

FIG. 1.2. Scanning electron micrograph of the endomysial connective tissue matrix within a skeletal muscle whose fibers were removed by acid digestion. (Courtesy of John Trotter, University of New Mexico.) Whole muscle structure should thus be viewed as muscle fibers embedded in a connective tissue matrix, and each fiber may not run from tendon plate to tendon plate. The mechanics of force transmission from muscle fibers to external tendons is thus not completely understood.

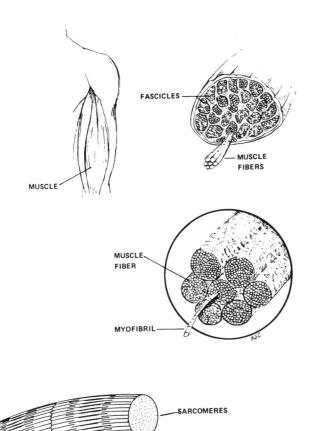

FIG. 1.3. Structural hierarchy of skeletal muscle. Whole skeletal muscles are composed of numerous fascicles of muscle fibers. Muscle fibers are composed of myofibrils arranged in parallel. Myofibrils are composed of sarcomeres arranged in series. Sarcomeres are composed of interdigitating actin and myosin filaments.

known as the M band. The distance from one Z band to the next is defined as the sarcomere length, which is an important variable relative to force generation.

Myosin Is the Motor in Skeletal Muscle

The myosin-containing filament is a polymer of molecules that are relatively large proteins (about 230 kDa) known as the myosin heavy chain (MHC) along with smaller proteins associated with each MHC molecule known as the myosin light chain (7). The MHC is one of the most widely studied proteins in all of biology because it is found in all cells (8,9) and is the motor that drives muscle contraction, drives other cellular motile processes such as cytokinesis (cell division), and is even involved in hearing transduction. Most definitions of muscle fiber types are based primarily on the cellular expression of a particular MHC isoform, with slow (type 1) muscle fibers expressing a slow-

contracting myosin and faster contracting fibers expressing one or more types of fast-contracting (type 2) MHC (see below).

Actin Regulates Muscle Contraction

The structure of the actin-containing filament is equally as elegant as that of the myosin filament. Whereas the myosin-containing filament *generates* tension during muscle contraction, the actin-containing filament *regulates* tension generation. (Not all muscle systems are regulated by the actin-containing filament. In several invertebrate systems, force regulation and generation are both performed on the myosin-containing filament [10]. These so-called thick-filament–regulated systems are actually quite common. However, mammals use only thin-filament–based regulation.) The actin filament is composed of a long α-helical arrangement of actin monomers, each of molecular weight approximately 40 kDa (Fig. 1.4).

Actin is a ubiquitous protein found in virtually all cells as part of the intermediate filament network—part of the cell's cytoskeleton. As a result of their helical arrangement, a long groove is created along the fila-

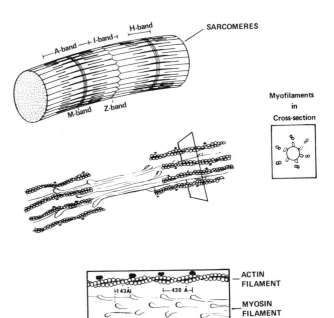

FIG. 1.4. Hexagonal array of interdigitating myosin and actin filaments, which comprise the sarcomere. The myosin filament is composed of myosin molecules, and the actin filament is composed of actin monomers. Arranged at intervals along the actin filament are the regulatory proteins troponin and tropomyosin.

ment's length. The regulatory protein, tropomyosin, fits nicely into this groove along the filament length (Fig. 1.4). At intervals along the filament (every seven actin monomers), the troponin protein is located. Troponin is a protein complex that is responsible for turning on contraction. Troponin (Tn) is composed of three subunits: Tn-I, Tn-C, and Tn-T. Tn-T binds troponin to tropomyosin (hence "T"), Tn-C binds calcium during contraction (hence "C"), and Tn-I exerts an inhibitory influence on tropomyosin when calcium is not present (hence "I").

The Muscle Cytoskeleton

Based on a huge volume of experimental evidence, it is well established that actin–myosin interaction is responsible for force generation in skeletal muscle. However, there is growing evidence that force transmission from actin and myosin outward to the extracellular matrix is more complicated than previously thought. Force transmission from the myosin filaments to the Z disk is mediated both by the actin filament and by the huge intrasarcomeric cytoskeletal protein, titin (see below). Lateral force transmission to adjacent sarcomeres via the intermediate filament system is likely to be important when muscle cells are injured and still required to perform work. The major intermediate filament protein in adult skeletal muscle is desmin (for a recent review, see reference 11). These proteins interconnect adjacent myofibrils and then form connections with the cell surface membrane via specialized focal adhesion sites known as "costameres" along the fiber length and at the muscle–tendon junction. The most widely studied protein located in the costamere is dystrophin, the protein product absent in muscles suffering from muscular dystrophy (12). Muscular dystrophy represents a family of approximately 10 disorders involving a primary myopathy. Symptoms of the disorder include false hypertrophy of the muscles (especially the calves), mental retardation, and quadriceps femoris muscle atrophy. The disorder is X-linked and thus primarily affects young males, with death usually occurring by age 14 secondary to respiratory muscle failure (in Duchenne muscular dystrophy).

Because dystrophic muscle demonstrates signs of degeneration and is more vulnerable to physical stress, dystrophin is believed to be important in maintaining muscle fiber integrity. However, the mechanism by which this is accomplished is not known. There is evidence that dystrophin may behave as a stabilizer of integral membrane ion channels or that it may stabilize folds in the membrane to prevent membrane disruption that could result from loading. Whatever the mechanism, it is clear that cells lacking the dystrophin gene product are more vulnerable to mechanical damage (13).

Membrane Components Activate Muscle

In addition to the well-defined arrangement of force-generating components present in muscle cells, an intricate system exists for activating these force generators. The membrane system present is actually a specially designed version of the membrane systems within normal cells. The two main components of this system are the transverse tubular system (T system) and the sarcoplasmic reticulum (SR). The T system begins as an array of invaginations of the surface membrane and is therefore physically contiguous with the sarcolemma (Fig. 1.1). These invaginations extend transversely across the long axis of the muscle fiber (hence their name). The function of the T system is to convey the activation signal to the myofibrils, which are themselves not in direct contact with the motoneuron. The T system thus acts as an electrical conduit for the nervous signal that reaches deep into the fiber. This provides a means of myofibrillar activation that is much faster than, say, diffusion of molecules from the cell surface deep into the fiber. The SR is a much more complex membrane system whose main function is to release and take up calcium during contraction and relaxation, respectively. As such, the SR envelops each myofibril to permit intimate contact between the activation and force-generation systems. The SR is also in contact with the T system and therefore acts a type of "middleman" in skeletal muscle activation and relaxation. Physical structures that link the T system to the SR have been identified and termed the "junctional feet" of the SR (14).

SKELETAL MUSCLE ARCHITECTURE

Skeletal muscle is not only highly organized at the microscopic level; the *arrangement* of the muscle fibers at the macroscopic level also demonstrates a striking degree of organization. In making functional comparisons among muscles, certain factors such as fiber type distribution are important, but there is no question that a most important factor in determining a whole muscle's contractile properties is the muscle's architecture.

Skeletal muscle architecture is defined as "the arrangement of muscle fibers relative to the axis of force generation." Although muscle fibers have a relatively consistent fiber diameter between muscles of different sizes, the arrangement of these fibers can be quite different. The various types of fiber arrangement are as numerous as the muscles themselves, but for convenience we present three general types of muscle architecture. Muscles with fibers that extend parallel to the muscle force-generating axis are termed parallel or longitudinally arranged muscles (Fig. 1.5A). Although the fibers extend parallel to the force-generating axis, they do not extend the entire muscle length. Muscles with fibers that are oriented at a single angle relative to the force

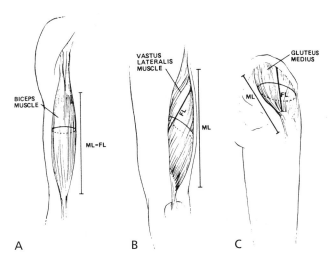

FIG. 1.5. Three general types of architecture that can be used to describe skeletal muscles. **A:** Longitudinal architecture, where muscle fibers run parallel to the axis of muscle force generation. **B:** Pennate architecture, where the muscle fibers run at a fixed angle (usually less than 30 degrees) relative to the axis of muscle force generation. **C:** Multipennate, where muscle fibers run at two or more angles relative to the axis of force generation.

generating axis are termed unipennate muscles (Fig. 1.5B). The angle between the fiber and the force-generating axis generally varies from 0 to 30 degrees. It is obvious when preparing muscle dissections that most muscles fall into the most general category, multipennate muscles—muscles composed of fibers that are oriented at several angles relative to the axis of force generation (Fig. 1.5C). An understanding of muscle architecture is critical to understanding the functional properties of different sized muscles.

Experimentally, muscle fiber length is determined by microdissection of individual fibers from fixed tissues. Unless investigators are explicit, when they refer to muscle fiber length, they are usually referring to muscle fiber *bundle* length. It is extremely difficult to isolate intact fibers, which run from origin to insertion, especially in mammalian tissue (2,3,15,16). The functional significance of muscle fiber length is that muscle excursion and contraction velocity are proportional to fiber length. This, of course has implications not only for understanding normal muscle function but for making surgical decisions regarding the appropriate muscle to use in a reconstructive procedure.

Physiologic cross-sectional area (PCSA) is the other extremely important architectural parameter calculated based on measurement of muscle mass and fiber length. This value is almost never the cross-sectional area of the muscle that would be measured in any of the traditional anatomic planes, using a noninvasive imaging method such as magnetic resonance imaging or computed tomography. Theoretically, PCSA represents the sum of the cross-sectional areas of all the muscle fibers within the

muscle. It is calculated using the following equation, where ρ represents muscle density (1.056 g/cm^3 for mammalian muscle) and $\emptyset$ represents surface pennation angle:

$$PCSA\ (cm^2) = \frac{Muscle\ Mass\ (g) \cdot Cos}{P(g/cm^3) \cdot fiber\ length\ (cm)}$$

The accuracy of this equation was recently highlighted in an experimental comparison between the *estimated* maximum muscle tetanic tension (based on PCSA calculations) and *measured* maximum tetanic tension (measured using traditional physiologic testing techniques) (17). These investigators found that estimations and predictions agreed within experimental error, providing strong evidence that calculation of PCSA provides an excellent prediction of a muscle's maximum tension generating ability. The only exception to that conclusion was that the soleus muscle did not seem to agree with this general paradigm. Interestingly, this was the only muscle tested that contained a large proportion of slow muscle fibers. These data may suggest that slow fibers generate less tension than fast fibers, but the precise explanation is not known.

It is important to highlight the observation that PCSA (and therefore maximum muscle tension) is not simply proportional to muscle mass (as is clear from the equation). In other words, given information on muscle mass or on muscle mass change (say, due to immobilization or spinal cord injury), we can make no statement with respect to muscle force. This is another way of saying that although mass is proportional to the amount of contractile material in the muscle, the arrangement of that material is of critical importance. In some pathologic conditions, mass may change due to noncontractile proteins (e.g., increased connective tissue or massive infiltration of inflammatory cells). In such cases, PCSA will not accurately predict tetanic tension.

Architecture of Muscles of the Lower Limb

Several architectural investigations have been performed in human lower limbs (18,19). Although each muscle within the lower limb is unique in terms of its architecture, taken as functional groups (e.g., hamstrings, quadriceps, dorsiflexors, plantarflexors), a number of generalizations can be made (Fig. 1.6). The quadriceps femoris are characterized by their relatively high pennation angles, large PCSAs, and short fibers. In terms of design, these muscles appear suited for the generation of large forces. The hamstrings, on the other hand, by virtue of their relatively long fibers and intermediate PCSAs, appear to be designed for large excursions. A very general conclusion might be that the antigravity extensors are more designed toward force production, whereas the flexors are more designed for high excursions.

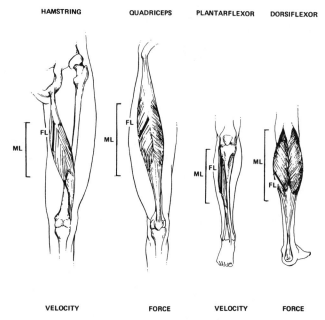

FIG. 1.6. General architectural design of lower limb muscles. Plantarflexors and quadriceps have an architectural design that favors force production, whereas dorsiflexors and hamstrings have an architectural design that favors excursion (or velocity).

Because the two most important muscle architectural parameters are muscle PCSA (which is proportional to maximum muscle force) and muscle fiber length (which is proportional to maximum muscle excursion), these two parameters are shown in graphic form for each muscle (Fig. 1.7) and can be used to make general comparisons between muscles in terms of design. For example, note that the sartorius, semitendinosus, and gracilis muscles have extremely long fiber lengths and low PCSAs, permitting long excursions at low forces, whereas at the other end of the spectrum is the soleus muscle, with its high PCSA and short fiber length, suitable for generating high forces with small excursions.

Architecture of Muscles of the Upper Limb

As might be expected, a high degree of architectural specialization is present in upper limb muscles as well (20–23). For example, the superficial and deep digital flexors are similar to one another but very different from the digital extensors (Fig. 1.8). The flexor carpi ulnaris is clearly the strongest wrist extensor. The extensor carpi radialis longus and brevis have clearly distinct architectures despite being synergistic (24). This type of scatter plot can be used to compare functional properties between muscles of the forearm not only to understand the normal design of these muscles but to assist in the decision-making process during planning of tendon transfer surgery (23). One might expect that when a muscle is surgically transferred to perform the function of another muscle whose function has been lost, matching of architectural properties may prove beneficial.

In terms of motor control, by virtue of architectural specialization, it is clear that the neuromuscular system does not simply modify muscular force and excursion

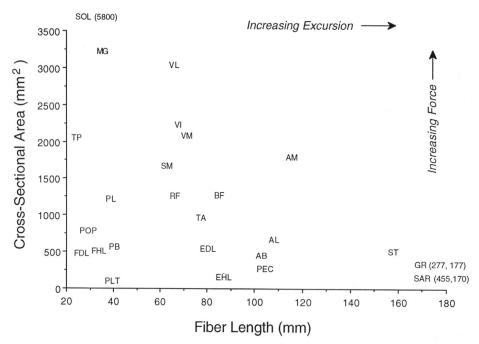

FIG. 1.7. Scatter plot of fiber length and physiologic cross-sectional area of the lower limb muscles. Because fiber length is proportional to muscle excursion and cross-sectional area proportional to force production, this graph represents the excursion and force-generating ability of each muscle.

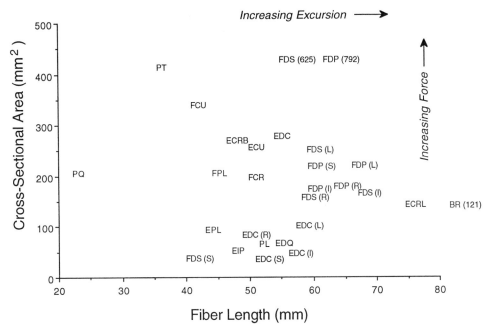

FIG. 1.8. Scatter plot of fiber length and physiologic cross-sectional area of the upper limb muscles. Because fiber length is proportional to muscle excursion and cross-sectional area proportional to force production, this graph represents the excursion and force-generating ability of each muscle.

only by changing the nervous input to the muscles. Muscles are *designed* for a specific function—large excursion, for example. The nervous system provides the signal for the muscle to "act" but does not necessarily specify the details of that action. It is as if the nervous system acts as the central controller, whereas the muscle interprets the control signal into an external action by virtue of its intrinsic design.

EXCITATION—CONTRACTION COUPLING

It is well known that peripheral nerves innervate skeletal muscles and that neural activation precedes muscle contraction. The precise process by which this neural activation signal culminates in muscle contraction is known as excitation–contraction (EC) coupling (Fig. 1.9). EC coupling is viewed as a sequence of events, each of which is necessary for contraction to occur. If any single step of EC coupling is impaired, muscle contraction does not occur normally. This impairment might be interpreted as muscle paralysis or fatigue. However, such a general classification in not useful unless the underlying cause is known (10).

The first step in the EC coupling chain is the generation of the peripheral nerve action potential. The action potential results from depolarization of the peripheral nerve axon that innervates the muscle. In addition to a signal from the central nervous system, the axon may be depolarized in a number of ways, including trauma to the peripheral nerve or application of an external electrical stimulating device. In any case, the resulting action potentials that propagate down the peripheral nerve are identical. The action potential arrives at the neuromuscular junction, the interface between muscle and nerve. The end of the nerve contains packets of the neurotransmitter acetylcholine (ACh), which causes muscle fiber excitation. ACh is synthesized by the cell body of the motor nerve and transported down the axon where it is stored at nerve endings for later use. After nerve depolarization, a quantum or unit of ACh is released into the small space between the muscle and nerve, the synaptic cleft. ACh then diffuses across the synaptic cleft and binds to the ACh receptor, which is integrated into the muscle membrane. ACh binding results in depolarization of the muscle fiber sarcolemma and an action potential that propagates from the neuromuscular junction outward in all directions.

As discussed above, at various intervals along the fiber surface, the action potential encounters invaginations of the sarcolemma that extend into the fiber—the T system. The action potential is conducted deep into the fiber by the T system. After the T system signals the SR, the SR releases calcium ions in the region of the myofilaments (Fig. 1.9). This release process is extremely fast. The calcium ions bind to troponin, the actin filament regulatory protein, which in turn releases the inhibition on the actin filament, permitting interaction with the myosin filament and resulting in cross-bridge cycling (i.e., force generation).

As long as neural impulses arrive at the neuromuscular junction and therefore calcium concentrations remain high in the region of the myofilaments, force gener-

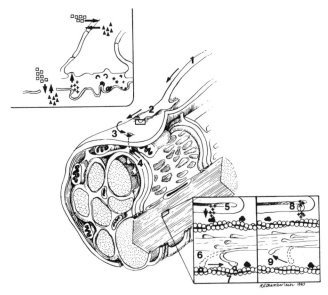

FIG. 1.9. Steps involved in skeletal muscle excitation–contraction coupling. *(1)* Generation of the action potential; *(2)* release of the neurotransmitter, acetylcholine, at the neuromuscular junction; *(3)* depolarization of the muscle fiber membrane; *(4)* conduction of the fiber action potential within the T tubules; *(5)* release of calcium from the sarcoplasmic reticulum (SR) and binding of calcium to the troponin regulatory protein; *(6)* binding of myosin to acting; *(7)* muscle force generation; *(8)* active transport of calcium back into the SR; and *(9)* muscle fiber relaxation.

ation continues. However, when the impulses cease, calcium is pumped back into the SR by the calcium-activated adenosine triphosphatase (ATPase) enzyme. The calcium-activated ATPase enzyme is an integral protein that is embedded in the bilayer of SR membrane. The mechanism of action of this enzyme has been thoroughly studied and is one of the best understood of the ion transport enzymes (25). The calcium pumping process is energy dependent and requires ATP. When calcium levels in the region of the myofilaments drop below a critical level, thin filament inhibition again resumes, and actin–myosin interaction is prevented. This inhibition is manifest externally as muscle fiber relaxation.

TEMPORAL SUMMATION

A well-known physiologic property follows directly from an understanding of the EC coupling sequence presented above. It should be obvious that the time required for activation, contraction, and then relaxation to occur is finite. That is, excitation (with accompanying calcium release) is relatively rapid (on the order of a few milliseconds), whereas contraction and relaxation are relatively slow (on the order of 100 ms). The mechanical consequence of the activation process (i.e., the muscle twitch) lags far behind the activation process itself. It is possible for two discreet activation pulses to

reach the muscle fiber before the mechanical event is completed, and thus the second impulse will be superimposed somewhat on the first one, resulting in summation. Because the two events have summated due to their relative temporal relationship, this process is referred to as temporal summation.

The physiologic effects of temporal summation are quite dramatic. If a "train" of pulses (say, 50 pulses in a row) is delivered to the muscle, separated in time by different amounts, this results in a tetanic contraction, and the resulting force is quite different (Fig. 1.10). Higher forces result when stimuli are delivered at higher frequencies because there is less time for relaxation. At relatively low frequencies (e.g., 10 Hz), the contractile record almost completely relaxes between successive pulses, whereas as stimulation frequency increases, the tetanic record becomes more fused until at very high frequencies (e.g., 100 Hz) the contractile record becomes a *fused contraction*. A fused tetanic contraction appears as such because the repeated calcium release onto the myofilaments is much faster than the rate at which the myofilaments can relax. This basic contractile property has significant implications in the use of isometric electrical stimulation for strengthening of quadriceps muscles after knee surgery. Because muscle strengthening depends on the force imposed on the muscle, higher stimulation frequencies are typically more effective in strengthening muscle (26).

MUSCLE MECHANICAL PROPERTIES

Active Length–Tension Relationship

Since the late 1800s (27), it has been known that the force developed by a muscle during isometric contraction (i.e., when the muscle is not allowed to shorten) varies with starting length. The isometric length–tension

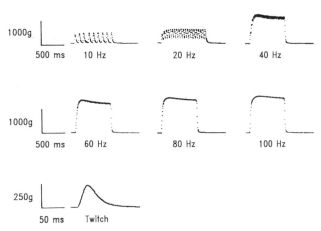

FIG. 1.10. Muscle force generated as a function of stimulation frequency. Tetanic force increases with stimulation frequency because the mechanical events fuse together in time in a phenomenon known as temporal summation. Actual data were obtained from a rabbit tibialis anterior muscle.

curve is generated by maximally stimulating a skeletal muscle at a variety of discrete lengths and measuring the tension generated at each length. When maximum tetanic tension is plotted against each length, a relationship such as that shown in Fig. 1.11 is obtained. Although a general description of this relationship was established early in the history of biologic science, the precise structural basis for the length–tension relationship in skeletal muscle was not elucidated until the sophisticated mechanical experiments of the early 1960s were performed (28,29). It was these experiments that defined the precise relationship between myofilament overlap and tension generation, which we refer to today as the length–tension relationship. In its most basic form, the length–tension relationship states that tension generation in skeletal muscle is a direct function of the magnitude of overlap between the actin and myosin filaments.

In frog muscle, where this relationship has been studied in detail, as a muscle is highly stretched to a sarcomere length of 3.65 μm, the fiber develops no active force. This is because the myosin filament is 1.65 μm long and the actin filament is 2.0 μm in length, so that at a sarcomere length of 3.65 μm, there is no overlap (interdigitation) between the actin and myosin filaments. Therefore, although EC coupling might *permit* actin–myosin interaction by removing the inhibition of the actin filament, because no myosin cross-bridges are in the vicinity of the actin active sites, no force generation can occur.

As the fiber is allowed to shorten, overlap between actin and myosin increases and the amount of force generated by the fiber increases until the fiber reaches a sarcomere length of 2.2 μm. As sarcomere length changes from 2.0 to 2.2 μm, muscle force remains because, at the center of the myosin filament, a bare region of the myosin molecule exists that is devoid of crossbridges. Although sarcomere length shortening over the range of 2.2 to 2.0 μm results in greater filament overlap, it does not result in increased force generation because no additional cross-bridge connections are made. The maximum tetanic tension of the muscle in this region is abbreviated P_o. The length at which P_o is attained is known as optimal length and is abbreviated L_o. At a sarcomere length of 2.0 μm, the actin filaments from one side of the sarcomere juxtapose the actin filaments from the opposite side of the sarcomere (Fig. 1.11), and as sarcomere length decreases below the plateau region, actin filaments from one side of the sarcomere double overlap with actin filaments on the opposite side of the sarcomere, resulting in decreased muscle force output. This region is known as the ascending limb of the length–tension curve.

Passive Length–Tension Relationship

The thin solid line in Fig. 1.11 represents the tension borne by a muscle when it is stretched to various lengths without stimulation. Near optimal length in frog muscle, passive tension is near zero. However, as the muscle is stretched to longer lengths, passive tension increases dramatically. These relatively long lengths can be attained physiologically, and therefore passive tension may play a role in providing resistive force even in the absence of muscle activation. Recent studies performed have shown that the origin of passive muscle tension is actually *within* the myofibrils themselves (30–33). A novel structural protein has been identified, which is the source of this passive tension and is named "titin" because of its extremely large size (3 MDa). Titin connects the thick myosin filaments from the middle of the M band to the Z band. In addition to passively supporting the sarcomere, titin stabilizes the myosin lattice so that high muscle forces do not disrupt the orderly hexagonal array. If titin is selectively destroyed, normal muscle contraction causes significant myofibrillar disruption (31). The molecular basis for this passive tension was subsequently identified as coming from the titin protein—a giant molecular "spring" (33).

Human titin was recently cloned (34), and the sequence provided great insights into its function. A most interesting observation was that muscles of different passive stiffnesses and resting sarcomere lengths contained a so-called PEVK region (named for the predominant amino acids) of differing lengths. Because the length of the PEVK region correlated well with muscle passive stiffness and was located in the I-band region of the sarcomere where it would be untethered by other

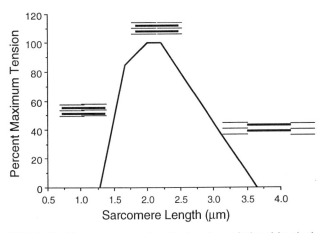

FIG. 1.11. The sarcomere length–tension relationship elucidated for frog skeletal muscle. Schematic filaments shown provide relative actin and myosin filament overlap at each of the sarcomere lengths shown. Maximum force is abbreviated P_o and exists when myofilament overlap is optimal. This length is abbreviated L_o. Thin line represents the passive tension of an unstimulated muscle obtained as muscle length is slowly increased. (From Gordon AM, Huxley AF, Julian FJ. The variation in isometric tension with sarcomere length in vertebrate muscle fibres. *J Physiol* (*Lond*) 1966;184:170–192, with permission.)

TABLE 1.1. *Definition of muscle length terms*

Optimal length	Length at which myofilament overlap is optimal and force is maximal (2.6–2.8 μm in human muscle; 2.0–2.2 μm in frog muscle).
Slack length	Length at which muscle force equals zero. This length is unknown for most human muscles but is the retracted length that a muscle becomes after cutting the tendinous insertion.
Resting length	A clear definition of this length is not possible because passive tension is variable between muscles and the resting condition is not well defined. Should not be used to describe an absolute length.
In situ length	Muscle length under a specified joint angle configuration. Should not be used to describe an absolute length.
In vivo length	Muscle length under a specified joint angle configuration. Should not be used to describe an absolute length.

sarcomeric proteins, it was suggested that this region acted as a molecular spring, conferring different passive properties on different muscles. For example, the psoas muscle, known to be passively stiff, has a PEVK region that is about 300 amino acids in length, whereas the more compliant lattisimus dorsi muscle has a PEVK region that is over 800 amino acids in length (34). This raises the intriguing possibility that various isoforms of titin might be expressed in different muscles or in pathologic conditions, thus conferring different passive mechanical properties on the muscles. Because the relationship between muscle force at zero tension and optimal sarcomere length is highly variable, there is much confusion in the literature regarding the terms optimal length, slack length, resting length, *in situ* length, and *in vivo* length, all of which are often incorrectly interchanged (Table 1.1).

One caution: Do not describe a shortening muscle using the length–tension relationship. One might be tempted to predict that as a muscle shortens from a long length, force increases. However, one must remember that the length–tension relationship is strictly valid only for *isometric* contractions, where muscle velocity is zero. Thus, the curve represents the artificial connection of individual data points from isometric experiments. To describe motion, an understanding of the force–velocity relationship is required.

Force–Velocity Relationship

Unlike the length–tension relationship, the force–velocity relationship does not have a simple anatomi-

cally identifiable basis. The force–velocity relationship describes the force generated by a muscle as a function of its velocity and has been ascribed to the physiologist A. V. Hill (see summary in reference 35).

Experimentally, the force–velocity relationship, like the length–tension relationship, is a curve that actually represents the results of many individual experiments plotted on the same graph. Experimentally, a muscle is stimulated maximally and allowed to shorten (or lengthen) against a constant load. The muscle velocity during shortening (or lengthening) is measured and plotted against the resistive force. The general form of this relationship is plotted in Fig. 1.12. When a muscle is activated and required to lift a load that is less than its maximum tetanic tension, the muscle begins to shorten. Contractions that permit the muscle to shorten are known as concentric contractions. As the load the muscle is required to lift decreases, contraction velocity increases. This occurs until the muscle finally reaches its maximum contraction velocity, V_{max}; V_{max} is a parameter that is used to characterize muscle and is related to both fiber type distribution and architecture. However, note for low velocities, force drops off rapidly as velocity increases. For example, in a muscle that is shortening at only 1% of its maximum contraction velocity (extremely slow), tension drops by 5% relative to maximum isometric tension. Similarly, as contraction velocity increases to only 10% maximum (easily attainable physiologically), muscle force drops by 35%. Even when muscle force is only 50% maximum, muscle velocity is still only 17% V_{max}.

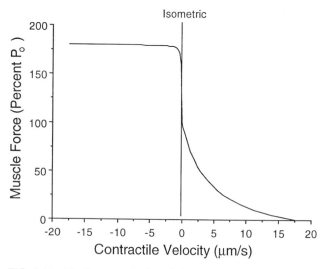

FIG. 1.12. The force–velocity relationship elucidated for skeletal muscle. To determine this relationship, initial shortening (or lengthening velocity) is plotted as a function of load. Note the familiar relationship demonstrating muscle force declines for shortening contractions and high forces obtained for eccentric contractions. (From Lieber RL. *Skeletal Muscle Structure and Function.* Baltimore; MD: Williams & Wilkins, 1992.)

As the load on the muscle increases, it reaches a point where the external load is greater than the force that the muscle itself can generate. Even though the muscle is activated, it is forced to lengthen due to the high external load. This is referred to as an eccentric contraction ("contraction" in this context does not necessarily imply shortening). There are two main properties of eccentric contractions. First, the absolute tensions are very high relative to the muscle's maximum tetanic tension-generating capacity. Second, absolute tension is relatively independent of lengthening velocity. This suggests that skeletal muscles are very resistant to lengthening, a property that is useful to control many normal movement patterns where skeletal muscles are required to brake movement.

Eccentric contractions are currently an active area of research for three main reasons. First, much of a muscle's normal activity occurs while it is actively lengthening, so that eccentric contractions are physiologically common. Second, muscle injury and soreness are selectively associated with eccentric contraction. Finally, muscle strengthening is greatest using exercises that involve eccentric contractions.

MECHANICAL PROPERTIES OF MUSCLES WITH DIFFERENT ARCHITECTURES

Even though one might understand the details of sarcomere structure and cross-bridge action, it is impossible to explain the force-generating properties of a whole muscle without an understanding of muscle architecture as described above. The main point regarding muscle architecture is that muscle force is proportional to PCSA, whereas muscle velocity (or excursion) is proportional to muscle fiber length.

Suppose that two muscles have identical fiber lengths and pennation angles, but one muscle has twice the mass (equivalent to saying that one muscle has twice the number of fibers and thus twice the PCSA). Let us examine the functional significance of such architectural differences.

As shown in Fig. 1.13, the only effect is to increase maximum tetanic tension so that the length–tension curve has the same basic shape but is simply amplified upward in the case of the heavier muscle. Similarly, the force–velocity curve simply changes the location of P_o, but the curve retains the same basic shape. Now consider the effects of architecture using an example of two muscles with identical PCSAs and pennation angles but different fiber lengths. As shown in Fig. 1.13, the effect is to increase the muscle velocity (or to increase the muscle excursion). The peak absolute force of the length–tension curves is identical, but the absolute muscle active range is different. For the same reason that fiber length increases the active muscle range of the

length–tension relationship, it causes an increase in the muscle's absolute maximum contraction velocity (V_{max}).

MUSCLE FIBER TYPES

To retain the view that all muscle fibers are the same is an oversimplification in light of the overwhelming evidence that skeletal muscle fibers are heterogeneous. In the early 1800s it was observed that the gross appearance of different skeletal muscles ranged in color from pale white to deep red. In fact, one of the earliest classification schemes for muscle was based on color, and thus muscles were classified as "red" or "white." However, as experimental methods became more sophisticated, it became clear that numerous other differences existed between muscles. Using traditions staining methods (hematoxylin and eosin), muscle fibers appear in cross-section as tightly packed polygonal fibers (Fig. 1.14A). The subsarcolemmal region of these fibers localizes the dystrophin protein so important for structural integrity (Fig. 1.14B). However, despite these similarities between fibers, the current view of muscle fiber types is that skeletal muscle fibers possess a wide and nearly continuous spectrum of morphologic, contractile, and metabolic properties. The appropriate view of any classification scheme, therefore, is that it is an artificial system superimposed on a continuum for our convenience.

Muscle Fiber Typing by Combined Histochemistry

One of the most widely used methods for describing animal muscle is the so-called metabolic classification scheme in which physiologic, biochemical, and histochemical experiments were combined to develop a scheme consistent across methodologies (36).

In the metabolic method, three fundamental muscle fiber properties are estimated using histochemical methods: speed, oxidative capacity, and glycolytic capacity. First, the histochemical assay for myofibrillar ATPase activity is used to distinguish between fast- and slow-contracting muscle fibers. Because myosin ATPase activity is positively correlated with muscle contraction velocity, measures of ATPase activity can be interpreted in terms of contraction speed. Thus, when given equivalent times, under alkaline conditions, fast-contracting fibers appear dark histochemically and slow-contracting fibers appear light (Fig. 1.14D), whereas under acidic conditions, these relationships reverse (Fig. 1.14C). In this manner, the myosin ATPase assay can be used to distinguish between fast- and slow-contracting muscle fibers as could an antibody stain for MHC (Fig. 1.14E).

The histochemical assay for succinate dehydrogenase (SDH) is used to distinguish between highly oxidative and less oxidative fibers. Similar to the ATPase assay, fibers rich in SDH (and thus rich in mitochondria) stain

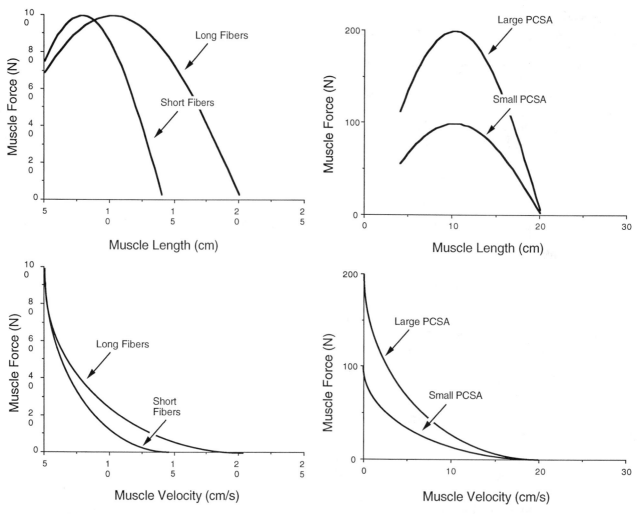

FIG. 1.13. Schematic muscle length–tension and force–velocity relationship illustrated for two muscles of different architectures.

with a speckled pattern of the mitochondria, proportional to the number of mitochondria and the SDH activity within them (Fig. 1.14F). Oxidative fibers have a relatively dense, purple, speckled appearance, whereas nonoxidative fibers have only scattered purple speckles. Therefore, this histochemical assay reflects the relative oxidative potential of muscle fibers. Finally, the enzyme α-glycerophosphate dehydrogenase is used to distinguish fibers based on their relative glycolytic potential. The chemical reactions involved in glycolysis take place in the muscle cell cytoplasm. As such, the α-glycerophosphate dehydrogenase stain is not confined to a specific cellular organelle as is the SDH stain, and the appearance is much more homogeneous across the cell. This assay can thus distinguish between glycolytic and nonglycolytic fibers. In practice, over 95% of normal muscle fibers can be classified into one of three categories (Table 1.2). These fiber types, named for the particular property measured, are grouped into types: fast glyco-

lytic (FG), fast oxidative glycolytic (FOG), and slow oxidative (SO).

Muscle Fiber Typing by ATPase Histochemistry Alone

A scheme used often in human muscle pathology is the so-called ATPase-based classification scheme (37). In this scheme, several repetitions of the ATPase assay mentioned above are carried out on serial sections of muscle. However, whereas the routine ATPase assay is carried out under alkaline conditions (pH 9.4), in the ATPase-based classification scheme, several other assays are performed under increasingly acidic conditions (at pH 4.0), and optical density is observed. Thus, the assay determines the sensitivity of the ATPase enzyme to the pH of the medium. Fast muscle myosin has a different pH sensitivity than slow myosin. Thus, at acid pH, slow fibers stain more darkly than fast fibers,

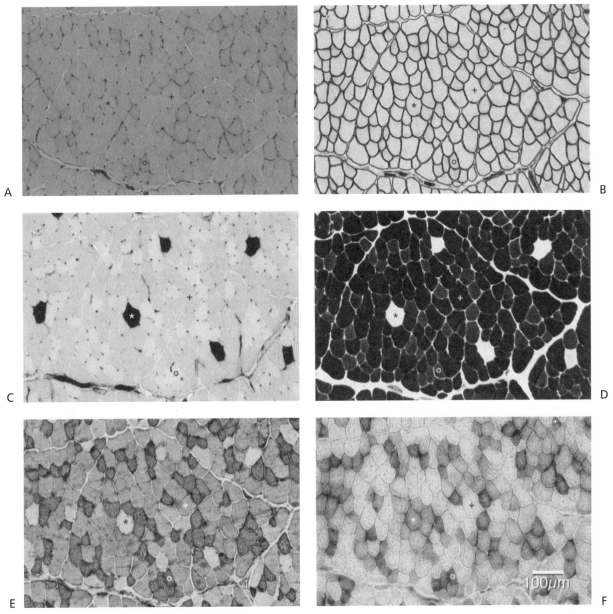

FIG. 1.14. Cross-sections of rabbit tibialis anterior skeletal muscles under various staining conditions. **A:** Hematoxylin and eosin, demonstrating general muscle fiber morphology. **B:** Dystrophin immunohistochemistry showing the subsarcolemmal nature of this protein. **C:** Myofibrillar ATPase under acid preincubation conditions. Under these conditions, slow fibers stain darkly as do the extracellular capillaries and fast fibers stain lightly. **D:** Myofibrillar ATPase under alkaline preincubation conditions. Under these conditions, slow fibers stain lightly, whereas fast fibers stain darkly. Note that in both C and D, fast fiber staining intensity occurs at two levels. **E:** Immunohistochemical reaction for fast myosin heavy chain antibody. In rat skeletal muscle, this antibody (F71) stains type 2A fibers darkly and type 2X fibers more lightly and is negative for type 1 fibers. In the rabbit tibialis anterior, based on ATPase reactions, this reactivity is probably the same. **F:** Succinate dehydrogenase used to demonstrate muscle fiber oxidative capacity. Note that the slow fibers (*) and the type 2A fast fibers (°) have higher oxidative capacity compared with the type 2X fibers (+).

TABLE 1.2. *Three fiber types obtained by histochemical assay*

Fiber type designation	ATPase activity (fast or slow)	SDH activity (oxidative)	α-GP activity (glycolytic)
FG	High	Low	High
FOG	High	High	High
SO	Low	High	Low

SDH, succinate dehydrogenase; α-GP, α-glycerophosphate dehydrogenase; FG, fast glycolytic; FOG, fast oxidative glycolytic; SO, slow oxidative.

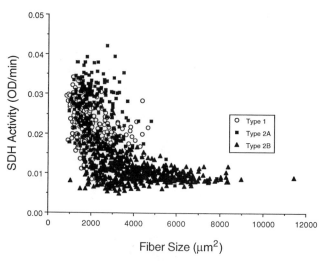

FIG. 1.15. Relationship between fiber type, fiber size, and oxidative capacity in single typed muscle fibers of the rabbit extensor digitorum longus muscle. ○, type 1 fiber; ▲, type 2A fiber; ■, type 2B fiber.

whereas at alkaline pH the opposite is true. In fact, the scheme takes this differential pH sensitivity a step further. Fast fibers themselves can be subdivided based on differential pH sensitivity over the range of pH 4.3 to 4.6. This classification scheme can thus differentiate between fast fibers (termed type 2) and slow fibers (termed type 1) and between (at least) two fast fiber *subtypes* (termed type 2A and type 2B). Table 1.3 presents the definitions of type 1, 2A, and 2B fibers based on the ATPase scheme. Note that this technique must be fine tuned to accurately and repeatedly obtain valid results on various tissues.

It has been shown that type 2A fibers have a greater oxidative capacity than type 2B fibers, and therefore many equate them (incorrectly) with type FOG fibers. A number of studies have directly demonstrated that the metabolic scheme does not correlate well with the ATPase-based scheme. This should not be surprising based on an understanding of what the two schemes measure. It is not necessary that the pH sensitivity of the myosin ATPase enzyme is related to the oxidative or glycolytic capacity of the cell. A relationship *may* exist in general, because most cellular metabolic processes are complimentary. However, the relationships may not hold after a perturbation of the cellular environment and therefore must be used with great caution.

Muscle Fiber Classification by Immunohistochemistry

Although histochemical fiber type identification can yield valuable insights into muscle function, it is limited in its ability to identify specific cellular proteins. For this purpose, we must use specific identification methods that identify a particular region (epitope) of a particular

protein. The most common protein used to distinguish among fiber types is the MHC. This is logical because MHC is the molecular motor that drives muscle contraction. Thus, to a large extent, muscle fibers that are classified using the metabolic scheme will show parallel classifications using MHC immunohistochemistry (Fig. 1.14E). In practice, the method used for fiber typing should be related to the goals of the study. If knowledge of a particular protein is necessary, immunohistochemistry must be used. Otherwise, histochemical methods may suffice.

Relationship Between Fiber Type and Fiber Size

Coordination between muscle fiber size and type is apparent when fiber size and fiber oxidative capacity are plotted in scatter graph format and separated by fiber type (Fig. 1.15) (38). The largest, fastest, and lowest oxidative capacity fibers are the type 2B or type FG fibers within a muscle. This suggests that type 2B fibers are used only occasionally for activities requiring high force production. At the other extreme are the smallest, slowest, and highest oxidative capacity fibers, the type 1 or SO fibers. This relationship suggests that these fiber types are used on a regular basis for relatively low force-requiring activities. The fact that fiber type and fiber size are related indicates a tightly regulated system where cellular structure is matched to cellular function.

PHYSIOLOGIC PROPERTIES OF MUSCLE FIBER TYPES

The best information regarding the physiologic properties of different fiber types comes from physiologic ex-

TABLE 1.3. *Fiber types definition using the ATPase assay*

Preincubation pH	Type 1	Type 2A	Type 2B
9.4	Light	Dark	Dark
4.6	Dark	Light	Medium
4.3	Dark	Light	Medium

periments on muscles composed *mainly* of one fiber type. Many animal muscles fulfill this criterion, whereas very few human muscles do. The problem with this approach is that it assumes that a muscle's properties are simply the sum of all the available fibers in the muscle and that each fiber exerts the same relative influence. The force–velocity relationship described previously provides a convenient tool for muscle fiber type-specific characterization of "speed." The parameter V_{max} can be compared between muscles that have large differences in fiber type distribution to measure fiber type-specific values for V_{max}. Muscle architecture has a profound influence on absolute contraction velocity, and therefore all velocities measured experimentally must be expressed in terms of a normalized velocity such as fiber lengths per second or sarcomere lengths per second to determine the intrinsic V_{max} value for a fiber. Fast-contracting muscle fibers shorten two to three times faster than slow-contracting fibers at V_{max} (39). This is actually not a large difference and probably has very little overall influence on performance in sports or in rehabilitation. Despite the popular discussion of fiber type distribution, it probably has very little to do with performance.

In a manner similar to that used for measurement of V_{max}, maximum tetanic tension can be measured in muscles of different fiber type distributions. Again, one must account for differences in architecture to attribute differences in force to fiber type differences and not to architectural differences (i.e., PCSA). This value is then normalized to the PCSA of the muscle studied to yield the value known as "specific tension" or force of contraction per unit area of muscle. In measuring the specific tension of whole skeletal muscle, most investigators find that muscles composed mainly of fast fibers have a greater specific tension than muscles composed mainly of slow fibers. The typical value for specific tension of fast muscle is approximately 22 N/cm², whereas that for slow muscle is 10 to 15 N/cm². The common interpretation of these whole-muscle experiments has been that fast muscle fibers have a greater specific tension than slow muscle fibers. The problem with this interpretation is that it assumes that a muscle fiber from a mixed muscle has the same properties as a muscle fiber of the same type that is in a homogeneous muscle. This assumption may not be true.

The best estimates of specific tension come from isometric contractile experiments of single motor units. The advantage of this approach is that the contractile properties are measured from the same fiber type because a single axon innervates the different fibers. The problem with this approach in calculating specific tension is that measurement of motor unit PCSA is technically difficult. Generally, methods used for motor PCSA determination are indirect, relying on a series of questionable assumptions. The best data from such experi-

ments showed that fast muscle fibers develop just *slightly* more tension than slow muscle fibers (40).

The endurance (or its opposite, fatigue) of muscle fibers is more difficult to define precisely compared with speed or strength. This is because endurance depends on the type of work the muscle is required to perform. For example, if the work load is extremely light, there is almost no difference between fiber types. If the work load is extremely heavy, the muscle fibers themselves do not fatigue; rather, the neuromuscular junction fatigues, and again, there is no difference between types. Because EC coupling involves a chain of events, it is possible to produce fatigue by interrupting any point in the chain. Thus, a danger exists in simply ascribing a force drop to muscle fiber fatigue without understanding the basis for the drop. Endurance of the various motor units (and muscle fiber types) differs considerably. However, it is difficult to give a quantitative difference unless the work conditions are known. Generally, SO fibers have the greatest endurance, followed by FOG fibers, and finally FG fibers (corresponding to types S (slow), FR (Fast Fatigue-resistant) and FF (Fast Fatigable), FR, and FF motor units, respectively) (41). This is not surprising in that we have seen that FG fibers have the lowest oxidative capacity and SO fibers the highest.

MORPHOLOGIC PROPERTIES OF DIFFERENT MUSCLE FIBER TYPES

Contractile Protein Differences Between Fiber Types

We have seen repeatedly that myosin differs considerably between fast and slow muscle fibers. Although this difference is profound functionally, there is really not a large structural difference between the different myosins as determined by electron microscopy and x-ray diffraction (42). In fact, in terms of sarcomere force-generating components, although the proteins have very different functional properties, structurally they are quite similar. Fast and slow myosin have approximately the same mass and shape. Muscles composed of either fast or slow sarcomeres have approximately the same filament spacing and cross-bridge density. However, it has been demonstrated in a number of systems that different fiber types contain different isoforms of the MHC, which has a significant effect on contractile performance. In studies performed on isolated rat muscle fibers, it was shown that type 1 fibers had a V_{max} that was much less than any of the fast fiber types, but within the fast fiber family, V_{max} progressed in the order type 2B > type 2X > type 2A (43–45).

Metabolic Differences Between Fiber Types

Clearly, the large difference in oxidative and glycolytic capacity is represented in the cell as large differences

TABLE 1.4. *Differences between fiber types*

Parameter	SO	FOG	FG
T/SR system quantity	Little	Much	Much
Z-disk width	Wide	Intermediate	Narrow
Contractile speed	Slow	Fast	Fast
Mitochondrial density	High	Moderate	Low
Lipid droplets	Many	Few	None
Glycogen granules	Few	Many	Many
Endurance	High	Moderate	Low

SO, slow oxidative; FOG, fast oxidative glycolytic; FG, fast glycolytic; T/SR, transverse tubular system, sarcoplasmic reticulum.

in the concentration of the metabolic enzymes (Table 1.4). For example, in fast fibers, the cytoplasm has a much higher concentration of all the glycolytic intermediates. Similarly, all the oxidative fibers (FOG and SO) have a much higher concentration of oxidative enzymes. Because oxidative phosphorylation occurs in the mitochondria, oxidative fibers have a higher mitochondrial density than nonoxidative fibers. In a detailed quantitative study of the ultrastructure of the various fiber types, it was shown that highly oxidative fibers may have a concentration of mitochondria of up to 25% and may contain twice the volume fraction of lipid (46). This alone is one reason why it is difficult to compare the specific tension of the various fiber types even if it were possible to isolate intact single fibers. Not all the space within the fiber is contractile material, and the difference between the fibers in the amount that is contractile material is type specific.

Membrane Differences Between Fiber Types

The T system and SR are involved in the excitation portion of EC coupling. It makes sense that muscles required to respond rapidly (fast fibers) would have a well-developed membranous activation system as shown biochemically. The SR and T system of fast fibers may occupy two to three times more volume in fast fibers than slow fibers. Thus, differences in speed between fast and slow fibers result from differences in cross-bridge cycling rates and differences in activation speed.

A final interesting structural difference between fiber types that is very useful but poorly understood is the difference between muscle fiber type Z-disk thickness (47). It was shown that FG fibers have the most narrow Z disks (60 nm), whereas SO fibers have the widest Z disks (150 nm). The thickness of the Z disk in FOG fibers is intermediate (80 nm). The reason for this difference is not clear.

SUMMARY

The structural and functional specialization of skeletal muscle to perform work has been reviewed. At the cellular level, muscle cells are constantly attempting to match their protein components to the type of work required. This is true of the contractile and metabolic proteins expressed. It is possible that we will soon understand the cytoskeletal protein arrangement and its suitibility to perform force transmission within the cell. At the whole organ level, the muscles themselves are suited to particular tasks based on their architectural design, innervation pattern, and microcirculation. These studies suggest that a knowledge of this cellular and tissue organization may ultimately be used to improve our ability to optimize muscle performance as a result of particular training protocols or to improve our ability to treat injured and diseased muscle.

ACKNOWLEDGMENTS

Much of the work described in this chapter was supported by the Department of Veterans Affairs and National Institutes of Health grants AR40050 and AR35192. I very much appreciate the technical support over the past 10 years of Denise Cuizon, who carefully prepared Fig. 1.14.

REFERENCES

1. Alway SE, Gonyea WJ, Davis ME. Muscle fiber formation and fiber hypertrophy during the onset of stretch-overload. *Am J Physiol* 1990;259:C92–C102.
2. Loeb GE, Pratt CA, Chanaud CM, et al. Distribution and innervation of short, interdigitated muscle fibers in parallel-fibered muscles of the cat hindlimb. *J Morphol* 1987;191:1–15.
3. Ounjian M, Roy RR, Eldred E, et al. Physiological and developmental implications of motor unit anatomy. *J Neurobiol* 1991;22:547–559.
4. Street SF. Lateral transmission of tension in frog myofibers: a myofibrillar network and transverse cytoskeletal connections are possible transmitters. *J Cell Physiol* 1983;114:346–364.
5. Trotter JA. Interfiber tension transmission in series-fibered muscles of the cat hindlimb. *J Morphol* 1990;206:351–361.
6. Peachey LD, Eisenberg BR. Helicoids in the T system and striations of frog skeletal muscle fibers seen by high voltage electron microscopy. *Biophys J* 1978;22:145–154.
7. Staron RS, Pette D. The multiplicity of combinations of myosin light chains and heavy chains in histochemically typed single fibres. Rabbit soleus muscle. *Biochem J* 1987;243:687–693.
8. Emerson CP Jr, Bernstein SI. Molecular genetics of myosin. *Annu Rev Biochem* 1987;56:695–726.
9. Pollard TD, Doberstein SK, Zot HG. Myosin-l. *Annu Rev Physiol* 1991;53:653–681.
10. Ebashi S. Excitation-contraction coupling. *Annu Rev Physiol* 1976;38:293–313.
11. Patel TJ, Lieber RL. Force transmission in skeletal muscle: from actomyosin to external tendons. *Exerc Sport Sci Rev* 1997;25:321–363.
12. Campbell KP. Three muscular dystrophies: loss of cytoskeletal-extracellular matrix linkage. *Cell* 1995;80:675–679.
13. Petrof BJ, Shrager JB, Stedman HH, et al. Dystrophin protects the sarcolemma from stresses developed during muscle contraction. *Proc Natl Acad Sci USA* 1993;90:3710–3714.

14. Peachey LD, Franzini-Armstrong C. Structure and function of membrane systems of skeletal muscle cells. In: Peachey LD, ed. *Handbook of physiology.* Baltimore, MD: American Physiological Society, 1983:23–73.
15. Lieber RL, Blevins FT. Skeletal muscle architecture of the rabbit hindlimb: functional implications of muscle design. *J Morphol* 1989;199:93–101.
16. Sacks RD, Roy RR. Architecture of the hindlimb muscles of cats: functional significance. *J Morphol* 1982;173:185–195.
17. Powell PL, Roy RR, Kanim P, et al. Predictability of skeletal muscle tension from architectural determinations in guinea pig hindlimbs. *J Appl Physiol* 1984;57:1715–1721.
18. Friederich JA, Brand RA. Muscle fiber architecture in the human lower limb. *J Biomech* 1990;23:91–95.
19. Wickiewicz TL, Roy RR, Powell PL, et al. Muscle architecture of the human lower limb. *Clin Orthop* 1983;179:275–283.
20. Brand PW, Beach RB, Thompson DE. Relative tension and potential excursion of muscles in the forearm and hand. *J Hand Surg* 1981;3:209–219.
21. Jacobson MD, Raab R, Fazeli BM, et al. Architectural design of the human intrinsic hand muscles. *J Hand Surg* 1982;17:804–809.
22. Lieber RL, Fazeli BM, Botte MJ. Architecture of selected wrist flexor and extensor muscles. *J Hand Surg* 1990;15A:244–250.
23. Lieber RL, Jacobson MD, Fazeli BM, et al. Architecture of selected muscles of the arm and forearm: anatomy and implications for tendon transfer. *J Hand Surg* 1992;17A:787–798.
24. Lieber RL, Ljung B-O, Fridén J. Intraoperative sarcomere measurements reveal differential musculoskeletal design of long and short wrist extensors. *J Exp Biol* 1997;200:19–25.
25. Entman ML, Van Winkle WB. *Sarcoplasmic reticulum in muscle physiology.* Boca Raton, FL: CRC Press, 1986.
26. Cyriax JH. The pathology and treatment of tennis elbow. *J Bone Joint Surg Am* 1936;18:921–940.
27. Blix M. Die lange und die spannung des muskels. *Skand Arch Physiol* 1895;5:150–172.
28. Edman K. The relation between sarcomere length and active tension in isolated semitendinosus fibres of the frog. *J Physiol (Lond.)* 1966;183:407–417.
29. Gordon AM, Huxley AF, Julian FJ. The variation in isometric tension with sarcomere length in vertebrate muscle fibres. *J Physiol (Lond)* 1966;184:170–192.
30. Granzier H, Irving T. Passive tension in cardiac muscle: contribution of collagen, titin, microtubules, and intermediate filaments. *Biophys J* 1995;68:1027–1044.
31. Horowits R, Podolsky RJ. The positional stability of thick filaments in activated skeletal muscle depends on sarcomere length: evidence for the role of titin filaments. *J Cell Biol* 1987;105:2217–2223.
32. Magid A, Law DJ. Myofibrils bear most of the resting tension in frog skeletal muscle. *Science* 1985;230:1280–1282.
33. Wang K, McCarter R, Wright J, et al. Viscoelasticity of the sarcomere matrix of skeletal muscles. The titin-myosin composite filament is a dual-stage molecular spring. *Biophys J* 1993;64:1161–1177.
34. Labeit S, Kolmerer B. Titins: giant proteins in charge of muscle ultrastructure and elasticity. *Science* 1995;270:293–296.
35. Hill AV. *First and last experiments in muscle mechanics.* New York: Cambridge University Press, 1970.
36. Peter JB, Barnard RJ, Edgerton VR, et al. Metabolic profiles on three fiber types of skeletal muscle in guinea pigs and rabbits. *Biochemistry* 1972;11:2627–2733.
37. Brooke MH, Kaiser KK. Muscle fiber types: how many and what kind? *Arch Neurol* 1970;23:369–379.
38. Martin TP, Vailas AC, Durivage JB, et al. Quantitative histochemical determination of muscle enzymes: biochemical verification. *J Histochem Cytochem* 1985;33:1053–1059.
39. Close RI. Dynamic properties of mammalian skeletal muscles. *Physiol Rev* 1972;52:129–197.
40. Bodine SC, Roy RR, Eldred E, et al. Maximal force as a function of anatomical features of motor units in the cat tibialis anterior. *J Neurophysiol* 1987;6:1730–1745.
41. Burke RE, Levine DN, Tsairis P, et al. Physiological types and histochemical profiles in motor units of the cat gastrocnemius. *J Physiol (Lond)* 1973;234:723–748.
42. Haselgrove JC. Structure of vertebrate striated muscle as determined by x-ray-diffraction studies. In: Peachey LD, ed. *Handbook of physiology.* Bethesda, MD: American Physiological Society, 1983:143–171.
43. Bottinelli R, Schiaffino S, Reggiani C. Force-velocity relations and myosin heavy chain isoform compositions of skinned fibres from rat skeletal muscle. *J Physiol (Lond)* 1991;437:655–672.
44. Bottinelli R, Betto R, Schiaffino S, et al. Maximum shortening velocity and coexistence of myosin heavy chain isoforms in single skinned fast fibres of rat skeletal muscle. *J Muscle Res Cell Motil* 1994;15:413–419.
45. Bottinelli R, Betto R, Schiaffino S, et al. Unloaded shortening velocity and myosin heavy chain and alkali light chain isoform composition in rat skeletal muscle fibres. *J Physiol (Lond)* 1994;478:341–349.
46. Eisenberg BR. Quantitative ultrastructure of mammalian skeletal muscle. In: Peachey LD, Adrian RH, Geiger SR, eds. *Skeletal muscle.* Baltimore, MD: American Physiological Society, 1983:73–112.
47. Eisenberg BR, Kuda AM. Retrieval of cryostat sections for comparisons of histochemistry and quantitative electron microscopy in a muscle fiber. *J Histochem Cytochem* 1977;25:1169–1177.

Principles and Practice of Orthopaedic Sports Medicine,
edited by William E. Garrett, Jr., Kevin P. Speer, and Donald T. Kirkendall.
Lippincott Williams & Wilkins, Philadelphia © 2000.

CHAPTER 2

Basic Science of Tendons

Pekka Kannus, Laszlo Jozsa, and Markku Järvinen

TENDON ANATOMY AND PHYSIOLOGY

Full understanding of the structure and metabolism of normal tendons is required for full understanding of tendon injuries. This knowledge is important in planning treatment and rehabilitation for the patient with specific tendon problems (1).

Macroscopic Structure of Tendons

Tendons transmit force created in the muscle to bone, making joint movement possible. Basically, each muscle has two tendons, proximal and distal connected with muscle at the myotendinous junction (MTJ), with bone at the osteotendinous junction (OTJ). The attachment of the proximal tendon of a muscle to bone is called the muscle origin and the distal tendon the insertion.

Healthy tendons are brilliant white in color and fibroelastic in texture, showing great resistance to mechanical loads. They may vary considerably in shape ranging from wide and flat tendons to cylindrical, fan-shaped, and ribbon-shaped tendons. Muscles that create powerful resistive forces, like the quadriceps and triceps brachii muscles, have short and broad tendons. Contrast these to muscles that carry out subtle and delicate movements, like the finger flexors that have long and thin tendons.

The MTJ varies from muscle to muscle. End-to-end attachment is typical for wide muscles such as the abdominal muscles, whereas lateral attachment (the muscle belly joints the tendon obliquely) is characteristic for long muscles such as the biceps brachii.

The surrounding structures of the tendons can be divided into five categories. The fibrous sheaths or retinacula are the canals through which the (usually long) tendons glide during their course. Without bony grooves and notches, friction could impair tendon gliding. The grooves and notches are usually lined with a fibrocartilage and covered with this fibrous sheath or retinaculum. A characteristic example is the retinacula of the extensors and flexors of the hand and feet. The *reflection pulleys* are the anatomic reinforcements of the fibrous sheaths in places where there are curves along the course of the tendon. Their task is to keep the tendon inside its sliding bed.

The *synovial sheaths* are access tunnels for tendons at bone surfaces or other anatomic structures that might cause friction. They can be found around the tendons of the hand and feet. Under a fibrous layer, there are the thin parietal and visceral serous sheaths that form a closed duct containing peritendinous fluid for lubrication. In tendons that do not have a true synovial sheath, there can be a *peritendinous sheath* (paratenon) to reduce friction. It is composed of loose fibrillar tissue and functions as an elastic sleeve permitting free movement of the tendon against surrounding tissues. The Achilles tendon has a well-identifiable paratenon with thin gliding membranes (1).

The *tendon bursae* are the fifth extratendinous structure and are located where a bony prominence might otherwise compress and wear the tendon. Typical examples are the subacromial, deep trochanteric, pes anserinus, infrapatellar, and retrocalcaneal bursae.

Tendon Sheath

The tendon sheaths are commonly seen around the tendons of the hands and feet located in the areas of curved long excursion (such as carpal or tarsal tunnels) and in

P. Kannus: Accident & Trauma Research Center and Tampere Research Center of Sports Medicine, UKK Institute, FIN-33500 Tampere, Finland.

L. Jozsa: Department of Morphology, National Institute of Traumatology, H-1 430 Budapest, Hungary.

M. Järvinen: Medical School and Department of Surgery, Tampere University and University Hospital, FIN-335201, Tampere, Finland.

the areas of the fingers and toes. Their main function is to minimize the friction between the tendon and its surrounding structures.

The tendon sheath has two layers. The outer layer is the *fibrotic sheath* and the inner layer, consisting of the parietal and visceral sheets, is called the *synovial sheath.* The fibrotic sheath consists of spongylike fibril network of collagen that are oriented longitudinally, obliquely, or circularly with respect to the long axis of the tendon.

The internal surface of the fibrotic layer is covered with the lining synovial cells of the parietal synovial sheet and the tendon surface with the lining cells of the visceral sheet. The cavity between these two sheets contains a thin film of fluid whose chemical composition is similar with the composition of synovial fluid. The synovial lining cells are covered with fine collagen fibrils in a wavy pattern and hemispherical villi (2).

The main functions of the tendinous synovial fluid are to improve lubrication and help in tendon nutrition. Lundborg (3) suggested that synovial fluid provides an important route for nutrient transportation to tendon tissue.

The mesotenon (vincula) is characteristic to tendons of the hand and foot and has two functions. First, it anchors the tendon and prevents it from excess rotation. Second, it provides the patch for the vessels and nerves to enter the tendon tissue. Mesotenon is also lined by the two-layer synovial sheath.

Paratenon and Epitenon

Only parts of a few tendons in the hands and feet are provided with the two-layer tendon sheaths. True tendon sheaths can only be found in the areas where a change of direction and increase in friction necessitate very efficient lubrication. Instead, many of our tendons are surrounded by loose areolar connective tissue called paratenon.

The collagenous fiber system of the paratenon is well defined. The main components of the paratenon are the type I and type III collagen fibrils and elastic fibrils (4), and the paratenon is lined on its inner surface by synovial cells (5).

Paratenon functions as an elastic sleeve (although probably not so effectively as a true tendon sheath), permitting free movement of the tendon against the surrounding tissues (6). Under the paratenon, the entire tendon is surrounded by a fine connective tissue sheath called *epitenon.* The epitenon is contiguous on its outer surface, with the paratenon and on its inner surface with the endotenon. Inside the tendon, the endotenon invests each tendon fiber and binds individual fibers, and in larger units fiber bundles, together (7,8).

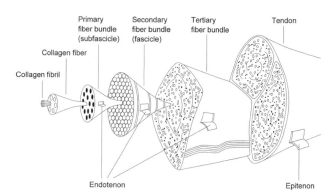

FIG. 2.1. The organization of tendon structure from collagen fibrils to the entire tendon. (From Jozsa L, Kannus P. *Human tendons. Anatomy, physiology, and pathology.* Champaign, IL: Human Kinetics, 1997, with permission.)

The epitenon has a relatively dense fibrillar network of collagen strands 8 to 10 nm in thickness. This network contains longitudinal, oblique, and transverse fibrils. It shows little variation in density or fibril orientation. Occasionally, epitenon fibrils are fused with superficially located tendon fibrils (8).

Endotenon

Inside the tendon, the endotenon is a thin reticular network of connective tissue with a well-developed crisscross pattern of collagen fibrils (7,9,10). The endotenon fibrils invest tendon fibers and binds fibers together (Figs. 2.1 and 2.2). A bunch of tendon fibers forms a

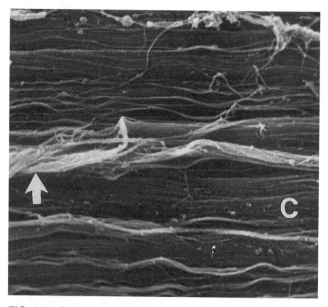

FIG. 2.2. Scanning electron micrograph (×350) of the internal structure of a human tibialis anterior tendon. *C,* collagen fibers; *arrow,* endotenon fibrils.

primary fiber bundle (subfascicle), and groups of these bundles form secondary bundles (fascicles). A group of secondary bundles forms a tertiary bundles, which make up the tendon. The endotenon surrounds the primary, secondary, and tertiary bundles (Fig. 2.1).

To improve binding, there is a high degree of hydralation of proteoglycan components between the endotenon and the surface of the tendon fascicles (10). Along with its important functions of binding, the endotenon network allows the fiber groups to glide on each other and carries blood vessels, nerves, and lymphatics to the deeper portion of the tendon (6,7).

Fiber Orientation

The divergent spiral arrangement of fibers of the flexor digitorum superficialis tendon that encircle the tendon was illustrated by Leonardo da Vinci (1452 to 1519) in his earliest studies of the mechanism of the hand in the 15th century. With the current use of transmission and scanning electron microscopes, it is well documented that the collagen fibrils are oriented not only longitudinally but also transversely and horizontally, with the longitudinal fibrils crossing each other, forming spirals and plaits (8,11). This complex ultrastructure of tendons provides good buffer against longitudinal, transverse, horizontal, and rotational forces during movement and activity.

Although the fiber orientation of the Achilles tendon and hand tendons has been studied in detail, the three-dimensional macrostructure of other tendons is poorly understood (12). The rotator cuff tendons have multidirectional orientation of collagen fibers (11), and there is great tendon-to-tendon, and within tendon site-to-site, variation in collagen content and type distribution (13). It seems likely that a specific structure and organization exist in these other tendons too. A systematic approach using a minute dissection technique is needed to understand the mechanical behavior of each tendon. The frequently observed twists and intertextures of the tendon fibers are likely to be related to optimal transmissions of muscle forces by increasing the tensile strength of the tendon in general and in certain anatomic points.

Internal Architecture of Tendons

Tendons consist of collagen (mostly type I collagen) and elastin embedded in a proteoglycan–water matrix with collagen accounting for 65% to 80% and elastin approximately 2% of the dry mass of the tendon (6,14–17). These elements are produced by tenoblasts and tenocytes, the elongated fibroblasts and fibrocytes that lie between the collagen fibers, and organized in a complex hierarchical scheme to form the tendon proper (6). Soluble tropocollagen molecules form cross-links to create insoluble collagen molecules that aggregate in definable and (under the electron microscopy) clearly visible units (Fig. 2.1).

Collagen Fibers, Fiber Bundles, and Fascicles

A bunch of collagen fibrils forms a collagen fiber, which is the basic unit of a tendon (Figs. 2.1 and 2.2). It is the smallest tendon unit visible using light microscopy (14). A fiber, aligned from end to end in a tendon, represents the smallest collagenous structure that can be tested mechanically. There is no standard nomenclature for aggregations of collagen fibrils within the tendon, perhaps because of their great variability (7,14). Therefore, the classification presented here is not the only possible but represents the system the authors prefer.

In human tendons, the diameter of the tertiary bundles varies from 1 to 3 mm. The diameter of the secondary bundles ranges from 150 to 1,000 μm. The diameter of both types of bundles is directly related to the macroscopic size of the tendon. The smallest bundle diameters are seen in the small tendons, such as the flexors and extensors of the fingers and toes, and the largest bundle diameters are in the big tendons, such as the Achilles, tibialis anterior, and extensor hallucis longus tendons.

In transverse sections, the profile of the primary fiber bundles or subfascicles (15 to 400 μm in diameter) is usually triangular with relatively sharp corners. This shape is influenced, but not completely determined, by compression from the surrounding structures or by the presence of neighboring fascicles. One fascicle usually has three or four subfascicles, although Kastelic et al. (9) reported that tendon fascicles may have up to 10 to 12 subfascicles. From our experience, the number of subfascicles varies from tendon to tendon and occasionally even within the same tendon (1). The same concerns the diameters of the fascicles and subfascicles. Both the fascicles and tertiary tendon bundles frequently show spiral formation along the course of the tendon.

Either within one fascicle or between different fascicles, crimping or wavy formation of the collagen fibers is a characteristic phenomenon (Fig. 2.3). Along the course of the fibers or between the fibers, crimping is a varied irregular phenomenon with the crimp angle varying between 0 and 60 degrees. This may be due to varying contribution of the proteoglycan cross-linking to the crimp. The direction of the fiber crimping or the phase of the wave pattern may be completely reversed between the front and back surfaces of the fascicles and subfascicles. Rotation of the subfascicles demonstrates the diversity of crimp patterns within just a short length of the tendon.

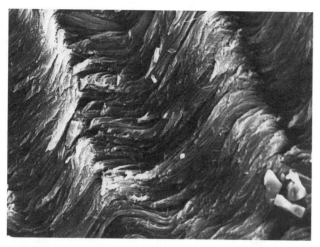

FIG. 2.3. In a resting state, the collagen fibers of an intact human Achilles tendon show regular wavy formation (scanning electron micrograph, ×4,600).

Collagen Fiber

The number of collagen fibers in each primary bundle (subfascicle) may vary considerably from tendon to tendon. The collagen fiber diameter also shows variation, with diameters ranging from 5 to 30 μm in the rat tail tendon (18). In human tendons, the fiber diameter can be as high as 300 μm (7). Collagen concentration in each fiber is directly related to the fiber diameter, which in turn depends on the number, rather than size, of its constituent fibrils (7).

In the resting state, collagen fibers and fibrils tendon show a wavy configuration that appears as regular bands across the fiber surface (Fig. 2.3). The fiber orientation is well definable (10). This configuration disappears if the tendon is stretched slightly corresponding to a straightening of the collagen fibers (6,7). When the tensile force is released, the tendon resumes its normal wavy appearance. Below about 4% elongation, the stress–strain curve of a tendon is reproducible by a sequence of stretches, but as soon as this limit is exceeded, the wavy form will not reappear and subsequent deformations will not reproduce the original curve. If an acute stress causes an elongation of 8% or more, the tendon is likely to rupture.

The running of collagen fibers along the course of the tendon is not only parallel. Under a polarized light microscope, four types of fiber crossing can be demonstrated (19): simply crossing two fibers, crossing of two fibers with one straight-running fiber, a plait formation with three fibers, and up-tying of parallel running fibers with one fiber. Along the whole length of tendons, the ratio of longitudinally to transversely (or horizontally) running fibers ranges between 10:1 and 26:1 (8). In addition, all these fibers form spirals (8–10).

Collagen Fibrils

A collagen fiber consists of a various number of fibrils. The diameter of fibrils varies from 20 to 150 nm (19,20). In the human Achilles tendon, the fibrils are between 30 and 130 nm in diameter (most of them between 50 and 90 nm), whereas in the flexors and extensors of the fingers and toes, the diameter is 20 to 60 nm. We observed that the fibril thickness of healthy human Achilles and biceps brachii tendons was between 30 and 80 nm (Fig. 2.4) (19).

The quantitative morphometric analysis have confirmed that the collagen fibril diameter increases from birth to maturity in animals and that the mean diameter of fibrils is different in different tendons (21). However, within one tendon, the proximal and distal parts, or the central and peripheral regions, do not show clear differences in fibril thickness as evidenced by electron microscopy (20).

The three-dimensional ultrastructure of a tendon fiber is complex. Within one collagen fiber, the fibrils are oriented not only longitudinally but also transversely and horizontally. The longitudinal fibers do not run only parallel but also cross each other, forming spirals. Some individual fibrils and fibril groups form spiral-type plaits, as demonstrated by an electron microscope (8). On the surface of fibrils, a sequence of elevated and depressed segments with diversed molecular density can be observed (22).

Importance of the Complex Three-dimensional Structure of a Tendon

The basic function of the tendon is to transmit the force created by muscle to bone to make joint movement

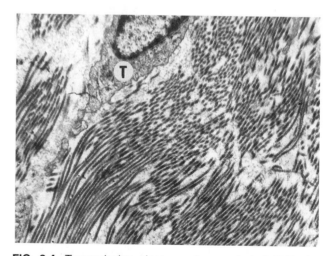

FIG. 2.4. Transmission electron micrograph (×6,600) of a dense collagen fibril network of an intact human Achilles tendon. The fibrils are uniform in diameter. *T*, tenocyte.

possible. The complex macro- and microstructure of tendons and tendon fibers are made for this purpose. During various phases of movements, the tendons are exposed not only to longitudinal but also to transverse and rotational forces. In addition, they must be prepared to withstand direct contusions and pressures. The three-dimensional internal structure of the fibers forms a buffer against forces of various directions, preventing damage and disconnection of the fibers (1).

Myotendinous Junction

In the MTJ (Fig. 2.5), the tension generated by muscle fibers is transmitted from intracellular contractile proteins to extracellular connective tissue proteins (collagen fibrils) of the tendon (23–26). Morphologic studies have demonstrated that at the MTJ, the tendinous collagen fibrils insert into deep recesses that are formed between the fingerlike processes (endings) of the muscle cells (Fig. 2.6) (23,27). By this type of folding of the basal membrane of the muscle cell endings, the contact area between the muscle fibers and tendon collagen fibers is markedly increased 10- to 20-fold (27). This significantly reduces the force applied per surface unit of the MTJ during muscle contraction (23).

The fingerlike processes of the muscle cells are 1 to 8 μm long, usually incompletely separated from each other with perforations that the tendinous collagen fibrils penetrate. In both type 1 and 2 muscle fibers, the

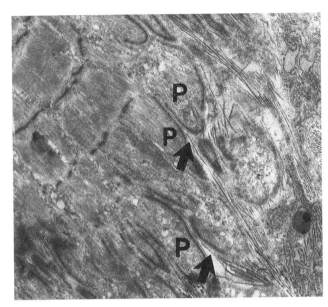

FIG. 2.6. At the myotendinous junction, the tendinous collagen fibrils (*arrows*) insert into deep recesses that are formed between the fingerlike processes (*P*) of the muscle cells (transmission electron micrograph, ×12,000).

basal lamina of the MTJ is approximately three times thicker compared with that on the longitudinal sites of the muscle cells.

The macromolecular composition of the basal lamina of the MTJ is similar in type 1 and type 2 muscle fibers. The basal membrane of the muscle cell processes contain proteoglycans and glycosaminoglycans (GAGs), especially heparin sulfate, chondroitin-4-sulphate, and dermatan sulfate (23,28). Fibronectin, laminin, and tenascin can be detected in large amounts on the membranous endings of the muscle cells (Fig. 2.7). The main collagenous component in the MTJ is type I collagen (Fig. 2.8). Small amounts of type III collagen can be detected on the muscular site of the junction.

On the tendinous side of the junction, the type I collagen fibrils are a thin (10 to 20 nm in diameter) and composed of dense fibrillar network. The matrix at the tendinous part is rich in GAGs and proteoglycans.

It is very likely that the various glycoproteins and GAGs found at the MTJ have a joint function in helping to transmit the forces between the muscle cell membrane and tendinous collagen fibrils. The high concentration of these polysaccharides possibly increases the adhesive forces between the two structures (the glue effect) and may be important in improving the elastic buffer capacity of the MTJ against loading. Chondroitin and dermatan sulfates may possess adhesive function (29).

However, despite membrane folding and specific mac-

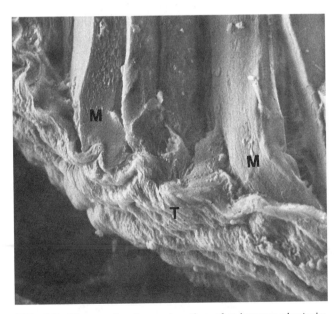

FIG. 2.5. The myotendinous junction of a human plantaris muscle. *T,* tendon collagen fibers; *M,* muscle cells (scanning electron micrograph, ×2,400).

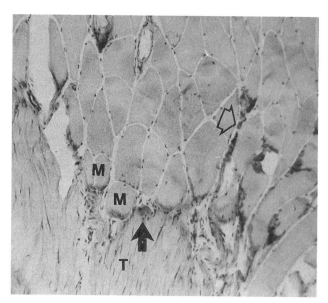

FIG. 2.7. Tenascin can be seen on the tips of the muscle cell processes (*closed arrow*) and microtendons (*open arrow*) of the myotendinous junction of a rat gastrocnemius–Achilles unit. Microtendons are slim and long extensions of the tendon collagen fibers and are located between the muscle cell processes. *T*, tendon; *M*, muscle cells (tenascin immunostaining, ×200).

romolecular composition, the MTJ is the weakest point in the muscle–tendon unit, making it susceptible to strain injuries (28,30,31). Therefore, this area is clinically very important and of special interest in sports medicine.

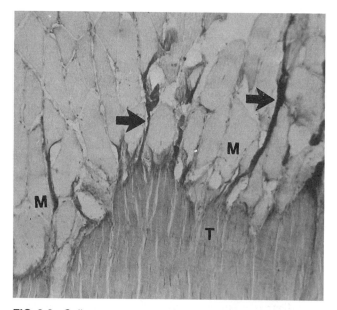

FIG. 2.8. Collagen structure of the myotendinous junction of a rat gastrocnemius–Achilles unit. The microtendons protrude between the muscle cell processes (*arrows*). *T*, tendon; *M*, muscle cells (type I collagen immunostaining, ×200).

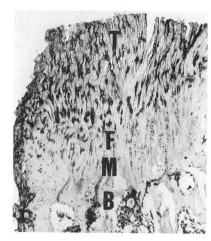

FIG. 2.9. The histology of the osteotendinous junction. Insertion of the rat quadriceps tendon into the patella. *T*, tendon tissue; *F*, fibrocartilage; *M*, mineralized fibrocartilage; *B*, bone (tenascin immunostaining, ×100).

Osteotendinous Junction

Insertion of a tendon to bone, the OTJ, is a very specialized region in the muscle–tendon unit. In the OTJ, the viscoelastic tendon transmits the muscular force to a rigid bone. The first comprehensive presentation on the anatomy of the OTJ was given by Dolgo-Saburoff (32). Based on the observations with a cat quadriceps tendon, he divided the junction to four light microscopic zones: tendon, fibrocartilage, mineralized fibrocartilage, and bone (Fig. 2.9). He also noted that specific tendinous fibers (Sharpey's fibers) perforated the periosteum at insertion.

At the Achilles tendon insertion onto the calcaneus, the retrocalcaneal bursa intervenes between it and the bone immediately proximal to the enthesis (33). If the calcaneus shows a prominent superior tuberosity, the walls of the bursa are fibrocartilaginous, but otherwise are not (33).

Tendon Zone

The tendinous part of the OTJ consists of dense collagen bundles with interspersed elongated tenoblasts. The collagen fibers are 10 to 55 μm in diameter with fibrils of 25 to 100 nm in thickness containing granular and filamentous material. In some regions, elastic fibers can also be seen. Toward the fibrocartilage layer, the amount of noncollagenous matrix increases. Between the fibrils and fibril bundles, a great amount of glycosaminoglycans, especially chondroitin sulfate, can be demonstrated (1).

Fibrocartilage

Seen under the light microscope, the transition from the tendon tissue to fibrocartilage is gradual. This zone is clearly thicker in children (1 to 2 mm) than in adults (usually between 150 and 400 μm, ranging from approximately 10 to 1,000 μm). Gradually, the cells lose their elongated appearance, becoming round, and begin to look like the chondrocytes. They lie in pairs or rows surrounded by a lacunar space of the extracellular matrix. The cytoplasmic processes are short. In the cytoplasm, the rough endoplasmic reticulum, the Golgi apparatus, the lysosomes, and the lipid cells all increase. The cells also have vesicles full with granular material.

Around the chondrocytes, 10- to 30-nm tendinous collagen fibrils can be seen. Immunohistochemical studies have shown that they are type II collagen, which is the main collagen of articular cartilage (34).

Mineralized Fibrocartilage

The fibrocartilage is separated from the mineralized (calcified) fibrocartilage by a distinct border named as the "cementing" or "blue" line (when stained with hematoxylin and eosin). The transition to mineralized fibrocartilage can be abrupt, although routine electron microscopic techniques do not reveal anything special that would correspond to the blue line in light microscopy.

The width of the mineralized fibrocartilage is 100 to 300 μm. The cells in this region are similar to the chondrocytes of the fibrocartilage, meaning that many of these cells remain alive although surrounded by mineralized tissue. Cell degeneration is not, however, a rare phenomenon. At the same time, the amount of ground substance rich in chondroitin sulfate increases.

The collagen fibers of the tendon reach this region. Two patterns and areas of collagen fiber calcification can be distinguished. Mineralization takes place either as fine granular deposition on the C2, D, E, and A bands of the fibrils or as hydroxyapatite crystals (1). When the first hydroxyapatite crystals appear, they are found between and, somewhat later, on the collagen fibrils. The diameter of this layer is 5 to 20 nm. Deeper in this zone, the crystals start to show up in fine granular or cloudlike forms that are also within the fibers and fibrils.

Bone

As is the case with tendon and fibrocartilage, the boundary between mineralized fibrocartilage and bone is gliding when examined under light and electron microscopes. The bone tissue shows no special features that would separate it from normal bone.

Depending on the directions of the transmitting forces, the collagen fiber architecture of the OTJ varies considerably. In the fibrocartilage and its mineralized counterpart, the fibers criss-cross around the chondrocytes (34). Along with a high concentration of gluelike GAGs, this arrangement is likely to have an important cushioning role in improving the elastic buffer capacity of the OTJ against loading. The fibrocartilage also permits bone growth at the point of insertion as the body grows.

In general, little is known about the functional behavior of the OTJ under various loading conditions *in vivo*. Thus, very little is known about the pathogenesis and mechanisms of the tendon avulsion fractures and overuse-induced apophysitises.

Elastic Fibers

The extracellular tendon matrix is composed of the collagen fibers, elastic fibers, the ground substance, and anorganic components. As previously discussed, collagen constitutes approximately 90% of the total protein of tendons, or 65% to 80% of the dry mass of tendons. Elastic fibers, in turn, account for approximately 2% of the dry mass of a tendon (6,15), whereas in the aorta, elastic fibers make up 30% to 60% of dry weight (35).

The mechanical stability of the tendinous collagen is the most important factor for the mechanical strength of a tendon. The function of elastic fibers is not entirely clear, but they may contribute to the recovery of the wavy configuration of the collagen fibers after tendinous stretch (36).

The tendinous ground substance, which surrounds the collagen, consists of proteoglycans, GAGs, structural glycoproteins, and a vide variety of other small molecules. It is a hydrophilic gel and can vary in consistency depending on the relative proportions of hyaluronic acid and chondroitin sulfate present (37). The water-binding capacity of these macromolecules (proteoglycans and GAGs) is considerable and improves the elasticity of a tendon against shear and compressive forces. They are also important for stabilizing the whole collagenous system of connective tissue and for maintenance of ionic homeostasis and collagen fibrillogenesis.

Elastic fibers are scarcely present in human tendons (38). We found that elastic fibers were actually demonstrable in only 10% of healthy human tendons (39). Elastic fibers have been observed in the Achilles tendons of young and old rabbits (40) and in the tendons of rats (41). In some pathologic conditions of humans, such as Ehlers-Danlos syndrome and chronic uremia, the number and volume of the tendinous elastic fibers are clearly increased. In addition, the fibrocartilage and mineralized fibrocartilage zones of the OTJ contain elastic fibers (34). Electron microscopy reveals that elastic fibers are approximately 0.3 to 2.0 μm in diameter and consists of two distinct morphologic components: an amorphous central bulk (core) and electrodense filaments.

Ground Substance

The macromolecules that comprise the great majority of the extracellular substance of tendons can be classified into three groups: fibril-forming collagen, proteoglycans, and matrix glycoproteins.

Proteoglycans

Proteoglycans are composed of a protein core in which one or more GAG are covalently attached. They are large (molecular mass, 106 Da) negatively charged hydrophilic molecules that can entrain water 50 times their weight. The are mostly entrapped within and between collagen fibrils and fibers. By virtue of their high fixed charge density and charge-to-charge repulsion force, proteoglycans are stiffly extended, providing the collagen fibrils a high capacity to resist high compressive and tensile forces. The mechanism is accentuated by the fact that these molecules are compressed about 20% of their natural solution domain during stress. The proteoglycans also enable rapid diffusion of water-soluble molecules and migration of cells. In addition, the presence of the negatively charged groups attracts many positive counterions in this aqueous surrounding, thus creating a Donnan effect.

The concentration of GAGs is considerably smaller in tendon than in cartilage or other types of connective tissue. The tensional zone of a tendon includes approximately 0.2% GAG (dry mass) of which 60% is dermatan sulfate, whereas the pressure zone and especially the insertion area include up to 3.5 to 5.0% GAG of which 65% is chondroitin sulfate (42). Hyaluronic acid constitutes about 6% of the total GAG. Heparan sulfate can be found at the MTJ (23,28). Neither keratan sulfate nor heparin can be demonstrated in tendon tissue (43).

Matrix Glycoproteins

The glycoproteins are macromolecules that consist of a large protein fraction and a small glycidic component. They have a relatively low molecular mass between 50 and 100 kDa. Glycoproteins have quantitative differences in the protein-to-carbohydrate ratio and qualitative differences in the composition of glycidic radicals. In glycoproteins, the glycidic chains are very short.

Tendon tissue contains various noncollagenous proteins whose identities and functions are not yet well established. Among others, they include the link protein that stabilizes proteoglycan–hyaluronic acid aggregates and a 116-kDa protein of unknown function. In tendon, there is a close relationship between collagen and the glycoproteins (44).

The so-called adhesive glycoproteins form an interesting subgroup of the matrix glycoproteins. These macromolecules either bind other macromolecules or cell surfaces together. Two such molecules have been identified from tendon tissue: fibronectin (43) and thrombospondin (45). Laminin, another candidate, can be found in the vascular walls of the tendons (43) and in great amounts at the MTJ (23,28). Fibronectin—like the other adhesive glycoproteins—participates in both degenerative and repair processes of tendon (43). Thrombospondin, like laminin, is a multidomain adhesive glycoprotein that can interact with fibrinogen, fibronectin, plasminogen, glycolipids, and calcium (46). Thrombospondin is a good candidate for the mediator of or cell–matrix interactions that occur in normal homeostasis and in repair and regeneration.

Anorganic Components

In human tendons, the dry mass is approximately 30% of the total mass of the tendon (7). Collagen comprises approximately 65% to 75% of the tendinous dry mass. Of the remaining substances, most are proteoglycans, approximately 2% are noncollagenous proteins (elastin), and less than 0.2% are anorganic components.

In general, the anorganic components are known to be intimately involved in growth, development, and normal metabolism of musculoskeletal structures (47). For example, copper has an important role in the formation of collagen cross-linking (48), manganese is required for several enzymatic reactions during the synthesis of connective tissue molecules, and calcium has a key role in the development of the OTJ.

In tendons, a wide variety of anorganic components have been detected (49). Calcium is found in the highest concentrations (0.001% to 0.01% of tendon dry mass in the tensional area of a normal tendon and 0.05% to 0.1% in the insertion). In pathologic conditions such as calcifying tendinopathy, 10- to 20-fold increases can be detected (15). Other detected components have been magnesium, manganese, cadmium, cobalt, copper, zinc, nickel, lithium, lead, fluoride, phosphor, and silicon. The trace elements are usually in concentration of 0.02 to 120 ppm in tendon tissue (50). With the exception of copper, manganese, zinc, and calcium, the biochemical and functional role of the trace elements in tendons is unknown.

Tenoblasts and Tenocytes

The tendon cells, the tenoblasts and tenocytes, comprise about 90% to 95% of the cellular elements of the tendon. The other 5% to 10% includes the chondrocytes at the pressure and insertion sites, the synovial cells of the tendon sheath on the tendon surface, and the vascular cells (such as capillary endothelial cells and smooth muscle cells of the arterioles) in the endo- and epitenon. In pathologic conditions, many other types of cells, such as inflammatory cells, macrophages, and myofibroblasts, can be observed in the tendon tissue (1).

Tendon Cell Morphology

The newborn tendon has a very high cell-to-matrix ratio. The cells (tenoblasts) are arranged in long parallel chains (40) of different shapes and sizes. Some are elongated, others rounded, and still others polygonal. In young individuals, a gradual decrease in the cell-to-matrix ratio occurs and the spindle-shaped tenoblasts start to resemble each other. In adults, the cell-to-matrix ratio further decreases and the cells (now called tenocytes) are very elongated.

The size of tenoblasts varies, the length from 20 to 70 μm and the width from 8 to 20 μm. The shape of the nuclei varies from ovoid to very long spindle-shaped nuclei. Although the rough endoplasmic reticulum and the Golgi apparatus are well developed, few mitochondria are seen in the cytoplasm.

In tenoblasts, pinocytotic vesicles and few lysosomes can be observed in the peripheral parts of the cytoplasm. Numerous long and slender cytoplasmic processes extend into the matrix. They contain a remarkable number of cytoplasmic organs and establish the intercellular contacts that can be desmosomal junctions, tight junctions, or gap junctions.

The immature elastic fibers with well-developed amorphous central cores seem to be in close contact with the tenoblast plasma membrane. Around the tenoblasts, granular (amorphic) electrodense material can be also found bearing resemblance to matrix proteoglycans. All these morphologic features of young tenoblasts support the concept of the high metabolic activity of these cells (i.e., intense synthesis of the matrix components).

As the cell-to-matrix ratio gradually decreases with age, many other changes occur inside the tendon cells. The tenoblasts transform to tenocytes (and occasionally vice versa) and become very elongated from 80 to 300 μm in diameter (Fig. 2.4). The nucleus-to-cytoplasm ratio increases, and the cellular processes (2 to 10 μm in diameter) become longer and thinner, extending far from the main body of the cell. The tenocytes, therefore, look like spiders. The long cell processes are needed to keep the close contact between the cells and the matrix components to compensate the decreasing number of cells and increasing amount of tendon matrix during aging.

The nucleus of a tenocyte is elongated, occupying almost entirely the length of the cell. The nuclear chromatin condenses to the margins of the nuclear membrane. The intracytoplasmic actin and myosin filaments and pinocytotic vesicles can be still detected.

Ultrastructural analysis confirms the impression that tenocytes are metabolically active cells, although not in the same level as the tenoblasts. Rough endoplasmic reticulum and Golgi apparatus are still well developed, and the cytoplasm has high quantities of free ribosomes. Mitochondria are few in number but have well-defined cristae. Lysosomes can be identified in varying numbers.

Tendon Cell Metabolism

Today it is well known that tendon cells are active in both energy production and biosynthesis of collagen and other matrix components (16). Animal tendon cells have the enzyme chains for all three main pathways of energy metabolism: the aerobic Krebs cycle, the anaerobic glycolysis, and the pentose phosphate shunt (17,51,52). We showed that the three major pathways of energy metabolism also existed in the tenocytes and peritendinous cells of a human tendon (Fig. 2.10) (51,53).

During the highest growth rate of a young tendon, all three pathways of energy production are highly active. With increasing age, activity of the Krebs cycle and the pentose phosphate shunt decreases, whereas the anaerobic glycolysis remains more or less constant. In other words, the metabolic pathways shift from aerobic to more anaerobic energy production (6,54).

In matrix metabolism, the tendon cells are able to synthesize all components of the tendon matrix, that is, the collagen and elastic fibers, proteoglycans, and structural glycoproteins (14). In general, the synthetic activity is high during growth and declines with age. However, the activity pattern may change drastically in many pathological conditions.

The studies of tendon matrix metabolism have been almost exclusively concerned with collagen metabolism. The literature provides little information about the turnover of the other components of tendon matrix. Concerning collagen metabolism in tendons, three conclusions can be drawn. First, in neonate tendon the collagen

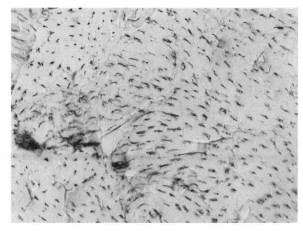

FIG. 2.10. The tenocytes (*black spots*) reveal intense lactate dehydrogenase (LDH) activity in an intact human Achilles tendon (LDH enzyme reaction, ×100).

synthesis rate is relatively high but reduces drastically with age. Second, collagen turnover (synthesis and catabolism) of an adult tendon is fairly low, compared with ligamentous tissue. Finally, the metabolically most active collagen is the most newly synthetized, soluble collagen.

The low metabolic rate of tendon tissue and its well-developed anaerobic energy production is essential if the tendon is to carry loads and remain in tension for periods of time without the risk of ischemia and necrosis. The tendon tolerates low oxygen tension well without injury. However, inevitable drawback of this low metabolic rate is the slow rate of recovery after activity and of healing after injury (5).

The synthesis of the proteoglycans and glycoproteins occur in two places of a tendon cell. The protein component is synthesized at the rough endoplasmic reticulum, but the glycidic part is synthesized in the Golgi apparatus (55). After the protein component has been formed in the rough endoplasmic reticulum, a series of several enzymes in the cisternae of the Golgi apparatus conjugate and sulfate the glycidic radicals. Once the synthesis is complete, the protein–polysaccharide complex is carried through the Golgi apparatus to the plasma membrane to be secreted out of the cell. Again, the literature provides little information about the turnover rates of tendinous proteoglycans and glycoproteins in health or disease.

Compared with the knowledge on the biosynthesis of tendon components, little is know about the anatomic sites and mechanisms of matrix catabolism of a tendon. According to studies from other connective tissue matrices, two methods of degradation seem possible. In one method, the tenocytes produce degradative enzymes and secrete them into extracellular space where degradation of the matrix components occurs. In the second method, the degradation of tendon matrix occurs through direct cellular phagocytosis and pinocytosis, much like osteoclasts in bone (1).

Blood Supply of Tendons

It has been stated that the major blood supply of the tendon is provided through vessels surrounding the tendon and that tendon can not receive the entire circulation required from its proximal or distal attachments (56). In the Achilles tendon, for example, a zone of relative avascularity is between 2 and 6 cm proximal to the tendon insertion (57–59).

At the MTJ, the perimysial blood vessels of the muscle continue between the fasciculi of the tendon and are of the same size as its vessels elsewhere. Other small vessels enter by the paratenon, branching several times in the long axis of the tendon, and where there is a synovial sheath, a plexus transverses the mesotenon or vincula (7). According to Edwards (60), the OTJ is not an important site of entry.

Synovial Sheath

The parietal sheet of the synovial sheath receives most of its vessels directly from the surrounding tissues. However, some vessels of this sheet originate from the branches of the vessels of the mesotenon or vincula. The visceral sheet, in turn, receives its blood supply from the arches of vessels that originate from the major vessels that pass through the mesotenon (1).

In the mesotenon, the vessels are organized in arches like the mesentery of the intestine. In the visceral sheet, these vessels form a vascular plexus similar to that of the peritoneum. The superficial parts of the tendon are supplied by this vessel plexus while part of the mesotenon vessels perforate the epitenon, run in the endotenon septae, and in this way form a connection between the peri- and intratendinous vascular networks.

At each end of the synovial sheath, the visceral and synovial sheaths and their vascular beds join together. The vessels originating from the parietal sheet penetrate into the intratendinous septae, ensuring adequate blood supply for the internal structures of the tendon (60).

Paratenon

In the sites where there is no synovial sheath, the vascular network of paratenon is a very important source of blood for a tendon. The vessels that come into the paratenon usually run transversely through the paratenon (61). These then branch repeatedly, becoming longitudinally and transversely oriented along the fascicles of the tendon to form the vascular network of paratenon.

The arrangement of the vascular network of the paratenon shows great variation from tendon to tendon and even within one tendon. It may look like a regular or irregular mesh, or the vessels can be randomly arranged (62). The arteries of the paratenon are small or medium in diameter, each of them accompanied by one or two veins. The branches of the arteries then penetrate the epitenon and run into the endotenon septae to form the intratendinous vascular network.

Intratendinous Vascular Network

The endotenon carries the blood vessels, nerves, and lymphatics (6–8). The intratendinous network of vessels consists of longitudinally arranged vessels with one artery followed by two veins. These vessels communicate with each other through transverse anastomoses (60). Some of these arteries are greater in diameter than others, sometimes called the main arteries of the intratendinous vascular bed.

The small arterioles and capillaries that originate from the longitudinal arteries form the three types of microvascular units of the tendon tissue. In the first type, where one arteriole supplies several capillaries, each capillary runs parallel with the long axis of the tendon and then loops back to end flowing into a venule. In the second type, the capillaries are looped or irregular in shape. In the third type, the capillaries are very short, run straight, and most likely function as arteriovenous shunts. Because each microvascular unit has a limited capacity and area for efficient gas and metabolite exchange, this overlapping complex vascular system is needed to ensure undisturbed metabolism in all parts of the fiber fascicles.

Myotendinous Junction

At the MTJ, the perimysial blood vessels of the muscle continue between the fasciculi of the tendon and are of the same size as its vessels elsewhere (7). Peacock (63) stated that the blood vessels originating from the muscle do not run beyond the proximal one third of the tendon. A similar finding was made by Carr and Norris (57), who studied the microvascular anatomy of cadaver Achilles tendons by injecting barium sulfate and India ink. When the Achilles paratenon was removed from the limbs, the number of vessels was markedly reduced so that the only vessels still visible were in the MTJ and OTJ.

The abrupt transition at the MTJ is quite clear from the very rich vascular network of the muscle to the relatively poor vascular network in tendon. Many capillaries in the muscle run along the fibers at the MTJ then loop and run backward. There is, however, vascular communication between the perimyseal and tendinous vessels and between vessels at the endomysial and intratendinous levels.

In a rat gastrocnemius–Achilles unit, the MTJ has a vascular organization of the so-called capillary–arteriole–capillary system (64). In this system, capillaries join into small arterioles, the arterioles penetrate the junction, and, on the tendon site, the arterioles again dissolve into capillaries. However, some muscular capillaries penetrate the junction independently and directly. It is not well known if such a system exist in human MTJs, but the system seems to be protecting the blood supply against injuries and other pathologic conditions (64).

Osteotendinous Junction

It is not entirely clear whether or not the intratendinous vessels anastomose with the intraosseus circular network. However, there is good agreement that the vessels of the paratenon or synovial sheath communicate with those of the periosteum at the OTJ (57). The blood supply from the OTJ to the tendon is rather sparse and limited to the insertion zone of the tendon only, and thus this blood supply does not contribute to the vascularity of the main body of the tendon.

Innervation of Tendons

Stillwell (65) described the sensory innervation of tendons as derivations of neighboring muscular, cutaneous, peritendinous, or deep nerve trunks and consisting of a longitudinal plexus with terminations lying mainly near the MTJ. Those from the MTJ cross the junction and continue into the endotenon septae. Those from the paratenon form rich plexuses, send penetrating branches to the epitenon and anastomose with the branches of muscular origin. Where the tendon has a synovial sheath, the nerves go through the mesotenon, branch out into the visceral sheet of the synovial sheath, then penetrate into the tendon. Many nerve fibers do not go inside the tendon but terminate in the sensory nerve endings on the surface of the tendon. Inside a tendon, the scarce nerves follow the vascular channels that run along the long axis of the tendon and finally terminate in the sensory nerve endings.

According to anatomic and functional differences, the nerve endings in tendons, ligaments, and joint capsules can be classified into four categories: type I endings or Ruffini corpuscles, type II endings or Vater-Pacini corpuscles, type III endings or Golgi tendon organs, and type IV free nerve endings. Types I to III are mechanoreceptors that function as transducers converting physical energy, expressed as pressure or tension, into afferent nervous signals (66). Thus, they play a significant role in the organization of the afferent sensory neuron system controlled by the central nervous system (67,68). Their structure in tendons is similar with that in ligaments, capsules, skin, and deep connective tissue. They are found both at the surface and inside the tendon (66). The type IV endings are pain receptors (1,16).

FUNCTION AND BIOMECHANICS OF TENDONS

Basic Tendon Function

The basic function of the tendons is to transmit the force created in the muscle to bone and to make joint and limb movement possible (1). Functional and mechanical behavior of tendons differ from that of a ligament considerably because tendons have the active component (i.e., muscle), whereas ligaments are passive structures subject to external forces only. In fact, tendon function and biomechanics should not be separated from that of the whole muscle–tendon unit (35,36,69,70).

To transmit force effectively, tendons must be capable of resisting high tensile forces with limited elongation

(35,71). In other words, tendons are designed to transmit loads with minimal energy loss and deformation. A tendon is not, however, an entirely inextensible cable that directly transfers the length change or force of a contracting muscle to the bone. Tendon shows an elastic component as well, being capable of deforming and returning to its original length. In this respect, the MTJ and OTJ are very important parts of the muscle–tendon unit.

The physical characteristics of tendons include great tensile strength (which is in part the property of the molecular and supramolecular structure of collagen), good flexibility (which is the property of the elastic fiber), and considerable inextensibility (that means poor, but optimal, elasticity) (7,35,72,73). Compared with their ability to withstand tensile, or stretching, forces, tendons are less able to withstand the shear and compressive forces transmitted by the muscles (6,35). However, because tendons are highly resistant to extension but flexible, they can change the direction of pull (72). In the tendons where tension is exerted in all directions, the fiber bundles are interwoven without regular orientation and the tissues are irregularly arranged (72). If tension is in only one direction, the collagen fibers have an orderly more parallel orientation. In other words, fusiform muscles exert greater tensile force on their tendons than do pennate muscles, because all the force is applied in series with the longitudinal axis of the tendon. The more oblique the muscle fibers, the more force is dissipated laterally, relative to the axis of the tendon (72). The greater the tissue cross-sectional area, the larger the load applied before failure (increased tissue strength and stiffness); the longer the tissue fibers, the greater is the fiber elongation before failure (decreased tissue stiffness with unaltered strength) (36).

Tendon rotation, if present, plays an important role in tendon mechanics and function (12). The Achilles tendon, for example, twists as it descends. Rotation begins above the region where the soleus joins, and the degree of rotation is greater if there is minimal fusion. This twisting may produce areas of high stress concentration on the tendon (74), most severely 2 to 5 cm above the insertion (75). Interestingly, this is also the area where many Achilles tendon ruptures are seen. Also, the Achilles tendon absorbs forces in two planes: the sagittal plane (plantarflexion and dorsiflexion) and the frontal plane (inversion and eversion). These combined stresses create unequal tensile forces on different parts of the tendon (61). This relates to the torsional ischemic "wringing out" (76,77).

In addition to transmitting the force developed by a muscle, a tendon possesses certain secondary functions. For instance, the tendon eliminates the need of any unnecessary length of muscle between origin and insertion and enables the muscle belly to be at a convenient distance from the joint over which it acts while concentrating its pull onto a relatively small area of bone (7). In addition to this load-transmitting role, tendons satisfy both kinematic (they must be flexible enough to bend at joints) and damping requirements (they must absorb sudden shock to limit damage to muscle) (71). The collagenous elements that are not forming the parallel organized tendon fibers (i.e., criss-crossing of fiber bundles and the delicate fibers that form the endotendon and epitenon) can alter tendon course and modify the action of the muscle over one or more joints. Also, tendon tissue carries out a kind of modulation on muscle contraction in such a way as to cushion abrupt, unexpected, and violent motor stimuli (tissue protection) and while accentuating weak subliminal contractions that are functionally insufficient. This modulation derives from the action of the noncollagenous components of the tendon, that is, the action of the elastic fibers, proteoglycan–water matrix, and the tenocytes. There is also evidence that the mechanical properties of collagenous tissues depend not only on the amount and orientation of the collagen but also on the maintenance of cohesion by these interfibrillar substances (7).

Tendon Biomechanics

The mechanical properties of isolated tendons are normally determined by *in vitro* tensile tests. The tissue is elongated to failure at a prescribed rate while the changes in force are recorded. The force is plotted against time, but because a constant strain rate is normally used, the time axis is proportional to elongation. The parameters that are measurable from this force–elongation curve include stiffness (slope) in the linear region, linear load (end of linear region), maximum load, strain (time) to maximum load, strain to failure, and energy to failure (area beneath the entire curve) (36).

However, because tissue dimensions (cross-sectional area and length) affect the shape of the force–elongation curve, the force–elongation curves have been adjusted by dividing force by original cross-sectional area (tensile stress) and elongation by initial length (tensile strain) (78,79). This passive stress–strain curve provides mechanical parameters that are independent of tissue dimensions (Fig. 2.11) (36). The curve is quite similar in shape with the force–elongation curve and has been a valuable tool in studying the mechanical properties of connective tissue (78). It must be remembered that the conditions in the *in vitro* experiments are always more or less artificial.

The mechanical behavior of collagen during a tensile stress is ultimately dependent on the number, types, and sites of the intramolecular and weaker intermolecular bonds (79,80). The molecular alterations that occur during stretching happen not only in transversal (intramo-

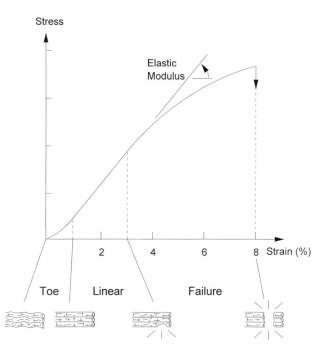

FIG. 2.11. A stress–strain curve of a tendon.

lecular bonds) but especially in longitudinal (intermolecular cohesion) dimensions (81–83).

The intratendinous tension increases at the beginning of the stretch but decreases when the interfibrillar slipping starts even though the fibers continue to stretch. The tension-induced increase in the D period of the fibrils (the cross-striated long periods of the fibrils) from 67 to 70 nm represents the fibril-specific loading limit, an age-dependent phenomenon (82). Electron microscopic investigations first show longitudinal disintegration of the fibrils after which the damage profile bears resemblance to the so-called Knick deformation, a characteristic folding of the surface of the collagen fibrils in the inner curve of the angulated fibrils (84). This damage is preceded by intrafibrillar sliding that occurs at the fiber-specific loading maximum before the beginning of the macroscopic slipping (83). This process of the fibrils is irreversible and must be differentiated from the earlier occurring molecular sliding of the triple helices of collagen, which is a reversible phenomenon (84).

The higher rate of tendon ruptures can be expected to occur in tendons that undergo the above-described structural destabilization as a trigger to the subsequent rupture. Therefore, tendon rupture is the consequence of fibrillar damage of mechanical origin. A quick stretch causes greater molecular and supramolecular deformations than further stretching of the same magnitude and may lead to disordered domain in the tendon structure.

A tissue is said to be elastic if it returns to its original geometric shape after the stress has been removed. If it does not return, the tissue is viscous (79). A tendon

is perfectly elastic as long as the strain does not exceed 4%, after which the viscous range commences. Dunn and Silver (85) hypothesized that the elastic fraction is related to the type of fiber loading and the tissue geometry. Against force, elasticity is a time-independent phenomenon and the viscosity, a time-dependent phenomenon. The elastic fraction (equilibrium force/initial force) at a given strain represents the fraction of the strain energy that is stored reversibly. The elastic component is consistently greater than the viscous component of the tendon (85). The stress deformation of tendon tissue may involve either viscous sliding of the fibrils by their nearest neighbors, viscous rearrangement of material between the fibrils, or both.

Thus, tendons are viscoelastic materials and display a sensitivity to different strain rates. Also, they undergo force relaxation, creep, and hysteresis. Force relaxation (stress relaxation) means that with the same degree of deformation, with time there is a decrease in the load required to maintain that extension (71,80). Creep means that with a constant load, there is an increase in deformation over time. Hysteresis loop (area between the loading and unloading force-displacement curves) is a measure of the energy dissipated or lost during the loading–unloading test and is an indication of the viscous properties of the tissue (36).

At low rates of loading, tendons are more viscous, and therefore they absorb more energy, which is less effective at moving loads. At high rates of loading, tendon absorbs less energy and is more effective at moving heavy loads (80). A short tendon is strong but absorbs less total energy than a long tendon, although its energy-absorbing capacity per unit volume is higher than that of a long tendon.

Stress–Strain Curve of Tendons

In the resting state, the collagen fibers and fibrils of a tendon show a wavy crimped configuration (Fig. 2.3). This configuration disappears when the tendon is stretched by 2%, straightening the fibers (6,7). When the tensile force is released, the tendon resumes its normal wavy appearance.

The initial concave portion of the stress–strain curve (region I) has been termed the "toe" region (7,36,86) (Fig. 2.11). This portion results when the fiber bundle waviness straightens out (14,71). In this region, continued elongation produces stiffer tissue; that is, greater increases in force are needed for equivalent elongations. The strain or relative elongation of the tissue at the end of this region has been reported to be between 1.5% and 4% (36,86). *In vitro* and *in vivo* alterations are similar (87).

Following the toe region, the tendon shows a relatively linear response to stress (region II). The fibers become more parallel and have lost their crimped appearance (88). The slope of this region of the curve is often referred to as the elastic stiffness of the tendon (71). If collagen fibers are tested alone, the strain limits of this region seems to be from 2% to 5% (7,36). Microfailure of fibers occurs at the end of this linear loading region, which may explain the small force reduction that is sometimes seen in this part of the curve. If the tendon is not stressed more than 4%, it will return to its original length (74). When whole ligaments or tendons are tested, the linear region may extend to much higher strain levels—as high as 20% to 50% (89). This is thought to be due to the three-dimensional organization of the fiber bundles within the whole tissue (36).

Beyond linear load (region III), additional fiber failure occurs in unpredictable fashion (36). This region corresponds to strains of 3% to 8% when collagen fibers slide past one another as cross-links fail (72).

In the fourth part of the curve (region IV), macroscopic failure occurs because of the tensile and shear failure between the fibers (72). Once the maximum load is attained, complete failure occurs rapidly and the load-supporting ability of the tendon is lost. Upon failure, the fibers recoil and blossom into a tangled bud at the ruptured end (71).

The above-mentioned passive stress–strain curve represents a simple "stretching to failure" experiment. Improved study design can be reached when the whole muscle–tendon unit is stretched. Using this technique, Nikolau et al. (31) showed with experimental animals that the MTJ is the weakest point in the unit, making is susceptible to strain injuries. True active stress–strain curves can be accomplished using muscle–tendon preparations where the muscle is electrically stimulated at the appropriate time (90).

Tensile Strength of Tendons

Tendons are remarkably strong. As reported by Elliott (7), their *in vitro* tensile strength is about 50 to 100 N/mm^2 (or 5.0 to 10.0 kN/cm^2). Thus, a tendon with a cross-section area of 1 cm^2 is capable of supporting a weight of 500 to 1,000 kg. The tensile strength of compact bone is less than that of tendons (91).

The tensile strength of healthy tendons increases during childhood and adolescence, being highest between 25 to 35 years of age. Thereafter, it slowly decreases. Children's and adolescents' tendons are weaker but more elastic than those of adults. When calculated per cross-section area, there is no gender differences in the tensile strength of human tendons (34).

Inside a resting tendon there is a certain hydrostatic pressure caused by the traction of the elastic fibers (92). Under loading, this pressure increases considerably. According to Ehricht and Passow (93), in the Achilles tendon the pressure is about 7 mm Hg, whereas at maximal loading the pressure may reach 125 mm Hg.

The absolute strength of a tendon is determined by its thickness and internal structure. In this respect, fibrillar organization is of great importance (73). We observed that the finger flexors are stronger than finger extensors, most probably due to their plait-forming spiral structure (94). We also demonstrated that the tensile strength of the common toe extensor tendons differed from that of the common flexor tendons. In both groups, however, the following toe ranking in tendon strength could be seen: toe IV > toe II > toe III > toe V (95).

The close functional relationship between muscle and tendon, the intimate nature of their junction, and the relationship between their longitudinal growth rates would suggest good correlation between the size of the muscle and the girth of its tendon (7). However, in adult rabbits there is no direct relationship between tendon thickness and the contraction force of a corresponding muscle (96). There is about a threefold increase in the weight of the rat Achilles tendon during growth, whereas its muscle weight increases as much as fivefold. Also, muscle type (penniform or fusiform) and durations of characteristic muscular contractions (a slow-twitch or fast-twitch muscle) influence the relationship. In general, the strength of a tendon is related to its thickness and collagen content, not to the maximum tension its muscle can exert (80). Usually, the tensile strength of a healthy tendon is greater than twice the strength of its attached muscle (92,97).

There is a large gap between physiologic loads (less than 4% strains) and the stress that causes tendon failure (98). Tendon is probably never stressed more than a quarter of its ultimate tensile strength during normal activities (7,99). However, Wahrenberg et al. (100) estimated patellar tendon forces up to 5.2 kN during kicking, and it has been estimated that biomechanical forces within this tendon may reach 0.5 kN during level walking, 8.0 kN when landing from a jump, up to 9.0 kN during fast running, and 14.5 kN during competitive weight lifting (14,101).

In Vivo Tensile Forces of Tendons

It has been difficult to determine the tensile forces of tendons *in vivo* (70) or at the time of the tendon injury (72). The accurate determination of *in vivo* functional forces and deformations is, however, a goal of biomechanical research.

Komi (69) and Komi et al. (70,102) were the first to study *in vivo* Achilles tendon forces in humans using the buckle transducers during a wide range of performances in walking, running, jumping, hopping, and bicycling. Their results showed that in many activities the peak Achilles tendon forces (e.g., in running, 9 kN corresponded to 12.5 times body weight, or 11.0 kN/cm^2) were very individual and well above the range of the single-load ultimate tensile strength of the tendon

(7,36). Thus, they demonstrated the limited value of *in vitro* tests for *in vivo* situations. Komi et al. (70) suggested that for injury mechanism, the rate of force increase during the breaking phase of the loading may be much more related to tissue rupture and overuse than the simple loading amplitudes.

In rare cases, estimates of traumatic loads on tendons or ligaments have been reported for actual injuries. Zernicke et al. (101) estimated that 14 to 17 body weight forces acted on the patellar tendon of a skilled weight lifter at the moment of tendon rupture. Usually, the spontaneously ruptured tendons are degenerated and weakened before the rupture (54,103–105), but even a healthy tendon may tear under unfavorable circumstances (72,106).

Forces that place highest stress on the tendon occur during the eccentric muscle contractions (80,98,107). Concerning the Achilles tendon, examples of these include pushing off the weight-bearing foot while simultaneously extending the knee (uphill running), sudden ankle dorsiflexion that occurs unexpectedly (stepping up and then slipping off a step with the heel dropping), and rapid involuntary dorsiflexion of a plantarflexed foot (74). Barfred (75) stated that the tendon is at risk most when tension is applied quickly and obliquely if the tendon is tense before injury, if the tendon is weak in comparison with its muscle, or if the muscle group is stretched by external stimuli such as electrical stimulation. These situations should be avoided to prevent tendon ruptures.

ACKNOWLEDGMENTS

We thank the Medical Research Fund of the Tampere University Hospital, Tampere, Finland, for financial support of the studies.

REFERENCES

1. Jozsa L, Kannus P. *Human tendons. Anatomy, physiology, and pathology.* Champaign, IL: Human Kinetics, 1997.
2. Takahashi M. Microconstructive studies of human digital flexor tendon and tendon sheath. Observation by scanning electron microscope and light microscope. *J Jpn Orthop Assoc* 1982; 56:133.
3. Lundborg G. Experimental flexor tendon healing without adhesion formation—a new concept of tendon nutrition and intrinsic healing mechanism. *Hand* 1976;8:235.
4. Kvist M, Jozsa L, Järvinen M, et al. Fine structural alterations in chronic Achilles paratenonitis in athletes. *Pathol Res Pract* 1985;180:416.
5. Williams JGP. Achilles tendon lesions in sport. *Sports Med* 1986;3:114.
6. Hess GP, Cappiello WL, Poole RM, et al. Prevention and treatment of overuse tendon injuries. *Sports Med* 1989;8:371.
7. Elliott DH. Structure and function of mammalian tendon. *Biol Rev* 1965;40:392.
8. Jozsa L, Kannus P, Balint BJ, et al. Three-dimensional ultrastructure of human tendons. *Acta Anat* 1991;142:306.
9. Kastelic J, Galeski A, Baer E. The multicomposite structure of tendon. *Connect Tissue Res* 1978;6:11.
10. Rowe RWD. The structure of rat tail tendon fascicles. *Connect Tissue Res* 1985;14:21.
11. Chansky HA, Iannotti IP. The vascularity of the rotator cuff. *Clin Sports Med* 1991;10:807.
12. van Gils CC, Steed RH, Page JC. Torsion of the human Achilles tendon. *J Foot Ankle Surg* 1996;35:41.
13. Fan L, Sarkar K, Franks DJ, et al. Estimation of total collagen and types I and III collagen in canine rotator cuff tendons. *Calcif Tissue Int* 1997;60:223.
14. Curwin S. Biomechanics of tendon and the effects of immobilization. *Foot Ankle Clin* 1997;2:371.
15. Jozsa L, Lehto M, Kvist M, et al. Alterations in dry mass content of collagen fibers in degenerative tendinopathy and tendon rupture. *Matrix* 1989;9:140.
16. O'Brien M. Structure and metabolism of tendons. *Scand J Med Sci Sports* 1997;7:55.
17. Tipton CM, Matthes RD, Maynard JA, et al. The influence of physical activity on ligaments and tendons. *Med Sci Sports Exerc* 1975;7:165.
18. Angel G, Georghe V. Interferometric evaluation of collagen concentration in tendon fibers. *Connect Tissue Res* 1985;13:323.
19. Jozsa L, Reffy A, Balint BJ. Polarization and electron microscopic studies on the collagen of intact and ruptured human tendons. *Acta Histochem* 1984;74:209.
20. Dyer RF, Enna CD. Ultrastructural features of adult human tendon. *Cell Tissue Res* 1976;168:247.
21. Moore MJ, De Beaux A. A quantitative ultrastructural study of rat tendon from birth to maturity. *J Anat* 1987;153:163.
22. Marchini M, Morocutti M, Castellani PP, et al. The banding pattern of rat tail tendon freeze-etched collagen fibrils. *Connect Tissue Res* 1983;11:175.
23. Kvist M, Jozsa L, Kannus P, et al. Morphology and histochemistry of the myotendinous junction of the rat calf muscles. Histochemical, immunohistochemical and electron microscopic study. *Acta Anat* 1991;141:199.
24. Michna H. A peculiar myofibrillar pattern in the murine muscle-tendon junction. *Cell Tissue Res* 1983;233:227.
25. Tidball JG, Daniel TL. Myotendinous junction of tonic muscle cells: structure and loading. *Cell Tissue Res* 1986;245:315.
26. Trotter JA, Baca JM. A stereological comparison of the muscle-tendon junction of fast and slow-fibers in chicken. *Anat Rec* 1987;218:256.
27. Tidball JG. Myotendinous junction injury in relation to junction structure and molecular composition. *Exerc Sport Sci Rev* 1991;19:419.
28. Järvinen M, Kannus P, Kvist M, et al. Macromolecular composition of the myotendinous junction. *Exp Mol Pathol* 1991; 55:230.
29. Jozsa K, Kannus P, Järvinen M, et al. Denervation and immobilization induced changes in the myotendinous junction. *Eur J Exp Musculoskel Res* 1992;1:105.
30. Garrett WE. Muscle strain injuries: clinical and basic aspects. *Med Sci Sports Exerc* 1990;22:436.
31. Nikolau PK, McDoland BL, Glisson RR, et al. Biomechanical and histological evaluation of muscle after controlled strain injury. *Am J Sports Med* 1987;15:9.
32. Dolgo-Saburoff G. Über Ursprung und Insertion der Skelettmuskeln. *Anat Anz* 1929;68:30.
33. Rufai A, Ralphs JR, Benjamin M. Structure and histopathology of the insertional region of the human Achilles tendon. *J Orthop Res* 1995;13:585.
34. Becker W, Krahl H. *Die Tendopathien.* Stuttgart: G. Thieme, 1978.
35. Kirkendall DT, Garrett WE. Function and biomechanics of tendons. *Scand J Med Sci Sports* 1997;7:62.
36. Butler DL, Grood ES, Noyes FR, et al. Biomechanics of ligaments and tendons. *Exerc Sport Sci Rev* 1978;6:125.
37. Karpakka J. Effects of physical activity and inactivity on collagen synthesis in rat skeletal muscle and tendon. *Acta Univ Oul D* 1991;231:1.
38. Carlstedt CA. Mechanical and chemical factors in tendon healing. *Acta Orthop Scand Suppl* 1987;224:13.
39. Jozsa L, Balint BJ. The architecture of human tendons. II. The

peritenonium and so-called surface phenomenon. *Traumato-logia* 1978;21:293.

40. Ippolito E, Natali PG, Postacchini F, et al. Morphological, immunochemical and biochemical study of rabbit Achilles tendon at various ages. *J Bone Joint Surg Am* 1980;62:583.

41. Greelee TK, Pike D. Studies of tendon healing in the rat. *Plast Reconstr Surg* 1971;48:260.

42. Merrilees MJ, Flint MH. Ultrastructural study of tension and pression zones in a rabbit flexor tendon. *Am J Anat* 1980;157:87.

43. Jozsa L, Kvist M, Kannus P, et al. Structure and macromolecular composition of the myotendinous junction. *Acta Morphol Hung* 1991;39:287.

44. Anderson JC. Glycoproteins of the connective tissue matrix. *Int Rev Connect Tissue Res* 1976;7:251.

45. Miller RR, McDevitt CA. The presence of thrombospondin in ligament, meniscus and intervertebral disc. *Glycoconjugate* 1988;5:312.

46. Lawler JW. The structural and functional properties of thrombospondin [Review]. *Blood* 1986;67:1192.

47. Schor RA, Prussin SG, Jewett DL, et al. Trace levels of manganase, copper and zinc in rib cartilage as related to age in humans and animals both normal and dwarfed. *Clin Orthop* 1973;93:346.

48. Minor RR. Collagen metabolism. *Am J Pathol* 1980;98:227.

49. Lappalainen R, Knuottila M, Lammi S, et al. Zn and Cu content in human cancellous bone. *Acta Orthop Scand* 1982;53:51.

50. Spadaro JA, Becker RO, Bachman CH. The distribution of trace metal ions in bone and tendon. *Calcif Tissue Res* 1970;6:49.

51. Jozsa L, Balint BJ, Reffy A, et al. Histochemical and ultrastructural study of adult human tendon. *Acta Histochem* 1979;65:250.

52. Tipton CM, Vailas AC, Laughlin HM, et al. Aerobic characteristics of isolated ligaments and tendons. *Physiologist* 1975;14:422.

53. Kvist M, Jozsa L, Järvinen M, et al. Chronic Achilles paratenonitis in athletes: a histological and histochemical study. *Pathology* 1987;19:1.

54. Kannus P, Jozsa L. Histopathological changes preceding spontaneous rupture of a tendon. A controlled study of 891 patients. *J Bone Joint Surg Am* 1991;73:1507.

55. Gallop PM, Blumenfield OO, Seifter S. Structure and metabolism of connective tissue proteins. *Annu Rev Biochem* 1972; 41:617.

56. Archambault JM, Wiley JP, Bray RC. Exercise loading of tendons and the development of overuse injuries. *Sports Med* 1995;20:77.

57. Carr AJ, Norris SH. The blood supply of the calcaneal tendon. *J Bone Joint Surg Br* 1989;71:100.

58. Håstad K, Larsson LG, Lindholm Å. Clearance of radiosodium after local deposit in the Achilles tendon. *Acta Chir Scand* 1958 & 1959;116:251.

59. Lagergren C, Lindholm Å. Vascular distribution in the Achilles tendon. An angiographic and microangiographic study. *Acta Chir Scand* 1958 & 1959;116:491.

60. Edwards DAW. The blood supply and lymphatic drainage of tendons. *J Anat* 1946;80:147.

61. Reynolds NL, Worrell TW. Chronic Achilles peritendinitis: etiology, pathophysiology, and treatment. *J Orthop Sports Phys Ther* 1991;13:1716.

62. Brockis JG. The blood supply of the flexor and extensor tendons of the fingers in man. *J Bone Joint Surg Br* 1953;35:131.

63. Peacock EE. A study of the circulation in normal tendons and healing grafts. *Ann Surg* 1959;149:415.

64. Kvist M, Hurme T, Kannus P, et al. Vascular density at the myotendinous junction of the rat gastrocnemius muscle after immobilization and remobilization. *Am J Sports Med* 1995; 23:359.

65. Stillwell DL. The innervation of tendons and aponeuroses. *Am J Anat* 1957;100:289.

66. Jozsa L, Balint J, Kannus P, et al. Mechanoreceptors in human myotendinous junction. *Muscle Nerve* 1993;16:453.

67. Jozsa L, Kvist M, Kannus P, et al. The effect of tenotomy and immobilisation on muscle spindles and tendon organs of the rat calf muscles. *Acta Neuropathol* 1988;76:465.

68. Katonis PG, Assimakopoulos AP, Agapitos MV, et al. Mechanoreceptors in the posterior cruciate ligament. *Acta Orthop Scand* 1991;62:276.

69. Komi PV. Relevance of in vivo force measurements to human biomechanics. *J Biomech* 1990;23:23.

70. Komi PV, Fugashiro S, Järvinen M. Biomechanical loading of Achilles tendon during normal locomotion. *Clin Sports Med* 1992;11:521.

71. Best TM, Garrett WE. Basic science of soft tissue: muscle and tendon. In: DeLee JC, Drez D, eds. *Orthopaedic sports medicine.* Philadelphia: W.B. Saunders, 1994:1.

72. O'Brien M. Functional anatomy and physiology of tendons. *Clin Sports Med* 1992;11:505.

73. Oxlund H. Relationships between the biomechanical properties, composition and molecular structure of connective tissues. *Connect Tissue Res* 1986;15:65.

74. Curwin S, Stanish WD. *Tendinitis: its etiology and treatment.* Lexington, MA: Collamore Press, 1984.

75. Barfred T. Experimental rupture of Achilles tendon. *Acta Orthop Scand* 1971;42:528.

76. Clement D, Taunton J, Smart G. Achilles tendinitis and peritendinitis: etiology and treatment. *Am J Sports Med* 1984;12:179.

77. Smart G, Taunton J, Clement D. Achilles disorders in runners—a review. *Med Sci Sports Exerc* 1980;12:231.

78. Stone MH. Connective tissue and bone response to strength training. In: Komi PV, ed. *Strength and power in sport.* Oxford: Blackwell, 1992:279.

79. Viidik A. Biomechanics and functional adaptation of tendons and joint ligaments. In: Evans GF, ed. *Studies on the anatomy and function of bone and joints.* New York: Springer, 1966:17.

80. Fyfe J, Stanish WD. The use of eccentric training and stretching in the treatment and prevention of tendon injuries. *Clin Sports Med* 1992;11:601.

81. Kuhnke E. The fine structure of collagen fibrils as the basis for functioning for tendon tissue. In: Ramanathan N, ed. *Collagen.* New York: Interscience Publishers, 1962:479.

82. Nemetschek T, Riedl H, Jonak H, et al. Die Viskoelastizität parallelsträngingen Bindegewebes und ihre Bedeutung für die Funktion. *Virchows Arch A* 1980;386:125.

83. Knörzer E, Folkhard W, Greeken W, et al. New aspects of the etiology of tendon rupture: an analysis of time-resolved dynamic-mechanical measurement using synchroton radiation. *Arch Orthop Trauma Surg* 1986;105:113.

84. Mösler E, Folkahard W, Knörzer F, et al. Stress-induced molecular rearrangement in tendon collagen. *J Mol Biol* 1985; 182:589.

85. Dunn MG, Silver FH. Viscoelastic behaviour of human connective tissues: relative contribution of viscous and elastic components. *Connect Tissue Res* 1983;12:59.

86. Viidik A. Functional properties of collagenous tissues. *Int Rev Connect Tissue Res* 1973;6:127.

87. Whittager P, Canham PB. Demonstration of quantitative fabric analysis of tendon collagen using two-dimensional polarized light microscopy. *Matrix* 1991;11:56.

88. Zernicke RF, Loitz BJ. Exercise-related adaptations in connective tissue. In: Komi PV, ed. *Strength and power in sport. The encyclopaedia of sports medicine.* Oxford: Blackwell, 1992:77.

89. Kennedy JC, Hawkins RJ, Willis RB, et al. Tension studies of human knee ligaments. *J Bone Joint Surg Am* 1976;58:350.

90. Garrett WE, Safran MR, Seaber AV, et al. Biomechanical comparison of stimulated and nonstimulated skeletal muscle pulled to failure. *Am J Sports Med* 1987;15:448.

91. Barnett CH, Davies DV, MacConaill MA. *Synovial joints: their structure and mechanics.* London: Longmans, 1961:82.

92. Kvist M. Achilles tendon overuse injuries. Academic Thesis. Turku, Finland: University of Turku, 1991:1.

93. Ehricht H-G, Passow G. Achillodynie-Achilles-sehnenruptur: Genese, Klinik, Therapie, Prophylaxe und Metaphylaxe. *Med Sport* 1972;12:333.

94. Jozsa L. Architecture of flexor tendons of digits. In: Endrödi J, Simonka JA, eds. *Surgery of flexor tendons.* Szeged: University Press, 1980:7.

95. Jozsa L. The biology of tendon. In: Csaba GY, ed. *Actual problems in biology.* Budapest: Medicina, 1983:101.

96. Elliott DH, Crawford GNC. The thickness and collagen content

of tendon relative to the strength and cross-sectional area of muscle. *Proc R Soc Med* 1965;B162:137.

97. Frey C, Shereff M. Tendon injuries about the ankle in athletes. *Clin Sports Med* 1988;7:103.

98. Stanish WD, Curwin S, Rubinovich M. Tendinitis: the analysis and treatment for running. *Clin Sports Med* 1985;4:593.

99. Walker LB, Harris EH, Benedict JV. Stress-strain relationships in the human plantaris tendon: a preliminary study. *Med Biol Eng* 1964;2:31.

100. Wahrenberg H, Lundbeck L, Ekholm J. Dynamic load in human knee during voluntary active impact to lower leg. *Scand J Rehabil Med* 1978;10:93.

101. Zernicke RF, Garhammer J, Jobe FW. Human patellar-tendon rupture. *J Bone Joint Surg Am* 1977;59:179.

102. Komi PV, Salonen M, Järvinen M, et al. In vivo registration of Achilles tendon forces in man. I. Methodological development. *Int J Sports Med* 1987;8:S3.

103. Kannus P, Jozsa L, Järvinen M. Epidemiology and histology of Achilles tendon rupture. *Foot Ankle Clin* 1997;2:475.

104. Kannus P, Natri A, Jozsa L. Aetiology and pathogenesis of chronic tendon injuries in sports. *Baillieres Clin Orthop* 1997; 2:25.

105. Movin T, Guntner P, Gad A, et al. Ultrasonography-guided percutaneous core biopsy in Achilles tendon disorder. *Scand J Med Sci Sports* 1997;7:244.

106. Plecko M, Passl R. Ruptures of the Achilles tendon: Causes and treatment. *J Finn Orthop Trauma* 1991;14:201.

107. Komi PV. Physiological and biomechanical correlates of muscle function: effects of muscle structure and stretch-shortening cycle on force and speed. *Exerc Sports Sci Rev* 1984;12:81.

Principles and Practice of Orthopaedic Sports Medicine,
edited by William E. Garrett, Jr., Kevin P. Speer, and Donald T. Kirkendall.
Lippincott Williams & Wilkins, Philadelphia © 2000.

CHAPTER 3

Biomechanics of Ligaments: Healing and Reconstruction

Savio L-Y. Woo, C. Benjamin Ma, Eric K. Wong, and Akihiro Kanamori

ANATOMY

Ligaments are highly specialized dense connective tissue that connect bones and support viscera. Grossly, they are white, shiny, bandlike structures. Besides water (which comprises 65% to 70% of the ligament's weight), ligaments are composed predominantly of matrix substance. Ligaments are also relatively hypocellular, with fibroblastic cells interspersed in the tissue matrix. Microscopically, the extracellular matrix is highly organized with fiber bundles composed primarily of type I collagen.

Ligaments attach to bones through direct or indirect insertions (1). For direct insertions, there are four distinct zones of transition: ligament, uncalcified fibrocartilage, calcified fibrocartilage, and bone. For indirect insertions, the surface of the ligament connects with the periosteum, whereas the deeper layers connect to bone via Sharpey fibers. A prime example of a ligament that exhibits both types of insertion is the medial collateral ligament (MCL). Its femoral insertion is direct, whereas the tibial insertion is indirect (2,3).

Ligaments are important structures that bear tensile loads in the joints. Their behavior governs the complex joint motion and helps to distribute load to other structures in the joint. In this chapter, we focus on the biomechanical properties, healing potential of knee ligaments, and the current concepts of evaluating ligament reconstructions. An understanding of these properties is important in preventing injuries and improving outcomes of ligament injuries.

TENSILE PROPERTIES OF LIGAMENTS

Ligaments consist of densely packed collagen fibers that are nearly parallel with the long axis of the ligament. Under polarized light microscopy, the fibrils comprising ligaments have a microstructural form with a sinusoidal wave pattern (crimp). Crimping is thought to have significant importance on the biomechanical behavior of ligaments. This can be demonstrated by examining the structural properties obtained from tensile testing of a bone–ligament–bone complex. Structural properties of a complex include the ultimate tensile load, stiffness, and energy absorbed to failure. As a tensile load is applied, the relationship between the load and elongation of the ligament is initially nonlinear. This nonlinear region is referred to as the toe region (T in Fig. 3.1A) and is characterized by large elongations with only small increases in load. Physically, this behavior is thought to be due to the straightening of crimped collagen fibrils. Typically, the toe region is defined as less than 3% strain. As the applied load continues to increase, the fibrils become taut, the stiffness (defined as the slope of the curve) increases, and the load versus elongation plot becomes more linear (S in Fig. 3.1A). A third region of the load–elongation curve shows a slight decrease in stiffness as individual fibers start to fail (Y in Fig. 3.1A). This region is followed by failure of the structure after the ultimate load is reached (U in Fig. 3.1A). The area under the entire curve constitutes the energy absorbed to failure of the structure (W in Fig. 3.1A).

To determine the quality of the ligament substance, its mechanical properties could be determined from the stress–strain curve. The stress–strain curve can be derived from the load–elongation relationship of the ligament. The stress in a ligament is defined as load per cross-sectional area (N/mm^2), whereas strain is defined as the change in length divided by the resting length of a ligament. Similar to the load–elongation curve, the

SL-Y. Woo, C. B. Ma, E. K. Wong, and A. Kanamori: Musculoskeletal Research Center, Department of Orthopaedic Surgery, University of Pittsburgh, Pennsylvania, 15213.

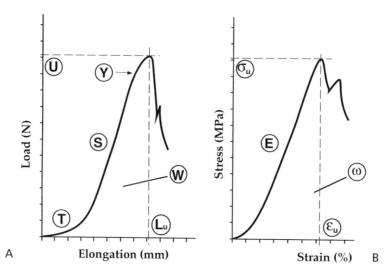

FIG. 3.1. A: Schematic load–elongation curve obtained from tensile testing of a muscle–tendon–bone or bone–ligament–bone complex. **B:** The corresponding stress–strain curve of the ligament or tendon substance.

stress–strain curve is also nonlinear. From the stress–strain curve, one may obtain parameters such as modulus (slope of the stress–strain curve, E in Fig. 3.1B), tensile strength (stress at which the tissue substance fails, σ_u in Fig. 3.1B), and ultimate strain (strain at which the tissue fails, ε_u in Fig. 3.1B). The area under this curve is called the strain energy density of the ligament (ω in Fig. 3.1B).

Bone–Ligament–Bone Complex

Several factors have been known to change the structural properties of a bone–ligament–bone complex. For

the human femur–anterior cruciate ligament–tibia complex (FATC), the effects of age and direction of load application on its structural properties have been evaluated (4,5). Linear stiffness, ultimate load, and energy absorbed to failure decreased significantly with specimen age. For the human FATC, the specimens tested in the anatomic orientation (tensile load aligned with the anatomic orientation of the anterior cruciate ligament [ACL]) had higher values for structural properties than specimens tested in the tibial orientation (tensile load applied along the long axis of the tibia) (6) (Fig. 3.2). In fact, in the younger specimens (22 to 35 years) tested in the anatomic orientation, linear stiffness was found

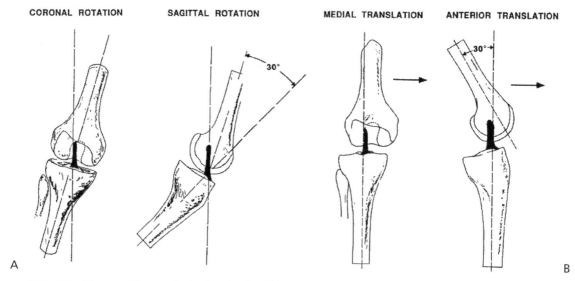

FIG. 3.2. Alignment for tensile testing for the **(A)** anatomic orientation and the **(B)** tibial orientation of the human femur–anterior cruciate ligament–tibia complex. (From Woo S.L-Y, Hollis JM, Adams DJ. Tensil properties of the human femur–anterior cruciate ligament–tibia complex: the effect of specimen age and orientation. *Am J Sports Med* 1991;19:217–225, with permission.)

to be 242 N/mm and ultimate load was 2,160 N. These values were approximately 20% higher than the results obtained from tensile loading of the FATC in the tibial orientation (7). This new result obtained from the anatomic position should be considered as the stiffness and ultimate tensile load of the human ACL.

Homogeneity

Ligaments can be subdivided into bundles with specific fiber orientations. The human ACL consists of two distinct bundles, the anteromedial and posterolateral bundles, whereas the posterior cruciate ligament consists of the anterolateral and posteromedial bundles (8–10). These bundles have significantly different orientations and are named with respect to their tibial insertions. Previous studies have shown that different bundles within the ligament resist different loads (8–12) and thus are of great importance when performing cruciate ligament reconstructions. However, the complex geometry of these ligaments makes the determination of the mechanical properties of the ligament substance difficult. To determine the mechanical properties of the ligament, the individual bundles have to be evaluated separately. In the rabbit ACL, the mechanical properties of the medial and lateral bundles were evaluated (13) and were found to be similar. For instance, the moduli of the medial and lateral bundles were 516 ± 64 and 516 ± 69 MPa, respectively. Butler et al. (14) subdivided the human ACL into three bundles and examined the mechanical properties of the anteromedial, anterolateral, and posteriolateral bundles of the human ACL. They noted higher values for modulus, tensile strength, and strain energy in the anterior bundles when compared with those of the posterior bundle.

Effect of Strain Rate

Historically, it has been thought that strain rate would play a significant role in the mechanical properties of ligaments; however, careful studies revealed that strain rate actually plays a relatively minor role (15–19). The mechanical properties of rabbit ACL (medial portion) and patellar tendon (middle third) over a wide range of strain rates were also studied (18). Results showed that the modulus of rabbit ACL increased minimally with higher strain rates. Moreover, the modulus of the rabbit patellar tendon was slightly more sensitive over 4.5 decade difference in strain rates.

Homeostasis

The immobilization of a joint for injured ligaments has significant effects on its mechanical properties (3,20–25). The healed ligament from an isolated injury treated with immobilization is known to be less stiff and less

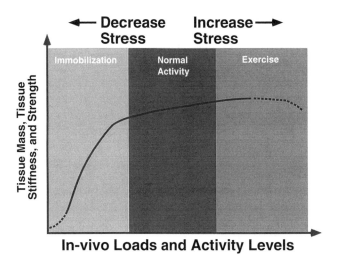

FIG. 3.3. Hypothetical response of ligaments to levels of stress.

strong than the ligament in joints that have been allowed to move (Fig. 3.3). In a canine study, long-term results of the healed MCL were compared between the nonrepaired mobilized group and suture-repaired immobilized group. At 48 weeks, the ultimate load and modulus of the MCL from the nonrepaired mobilized group was stronger than the repaired and immobilized group. Results of this study suggest that prolonged immobilization after ligament injury may be harmful to the ligament itself. However, motion that is too early and excessive may elongate or disrupt the healed ligament, especially in cases involving multiple ligament injury. This effect has been proven by a rabbit study in which osteoarthritic changes were observed in a combined ligament injury model.

Viscoelastic Properties of Ligaments

The time- and history-dependent viscoelastic behavior of ligaments (including creep, stress relaxation, and hysteresis) may explain the postoperative changes observed in graft properties (26–28). Stress relaxation is defined as the decrease in load (or stress) of a viscoelastic material when subjected to constant elongation (Fig. 3.4A). Similarly, creep is defined as the time-dependent elongation of a tissue subjected to a constant load (or stress) (Fig. 3.4B). This viscoelastic behavior will cause a hysteresis loop between each cycle of loading and unloading of a ligament between two limits of elongation. The area between the loading and unloading curves represents the energy losses during each cycle (Fig. 3.5). Because of stress relaxation, the peak load at the same elongation decreases with each cycle. Over the course of several cycles, the area of hysteresis is reduced and the curves are subsequently more repeatable. This phe-

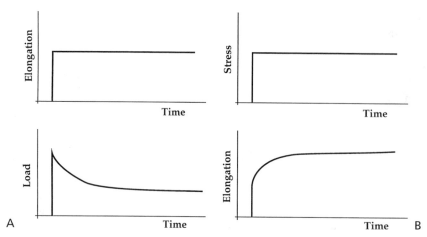

FIG. 3.4. (A) Stress relaxation under a constant elongation and **(B)** creep under a constant load.

nomenon provides the rationale for preconditioning tissue before performing tensile testing.

Clinically, the phenomenon of stress relaxation suggests that the initial tension applied to fix a graft at a set length (elongation) during ACL reconstruction can significantly decrease over time. Graf et al. (29), using primate patellar tendon grafts, noted that preconditioned specimens experienced a significant reduction in stress relaxation when compared with unpreconditioned specimens (*i.e.*, a 30.2% ± 11.5% drop in initial load over 10 minutes versus a 69.8 ± 7.2% drop). This study demonstrated that intraoperative graft preconditioning before fixation could minimize the amount of stress relaxation of the graft after fixation.

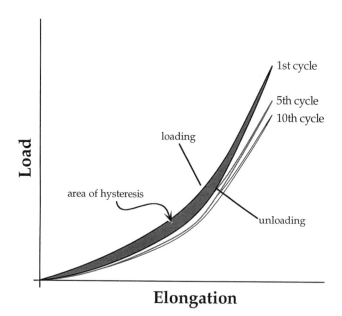

FIG. 3.5. Cyclic loading–unloading curves for ligaments. Both the area of hysteresis and the peak load reduce with the number of cycles.

Cyclic stress-relaxation behavior also plays a role in preventing ligament injury as it undergoes an extensive number of cyclic elongations during the performance of daily activities. These repetitive subfailure stresses have the potential to cause fatigue failure. However, cyclic stress relaxation that results in a reduction in stress with each elongation cycle could prevent fatigue failure of a ligament. Cyclic stress relaxation (or creep) can also be translated to explain the importance of stretching or warm-up exercises before vigorous physical activity to decrease maximal tissue stresses.

Static and cyclic stress-relaxation and creep tests can be used to formulate mathematical descriptions that characterize or predict the viscoelastic response of a tissue. The quasilinear viscoelastic theory developed by Fung (30,31) has been useful in describing and predicting the time- and history-dependent viscoelastic properties of ligaments (24,27,32). In this theory, five constants are determined and can then be used to predict the stresses in a tissue at any time. A more general, nonlinear, single-integral finite strain viscoelastic theory to model the behavior of ligaments and tendons has also been used (33,34). This theory can describe the finite deformation of a three-dimensional nonlinearly viscoelastic continuum and follows the work on general integral series representations by Pipkin and Rogers. The single-integral finite strain theory can also be used to describe the viscoelastic behavior of tissues subjected to more complex loading conditions than uniaxial tension. In the limited case of infinitesimal strain under uniaxial tension, the single-integral finite strain theory is reduced to the quasilinear viscoelastic theory (33).

LIGAMENT HEALING

Different ligaments have different potential to heal with injury. Clinically, injury to the MCL could heal without significant dysfunction, whereas injury to the ACL has significantly worse outcomes when these injuries are treated nonoperatively. Healing of isolated injuries of the ACL and MCL has been well studied in animal models (35–47). There are a number of differences between the ACL and MCL. The MCL is an extraarticular ligament, whereas the ACL is an intraarticular ligament located in the synovial joint space. Cell morphology (48), cell proliferation (49), biomechanical properties (2), biochemical properties (50), and the stress that the ligaments resist (51) are also markedly different.

Similar to wound healing, ligament healing follows the process of producing extracellular matrix to fill the ruptured site (52). The first phase of healing (hemorrhagic phase) occurs within minutes to hours postinjury with bleeding and clot formation at the site of injury. Polymorphonuclear cells and lymphocytes appear at the injured area within a few hours. The second phase (inflammatory phase) follows with the migration of monocytes to the injured area. Monocytic cells are present within 24 hours and become the predominant cell type over the next few days. The monocytic cells are engaged in phagocytosis of necrotic tissue and cellular debris. At the end of the second phase, a few days after injury, fibroblasts are evident and are producing extracellular matrix. The third phase (proliferative phase) is marked by the beginning of cellular and matrix proliferation. During this stage, new vessels are formed and fibroblasts produce extracellular matrix actively. The final stage, the remodeling phase, comes several weeks after injury. There is an increase in collagen matrix, and collagen fibers become better aligned along the long axis of the ligament. This matrix continues to improve the biomechanical properties of the healing ligament over the next few months and years.

Healing of the Medial Collateral Ligament

Using animal models for MCL injuries, various factors that affect healing have been studied (35–47). Injuries to the MCL have been shown to heal spontaneously without surgical intervention; however, the healed tissue remains abnormal postinjury even after a long period of time. Biomechanical studies using the canine model have shown that the stiffness and strength of the MCL remain inferior to those for the normal MCL even at 48 weeks postinjury (53). In contrast, knee kinematics improve in a significantly shorter period of time. The varus-valgus laxity of the MCL injured knee, under ideal conditions (isolated injury with proper mobilization), recovers almost completely in 12 weeks, and this improvement continues up to 48 weeks (3,53). Healed MCL also has very different collagen composition. The distribution of collagen types (i.e., types I and III) resembles that of normal ligaments by 1 year (52); however, the mature collagen cross-links remain low (54).

The diameters of the collagen fibrils in the healed ligament are also significantly smaller than the normal ligament (52).

In the past, there has been a lot of controversy regarding surgical or conservative treatments for isolated MCL ruptures. Isolated MCL ruptures have been studied using the canine and rabbit models, and these studies demonstrated that the histologic appearance of both the surgical and conservative treatment groups were similar to the normal MCL at 48 weeks. However, the biomechanical properties of the unrepaired ligament were better at all time periods (55). Clinical studies also confirmed this observation for nonoperative treatment of complete MCL ruptures. Patients who received conservative treatment had similar or better results, suggesting that surgical repair is not needed (56). With our current knowledge, the optimal treatment for isolated MCL injury has been nonoperative treatment with early motion and functional rehabilitation.

Healing of the Anterior Cruciate Ligament

The healing process of ACL injuries has also been studied in animal models (40–42,47,57,58); however, the results were not the same as MCL injuries (59). In general, studies have shown that a midsubstance ACL tear does not heal with conservative treatment or primary surgical repair (40,60,61). In the canine model, resorption of the repaired ACL stump was seen frequently, resulting in poor surgical outcomes (60,61). For primary repair of the ACL using sutures, the ACL stump was reabsorbed in 40% of the specimens. Although some repairs have failed, even those that went on to heal had poor biomechanical properties.

A number of theories have been proposed for the poor healing potential of the ACL. One theory was that the ACL is an intraarticular ligament surrounded by synovial fluid that contains aggressive enzymes (62). However, a number of in vitro studies have shown the positive effect of synovial fluid on ligament cell proliferation (52). Another theory for poor healing potential involves the synovium that covers the intact ACL. The synovium is highly vascularized with blood vessels that originate from the ligamentous branch of the middle geniculate artery (63,64). It has been proposed that when the ACL is ruptured, the surrounding synovial membrane is simultaneously ruptured, disrupting the blood supply to the ligament. Thus, poor vascular supply may be the cause for the poor potential for healing of the ACL. Others have suggested that the important role of the ACL, especially in resisting anterior tibial load (12), might affect its healing. These authors proposed that the injured ACL may be under too much stress to allow adequate healing to take place (65,66). With the poor healing potential of ACL injuries, biologic or synthetic grafts are currently being used for ACL reconstructions to restore normal knee function.

Combined Injury of the Anterior Cruciate Ligament and the Medial Collateral Ligament

In multiple ligament injuries such as the combined ACL+MCL injury, the healing potential of individual ligaments is significantly different than isolated ligament injuries. Contrary to an isolated MCL injury where other ligaments could effectively distribute the load to allow MCL healing (65), the healing potential of the MCL is significantly worsened in combined ACL+MCL injuries. In a canine study on the combined MCL+ACL injury, the stiffness and strength of the healed MCL after an untreated combined ACL+MCL injury is significantly lower than that of the healed MCL after an isolated MCL injury (47). It has been proposed that the ACL contributes resistance to valgus stress to the knee, especially in the MCL-deficient state (67). Thus, when a combined ACL+MCL injury occurs, the injured knee will not be able to redistribute the load, especially valgus load, which is previously resisted by the MCL. This results in high stress on the healing ligament and poor healing conditions. Animal studies have shown that ACL reconstruction can have a beneficial effect on MCL healing when the valgus instability is corrected (42).

As ACL reconstruction is recommended in combined ACL+MCL injury, controversy remains with whether the MCL injury requires any surgical intervention. In a combined ACL+MCL rabbit injury model, suture repair of the MCL with ACL reconstruction resulted in less valgus instability than ACL reconstruction alone at 12 weeks (42). However, at 52 weeks, no significant differences were demonstrated between the two groups for knee laxity and ultimate failure load of the injured ligaments (58). This result demonstrated that suture repair of the MCL produced little or no improvements in the healing of MCL. With the knowledge from animal studies regarding ACL and MCL healing, as well as improved techniques of ACL reconstruction and postoperative rehabilitation protocols, the recommended clinical treatment of combined ACL+MCL injury has also been revised (68).

Potential Use of Growth Factors

Increasing interest in molecular biology and improvement in cell studies have led to significant research efforts on the effect of growth factors on ligament healing (46,69–76). Growth factors are proteins that are detected during the early phase of ligament healing. Investigators believe that these factors play a major regulatory role in the healing process, such as cell proliferation, matrix synthesis, and secretion of other growth factors. Cell culture studies have shown that a number of these

growth factors have positive effects on the healing process, including MCL and ACL fibroblasts (49,70,77). Recently published *in vivo* studies have also suggested that the application of growth factors can enhance the structural and mechanical properties of the healed MCL (71,76). However, other studies have failed to show the beneficial effect of growth factors in ligament healing (78,79). Thus, the application of growth factors to enhance ligament healing remains an exciting field in medicine that will require more studies to determine its mechanism and its long-term benefits.

LIGAMENT RECONSTRUCTION

With the increasing emphasis in sports and higher incidence of high-energy trauma, the number of ligament injuries has also increased accordingly. The cruciate ligaments, also known as the crucial ligaments in the knee, are commonly injured. Their deficiency may lead to knee instability and early degeneration of other knee structures.

Since 1917 when Hey Groves (80) first published his method of ACL reconstruction using tensor fascia latae, various methods and replacement grafts have been sed for ACL reconstructions. Patellar tendon (81–87), semitendinosus tendon (88–91), gracilis tendon, tensor fascia latae (80), and quadriceps tendon (92–94) are common replacement grafts; however, before determining the appropriate graft and reconstructive procedure, studies have to be performed to determine the importance of the intact ligament within the knee. For the past 20 years, much research has been devoted to characterizing the biomechanical behavior of knee ligaments.

Six Degrees of Freedom of Knee Motion

The knee joint is a complex diarthrodial joint that has six degrees of freedom (DOFs): three translations and three rotations. The knee has three axes that can be defined by the femoral shaft axis, mid-epicondylar axis, and the floating axis perpendicular to the two axes, also know as the anterior–posterior axis. Translation along these three axes will lead to distraction–compression, medial–lateral translation, and anterior-posterior translation, respectively. Rotation about these axes will lead to internal–external tibial rotation, flexion–extension, and varus–valgus rotation, respectively (Fig. 3.6). The six DOFs together with the knee's anatomy led to the complex motion of this diarthrodial joint.

Early studies on the function of knee ligaments simplified the complex motion of the knee joint. When evaluating the function of a ligament, kinematic changes of the joint in one DOF were measured in response to applied loads before and after sectioning of a ligament.

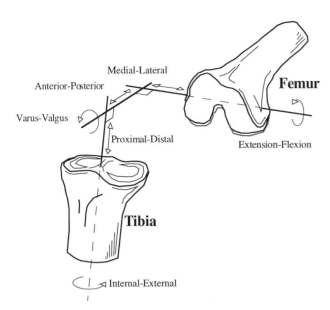

FIG. 3.6. Six degrees of freedom of the human knee joint. Three main axes are shown: the femoral axis, the tibial axis, and the floating varus–valgus axis. (From Wou S.L-Y, Livesay GA, Smith BA. Kinematics. In: *Knee surgery.* Baltimore, MD: Williams & Wilkins, 1994:173–187, with permission.)

For example, the anterior–posterior translation of the knee was measured before and after the transection of the ACL in response to an anterior–posterior load. When performing these experiments, the other DOFs were constrained and were not studied. Fukubayashi et al. (95) later developed a testing apparatus that could accommodate multiple DOF tests. By increasing the DOF, the investigators were able to recognize the importance of coupled motion. When an anterior load was applied to the tibia, the knee responded with anterior translation and coupled internal rotation. This coupled motion is a result of the complex geometry of the joint and various orientations of load-bearing structures. The concept of multiple DOF tests is important to increase the accuracy of studying the function of ligaments and understanding the complexity of knee motion.

In the laboratory, biomechanical tests are usually performed with the knee in five DOF, constraining the flexion angle. Under these conditions, investigators are able to simulate clinical tests like the Lachman and anterior drawer test when the patient's knee is examined at certain flexion angles.

In Situ Forces in the Ligament

To further identify the role played by ligaments, it is necessary to determine the amount of force carried by the ligaments in response to external loads. The Latin term "*in situ*" force was used to describe the force carried by the ligament in its normal position and environment in the knee. Knowledge of the *in situ* forces in the

ACL is important for the understanding of the function of the ACL and for improving ACL reconstructions. Moreover, one can identify loading conditions that will adversely load the ACL and ACL replacement grafts. This information is useful for designing postoperative rehabilitation exercises.

Several techniques have been developed to measure the *in situ* force in ligament; they could be categorized mainly into contact and noncontact methods. Contact methods involve making direct mechanical contact with the ligament midsubstance by a force-measuring device. These methods include the use of buckle transducers (96–99) and implantable transducers (100–106). Noncontact methods include the placement of strain gauges near the ligament insertion site, linkage systems (107,108), the placement of in-line external force transducers (109), and the use of x-rays to make kinematic calculations (110,111).

Use of Robotic/Universal Force-moment Sensor Technology in Biomechanics

Robotic technology has recently been introduced to the study of knee kinematics and the *in situ* forces in ligaments. The robotic/universal force-moment sensor (UFS) system consists of a robotic manipulator with a UFS mounted to its end effector (Fig. 3.7) (112–114). This innovative system enabled highly accurate kinematic measurements and direct measurement of the force in a ligament without physical contact of the ligament or significant dissection of the joint. Besides being used to study the biomechanics of the knee, this technology has also been extended to the characterization of the glenohumeral joint and spine mechanics (115,116).

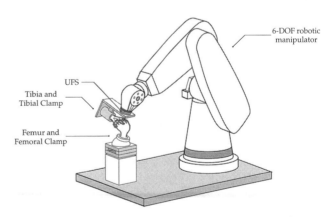

FIG. 3.7. Robotic/universal force-moment sensor (UFS) test system with a knee specimen mounted. Note that the tibia is fixed through the UFS to the manipulator. (From Livesay GA, Rudy TW, Wou S.L-Y, et al. *Evaluation of the effect of joint constraints on the in situ force distribution in the anterior cruciate ligament. J Orthop Res* 1997;15:278–284, with permission.)

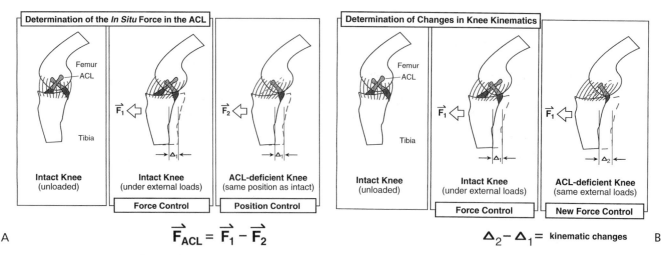

FIG. 3.8. A: Calculation of the *in situ* force in the anterior cruciate ligament (ACL) using a side view of the knee. The force in the ACL is obtained by comparing the forces measured for the intact joint with forces measured for the ACL-deficient joint in the same position as the intact knee. (Note: The displacement has been exaggerated to illustrate this idea.) B: Force-control mode of the Robotic/ universal force-moment sensor testing system. Changes in kinematics of the knee can be determined by applying the same external loading condition (anterior 110 N) and comparing the differences in the resulting motions. (Note: The displacements have been exaggerated to illustrate this idea.)

The robotic manipulator is a position-control device, which enables accurate recording and a high degree of repeatability of positions in space. In combination with the UFS, which records three forces and three moments, the system is also capable of force-control. The robot can apply a desired force or moment target and allow the knee to move in space until the target is reached.

When investigating the *in situ* force in the ligament at certain loading conditions, the external load is applied to the knee at desired flexion angles while the robot records the positions of the knee in space. The ligament is then transected or removed and the robot reproduces the same positions. Because the robot can repeat the identical kinematics of the knee before and after the ligament is sectioned, the change in forces and moments measured by the UFS can be attributed to the *in situ* force in the ligament using the principle of superposition (Fig. 3.8A). To determine the kinematic changes of the knee after the removal of the ligament, the external loads are applied again to the ligament-deficient knee and the resulting kinematics can be recorded (Fig. 3.8B).

With this technology, the *in situ* force in the ligament can be determined with minimal dissection and manipulation of the joint. When determining the *in situ* forces in cruciate ligaments, the ligaments are usually transected arthroscopically. Moreover, the *in situ* force in multiple ligaments and loading conditions can be studied in the same specimen, thus minimizing interspecimen variations. Specifically, Sakane et al. (12) measured the *in situ* force of the two bundles in the human ACL. The

study revealed that the two ACL bundles are under different tension at various flexion angles of the knee: The posterolateral bundle has a higher *in situ* force at low flexion angles, whereas the anteromedial bundle has a rather constant *in situ* force throughout the range of motion (Fig. 3.9).

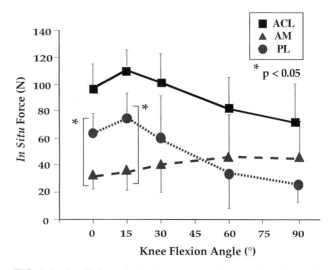

FIG. 3.9. *In situ* force in the human anterior cruciate ligament and its AM Anteromedial and PL Posterolateral bundles when the knee is subjected to 110 N anterior tibial loading ($n = 9$, mean ± SD). (From Sakane M, Fox RJ, Woo S.L-Y, et al. In situ Foras in the anterior cruciate ligament and its bundles in response to anterior tibial loads. *J Orthop Res* 1997;15:285–293, with permission.)

Anterior Cruciate Ligament Reconstruction: Bone–Patellar Tendon–Bone Graft versus Quadruple Hamstring Graft

With the robotic/UFS technology, reconstructions using the central third bone–patellar tendon–bone (BPTB) and quadruple semitendinosus/gracilis graft in cadaveric knees have been compared (117). Patellar tendon (81–87) and quadruple hamstring grafts (88–91) are two common ligament grafts that have been used for ACL reconstruction. The two reconstructions were performed on the same cadaveric knee and the kinematics and *in situ* forces were compared with the intact ACL under various loading conditions. The results showed that both reconstructions were similar in restoring intact knee kinematics; however, the quadruple semitendinosus and gracilis graft better reproduced the *in situ* forces in the intact ACL. It has been postulated that the multiple bundle hamstring graft could better restore the *in situ* forces in the two-bundle ACL than the single bundle BPTB.

Graft Incorporation

Although most kinematic studies were performed on cadavers, ligament reconstructions also involve healing of the ligament replacement grafts. Graft incorporation is different from ligament healing because the graft usually has different biochemical and biomechanical properties from the intact ligament. In 1986, Amiel et al. (118) reported the changes with time observed for an autogenous patellar tendon graft when used as an ACL replacement in the rabbit model. They reported changes of cell morphology within the ACL replacement graft to a ligamentous appearance. Moreover, there was an increase in type III collagen in the graft that was seen in the normal ACL but not in the patellar tendon. They reported the completion of this phenomenon at 30 weeks after transplantation. In general, graft incorporation involves an initial phase of ischemic necrosis, followed by revascularization. Remodeling and maturation include a transition of cellularity, distribution of collagen types, fiber size and alignment, and biochemical characteristics that are more ligament-like. Initially, failure after replacement surgery is at the fixation sites. As these attachments heal, failure is more likely to occur within the graft substance, specifically within the intraarticular portion.

Graft Insertion Healing

With the recent interest in semitendinosus and gracilis graft and quadriceps graft for ligament reconstruction, questions were raised regarding the healing of the ligament replacement graft at its new insertion site. For the central third patellar tendon graft, the tendon insertion sites are left intact with the bone block upon harvest, and healing of the replacement graft within the femoral and tibial bone tunnel is believed to be bone-to-bone healing, similar to fracture healing. However, for soft tissue grafts without bony insertions, like the semitendinosus and gracilis tendon, the healing of the graft inside the bone tunnel remains unknown.

Rodeo et al. (119) used a canine extraarticular model to study healing of tendon inside a bone tunnel. The authors transected the long extensor tendon of the leg and redirected the tendon through a tibial bone tunnel. Their results demonstrated that ligament healing within bone tunnel took 6 to 8 weeks before strength of the graft increased. They also reported appearance of "bony spicules" that resemble tendon insertions at 6 weeks.

Grana and coworkers (120,121) used a rabbit intraarticular model for ACL reconstruction. The authors used a single-strand semitendinosus tendon for ACL reconstruction. Their results showed a gradual increase of graft strength with time. However, at 1 year after operation, the graft still did not restore the strength of the intact ligament.

Soft Tissue Fixation

To have adequate tendon–bone healing in ligament reconstruction, initial fixation of the tendon replacement graft is important. These replacement grafts, like semitendinosus, gracilis, and quadriceps, do not have rigid bone blocks at their ends, and alternative fixation methods have to be used. A number of methods have been recommended for soft tissue fixation, namely soft tissue washers (122,123), staples, bioabsorbable screws, and titanium button/polyester tape fixations (124–126). Most of these fixation methods have undergone tensile testing to determine their stiffness and ultimate tensile load at failure (127).

The goal of ACL reconstruction by replacement grafts is to have the graft behave as cloesly as possible to the native ACL. Therefore, the two should have similar biomechanical properties (i.e., the stiffness of the graft construct, the ultimate tensile load at failure, and the energy absorbed to failure). Stiffness of the graft construct is significant because it can be a complex structure, including tape, sutures, screws, and other devices for the graft tissue to be fixed to the bone. To date, laboratory data have clearly shown that the stiffness of the graft construct is well below those of the graft and the intact ACL (128–130).

Höher et al. (131) studied the amount of motion of the semitendinosus/gracilis tendon within the femoral bone tunnel when using the titanium button/polyester tape fixation technique, a popular soft tissue fixation method. The investigators labeled this motion as graft–tunnel motion. The motion between the graft and osseous tunnel was tracked with reflective markers while

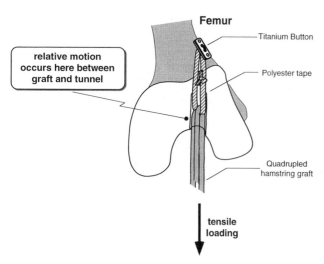

FIG. 3.10. Graft–tunnel motion as it may occur in hamstring grafts with titanium button/polyester tape fixation. Cyclic tensile loading of the graft results in motion at the tendon–bone interface in the femoral tunnel.

the construct was subjected to cyclic loading (Fig. 3.10). Results of the study demonstrated that significant graft–tunnel motion, which ranged from 0.7 to 3.3 mm, occurred within the physiologic load range of 50 to 300 N. These results suggest that when using this technique for hamstring fixation, motion of the graft inside the bone tunnel should be considered and moderate rehabilitation is recommended during the early postoperative period.

Besides stiffness and ultimate load at failure, the viscoplastic behavior of a graft construct can be a key to success or failure for an ACL replacement graft. Viscoplastic properties are defined as the combined viscoelastic properties and plastic deformation of a graft construct at the end of a series of cyclic loadings. Plastic, or residual, deformation of a graft construct can be a result of a knot tightening under cyclic tension, slippage from a staple, tightening of the sutures placed on the soft tissue, or other unknown reasons (130,132,133). This permanent lengthening of the construct can be detrimental to the ACL reconstruction because the tension in the graft is now decreased or has completely disappeared. Thus, the normal stability of the knee is also gone. Adequate preconditioning of the graft construct, which reduces its viscoplastic behavior (134,135), or improved fixation methods should be explored to minimize this undesirable effect.

Autograft versus Allograft

Besides prosthetic ligaments, autografts have been the only other graft substitute available until the organization of tissue banks that provided the use of allografts. The advantage of using autograft is the absence of ad-

verse inflammatory response and risk of disease transmission (136,137). However, the use of autograft has been associated with some donor site morbidity. Patients that underwent autogenous central third patellar tendon ACL reconstruction occasionally complain of patellofemoral symptoms. There are also reported complications of patella fracture after the harvest of the BPTB. For autogenous semitendinosus and gracilis ACL reconstruction, most patients complain of less donor site morbidity; however, there have been reports of hamstring weakness at extreme knee flexion (138).

Allografts have become a popular alternative for ligament reconstruction because patients would have no donor site morbidity (139,140). Allografts are also extremely useful in revision ligament reconstructions. Allografts are usually preserved by the deep-freezing or freeze-drying techniques, whereas sterilization is achieved using cobalt irradiation or cold ethylene oxide gas.

Deep freezing without drying has little or no effect on the mechanical properties of the ligament or tendon. No significant differences in the ultimate load, stiffness, or modulus were noted between the treated and control ligaments 26 weeks after treatment (141). Sterilization with cold ethylene oxide gas and low-dosage irradiation (2 Mrad) does not appear to change the mechanical properties of allografts, whereas sterilization with greater than 3 Mrad irradiation does. Significantly reduced ultimate tensile strength was noted with 3 Mrad of cobalt irradiation (142). Irradiation also alters tissue morphology. After 2 Mrad irradiation, human patellar tendons were visibly crimped, and the collagen fascicles were separated. Ethylene oxide sterilization is not well accepted by the host, and the use of fresh tissue, without freezing, results in a substantial inflammatory response (143). Fresh-frozen tissue and low-dose irradiation are currently the most accepted methods, and rejection and infection have not been substantial problems.

Although allografts are great alternatives for graft materials, some studies have demonstrated that the mechanical behavior of allograft is inferior to autogenous tissue after transplantation in a goat ACL reconstruction model (144). At 6 months after reconstruction, the autografts have less anterior–posterior laxity and higher ultimate tensile strength and cross-sectional area when compared with allografts. The authors also reported prolonged inflammation after allograft ACL reconstructions allograft transplants.

FUTURE DIRECTIONS

With the growing interest in ligament healing and reconstruction, significant advances have been made to characterize the function and understand the properties of ligaments. Current knowledge of ligament healing has led to significant improvement in the treatment of ligament injuries. Although cruciate ligament reconstructions are considered fairly successful, significant research is still devoted to improved surgical outcomes. Research on the molecular level of cell repair and cell communication has led to the possibility of applying growth factors to enhance recovery from ligament injuries. However, significant effort is needed to transform observations on the molecular or cellular level to clinical application. Regarding surgical reconstructions, the ideal graft fixation, tunnel position, and graft choices remain unknown for cruciate ligament reconstructions. Although many studies have compared different reconstruction technique in cadaveric models, *in vivo* animal studies or long-term prospective clinical trials are needed to validate the results shown in cadaveric studies. Advances in computer simulation of joint motion and visualization also have tremendous potential for surgical planning and injury modeling. With more precise and accurate methods of characterizing the function of ligaments and their reconstructions, we believe that there will be more successful long-term outcome of ligament injuries in the future.

REFERENCES

1. Woo SL-Y, Maynard J, Butler D, et al. Normal ligament: structure, function and composition. In: Woo SL-Y, Buckwalter JA, eds. *Injury and repair of musculoskeletal soft tissues.* Chicago: American Academy of Orthopedic Surgery, 1988:103.
2. Woo SL-Y, An K-A, Arnoczky SP, et al. Anatomy, biology, and biomechanics of tendon, ligament, and meniscus. In: Simon SR, ed. *Orthopaedic basic science,* American Academy of Orthopaedic Surgery, 1993:45–87.
3. Woo SL-Y, Gomez MA, Sites TJ, et al. The biomechanical and morphological changes in the medial collateral ligament of the rabbit after immobilization and remobilization. *J Bone Joint Surg Am* 1987;69:1200.
4. Figgie HE, Bahniuk EH, Heiple KG, et al. The effects of tibial-femoral angle on the failure mechanics of the canine anterior cruciate ligament. *J Biomech* 1986;19:89.
5. Noyes FR, Grood ES. The strength of the anterior cruciate ligament in humans and rhesus monkeys. *J Bone Joint Surg Am* 1976;58:1074.
6. Woo SL-Y, Hollis JM, Adams DJ, et al. Tensile properties of the human femur-anterior cruciate ligament-tibia complex: the effect of specimen age and orientation. *Am J Sports Med* 1991;19:217.
7. Noyes FR, Butler DL, Grood ES, et al. Biomechanical analysis of human ligament grafts used in knee-ligament repairs and reconstructions. *J Bone Joint Surg Am* 1984;66:344.
8. Fuss FK. Anatomy of the cruciate ligaments and their function in extension and flexion of the human knee joint. *Am J Anat* 1989;184:165.
9. Harner CD, Xerogeanes JW, Livesay GA, et al. The human posterior cruciate ligament complex: an interdisciplinary study. *Am J Sports Med* 1995;23:736.
10. Race A, Amis AA. The mechanical properties of the two bundles of the human posterior cruciate ligament. *J Biomech* 1994;27:13.
11. Girgis FG, Marshall JL, Al Monajem ARS. The cruciate ligaments of the knee joint: anatomical and experimental analysis. *Clin Orthop Rel Res* 1975;106:216.
12. Sakane M, Fox RJ, Woo SL-Y, et al. In situ forces in the anterior cruciate ligament and its bundles in response to anterior tibial loads. *J Orthop Res* 1997;15:285.
13. Woo SL-Y, Newton PO, MacKenna DA, et al. A comparative

14. Butler DL, Guan Y, Kay MD, et al. Location-dependent variations in the material properties of the anterior cruciate ligament. *J Biomech* 1992;25:511.
15. Blevins FT, Hecker AT, Bigler GT, et al. The effects of donor age and strain rate on the biomechanical properties of bone-patellar tendon-bone allografts. *Am J Sports Med* 1994;22:328.
16. Butler DL, Grood ES, Noyes FR, et al. Effects of structure and strain measurement technique on the material properties of young human tendons and fascia. *J Biomech* 1984;17:579.
17. Danto MI, Hacker SA, MacKenna DA, et al. Effect of strain rate on the mechanical properties of rabbit anterior cruciate ligament (ACL) and patellar tendon (PT). *Trans Orthop Res Soc* 1991;16:233.
18. Danto MI, Woo SL-Y. The mechanical properties of skeletally mature rabbit anterior cruciate ligament and patellar tendon over a range of strain rates. *J Orthop Res* 1993;11:58.
19. Neumann P, Keller TS, Ekstrom L, et al. Effect of strain rate and bone mineral on the structural properties of the human anterior longitudinal ligament. *Spine* 1994;19:205.
20. Amiel D, Woo SL-Y, Harwood FL, et al. The effect of immobilization on collagen turnover in connective tissue: a biochemical-biomechanical correlation. *Acta Orthop Scand* 1982;53:325.
21. Binkley JM, Peat M. The effects of immobilization on the ultrastructure and mechanical properties of the medial collateral ligament of rats. *Clin Orthop Rel Res* 1986;203:301.
22. Bray RC, Shrive NG, Frank CB, et al. The early effects of joint immobilization on medial collateral ligament healing in an ACL-deficient knee: a gross anatomic and biomechanical investigation in the adult rabbit model. *J Orthop Res* 1992;10:157.
23. Kamps BS, Linder LH, DeCamp CE, et al. The influence of immobilization versus exercise on scar formation in the rabbit patellar tendon after excision of the central third. *Am J Sports Med* 1994;22:803.
24. Woo SL-Y, Gomez MA, Woo Y-K, et al. Mechanical properties of tendons and ligaments II: the relationships of immobilization and exercise on tissue remodeling. *Biorheology* 1982;19:397.
25. Woo SL-Y, Kuei SC, Gomez MA, et al. The effect of immobilization and exercise on the strength characteristics of bone-medial collateral ligament-bone complex. In ASME Biomechanics Symposium, 1979.
26. Haut RC, Powlison AC. The effects of test environment and cyclic stretching on the failure properties of human patellar tendons. *J Orthop Res* 1990;8:532.
27. Johnson GA, Tramaglini DM, Levine RE, et al. Tensile and viscoelastic properties of human patellar tendon. *J Orthop Res* 1994;12:796.
28. Schwerdt H, Constantinesco A, Chambron J. Dynamic viscoelastic behaviour of the human tendon in vivo. *J Biomech* 1980;13:913.
29. Graf BK, Vanderby RJ, Ulm MJ, et al. Effect of preconditioning on the viscoelastic response of primate patellar tendon. *Arthroscopy* 1994;10:90.
30. Fung YCB. Elasticity of soft tissues in simple elongation. *Am J Physiol* 1967;213:1532.
31. Fung YCB. *Biomechanics: mechanical properties of living tissues,* 2nd ed. New York: Springer, 1993:568.
32. Woo SL-Y, Gomez MA, Akeson WH. The time and history-dependent viscoelastic properties of the canine medial collateral ligament. *J Biomech Eng* 1981;103:293.
33. Johnson GA, Livesay GA, Woo SL-Y, et al. A single integral finite strain viscoelastic model of ligaments and tendons. *J Biomech* 1996;118:221.
34. Woo SL-Y, Johnson GA, Smith BA. Mathematical modeling of ligaments and tendons. *J Biomech Eng* 1993;115:468.
35. Bray RC, Rangayyan RM, Frank CB. Normal and healing ligament vascularity: a quantitative histological assessment in the adult rabbit medial collateral ligament. *J Anat* 1996;188:87.
36. Engle CP, Noguchi M, Ohland KJ, et al. Healing of the rabbit medial collateral ligament following an O'Donoghue triad injury: effects of anterior cruciate ligament reconstruction. *J Orthop Res* 1994;12:357.

evaluation of the mechanical properties of the rabbit medial collateral and anterior cruciate ligaments. *J Biomech* 1992;25:377.

37. Frank C, Amiel D, Akeson WH. Healing of the rabbit medial collateral ligament of the knee. A morphological and biochemical assessment in rabbits. *Acta Orthop Scand* 1983;54:917.

38. Frank C, Woo SL-Y, Amiel D, et al. Medial collateral ligament healing: a multidisciplinary assessment in rabbits. *Am J Sports Med* 1983;11:379.

39. Hart DP, Dahners LE. Healing of the medial collateral ligament in rats: the effects of repair, motion, and secondary stabilizing ligaments. *J Bone Joint Surg Am* 1987;69:1194.

40. Hefti FL, Kress A, Fasel J, et al. Healing of the transected anterior cruciate ligament in the rabbit. *J Bone Joint Surg Am* 1991;73:373.

41. Kobayashi D, Kurosaka M, Yoshiya S, et al. The effect of basic fibroblast growth factor on primary healing of the defect in anterior cruciate ligament. *Trans Orthop Res Soc* 1995;20:630.

42. Ohno K, Pomaybo AS, Schmidt CC, et al. Healing of the medial collateral ligament after a combined medial collateral and anterior cruciate ligament injury and reconstruction of the anterior cruciate ligament: comparison of repair and nonrepair of medial collateral ligament tears in rabbits. *J Orthop Res* 1995;13:442.

43. Weiss JA, Ohland KJ, Newton PO, et al. A new injury model to study medial collateral ligament healing. *Trans Orthop Res Soc* 141989.

44. Weiss JA, Woo SL-Y, Ohland KJ, et al. Evaluation of a new injury model to study medial collateral ligament healing: primary repair versus nonoperative treatment. *J Orthop Res* 1991;9:516.

45. Woo SL-Y, Schmidt CC, Taylor BJ, et al. The effects of EGF and TGF-β on the biomechanical properties of the healing rabbit medial collateral ligament. In ASME, San Francisco, CA, 1995.

46. Woo SL-Y, Taylor BJ, Schmidt CC, et al. The effect of dose levels of growth factors on the healing of the rabbit medial collateral ligament. *Trans Orthop Res Soc* 1996;21:97.

47. Woo SL-Y, Young EP, Ohland KJ, et al. The effects of transection of the anterior cruciate ligament on healing of medial collateral ligament: a biomechanical study of the knee in dogs. *J Bone Joint Surg Am* 1990;72:382.

48. Lyon RM, Akeson WH, Amiel D, et al. Ultrastructural differences between the cells of the medial collateral and the anterior cruciate ligaments. *Clin Orthop Rel Res* 1991;272:279.

49. Schmidt CC, Georgescu HI, Kwoh CK, et al. Effect of growth factors on the proliferation of fibroblasts from the medial collateral and anterior cruciate ligament. *J Orthop Res* 1995;13:184.

50. Amiel D, Frank C, Harwood F, et al. Tendons and ligaments: a morphological and biochemical comparison. *J Orthop Res* 1984;1:257.

51. Sakane M, Fox RJ, Rudy TW, et al. The importance of the medial collateral, the posterolateral structures, and bony contact in knee stability. *Trans Orthop Res Soc* 1997;22:871.

52. Frank CB, Bray RC, Hart DA, et al. Soft tissue healing. In: Fu FH, Harner CD, Vince KG, eds. *Knee surgery.* Baltimore, MD: Williams & Wilkins, 1994:189.

53. Inoue M, Woo SL-Y, Amiel D, et al. Effects of surgical treatment and immobilization on the healing of the medial collateral ligament: a long-term multidisciplinary study. *Connect Tissue Res* 1990;25:13.

54. Frank C, McDonald D, Wilson J, et al. Rabbit rabbit medial collateral ligament scar weakness is associated with decreased collagen pyridinoline crosslink density. *J Orthop Res* 1995;13:157.

55. Woo SL-Y, Inoue M, McGurk-Burleson E, et al. Treatment of the medial collateral ligament injury. II. Structure and function of canine knees in response to differing treatment regimens. *Am J Sports Med* 1987;15:22.

56. Indelicato PA. Isolated medial collateral ligament injuries in the knee. *J Am Acad Orthop Surg* 1995;3:9.

57. Woo SL-Y, Niyibizi C, Matyas J, et al. Medial collateral knee ligament healing: combined rabbit medial collateral and anterior cruciate ligaments injuries studied in rabbits. *Acta Orthop Scand* 1997;68:142.

58. Yamaji T, Levine RE, Woo SL-Y, et al. Medial collateral ligament healing one year after a concurrent medial collateral ligament and anterior cruciate ligament injury: an interdisciplinary study in rabbits. *J Orthop Res* 1996;14:223.

59. Johnson RJ, Beynnon BD, Nicholas CE, et al. Current concept review: the treatment of injuries to the anterior cruciate ligament. *J Bone Joint Surg Am* 1992;74:140.

60. O'Donoghue DH, Frank CG, Jeter GL, et al. Repair and reconstruction of the anterior cruciate ligament in dogs: factors influencing long-term results. *J Bone Joint Surg Am* 1971;53:710.

61. O'Donoghue DH, Rockwood CC Jr, Frank GR. Repair of anterior cruciate ligament in dogs. *J Bone Joint Surg Am* 1966;48:503.

62. Neurath MF, Printz H, Stofft E. Cellular ultrastructure of the ruptured anterior cruciate ligament. *Acta Orthop Scand* 1994;65:71.

63. Arnoczky SP. Anatomy of the anterior cruciate ligament. *Clin Orthop Rel Res* 1983;172:19.

64. Kennedy JC, Weinberg HW, Wilson AS. The anatomy and function of the anterior cruciate ligament: as determined by clinical and morphological studies. *J Bone Joint Surg Am* 1974;56:223.

65. Frank CB. Ligament healing: current knowledge and clinical applications. *J Am Acad Orthop Surg* 1996;4:74.

66. Woo SL-Y, Hildebrand KA, Healing of ligament injuries: from basic science to clinical practice. International practice and research. *Baillieres Clin Orthop* 1997;2:63.

67. Inoue M, McGurk-Burleson E, Hollis JM, et al. Treatment of the medial collateral ligament injury. I. The importance of anterior cruciate ligament on the varus-valgus knee laxity. *Am J Sports Med* 1987;15:15.

68. Shelbourne KD, Patel DV. Management of combined injuries of the anterior cruciate and medial collateral ligaments. *J Bone Joint Surg Am* 1995;77:800.

69. Amiel D, Nagineni CN, Choi SH, et al. Intrinsic properties of ACL and MCL cells and their responses to growth factors. *Med Sci Sports Exerc* 1995;27:884.

70. DesRosiers EA, Yahia L, Rivard C-H. Proliferative and matrix synthesis response of canine anterior cruciate ligament fibroblasts submitted to combined growth factors. *J Orthop Res* 1996;14:200.

71. Hildebrand K, Woo S-Y, Smith D, et al. Growth factors can improve MCL healing in vivo. *Trans AOSSM* 1997;23:739.

72. Lee J, Green MH, Amiel D. Synergistic effect of growth factors on cell outgrowth from explants of rabbit anterior cruciate and medial collateral ligaments. *J Orthop Res* 1995;13:435.

73. Scherping SC Jr, Schmidt CC, Georgescu HI, et al. Effect of growth factors on the proliferation of ligament fibroblasts from skeletally mature rabbits. *Connect Tissue Res* 1997;36:1.

74. Scherping SC, Schmidt CC, Georgescu HI, et al. The effect of aging on the proliferative response of anterior cruciate and medial collateral ligament fibroblasts to growth factors. *Trans Orthop Res Soc* 1995;20:92.

75. Schmidt CC, Georgescu HI, Kwoh CK, et al. The effect of growth factors on medial collateral and anterior cruciate ligament fibroblast proliferation. *Trans Orthop Res Soc* 1994.

76. Weiss JA, Beck CL, Levine RE, et al. Effects of platelet-derived growth factor on early medial collateral ligament healing. *Trans Orthop Res Soc* 1995;20:159.

77. Marui T, Niyibizi C, Georgescu HI, et al. The effect of growth factors on matrix synthesis by ligament fibroblasts. *J Orthop Res* 1997;15:18.

78. Spindler KP, Mayes CE, Miller RR, et al. Regional mitogenic response of the meniscus to platelet-derived growth factor (PDGF-AB). *J Orthop Res* 1995;13:201.

79. Stahlman G, Spindler K, Dawson J, et al. Do the growth factors TGF-b2 and PDGF-AB affect the structural properties of the healing medial collateral ligament? *Trans AOSSM* 1994;20:121.

80. Hey Groves E. Operation for the repair of the cruciate ligaments. *Lancet* 1917;2:674.

81. Barrett GR, Field LD. Comparison of patellar tendon versus patellar tendon/Kennedy ligament augmentation device for anterior cruciate ligament reconstruction: study of results, morbidity, and complications. *Arthroscopy* 1993;18:624.

82. Buss DD, Warren RF, Wickiewicz TL, et al. Arthroscopically assisted reconstruction of the anterior cruciate ligament with use of autogenous patellar-ligament grafts. *J Bone Joint Surg Am* 1993;75:1346.

83. Clancy WG, Nelson DA, Reider B, et al. Anterior cruciate ligament reconstruction using one-third of the patellar ligament,

augmented by extra-articular tendon transfers. *J Bone Joint Surg Am* 1982;64:352.

84. Jones KG. Reconstruction of the anterior cruciate ligament using the central one-third of the patellar ligament. *J Bone Joint Surg Am* 1970;52:838.

85. Jones KG. Results of the use of the central one-third of the patellar ligament to compensate for anterior cruciate ligament deficiency. *Clin Orthop Rel Res* 1980;147:39.

86. Kurosaka M, Yoshiya S, Andrish JT. A biomechanical comparison of different surgical techniques of graft fixation in anterior cruciate ligament reconstruction. *Am J Sports Med* 1987;15:225.

87. Shelbourne KD, Klootwyk TE, DeCarlo MS. Update on accelerated rehabilitation after anterior cruciate ligament reconstruction. *J Orthop Sports Phys Ther* 1992;15:303.

88. Brown CHJ, Steiner ME, Carson EW. The use of hamstring tendons for anterior cruciate ligament reconstruction: technique and results. *Clin Sports Med* 1993;12:723.

89. Cho KO. Reconstruction of the anterior cruciate ligament by semitendinosis tenodesis. *J Bone Joint Surg Am* 1975;57:608.

90. Johnson LL. The outcome of a free autogenous semitendinosus tendon graft in human anterior cruciate reconstructive surgery: a histological study. *Arthroscopy* 1993;9:131.

91. Sgaglione NA, Del Pizzo W, Fox JM, et al. Arthroscopically assisted anterior cruciate ligament reconstruction with the pes anserine tendons: comparison of results in acute and chronic ligament deficiency. *Am J Sports Med* 1993;21:249.

92. Howe JG, Johnson RJ, Kaplan MJ, et al. Anterior cruciate ligament reconstruction using quadriceps patellar tendon graft. Part 1. Long-term follow-up. *Am J Sports Med* 1991;19:447.

93. Kornblatt I, Warren RF, Wickiewicz TL. Long-term follow-up of anterior cruciate ligament reconstruction using the quadriceps tendon substitute for chronic anterior cruciate ligament insufficiency. *Am J Sports Med* 1988;16:444.

94. Yasuda K, Tomiyama Y, Ohkoshi Y, et al. Arthroscopic observations of autogeneic quadriceps and patellar tendon grafts after anterior cruciate ligament reconstruction of the knee. *Clin Orthop Rel Res* 1989;246:217.

95. Fukubayashi T, Torzilli PA, Sherman MF, et al. An in-vitro biomechanical evaluation of anterior-posterior motion of the knee: tibial displacement, rotation, and torque. *J Bone Joint Surg Am* 1982;64:258.

96. Ahmed AM, Burke DL, Duncan NA, et al. Ligament tension pattern in the flexed knee in combined passive anterior translation and axial rotation. *J Orthop Res* 1992;10:854.

97. Ahmed AM, Hyder A, Burke DL, et al. In-vitro ligament tension pattern in the flexed knee in passive loading. *J Orthop Res* 1987;5:217.

98. An K-N, Berglund L, Cooney WP, et al. Direct in-vivo tendon force measurement system. *J Biomech Eng* 1990;23:1269.

99. Lewis JL, Lew WD, Schmidt J. A note on the application and evaluation of the buckle transducer for knee ligament force measurement. *J Biomech Eng* 1982;104:125.

100. Beynnon BD, Fleming BC, Johnson RJ, et al. Anterior cruciate ligament graft elongation at the time of implantation and one year postoperatively. *Trans Orthop Res Soc* 1994;40:612.

101. Beynnon BD, Fleming BC, Johnson RJ, et al. Anterior cruciate ligament strain behavior during rehabilitation exercises in vivo. *Am J Sports Med* 1995;23:24.

102. Beynnon BD, Johnson RJ, Fleming BC, et al. The measurement of elongation of anterior cruciate-ligament grafts in-vivo. *J Bone Joint Surg Am* 1994;76:520.

103. Beynnon BD, Stankevich CJ, Fleming BC, et al. The development and initial testing of a new sensor to simultaneously measure strain and pressure in tendons and ligaments. Combined ORS—USA, Japan, and Canada, Banff, Canada 1991;1:104.

104. Glos DL, Holden JP, Butler DL, et al. Pressure versus deflected beam force measurement in the human patellar tendon. *Trans Orthop Res Soc* 1990;15:490.

105. Henning CE, Lynch MA, Glick KR Jr. An in-vivo strain gauge study of elongation of the anterior cruciate ligament. *Am J Sports Med* 1985;13:22.

106. Holden JP, Grood ES, Korvick DL, et al. In vivo forces in the anterior cruciate ligament: direct measurements during walking and trotting in a quadruped. *J Biomech* 1994;27:517.

107. Takai S, Adams DJ, Livesay GA, et al. Effects of knee motion and external loading on the loads within the anterior cruciate ligament (ACL): a kinematic study. *First World Congr Biomech* 1:51, 1990.

108. Takai S, Adams DJ, Livesay GA, et al. Determination of loads in the human anterior cruciate ligament. *Trans Orthop Res Soc* 1991;16:235.

109. Markolf KL, Gorek JF, Kabo JM, et al. Direct measurement of resultant forces in the anterior cruciate ligament. *J Bone Joint Surg Am* 1990;72:557.

110. Lange Ad, Huiskes R, Kauer JMG. Measurement errors in roentgen-stereophotogrammetric joint-motion analysis. *J Biomech* 1990;23:259.

111. Lange Ad, van Dijk R, Huiskes R, et al. Three-dimensional experimental assessment of knee ligament length patterns in-vitro. *Trans Orthop Res Soc* 1983;8:10.

112. Fujie H, Livesay GA, Kashiwaguchi S, et al. Determination of in-situ force in the human anterior cruciate ligament: a new methodology. *ASME Adv Bioeng BED* 1992;22:91.

113. Fujie H, Mabuchi K, Woo SL-Y, et al. The use of robotics technology to study human joint kinematics: a new methodology. *J Biomech Eng* 1993;115:211.

114. Rudy TW, Livesay GA, Woo SL-Y, et al. A combined robotics/universal force sensor approach to determine in-situ forces of knee ligaments. *J Biomech* 1996;29:1357.

115. Debski RE, Wong EK, Sakane M, et al. In-situ forces in the glenohumeral ligaments during anterior loading. *Trans Orthop Res Soc* 1998;23:1031.

116. Gilbertson LG, Doehring TC, Nishida K, et al. Delineation of whole cervical spine (C0-T1) in-vitro kinematics using a robotics-based testing system. *Trans Orthop Res Soc* 1998;23:1057.

117. Woo SL-Y, Fox RJ, Sakane M, et al. Force and force distribution in the anterior cruciate ligament and its clinical implications. *Sportorthop Sporttraumatol* 1997;13:37.

118. Amiel D, Kliener JB, Roux RD, et al. The phenomenon of "ligamentization": anterior cruciate ligament reconstruction with autogenous patellar tendon. *J Orthop Res* 1986;4:162.

119. Rodeo SA, Arnoczky SP, Torzilli PA, et al. Tendon-healing in a bone tunnel: a biomechanical and histological study in the dog. *J Bone Joint Surg Am* 1993;75:1795.

120. Blickenstaff K, Grana W, Egle D. Analysis of a semitendinosus autograft in a rabbit model. *Am J Sports Med* 1997;25:554.

121. Grana WA, Egle DM, Mahnken R, et al. An analysis of autograft fixation after anterior cruciate ligament reconstruction in a rabbit model. *Am J Sports Med* 1994;22:344.

122. Friedman MJ. Arthroscopic semiteninosus (gracilis) reconstruction for anterior cruciate ligament deficiency. *Techniques Orthop* 1988;2:74.

123. Sisk TD. Knee injuries. In: Crenshaw AB, ed. *Campbell's operative orthopaedics,* 7th ed., Vol. 3. St. Louis, MO: CV Mosby, 1987:2283.

124. Maeda A, Shino K, Horibe S, et al. Anterior cruciate ligament reconstruction with multistranded autogenous semitendinosus tendon. *Am J Sports Med* 1996;24:504.

125. Rosenberg TD. Technique for endoscopic method of ACL reconstruction. *Acufex Microsurgical Technical Bulletin,* 1993.

126. Swenson TM, Harner CD, Fu FH. Endoscopic ACL reconstruction using a quadrupled semitendinosus graft. *Pittsburgh Orthop J* 1995;6:25.

127. Ivey M, Li F. Tensile strength of soft tissue fixations about the knee. *Am J Knee Surg* 1991;4:18.

128. Steiner ME, Hecker AT, Brown CH Jr, et al. Anterior cruciate ligament graft fixation: comparison hamstring and patellar tendon graft. *Am J Sports Med* 1994;22:240.

129. Rowden NJ, Shaw D, Rogers GJ, et al. Anterior cruciate graft fixation: initial comparison of patellar tendon and semitendinosus autografts in young fresh cadavers. *Am J Sports Med* 1997;25:472.

130. Hoher J, Sakane M, Vogrin TM, et al. Viscoplastic elongation of a quadruple semitendinosus graft construct with tape and suture fixation in response to cyclic loading. *Arthroskopie* 1998;11:52.

131. Hoher J, Withrow JD, Livesay GA, et al. Hamstring graft motor in the femoral bone tunnel when using titanium button/polyester tape fixation. *Knee Surg, Sports Traumatol, Arthrosc* 1990;4:215.

132. Havig MT, Paulos LE, Weiss J, et al. Interference screw fixation of soft tissue ACL grafts: effects of cyclic loading on initial fixation strength. *Trans AOSSM* 1999;28.

133. Weiler A, Hoffman RF, Stahelin AC, et al. Hamstring tendon fixation using interference screws: a biomechanical study in calf tibial bone. *Arthroscopy* 1998;14:29.

134. King GJ, Edwards P, Brant RF, et al. Intraoperative graft tensioning alters viscoelastic but not failure behaviors of rabbit medial collateral ligament autografts. *J Orthop Res* 1995; 13:915.

135. Levine RE, Simonian PT, Wright TM, et al. Response of hamstring and patellar tendon grafts for anterior cruciate ligament reconstruction during cyclic tensile loading. *Trans Orthop Res Soc* 1998;23:620.

136. Arnoczky SP, Dipl DVM, Warren RF, et al. Replacement of the anterior cruciate ligament using a patellar tendon allograft. *J Bone Joint Surg Am* 1986;68:376.

137. Eastland T. Infectious disease transmission through tissue transplantation: reducing the risk through donor selection. *J Transplant Coord* 1991;1:23.

138. Marder TA, Raskind JR, Carroll M. Prospective evaluation of arthroscopically assisted anterior cruciate ligament reconstruction: Patellar tendon versus semitendinosus and gracilis tendons. *Am J Sports Med* 1991;19:478.

139. Shino K, Inoue M, Horibe S, et al. Reconstruction of the anterior cruciate ligament using allogenic tendon. *Am J Sports Med* 1990; 18:457.

140. Shino K, Inoue M, Horibe S, et al. Maturation of allograft tendons transplanted into the knee. *J Bone Joint Surg Br* 1988; 70:556.

141. Butler DL, Noyes FR, Walz KA, et al. Biomechanics of human knee ligament allograft treatment. *Trans Orthop Res Soc* 1987;12:128.

142. Gibbons MJ, Butler DL, Grood ES, et al. Dose dependent effects of gamma irradiation on the material properties of frozen bone-patellar tendon-bone allografts. *Trans Orthop Res Soc* 1989; 14:513.

143. Jackson D, Windler G, Simon T. Intraarticular reactions associated with the use of freeze-dried, ethylene oxide sterilized bone-patellar tendon-bone allografts in the reconstruction of the anterior cruciate ligament. *Am J Sports Med* 1990;18:1.

144. Jackson DW, Grood ES, Goldstein JD, et al. A comparison of patellar tendon autograft and allograft used for anterior cruciate ligament reconstruction in the goat model. *AJSM* 1993;21.176.

Principles and Practice of Orthopaedic Sports Medicine,
edited by William E. Garrett, Jr., Kevin P. Speer, and Donald T. Kirkendall.
Lippincott Williams & Wilkins, Philadelphia © 2000.

CHAPTER 4

Structure and Function of Articular Cartilage

Farshid Guilak, Lori A. Setton, and Virginia B. Kraus

Articular cartilage is the thin layer of deformable load-bearing material that lines the bony ends of all diarthrodial joints (Fig. 4.1). The primary functions of this tissue are to support and distribute forces generated during joint loading and to provide a lubricating surface to prevent wear of the joint. Under normal physiologic conditions, articular cartilage can perform these essential biomechanical functions with little damage or wear over the human life span. However, injury of the cartilage due to trauma, progressive degenerative joint diseases, or genetic mutations influencing structural components in cartilage can impair the biomechanical capabilities of the tissue, leading to pain and loss of joint function. There are currently few clinical options for treatment of end-stage joint disease other than total joint replacement.

Articular cartilage is a metabolically active tissue that under normal conditions is maintained in a state of constant turnover by a sparse population of specialized cells (chondrocytes) distributed throughout the tissue. Despite the activity of these cells, articular cartilage exhibits a limited capacity for self-repair. Recent advances in cartilage research have greatly improved our understanding of the physiology, ultrastructure, and biomechanical properties of articular cartilage in both normal and pathologic conditions. These advances have provided an improved understanding of the etiopathogenesis of joint diseases and offer hope in the development of new clinical modalities for the prevention or treatment of various conditions. Whether they are based on pharmaceutical, surgical, biophysical, or tissue engineering approaches, development of new treatment modalities requires a thorough understanding of the structure, function, and biology of normal and diseased cartilage. This chapter presents a review of current understanding of articular cartilage physiology and pathophysiology, including cartilage structure, composition, metabolism, and biomechanics.

COMPOSITION AND ORGANIZATION OF NORMAL ARTICULAR CARTILAGE

Articular cartilage consists of a large organic extracellular matrix that is saturated with water and a small volume fraction of cells (Table 4.1). The water phase of cartilage constitutes from 65% to 85% of the total tissue weight and plays an important role in controlling many physical properties and the transport of nutrients, metabolites, and soluble mediators (1–4). The dominant structural components of the solid matrix are the collagen molecules (75% by dry tissue weight) and the negatively charged proteoglycans (20% to 25% by dry tissue weight). Several other minor collagen species, smaller proteoglycans, and other proteins are present in the tissue.

Water

Water forms most of the wet weight of articular cartilage (1,5). A fraction of this water is contained in the intracellular space, whereas most is contained in the molecular pore space of the extracellular matrix. The water in articular cartilage is dissolved with inorganic salts such as sodium, calcium, chloride, and potassium. Most water in cartilage is "movable" (6,7) and can be transported through the tissue or exuded by applying a pressure gradient across the tissue or by compressing the solid matrix (1,4). Because the frictional resistance between

F. Guilak: Division of Orthopaedic Surgery, Department of Surgery, Duke University Medical Center, Durham, North Carolina 27710.
L. A. Setton: Department of Biomedical Engineering, Duke University, Durham, North Carolina 27710.
V. B. Kraus: Division of Rheumatology, Allergy, and Clinical Immunology, Department of Medicine, Duke University Medical Center, Durham, North Carolina 27710.

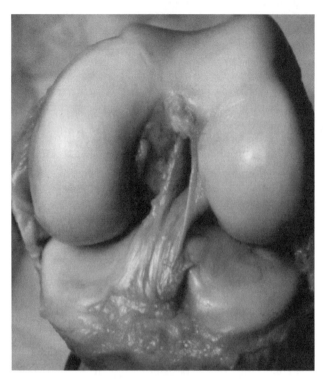

FIG. 4.1. Articular cartilage of the knee joint. Articular cartilage is the thin layer of deformable load-bearing material that lines the bony ends of all diarthrodial joints. Normal cartilage exhibits a smooth, white, translucent appearance.

TABLE 4.1. *Composition of articular cartilage*

Major constituents	Wet weight	Quantitatively minor constituents (<5%)
Water	65–80%	Electrolytes (e.g., Na⁺, Ca²⁺, K⁺, Cl⁻)
Type II collagen	10–20%	Other collagens (types V, VI, IX, X, and XI)
Aggrecan	4–7%	Proteoglycans (biglycan, decorin, (fibromodulin)
Cellular constituents	1–10%	Fibronectin Hyaluronate Link protein Cartilage oligomeric protein Thrombospondin Matrix-GLA (glycine-leucine-alanine) protein Chondrocalcin Tenascin GP-39 Lipids Calcium phosphate crystals

the water and solid matrix is relatively high, the hydraulic permeability of cartilage is low, and high pressures are required to cause interstitial fluid flow. Because of this characteristic, mechanical compression of the cartilage matrix results in rapid pressurization of the interstitial water, which in turn serves to support the applied load (8). The pressurization of the water in the cartilage extracellular matrix is an important mechanism (9) that allows cartilage to withstand repeated loading at very high joint stresses of up to 18 MPa (1 MPa = 145 pounds per square inch) (10). The flow of water through the tissue and across the articular surface is also believed to increase the transport of nutrients and waste products and thus may contribute to the overall regulation of cellular activity (11,12).

Collagen

Collagen is the major constituent of the solid fraction of the extracellular matrix and is responsible for providing the primary structure of articular cartilage (13–16). Collagen molecules are found throughout the body and serve a primary structural role in most connective tissues (13,16–18). They are characterized by a repeating sequence of amino acids (generally glycine, proline, and other amino acids such as hydroxyproline) and contain a characteristic triple helix structure over all or a portion of their length. Over 19 collagen types have presently been identified, and there is additional evidence for other variants of these collagen molecules (19,20). The predominant collagen type in articular cartilage is type II, which constitutes over half the dry weight of the tissue (21). Type II collagen molecules assemble to form small fibrils and larger fibers with an orientation and dimension that vary throughout the depth of the cartilage layer (16,22,23). These fibers may be additionally stabilized by trivalent hydroxypyridinium cross-links (24,25) that are believed to contribute to mechanical stiffness and strength for the collagen network. The first direct evidence for genetic etiologies of osteoarthritis was the discovery of mutations in type II collagen in families with early-onset generalized osteoarthritis and mild spondylepiphyseal dysplasia (26).

Cartilage also contains appreciable amounts of other fibrillar and globular collagen types, including types V, VI, IX, X, and XI (27). Collagen types IX and XI are codistributed with the fibrillar collagen type II within the cartilage extracellular matrix, whereas type VI collagen is mostly localized to the pericellular matrix of the chondrocyte (13,28–32). Although the precise roles of these collagens are not yet known, these collagens are believed to play important roles in promoting intermolecular interactions and in controlling the fibrillar structure of collagen type II. Mutations in type IX collagen are associated with epiphyseal dysplasias of cartilage, providing compelling evidence for an integral role of a quantitatively minor cartilage collagen in the overall structural integrity of the cartilage matrix (33). Type VI collagen may contribute to the mechanical properties of the pericellular matrix and may also regulate interactions between the chondrocyte and the extracellular matrix (34–36). Type X collagen is generally found in the zone of calcified cartilage and seems to play a role in the mineralization of cartilage that occurs at the interface with the subchondral bone (37). Together these collagens form a highly cross-linked network with a specialized structure and organization that predominantly determines the tissue's tensile and shear behaviors.

Proteoglycans

Proteoglycans are large complex macromolecules that consist of a protein core to which polysaccharide (glycosaminoglycan) chains are attached. The predominant proteoglycan of articular cartilage is aggrecan, a large polymer consisting of many aggregating macromolecules (38–41). A single aggrecan molecule consists of a large protein core and numerous glycosaminoglycan side chains. Chondroitin and keratan sulfates are the dominant side chains for most aggrecan in mature articular cartilage (38). Significant variations exist in the number, size, sulfation pattern, and charge density of the glycosaminoglycans of the cartilage proteoglycans with development, aging, and disease (42). The protein core contains several distinct globular and extended domains to which the glycosaminoglycans are attached (43). The function of one specific globular domain is to attach to hyaluronan, a bond that is stabilized by a link protein. Most aggrecan molecules are further bound to a single long chain of hyaluronan to form large proteoglycan aggregates of up to 200 aggrecan molecules, which results in an overall molecular weight of 50 to 100 $\times 10^6$ Da (41,44). The large size and complex structure of the proteoglycan aggregate function to immobilize and restrain it within the collagen network.

The proteoglycans are negatively charged due to the presence of carboxyl and sulfate groups on the glycosaminoglycans and thus confer a net negative charge on the cartilage extracellular matrix known as a "fixed charge density" (45). As a result, cartilage is highly hydrophilic, with a tendency to imbibe fluid and "swell" to maintain a physicochemical and mechanical equilibrium (46–48). This property significantly contributes to the mechanical function of articular cartilage by generating a large swelling pressure that facilitates load support and tissue recovery from deformation. This swelling pressure largely arises from a Donnan osmotic pressure effect due to the high concentration of counterions (e.g., Ca^{2+}, Na^+, K^+) required to neutralize the negative charges of the proteoglycans. An entropic tendency of the proteoglycan exists to increase in volume when in solution due to its large molecular weight and polymeric structure. This phenomenon may further contribute to the swelling effects in cartilage. The total hydration of the tissue is determined by a balance of the swelling pressures against the elastic restraint of the collagen network (49,50). Under normal physiologic conditions, the cartilage extracellular matrix is in a state of "prestress," or internal stress, that places the surface zone of the tissue in tension (51). Thus, one of the first characteristics observed with damage or disruption of the surface zone is an increase in water content of the tissue as the balance of restraining forces and swelling pressure is altered (48,49,52).

Articular cartilage also contains lesser amounts of other proteoglycan species, such as biglycan, decorin, and fibromodulin, which may play important structural roles in the tissue (39,41,53). These molecules are characterized by a core protein that is significantly smaller than that of aggrecan and by the presence of distinctly different glycosaminoglycan species such as dermatan sulfate. The precise function of the smaller proteoglycans is not fully understood, although it has been hypothesized that they play a role in fibrillogenesis and matrix assembly.

Other Components of Cartilage

A large number of noncollagenous proteins are additionally present in the cartilage extracellular matrix, including fibronectin, cartilage oligomeric protein (COMP), thrombospondin, tenascin, matrix-GLA (glycine-leucine-alanine) protein, chondrocalcin, glycoprotein-39 (54), and superficial zone protein (55,56), a multifunctional proteoglycan with growth-promoting and lubricating properties. Although many of these proteins are present at relatively high concentrations of up to 1 mg/mL, their contribution to the function and maintenance of the extracellular matrix may not be fully understood at this point. It is hypothesized that some of these proteins may influence intermolecular interactions, whereas other proteins may function in intercellular communication and intracellular signaling. Importantly, the concentrations of several of these components (e.g., COMP, fibronectin, and tenascin) increase with osteoarthritis, suggesting their potential utility as catabolic or anabolic markers of a degenerative or regenerative state, respectively (57–59).

In addition to these matrix proteins, cartilage contains several other classes of molecules, including lipids, phospholipids, glycoproteins, and inorganic crystal compounds (e.g., calcium phosphate) (54,60–62). A major glycoprotein constituent of articular cartilage is hyaluronan, an unbranched high-molecular-weight nonsulfated polysaccharide (63). Hyaluronan is the major determinant of synovial fluid viscoelastic properties (64) and mediates aggregation of proteoglycan monomers by their noncovalent attachment to the hyaluronan filament (65). Studies of the exact function of these matrix components is ongoing, although it is known that their composition and distribution may vary with age and the presence of osteoarthritis.

Cartilage Structure

The solid matrix of articular cartilage has a highly specific ultrastructure that varies with depth from the cartilage surface to the subchondral bone (66). In this regard, the tissue may be divided into a number of successive "zones" based on extracellular matrix structure and composition and on cell shape and cell arrangement (67,68) (Fig. 4.2). Collagen fibers in the superficial-most zone of cartilage are of small diameter, densely packed, and oriented parallel to the articular surface (69). This surface zone is also characterized by a relatively low proteoglycan content and a low permeability to fluid flow (16,47). In the middle or transitional zone, the collagen fibers form a well-characterized arcadelike structure upon which is superimposed a randomly arranged one (66). The proteoglycan concentration is at a maximum in this region (70). In the deep zone, adjacent to the zone of calcified cartilage and subchondral bone, the collagen fibers are larger and form bundles that are oriented perpendicular to the bone, and the proteoglycan content is again low (16,70). Chondrocyte density is highest in the surface zone and decreases

exponentially with depth (71). Chondrocyte shape seems to reflect the local collagen fiber orientation with a flattened discoidal shape in the surface zone, to nearly spherical in the middle zone, and slightly elongated in a columnar arrangement in the deep zones (68). The zone of calcified cartilage separates the hyaline articular cartilage from the subchondral bone, and the deep zone of the articular cartilage is distinguished from the calcified zone by a thin line termed the "tidemark" (72–74). This transition layer of calcified cartilage, of stiffness intermediate to that of articular cartilage and that of the subchondral plate, is hypothesized to serve as a tethering mechanism for collagen fibers (73) and is believed to minimize the stiffness gradient and therefore the shear stresses at the subchondral interface (75). Matrix vesicles are another feature of the cartilage extracellular matrix. These vesicles are extracellular organelles associated with calcification (76). Matrix vesicles exist in articular cartilage and generate calcium pyrophosphate dihydrate-like or apatite-like mineral (77). The vesicle composition or attached matrix components differ from zone to zone and may regulate the zonal differences in mineral deposition (78).

In addition to zonal variations with depth from the cartilage surface, articular cartilage contains several distinct matrix "compartments" that are defined by the proximity to the cell (79). These regions have significantly different composition, structure, and mechanical properties as compared with bulk extracellular matrix

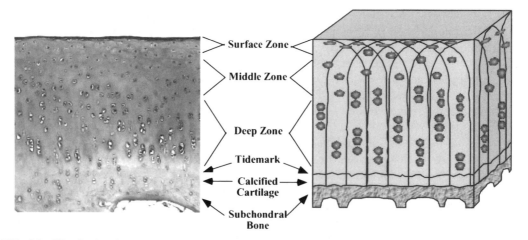

FIG. 4.2. Histologic micrograph **(left)** and schematic **(right)** of the structural arrangement of articular cartilage. Articular cartilage can be divided into four morphologic layers based on structure, composition, and cell shape. In the surface zone (top 50 to 100 μm of the tissue), collagen content is the highest and collagen fibers are oriented in a plane parallel to the tissue surface. This zone is also referred to as the "superficial," "tangential," or "gliding" zone. Chondrocytes have a flattened shape in the surface zone and seem to conform to the local collagen architecture. In the middle zone, collagen fibers are oriented in multiple directions and proteoglycan content is increased as compared with the surface zone. Chondrocytes are more spherical in shape. In the deep zone, collagen fibers are oriented radially or perpendicular to the cartilage surface. Chondrocytes are found in a columnar arrangement that parallels the collagen fiber architecture. Collagen fibers attach to the subchondral bone after transition through the zone of calcified cartilage.

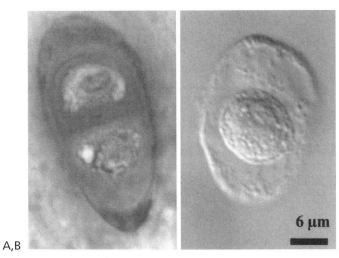

A,B

6 µm

FIG. 4.3. The pericellular matrix of articular cartilage. Chondrocytes are surrounded by a pericellular matrix that is rich in type VI collagen and proteoglycans. The "interterritorial" matrix makes up most of the cartilage extracellular tissue. The chondrocyte, its pericellular matrix, and a surrounding capsule have been termed the "chondron." **A:** Toluidine blue staining of a section of human articular cartilage, indicating the presence of a proteoglycan-rich pericellular region. **B:** Differential interference contrast microscopy of an enzymatically isolated chondron from human articular cartilage. (From Guilak F, Jones WR, Ting-Beall HP, et al. The deformation behavior and mechanical properties of chondrocytes in articular cartilage. *Osteoarthritis Cartilage* 1999;7:59–70, with permission.)

(34,80,81) (Fig. 4.3). Chondrocytes are immediately surrounded by a region termed the pericellular matrix, which is demarcated by the presence of high concentrations of proteoglycans, fine collagen fibers, and the presence of type VI collagen and fibronectin (31,82). The chondrocyte and its pericellular matrix, together with a surrounding membrane of type II collagen, have been termed the "chondron" (83). Farther away from the cell, the interterritorial matrix forms most of the extracellular matrix of articular cartilage and is generally believed to provide for the mechanical properties of the tissue. It encompasses all of the matrix between the pericellular and territorial matrices of the individual cells or clusters of cells and contains large type II collagen fibers and most of the proteoglycans (68).

Age-related Changes in Cartilage Structure and Composition

With age, the structure and composition of articular cartilage change significantly. Decreases in cartilage thickness have been noted with age, but these are most likely due to an erosive loss of cartilage from osteoarthritis but not aging (84–87). The predominant changes occur in the ultrastructure of the collagen matrix. Young immature cartilage is significantly thicker than adult articular cartilage and is generally more uniform in structure and composition than adult cartilage. The cell density is also much higher in young cartilage and is fairly uniform with depth. Although young cartilage generally possesses a "surface" or "tangential" zone, significant differences are apparent in the structure and cellular arrangement of the deep zones. With age, cartilage acquires a stratified structure and cellular density decreases in the deeper zones, and cells become aligned in the characteristic columnar arrangement (68).

Cartilage composition also changes with age. Water content is generally believed to decrease with age (47,88). Collagen content and collagen cross-linking have been shown to increase with skeletal maturity (89). Several changes in proteoglycan composition and structure occur with age observed as a decreased length for the protein core and changes in the pattern of glycosylation (90–93). High concentrations of chondroitin 4-sulfate are present in immature cartilage but decrease rapidly with age as the concentration of keratan sulfate increases. Moreover, the nonreducing terminal residues on aggrecan chondroitin sulfate are specific and distinguishing features of aggrecan before and after skeletal maturity. In growth cartilage, the termini are almost exclusively chondroitin 4-sulfate, whereas in mature cartilage, about 50% are 4-monosulfated and 50% 4,6-disulfated (94). Whereas chondroitin sulfate is concentrated in the territorial matrix and decreases with aging, keratan sulfate is concentrated in the interterritorial matrix and increases with aging (36). The ratio of chondroitin sulfate to keratan sulfate concentration falls until approximately age 30 in humans and is believed to be constant thereafter. The structure of smaller proteoglycan components is also altered (95). Furthermore, the overall biosynthetic and proliferative activity of the chondrocytes, as well as their responsiveness to growth factors, is diminished with age (96–98), suggesting a compromised ability to maintain and repair the extracellular matrix for aged cartilage. Although the incidence of degenerative changes indeed increases with age, many of these changes in cartilage composition, structure, and biosynthesis reported for aged cartilage are markedly different from those observed in osteoarthritis and joint degeneration. For example, sulfation patterns of the terminal residues of chondroitin sulfate in osteoarthritic cartilage are altered, showing an increase in 4-monosulfation and a decrease in 4,6-disulfation relative to mature normal cartilage (94). Other changes associated with osteoarthritis are discussed further below.

BIOMECHANICS OF ARTICULAR CARTILAGE

Articular cartilage functions as a smooth wear-resistant surface facilitating load support, load transfer, and translation and rotational motions between the bones of the skeleton. When an external load is applied to a joint, articular cartilage will deform (99), which may be favorable for increasing joint contact areas while decreasing contact stresses. Loading and deformation of cartilage will generate a combination of tensile, compressive, and shear stresses within the tissue. The mechanical response of cartilage to these stresses is highly specialized due to the tissue's unique composition and structural organization. Furthermore, the tissue exhibits viscoelastic properties so that loading is associated with time-dependent effects such as creep, stress relaxation, and energy dissipation (100–102). These viscoelastic behaviors arise from both interstitial fluid flow through the porous-permeable solid matrix and from physical interactions between the solid matrix constituents (e.g., collagen and proteoglycan). In a healthy joint, these characteristics contribute to load bearing, energy dissipation, and joint lubrication over the lifetime of the joint. With injury or degeneration related to osteoarthritis, cartilage changes will occur that are associated with significant loss of mechanical function and the potential to cause further progressive degeneration of the joint.

Articular cartilage can be viewed as a fiber-reinforced, porous, and permeable composite matrix that is saturated with fluid (4,8). In terms of material behavior, these characteristics result in a highly complex material whose properties are viscoelastic (time or rate dependent), anisotropic (dependent on direction), and nonlinear (dependent on magnitude of strain). Accordingly, the biomechanics of cartilage has been widely studied using models that account for the multiple phases (collagen solid matrix, interstitial fluid, and mobile and "fixed" ionic groups) and the interactions between these phases. Such model development, in combination with experimental testing of material properties, are important for understanding the mechanisms by which cartilage provides its functions within the joint and the associated changes in its function with degeneration and aging.

Tension

When cartilage is loaded or stretched in tension, the collagen fibrils and entangled proteoglycan molecules will align and stretch along the axis of loading. For small deformations, the collagen fibers are believed to align and orient with the applied tractions, whereas at larger deformations the collagen fibers themselves may stretch. Because of the high intrinsic stiffness of the cross-linked collagen fiber, this phenomenon gives rise to a greater tensile Young's modulus (i.e., ratio of stress to strain for a linear material) at higher strains (103–107). In general terms, the Young's modulus is a measure of the intrinsic stiffness of the collagenous solid matrix, and it will depend on the density of collagen fibers, the fiber

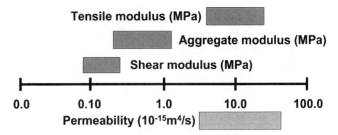

FIG. 4.4. Elastic mechanical properties and permeability of articular cartilage. Cartilage possesses significantly different properties in tension, compression, and shear. The moduli control the response of the tissue in various modes of mechanical loading. The low hydraulic permeability of cartilage is responsible for restricting fluid flow through the tissue and thus allowing significant support of matrix loading by a hydrostatic pressurization of the interstitial fluid.

diameter, the type or amount of collagen cross-linking, and the strength of ionic bonds and frictional interactions between the collagen network and the entangled proteoglycan network (14,105). In general, the tensile modulus of healthy human cartilage varies from 5 to 25 MPa (Fig. 4.4) depending on the location on the joint surface (e.g., high and low weight-bearing regions) and depth and "orientation" of the test specimen relative to the joint surface (103,106,108). For skeletally mature tissue, surface zone articular cartilage is much stiffer than middle and deep zone cartilage, and the tensile stiffness is larger in samples oriented parallel to the local "split-line" direction at the articular surface (i.e., the predominant collagen fiber orientation at the articular surface) (107,108).

Studies have demonstrated the strong dependence of the tensile properties of cartilage on the collagen content and structure. Correlative studies have demonstrated direct relationships between the tensile modulus, stiffness, and failure stress of cartilage and collagen content, and ratio of collagen to proteoglycan contents in samples of human cartilage (14,108). Reductions in tensile stiffness and tensile failure stress of cartilage were observed after treatment with enzymes to disrupt collagen cross-linking (i.e., elastase), clearly demonstrating that collagen cross-linking and fibrillar organization are significant determinants of the tensile properties of cartilage (109–111). Changes in the viscoelastic behavior of cartilage have also been observed after enzymatic extraction of glycosaminoglycans, including a significant increase in the rate of collagen alignment, and therefore the rate of deformation, or creep of cartilage samples in tension (105). Although proteoglycan–collagen interactions appear to govern transient phenomena, it is the intrinsic stiffness of the collagenous solid network that most significantly contributes to the stress–strain behavior and failure properties of cartilage in tension.

Shear

Articular cartilage responds to shearing forces by both stretching and deformation of the collagen–proteoglycan network. Under conditions of pure shear, the tissue will deform with no change in volume (i.e., equivoluminal deformation) and therefore with no significant interstitial pressure gradient or fluid flow through the matrix (100). Therefore, shear studies are useful for characterizing the nature of physical interactions between molecules of the cartilage solid matrix. The shear modulus of articular cartilage has been found to vary from 0.05 to 0.25 MPa for healthy human, bovine, and canine articular cartilages (112–114) (Fig. 4.4). These lower values for the shear modulus, as compared with the tensile modulus, demonstrate the importance of the proteoglycan matrix in contributing to the torsional shear behaviors of articular cartilage.

Dynamic shear experiments have been used to quantify the dissipation resulting from frictional interactions between macromolecules in articular cartilage. In these experiments, cartilage is subjected to an oscillatory torsional strain over a range of frequencies and the dynamic shear modulus (G*) and loss angle (γ) are measured. The magnitude of the dynamic shear modulus ($|G*|$) reflects contributions to the stiffness associated with both elastic and viscous matrix effects, whereas the loss angle (γ) is a measure of the internal frictional dissipation. The loss angle γ ranges from 0 degrees for a perfectly elastic material to 90 degrees for a perfectly dissipative material (e.g., purely viscous fluid). Values for $|G*|$ of healthy cartilage are rate sensitive and fall in the range of 0.2 to 2.0 MPa (Fig. 4.4). Although the shear behavior of cartilage clearly depends on both collagen and proteoglycan molecular species, the relatively small loss angle (γ approximately 10 degrees) and large shear modulus ($|G*|$ approximately 1 MPa) compared with that for solutions of proteoglycan networks alone (γ approximately 70 degrees and $|G*|$ approximately 10 Pa) suggest that the density and integrity of the proteoglycan–collagen network is sufficient to generate significant solidlike behaviors for the material in shear (114–116).

Compression

When cartilage is loaded in compression, volumetric changes may occur due to fluid exudation from the tissue and/or fluid redistribution within the tissue. Fluid movements are governed by the hydraulic permeability of the solid matrix, which is related to the extracellular matrix pore structure and their apparent size and connectivity (4,117–121). Fluid movements in cartilage give rise to significant time-dependent viscoelastic behaviors such as creep and stress relaxation (8). Further, the movement of the interstitial fluid is associated with very high drag forces as the low permeability of the cartilage solid matrix will resist this fluid movement. This phenomena will give rise to very high interstitial fluid pressures in articular cartilage that may be a very significant mechanism for load support (4,119,120,122). As fluid is redistributed within the tissue, there are associated time-dependent changes in fluid pressurization and fluid flow that contribute to "flow-dependent" viscoelastic effects in the tissue. Importantly, as fluid pressure decreases with time, more of the load will be supported by the cartilage solid matrix, giving rise to time-dependent deformations, or creep. At equilibrium when no fluid flow or pressure gradients exist within the tissue, the entire load will be borne by the solid matrix. Upon removal of the compressive load or deformation, articular cartilage will "recover" its initial dimensions, largely through elasticity of the solid matrix and imbibition and redistribution of fluid within the interstitium (1,4). In compression, the frictional drag associated with interstitial fluid flow through the porous and permeable solid matrix is the dominant dissipative mechanism for cartilage. However, the importance of this effect may be governed by the existence of an intact surface zone (101). Additional phenomena may contribute to a dissipative mechanism for cartilage in compression, including contributions from flow-independent interactions between macromolecules of the solid matrix (100–102).

To understand the mechanisms governing physical interactions between fluid and solid phases within cartilage, it is useful to consider a biphasic model for cartilage as an interacting mixture of fluid and solid phases (8). This biphasic model has served as an important tool to date for determining the material properties of articular cartilage in compression (e.g., 123,124). Theoretical predictions of the compressive creep and stress-relaxation experiments have been obtained and matched to experimental data to obtain measures of the hydraulic permeability coefficient (k), equilibrium compressive modulus (H_A), and Poisson's ratio (ν_s). Typical values of k range from 0.5 to 5.0 $\times 10^{-15}$ m^4/N-s and are extremely small, indicating that very large interstitial fluid pressures and drag-induced dissipations are occurring in normal articular cartilage during compressive loading. These mechanisms for fluid pressurization and flow-dependent energy dissipation provide an efficient method to shield the solid matrix of cartilage from the high stresses and strains associated with joint loading, as the pressurized fluid component will provide for most load bearing in the cartilage layer (125). Values of the equilibrium compressive modulus (H_A, 0.4 to 1.0 MPa) and Poisson's ratio (ν_s, 0.0 to 0.4) of healthy cartilage have been found to vary with site on the joint surface and between species (123).

The generally low values for the compressive modulus, as compared with that for cartilage in tension, reflects the importance of the proteoglycan matrix in contributing to the tissue's compressive behavior. This is partly demonstrated in the repeated findings of a direct relationship between measures of the compressive stiffness of articular cartilage and its proteoglycan and water contents (88,110,126–129). The coincident dependence of the compressive stiffness on water and proteoglycan contents points to the physicochemical properties of the proteoglycans as important in influencing the compressive behaviors of cartilage. The negatively charged proteoglycans are strongly hydrophilic and so are important for providing cartilage with water retention and imbibition mechanisms during load support and recovery of tissue dimensions after removal of joint loading. Furthermore, the proteoglycans may directly contribute to resistance to fluid flow within the cartilage solid matrix (130), which will additionally support the fluid pressurization mechanism for load support and apparent compressive stiffness of cartilage. During compression, tissue compaction will be associated with an increase in fixed charge density resulting in an increased swelling pressure and associated propensity to imbibe fluid (46,47,131). This elevated swelling pressure is associated with an apparent "stiffening" effect for the cartilage matrix in compression. Therefore, biologic factors that contribute to a lower fixed charge density, such as a higher water or lower glycosaminoglycan content, will give rise to a tissue that effectively has a lower modulus in compression.

Swelling

Changes in the hydration of articular cartilage, or "edema," are some of the first effects to be detected in cartilage degeneration and osteoarthritis (48,49,52,88). With aging, there is evidence of a slight decrease in hydration, so that swelling may be a distinguishing characteristic of cartilage degeneration and osteoarthritis. As explained above, swelling in cartilage arises from the presence of a high density of negatively charged proteoglycan molecules. An excess of mobile counterions gives rise to an interstitial osmotic pressure that contributes to a swelling pressure in articular cartilage. Because the proteoglycan molecules in cartilage are complex, polymeric structures constrained to occupy a small volume (one fifth of that in free solution), it is believed that there may be an additional "excluded volume" or entropic contribution to the swelling effects observed in cartilage (46,132).

At equilibrium, the swelling pressure in articular cartilage will be balanced by tensile forces generated in the collagen network and by the swelling stresses developed in the solid matrix (50,51,133–135). Therefore, at physiologic concentrations the solid matrix of cartilage, even when unloaded, is in a state of prestress (46,136). Changes in the internal swelling pressure arising from altered glycosaminoglycan or counterion concentrations

will directly result in changes in tissue prestress and hence tissue hydration, dimensions, and mechanical function. Similarly, it is a nonuniformity in the glycosaminoglycan concentration and matrix stiffness with depth through the cartilage layer that gives rise to the nonuniform swelling and dimensional changes in cartilage upon excision from the surface, known as a "warping" or "curling" effect *ex situ* (135). Importantly, loss of the structure of the collagen matrix due to osteoarthritic changes, or mechanical or enzymatic disruption, has been shown to cause an increase in swelling effects for cartilage (51,133,137–142). The integrity of the collagen network is critical for resisting the swelling pressures in articular cartilage, so that a damaged collagen network would be associated with increased hydration.

As with the biphasic model descriptions, a triphasic constitutive model exists for articular cartilage to describe the important physicochemical effects of proteoglycan-associated negative charge groups, including swelling pressure, streaming potentials, streaming currents, and osmosis (46,130,143). This model provides for explicit mathematical relationships between the material coefficients of cartilage and the fundamental physicochemical parameters such as hydration, fixed charge density, electrical conductivity of cartilage, and the frictional drag coefficients between water and solid or between ions and water. This theory has been useful for verifying the experimental observations of a direct relationship between the hydraulic permeability and water content of articular cartilage and the nonlinear electrokinetic effects in cartilage such as flow-induced streaming potentials (117,143). Ongoing studies of these phenomena will be increasingly important for understanding the mechanisms by which articular cartilage so successfully performs its functions as a load-bearing and wear-resistant material.

Friction

One of the most unique characteristics of the diarthrodial joint is the ability to provide a wear-resistant surface that is capable of withstanding repeated loadings of up to 10 times body weight and for up to eight decades of life. This property is provided by the extremely low coefficient of friction of cartilage moving against another cartilage surface. The coefficient of friction represents the ratio of the tangential frictional force to the compressive load acting between two surfaces. The coefficient of friction of cartilage on cartilage has been reported to be approximately 0.002 to 0.005, which is nearly an order of magnitude lower than any contacting synthetic bearing (144–146) (Table 4.2). Several mechanisms contribute to this important characteristic, including the lubricating properties of the synovial fluid and the presence of lubricating glycoproteins on the cartilage surface (147). Increasingly, there is evidence that

TABLE 4.2. *Coefficients of friction of various materials*

Materials	Coefficient of friction
Rubber tire on dry road	~1
Nylon on steel	0.3
Steel on oiled bronze	0.2
Teflon on teflon	0.07
Hydrodynamic oil bearing	0.05
Artificial joint (UHMWPE on metal)	0.05
Cartilage on glass	0.05
Cartilage on cartilage	0.002

UHMWPE, ultra-high molecular weight polyethylene.
From Dowson D. Basic tribology. In: Dowson D, Wright eds. *Introduction to the biomechanics of joints and joint replacements.* London: Mechanical Engineering Publications, 1981:49–60.

the predominant mechanism responsible for the frictional properties of cartilage is the pressurization of the interstitial water within the tissue that occurs immediately in response to joint loading (9,148). In this manner, most of the joint load (up to 90%) is carried not by the solid matrix of the cartilage but by a "pressurized" fluid phase. This mechanism significantly decreases the effective load placed on the solid matrix and therefore the apparent coefficient of friction.

PHYSIOLOGY OF ARTICULAR CARTILAGE CHONDROCYTES

Chondrocytes and Cartilage Metabolism

Articular cartilage is maintained in a constant state of turnover through a homeostatic balance of the anabolic and catabolic activities of the chondrocytes. Under normal conditions, the rate of synthesis of extracellular matrix components is close or equal to their rate of breakdown. After injury or with disease, an imbalance of anabolic and catabolic activities occurs that may contribute to the progressive nature of cartilage degeneration (149). The activities of the cells within cartilage are influenced by a number of factors, including genetic coding, environmental factors such as soluble mediators (e.g., growth factors, cytokines), extracellular matrix composition, and biophysical factors such as mechanical stress. Chondrocytes are believed to receive their nutrition through diffusion from the synovial fluid, and their activity may therefore be influenced in part by systemic factors. However, it is generally accepted that the predominant endocrine and paracrine regulation of chondrocyte metabolism occurs due to more "local" signaling from chondrocytes or cells from other tissues in the joint. An important component of the local regulation of cellular activity appears to be mechanical stimuli such as stress, strain, and pressurization and associated electrokinetic effects and physicochemical changes, which are engendered by joint loading (150).

Nutrition and Metabolite Clearance

Adult articular cartilage is avascular, aneural, and alymphatic, indicating that nutrient and metabolite transport must occur by diffusion through the tissue surface or from the subchondral bone. Although there is some evidence that small molecules may diffuse through the underlying bone and zone of calcified cartilage in immature cartilage, it is generally believed that articular cartilage receives most of its nutrition from the synovial fluid within the joint (151,152). The diffusion times for transport of nutrients from the cartilage to the deep zone can be appreciable, ranging from seconds to hours, depending on the size, structure, and charge of the diffusing molecule (151–154). Solutes and nutrients may move through the cartilage matrix by diffusion or by convection as the interstitial water moves through the extracellular matrix during loading. It has been shown that small solutes (e.g., inorganic ions, oxygen, glucose, free sulfate) move freely through the extracellular matrix and their transport is not enhanced by mechanical loading. However, cyclic loading, which causes significant fluid movement, is believed to enhance the transport of larger molecules such as enzymes, growth factors, and cytokines (12,143,154,155).

Synthesis of Matrix Molecules

Chondrocytes are metabolically active cells that occupy only a small fraction (1% to 10%) of the extracellular matrix of articular cartilage. As the only cell population in articular cartilage, chondrocytes are responsible for the synthesis of matrix macromolecules of articular cartilage. The overall process of matrix biosynthesis requires several steps, including transcription of a gene to form messenger RNA (mRNA) for a specific molecule, translation of that mRNA to generate the molecule or parts of the molecule, posttranslational modifications, and finally secretion and matrix assembly. Aggrecan mRNA, for example, is transcribed in the chondrocyte nucleus and is transported to the endoplasmic reticulum where the mRNA is then translated by ribosomes to produce the protein core. The glycosaminoglycan chains are then added to the protein core within the Golgi complex (156,157). After sulfation of the disaccharide units, the proteoglycan is secreted by the cell into the pericellular space via secretory vesicles. The formation of aggrecan, the high-molecular-weight aggregate molecule, occurs extracellularly via interactions with hyaluronan and link protein.

Collagen II is a triple helical structure composed of three identical α chains. These α chains contain the signal peptide, the collagenous and noncollagenous domains, and the N- and C-terminal ends of the molecule (20). After removal of the signal peptide, the triple helix is formed as disulfide bonds are created starting at the carboxy-terminal end. The procollagen molecule is modified in the Golgi and then secreted extracellularly, at which point the nonhelical domains at the ends of the molecule are cleaved from the helical domain (18). After this process, the tropocollagen molecules assemble into a quarter-staggered array of collagen fibrils. Covalent cross-links are then formed between different collagen fibrils, primarily via the 3-hydroxypyridinium residue.

The synthesis, secretion, and assembly of other extracellular matrix macromolecules is the subject of ongoing studies but most likely involves a similar sequence of events from nuclear transcription to posttranslational modifications both within and outside of the cell.

Degradation of Matrix Molecules

Enzymatic degradation of matrix components is one of the steps involved in the normal maintenance of articular cartilage. The turnover is initiated and regulated by various proteolytic and glycosidic enzymes that are synthesized and activated by the chondrocytes and potentially by other cell populations within the synovial joint. Several classes of enzymes are known to be active within articular cartilage, including the metalloproteinases (MMPs), serine proteinases, the cysteine proteinases (cathepsins), the ADAMs ("a disintegrin and MMP" containing enzyme), and the ADAMTS proteinases (ADAMs containing thrombospondin domains) (158–168). Of particular interest are the MMPs that may have important specific and nonspecific activities on cartilage extracellular matrix proteins. MMPs are a set of zinc-dependent endopeptidases whose activity depends on their synthesis, activation, and inhibition by other molecules such as tissue inhibitor of metalloproteinase and other protease inhibitors. Collagenase 1 (MMP1) has specific activity on fibrillar collagens and acts to cleave the triple helix at a single site on the molecule. Gelatinase (MMP2) acts to cleave individual α chains that have been exposed by the activity of MMP1. Stromelysin (MMP3) has been shown to act on type II and type IX collagen and on aggrecan, cleaving the core protein between the G1 and G2 domains. There is also evidence for the important actions of other MMPs such as MMP8 (neutrophil collagenase or collagenase 2), MMP9, and MMP13 (collagenase 3) (160–165). MMPs are generally synthesized in an inactive pro form and then cleaved to remove a cysteine in the propeptide domain, thus generating a mature active enzyme. Although many of these MMPs are constitutively expressed by chondrocytes for the maintenance of the cartilage extracellular matrix, others such as MMP9 and MMP13 may be present only under pathologic condition leading to cartilage degeneration. The activities of these MMPs are believed to significantly contribute to both the initiation and progression of cartilage degeneration in osteoarthritis and after injury.

ADAMs are a new class of proteases closely related to the MMPs. Members with one or more thrombospondin domains are referred to as ADAMTS proteins. Recent studies have determined the aggrecan-degrading MMP, termed "aggrecanase," to be a member of the ADAMTS class (167), and it is likely a family of enzymes exists with aggrecanase activity. This enzyme cleaves aggrecan at a distinct site as compared with the action of other MMPs (161,169).

Physical Regulation of Cartilage Metabolism

A number of *in vivo* investigations have demonstrated that biophysical factors, in addition to biochemical factors, have an important effect on the physiologic activity of the chondrocytes. In particular, there is compelling evidence that "abnormal" joint loading, defined as changes in the magnitude, distribution, or frequency of joint loading, can significantly affect the composition, structure, metabolic activity, and mechanical properties of articular cartilage and other joint tissues (170,171). Experimental models of altered joint loading have been developed for studies of cartilage degeneration in response to observations of natural cartilage degeneration in the human joint after traumatic loading, joint instability, joint immobilization, or isolated injury. These experimental studies have provided a means for tracking the time sequence of events in cartilage that occur with degeneration and also provide an important tool for isolating aging changes from the degenerative process of osteoarthritis.

In one experimental model, disuse of the knee joint achieved through immobilization, casting, or muscle transection may result in changes in cartilage composition and mechanical behavior that are characteristic of degeneration. Important changes observed in the cartilage include a loss of proteoglycans and changes in proteoglycan conformation, a decrease in cartilage thickness, and material property changes including a decreased compressive stiffness and increased tensile stiffness (172–176). In addition, there is direct evidence of decreased proteoglycan and collagen biosynthesis and elevated levels of MMPs suggesting an altered metabolic balance after periods of joint unloading in both human and experimental animal tissue (172,174,177,178). Many of these changes are localized to specific sites and depths in the cartilage layer, and some of these changes have been shown to be partly reversible with remobilization of the joint (173,174,179). In contrast to studies of joint disuse, moderate exercise seems to have few deleterious effects on the cartilage and does not seem to influence the induction or progression of joint disease unless there are abnormalities present or the exercise involves repetitive high levels of impact (180–184).

Damage to the pericapsular and intracapsular soft tissues, such as ligaments and menisci, has been often observed to produce degenerative changes in the knee joint under both clinical and experimental conditions. The menisci and ligaments are important force attenuating and stabilizing structures in the joint, so that damage to either menisci or ligaments will alter the magnitude and distribution of forces applied to the cartilage layers *in vivo*. It has been well documented that the clinical phenomena of "joint laxity" and "joint instability" lead to alterations in contact areas and stresses (185,186), and therefore surgically induced "joint instability" has been used as an animal model to study the effects of altered joint loading on cartilage degeneration. Transection of the anterior cruciate ligament has been the most widely used model for studying degenerative changes in articular cartilage that occur after destabilization of the joint (112,129,139,187–194). This model was studied over an extended time course of 54 months and was found to produce degenerative changes in the joint similar to those of human osteoarthritis (188). Morphologic and histologic changes include fibrillation of the articular surface, loss of proteoglycan content and collagen fibril organization, increased cellularity, meniscal changes, and joint capsule thickening. Compositional and metabolic changes include an increase in water content, increased rates of proteoglycan and collagen synthesis, decreased concentration of collagen cross-links, decreased content of hyaluronic acid, and alterations in the number and size of proteoglycan aggregates (189,191,195–199). These structural and compositional changes are accompanied by distinct changes in the biomechanical properties of the articular cartilage, including a decrease in the tensile, compressive, and shear moduli; increased evidence of swelling behavior; and increased hydraulic permeability of the tissue (112,126, 129,187,191).

Surgical resection of the meniscus has also proved to be a valuable experimental system for studying altered joint loading, and cartilage degeneration, in a number of animal models (192,200–204). Degenerative changes after meniscectomy are observed in the articular cartilage, including signs of cartilage fibrillation (i.e., a roughening of the cartilage surface as collagen fiber bundles become frayed), increased hydration and decreased proteoglycan content of the extracellular matrix, and elevated collagen and proteoglycan synthesis rates (201,202,204–206). In addition, changes in the mechanical behavior of the cartilage layer have been observed, including alterations in the magnitude of streaming potentials and changes in both the compressive and tensile properties (128,202,207,208). As with the experimental models of impact loading or ligament transection, it is unclear which mechanical stimuli is most significant for

initiating the cascade of degenerative changes. Furthermore, the specific role of the chondrocytes in eliciting these changes in cartilage composition and mechanical behavior are not fully understood. There are numerous ongoing studies of cartilage metabolism *in vitro* with a focus on the role of physical factors in controlling this metabolism to more fully understand the mechanisms for the chondrocytes' role in controlling homeostasis and degeneration in articular cartilage (209).

These *in vivo* studies emphasize the relationship between joint loading and the function of articular cartilage and suggest that the chondrocyte population plays an active role in maintaining this relationship. It appears that a critical level and manner of joint loading is required to send the appropriate physical signals to the chondrocyte for maintenance of the composition, material properties, and mechanical function of the cartilage extracellular matrix.

INTRINSIC REPAIR CAPABILITIES

Adult articular cartilage has a limited capacity to repair its matrix in response to injury or disease (210–213). In particular, spontaneous repair is rarely observed with superficial lacerations and is virtually nonexistent with large defects, whether they penetrate through the full or partial thickness of the cartilage. Several factors have been implicated in this poor repair response, including a lack of blood supply, a lack of an undifferentiated cell population, and a relatively harsh mechanical environment. In general, tissue repair and regeneration in the body requires formation of a fibrin clot at the site of damage, which is then infiltrated by inflammatory cells. Inflammatory cells are responsible for the removal of necrotic cells and tissue and for the promotion of migration and proliferation of undifferentiated "progenitor" cells that then regenerate new matrix. In fact, several surgical techniques for promoting cartilage repair rely on drilling or abrasion of the subchondral bone in an effort to provide an intrinsic blood supply and source of undifferentiated mesenchymal cells to the site of injury (214,215). However, it has been shown repeatedly that the cells that repopulate a site of injury are unable to restore the normal composition, structure, or mechanical properties of the normal cartilage extracellular matrix. In particular, the repair tissue often consists of fibrocartilage, which contains predominantly type I collagen and has little if any of the complex organization and structure of hyaline articular cartilage (212). Fibrocartilaginous repair tissue does not seem to restore the functional characteristics of normal cartilage (216) and often fails within a short period of time. Clinical evidence and experimental animal studies suggest that repair tissue has inadequate mechanical properties as compared with normal cartilage.

MECHANICAL INJURY OF ARTICULAR CARTILAGE

Injury to articular cartilage is most often attributed to a single or repeated impact loading condition. Impact loading (i.e., a rapid increase of force across the joint) can be expected to produce a highly nonuniform combination of tensile, compressive, and shear stresses and strains, as well as very high hydrostatic pressures, through the cartilage layer (217). Impact loading has been shown to cause both immediate and progressive damage to articular cartilage of the knee joint (217–224). Studies have used single or repetitive impact loading to emulate different loading conditions in the human related to injury or repetitious daily activity, respectively. In studies of the canine or porcine patellofemoral joint after isolated impact, cartilage changes included altered cellular activity and histologic appearance and increased hydration and proteoglycan content within 2 weeks after loading (217,218). Subfracture impact loads also cause a significant decrease in the tensile stiffness of the surface zone cartilage but no detectable changes in either the compressive modulus or hydraulic permeability of the cartilage (217).

Cartilage "delamination," or separation from the subchondral bone, is believed to be caused by high shear stresses at the tidemark due to a rapid lateral expansion of the articular cartilage in response to impact loading. In this situation, the high rate of loading does not allow time for fluid exudation from the tissue, and cartilage behaves as an incompressible elastic material, resulting in high shear stresses at the subchondral bone interface (9,225,226). Given the poor repair capacity of articular cartilage, this type of injury generally does not repair spontaneously and may require surgical intervention to resect the damaged tissue (227).

Of particular importance is the cascade of degenerative events that follows posttraumatic injury, which may lead to osteoarthritis (218,223,228). Although there is clearly a biologic response to the impact load, it is not yet clear which biomechanical stimuli is most important for initiating the cascade of degenerative changes. It is certain, however, that the changes in the mechanical environment due to impact loading may serve to directly induce matrix damage and transduce cellular signals that result in altered biosynthetic activities.

OSTEOARTHRITIS AND CARTILAGE DEGENERATION

Osteoarthritis is the most prevalent form of joint disease and affects an estimated 20,000,000 individuals in the United States (229). Osteoarthritis manifests itself as a slowly progressing debilitating disease that affects one or more joints of the body. Clinical signs include pain, swelling, enlargement of the joints, and decreased range of joint motion. Radiographic changes are often apparent, such as narrowing of the joint space and formation of osteophytes. The primary pathologic changes of osteoarthritis are fibrillation and loss of the articular cartilage, accompanied by thickening and remodeling of the subchondral bone. Osteoarthritis seems to be the common end point of a number of potentially independent pathogenetic processes that culminate in a failure of the joint (230,231). The important radiographic, histologic, biomechanical, and biochemical characteristics of osteoarthritis have been carefully studied and are well documented in several volumes (232–234). In this section, we present a brief introduction to the pathology of osteoarthritis with a focus on the known changes in articular cartilage.

Cartilage Morphology and Histology with Osteoarthritis

Osteoarthritis is a condition of the diarthrodial joint that involves the articular cartilage, the underlying bone, and the capsular tissues (235). However, it is still unclear whether cartilage and bone pathology occur concomitantly or whether one tissue is the predominant side where osteoarthritis is initiated. In its early stages, osteoarthritis is characterized by fibrillation and irregularity and lesions of the cartilage surface (Fig. 4.5). Histologic analysis at this stage often reveals a loss of metachromatic staining in the surface zone of the tissue. In the intermediate stage, osteoarthritis is characterized by focal regions of cartilage loss and clefts and fissures that extend partially or fully through the thickness of the tissue. Histologic changes in this stage may reveal a loss of staining that extends into the middle and deep zones. At this stage, significant changes in the tidemark and calcified cartilage layer are generally observed, including reduplication and other irregularities of the tidemark (74). In many cases, vascular invasion is observed such that blood vessels penetrate the subchondral bone and thereby form a connection between the marrow cavity and the articular cartilage. Chondrocyte "clones" may be observed in the surface zone, which are clusters of chondrocytes that have presumably undergone proliferation. In late-stage osteoarthritis, the loss of articular cartilage can extend to the subchondral bone, and in many cases, little if any cartilage remains.

Although there is no universally accepted classification system to measure the morphologic and histologic changes with osteoarthritis, several different "grading" schemes have been developed in an effort to characterize and in some cases quantify the extent of morphologic and histologic changes with osteoarthritis. Macroscopic grading schemes generally use a visual scale between 0 and 4 to rate the extent of gross morphologic changes, where 0 represents normal articular cartilage and 4 represents severe osteoarthritic changes that expose the

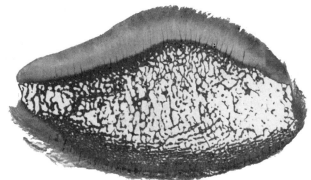

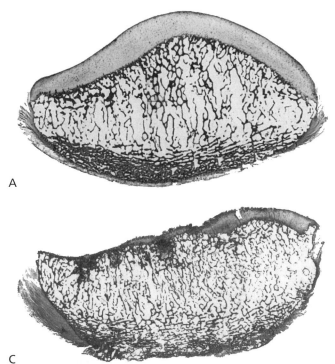

A

B

C

FIG. 4.5. Histologic micrographs of the cross-sections of human patellae in health and disease. **A:** Normal healthy patella showing no fibrillation, osteophytes, cartilage loss, or other gross signs of osteoarthritis. **B:** Early-stage osteoarthritis is characterized by fibrillation and horizontal splitting of the cartilage surface and remodeling and thickening of the subchondral bone. **C:** Late-stage osteoarthritis is characterized by extensive loss of cartilage and remodeling of the underlying bone, osteophytes, cellular cloning, and the presence and bone cysts. (Photographs courtesy of Dr. Leon Sokoloff.)

subchondral bone. Variations of this concept exist, and a recent study has shown that the "SFA" score (Société Française Arthroscopie) provides a relatively precise and accurate macroscopic measure of osteoarthritic degeneration by factoring in the size and the depth of lesions (236–238). Histologic grading has also been commonly used to evaluate cartilage degeneration (239,240). The "Mankin" grading scheme, as well as modifications of this scheme, use histologic changes in the cartilage to rank features such as structural changes, chondrocyte cloning, subchondral bone thickening, and more to form an aggregate score that represents the overall disease state (241). Because the relative importance and weighting of individual variables to an overall histologic score is not apparent *a priori,* statistical methods such as principal components analysis are valuable in that they can be used to combine these several types of variables, with potential interrelationships, into a reduced number of "factors" without assumptions as to their relative importance (239). These statistical factorial analyses have been useful for demonstrating important relationships between histologic evidence of cartilage degeneration and biochemical and biomechanical markers of osteoarthritis (242).

Cartilage Composition with Osteoarthritis

Osteoarthritic cartilage also exhibits compositional changes relative to the nondegenerate tissue. One of the earliest events in osteoarthritis seems to be an increased

"swelling" or water content of the cartilage, which reflects damage or "disruption" of the collagen matrix (133,243). Increases in cartilage hydration have also been observed in middle- and late-stage osteoarthritis, in contrast to a slight decline in water content that occurs in normal cartilage with aging. Consequently, in most stages of osteoarthritis, many studies have observed a decrease in collagen and proteoglycan content on a wet weight basis, due to the increase in water content (244). However, in early osteoarthritis, it is not clear whether there is an intrinsic change in the composition of any particular extracellular matrix constituent. There is, however, evidence for enzymatic activities such as aggrecanase and collagenase, resulting in cleavage of aggrecan and collagen, respectively, with appearance of catabolic "neoepitopes," newly generated epitopes as a result of the metabolic degradative process (162,245). As the disease progresses, a significant loss of extracellular matrix may occur, however, leading to focal erosion as described above.

Important changes occur in the structure of the macromolecules that form the cartilage matrix with osteoarthritis. Previous studies have reported changes in proteoglycan size, glycosaminoglycan chain length, and proportions of the different glycosaminoglycans with osteoarthritis (244). In many cases, the size and sulfation pattern of the proteoglycans may revert to that of immature or even fetal cartilage (94). Although few changes have been observed in total collagen content in early osteoarthritis, several studies have shown important alterations in the distribution of collagen types within the cartilage layer. Increases in collagen types VI, IX, X, and XI have been shown to occur in later stages of osteoarthritis (244), which is consistent with findings of elevated collagen synthesis rates in osteoarthritic cartilage. Some structural changes are observed in the collagen, such as changes in the size and arrangement of the individual fibers. Early osteoarthritis is also characterized by a decrease in the concentration of hydroxypyrodinoline cross-links per mole of collagen, presumably due to the presence of newly synthesized immature collagen (191).

Osteoarthritic cartilage is also characterized by an increase in the concentration of several matrix components, such as COMP, tenascin, and fibronectin. The increased concentration of these matrix macromolecules in the tissue and the presence of alterations in the structure of proteoglycans and collagens have led to the investigation of the potential of these molecules within the cartilage tissue, the synovial fluid, serum, and urine to serve as biologic markers ("biomarkers") of the presence and severity of osteoarthritis and response to therapy (59,246–251). Promising results have been yielded from efforts to apply principle components analysis, a means of separating factors into rational groups on the basis of their covariance, to the study of biomarkers in osteoarthritis. Based on an analysis of 14 biomarkers in one study, better than 90% discrimination between osteoarthritic and normal subjects could be obtained using one marker from each of three groups: a marker of inflammatory activity (tumor necrosis factor type II receptor), a marker of cartilage biosynthesis (846), and a marker of cartilage turnover (COMP) (252). It is therefore likely that panels of discriminant biomarkers, including imaging modalities, may be used to more sensitively identify and distinguish normal from pathological cartilage.

Cartilage Mechanics with Osteoarthritis

In early studies of human cartilage, osteoarthritis was associated with decreased tensile stiffness and failure stress in the cartilage from hip or knee joints (108,253). Decreases in the tensile modulus of cartilage were observed both in cartilage samples with osteoarthritis and in those with signs of mild fibrillation. The disorganization and disruption of the fibrillar collagen network that occurs with osteoarthritis thus manifests as a significant decrease in both tensile stiffness and strength of cartilage. These findings have been repeated in experimental studies of animal models of osteoarthritis (112,191,254). Age-related changes have also been reported in the tensile properties of human cartilage, including a decrease in the tensile stiffness and fracture stress of cartilage (104,255), but are generally less severe than osteoarthritic changes. Aging changes have been attributed

to alterations in collagen density or structure that may be distinct from the "unwinding," "fibrillation," or loss of collagen cross-linking associated with osteoarthritis and progressive degeneration (191,256). Damage to the collagenous cartilage matrix with osteoarthritis is consistent with findings for increased shear compliance of human degenerate cartilage (100) and with similar findings for reductions in the shear modulus in a canine model of osteoarthritis (112,128).

Osteoarthritis is also associated with altered compressive behaviors of human articular cartilage, with a direct relationship observed between changes in cartilage properties, and with increasing severity of degeneration (88). Cartilage degeneration is associated with decreases in the compressive modulus and increases in the hydraulic permeability, both changes that have been supported by findings of experimental models of osteoarthritis (126,128,129). These particular changes in the compressive properties suggest a compromised ability of the tissue to support loads through fluid pressurization. This may be important for explaining the progressive nature of the cartilage changes, because this initial damage to the cartilage will be associated with a shift in mechanical behaviors toward increased matrix deformations, decreased fluid pressures, and altered areas of contact during joint loading. These shifts in the mechanical environment within the cartilage extracellular matrix may be considered to be deleterious and may lead to altered cellular signals and direct damage to the cartilage matrix.

Cartilage Metabolism with Osteoarthritis

Chondrocytes from osteoarthritic articular cartilage show significantly higher metabolic and proliferative activity than normal cells. Increased DNA synthesis is observed in nearly all stages of osteoarthritic cartilage, and increased rates of biosynthesis and degradation have been observed for many constituents of the extracellular matrix. Increased rates of matrix synthesis are often concomitant with a net loss of concentration of specific matrix components such as aggrecan, suggesting that rates of degradation may exceed increased rates of biosynthesis. Proteoglycan turnover rates are elevated in osteoarthritis in what is believed to be an effort by the chondrocytes to "repair" the surrounding articular cartilage. The structure of the newly synthesized proteoglycans shows both major and minor differences as compared with normal proteoglycans, such as changes in aggregate size and glycosaminoglycan chain lengths and sulfation patterns (38). Of particular interest has been the discovery of various proteoglycan anabolic "neoepitopes" via monoclonal antibodies that have revealed subtle but distinct changes in the structure of newly synthesized proteoglycans (245). The rate of degradation of proteoglycan is also significantly increased by the action of various proteolytic enzymes such as the MMPs, cathepsins, and aggrecanase. Despite the elevated rates of proteoglycan synthesis, increased degradation leads to a net decrease of proteoglycan concentration in the tissue. The newly synthesized proteoglycans and the proteolytic fragments have been found in increased concentration in both the synovial fluid and the serum (246,247), suggesting that these molecules may represent an objective means to diagnose and monitor osteoarthritic changes in a minimally invasive manner.

Increased collagen turnover has also been observed in osteoarthritis. Under normal circumstances, the turnover of type II collagen in articular cartilage is relatively slow, with a half-life on the order of years as opposed to months for proteoglycans. Collagen synthesis rates are increased with osteoarthritis, although it seems that the newly synthesized molecules may not be able to reverse the concomitant increase in collagen breakdown due to increased MMP activity. Because the collagen fibers are self-assembled extracellularly, it is believed that any degradative damage (enzymatic or mechanical) to the collagen network requires significant time to repair.

CLINICAL MODALITIES FOR CARTILAGE REPAIR

Articular cartilage has a limited capacity for repair, and thus even minor lesions or injuries may lead to progressive damage and joint degeneration. Isolated chondral and osteochondral lesions are also a significant source of pain and loss of function and will rarely, if ever, heal spontaneously. Several methods have been used clinically to promote cartilage repair in cases of injury and arthritis, albeit with inconsistent or undocumented success (214,215). One of the potential explanations for the poor repair response of articular cartilage is the lack of a blood supply or a source of undifferentiated cells that can promote repair. For these reasons, many clinicians have used different means of penetrating the subchondral bone to induce bleeding in a repair site in the cartilage. These techniques have included drilling, abrasion, and microfracture of the subchondral bone, often times in a manner that penetrates to the marrow cavity. This methods generally lead to the formation of a fibrocartilaginous repair tissue that in some cases is satisfactory and decreases pain and disability. In general, however, fibrocartilaginous repair tissue does not have the same mechanical properties of normal articular cartilage and does not seem to function effectively as a replacement for normal cartilage.

Recent advances in biology and engineering have introduced the concept of "tissue engineering," whereby novel technologies are used to promote tissue repair or replacement (e.g., 257–261). At this writing, there is one cell-based repair procedure available for clinical use, which involves the isolation and amplification of autologous chondrocytes, followed by reimplantation of cells into the cartilage defect that is covered by a flap of autologous periosteal tissue (262–264). The long-term success of this technique has not been shown in animals models, although clinical outcomes are initially satisfactory. Many other such techniques are being currently explored and involve a range of synthetic and biologic matrices that may be coupled with cell supplementation to enhance repair. Such technologies may also be augmented by various growth factors, such as transforming growth factor β, bone morphogenetic protein 6, basic fibroblast growth factor, and insulin growth factor, which have been shown to promote chondrogenic potential (265–267). The combination of living tissue substitutes coupled with the identification of chondrogenic growth factors will hopefully introduce many new cartilage repair options in the near future.

REFERENCES

1. Linn FC, Sokoloff L. Movement and composition of interstitial fluid of cartilage. *Arthritis Rheum* 1965;8:481–494.
2. Mankin HJ, Thrasher AZ. Water content and binding in normal and osteoarthritic human cartilage. *J Bone Joint Surg Am* 1975;57A:76–79.
3. Maroudas A. Physicochemical properties of cartilage in the light of ion exchange theory. *Biophys J* 1968;8:575–595.
4. Mow VC, Holmes MH, Lai WM. Fluid transport and mechanical properties of articular cartilage: a review. *J Biomech* 1984;17:377–394.
5. Maroudas A, Evans H, Almeida L. Cartilage of the hip joint. Topographical variation of glycosaminoglycan content in normal and fibrillated tissue. *Ann Rheum Dis* 1973;32:1–9.
6. Maroudas A, Schneiderman R. "Free" and "exchangeable" or "trapped" and "non-exchangeable" water in cartilage. *J Orthop Res* 1987;5:133–138.
7. Torzilli PA, Dethmers DA, Rose DE, et al. Movement of interstitial water through loaded articular cartilage. *J Biomech* 1983;16:169–179.
8. Mow VC, Kuei SC, Lai WM, et al. Biphasic creep and stress relaxation of articular cartilage in compression: theory and experiments. *J Biomech Eng* 1980;102:73–84.
9. Ateshian GA, Lai WM, Zhu WB, et al. An asymptotic solution for the contact of two biphasic cartilage layers. *J Biomech* 1994;27:1347–1360.
10. Hodge W, Fijan R, Carlson K, et al. Contact pressures in the human hip joint measured in vivo. *Proc Natl Acad Sci USA* 1986;83:2879–2883.
11. Maroudas A. Mechanisms of fluid transport in cartilaginous tissues. In: Freeman M, ed. *Adult articular cartilage,* 1st ed. Tunbridge Wells: Pitman Medical, 1973:47–72.
12. O'Hara BP, Urban JP, Maroudas A. Influence of cyclic loading on the nutrition of articular cartilage. *Ann Rheum Dis* 1990;49:536–539.
13. Eyre DR, Wu J-J, Woods P. Cartilage specific collagens: structural studies. In: Kuettner KE, Schleyerbach R, Peyron JG, Hascall VC, eds. *Articular cartilage and osteoarthritis.* New York: Raven Press, 1992:119–131.
14. Kempson GE, Muir H, Pollard C, et al. The tensile properties of the cartilage of human femoral condyles related to the content of collagen and glycosaminoglycans. *Biochim Biophys Acta* 1973;297:456–472.
15. Miller EJ, Van der Korst JK, Sokoloff L. Collagen of human articular and costal cartilage. *Arthritis Rheum* 1969;12:21–29.
16. Muir H, Bullough P, Maroudas A. The distribution of collagen

in human articular cartilage with some of its physiological implications. *J Bone Joint Surg Br* 1970;52:554–563.

17. Burgeson RE, Nimni ME. Collagen types. Molecular structure and tissue distribution. *Clin Orthop* 1992;282:250–272.

18. Nimni ME. Collagen: structure, function, and metabolism in normal and fibrotic tissues. *Semin Arthr Rheum* 1983;13:1–86.

19. Myers JC, Yang H, D'Ippolito JA, et al. The triple-helical region of human type XIX collagen consists of multiple collagenous subdomains and exhibits limited sequence homology to alpha 1 (XVI). *J Biol Chem* 1994;269:18549–18557.

20. Sandell LJ, Goldring MB, Zamparo O, et al. Molecular biology of type II collagen: new information in the gene. In: Kuettner KE, Schleyerbach R, Peyron JG, Hascall VC, eds. *Articular cartilage and osteoarthritis.* New York: Raven Press, 1992:81–94.

21. Deshmukh K, Nimni ME. Isolation and characterization of cyanogen bromide peptides from the collagen of bovine articular cartilage. *Biochem J* 1973;133:615–622.

22. Clark JM. The organisation of collagen fibrils in the superficial zones of articular cartilage. *J Anat* 1990;171:117–130.

23. Weiss C, Rosenberg LC, Helfet AJ. An ultrastructural study of normal young adult human articular cartilage. *J Bone Joint Surg Am* 1968;50A:663–674.

24. Eyre DR, Oguchi H. The hydroxypyridinium cross-links of skeletal collagens: their measurement, properties and a proposed pathway of formation. *Biochem Biophys Res Commun* 1980;92:403–410.

25. Eyre DR, Koob TJ, Van Ness KP. Quantitation of hydroxypyridinium cross-links in collagen by high-performance liquid chromatography. *Anal Biochem* 1984;137:380–388.

26. Knowlton RG, Katzenstein PL, Moskowitz RW, et al. Genetic linkage of a polymorphism in the type II procollagen gene (COL2A1) to primary osteoarthritis associated with mild chondrodysplasia. *N Engl J Med* 1990;322:526–530.

27. Eyre DR, Wu JJ. Collagen structure and cartilage matrix integrity. *J Rheumatol* 1995;43[Suppl]:82–85.

28. Eyre DR. Collagen structure and function in articular cartilage: metabolic changes in the development of osteoarthritis. In: Kuettner KE, Goldberg VM, eds. *Osteoarthritic disorders.* Rosemont, IL: American Academy of Orthopaedic Surgeons, 1994:219–227.

29. Olsen BR. New insights into the function of collagens from genetic analysis. *Curr Opin Cell Biol* 1995;7:720–727.

30. Poole CA, Glant TT, Schofield JR. Chondrons from articular cartilage. IV. Immunolocalization of proteoglycan epitopes in isolated canine tibial chondrons. *J Histochem Cytochem* 1991;39:1175–1187.

31. Poole CA, Ayad S, Schofield JR. Chondrons from articular cartilage. I. Immunolocalization of type VI collagen in the pericellular capsule of isolated canine tibial chondrons. *J Cell Sci* 1988;90:635–643.

32. Wu JJ, Eyre DR. Covalent interactions of type IX collagen in cartilage. *Connect Tissue Res* 1989;20:241–246.

33. Holderbaum D, Haqqi TM, Moskowitz RW. Genetics and osteoarthritis: exposing the iceberg. *Arthritis Rheum* 1999;42:397–405.

34. Guilak F, Jones WR, Ting-Beall HP, et al. The deformation behavior and mechanical properties of chondrocytes in articular cartilage. *Osteoarthritis Cartilage* 1999;7:59–70.

35. McDevitt CA, Marcelino J, Tucker L. Interaction of intact type VI collagen with hyaluronan. *FEBS Lett* 1991;294:167–170.

36. Poole CA. Chondrons, the chondrocyte and its pericellular microenvironment. In: Kuettner KE, Schleyerbach R, Peyron JG, Hascall VC, eds. *Articular cartilage and osteoarthritis.* New York: Raven Press, 1992:201–220.

37. Aigner T, Reichenberger E, Bertling W, et al. Type X collagen expression in osteoarthritic and rheumatoid articular cartilage. *Virchows Arch B Cell Pathol Mol Pathol* 1993;63:205–211.

38. Hardingham TE, Fosang AJ, Dudhia J. The structure, function and turnover of aggrecan, the large aggregating proteoglycan from cartilage. *Eur J Clin Chem Clin Biochem* 1994;32:249–257.

39. Heinegård D, Oldberg A. Structure and biology of cartilage and bone matrix noncollagenous macromolecules. *FASEB J* 1989;3:2042–2051.

40. Neame PJ, Sandy JD. Cartilage aggrecan. Biosynthesis, degradation and osteoarthritis. *J Flor Med Assoc* 1994;81:191–193.

41. Roughley PJ, Lee ER. Cartilage proteoglycans: structure and potential functions. *Microsc Res Tech* 1994;28:385–397.

42. Plaas AH, Wong-Palms S, Roughley PJ, et al. Chemical and immunological assay of the nonreducing terminal residues of chondroitin sulfate from human aggrecan. *J Biol Chem* 1997;272:20603–20610.

43. Hardingham TE, Fosang AJ, Dudhia J. Aggrecan: the chondroitin sulfate/keratan sulfate proteoglycan from cartilage. In: Kuettner KE, Schleyerbach R, Peyron JG, Hascall VC, eds. *Articular cartilage and osteoarthritis.* New York: Raven Press, 1992:5–20.

44. Watanabe H, Yamada Y, Kimata K. Roles of aggrecan, a large chondroitin sulfate proteoglycan, in cartilage structure and function. *J Biochem* 1998;124:687–693.

45. Maroudas A, Muir H, Wingham J. The correlation of fixed negative charge with glycosaminoglycan content of human articular cartilage. *Biochim Biophys Acta* 1969;177:492–500.

46. Lai WM, Hou JS, Mow VC. A triphasic theory for the swelling and deformation behaviors of articular cartilage. *J Biomech Eng* 1991;113:245–258.

47. Maroudas A. Physicochemical properties of articular cartilage. In: Freeman M, ed. *Adult articular cartilage.* Tunbridge Wells: Pitman Medical, 1979:215–290.

48. Maroudas A, Ziv I, Weisman N, et al. Studies of hydration and swelling pressure in normal and osteoarthritic cartilage. *Biorheology* 1985;22:159–169.

49. Brocklehurst R, Bayliss MT, Maroudas A, et al. The composition of normal and osteoarthritic articular cartilage from human knee joints. With special reference to unicompartmental replacement and osteotomy of the knee. *J Bone Joint Surg Am* 1984;66:95–106.

50. Maroudas A. Balance between swelling pressure and collagen tension in normal and degenerate cartilage. *Nature* 1976;260:808–809.

51. Narmoneva DA, Wang JY, Setton LA. Nonuniform swelling-induced residual strains in articular cartilage. *J Biomech* 1999;32:401–408.

52. Akizuki S, Mow VC, Muller F, et al. Tensile properties of human knee joint cartilage. II. Correlations between weight bearing and tissue pathology and the kinetics of swelling. *J Orthop Res* 1987;5:173–186.

53. Rosenberg LC. Structure and function of dermatan sulfate proteoglycans in articular cartilage. In: Kuettner KE, Schleyerbach R, Peyron JG, Hascall VC, eds. *Articular cartilage and osteoarthritis.* New York: Raven Press, 1992:45–63.

54. Heinegård D, Lorenzo P, Sommarin Y. Articular cartilage matrix proteins. In: Kuettner KE, Goldberg VM, eds. *Osteoarthritic disorders.* Rosemont, IL: American Academy of Orthopaedic Surgeons 1995.

55. Flannery CR, Hughes CE, Schumacher BL, et al. Articular cartilage superficial zone protein (SZP) is homologous to megakaryocyte stimulating factor precursor and is a multifunctional proteoglycan with potential growth-promoting, cytoprotective, and lubricating properties in cartilage metabolism. *Biochem Biophys Res Commun* 1999;254:535–541.

56. Schumacher BL, Block JA, Schmid TM, et al. A novel proteoglycan synthesized and secreted by chondrocytes of the superficial zone of articular cartilage. *Arch Biochem Biophys* 1994;311:144–152.

57. Chevalier X, Groult N, Larget-Piet B, et al. Tenascin distribution in articular cartilage from normal subjects and from patients with osteoarthritis and rheumatoid arthritis. *Arthritis Rheum* 1994;37:1013–1022.

58. Lust G, Burton-Wurster N, Leipold H. Fibronectin as a marker for osteoarthritis. *J Rheumatol* 1987;14:28–29.

59. Heinegård D, Saxne T. Macromolecular markers in joint disease. *J Rheumatol* 1991;27[Suppl]:27–29.

60. Boskey AL. Current concepts of the physiology and biochemistry of calcification. *Clin Orthop* 1981;157:225–257.

61. Poole AR, Matsui Y, Hinek A, et al. Cartilage macromolecules and the calcification of cartilage matrix. *Anat Rec* 1989;224:167–179.

62. Pritzker KP, Cheng PT, Renlund RC. Calcium pyrophosphate crystal deposition in hyaline cartilage. Ultrastructural analysis and implications for pathogenesis. *J Rheumatol* 1988;15:828–835.

63. Asari A, Miyauchi S, Kuriyama S, et al. Localization of hyaluronic acid in human articular cartilage. *J Histochem Cytochem* 1994;42:513–522.

64. Gomez JE, Thurston GB. Comparisons of the oscillatory shear viscoelasticity and composition of pathological synovial fluids. *Biorheology* 1993;30:409–427.

65. Brandt KD, Palmoski MJ, Perricone E. Aggregation of cartilage proteoglycans. II. Evidence for the presence of a hyaluronate-binding region on proteoglycans from osteoarthritic cartilage. *Arthritis Rheum* 1976;19:1308–1314.

66. Hunziker EB, Michel M, Studer D. Ultrastructure of adult human articular cartilage matrix after cryotechnical processing. *Microsc Res Tech* 1997;37:271–284.

67. Buckwalter JA, Hunziker E, Rosenberg L, et al. Articular cartilage: composition and structure. In: Woo SL-Y, Buckwalter JA, eds. *Injury and repair of the musculoskeletal soft tissues.* Park Ridge, IL: American Academy of Orthopaedic Surgeons, 1988:405–430.

68. Eggli PS, Hunziker EB, Schenk RK. Quantitation of structural features characterizing weight- and less-weight-bearing regions in articular cartilage: a stereological analysis of medial femoral condyles in young adult rabbits. *Anat Rec* 1988;222:217–227.

69. Meachim G, Roy S. Surface ultrastructure of mature adult human articular cartilage. *J Bone Joint Surg Br* 1969;51B:529–539.

70. Venn M, Maroudas A. Chemical composition and swelling of normal and osteoarthrotic femoral head cartilage. I. Chemical composition. *Ann Rheum Dis* 1977;36:121–129.

71. Stockwell RA, Meachim G. The chondrocytes. In: Freeman MAR, ed. *Adult articular cartilage.* London: Pitman Medical, 1973:51–99.

72. Meachim G, Allibone R. Topographical variation in the calcified zone of upper femoral articular cartilage. *J Anat* 1984;139:341–352.

73. Redler I, Mow VC, Zimny ML, et al. The ultrastructure and biomechanical significance of the tidemark of articular cartilage. *Clin Orthop* 1975;112:357–362.

74. Oegema TR Jr, Thompson RC Jr. Cartilage-bone interface (tidemark). In: Brandt KD, ed. *Cartilage changes in osteoarthritis.* Indianapolis, IN: Indiana University School of Medicine, 1990:43–52.

75. Radin EL, Rose RM. Role of subchondral bone in the initiation and progression of cartilage damage. *Clin Orthop* 1986;213:34–40.

76. Schwartz Z, Swain L, Sela J, et al. In vivo regulation of matrix vesicle concentration and enzyme activity during primary bone formation. *Bone Miner* 1992;17:134–138.

77. Derfus B, Kranendonk S, Camacho N, et al. Human osteoarthritic cartilage matrix vesicles generate both calcium pyrophosphate dihydrate and apatite in vitro. *Calcif Tissue Int* 1998;63:258–262.

78. Camacho N, Long C, Derfus B. Zonal heterogeneity of articular cartilage vesicle mineralization is confirmed by FT-IR spectroscopy. *Trans Orthop Res Soc* 1996;21:591.

79. Hunziker EB, Herrmann W. In situ localization of cartilage extracellular matrix components by immunoelectron microscopy after cryotechnical tissue processing. *J Histochem Cytochem* 1987;35:647–655.

80. Lee GM, Poole CA, Kelley SS, et al. Isolated chondrons: a viable alternative for studies of chondrocyte metabolism in vitro. *Osteoarthritis Cartilage* 1997;5:261–274.

81. Poole CA, Flint MH, Beaumont BW. Chondrons extracted from canine tibial cartilage: preliminary report on their isolation and structure. *J Orthop Res* 1988;6:408–419.

82. Hunziker EB, Herrmann W, Schenk RK. Ruthenium hexamine trichloride (RHT)-mediated interaction between plasmalemmal components and pericellular matrix proteoglycans is responsible for the preservation of chondrocytic plasma membranes in situ during cartilage fixation. *J Histochem Cytochem* 1983;31:717–727.

83. Poole CA, Flint MH, Beaumont BW. Chondrons in cartilage: ultrastructural analysis of the pericellular microenvironment in adult human articular cartilages. *J Orthop Res* 1987;5:509–522.

84. Gannon FH, Sokoloff L. Histomorphometry of the aging patella:

85. the histologic criteria and normals. *Osteoarthritis Cartilage* 1999;7:173–181.

85. Karvonen RL, Negendank WG, Teitge RA, et al. Factors affecting articular cartilage thickness in osteoarthritis and aging. *J Rheumatol* 1994;21:1310–1318.

86. Meachim G, Bentley G, Baker R. Effect of age on thickness of adult patellar articular cartilage. *Ann Rheum Dis* 1977;36:563–568.

87. Meachim G. Effect of age on the thickness of adult articular cartilage at the shoulder joint. *Ann Rheum Dis* 1971;30:43–46.

88. Armstrong CG, Mow VC. Variations in the intrinsic mechanical properties of human articular cartilage with age, degeneration, and water content. *J Bone Joint Surg Am* 1982;64:88–94.

89. Moriguchi T, Fujimoto D. Age-related changes in the content of the collagen cross-link, pyridinoline. *J Biochem* 1978;84:933–935.

90. Buckwalter JA, Kuettner KE, Thonar EJ. Age-related changes in articular cartilage proteoglycans: electron microscopic studies. *J Orthop Res* 1985;3:251–257.

91. Flannery CR, Urbanek PJ, Sandy JD. The effect of maturation and aging on the structure and content of link proteins in rabbit articular cartilage. *J Orthop Res* 1990;8:78–85.

92. Hardingham T, Bayliss M. Proteoglycans of articular cartilage: changes in aging and in joint disease. *Semin Arthr Rheum* 1990;20:12–33.

93. Roughley PJ. Structural changes in the proteoglycans of human articular cartilage during aging. *J Rheumatol* 1987;14:14–15.

94. Plaas AH, West LA, Wong-Palms S, et al. Glycosaminoglycan sulfation in human osteoarthritis. Disease-related alterations at the non-reducing termini of chondroitin and dermatan sulfate. *J Biol Chem* 1998;273:12642–12649.

95. Roughley PJ, White RJ, Magny MC, et al. Non-proteoglycan forms of biglycan increase with age in human articular cartilage. *Biochem J* 1993;295:421–426.

96. Barone-Varelas J, Schnitzer TJ, Meng Q, et al. Age-related differences in the metabolism of proteoglycans in bovine articular cartilage explants maintained in the presence of insulin-like growth factor I. *Connect Tissue Res* 1991;26:101–120.

97. Brand HS, de Koning MH, van Kampen GP, et al. Age related changes in the turnover of proteoglycans from explants of bovine articular cartilage. *J Rheumatol* 1991;18:599–605.

98. Livne E, Weiss A, Silbermann M. Articular chondrocytes lose their proliferative activity with aging yet can be restimulated by PTH-(1-84), PGE$_1$, and dexamethasone. *J Bone Miner Res* 1989;4:539–548.

99. Armstrong CG, Bahrani AS, Gardner DL. Changes in the deformational behavior of human hip cartilage with age. *J Biomech Eng* 1980;102:214–220.

100. Hayes WC, Mockros LF. Viscoelastic properties of human articular cartilage. *J Appl Physiol* 1971;31:562–568.

101. Setton LA, Zhu W, Mow VC. The biphasic poroviscoelastic behavior of articular cartilage: role of the surface zone in governing the compressive behavior. *J Biomech* 1993;26:581–592.

102. Mak AF. The apparent viscoelastic behavior of articular cartilage—the contributions from the intrinsic matrix viscoelasticity and interstitial fluid flows. *J Biomech Eng* 1986;108:123–130.

103. Kempson GE, Freeman MA, Swanson SA. Tensile properties of articular cartilage. *Nature* 1968;220:1127–1128.

104. Roth V, Mow VC. The intrinsic tensile behavior of the matrix of bovine articular cartilage and its variation with age. *J Bone Joint Surg Am* 1980;62:1102–1117.

105. Schmidt MB, Mow VC, Chun LE, et al. Effects of proteoglycan extraction on the tensile behavior of articular cartilage. *J Orthop Res* 1990;8:353–363.

106. Woo SL, Akeson WH, Jemmott GF. Measurements of nonhomogeneous, directional mechanical properties of articular cartilage in tension. *J Biomech* 1976;9:785–791.

107. Woo SL, Lubock P, Gomez MA, et al. Large deformation nonhomogeneous and directional properties of articular cartilage in uniaxial tension. *J Biomech* 1979;12:437–446.

108. Akizuki S, Mow VC, Muller F, et al. Tensile properties of human knee joint cartilage. I. Influence of ionic conditions, weight bearing, and fibrillation on the tensile modulus. *J Orthop Res* 1986;4:379–392.

109. Bader DL, Kempson GE, Barrett AJ, et al. The effects of leuco-

cyte elastase on the mechanical properties of adult human articular cartilage in tension. *Biochim Biophys Acta* 1981;677:103–108.

110. Kempson GE, Tuke MA, Dingle JT, et al. The effects of proteolytic enzymes on the mechanical properties of adult human articular cartilage. *Biochim Biophys Acta* 1976;428:741–760.

111. Kempson GE. The effects of proteoglycan and collagen degradation on the mechanical properties of adult human articular cartilage. In: Burleigh P, Poole A, eds. *Dynamics of connective tissue macromolecules.* Amsterdam: North-Holland, 1975:277–307.

112. Setton LA, Mow VC, Howell DS. Mechanical behavior of articular cartilage in shear is altered by transection of the anterior cruciate ligament. *J Orthop Res* 1995;13:473–482.

113. Simon WH, Mak A, Spirt A. The effect of shear fatigue on bovine articular cartilage. *J Orthop Res* 1990;8:86–93.

114. Zhu W, Mow VC, Koob TJ, et al. Viscoelastic shear properties of articular cartilage and the effects of glycosidase treatments. *J Orthop Res* 1993;11:771–781.

115. Zhu W, Lai WM, Mow VC. The density and strength of proteoglycan-proteoglycan interaction sites in concentrated solutions. *J Biomech* 1991;24:1007–1018.

116. Zhu W, Mow VC, Rosenberg LC, et al. Determination of kinetic changes of aggrecan-hyaluronan interactions in solution from its rheological properties. *J Biomech* 1994;27:571–579.

117. Gu WY, Lai WM, Mow VC. Transport of fluid and ions through a porous-permeable charged-hydrated tissue, and streaming potential data on normal bovine articular cartilage. *J Biomech* 1993;26:709–723.

118. Lai WM, Mow VC, Roth V. Effects of nonlinear strain-dependent permeability and rate of compression on the stress behavior of articular cartilage. *J Biomech Eng* 1981;103:61–66.

119. Lai WM, Mow VC. Drag-induced compression of articular cartilage during a permeation experiment. *Biorheology* 1980;17:111–123.

120. Mansour JM, Mow VC. The permeability of articular cartilage under compressive strain and at high pressures. *J Bone Joint Surg Am* 1976;58:509–516.

121. Maroudas A, Bullough P, Swanson SA, et al. The permeability of articular cartilage. *J Bone Joint Surg Br* 1968;50:166–177.

122. Maroudas A. Proteoglycan osmotic pressure and the collagen tension in normal, osteoarthritic human cartilage. *Semin Arthr Rheum* 1981;11:36–39.

123. Athanasiou KA, Rosenwasser MP, Buckwalter JA, et al. Interspecies comparisons of in situ intrinsic mechanical properties of distal femoral cartilage. *J Orthop Res* 1991;9:330–340.

124. Setton LA, Zhu W, Mow VC. The biphasic poroviscoelastic behavior of articular cartilage: role of the surface zone in governing the compressive behavior. *J Biomech* 1993;26:581–592.

125. Ateshian GA, Kwak SD, Soslowsky LJ, et al. A stereophotogrammetric method for determining in situ contact areas in diarthrodial joints, and a comparison with other methods. *J Biomech* 1994;27:111–124.

126. Sah RL, Yang AS, Chen AC, et al. Physical properties of rabbit articular cartilage after transection of the anterior cruciate ligament. *J Orthop Res* 1997;15:197–203.

127. Bader DL, Kempson GE, Egan J, et al. The effects of selective matrix degradation on the short-term compressive properties of adult human articular cartilage. *Biochim Biophys Acta* 1992; 2:147–154.

128. LeRoux MA, Arokoski J, Vail TP, et al. Simultaneous changes in the mechanical properties, quantitative collagen organization, and proteoglycan concentration of articular cartilage following canine meniscectomy. *J Orthop Res* in press 2000.

129. Setton LA, Mow VC, Muller FJ, et al. Mechanical properties of canine articular cartilage are significantly altered following transection of the anterior cruciate ligament. *J Orthop Res* 1994;12:451–463.

130. Gu W, Lai WM, Mow VC. Theoretical basis for measurements of cartilage fixed-charge density using streaming current and electro-osmosis effects. *ASME Adv Bioeng* 1993;26:55–58.

131. Gray ML, Pizzanelli AM, Grodzinsky AJ, et al. Mechanical and physiochemical determinants of the chondrocyte biosynthetic response. *J Orthop Res* 1988;6:777–792.

132. Urban JPG, Maoudas A, Bayliss MT, et al. Swelling pressures of proteoglycans at the concentrations found in cartilaginous tissues. *Biorheology* 1979;16:447–464.

133. Maroudas A, Mizrahi J, Katz EP, et al. Physicochemical properties and functional behavior of normal and osteoarthritic human cartilage. In: Kuettner KE, Schleyerbach R, Hascall VC, eds. *Articular cartilage biochemistry.* New York: Raven Press, 1986:311–329.

134. Mizrahi J, Maroudas A, Lanir Y, et al. The "instantaneous" deformation of cartilage: effects of collagen fiber orientation and osmotic stress. *Biorheology* 1986;23:311–330.

135. Setton LA, Tohyama H, Mow VC. Swelling and curling behaviors of articular cartilage. *J Biomech Eng* 1998;120:355–361.

136. Setton LA, Gu WY, Mow VC, et al. Predictions of the swelling-induced prestress in articular cartilage. In: Selvadurai A, ed. *Mechanics of poroelastic media.* Dordrecht: Kluwer Academic Publishers, 1995:299–322.

137. Adams ME. Cartilage hypertrophy following canine anterior cruciate ligament transection differs among different areas of the joint. *J Rheumatol* 1989;16:818–824.

138. Altman RD, Dean DD, Muniz OE, Howell DC. Prophylactic treatment of canine osteoarthritis with glycosaminoglycan polysulfuric acid ester. *Arthritis & Rheumatism* 1989;32:759–66.

139. McDevitt CA, Muir H. Biochemical changes in the cartilage of the knee in experimental and natural osteoarthritis in the dog. *J Bone Joint Surg Br* 1976;58B:94–101.

140. Maroudas A, Venn M. Chemical composition and swelling of normal and osteoarthrotic femoral head cartilage. II. Swelling. *Ann Rheum Dis* 1977;36:399–406.

141. Narmoneva DA, Wang JY, Patel S, et al. Altered swelling-induced strain fields in articular cartilage following immobilization. In: Simon B, ed. *1997 Advances in Bioengineering.* Vol. 36. New York: American Society of Mechanical Engineers, 1997:125–126.

142. Narmoneva DA, Guilak F, Vail TP, et al. Quantitation of swelling effects in articular cartilage following meniscectomy in a canine model. *Trans Orthop Res Soc* 1998;23:480.

143. Gu WY, Lai WM, Mow VC. A triphasic analysis of negative osmotic flows through charged hydrated soft tissues. *J Biomech* 1997;30:71–78.

144. Mow VC, Ateshian GA. Lubrication and wear of diarthrodial joints. In: Mow VC, Hayes WC, eds. *Basic orthopaedic biomechanics,* 2nd ed. Philadelphia: Lippincott-Raven, 1997:275–315.

145. Wright V, Dowson D. Lubrication and cartilage. *J Anat* 1976;121:107–118.

146. Unsworth A. Tribology of human and artificial joints. Proceedings of the Institution of Mechanical Engineers Part H. *J Eng Med* 1991;205:163–172.

147. Williams PFD, Powell GL, LaBerge M. Sliding friction analysis of phosphatidylcholine as a boundary lubricant for articular cartilage. Proceedings of the Institution of Mechanical Engineers Part H. *J Eng Med* 1993;207:59–66.

148. Ateshian GA. A theoretical formulation for boundary friction in articular cartilage. *J Biomech Eng* 1997;119:81–86.

149. Poole AR, Rizkalla G, Ionescu M, et al. Osteoarthritis in the human knee: a dynamic process of cartilage matrix degradation, synthesis and reorganization. *Agents Actions* 1993; 39[Suppl]:3–13.

150. Mow VC, Bachrach N, Setton LA, et al. Stress, strain, pressure, and flow fields in articular cartilage. In: Mow VC, Guilak F, Tran-Son-Tay R, Hochmuth R, eds. *Cell mechanics and cellular engineering.* New York: Springer-Verlag, 1994:345–379.

151. Maroudas A, Bullough P. Permeability of articular cartilage. *Nature* 1968;219:1260–1261.

152. Maroudas A. Physical chemistry and the structure of cartilage. *J Physiol (Lond)* 1972;223:21P–22P.

153. Garcia AM, Lark MW, Trippel SB, et al. Transport of tissue inhibitor of metalloproteinases-1 through cartilage: contributions of fluid flow and electrical migration. *J Orthop Res* 1998; 16:734–742.

154. Torzilli PA, Grande DA, Arduino JM. Diffusive properties of immature articular cartilage. *J Biomed Mater Res* 1998;40:132–138.

155. Garcia AM, Frank EH, Grimshaw PE, et al. Contributions of fluid convection and electrical migration to transport in cartilage: relevance to loading. *Arch Biochem Biophys* 1996;333:317–325.

156. Vertel BM, Walters LM, Flay N, et al. Xylosylation is an endoplasmic reticulum to Golgi event. *J Biol Chem* 1993;268:11105–11112.

157. Zheng J, Luo W, Tanzer ML. Aggrecan synthesis and secretion. A paradigm for molecular and cellular coordination of multiglobular protein folding and intracellular trafficking. *J Biol Chem* 1998;273:12999–13006.

158. Ehrlich MG. Degradative enzyme systems in osteoarthritic cartilage. *J Orthop Res* 1985;3:170–184.

159. Woessner JF. Imbalance of proteinases and their inhibitors in osteoarthritis. In: Kuettner KE, Goldberg VM, eds. *Osteoarthritic disorders*. Rosemont, IL: American Academy of Orthopaedic Surgeons Publishers, 1995:281–290.

160. Billinghurst RC, Dahlberg L, Ionescu M, et al. Enhanced cleavage of type II collagen by collagenases in osteoarthritic articular cartilage. *J Clin Invest* 1997;99:1534–1545.

161. Fosang AJ, Last K, Neame PJ, et al. Neutrophil collagenase (MMP-8) cleaves at the aggrecanase site E373-A374 in the interglobular domain of cartilage aggrecan. *Biochem J* 1994;304: 347–351.

162. Huebner JL, Otterness IG, Freund EM, et al. Collagenase 1 and collagenase 3 expression in a guinea pig model of osteoarthritis. *Arthritis Rheum* 1998;41:877–890.

163. Mohtai M, Smith RL, Schurman DJ, et al. Expression of 92-kD type IV collagenase/gelatinase (gelatinase B) in osteoarthritic cartilage and its induction in normal human articular cartilage by interleukin 1. *J Clin Invest* 1993;92:179–185.

164. Shlopov BV, Lie WR, Mainardi CL, et al. Osteoarthritic lesions: involvement of three different collagenases. *Arthritis Rheum* 1997;40:2065–2074.

165. Tsuchiya K, Maloney WJ, Vu T, et al. Osteoarthritis: differential expression of matrix metalloproteinase-9 mRNA in nonfibrillated and fibrillated cartilage. *J Orthop Res* 1997;15:94–100.

166. Black RA, White JM. ADAMS: focus on the protease domain. *Curr Opin Cell Biol* 1998;10:654–659.

167. Tortorella MD, Burn TC, Pratta MA, et al. Purification and cloning of aggrecanase-1: a member of the ADAMTS family of proteins. *Science* 1999;284:1664–1666.

168. Chubinskaya S, Cs-Szabo G, Kuettner KE. ADAM-10 message is expressed in human articular cartilage. *J Histochem Cytochem* 1998;46:723–729.

169. Hughes C, Caterson B, Fosang A, et al. Monoclonal antibodies that specifically recognize neoepitope sequences generated by "aggrecanase" and matrix metalloproteinase cleavage of aggrecan: application to catabolism in situ and in vitro. *Biochem J* 1995;305:799–804.

170. Helminen HJ, Jurvelin J, Kiviranta I, et al. Joint loading effects on articular cartilage: A historical review. In: Helminen HJ, Kiviranta I, Tammi M, et al., eds. *Joint loading: biology and health of articular structures*. Bristol: Wright and Sons; 1987:1–46.

171. Tammi M, Paukkonen K, Kiviranta I, et al. Load induced alteration in articular cartilage. In: Helminen HJ, Kiviranta I, Tammi M, et al., eds. *Joint loading: biology and health of articular structures*. Bristol: Wright and Sons, 1987:64–88.

172. Caterson B, Lowther DA. Changes in the metabolism of the proteoglycans from sheep articular cartilage in response to mechanical stress. *Biochim Biophys Acta* 1978;540:412–422.

173. Jurvelin J, Kiviranta I, Saamanen AM, et al. Partial restoration of immobilization-induced softening of canine articular cartilage after remobilization of the knee (stifle) joint. *J Orthop Res* 1989;7:352–358.

174. Palmoski MJ, Perricone E, Brandt KD. Development and reversal of a proteoglycan aggregation defect in normal canine knee cartilage after immobilization. *Arthritis Rheum* 1979;22:508–517.

175. Saamanen AM, Tammi M, Jurvelin J, et al. Proteoglycan alterations following immobilization and remobilization in the articular cartilage of young canine knee (stifle) joint. *J Orthop Res* 1990;8:863–873.

176. Setton LA, Mow VC, Muller FJ, et al. Altered material properties of articular cartilage after periods of joint disuse and joint disuse followed by remobilization. *Osteoarthritis Cartilage* 1997.

177. Tammi M, Kiviranta I, Peltonen L, et al. Effects of joint loading on articular cartilage collagen metabolism: assay of procollagen prolyl 4-hydroxylase and galactosylhydroxylysyl glucosyltransferase. *Connect Tissue Res* 1988;17:199–206.

178. Cheung HS, Setton LA, Guilak F, et al. Upregulation of metalloproteinases in articular cartilage resultant from disuse immobilization, as well as subsequent vigorous exercise. *Trans Orthop Res Soc* 1999;24:40.

179. Kiviranta I, Tammi M, Jurvelin J, et al. Articular cartilage thickness and glycosaminoglycan distribution in the young canine knee joint after remobilization of the immobilized limb. *J Orthop Res* 1994;12:161–167.

180. Buckwalter JA, Lane NE. Athletics and osteoarthritis. *Am J Sports Med* 1997;25:873–881.

181. Lane NE. Physical activity at leisure and risk of osteoarthritis. *Ann Rheum Dis* 1996;55:682—684.

182. Jurvelin J, Kiviranta I, Saamanen AM, et al. Indentation stiffness of young canine knee articular cartilage—influence of strenuous joint loading. *J Biomech* 1990;23:1239–1246.

183. Kiviranta I, Tammi M, Jurvelin J, et al. Articular cartilage thickness and glycosaminoglycan distribution in the canine knee joint after strenuous running exercise. *Clin Orthop* 1992;283:302–308.

184. Lammi MJ, Hakkinen TP, Parkkinen JJ, et al. Adaptation of canine femoral head articular cartilage to long distance running exercise in young beagles. *Ann Rheum Dis* 1993;52:369–377.

185. Kurosawa H, Fukubayashi T, Nakajuma H. Load-bearing mode of the knee joint: physical behavior of the knee joint with or without menisci. *Clin Orthop* 1980;149:283–290.

186. Levy IM, Torzilli PA, Fisch ID. The contribution of the menisci to the stability of the knee. In: Mow VC, Jackson DW, Arnoczky SP, eds. *Knee meniscus: basic and clinical foundations*. New York: Raven Press, 1992:107–115.

187. Altman RD, Tenenbaum J, Latta L, et al. Biomechanical and biochemical properties of dog cartilage in experimentally induced osteoarthritis. *Ann Rheum Dis* 1984;43:83–90.

188. Brandt KD, Myers SL, Burr D, et al. Osteoarthritic changes in canine articular cartilage, subchondral bone, and synovium fifty-four months after transection of the anterior cruciate ligament. *Arthritis Rheum* 1991;34:1560–1570.

189. Carney SL, Billingham ME, Muir H, et al. Demonstration of increased proteoglycan turnover in cartilage explants from dogs with experimental osteoarthritis. *J Orthop Res* 1984;2:201–206.

190. Gilbertson EMM. Development of periarticular osteophytes in experimentally induced osteoarthrosis in the dog. *Ann Rheum Dis* 1975;34:12–25.

191. Guilak F, Ratcliffe A, Lane N, et al. Mechanical and biochemical changes in the superficial zone of articular cartilage in canine experimental osteoarthritis. *J Orthop Res* 1994;12:474–484.

192. Moskowitz RW, Davis W, Sammarco J. Experimentally induced degenerative joint lesions following partial meniscectomy in the rabbit. *Arthritis Rheum* 1973;16:397–405.

193. Pond MJ, Nuki G. Experimentally induced osteoarthritis in the dog. *Ann Rheum Dis* 1973;32:387–388.

194. Stockwell RA, Billingham MEJ, Muir H. Ultrastructural changes in articular cartilage after experimental section of the anterior cruciate ligament of the dog knee. *J Anat* 1983;136:425–439.

195. Eyre DR, McDevitt CA, Billingham ME, et al. Biosynthesis of collagen and other matrix proteins by articular cartilage in experimental osteoarthrosis. *Biochem J* 1980;188:823–837.

196. Manicourt DH, Thonar EJ-M, Pita JC, et al. Changes in the sedimentation profile of proteoglycan aggregates in early experimental canine osteoarthritis. *Connect Tissue Res* 1989;23:33–50.

197. McDevitt C, Gilbertson E, Muir H. An experimental model of osteoarthritis: early morphological and biochemical changes. *J Bone Joint Surg Br* 1977;59B:24–35.

198. Ratcliffe A, Billingham ME, Saed-Nejad F, et al. Increased release of matrix components from articular cartilage in experimental canine osteoarthritis. *J Orthop Res* 1992;10:350–358.

199. Sandy JD, Adams ME, Billingham ME, et al. In vivo and in vitro stimulation of chondrocyte biosynthetic activity in early experimental osteoarthritis. *Arthritis Rheum* 1984;27:388–397.

200. Arnoczky SP, Warren RF, Kaplan N. Meniscal remodeling following partial meniscectomy—an experimental study in the dog. *Arthroscopy* 1985;1:247–252.

201. Floman Y, Eyre DR, Glimcher MJ. Induction of osteoarthrosis

in the rabbit knee joint: biochemical studies on the articular cartilage. *Clin Orthop* 1980;147:278–286.

202. Hoch DH, Grodzinsky AJ, Koob TJ, et al. Early changes in material properties of rabbit articular cartilage after meniscectomy. *J Orthop Res* 1983;1:4–12.

203. Jackson DW, McDevitt CA, Simon TM, et al. Meniscal transplantation using fresh and cryopreserved allografts. An experimental study in goats. *Am J Sports Med* 1992;20:644–656.

204. Shapiro F, Glimcher MJ. Induction of osteoarthrosis in the rabbit knee joint. Histologic changes following meniscectomy and meniscal lesions. *Clin Orthop* 1980;147:287–295.

205. Berjon JJ, Munera L, Calvo M. Degenerative lesions in articular cartilage after meniscectomy. *J Traumatol* 1991;31:342–350.

206. Lufti AM. Morphological changes in the articular cartilage after meniscectomy: an experimental study in the monkey. *J Bone Joint Surg Br* 1975;57B:525–528.

207. Elliott DM, Guilak F, Vail TP, et al. Tensile properties of articular cartilage are altered by meniscectomy in a canine model of osteoarthritis. *J Orthop Res* 1999;17:503–508.

208. Lane JM, Chisena E, Black J. Experimental knee instability: Early mechanical property changes in articular cartilage in a rabbit model. *Clin Orthop* 1979;140:262–265.

209. Guilak F, Sah RL, Setton LA. Physical regulation of cartilage metabolism. In: Mow VC, Hayes WC, eds. *Basic Orthopaedic Biomechanics,* 2nd ed. Philadelphia: Lippincott-Raven, 1997: 179–207.

210. Amiel D, Coutts RD, Abel M, et al. Rib perichondral grafts for the repair of full-thickness articular-cartilage defects. A morphological and biochemical study in rabbits. *J Bone Joint Surg Am* 1985;67:911–920.

211. Green WT Jr. Articular cartilage repair. Behavior of rabbit chondrocytes during tissue culture and subsequent allografting. *Clin Orthop* 1977;124:237–250.

212. Ghadially JA, Ghadially R, Ghadially FN. Long-term results of deep defects in articular cartilage. A scanning electron microscope study. *Virchows Archiv B Cell Pathol* 1977;25:125–136.

213. Mankin HJ. Current concepts review: the response of articular cartilage to mechanical injury. *J Bone Joint Surg Am* 1982;64A:460–466.

214. Gilbert JE. Current treatment options for the restoration of articular cartilage. *Am J Knee Surg* 1998;11:42–46.

215. Menche DS, Frenkel SR, Blair B, et al. A comparison of abrasion burr arthroplasty and subchondral drilling in the treatment of full-thickness cartilage lesions in the rabbit. *Arthroscopy* 1996;12:280–286.

216. Mow VC, Ratcliffe A, Rosenwasser MP, et al. Experimental studies on repair of large osteochondral defects at a high weight bearing area of the knee joint: a tissue engineering study. *J Biomech Eng* 1991;113:198–207.

217. Armstrong CG, Mow VC, Wirth CR. Biomechanics of impact-induced microdamage to articular cartilage: A possible genesis for chondromalacia patella. In: Finerman G, ed. *AAOS Symposium on Sports Medicine: The Knee.* St. Louis; W.B. Saunders, 1985:70–84.

218. Donohue JM, Buss D, Oegema TR Jr, et al. The effects of indirect blunt trauma on adult canine articular cartilage. *J Bone Joint Surg Am* 1983;65:948–957.

219. Oegema TR Jr, Lewis JL, Thompson RC Jr. Role of acute trauma in development of osteoarthritis. *Agents Actions* 1993;40: 220–223.

220. Radin EL, Parker GH, Pugh JW, et al. Response of joints to impact loading. III. Relationship between trabecular microfractures and cartilage degeneration. *J Biomech* 1973;6:51–57.

221. Radin EL, Paul IL. Response of joints to impact loading. I. In vitro wear. *Arthritis Rheum* 1971;14:356–362.

222. Repo RU, Finlay JB. Survival of articular cartilage after controlled impact. *J Bone Joint Surg Am* 1977;59A:1068–1076.

223. Thompson RC Jr, Oegema TR Jr, Lewis JL, et al. Osteoarthrotic changes after acute transarticular load. An animal model. *J Bone Joint Surg Am* 1991;73:990–1001.

224. Vener MJ, Thompson RC Jr, Lewis JL, et al. Subchondral damage after acute transarticular loading: an in vitro model of joint injury. *J Orthop Res* 1992;10:759–765.

225. Anderson DD, Brown TD, Yang KH, et al. A dynamic finite element analysis of impulsive loading of the extension-splinted rabbit knee. *J Biomech Eng* 1990;112:119–128.

226. Eberhardt AW, Lewis JL, Keer LM. Normal contact of elastic spheres with two elastic layers as a model of joint articulation. *J Biomech Eng* 1991;113:410–417.

227. Levy AS, Lohnes J, Sculley S, et al. Chondral delamination of the knee in soccer players. *Am J Sports Med* 1996;24:634–639.

228. Newberry WN, Zukosky DK, Haut RC. Subfracture insult to a knee joint causes alterations in the bone and in the functional stiffness of overlying cartilage. *J Orthop Res* 1997;15:450–455.

229. Praemer A, Furner S, Rice DP. *Musculoskeletal conditions in the United States.* Park Ridge, IL: American Academy of Orthopaedic Surgeons, 1992.

230. Howell DS, Treadwell BV, Trippel SB. Etiopathogenesis of osteoarthritis. In: Moskowitz RW, Howell DS, Goldberg VM, Mankin HJ, eds. *Osteoarthritis, diagnosis and medical/surgical management,* 2nd ed. Philadelphia: W.B. Saunders, 1992:233–252.

231. Kraus VB. Pathogenesis and treatment of osteoarthritis. *Med Clin North Am* 1997;81:85–112.

232. Moskowitz RW, Howell DS, Goldberg VM, et al., eds. *Osteoarthritis: diagnosis and medical/surgical management,* 2nd ed. Philadelphia: W.B. Saunders, 1992.

233. Kuettner KE, Schleyerbach R, Peyron JG, et al., eds. *Articular cartilage and osteoarthritis.* New York: Raven Press, 1992.

234. Brandt KD, Doherty M, Lohmander LS, eds. *Osteoarthritis.* New York: Oxford University Press, 1998.

235. Sokoloff L. *The biology of degenerative joint disease.* Chicago: University of Chicago Press, 1969:162.

236. Ayral X, Gueguen A, Ike RW, et al. Inter-observer reliability of the arthroscopic quantification of chondropathy of the knee. *Osteoarthritis Cartilage* 1998;6:160–166.

237. Bello AE, Garrett WE Jr, Wang H, et al. Comparison of synovial fluid cartilage marker concentrations and chondral damage assessed arthroscopically in acute knee injury. *Osteoarthritis Cartilage* 1997;5:419–426.

238. Dougados M, Ayral X, Listrat V, et al. The SFA system for assessing articular cartilage lesions at arthroscopy of the knee. *Arthroscopy* 1994;10:69–77.

239. Carlson CS, Loeser RF, Jayo MJ, et al. Osteoarthritis in cynomolgus macaques: a primate model of naturally occurring disease. *J Orthop Res* 1994;12:331–339.

240. Van der Sluijs JA, Geesink RGT, van der Linden AJ, et al. The reliability of the Mankin score for OA. *J Orthop Res* 1992;10:58–61.

241. Mankin HJ, Dorfman H, Lippiello L, et al. Biochemical and metabolic abnormalities in articular cartilage from osteo-arthritic human hips. II. Correlation of morphology with biochemical and metabolic data. *J Bone Joint Surg Am* 1971;53:523–537.

242. Carlson CS, Kraus VB, Vail TP, et al. Articular cartilage damage following medial meniscectomy in dogs is predicted by synovial fluid biomarker levels. *Trans Orthop Res Soc* 1999;24:194.

243. Basser PJ, Schneiderman R, Bank RA, et al. Mechanical properties of the collagen network in human articular cartilage as measured by osmotic stress technique. *Arch Biochem Biophys* 1998;351:207–219.

244. Mankin HJ, Brandt KD. Biochemistry and metabolism of articular cartilage in osteoarthritis. In: Moskowitz RW, Howell DS, Goldberg VM, Mankin HJ, eds. *Osteoarthritis: diagnosis and medical/surgical management.* Philadelphia: W.B. Saunders, 1992:109–154.

245. Caterson B, Hughes CE. Anabolic and catabolic markers of proteoglycan metabolism in arthritis. In: Kuettner KE, Goldberg VM, eds. *Osteoarthritic disorders.* Rosemont, IL: American Academy of Orthopaedic Surgeons, 1995:315–328.

246. Lohmander LS, Ionescu M, Jugessur H, et al. Changes in joint cartilage aggrecan after knee injury and in osteoarthritis. *Arthritis Rheum* 1999;42:534–544.

247. Lohmander LS, Felson DT. Defining the role of molecular markers to monitor disease, intervention, and cartilage breakdown in osteoarthritis. *J Rheumatol* 1997;24:782–785.

248. Slater RR Jr, Bayliss MT, Lachiewicz PF, et al. Monoclonal antibodies that detect biochemical markers of arthritis in humans. *Arthritis Rheum* 1995;38:655–659.

249. Lindhorst E, Vail TP, Guilak F, et al. Longitudinal characteriza-

tion of synovial fluid biomarkers in the canine meniscectomy model of osteoarthritis. *J Orthop Res* 2000;18:269–280.

250. Thonar EJ, Lenz ME, Klintworth GK, et al. Quantification of keratan sulfate in blood as a marker of cartilage catabolism. *Arthritis Rheum* 1985;28:1367–1376.

251. Kraus VB, Gell N, Blumenthal J. The effect of chronic exercise on circulating biomarkers in individuals with musculoskeletal disease. *Clin Exerc Phys* 1999;1:17–23.

252. Otterness IG, Zimmerer RO, Swindell AC, et al. An examination of some molecular markers in blood and urine for discriminating patients with osteoarthritis from healthy individuals. *Acta Orthop Scand* 1995;68:148–150.

253. Kempson GE, Spivey CJ, Swanson SA, et al. Patterns of cartilage stiffness on normal and degenerate human femoral heads. *J Biomech* 1971;4:597–609.

254. Elliott DM, Setton LA, Shah MP, et al. Effects of meniscectomy on the tensile properties of articular cartilage. *Adv Bioeng* 1996;33:247–248.

255. Kempson GE. Relationship between the tensile properties of articular cartilage from the human knee and age. *Ann Rheum Dis* 1982;41:508–511.

256. Dodge GR, Poole AR. Immunohistochemical detection and immunochemical analysis of type II collagen degradation in human normal, rheumatoid, and osteoarthritic articular cartilages and in explants of boving articular cartilage cultured with interleukin 1. *J Clin Invest* 1989;83:647–661.

257. Coutts RD, Woo SL, Amiel D, et al. Rib perichondrial autografts in full-thickness articular cartilage defects in rabbits. *Clin Orthop* 1992;275:263–273.

258. Grande DA, Pitman MI, Peterson L, et al. The repair of experimentally produced defects in rabbit articular cartilage by autologous chondrocyte transplantation. *J Orthop Res* 1989;7:208–218.

259. O'Driscoll SW, Keeley FW, Salter RB. The chondrogenic potential of free autogenous periosteal grafts for biological resurfacing of major full-thickness defects in joint surfaces under the influence of continuous passive motion. An experimental investigation in the rabbit. *J Bone Joint Surg Am* 1986;68:1017–1035.

260. Sams AE, Nixon AJ. Chondrocyte-laden collagen scaffolds for resurfacing extensive articular cartilage defects. *Osteoarthritis Cartilage* 1995;3:47–59.

261. Wakitani S, Goto T, Pineda SJ, et al. Mesenchymal cell-based repair of large, full-thickness defects of articular cartilage. *J Bone Joint Surg Am* 1994;76:579–592.

262. Brittberg M, Lindahl A, Nilsson A, et al. Treatment of deep cartilage defects in the knee with autologous chondrocyte transplantation. *N Engl J Med* 1994;331:889–895.

263. Gillogly SD, Voight M, Blackburn T. Treatment of articular cartilage defects of the knee with autologous chondrocyte implantation. *J Orthop Sports Phys Ther* 1998;28:241–251.

264. Minas T, Nehrer S. Current concepts in the treatment of articular cartilage defects. *Orthopedics* 1997;20:525–538.

265. O'Driscoll SW, Recklies AD, Poole AR. Chondrogenesis in periosteal explants. An organ culture model for in vitro study. *J Bone Joint Surg Am* 1994;76:1042–1051.

266. Trippel SB. Growth factor actions on articular cartilage. *J Rheumatol* 1995;43:129–132.

267. Toolan BC, Frenkel SR, Pachence JM, et al. Effects of growth-factor-enhanced culture on a chondrocyte-collagen implant for cartilage repair. *J Biomed Mater Res* 1996;31:273–280.

268. Dowson D. Basic tribology. In: Dowson D, Wright V, eds. *Introduction to the biomechanics of joints and joint replacements.* London: Mechanical Engineering Publications, 1981:49–60.

Principles and Practice of Orthopaedic Sports Medicine,
edited by William E. Garrett, Jr., Kevin P. Speer, and Donald T. Kirkendall.
Lippincott Williams & Wilkins, Philadelphia © 2000.

CHAPTER 5

Bone Adaptation to Exercise in the Basic Science of Sports Medicine

Bert R. Mandelbaum, Luc Teurlings, and Joseph A. Buckwalter

The ability of bone to adapt to exercise makes it possible for individuals to increase their level of physical activity. Failure of bone to adapt to increasing mechanical demands leads to stress fractures, and the changes in bone that occur with decreased levels of physical activity increase the risk of fractures during participation in sports. For these reasons, understanding of how bone adapts to exercise is critical for the practice of sports medicine.

At one time, scientists believed that bone was an inert material and did not respond to mechanical stimuli. It was not until 1892 that Wolff postulated and eventually popularized the concept that mechanical force applied to bone resulted in adaptation. It is only in recent years that the sophistication of biochemical and other laboratory techniques have allowed us to characterize, define, and quantify the responses of bones to these stimuli. We now understand that bone is a complex composite structure that responds to changes in physical activity with a gain or loss of density, mass, and strength. Analogously, the science of connective tissue physiology and biochemistry have been in embryonic stages and in fact may be at the same stage as cardiovascular physiology earlier in this century. Thus, with the development of new assessment techniques combined with objectively quantifiable methods of directing exercise specificity, the clinician can better define bone structure and function and can understand the impact of multiple modulation factors and local, regional, and systemic levels. This understanding is vital, given that a bone stress injury can result in pain, diminution of performance, and inability to participate. These are the specific clinical problems that are significant to the physician, athlete, and parent. In view of this, the goals of the health care team include maximizing performance, minimizing morbidity, and preventing injury. Consequently, it is imperative that the connective tissue scientist, in collaboration with the clinician, develop a sophisticated understanding of the complex dose–response relationships that exist between exercise and bone strength. The purpose of this chapter is to introduce bone structure and physiology and specifically focus on the adaptive response of bone. This includes biochemical, nutritional and mechanical factors. Finally, we focus on the maladaptive response and stress injury in the young and mature athlete and how to diagnose, treat, and prevent these problems.

BONE STRUCTURE

Bones can be classified by their shape into three groups: short, flat, and long or tubular. Short bones, like the tarsals and carpals, are approximately the same length in all directions and have trapezoidal, cuboidal, cuneiform, or irregular shapes. These bones have relatively thin cortices. Flat bones have one dimension that is much shorter than the other two. The larger flat bones form the cranial vault, the scapula and wing of the ileum. Long or tubular bones, including the femur, tibia, or humerus, have an expanded metaphysis and an epiphysis at either end of a thick-walled tubular diaphysis. Like the larger limb bones, metacarpals, metatarsals, and phalanges have the form of long or tubular bones.

B. R. Mandelbaum and L. Teurlings: Santa Monica Orthopaedic and Sports Medicine Group, Santa Monica, California 90404.

J. A. Buckwalter: Department of Orthopaedics, University of Iowa Hospital, Iowa City, Iowa 52242.

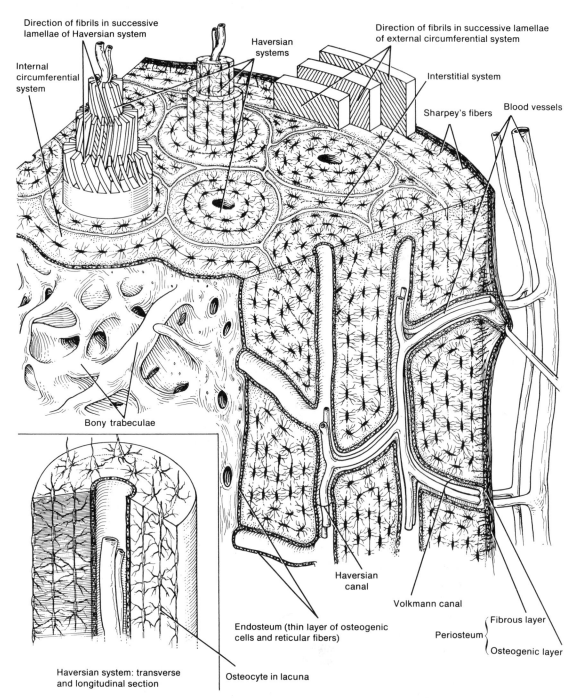

Direction of fibrils in successive lamellae of Haversian system

Internal circumferential system

Haversian systems

Direction of fibrils in successive lamellae of external circumferential system

Interstitial system

Sharpey's fibers

Blood vessels

Bony trabeculae

Haversian canal

Volkmann canal

Endosteum (thin layer of osteogenic cells and reticular fibers)

Periosteum {
Fibrous layer
Osteogenic layer

Haversian system: transverse and longitudinal section

Osteocyte in lacuna

FIG. 5.1. Structure of cortical bone, showing the types of cortical lamellar bone: the internal circumferential system, interstitial system, osteonal lamellae, and outer circumferential system. Intraosseous vascular system is also shown that serves the osteocytes and connects the periosteal and medullary blood vessels. The haversian canals run primarily longitudinally through the cortex, whereas the Volkman canals create oblique connections between the haversian canals. Cement lines separate each osteon from the surrounding bone. Periosteum covers the external surface of the bone and consists of two layers: the osteogenic (inner) cellular layer and a fibrous (outer) layer. (From Kessel RG, Kardon RH. *Tissues and organs: a text atlas of scanning microscopy.* New York: W.H. Freeman, 1979:25, with permission.)

Mature bones consist of hemopoietic marrow that is supported and surrounded by bone tissue covered with periosteum. Blood vessels in the marrow form a critical part of the circulatory system in bone, and disorders or mechanical disruption of marrow can affect the activities of bone and periosteal cells. There are two forms of bone tissue: cortical (compact) bone (Fig. 5.1) and cancellous (trabecular) bone (1–4). Although cortical and cancellous bone have the same matrix composition and structure, the mass of cortical bone matrix per unit volume is much greater. As a result, the modulus of elasticity and the ultimate compressive strength of cortical bone is as much as 10 times greater than those of cancellous bone (1,5–7). The structure of both cancellous and cortical bone changes in response to applied load, immobilization, hormonal influences, and other factors (1,5–9). Cancellous bone has 20 times more surface area than cortical bone. The cells lie primarily between lamellae or on the surface of the trabeculae where they can directly be influenced by adjacent bone marrow cells (3,10,11). In contrast, a higher proportion of the cell population of cortical bone is completely surrounded by matrix (3,10,11). Cancellous bone has a higher rate of metabolic activity remodeling and appears to respond more rapidly to changes in mechanical loads than does cortical bone. This can be observed after immobilizing a limb due to significant bone atrophy and osteopenia.

Cortical or cancellous bone may consist of woven (fiber or primary) or lamella (secondary) bone (1,3,12). Woven bone forms the embryonic skeleton and is then resorbed and replaced by mature bone as the skeleton develops. Fracture callous follows the same sequence (13). Woven and lamellar bone differ with respect to the formation, composition, organization, and mechanical properties. Woven bone, in irregular collagen fiber orientation, high cell and water content, and irregular pattern of mobilization, is more flexible, more easily deformed, and weaker than lamellar bone. Lamellar bone mechanical properties differ depending on the orientation of applied forces. For these reasons, the restoration of normal mechanical properties to bone tissue at the site of healing fracture requires eventual replacement of woven bone of the fracture callous with mature lamellar bone (4).

There are four forms of lamellar bone in mature long bones: trabecular lamellae of cancellous bone, the inner and outer circumferential lamellae of cortical bone, interstitial lamellae of cortical bone, and lamellae of osteons (4,10,14). Each lamella consists of highly oriented densely packed collagen fibrils. The fibrils and adjacent lamellae run in different directions, similar to the alternating directions of wood grain in plywood.

Osteons form the bulk of the diaphyseal cortex of the mature skeleton (Fig. 5.2) (4,10,11,14). They consist of

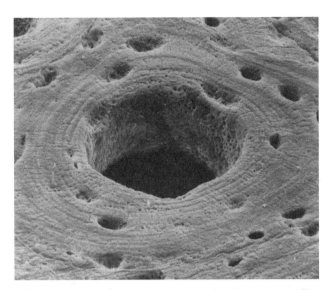

FIG. 5.2. Scanning electron micrograph of an osteon. The grooves in the bone matrix forming concentric circles around the central canal separate adjacent lamellae. Lacunae, the spaces occupied by osteocytes in living cells, appear as depressions or holes in the matrix. The canaliculi that contain osteocyte cell processes in living cells appear as fine grooves radiating from the central canal. Note the canaliculi that open into the central canal. (From Kessel RG, Kardon RH. *Tissues and organs: a text-atlas of scanning microscopy.* New York: W.H. Freeman, 1979:28, with permission.)

irregularly branching and anastomosing longitudinally running cylinders that spiral around the diaphysis. These central canals of osteons contain blood and lymphatic vessels and occasionally nerves. Canaliculi containing the cell processes of osteocytes extend in a radial pattern from the central canal like the spokes of a wheel. The cells depend on the canaliculi for the delivery of metabolic requirements. Cement lines define the outer boundary of each osteon. These thin layers of organic matrix, the composition of which is similar to that of osteoid, mark sites where resorption of bone stops and new bone formation begins. It is generally the cell processes of canaliculi and the collagen fibers of osteons that do not cross cement lines, so each osteon is left in isolation from adjacent ones. For this reason, cracks in the bone matrix tend to follow cement lines rather than to cross osteons. This deflection of a crack propagation may prevent fatigue cracks from extending rapidly across the bone, allowing the bone cells to repair the cracks before a complete fracture. Complex internal network of canals, lacunae, and canaliculi forms one of the most remarkable structural features of mature lamellar cortical bone. Osteonal central canals branch and anastomose and join obliquely oriented vascular canals referred to as Volkmann canals (Fig. 5.1) (4). This elaborate network of interosseous canals next to the periosteal surface thereby creates channels between marrow and periosteum. Network of canals and lacunae within bone form an extensive extravascular space where ions and fluid can flow freely directly adjacent to the mineralized matrix (4) and decimation of bone pride loads causes fluid and ionic flows that generate electric potentials (4,15).

Periosteum covers the external surfaces of bone and contributes an important part to the blood supply of bone. Periosteal cells can resorb and form bone in response to local and systemic stimuli and may have important roles in bone metabolism. The periosteum consists of two layers: an outer layer that is dense and fibrous and an inner layer that is looser, more vascular, and is referred to as a cambium layer. This layer contains cells that are capable of becoming osteoblasts and forming bone. In addition, these cells can form hyaline cartilage under appropriate circumstances and help to form extraosseous callus during fracture healing (4). Over time and with age, the periosteum becomes thinner and less cellular (16).

Mature bones have an elaborate vascular system that supplies the cells of the marrow and bone tissue and periosteum (Fig. 5.1) (3,14,16–20). Obstructions of the blood supply of bone caused by disease, injury, or surgical procedures can cause necrosis and impaired healing. Overall, all long bones have the same general pattern consisting of two circulatory systems: the periosteal diaphyseal metaphyseal system and the epiphyseal physeal system. These two systems form anastomoses on or within the periosteum and across the physis (16). The understanding of the dual circulatory system explains why diaphyseal metaphyseal bone can remain viable and fractures can heal after medullary reaming or periosteal stripping.

The bone cells are important to manifest diverse functions of bone formation and resorption, mineral homeostasis, and bone repair. These cells are distinguished by morphology, function, and characteristic location. They originate from two cell lines, mesenchymal stem cell line and hematopoietic stem cell line. Mesenchymal stem cell line consists of undifferentiated cells or preosteoblasts, osteoblast bone lining cells, and osteocytes. The hematopoietic stem cell line consists of marrow monocytes, preosteoclasts, and osteoclasts.

The undifferentiated mesenchymal cells have the potential of becoming osteoblasts. They reside in bone canals, endosteum, periosteum, and marrow. Fracture healing depends on the migration, proliferation, and differentiation of these undifferentiated cells into osteoblasts.

The osteoblasts line the surfaces of bone and pack tightly against adjacent osteoblasts (4,10,14,21,22). The most apparent function of the osteoblast is the synthesis and secretion of organic matrix of bone, and these cells may have a role in controlling electrolyte fluxes between

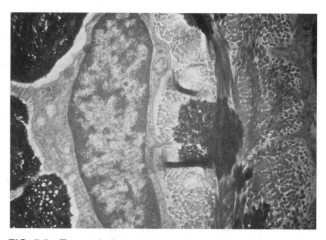

FIG. 5.3. Transmission electrom micrograph showing an osteoblast becoming an osteocyte. The cell has surrounded itself with matrix that has become mineralized on one side of the cell (*M*) and partially mineralized (*P*) on the other. Cell processes extend from the cell into the mineralized matrix. (From Buckwalter JA, Cooper RR. Bone structure and function. In: Griffin PP, ed. *Instructional course lectures XXXVI*. Park Ridge, IL: American Academy of Orthopaedic Surgeons, 1987:27–48, with permission.)

the extracellular fluid and influence mineralization of bone. In addition, systemic hormones, including parathyroid hormone and local cytokines, may stimulate the osteoblasts to release mediators that activate theosteoclasts.

Bone lining cells lie directly against the bone matrix. They are sometimes referred to as resting osteoblasts on surface osteocytes. When exposed to parathyroid hormone, lining cells contract and secrete enzymes that remove the thin layer of osteoid that covers the mineralized matrix (21,23). These are the first actions that allow osteoclasts to attach to the surface of bone and begin resorption.

More than 90% of bone cells in mature human skeleton are osteocytes (Fig. 5.3) (4,10,14,18,24). They surround themselves with organic matrix that can mineralize, and together with the periosteal and endosteal cells they cover the matrix. A large complex network of cells that cover the internal and external surfaces of bone may be extremely sensitive to stresses on the bone and also may be able to control the movements of ions in and out of the mineralized matrix.

Unlike the other bone cells, osteoclasts share a hemopoietic stem cell precursor with the cells of the monocyte family (Fig. 5.4). These large multinucleate cells can rapidly degrade and remove bone matrix. Specific hormones and growth factors influence the monocytic stem cells that develop into osteoclasts; as they proliferate, they fuse to form large multinucleated osteoclasts. On cancellous or periosteal surfaces osteoclasts create a

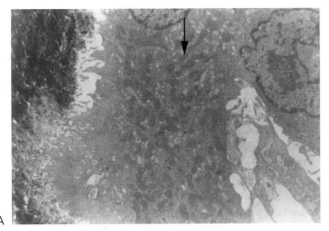

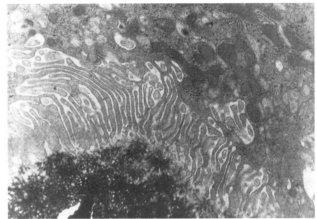

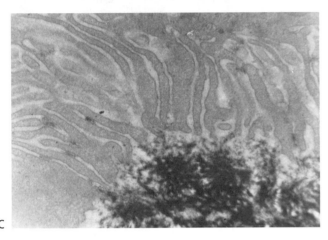

FIG. 5.4. Transmission electron micrographs of osteoclasts. **A:** The osteoclast has applied itself to the surface of the mineralized bone matrix. Note the multiple nuclei, the large number of mitochondria (oval or ellipsoidal membrane-bound organelles that serve as the cells' principal source of energy) (*arrow*), and the formation of a ruffled cell border in the region of resorption. **B:** An osteoclast brush border. Note the complex folding of the cell membrane and the direct application of the brush border to the mineralized matrix. **C:** High magnification micrograph of the brush border applied to the mineralized matrix. (From Buckwalter JA, Cooper RR. Bone structure and function. In: Griffin PP, ed. *Instructional course lectures XXXVI*. Park Ridge, IL: American Academy of Orthopaedic Surgeons, 1987:27–48, with permission.)

characteristic depression referred to as a Howship's lacunae. In dense cortical bone they lead osteonal cutting cones that tunnel through the bone, creating resorption cavities.

The bone matrix makes 90% of the volume of bone with the remainder mostly cells, cell processes, and blood vessels (25). The bone matrix is a composite material consisting of organic and inorganic components (25,26). The remaining 65% of it is inorganic, 20% is organic, and 10% is water. Organic components, primarily collagen, give bone its form and contribute to its ability to resist tension, whereas the inorganic or mineral component primarily resists compression. The organic matrix resembles that of other connective tissue structures such as tendons, ligaments, and capsules. In bone, the collagens are predominantly type I, but also types V and VII make up the bone matrix. Collagen type I is distinguished from other collagens by its relatively large diameter of its fibrils and is most helpful in structures that require large tensile loads. Other noncollagenous proteins of bone include osteocalcin, osteonectin, bone sialoprotein, bone phosphoproteins, and small

protealglycan (2,25,27). In bone there are other growth-stimulating factors, including growth factor B family, insulin growth factor-1, insulin growth factor-2, bone morphogenic proteins, platelet-derived growth factors, interleukin-1, interleukin-6, and colony-stimulating factors.

The inorganic matrix or mineral phase performs two essential functions: It serves an ion reservoir and gives it most of its stiffness and strength. Approximately 90% of the body's calcium, approximately 85% of the phosphorus, and between 40% and 60% of the total body sodium and magnesium are associated with bone mineral crystals, the major source for transport of these ions to and from the extracellular fluid (26). The inorganic matrix of bone maintains the extracellular fluid concentrations within the range necessary for critical physiologic functions, including nerve conduction, muscle contraction, and biochemical reactions.

Mineralization of bone is a phase transformation of soluble calcium and phosphate into the formation of solid calcium phosphate. With increasing mineralization and organization of the matrix, maturation of bone crystals, and replacement of woven bone by lamellar bone, the stiffness of bone increases (4). Maturational changes in bone matrix explain why bones in children differ from adults with respect to patterns of fracture.

BONE ADAPTIVE RESPONSE

In recent years, researchers have begun to understand how bone adapts to changes in physical activity. In the past, there has been a dearth of sensitive, accurate, and reproducible techniques to identify various components and how they respond to physical, mechanical, and biochemical stimuli. Existing parameters followed the four groups of physical, inorganic, organic, and strength. Physical parameters include measurements of bone size, length, cortical diameter, and width. The inorganic fraction is best measured with total body calcium, bone mineral density, and bone mineral concentration. The organic fraction can be assayed through metabolites of collagen metabolism, including hydroxyproline and respective cross-links. Tests of bone strength have been limited to tensile strength in animal studies and fracture rate and fracture details in human studies. Because assay techniques are now more sensitive, we can evaluate Wolff's law, which states (in translation) that every "change in form of function or bone results in a change in internal architecture" (28). Before Wolff's observations, Galileo noted a correlation existed between bone size, body weight, and activity. Experimental studies have verified the existence of Wolff's law by showing that bone modeling and remodeling can be adaptive response to a change in cyclical loading even in the mature skeleton (4). These investigations have demonstrated that maintenance of normal bone density requires repetitive loading.

To this end, evaluation of the dose of specific activity and response is analogous to a pharmacologic evaluation of a drug dose and consequent response. The dose involves a spectrum of factors, such as the duration, intensity and frequency and the activity itself (which can range from weightlessness in space to bedrest immobilization). In addition, the assessment must consider the specific athletic activity and how the respective activity is administered. Therefore, the system must be remodeled after the work of the pharmacologist, who interprets a drug and its impact on the organism as a dose–response curve. The route of administration, mechanism, the age of the organism, and other details define the athlete's response to the dose for the spectrum from immobilization to strenuous exercise. Therefore, it is imperative that the spectrum be developed from zero loading, which includes weightlessness in space, to immobilization, low-intensity exercise and high-intensity exercise, and the consequent responses.

Space Flight and Weightlessness

Animal studies conducted with rats during the various Cosmos and Space Lab III flights demonstrate that weightlessness decreases (8) bone mass, periosteal new bone formation, and physical parameters of strength and stiffness (29,30).

Allison and Brooks (5) demonstrated that immobilization decreases overall length in bones and increases the canal diameter. Steinberg and Trueta (31) demonstrated in immature rats that immobilization decreases whole body weight and length, thickness, and mass of long bones; articular surfaces and epiphyseal lines where regular bone formation was retarded and the circulation to the femoral head was diminished. Reactivation of these in animals resulted in increases in weight and length, thickness, and mass of the bone. Immobilization in mature animals led to a decrease in bone mass, whereas activity resulted in an increase. Allison and Brooks (5) reported that immobilizing the extremities (in calves of immature dogs) resulted in decreased length and increased canal diameter. Laros et al. (32) demonstrated that immobilization of pig tibias resulted in decreased bone mass; the histologic changes included increased skeleton and an increased number of osteoclasts. Gillespie in 1954 (33) demonstrated increased muscle and bone mass in immobilized rats.

Vogel and Whittle (34) demonstrated that immobilization resulted in atrophy of muscle and bone. Dietrich et al. (12) demonstrated immobilization resulted in increased hydroxyproline and calcium excretion. In addition, there is an increase in osteoclast number and release of organic and inorganic phases, which results in a net bone resorption relative to a decreased bone formation. Thus, immobilization results in a decrease in mineral organic phases of bone. This appears to result in a net resorption and decreased bone mass. Historically, exercise was thought to exert a positive effect on bone. Sayille and colleagues (35,36) created a bipedal rat model that resulted in increased size of the femur and increased breaking strength. Chamay and Tschantz (8) excised a dog radius, which resulted in ulna hypertrophy. Goodship et al. (37) excised pig ulna, resulting in radial hypertrophy.

Low-intensity Exercise

Wood in 1981 (38), using a pig treadmill study (Fig. 5.5), documented increased cortical thickness as a result of exercise as a discrete entity; there were also increases in the mineral and organic phases (38). Vailas et al. (39), in a running model, demonstrated an increase in glycosaminoglycans. Heikkinen and Vuori (40), using a growing mice training model, demonstrated increased collagen metabolism. Liu and McCay (41), in a running

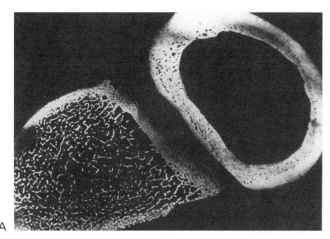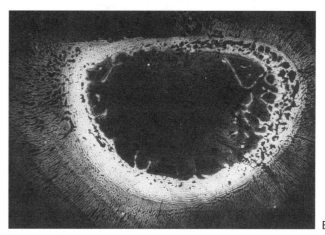

A   B

FIG. 5.5. Microradiograph of pig forelimb bones. **A:** Mid-diaphyseal sections of the radius and ulna from a normal animal. **B:** Mid-diaphyseal section of the radius 3 weeks after resection of the ulnar diaphysis. There is spectacular growth of radially oriented trabeculae formed by periosteum and extensive remodeling of the cortical bone. (From Goodship AE, Lanvon KF, McFie H. Functional adaptation of bone to increased stress: an experimental study. *J Bone Joint Surg Am* 1979;61A:539–546, with permission.)

dog model, demonstrated that on the days the animals were run, calcium excretion in the urine decreased. Thus, animal studies show that bone response with exercise typically increases in physical size and also positively affects the mineral and organic phases, thus increasing the material properties and the strength of bone.

High-intensity Exercise

Booth and Gold hypothesized that low-intensity exercise increased bone length and growth, whereas high-intensity exercise may inhibit bone growth. Relating to the Hueter–Volkmann principle of epiphyseal pressures, there is an inverse relationship between the status of compressive forces parallel to the axis of epiphyseal growth and the rate of growth of that cartilage. Furthermore, via Wolff's law transformation (28), physical load stimulates hypertrophy of growing bone with direct response to additional strain. Gelbke (42), using a dog model, concluded that strong compressive forces resulted in increase in chondral ossification. In addition, the extremes of tension and pressure caused a disappearance of epiphyseal growth plate and diminution of growth. The Hueter–Volkmann principle further states that compression stimulates longitudinal growth of the epiphysis. However, excessive compressive forces can diminish growth.

In 1978, Simon (43), using a bipedal fifth metatarsal amputation model, illustrated increased compressive load of intermittent dynamic loading. As a consequence, he demonstrated inverse U curves such that low levels

of compression were essential to stimulate accelerated physeal growth; however, when the threshold was obtained, compressive forces caused suppression of physeal cartilage and consequent compressive forces caused suppression of the physeal cartilage and subsequent enchondral ossification. In addition, cell proliferation rate in the growth plate decreased with increasing progressive stress, which parallels the decrement in long bone growth (44). Vasan showed in rats that training at a very low dose and low intensity had actually no effect on bone. Sayille and Smith (35) corroborated this finding 4 years later with a rat model.

Kiskinnen and Heikkinen in 1973 (45,46) and Kiskinnen in 1977 (47) demonstrated in growing mice that increasing intensity resulted in longer heavier bones. In addition, increasing duration caused typically shorter and lighter bones. Matsuta et al. in 1986 (48), studying immature growing chickens, demonstrated that very strenuous high-level intensive exercise decreased size and strength of bones and biochemically decreased nonreducible cross-link collagen byproducts. Vailas et al. in 1987 (30), studying 3-week-old chicks on a treadmill, demonstrated decreased long bone growth in the tarsal metatarsal and increased physeal height of 42%. Observing increased cellularity and decreased chondrocyte mitosis, they concluded there was retardation of maturation with very intense exercise. Pedrini-Mille et al. in 1986 (49), using very intense exercise in 4-week-old chicks, demonstrated decreased proteoglycans, decreased matrix, and a widened physis. These material properties of bone, including bending stiffness and overall strength, were also increased. Therefore, it appears that the physis has a degree of susceptibility to the dose of mechanical load in which the qualitative and quantitative factors may be significant.

Response Modulators

Physeal susceptibility may depend on dose factors and also on response modulators. These modulators may include endocrine and nutritional factors.

Endocrine Factors

Van Buul-Offers et al. in 1984 (50) illustrated that growth hormone and thyroxine influenced thickness of various zone layers of the physis. Growth hormone increased the thickness of both the proliferating and the hypertrophic cell layers, whereas thyroxine stimulated primarily the resting zone. Patients with growth hormone secretory function show low bone mass, and recent studies indicated that growth hormone replacement in such patients promotes significant increases in both axial and peripheral bone mineral density. Because healthy elderly men and women also show low circulatory growth hormone and insulin growth factor-1 and deficient growth hormone responses to a physiologic stimuli, there has been considerable interest in the possibility that growth hormone replacement would restore bone mass in such individuals. Sustained treatment with growth hormone does not initiate bone remodeling activity.

Burch in 1984 (6) found that calcitonin increases cartilage growth primarily via cell hypertrophy rather than hyperplasia. In addition, calcitonin was determined to increase matrix formation. It appears that cortisol increases a rate of collagen synthesis in the short term; however, prolonged glucocorticoid treatment decreases collagen synthesis. This may be quite a significant factor, given that research has shown that mammals' levels of glucocorticoids increases with high-intensity exercise (6,50). This may explain why there is a decreased collagen synthesis and suppression of long bone growth in transition from moderate to heavy very intense exercise, and it further supports the theory that increased physeal susceptibility with increasing intensity of activities and the increased sensitivity to complex endocrinologic milieu of simulators.

Acaney supports a critical role for gonadal function in the acquisition and maintenance of bone mass. Hypogonadal boys and girls show deficits in cortical and trabecular bone mineral, but loss of endogenous sex steroids in adult life regularly leads to accelerated bone loss of bone mineral and effect that is primarily striking when it occurs at an early age. Of particular importance for bone acquisition is 17 mid estradiol. In women, loss of estrogen has dual effects: Decreased efficiency of intestinal and renal calcium handling increases the level of calcium necessary to maintain neutral calcium balance. In addition, estrogen directly affects bone cell function. In animal models, strong evidence indicates that estrogen directly regulates osteoblast production of interleukin-6 and potential regular osteoclast recruitment. The precise details of estrogen regulation of skeletally active cytokines in humans is unclear, but such interactions are thought to underlie the accelerated bone loss of early estrogen deficiency. This may lead to perforation and elimination of entire trabecular elements so that no scaffold remains for initiation of bone formation. For women at menopause, the most important influence on bone mass is clearly estrogen deprivation. No amount of exercise or dietary excess can likely overcome accelerated loss of bone specifically due to estrogen withdrawal. Menopausal estrogen replacement can serve to improve bone mass and, if continued for 5 years or more, results in a 60% reduction in risk for osteoporotic fracture.

Nutritional Factors

Nutritional factors have a direct impact on physeal and bone-growing activities. Nutritional integrity depends on adequate levels of protein, calories, trace elements, and vitamins. A deficiency in any one of these components may significantly impact the modulatory response of bone adaptation during exercise. Severe protein deficiency in prisons of war and in patients with anorexia nervosa has been associated with significantly decreased growth rate, decreased cortical thickness, and increased endosteal bone resorption. These osseous changes only occur when protein deficiency less than the 15th percentile is reached. Caloric intake does have indirect effects on bone adaptive responses. Specifically, adipose tissue is responsible for the conversion of androstenedione to estrogen. Therefore, adipose tissue is involved in peripheral conversion of adrenal steroid precursors to estrogen. In addition, body weight directly correlates to estrogen production and directly relates to menstrual abnormalities.

Calcium, in view of its direct role in the mineral phase of bone, is significant and has a direct impact on growth, growth development adaptive response, and maintenance of integrity. Studies indicate that calcium intake is directly proportional to the maintenance of positive calcium balance. In addition, positive calcium balance is proportional to bony adaptation and the ability of bone to respond to stress. Poor calcium dietary intake is directly proportional to bony maladaptation. Studies indicate that lactase-deficient patients and patients with low calcium intake suffer significantly increased fracture rate and low bone mineral intensities. Therefore, positive calcium balance is essential at all ages to ensure normal growth and development and to maintain an adequate bone density and therefore mechanical strength of bone relative to its important functions of support, protection, and mineral storage.

Several trace elements may have significant impact in bone adaptation and maladaptation. Zinc impacts the musculoskeletal system on multiple levels, including growth development and adaptive response to bone and stress. It has been shown that zinc-deficient rats had tibial epiphyses that were narrower and thinner than those in normal rats. In addition, the trabecula of test rats were thinner and had less hypertrophy of cells and osteoblasts. It has been demonstrated that zinc-deficient chickens had significant collagenase deficiency and a decrement in collagen turnovers resulting in a tibial deformity called terosis. This decrement in collagen synthesis was associated with decreased alkaline phosphatase activity and decreased tibial collagenase. A study using a rat tibia fracture model demonstrated the effect of zinc deficiency and supplementation on fracture healing. Zinc contributed to a more proliferative callous but did not significantly affect the time of fracture healing. A study using a rat femur model demonstrated that zinc was necessary for osteogenesis and that the strength of cancellous bone was directly proportional to zinc intake. In addition, zinc was found to accumulate at the sites of osteogenesis, and this accumulation could be accelerated by increasing zinc intake. These studies identify the importance of zinc in bone growth, the adaptive response, and healing.

Alkaline phosphatase is a zinc-dependent metalloenzyme and therefore dependent on accumulation of this trace element. Human studies have concentrated less on the effects of growth and osteogenesis and more on dietary intake in population studies. It is essential to define adequate levels of zinc to the target tissue of bone to maintain adequate hemostasis in positive zinc balance. In recent years, changes in the American diet, especially in younger athletes, have resulted in decreasing intake. The collegiate athlete commonly who consumes a diet devoid of beef and other meat may be 50% short of recommended dally allowance of zinc. Thus, dietary zinc is being decreased concomitant with an increase in physical and physiologic requirements. This ongoing deficit may result in bone maladaptation and theoretically may increase physeal susceptibility to injury. Zinc homeostasis can be corrected by supplementation that has significantly positive implications. Therefore, early nutritional integrity appears to be a central component of bone's response to stress.

Deficiencies in protein, calories, and specifically trace elements may impact that adaptive response. Nutritional elements that relate to this modulation include calcium phosphate, magnesium, zinc, and manganese. Those nutritional elements that have no relationship

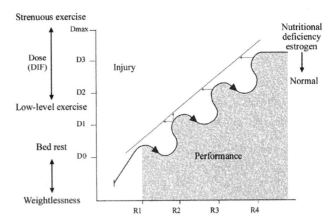

FIG. 5.6. Dose–response curve.

include sodium fluoride, fiber, and vitamin B. There are several other possible modulators of bone adaptation, including the maximum oxygen capacity and degree of aerobic fitness. An important implication is that bone has a degree of "contractility," which means that there is a cyclical integration of modulators that allows the progressive increased responsiveness to increasing doses of exercise and training. This concept is illustrated by Fig. 5.6, which shows a dose–response curve. The x-axis illustrates the responsive adaptation; the y-axis represents activity dose relative to weightlessness; bedrest; and duration, intensity, and frequency of exercise. On the spectrum of the curve between weightlessness and bedrest, which both lack ground reactive forces, performance negatively adapts and results in decreased bone mineral density, decreased tensile strength, and decreased new periosteal bone formation. The exercise portion of the curve demonstrates that it is essential that bone adapt in a cyclically progressive fashion. All points below the curve allow a positive adaptation that prevents the athlete from injury.

Increasing the activity dose in a way inconsistent with the athlete's pattern and quantity response adaptation, such as those practiced in a progressive training program, results in a maladaptive response and injury. In addition, in moderate and high doses of exercise, dose–response is key. In any specific training program, an understanding integrates details of the adaptive response. This includes not only quality and quantity but also the temporal relationships. Negative modulation such as hormonal deficiency; nutritional deficiency; or increase in the duration, intensity, and frequency outside the temporal response will also cause the negative response adaptation. When the maximal dose is exceeded, there will be a negative response and maladaptation, as demonstrated by Simon in 1978 (43). Based on animal studies, it appears that the dose–response curve and the cyclic progression curve may comprise an appropriate working hypothesis from which new concepts can be generated and developed.

SUMMARY

Bone is a complex, highly organized, constantly changing tissue. Understanding of the adaptive response to bone is necessary for optimal care of athletes. In normal individuals, a regimen of increasing cyclic loading of bone will increase bone density, mass, and strength. These changes make it possible to continue to improve physical performance. Failure of bone adaptation to increased loading leads to stress fractures. Better understanding of the relationships between exercise and bone adaptation will decrease the risk of stress fractures.

REFERENCES

1. Canalis E, McCarthy T, Centrella M. Growth factors and the regulation of bone remodeling. *J Clin Invest* 1988;81:277.
2. Boskey AL. Noncollagenous matrix proteins and their role in mineralization. *Bone Miner* 1989;6:111.
3. Brookes M. *The blood supply of bone: an approach to bone biology.* London: Butterworth, 1971.
4. Buckwalter JA, Glimcher MJ, Cooper RR, et al. Instructional course lectures, Vol. 45, 1996.
5. Allison N, Brooks B. Bone atrophy. *Surg Gynecol Obstet* 1921;33:250.
6. Burch WM. Calcitonin stimulates growth and maturation of embryonic chick pelvic cartilage in vitro. *Endocrinology* 1984;114:1196.
7. Centrella M, McCarthy TL, Canalis E. Transforming growth factor-beta and remodeling of bone. *J Bone Joint Surg Am* 1991;73A:1418.
8. Chamay A, Tschantz P. Mechanical influences in bone remodeling: experimental research on Wolff's law. *J Biol Mechan* 1972; 51:173.
9. Currey J, ed. *The mechanical adaptations of bones.* Princeton, NJ: Princeton University Press, 1984.
10. Buckwalter JA. Musculoskeletal tissues and the musculoskeletal system. In: Weinstein SL, Buckwalter JA, eds. *Turak's orthopaedics: principles and their application,* 5th ed. Philadelphia: J. B. Lippincott, 1994:13.
11. Cooper RR, Misol S. Tendon and ligament insertion: a light and electron microscopic study. *J Bone Joint Surg Am* 1970; 52A:1.
12. Deitrick JE, Whedon GD, Schorre E. Effects of immobilization upon various metabolic and physiologic functions in normal men. *Am J Med* 1984;4:3.
13. Cowin SC. Properties of cortical bone and theory of bone remodeling. In: Mow VC, Ratcliffe A, Woo SL-Y, eds. *Biomechanics of diarthrodial joints.* Vol. 2. New York: Springer-Verlag, 1990:119.
14. Buckwalter JA, Cooper RR. Bone structure and function. In: Griffin PP, ed. *Instructional course lectures XXXVI.* Park Ridge, IL: American Academy of Orthopaedic Surgeons, 1987:27.
15. Hastings GW, Mahmud FA. Electrical effects in bone. *J Biol Med Eng* 1988;10:515.
16. Whiteside L. Circulation in bone. In: Evarts CM, ed. *Surgery of the musculoskeletal system.* New York: Churchill Livingstone, 1983:51.
17. Arlet J, Ficat RP, Hungerford DS, eds. *Bone circulation.* Baltimore, MD: Williams & Wilkins, 1984.
18. Matthews JL. Bone structure and ultrastructure. In: Urist MR, ed. *Fundamental and clinical bone physiology.* Philadelphia: J. B. Lippincott, 1980:4.
19. Trueta J, Caladias AX. A study of the blood supply of the long bones. *Surg Gynecol Obstet* 1964;118:485.
20. Rhinelander FW. Circulation in bone. In: Bourne GH, ed. *The biochemistry and physiology of bone,* 2nd ed. Vol. 2. New York: Academic Press, 1972:2.
21. Recker RR. Embryology, anatomy, and microstructure of bone. In: Coe FL, Favus MJ, eds. *Disorders of bone and mineral metabolism.* New York: Raven Press, 1992:219.
22. Rodan GA. Introduction to bone biology. *Bone* 1992;13 [Suppl 1]:S3.
23. Helfrich MH, Mieremet RH, Thesings CW. Osteoclast formation in vitro from progenitor cells present in the adult mouse circulation. *J Bone Miner Res* 1989;4:325.
24. Revell PA. Normal bone. In: Revell PA, ed. *Pathology of bone.* Berlin: Springer-Verlag, 1986:1.
25. Triffitt JT. The organic matrix of bone tissue. In: Urist MR, ed. *Fundamental and clinical bone physiology.* Philadelphia: J. B. Lippincott, 1980:45.
26. Glimcher MJ. The nature of the mineral component of bone and the mechanisms of calcification. In: Coe FL, Favus MJ, eds. *Disorders of bone and mineral metabolism.* New York: Raven Press, 1992:265.
27. Young MF, Kerr JM, Ibaraki K, et al. Structure, expression, and regulation of the major noncollagenous matrix proteins of bone. *Clin Orthop* 1992;281:275.
28. Wolff J. *Das gesetz der transformation der knochen.* Berlin: Hirschwald, 1892.
29. Shaw SR, Vailas AC, Grindeland RE, et al. Effects of a one week space flight on the morphological and mechanical properties of growing bone. *Am J Physiol* 1988;254:R78.
30. Vailas AC, Martinez D, Shaw S, et al. Biochemical morphological and mechanical characteristics of corical bone in young growing rats exposed to seven days of space flight: results from the SL-3 flight mission. *NASA Life Sci* 1987;1:173.
31. Steinberg ME, Trueta J. The effects of activity on rate bone growth. *Clin Orthop* 1981;56:52.
32. Laros GS, Tipton CM, Cooper RR. Influence of physical activity on ligament insertions in the knees of dogs. *J Bone Joint Surg Am* 1971;53A:275.
33. Gillespie JA. The nature of the bone changes associated with nerve injuries and disuse. *J Bone Joint Surg Br* 1954;36B:464.
34. Vogel JM, Whittle MW. Bone mineral changes. The second manned skylab mission. *Aviat Environ Med* 1976;47:396.
35. Sayille PD, Smith RE. Bone density: breaking force and leg muscle mass as functions of weight in bipedal rats. *Am J Phys Anthr* 1996;25:35.
36. Sayille PD, Whyte MP. Muscle and bone hypertrophy: positive effect of running exercise in the rat. *Clin Orthop* 1969;65:81.
37. Goodship AE, Lanyon LE, McFieh H. Functional adaptation of bone to increased stress. *J Bone Joint Surg Am* 1979;61A: 539.
38. Wood SL, Kuei SC, Amiel D, et al. The effect of prolonged physical training on the properties of long bone: a study of Wolff's law. *J Bone Joint Surg Am* 1981;63A:780.
39. Vailas, AC, Deluna DM, Lewis LL, et al. Adaptation of bone and tendon to prolonged hind limb suspension in rats. *J Appl Physiol* 1988;65:373.
40. Heikkinen E, Vuori I. Effect of physical activity of collagen in aged mice. *Acta Physiol Scand* 1972;81:543.
41. Liu CH, McCay CM. Studies of calcium metabolism in dogs. *J Gerontol* 1953;8:264.
42. Gelbke H. Tierexperimentelle. Unterbuchugen zur Frage des enthandralen Knochenwaschstums unter zug. *Arch Duetsch Ztschr Chir* 1950;266:271.
43. Simon MR. The effect of dynamic loading on the growth of epiphyseal cartilage in the rat. *Acta Anat* 1978;102:176.
44. Shinozuka M, Tsurui A, Nagumuma T, et al. A stochastic-mechanical model of longitudinal long bone growth. *J Theor Biol* 1984;108:413.
45. Kiiskinen A, Heikkinen E. Effects of physical training on development and strength of tendons and bones in growing mice. *Scand J Clin Lab Invest* 1973;29 [Suppl 123]:20.
46. Kiiskinen A, Heikkinen E. Effect of prolonged physical training on the development of connective tissues in growing mice [Ab-

stract]. Proceedings of the International Symposium on Exercise Biochemics, 2nd ed. 1973:25.

47. Kiiskinen A. Physical training and connective tissues in young mice-physical properties of Achilles tendons and long bones. *Growth* 1977;41:123.

48. Matsuda JJ, Zernicke RF, Vailas AC, et al. Structural and mechanical adaptation of immature bone and strenuous exercise. *J Appl Physiol* 1986;60:2028.

49. Pedrini-Mille A, Peprini VA, Maynard JA, et al. Effects of strenuous exercise on physes and bones of growing animals. *Orthop Trans* 1986;11:164.

50. Van Buul-Offers S, Smeets T, Van den Brande JL. Effects of growth hormone and thyroxine on the relation between tibial length and the histological appearance of the proximal tibial epiphysis in Snell dwarf mice. *Growth* 1984;48:166.

Principles and Practice of Orthopaedic Sports Medicine,
edited by William E. Garrett, Jr., Kevin P. Speer, and Donald T. Kirkendall.
Lippincott Williams & Wilkins, Philadelphia © 2000.

CHAPTER 6

Acute and Chronic Compartment Syndromes

Robert A. Pedowitz and Alan R. Hargens

A compartment syndrome is defined as a condition of elevated pressure within a space bounded by bone and/or fascia that results in decreased perfusion of tissues within the compartment (1). The late sequelae of an undiagnosed or undertreated compartment syndrome may be the dreaded Volkmann's ischemic contracture, with myonecrosis, decreased extremity function, and permanent deformity. Compartment syndromes may occur in sports and exercise either acutely (acute compartment syndrome [ACS]) or in an intermittent exertional form (chronic compartment syndrome [CCS]). Clinical diagnosis and treatment of compartment syndrome should be based on a clear understanding of the pathophysiology of this potentially devastating disorder.

Upper and lower extremity compartments are defined by local osseofascial anatomy. Because bone and fascia are relatively inelastic, relatively small increases in intracompartmental volume may lead to large increases of intracompartmental pressure. Each osseofascial compartment has its own unique pressure-volume relationship. However, it is useful conceptually to view each compartment as a closed space. The contents within this three-dimensional space can be pressurized either by increasing the internal volume (e.g., by muscle hypertrophy or acute hemorrhage) or by extrinsic compression of the compartment (e.g., by a constrictive cast). In either case, increased pressure within the compartment interferes with microvascular perfusion with resultant tissue ischemia (Figs. 6.1 and 6.2).

In the earliest phases, ischemia is associated with pain (in a normal conscious patient), but in the later stages ischemia causes tissue necrosis. Broad pressure-time thresholds for permanent tissue injury are difficult to define, because each musculoskeletal tissue has its own sensitivity and because antecedent condition of the tissue and comorbid factors affect subsequent tissue damage with compression and ischemia (e.g., hypotension, muscle trauma, etc.). Therefore, it is critical for the treating clinician to understand the essential factors that can be used for clinical decision making and then apply this knowledge to each individual clinical situation.

Virtually all muscles of the extremities and axial skeleton can be affected by ACS or CCS. However, certain anatomic locations are obviously predisposed to this disorder, with the four compartments of the leg most commonly involved. Some authors consider the deep posterior compartment of the leg to be functionally subdivided into two or even three subcompartments (2,3). This concept has been further supported by recent anatomic dissections that demonstrate variable proximal and distal subcompartments of the deep posterior compartment of the leg (4). This type of anatomic variability must be taken into account for diagnosis and surgical treatment of compartment syndrome. The other compartments of the leg are defined as the anterior, lateral, and superficial posterior.

The thigh compartments are generally divided into the anterior (quadriceps), posterior (hamstrings), and abductor groups. The arm is defined by the deltoid, anterior (biceps brachialis), and posterior (triceps) compartments. The forearm is comprised of volar and dorsal compartments, and some consider the mobile wad to be functionally separate. The carpal tunnel is considered by most to be functionally distinct from the forearm and hand, with the hand separated into thenar, hypothenar, and interosseous groups. Similarly, the foot can be divided into medial, lateral, central, and intraosseous compartments.

In the axial skeleton, the paraspinal musculature may be anatomically subdivided, and the muscles of the internal and external pelvis and the gluteal muscles are considered functionally separate. This functional anatomic approach has even been extended to the abdo-

R. A. Pedowitz and A. R. Hargens: Department of Orthopaedics, University of California, San Diego 92103-8894.

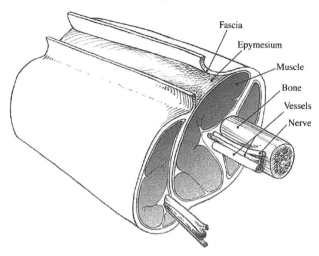

FIG. 6.1. Extremity compartments are surrounded by relatively inelastic fascia connected to the bone. This osseofascial envelope contains muscle and neurovascular structures.

men, whereby increased abdominal pressure produces organ ischemia and significant consequent morbidity (5,6). An understanding of three-dimensional anatomy is critical not only to appreciate the various potential locations for compartment syndrome but also for the safe placement of invasive pressure measurement devices that may penetrate local neurovascular structures.

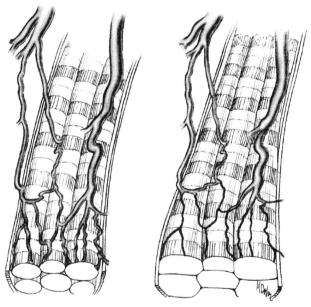

FIG. 6.2. Schematic of normal muscle fibers and vasculature (**left**). A compartment syndrome may be caused by fiber swelling that elevates intracompartmental pressure (**right**). This causes ischemia due to microvascular occlusion at the capillary level. Note that major vessels usually remain open with preservation of distal pulses.

PATHOPHYSIOLOGY OF COMPARTMENT SYNDROMES

Although the common feature of compartment syndrome is elevated pressure within the osseofascial compartment that causes ischemia and possible necrosis, the basic pathophysiology of this syndrome is still not completely understood. Tissue viability depends on capillary perfusion. The delicate balance of intravascular and extravascular fluid dynamics that affect transcapillary flow are defined by the Starling equation (7). This relationship considers hydrostatic factors (intravascular and interstitial fluid pressures), colloid osmotic factors (plasma and interstitial colloid osmotic pressures), and permeability factors (capillary surface area and water conductivity) (7). In normotensive humans, capillary blood pressure ranges between 20 and 30 mm Hg. Thus, elevation of interstitial fluid pressure above 30 mm Hg in a normotensive individual results in progressive decrease of capillary perfusion. It should be emphasized that this pressure threshold marks the beginning of capillary hypoperfusion and may not reflect the threshold for overt compartmental necrosis. However, it seems reasonable to use 30 mm Hg as a conceptual threshold for the normotensive patient that should significantly raise clinical concern. Systemic hypotension decreases the critical compartment pressure thresholds for tissue liability because the driving force for local perfusion is decreased (see below).

Various theories exist for the specific anatomic basis of microvascular dysfunction in compartment syndrome. Early reports (8) suggested that increased intracompartmental pressure causes reflex arterial spasm with consequent tissue ischemia. However, more recent descriptions focus on the effects of increased compartment pressure on the microvasculature. Burton (9) and Eaton et al. (10) proposed the critical closure theory that suggested that microvascular occlusion occurs when tissue pressure exceeds arterial or transmural pressure. This concept predicts that microvascular occlusion would be exacerbated by either increased tissue pressure or by decreased systemic blood pressure. Matsen (11) suggested that increased intracompartmental pressure leads to increased venous pressure, which produces a drop in the arterial venous pressure gradient. The arterial venous gradient is the critical driving force for blood flow across the capillary bed. Hargens et al. (12) suggested that increased compartmental pressure leads to collapse and then occlusion of the thin-walled capillary vessels. Direct measurements of intracapillary pressures in normotensive dogs demonstrated intracapillary pressures between 20 and 30 mm Hg. These observations correlate well with a compartment pressure threshold of 30 mm Hg for observation of the earliest ischemic changes with compartment syndrome.

In an ACS, increased intracompartmental pressure

leads to tissue ischemia, which may initiate a vicious cycle that can only be reversed by surgical decompression. Increased intracompartmental pressure may cause ischemia that produces increased microvascular permeability with increased tissue fluid accumulation and increased pressure, and so on. Once this vicious cycle is firmly developed, emergent fasciotomy is clearly indicated. However, in some cases of borderline ACS, other variables may be controlled that could potentially reverse the cycle. Such variables include elevation of systemic blood pressure in the hypotensive patient, facilitation of edema reduction with a venous foot pump, or in experimental conditions administration of hypobaric oxygen. The opportunity to intervene in borderline cases to reverse the compartment syndrome without surgical fasciotomy is, of course, appealing due to the inherent morbidity of fasciotomy and the need for subsequent surgical procedures to close the wound. Such approaches must be tempered by the patient's clinical condition (i.e., the ability to perform an accurate physical examination, which could be obviated by head injury or drug or alcohol abuse) and by other clinical conditions that may make nonoperative treatment extraordinarily risky (i.e., polytrauma with concomitant surgical procedures). Under no circumstance should the end point of an ACS (i.e., myonecrosis) be used as the clinical indication for surgical treatment, because that event marks a missed opportunity for treatment.

In contrast to ACS, CCS is defined by intermittent elevation of tissue pressure associated with exertion that reverses when the exercise is stopped. There are currently no definitive unifying concepts of the basic etiology of CCS. During normal vigorous skeletal muscle contractions, high intramuscular pressures are generated, over 500 mm Hg (13,14). Because such high pressures are generated during muscle contraction, tissue perfusion must occur during the periods between contractions. This situation is analogous to the perfusion of cardiac muscle that occurs during diastole, because cardiac transmural pressures are normally sufficient to occlude microvascular flow during systole. Elevation of muscle relaxation pressure (the interval between contractions) is associated with CCS (see below).

Styf and Körner (15,16) suggested that CCS of the anterior leg may be due to occlusion of large vessels by local muscle herniation as they transverse the interosseous membrane. Martens and Moeyersoons (17) reported that CCS is usually caused by noncompliant fascia that does not accommodate the increase in muscle volume that occurs normally during exercise. Intracompartmental volume may increase up to 20% over baseline values during vigorous exercise (18). Detmer et al. (19) noted increased fascial thickness in 25 of 26 samples taken from leg compartments in patients with CCS. These abnormalities may be the cause or the effect of chronic elevated intramuscular pressure. Other authors note anatomic abnormalities that could predispose a compartment to development of exertional compartment syndrome (20–23). However, specific anatomic abnormalities have not been observed consistently in patients diagnosed with CCS.

Although ischemia is clearly implicated in ACS, the role of muscle ischemia in CCS is more controversial. Amendola et al. (24) could not demonstrate consistent ischemic changes by magnetic resonance imaging in clinic patients with CCS. Balduini et al. (25) were also unable to demonstrate ischemic changes by nuclear magnetic resonance spectroscopy in 21 of 23 patients with CCS. However, Takebayashi et al. (26) observed decreased thallium-201 distribution in muscles affected by CCS using single-photon emission computed tomography. In addition, Mohler et al. (27) observed greater relative deoxygenation, as well as delayed re-oxygenation, after exercise in patients with CCS using near infrared spectroscopy. These recent articles suggest that pain with CCS probably does correlate with intramuscular ischemia. Better definition of the underlying cause of this intermittent ischemia could lead to nonsurgical strategies for treatment of CCS.

CLINICAL PRESENTATION OF ACUTE COMPARTMENT SYNDROME

ACS is usually caused by increased intracompartmental volume, resulting in increased pressure. Fractures are the most common etiology of ACS (1). Tibia fractures are the most common cause of ACS in adults, whereas femur fractures are the most common source in children. Soft tissue injury from contusion and postischemic swelling are other causes of ACS. Burns, snakebites, and prolonged compression (i.e., with drug or alcohol overdose) may also cause ACS. Compartment syndrome can be caused either by direct hemorrhage into the compartment driven by arterial inflow pressure, by interstitial edema due to increased capillary permeability, or by intracellular edema formation. Manipulation of capillary permeability and intracellular edema reduction are targets for future pharmacologic intervention.

ACS can also be caused or exacerbated by extrinsic compression. Circumferential dressing with a cast or tight-fitting dressing may be the offending agent, and simply splitting or removing the dressing may decrease intracompartmental pressure significantly. Burns may also cause ACS due to constriction by a restrictive eschar, and escharotomy may be indicated in these cases. Compartment volume may also be decreased iatrogenically by closure of fascial defects (1,28). Therefore, closure of fascial defects is generally contraindicated.

A number of recent reports of ACS are of specific interest to physicians caring for athletes. Gwynne Jones and Theis (29) describe ACS due to closed rupture of the peroneus longus midbelly. Willy et al. (30) reported delayed diagnosis of ACS of the anterior tibial compartment after only 5 minutes of soccer play in a relatively untrained individual. Chautems et al. (31) observed spontaneous anterior and lateral ACS of the leg in a diabetic patient after just a 5-minute walk. Richards and Moss (32) described a patient with compartment syndrome of the upper arm due to rupture of the long head of the biceps. Weber and Churchill (33) treated a patient with ACS of the anterior leg after an athlete played squash in an unusually warm environment. This case was actually associated with significant rhabdomyolysis, but fortunately good recovery was noted 10 months after fasciotomy. Goldfarb and Kaeding (34) described a college football player with a 1-year history of recurrent anterolateral leg pain (presumed to be CCS) that converted to ACS after practice for a bowl game. Krome et al. (35) observed a 43-year-old man with a rupture of a Baker's cyst that caused an ACS of the leg. Wise and Fortin (36) reported a case of bilateral thigh compartment syndrome that was diagnosed approximately 12 hours after intense weight training. Bidwell et al. (37) described a 16-year-old boy with ACS of the anterior thigh diagnosed 2 days after intense quadriceps exercise with weight lifting. These recent reports emphasize that ACS may occur during or after exercise. Sports medicine providers must maintain a very high index of suspicion for ACS because missed diagnosis has a high probability of long-term morbidity.

Patients with ACS typically present with severe pain as their chief complaint. Often their description of pain is out of proportion to the severity of the associated injury. The hallmarks of ACS (the "p's") include *pain* out of *proportion, pain* with *passive* stretch, a *pink* extremity, *palpable pulses,* and (in the later phases) *paresthesias* and *paresis.* It is critical to emphasize that pain with passive stretch is the hallmark of ischemic conditions of muscle, regardless of etiology. However, ischemia with arterial injury is distinguished from ACS by the presence of palpable or dopplerable pulses in compartment syndrome. In addition, the skin overlying and distal to a compartment with ACS is usually pink, whereas lack of arterial inflow typically causes pallor. It should also be noted that paresthesias and paralysis are late findings and may suggest impending compartment necrosis. In some situations, the clinical picture is so clear that ACS diagnosis may be made on clinical grounds alone. In these extremely clear cases, it is reasonable to proceed directly to surgical decompression. However, clinical estimation of intracompartmental pressure is notoriously unreliable, and therefore objective assessment by intracompartmental pressure measurement is very helpful for documentation and clinical decision making. These techniques are described below.

ACS may also be precipitated by surgical interventions. Compartment syndrome has been observed after arthroscopic surgery of the knee (38). Patients may be particularly at risk if extremely high pump pressures are used for joint distention. Use of a high-pressure pump is particularly risky when the capsule has been traumatically ruptured (e.g., after knee dislocation) or after intraarticular fracture (e.g., tibial plateau fracture). Some authors suggest that ACS associated with arthroscopic surgery may be treated nonoperatively (38,39). It may be reasonable to observe these patients for a short period of time if the elevated pressure has been present for short duration, as long as the patient remains in an environment that facilitates careful observation. However, a trend to higher intracompartmental pressure, worsening symptoms, or severe pain should prompt surgical fasciotomy (if necessary).

ACS may also be precipitated by prolonged or by extremely high-pressure tourniquet application. In these situations, muscle injury may be caused by direct crush of the tissue underneath the tourniquet cuff and result in myonecrosis or by postischemic reperfusion when extremely long tourniquet times are used. Iatrogenic compartment syndromes should obviously be treated aggressively by surgical fasciotomy but are best avoided by appreciation of the detrimental effects of high-pressure joint distention, prolonged tissue compression, and tourniquet ischemia.

CLINICAL PRESENTATION OF CHRONIC COMPARTMENT SYNDROME

Most information regarding clinical presentation of chronic exertional compartment syndrome relates to patients with the syndrome in the lower leg. Presumptive diagnosis of CCS requires a high index of suspicion in patients with exertional extremity pain. Unfortunately, patients with the syndrome often present without the classic constellation of symptoms.

The hallmark of CCS is pain induced by exercise that resolves quickly on cessation of exercise. Most cases of CCS are associated with running, but nonrunning activities may be implicated as well. Recreational and elite athletes may be affected. Some investigators report equal sex distribution (19,40), whereas others report male sex predilection (17,41). Patients are typically young active adults, but CCS has been diagnosed in adolescents and elderly patients as well (40).

If CCS is in the differential diagnosis, the athlete should be carefully questioned about the character and pattern of pain. Pain may be described as a sensation of muscle tightness, cramping, or swelling or may cause feelings of weakness or numbness when the pain is severe. The symptoms may be achy, sharp, dull, or diffuse. Some patients note loss of muscle control, such as a slap foot or altered distal sensation during exercise.

Symptoms may be unilateral or bilateral and may be brought about by light or heavy exercise. However, the pattern of pain production in terms of duration of exercise is fairly consistent for a given athlete. Similarly, resolution of symptoms usually follows a relatively consistent pattern over minutes to hours and rarely days after exercise. It should be remembered that CCS may coexist with other forms of exercise-induced extremity pain, and these coexistent problems significantly blur the clinical presentation (see Differential Diagnosis, below). Although CCS of the leg is most common, any muscle compartment may be affected by the syndrome. CCS has been observed in the thigh, feet, lumbar paraspinal muscles, dorsal and volar forearm compartments, and in the intraosseous compartments of the hand (18,21,42–52). We have also diagnosed a case of CCS of the biceps compartment in a manual laborer (unpublished data, R.A.P., 1997).

CCS of the leg usually involves the anterior and/or lateral compartments. The superficial posterior compartment is much less commonly involved, probably because of its relatively high compliance compared with the other compartments of the leg. Deep posterior CCS is a subject of controversy. Melberg and Styf (53) suggest that CCS of the deep posterior compartment was, at best, extremely rare. These investigators were unable to demonstrate elevation of muscle relaxation pressure during or after exercise in the tibialis posterior or flexor digitorum longus muscles. However, Martens and Moeyersoons (17) described 63 cases of deep posterior CCS, and Pedowitz et al. (40) reported 15 cases of CCS of the deep posterior compartment of the leg. Davey et al. (2) observed that the tibialis posterior compartment may be a site of unrecognized cases of exertional compartment syndrome because of its anatomic and functional separation from the rest of the deep posterior compartment. These concerns were recently validated by anatomic dissections (4). It appears, therefore, that any muscle compartment may be involved by CCS. The most important factor, therefore, remains an adequate index of suspicion. Unfortunately, objective diagnosis by direct compartmental pressure measurement in these atypical locations may be difficult because pressure criteria for one compartment are not necessarily directly applicable to other muscle compartments (see Objective Assessment, page 92).

The physical examination of patients with CCS should focus on ruling out other possibilities in the differential diagnosis. Pedowitz et al. (40) reported that the only feature that distinguished CCS from other causes of exertional leg pain was the increased prevalence of fascial hernias, noted in 46% of CCS patients compared with 13% of non-CCS patients. Other authors have noted a 20% to 60% instance of fascial defects in patients with CCS (1,17,28,54). The neurovascular examination is usually normal. Bony or periosteal tenderness suggests other etiologies of exertional leg pain.

DIFFERENTIAL DIAGNOSIS OF ACUTE COMPARTMENT SYNDROME

The major disorder that leads to ACS is usually quite obvious, for example, fracture or massive soft tissue injury from contusion. In fact, these disorders may distract the clinician from the possibility of ACS. However, there is an extended differential diagnosis for a painful swollen extremity that includes deep venous thrombosis, infection, stress fracture, tenosynovitis, or vascular abnormalities such as an aneurysm. Most of these disorders do not precipitate ACS and are not associated with ischemic pain. Deep venous thrombosis, however, may be particularly problematic because it may present with swelling and associated fullness of the compartment and pain with passive stretch of the calf (a positive Homan's sign). Ultrasonography or venography may be helpful for differentiation.

Acute ischemic pain due to arterial occlusion may be distinguished from ACS by the absence of palpable or dopplerable pulses. In such instances, arteriography is diagnostic. In some cases, an acute vascular abnormality may cause a secondary ACS (55). Prophylactic fasciotomy may be indicated after a prolonged period of acute ischemia treated by revascularization.

Certain clinical situations are particularly problematic in the diagnosis of ACS. Children with elbow, forearm, or other fractures may be extremely difficult to examine with a detailed neurovascular examination. These injuries are often associated with significant extremity swelling even if a compartment syndrome is not present. Similarly, adults who are under the influence of alcohol and drugs can be very hard to examine clinically. Obviously, patients who are comatose on admission or are extremely sedated or paralyzed for therapeutic reasons require an extremely high index of suspicion for ACS, because they will obviously not complain of pain. Pain will also not be a useful sign in patients with proximal nerve injuries (i.e., traumatic laceration or after severe neuropraxia). All these clinical situations require diligence and measurement of intracompartmental pressure.

DIFFERENTIAL DIAGNOSIS OF CHRONIC COMPARTMENT SYNDROME

CCS is particularly difficult to diagnose on clinical grounds alone because the signs and symptoms overlap with other etiologies of exertional leg pain. Detmer et al. (19) used a particularly applicable classification system for categorizing patients with exertional leg pain; the most common diagnoses that should be considered, at least in the leg, are stress fracture (type I), medial tibial periostalgia (type II), and CCS (type III). Other considerations include tendinitis, nerve entrapment disorders, vascular or neurogenic claudication, and venous stasis. Much less common considerations are occult infection, metabolic bone disease, or neoplastic processes.

Vascular abnormalities may be confused with CCS. Popliteal artery entrapment syndrome may cause intermittent distal ischemia (56). A similar situation was recently described by Sammarco et al. (57) involving the superficial femoral artery in the adductor canal. Knight et al. (58) described a 48-year-old man with symptoms consistent with CCS who was subsequently diagnosed with a popliteal artery aneurysm. This case is particularly important, because he underwent fasciotomy for the presumed CCS with recurrence of symptoms and eventual diagnosis by angiography 3 years after initial presentation. It is clear that various diagnostic tests may be needed to work through this complex differential diagnosis. These studies may include bone scintigraphy, magnetic resonance imaging, angiography, or electromyography. These challenges also emphasize the importance of objective diagnostic methods for definitive diagnosis of CCS.

OBJECTIVE ASSESSMENT

The hallmark of objective assessment of ACS and CCS is direct measurement of intracompartmental pressure. Noninvasive techniques such as magnetic resonance spectroscopy (59,60), thallium-201 single-photon emission computed tomography (61), and near infrared spectroscopy (62) or other methods will hopefully emerge as useful diagnostic modalities. However, done properly, intracompartmental pressure measurement can be performed safely and with a relatively small degree of pain. Intracompartmental pressure measurement must be considered the gold standard for comparison with newer methodologies.

Intracompartmental pressure measurement can be broadly divided into techniques that are "indirect" and those that are more "direct." The indirect techniques involve transmission of fluid pressure from the muscle level to a remote transducer, whereas the direct methods place a miniature pressure transducer directly at the tissue level.

Early attempts at measurement of tissue pressure used a fine needle inserted into the interstitium. Intermittent injection or continuous infusion of fluid was needed with these techniques to keep the needle tip from occluding with muscle; however, excessive fluid administration could artificially increase pressure recordings or even precipitate an ACS. Mubarak et al. (63) described the wick catheter for clinical assessment of ACS. This technique was first described by Scholander et al. (64) for animal studies. The wick catheter

uses Dexon fibers that are fixed at the tip of the fluid-filled polyethylene catheter. These fibers minimize tip occlusion and increase the surface area at the catheter-tissue interface. The slit catheter subsequently replaced the wick catheter by creation of small slits in the polyethylene tubing catheter (65). This catheter became very popular for clinical application because it eliminated the risk of retained wick material and gave more rapid response. These catheter systems involve transmission of fluid pressure to a remote transducer that must be carefully "zeroed" to the level of the planned pressure measurement. Measurement of intracompartmental pressure may be simplified by use of a handheld device with the pressure transducer included (Stryker Surgical, Kalamazoo, MI). The transducer is connected to a needle with multiple side ports that limits occlusion by muscle. The system is simple to use but must be applied carefully to avoid false readings.

Styf and Körner (15) described the microcapillary infusion technique for measurement of intracompartmental pressure during exercise. This technique uses a Teflon catheter (Atos Medical Inc., Moorby, Sweden) with constant fluid infusion rates of 0.2 mL/h or less. The catheter tip has multiple side holes, and the very slow constant infusion keeps the tip open. The result is a system that has very high dynamic response for exercise studies but is still fraught with the artifacts caused by changing levels of a hydrostatic fluid column.

Other systems are available for *direct* measurement of intracompartmental pressure with transducer tip catheters. These systems are advantageous because they are not affected by variable height of the hydrostatic column with the indirect methods. Crenshaw et al. (66) studied a transducer-tipped fiberoptic catheter and noted good accuracy and dynamic characteristics. However, the catheter may underestimate muscle relaxation pressure and muscle rest pressure after exercise. Miniaturization techniques have also resulted in solid state transducer-tipped catheters that have high accuracy and frequency response (67). The authors expect that in the future, miniaturized solid state catheter systems will be developed that will be less invasive and therefore more comfortable for acute and chronic measurement of intracompartmental pressure at rest and during exercise. Regardless of the method chosen, intracompartmental pressure assessment should be performed using sterile technique and small amounts of local anesthesia. The skin, subcutaneous tissues, and fascia can be anesthetized without fear of elevating intramuscular pressure, but large volumes of anesthetic should not be infiltrated directly into the muscle compartment of question. Placement of the catheter or needle must be made with appropriate respect for the overlying and adjacent neurovascular anatomy. Specific techniques for catheter placement are described in detail previously (1).

In contrast to ACS assessment, where the patient

is typically supine and stationary, assessment of CCS usually requires exercise by the subject to elicit symptoms and correlate changes in intracompartmental pressure. For the measurement of CCS, pressures may be measured before, during, and after exercise. Pre- and postexercise pressures are essentially static assessments that can use the same techniques that are described for ACS measurement. However, to monitor pressures during exercise, systems with high-frequency response are needed to pick up the rapid changes in intramuscular pressure that are encountered during and between contractions. In addition, the changing hydrostatic columns that are induced by exercise protocols may introduce substantial artifact for systems that involve transmission along the fluid column to a separate transducer. These considerations have lead most investigators to use static measurements before and after exercise for diagnostic purposes (see Diagnostic Criteria, below).

Regardless of the catheter technique selected, it is very important to reproduce the patient's symptoms during assessment of CCS. Although a variety of exercise protocols have been described, including resisted ankle plantar and dorsiflexion, cycling on an ergometer, or treadmill running, ultimately it may be necessary to have the subject perform the specific activity that typically elicits their pain (68). It is important to reproduce the subject's symptoms during the assessment, because if the pain is not reproduced and the pressures are low, a false-negative diagnosis could result. Therefore, the authors usually recommend that the subject exercise in the days to weeks before the testing session to maximize the possibility of reproduction of typical symptoms.

DIAGNOSTIC CRITERIA FOR ACUTE COMPARTMENT SYNDROME

Intracompartmental pressure measurement is an important adjunct for diagnosis of ACS; however, pressure studies must be used in the context of a given patient's injury and comorbidities. In certain circumstances, fasciotomy would be indicated based on clinical grounds alone due to either an extremely high index of suspicion or because of other factors. For example, revascularization after a long warm ischemia time should be managed by prophylactic fasciotomy to decrease the probability of adverse sequelae. However, there are many situations where intracompartmental pressure measurement is the critical factor for surgical decision making. Unfortunately, considerable controversy exists regarding the optimal pressure level for diagnosis of compartment syndrome.

A series of laboratory and clinical studies by Hargens et al. (69) led to development of specific diagnostic pressure criteria (>30 mm Hg) in the presence of appropriate clinical findings for ACS. This pressure criteria

correlates well with the extravascular pressure needed to collapse capillaries and interfere with nutritive blood flow. However, other investigators found that higher intramuscular pressures may be tolerated in humans without permanent adverse sequelae. Matsen et al. (70) suggested that the critical pressure threshold was greater than 45 mm Hg in patients. This controversy is probably a reflection of the fact that soft tissue injury from compression and ischemia is a function of magnitude, duration, and distribution of pressure and the premorbid status of the tissues.

Whitesides et al. (71) reported that muscle perfusion was significantly decreased when intracompartmental pressure was within 10 to 30 mm Hg of diastolic blood pressure. Reneman et al. (72) noted similar phenomenon when tissue pressure was within 30 to 35 mm Hg of mean arterial blood pressure. More recently, Heppenstall et al. (73–75) performed a series of studies using magnetic resonance spectroscopy and have extended this concept of a physiologically based pressure threshold defined by the difference between mean arterial blood pressure and intracompartmental pressure (the "delta P"). These studies suggest that in tissue that has been traumatized bluntly or subjected to antecedent ischemic trauma, fasciotomy should be considered when delta P is no more than 40 mm Hg. Noninjured muscle may tolerate a delta P within 30 mm Hg, but this is a scenario that is rarely encountered clinically. This approach takes into consideration changes in systemic blood pressure (e.g., with hypotension after trauma). It should be emphasized again, however, that pressure criteria should be used as an adjunct to clinical decision making. Clinical situations occur when compartment syndrome may be suspected very strongly but the pressure measurements do not quite "fit." In these situations, it is essential that the clinician trust his or her judgment and question the validity of pressure measurements due to technical problems with the monitoring techniques.

DIAGNOSTIC CRITERIA FOR CHRONIC COMPARTMENT SYNDROME

Considerable controversy exists regarding the optimal pressure criteria for diagnosis of CCS. Criteria are described for pressures before, during, and after exercise. Pressure criteria during exercise are particularly problematic because accurate assessment requires pressure transducers with extremely high-frequency response that are not affected by changes in hydrostatic columns. In addition, intramuscular pressures normally become high during active muscle contraction. Therefore, peak intramuscular pressures and mean intramuscular pressures (calculated from peak pressure) during exercise should not be used for diagnostic purposes. Styf et al. (76) noted that the muscle relaxation pressure (the intramuscular pressure between contractions) increases in patients with CCS. These authors note that when muscle relaxation pressure exceeds 35 mm Hg, patients with CCS complain of pain and swelling associated have decreased muscle blood flow. In addition, Styf and Körner (77) were particularly concerned about the use of intramuscular pressure before exercise, because these investigators noted that some patients have a generalized increase of muscle tension at rest (coined the "muscle hypertension syndrome"). Some patients with muscle hypertension syndrome also have elevated pressures after exercise due to their inability to relax, which could lead to false-positive diagnosis of CCS. However, use of muscle relaxation pressure for diagnosis has not been widely adopted because of the inherent difficulties outside of the clinical research laboratory, even though the approach is justified physiologically.

Thus, objective diagnosis of CCS has focused on measurements of resting pressures before and after exercise due to the relative simplicity of this approach. Pedowitz et al. (40) studied 210 leg compartments in patients with exertional pain who were thought not to have CCS. Pressure distribution in these patients tended to be distributed normally, and therefore these studies were used to define confidence intervals for diagnostic purposes. The diagnostic pressure thresholds were set at greater than two standard deviations over the mean for this reference population (using slit catheters). Based on these data, diagnostic pressures of at least 15 mm Hg at rest, at least 30 mm Hg 1 minute after exercise, and/ or at least 20 mm Hg 5 minutes after exercise were believed to be diagnostic of CCS. However, it should be noted that these criteria varied somewhat according to the specific leg compartment studied. For example, the 95% upper limit for the anterior compartment was 28.2 mm Hg compared with 16.5 mm Hg for the superficial posterior compartment 1 minute after exercise. These differences probably reflect unique physiologic characteristics of the specific compartments due to their anatomy and local compliance. Therefore, pressure criteria established for one region may not be necessarily applicable to other more unusual sites of CCS.

Other investigators (15,65,72,78–81) note that the return to baseline after cessation of exercise is delayed in patients with CCS. In general, intramuscular pressure should return to baseline within 5 ot 6 minutes and certainly within 10 minutes after completion of the exercise bout. This phenomenon may be useful in assessment of borderline cases.

Recently, Mohler et al. (27) described noninvasive assessment of CCS of the anterior compartment of the leg using near infrared spectroscopy. This noninvasive technique assesses the relative concentration of oxygenated versus deoxygenated blood within the muscle based on the different absorbance characteristics of oxyhemoglobin and deoxyhemoglobin. Definitive diagnosis was established by intracompartmental pressure measurement as described previously (40). Patients with CCS had greater relative deoxygenation and significantly longer interval to recovery of preexercise oxygenation than patients who did not have the syndrome. In the future, we expect that noninvasive techniques will be perfected that will facilitate the accurate noninvasive diagnosis of CCS.

TREATMENT OF ACUTE COMPARTMENT SYNDROME

Once the diagnosis of ACS is established, most patients should be treated by decompressive surgical fasciotomy. Occasionally, a patient will be encountered who has borderline pressures and is suitable for close observation of symptoms and trends in pressure. Repeated clinical evaluation and perhaps indwelling monitoring of interstitial pressure are indicated. This approach is not recommended for patients who are unable to cooperate with close repeated physical examination.

Surgical fasciotomy for ACS should be performed through relatively large skin incisions. Garfin et al. (82) studied the decrease in intracompartmental pressure after fasciotomy with sequential enlargement of dermotomy and noted that a skin incision of at least 12 cm was needed to achieve adequate decompression in most cases of ACS. Although the cosmetic result after wide dermotomy may be unappealing and often requires skin grafting, inadequate decompression may lead to significant adverse sequelae due to unrelieved pressure. After fasciotomy, the muscle should be observed for signs of viability and reperfusion. Muscle viability may be tested by gentle pinch or cautery stimulation to look for contractility. Sometimes it is very difficult to decide acutely whether the muscle will recover, and in such circumstances repeat trips to the operating room and, if necessary, multiple surgical debridements may be needed to limit the chances of sepsis.

In very rare cases, ACS may be better treated without fasciotomy. ACS due to rattlesnake bite may not benefit from fasciotomy because venom inoculation into the compartment causes such extensive myonecrosis that fasciotomy rarely changes the ultimate result. However, it is very difficult in the clinical setting to not intervene in the face of an extremely tense and swollen compartment shortly after snakebite. Another extremely difficult clinical situation involves management after long-standing ACS. This may occur if a patient was comatose from drug overdose or immobilized after a building collapse, thereby sustaining a prolonged crush injury. In such situations, intracompartmental pressure may be elevated but may already be on the descending limb at the time of presentation. In this circumstance, the compartments may already be extensively necrotic as reflected by an increase in serum creatine phosphokinase or early renal compromise. In this difficult circumstance, it may actually be better to leave the compartment closed to limit the likelihood of gross infection.

TREATMENT OF CHRONIC COMPARTMENT SYNDROME

Patients with CCS may be treated conservatively because the syndrome is not life or limb threatening. Nonsurgical management includes activity modification and conditioning, taping, use of orthotics, stretching, and nonsteroidal anti-inflammatory administration. Unfortunately, most patients with CCS do not achieve adequate relief of symptoms with this approach. Definitive treatment of CCS involves decompressive fasciotomy, but in contrast to ACS, fasciotomy may be performed through relatively limited skin incisions. It may be appropriate to decompress the superficial peroneal nerve as it exits the fascial defect between the anterior and lateral compartments at the same time as a fasciotomy. Closure of such defects is not indicated because ACS may be precipitated. Specific details of decompression for the various compartments have been described previously (1,83).

Adequate release for CCS may be achieved through one moderately sized longitudinal dermotomy or through multiple small transverse incisions. Good cosmetic result can be achieved in either case, but care must be used to avoid injury to neurovascular structures because these methods are relatively "blind." Decompression of the deep posterior compartment may be somewhat more difficult. Recent descriptions of the varied anatomy and subcompartmentation of the deep posterior compartment suggests greater visualization, and careful decompression are indicated in this area (see above). Postoperatively, patients with CCS may be placed in a light compressive dressing with return to weight bearing as tolerated. Gradual strengthening and return to sports are allowed after wound healing is achieved.

Most patients have significantly less pain, improved function, and return to higher level of sports participation after fasciotomy for CCS. One theoretic concern involves potential adverse effects of fasciotomy upon muscle function. The intact fascia does play an important biomechanical role for force production, as demonstrated by Garfin et al. (82) in studies of tibialis anterior contractile force after fasciotomy in dogs. These theoretic concerns have not been borne out in clinical situations, because most patients recover good strength with adequate rehabilitation after decompressive fasciotomy.

Poor results after fasciotomy may reflect either incomplete decompression or incorrect diagnosis. If fasciotomy fails, clinicians should carefully review the clinical situation to ensure that another condition was not missed. It may be necessary to repeat the diagnostic pressure studies to rule out recurrent CCS. Occasionally, a true recurrence of the syndrome will be observed due to restrictive scarring at the fasciotomy site. In this situation, repeat fasciotomy or partial fasciectomy may be considered.

CONCLUSION

ACS and CCS continue to be important clinical concerns due to the substantial associated morbidity. The essential feature of compartment syndrome involves increased intracompartmental pressure that decreases tissue perfusion and causes ischemic pain. Although presumptive diagnosis can be made on clinical grounds, definitive diagnosis continues to be based on direct measurement of intracompartmental pressure. Newer techniques are evolving for noninvasive diagnosis of ACS and CCS. At present, the mainstay of treatment continues to be decompressive fasciotomy.

REFERENCES

1. Mubarak SJ, Hargens AR. *Compartment syndromes and Volkmann's contracture.* Philadelphia: W.B. Saunders, 1981.
2. Davey JR, Rorabeck CH, Fowler PJ. The tibialis posterior muscle compartment. An unrecognized cause of exertional compartment syndrome. *Am J Sports Med* 1984;12:391.
3. Matsen FA III, Clawson DK. The deep posterior compartmental syndrome of the leg. *J Bone Joint Surg Am* 1975;57A:34.
4. Kwiatkowski TC, Detmer DE. Anatomical dissection of the deep posterior compartment and its correlation with clinical reports of chronic compartment syndrome involving the deep posterior compartment. *Clin Anat* 1997;10:104.
5. Schein M, Wittmann DH, Aprahamian CC, et al. The abdominal compartment syndrome: the physiological and clinical consequences of elevated intraabdominal pressure. *J Am Coll Surg* 1995;180:745.
6. Reeves ST, Pinosky ML, Byrne TK, et al. Abdominal compartment syndrome. *Can J Anaesth* 1997;44:308.
7. Hargens AR, Villavicencio JL. Mechanics of tissue/lymphatic transport. In: Bronzino JD, eds. *Biomedical engineering handbook.* Boca Raton, FL: CRC Press, 1995:493.
8. Griffiths DL. Volkmann's ischaemic contracture. *Br J Surg* 1940;28:239.
9. Burton AC. On the physical equilibrium of small blood vessels. *Am J Physiol* 1951;1674:319.
10. Eaton RG, Green WT, Stark HA. Volkmann's ischemic contracture in children. *J Bone Joint Surg Am* 1965;47A:1289.
11. Matsen FA. Etiologies of compartment syndromes. In: *Compartmental syndromes.* Matsen FA, ed. New York: Grune & Stratton, 1980.
12. Hargens AR, Akeson WH, Mubarak SJ, et al. Fluid balance within the canine anterolateral compartment and its relationship to compartment syndromes. *J Bone Joint Surg Am* 1978;60A:499.
13. Sejersted OM, Hargens AR, Kardel KR, et al. Intramuscular fluid pressure during isometric contraction of human skeletal muscle. *J Appl Physiol* 1984;56:287.
14. Styf JR. Intramuscular pressure measurements during exercise. *Oper Tech Sports Med* 1995;3:243.
15. Styf JR, Körner LM. Microcapillary infusion technique for measurement of intramuscular pressure during exercise. *Clin Orthop* 1986;207:253.
16. Styf JR, Körner LM. Chronic compartment syndrome of the leg. Results of treatment by fasciotomy. *J Bone Joint Surg Am* 1986;68A:1338.
17. Martens MA, Moeyersoons JP. Acute and effort-related compartment syndrome in sports. *Sports Med* 1990;9:62.

18. Raether PM, Lutter LD. Recurrent compartment syndrome in the posterior thigh. *Am J Sports Med* 1982;10:40.
19. Detmer DE, Sharpe K, Sufit RL, et al. Chronic compartment syndrome: diagnosis, management, and outcomes. *Am J Sports Med* 1985;13:162.
20. Soffer SR, Martin DF, Stanish WD, et al. Chronic compartment syndrome caused by aberrant fascia in an aerobic walker. *Med Sci Sports Exerc* 1991;23:304.
21. Pedowitz RA, Toutounghi FM. Chronic exertional compartment syndrome of the forearm flexor muscles. *J Hand Surg* 1988; 13A:694.
22. Kutz JE, Singer R, Lindsay M. Chronic exertional compartment syndrome of the forearm: a case report. *J Hand Surg* 1985;10A:302.
23. Styf JR, Körner LM. Diagnosis of chronic anterior compartment syndrome in the lower leg. *Acta Orthop Scand* 1987;58:139.
24. Amendola A, Rorabeck CH, Vellett D, et al. The use of magnetic resonance imaging in exertional compartment syndromes. *Am J Sports Med* 1990;18:29.
25. Balduini FC, Shenton DW, O'Connor KH, et al. Chronic exertional compartment syndrome: correlation of compartment pressure and muscle ischemia utilizing ^{31}P-NMR spectroscopy. *Clin Sports Med* 1993;12:151.
26. Takebayashi S, Takazawa H, Sasaki R, et al. Chronic exertional compartment syndrome in lower legs: localization and follow-up with thallium-201 SPECT imaging. *J Nucl Med* 1997;38:972.
27. Mohler LR, Styf JR, Pedowitz RA, et al. Intramuscular deoxygenation during exercise in patients who have chronic anterior compartment syndrome of the leg. *J Bone Joint Surg Am* 1997;79A:844.
28. Fronek J, Mubarak SJ, Hargens AR, et al. Management of chronic exertional anterior compartment syndrome of the lower extremity. *Clin Orthop* 1987;220:217.
29. Gwynne Jones DP, Theis JC. Acute compartment syndrome due to closed muscle rupture. *Aust N Z J Surg* 1997;67:227.
30. Willy C, Becker H-P, Evers B, et al. Unusual development of acute exertional compartment syndrome due to delayed diagnosis. *Int J Sports Med* 1996;17:458.
31. Chautems RC, Irmay F, Magnin M, et al. Spontaneous anterior and lateral tibial compartment syndrome in a type I diabetic patient: a case report. *J Trauma* 1997;43:140.
32. Richards AM, Moss ALH. Biceps rupture in a patient on long-term anticoagulation leading to compartment syndrome and nerve palsies. *J Hand Surg* 1997;22B:411.
33. Weber AB, Churchill JO. Compartment syndrome after squash. *Aust N Z J Surg* 1996;66:771.
34. Goldfarb SJ, Kaeding CC. Bilateral acute-on-chronic exertional lateral compartment syndrome of the leg: a case report and review of the literature. *Clin J Sports Med* 1997;7:59.
35. Krome J, de Araujo W, Webb LX. Acute compartment syndrome in ruptured Baker's cyst. *J South Orthop Assoc* 1997;6:110.
36. Wise JJ, Fortin PT. Bilateral, exercise-induced thigh compartment syndrome diagnosed as exertional rhabdomyolysis. *Am J Sports Med* 1997;25:126.
37. Bidwell JP, Gibbons CER, Godsiff S. Acute compartment syndrome of the thigh after weight training. *Br J Sports Med* 1996;30:264.
38. Kaper BP, Carr CF, Shireffs TG. Compartment syndrome after arthroscopic surgery of knee. *Am J Sports Med* 1997;25:123.
39. Ekman EE, Poehling GG. An experimental assessment of the risk of compartment syndrome during knee arthroscopy. *Arthroscopy* 1996;12:193.
40. Pedowitz RA, Hargens AR, Mubarak SJ, et al. Modified criteria for objective diagnosis of chronic compartment syndrome of the leg. *Am J Sports Med* 1990;18:35.
41. Styf J. Diagnosis of exercise-induced pain in the anterior aspect of the lower leg. *Am J Sports Med* 1988;16:165.
42. Lokiec F, Sievner I, Pritsch M. Chronic compartment syndrome of both feet. *J Bone Joint Surg Br* 1991;73B:178.
43. Manoli A. Compartment syndromes of the foot: current concepts. *Foot Ankle* 1990;10:340.
44. Myerson MS. Management of compartment syndromes of the foot. *Clin Orthop* 1991;271:239.
45. Carr D, Gilbertson L, Frymoyer J, et al. Lumbar paraspinal compartment syndrome. A case report with physiologic and anatomic studies. *Spine* 1985;10:816.
46. Styf J, Lysell E. Chronic compartment syndrome in the erector spinae muscle. *Spine* 1987;12:680.
47. Styf J. Pressure in the erector spinae muscle during exercise. *Spine* 1987;12:675.
48. Tompkins DG. Exercise myopathy of the extensor carpi ulnaris muscle: report of a case. *J Bone Joint Surg Am* 1977;59A:407.
49. Rydholm U, Werner C, Ohlin P. Intracompartmental forearm pressure during rest and exercise. *Clin Orthop* 1983;175:213.
50. Reid RL, Travis RT. Acute necrosis of the second interosseous compartment of the hand. *J Bone Joint Surg Am* 1973;55A:1095.
51. Kutz JE, Singer R, Lindsay M. Chronic exertional compartment syndrome of the forearm: a case report. *J Hand Surg* 1985;10A:302.
52. Styf J, Forssblad P, Lundborg G. Chronic compartment syndrome in the first dorsal interosseous muscle. *J Hand Surg* 1987;12A:757.
53. Melberg P-E, Styf J. Posteromedial pain in the lower leg. *Am J Sports Med* 1989;17:747.
54. Reneman RS. The anterior and the lateral compartmental syndrome of the leg due to intensive use of muscles. *Clin Orthop* 1975;118:69.
55. Seybold EA, Busconi BD. Traumatic popliteal artery thrombosis and compartment syndrome of the leg following blunt trauma to the knee: a discussion of treatment and complications. *J Orthop Trauma* 1996;10:138.
56. Darling RC, Buckley CJ, Abbott WM. Intermittent claudication in young athletes: popliteal artery entrapment syndrome. *J Trauma* 1974;14:543.
57. Sammarco GJ, Russo-Alesi FG, Munda R. Partial vascular occlusion causing pseudocompartment syndrome of the leg. A case report. *Am J Sports Med* 1997;25:409.
58. Knight JL, Au K, Whitley MA. Popliteal aneurysm presenting as chronic exertional compartment syndrome. *Orthopedics* 1997; 20:166.
59. Chance B, Eleff S, Leigh JJ. Noninvasive, nondestructive approaches to cell bioenergetics. *Proc Natl Acad Sci USA* 1980; 77:7430.
60. Bernot M, Gupta R, Dobrasz J, et al. The effect of antecedent ischemia on the tolerance of skeletal muscle to increased interstitial pressure. *J Orthop Trauma* 1996;10:555.
61. Takebayashi S, Takawaza H, Sasaki R, et al. Chronic exertional compartment syndrome in lower legs: localization and follow-up with thallium-201 SPECT imaging. *J Nucl Med* 1997;38:972.
62. Mohler LR, Styf JR, Pedowitz RA, et al. Intramuscular deoxygenation during exercise in chronic anterior compartment syndrome of the leg. *J Bone Joint Surg* 1997;79A:844.
63. Mubarak SJ, Hargens AR, Owen CA, et al. The wick catheter technique for measurement of intramuscular pressure: a new research and clinical tool. *J Bone Joint Surg Am* 1976;58A:1016.
64. Scholander PF, Hargens AR, Miller SL. Negative pressure in the interstitial fluid of animals. *Science* 1968;161:321.
65. Rorabeck CH, Hardie PC, Logan J. Compartmental pressure measurement: an experimental investigation using the slit catheter. *J Trauma* 1981;21:446.
66. Crenshaw AG, Styf JR, Mubarak SJ, et al. A new "transducer-tipped" fiber optic catheter for measuring intramuscular pressures. *J Orthop Res* 1990;8:464.
67. Hargens AR, Ballard RE. Basic principles for measurement of intramuscular pressure. *Oper Tech Sports Med* 1995;3:237.
68. Padhiar N, King JB. Exercise induced leg pain–chronic compartment syndrome. Is the increase in intra-compartment pressure exercise specific? *Br J Sports Med* 1996;30:360.
69. Hargens AR, Schmidt DA, Evans KL, et al. Quantitation of skeletal-muscle necrosis in a model compartment syndrome. *J Bone Joint Surg Am* 1981;63A:631.
70. Matsen FA III, Winquist RA, Krugmire RB. Diagnosis and management of compartmental syndromes. *J Bone Joint Surg Am* 1980;62A:286.
71. Whitesides TE, Haney TC, Morimoto K, et al. Tissue pressure measurements as a determinant for the need of fasciotomy. *Clin Orthop* 1975;118:43.
72. Reneman RS, Slaff DW, Lindbom L, et al. Muscle blood flow disturbances produced by simultaneously elevated venous and total muscle pressure. *Microvasc Res* 1980;20:307.
73. Heppenstall RB, Sapega AA, Izant T, et al. Compartment syndrome: a quantitative study of high-energy phosphorus com-

pounds using ^{31}P-magnetic resonance spectroscopy. *J Trauma* 1989;29:11139.

74. Heppenstall RB, Scott R, Sapega A, et al. A comparative study of the tolerance of skeletal muscle to ischemia. Tourniquet application compared with acute compartment syndrome. *J Bone Joint Surg Am* 1986;68A:820.

75. Heppenstall RB, Sapega AA, Scott R, et al. The compartment syndrome. An experimental and clinical study of muscular energy metabolism using phosphorus nuclear magnetic resonance spectroscopy. *Clin Orthop* 1988;226:138.

76. Styf J, Körner L, Suurkula M. Intramuscular pressure and muscle blood flow during exercise in chronic compartment syndrome. *J Bone Joint Surg Br* 1987;69B:301.

77. Styf JR, Körner LM. Diagnosis of chronic anterior compartment syndrome in the lower leg. *Acta Orthop Scand* 1987;58:139.

78. Mannarino F, Sexson S. The significance of intracompartmental pressures in the diagnosis of chronic exertional compartment syndrome. *Orthopedics* 1989;12:1415.

79. McDermott APG, Marble E, Yabsley RH, et al. Monitoring dynamic anterior compartment pressure during exercise: a new technique using the STIC catheter. *Am J Sports Med* 1982; 10:83.

80. Turnipseed W, Detmer DE, Girdley F. Chronic compartment syndrome. An unusual cause for claudication. *Ann Surg* 1989;210:557.

81. Wallenstein R. Results of fasciotomy in patients with medial tibial stress syndrome or chronic anterior compartment syndrome. *J Bone Joint Surg Am* 1983;65A:1252.

82. Garfin SR, Tipton CM, Mubarak SJ, et al. Role of fascia in maintenance of muscle tension and pressure. *J Appl Physiol* 1981; 51:317.

83. Mubarak SJ. Surgical management of chronic compartment syndrome of the leg. *Oper Tech Sports Med* 1995;3:259.

Principles and Practice of Orthopaedic Sports Medicine,
edited by William E. Garrett, Jr., Kevin P. Speer, and Donald T. Kirkendall.
Lippincott Williams & Wilkins, Philadelphia © 2000.

CHAPTER 7

Impact of Magnetic Resonance Imaging in Sports Medicine

Charles E. Spritzer

Not since the advent of the x-ray has an imaging modality so profoundly affected the field of sports medicine. Magnetic resonance imaging (MRI) has improved our diagnostic capabilities, significantly changed our diagnostic algorithms, and in many cases has altered, and hopefully improved, our understanding of many sports-related injuries. Indeed, whereas ultrasound and computed tomography (CT) continue to be used in specific applications, the general imaging algorithm in the workup of an acute injury is typically plain films followed by an MRI.

It is important to state that MRI has not replaced either the plain film or the physical examination but rather compliments these steps in the workup of a patient with an acute injury. Often, it is the plain film that facilitates interpretation of observations detected on the MR examination. For example, a calcific deposit can be better appreciated on the plain film than on the MRI. More importantly is the interpretation of the knowledge of the clinical examination that allows one to assign importance to observations seen with MRI. It is well appreciated that many patients have meniscal tears that are incidentally discovered with MRI. Whether intervention is warranted rests solely with the patient's symptoms and clinical examination.

The objectives of this chapter are fairly broad and to some extent unachievable. I intend to provide a rudimentary understanding of the physics and terminology associated with MRI, the necessary pulse sequences required to optimally image sports-related injuries, and a brief discussion of practical safety considerations. Most importantly, an overview of the capabilities and limitations of MR as applied to the field of sports medicine is provided. By necessity, this is not a complete accounting of entities that can or cannot be diagnosed by MRI in various anatomic locations, but rather this chapter is intended to provide the reader with a feeling for the general capabilities of the imaging modality.

MAGNETIC RESONANCE IMAGING SAFETY

The literature is replete with literally hundreds of articles addressing the potential biologic effects of static and time-varying magnetic and radiofrequency (RF) fields and their potential impact on MRI. A comprehensive review of this subject is beyond the scope of this chapter, and the reader is referred to works by Shellock, Kanal, Beers, and others for a more comprehensive overview (1–3).

In brief, it is not unreasonable to state that MRI is considered to be a safe noninvasive imaging modality. More pragmatic than theoretic concerns of RF power deposition and exposure to electromagnetic fields is the status of hardware in and on the patient. Magnets currently in operation have field strengths that are 6 to 30 thousand times greater than the earth's magnetic field. Even with the weakest clinical scanners, the attractive force of the magnet is sufficient to cause patient injury. Because of the strong magnetic field, there are several absolute contraindications: cardiac pacemakers and similar devices, ferrous intracranial aneurysm clips, cochlear implants, and metal in the eye. Neurostimulators are somewhat controversial; however, most sites will not image these devices. Hardware on the patient, such as an external fixator or halo, must be assessed on an individual basis. Not only do these devices have the potential to be attracted to the magnet, but they may create a current loop, causing burns to the patient (3).

As a rule, most surgical hardware is considered MRI

C. E. Spritzer: Department of Radiology, Duke University Medical Center, Durham, North Carolina 27710.

compatible after it has been in place 6 weeks. It is believed that by this point sufficient fibrosis or bony healing has occurred to prevent even ferrous hardware from torquing and causing damage. Again, however, there are exceptions, and often these must be assessed on an individual basis. Of a practical concern, selection of hardware may determine whether the MRI examination is diagnostic. For example, a stainless steel screw may cause greater artifact than one made of titanium.

PHYSICS AND TERMINOLOGY

MRI is an extrapolation of the nuclear magnetic resonance techniques first described in the 1940s. The first clinical images were produced in the late 1970s and early 1980s. Although other nuclei can be imaged, it is the hydrogen atom that clinical scanners use to produce MR data given their intrinsic signal and abundance in the body. Hydrogen nuclei can be thought of as having a spin and a magnetic moment. Normally, these nuclei are randomly oriented. With the application of a uniform external magnetic field, hydrogen nuclei align in the direction of the applied field because this is the lowest energy state obtainable. These nuclei will spin or precess about the magnetic field at a frequency that depends on the applied magnetic field. The stronger the field, the faster the rate of precession. It is the magnetic moment of multiple similarly aligned nuclei that produces the MRI signal known as the net magnetic moment vector. These protons are brought to a higher energy state by applying an RF electromagnetic field (B_1) orthogonal to the main magnetic field at a frequency equal to the precession frequency of the protons. With the application of this resonant electromagnetic field, the net magnetic moment vector will rotate about the original magnetic field. The degree of rotation will be determined by the strength and duration of the applied electromagnetic field. If one assumes that B_0 is oriented in the z direction, the net magnetic moment vector is usually rotated 90 degrees into the xy plane. With termination of the B_1 RF field, the protons will precess in the transverse or xy plane. Because these are charged particles, they will induce a current in loops of wires that are aligned with the transverse plane, producing the MR signal.

After excitation, the nuclei precess coherently within the xy plane. However, fluctuations in the magnetic field caused by other nearby nuclei result in energy being transferred from one nucleus to another. With this transfer of energy, the coherence of the precession is lost. The result is loss of the net magnetic moment vector over time and a corresponding loss of signal. The rate of this signal loss is called spin-spin relaxation or T2 relaxation. This is an intrinsic property of each tissue.

Because the spins are in a high-energy state, there is a subsequent attempt to lose energy to the surrounding tissue (the lattice) and for the spins to return to a low-energy state by realigning with the main magnetic field. This spin-lattice or T1 relaxation time is also a unique property of the tissue. Tissues with short T1 relaxation times recover more quickly and have more signal available for the next excitation. This process of excitation and subsequent T2 and T1 relaxation is repeated multiple times to provide spatial localization of the signal arising from various tissues.

The difference in the T1 and T2 relaxation times between different tissues is contrast. It is in contrast that MRI excels over other imaging modalities. Because the density of ligaments and muscles are similar, CT affords almost no distinction between the two. On MRI, the two are readily discernible, and injuries of both structures are easily detected.

The general MRI strategy is accordingly very straightforward: Images are obtained that maximize contrast based on T1 or spin-lattice relaxation, so-called T1-weighted images, and images are obtained that accentuate contrast based on T2 or spin-spin relaxation mechanisms, so-called T2-weighted images. Table 7.1 shows the signal intensities of normal tissues.

Most abnormal tissues parallel the signal intensity of fluid. In other words, the tissues are dark on T1-weighted images and bright with more T2 weighting. The exceptions are few but notable. Clearly, fatty tu-

TABLE 7.1. *Signal intensity of tissue*

Tissue	T1-weighted image	Proton density-weighted image	T2-weighted image	STIR
Fat	B	B	I	D
H_2O	D	I	B	VB
Muscle	I	I	D	DI
Cortical bone (calcium)	D	D	D	D
Blood (hematoma)	D or B	D or B	D or B	D or B
Fibrous tissue	D	D[a]	D[a]	D[a]

[a]May occasionally show high signal.
VB, very bright; B, bright; I, intermediate; D, dark; DI, dark to intermediate.

mors will follow the signal intensity of fat (i.e., bright with T1 weighting and slightly darker with more T2 weighting). Hemorrhagic lesions can have both high and low signal on either T1- or T2-weighted images. Fibrous tissue is typically dark on all pulse sequences. Calcium, and therefore cortical bone, typically shows no signal on MRI. This is clearly a major limitation when characterizing bony tumors.

There are numerous approaches to exciting the tissue of interest in generating an MR signal. These various techniques are called pulse sequences and are designed to accentuate T1 or T2 mechanisms of contrast, look at flow in vessels, or look at other properties, including the density of the tissue, diffusion, and profusion.

Until recently, the mainstay of musculoskeletal imaging has been the spin echo pulse sequence. In this pulse sequence, an initial 90-degree RF pulse excitation is applied and is subsequently followed by a second 180-degree RF pulse. The 180-degree RF pulse corrects for imperfections in the main magnetic field that tend to degrade the MR signal. Spin echo sequences are capable of producing both T1- and T2-weighted images. The principal advantage of the spin echo technique is that it is robust, easily implemented, and provides images of high tissue contrast, either T1 or T2 weighted.

In addition to producing T1- and T2-weighted images, spin echo imaging is able to produce a "proton density" image. This image provides a high signal-to-noise ratio but generally has limited soft tissue contrast. The notable exceptions are menisci and ligaments where proton density images excel over other options.

The major disadvantage of spin echo imaging is that the acquisition time is lengthy for T2-weighted images, typically on the order of 10 to 15 minutes. As such, multiple pulse sequences have been developed to either reduce scan time or supplement perceived weaknesses of the spin echo sequence. As the saying goes, there is no free lunch, and although each of these newer sequences may have a speed advantage over conventional spin echo, there is often an associated disadvantage. To compensate for these disadvantages, most studies contain multiple pulse sequences, often in multiple planes.

The most important new pulse sequence for musculoskeletal imaging is Rapid Acquisition with Relaxation Enhancement (RARE) and its derivatives turbo-spin echo or fast spin echo. These pulse sequences are capable of producing T2-weighted images that appear very similar to conventional T2-weighted spin echo images but are much faster. Depending on the particular hardware, the acquisition time may be reduced by 75% or more. The major difference is that with fast spin echo imaging, the fat appears brighter than on a similar conventional spin echo image. However, it is possible to suppress the signal from fat and actually improve the pulse sequence sensitivity for detecting marrow and soft tissue abnormalities.

Sequences that do not use the 180-degree RF pulse, so-called gradient recalled echo sequences (GRE), such as Gradient-Recalled Acquisition in the Steady State (GRASS), Fast Low-Angle Shot (FLASH), or Fast Imaging with Steady Precession (FISP), are capable of producing both T1- and T2-weighted information in seconds compared with minutes using conventional spin echo imaging. These sequences are quite sensitive to flowing blood and are used extensively in vascular imaging. In addition, the rapid acquisition of data allows volume imaging with the inherent advantage of producing contiguous slices and multiplanar reformations, albeit with long imaging times. Selected GRE sequences are also useful in cervical spine imaging and show promise in assessing menisci and cartilage abnormalities. Despite being able to acquire images in seconds, the sequences suffer from several major disadvantages. The foremost is the limited contrast available for a given set of imaging parameters. For example, it is possible to optimize visualization of the menisci but not to simultaneously see the articular cartilage. The second major disadvantage of this sequences is its poor visualization of marrow abnormalities. Susceptibility artifacts from the trabecula obscure lesions within the marrow. These susceptibility artifacts result in apparent enlargement of cortical bone when compared with spin echo imaging. In spinal acquisitions, this may result in an overestimation of neural foraminal stenosis. Finally, artifacts due to metallic hardware are significantly worse than with conventional spin echo imaging.

Short tau inversion recovery (STIR) imaging combines both T1 and T2 information in a single acquisition. It is a robust means of suppressing fat as well. If an abnormality has both long T1 and T2 relaxation times, STIR images are considered the most sensitive for detecting marrow or soft tissue abnormalities. The major limitation of the technique is that the signal-to-noise ratio is poor and it is relatively slow. More recently, fast STIR techniques have become available. Much like fast spin echo, the images are acquired in a fraction of the time necessary to produce an inversion recovery image. However, when compared with spin echo and fast spin echo, the signal-to-noise ratio remains low and tissue characterization is more limited.

New techniques are continually being developed, each of which reports significant advantages over conventional spin echo. It must be cautioned that validation of these pulse sequences may require years of careful scrutiny.

Appropriate pulse sequence selection and attention to the details of the actual acquisition (e.g., field of view, slice thickness, matrix, etc.) are critical for achieving maximum accuracy. Particularly illustrative in this regard is an article by Fischer et al. (4) that evaluated the ability of MRI to assess meniscal pathology. Examinations were performed at several centers, and results were reported using arthroscopy as the reference standard. Accuracies ranged from 64% to 95% for assessing the medial meniscus, lateral meniscus, and anterior cruciate ligaments (ACLs). However, when the data are broken down by center and by field strength (and, in reality, technique), several sites consistently reported accuracies at the 95% level. Those sites using relatively poor technique (i.e., thick slices, large interspace gap) consistently reported unacceptable results. Of note, one site changed their scanner and technique during the study with a marked improvement in accuracy.

MAGNETIC RESONANCE IMAGING OF THE KNEE

It may be unequivocally stated that MRI is the noninvasive method of choice for evaluating internal derangements of the knee. After plain films, MRI is the next examination in the imaging algorithm of injury to the knee.

Meniscal Injuries

A large number of studies attest to the accuracy of MRI in the detection of meniscal abnormalities (5–8). Using state of the art techniques, including dedicated knee surface coils and high-resolution thin sections (3.0 to 3.5 mm), accuracies in the 90% to 98% range are achievable. If present, the precise location of a meniscal tear (i.e., anterior horn, posterior horn, or body, inner, or outer one third of the meniscus) may be conveyed to the arthroscopist.

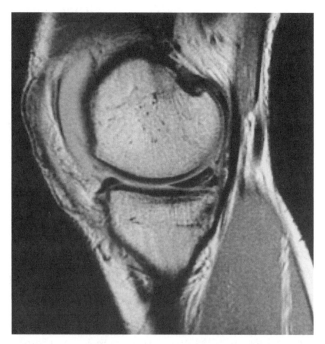

FIG. 7.1. A 21-year-old man with medial joint line tenderness. Sagittal proton density spin echo image shows a linear degenerative tear of the posterior horn of the medial meniscus extending to the inferior articular surface.

In addition to identifying the presence of a tear, MRI can categorize the tears into those that are likely to be asymptomatic degenerative tears versus those that are causing mechanical symptoms such as a radial tear or a bucket-handle tear. This is especially important in light of studies suggesting a relatively high prevalence of meniscal tears in asymptomatic middle-aged people (6,9) (Figs. 7.1 and 7.2).

Given the sensitivity to internal changes in meniscal structures, one place where MRI has been considered relatively insensitive is in the ability to distinguish post-surgical scarring of a meniscus from a true recurring meniscal tear. The difficulty lies in the fact that the "healing" of a meniscal tear is done with a fibrocartilage different from that originally present. As such, the sensitivity of MR is reduced. This is one of the few MRI indications where intraarticular contrast agents have been advocated.

The second weakness of MRI is in the assessment of meniscal capsular separation. Although criteria have certainly been promoted as being useful for detecting meniscal capsular injury, a recent study has shown them to be inaccurate (10).

Ligamentous Injury

MRI has been shown to be equally useful for assessing the ligamentous structures of the knee. The Anterior Cruciate Ligament (ACL) is one of the most important of the knee stabilizers and is unfortunately the most frequently injured. Multiple mechanisms have been shown to cause ACL injury (11). Often, clinical examination is suboptimal in the acute setting, with accuracies of as low as 50% reported (12). Discontinuity of the ACL on MR images clinches the diagnosis. There is often an associated soft tissue mass reflecting hemorrhage and edema.

Associated injuries, including lateral femoral condyle and posterior capsular bone bruises, and medial collateral ligament (MCL) injuries are routinely visualized. However, these and other ancillary findings have not improved the accuracy of ACL injury detection (7,13,14). One reported weakness of MRI in the acute ACL injury setting is the relative insensitivity of posterior horn lateral meniscal injuries (15) (Fig. 7.2).

MRI has been shown to be equally useful in the assessment of MCL, Lateral Collateral Ligament (LCL) and Posterior Collateral Ligament (PCL) injuries. Because both the MCL and LCL are extracapsular and often not repaired in isolation or even when associated with ACL injury, true accuracy is difficult to ascertain. Nonetheless, MRI is considered the reference standard for such abnormalities (Fig. 7.2).

MRI readily visualizes medial retinacular complex injuries (16–20). Characteristic findings associated with patellar dislocation include lateral femoral condyle bone

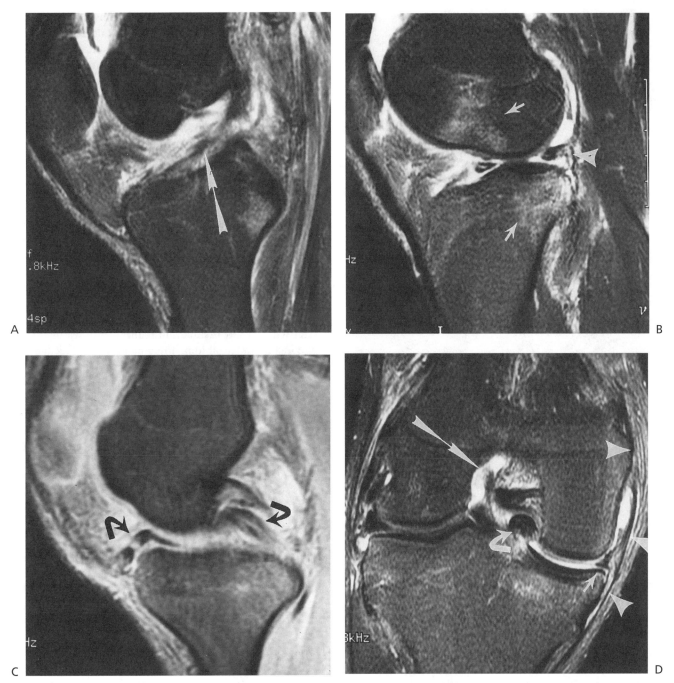

FIG. 7.2. Anterior cruciate ligament (ACL) tear and bucket-handle tear of the medial meniscus in a 31-year-old man with acute injury to knee. **A:** Sagittal T2-weighted fast spin echo image shows complete disruption of the ACL (*large arrow*). **B:** Osseous injuries of the femoral condyle and at the insertion of the lateral capsule on the tibia (*arrows*) are shown in the lateral femoral condyle on this sagittal fast spin echo image. The posterior horn of the lateral meniscus (*arrowhead*) appears somewhat truncated on this sequence, indicative of tear. **C:** Sagittal proton density spin echo image shows a flipped meniscal fragment anteriorly and a portion of the displaced medial meniscus beneath the Posterior Collateral Ligament (PCL) (double PCL sign) posteriorly (*curved arrows*). **D:** Coronal fast spin echo image shows the truncated medial meniscus (*small arrow*), displaced meniscus within the intercondylar notch (*curved arrow*), injury to the MCL (*arrowheads*), and the torn ACL (*large arrow*).

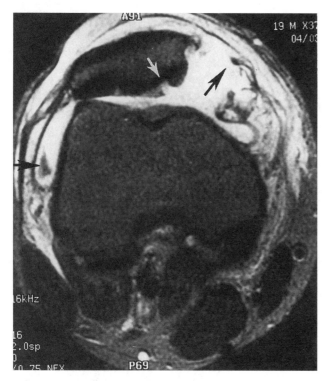

FIG. 7.3. A 19-year-old man with acute patellar dislocation. Axial T2-weighted fast spin echo image shows complete disruption of the medial patellofemoral ligament (*large arrow*). A chondral defect of the patella is also noted (*small arrow*). The free cartilage fragment is seen laterally (*arrowhead*).

bruise, patellar bone bruise or fracture, injury to the medial patellofemoral ligaments, increased signal on T2-weighted images in the tissues adjacent to the adductor tubercle, and increased signal on T2-weighted images in the posterior aspect of the vastus medialis muscle (Fig. 7.3). Recent studies report that tears of the medial patellofemoral ligament, the primary support of the medial retinacular complex, occur not only at the patellar attachment but at the adductor tubercle attachment and within the substance of the ligament. MRI is uniquely capable of assessing the location of the tear. In addition to confirming the diagnosis of the patellar dislocation, identification of the sites of ligamentous injury appear to have important interventional consequences. Sallay et al. (21) suggested that the high percentage of subsequent patellar dislocation after traditional intervention relates to tears near the adductor tubercle that are not being addressed. In their preliminary series, the incidence of subsequent patellar dislocation appears to be significantly reduced.

Patellar tendinosis (i.e., jumper's knee) is readily assessed by MRI. Histologically, there is expansion of the tendinous tissue with associated mucoid degeneration and separation of the collagen bundles when imaged with polarized light and increased cellularity and vascu-

larity. Typically, there is an abrupt transition from normal to abnormal tendon. MRI readily detects these abnormalities, showing increased signal with STIR, fast spin echo, and T2*-weighted GRE imaging (22). Nonetheless, Schweitzer et al. (23) reported that in asymptomatic patients, almost 75% have some signal abnormality within the patellar tendon. As such, awareness of the patient's clinical status is critical to ascribe significance to the MRI observations.

Chondral and Osteochondral Injuries

In patients with acute or chronic knee injury, detection of articular cartilage abnormalities is important for optimal patient management. Untreated, cartilage damage may prolong patient recovery. The reported incidence of articular cartilage injury varies from a low of 4% to a high of 20% (24). Unfortunately, the clinical diagnosis of chondral lesions is difficult. Numerous investigators have attempted to access cartilage abnormalities using MRI with varied results. Difficulties in assessing cartilage include a variable histologic and biochemical composition from its surface to its osseous attachment (25,26); spatial resolution issues, especially true of the tibial plateau; artifact issues inherent in the MRI acquisition, including chemical shift and magic angle effects; and variability in the anatomic appearance of the cartilage abnormalities (i.e., softening and blistering vs. full thickness defects).

Early works (24,27–29) assessing cartilage showed MRI to be less than optimal. Speer et al. (24), using multiplanar spin echo imaging supplemented with a three-dimensional GRE technique, reported a retrospective sensitivity for detecting a full thickness cartilage injury in 83% and a partial thickness injury sensitivity of 55% in 28 knees. Others have reported similar observations using GRE acquisitions (28). When specifically addressing chondromalacia patellae, sensitivities ranging from 52% to 100% with specificities ranging from 50% to 76% have been reported using spin echo imaging (27,30,31).

Some investigators have advocated instilling dilute gadolinium intraarticularly, either via direct injection or via a venous route as a means of improving the accuracy of MRI for the detection of cartilage abnormalities. Gagliardi et al. (32) compared T1- and T2-weighted spin echo imaging with fat-suppressed Spoiled Grass (SPGR) acquisitions, MR arthrography, and CT arthrography. Their conclusions were that none of the techniques were sensitive for detecting grade I or grade II chondromalacia but both the arthrography sequences and T2-weighted spin echo were sensitive for detecting grade IV and, to a lesser extent, grade III chondromalacia. The authors also concluded that both MR and CT arthrography were the techniques of choice in assessing chondromalacia patella given that T2-weighted spin echo imaging tended to have more false positives. However, newer pulse sequences appear promising and less invasive (33,34). Magnetization transfer acquisitions, fat-suppressed three-dimensional volume GRE imaging, and fast spin echo techniques have all been advocated as accurate methods of assessing articular cartilage.

Disler et al. (35,36) in several publications suggested that fat-suppressed three-dimensional spoiled gradient echo MRI is superior to conventional spin echo imaging in the detection of cartilage abnormalities. Their largest study demonstrated a sensitivity of 85% and a specificity of 97% compared with 38% and 97%, respectively, with spin echo imaging in 114 consecutive patients.

Brodrick et al. (37) evaluated the utility of fast spin echo imaging for assessing cartilage abnormalities. In this preliminary work of 23 subjects, MR arthroscopy provided the same grade in 68% (93 of 137 joint surfaces) as arthroscopy. Ninety percent of the joint surfaces evaluated were graded the same or differed by one grade between the two techniques. In addition to detecting cartilage lesions, fast spin echo also has the added advantage of being extremely sensitive to marrow abnormalities (Fig. 7.4). Although these techniques are promising, confirmation from other sites with larger numbers will be necessary to substantiate their utility for the assessment of chondral defects.

Osteochondral injuries are more readily detected and characterized by MRI than plain film (38) (Fig. 7.5). Mesgarzadeh et al. (38) reported that MRI was able to predict fragment instability with a sensitivity of 92%

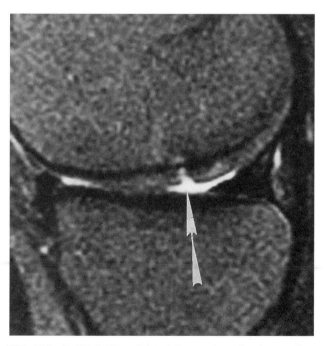

FIG. 7.4. Sagittal T2-weighted fast spin echo image that shows a focal full-thickness cartilage injury in a patient with medial pain with activity.

and specificity of 90%. Important was the appearance of high signal around the osseous fragment that corresponds to granulation tissue. As is true of cartilage lesion detection elsewhere, the accuracy of assessing the overlying cartilage with spin echo images was less than optimal.

Clinical Utility

Perhaps the most important utility of MRI of the knee is to direct appropriate clinical management. MRI is capable of distinguishing between meniscal tears and osseous infractions or bone bruises that may mimic meniscal pathology. In the acute situation where assessment of the ACL is difficult, MRI provides reliable data and complete assessment of other suspected or unsuspected pathologies. In addition to enhancing our understanding of internal derangements of the knee, MRI has been shown to be cost effective in the workup of sports and other traumatic injuries (39–41).

MAGNETIC RESONANCE IMAGING OF THE SHOULDER

Rotator Cuff Tears

MRI accurately depicts rotator cuff pathology. Evancho et al. (42) studied 31 patients and concluded that for complete tears, MRI was 80% sensitive, 94% specific, and 89% accurate (42). When compared with arthrography (38 cases), sonography (23 cases), and surgery (16 cases), Burk et al. (43) concluded that MRI and arthrography were equivalent, both having a sensitivity of 92%, specificity of 100%, and accuracy of 94%. Both techniques missed a small (less than 1 cm^2) tear and overcalled a partial thickness tear as being full thickness. In this series it was concluded that both MRI and arthrography were superior to ultrasound at a statistically significant level (MRI and arthrography sensitivity was 88%, specificity 100%, and accuracy 90% compared with sonography 63%, 50%, and 60%, respectively), although only a small number of patients were studied by all three modalities.

Zlatkin et al. (44), in a study of 32 patients who underwent surgery, concluded that MRI was superior to arthrography for the detection of both partial and full-thickness tears. MRI was 91% sensitive and 88% specific, whereas the corresponding sensitivity and specificity of arthrography was 71% and 71%, respectively. With the implementation of an objective scoring system, Zlatkin et al. suggested that MRI's sensitivity and specificity could be increased to 100% and 92% (44).

In addition to identifying the presence or absence of rotator cuff injury, MRI may size the cuff tear and, more importantly, assess the quality of the residual tendon and muscle. Such information is considered crucial in

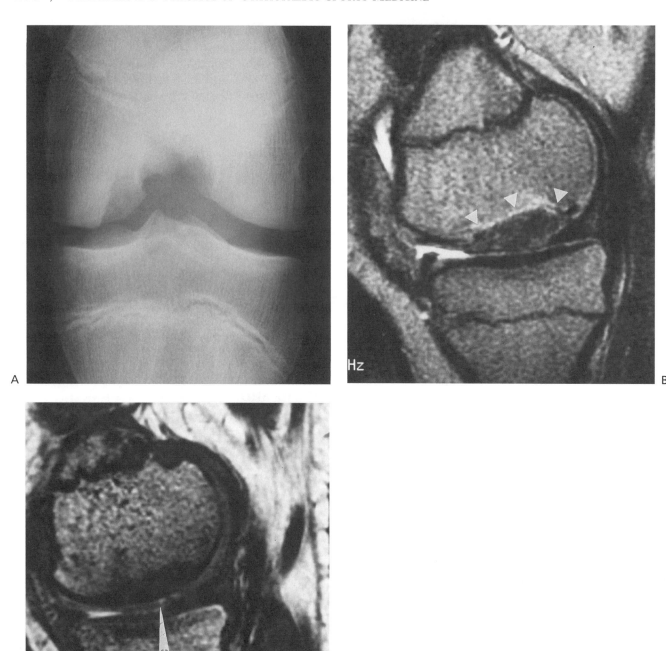

FIG. 7.5. Osteochondritis dissecans in an 18-year-old man. **A:** Plain film shows a defect in lateral aspect of medial femoral condyle. **B:** Sagittal T2-weighted spin echo image showing slightly increased signal around the osteochondral fragment suggesting loosening (*arrowheads*). **C:** Sagittal gradient-recalled echo sequence shows overlying cartilage injury (*arrow*).

terms of patient prognosis and management (Figs. 7.6 to 7.8).

It is commonly accepted that increased signal seen by MRI within the rotator cuff represents fluid within the rent of the rotator cuff tendon. More problematic are those rotator cuffs that do not show markedly increased signal but with findings suggestive of tendon disruption. It has been suggested that these abnormal areas may represent areas of granulation tissue that obscure the defect in the rotator cuff tear and prevent fluid from entering the tear. Zlatkin et al. (44) attributed the increased accuracy of MRI over arthrography in their series to this explanation.

Perhaps the most significant improvement in evaluat-

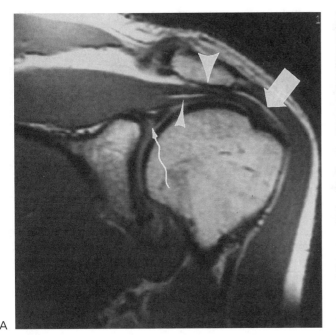
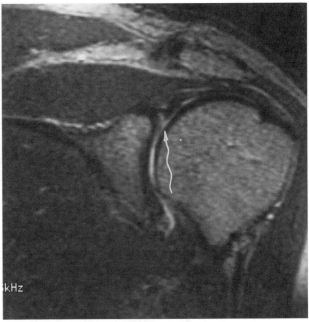

A   B

FIG. 7.6. A 54-year-old patient with chronic left shoulder pain and no antecedent trauma. **A:** Oblique coronal T1-weighted spin echo image shows the supraspinatus is intact (*arrow*). There is mild impingement by the clavicle (*arrowhead*) on the supraspinatus tendon with a suggestion of minimal fatty infiltration (*small arrowhead*). **B:** T2-weighted spin echo image showing similar findings. In both A and B there is irregularity of the superior labrum consistent with a grade 1 Superior Labrum Anterior Posterior (SLAP) lesion (*wavy arrow*).

ing the rotator cuff has been the introduction of fast spin echo (turbo spin echo, RARE) sequences into shoulder protocols. Carrino et al. (45) reported a comparison of fast spin echo with and without fat saturation with conventional spin echo. Their study included the evaluation of 126 patients. In essence, correlation between the various techniques was greater than 92% in each instance (with a kappa of greater than 0.73). Impor-

tantly, scan times were reduced from nearly 9 minutes to 3.5 minutes for each T2-weighted sequence.

Shoulder Instability

Shoulder stability is maintained by both the anterior and posterior capsular mechanisms. MRI is capable of visualizing glenohumeral ligaments, labrum, subscapu-

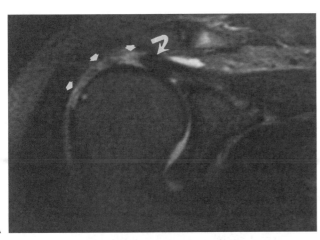
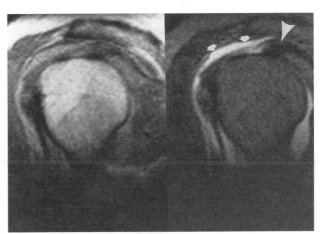

A   B

FIG. 7.7. A 45-year-old man who felt a pop in his shoulder. **A:** Oblique coronal T2-weighted spin echo image shows a rotator cuff discontinuity (*arrows*) with 3- to 4-cm retraction of the supraspinatus tendon (*curved arrow*). **B:** Oblique sagittal proton density and T2-weighted images show tear of supraspinatus (*arrows*). The infraspinatus is relatively preserved (*arrowhead*).

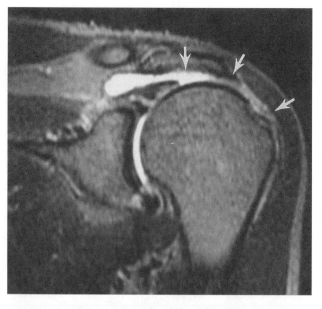

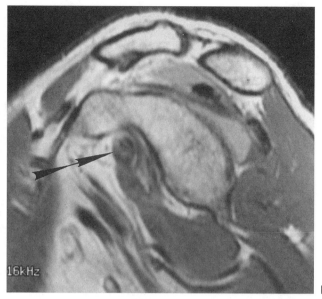

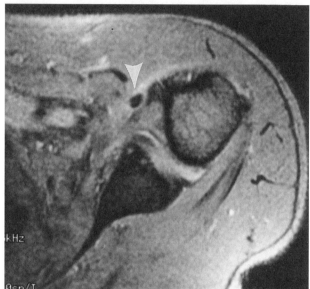

FIG. 7.8. A 51-year-old man with right shoulder injury status post-motor vehicle accident (post-MVA). **A:** Coronal T2-weighted spin echo image shows complete tear of the supraspinatus tendon (*arrows*). **B:** Sagittal proton density image shows injury to the subscapularis tendon (*large arrow*). **C:** Axial gradient-recalled echo image. The biceps tendon is dislocated anteriorly (*arrowhead*).

laris muscle and tendon, and capsule. Posteriorly, the infraspinatus and teres minor and the capsule can all be imaged by MRI. Biceps subluxation/dislocation and tendinopathy are also readily identified (Fig. 7.8).

Much debate centers on the significance of the labrum for maintaining shoulder stability. The significance is important in that numerous, but by no means all, authors have shown MRI to be insensitive in the detection of labral tears (46,47). Garneau et al. (46) (two readers) showed poor sensitivity, specificity, and reproducibility when assessing 15 patients with potential labral abnormalities. There was agreement between two readers in only three of nine true positives and two of six true negatives in this study.

In contradistinction, Iannotti et al. (48), Kieft et al. (49), and Seeger et al. (50) reported sensitivities and

specificities well above 85%. More recent data suggest even higher accuracies in the detection of labral injuries. Gusmer et al. (51) reported 103 patients with suspected labral disease who underwent arthroscopy or surgery. They were studied by a combination of high-resolution axial multiplanar gradient echo sequence and axial fast spin echo images. The authors reported for anterior, superior, and posterior labral tears sensitivities of 100%, 86%, and 74%, respectively. The corresponding specificities were 95%, 100%, and 95%. The authors concluded that unenhanced MRI was 95% accurate in the detection of labral injuries (Fig. 7.6).

Despite such optimism, mainstream consensus suggests MR arthrography is required to optimally assess labral abnormalities. Chandnani et al. (52) compared MR, MR arthrography, and CT arthrography for the detection of labral abnormalities in 30 patients. MRI detected 26 lesions (93%), MR arthrography detected 27 lesions (96%), and CT arthrography detected only 19 lesions (73%). Interestingly, MR arthrography was significantly superior to CT arthrography ($p = 0.014$).

MR arthrography was also superior to conventional MRI and CT arthrography for detecting fragment detachment with sensitivities of 96%, 46%, and 52%, respectively. MR arthrography was also more sensitive in detecting nondetached tears. Degeneration of the labrum was poorly identified in all instances, but MR arthrography was superior in 10 of 18 cases (56%) versus 2 cases with MRI (11%) and 4 cases (24%) with CT arthrography.

Palmer and Caslowitz (53), in 121 patients with arthroscopic or open surgical confirmation, concluded that MR arthrography was 92% sensitive and 92% specific in diagnosing labral tears using fat-suppressed short TR/TE images (450/18, 3 mm/0 thickness gap, 16-cm field of view, 256 × 256 or 192 matrix, 2 nex) (Fig. 7.9). Despite the high accuracy touted in the literature, numerous musculoskeletal radiologists suggest that accurately diagnosing labral pathology is problematic at best.

MR arthrography is considered less capable of identifying anterior shoulder instability. Palmer and Caslowitz (53) reported that the most useful predictor of anterior shoulder instability was inferior labral/glenohumeral

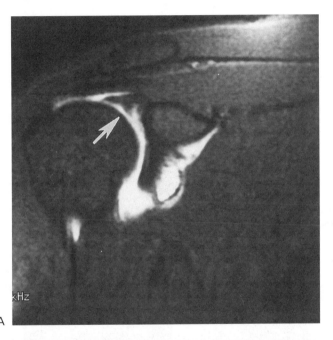

A

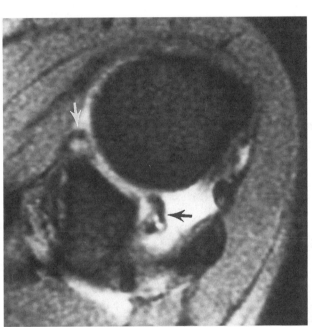

B

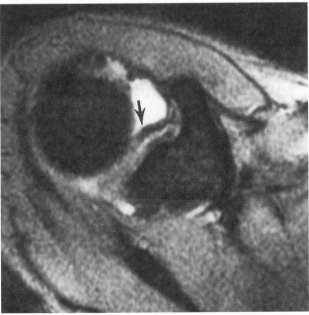

C

FIG. 7.9. A 16-year-old competitive swimmer with right shoulder pain for several months. **A:** Fat-suppressed T1-weighted spin echo image status after arthrogram that shows irregularity of the inferior surface of the superior labrum consistent with Superior Labrom Anterior Posterior (SLAP) lesion (*arrow*). **B and C:** Gradient-recalled echo sequences showing irregularity of the superior, anterior, and posterior labrum (*arrows*).

ligamentous abnormalities. In their series, MR arthrography had a diagnostic sensitivity of 76% and a specificity of 98% for predicting such instability by the identification of inferior labral and glenohumeral ligamentous injuries. The reduced sensitivity of MR arthrography was ascribed to the inability to identify capsuloligamentous laxity.

Although uncommon, chondral abnormalities do occur at the glenohumeral articulation. The current selection of imaging techniques are not generally optimized for such evaluation. Consequently, the sensitivity of MRI for their detection is considered poor (47).

MAGNETIC RESONANCE IMAGING OF THE FOOT AND ANKLE

As in other joints, the utility of MR stems from its ability to image the muscles, soft tissues, ligaments and tendons, and osseous structures and joints simultaneously.

Ligamentous Injury

Perhaps the earliest application of MRI in sports medicine was the assessment of Achilles tendon injuries. Although such injuries may be correctly diagnosed clinically, up to 25% of Achilles injuries are inadequately assessed before surgery or imaging. This is especially true in injuries where hematomas obscure tendinous defects. MRI is capable of distinguishing complete from partial tears and delineating the distance between the two tendon fragments, the orientation of the tendon fibers, and the quality of the tendon and the musculotendinous junctions above and below the torn tendon. Although treatment of an Achilles tear is controversial, MRI provides the information necessary for the treating physician to decide how to care for his or her patient.

Tendinopathy may also develop within the Achilles tendon. In such instances, the tendon shows either diffuse or focal thickening. The mucinous or myxoid degeneration appears as slightly increased signal within the tendon compared with the uniformly decreased signal seen normally. This appearance is often identical to that seen in partial tears. Accordingly, distinguishing tendinopathy and a partial tear may be impossible without clinical history.

Posterior tibial tendon injury is also well delineated by MRI (Fig. 7.10). Although the diagnosis is usually clinically apparent, the utility of MRI rests in its ability to afford a more detailed look at the tendon, fluid within the sheath, edema, fibrosis from adjacent tissues, and associated abnormalities such as sinus tarsi syndrome, subtalar arthritis, subluxation, and dislocation. It has been suggested that MRI is a more accurate predictor of surgical outcome than intraoperative evaluation of the torn posterior tibialis tendon itself (54).

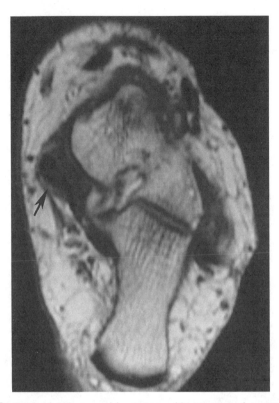

FIG. 7.10. A 58-year-old woman with suspected posterior tibial tendon injury. Axial T1-weighted spin echo image shows enlargement of the posterior tibial tendon with increased signal (*arrow*), consistent with a partial tear. Tendon injury extended along the entire course of the tendon on other images (not shown).

Although the peroneus brevis tendon is considered more likely to be injured, both the peroneus longus and brevis tendons may be damaged. MRI is useful in distinguishing injury to one or both of these tendons from other potentially confusing entities, including lateral collateral ligament injury, sinus tarsi syndrome, subtalar arthritis, and even hind foot valgus.

In addition to identifying frank peroneus brevis tendon tears, the conditions associated with injury of this tendon may be evaluated. These include a convex retromalleolar groove, a lax superior peroneal retinaculum, a low-lying peroneus brevis muscle belly, and a peroneus quartus muscle (55–58).

Osteochondral Injury

Osteochondral lesions (osteochondritis dissecans) of the talus are seen on both the medial and the lateral aspects of the talar dome. The medially located lesions occur more posteriorly. They are caused by inversion of the foot with plantar flexion and lateral rotation of the tibia. Lateral talar dome lesions are located more anteriorly and are associated with inversion injuries with the foot in dorsiflexion. Acute osteochondral injuries

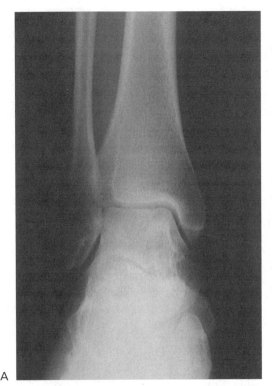
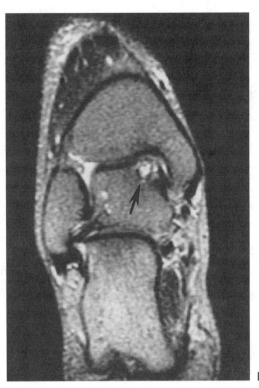

FIG. 7.11. A 51-year-old woman with chronic ankle pain. **A:** AP radiograph shows no obvious abnormality. **B:** T2-weighted spin echo coronal image shows an osteochondral injury in the medial dome of the talus (*arrow*).

typically occur laterally and are often identified on plain radiographs. In contrast, medial osteochondral fractures occur in patients with chronic pain and are associated with negative radiographs (59). Magee and Wong (60) reported that 17 or 30 patients with persistent ankle pain at 6 weeks had chondral injuries of the talar dome despite normal conventional radiographs (Fig. 7.11).

MRI appears to be the most sensitive and specific imaging technique available for use in assessing osteochondral lesions of the talus. Radionuclide scintigraphy, although sensitive, lacks the specificity of MRI. In particular, avascular necrosis, neoplasm, and infection cannot be excluded. In cases with positive plain radiographs, CT is comparable with MRI. However, in cases with negative plain radiographs, MRI is more sensitive than CT. In a study by Andresen et al. (61), CT did not depict 5 of 15 abnormalities seen on MR images; in all 5 cases, subchondral trabecular compression was present.

Osteochondral fragment stability is readily evaluated with MRI. Partially attached fragments have slightly to moderately increased signal intensity at the fragment-talus interface on T2-weighted images, whereas stable fragments do not demonstrate such increased signal intensity. In cases with complete fragment dissociation, displacement and/or fluid surrounding the loose body is readily present. Histologically, these areas of increased signal intensity between the bone fragment and the parent bone represent granulation tissue and/or fibrocartilage (62). Fragment signal intensity is variable and of no diagnostic significance. MRI may also be useful for assessing the cartilage overlying osteochondral injuries. In a study by Yulish et al. (63), MRI correctly depicted cartilage abnormalities in eight patients and enabled identification of cartilage disruption in four of five instances.

Although data are relatively preliminary, MRI has been useful in the assessment of anterolateral impingement, sinus tarsi syndrome, medial and lateral collateral ligamentous injuries, plantar fasciitis, tarsal tunnel syndrome, and stress fractures (64–66) (Fig. 7.12).

The utility of MRI in the ankle in part stems from its ability to assess all structures simultaneously. Yu and Long (67), looking at 200 patients with persistent ankle pain after sustaining trauma, found medial and lateral collateral ligamentous abnormalities in 125 patients. Clinically unsuspected peroneus brevis and longus tendon abnormalities were identified in 20 and 13 patients, respectively. Of equal importance, there were 35 talar dome fractures, 21 of which were unsuspected.

MRI evaluation of the ankle has been shown to affect clinical management (68). In a study of 81 patients who underwent MRI, there was a 47% pre- and post-MRI

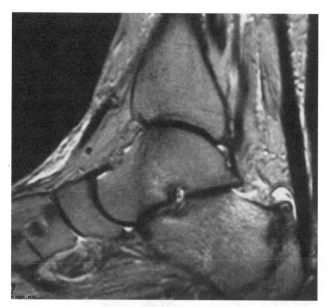

FIG. 7.12. A 38-year-old woman with heel pain and normal radiographs (not shown). Sagittal T2-weighted spin echo image shows an area of linear decreased signal with some surrounding edema consistent with stress fracture.

mismatch of diagnoses by the referring physicians, all of whom were experienced in assessing the foot and ankle. Equally important, treatment plans were changed after the MRI in approximately one third. Even in those cases where MRI did not change the diagnosis, MRI aided surgical planning in 35%. MRI has become a valuable modality for assessing the foot and ankle. The indications for such an examination continue to increase as the ability to diagnose more subtle abnormalities advances.

MAGNETIC RESONANCE IMAGING OF THE HIP AND PELVIS

Pubalgia or groin pain is a common athletic disability. Although it may be seen in most athletic endeavors, hockey and soccer players are considered to be at even greater risk (69–71). The most common entities involve musculotendinous injury of the gracilis, adductor, and obturator muscle groups. However, the differential is much broader and in the athlete would include hernias, sacroiliitis, and osseous fractures of the pelvis and femur among others (Fig. 7.13). Although many of these may be suggested on the basis of history and physical examination, MRI is capable of elucidating the precise cause of pain (69–79).

Osteitis pubis is another cause of groin pain and has been reported in association with multiple activities, including soccer, football, ice hockey, weight lifting, and long distance running (80,81). It has been suggested by Albers et al. (72) that osteitis pubis, musculotendinous

injuries of the obturator gracilis and adductor muscles, and abdominal wall weakness may be part of a related complex. As such, optimal treatment would necessitate examination of all these structures, a task easily accomplished with a single MRI examination.

MRI will identify sacral, acetabular, and pubic rami insufficiency fractures (82–86). In a similar fashion, MRI has been shown to be an accurate and cost-effective method for assessing occult fractures and stress fractures of the proximal femur (84,87–90). It should be noted that the utility of MRI rests in the detection of occult or subtle fractures. In cases of major trauma, MRI offers no advantages when compared with CT, and it has been suggested that free fragments are less well visualized on MRI (91).

Although relatively little has been written specifically addressing athletes, MRI has been shown to be an accurate means of assessing marrow abnormalities of the hip and pelvis (92–95). MRI is the study of choice for assessing avascular necrosis of the femoral head (Fig. 7.14). It is considered to be the most sensitive and specific noninvasive method for making this determination (93,94). MRI is considered to be insensitive for acutely diagnosing avascular necrosis in cases of fracture dislocation. However, follow-up studies in 6 weeks to 3 months will depict areas of infarction before radiographic changes (96,97). Alternative, a preliminary study by Lang et al. (98) suggested the use of dynamic gadolinium enhancement may show lack of femoral head perfusion in patients at risk for developing avascular necrosis before the development of classic MRI changes.

Although not considered to be a traumatic lesion per se, transient osteoporosis of the hip and transient bone marrow edema of the hip are associated with active middle-aged men and are readily apparent with fat-suppressed T2-weighted MR images. In both these entities, there is acute onset of pain without antecedent trauma or infection. The distinction between the two entities is the development of plain film signs of radiographic osteopenia, some 6 to 8 weeks after the onset of pain. These entities may be different manifestations of reversible ischemia of bone marrow (99–102). In distinguishing between transient bone marrow edema and early avascular necrosis, the intravenous infusion of gadolinium may be useful. Otherwise, follow-up studies will show resolution of the marrow abnormality in cases of transient bone marrow edema syndrome, whereas the more classic changes of avascular necrosis will become apparent in cases of bone infarction.

Bursitis is a common malady in the athlete. In the hip region, bursal inflammation is typically secondary to direct injury or excessive activity. The trochanteric, ileopsoas, and ischial gluteal bursae are most frequently affected (85). The use of T2-weighted spin echo, fast spin echo, or STIR images can readily identify these

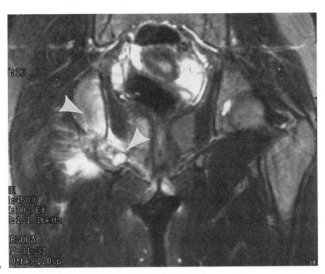
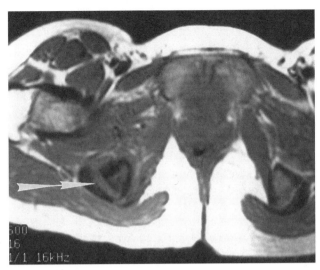

FIG. 7.13. A 13-year-old girl with recent injury and right hip pain. **A:** Coronal T2-weighted fast spin echo image shows edema in the muscles consistent with injury. There is increased signal within the ilium and ischium (*arrowheads*) consistent with osseous injury. **B:** Axial T1-weighted spin echo image shows avulsion of the right ischial tuberosity (*arrow*).

bursal fluid collections. In addition, associated "inflammation" in the adjacent soft tissue and tendons may be simultaneously assessed.

Until recently, MRI has not been considered useful for assessing the labrum or cartilage of the hip. As in the knee, assessment of cartilage has been difficult given the lack of an optimal pulse sequence. Additionally, geometric and anatomic considerations render the

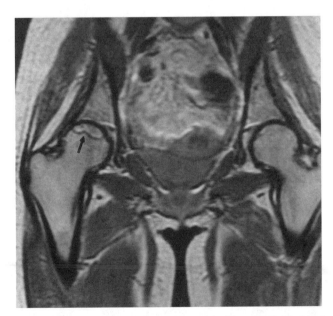

FIG. 7.14. A 24-year-old woman on steroids with right-sided hip pain. Coronal T1-weighted spin echo image shows avascular necrosis of the right femoral head. Plain films, not shown, were negative.

hip less favorable than the knee for high-resolution imaging. However, with the introduction of MR arthrography, labral and chondral visualization has significantly improved (103,104). Unfortunately, such techniques do not improve assessment of labral degeneration and are complicated by marked anatomic variation of the labrum (105).

Although other modalities may be useful in assessing athletes with hip pain, MRI provides the most information from a single study. In a recent study reported by Shin et al. (106), 19 military subjects undergoing endurance training developed hip pain and had negative radiographs. Twenty-two hips were considered to have femoral neck stress fractures by radionuclide imaging. MRI was able to separate patients with true stress fractures from those with other causes, including muscle and tendinous injury, avascular necrosis, and a solitary unicameral cyst. Based on follow-up radiographs and clinical outcome, MRI was considered to be 100% accurate compared with an accuracy of 68% for radionuclide bone scan imaging.

MAGNETIC RESONANCE IMAGING OF THE ELBOW

Loose bodies occur commonly in the elbow, second only to the knee in frequency. Besides alleviating pain, loose bodies are removed because of their mechanical restriction of joint motion and their propensity to accelerate degenerative changes (107,108). The overall accuracy of MRI for detecting loose bodies is poorly documented. Quinn et al. (109) in a study involving 20 patients concluded that MRI was 100% sensitive with a specificity of 67% when compared with arthroscopy. For MRI to be accurate, however, a joint effusion needs to be present (109). At our institution, MR arthrography is typically performed for the assessment of loose bodies to ensure adequate joint distention (Fig. 7.15).

The MCL complex, the common flexor tendon origin, the origin of the pronator teres, and the ulnar nerve are easily visualized with MRI. MRI is uniquely suited to differentiate MCL injury from medial epicondylitis and ulnar nerve entrapment (110). Acute injury of the MCL is detectable with conventional MRI (110–113). However, for subtle tears and partial detachment of the deep undersurface fibers, MR arthrography is considered to be superior to noncontrast imaging (112,114–117) (Fig. 7.16). Timmerman et al. (112,114) were the first to point out the utility of the T sign reflecting partial injury to the ulnar collateral ligament, typically described in baseball pitchers. Thickening of the MCL secondary to scarring as a consequence of chronic degeneration may also be evaluated (111).

In patients with suspected medial epicondylitis, MRI may directly visualize the common flexor tendon origin and may distinguish a strain or partial tear from a full thickness tendon disruption (102,118,119). In addition to visualizing muscle injury and discontinuity, reactive changes in the epicondyle may also be identified.

Cubital tunnel syndrome is another cause of medial pain that may be assessed by MRI. Pain and parathesia due to repetitive valgus stress may cause inflammation

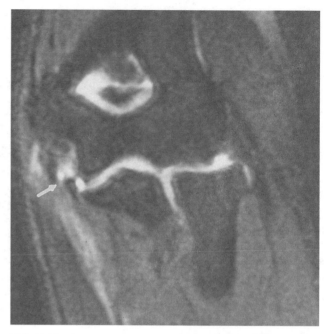

FIG. 7.16. A 20-year-old pitcher who experienced acute elbow pain while pitching. Coronal MR arthrogram shows extravasation of contrast through a torn ulnar collateral ligament.

of the ulnar nerves as it passes through the cubital tunnel. The inflammation within the cubital tunnel, increased signal within the nerve, and nerve enlargement are readily detected by MRI (119,120). Britz et al. (121) in a recent study concluded that with STIR imaging, there is increased signal in the ulnar nerve in 90% (30/31) of patients with ulnar nerve entrapment; 74% also showed enlargement of the ulnar nerve.

Although objective data are scant, MRI is considered the study of choice for assessing lateral elbow pain caused by injury to the common extensor tendon (119,122,123) (Fig. 7.17). In addition to expected findings of an injured common extensor tendon and reactive changes in the lateral epicondyle, one study suggested abnormal signal in the anconeus muscle. The authors are unclear whether this is a cause or effect of the lateral epicondylitis.

Originally described by O'Driscoll (124), posterolateral rotary instability of the elbow is due to injury of the lateral ulnar collateral ligament. Potter et al. (123) in a recent study have suggested that MRI can accurately assess this derangement as well.

Osseous injuries, including osteochondritis dissecans, lateral impaction, posteromedial impingement, and Panner's disease, have all been described as being amenable to diagnosis by MRI (110,119,122,125). It must be cautioned that such reports are generally anecdotal, and the true accuracy of MRI in such situations remains to be determined.

Although originally thought to be uncommon, bicepi-

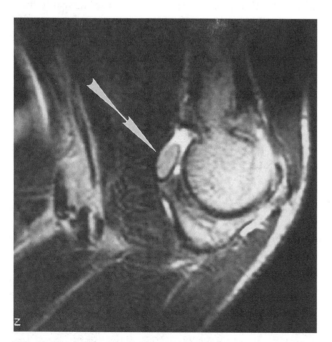

FIG. 7.15. A 29-year-old mam with elbow pain and limited range of motion. Oblique sagittal T2-weighted spin echo image demonstrates a loose body adjacent to the capitellum (*arrow*).

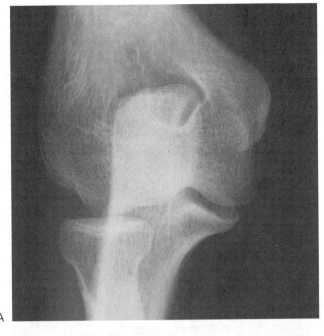

A

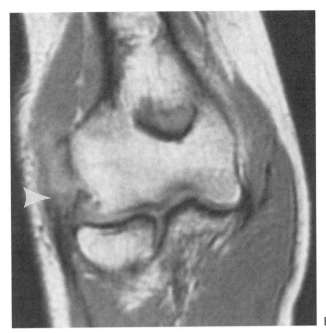

B

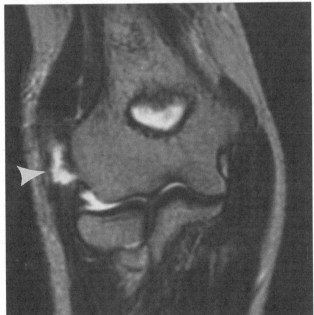

C

FIG. 7.17. A 41-year-old woman with radial elbow pain. **A:** Frontal radiograph shows subtle calcification adjacent to the lateral epicondyles. Coronal proton density **(B)** and fast spin echo **(C)** images demonstrate a tear of the common extensor muscle group near the insertion on the humerus (*arrowheads*).

tal tendon injuries are increasingly being reported (126,127). With the advent of MRI, it is also evident that partial bicipital tears, although unusual, are more common than previously recognized. In addition to evaluating the musculotendinous junction and the tendon as it attaches to the radial tuberosity, assessment of the biceps aponeuroses is possible. Fitzgerald et al. (127), in a study of 21 patients, reported that MRI and surgical findings agreed in 100%. More importantly, the MRI changed patient management in eight patients (38%). As with other tendon abnormalities, increased signal

seen on proton density and T2-weighted images was critical for making the diagnosis.

MAGNETIC RESONANCE IMAGING OF THE WRIST AND HAND

Of all the regions of the body subject to athletic injuries, the hand and wrist are probably the areas least imaged by MRI. In part, the paucity of imaging in this region may be accounted for by the technical limitations of the modality. High resolution, often at the extreme capability of the scanner, is required. Structures are minute and often poorly differentiated from one another. This being said, there are two areas where MRI seems to be useful: occult osseous abnormalities and injury to the ulnar collateral ligament of the thumb. MRI evaluation of injury to the various tendons, Triangular Fibrocartilage Complex (TFCC), and intraosseous ligaments, although promising, are not routinely performed at most institutions.

The most frequently injured carpal bone is the scaphoid. For optimal patient outcome, it is imperative that a nondisplaced scaphoid fracture is not missed. Unfortunately, avascular necrosis is the sequela in up to 30% of fractures through the waist of the bone (128). Other complications include delayed union, incomplete healing, and nonunion with the development of posttraumatic degenerative changes (129). As such, radionuclide imaging, CT, and MRI all have been suggested for immediate diagnosis.

As expected, acute fractures are depicted by MRI as areas of increased signal with T2 weighting and decreased signal with T1 weighting, often with the fracture line being visualized as a discrete band of absent signal (128,130,131). Equally important is the ability of MRI to not only identify the occult fracture of the scaphoid but to detect other fractures not clinically apparent. Breitenseher et al. (130), in a study of 42 patients with suspected scaphoid fractures, found scaphoid fracture in one third of patients and fractures in other bones in almost 20%.

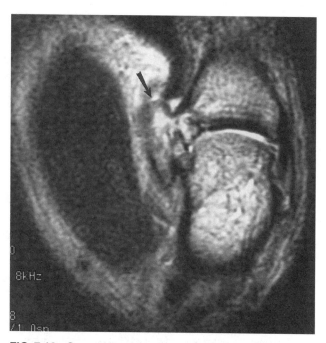

FIG. 7.18. Coronal T2-weighted spin echo image shows avulsion of the ulnar collateral ligament. Residual of the ulnar collateral ligament appears superficial to the adductor aponeurosis (*arrow*).

Injury of the ulnar collateral ligament, so-called gamekeeper's thumb, has been evaluated by MRI (132–134). Rupture of the ulnar collateral ligament is caused by abnormal abduction. Management of such injuries rests solely with the residing position of the ulnar collateral ligament after injury. If the torn ulnar collateral ligament remains in anatomic position (i.e., beneath the adductor aponeurosis), conservative management will be satisfactory. If, however, the ulnar collateral ligament is displaced and lies superficial to the aponeurosis (a so-called Stener lesion), surgical intervention is required. High-resolution MRI can accurately make such a distinction (132–134) (Fig. 7.18).

MAGNETIC RESONANCE IMAGING OF MUSCLE AND TENDON INJURIES

When a muscle injury does not respond to conservative therapy, MRI is the study of choice for further evaluation (135,136). The modality can detect subtle abnormalities and, more importantly, define the severity and anatomic extent of injuries. As such, prognosis and therapy may be more appropriately tailored to the patient. In addition to anatomic images, T1-weighted fat-suppressed spin echo or STIR imaging is critical for optimum sensitivity.

In the setting of recurrent trauma, MRI can assess complete muscle tears. MRI provides useful information concerning the degree of fibrous disruption and hemorrhage. A strain occurring at the musculotendinous junction is also readily detected by MRI (Figs. 7.13 and 7.19). Interestingly, some strains can remain positive on MRI for prolonged periods of time even after clinical resolution (137,138).

The sequela of chronic muscle injury, including atrophy and compensatory hypertrophy, may be detected by MRI. A potential weakness of MRI is that chronic fibrous scarring is dark on all pulse sequences and may be difficult to distinguish from normal adjacent tissue.

Hematomas are readily diagnosed by MR. The signal intensity on T1- and T2-weighted images is variable and also depends on field strength. Acutely, however, areas of increased signal are typically seen with T1-weighted images (Fig. 7.20). Compartment syndromes can be identified based on an increase in size and signal intensity of muscles with STIR and T2-weighted images. It has been suggested that the intravenous administration of gadolinium can assess perfusion of the affected muscle (139,140). Fascial herniation such as those seen in the anterior tibialis muscle may also be diagnosed (141).

Compressive or entrapment neuropathies have been studied with MRI. Although CT and plain films can exclude osseous abnormalities, MRI has become the mainstay of such an evaluation (120,142,143). The utility of MRI rests principally with the exclusion of mechanical compression or compartment syndrome. In addition,

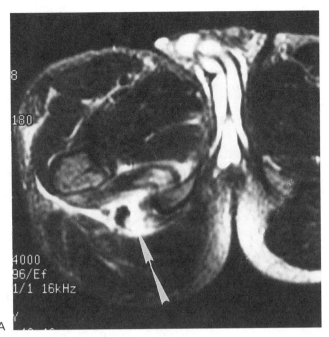 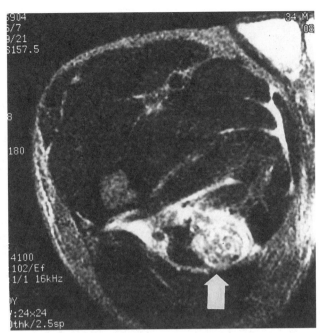

FIG. 7.19. A 34-year-old man who injured his hamstrings while water skiing. **A:** Axial fast spin echo shows avulsion of the hamstrings of the ischial tuberosity (*arrow*). **B:** Hemorrhage and hematoma are seen in the mid-thigh (*thick arrow*).

other lesions that may mimic these neuropathies can often be excluded.

The major limitation of MRI in the assessment of muscle and tendon abnormalities is its relative nonspecificity. Without clinical history, contusions, sprains, compartment syndrome, denervation, infection, necrosis, and even hematomas and tumors can be difficult to distinguish. Because MRI is insensitive to calcification,

it may also be problematic in distinguishing myositis ossificans from other etiologies.

SUMMARY

MRI has radically altered the evaluation of patients with sports-related injuries. After the clinical examination and often the acquisition of plain films, MRI is often the next and only imaging procedure required.

MRI excels at detecting subtle osseous abnormalities, and it is the study of choice for assessing muscle and ligamentous injuries. The advent of MR arthrography has further extended the utility of MRI. The weaknesses of the modality stem from its inability to visualize cortical bone and calcium. Although cartilage assessment still remains problematic, new imaging techniques show promise.

Despite its expense, the ability of MRI to clarify diagnostic dilemmas, guide therapeutic management, and prognosticate clinical outcome ensure an ever-increasing role for the modality in the assessment of sports-related injuries.

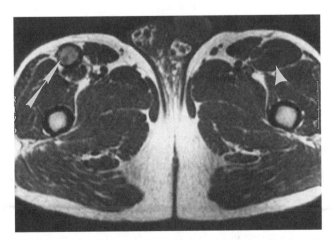

FIG. 7.20. Patient with long-standing weakness of his right leg. Axial non–fat-suppressed fast spin echo imaging shows avulsion of the right rectus muscle (*arrow*) when compared with the left (*arrowhead*). Hematoma is seen within the right rectus tendon sheath.

REFERENCES

1. Beers GJ. Biological effects of weak electromagnetic fields from 0 Hz to 200 MHz: a survey of the literature with special emphasis on possible magnetic resonance effects. *Magn Reson Imaging* 1989;7:309–331.
2. Kanal E, Shellock FG, Talagala L. Safety considerations in MR imaging. *Radiology* 1990;176:593–606.

3. Shellock FG. *Pocket guide to MR procedures and metallic objects: update 1997.* Philadelphia: Lippincott-Raven, 1997.

4. Fischer SP, Fox JM, Pizzo WD, et al. Accuracy of diagnoses from magnetic resonance imaging of the knee. *J Bone Joint Surg Am* 1991;73A:2–10.

5. Crues JV III, Mink JH, Levy TL, et al. Meniscal tears of the knee: accuracy of MR imaging. *Radiology* 1987;164:445–448.

6. Stoller DW, Martin C, Crues JV III, et al. Meniscal tears: pathologic correlation with MR imaging. *Radiology* 1987;163:731–735.

7. Mink JH, Levy T, Crues JV. Tears of the anterior cruciate ligament and menisci of the knee. MR imaging evaluation. *Radiology* 1988;167:769–774.

8. Spritzer CE, Vogler JB, Martinez S, et al. MR imaging of the knee: preliminary results with a three-dimensional FT GRASS pulse sequence. *AJR* 1988;150:597–603.

9. Kornick J, Trefelner E, McCarthy S, et al. Meniscal abnormalities in the asymptomatic population [Abstract]. *Radiology* 1989; 173:232.

10. Rubin DA, Britton CA, Towers JD, et al. Are MR imaging signs of meniscocapsular separation valid? *Radiology* 1996;201: 829–836.

11. Feagin JA. *The crucial ligaments: diagnosis and treatment of ligamentous injuries about the knee,* 2nd ed. New York: Churchill Livingstone, 1994.

12. Dupont JY. Evolution of lesions and symptoms after ACL injury. In: Feagin JA, ed. *The crucial ligaments: diagnosis and treatment of ligamentous injuries about the knee,* 2nd ed. New York: Churchill Livingstone, 1994:239–268.

13. Lee JK, Yao L, Phelps CT, et al. Anterior cruciate ligament tears: MR imaging compared with arthroscopy and clinical tests. *Radiology* 1988;166:861–864.

14. Barry KP, Mesagarzadeh M, Moyer R, et al. Patterns and accuracy of diagnosis of anterior cruciate ligament tears with MR imaging. *Radiology* 1991;181:303–305.

15. DeSmet AA, Graf BK. Meniscal tears missed on MR imaging: relationship to meniscal tear patterns and anterior cruciate ligament tears. *AJR* 1994;162:905–911.

16. Courneya CA, Spritzer CE, Burk DL, et al. MR imaging of patellofemoral ligament avulsion: a newly recognized medial retinaculum injury [Abstract]. *Radiology* 1994;193:289.

17. Kirsch M, Fitzgerald S, Friedman H, et al. Transient patellar dislocation: diagnosis with MR imaging. *AJR* 1993;161:109–113.

18. Quinn SF, Brown T, Demlow T. MRI of patellar retinacular ligament injuries. *J Magn Reson Imaging* 1993;3:843–847.

19. Virolainen H, Visuri T, Kuusella T. Acute dislocation of the patella: MR findings. *Radiology* 1993;189:243–246.

20. Spritzer CE, Courneya DL, Burk DL, et al. Medial retinacular complex injury in acute patellar dislocation: MR findings and surgical implications. *AJR* 1997;168:117–122.

21. Sallay PI, Poggie J, Speer KP, et al. Acute dislocation of the patella: a correlative pathoanatomic study. *Am J Sports Med* 1996;24:52–60.

22. Khan KM, Bonar F, Desmond PM, et al. Patellar tendinosis (jumper's knee): findings at histopathologic examination, US, and MR imaging. *Radiology* 1996;200:821–827.

23. Schweitzer ME, Mitchell DG, Dhrlich SM. The patellar tendon: hickening, internal signal buckling, and other MR variants. *Skeletal Radiol* 1993;22:411–416.

24. Speer KP, Spritzer CE, Goldner JL, et al. Magnetic resonance imaging of traumatic knee articular cartilage injures. *J Bone Joint Surg Am* 1998;72:98–103.

25. Lehner KB, Rechl HP, Gmeinwieser JK, et al. Structure, function, and degeneration of bovine hyaline cartilage: assessment with MR imaging in vitro. *Radiology* 1989;170:495–499.

26. Burk DL Jr, Kanal E, Brunberg JA, et al. 1.5-T surface-coil MRI of the knee. *AJR* 1985;147:293–300.

27. Handelberg F, Shahabpour M, Casteleyn PP. Chondral lesions of the patella evaluated with computed tomography, magnetic resonance imaging, and arthroscopy. *Arthroscopy* 1990;6:24–29.

28. Tyrrell RL, Gluckert K, Pathria M, et al. Fast three-dimensional MR imaging of the knee: comparison with arthroscopy. *Radiology* 1988;166:865–872.

29. Wojtys E, Wilson M, Buckwalter K, et al. Magnetic resonance imaging of knee hyaline cartilage and intraarticular pathology. *Am J Sports Med* 1987;155:455–463.

30. Yulish BS, Montanez J, Goodfellow DB, et al. Chondromalacia patellae: assessment with MR imaging. *Radiology* 1987;164: 763–766.

31. Barronian AD, Zoltan JD, Bucon KR. Magnetic resonance imaging of the knee: correlation with arthroscopy. *Arthroscopy* 1989;5:187–191.

32. Gagliardi JA, Chung EM, Chandnani VP, et al. Detection and staging of chondromalacia patellae: relative efficacies of conventional MR imaging, MR arthrography, and CT arthrography. *AJR* 1994;163:629–636.

33. Gylys-Morin VM, Hajek PC, Sartoris DJ, et al. Articular cartilage defects: detectability in cadaver knees with MR. *AJR* 1987; 148:1153–1157.

34. Hajek PC, Baker LL, Sartoris DJ, et al. MR arthrography: anatomic pathologic investigation. *Radiology* 1987;163:141–147.

35. Disler DG, McCauley T, Wirth CR, et al. Detection of knee hyaline cartilage defects using fat-suppressed three-dimensional spoiled gradient-echo MR imaging: comparison with standard MR imaging and correlation with arthroscopy. *AJR* 1995;165:377–382.

36. Disler DG, McCauley TR, Kelman CG, et al. Fat-suppressed three-dimensional spoiled gradient-echo MR imaging of hyaline cartilage defects in the knee: comparison with standard MR imaging and arthroscopy [see comments]. *AJR* 1996;167:127–132.

37. Broderick LS, Turner DA, Renfrew DL, et al. Severity of articular cartilage abnormality in patients with osteoarthritis: evaluation with fast spin echo MR vs arthroscopy. *AJR* 1994;162: 99–103.

38. Mesgarzadeh M, Sapega AA, Bonakdarpour A, et al. Osteochondritis dissecans: analysis of mechanical stability with radiography, scintigraphy, and MR imaging. *Radiology* 1987;165:775–780.

39. Williams RL, Williams LA, Watura R, et al. Impact of MRI on a knee arthroscopy waiting list. *Ann R Coll Surg Engl* 1996; 78:450–452.

40. Rappeport ED, Mehta S, Wieslander SB, et al. MR imaging before arthroscopy in knee joint disorders? *Acta Radiol* 1996; 37:602–609.

41. Bui-Mansfield LT, Youngberg RA, Warme W, et al. Potential cost savings of MR imaging obtained before arthroscopy of the knee: evaluation of 50 consecutive patients. *AJR* 1997;168: 913–918.

42. Evancho AM, Stiles RG, Fajman WA, et al. MR imaging diagnosis of rotator cuff tears. *AJR* 1988;151:751–754.

43. Burk DL Jr, Karasick D, Kurtz AB, et al. Rotator cuff tears: prospective comparison of MR imaging with arthrography, sonography, and surgery. *AJR* 1989;153:87–92.

44. Zlatkin MB, Iannotti JP, Roberts MC, et al. Rotator cuff tears: diagnostic performance of MR imaging. *Radiology* 1989;172: 223–229.

45. Carrino JA, McDauley TR, Katz LD, et al. Rotator cuff: evaluation with fast spin echo versus conventional spin echo MR imaging. *Radiology* 1997;202:533–539.

46. Garneau RA, Renfrew DL, Moore TE, et al. Glenoid labrum: evaluation with MR imaging. *Radiology* 1991;179:519–522.

47. Davidson JJ, Spritzer CE, Speer KP. Diagnosing labral and chondral lesions in the shoulder by MRI and MR arthrography. (abstract). American Orthopaedic Society, Atlanta, Georgia, 1996.

48. Iannotti JP, Zlatkin MB, Esterhai SL, et al. Magnetic resonance imaging of the shoulder. *J Bone Joint Surg Am* 1991;73A:17–29.

49. Kieft GJ, Bloem JL, Rozing PM, et al. Rotator cuff impingement syndrome: MR imaging. *Radiology* 1988;166:211–214.

50. Seeger LL, Gold RH, Bassett LW. Shoulder instability: evaluation with MR imaging. *Radiology* 1988;168:695–697.

51. Gusmer PB, Potter HG, Schatz JA, et al. Labral injuries: accuracy of detection with unenhanced MR imaging of the shoulder. *Radiology* 1996;200:519–524.

52. Chandnani VP, Yeager TD, DeBerardino T, et al. Glenoid labral tears: prospective evaluation with MR imaging, MR arthrography, and CT arthrography. *AJR Am J Roentgenol* 1993;161:1229–1235.

53. Palmer WE, Caslowitz PI. Anterior shoulder instability: diagnos-

tic criteria determined from prospective analysis of 121 MR arthrograms. *Radiology* 1995;197:819–825.

54. Conti S, Michelson J, Jahss M. Clinical significance of magnetic resonance imaging in preoperative planning for reconstruction of posterior tibial tendon ruptures. *Foot Ankle* 1992;13:208–214.

55. Tjin A, Schweitzer ME, Karasick D. MR imaging of peroneal tendon disorders. *AJR* 1997;168:135–140.

56. Sammarco GJ. Peroneus longus tendon tears: acute and chronic. *Foot Ankle Int* 1995;16:245–253.

57. Rosenberg ZS, Beltran J, Cheung YY, et al. MR features of longitudinal tears of the peroneus brevis tendon. *AJR* 1997;168:141–147.

58. Khoury NJ, el-Khoury GY, Saltzman CL, et al. Peroneus longus and brevis tendon tears: MR imaging evaluation. *Radiology* 1996;200:833–841.

59. Anderson IF, Crichton KJ, Grattan-Smith T, et al. Osteochondral fractures of the dome of the talus. *J Bone Joint Surg Am* 1989;71A:1143–1152.

60. Magee TH, Wong JS. MR utility in the acutely injured ankle [Abstract]. *AJR* 1997;168:(3)25.

61. Andresen R, Radmer S, Konig H, et al. MR diagnosis of retropatellar chondral lesions under compression. A comparison with histological findings. *Acta Radiol* 1996;37:91–97.

62. DeSmet AA, Fisher DR, Burnstein MI, et al. Value of MR imaging in staging osteochondral lesions of the talus (osteochondritis dissecans): results in 14 patients. *AJR* 1990;154:555–558.

63. Yulish BS, Mulopulos GP, Goodfellow DB, et al. MR imaging of osteochondral lesions of talus. *J Comput Assist Tomogr* 1987;11:296–301.

64. Cooperman AE, Helms CA, Collins AJ, et al. Magnetic resonance imaging findings in anterolateral impingement of the ankle [Abstract]. *AJR* 1997;168:(3)25.

65. Klein M, Spreitzer AM. MR imaging of the tarsal sinus and canal: normal anatomy, pathologic findings, and features of the sinus tarsi syndrome. *Radiology* 1993;186:233–240.

66. Ho VW, Peterfy C, Helms CA. Tarsal tunnel syndrome caused by strain of an anomalous muscle: an MRI specific diagnosis. *J Comput Assist Tomogr* 1993;17:822–823.

67. Yu JS, Long D. Persistent post-traumatic ankle pain: MR imaging observations [Abstract]. *AJR* 1997;168:(3)25.

68. Anzilotti K, Schweitzer ME, Hecht P, et al. Effect of foot and ankle MR imaging on clinical decision making. *Radiology* 1996;201:515–517.

69. Ekberg O, Persson NH, Per-Anders A. Longstanding groin pain in athletes: a multidisciplinary approach. *Sports Med* 1988;6:56–61.

70. Smodlaka VN. Groin pain in soccer players. *Phys Sports Med* 1980;8:57–61.

71. Renstrom P, Peterson L. Groin injuries in athletes. *Br J Sports Med* 1980;14:30–36.

72. Albers SL, Spritzer CE, Garrett WE Jr, et al. MRI evaluation of groin pain (pubalgia) in athletes. *Radiology* 1996;20:199.

73. Brunett B, Brunet-Geudj E, Genety J, et al. La pubalgie: syndrome "fourretout" pour une plus grande rigueur diagnostique et therapeutique. *Intantanes Med* 1984;55:25–30.

74. Casey D, Mirra J, Staple TW. Parasymphyseal insufficiency fractures of the os pubis. *AJR* 1984;147:581–586.

75. Nicholas JJ, Haidet E, Helfrich D. Groin and hip pain due to fractures at or near the pubic symphysis. *Arch Phys Med Rehabil* 1989;70:696–698.

76. Middleton RG, Carlile RG. The spectrum of osteitis pubis. *Compr Ther* 1993;19:99–102.

77. Sequeira W. Diseases of the pubic symphyis. *Semin Arthritis Rheum* 1986;16:11–21.

78. Taylor DC, Meyers WC, Moylan JA, et al. Abdominal musculature abnormalities as a cause of groin pain in athletes: inguinal hernias and pubalgia. *Am J Sports Med* 1991;19:239–243.

79. Wiley JJ. Traumatic osteitis pubis: the gracilis syndrome. *Am J Sports Med* 1983;11:360–363.

80. Schneider R, Kaye JJ, Ghelman B. Adductor avulsive injuries near the symphysis pubis. *Radiology* 1976;120:567–569.

81. Koch RA, Jackson DW. Pubic symphysitis in runners. A report of two cases. *Am J Sports Med* 1981;9:62–63.

82. Otte MT, Helms CA, Fritz RC. MR imaging of supra-acetabular insufficiency fractures. *Skeletal Radiol* 1997;26:279–283.

83. Bogost GA, Lizerbram EK, Crues JV. MR imaging in evaluation of suspected hip fracture: frequency of unsuspected bone and soft tissue injury. *Radiology* 1995;197:263–267.

84. Guanche CA, Kozin SH, Levy AS, et al. The use of MRI in the diagnosis of occult hip fractures in the elderly: a preliminary review. *Orthopaedics* 1994;17:327–330.

85. Kerr R. MR imaging of sports injuries of the hip and pelvis. *Semin Musculoskel Radiol* 1997;1:65–82.

86. Major NM, Helms CA. Pelvic stress injuries: the relationship between osteitis pubis (symphysis pubis stress injury) and sacroiliac abnormalities in athletes. *Skeletal Radiol* 1997;26:711–717.

87. Evans PD, Wilson C, Lyons K. Comparison of MRI with bone scanning for suspected hip fracture in elderly patients. *J Bone Joint Surg Br* 1994;76:158–159.

88. Ingari JV, Smith DK, Aufdemorte T, et al. Anatomic significance of magnetic resonance imaging findings in hip fracture. *Clin Orthop* 1996;209–214.

89. Rafii M, Mitnick H, Klug J, et al. Insufficiency fracture of the femoral head: MR imaging in three patients. *AJR* 1997;168:159–163.

90. Stiris MG, Lilleas F. MR findings in cases of suspected impacted fracture of the femoral neck. *Acta Radiol* 1997;38:863–866.

91. Potter HC, Montgomery KD, Heise C, et al. MR imaging of acetabular fractures: value in detecting femoral head injury, intraarticular fragments, and sciatic nerve injury. *AJR* 1994;163:881–886.

92. Glickstein MF, Burk LD, Schiebler ML, et al. Avascular necrosis vs other diseases of the hip: sensitivity of MR imaging. *Radiology* 1988;169:213–215.

93. Coleman BG, Kressel HY, Dalinka M, et al. Radiographically negative avascular necrosis: detection with MR imaging. *Radiology* 1988;168:525–528.

94. Mitchell D, Rao V, Dalinka M, et al. Femoral head avascular necrosis: correlation of MR imaging, radiographic staging, radionuclide imaging, and clinical findings. *Radiology* 1987;162:709–715.

95. Mitchell MD, Kundel HL, Steinberg ME, et al. Avascular necrosis of the hip: comparison of MR, CT, and scintigraphy. *AJR* 1986;147:67–71.

96. Poggi JJ, Callaghan JJ, Spritzer CE, et al. Prospective serial evaluation of MRI changes following traumatic hip dislocation. *Clin Orthop Relat Res* 1995;319:249–259.

97. Sugano N, Masuhara K, Nakamura N, et al. MRI of early osteonecrosis of the femoral head after transcervical fracture. *J Bone Joint Surg Br* 1996;78:253–257.

98. Lang P, Mauz M, Schorner W, et al. Acute fracture of the femoral neck: assessment of femoral head perfusion with gadopentetate dimeglumine-enhanced MR imaging. *AJR* 1993;160:335–341.

99. Wilson AJ, Murphy WA, Hardy DC, et al. Transient osteoporosis: transient bone marrow edema? *Radiology* 1988;167:757–760.

100. Hayes CW, Conway WF, Daniel WW. MR imaging of bone marrow edema pattern: transient osteoporosis, transient bone marrow edema syndrome, or osteonecrosis. *Radiographics* 1993;13:1001–1011.

101. Vande Berg BE, Malghem JJ, Labaisse M, et al. MR imaging of avascular necrosis and transient marrow edema of the femoral head. *Radiographics* 1993;13:501–520.

102. Guerra JJ, Steinberg ME. Distinguishing transient osteoporosis from avascular necrosis of the hip. *J Bone Joint Surg [Am]* 1995;77:616–624.

103. Leunig M, Werlen S, Ungersbock A, et al. Evaluation of the acetabular labrum by MR arthrography [published erratum in *J Bone Joint Surg Br* 1997;79:693]. *J Bone Joint Surg Br* 1997;79:230–234.

104. Hodler J, Yu JS, Goodwin D, et al. MR arthrography of the hip: improved imaging of the acetabular labrum with histologic correlation in cadavers [published erratum appears in *AJR* 1996;167:282]. *AJR* 1995;165:887–891.

105. Lecouvet FE, Vande Berg BC, Malghem J, et al. MR imaging of the acetabular labrum: variations in 200 asymptomatic hips. *AJR* 1996;167:1025–1028.

106. Shin AY, Morin WD, Gorman JD, et al. The superiority of

magnetic resonance imaging in differentiating the cause of hip pain in endurance athletes. *Am J Sports Med* 1996;24:168–176.

107. Ogilvie-Harris DJ, Schmeitsch E. Arthroscopy of the elbow for removal of loose bodies. *Arthroscopy* 1993;9:5–8.

108. O'Driscoll SW, Morrey BF, Korinek S, et al. Elbow subluxation and dislocation. A spectrum of instability. *Clin Orthop* 1992;280:186–197.

109. Quinn SF, Haberman JJ, Fitzgerald SW, et al. Evaluation of loose bodies in the elbow with MR imaging. *J Magn Reson Imaging* 1994;4:169–172.

110. Gaary EA, Potter HG, Altchek DW. Medial elbow pain in the throwing athlete: MR imaging evaluation. *AJR* 1997;168:795–800.

111. Fritz RC. MR imaging of osteochondral and articular lesions. The elbow. *Magn Reson Imag Clin North Am* 1997;5:579–602.

112. Timmerman LA, Schwartz ML, Andrews JR. Preoperative evaluation of the ulnar collateral ligament by magnetic resonance imaging and computed tomography arthrography. Evaluation in 25 baseball players with surgical confirmation. *Am J Sports Med* 1994;22:26–31; discussion 32,

113. Hergan K, Mittler C, Oser W. Ulnar collateral ligament: differentiation of displaced and nondisplaced tears with US and MR imaging. *Radiology* 1995;194:65–71.

114. Timmerman LA, Andrews JR. Undersurface tear of the ulnar collateral ligament in baseball players. A newly recognized lesion. *Am J Sports Med* 1994;22:33–36.

115. Nakanishi K, Masatomi T, Ochi T, et al. MR arthrography of elbow: evaluation of the ulnar collateral ligament of elbow. *Skeletal Radiol* 1996;25:629–634.

116. Schwartz ML, al-Zahrani S, Morwessel RM, et al. Ulnar collateral ligament injury in the throwing athlete: evaluation with saline-enhanced MR arthrography. *Radiology* 1995;197:297–299.

117. Cotten A, Jacobson J, Brossmann J, et al. MR arthrography of the elbow: normal anatomy and diagnostic pitfalls. *J Comput Assist Tomogr* 1997;21:516–522.

118. Ho CP. Sports and occupational injuries of the elbow: MR imaging findings. *AJR* 1995;164:1465–1471.

119. Patten RM. Overuse syndromes and injuries involving the elbow: MR imaging findings. *AJR* 1995;164:1205–1211.

120. Beltran J, Rosenberg ZS. Diagnosis of compressive and entrapment neuropathies of the upper extremity: value of MR imaging. *AJR* 1994;163:525–531.

121. Britz GW, Haynor DR, Kuntz C, et al. Ulnar nerve entrapment at the elbow: correlation of magnetic resonance imaging, clinical, electrodiagnostic, and intraoperative findings. *Neurosurgery* 1996;38:458–65; discussion 465.

122. Fritz RC. MR imaging in sports medicine: the elbow. *Magn Reson Imag Clin North Am* 1997;5(3):29–50.

123. Potter HG, Weiland AJ, Schatz JA, et al. Posterolateral rotatory instability of the elbow: usefulness of MR imaging in diagnosis. *Radiology* 1997;204:185–189.

124. O'Driscoll SW. Classification and spectrum of elbow instability: recurrent instability. In: Morrey BF, ed. *The elbow and its disorders*. Philadelphia: W.B. Saunders, 1993:453–463.

125. Stoane JM, Poplausky MR, Haller JO, et al. Panner's disease: x-ray, MR imaging findings and review of the literature. *Comput Med Imaging Graph* 1995;19:473–476.

126. Falchook FS, Zlatkin MB, Erbacher GE, et al. Rupture of the distal biceps tendon: evaluation with MR imaging. *Radiology* 1994;190:659–663.

127. Fitzgerald SW, Curry DR, Erickson SJ, et al. Distal biceps tendon injury: MR imaging diagnosis. *Radiology* 1994;191:203–206.

128. Munk PL, Lee MJ, et al. Scaphoid bone waist fractures, acute and chronic: imaging with different techniques. *AJR* 1997;168:779–786.

129. Sakuma M, Nakamura R, Imade T. Analysis of proximal fragment sclerosis and surgical outcome of scaphoid non-union by magnetic resonance imaging. *J Hand Surg* 1995;20B:201–205.

130. Breitenseher MJ, Metz VM, Gilula LA, et al. Radiographically occult scaphoid fractures: value of MR imaging in detection. *Radiology* 1997;203:245–250.

131. Hunter JC, Escobedo EM, Wilson AJ, et al. MR imaging of clinically suspected scaphoid fractures. *AJR* 1997;168(5):1287–1293.

132. Hinke DH, Erickson SJ, Chamoy L, et al. Ulnar collateral ligament of the thumb: MR findings in cadavers, volunteers, and patients with ligamentous injury (gamekeeper's thumb). *AJR* 1994;163:1431–1434.

133. Hergan K, Mittler C, Oser W. Ulnar collateral ligament: differentiation of displaced and nondisplaced tears with US and MR imaging. *Radiology* 1995;194:65–71.

134. Spaeth HJ, Abrams RA, Bock GW, et al. Gamekeeper thumb: differentiation of nondisplaced and displaced tears of the ulnar collateral ligament with MR imaging. *Radiology* 1993;188:553–556.

135. Speer KP, Lohnes H, Garrett W. Radiographic imaging of muscle strain injury. *Am J Sports Med* 1993;21:89–95.

136. Steinbach LS, Fleckenstein JL, Mink JH. MR imaging of muscle injuries. *Semin Musculoskel Radiol* 1997;1:127–142.

137. Fleckenstein JL, Weatherall PT, Parkey RW, et al. Sports related muscle injuries: evaluation with MR imaging. *Radiology* 1988;172:793–798.

138. Shellock FG, Fukunaga T, Mink JH, et al. Acute effects of exercise on skeletal muscle: concentric vs eccentric actions. *AJR* 1991;156:765–768.

139. Fleckenstein JL, Weatherall PT, Bertocci LA, et al. Locomotor system assessment by muscle magnetic resonance imaging. *Magn Reson Q* 1991;7:79–103.

140. Fleckenstein JL, Shellock FG. Exertional muscle injuries: MRI evaluation. *Top Magn Reson Imaging* 1991;3:50–70.

141. Zeiss J, Ebraheim NA, Woldenberg LS. Magnetic resonance imaging in the diagnosis of anterior tibialis muscle herniation. *Clin Orthop Relat Res* 1989;244:249–253.

142. Linker CS, Helms CA, Fritz RC. Quadrilateral space syndrome: findings at MR imaging. *Radiology* 1993;188:675–676.

143. Fritz RC, Helms CA, Steinbach LS, et al. Suprascapular nerve entrapment: evaluation with MR imaging. *Radiology* 1992;182:437–444.

Principles and Practice of Orthopaedic Sports Medicine,
edited by William E. Garrett, Jr., Kevin P. Speer, and Donald T. Kirkendall.
Lippincott Williams & Wilkins, Philadelphia © 2000.

CHAPTER 8

Statistical Practices in Sports Medicine

Mary Lou V. H. Greenfield

More than ever before, physicians today must be able to interpret medical research, even if they are not researchers themselves. Both colleagues and patients expect sports medicine physicians to be knowledgeable about current orthopedic and sports medicine issues and more general medical issues. Patients often query their physicians about medical stories from supermarket tabloids: "Doctor, I wonder if shark cartilage will help my throwing shoulder?" or "I read that laser surgery is the latest thing for fixing knee injuries." Some of these lay reports are based loosely on legitimate medical reports, and patients expect their doctors to know something about these topics, if only to indicate that initial results were inconclusive. Editorials and reviews are helpful ways to keep up with medical research in a particular field, but we cannot depend entirely on these sources. If we want to do more good than harm to our patients, we need skills to evaluate primary research articles and judge their value.[1] Such evaluations allow us to incorporate only those sports medicine treatments that are both sound and consistent with valid scientific research (1).

Unfortunately, it is easy to become overwhelmed by the volume of published material that arrives in medical libraries and in mailboxes every day. The number of research articles published each year is vast, and many of us are intimidated by the statistical analyses presented in such publications. Our task is further complicated because much of the medical literature reports numerical data that contain statistical errors and faulty research design (2–13). Even peer reviewers do not always detect these errors (12). Everything you read should be sus-

pect, because even highly regarded expert investigators can make mistakes with their data and report biased interpretations (14).

Further, we must recognize that errors in statistical practices are not limited solely to errors in statistical analyses. Errors of statistical practices include such problems as lack of a clearly defined study question or hypothesis, inappropriate study design for the question being asked, absent measures of validity or reliability in key measurements, misclassification of types of data, confusion regarding assumptions of independence among the data, failure to report how the sample was chosen, bias, inappropriate summary of patient characteristics, lack of reporting of specific statistical tests used, failure to report exact P values associated with the test chosen, failure to report confidence intervals, and lack of generalizability of study findings (2–5,7,8,10–12).

Misuse of statistical practices in the medical literature and a willingness to believe interpretations couched in mysterious-sounding statistical terminology often lead physicians to ignore their own clinical judgment and experience (15). Our blind acceptance of study findings and conclusions without a thoughtful evaluation of the statistical practices used may place both the truth and the well-being of our patients at risk (1,16). Physicians need to apply critical reasoning, common sense, and a healthy skepticism to their reading of the research literature (17).

Even very good studies can have some flaws. One must always ask the following questions: Are the flaws avoidable or unavoidable? How valid is the study with such flaws present? To what extent do these flaws distort the study's findings? On some occasions, "hypotheses are proven, despite imperfect design or data" (18). We do not want to underrate the value of any single study, and in fairness to our patients, we must evaluate all studies critically.

The goal of this chapter is to provide physicians with a guide for evaluating statistical practices in the sports medicine literature so that they can recognize misuses

---

[1] Although we refer to published reports of medical research, the methodologies described in this chapter apply equally well to podium and poster presentations of research.

M. L.V. H. Greenfield: Department of Anesthesiology, University of Michigan, Ann Arbor, Michigan 48109.

(1) What is the study question and the hypothesis to be tested?

(2) What is the study design?

(3) How is the sample selected?

(4) What background information is presented in each of the study and control groups?

(5) What are the statistical tests chosen?

(6) How are the data analyzed?

(7) How do you interpret the study results?

(8) How do the study findings apply to your practice of medicine?

FIG. 8.1. Key questions to ask when evaluating a research study.

of statistics and critically evaluate study findings. Very few (if any) published research studies are perfect. The trick is to identify which studies have real scientific merit (despite flaws and imperfections) to derive maximum benefit from the research presented. It is not necessary to be a statistician to accomplish this task. This chapter presents no statistical formulas, as we are more interested in conveying an inferential understanding of statistical practices. (We do assume a knowledge of basic statistics.) This chapter considers eight key questions to ask as you review any research study (12,19–25) (Fig. 8.1). How these questions are answered will have an impact on the validity of the study and its usefulness to you and your patients. Complex statistical procedures cannot make up for poor research design, faulty sample selection, and inappropriate statistical tests. Identifying key statistical practices in sports medicine research requires knowing what to look for in research articles, an understanding of basic statistical principles, and an integration of logic, experience, clinical judgment, and common sense.

QUESTION 1: WHAT IS THE STUDY QUESTION?

What was the driving force behind the study under review? What did the authors want to study? Underlying questions directed the investigators' work and led them to their study objectives. These objectives were the basis for their study outcomes and achievement of study outcomes. Clear questions lead to clear answers.

Most readers skim the titles of studies and scan the abstracts to see if an article is worth reading at all. They do not continue if the study has no relevance to their individual practice or seems too obscure. This is part of the "so what" test referred to by Huth (26). The so what test is a crude but powerful measure of the importance and clinical relevance of any study. It helps the reader to determine the effect of the study's message and whether it will change the reader's current practice or perception of a particular concept.

Once the reader has determined which studies might

be of interest, the merits of the study can be examined more closely. The first thing the reader should identify is the underlying study question and the study objective. A study question is the hallmark of an honest well-planned investigation. The more circumscribed the question, the more likely the investigator will reach an unequivocal answer (27,28). Meaningful answers to clinical questions do not come from arcane statistical analyses. Rather, meaningful answers come from questions that have direct applicability to patients in the reader's clinical practice and have high scientific merit (8,29). The reader should be able to find the study question and the resulting objective well-described somewhere in the Introduction of the article. The Introduction will also contain background information and historical developments that help the reader understand the origin and the context of the question without having to refer to earlier publications (30). The Introduction provides information about the impetus for the study, whereas the study question is the driving force behind the entire study. A clearly stated study question is followed by a clearly stated objective. The study question and objective(s) let the reader know exactly what it is that the author is trying to accomplish in the study. We should also ask ourselves the following questions: Does the underlying question make sense? What does the author plan to accomplish in this study? What specific outcome is going to be measured? In what population? How or by what means?

Consider the following hypothetical example of a clearly stated study question and a well-defined study objective:

Is there a relationship between the menstrual cycle and anterior cruciate ligament (ACL) injuries in female athletes? The following study was done to ascertain whether urinary estrogen, progesterone, and luteinizing hormone levels within 24 hours of noncontact ACL injuries are associated with noncontact ACL injuries in Big 10 female soccer players.

In addition to a clear statement of the study question, the objective flows naturally from the question raised:

It identifies the study population and the specific methods for evaluating the association.

Consider an example of a clearly stated question but a poorly defined objective for a similar study: "Is there a relationship between the menstrual cycle and ACL injuries in female athletes? We studied hormone levels of female athletes with ACL injuries." In this example, the study question is clear enough, but the objective is too general and vague: We do not know whether the target population is high school or college or recreational athletes, we do not know specifically what the investigators are planning to study, and we have no idea of how they will measure the success of their study. If the authors do not outline how they will measure their success, how will we? Missing in this poorly stated objective are the criteria to measure the relationship between the menstrual cycle and ACL injury rates. Also missing is any hint of how the authors can measure hormone levels in ways that are standard for all study participants. For example, an investigation such as this one might use self-report by the athlete, urinary hormone levels, or serum hormone levels to ascertain where the athlete was in her menstrual cycle at the time of the ACL injury. If the authors relied on a combination of these methods for determining points in the menstrual cycle, the findings would be suspect because they were not standardized for all study participants.

Some studies have no identifiable study question and very cryptic study objectives. Consider this example in which no study question is expressed: "We studied ACL injuries in female athletes." We have no idea of the authors' intention or objective or specific aim. And, if we do not know what the question and resulting objectives are, how can we be sure that the study methods or conclusions are warranted, correct, or even appropriate (30)? Clearly stated questions and objectives lead to an appropriate and workable study design; study design flows from careful consideration of the study question and objective (28).

If the study question is missing or the objective is poorly worded, or both, the reader cannot know what is driving the study. We cannot evaluate study methods and their effect on study findings. Is there some unknowable question that the author is seeking to answer by this study, or is the author simply presenting an exploratory study with many probes into the data? Without an identifiable study objective, we are left wondering if the authors have been driven simply by the adage "I have so much data. There must be something here." Study conclusions then become suspect.

Concise objectives are the basis for hypothesis testing and statistical tests of significance. For a study to be sound, all hypotheses must be specified before the study begins and before statistical testing or analysis takes place. These hypotheses are derived from the specific aims or objectives of a study. Investigators frequently present study results with tests of statistical significance (and associated P values) but without prespecified hypotheses. Results of tests of statistical significance without an *a priori* hypothesis are strictly invalid (7,31). If the study hypothesis is not specified *a priori*, then the study can easily turn into an exercise in "fishing" characterized by "data trawling" (7), "data dredging" (28), or "data torturing" (5). Although the researcher may have many objectives in mind when attempting to answer the underlying study question, it should be clear to the reader that the researcher has prioritized objectives and outcomes and then specified one main outcome to be studied—with the remaining outcomes to be presented as exploratory (7). Otherwise, the researcher is like the Texas sharpshooter who shoots into the side of a barn and then draws targets around the holes (32). In trawling and dredging data without a specific question and hypothesis, the researcher is the sharpshooter and significant P values become the targets drawn around the findings.

Question 1 Bottom Line: Identify the Study Question and Objective

Even if the study question was not presented by the authors, ask yourself what the underlying question was behind this study. Use the study question and objectives to determine how successful the study was in answering the question and meeting these objectives. Be skeptical of studies with no clear study question, and vague and broadly worded study objectives.

QUESTION 2: WHAT IS THE STUDY DESIGN?

Assume the study under review puts forth a well-formulated study question and clearly specified objectives. Now the reader must ask, was the study design appropriate to answer the study question? The design of the study is the method by which the investigator attempts to answer the study question and to achieve the study objectives. Just as the study question is the driving force behind the study, the study design flows from careful consideration of the study question (28). The real test of the validity of the study lies in our ability to evaluate whether the investigators have an unbiased objective strategy for answering the study question (8). A careful description of this strategy should be contained in the Methods and Materials section of the article. Figure 8.2 presents a map of how studies may fall under two general research design categories: *descriptive* and *explanatory designs*.

Descriptive Designs

Descriptive designs include studies that record events, observations, and activities (21). Their main purpose is

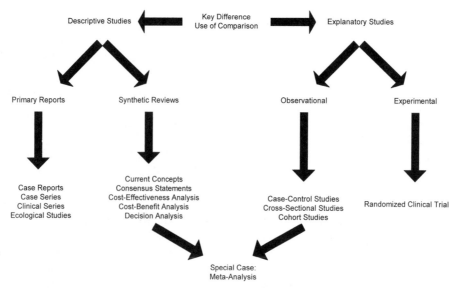

FIG. 8.2. Basic study designs.

to present accurate collections of data with regard to person, place, or time. In contrast to explanatory designs, descriptive designs do not provide explanations of cause-and-effect relationships because no variable has been actively manipulated and no experiment has taken place. However, descriptive designs are very important for characterizing patterns of disease or injury. They may be exciting documentaries that, once reported, provide the impetus for other research questions and investigations (21,33). Examples of descriptive research designs include the *case report* or *series, clinical series,* and *ecologic designs.*

Case Reports and Case Series

Case reports and case series are the most widespread examples of retrospective reviews in the medical literature (13). A case report describes the experience of a single patient with a specific diagnosis, whereas a case series describes the experience of a group of patients. Generally, the author identifies some uncommon feature of a disease or condition, or something unique in the patient's history that the author believes should be brought to the attention of colleagues (34). A case report documents an unusual finding and may be the first report of a new disease or new health hazard. Jogger's whiplash (35), space invaders' wrist (36), ulnar stress fracture in a bowler (37), and extrusion of the medial meniscus (38) are examples of case reports in which the authors examine new medical concerns or problems.

Case series, on the other hand, are characterized by a collection of case reports, frequently found by the authors within a relatively short period of time (33). The earliest epidemiologic studies were comprised of case series, and in our own time case series provide the basis for routine surveillance of new diseases or

conditions. Recent reports of double-layered lateral menisci (39), simultaneous rupture of the ACL and patellar tendon (40), nordic ski-jumping fatalities (41), and slot-machine tendonitis (42) are small collections of case reports.

The advantages of case reports and case series are that they alert the medical community to new diseases, unusual complications of illnesses, and adverse effects of medical treatments (21). The dissemination of these reports, in turn, may lead to further scientific inquiry with hypothesis generation. Descriptive data provide information for investigators to further study conditions that may result in confirmation and additional important findings. Case reports and case series must be interpreted with caution, however. The findings are reported by only one person, and such findings may be purely fortuitous. There is no comparison group in case reports or case series that permits exploration of associations. This lack of a comparison or control group may either obscure relationships that might truly exist or suggest associations that are coincidental. Case series and case reports should not, in general, be used for statistical association.

Clinical Series

A *clinical series* is a type of descriptive research in which the author reports on the outcome of a group of patients undergoing a new procedure or modification of currently used procedures. Clinical series are similar to case series except that clinical series do not occur in a short period of time. The emphasis in the clinical series is on the results of the procedure and patient follow-up. Reports of chronic painful ankle in skeletally immature athletes (43), acute and chronic ACL ruptures treated with arthroscopically assisted autogenous patellar tendon reconstruction (44), and long-term evaluation of the Elmslie-Trillat-Maquet procedure for patellofemoral dysfunction (45) are examples of clinical series.

The chief advantage of the clinical series is the cataloguing of the experience of the investigators for others to review (21). As in case series and case reports, the disadvantages of clinical series are that the findings are usually based on the experience of one person, and such findings may be coincidental, biased, or both. Again, the lack of a comparison group makes the clinical series generally inappropriate for testing of statistical associations.

Ecologic Studies

Ecologic studies examine some unique characteristic or feature—rate of cancer, hip fractures, injuries, and so forth. Unlike case series, however, which focus on individual subjects with a unique characteristic or feature, the ecologic study investigates entire populations for this unique characteristic and then links this characteristic with some other feature in the population, for example, age, diet, or gender. Ecologic studies use aggregate data in which no information is contained about individual persons, but only for groups. Cancer mortality and proximity to petrochemical plants (46), multiple sclerosis mortality and nutrition and latitude (47), and dental caries and community risk factors (48) are examples of ecologic studies. Each identifies a characteristic in a population (cancer mortality, multiple sclerosis mortality, and dental caries, respectively) and attempts to relate it to another characteristic (proximity to petrochemical plants, nutrition and latitude, and community risk factors, respectively).

Ecologic studies are relatively cheap, quick, and may use readily available pre-existing data (vital statistics, census information, and so forth). The chief advantage of the ecologic study is that it allows one to draw a relationship between a unique finding in the population and some other characteristic in that population. Specifically, the investigator may determine if the characteristic and feature are related linearly by use of the correlation coefficient (r). The correlation coefficient is a descriptive measure that indicates the strength of the linear relationship between two variables. (A further discussion of correlation coefficients is discussed under question 5.) Jacobsen et al. (49) used an ecologic study to report a relationship between hip fracture rates and exposure to fluoridated water in certain counties in Iowa. They found that communities with a longer duration of exposure to fluoridation had an increase in hip fracture rates. This represents a positive correlation between the two characteristics of interest. When communities with no fluoridation were excluded from the analysis, however, the correlation became negative (i.e., as the time of exposure to fluoridation decreased, the rate of hip fractures increased).

There are three chief disadvantages of ecologic studies. First, the relationships and associations discovered may not be applicable to individuals. For example, in the hip fracture–fluoridation study, the hypothesis was that there was a relationship between exposure to fluoridation and hip fracture rates. Although one of the analyses suggests that individuals with longer exposures to fluoridation may decrease their chances of a hip fracture, it is impossible to tell if the people who experienced a hip fracture were the same people who experienced a decreased exposure to fluoridation.

Second, ecologic studies lack the ability to control for *confounding*. Confounding refers to some factor other than the one(s) being studied that confuses the correct interpretation of the data; a confounder is, in some way, associated with both factors being studied (50). For example, there was a strong correlation between hip fracture rate and length of exposure to fluoridation. However, what remains unknown is if confounders such as age, nutritional status, smoking habits, and environmental conditions (ice, snow) played a role in the relationship between hip fracture rate and fluoridation. It is not possible to obtain this type of information from an ecologic study. For this reason, the presence (or absence) of statistical significance in ecologic studies must be viewed cautiously. As succinctly put by Hennekens and Buring (33) in their discussion of ecologic studies, "the presence of a correlation does not necessarily imply the presence of a valid statistical association. Conversely, the lack of a correlation in such studies does not necessarily imply the absence of a valid statistical association."

Finally, associations encountered in ecologic studies represent average exposures for the population, not individual values. Therefore, it is not possible to link a risk factor and disease in an individual person. For example, the average exposure to fluoridation in the hip fracture study is for the population and does not represent the actual exposure to fluoridation for any individual.

Synthetic Evaluations

Other types of *descriptive* studies frequently found in the medical literature are *synthetic evaluations*. Synthetic evaluations encompass a variety of techniques that interpret and integrate information obtained from primary descriptive and explanatory research (51). Synthetic evaluations include *decision analysis, cost-effective analysis, cost-benefit analysis, cost-identification studies, consensus statement papers,* and *current concepts* or *review articles*. Although the consensus statements, current concepts, and review articles are not generally characterized by a study question, a study question does generally distinguish various cost analyses and decision analyses.

Consensus Statements

Consensus statements are reports from a group of recognized experts from various fields related to a particular problem or concern. These experts come together to discuss and share experiences to form a group opinion or consensus. For example, in 1997 the American College of Sports Medicine presented a position statement on the Female Athlete Triad (52). This paper describes a syndrome occurring in young females and women who are physically active; it includes eating disorders, amenorrhea, and osteoporosis as a result of pressure to achieve unrealistically low body weight. This consensus statement by the American College of Sports Medicine describes a particular pattern of behaviors in these athletes and recommends a treatment plan.

Current Concepts and Review Articles

Review articles are intended to bring clinicians up to date on the state of the art of diagnosis, treatment, and medical or surgical management of patients. For example, in 1997 Wolf et al. (53) presented a review of amenorrhea in adolescent and adult female athletes. They summarized 36 related published articles and identified a potentially widespread problem of exploitation of young female athletes.

The advantage of review articles is that they are comprehensive, presenting a great deal of information from many sources in a condensed format, and saving the reader the time and effort of a literature search. Pitfalls of reviews include biases in selection of articles comprising the review and biases in interpretations brought by the author. Finally, be wary of reviews in "meta-analysis clothing." *Meta-analysis* is a distinct statistical overview and is not equivalent to a review (see A Special Case: Meta-analysis, under question 2).

Decision Analysis

Decision analysis is a set of techniques and strategies for modeling clinical decision making in the presence of uncertainty. It is an exercise in model building that allows the investigator to make a reasoned systematic decision so that readers may see how various opinions and uncertainty are combined in an explicit process. Information for the model is obtained from primary research findings in the medical literature. One characteristic of this type of analysis is that the problem is structured explicitly using a flow diagram or decision tree. The decision tree incorporates probabilities associated with different actions. Outcomes on decision trees are called utilities and reflect preferences for a combination of actions and events that lead to various outcomes. Because decision analysis is based on many assumptions, the investigator will conduct several analyses based on

variations of these assumptions to test the robustness of the model. In addition, decision analysis may consider economic factors such as direct and indirect costs. Decision analysis does not necessarily result in one best answer, because, in the face of uncertainty, there may not be an optimal decision. Rather, decision analysis can provide insight into the choices that must be made when outcomes are uncertain and risks are unavoidable (54).

Cost-effectiveness Analysis

Cost-effectiveness analysis is one of several types of economic analyses in which the investigator applies the tools of economics to the practice of medicine to examine and improve choices for health resource allocation. Physicians routinely make choices between interventions that cost more or less than comparative interventions that vary in their effectiveness. The most expensive intervention may or may not be the most effective for the greatest number of people. Because there are not enough resources to provide all the medical care that is technically possible, trade-offs and choices must be made. Cost-effectiveness analysis includes both the expected gain in healthy outcomes and the use of limited resources for individual patients to be used as a guide to medical decision making. The distinguishing feature of this type of economic analysis is that the health outcomes are converted to standardized units so that the value of various outcomes may be compared for various strategies. The standardized units are called utilities. Techniques for determining utilities include time trade-off, standard gamble, and ranking. A common method for expressing utilities in a cost-effectiveness analysis is quality-adjusted life-years or QALYs. Cost-effectiveness analysis compares the net cost of a health care intervention with a standardized measure of effectiveness, such as life-years saved or reduction in mortality rates (55).

Cost-Benefit Analysis

Cost-benefit analysis, in contrast to cost-effectiveness analysis, explicitly assesses whether the health outcomes are worth the cost (56). This is accomplished by measuring both the health care intervention and the health outcome in the same units. This generally means valuing the health outcome in currency. The cost-benefit analysis then compares intervention with outcomes "in terms of moneys lost to pay for a health care intervention compared with moneys gained from the use of an intervention" (55).

Cost-identification Studies

Unlike cost-effectiveness and cost-benefit analyses, a *cost-identification study* only identifies the costs of providing medical services with the implicit assumption that all medical outcomes considered in the study are equivalent. The goal of cost-identification studies is to find the least costly way of achieving an outcome; cost identification does not evaluate what the moneys spent may lead to in terms of health outcomes. Despite titles containing cost-effectiveness or cost-benefit, most studies in the sports medicine literature are really cost-identification studies.

It is important to note that these analyses rely on the use of primary research in their assumptions and models. In addition, the perspective taken (society's, the patient's, the physician's, or the insurance company's) will affect the results of the analysis. All economic analyses use specific terminology, and the words *effectiveness* and *benefit* have very specific economic meanings and should not be used interchangeably within the context of these analyses. In addition, how costs are determined in a particular study should be explicitly defined by the author because it greatly influences the ability of the reader to generalize findings of the analyses to individual practices, geographic locales, and institutions. Specific resources and guidelines for evaluating economic analyses in health and medicine are provided in Appendix 1.

Explanatory Designs

The distinguishing feature between descriptive and explanatory designs is the use of comparison. *Explanatory research designs* apply the strategy of comparison to examine etiology, cause, or efficacy of interventions (21,57). Explanatory studies are characterized by two major approaches: *observational or experimental.*

Observational Designs

In both observational studies and experimental studies, the investigator is seeking causes, predictors, or better treatments. The experimental study is characterized by the active manipulation by the investigator of an intervention or treatment. In the observational study, the investigator is relegated to the role of bystander and "observes nature" (21). There is no active manipulation of a treatment or intervention by the investigator. The investigator gathers information from a variety of sources such as vital statistics, census data, medical records, patients, health events, and so forth and then provides insights into the causes of disease or injury by making comparisons. Examples of observational study design include *cohort, case-control, and cross-sectional designs.*

Cohort Designs

The *cohort study* is also known as an *incidence study. Incidence* is the proportion of persons in a population who get a disease or injury for the first time during a specified period of time. All individuals in the population being studied are free of the disease of interest at the start of the study. (Incidence is distinguished from *prevalence*, which refers to the proportion of persons who already have the given disease at a specified point or period of time, divided by the number of individuals in the total population.) A cohort design is one in which the researcher starts with a group of people (cohort) who are free of disease or injury and then follows them over time to see if the subjects develop the disease or injury. Within the cohort, some subjects have been exposed to a particular risk factor and others have not. The subsequent incidence of the disease in both groups may be compared and attributed to the exposure. Researchers then may calculate the *relative risk* of developing a condition given the risk factor. The relative risk is the ratio of the incidence of the disease (or outcome of interest) in the group who have the risk factor compared with the incidence of the disease in the group who does not have the risk factor.

For example, in 1997 Kushi et al. (58) reported the results of a cohort study in which the outcome of interest was mortality from all causes and the exposure was physical activity. The cohort consisted of 40,417 postmenopausal women who were followed for 7 years. There were 2,260 all-cause deaths during this time period. The incidence of death in those women who reported no regular physical activity was 1,518 deaths per 157,379 person-years. Among those women who reported regular physical activity, the incidence was 742 deaths per 111,811 person-years. To diminish bias, investigators excluded women who reported baseline heart disease or cancer and who died in the first 3 years of follow-up. After adjustment for potential confounders, "women who reported regular physical activity were at a significantly reduced risk of death" (58). The relative risk was 0.77 (95% confidence interval, 0.66, 0.90). A relative risk of 0.77 indicates a protective effect of physical activity in this cohort. (A relative risk equal to 1.0 would have indicated an equivalent risk for mortality in both groups, and a relative risk greater than 1.0 would have indicated that increased physical activity was a risk factor for mortality.)

As this example illustrates, the main strength of a cohort study design is that it provides a powerful strategy for defining incidence of death, injury, disease, or any other outcome of interest defined by the investigators. Because the cohort study is a prospective study, the investigator has the opportunity to measure variables completely and accurately. This is particularly helpful if an investigator wants to accurately establish events that precede the outcome of interest; cohort studies can establish that the exposure or risk factor (e.g., lack of physical activity) indeed preceded the development of the outcome of interest (e.g., death).

Being able to identify the temporal sequence of events strengthens interpretations that the risk factor may cause the disease (59). For this reason, cohort designs are particularly good for studying rare exposures or risk factors.

Unfortunately, because the subjects in a cohort study are disease free at the time of entry into the study, they must be followed for a long enough period of time to develop the disease. That is, for meaningful comparisons to be made, the period of follow-up must be long enough to allow an adequate number of subjects to develop the outcome (33). As a result, cohort studies may be very expensive. Also, cohort designs are not appropriate for the study of rare diseases or conditions (even though they are great for studying rare exposures).

Case-Control

Investigators use case-control designs when they want to identify potential causes of some outcome of interest such as disease or injury. The investigator compares risk factors in a group of subjects (cases) with the outcome of interest to a group of subjects (controls) without the outcome. If the cases are determined to have a higher risk factor than the controls, this may suggest an association between exposure and outcome. For example, in 1997 Schieber et al. (60) reported the results of a case-control study examining the effectiveness of safety gear in preventing in-line skating injuries. The study sample was comprised of persons who sustained injuries from in-line skating and who sought medical attention at 1 of 91 hospital emergency departments that participated in the National Electronic Injury Surveillance System. Cases comprised those people who had injuries to the wrist, elbow, knee, or head. Controls were those skaters who suffered injuries to other parts of the body. The exposure was defined as protective safety gear consisting of knee pads, wrist guards, and helmets.

Advantages of case-control studies are that they save time, are relatively inexpensive to conduct, are appropriate for study of rare diseases or conditions (including diseases with long latency periods), and they allow the study of several risk factors or exposures simultaneously. Although case-control designs are good for rare diseases or outcomes, they are not appropriate for rare risk factors. And because the investigator selects cases based on the presence of the disease or condition, the researcher cannot obtain direct measures of incidence or prevalence. However, in case-control studies the investigator can calculate the odds of having a risk factor among the cases and the odds of having a risk factor among the controls. The ratio between these two odds is the *odds ratio*. For example, using the in-line skating data presented in Fig. 8.3, we can calculate that the odds of not wearing wrist guards among all the cases (who

	Cases	Controls
Wrist guard not worn	2 317	1 577
Wrist guard worn	154	1 356

FIG. 8.3. Wrist guard protection among cases and controls. (From ref #60.)

sustained wrist injuries) is 2,317/154 or 15.0; the odds of not wearing wrist guards among all the controls (who did not sustain wrist injuries) is 1,577/1,356 or 1.16. The odds ratio or the ratio between these two odds is 15.0/1.16 or 12.9. This odds ratio is interpreted as follows: The odds of developing a wrist injury if a skater was not wearing wrist guards is 12.9 times more likely than it is among skaters who did wear wrist guards. (The 95% confidence interval with this odds ratio is 4.5, 37.1. The association between not wearing wrist guards and sustaining a wrist injury is statistically significant using the chi-square test, $P < 0.001$.)

Case-control studies are particularly prone to both *selection bias and recall bias*. In case-control studies, the injury or disease and the exposure have already occurred at the time of selection or entry into the study. *Selection bias* is present because cases and controls have the potential for being selected differentially. For example, the investigator may unwittingly select sicker cases and healthier controls for the study. Or the investigator may select the cases that are the easiest to enroll, or cases that have the most information available. How the cases were chosen may affect the generalizability of the study. *Recall bias* may be likely in case-control studies because these studies are retrospective and must rely on differential recording of events in the medical records. Equivalent information may not be available for both cases and controls or it may not be of the same quality. Further, the investigator may be relying on the recall of the cases and controls, and both of these groups may be subject to recall biases. Although the potential for bias is real, it does not necessarily mean that the study is invalid. When evaluating a study that uses a case-control design, note whether the authors have considered the potential for bias in their study and how they have attempted to minimize or avoid these biases. Where bias cannot be avoided, how have the investigators discussed the impact of such biases on study conclusions? (Issues of bias are discussed further at the end of question 2.)

Cross-sectional Designs

Cross-sectional (or *prevalence*) studies examine a sample from a well-defined population for the presence of an existing disease, injury, or characteristic of interest. (Remember, *prevalence* is distinguished from *incidence,* which refers to the number of new cases of disease, injury, or characteristic of interest that develop during a specified period of time; prevalence refers to the *totality* of cases extant at a point in time.) The investigator in a cross-sectional study makes all the study measurements on a single occasion (59). Because this design provides information about prevalence, cross-sectional designs are particularly useful for planning how health resources should be allocated. Along with providing information about what disease or injury states are present at the point in time of interest, cross-sectional designs are also used to compare the presence or absence of disease or injury to one or more other variables (i.e., risk factors) at this same point in time (61). For example, in 1996 Williams (62) reported the results of a cross-sectional study investigating the relationship between high-density-lipoprotein (HDL) cholesterol levels and other risk factors for coronary heart disease in female runners. Subjects were recruited from national races and from a major running magazine; 1,837 female runners consented to complete a questionnaire on demographic characteristics, running history, weight history, menstrual history, hormone use, diet, tobacco use, family history of cancer and heart disease, and medications. In addition, these women agreed to allow investigators to obtain information from their physicians on such items as height, weight, plasma cholesterol and triglyceride concentrations, blood pressure, and resting heart rate. Specifically, the investigators compared the number of kilometers run per week (as reported by the women) with the HDL cholesterol levels reported by their physicians. The authors concluded that risk factors for coronary heart disease tend to be decreased in women who run greater distances. That is, incremental increases in exercise were associated with significant increases in HDL cholesterol and estimated reductions in coronary heart disease risk.

A major strength of the cross-sectional study is that it is relatively fast and inexpensive and there is no follow-up of subjects required. Although a cross-sectional study may reveal associations between risk factors and disease, a weakness of this design is that we cannot be sure which of these two comes first. That is, because risk factor and disease are studied at the same point in time, we cannot discern if the risk factor preceded the development of the disease or if the disease somehow affected a person's level of risk (33). For example, in the cross-sectional study of female runners, a reduction in the risk of heart disease is associated with greater distances run. However, we cannot be absolutely certain that a decrease in risk factors is a result of running. As the authors emphasize, "the cross-sectional associations in this report do not prove that running greater distances causes these reductions in risk factors" (62). It is possible that women with high HDL cholesterol may have chosen to run greater distances.

Experimental Designs

If the investigator manipulates the treatment or intervention, then the design is *experimental.* The main purpose of an experimental design is to provide understanding of scientific etiologies, treatment effects, hypothesis generation or clarification, and the refinement of causal relationships (57). Experimental designs may evaluate efficacy of therapeutic, educational, or administrative interventions, but the hallmark of this design is that the investigator actively manipulates the intervention. That is, whether the intervention is a surgical procedure, a drug, an educational method, or a prevention strategy, the assignment of subjects to the intervention is under the control of the investigator. The *randomized clinical trial* (RCT) uses an experimental research design.

Randomized Clinical Trial

In the RCT, members of a population are randomly assigned to a treatment or a control group. Both groups are then followed prospectively to see whether the groups subsequently differ on prespecified outcomes of interest. The RCT is considered the optimal standard of all research designs and capable of providing the most reliable evidence in research studies (8,33,59,63,64). The unique feature of randomization of subjects provides the basis for statistical significance tests at the end of the trial; randomization, on average, controls for all other factors (known and unknown) that might affect the outcome between subjects in the treatment and control groups, providing strong evidence for causal effects of the intervention; it is particularly the control of unknown factors that makes the RCT such an optimum research design (33). Readers should note, however, that randomization does not mean "haphazard" assignment, but rather that all subjects in the trial have an equal likelihood of being assigned to a group; a true random allocation should be outlined in the Methods and Materials section of the article, and the author should demonstrate that the allocation is tamper proof (59) (see question 3).

Another characteristic of the RCT that further strengthens the investigator's ability to draw causal inferences is *blinding or masking.* Blinding refers to participants in the study being unaware of treatment assignments. A study may be single blind (the subject does not know the treatment assignment) or double blind (neither the subject nor the investigator knows the treatment assignment). Blinding minimizes sources of bias and of confounding in studies. It is important to note that many studies cannot include blinding, for example, surgical trials (see question 4 for a discussion of blinding).

An example of an RCT is that reported by Brink et al. (65) in 1996. Stable lateral malleolar fractures were treated with two types of commercial braces. Sixty-six consecutive subjects were randomized using a random numbers table. Because of the highly visible nature of the treatment, blinding was not possible for the participants in this study. The authors concluded that either brace may be recommended because 3 months after injury "no differences were observed in grade of ambulation, pain, swelling, range of motion, or inflammatory score."

The major advantage of the RCT is that compared with all other study designs, it may produce the strongest evidence for cause and effect (59). There are, however, limitations to this design. Some important questions cannot be addressed by RCTs because outcomes are too rare. In addition, there may be ethical barriers (toxic or harmful side effects of treatment, treatment during pregnancy, and so forth). RCTs are very expensive, both in time and money. And finally, even the best controlled RCT is not able to prevent all sources of bias and confounding because not every behavior of the subject and investigator may be totally regulated by the study design (50).

A Special Case: Meta-analysis

"Meta-analysis is a collection of methods for combining information from single investigations for the purpose of reaching conclusions or addressing questions that were not possible on the basis of single investigations" (23). Meta-analysis is a distinct statistical overview using data from previous studies, which are generally small randomized clinical trials. These data are then pooled (66), and conclusions are drawn from the combined results. Such conclusions are not possible in the smaller studies by themselves because these smaller studies frequently lack sample size to detect meaningful differences. It is important to note that meta-analysis is not a review of the literature, with all studies on a particular subject synthesized for the reader in one concise report. Rather, meta-analysis uses specific exclusion criteria for studies, pools subjects, and uses specialized statistical techniques to determine outcome and treatment effects. Sachs et al. (66) list four purposes for meta-analysis: to increase the statistical power of studies to find meaningful differences, to resolve uncertainty when research studies show different findings, to improve effect size estimates, and to explore findings not specified at the beginning of individual trials.

For example, in 1995 Welton et al. (67) reported a meta-analysis of the effect of calcium on bone mass. The authors conducted this study because they believed that results of individual published reports of the relationship between bone mass and dietary calcium in young adults were inconsistent. They assessed the published reports from 1966 through 1994 on calcium intake and bone mass density in premenopausal women and adult men between the ages of 18 and 50. The quality of each study was evaluated. Those studies judged to be well designed based on predetermined objective criteria were combined and the data pooled to determine the effect of calcium intake on bone mass in men and women aged 18 to 50 years old. The authors concluded that those studies pooled in the meta-analysis seemed to offer overall evidence that calcium intake was positively associated with bone mass in premenopausal females. (There were too few studies of men [three] for meta-analysis to draw conclusions about men.)

The chief advantage of meta-analysis is that it may permit the investigators to detect meaningful effects of treatment by pooling many patients to create larger sample sizes in which true effects may be discovered. Thus, meta-analysis holds great promise for adding precision and power to estimates of treatment effects (21). However, the quality of the results of a meta-analysis relies heavily on the quality of the studies included. Studies combined should be similar in regard to diagnostic criteria, clinical severity, therapies or treatment rendered, and uniform outcome measures (21,33). For example, in the meta-analysis of the effect of calcium intake on bone mass, studies that included both perimenopausal and postmenopausal women were appropriately excluded; likewise, studies that included men and women but did not include a separate analysis for each gender were also excluded. If the investigators had included these latter studies they may have had dissimilar subjects and treatment in the meta-analysis—oranges and apples—resulting in a potentially distorted interpretation of a questionable effect.

We have stressed that a good study design is one that is not only appropriate to answer the study question but is also unbiased. How can we tell if a study is unbiased? To begin, bias is any systematic error in the design or conduct of a study (33,68). Bias can invalidate study results because it may cause us to see relationships, associations, and causation when none really exist. Although there are many kinds of bias, there are common sources of which we should be aware as we evaluate study designs and their potential to answer the study questions posed.

Selection Bias

This type of bias occurs when the criteria for entry into the study are different or noncomparable between groups. For example, the study group may be sicker than the control group, so that the chance for improvement after treatment is greater in the study group.

Researcher Bias

When researchers are combing the medical records of patients whom they know, looking in past histories for risk factors contributing to illness or injuries, which may also be known to the researcher, the investigators' objectivity may be suspect (21).

Recall Bias

This is a type of subject bias that may be present when groups of subjects are asked to recall events, and one group "remembers differently" than the other. Individuals with a particular exposure or injury are likely to remember their experiences differently from those who do not have this exposure or injury (33). The recall of subjects and controls may differ in both amount and accuracy (69). For example, mothers asked to recall pregnancy events before the birth of a child who has a birth defect may remember more exposures to potentially hazardous events (and a greater number of such events) than women with children without this birth defect.

Social Desirability Bias

This is another type of subject bias that occurs when subjects want to give the researcher "the right answer" for various reasons relating to "perceived good" or socially desirable behavior on the part of the patient. Such reasons might be a genuine concern that the investigator succeed, an interest in supporting research in important areas of study, and just wanting to feel good about having given a perceived "correct" answer. Also, this type of bias can be the result of perceived fear of retribution from the researcher if a particular answer is not forthcoming. The physician may be acting as researcher, but the subject is still a patient of the physician. The patient may fear giving the correct answer to the researcher because the correct answer is contrary to what the physician has recommended. For example, suppose the physician has recommended that a patient stop smoking, but the patient has not stopped smoking. The patient is participating in a study and is asked whether he or she smokes. The patient may not answer the question truthfully if he or she does not want the physician to know the truth, or if the patient in some way feels that his or her care will be affected by giving the truthful answer.

It is important to recognize that all studies may be affected by bias. We should expect researchers to identify potential sources of bias in their study design and to describe methods used to minimize or avoid this bias. It is more important to understand the concept of bias than it is to know the specific definition of every potential source of bias. We should assess not only whether the potential for bias exists but also the likelihood that its occurrence will affect the study results and conclusions (21). The presence of bias does not necessarily invalidate the results of a study, but conclusions and interpretations must be guarded. Readers should be skeptical if no discussion of design limitations is present in the paper.

We have presented various strategies to help the reader discern ways in which investigators design studies to answer specific research questions. These examples are meant to give the reader a taste of what study design is all about. Suggestions for further reading on this subject are included in Appendix 1. In summary, studies that are descriptive answer questions that provide new or additional information about a condition or disease or injury. They provide helpful information characterizing patterns of disease or injury and help to generate hypotheses for future studies. Another type of descriptive paper is the synthetic review. These reviews either serve to summarize findings from other descriptive studies or explanatory research or present information in fresh ways to assist in clinical decision making or policy-making. Explanatory studies are differentiated from descriptive studies by use of comparisons to answer the study question. Explanatory studies may be further categorized into observational and experimental, with the chief difference being that investigators in observational studies do not manipulate a key variable in the study.

Researchers may use a combination of design strategies to answer the study question. The choice of design may be influenced by time and money available, particular features of the injury or condition being studied, and the experiences of other investigators and reported research. The research design should be described by the authors in sufficient detail so that the reader is able to evaluate whether the study question may be answered using this design. Readers should consider the potential limitations of the study design and determine if these limitations may have an effect on the study conclusion and interpretation.

Question 2 Bottom Line

Was the chosen research design adequate to answer the study question? Were potential flaws or limitations inherent in the study design addressed by the authors? How might such weaknesses in the design affect study conclusions and inferences?

QUESTION 3: HOW IS THE SAMPLE SELECTED?

Assume that the study under review has a well-formulated study question and reflects good research design. The next question is, did the authors describe how the subjects for the study and control groups were selected?

It is important to know what the sample source for the study is. Readers should be able to determine from the Materials and Methods section of the article who the subjects were, why they were selected, where they came from, how they were recruited, and what sampling method was used to choose them. This information is important for two reasons. The reader should be able to first discern the underlying population that the study patients represent and second determine whether the study sample resembles the reader's clinical practice well enough that study findings can be generalized to it (9,30). Too often studies do not include the types of patients physicians see in clinical practice (70). And if the inclusion criteria and exclusion criteria are not specified (or are not clearly stated), the reader does not know whether the findings are generalizable to anyone but those people in the study sample (6). A statement of exclusion criteria is not simply restating the inclusion criteria in a negative fashion. An explicit statement of exclusion criteria permits the reader to evaluate the homogeneity of the sample, to decide if there are specific subsets of patients to which the study findings should not be extrapolated, and to determine with some degree of assurance that patient safety has been considered (30). "Male subjects, 18 years or older, and in good health" is a statement of inclusion criteria, whereas exclusion criteria for this same study might be "subjects requiring occasional use of inhaled steroids."

Control groups or comparison groups are often important parts of a study. They allow a researcher to compare findings in a study group with findings in a group that is very much like the study group, except for the treatment or condition of interest. If using a control group, the researcher should specify whether it is a concurrent, historical, or placebo control group. The researcher should also provide information that demonstrates that the control group is equivalent to the study group.

Assessing the process by which the study sample was selected is a very important part of study evaluation, because sample selection provides an opportunity to create, distort, or minimize potential bias. Study findings may be questionable if bias is present, because neither the reader nor the researcher can know for certain whether study conclusions are due to real differences between groups, due to biases in assignment to study treatments (selection bias), or due to biases in how the data are obtained (information bias) (22,61). The reader can evaluate how the sample was selected and how the study information was gathered to determine the effect of bias on study conclusions. Two chief ways that researchers try to minimize bias is through *randomization and blinding.*

Randomization ensures that the study groups are equivalent before introducing study treatments (71). It permits the investigators to establish equivalency be-

tween study groups so that the only difference between the groups is the treatment. If the patients were randomized, then the mechanism for generating the randomization schedule should be described. This assures the reader that the randomization is reliable. For example, were patients randomized by a coin toss, sealed envelopes, or random numbers generation? The word "random" has specific statistical meaning. Too often investigators equate the term random with "haphazard" and then proceed to haphazardly assign treatments to patients. The statistical meaning of the word random is that every subject has an independent and equal chance of being assigned to available treatments. Using methods such as coin tosses, birthdays, sealed envelopes, or zip codes appears to be reasonable, but such methods are easily interfered with (wittingly or unwittingly) and cannot always be verified if questions about them arise later (9). If study subjects were not randomized but instead volunteered or were part of a convenience sample, then the reader needs to consider whether this study sample is representative of the patients that are seen in his or her clinical practice (72). In nonrandomized studies, the reader needs to keep in mind that treatment outcomes may be affected by factors that are unrelated to the treatment (8).

Blinding (or masking) is another important tool the researcher can use to minimize bias. Although blinding is reported in many trials, it should be described sufficiently to let the reader know specifically who was blinded (9). For example, the study patients, the investigators, or the person making the final study assessment may all be blinded to treatment assignment. A study that is described as a single blind or double blind without regard to who actually was blinded leaves the reader guessing.

Finally, the size of the sample needs to be considered. Are there enough study subjects in the sample to detect a difference in treatments if a real difference exists? The investigators should describe power analysis and sample size estimates in their Materials and Methods section. Unfortunately, most trials do not specify an intended sample size (9). In addition, many times investigators do not discuss what an important (clinically meaningful) effect size might be for a study. We often see something like the following: "We studied 58 consecutive patients over a 2-year period." Where did this number come from and why did the authors stop at 58? What did the investigators hope to discover from these patients?

When there has been no power analysis and the investigators have concluded no statistical differences between groups, the reader is left to answer one of two questions: Was there, in fact, no difference or was the sample size simply too small to detect important differences (9)? A power analysis provides some degree of assurance that a type II error has not been committed.

(A type II error is failing to reject the null hypothesis when the null hypothesis is incorrect.) Even when there is a statistically significant finding, in the absence of a power analysis, the reader has no idea whether study results were reported at an arbitrary point because the data were analyzed at various points in time until a difference was found, or the study failed to achieve an intended sample size and the investigators decided to report findings anyway, or the study was extended beyond the intended recruitment for sample size to achieve better statistical power (7).

Question 3 Bottom Line

What was the source of the study sample? Were the eligibility and exclusion criteria clearly defined? Was the sample representative? Were randomization and blinding techniques used to reduce potential study bias? Was sample size projected through a power analysis?

QUESTION 4: WHAT BACKGROUND INFORMATION IS PRESENTED IN EACH OF THE STUDY AND CONTROL GROUPS?

Assume that the study under review has a well-formulated question, was well designed, and its sample assignment was well described. Now we must ask, did the authors provide summary results for each group studied? Before comparisons (statistical tests) can be made between the study group and control group, the researcher must assess the relevant characteristics and outcomes for each group. Observations and evidence gathered to answer the study question must be reliable and accurate so that any analyses conducted are relevant. This assessment precedes the statistical analysis. At this point, the reader should not necessarily be interested in whether the descriptive data answer the study question but rather are the outcomes of interest clear and concisely expressed and are they valid? For example, we are concerned with whether characteristics such as age, health status, gender, sociodemographics, and important outcome variables are clearly defined and measured consistently and accurately. In particular, we are interested in knowing how the investigators measured important variables. That is, are all measurement results reported appropriately? Have the investigators ensured the quality of the measurements and outcomes for each group, and what quality control measures have been used to ensure the reliability of these measures?

For example, suppose a researcher conducted an RCT of the effect of a particular drug on the outcome of plantar fasciitis in male recreational athletes. The outcome of interest is improvement in plantar fasciitis in two groups of men with and without drug treatment. There are two things that the researcher needs to demonstrate. First, the researcher needs to show that both groups indeed had plantar fasciitis. The diagnosis could be ascertained by physical examination, patient report, or some combination of these two. The researcher needs to establish that these two methods are part of generally accepted medical practice (standardized in some way). Second, the investigator needs to establish that the diagnosis is made consistently by each investigator in the study, that is, that the measurements themselves are reliable.

Reliability is a fundamental concept that characterizes measurement error. Some error, either systematic or random, is inherent in any measurement (73,74). The author needs to assure the reader that measurement error represents only a small fraction of the range of observations in a study. One way to do this is to contrast the degree of expected variation (biologic) among subjects with the expected subject variation plus the measurement error using *repeated-measures analysis of variance* (ANOVA). (ANOVA is discussed in further detail in question 5.) The total variance is derived using algebraic manipulations and results in a reliability coefficient that is the ratio of variance between patients to variance between patients plus error variance. This is one expression of an *intraclass correlation coefficient.* For example, if the reliability coefficient for a particular measurement score was 0.91, then the interpretation is that 91% of the variability in the scores results from true variation among the patients. The rest is measurement error.

There are two sources of measurement error. First, there is the error that occurs when a single observer or rater is measuring an item more than once. There are specific tests for determining how well the single rater is able to repeat the measurement of the item and "agree" with his or her original measure. These tests represent *intrarater or intraobserver reliability.* Second, there is also the error that results when two or more observers or raters are measuring the same item. Specific tests for determining how close the raters agree with one another in measuring the same item result in values that summarize *interrater or interobserver reliability.* Such measures of reliability or agreement are the *kappa coefficient, the weighted kappa, Cronbach's alpha,* and the methods proposed by Bland and Altman (75). If a nonstandard method of measuring is used in any area of the study, the reason why should be given, and the nonstandard method should be clearly described to the reader. What is important is that the author demonstrates that the measurements—upon which statistical tests are based—are reliable. If the measurements are not reliable, then study conclusions and interpretations based on these measurements are also not reliable.

Next, the researcher needs to establish the general characteristics of the recruited study groups to demonstrate that the groups are comparable in important baseline characteristics. Otherwise, we cannot be certain whether the treatment has an effect on the final outcome or whether the final outcome was due to some other underlying difference between study groups. In the planar fasciitis study, for example, did symptoms improve because of the treatment or because some patients never had plantar fasciitis in the first place? The investigators need to demonstrate that they are obtaining and measuring key characteristics in standard and reliable ways and that results are reproducible. Note that we have not yet addressed whether the study findings are statistically significant but rather whether the study findings are believable in terms of diagnosis, measurement of important variables, and agreement among study investigators. This is referred to as *internal validity*. Internal validity establishes for the readers and investigators alike that the study findings have been measured in such a way as to be true of the study subjects (61). (External validity, on the other hand, is present when the study findings can be generalized to persons not studied; see question 8.)

After deciding that methods for measuring important subject characteristics and key outcomes are made reliably and represent standard practice, the reader should look for a summary of patient characteristics, check for internal consistencies in numeric quantities, review the data for correct counts, and compare baseline values among study groups (76). We want to know what happened to everyone. First, note if the *response rate* is reported. The response rate is the number of patients who have agreed to participate from the larger group of eligible patients. Is there something different about the nonresponders? Are they sicker or healthier then those who agreed to participate? Researchers should account for all study patients. If study subjects are dropped from the analysis or subjects are lumped together in groups, the rationale should be given and the reader should evaluate how this affects the reliability and the generalizability of the study. Failure to report data can be a simple oversight. It can also be intentional if an investigator wants to obscure unfavorable results. Readers are urged to be suspicious, to be skeptical, and to bear in mind that it is their right to consider the latter when the author does not explain missing data (8,19,76). Were there dropouts? Did a high proportion of patients complete treatment? How compliant were patients with treatment? Were side effects or complications (both anticipated or unanticipated) reported? Were there any deaths? Were data missing for any reason? All of this information should be described by the investigators.

Finally, is all the evidence summarized well? Most authors will present some form of graphic report summarizing data. Tables and graphs contain statistics that summarize data, not necessarily answer questions (19). Tables help readers to form their own opinions from the recorded observations, to define their own questions, and to see "exceptions and individual peculiarities, so fundamental to medicine" (77). It is unrealistic to expect researchers to present all the raw data from their study. Instead, the reader should look for a few concise tables with supporting text (78). Tables should contain a careful reporting of units (e.g., kilograms or pounds) and frequencies, percentiles, or percentages (percentages should always be reported in such a way that the denominator can be determined easily) (79); the mean and standard deviation (SD) for appropriate variables should also be summarized. The SD is particularly important because it represents variability of the sample. Without variability, the reader can have difficulty interpreting the mean and estimating effect size of the study.

One important source of confusion to readers and authors alike is the difference between reporting *standard deviation and standard error of the mean* (SEM). The *SD* is the most commonly reported measure of variability seen in the literature. We can tell a great deal about the variability in the sample by the size of the SD. For a normally distributed variable, 95% of the observations in a population, on average, will fall within two SDs of the mean value of the observations. For example, if we say that the mean weight for 20 tenth grade boys on the lacrosse team was 140 ± 4 pounds (mean ± SD), we could surmise that about 95% of the boys' weights were between 132 and 148 pounds. The SD is specific to the sample in the particular study. The *SEM* (or commonly seen as *standard error or SE*), on the other hand, is a measure of the variability from statistic to statistic, usually from mean to mean (i.e., variation from sample to sample). The SEM provides an estimate of how the sample value means vary from sample to sample. The SEM is calculated by dividing the SD by the square root of the sample size, *n*. The SEM is used in calculations for Student's *t* tests, ANOVA, confidence intervals, regression, and so forth. The calculation for SEM indicates why mathematically the SEM will always be smaller than the SD. For example, in the lacrosse example, the SE is 0.89 pounds compared with the SD, which is 4 pounds. Authors who report a finding as a mean ± SEM rather than the mean ± SD may be trying to minimize the reader's ability to easily perceive a great deal of variability in the study data (80). Regardless of intent, this is a common error in the medical literature (2). Readers should be aware of the appropriate presentation of descriptive statistics.

Even if study methods are flawless and data are presented and summarized well, there is still plenty of potential for the distortion of study results (8). As discussed, distorting influences include problems with response rate, loss to follow-up, compliance, reliability, validity, and so forth. Generally authors will address these problems in terms of study limitations and offer explanations for why the study findings are still credible or why the influence of such distortions is only minimal. However, this is not always the case, and readers must be prepared to look for such limitations even when they are not identified by the authors. Without looking for a sophisticated statistical analysis, the reader can still determine if the study results are believable and whether these findings represent "truth."

Question 4 Bottom Line

Were the data for the study groups summarized appropriately? Were outcomes and characteristics important to the study question and design measured reliably? Did they seem valid? Were methods presented to indicate how the data quality was ensured? Were study groups comparable in baseline characteristics? Was the response rate reported? Were all patients who entered the study accounted for? Were there any anticipated or unanticipated side effects?

QUESTION 5: WHAT ARE THE STATISTICAL TESTS CHOSEN?

Assume that the study under review has a well-formulated question, reflects good research design, with appropriate sampling techniques, and provides important background information on each of the study groups. The next question is, did the investigators use appropriate statistical methods to evaluate the study question? Statistical techniques play an extremely important role in the planning of a good study. Just as the study design flows from careful consideration of the study question and objectives, the statistical analysis is uniquely determined by the study design (28,81). As emphasized earlier, no amount of clever analysis or "wizardry" by an investigator or statistician will be able to counteract major flaws in the study design (81,82). Statistical errors are common in the medical literature. Some experts report that almost half of published papers having numeric data contain statistical errors or design flaws (2–13). How can we evaluate the appropriateness of the statistical methods? We need to recall the purpose of statistical techniques, identify the type of data collected in the study, and be familiar with the commonly encountered statistical tests and techniques in the sports medicine literature. The mathematical calculations and formulas needed to perform these tests are not essential to the reader's understanding of their appropriateness. (Suggestions for texts containing common statistical tests are provided in Appendix 1.)

The real information in the study lies in the data. The overall purpose in using statistical techniques is to aid in data presentation and interpretation (28). More specifically, researchers use statistics to estimate the strength of relationships and magnitude of differences, for testing statistical significance to draw inferences about a population from information obtained from a sample (taking into consideration the role chance plays),

and to make adjustments for confounding variables on estimates and inferences (23).

Generally, there are two types of statistics: *Descriptive statistics* describe or characterize study samples or populations and *inferential statistics* infer or draw conclusions about populations based on the outcomes from samples studied (80). A study that presents descriptive statistics might include graphs and plots of the measures of central tendency, including the mean, the median, and the mode. It might also include measures of variation such as the range, the variance, the SD and the SE. Inferential statistics, on the other hand, are used to extrapolate information from a sample representative of the larger population. Statistical inference is the performance of statistical tests of significance to determine how well, and with some measure of confidence, the findings in the sample approximate those found in the population at large (80).

The choice of statistical test depends on the study design and the type of data collected. There are four types of data: nominal, ordinal, interval, and ratio data. *Nominal data* represent simple categories—frequently a dichotomy—such as male or female, dead or alive, drug or placebo treatment. Items are organized into mutually exclusive subgroups, so that an individual may belong to one and only one such group. The contingency table in Fig. 8.4 shows an example of how nominal data might be reported.

Ordinal data are ordered by degree of magnitude. There are still mutually exclusive subgroups but there is some inherent order or ranking in the data, and therefore the data must be assessed on a graded scale. For example, patients might be asked to report their pain as absent, mild, moderate, or severe. Other types of data that are ordinal might be surgical outcome (excellent, good, average, fair, poor) or socioeconomic status (low, medium, high). A key distinguishing feature of ordinal data is that distance between the rankings is not necessarily equal between categories. For example, the difference between mild and moderate pain is not necessarily equal to the difference between moderate and severe pain (80).

Interval data also have ordering, but the distance between rankings are equal. That is, as opposed to ordinal

	Ruptured ACL	Intact ACL
Females	154	400
Males	78	525

FIG. 8.4. Display of hypothetical data of anterior cruciate ligament injuries in males and females.

data, the distance between any given value and the next is the same and constant. The numbers have a defined unit of measurement and represent real numbers (80,83). Examples of interval data are the centigrade temperature scale, calendar days, and blood pressure measured in mm Hg. Interval data are what we most commonly see in the medical literature; such data can be either *continuous or discrete*. Discrete data can only be assigned integer values. Number of players injured in a season, heart beats per minute, and goals scored in a game are all examples of discrete data. Continuous data represent the highest degree of quantification. Each point lies somewhere on a continuum with theoretically infinite number of points (23). Examples of continuous data include height, age, and the times recorded in a mile race.

Ratio data are identical to interval data except that ratio data have a true absolute zero point. With ratio data, any two numbers have the same ratio regardless of the scale (83). For example, a basketball player is the same height whether she is measured in inches or feet. Other examples of ratio data are second, minutes, hours or centimeters, meters, kilometers.

Independence is another key characteristic of outcome measurements that the reader needs to consider carefully. It is very important because independence is an assumption required in many statistical tests, and readers should recognize when this assumption is violated. Independence means that the outcome of one measurement is not affected by any other outcome measurement in the study. When the researcher is studying groups of patients, generally the patients are independent. For example, the blood pressure measurement of one patient is not affected by the blood pressure measurement of another patient. However, if multiple observations are made on the same patient, these measurements are not independent—they are *dependent* (84). Consider an example in which a researcher wants to study the effect of a new treatment for knees in 50 patients at four points in time over a 2-year period; the researcher will have a final count of 400 observations. However, these observations are not independent. Violation of the assumption of independence is a frequent occurrence when investigators are studying a body part that happens to be paired. Two shoulders, for example, from the same subject may not be counted as two separate subjects; the shoulders are not independent and interpretations based on statistical tests in which the assumption of independence is violated are invalid.

Statistical tests are based on the general study design, the type of data, whether the data are independent, and whether the data have an underlying Normal (bell-shaped) distribution. Data that fit the criteria of Normality are usually analyzed with *parametric* tests. *Nonparametric* tests are used to analyze data that are based on

less specific assumptions regarding underlying distributions. The following section discusses the most common statistical tests likely to be found in the medical literature. If a little-known test is used, the reader should note if the author has specified why such a test has been used.

Parametric Tests

t Tests

A *one-sample Student's t test* is used when the investigator wants to compare a sample mean value of some variable with a hypothetical population value of this variable. This is accomplished by comparing the difference between the sample mean and this hypothetical population value, relative to the SE. (See discussion of SEM under question 4.) For example, the researcher might be interested in how close (or far) his or her team's mean weight is to the standard weight for high school football players in the country. The appropriate statistical test for this study is the one-sample *t* test (85).

The *independent two-sample t test* compares the mean values between two independent groups. If the researcher wants to compare the mean weight of the football players on two rival teams, the independent two-sample *t* test would be appropriate. Note that the groups are independent because none of the players on one team are also on the rival team. This is the assumption of independence emphasized earlier; it is critical for the two-sample *t* test to be valid. Unfortunately, this assumption is frequently violated. For example, if the investigators in the study of weight in football players compare the mean weight of players before and after the training program and apply the independent *t* test to their findings, the results would be invalid because the two groups of players are not independent—they are the same players measured at two different times (85).

When the samples are not independent, a *paired t test* is required. For example, the paired *t* test measures the difference in the weight of each individual before versus after training and then obtains the mean difference of each player. If the training has no effect, the mean difference in weight pre- and post-training would be zero. If an independent two-sample *t* test had been incorrectly used, the mean weight before and after training would not reflect the paired difference of each individual team member and could possibly result in the investigator erroneously concluding no training effect when there might be one, or vice versa (85).

Analysis of Variance

Analysis of Variance or *ANOVA* is an extension of the *t* test. In fact, when the means between two independent groups are compared, the conclusions from either the *t* test or ANOVA are identical; that is, either test may be used to determine statistical significance. However, ANOVA is used to determine a significant difference in mean values when there are more than two independent sample groups. Specifically, as its name suggests, ANOVA compares two sources of variation in the data. The first source of variation is that which summarizes the variability from mean to mean, that is, variation among groups of observations, or the *between-group variance.* The second source is called the *within-group variance,* representing the variation from individual to individual. ANOVA compares this calculated variance between the means of all the groups in the sample (the between-group variance) with the calculated variance pooled from within each group (the within-group variance). The ratio between these two variances is called the *F ratio or F statistic.* We would expect this ratio to be close to one (1.0) if there is no difference among the groups we are studying. If the F statistic resulting from the ANOVA is significant ($P < 0.05$), then we know that at least one of the group means is different (85).

For example, suppose a coach wants to study the weights of team members by year in school—9th, 10th, 11th, and 12th grade athletes. The weights of players from each of the four groups are measured and an ANOVA is computed for these data. The F statistic is associated with an overall *p* of 0.03: This indicates that at least one of the groups of players has a mean weight that is different from the other group means (85).

However, there is still a problem in the example, because the F statistic does not tell the coach which group mean is different from the other means or if all group means are different from the others, or anything in between. Several *posterior tests* are used to make specific comparisons between all possible pairs of means. For example, the coach can compare 9th to 10th graders, 9th to 11th graders, 9th to 12 graders, 10th to 11th graders, and so forth. Comparing two groups at a time is known as *pairwise comparisons.* The *P* value must be adjusted to account for these comparisons because the more comparisons that are made, the more likely the investigator is to find a statistically significant result due to chance alone. Examples of specific tests that adjust for these multiple comparisons include the *Bonferroni* method, the *Student-Newman-Keuls* procedure, the *Tukey* method, and the *Scheffé* method. The reader should look for these statistical adjustments whenever multiple comparisons are present. Unfortunately, these adjustments are not always made. As a rule of thumb, the reader can take the conventional *P* value of 0.05 and divide it by the number of comparisons made. The resulting number should then reflect the reader's adjusted cutpoint for statistical significance. For example, if there are four comparisons, then $P = 0.05/4$ or 0.0125.

So far this discussion of ANOVA using the example of weight and grade level has been limited to *one-way design or a one-way ANOVA;* this is because there is only one *factor* or characteristic—grade—that is being evaluated. Analyses that include more than one factor (e.g., grade and position played) are also available and may be referred to as *factorial ANOVA,* because more than one factor is being analyzed at the same time. Another type of ANOVA is a *repeated-measures ANOVA.* Repeated-measures ANOVA is used when measurements of the variable of interest are taken more than once for each individual (i.e., when measurements are not independent). For example, if the coach wanted to measure players' weights at several times throughout the season, a repeated-measures ANOVA would be an appropriate test to use.

Correlation and Regression

Correlation analysis gives a unitless number that summarizes the strength between two variables. In a correlation analysis, the investigator measures how two variables' values change together. The statistic that summarizes the strength of a linear relationship between the two variables is called the *correlation coefficient* (*r*). Correlation coefficients range from -1.0 to $+1.0$. The closer the *r* is to $+1.0$, the stronger the positive relationship. Likewise, the closer *r* is to -1.0, the stronger the negative relationship between two variables (86). There are various statistical tests to determine the correlation between two variables depending on distributional assumptions. The most common is the *Pearson product moment correlation,* which requires that the variables are Normal. In fact, this statistical procedure for correlation is so common that when we see a correlation analysis in a study, we can assume that, unless otherwise identified, the correlation test applied was the Pearson product moment correlation (87). Other types of correlation, such as *Spearman's or Kendall's,* are used when we cannot assume Normality for the distribution of variables, and when these types of correlations are used they should be specified by name. As with other statistical tests, there is a *P* value associated with *r.*

Correlation is part of a larger class of statistical techniques known as *regression analysis* (21). For example, in a correlation analysis, the value of the correlation coefficient, *r,* describes the strength of the relationship but not the magnitude of the change between the variables (21). Regression analysis uses the principles just described in correlation, but it does more than just describe the strength of a relationship between two variables. Regression analysis provides information about the magnitude of change between the variables. That is, it considers the effect of one or more variables to predict the change in a particular outcome of interest.[2]

---

[2] The predictor variable is also called the independent variable. The outcome variable is also called the dependent variable.

The relationship between variables and the outcome of interest can be linear or any of a number of other mathematical relationships (i.e., logarithmic, quadratic, and so forth). The slope of the regression line is the *regression coefficient,* and the closer the slope is to zero, the less likely there is a linear relationship between the dependent variable and the independent variable. *Simple linear regression* is characterized by the effect of one variable in predicting one continuous outcome variable. *Multiple regression* allows the investigator to assess the simultaneous effect of multiple variables on one continuous outcome variable. *Logistic regression* assesses the effect of one or more variables on one discrete outcome variable (e.g., life vs. death, injury vs. noninjury). Regression models have overall tests of significance. In many situations this is the F statistic, which has a *P* value associated with it. Individual regression coefficients in logistic and multiple regression analyses also have *P* values associated with all the independent variables in the models. In addition, regression coefficients have SEs, and confidence intervals can be calculated as well.

Frequently, authors will report the value of the *coefficient of determination,* also known as r^2. The coefficient of determination represents the amount (proportion) of the variation of the dependent variable that is associated with the independent variable. Consider an example of a relationship between percent body fat and number of injuries in hockey players and suppose that r^2 is 0.61. This means that 61% of the variation in this model can be accounted for by the relationship between percent body fat and injuries; 39% of the variation present is not accounted for by the relationship of the two variables to each other. That is, the relationship is not a perfect one. Although 61% does not explain as much variation as the researcher might hope, given the great variability within biologic data, this might be as good as the researcher is going to get.

There are several important concepts to be aware of when evaluating an author's report of a regression analysis. First, it is important for the reader to distinguish between r and r^2. Correlation and regression are two related but distinct statistical techniques with two different purposes. Correlation analysis assesses whether and how much the variables are related, whereas regression analysis is used to predict the dependent variable from the independent variable. These analyses result in two descriptors: r, which is a unit-free measure of the strength of a relationship, and r^2, which is useful in interpreting the proportion of variation in the dependent variable that is explained by the relation (regression) with the independent variable. The higher values of r should not be used in lieu of r^2 when making this interpretation in the regression model.

Second, note whether the author reports any outliers. Ideally, the data will be graphed, and outliers can be easily detected. Outliers can have an important impact on the regression equation and hence its interpretation. If outliers were observed, how were they treated in the analysis? Often, the researcher reports the results of analyses with and without outliers, and justification should be provided if outliers are excluded.

Third, authors should not predict relationships that go beyond the data collected. For example, suppose a study is reported of the relationship between age in years and points scored among young basketball players aged 7 to 14, and suppose that a simple regression analysis predicts that on average for each year older the child is, a point is scored. For example, a 7 year old scores five points, an 8 year old scores six points, a 9 year old scores seven points, and so forth up to 14 years old. The authors should not use this model to predict points scored for 17 year olds because they have no way of knowing if the relationship between age and points scored is linear in this range. Also, predictions outside of the range of the data can sometimes give rise to ridiculous figures: Will a 70 year old on average score 75 points? Will a 3 year old score one point? Will a 1 year old score minus one point?

Be clear on the interpretation of the regression model and do not confuse the relationship between the dependent and independent variables. For example, although age may predict the number of points scored in a game, the number of points scored in a game does not necessarily predict how old the player is.

Note that even if a statistical relationship between variables in a regression analysis is strong (large r^2) it does not necessarily indicate that such a relationship is causal (88). In the basketball example, age of players may be associated with higher points scored, but this does not necessarily mean that age causes more points to be scored.

Nonparametric Tests

Pearson Chi-square Test

When the investigator wants to answer questions about frequencies, proportions, or rates, chi-square tests may be used (89). The *Pearson chi-square test* (or simply the chi-square test) is used for determining statistical significance between two categorical variables. The hallmark of the chi-square test is that data are presented in a contingency table characterized by a format of rows (R) and columns (C), called an *R × C table.* Although an R × C table may have any number of rows and columns, the smallest and simplest R × C table is the 2 × 2 table. The chi-square test is one of the most commonly used tests in the medical literature and is popular because many people believe that it is a relatively easy calculation and because it can be expanded to analyze almost any number of rows and categories

(90). It is based on observed versus expected frequencies in the cells of the R × C table, with the investigator expecting at least one of the cells to be different (larger or smaller) from expected or predicted. (The expected count for each cell is calculated by multiplying the row total and the column total corresponding to each cell and then dividing that product by the total number of subjects.) The chi-square test is used only when the data in the cells are counts, not proportions or percentages. Consider and example from the case-control study of Schieber et al. (60) of in-line skating injuries and the use of wrist protection devices. The data are presented in the 2 × 2 table shown in Fig. 8.3. The P value associated with the resulting chi-square statistic is less than 0.001, suggesting a statistically significant difference between the observed wrist injury and the lack of wrist protection among the cases compared with what would be expected based on the experience among the controls.

Although we usually think of chi-square as being limited to discrete variables, continuous variables may be converted into categorical variables and then the chi-square statistical test may be applied. For example, age may be categorized as less than 17 or at least 17 years old. (Sometimes it is necessary to use age as a categorical variable because the sample size is too small to perform other statistical tests, but in general, creating a categorical variable from a continuous variable reduces the information content of the data [82].)

There are two misapplications of the chi-square test to be aware of as you review the medical literature (91). One error is that of using the chi-square tests when there are two few numbers in any cell. When determining the validity of a chi-square test, consider *Cochran's rule:* At least 80% of the expected frequencies should be greater than 5 and none should be less than 1 (92). Be suspicious of any data presented where the predicted or expected value in any cell of the R × C table is less than 5. Chi-square tests in these circumstances should be viewed with caution (90). (A test that may be appropriate when the expected value in any cell in a 2 × 2 table is less than 5 is the *Fisher test* [90,92].) The second error sometimes seen with chi-square tests is violation of the assumption of independence. As mentioned earlier, this is a subtle and unfortunately frequent occurrence in medical research where, for example, body parts of interest come in pairs. For example, if an investigator is interested in knee injuries, is the subject with two injured knees entered into the study twice as though each knee is independent? If so, this is a violation of independence. That is, the investigator cannot assume that the two knees are unrelated. The assumption of independence is a requisite of the chi-square test, and if this assumption is violated, then the conclusions are spurious.

The reader may see chi-square statistics presented with *Yates continuity correction.* Some statisticians argue that this correction should be used because it provides a more conservative P value (especially in tests of data from small samples) (93–97).

Nonparametric Substitutes for the t Test

The *Mann-Whitney U* test is used as a nonparametric substitute for the Student t test described earlier. Continuous data are converted to an ordinal scale and then a ranking procedure is used. All variables are ranked without regard to which group they belong. The test statistic in this procedure is called U (98). The advantage of the Mann-Whitney U test is that it does not rely on the underlying assumption that the data have the Normal distribution. The disadvantage is that it is less powerful than the t test when the underlying data are Normal, so that the t test detects smaller differences than the Mann-Whitney U. The Mann-Whitney U is almost as powerful as the t test for moderate or large sample sizes, but it is useless for small sample sizes (92). The *Wilcoxon two sample test* (also called *Wilcoxon rank sum test*) and the *Kendall Tau test* (also called *Kendall's S*) are identical to the Mann-Whitney U, and sometimes the names are used interchangeably (90,92,99,100).

Survival Analysis

In many studies, investigators will use simple proportions to describe an outcome, such as failure rate with a particular surgery or implant. For example, in a chi-square analysis of two types of total knee implants, the investigator records the number of failures and successes at 10 years after surgery. Whether a subject's knee fails at 2 years after operation or the day the study ends 10 years later, the data ignore the time that the subject had a working knee. Often the investigator is interested in the length of time that lapses before some event, for example, failure of a total hip arthroplasty. Survival analysis methods are used to analyze the length of time between entry into follow-up and an outcome event such as failure of a hip implant in a fixed population (71). The event may be any number of conditions; however, in many studies outside of the sports medicine literature, the event is death, and for this reason the analysis of such data has been called *survival analysis* (90,101). The survival of patients in terms of the event of interest is given by estimating the patient's probability of success or failure at each year and the cumulative probability of survival each year (92). Specifically, survival time is defined as the time between entry into the study and the development of an event (e.g., failure of an implant, full participation in sports, complete wound healing, death). Such data are often *censored.* That is, not all subjects who enter the study are followed long enough to observe the time of the outcome event. Such data often have highly skewed distributions, and special statistical methods are required to analyze such data (R. Wolfe, personal communication, 1997).

These data can be analyzed with *life-table methods* that consider the time to the outcome; this provides a more powerful estimate of survival than just a crude proportion of survivors at the end of a specified amount of time as in chi-square analysis (90,102). Survival analysis incorporates censored survival times into the analysis. Such censored survival times include the time patients were followed and were disease free. It also allows the contribution of disease-free time from patients who may have been lost to follow-up or patients who have not yet developed the outcome of interest at the time of the analysis (99,103,104). At the time of censoring, no new information may be added. The disease-free time up to the point of censoring is included in the analysis, and this produces a much more dynamic model than that of calculating proportions of success and failures at the end of a study.

Life tables are the most commonly used method of analyzing data in randomized clinical trials and in cohort studies. A plot of a life table provides the reader with a graphic representation and organization of data. Generally, the horizontal time axis measures time relative to entry into the study. The time origin could be, and often is, a different calendar date for each subject in the study. The time axis measures time from a well-defined event. The event may be, for example, time of surgery instead of a particular date that is the same for all subjects. The vertical axis generally measures the

fraction of the population that is event free. Life tables illustrate those factors that are important for prognosis. Plotting rates of failure year by year gives further insight into the process leading to failure, and this is the first step in looking at statistical models for survival (105). *Survival curves* are drawn to show the cumulative probability of the time to the development of the event or outcome of interest (Fig. 8.5). A *Kaplan-Meier survival curve* depicts the exact times of event occurrence and censoring (104). The *Kaplan-Meier estimate* is one common method of survival modeling.

Suppose a physician wished to study time to failure in a small cohort of former athletes and ballerinas after total hip arthroplasty. Each patient accrues success time from the beginning of the study (i.e., from the time of total hip arthroplasty) until the implant fails, patients are lost to follow-up (e.g., death unrelated to total hip arthroplasty, or patients simply lose study contact), or the study follow-up time is concluded without failure (71). Survival analysis takes into account the time that patient has a successful total hip arthroplasty, regardless of whether the hip ultimately fails or succeeds (71). A Kaplan-Meier statistic provides an estimate of the survivor function at various points in time.

When reviewing a study that uses survival analysis, there are several important points the reader should keep in mind. First, the investigators should have information in the life plots, allowing the reader to determine the number of individuals observed at each interval (23). Second, confidence intervals may be constructed around the survival probabilities so that the reader

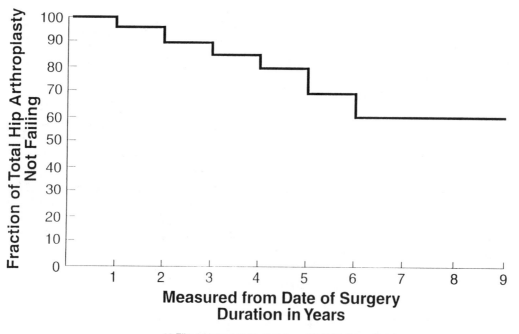

30 Elite Athletes Age 30-40 at time of THA (Ficticious Data)

FIG. 8.5. Kaplan-Meier Survival Curve

can see the degree of uncertainty that is accompanied by the estimated probability at any given time point. However, these estimates do not include all data; they estimate only those data up to that point in time and therefore are not a good method for comparing overall survival curves (104). Third, many life tables have a *plateau or flat phase,* which results because only a few individuals of the entire study group are actually monitored for the entire length of the study. This plateau should not be misinterpreted as a cure, unless there are many patients who have been observed for a long period of time (23).

Several tests of statistical significance are available for comparing survival curves, the best known of which is the *log rank test* (99,104). Another more sophisticated approach to comparing survival curves is the *Cox's proportional hazards model* (23,99). The Cox model permits the researcher to adjust the survival rates for covariates (see suggested readings in Appendix 1). All tests of significance in these models, however, need to be interpreted with caution. For example, if two groups of patients are being followed, remember that a statistically significant result means that one group has a better result than the other when taking into account both groups entire experience throughout the course of the study. Patients in one group may do better earlier in the study, only to do more poorly midway through, and then comparatively better at the end of the study. However, it is the overall experience that is important in the survival analysis. Thus, it is important to be aware of the natural history of the condition, treatment, or disease under study and the life expectancy of patients in the survival analysis. For example, in a study of total joint replacements, if patients are too old when they enter the study, they may not live long enough to develop a failure or demonstrate the success of the treatment because competing risks of diseases (such as coronary artery disease, cancer, and stroke) develop early in the follow-up period.

Evaluating the Diagnostic Value of a Test

Investigators are often interested in the usefulness of a particular medical test. Usefulness is described with the terms *sensitivity, specificity, positive predictive value, and negative predictive value.* Although these measures are not statistical tests *per se,* they do involve tools that are part of a general knowledge of statistical practices. Evaluating diagnostic tests is a useful way to determine the value of screening tools such as blood chemistries, physical examinations, or radiographs. (In addition to determining the sensitivity, specificity, positive predictive value, and negative predictive value, researchers are also interested in measures of validity and reliability of diagnostic tests; see question 4.) Sensitivity is the proportion of people with the condition or disease who

have a positive test—the number of true positives in the study. Specificity is the proportion of people without the condition or disease who have a negative test—the true negatives. The positive predictive value is the proportion of the people with a positive test who will actually have the condition or disease. And the negative predictive value is the proportion of people with a negative test who will not have the condition or disease.

Positive and negative predictive values are frequently more important in clinical practice than the sensitivity and specificity of the test. In a study by Liu et al. (105) in 1997, the authors were interested in comparing magnetic resonance imaging (MRI) and clinical examination to diagnose anterolateral ankle impingement. The MRI had sensitivity and specificity of 39% and 50%, respectively, whereas the clinical examination had sensitivity and specificity of 94% and 75%, respectively. Clearly, this study demonstrated that in this sample of patients, clinical examination was a much better test than the MRI. Given that the clinical examination remains the diagnostic tool of choice, when a patient presents with a potential anterolateral ankle impingement and the clinical examination is positive, we usually do not care about the sensitivity of the test. What we are really interested in is, in the presence of a positive clinical examination, how likely it is that your patient truly has anterolateral ankle impingement? Conversely, in the presence of a negative clinical examination, how likely is it that your patient does not have anterolateral ankle impingement? These last two questions are answered by the positive predictive value of the test and the negative predictive value of the test, respectively. In this study, the positive predictive value of the clinical examination was 94% and the negative predictive value was 75%. (The positive predictive value of the MRI was 78% and the negative predictive value was 15%.) A representation of these tests in terms of a contingency table is presented in Fig. 8.6A and B.

Question 5 presents a selection of the most common statistical tests. More complex or less commonly used tests are usually accompanied by an explanation of the tests and the reason why such tests were chosen over more commonly used techniques.

Question 5 Bottom Line

Were descriptive statistics or inferential statistics (or both) required to answer the study question? Was the type of statistics consistent with the study design and the best way to answer the study question? If more than one statistical test could have answered the study question, is the reason for using a specific test provided? Remember the common mistakes that are sometimes associated with the particular statistical test chosen:

MRI

	Impingement	No Impingement
Positive	7 (a)	2 (b)
Negative	11 (c)	2 (d)

Sensitivity $= \dfrac{[\,a\,]}{[\,a+c\,]} \times [100] = 7/(7+11) = 0.39$ or 39%

Specificity $= \dfrac{[\,d\,]}{[\,b+d\,]} \times [100] = 2/(2+2) = 0.5$ or 50%

Positive predictive value $= \dfrac{[\,a\,]}{[\,a+b\,]} \times [100] = 7/(7+2) = 0.78$ or 78%

Negative predictive value $= \dfrac{[\,d\,]}{[\,c+d\,]} \times [100] = 2/(12+2) = 0.15$ or 15%

A

Clinal Exam

	Impingement	No Impingement
Positive test	17 (a)	1 (b)
Negative test	1 (c)	3 (d)

Sensitivity $= \dfrac{[\,a\,]}{[\,a+c\,]} \times [100] = 17/(17+1) = 0.94$ or 94%

Specificity $= \dfrac{[\,d\,]}{[\,b+d\,]} \times [100] = 3/(1+3) = 0.75$ or 75%

Positive predictive value $= \dfrac{[\,a\,]}{[\,a+b\,]} \times [100] = 17/(17+1) = 0.94$ or 94%

Negative predictive value $= \dfrac{[\,d\,]}{[\,c+d\,]} \times [100] = 3/(1+3) = 0.75$ or 75%

B

FIG. 8.6. A: Example of the use of a contingency table for determining diagnostic values of magnetic resonance imaging. **B:** Example of the use of a contingency table for determining diagnostic values of a clinical examination. (From Liu SH, Nuccion SL, Finerman G. Diagnosis of anterolateral ankle impingement: comparison between magnetic resonance imaging and clinical examination. *Am J Sports Med* 1997;25:389–393, with permission.)

Know how these mistakes may potentially distort the interpretation and extrapolation of findings.

QUESTION 6: HOW ARE THE DATA ANALYZED?

Questions 5 and 6 are interrelated, because they focus on two parts of the same topic, statistical tests and procedures. Question 5 presents the statistical techniques to be considered when evaluating a research study, and question 6 discusses in more general terms how the reader should react to the statistical procedures used, considering what the results of the statistical procedures are in the study and control groups. That is, the reader must evaluate whether the statistics presented by the authors answered the study question. The investigator has presumably established the reliability and the validity of the study and control group observations, and now the investigator evaluates how the findings answer the study question. As readers, we are interested in the results of the comparisons of the group(s) in the study. The analysis should appear in the Results section of the study and should contain a clear concise description of the study results as they relate to the aims of the study and the study questions (18). These results may be presented in terms of univariate, bivariate, or multivariate statistical techniques. In particular, we are interested in the strength of association between variables in studies, the tests of statistical significance (where appropriate), the magnitude of the effect as expressed in confi-

dence intervals, and adjustments in the analysis for both the numbers of tests and for potential confounders.

Many studies require only descriptive statistics because they are exploratory in nature. The descriptive statistics may be both *univariate and bivariate*. Univariate statistics describe the completeness, measures of central tendency, and distribution of each study variable. Simple bivariate descriptive statistics present cross-tabulations, such as women's ages compared with men's or frequency of characteristics among groups (e.g., number of smokers among men and women) (18). Researchers also use statistical methods that demonstrate the strength of an association in a relationship. Relative risk and odds ratios are the chief measures used to quantitate data from cohort and case-control studies, respectively (23) (see question 2).

Descriptive studies such as case series, clinical series, and ecologic studies are examples of studies in which univariate and bivariate statistics may be presented. These are hypothesis-generating designs, and although simple statistical tests may be performed on data from these studies, care should be exercised when drawing inferences from the results of such statistical tests. This is because statistical analysis in a descriptive study is used to generate hypotheses, not to test hypotheses (18).

In observational or explanatory studies when a hypothesis has been specified *a priori*, statistical tests of significance are appropriate. The author should provide some evidence that the statistical assumptions of tests being used have not been violated. When statistical tests of significance are used, the author should also provide the specific test, the resulting test statistic, and the P value associated with the test statistic. The P value indicates how likely a study finding as extreme, or more extreme, than the one found is likely to be due to chance. Statistical significance testing only applies to the likelihood that a study finding is due to chance. It does not account for other sources of error that may be influencing the study result. That is, findings may also be due to bias or confounding, true treatment differences, chance, or any combination of these factors. By convention, P values of 0.05 or less are considered statistically significant. Suppose a coach wanted to compare preseason and postseason weights of a team of 20 female volleyball players. The research hypothesis is that there is a difference between pre- and postseason weights. Players are weighed before and after the season, and a paired t test is used to determine statistical significance. The average weight difference of a player before and after the season is 5 pounds. The t statistic is 2.861 and is associated with a P value equal to 0.01. This means that a finding as extreme as 5 pounds or more could be attributable to chance in 1 of 100 such studies. The rest of the time, such a finding would be due to either the treatment effect (a season of volleyball training and play) or to some other source, for example, the girls were weighed on different scales, the girls were weighed preseason after a heavy meal, or the scale was inaccurate. The P value only tells us the probability that a finding is due to chance. It does not take into account other explanations for the study finding. A significant P value is not "proof" of a difference; it is simply the likelihood that a difference is due to chance.

The reader is faced with many challenges when study results are reported only in terms of significance testing or P values. First, a finding may be statistically significant but may not be clinically relevant. For example, suppose the effects of two treatments (A and B) on the outcome of length of hospital stay resulted in a P value equal to 0.006—a highly statistically significant finding. However, the clinical result associated with treatment A results in an average length of stay of 6.2 days, whereas treatment B results in an average length of stay of 6.8 days. These results are biologically meaningless yet highly statistically significant. When large numbers are sampled, even small differences may take on statistical significance, even though clinically the results are not important (106). Readers should be very careful to ascertain that a study question is clinically and biologically meaningful, regardless of statistical significance (3,107,108).

Second, just because a study finding is not statistically significant does not mean that it is not clinically important. An excellent example of challenging the validity of conclusions based solely on P values is provided by Ebramzadeh et al. (109). The authors' example was a study of the effect of a new drug on infectious disease using a prospective randomized design. The outcomes in groups treated either with drug A (the experimental drug) or drug B (the conventional drug) were compared and at the end of the study there was a 30% higher rate of recovery in the experimental group. However, the corresponding P value was 0.11. The investigators concluded from this P value no statistical difference between the two drugs, and they recommended that conventional drug B should be used in future patients with this infectious disease. They publish their findings and recommendations, and other centers stop further use and study of drug A based on this study. Ebramzadeh et al. pointed out in their example that this conclusion represents a serious misuse of statistics. That is, if the experimental drug can save lives, even without statistical significance ($P = 0.11$), it should not be so readily dismissed.

Third, in addition to throwing out potentially important findings, another danger with undue reliance on P values is misinterpretation of findings associated with "nonsignificant" P values or P values > 0.05. Unfortunately, researchers and readers alike almost always interpret the absence of statistical significance to mean that a relationship does not exist (110). Freiman et al. (111) in a classic review of 71 studies demonstrated that in most cases, the absence of significance in studies has been interpreted by investigators as meaning that a treatment was not effective. A P value greater than 0.05 simply means a lack of evidence to reject the null hypothesis. Saying that there is no statistically significant evidence that two treatments are different does not mean that the investigators have established that the two treatments are the same, or equivalent (112). Put another way, "no proof of a difference is not equivalent to proof of no difference" (113).

Further, the lack of statistical significance may be related to sample size. That is, did the investigators plan their study to have enough subjects to find a difference, if such a difference truly exists? As mentioned under question 3, when there is no power analysis and the investigators' conclusions are that there are no statistical differences between groups, the reader needs to know that this is because there were, in fact, no differences and not because the sample size was too small to detect important differences (9). Failing to reject the null hypothesis when it should be rejected is a type II error.

Readers and investigators want to know not just whether a treatment has an impact or not but also how much impact (110). A P value cannot tell the reader anything about the magnitude of a difference between two treatments, nor can the P value tell the reader about the direction of the difference between two treatments (114). Assuming appropriate study design and research methods, a confidence interval can. A confidence interval provides a range of values that is based on a process whose prior probability is likely to capture the mean or proportion in the population.

Referring to the earlier hypothetical study example presented by Ebramzadeh et al. (109), a 95% confidence interval reveals that a 30% recovery rate is associated with limits of −15% to 75%. This means that in 100 samples drawn from the same population, 95 of these samples will capture the true recovery rate in the population. Thus, we are confident (with belief level of 95%) that our specific confidence interval, −15% to 75%, has in fact captured the true population recovery rate. In five of the samples drawn, the true recovery rate will lie outside the confidence limits determined for these samples. If the authors in this hypothetical example reject the study findings based on the P value ($P = 0.11$), it is possible that they are rejecting the potential for large important clinical improvement with the experimental drug. Instead, these authors should understand that the P value indicates slightly greater than a 1 in 10 ($P = 0.11$) chance that the 30% difference in survival rate occurred by accidental selection (chance) and that the experimental drug ought to be used while further studies are conducted.

If the author is attempting to answer the study question, then the numbers of statistical tests conducted should have been proposed *a priori*. Sometimes the main problem with an analysis is that it stems from too many analyses consisting of multiple end points, multiple time points, multiple subgroups analyses, and so forth (3). Be alert for excessive or unstructured use of significance testing (7). If study data are manipulated in enough different ways, eventually the data will prove whatever the investigator wants (5). It is easy for the reader to get lost in "a morass of subgroup analyses," especially if such analyses are not specified *a priori;* post hoc findings may represent a selective and distorted picture to the reader (7). This is why identifying the study question and study plan is so important. If the researcher is truly fishing, then this should be specified in the article so that the reader accepts the findings as exploratory and hypothesis generating. Not describing that the study is exploratory and then conducting multiple tests of statistical significance is analogous to the investigator who "goes fishing," catches a boot, and then tells us that the boot was what he was looking for.

Legitimate use of multiple tests of statistical significance requires a prespecified strategy for statistical analysis and appropriate adjustment of P values. The more comparisons that are made, the more likely the investigator is to find a statistically significant result due to chance alone. Unadjusted multiple tests of significance, therefore, increase the possibilities of a type I error (incorrectly rejecting the null hypothesis). For example, if 10 interim analyses on the same outcome measure are made during the course of a study, there is approximately a 20% chance of reaching a significance level of $P < 0.05$ even if the null hypothesis is true (7). Authors should indicate in their reports that they have made adjustments for multiple comparisons when many tests are used to assure themselves and their readers that study results are real.

Adjustment may also be required for potential confounders. Recall that if groups differ even in the absence of statistical significance, the investigator must consider that the difference between groups may be a result of confounding. For example, suppose that a study showed no statistical difference between surgical and nonsurgical treatment on the rerupture rate in a study of Achilles tendon treatment, but the investigator suspects that age may be confounding the study results. The investigator might subdivide the sample into patients older and younger than 40 years to determine if differences in rerupture rate exist when groups the same age are compared. Multivariable statistical techniques such as ANOVA and multiple regression analysis allow for reducing the effect of several potentially confounding variables at the same time (23).

Question 6 Bottom Line

Evaluate how the data were analyzed. Did descriptive studies use appropriate univariate and bivariate statistics? In explanatory studies, were appropriate measures of the strength of associations (odds ratios, relative risks) between groups reported? Were the results of hypothesis tests identified, with specific statistical procedures referenced, test statistics identified, and P values given? If multiple statistical tests were performed, were adjustments for type I errors identified? Were there any potential confounders to study findings, and did the investigators adjust for them in the analysis? Were confidence intervals reported for the main results?

QUESTION 7: HOW DO YOU INTERPRET THE STUDY RESULTS?

What findings did the researchers report at the conclusion of their study? Were any differences found between the experimental and control groups for participants in the study? How do you interpret the meaning of the study for the study's participants? So far we have identified key components of study implementation and analysis. We have determined whether the results were accurately summarized, and whether the study design and statistical analysis bear up under close scrutiny. We have determined whether all clinically relevant outcomes have been reported. We now want to evaluate the meaning of the study findings for the subjects who participated in the study. That is, what clinical significance do the study findings hold for the study participants? How do the authors interpret the results of their study?

To evaluate the authors' interpretation, go to the Discussion section of the article. It should include the implications of the study findings along with limitations of the study. The authors typically relate their observations with those of other relevant studies. The study conclusions are then linked to the study question and the study goals (115).

Readers are encouraged not to accept the Discussion section as the final explanation of the study's findings but rather to view it as an opportunity to either agree with or challenge the investigators' interpretations (1,8,76). If the tests are statistically significant, what explanation do the authors offer for such findings? Based on your own knowledge and experience, are there other explanations for these findings (20)? Remember that the P value is not the probability of making a mistake (2). Rather, it is the probability of obtaining a difference as extreme or more extreme than the one observed. If the P value associated with a study finding is not significant by conventional standards ($P > 0.05$), note carefully the authors' interpretation of this lack of statistical significance. More often than not, lack of statistical difference is due to inadequate power to detect meaningful differences (111). As emphasized earlier, "the absence of a proof of efficacy is not proof of an absence of efficacy" (116). Investigators should not interpret lack of statistical significance as meaning that a treatment or intervention is worthless, trivial, or not real (77). Nor should they erroneously claim that such a lack of a statistically significant difference means that the parameters being measured are equivalent and therefore conclude that both treatments are equally beneficial.

Researchers and readers also need to exercise care when interpreting results that have highly statistically significant findings as well. In the real world, would the difference found in the study be important? Remember that the P value is not a measure of the magnitude of the effect (2). Even though a statistical test is associated with a very low P value, it does not indicate any greater clinical importance. In a previous example, the difference between two treatments on hospital length of stay was 6.2 and 6.8 days in two groups. Whether the P value associated with these two findings based on a t test is 0.02 or 0.0002, it does not change the fact that such a difference is probably clinically meaningless. Also, watch for the use of the word "significance," because it is a commonly misused word in the medical literature. Careful researchers distinguish between statistical significance and clinical significance (117,118). For its meaning to be clear, *significance* ought to be preceded by one of two adjectives: clinical or statistical. As stressed throughout this chapter, clinical significance is not necessarily equivalent to statistical significance. No amount of statistical significance is going to make up for a clinically unimportant question or finding. And the absence of statistical significance does not mean that the study's findings are clinically unimportant.

Readers should also be aware of the meanings of the words "association" and "correlation," because these two words are often incorrectly used interchangeably. Association is a "usefully vague" word that suggests some sort of a relationship between or among variables. Correlation or correlated is a statistical term that refers to a specific way to measure association (i.e., correlation and correlated should only be used in a statistical sense) (118).

Readers should be alert for interpretations that conclude causality when statistical significance is present (e.g., from correlation or chi-square analysis) (79). For example, because there is a statistically significant correlation between the wearing of eye glasses and poor vision, this does not warrant the conclusion that wearing eye glasses causes poor vision.

Other interpretations to note are those based on the erroneous use of multiple t tests. It is incorrect to make comparisons between several groups' means with the use of t tests instead of using ANOVA with adjustments for comparisons. Likewise, when investigators take multiple looks at the data in hopes of identifying a significant finding earlier rather than later (without using appropriate statistical strategies), they are using incorrect statistical practices. Tests of hypotheses that were not decided in advance of the study should be considered exploratory. As discussed earlier, spurious statistically significant findings can be expected to occur due to chance alone in the presence of multiple tests and may pose considerable problems with study interpretation (79).

If a reader believed that the investigators have misinterpreted the data, the reader is urged to "reinterpret the misinterpretation" and then draw conclusions based on the reader's own interpretation (19). Even when flawless methods are used, there is still potential for distorting the results (8). Generally, such distortions are quite innocent and occur because authors are "unaware of their subconscious leaning" toward results that favor their hypotheses (8). That is, as emphasized under question 2, all studies may be affected by bias. We should expect researchers to identify potential sources of bias in the study design they have chosen and to describe the methods used to minimize or avoid it. To critically evaluate what we read, it is more important to understand the concept of bias rather than the specific definition of every potential source of bias. We should be assessing not only whether there is a potential that bias exists but also the likelihood of its occurrence or effect on the study (21). Remember that the potential for bias does not necessarily mean that the study is biased. However, authors and readers alike should assess the potential bias present within a study and should evaluate its impact on study results and conclusions.

Also, consider the biases that you as reader may bring to the interpretation. Owen (119), in a commentary in the *Journal of the American Medical Association,* proposed and described 25 types of reader bias, including prominent author bias, famous institution bias, rivalry bias, and friendship bias, to name a few. His point is that although the reader may identify sources of investigator bias, we cannot do anything to eliminate this bias. Our own biases, however, can be prevented or we can compensate for them. The reader is urged to avoid "overzealousness" in evaluating research articles, because the reader may underrate the value of an important article (76). Readers must recognize the limitations of a study and then put these limitations into perspective (23). Read with healthy skepticism but apply common sense (1,79). Many researchers have to "make do" with information that is reasonable and practical to collect. But even with less than perfect data, researchers should still indicate how valid their study is, how precise the estimates are, and the directions of any errors that may have distorted the data (18,81).

Evaluate whether the study conclusions are consistent with the study objectives and determine if the authors' interpretations support a reasonable answer to the study question for this group of study subjects. Even with flawless methods and no distortions, you have a "perfect right" to disagree with the authors' interpretations (21). That is, you may agree with the methodology and statistical analysis in the study and the study findings but disagree with the authors' opinions regarding the importance or meaning of such findings.

Question 7 Bottom Line

What was the author's interpretation of the study findings regarding the participants in the study? Were explanations given for the meaning of both statistically significant and nonsignificant findings? Regardless of statistical significance, were the results clinically important? Were both strengths and limitations of the study identified? Was the impact of limitations on the study findings discussed? Recognize both author biases and reader biases in interpreting the study. Within the bounds of the study, do the results represent the truth, are they believable, and are the conclusions based on these results appropriate?

QUESTION 8: HOW DO THE STUDY FINDINGS APPLY TO YOUR OWN PATIENTS AND PRACTICE OF MEDICINE?

We have just discussed the interpretation of results for the subjects that comprise the study sample. The reader evaluates the study findings to judge if the original research question posed by the author has been answered. The final step in evaluating a research article is to determine whether and to what extent the answer to the research question can be generalized to populations beyond the study sample (120). It is not enough to know that the findings are true. We must also determine whether the study findings, if true, are useful (1). Remember that the main purpose of statistics is to aid in inference making (121). An inference is a generalization derived from the evidence provided. Through its power to reduce data to manageable forms, statistics enable researchers to attach probability estimates to the inferences from the study data (120) and to then generalize findings to a larger population beyond the sample.

Extrapolation provides the link between the study sample and the population. To extrapolate the study findings and its interpretation to your practice of sports medicine, the data provided in the study must be *generalizable* to patients beyond those in the study sample. This is the definition of *external validity*. That is, are the results applicable to your practice of sports medicine? Will the patients you see and treat respond in the same way as those patients described in the study? Do the authors' interpretations extend beyond the study sample, and do the results given and interpreted by the authors support such extrapolation (21)?

For the study findings to be applied to your clinical practice, the study sample must share characteristics in common with your patients (68). As emphasized earlier, the criteria for inclusion and exclusion of patients should have been clearly defined. The clinical and sociodemographic characteristics of the patients in the study should have been reported in enough detail to enable you to determine if the study patients are comparable with those in your own practice (122). If patients were excluded from the analysis because they declined to participate, were noncompliant, or were lost to follow-up, then you cannot be sure that those patients who remained in the study and were analyzed were like or unlike your own patients. Further, you will not be sure whether the study findings can be applied to your practice of sports medicine. Even if the sample does resemble your patient population, if the size of the sample is insufficient (too small, low power), the results may not be generalizable.

Although the study findings may not be generalizable to your patients, they may still be generalizable to other important populations (120). For example, studies of patients over 50 years old with ankle injuries may have good external validity, great value, and practical use in the population over 50 years of age. But these study results may not be generalized to your practice of adolescent medicine.

In addition to evaluating the sample's comparability to other populations, the reader should evaluate whether the treatment methods in the study intervention are consistent with those typically used in current practice (20). Is the setting similar to your practice and are the people implementing procedures or treatments, conducting testing, or operating on patients similar in training and experience to those professionals in your practice performing these same tasks? Finally, is the treatment or intervention itself described in sufficient detail that it can be reproduced by other clinicians (22,25,69)?

Question 8 Bottom Line

Are the study results generalizable? Is there a link between the sample and the larger population of patients to which study results may be applied? Were the study's patients similar to your own patients? Are the patients you see and treat likely to respond in the same way as those described in the study? Were the treatments and interventions of the study similar to yours? Is the study conclusion feasible in your practice?

CONCLUSION

We have presented a guide for evaluating statistical practices in sports medicine research. They include eight questions to ask as you review any research study: What is the study question and the hypothesis to be tested, what is the study design, how is the sample selected, what are the study results in terms of the study participants, what is the statistical test chosen, how are the data analyzed, what is the meaning of the study findings for the study participants, and how do the study findings apply to your practice of medicine? In addition to using these questions as a guide for evaluating statistical practices, we urge that you read only what is interesting and useful, keeping in mind that complex statistical procedures do not compensate for a poorly designed and poorly executed study.

Reserve the right of final judgment: The ultimate interpretation and decision about the value of a study rests with you. Evaluating statistical practices is not just about juggling numbers and "doing the math." It requires using healthy skepticism and good judgment. Acknowledge imperfections in studies and decide whether, given limitations, the net effect of the work is valid and useful. Can you believe the results? Is the work applicable in your clinical practice with the kinds of patients you see? Your goal is not to find flaws but to find truth. Recognize problems and put them into perspective as you read the literature and apply what you read to your own practice of sports medicine. As emphasized at the beginning of this chapter, identifying key statistical practices in sports medicine research requires knowing what to look for in research articles, an understanding of simple and basic statistical principles, and an integration of logic, experience, clinical judgment, and common sense.

REFERENCES

1. Dept. of Clinical Epidemiology and Biostatistics, McMaster University Health Sciences Centre. How to read clinical journals. I. Why to read them and how to start reading them critically. *Can Med Assoc J* 1981;124:555–558.
2. Jamart J. Statistical tests in medical research. *Acta Oncol* 1992; 31:723–727.
3. Altman DG. Statistics in medical journals: developments in the 1980s. *Stat Med* 1991;10:1897–1913.
4. Murray GD. Statistical aspects of research methodology. *Br J Surg* 1991;78:777–781.
5. Mills JL. Data torturing. *N Engl J Med* 1993;329:1196–1199.
6. DerSimonian R, Charette LJ, McPeek B, et al. Reporting on methods in clinical trials. *N Engl J Med* 1982;306:1332–1337.
7. Pocock SJ, Hughes MD, Lee RJ. Statistical problems in the reporting of clinical trials: a survey of three medical journals. *N Engl J Med* 1987;317:426–432.
8. Pocock SJ. *Clinical trials—a practical approach.* Chichester: John Wiley & Sons, 1983.
9. Emerson JD, McPeek B, Mosteller F. Reporting clinical trials in general surgical journals. *Surgery* 1984;95:572–579.
10. Johnson T. Statistical guidelines for medical journals. *Stat Med* 1984;3:97–99.
11. Kuzon WM Jr, Urbanchek MG, McCabe S. The seven deadly sins of statistical analysis. *Ann Plast Surg* 1996;37:265–272.
12. Glantz SA. Biostatistics: how to detect, correct and prevent errors in the medical literature. *Circulation* 1980;61:1–7.
13. Fletcher RH, Fletcher SW. Clinical research in general medical journals: a 30-year perspective. *N Engl J Med* 1979;301:180–183.
14. Kraemer HC. "Lies, damn lies, and statistics" in clinical research. *Pharos* 1992;55:7–12.
15. Feinstein AR. Beyond statistics: what is really important in medicine? *Cleve Clin J Med* 1997;64:127–128.
16. Gaddis ML, Gaddis GM. Introduction to biostatistics. VI. Correlation and regression. *Ann Emerg Med* 1990;19:1462–1468.
17. Michels KB, Rosner BA. Data trawling: to fish or not to fish. *Lancet* 1996;348:1152–1153.
18. Bowker TJ. How to do a simple epidemiological study. II. Practice. *Int J Cardiol* 1996;57:197–205.
19. Yancey JM. Ten rules for reading clinical research. *Am J Surg* 1990;159:533–539.
20. Tanner CA. Evaluating research for use in practice: guidelines for the clinician. *Heart and Lung* 1987;16:424–431.
21. Gehlbach SH. *Interpreting the medical literature,* 3rd ed. New York: McGraw-Hill, 1993:1–31.
22. Girden ER. *Evaluating research articles—from start to finish.* Thousand Oaks: SAGE Publications, 1996.
23. Riegelman RK, Hirsch RP. *Studying a study and testing a test— how to read the health science literature,* 3rd ed. Boston: Little, Brown and Company, 1996:5.
24. Gardner MJ, Machin D, Campbell MJ. Statistics in medicine. Use of checklists in assessing the statistical content of medical studies. *Br Med J* 1986;292:810–812.
25. Dept. of Clinical Epidemiology and Biostatistics, McMaster University Health Sciences Centre. How to read clinical journals. V. How to distinguish useless or even harmful therapy. *Can Med Assoc J* 1981;124:1156–1162.
26. Huth EJ. *How to write and publish papers in the medical sciences,* 2nd ed. Baltimore: Williams & Wilkins, 1990:143–144.
27. Fredrickson DS. The field trial: some thoughts on the indispensable ordeal. *Bull NY Acad Med* 1968;44:985–993.
28. Schoolman HM, Becktel JM, Best WR, et al. Statistics in medical research: principles versus practices. *J Lab Clin Med* 1968;71: 357–367.
29. Haynes RB, McKibbon KA, Fitzgerald D, et al. How to keep up with the medical literature. I. Why try to keep up and how to get started. *Ann Intern Med* 1986;105:149–153.
30. Cuddy PG, Elenbaas RM, Elenbaas JK. Evaluating the medical literature. I. Abstract, introduction, methods. *Ann Emerg Med* 1983;12:549–555.
31. Jolley D. The glitter of the t table. *Lancet* 1993;342:27–29.
32. Rothman KJ. A sobering start for the cluster busters. *Am J Epidemiol* 1990;132:S6–S13.

33. Hennekens CH, Buring JE, eds. *Epidemiology in medicine.* Boston: Little, Brown and Company, 1987.
34. Hennekens CH, Buring JE. Methodologic considerations in the design and conduct of randomized trials: The U.S. Physicians' Health Study. *Controlled Clinical Trials* 1989;10:142s–150s.
35. Rosier RP, Lefer LG. Jogger's whiplash. *JAMA* 1978;239:2114.
36. McCowan TC. Space-invaders wrist. *N Engl J Med* 1981;304:1368.
37. Escher SA. Ulnar stress fracture in a bowler. *Am J Sports Med* 1997;25:412–413.
38. Pagnani MJ, Cooper DE, Warren RF. Extrusion of the medial meniscus. *Arthroscopy* 1991;7:297–300.
39. Suziki S, Mita F, Ogishima H. Double-layered lateral meniscus: a newly found anomaly. *Arthroscopy* 1991;7:267–271.
40. Levakos Y, Sherman MF, Shelbourne K, et al. Simultaneous rupture of the anterior cruciate ligament and patellar tendon. *Am J Sports Med* 1996;24:498–503.
41. Wright JR Jr. Nordic ski jumping fatalities in the United States: a 50-year summary. *J Trauma* 1988;28:848–851.
42. Neiman R, Ushiroda S. Slot-machine tendonitis. *N Engl J Med* 1981;304:1368.
43. Busconi BD, Pappas AM. Chronic, painful ankle instability in skeletally immature athletes: ununited osteochondral fractures of the distal fibula. *Am J Sports Med* 1996;24:647–651.
44. Noyes FR, Barber-Westin SD. A comparison of results in acute and chronic anterior cruciate ligament ruptures of arthroscopically assisted autogenous patellar tendon reconstruction *Am J Sports Med* 1997;25:460–471.
45. Naranja RJ Jr, Reilly PJ, Kuhlman JR, et al. Long-term evaluation of the Elmslie-Trillat-Maquet procedure for patellofemoral dysfunction. *Am J Sports Med* 1996;24:779–784.
46. Yang C, Chiu H, Chiu J, et al. Cancer mortality and residence near petrochemical industries in Taiwan. *J Toxicol Environ Health* 1997;50:265–273.
47. Esparza ML, Sasaki S, Kesteloot H. Nutrition, latitude, and multiple sclerosis mortality: an ecologic study. *Am J Epidemiol* 1995;142:733–737.
48. Amstutz RD, Rozier RG. Community risk indicators for dental caries in school children: an ecologic study. *Commun Dent Oral Epidemiol* 1995;23:129–137.
49. Jacobsen SJ, Goldberg J, Cooper C, et al. The association between water flouridation and hip fracture among white women and men aged 65 years and older. A national ecologic study. *Annals of Epidemiology* 1992;2:617–626.
50. Michael M III, Boyce WT, Wilcox AJ. *Biomedical bestiary: an epidemiologic guide to flaws and fallacies in the medical literature.* Boston: Little, Brown and Company, 1984.
51. Fineberg HV. Clinical evaluation: how does it influence medical practice? *Bull Cancer (Paris)* 1987;74:333–346.
52. Otis CL, Drinkwater B, Johnson M, et al. American College of Sports Medicine position stand. The female athlete triad. *Med Sci Sports Exerc* 1997;29:i–ix.
53. Wolf AS, Marx K, Ulrich U. Athletic amenorrhea. *Ann NY Acad Sci* 1997;816:295–304.
54. McNeil BJ, Pauker SG. Decision analysis for public health: principles and illustrations. *Annu Rev Public Health* 1984;5:135–161.
55. Udvarhelyi IS, Colditz GA, Rai A, et al. Cost-effectiveness and cost-benefit analyses in the medical literature: are the methods being used correctly? *Ann Intern Med* 1992;116:238–244.
56. Eisenberg JM. Clinical economics: a guide to the economic analysis of clinical practices. *JAMA* 1989;262:2879–2886.
57. Vrbos LA, Lorenz MA, Peabody EH, et al. Clinical methodologies and incidence of appropriate statistical testing in orthopaedic spine literature. Are statistics misleading? *Spine* 1993;18:1021–1029.
58. Kushi LH, Fee RM, Folsom AR, et al. Physical activity and mortality in postmenopausal women. *JAMA* 1997;277:1287–1292.
59. Hulley SB. *Designing clinical research: an epidemiologic approach.* Baltimore: Williams & Wilkins, 1988.
60. Schieber RA, Branche-Dorsey CM, Ryan GW, et al. Risk factors for injuries from in-line skating and the effectiveness of safety gear. *N Engl J Med* 1997;335:1630–1635.

61. Friedman GD. *Primer of epidemiology,* 4th ed. New York: McGraw-Hill, 1994.
62. Williams PT. High-density lipoprotein cholesterol and other risk factors for coronary heart disease in female runners. *N Engl J Med* 1996;334:1298–1303.
63. Friedman LM, Furberg CD, DeMets DL. *Fundamentals of clinical trials,* 3rd ed. St. Louis: Mosby, 1996.
64. Meinert C. *Clinical trials: design, conduct, and analysis.* New York: Oxford University Press, 1986.
65. Brink O, Staunstrup H, Sommer J. Stable lateral malleolar fractures treated with aircast ankle brace and DonJoy R.O.M.-Walker brace: a prospective randomized study. *Foot Ankle Int* 1996;17:679–684.
66. Sachs HS, Berrier MA, Reitman D, et al. Meta-analysis of randomized controlled trials. *N Engl J Med* 1987;316:450–455.
67. Welton DC, Kemper HC, Post GB. A meta-analysis of the effect of calcium intake on bone mass in young and middle aged females and males. *J Nutr* 1995;125:2802–2813.
68. Gross M. A critique of the methodologies used in clinical studies of hip-joint arthroplasty published in the English-language orthopaedic literature. *J Bone Joint Surg Am* 1988;70:1364–1371.
69. Sackett DL. Bias in analytical research. *J Chronic Dis* 1979;32:51–63.
70. Feinstein AR. Beyond statistics: what is really important in medicine? *Cleve Clin J Med* 1997;64:127–128.
71. Gottlieb M, Anderson G, Lepor H. Basic epidemiologic and statistical methods in clinical research. *Urol Clin North Am* 1992;19:641–653.
72. Albers LL, Murphy PA. Evaluation of research studies. III. Statistical significance testing. *J Nurse Midwife* 1993;38:51–53.
73. Streiner DL, Norman GR. *Health measurement scales: a guide to their development and use,* 2nd ed. Oxford: Oxford University Press, 1995.
74. DeVellis RF. *Scale development. Theory and applications: applied social research methods series.* Newbury Park, CA: Sage Publications, 1991.
75. Bland JM, Altman DG. Statistical methods for assessing agreement between two methods of clinical measurement. *Lancet* 1986;20:37–46.
76. Elenbaas JK, Cuddy PG, Elenbaas RM. Evaluating the medical literature. III. Results and discussion. *Ann Emerg Med* 1983;12:679–686.
77. Mainland D. Statistical ritual in clinical journals. I. Is there a cure? *Br Med J Clin Res Ed* 1984;288:841–843.
78. Morris RW. A statistical study of papers in the *Journal of Bone and Joint Surgery Br,* 1984. *J Bone Joint Surg Br* 1988;70:242–246.
79. Altman DG, Gore SM, Gardner MJ, et al. Statistical guidelines for contributors to medical journals. *Br Med J* 1983;286:1489–1493.
80. Elenbaas RM, Elenbaas JK, Cuddy PG. Evaluating the medical literature. II. Statistical analysis. *Ann Emerg Med* 1983;12:610–620.
81. Greenhouse JB, Yusif S, Wittes J. Practical Issues in the Synthesis of Clinical Trial Results. Preconference Workshop for the Society of Clinical Trials Annual Meeting, 1996.
82. Wolf JS Jr, Smith DS. Practical biomedical statistics: a guide to the selection of statistical tests. *Urology* 1996;47:2–13.
83. Niemcryk SJ, Kraus TJ, Mallory TH. Empirical considerations in orthopaedic research design and data analysis. II. The application of data analytic techniques. *J Arthroplast* 1990;5:105–110.
84. Santner TJ, Burstein AH. Fundamentals of statistics for orthopaedists. II. *J Bone Joint Surg Am* 1984;66:794–799.
85. Greenfield MLVH, Kuhn JE, Wojtys EM. A statistics primer: tests for continuous data. *Am J Sports Med* 1998;25:882–884.
86. Greenfield MLVH, Kuhn JE, Wojtys EM. A statistics primer: correlation and regression analysis. *Am J Sports Med* 1998;26(2):338–343.
87. Vogt WP. *Dictionary of statistics and methodology: a nontechnical guide for the social sciences.* Newbury Park, CA: Sage Publications, 1993.
88. Neter M, Wasserman W, Kutner MH. *Applied linear statistical models,* 3rd ed. Homewood. IL: Richard D. Irwin, Inc., 1990.
89. Gaddis GM, Gaddis ML. Introduction to biostatistics, V. Statisti-

cal inference techniques for hypothesis testing with nonparametric data. *Ann Emerg Med* 1990;19:1054–1059.

90. Armitage P, Berry G. *Statistical methods in medical research,* 3rd ed. Cambridge, MA: Blackwell Science, 1994.

91. Remington RD, Schork MA. *Statistics with applications to the biological and health sciences,* 2nd ed. Engelwood Cliffs, NJ: Prentice-Hall, 1970.

92. Bland M. *An introduction to medical statistics,* 2nd ed. Oxford: Oxford Medical Publications, 1995.

93. Conover WJ. Some reasons for not using the Yates continuity correction on 2 × 2 contingency tables. *Am J Public Health* 1997;69:374–376.

94. Mantel N. Some reasons for not using the Yates continuity correction of 2 × 2 contingency tables: comment and a suggestion. *Am J Public Health* 1974;69:378–380.

95. Gore SM. Assessing methods—survival. *Br Med J Clin Res Ed* 1981;283:840–843.

96. Starmer F, Grizzle JE, Sen PK. Some reasons for not using the Yates continuity correction of 2 × 2 contingency tables: comment. *Am J Public Health* 1997;69:376–378.

97. Miettinen OS. Some reasons for not using the Yates continuity correction of 2 × 2 contingency tables: comment. *Am J Public Health* 1974;69:380.

98. Conover WJ. Some reasons for not using the Yates continuity correction of 2 × 2 contingency tables: rejoinder. *Am J Public Health* 1974;69:382.

99. Hirsch RP, Riegelman RK. *Statistical first aid: interpretation of health research data.* Cambridge, MA: Blackwell Science, 1992.

100. Kirkwood BR. *Essentials of medical statistics.* Oxford: Blackwell Science, 1988.

101. Allison PD. *Survival analysis using the SAS® system: a practical guide.* Cary, NC: SAS Institute Inc., 1995.

102. Lachin JM. Introduction to sample size determination and power analysis for clinical trials. *Controlled Clin Trials* 1981;2:93–113.

103. Luus HG, Muller FO, Meyer BH. Statistical significance versus clinical relevance. III. Methods for calculating confidence intervals. *S Afr Med J* 1989;76:681–685.

104. Checkoway H, Pearce N, Dement JM. Design and conduct of occupational epidemiology studies. II. Analysis of cohort data. *Am J Ind Med* 1989;15:375–394.

105. Liu SH, Nuccion SL, Finerman G. Diagnosis of anterolateral ankle impingement: comparison between magnetic resonance imaging and clinical examination. *Am J Sports Med* 1997;25: 389–393.

106. Selvin S, White MC. Description and reporting of statistical methods. *Am J Infect Control* 1993;21:210–215.

107. Haupt HA, Rovere GD. Anabolic steroids: a review of the literature. *Am J Sports Med* 1984;12:469–484.

108. Lindgren BR, Wielinski CL, Finkelstein SM, et al. Contrasting clinical and statistical significance within the research setting. *Pediatr Pulmonol* 1993;16:336–340.

109. Ebramzadeh E, McKellop H, Dorey F, et al. Challenging the validity of conclusions based on *P*-values alone: a critique of contemporary clinical research design and methods. *Am Acad Orthop Surg* 1994;43:587–600.

110. Borenstein M. The case for confidence intervals in controlled clinical trials. *Controlled Clin Trials* 1994;15:411–428.

111. Freiman JA, Chalmers TC, Smith H, et al. The importance of beta, the type II error and sample size in the design and interpretation of the randomized control trial: survey of 71 "negative" trials. *N Engl J Med* 1978;299:690–694.

112. Greenfield MLVH, Kuhn JE, Wojtys EM. A statistics primer. *P* values: probability and clinical significance. *Am J Sports Med* 1996;24:863–865.

113. Gallagher EJ. Proof of a difference is not equivalent to proof of no difference. *J Emerg Med* 1996;12:525–527.

114. Gardner MJ, Altman DG. Confidence—and clinical importance—in research findings. *Br J Psych* 1990;156:472–474.

115. The International Committee of Medical Journal Editors: Harlem O, Huth EH, Lock SP, et al. Uniform requirements for manuscripts submitted to biomedical journals. *Ann Intern Med* 1982;96:766–771.

116. Detsky AS, Sackett DL. When was a "negative" clinical trial big enough? How many patients you needed depends on what you found. *Arch Intern Med* 1985;145:709–712.

117. Hanley JA. What statistical methods do journal readers need to understand? Do 75% of radiologists understand fewer statistical articals than the "average" radiologist? *AJR* 1994;163:716–718.

118. Bailar JC, Mosteller F. Guidelines for statistical reporting in articles for medical journals: amplifications and explanations. *Ann Intern Med* 1988;108:266–273.

119. Owen R. Reader bias. *JAMA* 1982;247:2533–2534.

120. Monsen ER, Cheney CL. Research methods in nutrition and dietetics: design, data analysis, and presentation. *J Am Diet Assoc* 1988;88:1047–1065.

121. Kerlinger FN. *Foundations of behavioral research,* 3rd ed. New York: Holt, Rinehart and Winston, 1986:175–176.

122. Raskob GE, Lofthouse RN, Hull RD. Methodological guidelines for clinical trials evaluating new therapeutic approaches in bone and joint surgery. *J Bone Joint Surg Am* 1985;67: 1294–1297.

APPENDIX 1: SUGGESTED READINGS

Clinical Trials

Friedman LM, Furberg CD, DeMets DL. *Fundamentals of clinical trials,* 3rd ed. St. Louis: Mosby, 1996.

Meinert C. *Clinical trials: design, conduct, and analysis.* New York: Oxford University Press, 1986.

Pocock SJ. *Clinical trials—a practical approach.* Chichester: John Wiley & Sons, 1983.

Cost-effectiveness Analysis and Decision Analysis

Drummond MF, Stoddart GL, Torrance GW. *Methods for the economic evaluation of health care programmes.* Oxford: Oxford Medical Publications, 1987.

Gold MR, Siegel JE, Russell LB, et al., eds. *Cost-effectiveness in health and medicine.* New York: Oxford University Press, 1996.

Sox HC Jr, Blatt MA, Higgins MC, et al. *Medical desision making.* Stoneham, MA: Butterworth Publishers, 1988.

Weinstein MC, Fineberg HV, Elstein AS, et al. *Clinical decision analysis.* Philadelphia, PA: W.B. Saunders, 1980.

Epidemiology

Friedman GD. *Primer of epidemiology,* 4th ed. New York: McGraw-Hill, 1994.

Hennekens CH, Buring JE. *Epidemiology in medicine.* Boston: Little, Brown and Company, 1987.

Hulley SB. *Designing clinical research: an epidemiologic approach.* Baltimore: Williams & Wilkins, 1988.

Sackett DL, Haynes RB, Guyatt GH, et al. *Clinical epidemiology—a basic science for clinical medicine,* 2nd ed. Boston: Little, Brown and Company, 1991.

Evaluation of Research Articles

Gehlbach SH. *Interpreting the medical literature,* 3rd ed. New York: McGraw-Hill, 1993.

Girden ER. *Evaluating research articles from start to finish.* Thousand Oaks: SAGE Publications, 1996.

Hirsch RP, Riegelman RK. *Statistical first aid: interpretation of health research data.* Cambridge, MA: Blackwell Science, 1992.

Riegelman RR, Hirsch. RP. *Studying a study and testing a test—how to read the health science literature,* 3rd ed. Boston: Little, Brown and Company, 1996.

Measurements for Reliability and Validity

DeVellis RF. *Scale development. Theory and applications: applied social research methods series.* Newbury Park, CA: Sage Publications, 1991.

Streiner DL, Norman GR. *Health measurement scales: a guide to their development and use,* 2nd ed. Oxford: Oxford University Press, 1995.

Statistics

Armitage P, Berry G. *Statistical methods in medical research,* 3rd ed. Cambridge, MA: Blackwell Science, 1994.

Bailar JC III, Mosteller F, eds. *Medical uses of statistics,* 2nd ed. Boston: New England Journal of Medicine Books, 1992.

Bland M. *An introduction to medical statistics,* 2nd ed. Oxford: Oxford Medical Publications, 1995.

Campbell MJ, Machin D. *Medical statistics—a commonsense approach.* Chichester: John Wiley & Sons, 1990.

Cohen J. *Statistical power analysis for the behavioral sciences,* 2nd ed. Hillsdale, NJ: Lawrence Erlbaum Associates, 1988.

Colton T. *Statistics in medicine.* Boston: Little, Brown and Company, 1974.

Fleiss JL. *Statistical methods for rates and proportions,* 2nd ed. New York: John Wiley & Sons, 1981.

Gardner MJ, Alman DG. *Statistics with confidence.* London: British Medical Journal, 1989.

Hosmer DW, Lemeshow S. *Applied logistic regression.* New York: Wiley, 1989.

Huff D. *How to lie with statistics.* New York: W.W. Norton, 1954.

Kirkwood BR. *Essentials of medical statistics.* Oxford: Blackwell Science, 1988.

Matthews DE, Farewell VT. *Using and understanding medical statistics,* 2nd ed. Basel, Switzerland: Karger, 1988.

Remington RD, Schork MA. *Statistics with applications to the biological and health sciences,* 2nd ed. Engelwood Cliffs, NJ: Prentice-Hall, Inc., 1970.

Snedecor GW, Cochran WC. *Statistical methods,* 7th ed. Ames, IA: Iowa State Unversity Press, 1980.

Writing Research

Day RA. *How to write and publish a scientific paper,* 3rd ed. Phoenix, AZ: Oryx Press, 1988.

Huth EJ. *How to write and publish papers in the medical sciences,* 2nd ed. Baltimore: Williams & Wilkins, 1990.

PART II

Torso and Axial Skeleton

Principles and Practice of Orthopaedic Sports Medicine,
edited by William E. Garrett, Jr., Kevin P. Speer, and Donald T. Kirkendall.
Lippincott Williams & Wilkins, Philadelphia © 2000.

CHAPTER 9

Intracranial and Cervical Spine Injuries

Joseph S. Torg and Thomas A. Gennarelli

The purpose of this chapter is to present clear concise guidelines for the classification, evaluation, and emergency management of injuries that occur to the head and neck as a result of participation in competitive and recreational activities. Although all athletic injuries require careful attention, the evaluation and management of injuries to the head and neck should proceed with particular consideration. The actual or potential involvement of the nervous system creates a high-risk situation in which the margin for error is low. An accurate diagnosis is imperative, but the clinical picture is not always representative of the seriousness of the injury at hand. An intracranial hemorrhage may present initially with minimal symptoms yet follow a precipitous downhill course, whereas a less-severe injury, such as neurapraxia of the brachial plexus associated with alarming paresthesias and paralysis, will resolve swiftly and allow a quick return to activity. Although the more severe injuries are rather infrequent, this low incidence coincidentally results in little if any management experience for the on-site medical staff.

EMERGENCY MANAGEMENT

Several principles should be considered by individuals responsible for athletes who may sustain injuries to the head and neck (1). The team physician or trainer should be designated as the person responsible for supervising the on-the-field management of the potentially serious injury. This person is the "captain" of the medical team. Planning must ensure the availability of all necessary emergency equipment at the site of potential injury. At

a minimum, this should include a spine board, stretcher, and equipment necessary for the initiation and maintenance of cardiopulmonary resuscitation. A properly equipped ambulance and a hospital equipped and staffed to handle emergency neurologic problems must be available. Also, the immediate availability of a telephone for communicating with the hospital emergency room, ambulance, and other responsible individuals in case of an emergency must be assured.

Managing the unconscious or spine-injured athlete is a process that should not be done hastily or haphazardly. Being prepared to handle this situation is the best way to prevent actions that could convert a repairable injury into a catastrophe. All the necessary equipment must be readily accessible and in good operating condition, and all assisting personnel must have been trained to use it properly. On-the-job training in an emergency situation is inefficient at best. Everyone should know what must be done beforehand so that on a signal the game plan can be put into effect.

A means of transporting the athlete must be immediately available in a high-risk sport such as football and "on call" in other sports. The medical facility must be alerted to the athlete's condition and estimated time of arrival so that adequate preparation can be made.

The availability of the proper equipment is essential. A spine board is necessary and is the best means of supporting the body in a rigid position. It is essentially a full body splint. By splinting the body, the risk of aggravating a spinal cord injury, which must always be suspected in the unconscious athlete, is reduced. In football, bolt cutters and a sharp knife or scalpel are also essential if it becomes necessary to remove the face mask. A telephone must be available to call for assistance and to notify the medical facility. Oxygen should be available and is usually carried by ambulance and rescue squads, although it is rarely required in an athletic setting. Rigid cervical collars and other external immobilization devices can be helpful if prop-

J. S. Torg: Department of Orthopedic Surgery, HCP Hahnemann School of Medicine, Philadelphia, Pennsylvania 19107.

T. A. Gennarelli: Department of Neurosurgery, Medical College of Wisconsin, Milwaukee, Wisconsin 53226.

erly used. Manual stabilization of the head and neck is recommended if no other means are available.

Prevention of further injury is the single most important objective. The first step should be to check for breathing, pulse, and level of consciousness. If the victim is breathing, simply remove the mouth guard, if present, and maintain the airway. It is necessary to remove the face mask only if the respiratory situation is threatened or unstable or if the athlete remains unconscious for a prolonged period. Leave the chin strap on.

Once it is established that the athlete is breathing and has a pulse, evaluate the neurologic status. The level of consciousness; response to pain; pupillary response; and any unusual posturing, flaccidity, rigidity, or weakness should be noted.

At this point, simply maintain the situation until transportation is available or until the athlete regains consciousness. If the athlete is face down when the ambulance arrives, change his or her position to face up by log rolling onto a spine board. Gentle longitudinal traction should be exerted to support the head without attempting to correct alignment. Make no attempt to move the injured person except to transport or to perform cardiopulmonary resuscitation if it becomes necessary.

If the athlete is not breathing or stops breathing, the airway must be established. If face down, he or she must be turned to a face-up position. The safest and easiest way to accomplish this is to log roll the athlete into a face-up position. In an ideal situation, the medical support team is made up of five members: the leader, who controls the head and gives the commands only; three members to roll; and another to help lift and carry when it becomes necessary. If time permits and the spine board is on the scene, the athlete should be rolled directly onto it. However, breathing and circulation are much more important at this point.

With all medical support team members in position, the athlete is rolled toward the assistants—one at the shoulders, one at the hips, and one at the knees. They must maintain the body in line with the head and spine during the roll. The leader maintains immobilization of the head by applying slight traction and by using the crossed-arm technique. This technique allows the arms to unwind during the roll.

The face mask must be removed from the helmet before rescue breathing can be initiated. The type of mask that is attached to the helmet determines the method of removal. Bolt cutters are used with the older single- and double-bar masks. The newer masks that are attached with plastic loops should be removed by cutting the loops with a sharp knife or scalpel. Remove the entire mask so that it does not interfere with further rescue efforts. Once the mask has been removed, initiate rescue breathing following the current stands of the American Heart Association.

Once the athlete has been moved to a face-up position, quickly evaluate breathing and pulse. If there is still no breathing or if breathing has stopped, the airway must be established. The jaw thrust technique is the safest approach to opening the airway of a victim who has a suspected neck injury because in most cases it can be accomplished by the rescuer grasping the angles of the victim's lower jaw and lifting with both hands, one on each side, displacing the mandible forward while tilting the head backward. The rescuer's elbows should rest on the surface on which the victim is lying.

If the jaw thrust is not adequate, the head tilt–jaw lift should be substituted. Care must be exercised not to overextend the neck. The fingers of one hand are placed under the lower jaw to help tilt the head back. The fingers must not compress the soft tissue under the chin, which might obstruct the airway. The other hand presses on the victim's forehead to tilt the head back.

The transportation team should be familiar with handling a victim with a cervical spine injury, and they should be receptive to taking orders from the team physician or trainer. It is extremely important not to lose control of the care of the athlete; therefore, be familiar with the transportation crew that is used. In an athletic situation, prior arrangements with an ambulance service should be made.

An appreciation of the controversy that currently exists between emergency medicine physicians and technicians on one hand and team physicians and athletic trainers on the other regarding helmet removal is in order. Existing emergency medical services guidelines mandate removal of protective headgear before transport of an individual suspected of having a cervical spine injury to a fixed medical installation. These guidelines were implemented with motorcycle helmets in mind to facilitate both airway accessibility and application of cervical spine-immobilizing devices. Clearly, such a procedure contradicts the long-standing principle adhered to by team physicians and athletic trainers of leaving the helmet in place on the football player suspected of having a cervical spine injury until he is transported to a definitive medical facility.

It must be emphasized that this particular problem is of more than academic interest. Specifically, there has been occasions where emergency medical technicians under the directions of emergency room physicians unfamiliar with the nuances of the relationship between helmet, shoulder pads, and the injured cervical spine have precipitated turf battles by refusing to move the injured player before helmet removal. Again, such episodes represent more than an honest difference of opinion. Such episodes are clearly detrimental to the health and well-being of the injured player. If is our view that removal of the football helmet and shoulder pads on site exposes the potentially injured spine to both unnecessary and awkward manipulation and disruption of the immobilizing capacity of the helmet and shoulder pads. Also, removal of the helmet alone subjects a potentially unstable spine to hyperlordotic deformity.

We are in agreement with the National Athletic Association Guidelines for helmet removal (2) as follows. Unless there are special circumstances such as respiratory distress coupled with an inability to access the airway, the helmet should never be removed during the prehospital care of the athlete with a potential head/neck injury unless

1. The helmet does not hold the head securely, such that immobilization of the helmet does not immobilize the head;
2. The design of the sport helmet is such that even after removal of the face mask, the airway cannot be controlled or ventilation provided;
3. After a reasonable period of time, the face mask cannot be removed;
4. The helmet prevents immobilization for transportation in an appropriate position.

When such helmet removal is necessary in any setting, it should be performed only by personnel trained in this procedure. If removal of the helmet is needed to initiate treatment or to obtain special x-rays, specific protocol needs to be followed. With the head, neck, and helmet manually stabilized, the chin strap can be cut. While maintaining stability, the cheek pads can be removed by slipping the flat blade of a screwdriver or bandage scissor under the pad snaps and above the inner surface of the shell. While another individual provides manual stability of the chin and neck, the persons stabilizing the head place their thumbs or index fingers into the earholes on both sides. By pulling both laterally and longitudinally, the helmet shell can be spread and eased off. If a rocking motion is necessary to loosen the helmet,

the head/neck unit must not be allowed to move. Those individuals participating in this important maneuver must proceed with caution and coordinate every move (Fig. 9.1A and B).

Supporting the concept of leaving the helmet on is the work of Swenson et al. (3) and Gastel et al. (4). Swenson et al. studied sagittal cervical alignment in live subjects with various combinations of helmets, shoulder pads, and no equipment. They concluded that football players with a potential cervical spine injury should be immobilized for transport with both their helmet and shoulder pads left in place, thereby maintaining the neck in a position most closely approximating "normal." Gastel et al. performed a similar study using stable and surgically destabilized cadaver spines. They concluded that to maintain a neutral position and minimize secondary injury to the cervical neural elements, the helmet and shoulder pads either should be both left on or both removed in the emergency setting.

Despite the advent of such "high-tech" imaging modalities as computed tomography (CT) and magnetic resonance imaging (MRI), the initial radiographic examination of a patient with suspected or actual cervical spine trauma remains a routine roentgenographic examination. The preliminary study, while immobilization of the head, neck, and trunk is maintained, includes an anteroposterior and lateral examination of vertebrae C1-7. If a major fracture, subluxation, dislocation or evidence of instability is not evident, the remainder of the routine examination, including open mouth and oblique views, should be obtained. Depending on the neurologic and comfort status of the patient, lateral flexion and extension views should be obtained at some point. CT and MRI may provide more detailed information; however, horizontally oriented fractures and subtle subluxations are best identified on the routine radio-

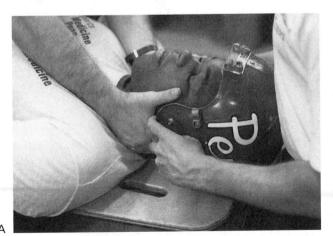
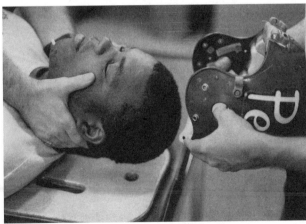

A   B

FIG. 9.1. A: The helmet should be removed only when permanent immobilization can be instituted. The helmet may be removed by detaching the chin strap, spreading the earflaps, and gently pulling the helmet off in straight line with the cervical spine. **B:** The head must be supported under the occiput during and after removing the helmet.

graphs. The choice of imaging technique will depend on the results of the routine examination, the neurologic status of the patient, the preference of the responsible physician, and the availability of the imaging modalities.

A study performed under the auspices of the National Institute of Neurological Disorders and Stroke showed that patients sustaining spinal cord injury demonstrated significant improvement in muscle function and sensation if administered methylprednisolone intravenously within 8 hours of injury (5). Specifically, the initial dose of methylprednisolone is administered in a bolus of 30 mg/kg body weight intravenously with an infusion pump for 15 minutes. Forty-five minutes after this, a maintenance dose of 5.4 mm/kg/h is administered intravenously with an infusion pump for 23 hours.

Although we do not propose that this regimen is initiated as an immediate on field emergency procedure, certainly those responsible for the spinal cord-injured athlete have an obligation to ensure that it is administered within the first 8 hours.

It is interesting to note that in the early 1970s Schneider (6) commented as follows:

> Currently there has been a major advance in the treatment of spinal cord injuries. It has been demonstrated definitely in the experimental animal, and is reasonably well supported in man, as of this writing, that the early use of steroids in the treatment of some spinal cord injuries will cause a diminution of swelling and destruction of the cord with the prevention of neurologic deficit. Experimental work has shown that the drug probably should be administered within 3 to 6 hours after the spinal cord is injured for the drug to be effective. Therefore the decision whether this form of medical therapy should be instituted should be made by the physician shortly after the player has been taken to the dressing room and the presence of spinal cord damage has been confirmed. It may be withheld if the patient definitely can be transported within 3 hours to the neurosurgeon so that he can make the decision. If the time interval is longer than this, then Decadron, 10 mg, should be administered intramuscularly and then 4 mg should be given every 6 hours.

INTRACRANIAL INJURIES

The athlete who receives a blow to the head or a sudden jolt to the body that results in a sudden acceleration-deceleration force to the head should be carefully evaluated. If the individual is ambulatory and conscious, the entire spectrum of intracranial damage, ranging from a grade 1 concussion to a more severe intracranial condition, must be considered. Initial on-field examination should include an evaluation of the following:

1. Facial expression;
2. Orientation to time, place, and person;
3. Presence of posttraumatic amnesia;
4. Presence of retrograde amnesia;
5. Abnormal gait.

Traumatic injuries to the brain can be classified as diffuse or focal. The immediate and definitive management of athletically induced trauma to the brain depends on the nature and severity of the injury. Those responsible for managing such injuries must understand the problems from the standpoint of basic pathomechanics.

Diffuse Brain Injuries

Diffuse brain injuries are associated with widespread or global disruption of neurologic function and are not usually associated with macroscopically visible brain lesions. Diffuse brain injuries result from shaking of the brain within the skull and thus are lesions caused by the inertial or acceleration effects of a mechanical input to the head. Both theoretic and experimental evidence points to rotational acceleration as the primary mechanism of injury in diffuse brain injuries.

Because diffuse brain injuries, for the most part, are not associated with visible macroscopic lesions, they have historically been lumped together to include all injuries not associated with focal lesions. More recently, however, diagnostic information has been gained from CT and MRI, as well as from neurophysiologic studies, that make it possible to define more clearly several categories within this broad group of diffuse brain injuries.

Three categories of diffuse brain injury are recognized (7–11):

1. Mild concussion: Several specific concussion syndromes involve temporary disturbances of neurologic function without loss of consciousness.
2. Classic cerebral concussion: This is a temporary reversible neurologic deficiency caused by trauma that results in temporary loss of consciousness.
3. Diffuse axonal injury: This takes the form of prolonged traumatic brain coma with loss of consciousness lasting more than 6 hours. Residual neurologic, psychologic, or personality deficits often result because of structural disruption of numerous axons in the white matter of the cerebral hemispheres and brainstem.

Mild Cerebral Concussion

The syndromes of mild cerebral concussion are included in the continuum of diffuse brain injuries; they represent the mildest form of injury in this spectrum. Mild concussion syndromes are those in which consciousness is preserved but some degree of noticeable temporary neurologic dysfunction occurs. These injuries are exceedingly common and, because of their mild degree, often are not brought to medical attention; however, they are the most common brain injuries encountered in sports medicine.

A grade 1 mild concussion, the mildest form of head injury, results in confusion and disorientation unaccompanied by amnesia. This temporary confusion, without loss of consciousness, lasts only momentarily after the injury. This concussion syndrome is completely reversible, and there are no associated sequelae. An individual with a grade 1 mild concussion is confused, has a dazed look, and may exhibit mild unsteadiness of gait. However, posttraumatic amnesia (forgetting events after the injury) and retrograde amnesia (forgetting the events before the injury) are not prominent features. This clinical picture is best described by the athletes themselves who say "I had my bell rung." Usually, the state of confusion is short-lived, and the athlete is completely lucid in 5 to 15 minutes. When the athlete's mind is clear, he or she may return to the former activity under the watchful supervision of the team physician or trainer. However, associated symptoms such as vertigo, headaches, photophobia, and labile emotions should preclude returning to the game.

A grade 2 mild concussion is characterized by confusion associated with retrograde amnesia that develops after 5 to 10 minutes. Again, this is an extremely frequent event. Athletes may experience a "ding," and although confused, they may continue coordinated sensorimotor activities after the injury. If examined immediately, these players have total recall of the events immediately before impact. However, retrograde amnesia develops 5 to 10 minutes later, and thereafter they do not remember the impact or events immediately before the impact. The amnesia usually covers only several minutes before the injury; it may diminish somewhat, but players always have some degree of permanent, through brief, retrograde amnesia despite resumption of completely normal consciousness. The confusion and disorientation completely resolve.

Individuals manifesting amnesia should not be permitted to return to play that day. These athletes require careful postinjury evaluation. They may develop the "postconcussion syndrome," characterized by persistent headaches, inability to concentrate, and irritability. In some instances, these symptoms may last for several weeks after the injury, and participation in the sport is precluded as long as symptoms are present.

As the mechanical stresses to the brain increase in grade 3 mild concussion, confusion and amnesia are present from the time of impact. Athletes can usually continue to play, although they have no recollection of previous events. By this stage, some degree of posttraumatic amnesia occurs in addition to retrograde amnesia. The confusion may last many minutes, but then the level of consciousness returns to normal, usually with some permanent degree of retrograde and posttraumatic amnesia.

These three syndromes of mild cerebral concussion have been frequently witnessed and described in detail.

Although consciousness is preserved, it is clear that some degree of cerebral dysfunction has occurred. The fact that memory mechanisms appear to be the most sensitive to trauma suggests that the cerebral hemispheres rather than the brainstem are the location of the mild injury forces. The degree of cerebral cortical dysfunction, however, is not sufficient to disconnect the influence if the cerebral hemispheres from the brainstem activating system, and therefore consciousness is preserved. Few cortical functions except memory seem to be in jeopardy, and the only residual deficit that patients with mild concussion syndromes have is the brief retrograde or posttraumatic amnesia. However, because definite alteration of brain function has occurred, athletes who sustain grades 2 and 3 mild cerebral concussions should not be permitted to participate in the remainder of the contest.

Classic Cerebral Concussion

Classic cerebral concussion is seen in the "knocked-out" player. This individual is in a paralytic coma, usually recovers after a few seconds or minutes, and then passes through stages of stupor, confusion with or without delirium, and finally an almost lucid state of automatism before becoming fully alert. Such an individual will most certainly have retrograde and posttraumatic amnesia. If the loss of consciousness last for more than several minutes or if there are other signs of a deteriorating neurologic state, the patient should be immediately transported to a hospital (12).

The athlete who has been rendered unconscious should be initially evaluated to determine whether he or she is breathing, whether there is a pulse, and the level of consciousness. If unobstructed respirations and an adequate pulse are present, there is no immediate need to do anything except keep in mind that head and neck injuries are frequently associated. Therefore, the player should be protected from injudicious manipulation or movement.

Such patients frequently remain semistuporous for more than several minutes. They should be removed from the field on a spine board or stretcher and should not be permitted to stagger off. An athlete who has been rendered unconscious for any length of time should not be allowed to return to contact activity that day, even if he or she is mentally clear. Overnight observation in a hospital should be considered for those who experience more than a transient loss of consciousness.

Insufficient attention has been given to the precise states of recovery from classic cerebral concussion. Although by definition loss of consciousness is transient and reversible, the sequelae of concussion are commonplace. Some sequelae such as headache or tinnitus may reflect injuries to the head, the inner ear, or other noncerebral structures. However, subtle changes in per-

TABLE 9.1. *Guidelines for return to play after concussion*

First concussion	Second concussion	Third concussion
Grade 1 (mild): may return to play if asymptomatic[a]	Return to play in 2 wk if asymptomatic at that time for 1 week	Terminate season; may return to play next season if asymptomatic
Grade 2 (moderate): return to play after asymptomatic for 1 wk	Minimum of 1 mo; may return to play then if asymptomatic for 1 wk; consider terminating season	Terminate season; may return to play next season if asymptomatic
Grade 3 (severe): minimum of 1 mo; may then return to play if asymptomatic for 1 wk	Terminate season; may return to play next season if asymptomatic	

[a]No headache, dizziness, or impaired orientation, concentration, or memory during rest or exertion.
Grade 1 (mild): no loss of consciousness or posttraumatic amnesia < 30 min; grade 2 (moderate): loss of consciousness < 5 min or posttraumatic amnesia > 30 min; grade 3 (severe): loss of consciousness > 5 min or posttraumatic amnesia > 24 hr.

sonality and in psychologic or memory functioning have been documented and must have a cerebrocortical origin. Thus, although most patients with classic cerebral concussion experience no sequelate other than amnesia for the events of impact, some individuals may have other long-lasting, although subtle, neurologic deficiencies that must be investigated further. Cantu, using a somewhat more simplified classification of cerebral concussion, developed criteria for return to play after concussion (Table 9.1) (13).

Second Impact Syndrome

Delayed brain swelling may occur after a concussion complicated by the postconcussion syndrome, that is, persistence of any symptoms such as of headache, vertigo, inability to concentrate, irritability, tenderness, or memory disturbance. Return to contact activity before complete resolution of a concussion and postconcussion syndrome can result in the second impact syndrome. The effects of delayed brain swelling associated with this phenomenon can be disastrous. The implications in making clinical decisions regarding the return of an individual to a contact activity are quite apparent (14).

Focal Brain Syndromes

In discussing the occurrence of intracranial hematoma resulting from athletic injury, two major points must be emphasized. First, due to recent developments in the clinical evaluation of patients and correlated animal research, there is now a satisfactory understanding of the mechanism of occurrence of focal intracranial hematoma, which is somewhat different from the older concepts of head injuries (15). Second, management of such patients has advanced rapidly and has changed dramatically during the last decade from what was accepted medical practice in the past.

The entire spectrum of traumatic intracranial hematomas occurs in sports injuries, including cerebral contusions, intracerebral hematomas, epidural hematomas,

and acute subdural hematomas. The presentation of athletes with head injuries who have had serious trauma is similar in most instances. Management depends on definitive diagnosis and varies according to the underlying pathologic process.

Intracerebral Hematoma and Contusion

These injuries occur in patients with a significant intracerebral pathologic condition who may not have suffered loss of consciousness or focal neurologic deficit but who do have a persistent headache or periods of confusion after a head injury and posttraumatic amnesia (16). As with any patient who has suffered a head injury, athletes with such symptoms should undergo a CT to permit early differentiation between solid intracerebral hematoma and hemorrhagic contusion with surrounding edema.

Epidural Hematoma

Epidural hematoma results when the middle meningeal artery, which is imbedded in a bony groove in the skull, tears as a result of a skull fracture crossing this groove. Because the bleeding in this instance is arterial, accumulation of clot continues under high pressure, leading to a potentially serious brain injury.

The classic description of an epidural hematoma is that of loss of consciousness at the time of injury, followed by recovery of consciousness in a variable period, after which the patient is lucid. This is followed by the onset of increasingly severe headache; decreased level of consciousness; dilation of one pupil, usually on the same side as the clot; and decerebrate posturing and weakness, usually on the side opposite the hematoma. In our experience, however, only one third of patients with epidural hematoma present with this classic history. Another third of patients do not become unconscious until late in the course of illness, and the remaining third are unconscious from the time of injury and remain unconscious throughout their course. The absence of a classic clinical picture of epidural hematoma cannot be relied on to rule out this diagnosis, and the best diagnostic test for evaluating these patients is a CT.

Acute Subdural Hematoma

Athletic head injuries result from inertial loading at a lower level than that associated with serious head injuries caused by vehicular accident or falling from heights. Also, acute subdural hematomas occur much more frequently than epidural hematomas in athletes. In patients with head injuries in general, approximately three times as many acute subdural hematomas occur as do epidural hematomas.

Two main types of acute subdural hematomas have been clearly identified: those with a collection of blood in the subdural space, apparently not associated with underlying cerebral contusion or edema, and those with collections of blood in the subdural space but associated with an obvious contusion on the surface of the brain and hemispheric brain injury with swelling. The mortality for simple subdural hematomas is approximately 20%, but this increases to more than 50% for subdural hematomas with an underlying brain injury.

Patients with an acute subdural hematoma typically are unconscious, may or may not have a history of deterioration, and frequently display focal neurologic findings. Patients with simple subdural hematomas are more likely to have had a lucid interval after their injury and are less likely to be unconscious at admission than patients with hemispheric injury and brain swelling. It is necessary to obtain a CT or MRI to diagnose an acute subdural hematoma. The size of the subdural clot relative to the size of the midline shift of the brain structures can be evaluated best by CT. Of patients with acute subdural hematoma, 84% also have an associated hemorrhagic contusion or intracerebral hematoma with associated brain swelling.

The term acute subdural hematoma raises the image of a large collection of clotted blood in the intracranial cavity, compressing the brain substance and causing brain compromise due to the space occupied by the hematoma. This is not an infrequent consequence of closed head trauma, but this type of subdural hematoma is more common in adults who have a degree of cortical atrophy.

Young athletes, and especially children, frequently develop only minimal subdural hematomas with underlying cerebral hemispheric swelling (17). This type of brain injury is not the result of a space-occupying mass resulting from clotted blood causing brain compression but rather swollen brain tissue causing a consequent rise in intracranial pressure. The advent of CT and MRI permits an accurate differential diagnosis between these two conditions, which frequently cause similar clinical pictures. The modalities of treatment for these two distinct types of acute subdural hematomas are quite different.

Brain Swelling

Brain swelling is a poorly understood phenomenon that can accompany any type of head injury. Swelling is not synonymous with cerebral edema, which refers to a specific increase in brain water. Such as increase in water content may not occur in brain swelling, and current evidence favors the concept that brain swelling is due in part to increased intravascular blood within the brain. This is caused by a vascular reaction to head injury that leads to vasodilation and increased cerebral blood volume. If this increased cerebral blood volume continues long enough, vascular permeability may increase, and true edema may result (18).

Although brain swelling may occur in any type of head injury, the magnitude of swelling does not correlate with the severity of the injury. Thus, both severe and minor head injuries may be complicated by brain swelling. The effects of brain swelling are thus additive to those of primary brain injury and may in certain instances be more severe than the primary injury itself.

Despite our lack of knowledge about the precise mechanism that causes brain swelling, it can be conceptualized in two general forms. It should be remembered that many difference types of brain swelling exist and that acute and delayed brain swelling represent phenomenologic rather than mechanistic entities.

Acute brain swelling occurs in several circumstances. Swelling that accompanies focal brain lesions tends to be localized, whereas diffuse brain injuries are associated with generalized swelling. Focal swelling is usually present beneath contusions but does not often contribute additional deleterious effects. On the other hand, the swelling that occurs with acute subdural hematomas, although principally hemispheric in distribution, may cause more mass effect than the hematoma itself. In such circumstances, the small amount of blood in the subdural space may not be the entire reason for the patient's neurologic state. If the hematoma is removed, the acute brain swelling may progress so rapidly that the brain protrudes through the craniotomy opening. Every neurosurgeon is all to familiar with the external herniation of the brain, which, when it occurs, is difficult to treat.

The more serious types of diffuse brain injuries are associated with generalized rather than focal acute brain swelling. Although not all patients with diffuse axonal injury have brain swelling, the incidence of swelling is higher than that in patients with either classic cerebral concussion or one of the mild concussion syndromes. Because of the serious nature of the underlying injury, it is difficult to determine the extent of swelling in these patients. The swelling, although widespread throughout the brain, may not cause a rise in intracranial pressure for several days. This late rise in pressure probably reflects the formation of true cerebral edema, and it may be that diffuse swelling associated with severe diffuse brain injuries is harmful because it produces edema. In any event, this type of swelling is different from the type of swelling associated with acute subdural hematomas.

Delayed brain swelling may occur minutes to hours after head injury. It is usually diffuse and is often associated with milder forms of diffuse brain injuries. Whether delayed swelling is the same or a different phenomenon from the acute swelling of the more serious diffuse injuries is unknown. However, in less severe diffuse injuries, there is a distinct time interval before delayed swelling becomes manifest, thus confirming that the primary insult to the brain was not serious. Considering the high frequency of mild concussions, the incidence of delayed swelling must be low. However, when it occurs, delayed swelling can cause profound neurologic changes or even death.

In its most severe form, severe delayed swelling can cause deep coma. The usual history is that of an injury associated with a mild concussion or a classic cerebral concussion from which the patient recovers. Minutes to hours later that patient becomes lethargic, then stuporous, and finally lapses into a coma. The coma may be either a light coma with appropriate motor responses to painful stimuli or a deep coma associated with decorticate or decerebrate posturing.

The key differences between these patients and those with diffuse axonal injury is that in the latter the coma and abnormal motor signs are present from the moment of injury, whereas with delayed cerebral swelling there is a time interval without these signs. This distinction is significant, however, because with diffuse axonal injury a certain amount of primary structural damage has occurred at the moment of impact, but this is not present in cases of pure delayed swelling. Therefore, the deleterious effects of delayed swelling should be potentially reversible, and if these effects are controlled the outcome should be good. However, such control may be difficult. Vigorous monitoring of and attention to intracranial pressure is required to control brain swelling. If this is accomplished successfully, the mortality from increased intracranial pressure associated with diffuse brain swelling should be low.

Principles of Management

As knowledge of physiology and pathophysiology has increased, so has the ability to resuscitate seriously ill or severely injured people successfully. The 1950s saw the start of successful treatment of acute respiratory and postoperative problems, followed by satisfactory cardiac resuscitation and emergency cardiac care in the 1960s. Innovations in critical care medicine were ex-

tended in the form of brain resuscitation in the 1970s. Such care is based on the concept that the degree of permanent neurologic, intellectual, and psychologic deficit after brain trauma with coma is only partly the result of the initial injury and is certainly in part due to secondary changes, which can be worsened or improved by the quality of the supportive care received. Head injuries by their very nature require resuscitation, that is, therapy initiated after the insult. The proper care of patients with head injuries, athletic or otherwise, depends on a full appreciation and use of brain resuscitation measures in an intensive care setting.

Treatment for focal intracranial hematoma consists of removal of the hematoma and recognition of and treatment for the underlying brain injury. Included in this concept is that of resuscitation of the brain, which is therapy designed to have specific neuron-saving potential once general resuscitation methods and supportive care have begun.

First aid should consist of getting the patient safely into a supine position and determining the vital signs and the significance of any associated injuries. Initial treatment should be to establish an adequate and useful airway and begin hyperventilation maneuvers. This can be accomplished by using a manual resuscitation bag with supplemental oxygen, if available. The patient should then be transferred as quickly as possible to a medical facility where diagnosis and treatment of brain injury can begin. Although these measures are important for all patients who have suffered concussion, they are vital for patients who remain comatose after trauma. Also, consideration must be given to the possibility of a concomitant cervical spine injury and appropriate measures taken. Once patients arrive in the emergency room and their cardiorespiratory status is determined to be stable, endotracheal intubation is immediately performed on comatose patients. CT or MRI is obtained as soon as possible to provide an immediate diagnosis of the intracranial condition. Patients are then categorized as either surgical or nonsurgical cases, depending on the size of the intracranial hematoma.

CERVICAL SPINE INJURIES

Athletic injuries to the cervical spine may involve the bony vertebrae; the intervertebral disks; the ligamentous supporting structures; the spinal cord, roots, and peripheral nerves; or any combination of these structures. The panorama of injuries observed runs the spectrum from the "cervical sprain syndrome" to fracture dislocations with permanent quadriplegia. Fortunately, severe injuries with neural involvement occur infrequently. However, those responsible for the emergency and subsequent care of the athlete with a cervical spine injury should possess a basic understanding of the variety of problems that can occur.

The various athletic injuries to the cervical spine and related structures are

1. Nerve root brachial plexus injury;
2. Stable cervical sprain;
3. Muscular strain;
4. Nerve root brachial plexus axonotmesis;
5. Intervertebral disk injury (narrowing herniation) without neurologic deficit;
6. Stable cervical fractures without neurologic deficit;
7. Subluxations without neurologic deficit;
8. Unstable fractures without neurologic deficit;
9. Dislocations without neurologic deficit;
10. Intervertebral disk herniation without neurologic deficit;
11. Unstable fracture with neurologic deficit;
12. Dislocation with neurologic deficit;
13. Quadriplegia;
14. Death.

Criteria for return to contact activities after congenital and traumatic problems of the cervical spine are included at the end of this chapter.

Nerve Root Brachial Plexus Injury

The most common and poorly understood cervical injuries are the pinch-stretch neurapraxias of the nerve roots and brachial plexus (Fig. 9.2). Typically, after contact with the head, neck, or shoulder, a sharp burning pain is experienced in the neck and on the involved side that may radiate into the shoulder and down the arm to the hand. There may be associated weakness and paresthesia in the involved extremity lasting from several seconds to several minutes. Characteristically, there is weakness of shoulder abduction (deltoid), elbow flexion (biceps), and external humeral rotation (spinatis). The key to the nature of this lesion is its short duration and the presence of a full pain-free range of neck motion. Although most of these injuries are short-lived, they are worrisome because of the occasional plexus axonotmesis that occurs. However, the youngsters whose paresthesia completely abates, who demonstrates full muscle strength in the intrinsic muscles of the shoulder and upper extremities, and who, most importantly, has a full pain-free range of cervical motion may return to his or her activity.

Persistence of paresthesia, weakness, or limitation of cervical motion requires that the individual is protected from further exposure and that he or she undergo neurologic, electromyographic, and roentgenographic evaluation. Persistent or recurrent episodes require a complete neurologic and radiographic imaging workup. If routine roentgenographic films of the cervical spine are negative and a preganglionic root lesion is suspected, MRI, plain myelography, or CT myelography should be considered.

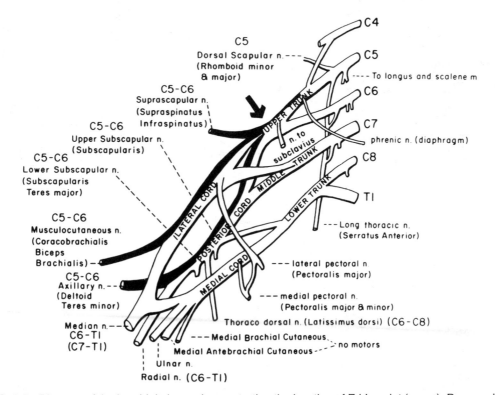

FIG. 9.2. Diagram of the brachial plexus demonstrating the location of Erb's point (*arrow*). Presumably, brachial plexus stretch injuries result from traction of the plexus at this joint. (From Torg JS. *Athletic injuries to the head, neck and face,* 2nd ed. St. Louis, MO: Mosby-Yearbook, 1991, with permission.)

Disk herniation, foraminal narrowing, and extradural intraspinal masses should be considered in the differential diagnosis. A complete electromyographic (EMG) examination, including both nerve conduction studies and a needle electrode examination, may be helpful. These studies should be delayed for 3 to 4 weeks from the time of the initial injury. Nerve conduction studies should include both routine conduction and sensory nerve action potential evaluations. Electrode evaluation of the cervical spine musculature will differentiate between preganglionic root injuries and plexus pathologies.

Brachial plexus injuries can be classified according to the staging system (19) described by Seddon (20). Neurapraxia is the mildest lesion and corresponds to a reversible aberration in the axonal function without intrinsic axonal disruption. The episode is transient and completely reversible, with resolution occurring almost immediately or within 2 weeks. The next level of nerve injury is axonotmesis, in which injury results in disruption of the axon and myelin sheath. The epineurium, however, remains intact. After injury, Wallerian degeneration occurs from the point of injury distally, and complete regeneration must occur for function to return.

The most severe injury, neurotmesis, results from an irreversible insult resulting in nerve laceration, crushing, or stretching such that the endoneurium, epineurium, and perineurium are all disrupted. Recovery does not occur. It should be noted that in the absence of frank shoulder dislocation or a penetrating injury, this lesion is rarely if even seen as a result of athletic activity.

The "burner" syndrome characteristically seen in contact activities such as football is generally believed to be a traction injury of the brachial plexus involving the upper trunk. The mechanism results from depression of the ipsilateral shoulder with forceful deviation of the head and cervical region to the opposite side. However, it is also quite apparent that a mechanism involving neck extension, ipsilateral rotation, and compression in individuals with intervertebral foraminal narrowing can result in root compression (21). This mechanism can be demonstrated by the Spurling maneuver, in which the head is extended, rotated toward the involved arm, and compressed. A positive test will reproduce the pain or symptoms.

With regard to management on the field of the athlete with a burner syndrome, generally, demonstrable weakness and anesthesia associated with burning pain are

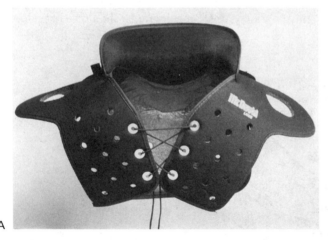

A

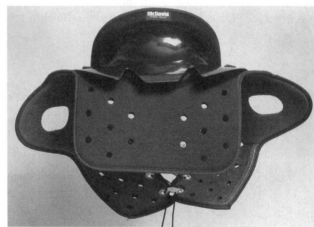

B

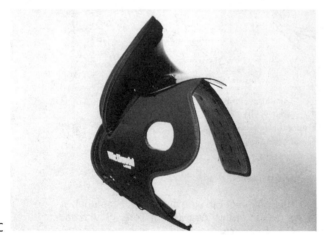

C

FIG. 9.3. (A) Frontal, (B) posterior, and (C) lateral views of the cowboy collar. This device, which is worn under the shoulder pads, effectively limits the extremes of extension and lateral bending of the cervical spine.

transient. If there is no associated neck pain or limitation of cervical motion, an asymptomatic individual may return to his or her activity. However, if examination reveals decreased neck motion and pain, the athlete should be removed from competition pending further evaluation. In individuals with persistent weakness, appropriate studies should be done as mentioned to rule out other significant cervical spine pathology. In most individuals, EMG will show an upper trunk plexopathy. The athlete's progress can be used as a guideline for return to activities. As stated by Hershman (22), "waiting for the EMG to return to normal is not an appropriate criteria for returning to activity." Although a mild degree of weakness may be tolerable if strength has been documented to be improving, weakness that will render the athlete unable to perform and protect him- or herself should preclude further activity. Those with recurrent burners may continue to participate as long as they have normal pain-free motion and full muscle strength. Prevention of recurrent plexus neurapraxia is based on a year-round neck and shoulder muscle strengthening program and appropriate "horse-collar" type neck rolls to prevent extreme neck deviation (Fig. 9.3A and B). Straps that bind the helmet to the shoulder pads should be prohibited.

Acute Cervical Sprain Syndrome

An acute cervical sprain is a collision injury frequently seen in contact sports. The patient complains of having "jammed" his/her neck with subsequent pain localized to the cervical area. Characteristically, the patient presents with limitation of cervical spine motion but without radiation of pain or paresthesia. Neurologic examination is negative, and roentgenograms are normal.

Stable cervical sprains and strains eventually resolve with or without treatment. Initially, the presence of a serious injury should be ruled out by performing a thorough neurologic examination and determining the range of cervical motion. Range of motion is evaluated by having the athlete perform the following actions: actively nod his head, touch his chin to his chest, extend his neck maximally, touch his chin to his left shoulder, touch his chin to his right shoulder, touch his left ear to his left shoulder, and touch his right ear to his right shoulder. If the patient is unwilling or unable to perform these maneuvers actively while standing erect, proceed no further. The athlete with less than a full pain-free range of cervical motion, persistent paresthesia, or weakness should be protected and excluded from activity. Subsequent evaluation should include appropriate roentgenographic studies, including flexion and extension views to demonstrate fractures and instability.

In general, treatment of athletes with "cervical sprains" should be tailored to the degree of severity of the injury. Immobilizing the neck in a soft collar and using analgesics and anti-inflammatory agents until there is a full spasm-free range of neck motion is appropriate. It should be emphasized that individuals with a history of collision injury, pain, and limited cervical motion should have routine cervical spine x-rays. Also, lateral flexion and extension roentgenograms are indicated after the acute symptoms subside. Marked limitation of cervical motion, persistent pain, or radicular symptoms or findings may require MRI to rule out an intervertebral disk or other injury.

Intervertebral Disk Injuries

Acute herniation of a cervical intervertebral disk associated with neurologic findings and occurring as an isolated entity is rare in the athlete. However, an acute onset of transient quadriplegia in an athlete who has sustained head impact but has negative cervical spine roentgenograms should prompt consideration of an acute rupture of a cervical intervertebral disk. The symptoms of acute anterior cervical spinal cord injury syndrome, as described by Schneider (6), may be observed in individuals with instability associated with acute disk herniation: "The acute anterior cervical spine cord injury syndrome may be characterized as an immediate acute paralysis of all four extremities with a loss of pain and temperature to the level of the lesion, but with preservation of posterior column sensation of motion, position, vibration and part of touch." The pressure of the disk is exerted on the anterior and lateral columns, whereas the posterior columns are protected by the denticulate ligaments. MRI or a CT myelogram should be performed to substantiate the diagnosis. Anterior diskectomy and interbody fusion for a patient with neurologic involvement or persistent disability because of pain should be considered.

Albright et al. (23) studied 75 University of Iowa freshman football recruits who had roentgenograms of their cervical spines after playing football in high school but before playing in college. Of this group, 32% had one or more of the following: "occult" fracture, vertebral body compression fractures, intervertebral disk-space narrowing, or other degenerative changes. Of this group, only 13% admitted to a positive history of neck symptoms. The development of early degenerative changes or intervertebral disk-space narrowing in this group was attributed to the effect of repetitive loading on the cervical spine as a result of head impact from blocking and tackling.

Acute and chronic intervertebral disk injury without frank herniation or neurologic findings occurs with considerable frequency in the athlete. Associated with a history of injury are neck pain and limited cervical spine motion. Roentgenograms may demonstrate disk-space narrowing and marginal osteophytes. MRI frequently demonstrates disk bulge without herniation. In general, management is conservative, withholding permission to engage in activity until the youngster is asymptomatic and has a full range of cervical spine motion.

Cervical Vertebral Subluxation Without Fracture

Axial compression–flexion injuries incurred by striking an object with the top of the head can result in disruption of the posterior soft tissue-supporting elements with angulation and anterior translation of the superior cervical vertebrae. Fractures of the bony elements are not demonstrated on roentgenograms, and the patient has no neurologic deficit. Flexion-extension roentgenograms demonstrate instability of the cervical spine at the involved level, manifested by motion, anterior intervertebral disk-space narrowing, anterior angulation and displacement of the vertebral body, and fanning of the spinous processes. Demonstrable instability on lateral flexion-extension roentgenograms in young vigorous individuals requires aggressive treatment. When soft tissue disruption occurs without an associated fracture, it is likely that instability will result despite conservative treatment. When anterior subluxation greater than 20% of the vertebral body is due to disruption of the posterior supporting structures, a posterior cervical fusion is recommended.

Cervical Fractures or Dislocations: General Principles

Fractures or dislocations of the cervical spine may be stable or unstable and may or may not be associated with neurologic deficit. When fracture or disruption of the soft tissue-supporting structure immediately violates or threatens to violate the integrity of the spinal cord, implementation of certain management and treatment principles is imperative:

1. Protection of the cord from further injury;
2. Expeditious reduction;
3. Attainment of rapid and secure stability;
4. Implementation of an early rehabilitation program.

The first goal is to protect the spinal cord and nerve roots from injury through mismanagement. It has been estimated that many neurologic deficits occur after the initial injury. That is, if a patient with an unstable lesion is carelessly manipulated during transportation to a medical facility or subsequently managed inappropriately, further encroachment on the spinal cord can occur.

Second, once appropriate roentgenograms have been obtained and qualified orthopedic and neurosurgical personnel are available, the malaligned cervical spine should be reduced as quickly and gently as possible. This will effectively decompress the spinal cord. When dislocation or anterior angulation and translation are demonstrated roentgenographically, immediate reduc-

tion is attempted with skull traction using Gardner-Wells tongs. These tongs can be easily and rapidly applied under local anesthesia without shaving the head in the emergency room or in the patient's bed. Because these tongs are spring loaded, it is unnecessary to drill the outer table of the skull for their application. The tongs are attached to a cervical traction pulley, and weight is added at a rate of 5 pounds per disk space or 25 to 40 pounds for a lower cervical injury. Reduction is attempted by adding 5 pounds every 15 to 20 minutes and is monitored by lateral roentgenograms.

Unilateral facet dislocations, particularly at the C3-4 level, are not always reducible using skeletal traction. In such instances, closed skeletal or manipulative reduction under nasotracheal anesthesia may be necessary. The expediency of early reduction or cervical dislocations must be emphasized (24,25).

It has been proposed that the presence of a bulbocavernosus reflex indicates that spinal shock has worn off and that, except for recovery of an occasional root at the site of the injury, neither motor or sensory paralysis will be resolved regardless of treatment. The bulbocavernosus reflex is produced by pulling on the urethral catheter. This stimulates the trigone of the bladder, producing a reflex contraction of the anal sphincter around the examiner's gloved finger. Although the presence of a bulbocavernosus reflex is generally a sign that there will be no further neurologic recovery below the level of injury, this is not always true. The presence of this reflex does not give the clinician license to handle the situation in an elective fashion. The malalignments and dislocations of the cervical spine associated with quadriparesis should be reduced as quickly as possible, by whatever means necessary, if maximum recovery is to be expected.

In most instances in which a vertebral body burst fracture is associated with anterior compression of the cord, decompression is logically effected through an anterior approach with an interbody fusion. Likewise, intervertebral disk herniation with cord involvement is best managed through an anterior diskectomy and interbody fusion. In patients with cervical fractures and dislocations, posterior cervical laminectomy is indicated only rarely when excision of foreign bodies or body alignment of the spine is the most effective method for decompression of the cervical cord.

Indications for surgical decompression of the spinal cord have been delineated. A documented increase in neurologic signs is the clearest mandate for surgical decompression. Further observation, expectancy, and procrastination in this situation are contraindicated. Persistent partial cord or root signs, with objective evidence of mechanical compression, are also an indication for surgical intervention.

The use of parenteral corticosteroids to decrease the inflammatory reactions of the injured cord and surrounding soft tissue structures is indicated in the management of acute cervical spinal cord injuries. The efficacy of methylprednisolone in improving neurologic recovery when given in the first 8 hours has been recently demonstrated. The recommended regimen is a bolus of 30 mg/kg body weight of methylprednisolone administered intravenously followed by an infusion of 5.4 mg/kg/h for 23 hours (26).

The third goal in managing fractures and dislocations of the cervical spine is to effect rapid and secure stability to prevent residual deformity and instability with associated pain and the possibility of further trauma to the neural elements. White et al. (27,28) recognized that the literature is neither always clear nor consistent in describing what constitutes an unstable cervical spine. Using fresh cadaver specimens, they performed load displacement studies on sectioned and unsectioned two-level cervical spine segments to determine the horizontal translation and rotation that occurred in the sagittal plane after each ligament was transected. The experiments constituted a quantitative biomechanical analysis of the effects of destroying ligaments and facets on the stability of the cervical spine below C2 in an attempt to determine cervical stability. The express purpose of the study was to establish indications for treatment methods to stabilize the spine. Although the intent of the study was to define clinical instability to formulate treatment standards and was not intended to establish criteria for a return to contact athletics, it appears that their findings are relevant to this latter issue.

White et al. described clinical stability as the ability of the spine to limit its patterns of displacement of physiologic loads to prevent damage or irritation of the spinal cord or the nerve roots. They delineated four important findings. First, in sectioning the ligaments, small increments of change in stability occur followed without warning by sudden complete disruption of the spine under stress. Second, removal of the facets alters the motion segment such that in flexion there is less angular displacement and more horizontal displacement. Third, the anterior ligaments contribute more to stability in extension than the posterior ligaments, and in flexion the posterior ligaments contribute more than the anterior ligaments. The fourth and most relevant finding from the standpoint of criteria for return to contact sports is as follows: The adult cervical spine is unstable, or on the brink of instability, when one or more of the following conditions is present: all the anterior or all the posterior elements are destroyed or are unable to function; more than 3.5-mm horizontal displacement of one vertebra exists in relation to an adjacent vertebra measured on lateral roentgenograms (resting or flexion-extension); or there is more than 11 degrees of rotation difference compared with that of either adjacent vertebra measured on a resting lateral or flexion-extension roentgenogram.

The method of immobilization depends on the postreduction status of the injury. Thompson et al. concisely delineated the indications for using nonsurgical and surgical methods for achieving stability (29). These concepts for managing cervical spine fractures and dislocations may be summarized as follows:

1. Patients with stable compression fractures of the vertebral body, undisplaced fractures of the lamina, or lateral masses or soft tissue injuries without detectable neurologic deficit can be adequately treated with traction and subsequent protection with a cervical brace until healing occurs.
2. Stable reduced facet dislocation without neurologic deficit can also be treated conservatively in a halo jacket brace until healing has been demonstrated by negative lateral flexion-extension roentgenograms.
3. Unstable cervical spine fractures or fracture dislocations without neurologic deficit may require either surgical or nonsurgical methods to ensure stability.
4. Absolute indications for surgical stabilization of an unstable injury without neurologic deficits are late instability after closed treatment and flexion-rotation injuries with unreduced locked facets.
5. Relative indications for surgical stabilization in patients with unstable injuries without neurologic deficit are anterior subluxation greater than 20%, certain atlantoaxial fractures or dislocations, and unreduced vertical compression injuries with neck flexion.
6. Cervical spine fractures with complete cord lesions require reduction followed by stabilization by closed or open means, as indicated.
7. Cervical spine fractures with incomplete cord lesions require reduction followed by careful evaluation for surgical intervention.

The fourth and final goal of treatment is rapid and effective rehabilitation started early in the treatment process.

A more specific categorization of athletic injuries to the cervical spine can be made. Specifically, these injuries can be divided into those that occur in the upper cervical spine, the midcervical spine, and the lower cervical spine.

Upper Cervical Spine Fractures and Dislocations

Upper cervical spine lesions involve C1 through C3. Although they rarely occur in sports, several specific injuries that can occur to the upper cervical vertebrae deserve mention. The transverse and alar ligaments are responsible for atlantoaxial stability. If these structures are ruptured from a flexion injury with translation of C1 anteriorly, the spinal cord can be impinged between a posterior aspect of the odontoid process and the posterior rim of C1. The patient gives a history of head trauma and complains of neck pain, particularly with nodding, and may or may not present with cord signs. Roentgenographically, lateral views of the C1-2 articulation demonstrate increase of the atlantodens interval. This interval is normally 3 mm in the adult. With transverse ligament rupture, it may increase up to 10 to 12 mm depending on the status of the alar and accessory ligaments. Note that increase in the atlantodens interval may only be seen when the neck is flexed. Fielding (30) stated that atlantoaxial fusion may be the "conservative" treatment of this lesion. He recommended posterior C1-2 fusion using wire fixation and an iliac bone graft.

Fractures of the atlas were described by Jefferson (31) in 1920. These may be of two types: posterior arch fractures and burst fractures. Posterior arch fractures are the more common of these two types, and with a brace support they go on to satisfactory fibrous or bony union. Burst fractures result from an axial load transmitted to the occipital condyles, which then disrupt the integrity of both the anterior and posterior arches of the atlas. Roentgenograms demonstrate bilateral symmetric overhang of the lateral masses of the atlas in relation to the axis, with an increase in the paraodontoid space on the open mouth view. Clinically, the patient characteristically has pain and imitates the nodding motion. These fractures are considered stable when the combined lateral overhang of the atlas measures less than 7 mm. When the transverse diameter of the atlas is 7 mm greater than that of the axis, a transverse ligament rupture should be suspected. Treatment, as recommended by Fielding, includes a head-halter traction until muscle spasm resolves, followed by a brace support. If flexion-extension roentgenograms subsequently demonstrate significant instability, fusion may be indicated.

Fractures of the odontoid have been classified into three types by Anderson and D'Alonzo (32). Type I is an avulsion of the tip of the odontoid at the site of the attachment of the alar ligament and is a rare and stable lesion. Type II is a fracture through the base at or just below the level of the superior articular processes. Type III involves a fracture of the body of the axis. When the odontoid is not displaced, planograms may be required to identify the lesion.

The mechanism of odontoid fractures has not been clearly delineated. However, they appear to be due to head impact. All routine cervical spine roentgenographic studies should include the open mouth view to identify lesions involving the odontoid and the atlas. If these are negative and if a lesion in this area is suspected, planograms or bending films may further delineate pathologic changes in this area.

Managing type II fractures is a problem. It has been reported that 36% to 50% of these lesions treated initially with plaster casts or reinforced cervical braces fail to unite. Cloward reported that 85% of his patients heal within 3 months when treated with the halo brace (33).

It is necessary to stabilize fibrous unions or nonunited fractures of the odontoid surgically if they are demonstrated to be unstable on flexion and extension views. Stabilization may be effected either through posterior C1-2 wire fixation and fusion or anterior fusion of C1-2 by a dowel graft through the articular facets, as described by Cloward.

Fractures through the arch of the axis are also known as traumatic spondylolisthesis of C2 or hangman's fractures. These are relatively rare lesions. The mechanism of injury is generally recognized to be by hyperextension. The injury is inherently unstable, but it has been shown to heal with predictable regularity without surgical intervention.

Midcervical Spine Fractures and Dislocations

Acute traumatic lesions of the cervical spine at the C3-4 level are rare and are generally not associated with fractures. These lesions are classified as follows: acute rupture of the C3-4 intervertebral disk, anterior subluxation of C3 on C4, unilateral dislocation of the joint between the articular processes, and bilateral dislocation of the joint between the articular processes (24,25).

An episode of transient quadriplegia in an athlete who has sustained head impact but has a negative cervical spine roentgenogram suggests acute rupture of the C3-4 intervertebral disk. The syndrome of acute anterior spinal cord injury, as described by Schneider et al., may be observed (34). A cervical myelogram or MRI will substantiate the diagnosis. Anterior diskectomy and interbody fusion may be the most effective treatment of this lesion.

Anterior subluxation of C3 on C4 is a result of a shearing force through the intervertebral disk space that disrupts the interspinous ligament and the posterior supporting structure. Roentgenograms demonstrate narrowing of the intervertebral disk space, anterior angulation and translation of C3 on C4, an increase in the distance between the spinous processes of the two vertebrae, and instability without fracture of the bony elements. Spinal fusion may be necessary for adequate stabilization in such cases, in contrast to cervical spine instability caused by fracture, in which adequate reduction and subsequent bony healing result in stability. When the patient has posterior instability, posterior fusion is preferable to an anterior body fusion.

Unilateral facet dislocation at C3-4 may result in immediate quadriparesis. This injury involves the intervertebral disk space, the interspinous ligament, the posterior ligamentous supporting structures, and the one facet with resulting rotatory dislocation of C3 on C4 without fracture. At this level, strong skeletal traction does not usually yield a successful reduction, and closed manipulation under general anesthesia is necessary to disengage the locked joint between the articular processes.

Bilateral facet dislocation at the C3-4 level is a grave lesion. Skeletal traction may not reduce the lesion, and the prognosis for this injury is poor.

Lower Cervical Spine Fractures and Dislocations

Lower cervical spine fractures or dislocations are those involving C4 through C7. In injuries resulting from various athletic endeavors, most fractures or dislocations of the cervical spine, with or without neurologic involvement, involve this segment. Although unilateral and bilateral facet dislocations occur, they are relatively rare. Most severe athletically incurred cervical spine injuries are fractures of the vertebral body with varying degrees of compression or comminution.

Unilateral Facet Dislocations

Unilateral facet dislocations are the result of axial loading flexion–rotation types of mechanisms. The lesion may be truly ligamentous without any associated vertebral fracture. In such instances, the facet dislocation is stable and is usually associated with neurologic involvement. Roentgenograms demonstrate less than 50% anterior shift of the superior vertebra on the inferior vertebra. Attempts should be made to reduce the facet dislocation by skeletal traction. However, as with similar lesions described at the C3-4 level, it may not be possible to effect a closed reduction. In this instance, open reduction under direct vision through a posterior approach with supplemental posterior element bone grafting should be performed.

Bilateral Facet Dislocations

Bilateral facet dislocations are unstable and are almost always associated with neurologic involvement. These injuries are associated with a high incidence of quadriplegia. Lateral roentgenograms demonstrate greater than 50% anterior displacement of the superior vertebral body on the inferior vertebral body. Immediate treatment, as previously described, consists of closed reduction with skeletal traction. Such lesions are generally reducible by skeletal traction and are then treated by halo-brace stabilization and posterior fusion. It should be noted that instability is directly related to the ease with which the lesion is reduced, because the easier it is to reduce, the easier it is to redislocate. If skeletal traction is unsuccessful, either manipulative reduction under sedation or general anesthesia or open reduction under direct vision is recommended. When the dislocation is reduced closed and the reduction is maintained, immobilization should be effected by use of the halo

brace for 8 to 12 weeks. Corrective bracing should continue for an additional 4 weeks.

Vertebral Body Compression Fractures

Compression fractures of the vertebral body are a result of axial loading. Vertebral body fractures of the cervical spine can be classified into five types.

Type I

Simple wedge or vertebral endplate compression fractures of the cervical vertebrae are common injuries that respond to conservative management and rarely if ever are associated with neurologic involvement. It is important to differentiate these lesions from compression fractures that are associated with disruption of the posterior element soft tissue supporting structures. The latter lesions are unstable and are frequently associated with neurologic involvement, including quadriplegia.

Type II

An isolated anterior-inferior vertebral body or "teardrop" fracture is without displacement, has intact posterior elements, and is not associated with neurologic involvement. This is a relatively stable fracture and may be treated conservatively.

Type III

Comminuted burst vertebral body fractures have intact posterior elements, but displacement of bony fragments into the vertebral canal may place the cord in jeopardy. Late settling of the fracture with deformity can occur. Surgical stabilization is recommended.

Type IV

The axial load three part–two plane vertebral body fracture consists of three fracture parts: an anteroinferior teardrop, a sagittal vertebral body fracture, and disruption of the posterior neural arch. This lesion is unstable and is almost always associated with quadriplegia. Careful evaluation of the routine anteroposterior roentgenogram or CT is necessary to appreciate the sagittal vertebral body fracture, a finding that portends a grave prognosis (Fig. 9.4).

Type V

This is a vertebral body three part–two plane compression fracture associated with disruption of posterior elements of an adjacent vertebra. This is an extremely unstable fracture.

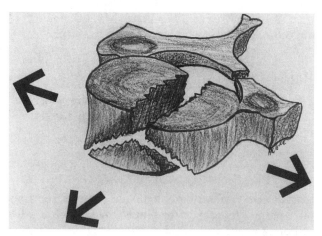

FIG. 9.4. The axial load teardrop fracture has a three part–two plane pattern. There is an anteroinferior corner fracture fragment, a sagittal fracture through the entire vertebral body, and a posterior arch fracture.

Cervical Spinal Stenosis with Cord Neurapraxia and Transient Quadriplegia

Characteristically, the clinical picture of cervical spinal cord neurapraxia with transient quadriplegia involves an athlete who sustains an acute transient neurologic episode of cervical cord origin with sensory changes that may be associated with motor paresis involving both arms, both legs, or all four extremities after forced hyperextension, hyperflexion, or axial loading of the cervical spine. Sensory changes include burning pain, numbness, tingling, or loss of sensation; motor changes consist of weakness or complete paralysis. The episodes are transient, and complete recovery usually occurs in 10 to 15 minutes, although in some cases gradual resolution does not occur for 36 to 48 hours. Except for burning paresthesia, neck pain is not present at the time of injury. There is complete return of motor function and full pain-free cervical motion. Routine x-ray films of the cervical spine show no evidence of fracture or dislocation. However, a demonstrable degree of cervical spinal stenosis is present.

In athletes with diminution of the anterior posterior diameter of the spinal canal, the cord can, on forced hyperextension and hyperflexion, be compressed, causing transient motor and sensory manifestations. The mechanics of cervical cord compression have been described by Penning (36) as the "pincer mechanisms" (Fig. 9.5). With hyperextension, the posterior inferior aspect of the superior vertebral body and the anterior superior aspect of the spinal laminar line of the subjacent vertebra approximate. In flexion, the spinal laminar line of the superior vertebra and the posterior superior aspect of the body of the subjacent vertebra approximate. In each situation, a rapid decrease occurs in the anteroposterior diameter of the canal with compression

of the spinal cord, resulting in a transient disturbance of sensory and/or motor function.

Determination of Spinal Stenosis: Method of Measurement

To identify cervical stenosis, a method of measurement is needed. The standard method, the one most commonly used for determining the sagittal diameter of the spinal canal, involves measuring the distance between the middle of the posterior surface of the vertebral body and the nearest point on the spinolaminar line. Using this technique, Boijsen (37) reported that the average sagittal diameter of the spinal canal from the fourth to the sixth cervical vertebra in 200 healthy individuals was 18.5 mm (range, 14.2 to 23 mm). The target distance he used was 1.4 m. Other have noted that values of less than 14 mm are uncommon and fall below the SD for any cervical segment. Other measurements reported in the literature vary greatly. It is the variations in the landmarks and the methods used to determine the sagittal distance and the use of different target distances for roentgenography that have resulted in inconsistencies in the so-called normal values. Therefore, the standard method of measurement for spinal stenosis is a questionable one.

An alternative way to determine the sagittal diameter of the spinal canal was devised by Pavlov et al. (38), called the ratio method. It compares the standard method of measurement of the canal with the anteroposterior width of the vertebral body at the midpoint of

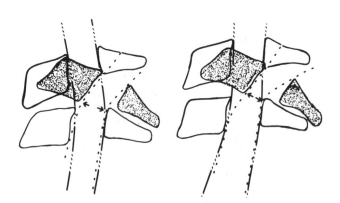

FIG. 9.5. The pincers mechanism, as described by Penning (36), occurs when the distance between the posteroinferior margin of the superior vertebral body and the anterosuperior aspect of the spinolaminar line of the subjacent vertebra decreases with hyperextension, resulting in compression of the cord. With hyperflexion, the anterosuperior aspect of the spinolaminar line of the superior vertebra would be the "pincers." (From Torg JS, Pavlov H, Gennario SE, et al. Neurapraxia of the cervical spinal cord with transient quadriplegia. *J Bone Joint Surg Am* 1986;68A:1354–1370, with permission.)

the corresponding vertebral body (Fig. 9.6). The actual measurement of the sagittal diameter in millimeters, as determined by the conventional method, is misleading both as reported in the literature and in actual practice because of variations in the target distances used for roentgenography and in the landmarks used for obtaining the measurement. The ratio method compensates for variations in roentgenographic technique because the sagittal diameter of both the canal and the vertebral body is affected similarly by magnification factors. The ratio method is independent of variations in technique, and the results are statistically significant. Using the ratio method of determining the dimension of the canal, a ratio of the spinal canal to the vertebral body of less than 0.80 is indicative of cervical stenosis. We believe that the ratio is a consistent and reliable way to determine cervical stenosis in those individuals who have experienced episodes of cervical cord neurapraxia. However, the ratio has a very low predictive value and should not be used as a screening tool.

On the basis of these observations, it may be concluded that the factor that explains the described neurologic picture of spinal cord neurapraxia is diminution of the anteroposterior diameter of the spinal canal, either as an isolated observation or in association with the intervertebral disk herniation, degenerative changes, posttraumatic instability, or congenital anomalies. In instances of developmental cervical stenosis, forced hyperflexion, or hyperextension of the cervical spine, further decreases the caliber of an already narrow canal, as explained by the pincer mechanism of Penning.

In patients whose stenosis is associated with osteophytes or a herniated disk, direct pressure can occur, again when the spine is forced in the extremes of flexion and extension. It is further postulated that with an abrupt but brief decrease in the anteroposterior diameter of the spinal canal, the cervical cord is mechanically compressed, causing transient interruption of either motor or sensory function, or both, distal to the lesion. The neurologic aberration that results is transient and completely reversible.

A review of the literature has revealed few reported cases of transient quadriplegia occurring in athletes. Attempts to establish the incidence indicate that the problem is more prevalent than may be expected. Specifically, in a population of 39,377 exposed participants, the reported incidence of paresthesia associated with transient quadriplegia was 1.3 per 10,000 in the one football season surveyed. From these data, it may be concluded that the prevalence of this problem is relatively high and that an awareness of the etiology, manifestations, and appropriate principles of management is warranted.

Characteristically, after an episode of cervical spinal cord neurapraxia with or without transient quadriplegia, the first question raised concerns the advisability of restricting activity. In an attempt to address this problem, 117 young athletes have been interviewed who sustained cervical spine injuries associated with complete permanent quadriplegia while playing football between the years 1871 and 1984. None of these patients recalled a prodromal experience of transient motor paresis. Conversely, none of the patients in this series who had experienced transient neurologic episodes subsequently sustained an injury that resulted in permanent neurologic injury. On the basis of these data, it is concluded that a young patient who has had an episode of cervical spinal cord neurapraxia with or without an episode of transient quadriplegia is not predisposed to permanent neurologic injury because of it.

With regard to restrictions on activity, no definite recurrent patterns have been identified to establish firm principles in this area. However, athletes who have this syndrome associated with demonstrable cervical spinal instability or with acute or chronic degenerative changes should not be allowed further participation in contact sports. Athletes with developmental spinal stenosis or spinal stenosis associated with congenital abnormalities should be treated on an individual basis. Of the six youngsters with obvious cervical stenosis who returned to football, three had a second episode and withdrew from the activity and three returned without any problems at 2-year follow-up. The data clearly indicate that

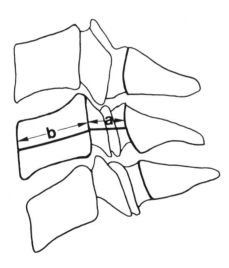

$$ratio = \frac{a}{b}$$

FIG. 9.6. The ratio of the spinal canal to the vertebral body is the distance from the midpoint of the posterior aspect of the vertebral body to the nearest point on the corresponding spinolaminar line (**a**) divided by the anteroposterior width of the vertebral body (**b**). (From Torg JS, Pavlov H, Gennario SE, et al. Neurapraxia of the cervical spinal cord with transient quadriplegia. *J Bone Joint Surg Am* 1986;68A:1354–1370, with permission.)

individuals with developmental spinal stenosis, with or without associated symptoms, are not predisposed to more severe injuries with associated permanent neurologic sequelae.

Subsequent to the description of neurapraxia of the cervical cord with transient quadriplegia, a number of issues concerning the disorder have arisen. An epidemiologic study performed to address these issues was published (39). Evaluation of 45 athletes who had an episode of transient neurapraxia of the cervical spinal cord revealed the consistent finding of developmental narrowing of the cervical spinal canal. The purpose of the study was to determine the relationship, if any, between a developmentally narrowed cervical canal and reversible and irreversible injury of the cervical cord with use of various cohorts of football players and a large control group. Cohort I was comprised of 227 college football players who were asymptomatic and had no known history of transient neurapraxia of the cervical cord. Cohort II consisted of 97 professional football players who also were asymptomatic and had no known history of transient neurapraxia of the cervical cord. Cohort III was a group of 45 high school, college, and professional football players who had at least one episode of transient neurapraxia of the cervical cord. Cohort IV was comprised of 77 individuals who was permanently quadriplegic as a result of an injury while playing high school or college football. Cohort V consisted of a control group of 105 male subjects who were not athletes and had no history of a major injury of the cervical spine, an episode of transient neurapraxia, or neurologic symptoms.

The mean and SD of the diameter of the spinal canal, the diameter of the vertebral body, and the ratio of the diameter of the spinal canal to that of the vertebral body were determined for the third through sixth cervical levels on the radiographs of each cohort. In addition, the sensitivity, specifically, and positive predictive value of the ratio of the diameter of the spinal canal to that of the vertebral body of 0.80 or less was evaluated. The findings of this study demonstrated that a ratio of 0.80 or less had a high sensitivity (93%) for transient neurapraxia. These findings also support the concept that the symptoms result from a transient reversible deformation of the spinal cord in a developmentally narrowed osseous canal. The low predictive value of the ratio (0.2%), however, precludes its use as a screening mechanism for determining the suitability of an athlete for participation in contact activities.

Axial load, the degree of instability, and the duration from the injury to the reduction have been implicated as factors in the occurrence of permanent neurologic injury in athletes who play tackle football (40). None of the 77 quadriplegic individuals (cohort IV) had an episode of neurapraxia of the spinal cord before the catastrophic injury. Also, none of the 45 high school,

college, and professional players who had an episode of transient neurapraxia (cohort III) became quadriplegic. These data, in combination with the absence of developmental narrowing of the cervical canal in the quadriplegic group (cohort IV), provide evidence that the occurrence of transient neurapraxis of the cervical cord and an injury associated with permanent catastrophic neurologic sequelae are unrelated (Fig. 9.7). Therefore, developmental narrowing of the cervical canal in a spine that has no evidence of instability is neither a harbinger of nor a predisposing factor for permanent neurologic injury.

The data did not reveal an association between developmental narrowing of the cervical canal and quadriplegia. The major factor in the occurrence of cervical quadriplegia in football players is a tacking technique in which the head is used as the primary point of contact, with resulting transmission of axial energy to, and subsequent failure of, the cervical spine. The findings of this study demonstrated the high sensitivity, low specificity, and low predictive value of the ratio of the diameter of the cervical spinal canal to that of the vertebral body, precluding its use as screening mechanism for determining the suitability of an individual for participation in contact sports. Developmental narrowing of the cervical canal without associated instability does not predispose an individual to permanent catastrophic neurologic injury and therefore should not preclude an athlete from participation in contact sports.

More recently, a group of 110 patients with cervical cord neurapraxia (CCN) has been studied. In this report, a classification system of CCN was developed, and clinical x-ray and MRI data using a new computerized measurement technique were analyzed (41).

CCN was classified according to the type of neurologic deficit: plegia for episodes with complete paralysis, paresis for episodes with motor weakness, and paresthesia for episodes that involve only sensory changes without any motor involvement. The CCN grade was defined by the length of time that the neurologic symptoms persisted: grade I, less than 15 minutes; grade II, greater than 15 minutes but less than 24 hours; and grade III, greater than 24 hours. The CCN pattern was defined by the anatomic distribution of all the neurologic symptoms: quad, episodes that involve all four extremities; upper, involving both arms; lower, episodes involving both legs; and hemi, episodes involving an ipsilateral arm and leg. Using this classification system, the incidence of CCN type was plegia in 44 cases (40%), paresis in 28 (25%), and paresthesia in 38 cases (35%). The incidence of CCN grade was grade I in 81 cases (74%), grade II in 17 (15%), and grade III in 12 cases (11%). The incidence of CCN pattern was quad in 88 cases (80%), upper in 17 (15%), lower in 2 cases (2%), and hemi in 3 cases (3%).

To analyze the relationship of the spinal cord to the

Profile Plot of Canal Size

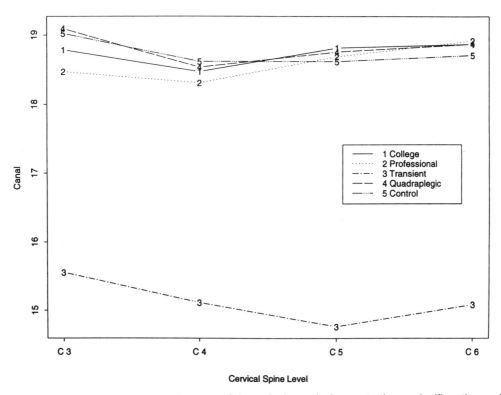

FIG. 9.7. Profile plot of the mean diameter of the spinal canal, demonstrating a significantly smaller value in cohort III compared with that in all other cohorts ($p < 0.05$). With the numbers available, no significant difference was found among cohorts I, II, IV, or V. (From Torg JS, Pavlov H, Gennario SE, et al. Neurapraxia of the cervical spinal cord with transient quadriplegia. *J Bone Joint Surg Am* 1996;178A:1308–1313, with permission.)

spinal canal, a computerized system was developed to analyze the MR images. This system consisted of a personal computer and a color scanner with a transparency adaptor. Images were digitized on the scanner and then uploaded using an imaging software package. The midsagittal T1- and T2-weighted images were digitized. Using a graphics digitizer pad with a resolution of 0.01 mm, the following measurements were made at levels C3-7: to quantify spondylitic narrowing, the disk level canal diameter was measured as the shortest distance between the intervertebral disk and the body posterior elements; the cord diameter was determined by measuring the transverse diameter of the spinal cord at the appropriate level; and the space available for the cord was calculated by subtracting the spinal cord diameter from the disk level canal diameter.

Follow-up evaluation was obtained by questionnaire mailing, telephone interview, or office evaluation and was available for 105 of the 110 cases. Sixty-three (57%) patients returned to contact activities after their first episode of CCN. Of this group, 35 patients (56%) experienced a second episode of CCN. Once again, there were no permanent or catastrophic neurologic injuries related

to the occurrence of CCN. Patients returning to football had a higher recurrence rate than those returning to other sports. Thirty-two (62%) of 52 football players who returned to the sport experienced a recurrence compared with 3 (27%) of 11 players who returned to other sports. All radiologic measurements except spinal cord diameter were predictive or recurrent. The patients' age, level of sports participation, radiographic findings, MRI findings, clinical CCN classification, and radiologic classification did not have predictive value in determining which patients were at risk of recurrence. The presence of disk herniation, cord compression, degenerative disk disease, or any other finding was not an indicator of whether patients would suffer future episodes of CCN. Based on the finding that narrowing of the canal is a causative factor of CCN, the recurrence and diameter data were analyzed and correlated. Graphic plots were constructed using logistic regression analysis or the percentage risk of recurrence versus the disk level canal diameter and the spinal canal/vertebral body (SC/VB) ratio. The plots demonstrated a strong inverse correlation between the risk of recurrence and the disk level canal diameter and SC/VB ratio (Fig. 9.8A and B).

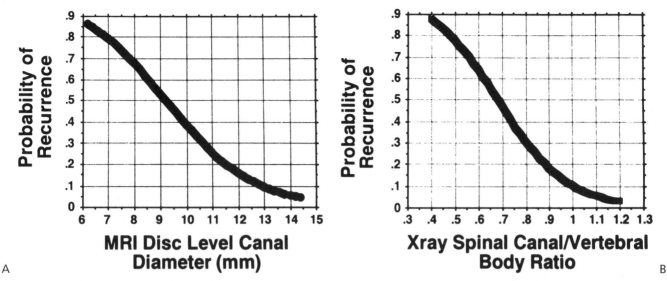

MRI Disc Level Canal Diameter (mm)

A

Xray Spinal Canal/Vertebral Body Ratio

B

FIG. 9.8. Graphs developed using regression analysis in which the risk of recurrence can be plotted as a function of the disk-level diameter measured on magnetic resonance imaging (**A**) and the SC/VB ratio calculated on the basis of x-ray films (**B**). The construction of these plots is based on the result that increased risk of recurrence is inversely correlated with canal diameter. Patients with cervical cord neurapraxia can be counseled regarding their individual risk of recurrence based on the particular size of their spinal canal.

PREVENTION

Athletic injuries to the cervical spine that result in injury to the spinal cord are infrequent but catastrophic events. Accurate descriptions of the mechanism or mechanisms responsible for a particular injury transcend simple academic interest. Before preventative measures can be developed and implemented, identification of the mechanisms involved in the production of the particular injury is necessary. Because the nervous system is unable to recover significant function after severe trauma, prevention assumes a most important role when considering these injuries.

Injuries resulting in spinal cord damage have been associated with football, water sports, wrestling (42), rugby (43–46), trampolining (46), and ice hockey (47). The use of epidemiologic data, biomechanical evidence, and cinematographic analysis has defined and supported the involvement of axial load forces in cervical spine injuries occurring in football, demonstrated the success of appropriate rule changes in the prevention of these injuries, and emphasized the need for employment of epidemiologic methods to prevent cervical spine and similar severe injuries in other high-risk athletic activities.

Data on cervical spine injuries resulting from participation in football have been compiled by a national registry since 1971 (48–50). Analysis of the epidemiologic data and cinematographic documentation clearly demonstrates that most cervical fractures and dislocations were due to axial loading. On the basis of these observations, rule changes banning both deliberate "spearing" and the use of the top of the helmet as the initial point of contact in making a tackle were implemented at the high school and college levels. Subsequently, a marked decrease in cervical spine injury rates has occurred. The occurrence of permanent cervical quadriplegia decreased from 34 in 1976 to 2 in the 1994 season (Fig. 9.9).

Identification of the cause of the cervical quadriplegia and prevention of cervical quadriplegia resulting from football involve four areas: the role of the helmet–face

Yearly Incidence of Permanent Quadriplegia Due to Football, 1975-1995

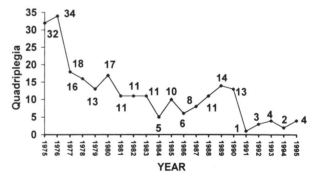

FIG. 9.9. Yearly incidence of permanent quadriplegia due to football, 1975–1995.

mask protective system; the concept of the axial loading mechanism of injury; the effect of the 1976 rule change banning spearing and the use of the top of the helmet as the initial point of contact in tackling; and the necessity for continued research, education, and enforcement of the rules.

The protective capabilities provided by the modern football helmet have resulted in the advent of playing techniques that have placed the cervical spine at risk of injury with associated catastrophic neurologic sequelae. Available cinematographic and epidemiologic data clearly indicate that cervical spine injuries associated with quadriplegia occurring as a result of football are not hyperflexion accidents. Instead, they are due to purposeful axial loading of the cervical spine as a result of spearing and head-first playing techniques. As an etiologic factor, the modern helmet–face mask system is secondary, contributing to these injuries because of its protective capabilities that have permitted the head to be used as a battering ram, thus exposing the cervical spine to injury (Fig. 9.10).

Classically, the role of hyperflexion has been emphasized in cervical spine trauma whether the injury was due to a diving accident, trampolining, rugby, or American

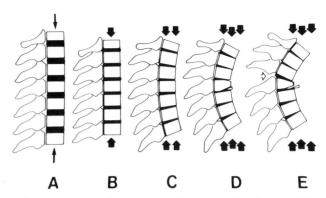

FIG. 9.11. An axial load energy input resulting in instability of the cervical spine. **A:** With the neck slightly flexed, the cervical lordosis is obviated and the straightened spine is subjected to an axial energy input. **B:** Compressive defamation occurs primarily in the intervertebral disk. **C:** Failure begins in a flexion mode. Bony **(D)** and ligamentous **(E)** failure occurs with resulting instability and injury to the cord.

football. Epidemiologic and cinematographic analyses have established that most cases of cervical spine quadriplegia that occur in football have resulted from axial loading. Far from being an accident or untoward event, techniques are deliberately used that place the cervical spine at risk of catastrophic injury. Recent laboratory observations also indicate that athletically induced cervical spine trauma results from axial loading (51–53).

In the course of a collision activity, such as tackle football, most energy inputs to the cervical spine are effectively dissipated by the energy-absorbing capabilities of the cervical musculature through controlled lateral bending, flexion, or extension motion. However, the bones, disks, and ligamentous structures can be injured when contact occurs on the top of the helmet when the head, neck, and trunk are positioned in such a way that forces are transmitted along the longitudinal axis of the cervical spine.

When the neck is in the anatomic position, the cervical spine is extended due to normal cervical lordosis. When the neck is flexed to 30 degrees, the cervical spine straightens. In axial loading injuries, the neck is slightly flexed, and normal cervical lordosis is eliminated, thereby converting the spine into a straight segmented column. Assuming the head, neck, and trunk components to be in motion, rapid deceleration of the head occurs when it strikes another object, such as another player, trampoline bed, or lake bottom. This results in the cervical spine being compressed between the rapidly decelerated head and the force of the oncoming trunk. When the maximum amount of vertical compression is reached, the straightened cervical spine fails in a flexion mode and fracture, subluxation, or unilateral or bilateral facet dislocation can occur (Fig. 9.11A through D).

Refutation of the "freak accident" concept with the

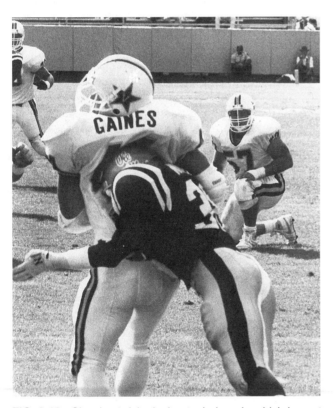

FIG. 9.10. Classic at-risk playing technique in which impact is made with the crown of the helmet. The head comes to an abrupt halt and the straightened cervical spine is subjected to an axial load with increased momentum of the body. This particular injury resulted in fractures of C4, C5, and C6 with associated quadriplegia.

more logical principle of cause and effect has been most rewarding in dealing with problems of football-induced cervical quadriplegia. Definition of the axial loading mechanism in which a football player, usually a defensive back, makes a tackle by striking an opponent with the top of the helmet has been a key element in this process. Implementation of rule changes and coaching techniques eliminating the use if the head as a battering ram have resulted in a dramatic reduction in the incidence of quadriplegia since 1976 (Fig. 9.9). We believe that most athletic injuries to the cervical spine associated with quadriplegia also occur as a result of axial loading (Fig. 9.10).

Tator et al. (54) studied 38 acute spinal cord injuries due to diving accidents and observed that "in most cases the cervical spine was fractured and the spinal cord crushed. The top of the head struck the bottom of the lake or pool." Scher, reporting on vertex impact and cervical dislocation in rugby players, observed that "when the neck is slightly flexed, the spine is straight (56). If significant force is applied to the vertex when the spine is straight, the force is transmitted down the long axis of the spine. When the force exceeds the energy-absorbing capacity of the structures involved, cervical spine flexion and dislocation will result." Tator and Edmonds (47) reported on the results of a national questionnaire survey by the Canadian Committee on the Prevention of Spinal Injuries due to hockey, which recorded 28 injuries involving the spinal cord, 17 of which resulted in complete paralysis. They noted that in this series the most common mechanism involved was a check in which the injured players struck the boards "with the top of their heads, while their necks were slightly flexed." Reports in the recent literature that deal with the mechanism of injury involved in cervical spine injuries resulting from water sports (diving), rugby, and ice hockey support our thesis.

CRITERIA USED TO GAUGE RETURN TO CONTACT ACTIVITIES AFTER CERVICAL SPINE INJURY

Injury to the cervical spine and associated structures as a result of participation in competitive athletic and recreational activities is not uncommon. It appears that the frequency of these various injuries is inversely proportional to their severity. Whereas Albright et al. (23) reported that 32% of college football recruits sustained "moderate" injuries while in high school, catastrophic injuries with associated quadriplegia occur in less than 1 in 100,000 participants per season at the high school level. As indicated, the variant of possible lesions is considerable and the severity variable. The literature dealing with diagnosis and treatment of these problems is considerable. However, conspicuously absent is a comprehensive set of standards or guidelines for estab-

lishing criteria for permitting or prohibiting return to contact sports (boxing, football, ice hockey, lacrosse, rugby, wrestling) after injury to the cervical spinal structures. The explanation for this void appears to be two-fold. First, the combination of a litigious society and the potential for great harm if things go wrong makes "no" the easiest and perhaps most reasonable advice. Second, and perhaps most important, with the exception of the matter of transient quadriplegia, there is a lack of credible data pertaining to postinjury risk factors. Despite a lack of credible data, this chapter attempts to establish guidelines to assist the clinician and the patient and family in the decision-making process.

Cervical spine conditions requiring a decision as to whether or not participation in contact activities is advisable and safe can be divided into two categories: congenital or developmental conditions and posttraumatic conditions. Each condition has been determined to present either no contraindication, relative contraindications, or an absolute contraindication on the basis of a variety of parameters. Information compiled from over 1,200 cervical spine injuries documented by the National Football Head and Neck Injury Registry has provided insight into whether various conditions may or may not predispose to a more serious injury. A review of the literature in several instances provides significant data for a limited number of specific conditions. Analysis of many conditions predicated on an understanding of recognized injury mechanisms has permitted categorization on the basis of "educated" conjecture. And last, much reliance has been placed on personal experience that must be regarded as anecdotal.

The structure and mechanics of the cervical spine enable it to perform three important functions. First, it supports the head and the variant of soft tissue structures of the neck. Second, by virtue of segmentation and configuration, it permits multiplanar motion of the head. Third, and most important, it serves as a protective conduit for the spinal cord and cervical nerve roots. A condition that impedes or prevents the performance of any of the three functions in a pain-free manner either immediately or in the future is unacceptable and constitutes a contraindication to participation in contact sports.

The following proposed criteria for return to contact activities in the presence of cervical spine abnormalities or after injury are intended only as guidelines. It is fully acknowledged that for the most part they are at best predicated on anecdotal experience, and no responsibility can be assumed for their implementation.

Critical to the application of these guidelines is the implementation of coaching and playing techniques that preclude the use of the head as the initial point of contact in a collision situation. Exposure of the cervical spine to axial loading is an invitation to disaster and makes all safety standards meaningless.

Congenital Conditions

Odontoid Anomalies

Hensinger (56) stated that "patients with congenital anomalies of the odontoid are leading a precarious existence. The concern is that a trivial insult superimposed on an already weakened or compromised structure may be catastrophic." This concern became a reality during the 1989 football season when an 18-year-old high school player was rendered a respiratory-dependent quadriplegic while making a head tackle that was vividly demonstrated on the game video. Postinjury roentgenograms revealed an os odontoidium with marked C1-2 instability. Thus, the presence of odontoid agenesis, odontoid hypoplasia, or os odontoidium are all absolute contraindications to participation in contact activities.

Spina Bifida Occulta

This is a rare incidental roentgenographic finding that presents no contraindication.

Atlantooccipital Fusion

This rare condition is characterized by partial or complete congenital fusion of the bony ring of the atlas to the base of the occiput. Signs and symptoms are referable to the posterior columns due to cord compression by the posterior lip of the foramen magnum and usually occur in the third or fourth decade. They usually begin insidiously and progress slowly, but sudden onset or instant death has been reported. Atlantooccipital fusion as an isolated entity or coexisting with other abnormalities constitutes an absolute contraindication to participation in contact activities.

Klippel-Feil Anomaly

This eponym is applied to congenital fusion of two or more cervical vertebrae. For purposes of this discussion, the variety of abnormalities can be divided into two groups: type I, mass fusion of the cervical and upper thoracic vertebrae, and type II, fusion of only one or two interspaces. To be noted, a variety of associated congenital problems have been associated with congenital fusion of the cervical vertebrae and include pulmonary, cardiovascular, and urogenital problems. Pizzutillo (57) pointed out that "children with congenital fusion of the cervical spine rarely develop neurologic problems or signs of instability." However, Pizzutillo further stated that "the literature reveals more than 90 cases of neurologic problems . . . that developed as a consequence of occipital cervical anomalies, late instability, disk disease, or degenerative joint disease." These reports included cervical radiculopathy, spasticity, pain, quadriplegia, and sudden death. Also, "more than two-thirds of the neurologically involved patients had single level fusion of the upper area, whereas many cervical patients with extension fusions of five to seven levels had no associated neurologic loss." Despite this, a type I lesion, a mass fusion, constitutes an absolute contraindication to participation in contact sports. A type II lesion with fusion of one or two interspaces with associated limited motion or associated occipitocervical anomalies, involvement of C2, instability, disk disease, or degenerative changes also constitutes an absolute contraindication to participation. On the other hand, a type II lesion involving fusion of one or two interspaces at C3 and below in an individual with a full cervical range of motion and an absence of occipitocervical anomalies, instability, disk disease, or degenerative changes should present no contraindication.

Developmental Conditions

Developmental Narrowing (Stenosis) of the Cervical Spinal Canal

This condition and its association with cervical cord neurapraxia and transient quadriplegia has been well defined (35). The definition of narrowing or stenosis as a cervical segment with one or more vertebrae that have a canal-vertebral body ratio of 0.8 or less is predicated on the fact that 100% of all reported clinical cases have fallen below this value at one or more levels. To be noted, 12% of asymptomatic control subjects also fell below the 0.8 level, as did 32% of asymptomatic professional and 34% of asymptomatic college players. In the group of reported symptomatic players, there was in every instance complete return of neurologic function, and in those who continued with contact activities, recurrence was not predictable.

Clearly, the presence of developmental narrowing of the cervical spinal canal does not predispose to permanent neurologic injury. Eismont et al. (58) indicated, on the basis of experience of cervical fractures or dislocations resulting from automobile accidents, that the degree of neurologic impairment was inversely related to the anteroposterior diameter of the canal. Due to the all or nothing pattern of axial load football spine injuries, this phenomenon has not been observed in sports-related injuries.

The presence of a canal-vertebral body ratio of 0.8 or less is not a contraindication to participation in contact activities in asymptomatic individuals. We further recommend against preparticipation screening roentgenograms in asymptomatic players. Such studies will not contribute to safety, are not cost effective, and will only contribute to the hysteria surrounding this issue.

In individuals with a ratio of 0.8 or less who experience either motor or sensory manifestations of cervical cord neurapraxia, there is a relative contraindication to return to contact activities. In these instances, each case must be determined on an individual basis depending on the understanding of the player and her parents and their willingness to accept any presumed theoretical risk.

An absolute contraindication to continued participation applies to those individuals who experience a documented episode of cervical cord neurapraxia associated with any of the following:

1. Ligamentous instability;
2. Intervertebral disk disease;
3. Degenerative changes;
4. MRI evidence of cord defects or swelling;
5. Symptoms or positive neurologic findings lasting more than 36 hours;
6. More than one recurrence.

"Spear Tackler's Spine"

Analysis of material recently received by the National Football Head and Neck Injury Registry has identified a subset of football players with "spear tackler's spine" (59). The entity consists of developmental narrowing

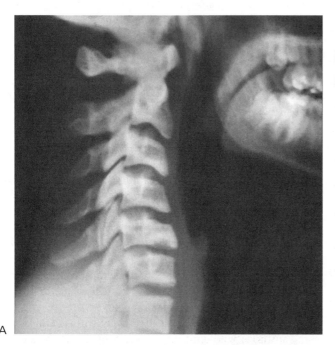

A

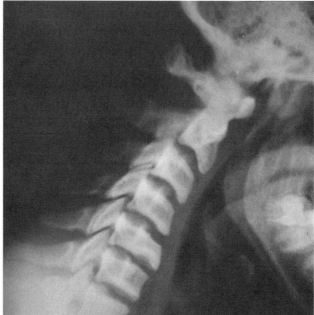

B

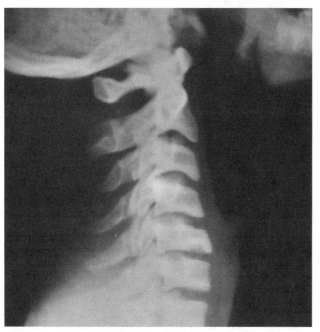

C

FIG. 9.12. Lateral neutral (**A**), flexion (**B**), and extension (**C**) views of a 19-year-old intercollegiate defensive back with spear tackler's spine. Note developmental stenosis and loss of normal cervical lordosis with virtually no motion on flexion and extension views, evidence of prior injury to C5. Player sustained a bilateral C3-4 facet dislocation with resulting quadriplegia as a result of a head impact axial loading injury.

(stenosis) of the cervical canal, persistent straightening or reversal of the normal cervical lordotic curve on an erect lateral roentgenogram obtained in the neutral position, concomitant preexisting posttraumatic roentgenographic abnormalities of the cervical spine, and documentation of the individual using the spear tackling technique (Fig. 9.12). In two instances in which preinjury roentgenograms and video documentation of axial loading of the spine due to spear tackling were available, a C3-4 bilateral facet dislocation resulted in one instance and C4-5 fracture dislocation in the other, both players being rendered quadriplegic. It is postulated that the straightened "segmented column" alignment of the cervical spine combined with head-first tackling techniques predisposed these individuals to an axial loading injury of the cervical segment. Thus, this combination of factors constitutes an absolute contraindication of further participation in collision sports.

Traumatic Conditions of the Upper Cervical Spine (C1-2)

The anatomy and mechanisms of the C1-2 segments of the cervical spine differ markedly from those of the middle or lower segments. Lesions with any degree of occipital or atlantoaxial instability portend a potentially grave prognosis. Thus, almost all injuries involving the upper cervical segment that involve a fracture or ligamentous laxity are an absolute contraindication to further participation in contact activities. Healed nondisplaced Jefferson fractures, healed type I and type II odontoid fractures, and healed lateral mass fractures of C2 constitute relative contraindications providing the patient is pain free, has a full range of cervical motion, and has no neurologic findings.

Because of the uncertainty of the results of cervical fusion, the gracile configuration of C1, and the importance of the alar and transverse odontoid ligaments, fusion for instability of the upper segment constitutes an absolute contraindication regardless of how successful the fusion appears roentgenographically.

Traumatic Conditions of the Middle and Lower Cervical Spine

Ligamentous Injuries

The criteria of White et al. (27,28) for defining clinical instability were intended to help establish indications for surgical stabilization. However, although the limits of displacement and angulation correlated with disruption of known structures, no one determinant was considered absolute. In view of the observations of Albright et al. (60) that 10% (7 of 75) of the college freshmen in their study demonstrated "abnormal motion," as well as on the basis of our own experience, it appears that in many instances some degree of "minor instability" exists in populations of both high school and college football players without apparently leading to adverse effects. The question, of course, is what are the upper limits of minor instability? Unfortunately, there are no data available relating this question to the clinical situation that allow reliable standards. Clearly, however, lateral roentgenograms that demonstrate more than 3.5 mm of horizontal displacement of either vertebra in relation to another, or more than 11 degrees of rotation than either adjacent vertebra, represent an absolute contraindication to further participation in contact activities. With regard to less degrees of displacement or rotation, further participation in sports enters the realm of "trial by battle," and such situations can be considered a relative contraindication depending on such factors as level of performance, physical habitus, position played (i.e., interior lineman vs. defensive back), and so on.

Fractures

An *acute fracture* of either the body or posterior elements with or without associated ligamentous laxity constitutes an absolute contraindication to participation.

The following healed stable fractures in an asymptomatic patient who is neurologically normal and has a full range of cervical motion can be considered to present *no contraindication* to participation in contact activities:

1. Stable compression fractures of the vertebral body without a sagittal component on anteroposterior roentgenograms and without involvement of either the ligamentous or the posterior bony structures;
2. A healed stable endplate fracture without a sagittal component on anteroposterior roentgenograms or involvement of the posterior or bony ligamentous structures;
3. Healed spinous process "clay shoveler" fractures.

Relative contraindications apply to the following healed stable fractures in individuals who are asymptomatic and neurologically normal and have a full pain-free range of cervical motion:

1. Stable displaced vertebral body compression fractures without a sagittal component on anteroposterior roentgenograms. The propensity for these fractures to settle causing increased deformity must be considered and carefully followed.
2. Healed stable fractures involving the elements of the posterior neural ring in individuals who are asymptomatic, neurologically normal, and have a full pain-free range of cervical motion. In evaluating radiographic and imaging studies to find the location and subsequent healing of a posterior neural ring fracture, it is important to understand that a rigid ring cannot break in one location. Thus, healing of paired fractures must be demonstrated.

Absolute contraindications to further participation in contact activities exist in the presence of the following fractures:

1. Vertebral body fracture with sagittal component;
2. Fracture of the vertebral body with or without displacement with associated posterior arch fractures or ligamentous laxity;
3. Comminuted fractures of the vertebral body with displacement into the spinal canal;
4. Any healed fracture of either the vertebral body or the posterior components with associated pain, neurologic findings and limitation of normal cervical motion;
5. Healed displaced fractures involving the lateral masses with resulting facet incongruity.

Invertebral Disk Injury

There is no contraindication to participation in contact activities in individuals with a healed anterior or lateral disk herniation treated conservatively or in those requiring an intervertebral diskectomy and interbody fusion for a lateral or central herniation who have a solid fusion, are symptomatic and neurologically negative, and have a full pain-free range of motion.

A *relative contraindication* exists in individuals with either conservatively or surgically treated disk disease with residual facet instability. An *absolute contraindication* exists in the following situations:

1. Acute central disk herniation;
2. Acute or chronic "hard disk" herniation with associated neurologic findings, pain, or significant limitation of cervical motion;
3. Acute or chronic hard disk herniation with associated symptoms of cord neurapraxia due to concomitant congenital narrowing (stenosis) of the cervical canal.

Status after Cervical Spine Fusion

A stable one-level anterior or posterior fusion in a patient who is asymptomatic, neurologically negative, and pain free and has a normal range of cervical motion presents no contraindication to continued participation in contact activities.

Individuals with a stable two- or three-level fusion who are asymptomatic and neurologically negative and have a pain-free full range of cervical motion have a relative contraindication. Because of the presumed increased stresses at the articulations of the uninvolved vertebrae and the propensity for development of degenerative changes at these levels, it appears to be the rare exception who should be permitted to continue contact activities.

In individuals with more than a three-level anterior or posterior fusion, an absolute contraindication exists as far as continued participation in contact activities.

SPINAL CORD RESUSCITATION

Twenty years ago it was neurosurgical practice to subject head-injured patients who were either deeply comatose or who showed signs of neurologic deterioration to burr-hole surgery. Often, bilateral burr holes were performed as an emergency procedure to assess and treat the possibility of significant intracranial hematoma. Patients were assumed, for all intents and purposes, to have subdural or epidural hematoma until proven otherwise.

Essentially, intracranial injury was thought to result from mechanical damage to the brain with subsequent neural insult. With improved diagnostic modalities and research findings, it became apparent that permanent brain injury was the result of both primary and secondary mechanisms.

Primary brain injury mechanisms produce mechanical damage to the brain by either the mechanical energy input or the effects of increased intracranial pressure. Fortunately, in most instances, the mechanical injury to the brain substance is not overwhelming. Secondary brain injury is caused by cerebral ischemia or hypoxia resulting from increased intracranial pressure, hemorrhage, brain swelling, or the indirect consequence of hypotension or respiratory compromise. Secondary brain injury has come to be recognized as the most important problem in the care and treatment of patients with closed head injuries. Thus, the major focus in the management of closed head injury now deals with implementation of the evolving principles of brain resuscitation.

It is proposed that with regard to resulting morbidity, the same pathophysiologic and mechanistic phenomena occur in acute spinal cord trauma. Specifically, it is secondary cord injury caused by hypoxia, edema, and aberrations in cell membrane potential that are largely responsible for resulting neurologic deficits. The concept of spinal cord resuscitation is proposed as an attempt to reverse secondary changes that occur to maintain neurologic recovery. Such measures include prompt relief of cord deformation, administration of intravenous corticosteroids, and initiation of measures to facilitate spinal cord perfusion.

Cervical cord injuries have resulted in reversible, incompletely reversible, and irreversible neurologic deficits. An explanation for this variable response to injury has been obtained from the study of the histochemical responses of a squid axon injury model to mechanical deformation (61). The spinal cord is considered an element with a low modulus of rigidity in which compressive macroscopic loads applied to the cord result in localized tension within the tissue. Various macroscopic deformations result in local elongation. With axial elongation of the cord, all elements experience stretch. With extension or flexion, the tension in the cord will vary across the diameter. Highly localized loadings such as shearing from subluxation of the vertebral elements or focal compressions, such as weight-drop experiment, result in elongation of the elements in the direction of the long axis of the cord. The effects of mechanical deformation of the axon membrane lead to an alteration in membrane permeability as a result of the development of nonspecific defects in the membrane. This allows calcium to flow into the cell and results in depolarization of the membrane.

The giant axon of the squid, *Loligo pealei,* was used as the tissue model to determine the effects of high-strain uniaxial tension to various degrees of stretch in concert with the changes of neurophysiology of the single axon. These experiments showed that the degree of mechanical injury to the axon influences the magnitude of the calcium insult and the time course of the recovery phase. A low rate of deformation produces only a small reversible depolarization. The axon responds to the increased intracellular calcium by pumping it extracellularly with no residual deficit. As the rate of loading was increased, the magnitude of the depolarization and the recovery time to the original resting potential increase in a nonlinear fashion. The axon may or may not fully recover depending on the ability of the cell to pump calcium. With a large influx of calcium, intracellular calcium pumps may be overwhelmed, resulting in irreversible injury. The excess intercellular calcium results in activation of calcium activated neutral proteases, which lead to cytoskeletal depolymerization and the accumulation of proteins intracellularly. The resulting increased osmotic pressure causes the cell to swell and eventually rupture (Fig. 9.13).

In addition to the immediate and direct effect of mechanical deformation on the cytosolic calcium concentration within the axon, it has been shown that high strain rate elongation of isolated venous specimens elicits a spontaneous constriction. The mechanically induced vasospasm has the effect of altering blood flow in various regions as a function of the level of vessel stretch. Ultimately, the outcome for the neural tissue will depend synergistically on the level of calcium introduced into the cytosol and the degree to which the metabolic machinery of the cell may be compromised by regional reduction in blood flow.

Clinical Correlation

The clinical evidence of varying degrees of recovery to cervical spine injury correlate with this model. Cord neurapraxia and transient quadriplegia, a completely reversible lesion, are associated with developmental narrowing of the cervical spine. Cord deformation must occur rapidly and is attributable to a hyperflexion or hyperextension mechanism. Disruption of cell membrane permeability leads to a small increase in intracellular calcium, but spinal stability and cell anatomy is not disturbed, and the deleterious effects of local anoxia secondary to venous spasm do not impede recovery of axonal function.

Cervical cord lesions with incomplete reversibility are often associated with instability such as seen with subluxation or unilateral facet dislocation where the cord undergoes maximal elastic deformation. It is proposed that lack of full recovery is attributable to prolonged duration of deformity when local anoxia inhibiting cell membrane function and a reduction of intracellular calcium concentrations. When unilateral facet dislocation is reduced within 3 hours of injury, significant neurologic recovery can occur.

Irreversible cord injury with a permanent quadriplegia results from an axial load mechanism that causes a

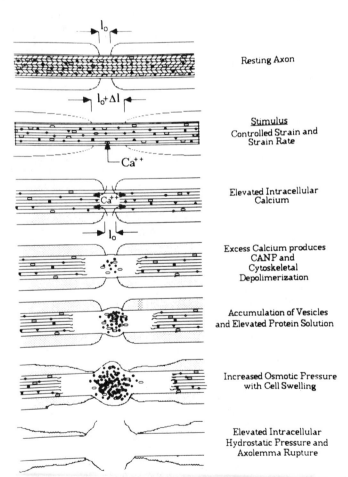

Resting Axon

Stimulus
Controlled Strain and
Strain Rate

Elevated Intracellular
Calcium

Excess Calcium produces
CANP and
Cytoskeletal
Depolimerization

Accumulation of Vesicles
and Elevated Protein Solution

Increased Osmotic Pressure
with Cell Swelling

Elevated Intracellular
Hydrostatic Pressure and
Axolemma Rupture

FIG. 9.13. Effects of elevated intracellular calcium concentration on cell viability. Specifically, elevated cytosolic-free calcium in excess of 50 μM will result in calcium activated neutral protease that can damage protein structures of the cell. (From Torg JS, Thibault HL, Snennett BJ, et al. The pathomechanics and pathophysiology of cervical spinal cord injury. *Clin Orthop* 1995;321:259–269, with permission.)

fracture or dislocation that renders the spine markedly unstable. The cord undergoes functional plastic deformation with anatomic disruption of axonal integrity.

Management Implications

These observations support the concept that acute spinal cord injury with concomitant subluxation and dislocation should be reduced promptly. This approach is at variance with previous approaches that recommended gradual reductions of cervical dislocations over a prolonged period of time. Recent studies have documented the efficacy of methylprednisolone in management of acute spinal cord injuries. These observations suggest the possible efficacy of other pharmacologic agents, such as agents that would increase vasodilation and local blood flow and counteract the effects of local cord anoxia or enhance the removal of intracellular calcium. Correlation of both reversible and irreversible spinal cord injury with the effect of neuronal and small vessel deformation have clearly indicated the potential for neurologic recovery by reversing the effects of increased intracellular calcium ion concentration and tissue anoxia. Presumably, these observations suggest that it is secondary cord injury caused by hypoxia and aberration in cell membrane potential that are largely responsible for irreversible neurologic deficits. Thus, the concept of spinal cord resuscitation is proposed as an attempt to reverse secondary changes that occur to obtain maximal neurologic recovery. Such measures would include prompt relief of cord deformation, administration of intravenous corticosteroids, measures to facilitate spinal cord profusion, and pharmacologic agents to facilitate the return of the calcium pump mechanism.

REFERENCES

1. Vegso JJ, Torg JS. Field evaluation and management of intracranial injuries. In: Torg JS, ed. *Athletic injuries to the head, neck and face,* 2nd ed. St. Louis: Mosby Year-Book, 1991.
2. National Collegiate Athletic Association Sports Medicine Handbook. *Guidelines for helmet fitting and removal in athletics.* Kansas: Overland Park, 1998.
3. Swenson TM, Lauerman WC, Blanc RO, et al. Cervical spine alignment in the immobilized football player. Radiographic analysis before and after helmet removal. *Am J Sports Med* 1997;25:226–230.
4. Gastel JA, Palumbo MA, Hulstyn MJ, et al. Emergency removal of football equipment: a cadaveric cervical spine injury model. *Ann Emerg Med* 1998;32:411–417.
5. Bracken MS, Shepard MJ, Collins WF, et al. A randomized, controlled trial of methylprednisolone or naloxone in the treatment of acute spinal cord injury. *N Engl J Med* 1990;322:1405–1411.
6. Schneider RC. *Head and neck injuries in football, mechanism, treatment, and prevention.* Baltimore: Williams & Wilkins, 1972: 183.
7. Gennarelli TA. Mechanisms and pathophysiology of cerebral concussion. *J Head Trauma Rehabil* 1986;1:23–29.
8. Gennarelli TA. Cerebral concussion and diffuse brain injuries. In: Cooper PR, ed. *Head injury.* Baltimore: Williams & Wilkins, 1987:108–124.
9. Gennarelli TA. Mechanisms of cerebral concussion, contusion,

and other effects of head injury. In: Youmans J, ed. *Neurological surgery.* Philadelphia: W.B. Saunders, 1990:1953–1964.
10. Gennarelli TA. Head injury mechanisms. In: Torg JS, ed. *Athletic injuries to the head, neck and face,* 2nd ed. St. Louis: Mosby Year-Book, 1991.
11. Gennarelli TA. Cerebral concussion and diffuse brain injuries. In: Torg JS, ed. *Athletic injuries to the head, neck and face,* 2nd ed. St. Louis: Mosby Year-Book, 1991.
12. Ommaya AK, Gennarelli TA. Cerebral concussion and traumatic unconsciousness. Correlation of experimental and clinical observations on blunt head injuries. *Brain* 1974;97:633–654.
13. Cantu RC. Criteria for return to competition after closed head injury. In: Torg JJ, ed. *Athletic injuries to the head, neck and face.* 2nd ed. St. Louis: Mosby Year-Book, 1991.
14. Saunders RL, Harbaugh RE. The second impact in catastrophic contact sports head trauma. *JAMA* 1984;252:538–539.
15. Thibault LE, Gennarelli TA. Biomechanics and craniocerebral trauma. In: Povlishock J, Becker D, eds. *Central nervous system trauma status report.* Bethesda, MD: NINCDS, 1985:370–390.
16. Bruno LA. Focal intracranial hematoma. In: Torg JS, ed. *Athletic injuries to the head, neck and face,* 2nd ed. St. Louis: Mosby Year-Book, 1991.
17. Bruce DA, Schut L, Bruno LA, et al. Outcome following severe head injuries in children. *J Neurosurg* 1978;48:679–688.
18. Langfitt TW, Tannenbaum HM, Kassell NF. The etiology of acute brain swelling following experimental head injury. *J Neurosurg* 1966;24:47–56.
19. Clancy WG. Brachial plexus and upper extremity peripheral nerve injuries. In: Torg JS, ed. *Athletic injuries to the head, neck and face,* 2nd ed. St. Louis: Mosby Year-Book, 1991.
20. Seddon H. Surgical disorders of the peripheral nerves. Edinburgh: Churchill, Livingstone, 1992.
21. Levitz CL, Reilly PJ, Torg JS. The pathomechanics of chronic recurring cervical nerve root neurapraxia. *Am J Sports Med* 1997;25:73–76.
22. Hershman EB. *Injuries to the brachial plexus.* In: Torg JS, ed. *Athletic injuries to the head, neck and face,* 2nd ed. St. Louis: Mosby Year-Book, 1991.
23. Albright JP, Moses JM, Feldich HG, et al. Non-fatal cervical spine injuries in interscholastic football. *JAMA* 1976;236:1243–1245.
24. Torg JS, Truex RC, Marshall J, et al. Spinal injury at the level of the third and fourth cervical vertebrae resulting from football. *J Bone Joint Surg Am* 1977;59A:1015.
25. Torg JS, Sennett BJ, Vegso JJ, et al. Axial loading injuries to the middle cervical spine segment: an analysis and classification of twenty-five cases. *Am J Sports Med* 1991;19:6–20.
26. Bracken MD, Shepard MJ, Collins WF, et al. A randomized, controlled trial of methylprednisolone or naloxone in the treatment of acute spinal cord injury. *N Engl J Med* 1990;322:1405–1411.
27. White AA, Johnson RM, Panjabi MM. Biomechanical analysis of clinical stability in the cervical spine. *Clin Orthop* 1975;109:85–96.
28. White AA, Punjab MM. *Clinical biomechanics of the spine.* Philadelphia: J.B. Lippincott, 1978.
29. Thompson RC, Morris JN, Jane JA. Current concepts in management of cervical spine fractures and dislocations. *Am J Sports Med* 1975;3:159.
30. Fielding JW, Fietti VG, Mardam-Bey TH, et al. Athletic injuries to the atlanto-axial articulation. *Am J Sports Med* 1978;6:226.
31. Jefferson G. Fracture of the atlas vertebra. *Br J Surg* 1920;7:407.
32. Anderson LD, D'Alonzo RT. Fractures of the odontoid process of the axis. *J Bone Joint Surg Am* 1974;56A:1663.
33. Cloward RB. Acute cervical spine injuries. *Clin Symp* 1980;32:2–32.
34. Scheider RC. The syndrome of acute anterior spinal cord injury. *J Neurosurg* 1955;12:95–123.
35. Torg JS, Pavlov H, Genuario SE, et al. Neurapraxia of the cervical spinal cord with transient quadriplegia. *J Bone Joint Surg Am* 1986;68A:1354–1370.
36. Penning L. Some aspects of plain radiography of the cervical spine in chronic myelopathy. *Neurology* 1962;12:513–519.
37. Boijsen E. The cervical spinal canal in intraspinal expansive processes. *Acta Radiol* 1954;42:101–115.
38. Pavlov H, Torg JS, Robie B, et al. Cervical spinal stenosis determi-

nation with vertebral body ratio method. *Radiology* 1987;164: 771–775.

39. Torg JS, Naranja RJ Jr, Pavlov H, et al. The relationship of developmental narrowing of the cervical spinal canal to reversible and irreversible injury of the cervical spinal cord in football players. *J Bone Joint Surg Am* 1996;78A:1308–1314.
40. Burstein AH, Otis JC, Torg JS. Mechanisms and pathomechanics of athletic injuries to the cervical spine. In: Torg JS, ed. *Athletic injuries to the head, neck, and face.* Philadelphia: Lea & Febiger, 1982:139–154.
41. Torg JS, Corcoran TA, Thihault LE, et al. Cervical cord neurapraxia and classification of pathomechanics, morbidity, and management guidelines. *J Neurosurg* 1997;87:843–980.
42. Wu WQ, Lewis RC. Injuries of the cervical spine in high school wrestling. *Surg Neurol* 1985;23:143–147.
43. Scher AT. The high rugby tackle—an avoidable cause of cervical spinal injury. *South Afr Med J* 1978;53:1015–1018.
44. Scher AT. Vertex impact and cervical dislocation in rugby players. *South Afr Med J* 1981;59:227–228.
45. Silver JR. Injuries of the spine sustained in rugby. *Br Med J* 1984;288:37–43.
46. Torg JS, Das M. Trampoline-related quadriplegia: a review of the literature and reflections on the American Academy of Pediatrics position statement. *Pediatrics* 1984;74:804–812.
47. Tator CH, Edmonds VE. National survey of spinal injuries to hockey players. *Can J Neurol Sci* 1984;11:34–41.
48. Torg JS, Truex RC Jr, Quedenfeld TC. The National Football Head and Neck Injury Registry. Report and conclusions. *JAMA* 1979;241:1477–1479.
49. Torg JS, Vesgo JJ, Sennett BJ. The National Football Head and Neck Registry: 14 year report on cervical quadriplegia 1971 to 1975. *JAMA* 1985;254:3439–3443.
50. Torg JS, Vegsgo JJ, O'Neill MJ, et al. The epidemiologic, patho-logic, biomechanical, and cinematographic analysis of football-induced cervical spine trauma. *Am J Sports Med* 1990;18:50–57.
51. Nightingale RW, McElhaney JH, Richardson WJ, et al. Experimental impact injury to the cervical spine: relating motion of the head and the mechanism of injury. *J Bone Joint Surg Am* 1996;78A:412–421.
52. Mertz HJ, Hodgson VR, Murray TL, et al. An assessment of compressive neck loads under injury-producing conditions. *Physician Sports Med* 1978;6:95–106.
53. Roaf R. A study of the mechanics of spinal injuries. *J Bone Joint Surg Am* 1960;42B:810–823.
54. Tator CH, Edmonds VE, New ML. Diving: a frequent and potentially preventable cause of spinal cord injury. *Can Med Assoc J* 1981;124:1323–1324.
55. Scher AT. Vertex impact and cervical dislocation in rugby players. *South Afr Med J* 1981;59:227–228.
56. Hensinger RN. Congenital anomalies of the odontoid. In: The Cervical Spine Research Society Editorial Committee, eds. *The cervical spine,* 2nd ed. Philadelphia: J.B. Lippincott, 1989:248–257.
57. Pizzutillo PD. Kipple-Feil syndrome. In: The Cervical Spine Research Society Editorial Committee, eds. *The Cervical spine,* 2nd ed. Philadelphia: J.B. Lippincott, 1987:258–271.
58. Eismont FJ, Clifford S, Goldberg M, et al. Cervical sagittal spinal canal size in spine injuries. *Spine* 1984;9:663–666.
59. Torg JS, Sennett BJ, Pavlov H, et al. Spear tackler's spine, an entity precluding participation in tackle football and collision activities that expose the cervical spine to axial energy inputs. *Am J Sports Med* 1993;21:640–649.
60. Albright JP, Moses JM, Feldick HG, et al. Nonfatal cervical spine injuries in interscholastic football. *JAMA* 1976;236:1243–1245.
61. Torg JS, Thibault L, Sennett BJ, et al. The pathomechanics and pathophysiology of cervical spinal cord injury. *Clin Orthop* 1995;321:259–269.

Principles and Practice of Orthopaedic Sports Medicine,
edited by William E. Garrett, Jr., Kevin P. Speer, and Donald T. Kirkendall.
Lippincott Williams & Wilkins, Philadelphia © 2000.

CHAPTER 10

Brachial Plexus/Stingers

Eliot Hershman and Jeffrey Berg

The brachial plexus is a complex structure that organizes the cervical roots into the defined nerves of the upper extremity. Athletic injuries to this structure are rare. Most occur in football, wrestling, and ice hockey (1). Typically these injuries are self-limiting. Occasionally, however, the outcome can be catastrophic. The results are dependent on such factors as the anatomic variation of the plexus, the mechanism and location of the injury, and the chosen mode of treatment. Acute injuries to the brachial plexus can be confused with a variety of other impairments of the upper extremity. To avoid misdiagnosis and ensure maximum recovery for the athlete, the physician must have a clear understanding of the plexus anatomy, mechanism of injuries, common findings of clinical evaluation and imaging modalities, and available preventative and treatment options.

EPIDEMIOLOGY

Brachial plexus injuries in athletics are uncommon. These injuries have been reported in football, wrestling, ice hockey, basketball, track, skiing, diving, horse and motorcycle riding, squash, judo, and hiking (1,2–5). Shukla and Green (6) have even reported brachial plexus injuries resulting from competitive bowling.

Sports-related injuries to the brachial plexus range from mild compression or traction neuropraxias to traction axonotmesis. Rarely, neurotmesis or root avulsions are encountered (2,7–10). Additionally, atraumatic brachial plexopathies have also been described in athletes (11).

Most sports-related brachial plexus injuries occur in those participating in American football in whom the transient, "burner" or "stinger" syndrome is the most common injury (7,12,13). Chrisman et al. (4) initially described this disorder in 22 athletes, with 17 occurring in those participating in football. Speer and Bassett (12) noted that during the 1987 season, 19 players on a NCAA division I football team experienced a burner injury. The total number of football players on the team was not provided, and so the overall incidence is indeterminate. Robertson et al. (10) reported that the incidence of University of Wisconsin football players experiencing one or more episodes of burner symptomology during a given season was approximately 50%. During a 4-year period, these authors treated 150 such cases in this group. Clancy et al. (7) reported comparable findings, with 33 of 67 football players sustaining these injuries during their career and 26 of these same 67 players having a burner injury in a single season. Sallis et al. (14) also noted a similar incidence. These authors interviewed 201 NCAA division III football players. Sixty-five percent had an episode of transient brachial plexopathy, 52% within a single season and 57% recurrently. Interestingly, 70% of the injured players had not previously reported these injuries to anyone on the medical staff.

A much lower, but still significant, single season incidence of 18 of 261 (6.9%) intramural or varsity tackle football players at the United States Military Academy was noted by Markey et al. (15). A similar incidence was noted by Meyer et al. (16) in their study of the University of Iowa football team. These authors evaluated 288 players of their team from 1987 to 1991 who were available for radiographic follow-up. Forty players (15%) during the study period reported symptoms consistent with a stinger. Of these, however, only 6 players (2.3%) sustained a brachial plexus traction injury, whereas the remaining 34 players sustained an extension–compression cervical spine injury. The authors noted that this incidence might have underestimated the true occurrence rate because patients with full uncomplicated recovery and no time loss from activity may have been overlooked (16).

E. Hershman and J. Berg: Department of Orthopaedic Surgery, Lennox Hill Hospital, New York, New York 10021.

Compression resulting from carrying heavy backpacks while hiking is another common cause of sports-related brachial plexus injuries (3,13,17). Hirasawa and Sakakida (13) reviewed 1,167 peripheral nerve injuries and noted that 66 (5.7%) were related to sports. Most were secondary to knapsack palsy and the most frequently involved location of injury was the brachial plexus.

Root avulsion and nerve transection typically result from violent traction injuries, as might occur in automobile or motorcycle accidents during racing competitions. Because of the significant forces involved, these injuries are often associated with various fractures and dislocations about the shoulder girdle, including glenohumeral dislocations (18–23), scapular fractures (19,24), humeral fractures (18–20,25), clavicular fractures (26–28), sternoclavicular dissociations (20,29), acromioclavicular separations (20,30), and scapulothoracic dissociations (24). Most reports are anecdotal, and therefore the incidence of athletic root avulsions and neurotmesis injuries is unknown, as is the incidence of related fractures and dislocations. They do, however, appear to be quite rare, and because of their severity, their prognosis is most guarded (17,31). Clancy (32) described one such injury occurring in a United States Naval Academy football player. After sustaining what appeared to be a simple burner, the patient's deltoid, supraspinatus, and infraspinatus weakness failed to fully resolve over a 1.5-year period of observation, at which time the patient was

lost to follow-up (32). Wilbourn (33) reported a single case occurring in a young boy who sustained multiple root avulsions after striking a pole while sledding. Root avulsions occurring during athletic competition have also been reported in a series by Bergfield et al. (34).

Acute brachial neuropathy (ABN) is a rare disorder that produces severe shoulder and arm pain associated with shoulder girdle weakness. Hershman et al. (11) reported this disorder in 5 of 78 (6.4%) athletes who were evaluated for brachial plexus problems. The overall occurrence in the general population appears to be extremely rare; however, the actual incidence is unknown.

PATHOANATOMY AND MECHANISM OF INJURY

Anatomy of the Plexus

The brachial plexus lies in the posterior triangle of the neck, between the clavicle and the posterior aspect of the inferior sternocleidomastoid (35). The *spinal nerves* divide into the dorsal and ventral rami as they exit from the intervertebral foramen. The dorsal rami proceed to innervate the paraspinal musculature, a fact that assists in localizing plexus injuries (36). The brachial plexus is then formed from the ventral rami of the fifth, sixth, seventh, and eighth cervical and first thoracic nerves (Fig. 10.1). In the case of the *prefixed* plexus, a contribution from the fourth cervical nerve exists, whereas in

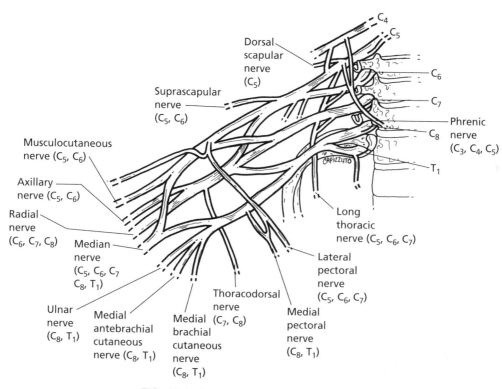

FIG. 10.1. Anatomy of the brachial plexus.

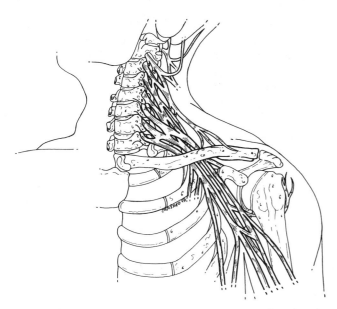

FIG. 10.2. The brachial plexus lies in the posterior triangle of the neck and runs posterior to the clavicle.

the *postfixed* plexus, a contribution from the second thoracic nerve exists (37). These arrangements are quite variable and have little clinical significance (36,38). In fact, variation in the manner that the individual ventral rami form the plexus occurs frequently (37). The most common pattern is as follows. The ventral rami of C5 and C6 unite to form the *upper trunk,* whereas the C7 ventral ramus continues as the *middle trunk* and the C8 and T1 ventral rami form the *lower trunk.* These trunks run laterally and inferiorly between the anterior and middle scalene muscles, running over the first rib and behind the clavicle (Fig. 10.2) (35). Before this, however, several supraclavicular branches arise. The dorsal scapular and a branch to the phrenic nerve originate from C5. The long thoracic nerve is formed from contributions of C5, C6, and C7. Branches of C5, C6, C7, and C8 innervate the longus colli and scalene muscles. Additionally, two branches arise from the upper trunk: the suprascapular nerve and the nerve to the subclavius muscle. The suprascapular nerve originates from the upper trunk at Erb's point (39).

Either just proximal to or behind the clavicle, each of the three trunks divide into an *anterior and posterior division.* No branches typically arise from these divisions. The divisions then unite in a specific pattern to form the *lateral, medial, and posterior cords,* so named to reflect their respective locations to the axillary artery. The anterior divisions of the upper and middle trunks form the lateral cord. The anterior division of the lower trunk continues as the medial cord and the posterior divisions of all three trunks unite to form the posterior cord. The cords lie behind the pectoralis minor. From the cords, multiple infraclavicular branches arise. The *lateral pectoral nerve* originates from the lateral cord.

The *medial pectoral, medial antebrachial cutaneous, and medial brachial cutaneous nerves* originate from the medial cord and the *superior, inferior subscapular, and thoracodorsal nerves* arise from the posterior cord. The individual cords then divide to form the remaining infraclavicular branches, the major nerves of the upper extremity. The lateral cord divides into the *musculocutaneous nerve* and one of the two branches to the *median nerve.* The medial cord produces the *ulnar nerve* and also provides the other branch to the median nerve, whereas the posterior cord divides into the *axillary and radial nerves* (37,40).

The plexus is well fixed to the surrounding structures that serve to protect it from traction. The spinal nerves of C5, C6, and C7 are attached to the transverse processes by fibrous bands of the epineurium and additionally to the cervical fascia, which forms a fibrous sheath surrounding the nerve. C8 and T1 are void of these reinforcements and are, therefore, more prone to avulsion injuries (17,41). The terminal branches also act to fix the plexus. The axillary nerve runs through the quadrilateral space, whereas the radial and ulnar nerves are strongly fixed as they wrap around the humerus and through the cubital tunnel, respectively. Additionally, the median and the musculocutaneous nerves serve to restrict the plexus via their adherence to the pronator teres and the corachobrachialis, respectively (41).

Root Anatomy

It is important to understand the composition of the roots, rami, and cords to differentiate between preganglionic and postganglionic sites of injury (Fig. 10.3). The sensory ganglion (the dorsal root ganglion) is located near or within the intervertebral foramen. Therefore, the sensory root is not a peripheral nerve until it leaves the intervertebral foramen. This differs from the motor roots, which have their ganglia (the anterior horn cells)

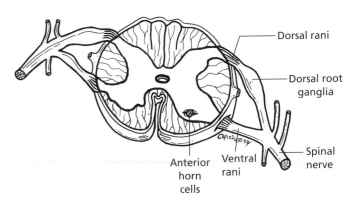

FIG. 10.3. Anatomy of the spinal nerve. Each spinal nerve is formed from a dorsal and ventral rami. The sensory ganglia (dorsal root ganglia) is located in the dorsal rami. The motor ganglia (anterior horn cells) are located in the gray matter of the ventral horn of the spinal cord.

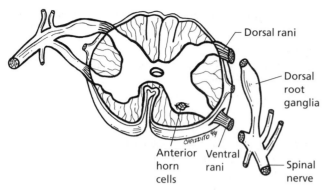

FIG. 10.4. Root avulsion. Ventral root avulsions are postganglionic and dorsal root avulsions are predominately preganglionic.

within the spinal cord and therefore are essentially peripheral nerves from that site distally. Root avulsions tend to be preganglionic lesions, that is, the injury occurs proximal to the dorsal root ganglia (Fig. 10.4). This injury produces Wallerian degeneration in the peripheral motor axon. However, because the sensory segment remains in continuity with its ganglion, degeneration will not occur in this component. Motor and sensory function is lost, the former because of separation from its ganglion and the latter because of separation from the cord. Additionally, the muscles and skin innervated by the posterior rami are also denervated. In postganglionic injuries, those occurring distal to the dorsal root ganglion, both motor and sensory peripheral axons are damaged, the paraspinal musculature and skin innervated by the posterior rami retain their innervation, and the potential for spontaneous recovery of motor and sensory function exists (1,17,39,42).

Microstructure

The microstructure of a peripheral nerve is complex (Fig. 10.5). Individual nerve fibers are surrounded by endoneurium and grouped together into fascicles. The fascicles, in turn, are then surrounded by perineurium.

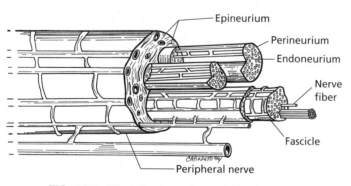

FIG. 10.5. Microstructure of a peripheral nerve.

Many fascicles are then combined to form the individual nerve. A layer of epineurium ultimately surrounds the nerve. The endoneurium, perineum, and epineurium are connective tissue layers of primarily a loose collagenous network that serves to support, nourish, and protect the neural structures (43–45).

Classification of Nerve Injuries

Nerve injuries and more specifically brachial plexus injuries can be grouped by the classification schema initially described by Seddon (46) and later modified by Sunderland (47). Seddon attempted to correlate histologic and clinical findings and prognostic factors with three stages of nerve injury. Sunderland expanded this classification to five stages or degrees. *Neuropraxia*, a first-degree injury, is the mildest form of injury. It describes a localized reversible interruption of nerve conduction at the site of injury. There is no Wallerian degeneration and generally motor and large myelinated fibers are more susceptible than sensory and fine nonmyelinated fibers. Recovery is predictable and usually is complete by 2 to 3 weeks (43,48–51).

Axonotmesis is a second-degree nerve injury. This stage represents severe injury or disruption of the axon itself and the surrounding myelin. The endoneural tube and the basal lamina of the Schwann cell remain intact, serving as conduits for nerve regeneration. Therefore, there is potential for full functional recovery (43,49,51–53). Typically, complete temporary loss of motor and sensory function occurs; however, because the axon distal to the injury site is initially intact, early on this segment can be electrically stimulated. Wallerian degeneration distal to the injury site then follows, and within 24 to 72 hours the ability to electrically stimulate this distal segment is lost. Electromyography (EMG) reveals fibrillation and positive waves, evidence of denervation, and the affected muscle begins to atrophy (38,43). Recovery is determined by the severity and level of the injury and the ability of the regenerating unit to elongate and reinnervate the appropriate end organ (43,53). In the adult, regeneration progresses at a rate of 1 mm/day (49).

Neurotmesis is the most severe form of nerve injury (49). This grade of injury represents a complete typically irreversible injury to the affected nerve. The endoneurium is disrupted and therefore functional regeneration is usually impossible, despite the ongoing process of Wallerian degeneration and sprouting (38,43,49,54). According to Sunderland (47), neurotmesis can be classified into three stages. In a third-degree injury, although the endoneurium is disrupted, the perineurium and epineurium remain intact (43,51). This leads to disturbance of the internal structure of the fascicles while maintaining the overall fascicular arrangement. In addition, retrograde injury to the proximal stump and the cell body occurs. This prolongs recovery. The prognosis for functional recovery is dependent on the extent of interfascicular fibrosis development and the ability of the regenerating unit to elongate and locate the appropriate end organ (43). A fourth-degree injury denotes disruption of the endoneurium and the perineurium. The epineurium remains intact, however. Because of the severity of this injury, a greater amount of proximal degeneration occurs and therefore the potential for functional recovery is even more limited. Typically, surgical repair of the damaged nerve segment is required to obtain any functional recovery (43). A fifth-degree injury results in discontinuity of the nerve itself. The endoneurium, perineurium, and epineurium are all disrupted. As in the case of a fourth-degree injury, surgical repair or nerve grafting is required if there is to be any chance of significant end-organ reinnervation (43,51,55).

CLINICAL CONDITIONS

Burner Syndrome

The most common brachial plexus injury in North American sports appears to be the burner syndrome. It has also been referred to as a stinger (2,15,16,56) or "pinched nerve" (5,7,38,42). This entity is so named because of its characteristic symptom pattern. Typically, the athlete sustains a collision involving his or her head, neck, or shoulder (1,2,7,10,54,57). Acute unilateral, radiating, sharp pain and dysesthesias, parasthesias, and anesthesias typically follow. These symptoms extend from the supraclavicular region, down the arm, to the finger tips (1,2,16,32,42,54,57). Motor weakness is often associated. Although it may not be present initially, weakness may be noted in follow-up (1,2,10,54,57). The spinatus, deltoid, biceps, and brachioradialis muscles are most often involved (33,57). The player characteristically walks on or off the field rubbing or shaking her arm or holding it at her side (Fig. 10.6) (42). Typically, resolution occurs over several seconds or minutes. Numbness tends to persist longer than weakness. In the chronic cases, symptoms of weakness and sensory loss may persist. In addition, pain may recur with further use of the affected extremity (58).

Clancy et al. (7) classified this disorder based on the rate of symptom resolution. Grade I lesions are those in which the athlete sustains a transitory motor and sensory loss that resolves by 2 weeks. Grade II lesions involve more extensive motor and occasionally sensory losses that persist beyond 2 weeks but ultimately resolve, whereas grade III lesions have motor and sensory deficits that persist for more than 1 year (35). The simple burner syndrome must be differentiated from the clinical entity presenting with bilateral upper extremity burning paresthesias and dysesthesias with or without motor or sensory loss. This constellation of symptoms

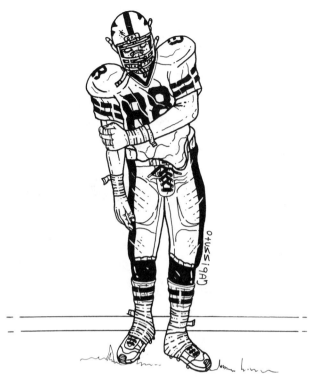

FIG. 10.6. Characteristic appearance of an athlete who just sustained a "burner."

more typically represents a cervical cord injury and requires much more vigilant management (59,60).

The etiology of the burner syndrome is somewhat controversial. The most common mechanism for producing this injury has been thought to be *traction* on the brachial plexus. This occurs when a force creating downward shoulder movement depresses the shoulder girdle. It is often associated with lateral flexion of the neck to the contralateral side, as occurs while tackling during North American football (Fig. 10.7) (1,5,35,61) or as might occur in wrestling during a take down (62,63). This mechanism is similar to that which causes acromioclavicular separations. Bergfield et al. (34) hypothesized that concomitant burners and acromioclavicular separations are rare because they differ in the area of shoulder contact during injury. The contact area is localized to the acromion in acromioclavicular separations and along the clavicle in burners (34). Nonetheless, this mechanism, it is hypothesized, results in a traction injury, producing a neuropraxia or a combination of neuropraxia and axonetmesis of the upper brachial plexus (5,7,42,64). Evidence that substantiates this mechanism is the high incidence among defensive football players who often tackle with their shoulder, consequently depressing the entire shoulder girdle. EMG data localizing the injury to the upper plexus also are consistent with a traction injury at the upper trunk area (10,38). Interestingly, a recent study using magnetic res-

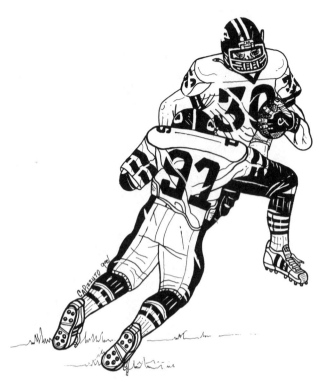

FIG. 10.7. Common mechanism for developing a "burner." Incorrect tackling technique often results in downward force on the shoulder associated with lateral flexion of the neck.

onance imaging (MRI) has consistently localized this injury to the division level of the plexus (65), whereas others have stated that the most common site of injury is at the root level within or near the vertebral foramina (62).

Other authors have argued that this is not the most common mechanism of injury (15,56). Some of these authors believe that a *direct compression* injury to the brachial plexus accounts for most cases. This injury mechanism is thought to occur after a blunt object, such as a player's shoulder pad, a hockey stick, or a karate chop, strikes Erb's point where the plexus is most superficial and therefore most vulnerable. In a prospective study of 14 tackle football players without a history of stinger syndrome and 18 players with a history of recurrent stinger syndrome, Markey et al. (15) used both clinical and electrodiagnostic data to show a high incidence of multiple peripheral nerve injuries at the plexus level. The authors hypothesized that a compression injury was more likely to explain this injury pattern than a traction injury. DiBenedetto and Markey (56), using electrodiagnostic data in 18 athletes, 16 football players, and 2 wrestlers with stinger syndrome symptoms of at least 3 months' duration, also concluded that the more common etiology for the plexopathy was compression. They did concede, however, that traction might have also played a part in these cases. Additional

evidence offered by both studies was the trend toward reduction in burner incidence among players using modified shoulder pads that prevented a compression mechanism (15,56).

Other common causes proposed are *radiculopathy* (2,12,54,56,58) and an *extension–compression* mechanism of the cervical spinal cord associated with cervical spine stenosis (16,61). Radiculopathy most often affects the C5 and C6 roots (2,58). Symptoms have been attributed to several factors such as scarring of the roots and fixation to the transverse processes or to hypertrophied scalene muscles often found in athletes (58). In addition, cervical flexion has also been implicated as a pathogenic element in symptoms occurring in this manner (2).

The extension–compression mechanism implicates the root level as the site of injury. Symptoms resulting from this mechanism have been attributed to degenerative changes of the cervical spine, most often occurring in chronic recurrent cases (54,62–64). Two potential etiologies have been blamed: degenerative disk disease (54) and foraminal narrowing secondary to facet joint subluxation (54,62–64). The degenerative changes are most frequently located at the C4-5, C5-6, and C6-7 levels (54). In addition, multiple authors have noted that athletes with symptoms resulting from an extension–compression mechanism possess a high incidence of central cervical stenosis, as measured by the method of Pavlov and Torg (see Chapter 11) (16,54,66,67). In fact, Meyer et al. (16) observed a three times greater incidence in stingers among those with extension–compression injuries and cervical stenosis than those with extension–compression injuries alone. In addition, cervical stenosis has also been observed to lead to a more complicated course (16) and have more frequent recurrences of stinger injuries (67).

From the data available, it appears that there are multiple causes of the symptomatology referred to as burner or stinger syndrome, although the predominant mechanism resulting in this clinical entity is not clear. Nonetheless, in the novice athlete, it appears that these symptoms are most often due to either a traction or acute compression injury, whereas in the older more experienced athlete, particularly those with chronic symptoms, occurrences more often result from a radicular or extension–compression mechanisms promoted by degenerative changes of the cervical spine.

Compression Injuries

Sports-related brachial plexus compression injuries present in two forms: rapid onset or delayed onset. No matter the presentation, however, the pathophysiology remains the same. The severity, conversely, may differ based on the magnitude and direction of the compression (68). The primary events appear to be direct disruption of intraneural blood flow and antegrade and retrograde axonal transport (50). As a result of intraneural blood flow impairment, intrafascicular anoxia and subsequent intrafascicular edema result. The increased edema's effect is twofold. It increases the intrafascicular pressure that further impairs axonal blood supply and it also increases the oxygen diffusion distance to the neural tissues. Both mechanisms serve to starve the axons of their essential nutrients and prevent removal of unnecessary waste materials (50). Direct disruption of axonal transport achieves this same end point. The ultimate result is disruption of the morphology and function of the nerve cell bodies, the nerves themselves, and the surrounding myelin and Schwann cells (50).

The mechanisms of injury of the rapid-onset compressive disorders have already been described earlier in this chapter. Classically, the so-called pack palsy defines the delayed-onset athletic compressive disorders (Fig. 10.8) (3). These lesions occur when heavy backpacks are carried using the axillary straps during extended hikes. The straps compress the plexus between the clavicle and the first rib. An additional traction component may result secondary to the posterior pull of the shoulder girdle due to the heavy pack. Injury isolated to the axillary and radial nerve produced by this same mechanism may occur as well (3,69).

Other mechanisms can also cause chronic compressive plexopathies. Neurogenic thoracic outlet syndrome is one such condition. Several entities are grouped under the heading of thoracic outlet syndrome, including cervical rib syndrome, Scalenius Anticus syndrome, Wright's hyperabduction syndrome, costoclavicular syndrome, and the so-called drooping shoulder syndrome (35,70). Most commonly, neurologic thoracic outlet syndrome occurs in women (71). Typically, affected females tend to be thin with drooping shoulders (35). The classical presentation is that of radiating pain along the side or back of the neck that extends into the shoulder and occasionally the proximal medial arm. Because this disorder is typically a lower plexopathy, paresthesias and hyposthesias of the ulnar aspect of the forearm and hand and weakness and atrophy of the intrinsic muscles often accompany these symptoms (35,71). Although occasionally present, concomitant venous congestion or arterial occlusion is fortunately rare (71). Athletes may note onset of symptoms when the upper extremity is in a variety of positions. For instance, repetitive hyperabduction, such as in swimming; elevation and hyperabduction, such as in swimming, serving, and throwing; and shoulder girdle depression, such as in overhead racquet sports and pitching, have all been noted to result in the characteristic symptoms (71–73).

Clavicle fractures and their treatment have also been implicated in the production of compressive brachial plexopathies. Healing fractures with exuberant callus, hypertrophic nonunions, and even figure-of-eight bandages occasionally used in the treatment of these fractures can result in a brachial plexus compression injury (26,27,74–77). Other causes reported are fractures of the first rib (21), space-occupying lesions (38), and even the use of body armor in soldiers while providing "top cover" (78).

Root Avulsion and Neurotmesis

Root avulsions and neurotmesis injuries are rare occurrences in sporting events. Most are limited to high-velocity trauma, such as that found in motorcycle or automobile racing (38). Frequently, these are associated with fractures or dislocations about the shoulder girdle (18).

In a scanning electron microscopy study performed on rats and a human cadaver by Bristol and Fraher (79), the injury site in avulsions was localized to the root-cord junction in most cases. Narakas (80) described six distinct mechanisms and correlated these with the injury patterns he found at surgery. A severe glenohumeral distraction may produce disruption of the terminal branches of the plexus. In addition, glenohumeral dislocation, rotator cuff or greater tuberosity avulsion, or a rupture of the axillary artery may be found. When the trauma to the plexus is due to scapulothoracic dissociation, one of two patterns may occur. Either an acromioclavicular separation or clavicle and scapular fracture associated with rupture or avulsion of the suprascapular, axillary, and musculocutaneous nerves and rupture of the axillary artery and possibly the median, ulnar, and musculocutaneous nerves may occur or a complete

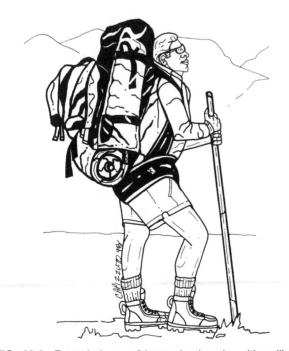

FIG. 10.8. Extended use of heavy backpacks with axillary straps is a common cause of compression plexopathy.

proximal plexus injury with lower root avulsions and injury to the subclavian artery occurs.

The most common mechanism of injury is often similar to that found in many burner injuries, that is, downward force to the shoulder along with contralateral head displacement. The impact in these injuries, however, is much more severe. The position of the arm at the time of impact determines the region of the cord most affected (9,81,82). If the arm is adducted and the head and shoulder are pushed far apart, then typically rupture of the upper trunk, rupture or avulsion of C7, root avulsion of C8 and T1, and possible palsies of the phrenic or long thoracic nerves will occur. If the arm is hyperabducted, then lower root avulsions with or without avulsion of the musculocutaneous and axillary nerves will occur. When the shoulder is violently forced downward, only upper root avulsions occur unless the force is severe enough to progress to the lower nerve roots as well (62,80). The arm may also be forced backward and upward, subsequently stressing the midportion of the plexus maximally. In this scenario, an isolated avulsion of C7 may occur. Furthermore, because of the violent unpredictable nature of these accidents, any combination of injuries may be seen (45,80,81).

Paralysis and anesthesia are immediate after the injury. The specific pattern of deficit is based on the severity and involvement of the various nerves. Because of the extreme forces required to produce these injuries and the subsequent severity of the injury, prognosis is generally poor (83–85).

Acute Brachial Neuropathy

ABN is a rare disorder responsible for severe shoulder pain associated with an episode of proximal upper extremity weakness. The syndrome was initially described by Feinberg (86) in 1897, and since that time numerous reports describing this entity have appeared in the literature (11,86–94). The same disorder has been referred to by a variety of names, including localized neuritis of the shoulder girdle (93), neuralgic amyotrophy (94), acute brachial radiculitis (89), Parsonage-Turner syndrome (95), paralytic brachial neuritis (88), and brachial neuritis (87). Males appear to be most often afflicted, and the most common age is during the third through sixth decades (88,95). The pathogenesis of ABN differs from most other plexus ailments in that its etiology appears to be atraumatic. Typically, the onset of pain is unprovoked and sudden, persisting despite cessation of activities. It often begins at the base of the neck and shoulder, only to later extend to the scapula and arm (35,89). Occasionally, the pain may cross the elbow and include the forearm (95). The pain usually subsides after a few hours to 2 to 3 weeks. Often, it is followed by proximal flaccid paralysis; however, weakness may begin with the initial symptoms or any time thereafter (88,89,94,95). Weakness, however, may be mild and only become clinically evident with strenuous athletic activity (38). The most current literature points to the C5 and C6 nerve roots and the axillary and suprascapular nerves as being most commonly involved. Therefore, the deltoid, supraspinatus, and infraspinatus are the muscles most often affected. The serratus anterior, biceps, triceps, and wrist and finger flexors are also often involved, however (88,94–96). Hyposthesias frequently occur and are most often localized to the shoulder region innervated by the axillary nerve and the regions of the upper extremity innervated by C5 and C6 (89,95). Hyperreflexia does not occur. In fact, hyporeflexia typically results from the existing muscle weakness (96).

Approximately 25% of cases are clinically bilateral, whereas approximately 50% show evidence of bilaterality on EMG studies (95,96). Despite numerous investigations, the etiology of this disorder remains elusive. Electron microscopy reveals a localized inflammatory process, perhaps implicating a viral or autoimmune pathogenesis (95). Evidence supporting the former is the frequency of onset after infections and immunizations (87,89,93,94). Evidence supporting the latter is the existence of a hereditary form of this disorder (95).

Most cases are sporadic and do not appear to occur as a result of any specific activities. However, cases occurring in athletes have been reported (11,35,61,96). Hershman et al. (11) presented five such cases in a group of 78 (6.4%) athletes evaluated for brachial plexus problems. Despite the rare occurrence of this disorder, the authors stressed the importance of including this diagnosis in the differential for acute shoulder pain and weakness when evaluating athletes with such symptoms. They listed five findings that should alert one to the possible presence of ABN: onset with noncontact and contact sports, acute onset of pain without trauma, persistent severe pain that continues despite rest, brachial plexus and/or peripheral nerve involvement, and dominant arm predominance (11).

CLINICAL EVALUATION

History

As with other musculoskeletal disorders, the history and physical examination are the most important components of the evaluation of an athlete with a presumed brachial plexus impairment. A complete medical history should always be obtained at initial evaluation. If possible, the exact mechanism of injury should be noted. This helps to differentiate between a true burner and other types of brachial plexus injuries. For instance, discerning the initiating mechanism will help to differentiate between the true burner injury and the potentially more serious spearing injury (97–99). In addition, as in the case of root avulsions and neurotmesis, recalling the precise mechanism of injury may help to identify the affected structures, that is, whether there is likely to be upper or lower cord involvement and/or associated neurovascular injuries (17,80).

Such factors as prior upper extremity pathology should also be sought. This will aid in determining acute from chronic pain, weakness, and sensory deficit. In the case of burner symptoms, it is also important to know if the athlete has experienced similar symptoms in the past and if so with what frequency. This information may dictate further evaluation and potential athletic restrictions (35). The history of recent infectious illness or immunization or a positive family history may aid in the diagnosis of ABN (35), whereas weight loss, lethargy, and malaise is indicative of compression of the plexus by a space-occupying tumor such as lymphoma or a metastatic, Pancoast, or superior sulcus tumor (38,42).

The patient's precise symptomology should also be ascertained. A burner will present with pain in the entire upper extremity in a circumferential stocking–glove distribution. Associated weakness, dysesthesias, or paresthesias are often immediate and diffuse after trauma and thereafter rapidly fleeting. In the case of root avulsions, complete paralysis and loss of sensation in the affected area are immediate and in a root distribution after trauma. These both contrast with ABN, where the pain typically is not associated with trauma or loss of sensation but rather with delayed development of proximal weakness.

In addition, if discomfort exists, its quality should be determined. As previously mentioned, spontaneous severe pain is often the first sign of ABN, whereas similar symptoms acutely after a traumatic injury often indicate root avulsions (100), and if occurring late after a traumatic injury, pain may actually be a sign of recovery (17). The presence of any significant neck pain should also be sought. Such a finding would require evaluation for cervical spine injury before resumption of play (1). Bilaterality of symptoms should be determined as well. In the case of atraumatic onset, this may indicate ABN, whereas if posttraumatic and particularly if associated with neck pain and lower extremity symptoms, transient quadriplegia, cervical spine fracture–dislocation, or disk herniation is more likely to be the cause (59,99,101).

Physical Examination

The physical examination is also essential to properly assess the patient with presumed brachial plexus pathology. A thorough examination will assist in appropriately defining the lesion, aid in choosing the appropriate treatment modalities, and better enable the physician to assess the potential for recovery. As with all disorders, the examination of brachial plexus injuries begins with inspection. The athlete should disrobe to fully expose his or her neck, both shoulders, axillas, and entire upper

extremities. Observation while the patient removes their shirt will allow assessment of the clinical limitations. Areas of atrophy and deformity should be identified. Malalignment of acute or healed fractures of the scapula, clavicle, and humerus should be noted. Likewise, dislocations of the glenohumeral, acromioclavicular, and sternoclavicular joints can be identified from careful clinical observation. The scapula should be assessed for winging as should the height of the shoulders relative to one another. The athlete should also be evaluated for any evidence of a Horner's syndrome, such as unilateral enophthalmos, partial ptosis, reactive miosis, and ipsilateral anhydrosis (102,103). This is often indicative of an avulsion injury of T1 and portends a worse prognosis (9,104).

Palpation of bony structures should then follow. Any crepitus or exuberant callus should be noted. Swelling, ecchymosis, masses, or a Tinel's sign in the supraclavicular fossa should be identified (17). Again, palpation over the acromioclavicular or sternoclavicular joints will help reveal dislocations at these sites.

The assessment of motor function is a critical part of the physical examination. Both active and passive range of motion of the neck, shoulders, scapula, elbows, wrists, and hands should be evaluated. Not only should function and range of motion be noted, but muscle strength should also be assessed and recorded. For objective determination of strength, dynamometers (such as the Cybex isokinetic equipment) or hand-held measuring devices (such as the Nicholas manual muscle tester) may be used (42). The importance of repeated testing cannot be overemphasized, particularly in the case of burner syndrome where weakness may present several hours to days after the injury. By closely identifying the weakened muscles, the location of injury can often be determined. For instance, because the diaphragm, rhomboids, and serratus anterior all receive their C5 contribution from the root proximal to Erb's point and just after it exits the intervertebral foramen, paralysis of these muscles is likely the result of an upper plexus root avulsion. Likewise, lesions involving the trunks, cords, and individual branches also give specific clinical pictures that can be delineated by careful examination (21).

Reflexes and sensory examination should be assessed. Reflexes of the upper extremity may be normal, absent, increased, or diminished by varying degrees. The precise quality should be noted. Sensory evaluation, like motor evaluation, will assist in localizing the lesion to a specific area of the plexus. Both pinprick and light touch sensory perception should be evaluated (17,36,105).

As previously mentioned, concomitant injuries to the brachial plexus and the axillary and subclavian vessels is possible, and therefore a vascular examination must always be performed (80). Arterial injury may be evidenced by weak or absent pulses, prolonged capillary refill, and pallor, whereas venous injury is often accompanied by edema and blanching.

Adjunctive Tests

Depending on the presumptive diagnosis, various additional clinical tests may be performed. A painful shoulder in an athlete frequently accompanies rotator cuff impingement or instability, and therefore in the appropriate setting, impingement and apprehension maneuvers should be performed (106–108). Spurling's maneuver or the modified Spurling's maneuver (109) (Fig. 10.9) can help identify degenerative disk disease of the cervical spine, whereas Wright's maneuver (103,110) may help to identify thoracic outlet syndrome.

In addition, various axonal reflex tests have been described to distinguish between preganglionic and postganglionic lesions in traction injuries of the brachial plexus (111). The histamine reflex test is one such method. This test requires a subcutaneous injection of 1% histamine. In normal skin and in anesthetic skin secondary to root avulsion (preganglionic lesion), a triple response of initial vasodilation, wheal formation, and a flare (further vasodilation) occurs. The flare response results because in both situations the cell body within the dorsal root ganglion is in continuity with the peripheral sensory receptors. In postganglionic lesions, however, the cell body and sensory receptor are structurally distinct, and therefore, after injection of histamine, the flare response will be absent (82). As a result

of difficulty in interpretation, the problems caused by pre- and postfixation of the plexus, the potential for allergic reaction to histamine, and the availability of more precise diagnostic aids, the use of this test is now discouraged (103,112).

Clinical Findings

Burner Syndrome

The athlete sustaining a burner injury typically will have unilateral pain, paresthesias, and anesthesias diffusely throughout the arm after the trauma (5,10,42,58,61). Symptoms are occasionally isolated to the regions innervated by roots C5 and C6 (12,14,58). These symptoms often resolve after several seconds or minutes (5,10,42,58). Usually, immediately after the injury, muscle strength will be normal. However, weakness and hyporeflexia often become apparent hours to days after the injury (5,42,57,61).

Compression Injuries

Pack palsy and other delayed compressive injuries typically present with diffuse upper extremity weakness. Because paralysis generally is short-lived, muscle tone usually remains normal. There is a conspicuous absence of pain, whereas parasthesia, anesthesia, and hyporeflexia are occasional findings. In the case of thoracic outlet syndrome, vascular abnormalities may be present as well (3).

Root Avulsion and Neurotmesis

Variable presentations of root avulsions and nerve disruptions can occur depending on the location and severity of the inciting force (9,81,103,113). Often there are associated injuries, and it is imperative that these be identified promptly. Typically, in the acute phase, the extremity displays paralysis and anesthesia in those areas innervated by the injured roots and nerves. The tendon reflexes are likewise absent. Only later do atrophy and contracture develop (9). Pain is a variable characteristic of this injury and tends to be an unfavorable prognostic sign in the acute phase and an encouraging sign if its initial onset is late (9,17). Sympathetic dysfunction, such as changes in the affected limb's color, sweat production, and temperature, and a Horner's syndrome may be present (104). Associated vascular injuries are common, and therefore careful evaluation of the arterial and venous systems must be undertaken (80).

Acute Brachial Neuropathy

ABN typically initiates with sudden severe pain about the shoulder girdle without antecedent trauma

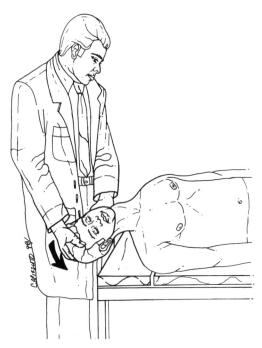

FIG. 10.9. Modified Spurling's maneuver. Symptoms are exacerbated with extension of the head accompanied by lateral flexion toward the affected side.

(90,93,95). Twenty-five percent to 50% of cases may be bilateral (88,90). Proximal weakness usually follows after 4 to 5 days; however, it may occur at any time during the clinical course of this disorder. Weakness is usually restricted to those muscles innervated by the axillary and suprascapular nerves, although the serratus anterior, biceps, triceps, and wrist and finger extensors may occasionally be affected as well (88,114). Atrophy of the affected muscles usually follows (90). Sensory changes are commonly limited to the region of the proximolateral arm innervated by the axillary nerve and those dermatomes innervated by C5 and C6 (95). The degree of deep tendon hyporeflexia is dependent on the degree of existing muscle weakness (114).

IMAGING

Radiography

Radiographs can be of great assistance in the diagnosis of brachial plexus and associated injuries (115,116). All athletes sustaining a severe acute injury to the brachial plexus, a persistent or recurrent burner injury, or burner symptoms associated with neck pain should have a complete radiographic evaluation of the cervical spine (38,117,118). In addition, as clinically indicated, radiographs of the shoulder girdle may also be needed (1,61,104,112).

Besides the obvious fractures, subluxations, and dislocations, which may be identified in either series, there are other more subtle findings that may indicate serious plexus injuries. Avulsions of the cervical transverse processes almost always indicate a severe traction injury to the plexus (17,20,96). Cervical scoliosis frequently is associated with multiple root avulsions (96,119). As previously mentioned, cervical canal stenosis may be associated with transient quadriplegia or a radicular injury (16,61,102). A C5 nerve root injury may be revealed by unilateral diaphragmatic palsy on a chest radiograph (116). The association of Horner's syndrome and a first rib avulsion often are evidence of T1, and possibly C8, root avulsions specifically (103,112). Additionally, the presence of a cervical rib should be noted; likewise, so should a clavicular malunion or hypertrophic nonunion, because these may be responsible for producing a thoracic outlet syndrome (112). Scapulothoracic dissociations are often associated with brachial plexus injuries, and therefore excessive lateral displacement of the scapula needs to be identified (24). Occasionally, to identify a superior sulcus or Pancoast tumor, a posterior–anterior chest radiograph or an apical lordotic view may be needed as well (38).

Many other radiographic modalities may provide additional useful information. Cervical myelography was initially shown by Murphy et al. (69) to be helpful in the diagnosis of brachial plexus injuries. These authors

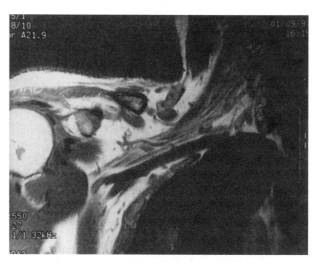

FIG. 10.10. T1-weighted coronal oblique magnetic resonance image of the normal brachial plexus. (Courtesy of Hollis G. Potter, M.D.)

noted "traumatic meningoceles," which have since been reported to be pathognomonic of a spinal root avulsion (120,121). Other authors, however, have disputed the accuracy of plain contrast myelography (103,122). For this reason, as well as the invasive nature of this study, other investigatory methods have been recommended. Computed tomography (CT) myelography, although no less invasive, seems to improve diagnostic accuracy, particularly at the C5 and C6 nerve roots (103,112,123). Pseudomeningoceles, absence of root shadows, and obliterated root pouches are all indicative of root avulsions in these studies (112). Additionally, although present experience is limited, MRI appears to have promise as a noninvasive accurate radiographic technique for evaluating brachial plexus injuries (Fig. 10.10) (38,42,68,65,124). In fact, some now believe it to be the imaging technique of choice for traumatic brachial plexus lesions (125,126). It is no doubt helpful, as is a cervical CT, in eliminating other potential causes of the athlete's symptoms, such as vertebral fracture–dislocation or cervical disk herniation (38). Cervical stenosis is also easily evaluated with MRI. In addition, MRI has been used to delineate the causes of brachial plexus compressive injuries after clavicle fractures (28).

Electrodiagnosis

Electrodiagnostic studies are very helpful in determining the diagnosis, location, and prognosis of brachial plexus lesions (33,49,103,127). These studies assess the changes in electrical responses that accompany nerve injury. There are essentially four studies that may be used: limb musculature EMG, paraspinal musculature EMG, motor and sensory nerve conduction evaluation, and motor and somatosensory evoked potentials, including F-wave responses (17,20,21,42,49,103,112,115, 116,128).

EMG is used to assess the electrical activity of both the active and resting muscle fiber. These studies are not only helpful in distinguishing between complete and partial injuries (presence of motor unit action potentials eliminate the diagnosis of complete nerve rupture or avulsion) and the status of recovery (small polyphasic potentials of reduced amplitude indicate ongoing recovery), but EMG can also be used to differentiate between root avulsions and more distal or peripheral nerve injuries (17,31,103,112,115,116,123,124,127). Normally, innervated muscle will illicit motor unit action potentials with volitional activity but possesses no spontaneous activity. Denervated muscle displays resting fibrillations and sharp positive waves at approximately 3 weeks after an injury (21,33,42,49,103,115,123,124). Recall that the nerve roots of C5-T1 divide into the dorsal rami, which innervate the paraspinal musculature and the ventral rami, which proceed to form the brachial plexus. Therefore, evidence of denervation of both the paraspinal musculature and the appendicular musculature is consistent with a proximal root avulsion, whereas denervation of the appendicular musculature alone signifies a more distal plexus or peripheral nerve injury (17,22,42,49, 103,112,115,116,123,128). EMG studies are also helpful in determining bilateral involvement in ABN. Although clinically undetectable weakness may occasionally occur in the so-called normal extremity, EMG evaluation often will be diagnostic (38,95,96).

Nerve conduction studies may also aid in differentiating between root avulsions and more peripheral nerve injuries (103,124). Both compound muscle and sensory nerve action potential evaluation should be conducted (32,42,103). As previously mentioned, the cell bodies of the sensory axons reside within the cord. For this reason, root avulsions result in the motor axon being separated from its cell body and undergoing subsequent Wallerian degeneration. This differs from the sensory axon, in which no proximal degeneration occurs because after root avulsions, axon–cell body continuity is maintained (103,116,124). Therefore, in these injuries, one will find normal sensory and absent motor conduction or, more importantly, normal sensory conduction in an insensate limb. In a peripheral injury, both sensory and motor conduction will be delayed (i.e., neuropraxic burner syndrome or compression neuropathy) or absent (i.e., neurotmesis), depending on the severity of the injury (33,64,98,103,111,116,124,127,129–132). Potential advantages of the nerve conduction studies over EMG studies in detection of lesions in the athlete are their noninvasive nature, effectiveness by 7 to 10 days, ability to assess both motor and sensory axonal injury, and superiority in identifying demyelination injuries (33).

Studies using somatosensory evoked potentials exploit these same principles. By stimulating peripheral nerves and subsequently monitoring cortical electrical activity, root avulsions can be differentiated from peripheral nerve injuries. In root avulsions, no cortical evoked potentials will be noted, despite normal peripheral nerve conduction (21,103,112,115,130). Motor evoked potentials used in conjunction with EMG has also shown to be an affective evaluation technique (124,128).

F-wave detection is another, albeit less precise, method for differentiating avulsions from peripheral nerve injuries. Supramaximal peripheral nerve stimulation produces antidromical impulses that travel toward the spinal cord. In an avulsion or proximal injury, the wave is absent or displays reduced conduction velocity, respectively. In injuries distal to the origin of the stimulation, the wave's conduction velocity is normal (43,49,103,115). These studies tend to be complex and are less useful in the diagnosis of most sports-related brachial plexus injuries. Their use is primarily limited to preoperative and intraoperative evaluation for other traumatic injuries (103,116,128,133,134).

TREATMENT

Most athletically sustained brachial plexus injuries are self-limiting, and therefore the treatment is usually preventative and rehabilitative. Occasionally, however, in the most severe cases surgical treatment may be required.

Burner Syndrome

The management of the burner syndrome begins at the time of injury. Initial examination must be performed meticulously to rule out a cervical spine injury. If a spinal injury is suspected due to cervical guarding, tenderness, or multiple extremity involvement, then the athlete must be treated with appropriate cervical immobilization and evacuation. Additionally, a full series of cervical radiographs, including flexion and extension views and if necessary additional studies (i.e., CT or MRI), must be obtained (14,38,61). If the symptoms are isolated to a unilateral upper extremity, then the athlete may resume play when his or her symptoms fully resolve (14,38,61). In this case, repeated examinations must be conducted periodically throughout the game and during the next several weeks, because occasionally weakness that can be absent initially may present late (32,39). If the symptoms are persistent or recurrent, a full cervical spine radiographic series must be obtained before resumption of play. Electrodiagnostic studies should be considered if symptoms last beyond 3 weeks (1,14 38,42,118).

The athlete who has been held from play due to persistent weakness may not return until full strength and mobility exists (1,7,34,38,60,118). Therefore, rehabilitative efforts should be initiated to strengthen and mobilize those muscle groups most affected, typically the supraspinatus, infraspinatus, teres minor, deltoid, biceps, and brachioradialis (33,38,57). Fibrillated potentials, noted on EMGs early after injury, resolve as acute nerve injury heals. Contrarily, long-term EMG findings demonstrate large motor unit potentials that are the result of "sprouting" of nerves to reinnervate "orphaned" motor units. Consequently, Bergfield et al. (34) noted that abnormal EMG findings may persist despite resolution of symptoms. Therefore, recovery should be based solely on clinical examination rather than EMG evaluation. In addition, to prevent repeated injury, a complete neck and shoulder flexibility and strengthening program that includes the trapezius muscle should be initiated (7,35,42). Strength training should include both isometric and isotonic exercises to maximize results (1,12,15).

Various equipment adjuncts and modifications have been recommended to prevent recurrences in football players. Unfortunately, however, most literature promoting these methods is anecdotal. Chrisman et al. (4) noted that burner injuries rarely recurred with the use of a padded horseshoe-shaped collar attached to the players shoulder pads. They developed this device based on their study that revealed an increased lateral cervical flexion in 22 previously injured athletes when compared with an uninjured control group. Markey et al. (15)

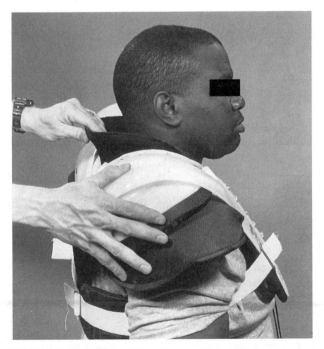

FIG. 10.11. A cowboy collar. The padded collar fits comfortably beneath standard shoulder pads. It helps to reduce both hyperextension of the neck and direct compression of the plexus by the medial border of the shoulder pads.

reported on five football players with a history of a prior burner injury who used a total-contact neck–shoulder–chest orthosis and a neck roll during an entire football season. Three athletes claimed that the orthoses had helped, and in the remaining two, each had one recurrent burner. In a recent study, Hovis and Limbird (135) evaluated three types of cervical orthoses, a foam collar, a cowboy collar (Fig. 10.11), and a custom-fitted cervicothoracic orthosis that had a high posterior rigid support. The study was conducted in a controlled manner using pulleys connected to the helmets of five athletes. All subjects wore shoulder pads as well. In this study, all the orthoses reduced neck extension significantly more than shoulder pads alone; however, no orthoses significantly reduced lateral flexion more than isolated shoulder pads. Cowboy collars (1,14,58,61) and neck rolls (12,14,42,64) have been promoted by other authors as well. In addition, various other adjuncts such as lifts under the shoulder pads (14,42,64) and restrictive shoulder pads (1,64) have also been recommended. Furthermore, most investigators agree that straps that bind the helmet to the shoulder pads should be avoided, because these tend to increase the axial forces on the cervical spine and therefore increase the risk of vertebral fracture and spinal cord injury (38,42,61).

Compression Injuries

Treatment of backpack palsy and other delayed-onset compression neuropathies, like that for burner syndrome, is mostly preventative and rehabilitative. Prevention in the case of pack paralysis includes well-padded shoulder straps and waist belts to reduce the downward and posterior forces on the plexus. Additionally, lighter packs and frequent rest periods during which the backpack is removed from the shoulders should be used. Preventative measures in clavicle fractures may include open reduction and internal fixation for highly comminuted patterns (28,42). Treatment of existing paralysis consists of removal of the offending object. Abstention from hiking in the case of pack palsy and operative decompression of the hypertrophic callus or displaced fragments after a clavicle fracture are examples (42).

Most forms of neurogenic thoracic outlet syndrome can often be treated nonoperatively (35,70,71,73). Of course, treatment must be based on the offending cause. A well-structured exercise program concentrating on the shoulder girdle musculature, particularly the trapezius, rhomboids, and levator scapulae, should be initiated. Upper extremity positions that produce symptoms should be avoided (71,73). Unfortunately, If there is severe outlet compression, conservative measures may not succeed and operative intervention might be necessary. Indications for surgical treatment are failure of appropriate trial of conservative measures, intractable pain, vascular compromise, or neurologic loss (35,71,73). Many decompressive procedures have been described; however, no consensus exists as to the most appropriate. Among those reported are scalenotomy, scalenectomy, first-rib resection, cervical rib resection, pectoralis minor tenotomy, claviculectomy, and various combinations of these procedures (8,71,73). No matter the operative technique used, appropriate strength and range of motion rehabilitation should follow (38).

Root Avulsion and Neurotmesis

The definitive treatment of brachial plexus root avulsions and nerve ruptures is primarily surgical (83). These procedures are technically demanding and therefore should be carried out only by those with special training in this area. Unless the lesion is associated with a vascular injury and an ischemic limb or results from a sharp penetrating injury, the surgical procedure should be delayed (31,104,113,131). Various lengths of delay have been proposed; consequently, the ideal delay remains controversial (131). The surgical procedures are typically performed before 6 months and should not be performed after 1 year except for palliative procedures (36,104,116,131,132). Initial treatment in most cases consists of splinting until the associated soft tissues and injured bony structures have healed. This is followed by physiotherapy stressing early range of motion (42,83,132,136). Available procedures consist of neurolysis (45,51,116,137,138), direct repair (31,36,51,83,112, 116,138), nerve grafting (31,36,45,51,116,132,137,138), and neurotization procedures (32,52,83,85,112,116,131 132,137,139,140), or a combination of these (112,134, 138). Typically, procedures use microscopic techniques (51,131,141). Often, intraoperative electrodiagnostic techniques are helpful (36,83,116). Careful preoperative planning of the procedures as dictated by clinical examination and electrodiagnostic and imaging studies must be performed to provide the best functioning limb. This frequently requires selective reinnervation of functionally important muscles (104). Additionally, surgical procedures such as muscle and tendon transfers, arthrodesis, and osteotomies may be used to further optimize function (51,83,100,104,112,132,142,143). Rarely, amputation of the involved limb and use of a prosthesis may provide a better functional result and is therefore occasionally recommended (100,136).

Acute Brachial Neuropathy

The treatment of ABN is nonoperative (35,42,57,95). Hershman et al. (11) divided it into two phases. The initial phase is from the onset of symptoms until the resolution of pain. Treatment during this time consists mostly of rest. A sling and analgesics are often required due to the severe pain frequently experienced in the early stages of this disorder (11). Other pain-relieving modalities, such as massage therapy and ultrasound, have been recommended. Corticosteroids have been used; however, they have not been shown to alter the disease's course (114,132). The second phase of treatment lasts from the resolution of pain until recovery from symptoms. Treatment during this phase consists mainly of rehabilitative efforts (11,132). Because subclinical weakness of distal muscles often exists, the rehabilitation program must include the entire upper extremity. Initial rehabilitation should concentrate on passive range of motion followed by active strengthening exercises (95). No strict guidelines for return to sport exist because so few cases occurring in athletes have been reported. Essentially, decisions need to be made on an individual basis, with return being delayed until strength is either full or has plateaued at an adequate level (35).

PROGNOSIS

Fortunately, most brachial plexus injuries in athletes have a favorable prognosis with full or nearly full recovery. However, in the rare case, the recovery may be incomplete, leaving the athlete disabled and preventing a return to his or her sport.

Burner Syndrome

Most athletes sustaining a burner injury will have full recovery of strength after only several seconds or minutes after the onset of symptoms. Therefore, a return to play is usually possible after only a brief rest (42,58). Occasionally, however, weakness or numbness may persist. Deficits lasting 2 to 3 weeks in the case of severe neuropraxia or even as long as 4 to 6 months, with associated axonetmesis, is not infeasible (7,61). Speer and Bassett (12) described this entity as the "prolonged burner syndrome." They noted players with persistent weakness and normal electrodiagnostic studies and those with normal strength and persistently abnormal electrodiagnostic studies. Bergfield et al. (34) observed similar findings. They evaluated 20 athletes who had sustained a burner, with an average follow-up of 4.25 years (range, 12 to 97 months). At follow-up, 65% had mild subjective complaints, primarily with overhead activities. Approximately one third had objective evidence of reduced but persistent weakness, most commonly affecting the deltoid. Despite the clinical improvement, EMG's remained abnormal in 80% of the athletes. Encouragingly, however, all but one athlete were able to return to competitive contact sports.

The greatest concern affecting the long-term prognosis of burner injuries is the potential for recurrences. Repeated injuries limit the athlete's effectiveness due to time loss from play required to allow recovery (16).

In addition, recurrent episodes may ultimately lead to permanent deficits (12,14). In a study by Sallis et al. (14), 201 players participating in Division III collegiate football were evaluated. Eighty-seven percent had sustained multiple injuries, with the average number of recurrences being 3.6 (range, 0 to 40). Various etiologies have been blamed for this high recurrence rate. Meyer et al. (16) and Castro et al. (67) noted statistically significant smaller Torg ratios in athletes sustaining recurrent burner episodes. Other authors (54,62–64) reported an increased incidence of recurrences associated with cervical degenerative disk disease. Moreover, additional investigators have attributed recurrences to body habitus (5), improper tackling and blocking techniques (1,15), and inadequate equipment (5,14,15,135). Various techniques to reduce the incidence of recurrent burners have been recommended (1,7,14,15,33,35,42) and have been discussed previously in this chapter.

Compression Injuries

As with most burner injuries, most compressive injuries in athletes have a favorable prognosis. Those having a short duration of symptoms have a better prognosis than those with more prolonged symptoms (144), although even after 2 years of symptoms cases of compressive neuropathies in athletes due to cervical ribs have been noted to fully recover after rib resection (8). The important factor in recovery of compressive injuries is the removal of the offending agent before permanent end organ damage occurs. In the case of backpack palsy, this simply requires more frequent resting or carrying lighter loads (3), whereas in cases of thoracic outlet syndrome, depending on the etiology, surgical excision of the offending structures or shoulder girdle strengthening to better protect the plexus may be required (8,27,71).

Root Avulsion and Neurotmesis

The prognosis for functional recovery of brachial plexus root avulsions or nerve ruptures in an athlete is likely to be grim. No series exists describing the outcome of this devastating injury in this specific population. However, results extrapolated from the nonathlete literature indicate that return to any form of competitive sports requiring the injured extremity would be unlikely. In fact, the usual goal of treatment of these lesions is simply to restore enough function to enable activities necessary for daily living. Leffert (132) stated that most adults with supraclavicular lesions will not be able to raise their arms overhead and only 75% of patients will be able to flex their elbow against gravity and resistance after reinnervation surgery. These findings have been substantiated by other authors as well (145). Nonetheless, the prognosis after properly timed surgery is considerably better than that after conservative care (22). In addition, the prognosis for infraclavicular lesions is somewhat better than for supraclavicular injuries (19,31,132,146,147). Other favorable prognostic findings in surgically treated lesions are younger age (19,148), an absence of a Horner's syndrome (9,104,121), surgery before 1 year postinjury (132,146,149), upper root surgery (31,83,116), lesions involving fewer roots (10), partial lesions (31,146), and short lesions or transections (83).

Acute Brachial Neuropathy

The prognosis for recovery from paralysis due to ABN is generally good. Functional recovery occurs in nearly 90% of those affected (90). Although weakness may begin to resolve after only a few days, most patients do not report improvement until after the first month of symptoms (87,90,94). Tsairis et al. (90) in a review of 99 cases of ABN noted that approximately 36% of their patients recovered within 1 year, 75% within 2 years, and 89% by 3 years.

Various prognostic factors have been identified. Those lesions involving predominantly the upper plexus tend to resolve more rapidly (87,90). Tsairis et al. (90) noted that lower plexus lesions took, on average, between 1.5 to 3 years to resolve, whereas 60% of upper plexus lesions resolved after only a year. Incomplete muscle paralysis is another favorable sign. Typically, full recovery can be expected within 6 months (94). Other encouraging findings are unilateral lesions and lesions associated with pain of a lesser severity or a shorter duration (87,90,94). Contrarily, those cases showing little or no improvement after 3 months or those with associated muscle atrophy have been shown to have a worse prognosis (87,88,114).

Although recurrences may occur up to several years after initial recovery, they tend to be rare (80,88,90,94). Tsairis et al. (90) noted only four recurrences of 84 cases. In addition, recurrences tend to be less severe and often last for a shorter duration (90,114).

Incomplete recovery tends to be a more common outcome than reoccurrence. Tsairis et al. (90) observed this phenomenon in 62% of the 16 patients they followed for 5 years, whereas, all five athletes with ABN that Hershman et al. (11) studied had residual weakness, including one patient followed for as long as 7 years. In addition, three of the five athletes had persistent EMG abnormalities at final follow-up. Encouragingly, all were able to return to competitive sports despite their deficits. This is typical for incomplete recovery, in which the persistent weakness is usually mild. Most commonly affected is the serratus anterior, characterized by persistent scapular winging (11,42,89,94). In addition to the persistent muscle weakness, sensory loss, muscle atrophy, and diminished deep tendon reflexes have been reported to occasionally persist as well (42,90,114).

AUTHOR'S PREFERENCES

Burners are by far the most common brachial plexus injuries we encounter. It has been our experience that most burners sustained by young athletes are the result of either plexus traction or acute compression, whereas those occurring in the older more experienced athlete often posses a component related to degenerative disease of the cervical spine.

We initiate the care of this injury immediately on the field or sideline. After excluding shoulder or other local noncervical injuries, we attempt to distinguish the burner from the more serious cervical spine injury. The existence of significant neck pain or multiple extremity neurologic abnormalities raises our concern. Patients with such symptoms are immediately stabilized with a cervical collar; undergo careful neurologic examination; and are assessed radiographically with anteroposterior, lateral, open mouth, and, when appropriate, active flexion–extension views of their cervical spine. In addition, CT and MRI studies are often necessary. The same evaluation is instituted for those athletes who experience recurrent burners and who have not undergone prior imaging assessment. Return to play for these athletes is not permitted until the presence of a cervical injury is excluded and the patient's symptoms fully resolve.

Athletes who experience isolated burner symptoms without cervical findings also undergo a complete on-field neurologic evaluation. Careful motor examination with particular attention to the deltoid, rotator cuff musculature, biceps, and wrist extensors and detailed sensory and reflex examinations are performed and recorded. Throughout the competition, the patient is periodically reassessed. Athletes with significant weakness are removed from participation. Once complete resolution of their neurologic deficits occurs, the athlete may return to play. This may take from a few minutes to many weeks depending on the nature of the injury.

We agree with those authors who have noted a delay in onset (7,32,39,61) or prolongation (12,34) of symptoms after a traction or compression injury to the plexus. Therefore, we clinically reassess the athletes at periodic follow-up visits. If symptoms persist longer than 3 weeks, electrodiagnostic studies may help localize the site of the lesion. If a root avulsion is suspected, sensory nerve action potential evaluation is obtained early after the injury. We do not, however, use electrodiagnostic studies to determine a players return to competition. Experience has shown us that these studies frequently remain abnormal despite clinical resolution of symptoms and a full return of strength.

Athletes with the burner syndrome are begun on a cervical, shoulder, and trapezius flexibility and strengthening program. In addition, football players who have sustained a burner injury will generally be instructed to wear a cervical orthosis during competition. We have found the cowboy collar to be very effective in this regard. For those athletes at risk of sustaining a recurrent traumatic compression injury, such as lacrosse players, local protective padding is often recommended. In the less experienced athlete, we have also found that additional instruction in technique, such as proper tackling training, can be quite helpful.

Our experience has been that most athletes who sustain a burner injury are able to return to full competition, usually within the same game. Additionally, with careful attention to proper rehabilitation and protection, the recurrence of these injuries may often be reduced.

In those rare cases of delayed-onset compression neuropathies, we recommend removal of the offending cause. This may simply require reducing the period or degree of exposure, as in the case of a pack palsy, or it may require surgical decompression, as in the case of exuberant callus formation after clavicular fracture malunion. It has been our experience that compression neuropathies of a short duration typically have an excellent prognosis with full resolution of symptoms, whereas protracted cases tend to have a less favorable outcome, often with some degree of weakness persisting due to irreversible neural injury.

Fortunately, we have had little personal experience with athletically sustained brachial plexus neurotmesis or avulsion injuries. Our care, however, follows that outlined in this chapter: assessment for other injuries, followed by immobilization and protection, subsequent passive mobilization and splinting, and then ultimate surgical intervention if deemed helpful. Referral to one who specializes in such severe injuries is recommended. Counseling becomes an important component in the care of athletes sustaining such disabling injuries, and therefore it should be initiated early in the treatment program.

Acute brachial neuritis is uncommon but should always be considered in the differential diagnosis of shoulder pain. It can occasionally present in an athlete and can be confused with a traumatic injury (11). The major dilemma in the care of this disorder is the differentiation from other causes of shoulder and arm pain and weakness. Because clinical and radiographic findings are either nonexistent or nonspecific, we use EMG to assist with this diagnosis. Once the diagnosis is confirmed, treatment proceeds in two phases, as outlined in this chapter. First, immobilization with a sling is instituted to help alleviate the characteristic severe pain often accompanying this disorder. Then, after the resolution of pain, mobilization and strengthening exercises are begun. Despite an often protracted course, we have found the prognosis of this disorder to generally be promising. Although mild weakness may frequently persist, it is typically not disabling. Consequently, most athletes are able to return to their respective sports. We permit this after resolution of pain and a return of adequate strength that enables safe competition.

SUMMARY

Athletic injuries to the brachial plexus are common in such sports such as football, lacrosse, and wrestling. Prompt identification of the lesion and careful neurologic evaluation will permit the athlete to return to competition at an appropriate time in a safe manner.

REFERENCES

1. Archambault JL. Brachial plexus stretch injury. *Injury* 1983;31:256–260.
2. Poindexter DP, Johnson EW. Football shoulder and neck injury: a study of the stinger. *Arch Phys Med Rehabil* 1984;65:601–602.
2. White HH. Pack palsy. A neurological complication of scouting. *Pediatrics* 1968;41:1001–1003.
3. Takazawa H, Sudo N, Akoi K, et al. Statistical observation of nerve injuries in athletes. *Brain Nerve Injury* 1971;3:11–17.
4. Chrisman OD, Snook GA, Stanitis JM, et al. Lateral-flexion neck injuries in athletic competition. *JAMA* 1965;192:117–119.
5. Bateman JE. Nerve injuries about the shoulder in sports. *J Bone Joint Surg Am* 1967;49A:785–792.
6. Shukla AY, Green JB. Bowling plexopathy. *N Engl J Med* 1994;324:928.
7. Clancy WG Jr, Brand RL, Bergfeld JA. Upper trunk brachial plexus injuries in contact sports. *Am J Sports Med* 1977;5:209–216.
8. Rayan GM. Lower trunk brachial plexus compression neuropathy due to cervical rib in young athletes. *Am J Sports Med* 1988;16:77–79.
9. Barnes R. Traction injuries of the brachial plexus in adults. *J Bone Joint Surg Br* 1949;31B:10–16.
10. Robertson WC, Eichman PL, Clancy WG. Upper trunk brachial plexopathy in football players. *JAMA* 1979;241:1480–1482.
11. Hershman EB, Wilbourn AJ, Bergfeld JA. Acute brachial neuropathy in athletes. *Am J Sports Med* 1989;17:655–659.
12. Speer KP, Bassett FH. The prolonged burner syndrome. *Am J Sports Med* 1990;18:591–594.
13. Hirasawa Y, Sakakida M. Sports and peripheral nerve injury. *Am J Sports Med* 1983;11:420–426.
14. Sallis RE, Jones K, Knopp W. Burners: offensive strategy for an underreported injury. *Phys Sportsmed* 1992;20:47–55.
15. Markey KL, Di Benedetto M, Curl WW. Upper trunk brachial plexopathy: the stinger syndrome. *Am J Sports Med* 1993;21:650–655.
16. Meyer SA, Schulte KR, Callaghan JJ, et al. Cervical spine stenosis and stingers in collegiate football players. *Am J Sports Med* 1994;22:158–166.
17. Leffert RD. Brachial plexus injuries. *N Engl J Med* 1974;291:1059–1066.
18. Coene LNJEM. Mechanisms of brachial plexus lesions. *Clin Neurol Neurosurg* 1993;95[Suppl]:531–540.
19. Leffert RD, Seddon HJ. Infraclavicular brachial plexus injuries. *J Bone Joint Surg Br* 1965;47B:9–22.
20. Ferenz CC. Review of the brachial plexus. Part I. Acute injuries. *Orthopaedics* 1988;11:479–486.
21. Davis DH, Onofrio BM, MacCarthy CS. Brachial plexus injuries. *Mayo Clin Proc* 1978;53:799–807.
22. Rorabeck CH, Harris WR. Factors affecting the prognosis of brachial plexus injuries. *J Bone Joint Surg Br* 1981;63B:404–407.
23. Rockwood CA Jr, Wirth MA. Subluxations and dislocations about the glenohumeral joint. In: Rockwood CA Jr, Green DP, Bucholz RW, et al., eds. *Fractures in adults,* 4th ed. Philadelphia: Lippincott-Raven, 1996.
24. Butters KP. Fractures and dislocations of the scapula. In: Rockwood CA Jr, Green DP, Bucholz RW, et al., eds. *Fractures in adults,* 4th ed. Philadelphia: Lippincott-Raven, 1996.
25. Bigliani LV, Flatow EL, Pollock RG. Fractures of the proximal humerus. In: Rockwood CA Jr, Green DP, Bucholz RW, et al. eds. *Fractures in adults,* 4th ed. Philadelphia: Lippincott-Raven, 1996.
26. Della Santa A, Narakas AO, Bonnard C. Late lesions of the brachial plexus after fracture of the clavicle. *Ann Hand Surg* 1991;10:531–540.
27. Matz SO, Welliver PS, Welliver DI. Brachial plexus neuropraxia complicating a comminuted clavicle fracture in a college football player: case report and review of the literature. *Am J Sports Med* 1989;17:581–583.
28. Craig EU. Fractures of the clavicle. In: Rockwood CA Jr, Green DP, Bucholz RW, et al., eds. *Fractures in adults,* 4th ed. Philadelphia: Lippincott-Raven, 1996.
29. Rockwood CA Jr, Wirth MA. Injuries to the sternoclavicular joint. In: Rockwood CA Jr, Green DP, Bucholz RW, et al., eds. *Fractures in adults,* 4th ed. Philadelphia: Lippincott-Raven, 1996.
30. Rockwood CA Jr, Williams GR, Young DC. Injuries to the acromioclavicular joint. In: Rockwood CA Jr, Green DP, Bucholz RW, et al., eds. *Fractures in adults,* 4th ed. Philadelphia: Lippincott-Raven, 1996.
31. Alnot JY. Traumatic brachial plexus lesions in the adult. *Hand Clin* 1995;11:623–631.
32. Clancy WG Jr. Brachial plexus and upper extremity peripheral nerve injuries. In: Torg JS, ed. *Athletic injuries to the head, neck, and face,* 1st ed. Philadelphia: Lea and Febiger, 1982.
33. Wilbaum AJ. Electrodiagnostic testing of neurologic injuries in athletes. *Clin Sports Med* 1990;9:229–245.
34. Bergfeld JA, Hershman EB, Wilbourn AJ. Brachial plexus injury in sports—a five year follow-up. *Orthop Trans* 1988;12:743–744.
35. Pianka G, Hershman EB. Neurovascular injuries. In: Nicholas JA, Hershman EB, eds. *The upper extremity and spine in sports medicine,* 2nd ed. St. Louis: Mosby, 1995.
36. McGillicuddy JE. Clinical decision making in brachial plexus injuries. *Neurosurg Clin North Am* 1991;2:137–150.
37. Williams PL, Warwick R. *Gray's anatomy,* 36th ed. Philadelphia: W.B. Saunders, 1980:1094–1096.
38. Hershman EB. Brachial plexus injuries. *Clin Sports Med* 1990;9:311–329.
39. McCann PD, Bidelglass DF. The brachial plexus: clinical anatomy. *Orthop Rev* 1991;December [Suppl]:64–70.
40. Anderson JA. *Grant's atlas of anatomy,* 8th ed. Baltimore: Williams & Wilkins, 1983.
41. Rozing PM. The topographical anatomy of the brachial plexus. *Clin Neurol Neurosurg* 1993;95[Suppl]:s12–s16.
42. Hershman EB. Injuries to the brachial plexus. In: Torg JS, ed. *Athletic injuries to the head, neck, and face,* 2nd ed. Philadelphia: Lea and Febiger, 1991.
43. Bodine SC, Liber RL. Peripheral nerve physiology, anatomy and pathology. In: Simon SR, ed. *Orthopaedic basic science.* Port City Press, 1994.
44. Meyers RR. Anatomy and microanatomy of peripheral nerve. *Neurosurg Clin North Am* 1991;2:1–20.
45. Szabo RM. Management of the peripheral nerve and brachial plexus palsy: neurolysis and nerve grafting. American Academy of Orthopaedic Surgeons, 64th Annual. Instructional Course lecture No. 206, 1997.
46. Seddon HJ. Three types of nerve injury. *Brain* 1943;66:237–288.
47. Sunderland S. A classification of peripheral nerve injuries producing loss of function. *Brain* 1951;74:491–516.
48. Tsairis P. Peripheral nerve injury in athletes. In: Jordan BD, Tsairis P, Warren RF, eds. *Sports neurology.* Rockville: Aspen, 1989.
49. Friedman WA. The electrophysiology of peripheral nerve injuries. *Neurosurg Clin North Am* 1991;2:43–56.
50. Dahlin LB. Aspects on pathophysiology of nerve entrapments and nerve compression injuries. *Neurosurg Clin North Am* 1991;2:21–28.

51. Millesi H. Surgical management of brachial plexus injuries. *J Hand Surg* 1977;2:367–378.
52. Denny-Brown D, Doherty MM. Effects of transient stretching of peripheral nerve. *Arch Neurol Psychiatry* 1948;51:116–129.
53. Liuzzi FJ, Tedeschi B. Peripheral nerve regeneration. *Neurosurg Clin North Am* 1991;2:31–42.
54. Levits CL, Reilly PJ, Torg JS. The pathomechanics of chronic, recurrent cervical root neuropraxia: the chronic burner syndrome. *Am J Sports Med* 1997;25:73–76.
55. Tsairis P. Peripheral Nerve Injury in Athletes. In: Jorden BD, Tsairis P, Warren RF, eds. *Sports neurology.* Maryland: Aspen, 1989.
56. DiBenedetto M, Markey K. Electrodiagnostic localization of traumatic upper trunk brachial plexopathy. *Arch Phys Med Rehabil* 1984;65:15–17.
57. Torg JS, Reilly PJ. Athletic injury to cervical nerve roots and brachial plexus. In: Torg JS, Shepard RJ, eds. *Current therapy in sports medicine,* 3rd ed. St. Louis: Mosby, 1995.
58. Rockett FX. Observations on the "burner": traumatic cervical radiculopathy. *Clin Orthop* 1982;164:18–19.
59. Maroon JC. "Burning hands" in football spinal cord injuries. *JAMA* 1977;238:2049–2051.
60. Griffin LY. *Orthopaedic knowledge update: sports medicine.* Rosemont: AAOS, 1994:153–177.
61. Garth WP. Evaluating and treating brachial plexus injuries. *J Musculosk Med* 1994;11:55–67.
62. Albright JP, Van Gilder J, El Khoury G, et al. Head and neck injuries in sports. In: Scott WN, Nisonson B, Nicholas JA, eds. *Principles of sports medicine.* Baltimore: Williams & Wilkins, 1984.
63. Wroble RR, Albright JP. Neck and low back injuries in wrestlers. *Clin Sports Med* 1986;5:295–325.
64. Watkins RG. Neck injuries in football players. *Clin Sports Med* 1986;5:215–246.
65. Dossett A, Dossett L, Weatherall P, et al. MRI localization of stinger injuries. Presented at the Annual Meeting of the American Orthopaedic Society for Sports Medicine, 1995.
66. Kelly JD, Clancy M, Marchetti PA, et al. The relationship of transient upper extremity parasthesias and cervical stenosis. *Orthop Trans* 1992;16:732.
67. Castro FP Jr, Ricciardi J, Brunet ME, et al. Stingers, the Torg ratio, and the cervical spine. *Am J Sports Med* 1997;25:603–608.
68. Lundborg G, Dahlin LB. Pathophysiology of nerve compression. In: Szabo RM, ed. *Nerve compression syndromes.* Thorofare, NJ: Slack, 1989.
69. Murphy F, Hartung W, Kirkh JW. Myelographic demonstration of avulsing injury of the brachial plexus. *AJR Am J Roentgenol* 1947;58:102–105.
70. Wilbourn AJ. Thoracic outlet syndrome: a plea for conservatism. *Neurosurg Clin North Am* 1991;2:235–245.
71. Leffert RD. Thoracic outlet syndrome. *J Acad Ortho Surg* 1994;2:317–325.
72. Strukel RJ, Garrick JG. Thoracic outlet compression in athletes. *Am J Sports Med* 1978;6:35–39.
73. Leffert RD. TOS. *Hand Clin* 1992;8:285–297.
74. Miller DS, Boswick JA Jr. Lesions of the brachial plexus associated with fractures of the clavicle. *Clin Orthop* 1969;64:144–149.
75. Kay SP, Eckhardt JJ. Brachial plexus palsy secondary to clavicular non-union. Case report and literature survey. *Clin Orthop* 1986;206:219–222.
76. Yates DW. Complications of fractures of the clavicle. *Injury* 1976;7:881–883.
77. Howard FM, Shafer SJ. Injuries to the clavicle with neurovascular complications: a study of fourteen cases. *J Bone Joint Surg Am* 1965;47A:1335–1346.
78. Bhatt BM. "Top cover neuropathy"—transient brachial plexopathy due to body armour. *J R Army Med Corps* 1990;136:53–54.
79. Bristol DC, Fraher JP. Experimental traction injuries of ventral spinal nerve roots. A scanning electron microscopic study. *Neuropathol Appl Neurobiol* 1989;15:549–561.
80. Narakas AO. Lesions found when operating on traction injuries of the brachial plexus. *Clin Neurol Neurosurg* 1993;95[Suppl]:s56–s64.
81. Tracy JF, Brannon EW. Management of brachial plexus injuries (traction type). *J Bone Joint Surg Am* 1958;40A:1031–1042.
82. Taylor PE. Traumatic intradural avulsion of the nerve roots of the brachial plexus. *Brain* 1962;85:579–601.
83. Kline DG. Perspectives concerning brachial plexus injury and repair. *Neurosurg Clin North Am* 1991;2:151–169.
84. Lusskin R, Campbell JB, Thompson WAC. Posttraumatic lesions of the brachial plexus: treatment by transclavicular exploration and neurolysis or autograft reconstruction. *J Bone Joint Surg Am* 1973;55A:1159–1176.
85. Friedman AH. Neurotization of elements of the brachial plexus. *Neurosurg Clin North Am* 1991;2:165–174.
86. Feinberg J. Fall von erb dlumpke scher lagming nach influenza. *Cent Ralbb* 1897;16:588.
87. Dillin L, Hoaglund FT, Scheck M. Brachial neuritis. *J Bone Joint Surg Am* 1985;67A:878–880.
88. Magee KR, DeJong RN. Paralytic brachial neuritis: discussion of clinical features with review of 23 cases. *JAMA* 1960;174:1258–1262.
89. Dixon GJ, Dick TBS. Acute brachial radiculitis: course and prognosis. *Lancet* 1945;2:707–708.
90. Tsairis P, Dyck PJ, Mulder DW. Natural history of brachial plexus neuropathy: report on 99 patients. *Arch Neurol* 1972;27:109–117.
91. Bradley WG, Madrid R, Thrush DC, et al. Recurrent brachial plexus neuropathy. *Brain* 1975;98:381–398.
92. Bale JF, Thompson JA, Petajan JH, et al. Childhood brachial plexus neuropathy. *J Pediatr* 1979;95:741–742.
93. Spillane JD. Localized neuritis of the shoulder girdle: a report of 46 cases in the MEF. *Lancet* 1943;Oct:532–535.
94. Parsonage MJ, Turner JWA. Neurologic amyotrophy: the shoulder-girdle syndrome. *Lancet* 1948;June:973–978.
95. Yang SS, Hershman EB. Idiopathic brachial plexus neuropathy: a review. *Crit Rev Phys Rehab Med* 1993;5:193–201.
96. Tindel NL, Hershman EB. Acute brachial neuropathy. In: Torg JS, Shepard RJ, eds. *Current therapy in sports medicine,* 3rd ed. St. Louis: Decker, 1995.
97. Torg JS, Sennet B, Pavlov H, et al. Spear tackler's spine. An entity precluding participation in tackle football and collision activities that expose the cervical spine to axial energy inputs. *Am J Sports Med* 1993;21:640–649.
98. Torg JS, Truex RC, Critchenfield T, et al. National Head and Neck Injury Registry: report and conclusions 1978. *JAMA* 1979;241:1477–1479.
99. Torg JS, Vegso JJ, Sennett B, et al. The National Football Head and Neck Injury Registry: 14-year report on cervical quadriplegia, 1971 through 1984. *JAMA* 1985;254:3439–3448.
100. Parry CBW. The Ruscoe Clarke Memorial Lecture, 1979: the management of traction lesions of the brachial plexus and peripheral nerve injuries to the upper limb. A study of teamwork. *Injury* 1979;11:265–285.
101. Torg JS, Pavlov H, Genuario SE, et al. Neuropraxia of the cervical spinal cord with transient quadriplegia. *J Bone Joint Surg Am* 1986;68A:1354–1370.
102. Wray SH. Disturbances of vision and ocular movements. In: Braunwald E, Isselbacher KJ, Petersdorf RG, et al. *Harrison's principles of internal medicine,* 11th ed. New York: McGraw-Hill, 1987.
103. Leffert RD. Clinical diagnosis, testing, and electromyographic study in brachial plexus traction injuries. *Clin Orthop* 1988;237:24–31.
104. Thameer RTWM. Recovery of brachial plexus injuries. *Clin Neurol Neurosurg* 1991;93:3–11.
105. Warren J, Gutmann L, Fiqueroa AF Jr, et al. Electromyographic changes of brachial root avulsions. *J Neurosurg* 1969;31:137–140.
106. Warren RF. Instability of shoulder in throwing sports. In: Stauffer ED, ed. *American Academy of Orthopaedic Surgeons instructional course lectures,* Vol. 34. St. Louis: Mosby, 1985.
107. Hawkins RJ, Hobeika PE. Impingement syndrome in the athletic shoulder. *Clin Sports Med* 1983;2:391–405.
108. Neer CS II. Impingement lesions. *Clin Orthop* 1983;173:70–77.
109. Levine MJ, Albert TJ, Smith MD. Cervical radiculopathy: diagnosis and nonoperative management. *J Am Acad Orthop Surg* 1996;4:305–316.

110. Wright IS. The neurovascular syndrome produced by hyperabduction of the arms. *Am Heart* 1945;29:1–19.
111. Bonney G. The value of axon responses in determining the site of lesion in traction injuries of the brachial plexus. *Brain* 1954;77:588–609.
112. Leffert RD. Lesions of the brachial plexus revisited. In: *American Academy of Orthopaedic Surgeons instructional course lectures,* Vol. 38. St. Louis: Mosby, 1989.
113. Wood MB. Diagnosis and clinical evaluation of the patient presenting with brachial plexus palsy, timing of surgical intervention. American Academy of Orthopaedic Surgeons, 64th Annual Meeting. Instructional Course Lecture No. 206, 1997.
114. Aymond JK, Goldner JL, Hardaker WT. Neurologic amyotrophy. *Orthop Rev* 1989;18:1275–1279.
115. Swash M. Diagnosis of brachial root and plexus lesions. *J Neurol* 1986;233:131–135.
116. Wilgis EF, Brushart TM. Brachial plexus and shoulder girdle injuries. In: Browner BD, Jupiter JB, Levine AM, et al., eds. *Skeletal trauma: fractures, dislocations and ligamentous injuries.* Philadelphia: W.B. Saunders, 1992.
117. Griffin LY. *Orthopaedic knowledge update: sports medicine.* Rosemont: AAOS, 1994:269–290.
118. Torg JS, Gennarelli TA. Head and cervical spine injuries. In: DeLee JC, Drez D Jr, eds. *Orthopaedic sports medicine: principles and practice.* Philadelphia: W.B. Saunders, 1994.
119. Roaf R. Lateral flexion injuries of the cervical spine. *J Bone Joint Surg Br* 1963;45B:36–38.
120. Tarlov TM. Myelography to help localize traction lesions of the brachial plexus. *Am J Surg* 1954;88:266–271.
121. Yeoman PM. Cervical myelography in traction injuries of the brachial plexus. *J Bone Joint Surg Br* 1968;50B:253–260.
122. Robles J. Brachial plexus avulsion: a review of diagnostic procedures and report of six cases. Presented at The Joint Meeting of the Mexican Society of Neurology and Psychiatry and the Minnesota Societies of Neurological Sciences and Psychiatry. 1967.
123. Bufalini C, Pescatori G. Posterior cervical electromyelography in the diagnosis and prognosis of brachial plexus injuries. *J Bone Joint Surg Br* 1969;51B:627–631.
124. Deletis V, Morota N, Abbott IR. Electrodiagnosis in the management of brachial plexus surgery. *Hand Clin* 1995;11:555–561.
125. Sherrier RH, Sostman HD. Magnetic resonance imaging of the brachial plexus. *J Thorac Imaging* 1993;8:27–33.
126. Panasci DJ, Holliday RA, Shpizner B. Advanced imaging techniques of the brachial plexus. *Hand Clin* 1995;11:545–553.
127. Parry GJ. Electrodiagnostic studies in the evaluation of peripheral nerve and brachial plexus injuries. *Neurol Clin* 1992;10:921–934.
128. Abbruzzese G, Morena M, Caponnetto C, et al. Motor evoked potentials following cervical electrical stimulation in brachial plexus lesions. *J Neurol* 1993;241:63–67.
129. Rubin M, Lange DJ. Sensory nerve abnormalities in brachial plexopathy. *Eur Neurol* 1992;32:245–247.
130. Zalis AW, Oester YT, Rodrquez AA. Electrophysiologic diagnosis of the cervical nerve root avulsion. *Arch Phys Med Rehabil* 1970;51:708–710.
131. Dobuisson A, Kline DG. Indications for peripheral nerve and brachial plexus surgery. *Neurol Clin* 1992;10:935–951.
132. Leffert RD. Neurologic problems. In: Rockwood CA Jr, Matsen FA, eds. *The shoulder.* Philadelphia: W.B. Saunders, 1990.
133. Flaggman PD, Lange DJ. Brachial plexus neuropathy. An electrophysiological evaluation. *Arch Neurol* 1980;37:160–164.
134. Landi A, Copeland SA, Parry CBW. The role of somatosensory evoked potentials and nerve conduction studies in the surgical management of brachial plexus injuries. *J Bone Joint Surg Br* 1980;62B:492–496.
135. Hovis WD, Limbird TJ. An evaluation of cervical orthoses in limiting hyperextension and lateral flexion in football. *Med Sci Sports Exerc* 1994;26:872–876.
136. Parry CBW. Thoughts on the rehabilitation of patients with brachial plexus lesions. *Hand Clin* 1995;11:657–675.
137. Narakas A. Brachial plexus surgery. *Orthop Clin North Am* 1981;12:303–323.
138. Millesi H. Brachial plexus injuries: management and results. *Clin Plastic Surg* 1984;11:115–120.
139. Nunley JA. Brachial plexus: neurotization. American Academy of Orthopaedic Surgeons, 64th Annual Meeting. Instructional Course Lecture No. 206, 1997.
140. Chuang DC-C. Neurotization procedures for brachial plexus injuries. *Hand Clin* 1995;11:633–645.
141. Simeson K. Microsurgery in brachial plexus lesions. *Acta Orthop Scand* 1985;56:238–241.
142. Benett JB. Tendon transfers about the shoulder and elbow in brachial plexus injury. American Academy of Orthopaedic Surgeons, 64th Annual Meeting. Instructional Course Lecture No. 206, 1997.
143. Bonnard C, Narakas A. Restoration of hand function after brachial plexus injury. *Hand Clin* 1995;11:647–656.
144. Sicuranza MJ, McCue FC. Compressive neuropathies in the upper extremities of athletes. *Hand Clin* 1992;8:263–273.
145. Simesen K, Haases J. Microsurgery in brachial plexus lesions. *Acta Orthop Scand* 1985;56:238–241.
146. Kline DG, Judice DJ. Operative management of selected brachial plexus lesions. *J Neurosurg* 1983;58:631–649.
147. Alnot JY. Traumatic brachial plexus palsy in the adult: retro- and infraclavicular lesions. *Clin Orthop* 1988;237:9–16.
148. Nagano A, Tsuyama N, Ochiai N, et al. Direct nerve crossing with intercostal nerve to treat avulsion injuries of the brachial plexus. *J Hand Surg* 1989;14A:980–985.
149. Solonen KA, Vastamaki M, Strom B. Surgery of the brachial plexus. *Acta Orthop Scand* 1984;55:436–440.

Principles and Practice of Orthopaedic Sports Medicine,
edited by William E. Garrett, Jr., Kevin P. Speer, and Donald T. Kirkendall.
Lippincott Williams & Wilkins, Philadelphia © 2000.

CHAPTER 11

Low Back and Lumbar Spine Injuries in the Athlete

William J. Richardson and Christopher G. Furey

A variety of conditions may cause disabling symptoms of low back pain and neurologic compromise in the athlete. Depending on the nature of the sporting activity, certain athletes are predisposed to particular pathologic conditions. Although their general excellent fitness makes high-caliber athletes better suited for recovery from injury, more emphasis is placed on rapid recovery and return to preinjury level of function. Athletes are less likely than others to tolerate prolonged recovery and place greater emphasis on timely evaluation and appropriate treatment of their particular conditions.

Acute mechanical low back pain, herniated lumbar disks, spondylolisthesis, and spondylolysis are the most common conditions that bring athletes to the attention of the specialty care provider. Although each of these conditions may have similar presentations, each is evaluated and treated in vastly different fashions.

Most conditions affecting the lumbar spine in the athlete are adequately treated nonoperatively, which does not mean they do not require aggressive attention and close follow-up. The sports medicine physician must be attuned to the varying causes of low back pain in the athlete, especially the young athlete. It is crucial to distinguish those individuals who may require more in-depth evaluation and treatment from most patients who can be treated with aggressive conservative therapy and rapid return to preexisting level of function.

ACUTE LOW BACK PAIN

Acute low back pain is ubiquitous in the general population, affecting 80% of individuals at some point in their lives. Thirty percent of athletes may experience acute low back pain at some point in time that is directly a result of their athletic pursuits (1). Although a specific pain generator cannot be determined in as many as 85% of cases, injuries of the soft tissue structures comprise most sources for acute low back pain (2). The paraspinal muscles and ligaments and the facet joints are the structures most frequently injured. Muscle strains are the most common source of pain and can occur in every athlete, regardless of particular sport. Strains may result from either repetitive mechanical overload of the low back or from an isolated more violent force. Similarly, injuries to the facet joint will produce pain, irritation of the posterior elements of the spine, and tend to occur in sports involving forceful repeated hyperextension.

Most studies of acute low back pain in laborers suggest that the incidence of returning to work is high (3), so that similar results could be expected with athletes who are generally well-motivated and eager to return to their sport. The major goal in managing athletes is to allow time for appropriate treatment and recovery to decrease risk for further more disabling injuries. Recurrence of low back pain often leads to a chronic problem, which as more caregivers realize has a vastly poorer prognosis for recovery.

Clinical Presentation

Typically, patients present with local persistent back pain of short duration, dating to a specific activity or injury. Mobility is limited in all directions secondary to exacerbation of pain. Symptoms are usually relieved with a recumbent posture, more so when a knee–chest position is assumed. Recumbence has been found to be associated with a more significant decrease in paravertebral muscle spasm than other positions (4).

W. J. Richardson and C. G. Furey: Division of Orthopedic Surgery, Duke University Medical Center, Durham, North Carolina 27710.

Radiculopathy is uncommon in episodes of acute low back pain. Less than 1% of all patients who present low back pain have symptoms of nerve root compression (5). If radicular symptoms are present and associated with focal neurologic deficits, suspicion should be raised about disk herniation.

Injury to the facet joints has a characteristic presentation often described as the facet syndrome. It is typified by acute low back pain, local tenderness lateral to midline corresponding to the location of the facets, and exacerbation of pain with hyperextension. Like other types of acute mechanical low back pain, symptoms are made worse with movement, especially when assuming an upright posture, and generally relieved with rest. As with muscle strain, nerve compression and radiculopathy are uncommon, and the neurologic exam is generally normal.

Imaging Studies

Radiographic imaging is generally not part of the initial evaluation of acute low back pain. The incidence of positive findings with plain x-rays in the setting of new onset back pain is low, generally 1% to 2% (6). Because only 10% to 20% of all patients with acute low back pain will ultimately be given a diagnosis, initial imaging studies should be discouraged. Persistence or worsening of symptoms, the development of neurologic deficits, or a history of a high energy injury are indications for obtaining imaging studies, beginning with plain radiographs and progressing to more in-depth imaging studies such as magnetic resonance imaging (MRI). A notable exception is the young athlete with new onset low back pain who is involved with hyperextension type activities. As discussed in depth, plain films at the time of initial evaluation are indicated to begin the evaluation for spondylolysis or spondylolisthesis.

Treatment

The goals of managing an athlete with acute low back pain are to decrease pain, maintain mobility and strength, assist with prompt return to full participation, and institute measures to prevent recurrence.

Treatment begins with rest and modification of activities, ice to the low back area, and nonsteroidal anti-inflammatory medication. If a patient's pain is severe enough, a short period of bedrest, generally no longer than 24 to 48 hours, may be warranted. Prolonged bedrest should be avoided, because it will exacerbate stiffness and can rapidly lead to deconditioning.

Initial rehabilitation should emphasize low-impact aerobic conditioning and simple stretching exercises that take the back through a pain-free range of motion. When initially severe pain begins to resolve, more aggressive range of motion and strengthening exercises

may be attempted. With the patient's symptoms as a guide, a regimen of specific exercises (either flexion or extension) should be determined and emphasized. Pool therapy, with walking, running, and range of motion exercises, can be particularly beneficial. The buoyancy of water unloads the normal stress across the spine while allowing most normal activities. Given the heightened fitness of most athletes, the requirements of an individual therapy program should be appropriately tailored for the athletic individual.

Because healing of acute low back injuries may occur over a 6- to 8-week period, loss of aerobic conditioning is a frequent occurrence. Efforts should be made to maintain cardiovascular and muscle tone. Stationary cycling and swimming are excellent means of doing so without aggravating the low back.

Specific physical therapy modalities such as ultrasound, electrical stimulation, iontophoresis, and deep massage may have a role in the subjective treatment of low back pain. However, as of now there is no scientific evidence to suggest that these measures expedite healing of soft tissue injuries of the low back.

Chiropractic management of acute low back pain has been shown by some investigators to provide temporary pain relief and decreased muscle spasm (7). However, excess manipulation of an acutely injured low back should be avoided because it may exacerbate both pain and inflammation.

With recurrence rates as high as 40% to 60% in athletic low back injuries, adequate recovery from injury and appropriate reconditioning and strengthening should be the cornerstone of all treatment programs (8). It is essential that the injured athlete complete an adequate rehabilitation program, so that they demonstrate full and pain-free range of motion with full exertion. Simulated participation in practice should be used before full competition, especially in contact sports, to adequately evaluate an athlete's functional status.

As with other conditions of the lumbar spine, when symptoms persist or exceed what might be expected of a simple muscular strain, further clinical and radiographic evaluation is warranted. The diagnosis of chronic low back sprain or recurrent backache must be used cautiously, especially in the young athlete. Relatively rare causes of low back pain, specifically spondylolysis, disk space infection, and benign bone tumor, should be part of a differential diagnosis in the adolescent and young adult. These entities can be effectively evaluated with a careful history and physical exam and appropriate radiologic evaluation.

Prevention of acute low back injuries is the best form of treatment. Identification of susceptible individuals and positive risk factors should be a responsibility of all coaches, trainers, and team physicians. Poor fitness and aerobic conditioning, decreased flexibility, and leg length inequalities have all been attributed to be risk factors for the development of low back pain in athletes (9–11). A study that prescreened college athletes suggested that females and those athletes with acquired lower extremity overuse and acquired ligamentous laxity are at increased risk of developing episodes of acute low back pain (12). Education of proper techniques, for example those involved in weight lifting may be taken for granted, but can avoid the disabling conditions of low back pain. A joint effort by the athlete and the athletic support staff should be made to appropriately educate all athletes and effectively intervene in those at-risk individuals.

Acute Skeletal Injuries of the Spinal Column

On rare occasions, fractures of the spinal column may occur and produce symptoms similar to those of an acute soft tissue injury of the low back. Fractures of the spinous process, transverse process, and vertebral endplate all may occur in the athletic individual. Fractures of the transverse process can occur after a direct blow to the back or as the result of a violent contracture of the psoas muscle, causing an avulsion fracture. Similarly, one or more spinous process fractures can occur as a result of a severe twisting or flexion injury or direct blow. Vertebral body endplate fractures occur in skeletally immature athletes after a significant compressive force. The cartilaginous endplate is weaker than the nucleus pulposus, so that with great force, the nucleus can fracture the endplate and be forced into the vertebral body.

Unlike burst fractures and fracture–dislocations of the spine that are high energy injuries occurring in falls and motor vehicle accidents, isolated process or endplate fractures do not cause spinal instability nor are they associated with neurologic deficits. Acute fractures of the pars interarticularis can also occur and are discussed along with other types of spondylolysis.

Fractures of the spinous and transverse process or vertebral endplate are often difficult to diagnosis with plain radiographs, often requiring a computed tomography (CT) to be adequately visualized. It is likely that some of these injuries are overlooked, because they are treated as contusions of the lumbar spine and have symptoms that resolve with time.

Treatment of these injuries is always conservative, with rest and restriction of activity. Symptomatic relief may be afforded with a lumbosacral corset. Like acute soft tissue injuries of the low back, maintenance of aerobic fitness and complete resolution of symptoms before return to competition are the cornerstones of a treatment program. As always, persistence of severe back pain or development of a neurologic deficit should trigger concern of a more severe injury and the use of more in-depth imaging modalities.

HERNIATED LUMBAR DISKS

Acute sciatica due a herniated nucleus pulposus (HNP) is an omnipresent condition, affecting as many as 1% of the population per year. In most patients it is a self-limited disease, with most individuals experiencing satisfactory resolution of symptoms with time. Sciatica in the athletic individual is a particularly challenging problem because of the disabling nature of its symptoms and frequently and the inability of the athlete to cope with the downtime inherent to an effective regimen of conservative therapy. To appropriately counsel and treat the athlete with acute sciatica, one must have a firm grasp of the natural history of the lumbar disk herniations and knowledge of both the conservative and surgical options that are available.

Although HNP and resultant sciatica do not seem to be more common in athletes, the approach to evaluation and treatment may differ considerably from the population in general. Conservative therapy is always the cornerstone of the initial treatment for symptomatic HNP. However, athletes, and in particular elite athletes, will likely place great emphasis on an expedient return to an active pain-free status. Athletes with documented herniated disks that appropriately correlate to their symptoms may require more aggressive surgical treatment than is generally the norm.

Pathophysiology

The intervertebral disk is composed of the inner nucleus pulposus and the outer annulus fibrosus. The nucleus pulposus is a complex of a randomly arranged collagen fibers and hydrated proteoglycans. The annulus is composed of collagen fibers arranged in concentric laminated bands; fibers within one band are identically oriented but in the opposite direction of the fibers in adjacent bands.

Disk pathology occurs as a spectrum from isolated annular tears, to contained nucleus pulposus herniation, complete extrusion, and finally sequestration of free disk fragments. The outer fibers of the annulus are well innervated, so that with local disruption the inflammatory response that is produced will trigger localized back pain. With extrusion of disk material, further inflammatory changes occur and impingement of nerve roots posterior to the intervertebral disk. Impingement produces radicular symptoms consisting of both pain and neurologic deficits.

Clinical Presentation

Acute HNP classically produces buttock and leg pain in a radicular fashion. Some degree of low back pain may be present as well. Appropriate history is required to correctly document the location and nature of the

TABLE 11.1. *Herniated lumbar disk clinical presentations*

Herniated disk	Nerve root affected	Muscles affected	Sensory deficit	Deep tendon reflex affected
L3-4	L-4	Tibialis anterior	Medial calf and foot	Patellar
L4-5	L-5	Ext. hallucis longus	Dorsal calf and foot	None
L5-S1	S-1	Peroneal longus and brevis	Lateral calf and foot	Achilles

symptoms. Careful physical exam is necessary to identify any muscle weakness, sensory deficits, or change in deep tendon reflexes. With widespread use of MRI and myelogram, there may be a tendency to rely solely on findings of imaging studies to guide the treatment plan. However, the cornerstone of appropriate diagnosis and treatment is correlating patient's symptoms and physical findings with associated pathologic lesions on the imaging study. The imaging study should be used to confirm a clinical suspicion of an HNP, not as the sole diagnostic tool.

Acute HNP occurs most commonly at the L4-5 and L5-S1 levels. The classic clinical scenarios are described in Table 11.1. A far lateral disk herniation may occur on occasion, with impingement of the nerve root that has exited from the more proximal level (e.g., far lateral HNP at L4-5 impinges the L-4 nerve root). Far lateral disks often have minimal associated low back pain, in distinction to most posterolateral lesions.

A cauda equina syndrome may develop from a large disk herniation that causes compression of neural elements, producing in part low back pain, unilateral or bilateral leg pain, perineal sensory disturbances, bowel and bladder dysfunction, and varying lower extremity weakness or sensory deficits, including paraplegia. A true cauda equina syndrome represents an absolute indication for decompression on an urgent, if not emergent, basis (13).

Radiographic Imaging

Although MRI is the imaging tool of choice for the diagnosis of sciatica-type pain, it is not routinely used as a screening tool on initial presentation. Because most acute episodes of sciatica resolve relatively quickly, a short course of conservative treatment is allowed before obtaining an MRI. However, for symptoms suggestive of a cauda equina syndrome, a progressive neurologic deficit, intractable or disabling pain, or associated constitutional symptoms suggestive of tumor or infection, more urgent assessment with MRI is indicated. Presentation in an elite athlete, in whom prompt return to high level of function is necessary, the threshold for obtaining an MRI will be lower.

The importance of correlation of clinical findings with imaging studies is essential, because incidental disk pa-

thology is frequently found with MRI. Boden et al. (14) studied asymptomatic individuals with MRI and found, in part, that in individuals aged 20 to 39, 21% had evidence of HNP (defined as focal extrusion of disk material beyond the margins of the vertebral endplates) and 56% had a disk bulge (defined as a nonfocal extension of disk material beyond the vertebral endplate). Conversely, not all patients will have anticipated positive findings on the imaging studies. The size, type, and location of herniated disk material does not always accurately correlate with true neurologic compromise (15). Modic et al. (16) reported on 25 patients with clinical diagnosis of acute lumbar radiculopathy, of whom only 18 had an HNP revealed by MRI.

Natural History

The true natural history of acute herniated disks continues to be a controversial topic. Because most patients have a favorable outcome in the long term, there is debate about the efficacy of either specific conservative treatment regimens or surgical decompression.

Comparative studies of conservative and surgical management of herniated disks in the population at large have suggested that surgically treated patients initially have a more favorable result than those treated conservatively but that with time the results may not be significantly different. Weber (17) followed 280 patients with radiculopathy and randomly assigned a portion of them into either surgical or conservative treatment groups. Although those treated surgically had more improvement at 1 year, they were no better than those treated conservatively at either a 4- or 10-year followup. Although Weber's study has been criticized as not a true natural history study, because those patients with profound motor weakness were removed from the randomization process, it remains the most often cited outcome study of acute herniated disks.

Hakelius (18) followed 583 patients treated either conservatively or surgically and found that immediately postoperatively, surgically treated patients were significantly better, but that within 6 months of presentation there was no significant difference than those treated conservatively. In the same study, by 7 years, the conservatively treated group did have more episodes of low back pain and recurrent sciatica and had lost more time from work (18).

Most studies suggest improved results after surgery in patients with predominantly radicular symptoms, no prior back surgeries, shorter duration of symptoms (generally 3 to 6 months), and no associated neurologic deficits (19–22). Occupations requiring heavy lifting, higher levels of education, and lack of pyschological disorders have similarly been associated with more favorable outcomes regardless of treatment (23). On the contrary, age greater than 50, lower education levels, associated worker's compensation litigation, and any psychological illnesses have been associated with less successful outcomes.

Conservative Treatment

The goals in managing acute sciatica are pain control, prevention of neurologic deficit, effective rehabilitation, and expedient return to premorbid level of function. In the athletic population, especially elite athletes, strong emphasis may be placed on expedient return to competition.

Most patients with sciatica can be treated effectively with a conservative approach. A typical conservative program consists of a short period of bedrest, antiinflammatory medication, and subsequent physical therapy regimens directed toward restoration of strength and flexibility followed by advancement of rehabilitation to sport-specific training activities. Bedrest of limited duration during the initial period of severe sciatica is thought to decrease mobility of the disk material and hence decrease pain and lessen the likelihood of progression of a neurologic deficit. Excessive bedrest (greater than 2 to 3 days) will rapidly cause deconditioning of muscle groups and further lengthen recovery periods. Exercise programs should emphasize aerobic conditioning initially and subsequently focus on increasing flexibility, trunk strength, balance, and coordination. Reports of serial imaging studies assessing acute HNP suggest the size of most herniations will decrease in part or entirely, with the largest herniations having the greatest tendency to shrink (22).

Several exercise programs have gained popularity in treating patients with low back pain and sciatica. The McKenzie exercises emphasize the use of certain postures and motion to centralize back and leg pain. Often mistakenly defined as solely an extension exercise program, the McKenzie approach consists of classification of low back disorders into specific categories, each having its specific stretching and postural treatment regimen (24). The importance of self-directed exercise is emphatically recommended (24).

The Williams flexion exercises are presumed to work by decreasing the load across the posterior portion of the intervertebral disk (and the site of herniation) and to increase the width of the neuroforamen (25). Specific exercises, including anterior and posterior pelvic tilts and double knee-to-chest position, are used for acute disk pathology in an effort to reduce the size of herniated fragments. These specific exercises may exacerbate symptoms related to spinal stenosis or degenerative conditions of the posterior elements (25).

Spine-stabilizing exercises emphasize the importance of attaining a neutral spine, which is the specific posture of the pelvis and spine that places the least amount of stress across the spine and its supporting soft tissue structures. Five components of back stabilization have been identified:

1. Increasing intraabdominal pressure via exertion against a closed glottis, so to decrease pressure across the spine, while increasing transmission of pressure within the abdomen.
2. Strengthening the thoracolumbar fascia, which are the muscular attachments of the latissimus dorsi, abdominal obliques, and gluteus maximus, which assist in spine stabilization.
3. Strengthening the erector spinae to produce a hydraulic amplifier effect they have upon the adjacent spinal column.
4. Involvement of the posterior spinal ligamentous structures.
5. Strengthening the support mechanism of the small intersegmental muscle that runs between the individual vertebral bodies.

Epidural steroid injections are frequently used in the management of acute sciatica despite controversy as to their true efficacy (26). Randomized control studies suggest that epidural steroids may provide short relief of leg pain and sensory deficits but do not have significant long-term effects nor decrease the need for surgical intervention in many patients (27). Jackson et al. (28), in a study of 32 high-level athletes with acute sciatica due to disk herniation, reported 44% had dramatic abatement of symptoms and a rapid return to competition after a single injection. Although successful in some athletes, they concluded these results were less impressive than those of series from the general population.

Surgical Treatment

Definite surgical indications include cauda equina syndrome, a rapidly progressive neurologic deficit, and severe incapacitating pain; these conditions represent some surgical candidates. The most common surgical indication is the persistence of symptoms despite adequate conservative therapy. Typically, conservative therapy should last for at least 6 weeks and generally not longer than 3 months (29). It is hypothesized that to avoid pathologic changes within a compressed nerve root, surgical decompression should occur no longer than 3 months after onset of symptoms (3).

In general, 85% to 90% of patients will have significant resolution of their radiculopathy. As noted, more favorable results occur with younger patients, those with radiculopathy as their primary symptoms, symptoms of less than 3 to 6 months duration, absence of neurologic deficits, and those with no prior back surgeries.

Standard laminectomy and diskectomy (macrodiskectomy) and microscopic diskectomy are the two major surgical options. The clinical outcome between the two does not seem to significantly differ. Instead, patient selection seems to be the primary factor in the outcome of surgically treated patients.

The main advantages of microscopic diskectomy are a smaller incision and less soft tissue dissection and superior visualization. It is hypothesized that the limited approach inherent to microdiskectomy forces the surgeon to examine the patient and their imaging studies with a more critical eye, avoiding a "seek and find" approach to addressing disk pathology (30). In any case, a diskectomy with minimal soft tissue dissection and boney resection whether using surgical loupes or a microscope is an attractive option for the athlete, in that minimally invasive surgery allows a more rapid recovery and return to prior activity level.

There have been no reports of large numbers of athletes treated for acute HNP, so treatment decisions are often anecdotal or based on the extensive literature addressing the natural history of conservative and surgically treated acute HNP treated in the general population. Sakou et al. (31) did report a series of 13 Japanese national-level athletes who were treated with percutaneous diskectomy, 9 of whom had a favorable outcome and were able to return to full competitive levels within 1 to 6 months. Similarly, Matsunanga et al. (32) described more satisfactory results in both athletes and laborers treated with percutaneous diskectomy versus standard diskectomy.

Illustrative Case 1

A 21-year-old Division I college football defensive lineman presented with a 1-month history of left buttock and leg pain after dead lifting 550 pounds. Within several days of the onset of leg pain, he developed weakness in the calf muscles. Exam revealed lumbar spasm, positive straight leg test, and a foot drop. MRI showed acute HNP at L5-S1 (Fig. 11.1). A short course of conservative therapy with rest, restriction of activities, nonsteroidal anti-inflammatory medication, and a single epidural steroid injection failed to relieve his symptoms or neurologic deficit. He underwent successful microscopic diskectomy with complete resolution of symptoms. He

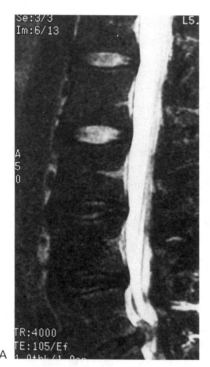 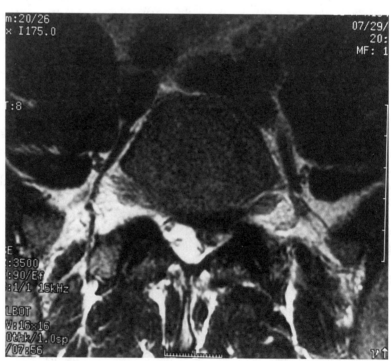

FIG. 11.1. Sagittal **(A)** and axial **(B)** magnetic resonance images of acute herniated nucleus pulposus at L5-S1.

returned to competitive football within 6 weeks of surgery.

SPONDYLOLYSIS AND SPONDYLOLISTHESIS

Spondylolysis is a defect in the pars interarticularis of the vertebral body, a portion of the lamina located between the superior and inferior articular facets. Spondylolisthesis is the forward displacement of a vertebral body on the immediately inferior body. Acquired pars defects are a frequent source of pain in the adolescent athlete and should always be considered when evaluating an active child complaining of back pain.

Wiltse et al. (33) comprehensively classified spondylolisthesis into six different categories:

1. Congenital spondylolisthesis;
2. Isthmic spondylolisthesis;
3. Lytic pars defect (presumably due to a stress fracture) and elongated but intact pars (likely to be a healed lytic defect);
4. Degenerative spondylolisthesis;
5. Posttraumatic spondylolisthesis: acute fracture or ligamentous injury at an area other than the pars interarticularis;
6. Pathologic spondylolisthesis.

The cause of spondylolisthesis in the athlete is most always due to an isthmic or lytic-type lesion of the pars interarticularis. As discussed, the mere presence of either a pars defect or spondylolisthesis does not predict the presence of symptoms or the progression of a slip.

Etiology

The etiology of spondylolisthesis is unclear, although it is likely to be multifactorial. A genetic susceptibility for a defect of the pars interarticularis is probable, but repetitive mechanical loading is necessary for the development of symptomatic spondylolysis and spondylolisthesis. Inheritance has been demonstrated by Wiltse (34), who identified 36 families in whom no one under age 5 had evidence of a pars defect, whereas there was a 40% incidence in those over age 10. Wynne-Davies and Scott (35), based on findings from a radiographic survey, suggested an autosomal dominance pattern with variable penetrance. As well, there is strong support for a mechanical etiology of spondylolysis and spondylolisthesis as fatigue fractures. It is theorized that pars defects are due to inherent stresses from bipedal locomotion occurring at a neural arch weakened by an inherited defect (36). It is clearly evident that spondylolisthesis does not occur in nonambulatory patients with cerebral palsy (37).

The cross-sectional area of cortical bone in the pars interarticularis is the focus of great stress loading and has the potential for fatigue failure (38). Once a pars defect is present, muscle forces acting on the posterior elements of the spine may cause continued displacement of the pars defect (39).

Spondylolysis is rarely due to a single traumatic event but rather represents a fatigue fracture due cyclical loading. Pars defect occur most commonly at L-5, due to the great change in stiffness that occurs at the lumbosacral junction, as transition is made from the mobile lumbar spine to the more rigid sacrum.

Participation in sports involving repetitive lumbar spine hyperextension and axial loading are clearly linked with a higher incidence of both spondylolysis and spondylolisthesis. Gymnasts, divers, football linemen, weight lifters, and pole vaulters all have been found to have an increased risk for development of a pars defect. Gymnasts routinely hyperextend and hyperflex and suffer significant shock from jumps and landings. As a result, there is clearly potential to both provoke symptoms from a preexisting structural abnormality or to produce the fatigue loading necessary to sustain a stress fracture *de novo* (38). Jackson et al. (40) found a fourfold increase in spondylytic defects in 100 young female gymnasts. Offensive and defensive linemen, in particular, have been noted to have a higher incidence of pars defects and spondylolisthesis thought to be due to the frequent stress they sustain while in a crouched position in addition to their penchant for heavy weight training. Ferguson et al. (41) reported a 50% incidence of pars defect in college football linemen. A review of radiographs of linemen attending two consecutive National Football League combines revealed a 10% incidence of either spondylolysis or spondylolisthesis (42). In contrast, other studies have not isolated linemen as being at higher risk than players with other positions (43,44). In a prospective study of college football players from the same Division I institution, McCarroll et al. (43) found a 15% incidence of pars defects, only some occurring in linemen. The hypothesis is that tackling, weight lifting, and certain training techniques in addition to blocking make all football players susceptible to pars injuries and spondylolisthesis, regardless of position.

Natural History

The incidence of spondylolysis in North American adolescents and young adults is 4% and increases to 6% in adults (45). The occurrence of spondylolysis and spondylolisthesis in children less than 5 years of age is exceedingly uncommon.

The probability of progression of a pars defect to spondylolisthesis depends on several factors. Slip progression occurs most commonly between ages 9 and 14, during the years of most rapid growth (46). Females have a greater propensity for slip progression, especially those with dysplastic spondylolisthesis (46,47). As skeletal maturity approaches, the probability of slip progression is markedly diminished. Symptomatic patients with spondylolisthesis are at a higher risk of progression, underscoring the importance of activity modification as the cornerstone of initial treatment (48).

As noted, certain sporting activities are associated with higher incidences of pars defects and spondylolisthesis. However, in the absence of symptoms, athletic activity has not been found to aggravate or precipitate progression of spondylolysis. In a retrospective study of adolescents enrolled in a school designed for elite competitive athletes, the incidental finding of spondylolysis or low-grade spondylolisthesis did not correlate with progression of either the pars defects or low-grade slip in asymptomatic athletes involved in high-level training and competition (49). Semon and Spengler (50) found no difference in time lost to participation in Division I football players with spondylolysis and nonprogressive episodes of back pain when compared with other players with low back pain and no radiographic evidence of pars defects.

Radiographic findings correlating with progression include a greater than 50% slip, convex sacral contour, spina bifida, and a high slip angle (48).

Clinical Presentation

Most adolescents with spondylolysis and low-grade spondylolisthesis remain asymptomatic. However, persistent low back pain in the active adolescent should be considered to be due to a pars defect until proven otherwise. Typically, a young athletic individual will participate in the offending activity until he or she is no longer able to continue because of pain. Pain is exacerbated with hyperextension and rotation of the lumbar spine. As noted, gymnasts, football lineman, pole vaulters, divers, weight lifters, and others who perform a significant amount of hyperextension are especially predisposed to this condition.

With mild pars defects or mild slips, the physical appearance of the spine and a child's gait generally appear normal. With increasing severity of a slip, there is increased flexion of both the hips and knees in addition to the development of a wide-based gait with a short stride length. Tight hamstrings are a common finding in both symptomatic and asymptomatic patients, thought to be due to a postural reflex stabilizing a painful lumbosacral junction. As a slip progresses, tight hamstrings function to adjust the anteriorly displaced center of gravity by extending the pelvis.

Radicular symptoms in the adolescent athlete are relatively uncommon. Young adults with higher grade spondylolisthesis may develop radiculopathy secondary

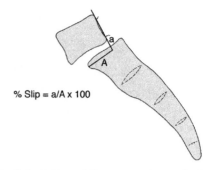

% Slip = a/A x 100

FIG. 11.2. Calculation of the percentage slip in spondylolisthesis.

to foraminal stances or hypertrophic callus emanating from a pars defect.

Radiologic Evaluation

Plain radiographs are the initial step in the evaluation of spondylolysis and spondylolisthesis and generally consist of weight-bearing AP lateral, and bilateral oblique films. Recumbent films may fail to detect a low-grade spondylolisthesis or not accurately reveal the true magnitude of a slip. Plain films are usually sufficient to visualize a pars defect and spondylolisthesis, if present. A lateral film is used to quantify the percentage of spondylolisthesis (Fig. 11.2). The Meyerding system is the most often used means of classifying the amount of vertebral displacement (51). Grade 0 is 0%, grade I 1% to 25%, grade II 26% to 50%, grade III 51% to 75%, and grade IV 76% to 100%. The lateral film also reveals the slip angle and degree of sacral inclination (Fig. 11.3). Oblique views can better visualize a pars defect as the well-known collar on the "Scotty dog."

If plain films do not reveal a suspected pars defect,

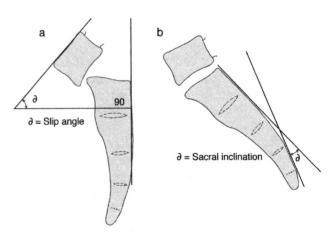

a   b

∂ = Slip angle

∂ = Sacral inclination

FIG. 11.3. Calculation of slip angle **(a)** and sacral inclination **(b)**.

bone scans are the next diagnostic study of choice. In addition to diagnosis of occult spondylolysis, nuclear bone scans also provide information about the healing capacity of a pars defect (52). Increased activity on bone scan has been shown to correlate with the healing potential of pars defects treated with activity modification and bracing (53). Single photon emission CT (SPECT) has surpassed standard technetium bone scans as a more sensitive tool to detect occult pars defects (54). Raby and Matthews (55) showed a positive correlation between a positive SPECT and persistent pain relief after successful fusion for spondylolisthesis.

CTs are the most useful modality to define the bony architecture of the pars interarticularis. CT should be used to clarify the cause of an abnormality of the pars detected by SPECT but not evident on plain film. CT can accurately confirm the finding of a pars defect and, unlike SPECT, can distinguish spondylolysis from facet arthritis, infection, or tumor. Additionally, with the use of contrast in a CT myelogram, central and foraminal stenosis causing compression of neural elements can be identified.

Treatment

Most patients with spondylolysis and isthmic spondylolisthesis are asymptomatic and thus do not require treatment. Nonetheless, athletes, parents, coaches, and trainers should all be educated about the nature of the disease and the importance of appropriate evaluation if symptoms arise.

In the asymptomatic adolescent who has an incidentally found pars defect or low-grade spondylolisthesis (grades I and II), no activity restrictions are placed, because the probability for the development of symptoms or progression of deformity are low. Periodic x-rays are recommended throughout the growth period, because this is clearly the period in which a treatable problem will develop (38).

In the symptomatic patient with a newly diagnosed pars defect or low-grade spondylolisthesis, activity modification is essential. In addition to cessation of all active sports participation, other conservative measures can be used. Heat and nonsteroidal anti-inflammatories can be used acutely to assist in controlling initial symptoms. Bracing and exercise programs have also been used with beneficial effects.

Bracing has been shown to be effective in both decreasing pain and healing pars defects. It must be emphasized that bracing is an adjunct to, and not a replacement for, activity modification. Braces are presumed to be effective by immobilizing the lumbar spine in a position of less lordosis, in addition to increasing intraabdominal pressure and thereby decreasing axial pressures across the lumbar (36). Steiner and Micheli (56) treated 52 teenagers and young adults

with symptomatic spondylolysis or grade I isthmic spondylolisthesis with a 6-month course of full-time Boston brace use and found a 78% incidence of resolution of pain and return to full activities. In this study, positive prognostic factors included young men with spondylolysis and those patients with acute onset of symptoms. Bell et al. (57) reviewed 28 teenagers with grades I and II isthmic or dysplastic spondylolisthesis treated with antilordotic thoracolumbosacral orthoses and found 100% resolution of pain and significant reduction of lumbar lordosis and increase in percentage of slip.

Exercise directed toward strengthening the abdominal and paraspinal muscles may play a role in pain reduction, when used in conjunction with restriction of offending activities and other conservative measures. A recent randomized controlled trial found exercises directed specifically at strengthening the deep abdominal lumbar multifidus muscles proximal to a pars defect to be superior to nonspecific aerobic conditioning programs in pain relief for patients with spondylolysis and low-grade spondylolisthesis (58).

Plain films generally will show evidence of healing within 3 months of the onset of symptoms if conservative treatment is to be effective. SPECT is a more sensitive means of following the healing of pars defect and should be used if there is any question after interpretation of the plain radiographs. Once symptoms have resolved and imaging studies reveal healing of the pars defect, a program for the return to competitive activity can be implemented. Completion of an adequate reconditioning and rehabilitation program is necessary, so that an athlete is pain free and at full strength before returning to active participation.

A small percentage of symptomatic patients with spondylolysis and spondylolisthesis will not respond to conservative therapy. If activity restriction, exercise programs, and bracing have failed to resolve symptoms or prevent progression of a deformity, surgical stabilization should be considered. As noted, risk factors for the progression of pars defects and spondylolisthesis include young age, occurrence before the growth spurt, female gender, higher grade slips, high slip angle, a rounded configuration of S1, and spina bifida occulta (45,47,59). Direct surgical repair of the pars defect and *in situ* fusion are the main surgical options available for spondylolysis and low-grade slips.

Surgical repair of the pars defect specifically addresses the pathologic lesion and presumably the primary source of pain. As well, direct surgical repair avoids the morbidity associated with the loss of a motion segment that occurs with a fusion, which may be especially important to the athletic individual. Buck (60) first described surgical repair of the pars, with the passage of a screw across the defect and local application of autologous bone graft. Roca et al. (61) reviewed 15 patients with spondylitic defects treated with screw fixation, 13 of whom solidly healed their defects and returned to full athletic competition by 1 year. Other techniques to directly fuse the pars include tension band wiring and a combination of screw and wire constructs (62,63). Biomechanical analysis suggests that screws, wires, and a combination of the two all effectively restore stiffness when compared with the intact spine (64).

In situ posterolateral fusion remains the most common surgical technique for symptomatic low-grade spondylolisthesis in adolescents and young adults who have failed conservative therapy. In general, single level L5-S1 fusion is satisfactory. Although a lumbar motion segment is sacrificed, the results are generally excellent with regard to pain relief, increase in mobility, and low rate of slip progression (65–67).

Patients with high-grade spondylolisthesis (grades III and IV), regardless of symptoms, should undergo posterolateral fusion. Likewise, the unusual instance of progression of a previously noted low-grade slip to one that is greater than 50% is a definite indication for surgical stabilization. If nerve root symptoms are present, decompression of the offending posterior elements is indicated. Decompression without fusion is contraindicated because of the likelihood of slip progression. Open instrumented reduction of high-grade spondylolisthesis has become an increasingly popular technique. The indication is improvement of a severe cosmetic deformity.

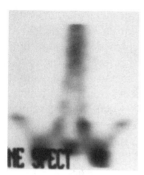

FIG. 11.5. Single photon emission computed tomography revealing increased uptake at left pars interarticularis.

However, because of a high incidence of associated neurologic complications, it should be reserved for marked deformities and surgeons familiar with the technique (68).

Illustrative Case 2

A 14-year-old boy who plays competitive soccer developed acute low back pain while extending to kick a ball toward the goal. Physical exam revealed lumbar spasm, pain with hyperextension, mild hamstring tightness, and a normal neurologic exam. Plain radiographs were normal. A technetium bone scan (Fig. 11.4) was normal. A SPECT study (Fig. 11.5) revealed uptake at the left pars interarticularis. A CT (Fig. 11.6) confirmed the left-sided pars defect.

He was treated with strict restriction of sports activities and a hyperextension brace (Boston brace). His pain resolved within 3 months, at which time he had a

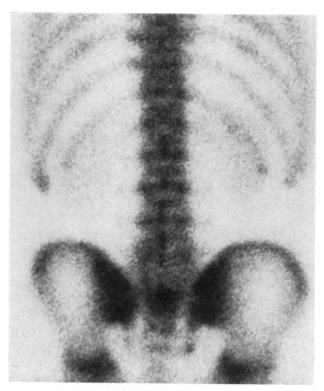

FIG. 11.4. A 14-year-old with acute low back pain (normal bone scan).

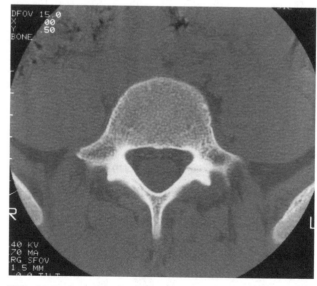

FIG. 11.6. Computed tomography revealing fracture of left pars interarticularis.

pain-free range of motion of his spine. His return to full activity was uneventful.

REFERENCES

1. Dreisinger TE, Nelson B. Management of back pain in athletes. *Injury Clin* 1996;21:313–320.
2. Nachemson A. Newest knowledge of low back pain. A critical look. *Clin Orthop* 1992;279:8–20.
3. Nachemson A. Advances in low back pain. *Clin Orthop* 1985;200:266–278.
4. Garfin SR, Pye SA. Bed design and its effect on chronic low back pain—a limited controlled trial. *Pain* 1981;10:87–91.
5. Frymoyer JW. Back pain and sciatica. *N Engl J Med* 1988; 318:291–300.
6. Curd JG, Thorne RP. The management of lumbar disc disease. *Hosp Pract* 1989;15:135–148.
7. Ohnmeiss DD, et al. Nonsurgical treatment of sports-related spine injuries. In: Hochschuler, ed. *The spine in sports.* Philadelphia: Hanley and Belfus, 1990:241–266.
8. Harvey J, Tanner S. Low back pain in young athletes. A practical approach. *Injury Clin* 1991;12:394–406.
9. Giles LG, Taylor JR. Low-back pain associated with leg length inequality. *Spine* 1981;6:510–521.
10. Kujala UM, Salminen JJ, Taimela S, et al. Subject characteristics and low back pain in young athletes and nonathletes. *Med Sci Sports Exerc* 1992;24:627–632.
11. Mierau D, Cassidy JD, Yong-Hing K. Low-back pain and straight leg raising in children and adolescents. *Spine* 1989;14:526–528.
12. Nadler SF, Wu KD, Galaski T, et al. Low back pain in college athletes: a prospective study correlating lower extremity overuse or acquired ligamentous laxity with low back pain. *Spine* 1998;23:828–833.
13. Delamarter RB, Sherman JE, Carr JB. Cauda equina syndrome: neurologic recovery after immediate, early, or late decompression. *Spine* 1991;16:1022–1029.
14. Boden SD, Davis DO, Dian TS, et al. Abnormal magnetic resonance scans of the lumbar spine in asymptomatic subjects. A prospective investigation. *J Bone Joint Surg Am* 1990;72:403–408.
15. Garfin SR, Rydevik BL, Brown RA. Compressive neuropathy of spinal nerve roots. *Spine* 1991;16:162–166.
16. Modic MT, Ross JS, Obuchowski NA, et al. Contrast-enhanced MR imaging in acute lumbar radiculopathy: a pilot study of the natural history. *Radiology* 1995;195:429–435.
17. Weber H. Lumbar disc herniation. A controlled, prospective study with 10 years of observation. *Spine* 1983;8:131–140.
18. Hakelius A. Prognosis in sciatica: a clinical follow-up of surgical and non-surgical treatment. *Acta Orthop Scand* 1970;129S:1–76.
19. Alaranta H, Hurme M, Einola S, et al. A prospective study of patients with sciatica. *Spine* 1990;15:1345–1349.
20. Dvorak J, Gauchat M-H, Valach L. The outcome of surgery for lumbar disc herniation. I. A 4–17 year follow-up with emphasis on somatic aspects. *Spine* 1988;13:1418–1422.
21. Herron LD, Turner J. Patient selection for lumbar laminectomy and discectomy with a revised objective rating system. *Clin Orthop* 1985;199:145–152.
22. Maigne J-Y, Rime B, Deligne B: Computerized tomographic follow-up study of 48 cases of non-operatively treated lumbar intervertebral disc herniation. *Spine* 1992;17:1071–1074.
23. Dvorak J, Valach L, Fuhrimann P, et al. The outcome of surgery for lumbar disc herniation. II. A 4–17 year follow-up with emphasis on psychological aspects. *Spine* 1988;13:1423–1427.
24. Donaldson R. The McKenzie approach to evaluating and treating low back pain. *Orthop Rev* 1990;29:681–686.
25. Young J, Press JM, Herring SA. The disc at risk in athletes: perspectives on operative and nonoperative care. *Med Sci Sports Exerc* 1997;29:S222–S232.
26. Koes BW, Scholten RJ, Mens JM, et al. Efficacy of epidural steroid injections for low back pain and sciatica: a systematic review of randomized clinical trials. *Pain* 1995;63:279–288.
27. Carette S, Leclaire R, Marcoux S, et al. Epidural corticosteroid injections for sciatica due to herniated nucleus pulposus. *N Engl J Med* 1997;336:1634–1640.
28. Jackson DW, Rettig A, Wiltse LL. Epidural steroid injections in the young athletic adult. *Am J Sports Med* 1980;8:239–243.
29. Saal JA. Natural history and nonoperative treatment of lumbar disc herniation. *Spine* 1996;24S:2S–9S.
30. McCulloch JA. Focus issue on lumbar disc herniation: macro- and microdiscectomy. *Spine* 1996;21:45S–56S.
31. Sakou T, Masuda A, Yone K, et al. Percutaneous discectomy in athletes. *Spine* 1993;18:2218–2221.
32. Matsunaga S, Sakou T, Taketomi E, et al. Comparison of operative results of lumbar disc herniation in manual laborers and athletes. *Spine* 1993;18:2222–2226.
33. Wiltse LL, Newman PH, MacNab I. Classification of spondylolysis and spondylolisthesis. *Clin Orthop* 1975;117:23–29.
34. Wiltse LL. Spondylolisthesis. Thesis for the American Orthopedic Association, 1958.
35. Wynne-Davies R, Scott JH. Inheritance and spondylolisthesis: a radiographic family survey. *J Bone Joint Surg Br* 1979;61:301–305.
36. Southern EP, An HS. Classification, diagnosis, radiographs, natural history, and conservative treatment of spondylolisthesis. *Semin Spine Surg* 1999;11:2–13.
37. Rosenberg NL, Bargar WL, Friedman B. The incidence of spondylolysis and spondylolisthesis in nonambulatory patients. *Spine* 1981;6:35–37.
38. Ciullo JV, Jackson DW. Pars interarticularis stress reaction, spondylolysis, and spondylolisthesis in gymnasts. *Clin Sports Med* 1985;4:95–110.
39. Krenz J, Troup JD. The structure of the pars interarticularis of the lower lumbar vertebrae and its relation to the etiology of spondylolysis. *J Bone Joint Surg Br* 1973;55:735–741.
40. Jackson DW, Wiltse LL, Cirincione RJ. Spondylolysis in the female gymnast. *Clin Orthop* 1976;117:68–73.
41. Ferguson RH, McMaster JH, Stanitski CL. Low back pain in college football lineman. *Am J Sports Med* 1974;2:63–69.
42. Speer KP, Warren RF, Pavlov H, et al. The cumulative effect of participation in college football on the lumbar spine. Presented to the AOSSM Meeting, June 1994.
43. McCarroll JR, Miller JM, Ritter MA. Lumbar spondylolysis and spondylolisthesis in college football players: a prospective study. *Am J Sports Med* 1986;14:404–406.
44. Shaffer B, Wiesel S, Lauerman W. Spondylolisthesis in the elite football player: an epidemiological study in the NCAA and NFL. *J Spinal Dis* 1997;10:365–370.
45. Fredrickson BE, Baker D, McHolick WJ, et al. The natural history of spondylolysis and spondylolisthesis. *J Bone Joint Surg* 1984;66:699–707.
46. Seitsalo S, Osterman K, Hyvarinen H, et al. Progression of spondylolisthesis in children and adolescents: a long term follow-up of 272 patients. *Spine* 1991;16:417–421.
47. Seitsalo S, Osterman K, Poussa M, et al. Spondylolisthesis in children under 12 years of age: long-term results of 56 patients treated conservatively or operatively. *J Pediatr Orthop* 1988; 8:516–521.
48. Thometz JG. Spondylolysis and spondylolisthesis in children. *Semin Spine Surg* 1999;11:22–27.
49. Muschik M, Hahnel H, Robinson PN, et al. Competitive sports and the progression of spondylolisthesis. *J Pediatr Orthop* 1996; 16:364–369.
50. Semon RL, Spengler D. Significance of lumbar spondylolysis in college football players. *Spine* 1981;6:172–174.
51. Meyerding HW. Spondylolisthesis. *Surg Gynecol Obstet* 1932;54:371–375.
52. Lusins JO, Elting JJ, Cicoria AD, et al. SPECT evaluation of lumbar spondylolysis and spondylolisthesis. *Spine* 1994;19: 607–612.
53. van den Oever M, Merrick MV, Scott JH. Bone scintigraphy in symptomatic spondylolysis. *J Bone Joint Surg Br* 1987;69:453–456.
54. Harvey CJ, Richenberg JL, Saifuddin A, et al. Pictorial review: the radiological investigation of lumbar spondylolysis. *Clin Radiol* 1998;53:723–728.
55. Raby N, Matthews S. Symptomatic spondylolysis: correlation of CT and SPECT with clinical outcome. *Clin Radiol* 1993;48:97–99.
56. Steiner ME, Micheli LJ. Treatment of symptomatic spondylolysis

and spondylolisthesis with the modified Boston brace. *Spine* 1985;10:937–943.

57. Bell DF, Erlich M, Zaleske DJ. Brace treatment for symptomatic spondylolisthesis. *Clin Orthop* 1988;236:192–198.

58. O'Sullivan PB, Phyty GD, Twomey LT, et al. Evaluation of specific stabilizing exercise in the treatment of chronic low back pain with radiologic diagnosis of spondylolysis and spondylolisthesis. *Spine* 1997;22:2959–2967.

59. Wiltse LL, Jackson DW. Treatment of spondylolisthesis in children. *Clin Orthop* 1976;117:92–100.

60. Buck JE. Direct repair of the defect in spondylolisthesis: preliminary report. *J Bone Joint Surg Br* 1970;52:432–437.

61. Roca J, Moretta D, Fuster S, et al. Direct repair of spondylolysis. Clin Orthop 1989;246:86–91.

62. Hambly M, Lee CK, Gutteling E, et al. Tension band wiring–bone grafting for spondylolysis and spondylolisthesis. A clinical and biomechanical study. *Spine* 1989;14:455–460.

63. Nicol RO, Scott JH. Lytic spondylolysis: repair by wiring. *Spine* 1986;11:1027–1030.

64. Deguchi M, Rapoff AJ, Zdeblick TA. Biomechanical comparison of spondylolysis fixation techniques. *Spine* 1999;24:328–333.

65. Frennereed AK, Danielson BI, Nachemson AL, et al. Midterm follow-up of young patients fused in situ for spondylolisthesis. *Spine* 1991;16:409–416.

66. Newton PO, Johnston CE. Analysis and treatment of poor outcomes after in situ arthrodesis in adolescent spondylolisthesis. *J Pediatr Orthop* 1997;17:754–761.

67. Pizzutillo PD, Mirenda W, MacEwen GD. Posterolateral fusion for spondylolisthesis in adolescence. *J Pediatr Orthop* 1986;6:311–316.

68. Petraco D, Spivak J, Cappadona J, et al. An anatomic evaluation of L5 nerve stretch in spondylolisthesis reduction. *Spine* 1996;21:1133–1139.

Principles and Practice of Orthopaedic Sports Medicine,
edited by William E. Garrett, Jr., Kevin P. Speer, and Donald T. Kirkendall.
Lippincott Williams & Wilkins, Philadelphia © 2000.

CHAPTER 12

Pelvis, Abdominal Wall, and Adductors

Scott A. Lynch and Per A.F.H. Renström

Pain in the lower abdomen, pelvis, and groin are common occurrences among athletes. As orthopedists we tend to think of pain and injuries as related to the musculoskeletal system, and indeed many of the causes of pain in these regions are related to the musculoskeletal system. However, most of the more serious and life-threatening problems are nonorthopedic. Therefore, we must be diligent in our history and examination to be sure that a medical problem is not causing musculoskeletal symptoms, as can occur when a pelvic tumor is irritating the iliopsoas muscle and mimicking groin pain. In such cases the correct diagnosis is often delayed many months. This has obvious potentially devastating consequences for the athlete.

Medical causes of pelvic pain can include bowel and intraabdominal problems such as appendicitis, bowel obstruction, Crohn's disease, and/or diverticulitis. In bowel-related problems, the athlete may present with lower abdominal and/or pelvic pain with a related change in his or her bowel habits and nausea and vomiting. When bowel problems are suspected, it is also important to perform a rectal exam with hemoccult analysis for blood in the stool.

The spondyloarthropathies are well-known causes of pelvic pain from sacroiliac joint inflammation and can include ankylosing spondylitis, Reiter's syndrome, and rheumatoid arthritis. In these cases it is important to elicit a history of other medical problems and a family history.

Pain related to the genitourinary system is also quite common in the athletic population. Kidney stones are not uncommon in the athletic age group. Urinary tract infections are quite common, particularly among the female population. Gynecologic complaints are quite common, with ovarian cysts and menstrual cramps being quite frequent problems among this age group. We must also remember that many athletes are in the most sexually active age group. Sexually transmitted diseases can cause pelvic pain from prostatitis in males or from pelvic inflammatory disease in females. Even pregnancy can present as pelvic pain. It is important to ask questions and to perform a thorough examination. This includes taking a history of sexual activity and a menstrual history in females.

It is evident that a good history is the key to making a correct diagnosis so that we do not overlook these important causes of lower abdominal, pelvic, and groin pain. We must ascertain the nature, type, duration, and inciting causes of the pain. Once we have answers to these important questions, a more focused history and examination can assist in determining the need for more specialized tests. These measures will assist in developing a correct diagnosis and treatment. With this in mind, the remainder of this chapter deals mainly with musculoskeletal causes of pelvic, abdominal wall, and adductor-related problems. Though it is somewhat artificial, because many problems cause pain in all three areas, the chapter is divided into the above three sections. We relate pelvic problems to the bony skeleton, whereas abdominal wall deals mainly with sports hernia and lower abdominal muscle injuries. The section on adductor injuries includes only injury and treatment of the adductors of the hip. We do not include other groin-related or hip problems in this chapter.

S. A. Lynch: Department of Orthopaedics and Rehabilitation, Penn State University College of Medicine, Hershey, Pennsylvania 17033.

P. A. F. H. Renström: Section of Sports Medicine, Department of Surgical Science, Karolinska Hospital, S-171 76 Stockholm, Sweden.

THE PELVIS

As mentioned above, pelvic injuries in this section deal with problems related to the bony pelvis. The pelvic bones and their ligamentous attachments are very strong, and it requires great forces to cause acute fractures or acute ligamentous injuries. These types of forces are uncommon in athletic participation, so most of the acute bony pelvic injuries are caused by high-energy trauma, as in motor vehicle accidents. Therefore, most injuries to the bony pelvis are problems of overuse. The one exception to this is avulsion fractures of the apophyses in adolescents. In this case, the relatively weak growth plate at the tendinous attachment of the strong muscles is the site of injury. Among the overuse injuries, stress fractures are the most common among athletes. Less commonly, but of significant occurrence, is osteitis pubis. It is interesting to note that many of these overuse problems seem to be particularly common among anorexic, amenorrheic, female endurance athletes. Therefore, it is again of paramount importance to take a dietary and menstrual history so that these problems can be addressed to aid in treatment and prevent recurrence.

Stress Fractures

The incidence of stress fractures is unknown, and it is likely that many stress fractures go unrecognized because the patient treats him- or herself by resting until the pain improves. The exact etiology of stress fractures is unknown, but they are generally believed to occur from a repetitive cyclic overload by submaximal forces. The rate of the cyclic forces causes breakdown of the bone that is faster than the bone's remodeling capacity, and this results in a stress fracture. Stress fractures most commonly affect the weight-loaded lower extremities, with the tibia being the most commonly affected bone. However, stress fractures of the pubic rami are common, especially among long distance running athletes. There also appears to be an association with anorexia and amenorrhea among female athletes. Barrow and Saha (1) reported that stress fractures occurred in 49% of collegiate female distance runners that had less than five menses per year. In addition, of those athletes that were amenorrheic, 47% had an eating disorder.

The most common presenting history for a stress fracture is that of an insidious onset of lower pelvic and groin pain that is worsened with weight-loading activities. Many times the pain will be worse just after running. The pain will gradually improve with rest. Often the athlete will report a recent increase in their training. Stress fractures can sometimes be seen on plain radiographs, but often they are not evident because of the lack of callous formation. Therefore, if a stress fracture is suspected, a bone scan or magnetic resonance imaging (MRI) is the test of choice (2).

The most common area of pelvic involvement is the inferior pubic rami, but stress fractures can also occur in other parts of the pelvis. Of particular concern, although not strictly part of the pelvis, are stress fractures of the femoral neck. An unrecognized stress fracture of the femoral neck can go on to complete fracture with the potential for avascular necrosis. This can have catastrophic consequences, so early recognition and treatment is the key. One study reported on 23 athletes with femoral neck stress fractures (3). Of the seven patients that developed complications, five had a displaced fracture. This stresses the importance of early recognition and treatment of these injuries to prevent displacement.

Treatment of stress fractures about the pelvis, except for femoral neck fractures, is relatively straightforward. This involves a period of rest, generally about 4 to 6 weeks, from the inciting activities followed by a gradual return to pain-free activities. Any dietary or hormonal issues must also be addressed to assist in healing and prevention of recurrence.

Treatment of femoral neck stress fractures is based on the displacement and location of the fracture (4). All displaced fractures require surgical treatment for anatomic reduction and fixation with cannulated screws. Among nondisplaced fractures, fractures that occur on the compression side of the bone, the inferior femoral neck, have a good potential to heal. Therefore, they can generally be treated nonoperatively. Activities should be restricted by pain. This may require a short period of protected weight bearing with crutches. This is followed by a gradual return to normal pain-free activities. It is important to stress that no activity should cause pain either during or after the activity. Progression of healing should be monitored with serial radiographs. Return to light running can usually begin at about 2 to 3 months as long as there is no pain and the radiographs show healing of the fracture.

Treatment of nondisplaced tension side fractures, those on the superior portion of the femoral neck, are best treated with surgical fixation using cannulated screws. This is because tension-sided fractures heal poorly and have a higher propensity to go on to complete fracture. As noted, if complete fracture occurs, avascular necrosis may develop with devastating consequences for the athlete. For nondisplaced fractures treated surgically, return to pain-free light running can begin at about 2 to 3 months.

Avulsion Fractures

Avulsion fractures about the pelvis occur almost exclusively in the adolescent population. This is due to the relatively weak connection that the apophysis makes with the central bony skeleton through the zone of provisional calcification of the growth plate. The powerful muscle contractions that are possible from the muscles about the hip and pelvis are occasionally able to overpower the growth plate and cause avulsion fractures.

There are three typical locations for avulsion fractures of the pelvis: anterior superior iliac spine, anterior inferior iliac spine, and ischial tuberosity. Avulsions from the anterior superior iliac spine typically occur from a strong contraction of the sartorius muscle during jumping in sports, such as in basketball. Anterior inferior iliac spine avulsions occur in kicking sports, such as soccer, resulting from a violent contraction of the rectus femoris muscle. Avulsions of the ischial tuberosity occur from hamstring contractions and are most frequently seen in running and hurdling sports. For avulsion fractures of the anterior superior iliac spine and anterior inferior iliac spine, most authors recommend nonoperative treatment that includes symptomatic activity restriction until the fracture heals. Although there are no large series in the literature, it does not appear that operative fixation offers any advantages over nonoperative treatment either in terms of return to activity or return of strength (5). The one area of controversy is in treatment of the ischial tuberosity avulsions. Though again there are no large series reported, some have indicated no functional deficits after nonoperative treatment (6), whereas others have reported a decrease in strength and function resulting from "widely displaced" fractures (7). In addition, these fractures can sometimes cause exuberant callus formation that can cause pain and can occasionally mimic an osteosarcoma (8). For these cases, some have advocated early surgical fixation (7), whereas others have indicated that late excision of the exuberant callus can be performed if necessary (5). We presently believe that large fragments that are displaced more than 1 to 2 cm warrant surgical reduction and fixation.

Osteitis Pubis

Osteitis pubis is a disorder of unknown cause. It is characterized by pain at the pubic symphysis that can be referred to the surrounding area to include the lower abdomen, hip, groin, scrotum, or perineum. The diagnosis is confirmed by the typical radiographic or bone scan findings.

The incidence of osteitis pubis among athletes is uncertain, but in one study of overuse injuries, osteitis pubis was implicated as the cause in 6.3% of the cases (9). In this series, men were affected twice as often as women, and most cases involved runners or soccer players. A second study of 59 patients with osteitis pubis found a male-to-female ratio of about 5 to 1 with an average age of presentation of about 30 years (10).

The exact etiology of osteitis pubis is undetermined. However, abnormal biomechanics of the pubic symphy-

sis has been implicated as the probable cause. In normal subjects it has been demonstrated that pubic symphysis movements are restricted to less than 2 mm (11). In one radiographic review, all patients that had greater than 2 mm of mobility had pubic symphysis pain (12). It is probable that stiffness and restricted motion from other joints about the pelvis contribute to increased motion and stress being placed on the pubic symphysis. Miller et al. (13) showed, in a cadaveric study, that fixation of the sacroiliac joint caused large increases in rotations and translations through the remaining joints. During sports-related weight-loading activities such as running and jumping, there is cyclic loading of the pubic symphysis. If the athlete has increased mobility of the pubic symphysis and/or stiffness of the hip joint or sacroiliac joint, the stresses across the pubic symphysis will be increased. This can lead to pain and radiographic changes about the joint.

As stated earlier, typical symptoms include pubic symphysis pain with pain also referred to the surrounding area. In the study by Fricker et al. (10), 80% of the patients had adductor pain, most often unilateral; 30% of patients had abdominal pain; and 12% had hip pain. Tenderness at the pubic symphysis was present in 70% of the cases. Typical radiographic changes were described by Harris and Murray (14): symmetric bone resorption, widening of the symphysis, and sclerosis along the rami. Differential diagnosis should include hyperparathyroidism, sarcoidosis, hemochromatosis, rheumatoid arthritis, and osteomyelitis.

Diagnosis can be assisted by technetium-99m isotope bone scanning that will show increased uptake at the pubic symphysis. Uptake will be greatest on the delayed views, indicating increased bone turnover. Fricker et al. (10), however, reported poor correlation between radiographic changes and clinical symptoms, with some symptomatic patients having no radiographic changes or isotope uptake on bone scan. In addition, radiographic changes and bone scan isotope uptake did not seem to correlate well with the duration or intensity of symptoms.

Given the above, it is evident that osteitis pubis is poorly understood, poorly defined, and may include several different etiologic processes. This makes the design of treatment protocols difficult. Despite this, the disease appears to be self-limiting. Therapies that may speed recovery have been advocated, although these have not been scientifically verified. The most obvious of these is reducing the athlete's activity level. Pounding type cyclic activities such as running should be substituted with nonpainful activities such as swimming. Appropriate stretching and strengthening exercises of the surrounding joints and musculature should be instituted. Particular attention should be paid to hip range of motion and adductor stretching and strengthening. Shock-absorbing shoes may also play an important role in reducing the shear forces across the symphysis.

Nonsteroidal anti-inflammatories may assist in recovery, but their utility has not been investigated. Corticosteroid injections may have a role in hastening the course of the disease. Holt et al. (15) reported good results after steroid injection, with most of their athletes returning to competition within 3 weeks of the injection. However, several athletes required repeat injections, and no noninjected control population was available. This makes interpretation of their results difficult, because osteitis pubis is a self-limited process that typically resolves without such measures. However, it is not unusual for conservative treatment to require a 6- to 9-month course for symptom resolution. The average time for return to sports in the study by Fricker et al. was 9.6 months (10). The relatively short duration of symptoms after steroid injection is encouraging.

ABDOMINAL WALL

Injuries about the abdominal wall fall into three basic categories: abdominal wall muscle and tendon injuries, sports hernia, and nerve compression injuries. Bear in mind that, as discussed previously, other more serious medical and intraabdominal problems can cause and/or mimic these orthopedic-related injuries. Therefore, it is important to take both a good medical and orthopedic history to obtain the correct diagnosis.

Abdominal Wall Muscle Strains

There is little discussion in the literature about abdominal muscle strains. This is surprising because these injuries seem to be fairly common among athletes and probably represent the most common athletic injury to the abdomen. The muscle groups that are susceptible to injury are the internal and external obliques, the rectus abdominus, and the iliopsoas. Injury to these muscles can take several weeks to improve. This is because it is difficult to completely rest these muscles because of their use in maintaining posture and controlling intraabdominal pressure for breathing and bowel and bladder control.

Most commonly, the athlete will implicate a specific event during which the injury occurred. This will be a violent contraction of the muscle against resistance with the muscle maximally stretched. Nearly all muscle strains occur just adjacent to the musculotendinous junction (16).

Injury to the oblique muscles of the abdomen will occur during twisting motions of the trunk. Sometimes the fibers that insert onto the anterior portion of the iliac crest can be disrupted, resulting in a "hip pointer." The athlete will have tenderness along the injured muscle, and iliac crest, if involved. Pain will be increased with passive stretch of the muscles by contralateral bending and by activation of the muscle by twisting and flexing the abdomen.

Similar problems result from strains of the rectus abdominus muscle. Although theoretically there should be less discomfort during trunk rotation, it is sometimes difficult to isolate the involved muscle group, and it is not uncommon to have injury to several muscle groups of the abdomen at the same time. Fortunately, treatment protocols are the same, so in practicality this is not of much concern.

Iliopsoas injuries occur during forceful resisted flexion of the hip. A sharp pain will occur in the groin region that may radiate up into the lower abdomen. Passive external rotation and hip extension and resisted hip flexion will cause pain. In adolescents, an avulsion fracture of the lesser tuberosity can occur, but in adults the same mechanism would cause an injury to the musculotendinous junction.

Treatment of musculotendinous injuries is outlined in detail in the section on adductor strains. In short, this is based on a graduated program of initially reducing inflammation and further injury, followed by range of motion exercises, and a step-wise return to activities that is limited by pain.

Sports Hernia

Sports hernia refers to a condition of chronic groin pain caused by a weakness of the posterior inguinal wall without a clinically obvious hernia. Because of the insidious onset and nonspecific nature of the symptoms, there is often a prolonged course before diagnosis. In one study, the average duration of symptoms was 20 months, with a range of 6 weeks to 5 years (17).

Athletes with a sports hernia will typically complain of an insidious onset of gradually worsening groin pain that he or she may attribute to repeated adductor strains. However, this pain is felt "deeper," slightly more proximal, and may be more intense. Kicking tends to increase the symptoms, as will endurance running. The pain tends to be diffuse with radiation along the inguinal ligament, the perineum, the rectus muscles, adductor muscles, and sometimes to the opposite side. Testicular pain is a component in about 30% male cases (18). A history of increased pain during maneuvers that cause increased intraabdominal pressure such as coughing, sneezing, or during bowel movements can assist in the diagnosis.

Physical findings are sometimes difficult to interpret. The patient will often have associated adductor spasm and may have tenderness of the surrounding area. The most specific signs, however, are tenderness and enlargement of the external ring of the inguinal canal and tenderness of the posterior wall of the inguinal canal.

The tenderness is worst at the posterior wall, and sometimes a bulge can be felt with increased intraabdominal pressure from coughing. In any case, the pain will be exacerbated during coughing. If the exam is questionable, an exam after vigorous exercise may be more helpful. The exam must be performed through the scrotum, so that all structures can be felt adequately. In addition, a scrotal and testicular exam are necessary to exclude tumors.

In cases with obvious clinical signs and symptoms, the diagnosis of a hernia is straightforward. This is usually not the case for sports hernias, however, and in those athletes with continued groin pain despite adequate rest and no obvious hernia, herniography can be of great value. Smedberg et al. (19) have shown that herniography is accurate in disclosing nonpalpable hernias. A typical positive herniographic radiograph is shown in Figure 12.1.

Herniography is performed by injecting contrast medium into the peritoneal cavity under local anesthesia (20). The contrast can be injected under fluoroscopic control to ensure correct positioning. After injection of the dye, the patient should be placed in the reverse Trendelenburg position so the dye pools to the inferior peritoneal cavity along the inguinal canal, and the athlete is then asked to perform a Valsalva maneuver. Radiographs of the lower pelvis are taken to detect bulging through the inguinal canal or contrast leaks extending through the canal and into the scrotum. Few complications have been reported with herniography (21). Puncture of the intestine with the small needle can occur, but as long as no aspiration occurs at that time, further problems are rare. Peritonitis from the contrast medium has been reported, but this is uncommon with the new

water-soluble contrasts (21). Herniography is contraindicated in patients with incarcerated hernias or a history of previous abdominal surgery or bowel obstruction. Incarcerated or irreducible hernias may give false-negative results because the contrast will be unable to leak through the defect.

If a true sports hernia is present, nonoperative treatment is rarely successful. The difficulty lies in making a correct diagnosis, and not all hernias are symptomatic. Therefore, it is always prudent to initially treat groin pain with a conservative approach. This includes a period of rest (for several weeks) followed by a gradual return to activities. If the pain continues despite these measures and no other problem is detected by exam or other tests, herniography may implicate sports hernia as the probable cause.

Treatment of painful sports hernia is by operative repair of the weak posterior inguinal wall. A variety of open procedures has been described to reinforce the posterior wall, either by plication and tightening of the existing tissue or by reinforcement with mesh. Results of these open procedures have been about the same, with about 90% success for full return to sports (18). Recently, laparoscopic procedures have been developed for hernia repair. This involves placement of synthetic mesh over the defect superficial to the peritoneum (22). Early results have been relatively encouraging with recurrence rates near open procedures (23,24). However, the procedure is technically difficult with a significant learning curve (25), and the procedure is much more costly than open procedures (23).

Nerve Compression

Nerve entrapment in the groin is a rare condition. When it occurs, pain is caused by the nerve being compressed as it passes through fibrous tunnels or between muscles. Extrinsic factors such as local edema, excess scar formation from previous surgical incisions, or compression due to clothing or equipment can contribute to nerve compression. Symptoms will be related to the nerve being compressed. The most commonly affected nerves in the abdomen and groin region are the ilioinguinal nerve, genitofemoral nerve, and the lateral cutaneous nerve of the thigh (26). The athlete will have tenderness at the site of compression, with pain radiating out to the area of the nerve's distribution (Fig. 12.2). Diagnosis can be verified by relief of symptoms after injection of local anesthetic at the compression site.

Treatment is by removal of external compressive sources by measures such as controlling edema and removing compressive equipment and clothing. Sometimes desensitization can occur by local massage, or the lesion will improve with time. If these measure fail, surgical neurolysis will relieve the pain.

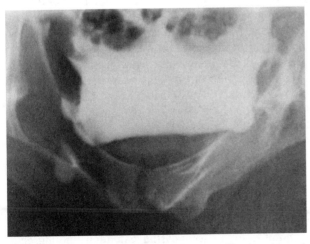

FIG. 12.1. Typical radiograph showing a positive herniograph revealing a direct hernia. (From Ekberg O, Kesek P, Besjakov J. Herniography and magnetic resonance imaging in athletes with chronic groin pain. *Sports Med Arthrosc Rev* 1997;5: 274–279, with permission.)

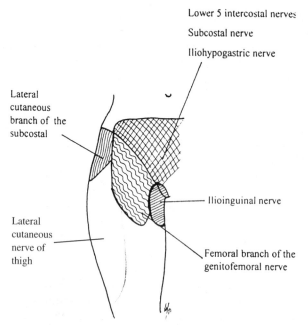

FIG. 12.2. Cutaneous nerve distribution around the groin. (From O'Brien M, Delaney M. The anatomy of the hip and groin. *Sports Med Arthrosc Rev* 1997;5:252–267, with permission.)

ADDUCTOR STRAINS

The exact incidence of groin pain in athletes is unknown. Prospective soccer studies in Scandinavia have reported groin injury rates of between 10 and 18 injuries per 100 soccer players (27,28). Renstrom and Peterson (29) found that 62% of groin injuries were from the adductor longus muscle–tendon unit (Fig. 12.3). Lovell (30) reported on 189 cases of chronic groin pain. He attributed 30% of the cases to adductor injuries and 20% of the cases to osteitis pubis. However, differentiating the two may be difficult, because adductor injury can have associated radiologic changes and osteitis pubis can have

associated adductor pain and/or tenderness. Determining which came first is problematic, and even developing a clear definition of each syndrome is difficult, because there is no real agreement in the literature. It is evident, however, that adductor pain is not uncommon in sports.

Several factors have been suggested as predisposing the adductors to injury (31). The muscles about the pelvis are subjected to very high loads and are partly responsible for maintaining stability of the hip. Anything that disturbs the muscular balance, such as unequal leg lengths or foot or lower leg malalignment syndromes, can increase the loads supported by the adductors. In addition, the tendon fibers insert into an area of poor blood supply, because of both the small insertion site and the relatively poor blood supply to the pubic bone itself.

The diagnosis of acute muscle strains is usually relatively straightforward. The athlete will present with a history of sudden injury to the groin. Often, as with most muscle strains, the injury occurs during a vigorous eccentric contraction, as can happen when two opposing soccer players try to kick the ball. The athlete will have pain and tenderness in the groin, and swelling and ecchymosis may be present. Occasionally, a defect in the muscle will be felt at the site of injury. The most common area of injury is just adjacent to the musculotendinous junction, although complete avulsions from the insertion do rarely occur. Typical adductor strains are easily diagnosed with clinical exam, and other studies are generally not needed. In unusual cases an ultrasound, computed tomography, or MRI will show the injury well.

Most adductor strains are incomplete strains and can be treated with nonoperative rehabilitation. Complete tears in athletes will generally do better with surgical repair, but this is rarely necessary. Treatment of partial acute adductor strains is based on the general biologic principles of healing. The rehabilitation protocol can be divided into four stages, as suggested by Sim and Scott (32). Stage I is based on limiting the swelling and preventing further injury. This involves rest, ice, and compression. Protected weight bearing may be necessary for a short period of time. Pain-causing activities must be avoided during this period. Stage I continues until the acute pain and swelling decrease; this is usually between 2 days to a week. Nonsteroidal anti-inflammatory medications can be used to control pain and to decrease swelling, but care should be exercised in their use due to their increased anticoagulatory effects and the delay that they cause in mature scar formation.

Stage II is based on limiting atrophy and restoring range of motion. This prevents the adverse effects of immobilization on joint cartilage, tendon, and musculature. Gentle passive and active assisted motion should begin. The range of motion exercises should be limited by pain. The athlete should begin to wean off of ambulatory assistive devices at this time. Physical therapy mo-

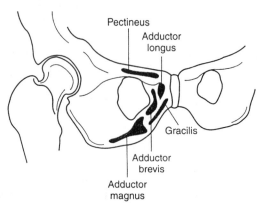

FIG. 12.3. Adductor muscle insertions onto the pelvis. (From Holmich P. Adductor-related groin pain in athletes. *Sports Med Arthrosc Rev* 1997;5:285–290, with permission.)

dalities can be added at this time, but their utility has not been scientifically verified.

Stage III begins when the athlete has nearly full pain-free range of motion. This phase is based on regaining strength, flexibility, and endurance. First isometric and then isokinetic exercises are begun, initially starting with low weight and many repetitions. The athlete can progress to heavier weight with fewer repetitions as his or her pain-free strength improves.

The final stage is based on returning the athlete to his or her sport. Exercises include proprioceptive and agility drills, with sport-specific training. This stage can usually begin when the athlete has reached about 70% of normal strength and is pain free.

Most athletes will do well after nonoperative therapy for acute adductor injuries. However, some athletes will develop chronic problems after acute injuries, and others will develop chronic pain without an known acute injury. These athletes are more difficult to treat. Athletes with chronic pain often have more diffuse pain that is difficult to attribute to specific structures. Indeed, the presentations for osteitis pubis, sports hernia, and chronic adductor pain are quite similar, and these entities can be present simultaneously. These symptoms include pain along the adductor tendon and insertion with radiation along the muscle. The pain will typically worsen with athletic activities, particularly when cutting and twisting movements are added. Imaging studies are sometimes helpful to eliminate other possible causes of the pain. These can include plain radiographs or a bone scan to show typical changes of osteitis pubis or herniography to rule out sports hernia. In addition, an ultrasound or MRI can evaluate the tendon structure for intrasubstance abnormalities.

Treatment of chronic groin pain is based on a graduated exercise and activity program (33). The first step of the program is to reduce the athlete's activity level to a nonpainful level. This means that the activity should not cause pain either during or after the exercise. This is sometimes hard to accomplish in a competitive athlete. Therefore, it is important to educate the athlete about the nature and suspected course of the problem. The next step in the process is to regain range of motion and flexibility. Once this is achieved, light strengthening activities can begin. The goal here is to reeducate the muscle and increase blood flow to the region to promote healing. This is achieved with low-resistance multiple-repetition exercises. Once pain-free exercises are achieved, higher resistance strengthening can progress with caution, and this should then go on to include eccentric muscle training. This should also be nonpainful during and after the exercise. The importance of addressing the surrounding muscle groups should also not be underestimated. For example, adductor training should also include exercises for abdominal and gluteal strengthening.

If the nonoperative therapy is unsuccessful after a minimum of several months of treatment, operative intervention can be considered. Before adductor surgery, other causes, such as sports hernia or osteitis pubis, should be ruled out. If the athlete meets these criteria, adductor tenotomy can improve the symptoms. Akermark et al. (34) performed adductor tenotomy on 16 athletes. All patients improved, with 10 returning to previous sports activities and 5 returning to sports at a lower level. Postoperatively, the patients did have decreased isokinetic strength compared with the normal side, but this did not seem to affect their ability to participate in athletics.

CONCLUSIONS

A high index of suspicion must be maintained for other nonorthopedic problems around the lower abdomen, pelvis, and groin. This will ensure that the more serious nonorthopedic diseases are not overlooked, and treatment is not delayed.

Management of pelvic, abdominal wall, and adductor injuries can be challenging. The overlap of symptoms between the different diagnoses is great, so this makes diagnosis of a specific injury difficult. This requires careful clinical exam and history taking and judicious use of special tests. Once a diagnosis is reached, aggressive nonoperative treatment should begin. Athletes who neglect or mismanage these injuries are at risk for developing chronic pain. Once the pain reaches this level, it becomes increasingly difficult to treat. Information about chronic groin problem is limited and based mostly on clinical experience. Controlled trials are needed to improve treatment protocols.

Fortunately, if treated early, most acute problems will heal well and the athlete will be able to return to his or her sport. However, problems in this anatomic region are notorious for taking a long time to heal, and therefore patience must be exercised to avoid returning to activities too early.

REFERENCES

1. Barrow G, Saha S. Menstrual irregularity and stress fractures in collegiate female distance runners. *Am J Sports Med* 1988;16: 209–216.
2. Norfray J, Schlaschter L, Kernahan W. Early confirmation of stress fractures in joggers. *JAMA* 1980;243:1647–1649.
3. Johansson C, Ekenman I, Tornkvist H, et al. Stress fractures of the femoral neck in athletes. *Am J Sports Med* 1990;18:524–528.
4. Devas M. *Stress fractures*. New York: Churchill Livingstone, 1975.
5. Gross M, Nasser S, Finerman G. Hip and pelvis. In: DeLee J, Drez J, eds. *Orthopaedic sports medicine*. Vol. 2. Philadelphia: W.B. Saunders, 1994:1063–1085.
6. Metzmaker J, Pappas A. Avulsion fractures of the pelvis. *Am J Sports Med* 1985;13:349–358.
7. Schlonsky J, Olix M. Functional disability following avulsion fracture of the ischial epiphysis. *J Bone Joint Surg Am* 1972;54A: 641–644.
8. Canale S, King R. Pelvic and hip fractures. In: Rockwood C,

Wilkins K, King R, eds. *Fractures in children.* Philadelphia: J.B. Lippincott, 1984:

9. Lloyd-Smith R, Clement D, McKenzie D, et al. A survey of overuse and traumatic hip and pelvic injuries in athletes. *Phys Sports Med* 1985;13:131–141.

10. Fricker P, Taunton J, Ammann W. Osteitis pubis in athletes: Infection, inflammation or injury? *Sports Med* 1991;12:266–279.

11. Walheim G, Olerun S, Ribbe T. Mobility of the pubic symphysis. Measurements by an electromechanical method. *Acta Orthop Scand* 1984;55:203–208.

12. Chamberlain W. The symphysis pubis in the roentgen examination of the sacro-iliac joint. *AJR Am J Roentgenol* 1930;24:621–625.

13. Miller J, Schultz A, Anderson G. Load-displacement behavior of sacroiliac joints. *J Orthop Res* 1987;5:92–101.

14. Harris N, Murray R. Lesions of the symphysis in athletes. *Br Med J* 1974;4:211–214.

15. Holt H, Keene J, Graf B, et al. Treatment of osteitis pubis in athletes. Results of corticosteroid injections. *Am J Sports Med* 1995;23:601–606.

16. Garrett W, Safran M, Seaber A, et al. Biomechanical comparison of stimulated and nonstimulated skeletal muscle pulled to failure. *Am J Sports Med* 1993;21:89–96.

17. Hackney R. The sports hernia. *Br J Sports Med* 1993;27:58–61.

18. Hackney R. The sports hernia. *Sports Med Arthrosc Rev* 1997;5:320–325.

19. Smedberg S, Broome A, Elmer O, et al. Herniography in primary inguinal and femoral hernia: an analysis of 283 operated cases. *Contemp Surg* 1990;36:48.

20. Smedberg S, Broome A, Elmer O, et al. Herniography in the diagnosis of obscure groin pain. *Acta Chir Scand* 1985;151:663–667.

21. Ekberg O. Complications after herniography in adults. *AJR Am J Roentgenol* 1983;140:491–495.

22. Smedberg S. Herniography and laparoscopic hernia surgery: developments in the diagnosis and treatment of hernias. *Sports Med Arthrosc Rev* 1997;5:313–319.

23. Payne J, Grininger L, Izawa M, et al. Laparoscopic or open inguinal herniorrhaphy? A randomized prospective trial. *Arch Surg* 1994;129:973–979.

24. Liem M, van der Graff Y, van Steensel C, et al. Comparison of conventional anterior surgery and laparoscopic surgery for inguinal hernia repair. *N Engl J Med* 1997;336:1541–1547.

25. Liem M, van Steensel C, Boelhouwer R, et al. The learning curve for totally extraperitoneal laparoscopic inguinal hernia repair. *Am J Surg* 1996;171:281–285.

26. Westlin N. Groin pain in athletes from southern Sweden. *Sports Med Arthrosc Rev* 1997;5:280–284.

27. Nielsen A, Yde J. Epidemiology and traumatology of injuries in soccer. *Am J Sports Med* 1989;17:803–807.

28. Engstrom B, Forssblad M, Johansson C, et al. Does a major knee injury definitely sideline an elite soccer player? *Am J Sports Med* 1990;18:101–105.

29. Renstrom P, Peterson L. Groin injuries in athletes. *Br J Sports Med* 1980;14:30–36.

30. Lovell G. The diagnosis of chronic groin pain in athletes: a review of 189 cases. *Aust J Sci Med Sport* 1995;27:76–79.

31. Holmich P. Adductor-related groin pain in athletes. *Sports Med Arthrosc Rev* 1997;5:285–290.

32. Sim F, Scott H. Injuries of the pelvis and hip in athletes. In: Nicholas J, Hershmann E, eds. *The lower extremity and spine in sports medicine.* St. Louis: C.V. Mosby, 1986:

33. Dahan R. Rehabilitation of muscle-tendon injuries to the hip, pelvis, and groin areas. *Sports Med Arthrosc Rev* 1997;5:326–333.

34. Akermark C, Johansson C. Tenotomy of the adductor longus in the treatment of chronic pain in athletes. *Am J Sports Med* 1992;20:640–643.

35. Ekberg O, Kesek P, Besjakov J. Herniography and magnetic resonance imaging in athletes with chronic groin pain. *Sports Med Arthrosc Rev* 1997;5:274–279.

36. O'Brien M, Delaney M. The anatomy of the hip and groin. *Sports Med Arthrosc Rev* 1997;5:252–267.

Principles and Practice of Orthopaedic Sports Medicine,
edited by William E. Garrett, Jr., Kevin P. Speer, and Donald T. Kirkendall.
Lippincott Williams & Wilkins, Philadelphia © 2000.

CHAPTER 13

Athletic Pubalgia and Groin Pain

William C. Meyers, Rocco Ricciardi, Brian D. Busconi,
Bert R. Mandelbaum, and Richard J. Waite

For years, lower abdominal pain has ended the careers of many gifted athletes. These injuries in Major League Soccer, the National Hockey League, and the National Football League have received much media attention. However, the pathophysiologic processes involved in these presumptive injuries have been poorly understood. In 1992 we reported success with an operation for a particular pattern of inguinal pain in a limited number of athletes (1). This success led to a much larger experience (2). We have also improved our knowledge in diagnosing this injury, differentiating it from other injuries and managing the associated symptoms more effectively.

PELVIC ANATOMY

The pelvic girdle (3) is made up of two paired innominate bones, the sacrum and the coccyx. The innominate bone is composed of the ileum, the ischium, and the pubis, which forms a portion of the acetabulum. In the normal state, there is little motion across the joints of the pelvis. However, athletes more commonly stretch these static joints and cause excessive motion at various sites within the pelvis (Fig. 13.1).

Several important structures insert onto the pelvis and its anterior attachment, the pubic symphysis, including the external oblique, internal oblique, transversus abdominis, and rectus abdominis (4). Structures inserting onto the inferior portion of the pelvis include the adductor muscles, pectineus, gracilis, obturator in-

ternus, quadratus femoris, and gluteus muscles. A series of ligamentous arches also exist between the pelvic bones, stabilizing the organ (5).

As stated earlier, athletes often exert considerable forces across the joints, muscles, tendons, and ligaments of the pelvis. With these destructive forces, damage can occur to any part of the athlete's pelvis, manifesting itself as groin pain. Even though a complete description of the anatomy of the pelvis is beyond the scope of this chapter, a thorough understanding of the anatomy is essential to diagnose and treat these injuries.

MECHANISM OF INJURY

The rectus tendon insertion on the pubis seems to be the primary site of pathology in athletic pubalgia. Most patients describe a hyperextension injury in association with hyper abduction of the thigh (Fig. 13.2). The pivot point seems to be the anterior pelvis and pubic symphysis. The location of pain suggests that the injury involves both the rectus abdominus and adductor longus muscles. Other tendinous insertion sites on the pubic bone may also be involved.

The location and progression of pain in these athletes suggests a disruption of the pivot apparatus and a redistribution of forces to other musculotendinous attachments during extremes of exercise. The accompanying inflammation includes osteitis, tendonitis, or bursitis, which contributes to the pain. This inflammation can often be corrected temporarily by injections or anti-inflammatory drugs. Deep massage therapy may also be effective. However, the lack of permanent relief by these methods suggests that the inflammation is not the primary problem and that stabilization of the anterior pelvis is necessary (6).

The pattern of symptoms in these patients, operative findings, and results of our studies all suggest that the

W. C. Meyers, R. Ricciardi, B. D. Busconi, R. J. Waite: Department of Surgery, University of Massachusetts Medical Center, Worcester, Massachusetts 01655.

B. R. Mandelbaum: Santa Monica Orthopaedic and Sports Medicine Group, Santa Monica, California 90404.

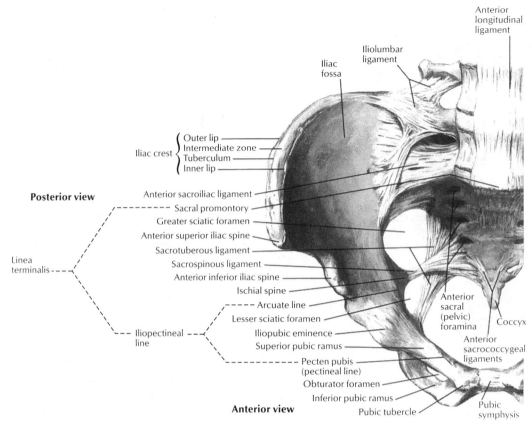

FIG. 13.1. The pelvic bones and ligamentous attachments. (From Netter FH. *Atlas of human anatomy.* New Jersey: CIBA Collection, 1989, plate 335, with permission.)

lower abdominal/inguinal pain in these patients is not due to occult hernia. By definition, none of the patients has evidence of a preoperative hernia, although some patients are found to have occult hernias at the time of surgery. Furthermore, when this did occur, the hernia was usually found on the side opposite the principal symptoms (7).

The principal complaint of hernia patients is usually a bulge with superior and lateral inguinal pain, consistent with the location of the internal ring. The pain in most pubalgia patients is near the pubis, far from the internal ring. In over 80% of pubalgia cases, the pain is also associated with an adduction of the hip against resistance. Progression of pain often involves the adductors, perineal regions, and eventually the opposite side. The combination of a distinct injury, localized pain, and progression suggests an initial injury with subsequent involvement of other structures adjacent to the injury. We doubt that the problem involves multiple different injuries, particularly because most of these patients often describe a single inciting injury.

DEFINITIONS AND EPIDEMIOLOGY

Many people are afflicted with groin pain, including athletes and nonathletes alike. The differential diagnosis in these patients is extremely important. In this chapter, we confine our comments primarily to abdominal/groin pain in athletes. The term "athlete" refers to patients actively or recently participating in competitive athletic

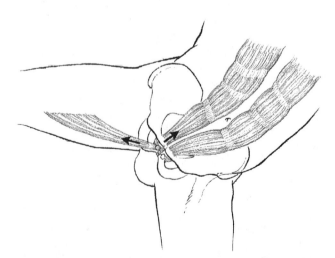

FIG. 13.2. The rectus abdominis and adductor longus tendon insertions on the pelvis. In athletic pubalgia, the typical injury pattern is a hyperextension of the abdomen with hyperabduction of the thigh.

activity as a livelihood or integral way of life. The term "athletic pubalgia" refers to chronic inguinal or pubic area pain in athletes, which is noted solely on exertion and not explainable preoperatively by demonstrable hernia or other medical diagnoses.

For the most part, patients that are afflicted with this injury are high-performance athletes. Although performance athletes and nonathletes have a similar potential for this syndrome, in general, nonathletes may not seek medical attention for what they perceive as minor problems. Most athletes examined have the potential to be pain free if they could become more sedentary. However, such a drastic life-style change is generally not in the best interest of these patients.

This injury seems to occur most commonly during autumn sports. The incidence is listed in decreasing order: soccer, hockey, football, track and field, baseball, basketball, racquet sports, and swimming. Over 90% of the patients that we have seen with this problem are male. Most females are found to have other causes for their pain (8). The other diagnosis that commonly causes this pain in women is endometriosis. We do not know the precise explanation for the difference in gender incidence. The observation seems attributable either to a relatively low participation (until recently) of females in highly competitive sports or a real difference in pelvic anatomy. Our thought is that the latter explanation is much more likely.

Data from eight trainers in Major League Soccer and the National Hockey League estimate that 9% of players on a given team suffer or will suffer from a syndrome consistent with athletic pubalgia. Another 12% of players have some minor degree of chronic discomfort, which is not disabling. Up to 18% of players had some type of "groin pull" in the past but with subsequent recovery (1). In another uncontrolled survey of one professional team, 4% of players over a 5-year period retired because of groin pain. This problem was the leading cause of injury-related retirement for that team (9).

The above surveys suggest that groin problems are extremely common in high-performance athletes and that roughly half the patients recover from acute injuries without significant sequelae; the other half of patients are divided into two groups, one in which the chronic pain is minor and the other group in which the pain is severe enough to require significant medical or surgical attention (10).

Over a 10-year time period we have seen this syndrome in only a small number of nonathletes. This small number represents less than 10% of cases that were evaluated for the suspicion of athletic pubalgia. Most nonathletes sought medical attention because of publicity related to successful repairs in athletes. In contrast with the 95% success rate in the athletes, successful repair occurred in less than half of the nonathletes who underwent similar operations. The operated nonathletes also had more diffuse symptoms and were more likely to be involved with legal claims and workman's compensation.

CLINICAL CONSIDERATIONS

Like other sports medicine physicians, we were slow to recognize that the syndrome of athletic pubalgia was surgically correctable. Prevalent attitudes of general surgeons had been against performing "hernia repairs" for inguinal pain in the absence of preoperatively detectable inguinal hernias (11). While we followed several patients with groin pain with conservative management in the mid-1980s, we heard reports from Nesovic (12) in Yugoslavia that suggested the problem was not occult hernia but instead secondary to an unstable pelvis. Therefore, an operation was devised to correct the problem by treating the instability.

The syndrome is apparently distinct in high-performance athletes. Most of these athletes face an end to their career because of groin pain. The syndrome's features include disabling lower abdominal/inguinal pain at extremes of exertion. The pain progresses over months to years and involves the adductor longus tendons and the contralateral inguinal or adductor regions. Occasionally, magnetic resonance imaging (MRI) or surgical pathologic findings actually demonstrate the disruption of the abdominal rectus muscle from the pubis, but generally the diagnosis is empiric.

Most patients remember a distinct injury during exertion. Usually, the abdominal pain involves the inguinal canal near the insertion of the rectus muscle on the pubis (1,13). The pain causes most patients to stop competing in sports.

The pain is noted to be minimal at rest and begins unilaterally but becomes bilateral within months or years if the injury is untreated. Concurrent problems on the opposite sides occur occasionally after repair, although subsequent contralateral involvement is infrequent (14). Two thirds of patients describe pain with an adduction of the hip, which can be more prominent than the abdominal findings. The pain may also be fleeting: appearing and disappearing on one or the other side or involving both abdominal and adductor components. Less than one fourth of patients have significant symptoms attributable to the posterior perineum. Interestingly, involvement of the posterior perineum is associated with a decreased likelihood of successful repair.

When examining a patient suspected of having athletic pubalgia, the physical exam must be directed to obtain key findings. Most patients exhibit pain with adduction of the hip against resistance (10). A fourth of patients have pubic or peripubic tenderness. A third of patients have some degree of subjective tenderness along the adductor tendons near the pubis. Superior inguinal or real abdominal tenderness is uncommon. By definition, no patients have hernias.

As mentioned, MRI findings are usually nonspecific. On the other hand, 12% of patients have MRI findings that clearly indicate a problem at the rectus insertion site. The relatively small incidence of a specific diagnosis by imaging studies suggests that the problem may be an attenuation of the muscle or tendon due to repeated microtrauma (10).

Nonspecific MRI findings, which occur frequently, do localize to the side or sides of injury in over 90% of patients. The nonspecific findings include focal osteitis and nonspecific abdominal wall, perineal, or adductor findings. The MRI findings of a patient with groin pain are depicted in Fig. 13.3.

Other common MRI findings include asymmetry, distinct inflammation, cortical irregularity, distinct fluid accumulation, irregularity of the rectus abdominis, atrophic changes, small pelvic avulsion fractures, or disruption of the pectineus muscle. It is possible that these nonspecific MRI findings may assist the surgeon in decision making, because MRI can often predict the side or sides of injury. In addition, the value of MRI has been noted in its demonstration of other severe problems as per the differential diagnosis (15).

Computed tomography and bone scans generally have no added value over MRI even if they show osteitis. In fact, we have seen a number of patients who were initially deemed nonsurgical candidates due to "osteitis pubis" who subsequently had surgery and did very well. Therefore, osteitis is no longer an automatic contraindication for surgery. On the other hand, there is a distinct population of patients who have severe primary osteitis.

They have continuous severe pain and tenderness at rest and/or exercise. This group of patients will not likely be helped by this operation.

OTHER CONSIDERATIONS IN MANAGEMENT

Key questions concerning the surgical management of these patients include the following. Does the patient have symptoms that qualify him or her for the syndrome? How disabling is the syndrome? Can the patient be treated nonoperatively? Can the patient be treated medically on a temporary basis to allow the athlete to finish the season? Should one perform unilateral or bilateral repairs? When should one perform an adductor release? What operations are likely to work? And what is the role of nonoperative therapy?

To answer these questions, definitions and presumptions need to be addressed. "Nonoperative therapy" refers to trials of prolonged rest, physical therapy, oral or injected steroids, or deep massage. The disabling pain has led to a curtailment or cessation of competitive athletic participation and diminution in his or her athletic ability. "Acute" injury refers to pain that has resolved or is clearly better within 2 weeks. "Recurrent acute" refers to evaluation within 2 weeks of a repeat groin injury after complete recovery from an initial episode. "Chronic" refers to the persistence of pain after 6 weeks without evidence of improvement at the time of evaluation.

Again, our data strongly suggest that the principal mechanism of athletic pubalgia is a disruption or attenuation of the rectus muscle insertion on the pubis. This disruption results in instability of the anterior pubis that is manifested by a rearrangement of focus to other mus-

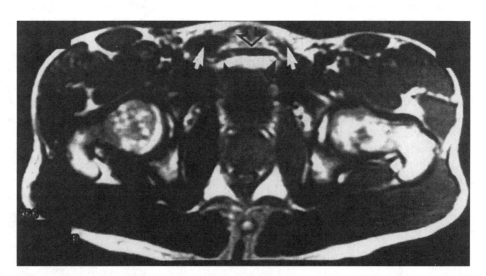

FIG. 13.3. Axial T1-weighted images through the level of the superior aspect of the symphysis pubis. The distal rectus abdominis tendon is noted by the *open black arrow.* There is mild relative enlargement of the right rectus abdominis fascia compared with the left. Also note the bulbous enlargement of the external opening of the right inguinal canal.

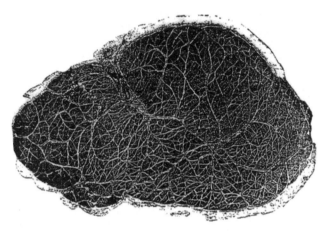

FIG. 13.4. Cross-sectional anatomy of a human sartorious muscle. The epimysium, made up of connective tissue, surrounds the entire muscle, whereas the perimysium surrounds individual muscle fiber. (From Heidenhain, 1911, Plasma and Zella 2 Leif. Jena.)

cular tendinous attachments of the pubis. Therefore, the best repair would be a broad surgical reattachment at the inferolateral edge of the rectus muscle with its fascial investments to the pubis and adjacent anterior ligaments. This is the operation we most commonly use for athletic pubalgia, and in most cases this repair significantly ameliorates or eliminates the adductor symptoms.

On a rare occasion, adductor symptoms may persist after pelvic floor repair and become particularly bothersome. This observation suggests that the adductor symptoms are most likely due to a secondary chronic inflammatory process involving the superior edge of the inferior pubic ramus. This jagged edge rubs on the adjacent soft tissues within the adductor compartment, causing inflammation and pain. The weakening of the anterior abdomen causes a kind of compartment syndrome.

During the evolution in treatment for this disease, it was suggested that an adductor release might help these patients. Thus, an anterior and lateral release of the epimysium of the adductor fascia is currently performed to expand this compartment. The epimysium is the layer of connective tissue that encloses the entire muscle (Fig. 13.4). During an epimysial release, the edema in the groin is noted to be released. This kind of fascial release is often very successful.

TREATMENT ALGORITHMS

We propose the attached algorithms for the treatment of patients diagnosed with athletic pubalgia. Algorithm 1 describes groin injury treatment during the season (Fig. 13.5), whereas algorithm 2 concentrates on treatment between seasons (Fig. 13.6). Generally, only treat the chronic or persistent acute recurrent problems surgi-

cally. Direct steroid injection into symptomatic bursas or other soft tissue sites may give enough temporary relief for patients to continue their season (16). When the process continues over several months and the athlete cannot return to previously expected activity because of pain, an operation should be considered. Deep massage therapy has a role in patients with equivocal symptoms or others in whom surgery for one reason or another is not favored. The effectiveness of deep massage cannot be explained.

RESULTS OF REPAIRS AND RELEASES

A success rate of 95% can be expected from surgical treatment in well-selected patients. This success was observed in 200 patients over a 3-year follow-up. We suggest operating only on the symptomatic side or sides. On the other hand, several patients with particularly severe MRI findings on the opposite side but without symptoms have also undergone bilateral repair with similar success rates.

Our data clearly indicate that many standard hernia repairs are inadequate in treating athletic pubalgia. In particular, laparoscopic hernia repair does not appear to be the correct solution for this problem. The laparoscopic repair emphasizes a "tension-free" mesh insertion that does not stabilize the anterior pelvis. We have seen several patients who have had unsuccessful laparoscopic repairs requiring reoperation.

The generally poor results of the laparoscopic repair and other hernia operations provide additional evidence that the mechanism of athletic pubalgia is not due to an occult hernia. However, a few patients have done well after hernia operations (17–19). The small success rates seem likely due to general fibrosis, which accompanies all operations and inadvertently stabilizes the anterior pelvis. The Cooper's ligament or McVay repair for inguinal hernia seems more likely to treat the problem but also stretches the anterior abdominal musculature down to the more posterior attachments of the pelvis. Therefore, this operation may not provide optimal anterior stabilization. We have seen inconsistent results with the McVay approach; thus, we recommend performing a rectus reattachment and adductor release to treat athletic pubalgia.

DIFFERENTIAL DIAGNOSIS

Several other diagnoses must be considered in patients with groin pain, including other musculoskeletal disorders and more severe visceral problems. Problems that we have encountered in athletes with inguinal pain include inflammatory bowel disease, prostatitis, aseptic necrosis of the hips, herpes, pelvic inflammatory disease, and rectal or testicular cancer (20). These other possible diagnoses emphasize the importance of a detailed care-

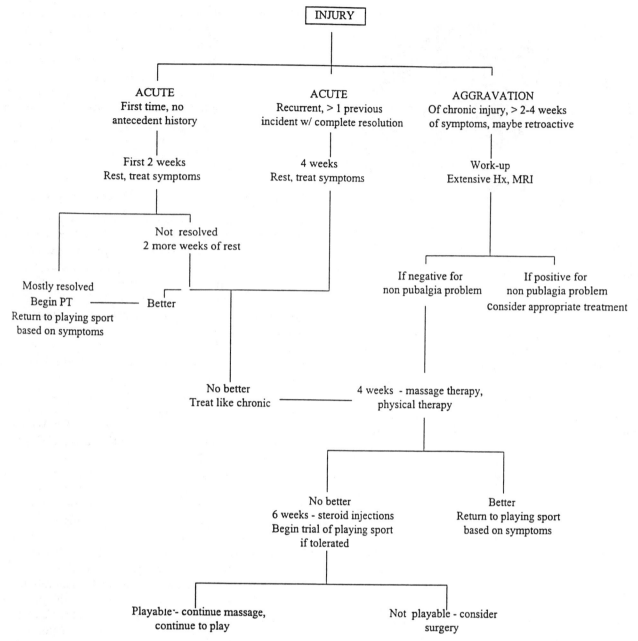

FIG. 13.5. Algorithm for groin injury treatment during the season.

ful history and physical examination and obtaining the appropriate imaging tests. Musculoskeletal syndromes commonly considered in the differential diagnosis of lower abdominal or groin pain in the athlete are discussed in more detail below.

OTHER ADDUCTOR INJURIES

The muscles of hip adduction are the adductor longus, magnus, brevis, and the pectineus muscles and the gracilis in the lower thigh and the gluteus maximus muscle. Each of these muscles has an ascribed syndrome (21).

However, the adductor longus is certainly the most frequently injured of the adductors.

Piriformis and Hamstring Syndromes

The piriformis syndrome is characterized as an evolving compression of the sciatic nerve by the piriformis muscle. The compression occurs where the sciatic nerve exits posterior to the named muscle (7,21). Puranen and Orava (22,23) described the hamstring syndrome, which is often confused with the piriformis syndrome. The syndrome is defined by entrapment of the sciatic nerve

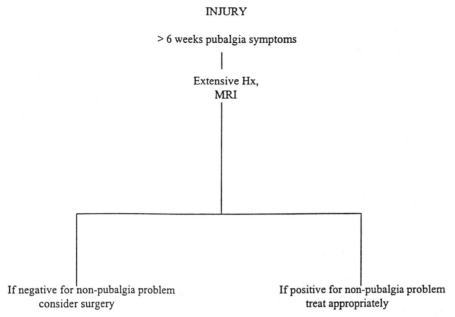

INJURY

> 6 weeks pubalgia symptoms

Extensive Hx,
MRI

If negative for non-pubalgia problem
consider surgery

If positive for non-pubalgia problem
treat appropriately

FIG. 13.6. Algorithm for groin injury treatment between seasons.

between the semitendinosus and biceps femoris by a fibrous band that constricts the two muscles.

Snapping Hip Joint

The "snapping hip joint" syndrome may be caused by a variety of extraarticular or intraarticular pathologies. Perhaps the most important syndrome to recognize is the "iliopsoas syndrome." In this syndrome, the snapping is caused by the iliopsoas tendon gliding over the iliopectineal eminence or lesser trochanter of the femur (20).

Iliopsoas Tendonitis and Iliotibial Band Syndrome

The iliacus and psoas tendons of the iliopsoas muscles conjoin and insert onto the lesser trochanter of the femur. Injuries to this tendon come from forceful contraction of the iliopsoas during flexion or extension (24). The iliotibial band syndrome may be caused by the iliotibial band crossing over the greater trochanter, usually in association with inflammation. Runners or cyclists who undergo repetitive knee flexion are commonly afflicted with this syndrome (21).

Sacroiliac Sprain

In general, the sacral iliac ligaments are strong and injury can only occur with violent contraction of the associated muscles or severe torsion. Bedrest, heat, analgesics, and oral anti-inflammatory agents are the principal methods of treatment (3).

Osteitis Pubis and the Gracilis Syndrome

We strongly believe that there is a primary osteitis pubis syndrome, which can be difficult to treat. On the other hand, most cases of osteitis pubis are secondary to another particular problem. For example, the disease may be related to a previous hernia repair in which infection occurred around sutures placed into the pubis. Traumatic osteitis pubis is a fatigue fracture involving the bony origin of the gracilis muscle at the pubic symphysis (25). When the bony lesion is due to trauma and located at the lower margin of the symphysis, the entity may be appropriately referred to as gracilis syndrome.

Simple Fractures and Stress Fractures

A wide variety of pelvic or hip fractures and other skeletal injuries may occur in the athlete. Pelvic fractures may occur in any area and are uncommon, of course, until the later adolescent years (20). Stress fractures should be considered in athletes who undergo a good deal of chronic repetitive motion, such as long distance runners. The common definition of a stress fracture is repetitive stress below the failure levels of bone in a period inadequate to allow for bony remodeling (26).

Intraarticular Pathology

Intraarticular hip pathology may be an important cause of groin or thigh pain. Some of the more important or more frequent diagnoses to consider include synovitis, loose congenital or traumatic bodies, septic or osteoarthritis, avascular necrosis, torn acetabular labrum, or a hypertrophied ligamentum teres (20,24).

Avascular Necrosis of the Femoral Head

Avascular necrosis in the athlete may occur in children and adults. Legg Calve Perthes disease is characterized by osteonecrosis of the ossific nucleus of the femoral head secondary to occlusion of the arterial or venous blood supply (27). The direct association with athletics is debatable.

Soft Tissue Injuries and Contusions

Soft tissue injuries are the most common injuries of the musculotendinous structures around the hip or pelvis (20). These injuries may result from repetitive microinjury or a specific macroinjury caused by an abnormal biomechanical force.

One should not forget that the most frequent hip, pelvic, or groin injury is a contusion. The most common contusions occur with contact sports, particularly football, but this entity often occurs in baseball when the player lands awkwardly on first base, trying to avoid a tag (24). The athlete should be reassured that he or she will do well with early activity, flexibility, and proper stretching.

Bursitis and Myositis Ossificans

Bursitis is usually the result of a direct blow or an associated hematoma (28). Myositis ossificans can occur with repetitive trauma, causing hematoma ossification and considerable inflammation of the muscle in association with calcification (3). The associated inflammation that causes the specific problem may subside with rest or steroid therapy. Occasionally, surgical treatment is indicated to remove a specific calcification.

CONCLUSIONS

Injuries to the abdomen and groin are common among athletes. Athletic pubalgia is a common chronic cause of inguinal groin pain that is often overlooked. Although the diagnosis of athletic pubalgia can be difficult, a working understanding of pelvic anatomy, mechanism of injury, and physical exam findings, as presented in this chapter, greatly assist the physician in diagnosis and treatment. The described surgical treatment of this disease is very effective because it directly treats the likely underlying pathology. Success rates of 95% can be achieved with proper selection of patients and a thorough understanding of surgical principles.

REFERENCES

1. Taylor DC, Meyers WC, Moylan JA, et al. Abdominal musculature abnormalities as a cause of groin pain in athletes. *Am J Sports Med* 1991;19:239.
2. Meyers WC, Foley DP, Mandelbaum BR, et al. Successful management of severe lower abdominal or inguinal pain in high performance athletes. *Am J Sports Med* 2000;28:2.
3. Gross ML, Nasser S, Finerman GAM. Hip and pelvis. In: DeLee JC, Drez DJ, eds. *Orthopaedic sports medicine.* Philadelphia: W.B. Saunders, 1994.
4. Anson BJ, Morgan EH, McVay CB. Surgical anatomy of the inguinal region. *Surg Gynecol Obstet* 1960;111:707.
5. Moore KL. *The abdomen and pelvis. Clinically oriented anatomy,* 3rd ed. Baltimore: Williams & Wilkins, 1985.
6. Ingoldby CJH. Laparoscopic and conventional repair of groin disruption in sportsmen. *Br J Surg* 1997;84:213.
7. Fishman LM, Zybert PA. Electrophysiologic evidence of piriformis syndrome. *Arch Phys Med Rehabil* 1992;73:359.
8. Hackney RG. The sports hernia: a cause of chronic groin pain. *Br J Sports Med* 1993;27:58.
9. Pro Hockey Athletic Trainers Meeting, Salt Lake City, Utah. June 21–24, 1997.
10. Smodlaka VN. Groin pain in soccer players. *Phys Sports Med* 1980;8:57.
11. Fredberg U, Kissmeyer-Nielson P. The sportsman's hernia—fact or fiction? *Scand J Med Sci Sports* 1996;6:201.
12. Zeitoun F, Frot B, Sterin P, et al. Pubalgia in sportsmen. *Ann Radiol* (Paris) 1995;38:244.
13. Williams P, Foster ME. Gilmore's groin—or is it? *Br J Sports Med* 1995;29:206.
14. Gilmore OJA. Gilmore's groin. *Sports Med & Soft Tissue Trauma* 1991;3:12.
15. Simonet WT, Saylor HL, Sim L. Abdominal wall muscle tears in hockey players. *Int J Sports Med* 1995;16:126.
16. Ashby EC. Chronic obscure groin pain is commonly caused by enthesopathy: "tennis elbow" of the groin. *Br J Surg* 1994;81:1632.
17. Ekberg O, Blomquist P, Olsson S. Positive contrast herniography in adult patients with obscure groin pain. *Surgery* 1981;89:532.
18. Polglase AL, Frydman GM, Farmer KC. Inguinal surgery for debilitating chronic groin pain in athletes. *Med J Austr* 1991; 155:674.
19. Smedberg SGG, Broome AEA, Gullmo A, et al. Herniography in athletes with groin pain. *Am J Surg* 1985;149:378.
20. Renstrom AFH. Tendon and muscle injuries in the groin area. *Clin Sports Med* 1992;11:815.
21. Griffin LH. *Sports medicine.* IL: American Academy of Orthopaedic Surgeons, 1994.
22. Puranen J, Orava S. The hamstring syndrome: a new diagnosis of gluteal sciatic pain. *Am J Sports Med* 1988;16:517.
23. Puranen J, Orava S. The hamstring syndrome: a new gluteal sciatica. *Ann Chir Gynaecol* 1991;80:212.
24. Busconi B, McCarthy J. Hip and pelvic injuries in the skeletally immature athlete. *Sports Med Arthrosc Rev* 1996;4:132.
25. Wiley JJ. Traumatic osteitis pubis: the gracilis syndrome. *Am J Sports Med* 1983;11:360.
26. Knapp TP, Mandelbaum BR. *Stress fractures.* In: The U.S. Soccer Sports Medicine Book. Baltimore: Williams & Wilkins, 1996.
27. Pavlov H. Roentgen examination of groin and hip pain in the athlete. *Clin Sports Med* 1987;6:829.
28. Renstrom P, Peterson L. Groin injuries in athletes. *Br J Sports Med* 1980;14:30.
29. Netter FH. *Atlas of human anatomy.* New Jersey: CIBA Collection, 1989.

PART III

Upper Extremity

Principles and Practice of Orthopaedic Sports Medicine,
edited by William E. Garrett, Jr., Kevin P. Speer, and Donald T. Kirkendall.
Lippincott Williams & Wilkins, Philadelphia © 2000.

CHAPTER 14

Hand Fractures

Robert J. Heaps and L. Scott Levin

Fractures and fracture–dislocations of the hand are common sports-related injuries. The exact incidence is difficult to determine but is likely underestimated, because many injuries go unreported (1). Fractures distal to the carpus often appear insignificant at the time of injury. However, if treated improperly, the injury can affect the long-term function of the hand.

Sports that require the competitor to frequently use an unprotected hand, including football, basketball, volleyball, gymnastics, handball, and wrestling, have a higher risk of hand injury. Patterns of sport-specific injuries often appear, such as metacarpal fractures in boxing and fractures and fracture–dislocations of the phalanges in baseball and basketball (1–4).

A spectrum of injury can be seen, ranging from simple nondisplaced fractures to complex open injuries of the hand. The basis for diagnosis includes a thorough history and a detailed examination of the entire extremity, with focus on the involved hand. Radiographs should include quality anteroposterior lateral and oblique views of the affected area. Though a global hand view may be adequate to identify the presence of a fracture, additional views focusing on the affected area are often needed to provide adequate information for proper treatment.

The athlete's desire to return quickly to competition should be considered when devising a treatment plan, especially at the higher levels of competition. Early surgical fixation of certain fractures and joint injuries may have better results. Postoperative rehabilitation and protection may also have to be individualized to the specific needs of the athlete (5).

In the younger athlete who is skeletally immature, physeal injuries present a unique group of considerations. The hand is the most common location for physeal injuries. Conversely, one third to one half of children's finger fractures involve the growth plate (6–8). Although there is often a greater remodeling capacity in the region of an intact physis, complete or partial growth arrest can occur, leading to a late deformity. Closed treatment is sufficient for most physeal injuries. Physeal injuries with intraarticular extension require anatomic reduction to avoid joint incongruity. A variation of Salter-Harris injuries that include Salter I through IV may be encountered in metacarpals and phalanges. Salter I is shifting of the epiphysis through the physeal plate. Salter II is fracture through the physeal plate into the metaphysis. Salter III involves disruption of the epiphysis. Salter IV includes disruption of the epiphysis and metaphysis. Salter V is an impaction fracture of the physis (9) Salter II fractures are the most frequently encountered (6–8). All pediatric fractures should be analyzed to evaluate for injury to physeal structures.

Fractures of the hand often require treatment of soft tissue and the bony injury. The skeleton acts as the foundation or platform against which motor-tendon units work to create function of the hand. In addition, secondary functions of the upper extremity skeleton provides the framework for which other soft tissues, such as skin, nerve, and vessels, can be suspended. One of the guiding principles in complex injuries of the hand is that a strong foundation (i.e., the correct alignment and rigid fixation of the skeleton) is essential to proceed with restoration of upper extremity function.

FRACTURE ANALYSIS

Decision making in fracture treatment relates to the following areas:

1. Location of the fracture (which bone[s] is broken)?
2. Where is the bone broken (proximal, middle, or distal)?
3. Is there articular involvement?

R. J. Heaps and L. S. Levin: Duke University Medical Center, Divisions of Orthopaedic and Plastic and Reconstructive Surgery, Durham, North Carolina 27710.

4. Is the fracture opened or closed?

5. Is there comminution associated with the fracture (mild, moderate, or severe)?

6. Is there vascular injury?

7. Is there contamination of the fracture?

8. Is there an overlying soft tissue defect?

9. How long has it been since the injury or fracture has been presented to the clinic or emergency room? What should be the timing of fixation (immediate, delayed, late)?

10. If fixation is to be used, how will this be accomplished?

11. Is opened or closed reduction necessary, or both?

12. What techniques of casting, splinting, or traction are required?

13. If internal fixation is selected, is it performed with Kirschner wires, either with open technique or percutaneous pinning? Are plates, screws, or intramedullary devices required? Are external fixators required for distraction or in combination with fixation devices?

14. If there is missing bone and requirement for fixation, is a temporary montage required such as a bridging plate, external fixator, or the placement of antibiotic beads or spacers with the realization that the surgeon will return in a second stage to reconstitute the intercalary defect in the hand skeleton.

15. Is the patient an adult or child? Are the physes opened or closed?

16. What is the displacement of the fracture in terms of its length, angulation of rotation, and displacement?

17. Are neurovascular structures involved?

18. Are ligaments torn or avulsed?

19. Are tendons lacerated?

20. Is there a compartment syndrome?

All these questions must be addressed on patient presentation because they serve as the basis for the principles of fracture repair.

The hand osseous structures that need to be analyzed for injuries include the metacarpals and phalanges. The carpus articulates with the metacarpals of the thumb, index, long, ring, and little fingers that subsequently articulate with the proximal distal phalanx of the thumb and digits proximal, proximal, middle, and distal phalanges. All fractures have the potential to heal provided alignment, appropriate stability, and appropriate blood supply are ensured. The lack of blood supply, lack of rigid fixation, and inappropriate alignment will lead to nonunion, malunion, and dysfunction. Each hand fracture below is reviewed referable to these principles.

IMPLANT SELECTION

Most hand fractures can be treated nonoperatively. For those that require operative intervention, there are several options (Fig. 14.1). Implants include K-wires, absorbable pins, screws, plates, external fixators, and a combination of all these. Most hand fractures requiring operative treatment can be adequately stabilized with K-wires, which can be placed across the fracture fragments, used as an intramedullary device, and, in treatment of metacarpal fractures, they can be placed into stable adjacent bones to maintain length and rotational control. Advantages of K-wires are that they are rapid, require minimal soft tissue dissection, and can be easily removed. Disadvantages are that they tend to tether motor tendon units (10–12).

Advantages of absorbable implants such as bioabsorbable pins are that they can be used on juxtaarticular fragments and osteochondral fragments that otherwise have no way of being captured. However, they are not as rigid as K-wires, especially in controlling torsional forces (13).

Screws are implants that can be used to provide interfragmentary compression. Principles of interfragmentary compression are as follows. The proximal bone is overdrilled relative to the distal bone so that the screw glides through the proximal fragment and engages the distal fragment. As the distal fragment becomes engaged, fracture fragments are drawn to one another and compressed.

Plates similarly can be used in a variety of modes, such as in compression plating, as spanning plates, as neutralization plates to resist torsional forces, or as but-

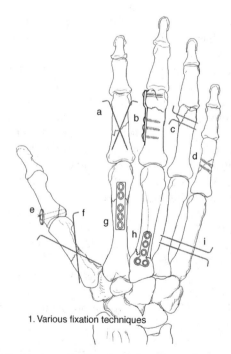

1. Various fixation techniques

FIG. 14.1. Various fixation techniques can be used in the fractured hand using Kirschner wires, minifragment screws, and plates to restore hand function.

tresses to support articular surfaces (14,15). Plates have a limited but useful role in the hand. They are better tolerated in the metacarpals than in the smaller phalanges, where there is less soft tissue coverage. There is a relatively high complication rate associated with the use of plates in the phalanges; however, their use is usually reserved for more serious injuries (16,17).

External fixators are often used when damage is severe to soft tissues and the skeletal part needs to be axially aligned. The external fixator can be used to maintain skeletal alignment in the instances where there is bone loss or significant contamination of bone that requires debridement, resulting in intercalary defect. The external fixator in this case is an excellent tool to allow soft tissues to heal and inflammatory mediators to resolve. Subsequently, a second stage reconstruction can be performed. One of the principles regarding external fixation is that if internal fixation is then subsequently to be considered, the external fixator should be removed for a period of time to allow the pin tracks to seal so that there can be no risk of contamination from the pin tracks. This is particularly true for the treatment of intercalary bone defects where nonvascularized bone is used for replacement after initial stabilization with the external fixator (18–21).

BONE GRAFTING

Bone grafting is done for a variety of reasons:

1. To substitute for comminuted bone that is removed during the treatment of the initial fracture;
2. To supplement fixation where there are bone defects on the basis of comminution;
3. To replace bone that is missing as the result of infection or injury and debridement.

Sources for bone include the iliac crest, distal radius, proximal ulna, bone bank, and a variety of bone substitutes (21–24). The gold standard is autogenous bone graft usually from the iliac crest. It can be harvested in the form of matchsticks, corticocancellous strips, or as cancellous bone alone. Often, structural cortical cancellous blocks can be harvested to substitute for intercalary defects in the metacarpals and phalanges. Conventional autogenous bone and vascularized bone is both osteoinductive and osteoconductive. Bone allograft is readily available. Its incorporation is slower and may carry the risk of disease transmission, although this is not likely. Bone substitutes such as hydroxyapatite, collagen hydroxyapatite, or coral bone are structural but, similar to allograft, they are only osteoconductive, not osteoinductive.

DISTAL PHALANX

Distal phalangeal fractures can be open or closed. Open injuries often involve a crush-type injury. Fractures can generally be classified into one of three types depending on location: tuft fractures, fractures of the shaft, and fractures of the base of the phalanx (25). Physeal injuries can also affect the distal phalanx.

Fractures involving the distal tuft usually are treated closed, with appropriate treatment of the nail bed. If nail-bed laceration is suspected, the nail plate is removed and the germinal and sterile matrix is repaired under loupe magnification with fine absorbable sutures. The nail is then replaced as a biologic stent or artificial material, such as plastic or suture packages, can be used to support the eponychial fold. The distal phalanx should be splinted. If there is severe open crush injury, small contaminated fragments that have no soft tissue attachments should be debrided; however, care should be taken to avoid excessive bony removal. If there is soft tissue loss, coverage with the appropriate local flap or skin graft is obtained. If there is inadequate bony support for the nail bed, a hooked or otherwise abnormal nail will be a likely result (25–28).

Distal phalangeal shaft fractures can be transverse or longitudinal (25). Nondisplaced fractures are inherently stable and need only splint immobilization. If there is significant displacement, the fracture may require pinning with a 0.028- or 0.035-inch K-wire to restore axial alignment. Other forms of treatment such as plates or screws are not usually practical due to the need for additional stripping of soft tissue.

Fractures at the base of the distal phalanx can be intra- or extraarticular. Intraarticular injuries may result in a disruption of the articular surface. Subsequently, treatment should be formulated to reconstitute the articular surface either with percutaneous pinning or open technique using miniscrews or K-wires. If the fracture can be reduced closed, then a percutaneous pinning through the pulp across the distal interphalangeal (DIP) joint is an acceptable way to hold the fracture in place until healing. Note that the x-ray often lags behind a clinical resolution of the fracture. Active flexion and extension of the proximal interphalangeal joint is begun immediately. The pin should be removed after a few weeks to prevent DIP joint stiffness and pin tract irritation (25,29).

The terminal extensor tendon of the digit inserts onto the proximal aspect of the distal phalanx dorsally, and improper care of such fractures may result in mallet deformity of the finger. A mallet fracture can be treated closed, similarly to a tendinous mallet (Fig. 14.2) (32). A transarticular K-wire crossing the DIP joint can be used as an internal splint in the athlete who requires a quick return to activities or when an external splint appears inadequate. If a substantial portion (more than 40% to 50%) of the articular surface is involved or if there is subluxation of the joint, then the fragment should be reduced with fixation achieved by a 1.5-mm minifragment screw or 0.045-inch K-wire (29,31).

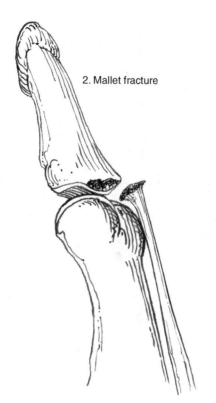

2. Mallet fracture

FIG. 14.2. A mallet fracture consists of a bony avulsion of the terminal extensor tendon at the base of the distal phalanx. If greater than 50% of the joint surface is involved, subluxation of the joint is likely to occur.

The flexor digitorum profundus (FDP) tendon inserts palmarly on the distal phalanx, distal to the attachment of the palmar plate. It is important to recognize that this fracture represents a tendinous avulsion (32,33). This injury often occurs in football or rugby when the player is grabbing the opponent's jersey, catching his or her finger. The distal phalanx gets extended while the FDP is flexing with maximal forces. Failure occurs at the bony insertion of the distal phalanx. The ring finger is involved most often, but all fingers have been implicated. The athlete may be able to bend his or her finger, but under closer examination, flexion occurs only at the PIP joint and not at the DIP joint. Depending on the size of the bony fragment, the tendon may retract to the level of the middle phalanx at the A4 pulley or at the level of the PIP joint. In contrast to a purely tendinous avulsion, which retracts into the palm, the vincular blood supply to the tendon is maintained (32,33). Treatment involves restoring the FDP to its insertion and restoring the articular surface of the DIP joint. A Brunner incision is used to expose the tendon sheath and the injury. Fixation can be achieved with a pullout suture technique using a nonabsorbable suture. Alternatively, if the fragment is large enough, fixation

can be achieved with a 1.5- or 2.0-mm minifragment screw.

In a child or adolescent, opened or closed injuries should be appropriately treated because this may involve the area of the growth plate of the distal phalanx. The younger child is likely to sustain a Salter-Harris type I or II fracture, whereas the adolescent presents with a type III fracture, resembling a mallet fracture. In the type III fracture with significant displacement, open reduction and K-wire fixation is indicated to restore articular congruity (6,34).

MIDDLE PHALANX

Fractures of the middle phalanx can occur at the base, shaft, or neck and condyles. Fractures along the shaft can be transverse, oblique, spiral, or comminuted. The major deforming forces, namely the central slip of the extensor tendon at the base dorsally and the flexor digitorum sublimis tendon with its more broad insertion along the palmar surface, increase angulation to less stable fractures. More proximal fractures tend to have apex dorsal angulation. Distal fractures tend to be angled palmarly.

The hand needs to be examined closely for malrotation. Whereas small amounts of angulation can be tolerated, rotation often is not. The fingernails should be observed with the hand in resting and partially flexed postures. Comparison is made with the opposite hand. Nondisplaced fractures of the shaft may be treated nonoperatively with splinting or buddy taping for protection. Some displaced but stable transverse fractures of the shaft can be reduced and splinted. In closed treatment of the middle phalanx, an outrigger hand-based splint can be used to create an appropriate means of stabilization. However, if prolonged immobilization is required to maintain acceptable alignment, percutaneous pinning should be considered. Unstable fractures should be addressed operatively. Treatment options include closed reduction with K-wire fixation and open reduction with internal fixation. The type of fixation depends on the fracture. Options include 0.045-inch K-wires, intraosseous wiring, or minifragment screw fixation. Fixation with minifragment screws combined with plating is used less often.

The approach to open reduction and internal fixation should be planned carefully. Approaches include a dorsal extensor splitting approach or an approach between the central slip and lateral band. In open injures, the opened wound can be extended to gain access to the phalanx for placement of a variety of implants or pins. The interval between the extensor mechanism and periosteum should be preserved to prevent adhesions. Periosteum stripping should be limited to what is necessary for visualization of the fracture fragments. The selection of plates can include microplates or miniplates, but the caveat is to avoid interruption of the extensor mechanism in open treatment of phalangeal fractures with rigid implants. Gliding can be impaired, resulting in an acceptable-looking x-ray but poor hand function (16,17).

Fractures of the condyles or neck of the middle phalanx or proximal phalanx should be approached with caution. Fractures of the neck of the phalanx occur more often in the younger athlete. Intraarticular condylar fractures can be mistaken for a neck fracture. These fractures often displace, and reduction is extremely difficult to maintain with closed methods. It is customary to fix these fractures early, even in the skeletally immature athlete, because remodeling is limited (34–36).

Fractures of one or both of the condyles of the proximal or middle phalanx are intraarticular and usually require internal fixation. Both separation and rotation of the fragments are commonly encountered. Closed reduction can be performed with bone reduction forceps. If anatomic reduction cannot be obtained under fluoroscopic assistance, the surgeon should proceed to an open reduction. K-wire fixation is often adequate. Alternatively fixation can be achieved with one or two 1.5-mm interfragmentary screws or a 1.5-mm minicondylar plate (14,37–39).

Fractures of the base of the middle phalanx often occur at the dorsal or palmar lip. A central articular disruption may also be seen. These are frequently associated with a dislocation of the PIP joint. The convention for dislocations includes naming of the displacements (dorsal or palmar) based on where the most distal aspect of the fracture occurs. For example, in the proximal lip fracture, dislocations are usually dorsal, implying that the middle phalanx displaces dorsally in relationship to the position of the proximal phalanx. These injuries are a result of an axial load in combination with flexion or extension force. It is critical that basilar fractures are identified and appropriately treated to avoid boutonniere or swan-neck deformities (40,41).

Fractures and fracture–dislocations of the dorsal lip represent an avulsion of the central slip of the extensor tendon (40–42). Subtle injuries can be missed if clinical suspicion is not heightened, because the PIP joint may be extended through the pull of the lateral bands. A maneuver described by Elson (43) consists of holding the PIP joint in approximately 90 degrees of flexion while the patient attempts to extend his or her finger. Absent extension of the PIP joint with strong fixed extension of the DIP in this position is a sign of a central slip avulsion. A neglected central slip avulsion will result in a boutonniere deformity. Closed treatment includes immobilization of the PIP joint in full extension for a minimum of 4 weeks, whereas flexion of the DIP joint is encouraged. Protected flexion and night splinting is continued for an additional 4 to 6 weeks. Larger displaced fragments may be associated with palmar subluxation of the PIP joint. In the acute injury, subluxation and joint incongruity is often corrected when the fracture is reduced. K-wire or screw fixation should be considered for larger displaced fragments with associated palmar subluxation (40–42).

More commonly, fractures and fracture–dislocations of the palmar lip are encountered (41). As a group, palmar lip fractures give the appearance of being a nuisance injury. However, the severity is more often underestimated, leading to suboptimal treatment. The simple palmar lip fracture can lead to a stiff joint with a pseudo-boutonniere or swan-neck deformity. Persistent subluxation, often leading to posttraumatic arthrosis, is a challenge to treat late if diagnosis is delayed. Open fracture–dislocations can be extremely problematic if not treated properly (39–41,44–47).

Pure extension injuries often produce a small avulsion fragment, representing a disruption of the palmar plate. There is minimal comminution. More often, extension is combined with an axial load injury, as in the typical jamming injury. The addition of an axial load contributes to a greater degree of joint involvement and increased comminution. When joint involvement approaches 30% to 40%, the PIP joint should be considered unstable (40,41,45).

A useful classification based on the stability of the joint as determined by radiographic and clinical means has been devised. It groups these fractures into one of three categories; stable, tenuous, and unstable. Type I or stable fractures involve less than 30% of the joint and do not sublux in full extension. Type II or tenuously stable injuries have 30% to 50% joint involvement, and reduction can be maintained with less than 30 degrees of flexion. Type III or unstable injuries involve greater than 50% of the joint surface or require greater than 30 degrees of flexion to maintain reduction (41).

Initial treatment should include closed reduction of the PIP joint if it has not already been done by the athlete or trainer. This is done after a metacarpal block with a local anesthetic. After reduction, a careful examination is performed to assess for stability and to check if the PIP joint hyperextends. Postreduction radiographs taken to confirm reduction can be helpful in formulating a treatment plan. Treatment can include static or dynamic splinting, extension block splinting, open reduction internal fixation, and palmar plate arthroplasty, described by Eaton (45).

Stable palmar lip fractures can be treated with buddy taping, which allows early motion of the affected finger. Dorsal extension block splinting can be used, starting with 20 to 30 degrees of flexion. The dorsal block is extended at weekly intervals. Active flexion of the PIP joint should be encouraged from the onset of treatment.

Fractures with tenuous stability can be treated with a dorsal extension block splint, as long as no more than 30 degrees of flexion is needed to maintain a reduced

PIP joint. Close follow-up is necessary. Alternatively, extension block pinning using a 0.035-inch K-wire for 5 to 6 weeks can also be used (44,50).

The management of an unstable palmar lip fracture–dislocation can be challenging. Primary treatment goals include elimination dorsal subluxation and avoiding prolonged immobilization. Anatomic restoration of the articular surface is desirable, but sometimes can only be achieved at the expense of a stiff joint and should be considered a secondary goal.

Dynamic traction with an external fixator or dynamic traction splint can be used to maintain joint congruity. The palmar plate arthroplasty described by Eaton reconstructs the palmar plate apparatus and provides an acceptable articular surface that is lost with significant impaction and comminution of the palmar lip (40,41,44–50).

PROXIMAL PHALANX

Fractures of the proximal phalanx may include the base, shaft, or head at the level of the PIP joint. Condylar fractures have been discussed above with their counterparts in the middle phalanx. The condyles are larger and are more amenable to K-wire or minifragment screw fixation (14,37–39).

Displaced fractures of the shaft more consistently display apex palmar angulation. The interosseous attaching proximally and the central extensor tendon attaching distally are the major deforming forces leading to the angulation. Angulation should be carefully assessed on the lateral radiograph, because an unrecognized deformity can lead to decreased finger flexion and extension. Closed reduction and splinting may be adequate for stable fractures with acceptable alignment as long as early mobilization can be achieved for 2 to 3 weeks (51). A splint or buddy taping can be used for protection during competition until complete union is confirmed. Spiral oblique fractures of the proximal phalanx are not uncommon, and early fixation should be considered because these fractures are prone to displace. Fixation can be achieved percutaneously with K-wires if closed reduction is satisfactory. Alternatively, if open reduction is required, the incision can be extended and fixation can be achieved either with two 1.5-mm interfragmentary compression screws or miniplates to provide fixation. A condylar blade plate described by Buchler and Fisher (37) is an alternative to dorsal plating and can be considered in juxtaarticular or shaft fractures.

Fractures to the base of the proximal phalanx often represent a collateral ligament injury in adults. The metacarpophalangeal joint should be assessed for stability. Small fractures with minimal displacement can be treated closed with a brief period of immobilization followed by early motion with buddy taping. Larger fractures that are displaced and are associated with joint

incongruity should be approached operatively. Closed reduction and percutaneous K-wire fixation can be attempted if congruity is achieved. Open reduction using a dorsal extensor splitting approach is followed by internal fixation with K-wires, tension band wiring, or minifragment screws (52).

Skeletally immature patients are susceptible to a physeal injury at the base of the proximal phalanx. A Salter-Harris type II fracture is most commonly seen. These are successfully treated with closed manipulation followed by splinting for 3 weeks. Remodeling can correct a small degree of angulation in the plane of motion of the joint; however, no rotational deformity is acceptable. Occasionally, a Salter-Harris III fracture of the proximal phalanx of the thumb occurs. This represents the equivalent of a bony gamekeeper's thumb. If the fracture is displaced or if there is significant laxity of the ulnar collateral ligament, an open reduction with internal fixation should be performed (6,53).

Treatment of fractures of the thumb phalanges is similar to the digits; however, the proximal phalanx of the thumb can be involved with radial or ulnar collateral ligament injuries. These must be recognized and appropriately treated to avoid late sequelae of pain and loss of grip strength. Fractures to the base of the proximal phalanx occur in 20% to 30% of ulnar collateral ligament injuries. Fractures that are nondisplaced can be treated closed in a thumb splint. Those that are significantly displaced or involving a significant portion of articular surface should be treated with open repair. If there is a rotational component to an otherwise minimally displaced avulsion, the surgeon should also consider open reduction internal fixation (5,53–56).

METACARPALS

Fractures of the metacarpal can include the base, shaft, neck, or articular surface. The ulnar metacarpals, the fourth and fifth, are mobile at the level of the carpometacarpal joint and subsequently a greater deal of deformity can be accepted in terms of angulation of the metacarpal in the flexion extension plane. Minimal deformity should be accepted in terms of rotation and radial ulnar deviation in any metacarpal because of the sequelae of scissoring of the hand skeleton during flexion and extension. Some shortening can be accepted in the metacarpals, particularly in rays 4 and 5 because of their mobility. In the index and long ray, angulation of the metacarpal heads should be avoided to evade metacarpalgia. Treatment of metacarpals includes closed reduction and casting, percutaneous pinning to adjacent metacarpals, rigid fixation with plates or interfragmentary screws, and, in the instances of open injury with segmental loss, treatment with external fixation (11,14,15,17–19).

Fractures of the metacarpal head are relatively uncommon intraarticular injuries and occur most often to the index metacarpal. The head can be split into two fragments or comminuted. Any displacement or step-off greater than 1 mm is an indication for Open Reduction Internal Fixation (ORIF). Large fragments can be stabilized with one or two 2.0-mm minifragment screws. If the fragments are small, K-wire fixation is sufficient. In the case of a significantly comminuted fracture, major fragments can be fixed to each other and to the shaft. Bony defects can be supported with bone graft (52).

Metacarpal neck fractures occur most often to the small finger metacarpal. They are usually a result of a direct blow to the metacarpal head. Apex dorsal angulation and palmar comminution is seen. A significant degree of angulation can be accepted, especially in the more mobile ring and small metacarpals. Rotation, however, is not well tolerated. Treatment for many fractures includes splinting for 2 to 3 weeks, followed by protection until healed. A reduction can be attempted but is usually lost to some degree with cast or splint immobilization. If angulation or rotation is unacceptable, closed reduction followed by K-wire fixation can be performed (5,57,58).

Shaft fractures can be transverse, oblique spiral, or comminuted. Transverse fractures usually occur from a direct blow to the hand. Apex dorsal angulation, a result of the deforming forces of the interossei, is encountered. Again, angulation can be tolerated but to a lesser degree than in the distal metacarpal neck. Rotation should be carefully assessed both clinically and on radiographs. Isolated transverse fractures are usually amenable to closed treatment. Closed reduction with crossed or intramedullary K-wire fixation is performed when casting is not an acceptable treatment. Open reduction internal fixation is reserved for multiple metacarpal fractures or when closed reduction is unacceptable. K-wire or minifragment plates may be used for stabilization. Spiral oblique fractures occur from a torsional injury. Rotation and shortening are common sequelae of inadequate treatment. A single spiral metacarpal fracture with no rotational deformity and less than 5 mm of shortening can be treated closed. Otherwise, closed reduction and pinning to the adjacent metacarpal or open reduction and internal fixation with K-wires, 2.0-mm screws, or a minifragment plate are performed. Open fractures or crush injuries may require internal fixation or external fixation if there is a significant soft tissue injury or segmental bony loss (11,14,15,17–19,57).

Fractures to the base of the metacarpal, excluding the thumb, are usually stable injuries. Adequate radiographs should exclude any associated dislocation of the Carpal Metacarpal Joint (CMC) joints. A displaced fracture of the base of the fifth metacarpal will shorten due to the pull of the extensor carpi ulnaris tendon. These injuries can be treated with closed reduction and either direct K-wire fixation or pinning the fifth metacarpal to

its adjacent metacarpal, thus maintaining length. Fracture–dislocation of the CMC joint requires reduction with fixation to the carpus and adjacent metacarpal (58,59).

A unique set of fractures is seen at the base of the thumb metacarpal. Basilar thumb fractures can be intraarticular or extraarticular. This is an important distinction because any significant incongruency to the first CMC joint will likely lead to painful arthrosis. Four types are seen: Bennett's fracture, Rolando's fracture, extraarticular fracture, and a physical injury in the skeletally immature (60).

A Bennett's fracture is sustained from a direct axial blow. The majority of the base is separated from a small palmar lip fragment. The deforming forces of the abductor pollicis longus tendon contribute to shortening of the metacarpal, resulting in further displacement (Fig. 14.3). Treatment of displaced fractures is operative. Closed reduction with percutaneous K-wire fixation to the carpus and adjacent metacarpal can be performed if the joint surface is restored. If an acceptable reduction cannot be performed closed, an open reduction with minifragment or alternatively K-wire fixation is used (61–63).

Rolando's fracture is seen less frequently. It has both palmar and dorsal fracture fragments and a greater degree of comminution. If fragments are large enough and a reasonable reduction can be obtained with traction, internal fixation is performed. Otherwise, percutaneous fixation to the adjacent metacarpal or external fixation is performed (61,64). Most extraarticular fractures are treated by closed means with a reduction and thumb spica casting. For the more unstable types, percutaneous K-wire fixation after closed reduction is performed.

Pediatric injuries to the metacarpal base can be either

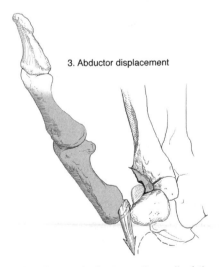

3. Abductor displacement

FIG. 14.3. In a Bennett's fracture, the pull of the abductor pollicis longus shortens and dorsally displaces the larger metacarpal fragment. Reduction and percutaneous or internal fixation is required to maintain articular congruity.

a Salter-Harris type II or III fracture or strictly metaphyseal. Most of these fractures can be managed closed because there is a significant capacity for remodeling in the extraarticular fracture. The exception is the Salter-Harris III fracture, which is the pediatric equivalent to the Bennett's fracture, requiring open reduction with K-wire fixation to restore the articular surface (6).

CONCLUSION

Management of the athlete's fractured hand requires prompt and accurate diagnosis and recognition of which fractures will benefit from primary operative intervention. Appropriate treatment should emphasize early return to competition, maximize long-term function, and prevent chronic deformity.

REFERENCES

1. Amadio P. Epidemiology of hand and wrist injuries in sports. *Hand Clin* 1990;6:379–381.
2. Dawson WJ. The spectrum of sports related interphalangeal injuries. *Hand Clin* 1994;10:315–326.
3. Linblad BE, Hoy K, Terkelsen CJ, et al. Handball injuries: an epidemiologic and socioeconomic study. *Am J Sports Med* 1992; 20:441–444.
4. Wilson RL, McGinty LD. Common hand and wrist injuries in basketball players. *Clin Sports Med* 1993;12:265–291.
5. Kahler DM, McCue FC. Metacarpophalangeal and proximal interphalangeal joint injuries of the hand, including the thumb. *Clin Sports Med* 1992;11:57–76.
6. Fischer MD, McElfresh EC. Physeal and periphyseal injuries of the hand. *Hand Clin* 1994;10:287–301.
7. Mizuta T, Benson W, Foster M. Statistical analysis of the incidence of physeal injuries. *J Pediatr Orthop* 1987;7:518–523.
8. Peterson C, Peterson H. Analysis of the incidence of injuries to the growth plate. *J Trauma* 1972;12:275–281.
9. Salter R, Harris W. Injuries involving the epiphyseal plate. *J Bone Joint Surg Am* 1963;45A:587–622.
10. Green D, Anderson J. Closed reduction and percutaneous pin fixation of fractured phalanges. *J Bone Joint Surg Am* 1973;55A: 1651–1654.
11. Grundberg A. Intramedullary fixation for fractures of the hand. *J Hand Surg* 1981;6A:568–573.
12. Baraty ME, Divelbiss B. Fixation of phalangeal fractures. *Hand Clin* 1997;13:541–555.
13. Fitoussi F, Lu W, Ip WY, et al. Biomechanical properties of absorbable implants in finger fractures. *J Hand Surg* 1998;23B: 79–83.
14. Hastings H II. Unstable metacarpal and phalangeal fracture treatment with screws and plates. *Clin Orthop* 1987;214:37–52.
15. Black D, Mann RJ, Constine R, et al. Comparison of internal fixation techniques in metacarpal fractures. *J Hand Surg* 1985; 10A:466–472.
16. Stern PJ, Weiser M, Reilly D. Complications of plate fixation in the hand skeleton. *Clin Orthop* 1987;214:58–65.
17. Page S, Stern PJ. Complications and range of motion following plate fixation of metacarpal and phalangeal fractures. *J Hand Surg* 1998;23A:811–820.
18. Ashmead D, Ruthkopf D, Walton R, Jupiter J. Treatment of hand injuries by external fixation. *J Hand Surg* 1992;17A:956–964.
19. Freeland A. External fixation for skeletal stabilization of severe fractures of the hand. *Clin Orthop* 1987;214:93–100.
20. Freeland AE, Jabaley ME. Stabilization of fractures in the hand and wrist with traumatic soft tissue and bone loss. *Hand Clin* 1988;4:425–436.
21. Freeland AE, Jabaley ME, Burkhalter WE, et al. Delayed primary bone grafting in the hand and wrist after traumatic bone loss. *J Hand Surg* 1984;9A:22–28.
22. Littler JW. Metacarpal reconstruction. *J Bone Joint Surg [Am]* 1947;29:723–737.
23. MacCollum MS. Cancellous bone grafts from the distal radius for use in hand surgery. *Plast Reconstr Surg* 1975;55:477–478.
24. Upton J, Glowacki J. Hand reconstruction with allograft demineralized bone: twenty-six implants in twelve patients. *J Hand Surg* 1992;17A:704–713.
25. Schneider LH. Fractures of the distal phalanx. *Hand Clin* 1988; 4:537–547.
26. Fassler P. Fingertip injuries: evaluation and treatment. *J Am Acad Orthop Surg* 1996;4:84–92.
27. Van Beek AL Kassan MA, Adson MH, et al. Management of acute fingernail injuries. *Hand Clin* 1990;6:23–35.
28. Zook EG, Guy RJ, Russell RC. A study of nail bed injuries: causes, treatment and prognosis. *J Hand Surg* 1984;9A: 247–252.
29. Lubahn JD, Hood JM. Fractures of the distal interphalangeal joint. *Clin Orthop* 1996;327:12–20.
30. Wehbe M, Schneider L. Mallet fractures. *J Bone Joint Surg Am* 1984;66A:658–669.
31. Damron T, Engber WD, Lange RH, et al. Biomechanical analysis of mallet finger fracture fixation techniques. *J Hand Surg* 1993; 18A:600–607.
32. Leddy JP, Packer JW. Avulsion of the profundus tendon insertion in athletes. *J Hand Surg* 1977;2A:66–69.
33. Leddy JP. Avulsions of the flexor digitorum profundus. *Hand Clin* 1985;1:77–83.
34. Hastings FM II, Simmons BP. Hand fractures in children. *Clin Orthop* 1984;188:120–130.
35. Leonard M, Dubravcik P. Management of fractured fingers in the child. *Clin Orthop* 1970;73:160–168.
36. Barton NJ. Fractures of the phalanges of the hand in children. *Hand* 1979;2:134–143.
37. Buchler V, Fisher T. Use of minicondylar plate for metacarpal and phalangeal periarticular injuries. *Clin Orthop* 1987;214: 53–58.
38. Schneider LH. Fractures of the distal interphalangeal joint. *Hand Clin* 1994;10:277–285.
39. Freeland AE, Benoist LA. Open reduction and internal fixation method for fractures at the proximal interphalangeal joint. *Hand Clin* 1994;10:239–250.
40. Agee JM. Unstable fracture dislocations of the proximal interphalangeal joint. *Clin Orthop* 1987;214:101–112.
41. Kiefhaber T, Stern P. Fracture dislocation of the proximal interphalangeal joint. *Hand Surg* 1998;23A:368–380.
42. Rosenstadt B, Glickel S, Lane L, et al. Palmar fracture dislocation of the proximal interphalangeal joint. *J Hand Surg* 1998;23A: 811–820.
43. Elson R. Rupture of the central slip of the extensor hood of the finger. *J Bone Joint Surg Br* 1986;68B:229–231.
44. McElfresh E, Dobyns J, O'Brien E. Management of fracture dislocation of the proximal interphalangeal joints by extension block splinting. *J Bone Joint Surg Am* 1972;54A:1705–1711.
45. Eaton R, Malerich M. Volar plate arthroplasty of the proximal interphalangeal joint: a review of ten years' experience. *J Hand Surg* 1980;5A:260–268.
46. Stern P, Lee A. Open dorsal dislocations of the proximal interphalangeal joint. *J Hand Surg* 1985;10A:364–370.
47. Isani A. Small joint injuries requiring surgical treatment. *Orthop Clin North Am* 1986;17:407–419.
48. Morgan J, Gordon D, Klug MS, et al. Dynamic digital traction for unstable comminuted intra-articular fracture-dislocations of the proximal interphalangeal joint. *J Hand Surg* 1995;20A: 565–573.
49. Schenck R. Dynamic traction and early passive movement for fractures of the proximal interphalangeal joint. *J Hand Surg* 1986;11A:850–858.
50. Viegas S. Extension block pinning for proximal interphalangeal joint fracture dislocation: preliminary report of a new technique. *J Hand Surg* 1992;17A:896–901.
51. Coonrad RW, Pohlman MH. Impacted fractures in the proximal

portion of the proximal phalanx of the finger. *J Bone Joint Surg Am* 1969;51A:1291–1296.

52. Light T, Bednar MS. Management of intra-articular fractures of the metacarpophalangeal joint. *Hand Clin* 1994;10:303–314.

53. Dinowitz M, Trumble T, Hanel D, et al. Failure of cast immobilization for thumb ulnar collateral ligament avulsion fractures. *J Hand Surg* 1997;22A:1057–1063.

54. Langford S, Whitaker J. Thumb injuries in the athlete. *Clin Sports Med* 1998;17:553–566.

55. Hintermann B, Holzach PJ, Schutz M, et al. Skier's thumb: the significance of bony injuries. *Am J Sports Med* 1993;21:800–804.

56. Smith RJ. Post-traumatic instability of the metacarpophalangeal joint of the thumb. *J Bone Joint Surg Am* 1977;59A:14–21.

57. Stern P. Fractures of the metacarpals and phalanges. In: Green DP, ed. *Operative hand surgery,* 3rd ed. New YorK: Churchill Livingstone, 1993.

58. Gunther SF. The carpometacarpal joints. *Orthop Clin North Am* 1984;15:259–277.

59. Rawles JG. Dislocations and fracture dislocations at the carpometacarpal joints of the fingers. *Hand Clin* 1988;4:103–112.

60. Green DP, O'Brien ET. Fractures of the thumb metacarpal. *South Med J* 1972;65:807–814.

61. Foster RJ, Hastings H II. Treatment of Bennett, Rolando, and vertical intraarticular trapezial fractures. *Clin Orthop* 1987;214:121–129.

62. Timmenga EJ, Blokhuis TJ, Maas M, et al. Long-term evaluation of Bennett's fracture. A comparison between open and closed reduction. *J Hand Surg* 1994;19B:373–377.

63. Kjaer-Petersen K, Langhoff O, Andersen K. Bennett's fracture. *J Hand Surg* 1990;15B:58–61.

64. Langhoff O, Andersen K, Kjaer-Petersen K. Rolando's fracture. *J Hand Surg* 1991;16B:454–459.

Principles and Practice of Orthopaedic Sports Medicine,
edited by William E. Garrett, Jr., Kevin P. Speer, and Donald T. Kirkendall.
Lippincott Williams & Wilkins, Philadelphia © 2000.

CHAPTER 15

Soft Tissue Injuries of the Hand

Richard S. Moore, Jr., Melissa Evans Talley, and James R. Urbaniak

Soft tissue injuries of the hand are common in athletes and often go unrecognized and untreated for significant periods of time. Neglect of these injuries can lead to chronic debilitating problems that are much more difficult to manage and have much less favorable outcomes than when treated acutely. Additionally, rehabilitation of the athlete's injured hand is a difficult task due to the pressure of coaches, trainers, and the athlete on him- or herself to return to play as quickly as possible. The role of the physician and therapist is to appropriately diagnose and devise a treatment plan that will both protect the healing tissue and limit time away from play. Cooperation of the athlete, coach, trainer, physician, and therapist is necessary to maximize the outcome of the injured athletic hand. The goal of this chapter is to address the diagnosis, treatment, and rehabilitation of select common soft tissue injuries in the athlete's hand.

LIGAMENTOUS INJURIES

Ligamentous injuries are perhaps the most common athletic hand injuries and are probably the most poorly treated. Most of these injuries occur during play and have no obvious deformity unless there is a dislocation. If evaluated, x-rays are usually negative and the injury is written off as a "sprain" with no definitive diagnosis or treatment. Most of these will then go on to chronic debilitating instability and may result in late functional limitations.

R. S. Moore, Jr.: Department of Surgery, Division of Orthopaedic Surgery, Duke University Medical Center, Durham, North Carolina 27710.

M. Evans Talley: Department of Physical and Occupational Therapy, Duke University Medical Center, Durham, North Carolina 27710.

J. R. Urbaniak: Division of Orthopaedic Surgery, Duke University Medical Center, Durham, North Carolina 27710.

A good understanding of the anatomy combined with a careful history and physical examination can nearly always localize the injury to a specific anatomic structure. Appropriate protection of this structure while preserving mobility in the remainder of the hand will maximize the functional outcome and limit time away from play. This section review the anatomy, mechanism of injury, treatment, and rehabilitation protocols for the most common ligamentous injuries in the hand.

Thumb Ligamentous Injuries

The metacarpophalangeal (MP) joint of the thumb is a multiaxial diarthrodial joint, which primarily allows flexion and extension with some variable degrees of adduction, abduction, and rotation (1). Stability at this joint is crucial for the thumb to properly function in its role of grip and pinch. The ulnar and radial collateral ligaments that extend from the condyles of the metacarpal to the volar portion of the proximal phalanx and volar plate are the primary stabilizers. Accessory collateral ligaments and the thenar musculature supplement the primary ligaments volarly. The role of the abductor and adductor brevis attachments on the dorsal aponeurosis has also been recognized (1).

The complexity of the interplay of these soft tissues and the significant stresses and demands placed on the thumb during play leave it especially vulnerable to injury. Ligamentous injuries of the thumb are perhaps the most common soft tissue injuries in the athlete's hand and can lead to chronic pain and disabling instability.

Ulnar Collateral Ligament of the Thumb

Ulnar stability of the thumb MP joint is crucial for grip and pinch, and the primary ulnar stabilizer is the large ulnar collateral ligament. Tears involving the ulnar collateral ligament are common in athletes and have classically been referred to as a "gamekeeper's thumb" due to the propensity for chronic ulnar instability in game-keepers of old (2). Today it is most commonly seen in skiers and ball-handling athletes (3–5).

The ulnar collateral ligament of the thumb is a broad thick ligament that extends from the ulnar aspect of the distal metacarpal to insert into the ulnar and volar base of the proximal phalanx. The ligament also inserts into the volar plate and is intimately associated with the capsule. The mechanism of injury is a forceful radial deviation of the proximal phalanx on the metacarpal head that results in loading of the soft tissues. Most commonly, the insertion of the ulnar collateral is avulsed from the base of the proximal phalanx. This tear may propagate into the volar plate. On some occasions a small fragment of bone may be avulsed in association with the ligament, resulting in what is commonly referred to as the "bony gamekeepers." Midsubstance tears and avulsions from the metacarpal head are less common, but they do occur.

The anatomy of the dorsal aponeurosis at the thumb MP is unique and plays a significant role in the management of these injuries. The ulnar expansion of the dorsal aponeurosis overlies the ulnar collateral ligament. With extreme radial deviation, the ligament is partially uncovered. With a significant radial load that results in avulsion of the ligamentous insertion, the adductor aponeurosis can actually become interposed between the ligament and its insertion, preventing the ligament from healing. Unless surgically managed, this results in chronic ulnar instability. This lesion was described by Stener in 1962 (6) and is classically referred to as the Stener lesion.

The diagnosis of an ulnar collateral ligament injury is made based on mechanism of injury and physical and radiographic evaluation. The injury is very common in skiers, racquet sports, and in ball-handling athletes when the thumb is loaded eccentrically, resulting in radial deviation at the MP joint. In most cases, the patient can recall the specific event and describe the mechanism in which they were injured clearly.

The physical examination is the most important element in the diagnosis and management of these injuries (7–9). Although in the acute phase there will often be significant swelling about the thumb MP joint, most symptoms will usually localize to the ulnar aspect. There will be tenderness directly over the ulnar collateral ligament, especially at its distal insertion site into the proximal phalanx. The tenderness will extend dorsally or volarly in association with dorsal capsular or volar plate injuries. There will usually be minimal discomfort with palpation over the radial collateral ligament. The extensor pollicis longus and flexor pollicis longus tendons should be tested to ensure that they are intact and functioning normally.

The critical element of the examination is evaluation of the stability of the MP joint. With complete injuries,

the thumb may appear supinated and radially deviated on presentation. Examination of ulnar collateral stability may be very uncomfortable and will often require a digital block before an adequate examination can be conducted. Stability should be tested with the thumb in approximately 30 degrees of flexion, neutral, and maximal extension to evaluate all components of the ulnar collateral ligament and associated soft tissues. Partial injuries will reveal some tenderness with increased laxity as opposed to the contralateral side; however, an end point will be present. In complete injuries the instability will be more significant. Radial deviation of greater than 35 degrees or 15 degrees greater than the contralateral thumb is indicative of a complete tear and suggestive of a Stener lesion (7,8). Additionally, a painful palpable mass at the base of the MP joint is essentially pathognomonic of a Stener lesion (10).

Radiographic views are necessary for the complete evaluation of this injury. The collateral ligament may be associated with an avulsion fracture on the base of the proximal phalanx. This usually represents a small fragment consisting of less than 10% of the articular surface; however, large fragments can occur. Occasionally, this fragment will be widely displaced, which is pathognomonic of a Stener lesion. Stress radiographs are often helpful and are routinely performed by the authors under fluoroscan in the office. Magnetic resonance imaging is only rarely indicated in the presence of an adequate physical and plain radiographic evaluation.

Treatment

Incomplete ulnar collateral ligament tears of the thumb can be managed by cast immobilization. We typically use a short-arm thumb spica cast with the thumb positioned at 30 degrees of palmar abduction and maintained for 3 to 4 weeks. Care must be taken in applying the cast to avoid radial deviation through the MP joint as the cast is molded, and a conscious effort to maintain the normal anatomic alignment is crucial. The thumb interphalangeal joint does not need to be included. Edema control and limitation of capsular tightness of the interphalangeal joint are the initial goals of therapy.

At 3 to 4 weeks, cast immobilization is discontinued and a removable hand-based thumb spica splint is fabricated (Fig. 15.1). Active range of motion exercises are initiated followed by passive range of motion. Strengthening of the entire hand with grippers, putty, weights, or Baltimore Therapeutic Equipment is initiated at 5 weeks. The physician, level of contact, and severity of the injury determines return to sports. With ball-handling sports, the athlete typically must refrain from play for 4 to 6 weeks. Non–ball-handling or racquet athletes may return earlier with protective immobilization, usually at 2 to 3 weeks. The authors typically fabricate a thumb spica cast from a rubber casting material (Soft-

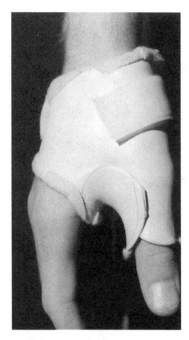

FIG. 15.1. Short opponens splint, which is initially worn for 4 or 5 weeks after injury of the metacarpophalangeal (MP) joint ulnar collateral ligament. The thumb is positioned in 30 to 40 degrees of palmar abduction with the MP joint in neutral to slight flexion. The interphalangeal joint and wrist are left free for normal range of motion.

Cast, 3M Healthcare, St. Pauls, MN) that is split with a single longitudinal dorsal cut (Fig. 15.2). The interphalangeal is included and the wrist is always crossed. The cast can be taped in place by the trainer for training or play. We typically recommend the use of this for 3 months after injury or repair. Patients should be educated about the chronicity of this problem and expect several months for absolute resolution of their symptoms.

Although some complete disruptions may heal adequately with immobilization alone, it is generally accepted that surgical management results in the most predictable outcome (5,8,9,11–13). The goal of surgery is primary repair of the ligament stump to its insertion at the base of the proximal phalanx. Our approach is through a curvilinear incision based over the ulnar collateral ligament. The dissection is carried through the subcutaneous tissues with careful attention to preserve any branches of the superficial radial nerve. The adductor aponeurosis is identified and incised longitudinally to expose the underlying ulnar collateral ligament. The ligament is repaired to its bed with a transosseous suture tied over a button or an incision can be made in the midlateral position, the radial digital nerve identified, and the suture tied directly over the periosteum. It is imperative that the radial neurovascular bundle is identified and protected if this technique is used. If the surgeon prefers not to use a transosseous technique, a su-

ture anchor can be placed in the base of the proximal phalanx and the ends woven through the ligament for repair. After the ligament is secure, any associated rents in the dorsal capsule or volar plate should be repaired. The adductor hood should be repaired over the ligament. Kirschner wire (K-wire) fixation of the joint is usually not necessary.

Postoperatively, the patient's thumb is placed in an initial well-padded thumb spica splint that is converted to a thumb spica cast at 7 to 10 days when sutures are removed. The patient's thumb remains in this cast for 4 weeks at which time a thermoplastic splint is used and pure flexion–extension exercises are initiated. Strengthening is begun at 6 to 8 weeks depending on the patient's pain. Protective splinting during physical activity continues for 3 months. Adhesive taping or soft neoprene splinting may be useful beyond this time. Although it provides minimal protection, it does remind the athlete of an injured digit and may provide some proprioceptive support.

Ulnar collateral tears that are associated with bony fragment are managed in much the same way (4). Small fragments that are nondisplaced or only minimally rotated can be managed with a period of cast immobiliza-

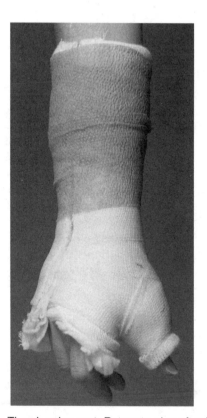

FIG. 15.2. Thumb spica cast. Return to play after injuries at the thumb metacarpophalangeal joint is facilitated by fabrication of a thumb spica cast from rubber casting material (Soft Cast, 3M Healthcare, St. Paul, MN) that is split longitudinally along the dorsum.

tion and followed by progressive range of motion as outlined above. Large fragments that are displaced or involve a significant portion of the joint surface should be reduced anatomically and fixed with a K-wire or screw depending on their size. Small fragments can be excised and the ligament repaired primarily to the bed as outlined above. The postoperative protocol is identical to that above.

Chronic reconstructions are much more challenging (1). Occasionally, the ligament can be elevated with a sleeve of periosteum and advanced for primary repair; however, it often must be supplemented. The most suitable substance for supplementation is a free tendon graft. If a palmaris longus is present, this is used. If the patient does not have a palmaris longus, a toe extensor is satisfactory. The tendon is passed through transverse drill holes in the base of the proximal phalanx and distal metacarpal in a figure-of-eight fashion, appropriately tensioned, and then sutured to itself. Long-term functional outcomes are not as satisfactory as with acute repairs, and this underscores the necessity for early recognition and treatment of these injuries (9).

Radial Collateral Ligament of the Thumb

Radial collateral ligament injuries of the thumb MP joint are much less common than ulnar collateral ligament injuries; however, if not recognized and inadequately treated, these can result in a significant functional impairment (11). The mechanism of radial collateral ligament injuries is a forced ulnar deviation or rotational deviation of the flexed MP joint. Unlike the ulnar collateral ligament, the point of avulsion is equally distributed between the origin on the metacarpal head and the insertion on the proximal phalanx. There is no equivalent to the Stener lesion on the radial side of the thumb.

The diagnosis of these injuries is made in much the same way as the ulnar collateral ligaments. The patient will have pain and swelling localized to the radial aspect of the thumb and pain with ulnar deviation. The patient will also often have a pronation deformity due to an associated dorsal capsular injury. With ulnar deviation there will be exacerbation of pain and instability. Stress radiographs are helpful.

Most radial collateral ligament injuries can be adequately managed with immobilization. The period of immobilization and subsequent rehabilitation protocol are identical to those for the ulnar collateral ligament. Surgical repair is rarely indicated unless there is significant displacement or subluxation. Surgical technique is similar to that for the ulnar collateral ligament (9,14).

Collateral Ligament Injuries of the Digits

The proximal interphalangeal (PIP) joint is a hinge joint with significant stability primarily derived from a strong volar plate and ligaments that are reinforced by the adjacent tendon and retinacular structures. The proximal phalanx articular surface consists of two concentric condyles with an intercondylar notch that articulates intimately with two depressions in the flat base of the middle phalanx. This high degree of articular congruency provides additional stability to lateral and rotational stress (15,16).

The collateral ligaments of the PIP are 2 to 3 mm thick and arise from a fossa on the lateral aspect of each condyle. They insert distally and volarly on the volar third of the middle phalanx and onto the volar plate. This conjoined attachment of the collateral ligaments and the volar plate is a crucial element in PIP joint stability. Any derangement can lead to altered mechanics and significant dysfunction (15–18).

Despite the stability of this complex, dislocations of the PIP joint are quite common. For the PIP joint to completely dislocate, disruption of two components of the complex is necessary (17). Dislocations can be classified as dorsal, volar, or rotatory and are described by the direction in which the middle phalanx is displaced in relation to the proximal phalanx. Each dislocation is associated with a specific soft tissue injury that requires a specialized course of therapy and rehabilitation that is described individually below.

Injuries to the ligaments that do not result in overt instability but do cause pain and swelling are very common and are often ignored. The mechanism of injury is radial or ulnar forced deviation and extension or a rotatory force. Ligamentous injuries are often found in conjunction with volar plate injuries due to the intimate association of these structures at their insertion (16).

Evaluation and management of ligament injuries is usually straightforward. The patient presents with concentric swelling of the joint, but tenderness will usually localize over a specific radial or ulnar collateral ligament. Pain will be accentuated with deviation of the PIP joint and stress on the affected collateral. Overt instability is uncommon with pure ligamentous injuries; however, mild subluxation can often be demonstrated on fluoroscan. Occasionally, a small bony fragment will be present with the avulsion.

Treatment of these injuries is primarily associated with edema control and protected range of motion. This can usually be accomplished with a course of buddy taping of the injured digit to the adjacent digit. If possible, the digit should be taped to the adjacent digit on the side of injury to prevent stress on the injured ligament. A gauze patch should be placed between the digits to prevent maceration and tape or velcro fasteners placed around the proximal and middle phalanges. This allows near complete range of motion with protection of the injured collateral. The patient should be encouraged to continue to work on passive range of motion daily to prevent fibrosis and joint stiffness.

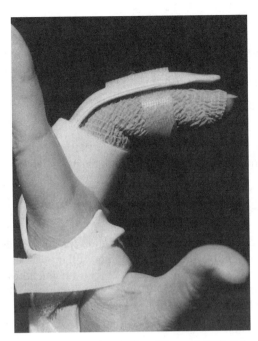

FIG. 15.3. Dorsal blocking splint. After a dorsal dislocation/volar plate rupture, a dorsal blocking splint with the proximal interphalangeal joint blocked at 20 to 30 degrees is used. The extension of the splint is incrementally increased until the patient is discharged to buddy taping.

Hyperextension injuries can produce pure volar plate injuries resulting in volar laxity and a sense of instability (19). If untreated, this will often result in a flexion contracture of the PIP joint. When recognized acutely, these injuries should be treated with graduated dorsal block splinting working from approximately 30 degrees of flexion to full extension over 3 to 4 weeks (Fig. 15.3). A short period of buddy taping is recommended with return to play for an additional 2 to 3 weeks. Volar plate injuries will often be associated with a small bony fragment avulsed from the middle phalanx that is usually of no significant consequence.

Proximal Interphalangeal Dislocations

Dorsal dislocations of the PIP joint usually result from a hyperextension injury associated with axial load. Eaton and Littler (17) have classified these injuries into three types. Type I injuries represent pure hyperextension. The volar plate is avulsed from the base of the middle phalanx and an incomplete longitudinal split occurs in the collateral ligaments. This results in the middle phalanx resting in a hyperextended position; however, the joint surfaces remain congruous. Type II injuries are associated with an avulsion of the volar plate accompanied by a complete bilateral split in the collateral ligaments. The middle phalanx displaces dorsally with the base of the middle phalanx resting on the dorsal aspect of the proximal phalanx. There is no articular contact.

Type III dislocations are actually a fracture dislocation with associated shear fracture or impaction of the volar base of the middle phalanx. The size of this fragment can range from a small inconsequential avulsion fracture to a significant fragment with associated impaction of the articular surface, resulting in joint instability.

Radiographic evaluation of these injuries is imperative even if the patient presents relocated. This allows evaluation of the articular congruency and assessment of any associated fractures. Dynamic fluoroscans are useful to evaluate stability through the entire range of motion, and stress views are helpful in defining the injury pattern. Type I fractures usually present in hyperextension and all easily reduce. Type II injuries most often present dislocated; however, patients will sometimes present with a history of having pulled the finger back into alignment.

These injuries are easily relocated under local anesthesia. The PIP joint is hyperextended with longitudinal traction placed on the middle phalanx and then flexed to allow the base of the middle phalanx to rearticulate with the condyles of the proximal phalanx. Occasionally, the volar plate will avulse and become interposed between the articular surface, making the dislocation irreducible. This is uncommon but does require open reduction when it occurs. Open dislocations should undergo copious irrigation and debridement and should be treated with an adequate course of antibiotics (20). After reduction, types I and II injuries are usually stable through the normal range of motion; however, as type II injuries come into full extension, they may become unstable and subluxate. The innate stability of the PIP allows treatment with a dorsal block splint and permits range of motion through a stable arc. Patients are initially immobilized in approximately 30 degrees of flexion and within 1 week are placed in a dorsal blocking splint and allowed to begin active flexion and extension limited at 30 degrees (Fig. 15.3). By 2 to 3 weeks this has been gradually increased to neutral, and the patient remains in a neutral blocking splint for 1 week. At that point, buddy taping can be resumed with activities. It is important to inform patients of residual swelling about the joint and a mild flexion contracture.

Stable type III injuries with a small volar fragment can be treated as type IIs. Type III injuries with a large volar fragment or impaction of the middle phalanx present a much more complicated clinical problem and require open reduction and internal fixation or some type of reconstruction. These procedures are beyond the scope of this chapter but are addressed in Chapter 16.

Volar Dislocations

Volar dislocations of the PIP joints are not as common as dorsal dislocations; however, they herald a much more significant injury pattern (21,22). The mechanism of injury is usually an axial load on a partially flexed PIP joint with some rotational component. The articular surface of the middle phalanx subluxates volarly with relation to the proximal phalanx. The condyles of the proximal phalanx then buttonhole through the extensor mechanism. With a pure volar dislocation this often results in avulsion of the central slip, resulting in a boutonniere deformity. If a rotatory component is involved, these injuries are usually associated with a unilateral disruption of a collateral ligament and a partial volar plate avulsion. As the middle phalanx subluxes, a condyle of the middle phalanx buttonholes between the central slip and lateral band. As the dislocation completes, the lateral band subluxes into the joint, becoming entrapped between the dorsal aspect of the middle phalanx and the volar aspect of the proximal phalanx. Flexion and longitudinal traction are necessary for reduction of most of these dislocations; however, with this injury pattern this maneuver creates a "Chinese finger trap" about the entrapped condyle, preventing reduction. These volar and rotatory dislocations have been previously described as irreducible requiring open reduction (23); however, longitudinal traction applied with the MP and PIP joints flexed and the wrist extended can be successful. This maneuver relaxes the extensor mechanism and allows reduction of the condyle and relocation of the lateral band (24).

After reduction of volar dislocations, it is crucial to assess the integrity of the central slip. In most of these injuries, a portion of the central slip and one lateral band will remain intact, allowing full active extension of the PIP joint. These patients can be treated with buddy taping and protected range of motion until comfortable but should be closely observed to ensure that a late boutonniere deformity does not occur. If patients lack full active extension after reduction, a central slip disruption must be assumed and the patient should be treated as if they have sustained a boutonniere injury. The treatment protocol for these injuries is outlined below.

Metacarpophalangeal Dislocations

Dislocation of the MP joint is not as common as the PIP joint. They usually occur in the thumb, index, or small finger and are very rare in the central digits. The mechanism is hyperextension of the proximal phalanx on the metacarpal head that results in rupture of the volar plate from its origin at the base of the metacarpal neck. The metacarpal head then buttonholes through the volar defect. The volar plate often comes to lie dorsal to the metacarpal head, the collateral ligaments around the metacarpal neck, the lumbrical muscle resting on the radial side, and the flexor tendons and their sheaths on the ulnar side (25,26). In the index and small finger, these dislocations are almost always irreducible,

even when using proper reduction technique. Under regional anesthesia, a single attempt at reduction can be performed. The described mechanism is hyperextension with an attempt to slide the proximal phalanx along the dorsum of the metacarpal and allow the interposed volar plate to reduce. If this is unsuccessful, open reduction through a volar (26) or dorsal (27) approach is recommended. Care should be taken in the volar approach to avoid the neurovascular bundles that will lie directly subcutaneous between the metacarpal head and the skin.

After reduction, the joint is usually stable. An initial compressive postoperative dressing is placed with the MPs in flexion to prevent edema. Two to 3 days postoperatively this is removed, the patient is placed in a dorsal blocking splint, and MP flexion and full interphalangeal motion is initiated. At 2 weeks this is advanced to neutral, and after 4 weeks of splinting the patients are advanced to a short period of buddy taping.

TENDON INJURIES

Tendon injuries in the hand are often associated with lacerations. This section deals primarily with closed injuries; however, open injuries deserve mention. On presentation, lacerations in the hand should undergo a thorough irrigation and debridement with a careful examination isolating each tendon individually. The physician should keep in mind the significant excursion of the tendinous structures in the hand resulting in seemingly remote injuries from the obvious zone of injury (28,29). A thorough neurovascular examination should be carried out as well. In the absence of vascular compromise, repair of tendon injuries is not emergent. At the time of injury, thorough irrigation and debridement with loose closure can be carried out and the hand splinted in a protected position. A thorough exploration of all tendinous and neurovascular structures near the zone of injury should be carried out at the time of definitive treatment. Partial injuries should be assessed and repaired as indicated. Complete lacerations should be fixed with a nonabsorbable grasping suture using standard techniques (30). Postoperatively, early range of motion should be initiated in a protected rehabilitation environment.

Extensor Tendon Injuries

Anatomy of the Extensor Mechanism

Perhaps one of the most complex and delicate structures in the human body is the extensor mechanism of the finger. A number of distinct muscular and tendonous units come together and through a complex interplay result in smooth and balanced digital function (Fig. 15.4). As the long extensor tendons pass across the dor-

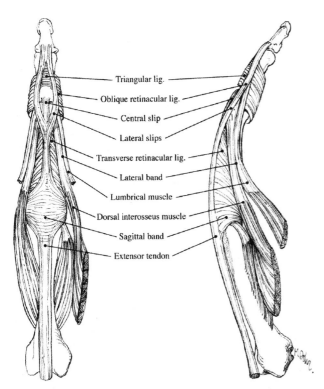

FIG. 15.4. Anatomy of the extensor mechanism.

Triangular lig.
Oblique retinacular lig.
Central slip
Lateral slips
Transverse retinacular lig.
Lateral band
Lumbrical muscle
Dorsal interosseus muscle
Sagittal band
Extensor tendon

Distal Interphalangeal Level

Injuries to the extensor mechanism at the level of the DIP joint are very common in athletes. Commonly referred to as mallet finger, baseball finger, or drop finger, this injury is the result of disruption of the terminal extensor tendon over the DIP joint. The injury is a result of forced flexion of the DIP joint while the extensor is actively contracting. Loss of continuity of the terminal extensor tendon results in an inability to extend the DIP joint and a fixed flexed posture.

Doyle (32) proposed a widely accepted classification of mallet finger deformities that aids in establishing a proper treatment plan. Type I injuries are the result of closed or blunt trauma with loss of tendon continuity. These injuries may be associated with a small avulsion fracture. Type II injuries are associated with a laceration at or proximal to the DIP joint with loss of tendon continuity. Type III injuries are the result of deep abrasions with loss of skin, subcutaneous cover, and tendon substance. Type IV injuries constitute a mallet fracture and are subdivided into three categories. Type IVA injuries are transepiphyseal plate fractures in children, type IVB are hyperflexion injuries with fracture of 20% or 50% of the articular surface, and type IVC are injuries of hyperextension with fracture of the articular surface usually involving more than 50% and with volar subluxation of the distal phalanx. Type I injuries are by far the most common in the athlete, and this section focuses primarily on the diagnosis and management of these closed injuries.

Diagnosis

The diagnosis of mallet finger is obvious from the clinical examination. The patient will usually present with a history of injury to the digit, most commonly an axial load applied by an oncoming ball, another player, or a fall onto the finger. These injuries are often painful, and tenderness will localize to the dorsum of the DIP. Although immediately after the injury the patient may have full extension, this will usually progress to an extensor lag that cannot be actively corrected. Passive motion is usually full.

X-rays are essential in the evaluation of mallet injuries to rule out a significant fracture. A large number of these injuries will be associated with a small avulsion from the dorsal aspect of the distal phalanx, but most of the articular surface will remain intact, and the joint will remain located. These fractures can be treated as pure tendinous injuries and will usually heal uneventfully with a good clinical result even if the fragment does not go on to radiographic union. Large fragments associated with disruption of a significant portion of the articular surface (usually greater than 30%) or with any joint subluxation should be treated operatively as any

sum of the hand to the level of the MP joint, they expand into "hoods" that cover the entire dorsum of the MP joints. These hoods pass radially and ulnarly to connect to the volar plates and transverse metacarpal ligaments and allow extension of the proximal phalanx. At this level, the extensor mechanism is joined by the interosseous and lumbrical tendons that combine to form a complex structure referred to as the extensor aponeurosis. These function to provide MP flexion and to contribute to PIP and distal interphalangeal (DIP) joint extension.

The extensor tendon continues beyond the MP to insert into the base of the middle phalanx as the central slip. On either side of the central slip, it also forms two lateral bands into which the lumbricals and interossei contribute. PIP extension is provided by the central slip with a contribution from the lateral bands. The lateral bands continue distally where they join just proximal to the distal interphalangeal joint to form a conjoined tendon that inserts into the base of the distal phalanx and provides DIP extension. The lateral bands are stabilized against volar subluxation by a triangular ligament overlying the middle phalanx. Each is also attached to a retinacular ligament laterally that allows proximal and distal migration but limits dorsal displacement. This transverse retinacular ligament is anchored volarly to the edge of the flexor tendon sheath at the PIP joint. The separate entities are delicately balanced, and injuries such as those discussed below will result in imbalance and profound functional deficits (31).

other intraarticular fracture. Restoration of a congruent joint is the primary goal in treatment of this type of injury.

Treatment

Closed zone I extensor tendon avulsion injuries can usually be managed nonoperatively. Treatment consists of 6 to 10 weeks of DIP joint immobilization in neutral to slight hyperextension (33–35). The position of immobilization is key to a good functional outcome. Excessive hyperextension places the dorsal skin at risk for necrosis because it compromises circulation by attenuating the blood supply to the volar fingertip that feeds the dorsal skin vessels (36,37). Aligning the joint to rest in the slightest bit of flexion will cause the tendon to heal in an elongated position, resulting in extensor lag (35).

Several splinting options are available: dorsal or volar aluminum padded splints, dorsal or volar custom-molded thermoplastic splints, and the Stack polyethylene splint (Warsaw Orthopaedics, Warsaw, IN). When treating the athlete's mallet finger, we prefer a custom thermoplastic dorsal padded splint secured with adhesive tape for play. This preserves fingertip sensory function and allows maximum PIP joint range of motion. Outside of sports activity, a volar static splint secured with tape is used. Alternating splints will prevent skin maceration, tape irritation, or local areas of pressure.

Achieving good results with mallet fingers depend on patient compliance. If the patient allows the fingertip to drop during the initial 6 weeks, then the splinting protocol must begin again from square one. Instruction on changing the splint when it becomes wet or for hygiene purposes must be given, and it is usually recommended that the patient seek help when donning and doffing the splint to ensure an extended DIP joint. Many authors advocate an additional 4 weeks of nighttime extension splinting plus intermittent splinting after the initial 6 weeks (34,35,38).

After the initial 6 weeks of extension splinting, unresisted flexion exercises within a range of 0 to 25 degrees are started. Exercising in a limited arc of motion is supported by Brand (39) calculations of the extensor strength to be less than one third that of the flexors. Hence, the flexor digitorum profundus (FDP) is a more powerful unit and may easily overcome the now weakened extensor tendon. During the seventh week, if full active extension is still present, flexion increments are increased to 35 to 40 degrees. Progressive template splints of 0 to 20, 0 to 30, and 0 to 40 degrees are used to ensure a controlled motion program. This is advanced weekly, and full flexion should be the goal at 3 months. If at any time the patient begins to develop an extensor lag, full-time splinting in extension is resumed for 1 week and the incremental motion protocol restarted.

Operative treatment is rarely indicated in closed zone I injuries. As previously stated, significant fractures involving greater than one third of the articular surface or associated with any joint subluxation require open reduction and internal fixation with congruent restoration of the joint surfaces (40,41). Rarely, K-wire fixation of the DIP joint in neutral is rarely recommended for closed tendinous injuries or those associated with a small avulsion fracture (42). This technique has been advocated for a patient whose livelihood is compromised by the use of a splint (i.e., surgeons and dentists). We do not recommend this treatment in the athlete because the DIP joint will still require splint protection to avoid the disastrous complication of bending or breakage of the K-wire at the DIP joint. If the treatment protocol is carefully outlined to the patient and the importance of compliance stressed, excellent results can be achieved with closed treatment alone (42).

Delayed presentation of mallet finger is not uncommon. If the patient has no secondary deformity or fixed contracture and the DIP is passively correctable, we recommend attempted closed management with the protocol outlined above. Because of the chronicity of the injury, splinting may need to be extended to 12 weeks before allowing progressive motion. Untreated mallet fingers will often result in a secondary swan-neck deformity (31). This deformity is characterized by hyperextension at the PIP with flexion at the DIP and is due to an imbalance in the extensor mechanism. With disruption of the terminal tendon, the extensor mechanism subluxates proximally, creating a hyperextension force at the PIP joint. This results in volar plate laxity and subsequently results in a hyperextension deformity. Over time, this can progress to a fixed deformity with degenerative changes in the joints (31). Although a swan-neck deformity can be functionally managed with splints, the deformity itself does not respond to conservative splinting and exercise programs due to the long-standing imbalance at the interphalangeal joints and the volar plate laxity. Multiple techniques for operative repair have been recommended but are beyond the scope of this chapter (31,43,44). Clearly, the best management for this secondary deformity is an early identification of the pathology and appropriate early conservative management.

Proximal Interphalangeal Level

Central slip injuries involve rupture of the central slip of the extensor mechanism as it inserts onto the base of the middle phalanx. These injuries can result from direct trauma to the dorsum of the PIP joint or acute flexion at the PIP while the extensor is contracting. As with mallet fingers, this injury is common in athletes struck by an oncoming ball, opposing player, or injured in a fall.

Central slip injuries can be very subtle in the acute

phase, and delayed treatment can result in a fixed deformity that is functionally debilitating and very difficult to manage nonoperatively (45). For this reason, early diagnosis and treatment is essential. A high index of suspicion is necessary to ensure that these injuries do not go unrecognized and untreated.

On presentation the athlete typically will have swelling and tenderness directly over the dorsal aspect of the PIP joint at the central slip insertion. A 15 to 20 degree or greater loss of active extension of the PIP joint when the wrist and MP are fully flexed has been reported as a useful test for early recognition of this lesion. Weak extension against resistance is also an excellent diagnostic sign and may be aided by placement of a digital block to alleviate pain.

The primary goal in treatment of a central slip injury is to prevent the development of a boutonniere deformity. Fresh cadaver studies have demonstrated that section of the central slip alone does not result in the development of boutonniere deformity (46,47). The boutonniere deformity occurs as the lateral bands tear away from the remaining fibers and migrate volarly while the disrupted ends of the central slip migrate proximally. As the lateral bands migrate volar to the axis of the

PIP joint, they begin to function as flexors. Proximal migration of the central slip leads to hyperextension at the DIP joint. As the central slip retracts further proximally, it concentrates its force on the MP joint, and a hyperextension posture is created at this level. If these deforming forces are left uncorrected, contractures of the ligamentous and capsular structures occur, making correction of this deformity even more difficult.

The treatment of acute central slip injuries is aimed at restoration of the normal tendon balance and length relationships of the central slip and lateral bands. This is achieved by splinting of the PIP in extension while leaving the DIP free for active range of motion (Fig. 15.5A and B). This has been shown to draw the lateral bands dorsally and to reduce the separation of the torn ends of the central slip of the extensor tendon, allowing the structures to heal in their anatomic positions (32). Some authors have advocated placement of a transarticular K-wire at the PIP; however, in the athlete this carries the same risk of hardware failure associated with pinning of mallet fingers and requires protective splinting during play.

Unfortunately, these injuries often go unrecognized

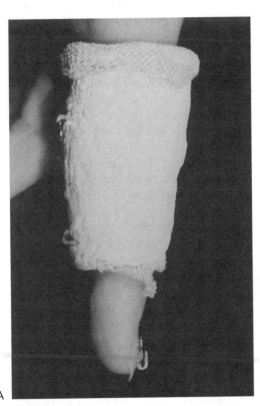 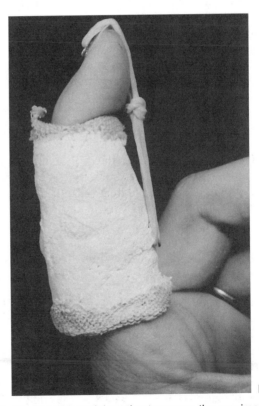

A

B

FIG. 15.5. A: Closed central slip ruptures are initially treated with serial casting to ensure the proximal interphalangeal joint rests at 0 degrees extension. Casts are usually changed every 2 to 3 days. **B:** Traction is applied to the distal interphalangeal joint to stretch the oblique retinacular ligaments of the extensor mechanism and maintain normal balance between the proximal and distal interphalangeal joints.

and will present to the physician with fixed contractures. If the PIP joint is passively correctable, the authors recommend initiating a course of splinting as outlined above for acute injuries. If there are fixed contractures, serial casting of the PIP joint is initiated until full extension is possible. This is then followed by PIP splinting with active DIP flexion.

After 3 to 4 weeks of immobilization, a volar flexion template is fabricated and gentle unresisted active flexion at the PIP is initiated. This allows some gliding of the lateral band, preventing adhesions. Nighttime splinting in full extension is continued. The treatment period for boutonniere deformities can be extended, often lasting anywhere from 3 to 6 months depending on the chronicity of the problem and the degree of contractures on presentation.

Operative treatment of acute central slip injuries is indicated in certain specific instances (45). Injuries associated with an avulsion of a significant portion of the base of the middle phalanx should be treated surgically with internal fixation or excision of the fragment and primary repair of the central slip to bone. In this instance, a transarticular pin should be placed for approximately 3 weeks, and after removal a course of progressive protected range of motion should be initiated using flexion templates.

Perhaps more so than with any other soft tissue injury of the hand, early diagnosis and appropriate management of central slip injuries is essential in preventing late secondary deformity that will always result in less satisfactory results. Knowledge of this injury and a high index of suspicion are necessary for any trainer, therapist, or physician treating athletes.

Metacarpophalangeal Level

Ruptures of the extensor hood at the MP level are uncommon injuries in the athlete; however, they can be significantly painful and debilitating (48,49). These injuries result from longitudinal tears in the oblique fibers of the extensor hood and usually occur after blunt trauma, although they can be spontaneous. The tears most often occur on the radial side, and the long finger is the most commonly involved.

The athletes will usually present with dorsal pain and swelling localized at the MP joint. The extensor tendon ulnarly subluxates into the sulcus between the two MP joints. An extensor lag is often present; however, the digit can be passively extended, and in the acute setting the extensor tendon will often localize over the MP joint with passive extension. With fixed subluxation there will often be ulnar deviation of the involved digit (33,50,51).

Acute injuries can usually be managed nonoperatively. If the extensor digitorum communis (EDR) tendon centralizes with the MP in extension, a splint can be fabricated to hold the MP in neutral or slight flexion

with the interphalangeals free. Active interphalangeal motion is encouraged to prevent stiffness. Splinting is maintained for 4 to 6 weeks with gradual progression of MP joint flexion. Full flexion by 12 weeks is the goal.

Chronic injuries in which the tendon will not centralize spontaneously require operative repair. Primary repair of the tear is sometimes possible after debridement of the granulation tissue if adequate structural integrity is present (49). If this repair alone is inadequate, it can be supplemented with a junctura tendonae or with a distally based slip of the extensor digitorum communis tendon (20,52). Postoperatively, the MP joints are casted in 20 degrees of flexion. Two weeks postoperatively, the patient begins PIP motion, and at 4 weeks MP motion is initiated and gradually progressed. Motion is protected for a minimum of 8 weeks with a goal of full motion by 12 weeks.

Flexor Tendon Injuries

Flexor Digitorum Profundus Avulsion

Avulsion of the FDP insertion on the distal phalanx is a common athletic injury. This is most common in contact sports when the athlete grasps the jersey or pants of an opposing player and the finger is forcibly extended while the FDP is contracting. This results in a disruption of the FDP at its insertion and is the etiology of its common name "jersey finger" (33,53–55).

FDP avulsions can occur in any digit; however, they are most commonly found in the ring finger. Multiple anatomic etiologies for the increased incidence in the ring finger have been suggested. Manske and Lesker (56) showed that the insertion of the profundus in the ring finger is weaker than that of the long finger. The common muscle belly of the profundus to the long, ring, and small fingers and tethering of the ring profundus in the palm by a bipennate lumbrical muscle may result in a more vulnerable ring finger (33). Leddy and Packer (57) showed that the small finger is more easily disengaged from an opponent's clothing, transferring most of the force to the ring finger, which remains entrapped.

As with many other soft tissue injuries in the athlete, FDP avulsions frequently go undetected and present late. Unlike mallet fingers and central slip injuries, no secondary deformities occur; however, with a delay in treatment, tendonous degeneration and adhesions often prevent primary repair and necessitate secondary reconstructive procedures. These classically have a less successful outcome than acute repairs.

The athlete typically presents with an inability to flex the DIP of the affected digit (Fig. 15.6). Superficialis function will be intact, but range of motion may often be limited by swelling or by mechanical blockage by the avulsed FDP tendon. Careful examination of each digit demonstrating function of both the FDP and flexor dig-

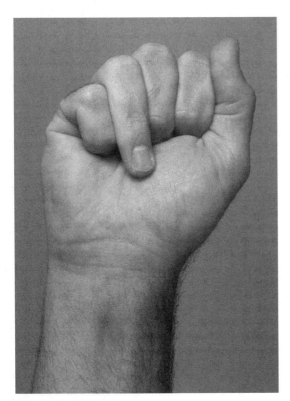

FIG. 15.6. Jersey finger. The classic clinical presentation of a flexor digitorum profundus avulsion in the athlete. Upon active flexion of the digits, the distal interphalangeal joint remains in an extended position.

itorum superficialis (FDS) tendon independently should be carried out because multiple fingers can be involved. Additionally, a careful examination of the extensor mechanism should be conducted. X-rays are mandatory because the avulsion can occur with a large bony fragment. The location of the avulsed tendon can often be identified by palpation along the tendon sheath for a prominence or a tender mass.

Leddy and Packer (57) classified FDP avulsions into three main categories (57): type I, the tendon retracts into the palm; type II, the tendon retracts to the level of the PIP joint; and type III, a bony fragment is avulsed, which usually becomes entrapped in the annular pulley at the level of the DIP. This classification system plays a role in treatment and prognosis. Type I injuries are the most severe injury. With proximal retraction into the palm, the tendon's blood supply from the vincular system is completely disrupted and synovial perfusion is absent. Type I injuries must be operatively repaired within 7 to 10 days or the tendon will become contracted and primary repair will be impossible.

In type II injuries, the tendon retracts to the PIP level where it is tethered by the long vinculum, which remains intact. The tendon thus remains within the sheath and is perfused through the intact vinculum. Although early repair within 7 to 10 days is recommended, type II avul-

sions have been successfully treated with primary repair as long as 3 months after injury (50).

Type III injuries behave similarly to type II injuries. Because the bony fragment is usually entrapped in the annular pulley at the level of the DIP joint, the vinculum remains intact and the tendon's nutritional supply is preserved. Avulsion of the profundus from the bony fragment has been reported, and therefore careful examination of the palm should be carried out even when x-rays demonstrate a bony fragment at the level of the DIP.

Treatment of the injury depends on time of presentation. Type II and type III injuries that are of less than 3 months' duration can usually be treated by advancement and primary repair of the FDP tendon. The tendon can be reinserted into the distal phalanx using a number of techniques. We prefer the use of a pull-out button with transosseous sutures tied over the nail. Successful use of suture anchors has been described. In type III injuries, the bony fragment can be repaired with a screw, fixed with a transosseous suture and button, or excised and the tendon primarily repaired to the defect if the bony fragment is too small for fixation. Type I injuries that are less than 2 weeks' duration can usually be repaired using these techniques.

The rehabilitation protocol for the athlete with jersey finger should not differ from the lay person. We use an early arc of motion based on Evans' work (58,59) for the zone I injuries that are repaired primarily end to end, advanced, or reinserted into bone. Wound care, edema reduction, protected splinting, patient education, and exercise should be initiated within 48 hours postoperatively. A dorsal protective splint is fabricated with joint angles of 30- to 40-degrees wrist flexion, 30- to 40-degrees MP flexion, the PIP at neutral, and the splint extending slightly beyond the fingertips. A second digital dorsal splint that holds the DIP joint in 40 degrees of flexion is also fabricated and used for the first 4 weeks after surgery (Fig. 15.7). The MP angle is 30 degrees rather than the traditional 60 degrees of flexion within the splint because at 30 degrees, the force of the lumbrical and the profundus is diminished. This position also allows the patient to perform a modified hook fist exercise that produces the greatest differential collide between the FDS and the FDP. The rationale for splinting the DIP joint in 40 degrees of flexion is to allow the profundus to heal proximal to its anatomic length by 3 to 4 mm. Recovering of excursion by stretching a repair site is an easier rehabilitative task than regaining proximal excursion.

The patient is instructed to exercise every waking hour with 20 repetitions of each exercise. These consist of passive DIP joint flexion from 40 degrees to full flexion (75 to 80 degrees), passive placement of the fingers in the modified hook fist position and composite flexion position, and active PIP joint extension with the

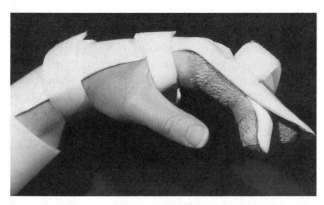

FIG. 15.7. Zone I splint. The zone I "jersey finger" requires protective splinting for the initial 21 days with the wrist positioned in 30 to 40 degrees of flexion, the metacarpophalangeal joints at 30 degrees, and the proximal interphalangeal joints at absolute zero. An additional dorsal splint is applied to the affected distal interphalangeal joint that holds it in 45 degrees of flexion but does not impede proximal interphalangeal joint flexion or extension.

MP joints held in maximum flexion. "Place and hold" active exercise for the involved digit superficialis is performed while the other digits are strapped to the roof of the splint in extension. During formal therapy sessions, controlled wrist tenodesis is performed along with the active hold component according to the short arc motion protocol. This exercise entails wrist extension at 30 degrees, MP joints at 75 to 80 degrees, PIP joints at 70 degrees, and the DIP joints at 40 degrees of flexion. The therapist positions these angles, and the patient is asked only to contract the muscles sufficiently to maintain this position. It is recommended practicing on the uninvolved hand first. This exercise requires the patient to attend formal therapy three to four times per week. Usually this is not a problem with the athlete because there is a high motivation to return to play.

The distal tip splint is removed 4 weeks postoperatively, but extension of the DIP joint is not used until week 5. If a flexion contracture of the DIP joint develops, static extension splinting may begin at 6.5 weeks. This is usually only a problem if the A5 and/or A4 pulleys are not intact. Secondary to increased tensile strength, greater flexion angles are encouraged with the active place and hold component. At our facility, if patients show a clear understanding of the rationale, can perform the program independently and correctly in therapy, and have proven themselves compliant, we will commence the active place and hold component in a controlled environment at home.

The protective splint is discharged at 6 to 7 weeks. This is one area in sports medicine where return to playing time varies among authors. If hand dexterity is not required in one's sport, then return to play with a mitten-type splint or cast is allowable 2 weeks postoper-

atively. Within the device, the wrist and digit should be flexed. In manual sports, return to play is delayed for 8 weeks until moderate tendon strength has returned. At that time, a blocking splint that prevents hyperextension is worn for an additional 4 weeks.

SUMMARY

Soft tissue injuries in the hand are common athletic injuries. When recognized acutely and appropriately treated, time lost from play can be limited and a good outcome anticipated. A delay in diagnosis or treatment often results in chronic debilitating deformities that are much more difficult to treat and have much less favorable outcomes. It is important that coaches, trainers, therapists, and physicians who are involved in the treatment of athletes recognize these injuries and the importance of early intervention.

REFERENCES

1. Coonrad RN, Goldner JL. A study of the pathological findings and treatment in soft tissue injury of the thumb metacarpophalangeal joint. *J Bone Joint Surg Am* 1968;50A:439.
2. Campbell CS. Gamekeeper's thumb. *J Bone Joint Surg Br* 1955;37B:148.
3. Browne EZ, Dunn HK, Snyder CC. Ski pole thumb injury. *Plast Reconstr Surg* 1976;58:19.
4. Husband JB, McPherson SA. Bony skier's thumb injuries. *Clin Orthop* 1996;327:79.
5. McCue FC, Hakala MW, Andrews JR, et al. Ulnar collateral ligament injuries of the thumb in athletes. *J Sports Med* 1974;2:70.
6. Stener B. Displacement of the ruptured ulnar collateral ligament of the metacarpophalangeal joint of the thumb. *J Bone Joint Surg Br* 1962;44B:869–879.
7. Heyman P, Gelberman RH, Duncan K, et al. Injuries of the ulnar collateral ligament of the thumb metacarpophalangeal joint. *Clin Orthop* 1993;292:165.
8. Louis DS, Huebner JJ, Hankin FM. Rupture and displacement of the ulnar collateral ligament of the metacarpophalangeal joint of the thumb. Preoperative diagnosis. *J Bone Joint Surg Am* 1986;68A:1320–1326.
9. Smith RJ. Post-traumatic instability of the metacarpophalangeal joint of the thumb. *J Bone Joint Surg Am* 1977;59:14–21.
10. Abrahamson SQ, Sollerman C, Lundborg G, et al. Diagnosis of displaced ulnar collateral ligament of the metacarpophalangeal joint of the thumb. *J Hand Surg* 1990;15A:457.
11. Frank WE, Dobyns JH. Surgical pathology of collateral ligamentous injuries of the thumb. *Clin Orthop* 1972;83:102.
12. Kessler I. Complete avulsion of the ulnar collateral ligament of the metacarpophalangeal joint of the thumb. *Clin Orthop* 1961;29:196.
13. Osterman AL, Haykne GD, Bora FWM. A quantitative evaluation of thumb function after ulnar collateral repair and reconstruction. *J Trauma* 1981;21:854.
14. Durham JW, Khuri S, Kim MH. Acute and late radial collateral ligament injuries of the thumb metacarpophalangeal joint. *J Hand Surg* 1993;18A:232–237.
15. Bowers WH, Wolf JW Jr, Nehil JL, et al. The proximal interphalangeal joint volar plate. I. An anatomical and biomechanical study. *J Hand Surg* 1980;5:79.
16. Kiefhaber TR, Stern PJ, Grood ES. Lateral stability of the proximal interphalangeal joint. *J Hand Surg* 1986;11A:661.
17. Eaton RG, Littler JW. Joint injuries and their sequelae. *Clin Plast Surg* 1976;3:85.
18. Rodriguez AL. Injuries to the collateral ligaments of the proximal interphalangeal joints. *Hand* 1973;5:55.
19. Bowers WH, Wolf JW Jr, Nehil JL, et al. The proximal interpha-

langeal joint volar plate. II. A clinical study of hyperextension injury. *J Hand Surg* 1981;6:77.

20. Wheeldon FT. Recurrent dislocation of extensor tendons. *J Bone Joint Surg Br* 1954;36B:612.

21. Palmer CA, Sullivan DJ, Wild DR. Palmer dislocation of the proximal interphalangeal joint. *J Hand Surg* 1984;9A:39.

22. Spinner M, Choi BY. Anterior dislocation of the proximal interphalangeal joint. *J Bone Joint Surg Am* 1970;52A:1329.

23. Green SM, Posner MA. Irreducible dorsal dislocations of the proximal interphalangeal joint. *J Hand Surg* 1985;10A:85.

24. Thompson JS, Eaton RG. Volar dislocation of the proximal interphalangeal joint. *J Hand Surg* 1977;2:232.

25. Green DP, Terry GC. Complex dislocation of the metacarpophalangeal joint. *J Bone Joint Surg Am* 1973;55A:1480.

26. Kaplan EB. Dorsal dislocation of the metacarpophalangeal joint of the index finger. *J Bone Joint Surg Am* 1957;39A:1081.

27. Becton JL, Christian JD, Goodwin HN, et al. A simplified technique for treating the complex dislocation of the index metacarpophalangeal joint. *J Bone Joint Surg Am* 1975;57A:696.

28. Wehbe MA, Hunter JM. Flexor tendon gliding in the hand I. In vivo excursions. *J Hand Surg* 1975;10A:570.

29. Wehbe MA, Hunter JM. Flexor tendon gliding in the hand. II. Differential gliding. *J Hand Surg* 1985;10A:570.

30. Urbaniak JR, Cahill JD, Mortenson RA. Tendon suturing methods: analysis of tensile strengths. In: American Academy of Orthopedic Surgeons, eds. *Symposium on tendon surgery of the hand.* St. Louis, MO: Mosby, 1975.

31. Smith RJ. Balance and kinetics of the fingers under normal and pathological conditions. *Clin Orthop* 1974;104:92.

32. Doyle JR. Extensor tendons-acute injuries. In: Green DP, ed. *Operative hand surgery.* New York: Churchill Livingstone, 1993:1925.

33. Rettig AC. Closed tendon injuries of the hand and wrist in the athlete. *Clin Sports Med* 1992;11:77.

34. Strickland J. The hand. *Orthop Sports Med* 1994;IB:945.

35. Evans RB. An update on extensor tendon management. In: Hunter JM, Mackin EJ, Callahan AD, eds. *Rehabilitation of the hand: surgery and therapy,* 4th ed. Vol. II. Philadelphia: Mosby, 1995:565–606.

36. Lovett WL, McCalla MA. Management and rehabilitation of extensor tendon injuries. *Orthop Clin North Am* 1983;44:811.

37. Macht SD, Watson HK. The Moberg volar advancement flap for digital reconstruction. *J Hand Surg* 1980;5:372.

38. Rosenthal EA. The extensor tendons: anatomy and management. In: *Rehabilitation of the hand: surgery and therapy,* 4th ed. Vol. II. Philadelphia: Mosby, 1995:519–564.

39. Brand PW. *Biomechanics of the hand.* St. Louis, MO: Mosby, 1985.

40. Stark HH, Gainor BJ, Ashworth CR, et al. Operative treatment of intra-articular fractures of the dorsal aspect of the distal phalanx of digits. *J Bone Joint Surg Am* 1987;69A:892.

41. Wehbe MA, Schneider LH. Mallet fractures. *J Bone Joint Surg Am* 1984;66A:658.

42. Stern PJ, Kastrup JJ. Complications and prognosis of treatment of mallet finger. *J Hand Surg* 1988;13A:329.

43. Litler JW. The finger extensor mechanism. *Surg Clin North Am* 1967;47:415.

44. Thompson JS, Littler JW, Upton J. The spiral oblique retinacular ligament. SORL. *J Hand Surg* 1978;3:482.

45. Coons MS, Green SM. Boutonniere deformity. *Hand Clin* 1995;11:387.

46. Harris C, Rutledge GL Jr. The functional anatomy of the extensor mechanism of the finger. *J Bone Joint Surg Am* 1972;54A:712.

47. Micks JE, Hager D. Role of the controversial parts of the extensor of the finger. *J Bone Joint Surg Am* 1973;55A:884.

48. Harvey FJ, Hume KF. Spontaneous recurrent ulnar dislocation of the long extensor tendons of the fingers. *J Hand Surg* 1980;5:492.

49. Kettlkamp DB, Flatt AE, Moulds R. Traumatic dislocation of the long finger extensor tendon: a clinical, anatomical, and biomechanical study. *J Bone Joint Surg Am* 1971;53A:229.

50. Rettig AC. Current concepts in management of sports injuries of the hand and wrist. *J Hand Ther* 1991;4:42.

51. Ritts GD, Wood MB, Engber WD. Nonoperative treatment of traumatic dislocations of the extensor digitorum tendon in patients without rheumatoid disorders. *J Hand Surg* 1985;10A:714.

52. McCoy FJ, Winsky AJ. Lumbrical loop operation for luxation of the extensor tendons of the hand. *Plast Reconstruc Surg* 1969;44:142.

53. Lunn PG, Lamb DW. "Rugby finger"—avulsion of profundus of ring finger. *J Hand Surg* 1984;9B:69.

54. McCue FC, Meister K. Common sports hand injuries—an overview of etiology, management, and prevention. *Sports Med* 1993;15:281.

55. Ruby LK. Common hand injuries in the athlete. *Orthop Clin North Am* 1980;11:819.

56. Manske PR, Lesker PA. Avulsion of the ring finger digitorum profundus tendon: an experimental study. *Hand* 1978;10:52.

57. Leddy JP, Packer JW. Avulsion of the profundus tendon insertion in athletes. *J Hand Surg* 1977;2:66.

58. Evans RB. A study of the zone I flexor tendon injury and implications for treatment. *J Hand Ther* 1990;3:133.

59. Evans RB. Rehabilitative techniques for applying immediate active tension to zone II and II flexor tendon repairs. *Techn Hand Upper Extrem Surg* 1997;1:286.

Principles and Practice of Orthopaedic Sports Medicine,
edited by William E. Garrett, Jr., Kevin P. Speer, and Donald T. Kirkendall.
Lippincott Williams & Wilkins, Philadelphia © 2000.

CHAPTER 16

Fractures of the Carpal Bones

Andrew E. Caputo and Richard D. Goldner

SCAPHOID FRACTURES

Epidemiology

The scaphoid is the most commonly fractured carpal bone, second only to the distal radius if all wrist fractures about the wrist are included (1). Scaphoid fractures occur most frequently in active young adult males who fall on the outstretched dorsiflexed hand, and it has been estimated that 1% of all college football players in the United States sustain a scaphoid fracture each year (2).

Anatomy

The scaphoid connects the proximal and distal carpal rows. It lies oblique to the longitudinal axis of the carpus on the radial aspect of the wrist. The largest articular surface is convex and articulates proximally with the radius. Distal articulation is with the trapezium and the trapezoid. The proximal ulnar surface articulates with the lunate, whereas the more distal ulnar articulation is with the capitate.

Approximately two thirds of the scaphoid surface is covered with articular cartilage, but the palmar concave surface is mostly nonarticular. With a fall on the dorsiflexed wrist, the scaphoid is tethered between the distal radius and the adjacent carpal bones. With force being applied to it by the radioscaphocapitate ligament, the scaphoid is particularly susceptible to fracture. The degree of radial or ulnar deviation and the amount of wrist dorsiflexion at the time of injury influence whether the fracture occurs proximal, distal, or at the waist of the scaphoid (3,4).

A. E. Caputo: Department of Orthopaedic Surgery, University of Connecticut Health Center, Farmington, Connecticut 06032.

R. D. Goldner: Division of Orthopaedic Surgery, Duke Medical Center, Durham, North Carolina 27710.

Scaphoid waist fractures have been created in a cadaveric model by applying a dorsiflexion load to the radial side of the palm. The palmar aspect of the scaphoid failed in tension, which was also transmitted dorsally (3). Osteotomy through the waist of the scaphoid in a cadaveric model resulted in volar angulation of the scaphoid (5). Clinically, this leads to collapse deformity of the wrist, with dorsiflexion of the lunate (dorsal intercalary segment instability) (6,7).

The major blood supply to the scaphoid is from branches of the radial artery that enter the bone at or distal to the waist, at the dorsal ridge. This blood supply accounts for 70% to 80% of the total interosseous vascularity and provides the sole blood supply to the proximal pole. Volar vessels enter through the tubercle and account for 20% to 30% of the internal vascularity of the distal aspect of the scaphoid (8,9). A fracture of the proximal third of the scaphoid can disrupt the arterial supply to the proximal pole, which enters the bone at or distal to the middle third.

Fracture Morphology

Scaphoid fractures can be divided into those occurring at the distal third (5% to 10%), middle third (65% to 75%), and proximal third (15% to 30%) (10). Dividing the fractures into these anatomic locations is relevant when deciding the most appropriate treatment modality for a given fracture. Tuberosity and distal third fractures heal the most quickly, often within 6 weeks. Proximal third fractures, in contrast, might take 6 months to revascularize, and small proximal pole fractures frequently develop osteonecrosis and delayed union or nonunion.

Russe (11) classified scaphoid fractures based on the direction of the fracture line relative to the long axis of the scaphoid. A middle third scaphoid fracture is most stable if the fracture lies perpendicular to the longitudinal axis of the bone (transverse). Horizontal oblique and vertical oblique fractures are subject to increased sheer forces when treated in a cast, take longer to heal, and have a higher incidence of nonunion than do transverse fractures.

An important factor in determining the most appropriate treatment of a scaphoid fracture is its stability; if treated nonoperatively, the unstable (displaced) fracture has a worse prognosis. A scaphoid fracture is considered unstable if displacement is 1 mm or greater or if a step-off is visible on any of the x-ray views. However, plain x-rays often demonstrate a gap of less than 1 mm when in fact the displacement is greater. Frequently,

fluoroscopy can demonstrate the true displacement of the fracture because the wrist can be positioned to view the fracture directly instead of obscuring it by an oblique projection. The most accurate determination of angulation and displacement of a scaphoid fracture is obtained by direct sagittal and coronal computed tomography (CT) (or direct sagittal and coronal polytomography) (Fig. 16.1).

In addition to fracture displacement, an unstable scaphoid fracture is suspected if the lunate capitate angle is greater than 15 degrees (as seen on the neutral

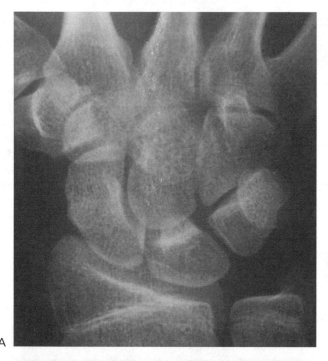

A

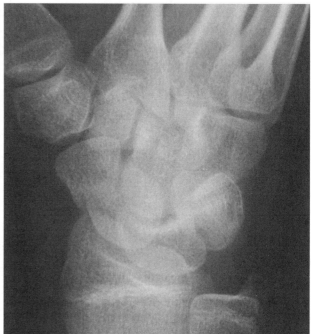

B

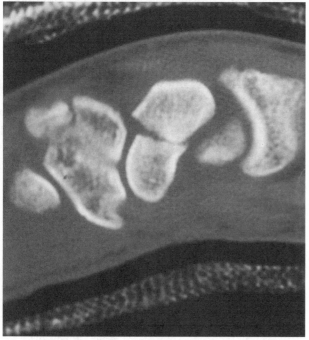

C

FIG. 16.1. A: Posteroanterior view of this 14-year-old girl's wrist does not reveal a scaphoid fracture. **B:** The oblique view, taken at the same time, demonstrates a cortical disruption on the radial aspect of the scaphoid. **C:** Sagittal computed tomography (CT) demonstrates significant displacement in addition to increased volar angulation of the scaphoid. Although x-rays are sufficient to diagnose certain scaphoid fractures, direct sagittal and coronal CT often give additional information regarding the displacement and angulation of the fracture. From the x-rays in A and B, cast treatment might have been recommended. The CT demonstrates a scaphoid fracture displaced sufficiently to indicate the need for open reduction and internal fixation.

lateral x-ray), if the radiolunate angle is greater than 15 degrees, or if the scapholunate angle is greater than 65 degrees (12). Any fracture in which both cortices are disrupted is at least potentially unstable. A completely nondisplaced hairline fracture detected only on CT might be considered stable, and an incomplete fracture is stable.

Despite the above distinction, certain "unstable" fractures do heal with cast treatment, whereas occasionally a completely nondisplaced fracture may develop a nonunion (Fig. 16.2). This inconsistency likely is related to the vascular insult caused by the fracture. Although a complete scaphoid fracture with less than 1 mm of displacement might heal with appropriate cast treat-

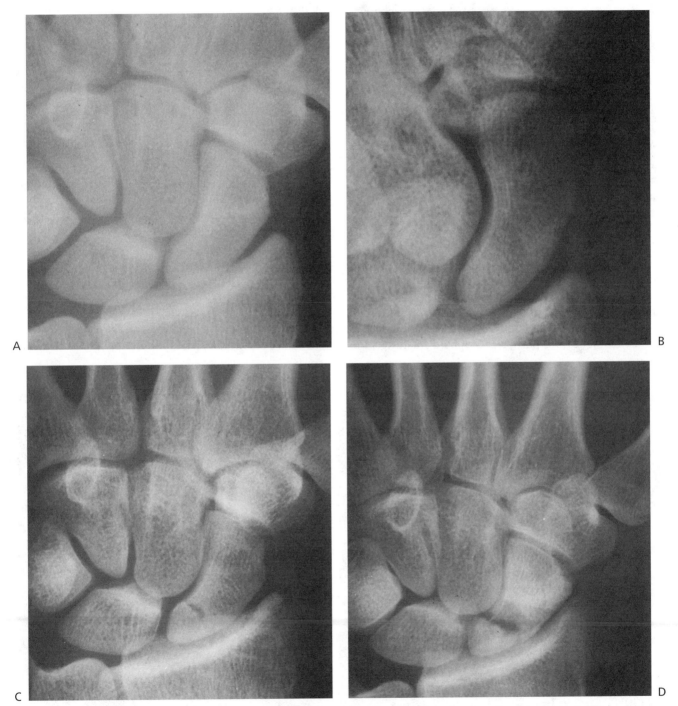

FIG. 16.2. A: This posteroanterior x-ray taken on the day of injury does not demonstrate a scaphoid fracture. **B:** This scaphoid view taken 2 months later suggests the possibility of a nondisplaced proximal third fracture. **C:** Posteroanterior x-ray taken at the same time as B clearly demonstrates the proximal pole fracture. **D:** Posteroanterior x-ray 2 years later demonstrates definite scaphoid nonunion.

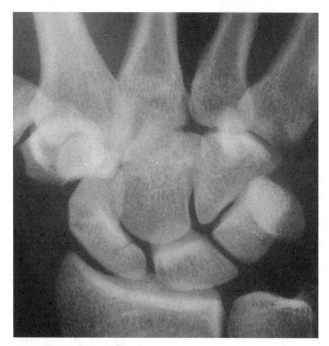

FIG. 16.3. This posteroanterior x-ray demonstrates an incomplete fracture of the proximal third of the scaphoid that healed with cast treatment alone.

time from the initial injury. The fracture is considered fresh if it is less than 3 weeks old, delayed union is suspected between 4 and 6 months after the injury, and nonunion is diagnosed greater than 4 to 6 months after the injury.

The fracture classification of Herbert and Fisher (13) is helpful in arriving at the appropriate treatment for a scaphoid fracture. This classification takes into account whether the fracture is stable or unstable; acute, delayed union, or established nonunion; complete or incomplete; whether the stable acute fracture involves the tubercle or is an incomplete waist fracture; whether the unstable acute fracture involves the distal, middle, or proximal pole; and whether there is ligamentous injury such as a transscaphoid perilunate fracture–dislocation. The type A fracture is stable and acute. It involves either the tubercle or an incomplete fracture and can be treated with cast immobilization (Fig. 16.3). Type B, unstable acute fractures, are treated more predictably by internal screw fixation than by cast immobilization (Fig. 16.4). Type C, delayed unions (Fig. 16.5), and type D, established nonunions (Fig. 16.6), are treated best operatively. Both internal screw fixation and bone grafting are appropriate for treatment of delayed unions and nonunions.

ment alone, internal fixation is more predictable, requires less time in cast immobilization, and often is the most appropriate treatment for the athlete.

One important factor to consider in determining the best treatment for a particular scaphoid fracture is the

Clinical Evaluation

The diagnosis of a scaphoid fracture should be suspected when a patient complains of wrist pain after a fall on

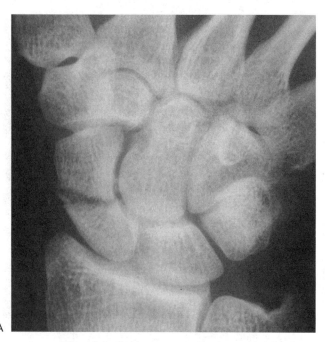
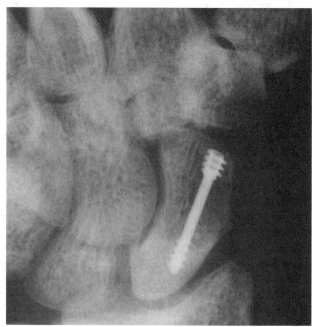

FIG. 16.4. A: Posteroanterior view taken the day of injury demonstrates a displaced scaphoid fracture. **B:** This was treated with Herbert screw fixation with subsequent healing.

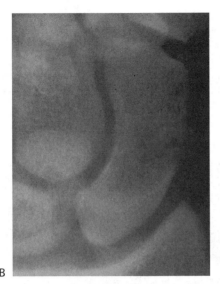
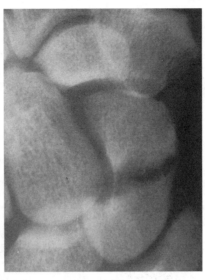
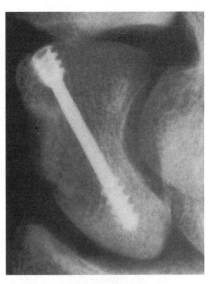

A,B   C

FIG. 16.5. A: Scaphoid view taken 2 months after injury, at which time the patient had persistent discomfort, suggests a nondisplaced fracture of the middle third of the scaphoid. **B:** Posteroanterior view taken at the same time as A reveals greater than 2-mm displacement between the fracture fragments and demonstrates a delayed union. **C:** This delayed union was treated with internal screw fixation and iliac crest bone graft.

the outstretched dorsiflexed hand. The physician should beware of diagnosing merely a "wrist sprain" and should have a high index of suspicion of a scaphoid fracture when dealing with wrist injuries.

Although various clinical signs have been reported as characteristic of scaphoid fractures, tenderness to palpation at the anatomic snuff box remains the principal diagnostic finding. However, pain can be present at the scaphoid tuberosity in the palm or at the scapholunate region just distal to Lister's tubercle on the dorsum of the wrist. Active wrist range of motion may be reduced, with pain present at extremes of motion. Initially, significant functional loss may be absent, and at times, the stoic athlete may continue to compete for weeks before realizing that he or she has sustained a significant injury. Swelling and ecchymosis usually are associated with more complex injuries such as carpal fracture dislocations. If an individual sustains a wrist injury and has tenderness to palpation in the anatomic snuff box, the physician should consider the diagnosis of scaphoid fracture.

Scaphoid Imaging

The initial imaging studies for a patient with a suspected scaphoid fracture should include the following wrist x-rays: posteroanterior (PA) in neutral position, PA in ulnar deviation, lateral with the wrist in neutral position, 45 degrees pronated oblique, 45 degrees supinated oblique, and anteroposterior clenched fist view. Ulnar deviation is important because it maxi-

mally extends the proximal carpal row, enabling full scaphoid visualization, which can be compromised by overlying shadows on the neutral PA and lateral views. In addition, the ulnar deviation view positions the long axis of the scaphoid more parallel to the x-ray plate and thus makes the fracture line more perpendicular to the x-ray beam. Finally, ulnar deviation tends to distract unstable fracture fragments and can facilitate visualization of the fracture line. Certain fractures can be demonstrated best on oblique views. The anteroposterior clenched fist view will enable assessment of the scapholunate gap and will help to exclude scapholunate dissociation that can occur in conjunction with a scaphoid fracture. At any time during the course of diagnosing or treating a scaphoid fracture, fluoroscopy can enable to wrist to be positioned so as to best visualize the scaphoid fracture and also can aid in assessing carpal ligament injuries.

If the patient is tender to palpation in the anatomic snuff box and if x-rays are normal, the wrist is immobilized in a thumb spica splint or cast for 10 to 14 days, and then x-rays are repeated. This allows bone resorption adjacent to the fracture site and enables nondisplaced fractures to be visualized more easily radiographically. If more urgent diagnosis is necessary to facilitate an athlete's return to competition, options for additional diagnostic studies include bone scan, magnetic resonance imaging (MRI), CT, or tomograms.

A technetium 99 bone scan is more sensitive than

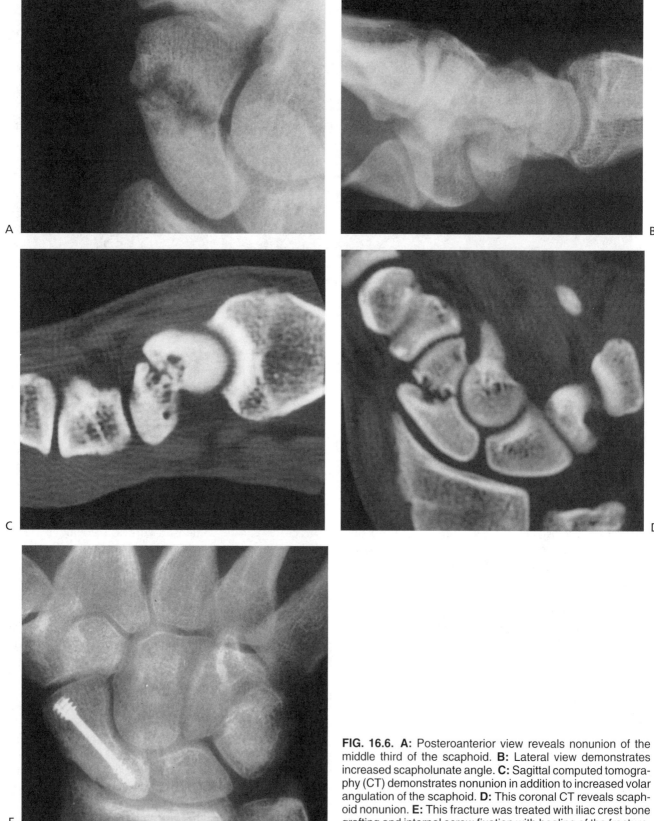

FIG. 16.6. A: Posteroanterior view reveals nonunion of the middle third of the scaphoid. **B:** Lateral view demonstrates increased scapholunate angle. **C:** Sagittal computed tomography (CT) demonstrates nonunion in addition to increased volar angulation of the scaphoid. **D:** This coronal CT reveals scaphoid nonunion. **E:** This fracture was treated with iliac crest bone grafting and internal screw fixation with healing of the fracture.

plain x-rays in detecting a scaphoid fracture (14) and generally is positive within 24 hours of the injury. Bone scans at 4 days after the injury have been shown to be accurate in ruling out scaphoid fractures but at the expense of a significant number of false-positive scans (15,16). Although the bone scan should demonstrate increased uptake if the scaphoid is fractured, it is non-specific and does not necessarily distinguish a scaphoid fracture from fracture of the adjacent radial styloid, for example.

MRI is best for imaging the marrow and will demonstrate abnormal signal intensity if the scaphoid is fractured. However, MRI is so sensitive that an abnormal signal may not clarify whether a fracture is unstable or not. Excellent sensitivity and specificity for MRI in the diagnosis of occult scaphoid fractures has been demonstrated in MRI's performed 2.8 days after initial trauma (17).

If either bone scan or MRI is positive or if precise anatomy of the scaphoid is required, CT is recommended. Direct sagittal and direct coronal CT performed in the longitudinal axis of the scaphoid (18) will provide more detail than sagittal and coronal computer reconstructions from axial images. Although polytomography can provide similar information, many radiology technologists are more familiar with CT than with tomography, and in many hospitals, a direct sagittal and direct coronal CT will provide more useful images than tomograms.

Direct sagittal and coronal CT in the plane of the scaphoid will give accurate detail of the anatomy of the fracture, whether it is complete or incomplete, whether comminution is present at the fracture site, and whether increased palmar flexion is present within the scaphoid (apex dorsal angulation, "humpback" deformity) (19). Usually, direct sagittal and coronal CT will provide the information necessary to make an appropriate decision regarding operative intervention.

In summary, if a fracture is suspected, plain x-rays are obtained. If these films demonstrate a fracture, neither bone scan nor MRI is needed. If the plain x-rays demonstrate a scaphoid fracture sufficiently displaced to require operative intervention, CT is not required unless additional information regarding the exact anatomy of the fracture is desired. If the fracture is not visible on plain x-rays, fluoroscopy with flexion, extension, radial and ulnar deviation, and rotation of the wrist sometimes can demonstrate the fracture. If the x-rays demonstrate a nondisplaced or incomplete fracture such that nonoperative treatment might be chosen, CT would not necessarily be mandatory, but a direct sagittal and coronal CT can be obtained to confirm if the fracture is incomplete or nondisplaced. If the fracture is not demonstrated by plain films or fluoroscopy, bone scan or MRI can be obtained. Alternatively, direct sagittal and coronal CT can be obtained instead of a bone scan or MRI to document the presence of a fracture and simultaneously to clarify the anatomy.

Treatment of Acute Scaphoid Fractures

Treatment of the acute nondisplaced fracture at the distal 20% of the scaphoid is accomplished appropriately by a short arm thumb spica cast for 6 to 8 weeks. This should allow sufficient healing for the individual to return to most sports. X-ray or fluoroscopy can be obtained at 3-, 6-, and 12-month intervals to make certain that there are no complications.

In contrast, fractures involving the proximal 20% of the scaphoid, even if nondisplaced, are treated most appropriately by open reduction and internal fixation (ORIF) (Fig. 16.7). The time for these fractures to heal in a cast is 3 to 6 months. This is too long to immobilize an athlete's wrist. Rigid fixation of an avascular proximal fragment may increase healing potential and may decrease symptomatic osteonecrosis. In addition, proximal pole fragments are usually avascular and commonly develop a nonunion that is even more difficult to treat than the acute fracture. Internal fixation of the acute scaphoid fracture is often less difficult than treating a nonunion or a malunion that might require removal of the sclerotic bone, repositioning of fragments, and bone grafting in addition to internal fixation. ORIF is the most predictable treatment for the proximal pole fracture, and even this does not guarantee a successful result.

Displaced unstable scaphoid fractures are treated best by ORIF. Dorsal or palmar approach can be chosen. If the Herbert screw is used with its accompanying jig, a palmar Russe approach is used. Alternatively, with the aid of an image intensifier, a cannulated screw can be inserted over a guidewire positioned from near the scaphotrapezoid trapezial joint. This can be done percutaneously if the fracture is nondisplaced. In addition, arthroscopically assisted insertion of cannulated screws is an option (20). If palmar comminution exists or if bone graft is required to reconstruct a humpback deformity, the palmar approach is used. Internal fixation of a very proximal pole fragment is accomplished best through a dorsal approach (21) with direct insertion of the screw or with the insertion of a cannulated screw (Fig. 16.7).

Although nonoperative treatment usually is successful in treating distal pole fractures and although ORIF is the recommended treatment for displaced scaphoid fractures and for fractures of the proximal pole, treatment of the nondisplaced middle third scaphoid fracture remains controversial. Some individuals favor cast immobilization, whereas others would choose ORIF.

Cast immobilization traditionally has been the accepted form of treatment for nondisplaced scaphoid

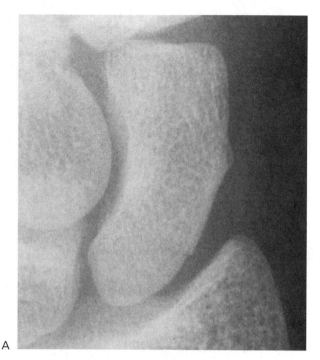

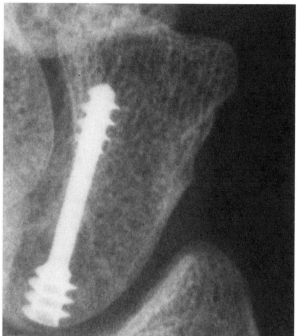

A

B

FIG. 16.7. A: This scaphoid view demonstrates a minimally displaced fracture of the proximal pole of the scaphoid. **B:** In view of the proximal location of this fracture, Herbert screw was inserted through a dorsal approach, in a retrograde fashion.

fractures, with reports suggesting approximately 95% union rate when treating acute nondisplaced fractures. However, we suspect that if sagittal and coronal CTs had been used instead of x-rays to assess healing, the 95% union rate with cast treatment of scaphoid fractures might not have been realized.

Cast treatment requires prolonged immobilization, it interferes with activities, and it should be changed frequently (2-week intervals) to maintain an adequate fit. The fracture can displace in the cast, and a displaced fracture has an increased rate of nonunion. In addition, assessing fracture healing with plain x-rays is difficult when a cast is in place (although direct sagittal and coronal CT can visualize a scaphoid fracture even though a cast is in place, as long as it is below the elbow so that the patient can pronate and supinate to assume the proper wrist position during the study).

The advantages of ORIF in treating nondisplaced middle third fractures include maintenance of articular congruity, rigid compression of fracture fragments, earlier rehabilitation, and earlier return to sports (if the athlete cannot play in a cast).

The disadvantages of ORIF include the anesthetic risk, infection risk, and cost. In the young healthy individual, anesthetic risk is minimal. In addition, the procedure can be done under axillary block to avoid general anesthesia. The risk of an axillary block (intraarterial or intravenous injection causing seizure or respiratory arrest; intraneural injection causing neurologic dam-

age), although it does exist, is small. Operative intervention carries with it a small risk of infection, although with proper skin preparation, perioperative antibiotics, proper surgical technique, and "clean air" in the operating environment, the risk is minimal. Iatrogenic injury is possible but should be rare. ORIF does carry with it a cost that is not present with cast treatment; however, in determining the cost of a particular treatment, one should include not only the cost of the procedure itself but also the cost to the patient if he or she develops a delayed union or a nonunion that precludes returning to sport or work.

Transverse waist fractures can heal in 6 to 10 weeks, and an oblique waist fracture in 8 to 12 weeks. However, if the average time for a fracture to heal is 10 weeks and if one heals in 6 weeks, then one will not heal for 14 weeks. The average time for healing of 100 nondisplaced scaphoid fractures treated within 1 week of injury was 12 weeks, but the actual time was extremely variable. Ten percent of the patients required 6 to 9 months in plaster (22). Even 3 months is often too long for a competitive athlete's wrist to be immobilized, and the possibility of immobilization lasting 6 to 9 months is usually unacceptable. Whether or not cast treatment is acceptable to a specific individual depends on the type of cast and the length of immobilization required. Even a nondisplaced fracture that completely traverses the scaphoid and could be treated with cast immobilization might be more appropriately internally fixed to allow

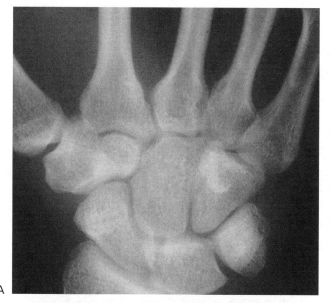

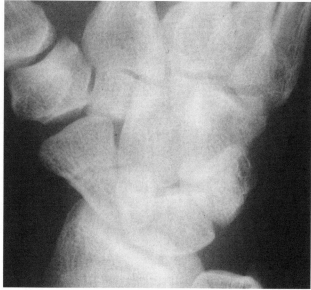

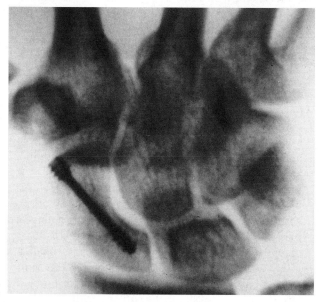

FIG. 16.8. A: This posteroanterior x-ray suggests the possibility of a fracture through the distal third of the scaphoid. **B:** This oblique view reveals an oblique fracture through the middle third of the scaphoid, minimally displaced. **C:** If computed tomography confirmed minimal displacement, this fracture might have been amenable to cast treatment, but internal screw fixation was chosen to provide rigid fixation of the fracture while minimizing cast treatment for this athlete.

the athlete to return to his or her sport more rapidly (Fig. 16.8).

Carter (23) summarized this well: "Because of the complexity, unpredictability, extended treatment and all too frequent failure of treatment of the established scaphoid nonunion, it is my opinion that even patients with nondisplaced fresh fractures in most cases should be stabilized with internal fixation. (Certainly the case for proximal one-third pole fractures is overwhelming.) Not only does this usually shorten treatment time but in those patients who are unfortunately born with a precarious blood supply, rigid fixation undoubtedly offers the best chance of union and reducing the sequelae of the ischemic proximal pole."

For those fractures chosen for cast treatment, controversy remains as to whether the cast should be above

the elbow or below, the exact position of the wrist, and whether the thumb interphalangeal joint should be included. Most physicians agree that if cast treatment is chosen for an unstable scaphoid fracture, a long arm cast is most appropriate, although generally this is not an issue because unstable scaphoid fractures in the athlete are best treated by screw fixation.

If cast treatment is chosen, the position of the wrist is debatable because palmar flexion and radial deviation reduces the fracture gap but causes collapse of the fracture. Ulnar deviation reduces the collapse deformity but causes increased distraction of the fracture.

A short arm thumb spica cast with the wrist positioned in volar flexion and radial deviation has been recommended for acute scaphoid fractures where no displacement of the fracture fragments or lunate dorsal tilting could be seen. One report indicated a 100% union of these nondisplaced fractures treated in this manner (10). Other authors reviewed 100 fractures immobilized alternatively in above and below elbow casts. Preventing pronation and supination of the forearm did not reduce the immobilization time, which, with either type of cast, averaged 7 weeks, after exclusion of the eight fractures that developed delayed union and were fixed with a lag screw (24). Other authors reported 45 patients of whom 6 (13%) had proximal third fractures, 35 (78%) had middle third fractures, and 4 (9%) had distal third fractures. Among the fractures of the middle third, 22 (63%) were displaced and 13 (37%) were undisplaced. Initial treatment was immobilization in a below elbow thumb spica cast. Thirty-five of the forty-five fractures healed. Ten patients after cast treatment required compression screw osteosynthesis. Plaster cast immobilization was satisfactory for treating the stable undisplaced fracture, but unstable displaced fractures were best treated by ORIF. Plaster casts were recommended for fractures involving the distal third of the scaphoid and for stable fractures of the middle and proximal thirds (25).

To make a decision between a long arm and short arm thumb spica, a prospective study of 51 patients who had nondisplaced scaphoid fractures was performed. These patients were assigned randomly to treatment with either a long arm or short arm thumb spica cast. The average follow up was 12 months. Twenty-eight fractures were treated with a long arm thumb spica and 23 with the short arm thumb spica. Hands that initially were treated with a long thumb spica were placed in a short thumb spica after 6 weeks. The fractures initially treated with a long thumb spica united in an average of 9.5 weeks, and those that were maintained in a short thumb spica healed at an average of 12.7 weeks. There were no nonunions and two delayed unions in the fractures that initially were treated with a long thumb spica cast, compared with two nonunions and six delayed unions in those that had only a short thumb spica. Fractures of the proximal or middle third of the scaphoid had significantly shorter time to union when they were treated initially in a long thumb spica cast. Fractures of the distal third did well regardless of type of immobilization (26).

If nonoperative treatment is chosen, fracture healing should be reassessed at about 6 weeks. If there is evidence of additional healing, cast treatment can be continued. If by 6 to 8 weeks there is evidence of increased cyst formation, increased sclerosis at the fracture site, or evidence of poor bony consolidation, then internal fixation with or without bone grafting should be considered rather than prolonging cast immobilization for additional months waiting for unpredictable scaphoid union (Fig. 16.5).

Occasionally, an individual will have a fracture that would be treated most predictably by operative intervention, but the patient refuses that treatment. In some of these patients, in addition to cast immobilization, noninvasive electrical stimulation might be used to augment the healing of a fracture that demonstrates evidence of delayed union.

Postoperative Rehabilitation

With internal screw fixation, if the fracture is not exceedingly comminuted and if the fixation device is in good position to provide stability of the fracture, postoperative bulky dressing with plaster splints remain in place for 5 to 7 days, after which a short arm thumb spica cast can be used for 2 additional weeks while soft tissues heal. Subsequently, a short arm thumb spica cast can be maintained, or, depending on the individual situation, a thermoplast splint can be applied and removed for gentle range of motion exercises. Grip and strengthening exercises may be started by 4 weeks. By 6 to 8 weeks after the operation, if the patient has regained enough flexibility and strength to protect the wrist and if x-rays demonstrate continued stable internal fixation and additional healing, contact sports might be resumed. If the athlete can participate in sports using a protective cast or splint, more rapid return to competition might be possible. Certain activities such as weight lifting, which place heavy loads across the scaphoid, would require longer healing times before resuming. Scaphoid fracture healing should not be jeopardized by allowing the athlete to return to sports prematurely.

One rehabilitation protocol is outlined below. At the initial therapy session, a thumb spica splint is fabricated with the wrist in neutral, the thumb carpometacarpal joint abducted and slightly extended, thumb metacarpophalangeal joint slightly flexed, and the interphalangeal joint free. The fingers are not included in the splint. If the patient is small, a circumferential 1/16th-inch thermoplastic material should be sufficient, but if the patient is large, a volar based thumb spica with 1/8th-inch material is preferable. The patient is instructed in application and removal of the splint and is warned to avoid forced thumb carpometacarpal adduction. Active range of motion of the thumb interphalangeal joint is stressed as is avoidance of strong pinch within the splint. Within the next couple of weeks or at the initial session, if appropriate for the specific fracture, the patient is instructed in active range of motion exercises, including wrist extension and flexion and radial and ulnar deviation. Sustained repetitions are emphasized, and these are to be done with gradual increased force. The exercises can be modified according to any increase in edema or discomfort.

Once the physician determines that the external splint is no longer needed, the patient is instructed in how to decrease the use of the splint gradually, according to symptoms, but may continue to wear it at night and in public and avoid heavy pinch and grip. The patient is instructed in pronation/supination, which usually is not difficult to regain. Light functional use out of the splint is permitted.

The next stage includes gentle passive range of motion for wrist and finger extension, possibly use of heat with gentle stretching. If range of motion, particularly wrist extension, is not improving, dynamic splinting is considered. A gentle stretching program for grip and pinch (usually putty initially, progressing to stronger equipment) and wrist extension/flexion (1-pound weight initially) are begun. The patient likely will be using a splint very little, and guidance is provided in appropriate functional activity. Subsequently, the patient is seen as needed to regain motion and strength to resume his or her activities and to address specific problems. Many athletes who have had scaphoid internal fixation will do well with only several therapy visits with more reliance on home exercises and splinting program.

Scaphoid fracture healing is suggested by absence of tenderness; disappearance of the fracture line with PA, lateral, internal and external oblique, and scaphoid views; and by assessing the scaphoid fracture in various positions under fluoroscopy. The most dependable method is direct sagittal and coronal CT. Healing is demonstrated by bridging bony trabeculae visible across the fracture site.

The use of plain films alone is not sufficient to determine healing of a scaphoid fracture. One study (27) compared the opinions of eight radiologists who reviewed 20 sets of good quality x-rays on two occasions separated by 2 months. There was poor agreement on whether trabeculae crossed the fracture line, whether there was sclerosis at or near the fracture, and whether the proximal part of the scaphoid was avascular. As a consequence, agreement on union also was poor. Their study suggests that x-rays taken 12 weeks after scaphoid fracture did not provide reliable and reproducible evidence of healing.

Results of Treatment

Custom-made silastic casts have been used to treat scaphoid fractures in the athlete (28). A retrospective review of 14 scaphoid fractures occurring in athletes competing in contact sports demonstrated that 10 of 11 middle third scaphoid fractures healed uneventfully. One nonunion did occur after a 7-week delay in diagnosis. Two of the three proximal third scaphoid fractures developed nonunion, whereas the third healed after a prolonged period of treatment. These data suggested that nondisplaced middle scaphoid fractures could be effectively immobilized for competition in contact sports with a custom-made silastic cast. At other times, either fiberglass or plaster short arm thumb spica is used. Rettig and Kollias (29) reported the treatment of 12

athletes with scaphoid waist fracture with Herbert screw fixation and an average return to sports at 5.8 weeks. At a 2.9-year follow-up, a clinical and radiographic union was noted in 11. They believed that internal fixation of scaphoid fractures allowed safe and early return to sports when a playing cast is not an acceptable option and when the athlete accepts the risk of surgery.

Rettig et al. (30) also compared the effectiveness of playing cast treatment versus ORIF of stable mid-third scaphoid fractures in in-season athletes. Return to sports averaged 8.0 weeks for the group treated with ORIF and 4.3 weeks for the group treated with a playing cast. Clinical and radiographic healing averaged 10.8 and 11.2 weeks for the group treated with ORIF and 13.7 and 14.2 weeks for those treated with playing casts. Their study confirms that in-season athletes with stable mid-third scaphoid fractures can safely achieve early return to sports with a playing cast or rigid internal fixation. Union rates were comparable with other series, and it appeared that the athletes were not at increased risks for malunion or nonunion.

Complex Fractures and Fracture–Dislocations

Transscaphoid perilunate fracture–dislocations are treated best with internal fixation of the scaphoid and ligament reconstruction with pinning of the carpal bones in anatomic position (Fig. 16.9). Scapholunate ligament injury can occur in conjunction with a "simple" scaphoid fracture, and the physician should not overlook this possibility (Fig. 16.10).

Complications

Osteonecrosis is seen in proximal pole fractures treated by casting alone, although it is not always prevented by internal fixation. Delayed union and nonunion often can be treated successfully by screw fixation and bone grafting (31). The bone graft used for treatment of nonunions consists of either two corticocancellous segments or one corticocancellous graft in which the cortical surface is placed palmar and the cancellous surface is in the medullary portion of the scaphoid (32). If there is excessive palmar flexion of the scaphoid (humpback deformity) or other type of malunion, this can be corrected and the appropriately contoured bone graft can be inserted (Fig. 16.6). Preoperative planning with direct sagittal and coronal CT is helpful in this regard. For persistent nonunion that has not responded to routine methods, a vascularized bone graft such as that described by Zaidemberg et al. (33) can be used.

Persistent nonunion or malunion with increased scaphoid palmar flexion (humpback deformity) can lead to dorsal intercalary segment instability (4), carpal collapse, and arthrosis, particularly between scaphoid and

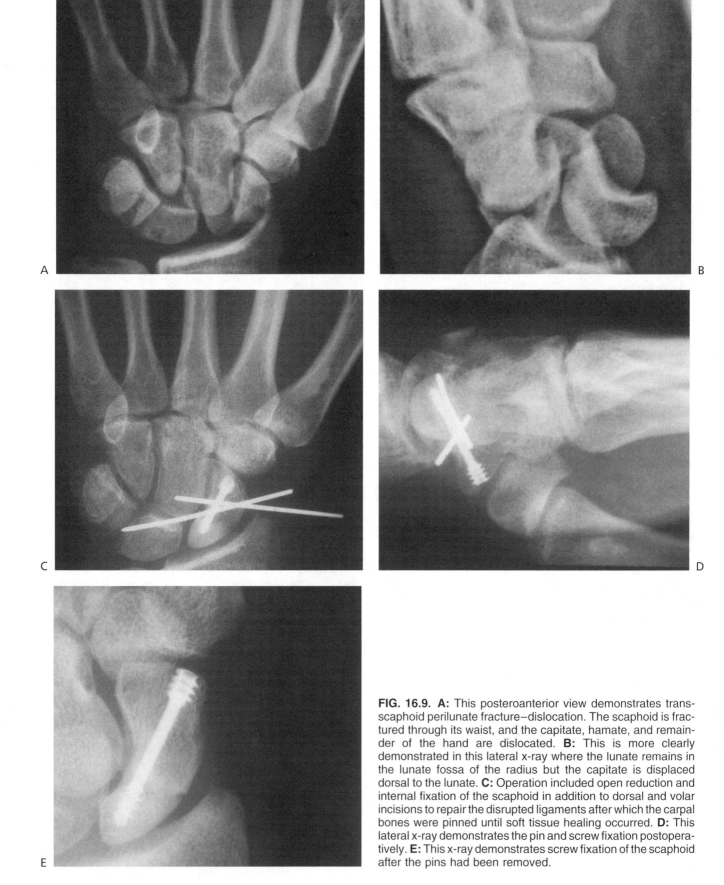

FIG. 16.9. A: This posteroanterior view demonstrates transscaphoid perilunate fracture–dislocation. The scaphoid is fractured through its waist, and the capitate, hamate, and remainder of the hand are dislocated. **B:** This is more clearly demonstrated in this lateral x-ray where the lunate remains in the lunate fossa of the radius but the capitate is displaced dorsal to the lunate. **C:** Operation included open reduction and internal fixation of the scaphoid in addition to dorsal and volar incisions to repair the disrupted ligaments after which the carpal bones were pinned until soft tissue healing occurred. **D:** This lateral x-ray demonstrates the pin and screw fixation postoperatively. **E:** This x-ray demonstrates screw fixation of the scaphoid after the pins had been removed.

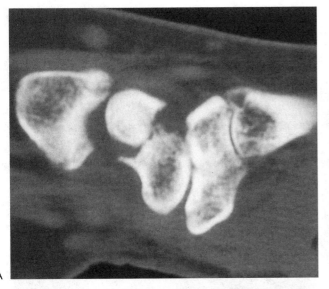

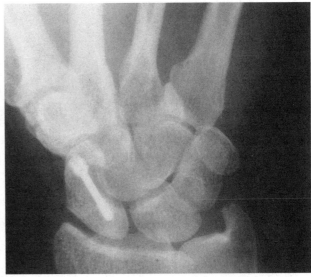

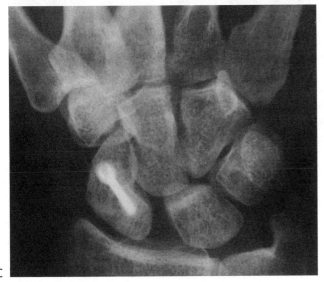

FIG. 16.10. A: This sagittal computed tomography demonstrates a displaced scaphoid fracture. **B:** Slightly oblique view taken several months after screw insertion suggests healing of the scaphoid fracture without definite evidence of scapholunate widening. **C:** This clenched fist view demonstrates widening at the scapholunate joint, indicating scapholunate ligament injury in addition to the scaphoid fracture.

radius and later between scaphoid and capitate (19). This results in decreased grip strength and pain. Eventually, this intercarpal arthritis, termed scaphoid nonunion advanced collapse, becomes diffuse. If symptoms are severe enough, treatment consists of scaphoid excision and four-corner fusion (capitate lunate hamate triquetrum) (34) (Fig. 16.11). Preferably, the scaphoid malunion can be identified and the malunion corrected and bone graft and screw fixation inserted to prevent chronic changes of arthrosis (35) (Fig. 16.12). Depending on the precise symptoms and degree of involvement, radial styloidectomy might be helpful, and certain situations are appropriate for proximal row carpectomy (36–40).

ACUTE LUNATE FRACTURES

Lunate fractures can involve the palmar pole, the dorsal pole, or a small marginal chip. They can involve the

body of the lunate in the coronal, sagittal, or transverse plain (41). A transverse fracture of the lunate is caused by wrist hyperextension that produces a tensile load within the palmar radiolunate (radiolunotriquetral) ligament. Subsequently, with continued load applied across the wrist, compression between the capitate and distal radius causes additional fracture displacement, separating the dorsal and palmar fracture fragments (42). The overlap of the lunate with the adjacent carpal bones makes these fractures difficult to see on PA and lateral views. Direct sagittal and coronal CT or transspiral tomography is used to make the diagnosis. ORIF is recommended for treatment of displaced palmar pole fractures.

Dorsal pole fractures occur as a result of avulsion by the dorsoradial lunotriquetral ligament or the dorsal portion of the scapholunate or lunotriquetral ligament. They also may be caused by wrist hyperextension, with

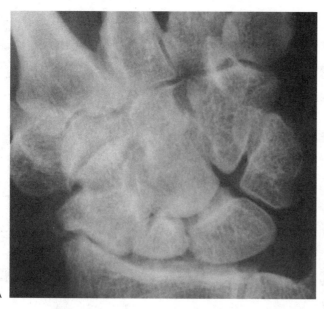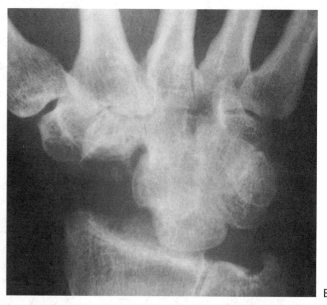

A   B

FIG. 16.11. A: This x-ray demonstrates scaphoid nonunion in addition to arthritis between scaphoid and radius and between scaphoid and capitate in addition to less severe changes between capitate and lunate. **B:** In view of this patient's severe pain and weakness, he was treated by excision of the scaphoid and four-corner fusion (capitate-lunate-hamate-triquetrum). Motion remains through the radiolunate joint, although it was decreased. His pain was relieved by the procedure.

the distal radius crushing the dorsal pole. If the fracture is not displaced, cast immobilization usually is sufficient. If the fracture is displaced, ORIF is indicated.

Osteonecrosis of the lunate can occur from either a single traumatic event or from less severe but repetitive trauma. Acute fractures of the lunate should be distin-

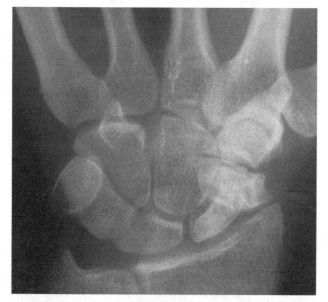

FIG. 16.12. This x-ray demonstrates scaphoid malunion. Arthritic changes are already present between the distal pole of scaphoid and the radial styloid. Proper diagnosis and treatment of scaphoid fractures should prevent this problem.

guished from Keinbach's disease, which is detected radiographically as osteonecrosis of the lunate.

FRACTURES OF THE TRIQUETRUM

Fractures of the triquetrum are the third most common carpal fracture (following scaphoid and lunate) (43). However, triquetrum fractures are more commonly associated with other carpal injuries such as transscaphoid transtriquetral perilunate fracture dislocations. The most common type of triquetral fracture is a dorsal cortical fracture. Controversy exists as to whether this dorsal chip fracture is caused by avulsion from the dorsal radiotriquetral or lunotriquetral ligament (44) or by impingement with either the hamate (43) or the ulnar styloid (45). Isolated fractures of the triquetral body are caused by a direct blow (46) and, if undisplaced, can be treated successfully by cast immobilization for 4 to 6 weeks. Displaced fractures of the body might require ORIF.

Standard PA and lateral x-rays may demonstrate a triquetral body fracture; however, a 45-degree oblique film is often necessary to reveal a dorsal chip fracture (46). Tomograms or CT may be necessary to demonstrate the fracture accurately.

FRACTURES OF THE PISIFORM

Fracture of the pisiform is uncommon and probably is caused by a direct blow on the hypothenar eminence.

A 30-degree supination oblique x-ray or a CT is used to demonstrate the fracture. Treatment of pisiform fractures is a short arm cast for 4 to 6 weeks. If nonunion or significant arthrosis occurs, excision of the pisiform is recommended (42) with repair of the flexor carpi ulnaris tendon.

FRACTURES OF THE TRAPEZIUM

Isolated fractures of the trapezium are infrequent and can occur either in the body of the trapezium or at the trapezial ridge. Trapezial ridge fractures are of two types (47). Type 1 injuries occur at the base, and type II injuries occur at the tip. If these fractures do not heal after 3 to 6 weeks with cast immobilization and if painful nonunion results, excision of the fragment is recommended.

Fractures of the body of the trapezium are treated by cast immobilization if they are not displaced. If displacement is greater than 1 mm, ORIF is considered.

FRACTURES OF THE CAPITATE

Capitate fractures often are associated with scaphoid fractures, thus the term naviculocapitate syndrome (48). In that situation, the capitate fracture involves the proximal pole. The head of the capitate can rotate 180 degrees with the articular surface of the proximal pole facing the fracture surface and the fracture surface of the proximal pole lying adjacent to the lunate. Although a nondisplaced fracture of the capitate can be treated with cast immobilization, displaced capitate fractures and those resulting in naviculocapitate syndrome require ORIF. The capitate fracture often is difficult to visualize on plain x-rays and direct sagittal and coronal CT or transspiral tomography may be required for adequate visualization.

FRACTURES OF THE HAMATE

Hamate fractures occur either within the body or the hook (hamulus) that projects downward into the palm. Both of these fractures are associated with discomfort in the ulnar aspect of the hand and wrist and tenderness to palpation over the hook of the hamate in the palm or over the dorsoulnar aspect of the hamate body.

Fractures of the hook of the hamate are particularly common in individuals whose sport involves gripping objects such as a club, racket, bat, or hockey stick (49–51). This injury should be suspected when a golfer or a tennis, baseball, squash, or lacrosse player has a deep ill-defined pain in the ulnar half of the wrist or tenderness over the hook of the hamate. The injury can occur when the handle of the club or racket strikes the hamate hook. To best visualize the hook of the hamate, a carpal tunnel view can be helpful, although CT or polytomography provides the most accurate diagnosis (Fig. 16.13). Because of the proximity of the flexor digitorum profundi of the little and ring fingers, rupture of these tendons can occur in conjunction with a fracture of the hook of the hamate (52,53). Sometimes a tendon rupture is detected before the diagnosis of hamate fracture (54). Because of the proximity of the ulnar nerve to the hook of the hamate, ulnar nerve symptoms may be present.

If diagnosed acutely, cast immobilization can permit some hook of hamate fractures to heal, although nonunion is common. Fractures identified late and nonunions are treated by surgical excision (55). Although ORIF can be considered for acute fractures of the waist or base of the hook of hamate, failures can occur, and most authors recommend excision of the symptomatic hook of hamate to return the athlete to participation as soon as possible (49). Less frequently, coronal dorsal fractures of the hamate body can occur (56). Often, these are associated with fourth and fifth carpo-metacarpal (CM) fracture–dislocations. If the hamate body frac-

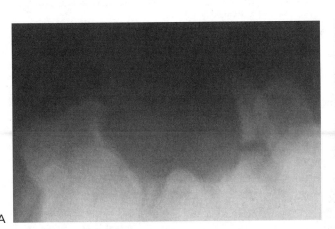
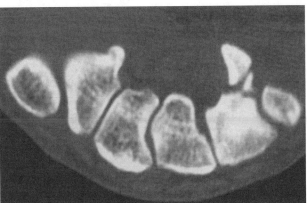

A   B

FIG. 16.13. Carpal tunnel view **(A)** and axial computed tomography **(B)** demonstrating fracture of the hook of the hamate.

ture is nondisplaced, cast immobilization for 4 to 6 weeks usually is sufficient. If the fracture is displaced or unstable, particularly when associated with proximal metacarpal dislocation, ORIF is recommended (42).

REFERENCES

1. Botte MJ, Gelberman RH. Fractures of the carpus, excluding the scaphoid. *Hand Clin* 1987;3:149–161.
2. Zemel NP, Stark HH. Fractures and dislocations of the carpal bones. *Clin Sports Med* 1986;5:709–724.
3. Weber ER, Chao EY. An experimental approach to the mechanism of scaphoid waist fractures. *J Hand Surg* 1978;3:142–148.
4. Weber ER. Biomechanical implications of scaphoid waist fractures. *Clin Orthop* 1980;149:83–89.
5. Smith DK, Cooney WP, An KN, et al. Effects of simulated unstable scaphoid fractures on carpal motion. *J Hand Surg* 1989; 14A:283–291.
6. Smith DK, Gilula LA, Amadio PC. Dorsal lunate tilt (DISI configuration): sign of scaphoid fracture displacement. *Radiology* 1990;176:497–499.
7. Fisk GR. Carpal instability and the fractured scaphoid. *Ann R Coll Surg Engl* 1970;46:63–76.
8. Taleisnik J, Kelly PJ. The extraosseous and intraosseous blood supply of the scaphoid bone. *J Bone Joint Surg Am* 1966;48A: 1125–1137.
9. Gelberman RH, Menon J. The vascularity of the scaphoid bone. *J Hand Surg* 1980;5A:508–513.
10. Cooney WP, Dobyns JH, Linscheid RL. Fractures of the scaphoid: a rational approach to management. *Clin Orthop* 1980;149:90–97.
11. Russe O. Fracture of the carpal navicular. Diagnosis, nonoperative treatment and operative treatment. *J Bone Joint Surg Am* 1960;42A:759–768.
12. Cooney WP, Dobyns JH, Linscheid RL. Non-union of the scaphoid: analysis of the results from bone grafting. *J Hand Surg* 1980; 5:343–354.
13. Herbert TJ, Fisher WE. Management of the fractured scaphoid using a new bone screw. *J Bone Joint Surg Br* 1984;66B:114–123.
14. Nielsen PT, Hedeboe J, Thommesen P. Bone scintigraphy in the evaluation of fracture of the carpal scaphoid bone. *Acta Orth Scand* 1983;54:303–306.
15. Murphy DG, Eisenhauer MA, Powe J, et al. Can a day 4 bone scan accurately determine the presence or absence of scaphoid fracture? *Ann Emerg Med* 1995;26:434–438.
16. Coupland DB. Determining the presence of scaphoid fracture with a day 4 bone scan. *Clin J Sports Med* 1996;6:137.
17. Gaebler C, Kukla C, Breitenseher M, et al. Magnetic resonance imaging of occult scaphoid fractures. *J Trauma* 1996;41:73–76.
18. Sanders WE. Evaluation of the humpback scaphoid by computed tomography in the longitudinal axial plane of the scaphoid. *J Hand Surg* 1988;13A:182–187.
19. Amadio PC, Berquist TH, Smith DK, et al. Scaphoid malunion. *J Hand Surg* 1989;14A:679–687.
20. Whipple TL. Stabilization of the fractured scaphoid under arthroscopic control. *Orthop Clin North Am* 1995;26:749.
21. dos Reis FB, Koeberle G, Leite NM, et al. Internal fixation of scaphoid injuries using the Herbert screw through a dorsal approach. *J Hand Surg* 1993;18A:792–797.
22. Dickinson JD, Shannon JG. Fractures of the carpal scaphoid in the Canadian army: review and commentary. *Surg Gynecol Obstet* 1944;79:225–239.
23. Carter P. Scaphoid fractures. Presented at the American Society for Surgery of the Hand, 1996 Specialty Day, Atlanta, GA, 1996.
24. Alho A, Kankaanpaa. Management of fractured scaphoid bone: a prospective study of 100 fractures. *Acta Orthop Scand* 1975; 46:737–743.
25. Khan FA, al Harby S. Fresh scaphoid fractures (analysis of 45 cases). *Afr J Med Sci* 1995;24:201–206.
26. Gellman H, Caputo RJ, Carter V, et al. Comparison of short and long thumb-spica casts for nondisplaced fractures of the carpal scaphoid. *J Bone Joint Surg Am* 1989;71A:354–357.
27. Dias JJ, Taylor M, Thompson J, et al. Radiographic signs of union of scaphoid fractures. An analysis of inter-observer agreement and reproducibility. *J Bone Joint Surg Br* 1988;70B:299–301.
28. Riester JN, Baker BE, Mosher JF, et al. A review of scaphoid fracture healing in competitive athletes. *Am J Sports Med* 1985; 13:159–161.
29. Rettig AC, Kollias SC. Internal fixation of acute stable scaphoid fractures in the athlete. *Am J Sports Med* 1996;24:182–186.
30. Rettig AC, Weidenbener EJ, Gloyeske R. Alternative management of mid-third scaphoid fractures in the athlete. *Am J Sports Med* 1994;22A:711–804.
31. Robbins RR, Ridge O, Carter PR. Iliac crest bone grafting and Herbert screw fixation of non-unions of the scaphoid with avascular proximal poles. *J Hand Surg* 1995;20A:818–831.
32. Green DP. The effect of avascular necrosis on Russe bone grafting for scaphoid non-union. *J Hand Surg* 1985;10A:597–605.
33. Zaidemberg C, Siebert JW, Angfigiani C. A new vascularized bone graft for scaphoid non-union. *J Hand Surg* 1991;16A:474–478.
34. Vender MI, Watson HK, Wiener BD, et al. Degenerative change in symptomatic scaphoid non-union. *J Hand Surg* 1987;12A: 514–519.
35. Fernandez DL. Anterior bone grafting and conventional lag screw fixation to treat scaphoid non-unions. *J Hand Surg* 1990;15: 140–147.
36. Tomaino MM, Miller RJ, Cole I, et al. Scapholunate advanced collapse wrist: proximal row carpectomy or limited wrist arthrodesis with scaphoid excision? *J Hand Surg* 1994;19A: 134–142.
37. Amadio PC, Taleisnik J. Fractures of the carpal bones. In: Green DP, Hotchkiss RN, Pederson WC, eds. *Green's operative hand surgery*, 4th ed. New York: Churchill-Livingstone, 1999.
38. Herndon JH, ed. *Scaphoid fractures and complications*. Rosemont, IL: Am Acad Ortho Surg, 1994.
39. Linscheid RL, Weber ER. Scaphoid fractures and non-union. In: Cooney WP, Linscheid RL, Dobyns JH, eds. *The wrist—diagnosis and operative treatment*. St. Louis: Mosby, 1998.
40. Ruby L. Fractures and dislocations of the carpus. In: Browner BD, Jupiter JB, Levine AM, et al., eds. *Skeletal trauma*. Philadelphia: W.B. Saunders, 1992.
41. Teisen H, Hjarbaek J. Classification of fresh fractures of the lunate. *J Hand Surg* 1988;13B:458–462.
42. Cooney WP. Isolated carpal fractures. In: Cooney WP, Linscheid RL, Dobyns JH, eds. *The wrist—diagnosis and operative treatment*. St. Louis: Mosby, 1998.
43. Bryan RS, Dobyns JH. Fractures of the carpal bones other than lunate and navicular. *Clin Orthop* 1980;149:107–111.
44. Bonnin JG, Greening WP. Fractures of the triquetrum. *J Surg* 1944;31B:278–283.
45. Garcia-Elias M. Dorsal fractures of the triquetrum-avulsion compression fractures? *J Hand Surg* 1987;12A:266–268.
46. Bartone NF, Grieco RV. Fracture of the triquetrum. *J Bone Joint Surg Am* 1956;38A:353–356.
47. Palmer AK. Trapezial ridge fractures. *J Hand Surg* 1981;6: 561–564.
48. Fenton RL. The naviculo-capitate fracture syndrome. *J Bone Joint Surg Am* 1956;38:681–684.
49. Parker RD, Berkowitz MS, Brahms MA, et al. Book of the hamate fractures in athletes. *Am J Sports Med* 1986;14:517–523.
50. Stark HH, Chao EK, Zemel NP, et al. Fracture of the hook of the hamate. *J Bone Joint Surg Am* 1989;71A:1202–1207.
51. Bishop AT, Beckenbaugh RD. Fracture of the hamate hook. *J Hand Surg* 1988;13A:135–139.
52. Crosby EB, Linscheid RL. Rupture of the flexor profundus tendon of the ring finger secondary to ancient fracture of the hook of the hamate. Review of the literature and report of two cases. *J Bone Joint Surg Am* 1974;56A:1076–1078.
53. Takami H, Takahashi S, Ando M. Rupture of flexor tendon associated with previous fracture of the hook of the hamate. *Hand* 1983;15:73–76.
54. Milek MA, Boulas HJ. Flexor tendon ruptures secondary to hamate hook fractures. *J Hand Surg* 1990;15A:740–744.
55. Carter PR, Eaton RG, Littler JW. Ununited fracture of the hook of the hamate. *J Bone Joint Surg Am* 1977;59A:583–588.
56. Roth JH, de Lorenzi C. Displaced intra-articular coronal fracture of the body of the hamate treated with a Herbert screw. *J Hand Surg* 1988;13A:619–621.

Principles and Practice of Orthopaedic Sports Medicine,
edited by William E. Garrett, Jr., Kevin P. Speer, and Donald T. Kirkendall.
Lippincott Williams & Wilkins, Philadelphia © 2000.

CHAPTER 17

Injuries to the Soft Tissues of the Wrist

James A. Nunley and Thomas Goetz

Injuries to the wrist are frequently seen with athletic activity and may occur as a result of exposure to a single uncontrolled force, such as a fall or collision, or as a result of repetitive loaded activity, such as occurs in racquet sports. These soft tissue injuries are often labeled "wrist sprains," and the competitive athlete may continue to play through the pain or will use splints or taping to limit movement or loading without first properly rehabilitating the injury. As with all athletic injuries, treatment of the elite athlete differs from the recreational athlete in that the elite athlete requires maximal performance and the earliest possible return to activity; therefore, prompt diagnosis is required to ensure early intervention and to allow maximal function as soon as possible. Thus, the treatment of soft tissue injuries forces the health care provider to balance the often conflicting objectives of satisfying the athlete's desire for early return to sporting activity while preventing long-term sequelae of the injury.

EPIDEMIOLOGY

The incidence of hand and wrist injuries in the sporting population has been reported to be as high as 25% to 30%; however, no reports describe the incidence and prevalence of soft tissue injuries to the wrist specifically (1,2). Unfortunately, both athletes and coaches frequently dismiss wrist injuries as "sprains" and tend to underplay their importance. The athlete will often continue to participate despite wrist injury, risking the development of a chronic problem. As well, difficulty in diagnosis and treatment of many soft tissue wrist injuries may lead to underreporting. Recent advances in the understanding, diagnosis, and treatment of soft tissue wrist injuries should improve our epidemiologic data; at present, data must be extrapolated from broader studies.

In a study of ice hockey injuries, it was found that athletes sustained an injury to the upper extremity at the rate of roughly 1 per 2,000 hours of play (3). In a study of 1,049 participants in a wrestling tournament, 21% of injuries were located in the upper extremity; however, many of these injuries were aggravations of old injuries, suggesting the need for adequate rehabilitation before return to competition (4).

A study of a professional football team over 15 years reported 46 major hand and wrist injuries. Most injuries involved the fingers, but nine wrist injuries were also noted: five fractures, two fracture dislocations, one dislocation, and one wrist sprain. Most injuries occurred during tackling, and these were sustained by defensive linemen (5).

A 1-year survey of all hand injuries seen at the Methodist Sports Medicine Center revealed that 213 injuries in 207 athletes had been treated; there was a relatively high incidence of wrist injuries in golf, gymnastics, and tennis. A higher percentage of injuries occurred during competition (41.1%) compared with practice (28.2%) and recreation (15.8%) (6).

Soft tissue injuries of the wrist can occur in any athletic activity but are more prevalent in certain sports (7). Injury may occur as a result of repetitive wrist motion characteristic of a sport, such as ulnar-sided wrist pathology found in racquet sports like tennis, or may occur when the wrist is subjected to an abnormally high-intensity stress or to a direct blow as is commonly seen in contact sports such as football and hockey. Sports in which the upper extremity is used for weight bearing, such as gymnastics, or repetitive heavy loading, such as weight lifting, expose the athlete to wrist injury as well. Linscheid and Dobyns (8) believed that most sport injuries were a result of a compressive load applied to

J. A. Nunley and T. Goetz: Department of Orthopaedic Surgery, Duke University Medical Center, Durham, North Carolina 27710.

the wrist while the hand was in some degree of extension.

The incidence and prevalence of wrist injuries seems to be highest in gymnasts. A study of wrist injuries on the varsity gymnastics team at UCLA revealed a prevalence of chronic wrist pain ranging from 17% to 43%, with nearly all gymnasts reporting upper extremity discomfort at some point in their careers (73% of men and 33% of women reported wrist pain). The difference between men and women was believed to be due to the high risk of injury with pommel horse exercises that involved high axial loading with rotation and are usually performed only by men (9).

Awareness of the nature of a sport and the common injury patterns helps the physician in establishing the diagnosis and assisting in the design of training and rehabilitation programs and splinting techniques.

EVALUATION OF THE PATIENT WITH AN INJURED WRIST

Assessment of the patient with an injured wrist requires a thorough history and directed physical examination; this cannot be overstated. Any ancillary investigations made become far less accurate and are less specific if a reasonable differential diagnosis is not first established. The "sprained" wrist should only be a diagnosis of exclusion. The history should ascertain the sporting activity because certain sports predispose to specific injuries; for instance, racquet sports can result in ulnar-sided wrist injuries such as lunotriquetral (LT) tears and triangular fibrocartilage injuries and tendonitis. Gymnasts are prone to distal radial deformities and ulnocarpal impaction. Contact sports expose the athlete to extension loading and injuries such as scaphoid impaction and scapholunate (SL) ligament injuries.

It is important to determine whether the injury is the result of a single traumatic episode or repetitive stress. This guides the differential diagnosis and also has a bearing on the treatment and the outcome. For example, chronic ulnocarpal impaction injury to the Triangular Fibrocartilage Complex (TFCC) secondary to repetitive loading is treated differently from a single episode that causes an acute tear of the TFCC.

It is important to determine whether the athlete is a hyperelastic individual because the susceptibility to recurrent injury and the outcome of surgical soft tissue repairs is affected by each individual's collagen pattern.

The physical examination must be methodical and thorough. It is important to examine the neck, shoulder, and elbow regions to exclude a proximal injury with distally referred pain. The vascular status of the limb should be examined carefully to determine presence of radial and ulnar pulses and adequate distal refill as determined by an Allen's test. The neurologic examination should ascertain motor function in all peripheral nerve groups, and the sensory examination should test

dermatomal and peripheral nerve sensory distributions. Moving and static two-point sensory testing and Semmes Weinstein monofilament testing should be performed if there are subjective sensory abnormalities. The location of tenderness and swelling should be noted and an effort made to localize it to a specific tendon, joint, or ligament if possible as soon after injury as possible.

In tendon-related disorders, symptoms are often reproduced with passive stretch of the muscle and isolated active contraction of the muscle–tendon unit against resistance. Capsuloligamentous injuries result in pain that is localized to the joint area, and the pain is worse at extremes of motion or with joint stress testing.

Specific tests are then performed according to suspected type of injury. These tests are described in each section, but it is beyond the scope of this chapter to discuss in detail the complex examination of the hand and wrist for all ligamentous injuries.

INJURIES TO THE CAPSULOLIGAMENTOUS STRUCTURES OF THE WRIST

Ligamentous injuries of the wrist, often described as wrist sprain, may ultimately be severe injuries and are often quite difficult to diagnose. Failure to recognize these injuries acutely may lead to chronic wrist pain or instability that is increasingly difficult to treat and may eventually lead to wrist arthritis (10–15).

A detailed discussion of the anatomy and biomechanics of the wrist is beyond the scope of this text; however, certain points bear mentioning. The wrist is composed of proximal and distal rows of carpal bones that have little stability under compression. Stability is provided by extrinsic capsular ligaments and intrinsic interosseous ligaments. The intrinsic interosseous ligaments are the strongest (13–20). They are intracapsular and, like the cruciate ligaments of the knee, they have little ability to heal spontaneously when injured.

The scapholunate (SL) interosseous ligament is critical in coordinating normal wrist motion, allowing the position of the scaphoid, which is unique in that it bridges both proximal and distal rows to control the position of the lunate (17,21,22). Radial-sided ligamentous wrist pain most commonly involves the SL ligament to some degree. This is one of the most common and, unfortunately, one of the most significant ligamentous injuries to occur in the wrist; the injury occurs with a reasonably predictable pattern of sequential tearing.

Injuries involving the ulnar side of the wrist frequently involve the lunatotriquefral (LT) ligament, the triangular fibrocartilage complex, or both. The triquetrohamate articulation controls the position of the triquetrum, which then helps to dictate lunate position through the LT ligament. The TFCC is a complex structure responsible for transmission of load through the ulnar side of the wrist and provides stability of the ulnar radiocarpal articulation (23).

The TFCC also plays a role in stability of the distal radioulnar joint. When approaching a wrist ligament injury, a careful history and physical examination can often ascertain whether the problem is predominantly radial or ulnar. This allows a narrowing of the diagnostic possibilities.

RADIAL-SIDED PAIN

Scapholunate Injury

Injury to the SL ligament commonly occurs in collisions in such contact sports as football or hockey.

Mechanism

SL ligament disruption occurs in hyperextension injuries of the wrist. Experimental studies by Mayfield et al. (24) suggest injury occurs with a force located on the radial side of the hand with the wrist in extension and the forearm in pronation. The force thus causes ulnar deviation, extension, and intercarpal supination.

SL ligament disruption is part of a spectrum of injury (25). It is described as the first stage of perilunate dislo-

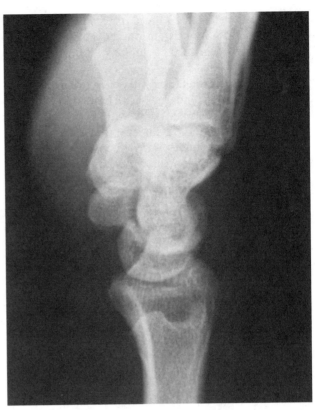

FIG. 17.2. Lateral radiograph of the wrist with scapholunate dissociation and dorsal intercalated segment instability. Note the dorsal tilting of the lunate with respect to the radius and the volar tilting of the scaphoid with respect to the lunate.

cation (24,26). Injury must occur to some degree to the radioscaphoid, radiocapitate, and radial collateral ligaments and the SL interosseous ligament. In complete disruption of the SL ligament accompanied by significant capsular ligamentous injury, the SL gap seen radiographically widens and the proximal pole of the scaphoid subluxes dorsally, which is easily seen radiographically (Fig. 17.1). With loss of this important strut (the scaphoid), the carpus shortens and collapses like an accordion, leading to dorsal intercalated segmental instability (DISI) patterns (Fig. 17.2), which is termed a static instability (11,13,26). Lesser degrees of injury to the SL ligament and extrinsic ligaments will not produce such gross disturbance in anatomy; however, under loaded conditions, the normal biomechanics will be disturbed, producing pain and dynamic instability. Diagnosis of dynamic instability requires synthesis of clinical impression with judicious and directed ancillary investigations.

Examination

Athletes may report a single hyperextension injury to the wrist; however, the exact mechanism or time of injury is often not remembered. The athlete will com-

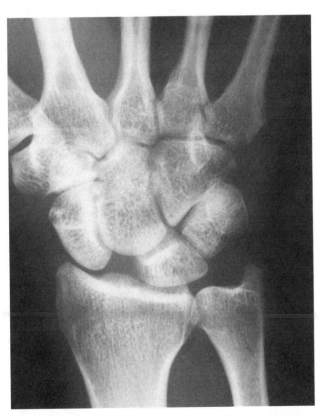

FIG. 17.1. Anteroposterior radiograph of the wrist demonstrating widened scapholunate interval known as Terry Thomas sign.

plain of pain referred to the dorsal radial SL interval that is aggravated by extension activities of the wrist and with grip. A history of clunking with wrist motion may also be elicited.

Acute injury examination will often reveal significant dorsal swelling and tenderness with limitation of motion and pain with attempted wrist extension. Tenderness will be present at the SL interval, and ballottment of the scaphoid and lunate will demonstrate tenderness and increased excursion when compared with the normal side.

The provocative scaphoid shift (Watson test) maneuver (Fig. 17.3) is performed by stabilizing the distal radius with the fingers of one hand while the thumb exerts pressure on the distal pole of the scaphoid as the other hand of the examiner moves the wrist from a position of ulnar deviation and slight extension to a position of radial deviation and flexion (27,28). This maneuver attempts to sublux the proximal pole of the

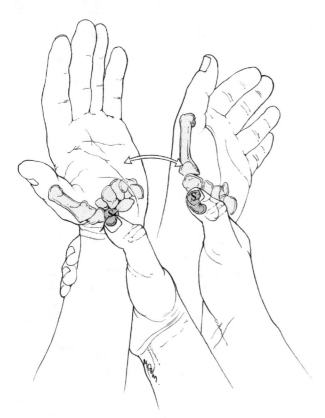

FIG. 17.3. The provocative scaphoid shift test as described by Watson. The examiner stabilizes the distal radius with the fingers of one hand while the thumb exerts pressure over the distal pole of the scaphoid. The examiner moves the wrist from a position of ulnar deviations and slight extension as seen on the right to a position of radial deviation and volar flexion as seen on the left. During this maneuver, one attempts to sublux the pole of the scaphoid within the radioscaphoid joint. A sensation of subluxation during the test with a reproducible clunk and production of pain is highly suggestive of dynamic scapholunate instability.

scaphoid within the radioscaphoid joint. A sensation of subluxation during the test or a reducing clunk with removal of thumb pressure suggests laxity of the scaphoid-stabilizing structures, especially when accompanied with pain that reproduces the patient's symptoms. Comparison with the uninjured extremity is important. Interpretation of the Watson test requires experience and should be viewed in light of the complete clinical picture. Easterling and Wolfe (29) found a 32% overall incidence and a 14% unilateral incidence of positive Watson test in asymptomatic individuals. Thus, the presence of a shift does not definitively establish a diagnosis.

Diagnostic Investigations

Plain Radiology

Plain radiographic wrist views should be the first imaging studies obtained; an anteroposterior view in full supination and a true lateral may show signs of a static SL dissociation (30–32). On the anteroposterior view, an SL gap of greater than 3 mm is believed to be diagnostic of dissociation (Fig. 17.1) (33). However, correlation with the opposite extremity is very helpful. The SL gap is very sensitive to radiographic technique and hand positioning (34).

On the anteroposterior view, the scaphoid may look foreshortened and a "cortical ring" sign may be present as a result of the scaphoid resting in a volar flexed position with the proximal pole subluxed dorsally. A lack of parallelism between opposing surfaces of the scaphoid and lunate may be noted. It is helpful to trace the arcs formed by the proximal and distal carpal rows. A step-off in these arcs is suggestive of ligament injury (35,36).

On the lateral view, palmar flexion of the scaphoid may be seen with increased SL and Radioscaphoid (R-S) angles; DISI deformity may also be seen (Fig. 17.1). Contralateral wrist views are extremely important; a gap not present on the uninjured extremity improves the physician's confidence in the diagnosis.

Special Views

Often, the plain radiographs will be normal, and in these cases stress views may reveal instability. The stress views frequently used are the clenched fist views in neutral and at extremes of radial and ulnar deviation and flexion and extension. These studies again must compare the injured with the uninjured side and are rarely truly diagnostic for a specific injury but will be helpful in the overall assessment.

Cineradiography

Availability of fluoroscopic machines in the clinic improves diagnostic accuracy, especially for dynamic instability patterns (37). Rotation of the wrist eliminates positioning errors in determination of the SL interval. Active, passive, and loaded examination of the wrist helps in determination of abnormal kinematics such as a sudden shift between the scaphoid and lunate occurring during radioulnar deviation motion (38). Office fluoroscopic examination has supplanted stress views and cineradiography in our hands for the diagnosis of most wrist injuries.

Arthrography

Traditionally, arthrography has played an important role in the diagnosis of ligamentous injuries of the wrist. Midcarpal arthrography is believed to be more sensitive than radiocarpal arthrography; however, Gilula (36) demonstrated that triple arthrography (distal radioulnar, radiocarpal, midcarpal) is the most sensitive and specific study to evaluate ligamentous injuries (39). Recent studies comparing arthrography with wrist arthroscopy suggest that arthrography may not be as sensitive or accurate as wrist arthroscopy in the hands of an experienced clinician (40,41).

Cantor et al. (42) analyzed results of bilateral arthrograms for Triangular Fibrocartilage (TFC) tears; they found that radial TFC tears were present in 88% of asymptomatic contralateral wrists, whereas 50% of LT tears and 57% of SL tears were bilateral. These data cast doubts on the accuracy of arthrography in establishing a definitive diagnosis.

Cooney (41) compared arthroscopy and arthrography and found arthroscopy to be more sensitive and specific, especially for the evaluation of the SL and LT ligaments. Weiss et al. (43) compared triple arthrography and arthroscopy in patients with wrist pain; they found that for all lesions, the arthrogram was 56% specific, 83% sensitive, and 60% accurate relative to arthroscopy. Eynde et al. (44) compared radiocarpal arthrography with radiocarpal arthroscopy and found sensitivity of arthrography was 52%, specificity was 50%, positive predictive value 92%, and negative predictive value only 8%.

Arthrography fails to demonstrate the degree and exact location of interosseous ligament damage, subtle ligamentous laxity, and the condition of the articular surfaces or synovitis, all of which may be viewed arthroscopically. In addition, arthrographic leaks can be seen on the normal uninjured side, leading same authors to recommend bilateral wrist arthrogram (45). Because of the lack of specificity and sensitivity, we stopped using wrist arthrography to evaluate ligamentous injuries in our practice.

Magnetic Resonance Imaging

Magnetic resonance imaging (MRI) of the wrist has become a source of intense research recently with the ongoing development of more accurate wrist coils. To date, MRI has been shown to image the TFCC and interosseous ligaments well; however, consistent and accurate descriptions of pathology are still being developed. MRI holds promise in imaging of extrinsic ligaments and capsule and in providing information about the osseous structures (46). Currently, its value in assessment of the injured athlete's wrist is confined to centers with the appropriate imaging coils and radiologists confident in interpreting the findings.

Wrist Arthroscopy

Increasingly, arthroscopy is becoming the diagnostic and therapeutic modality of choice in evaluating and treating wrist injuries. Arthroscopy allows accurate diagnosis of major wrist injuries and often allows concurrent treatment. Dautel et al. (47) reported improved diagnosis of SL tears with the use of dynamic maneuvers while performing arthroscopy. In athletic injuries, arthroscopy plays a very important role, allowing earlier diagnosis and treatment of subtle injuries that allow faster rehabilitation and return to sporting activities.

Our current protocol in suspected SL injury is to examine the wrist fluoroscopically initially. If no diagnosis is made, we obtain an MRI. If a diagnosis is still not made and a trial of conservative therapy has failed, we proceed to diagnostic and possibly therapeutic arthroscopy.

Differential Diagnosis

Other causes of radial-sided wrist pain should be considered besides SL ligament injury. Dorsal wrist ganglions, particularly the occult ganglion, may cause dorsal wrist pain and the sensation of swelling. It should be remembered that ganglions often arise from the SL ligament and may be secondary to a more severe wrist injury.

Chronic impingement of the scaphoid on the dorsal lip of the radius resulting from forced hyperextension may cause capsular and bony reaction; these are commonly seen in the young female gymnast. Chondral injuries can result in symptoms of wrist pain, occasionally with a click. These injuries may be seen in the radioscaphoid, radiolunate, or scaphotrapezial trapezoid joints. Arthroscopy allows diagnosis and usually treatment of these lesions as well.

Treatment

Nonoperative

In the patient where an SL injury is suspected but plain radiographic studies and fluoroscopy do not suggest a static separation of the ligaments, a trial of nonoperative treatment should be followed. In the athlete, the training program should be modified to one of relative rest, such that painful activity is avoided. The wrist should be splinted during activities. Conservative care should include ice after activity and nonsteroidal anti-inflammatory drugs (NSAIDs). Rehabilitation should include progressive passive and active range of motion followed by strengthening exercises when a full painless range of motion has been obtained.

The decision of when to proceed with arthroscopy should be tailored to the individual athlete and will depend on the type of the sport (whether wrist immobilization can be tolerated), the phase of the season, and the response to conservative therapy. Most authors suggest 3 months of conservative therapy before arthroscopy, but this will be unacceptable to the high-performance athlete who might miss an entire season (48).

Any evidence of static deformity in the acute wrist injury is a very serious condition that mandates immediate surgical intervention and will usually not do well with a period of conservative treatment.

Operative Treatment

With careful examination and radiographic studies that suggest SL injury, a diagnostic arthroscopy should be carried out; examination of both the midcarpal and radiocarpal joints should be performed so that the ligaments and alignment of the carpal bones can be seen from above and below (49).

Evidence of acute SL dissociation with static instability and complete SL tear probably mandates surgical treatment. Mayfield et al. (20) describes the paradox of closed reduction: Extension and ulnar deviation reduces the SL joint, whereas flexion and radial deviation will reapproximate the volar radial ligaments. This suggests that closed treatment will not be successful in restoration of normal anatomy.

Closed reduction and percutaneous pinning has been described either under image intensification or direct visualization at fluoroscopy; however, acute static SL instability is probably best treated by open reduction and pinning with repair of the dorsal SL ligament using the technique described by Lavernia et al. (50). The ligament is most commonly avulsed from the scaphoid and is sutured back through drill holes that exit through the waist of the scaphoid. Suture anchors can also be used to secure the ligament back to bone. It is important to reduce accurately and securely pin the scaphoid to the lunate to protect the repair. The pins are left in place and the wrist immobilized for 6 to 8 weeks.

Chronic SL disruptions are usually treated with some form of ligament reconstruction in addition to accurate pinning of the scaphoid to lunate. One of the most popular reconstructions is the Blatt procedure (51). This is a nonanatomic reconstruction that requires securing

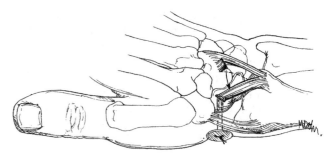

FIG. 17.4. The Blatt procedure. A strip of dorsal capsule approximately 5 mm wide is detached from the distal wrist but left attached to the distal radius. After correcting the volar flexed position of the scaphoid, this strip of capsule is passed through drill holes into or around the distal portion of the scaphoid and tied over a button on the volar thenar surface. This dorsal capsulodesis holds the scaphoid in an extended position and will not allow volar flexion, which is the controlling factor in dynamic scapholunate instability.

a proximally based flap of dorsal capsule to the dorsal and distal pole of the scaphoid while the scaphoid is held in an extended position (Fig. 17.4). The reconstruction is protected with Kirschner wires for 6 to 8 weeks. There is concern regarding the effect this reconstruction has on wrist motion, particularly wrist flexion. A recent study by Wintman et al. (52) on patients with dynamic SL instability reported good pain relief, increase in strength, decrease in clunking sensation, and loss of flexion averaging only 8 degrees; however, it must be remembered that their population was not athletes. It is not clear whether the Blatt procedure would provide sufficient pain relief to allow return to sporting activities in the elite athlete.

Weiss et al. (53) reported good results with arthroscopic debridement alone for ligament tears; in their patient there was a decrease in pain and improvement in grip strength. Their best results were for partial tears; the follow-up was short, only 2 years, and long-term results are not known. These same authors reported on the use of bone–retinaculum–bone for more severe SL instability (54). Many authors have reported short-term follow-up for the treatment of chronic SL Ligament tears, but no consensus has yet been obtained as to the best procedure for long-term restoration of the wrist (55–57).

Scaphoid Impaction Syndrome

This injury is caused by repeated hyperextension injury to the wrist with radial deviation; it is seen commonly in gymnasts using the pommel horse, in weight lifters, and in push-up enthusiasts. Weiker (58) believed there was an association with weak flexor strength in the fingers and wrist joints; thus, the limit to wrist hyperextension force then becomes the wrist ligaments and bony anatomy. Repeated dorsal impingement of the scaphoid on dorsal rim of the radius results in synovitis and reactive osteophyte formation.

The diagnosis of scaphoid impaction syndrome is made when the athlete has pain on hyperextension of the wrist with tenderness and swelling over the dorsoradial aspect of the wrist. Radiographs may reveal dorsal osteophyte formation.

Treatment rarely requires surgery and should include rest, activity modification with avoidance of hyperextension, and compression forces. Ice, NSAIDs, and other nonsurgical modalities can be used. A wrist orthosis that blocks hyperextension may allow early return to activity and is especially helpful in the gymnast. If nonoperative modalities fail, surgical exploration may reveal dorsal osteophytes, synovitis, and articular surface chondromalacia. Dobyns et al. (6) described performing a curative dorsal cheilectomy of the wrist.

ULNAR-SIDED WRIST PAIN

Lunotriquetral Ligament Injury

Injury to the LT ligament can be isolated or occur as a component of complex carpal dislocations or as part of advanced-stage TFCC injury and ulnocarpal impaction.

The triquetral–hamate joint plays an important role in controlling motion in radioulnar deviation; this joint complex secondarily controls the position of the lunate through the LT ligament. Loss of the LT ligament alone is insufficient to account for static carpal collapse and volar intercollated segment instability (VISI) deformity. There must be disruption of the LT and the dorsal radiotriquetral or LT plus volar ligaments to allow the wrist to collapse into a volar intercalated segment instability pattern in which the lunate is tilted in a volar direction on the lateral radiograph.

Mechanism of Injury

Actual mechanism of injury in the acute LT tear is poorly understood. There are three possible mechanisms. In the first, LT injury is believed to be a continuation of the spectrum of injury involved in the Mayfield spiral (Fig. 17.5); the wrist in a position of ulnar deviation and extension experiences a force located on the radial side of the hand and causes extension, ulnar deviation, and intercarpal supination. The second proposed mechanism is a fall on the outstretched hand positioned in extension and radial deviation with the force located on the hypothenar eminence, causing intercarpal pronation. The final proposed mechanism is a hyper–palmar–flexion injury.

Clinically, a spectrum of partial tears to complete disruption with static carpal collapse is seen. The athlete will complain of pain on the ulnar side of the wrist,

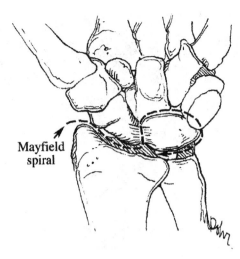

FIG. 17.5. The Mayfield spiral. The injury force to the wrist is initiated on the radial aspect. Ligamentous injury occurs across the scaphoid, and then the scapholunate ligament is disrupted. Next the capitate lunate area is disrupted, and finally the lunotriquetral ligament is divided. This can lead to a scapholunate dissociation, a perilunate dislocation if only part of the injury occurs, or a complete lunate dislocation if the spiral is completed.

especially in ulnar deviation and rotation of the wrist. There will be a loss in range of motion with weakness of grip. The patient may also complain of a clunking with motion from radial to ulnar deviation.

Examination must try to exclude all other causes of ulnar-sided wrist pain such as triquetral avulsion fractures, TFCC tears, and subluxation of the extensor carpi ulnaris (ECU) tendon. Usually, the point of maximal tenderness will be just distal to the TFCC at the location of the LT joint on the dorsum of the wrist. Ulnar deviation of the pronated hand while applying axial compression may reproduce pain and a clunk as the proximal carpal row reduces from VISI to DISI. Lateral compression of the wrist may cause pain as the LT joint is compressed. The shear or ballottment test involves stabilizing the lunate while the pisiform volarly and triquetrum dorsally are moved up and down relative to the stabilized lunate. This maneuver may reproduce the athlete's pain; it may reveal crepitus, and an impression of the relative mobility of the articulation can be compared with the normal side.

Plain radiographic views are usually normal; however, a disruption of the normal convex arc of the proximal carpal row may be noted with an LT step-off (35,36). An increase in the LT interval is not usually seen. In static instability, a VISI deformity may be noted but not always (Fig. 17.6). It is important to assess ulnar variance (the length of the distal ulna with respect to the sigmoid notch of the radius) for possible ulnocarpal abutment because this is related to acute and chronic LT ligament injury.

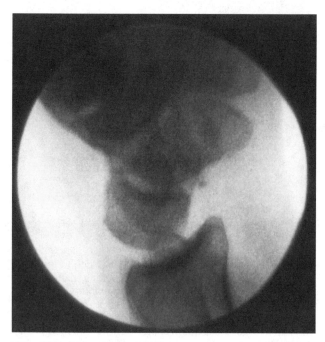

FIG. 17.6. Volar intercalated segment instability. Note the fact that the lunate is not colinear with the radius but rather is tipped in a volar direction. Nevertheless, the scapholunate angle is normal, indicating that this position is not secondary to wrist volar flexion but rather to injury, either through the lunotriquetral ligament of midcarpal joint. This patient was later reconstructed for a complete lunotriquetral ligament tear.

Fluoroscopy may reveal asynchronous motion between the lunate and the capitate or the triquetrum, especially with radial and ulnar deviation.

Arthrographic examination must be interpreted carefully and correlate with the clinical findings because of the frequent false-positive and -negative results at this articulation seen at arthrography (40,45). Bone scan is often extremely sensitive but not sufficiently specific; however, it may be a useful screening test, showing increased uptake in the lunate and triquetrum in this condition. If one elects to use arthrography, radiocarpal and midcarpal injection are advised to increase the accuracy.

The role of MRI for the LT joint is not well defined at this point. Arthroscopy can provide the diagnosis and allow debridement of the joint in partial tears or assist in pinning of the lunate to the triquetrum in acute tears.

Treatment

Initial treatment in the acute injury should be conservative, with casting or splinting. Molding of the cast to provide support volarly over the pisiform may help in maintaining the LT in an unstressed position. If there is a static VISI deformity, an LT ligament reconstruction or an LT fusion with ulnar recession if the patient is ulnar positive can give good results. If there is no static VISI deformity, an LT ligament repair with *in situ* pinning can be used.

Distal Radial Ulnar Joint Injury

Injury to the distal radial ulnar joint (DRUJ) is a common cause of ulnar-sided wrist pain in the athlete. Recent advances have improved diagnosis and treatment of conditions affecting the DRUJ and highlighted the importance of the TFCC and ulnar variance in pathogenesis of these disorders.

TFCC Injury

Mechanism

TFCC injuries can be classified as traumatic or degenerative. Acute athletic injuries usually occur with the wrist in a position of ulnar deviation. A compressive loading of the wrist with forearm rotation can tear the TFCC. Repetitive ulnar deviation and forearm rotation such as occurs in racquet sports may also lead to a tear.

Classification

Palmer (59) divided TFCC injuries into traumatic type 1 and degenerative type 2 lesions. Traumatic (type 1) lesions are subdivided into four types, according to the location of the tear (Fig. 17.7). The most common lesion (type 1A) occurs along the avascular origin of the articular disk along the radius. Type 1B is an avulsion of the TFCC attachment to the ulna. Avulsions of the palmar ulnocarpal ligaments, the ulnotriquetral and ulnolunate, are termed type 1C injuries. Avulsion of the entire TFCC from the sigmoid notch is a type 1D injury.

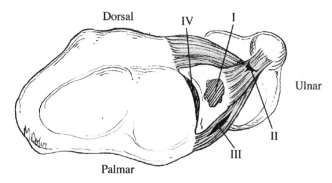

FIG. 17.7. Dorsal view of the distal end of the radius triangular fibrocartilage and ulnar styloid. Triangular Fibrocartilage Complex (TFCC) is depicted as the grayish structure attaching to the radius and subsequently the ulnar styloid. *I*, area of central perforation; *II*, area of attachment of the TFCC to the ulnar styloid; *III*, palmar ulnocarpal ligaments (ulnotriquetral and ulnolunate ligaments); *IV*, attachment of the TFCC to the radius and sigmoid notch. Any or all of these areas may be injured in traumatic type 1 or degenerative type 2 lesions.

Degenerative (type 2) lesions of the TFCC are believed to be secondary to ulnocarpal impaction. With repeated ulnar deviation, especially in association with a positive ulnar variance, perforation of the TFCC can occur. Palmer (59) described five stages of progression beginning with central wear of the articular disc (type 2A). This is followed by chondromalacia of the lunate and ulnar head (type 2B) and then perforation of the articular disc (type 2C). Partial tear of the LT ligament (type 2D) is followed by complete tear with ulnocarpal arthritis as the end stage in untreated cases.

Diagnosis

In traumatic injuries the patient may give a history of sudden pain with an ulnar deviation–extension loading of the wrist with forearm rotation. The patient may report pain with gripping in ulnar deviation during activities such as racquet sports. Examination reveals ulnar-sided tenderness. For type 1A and 1D lesions, the tenderness is often felt dorsally; for type 1B lesions it is located near the ulnar styloid, and for 1C lesions the tenderness is often located volarly over the distal ulna.

Pain may be reproduced by axially compressing the carpus with the wrist held in ulnar deviation while flexion–extension movements of the wrist are carried out. A click can often be produced during these maneuvers that will reproduce the patient's symptoms.

The DRUJ will be stable except in the 1C lesion, where palmar instability may be noted on stress testing.

Imaging Studies

Plain radiographs should include posteroanterior and lateral views of the wrist in neutral forearm rotation.

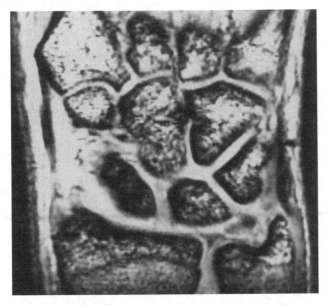

FIG. 17.8. Magnetic resonance imaging of the wrist demonstrating disruption of the central portion of the Triangular Fibrocartilage Complex (TFCC) (*arrow*).

Ulnar variance can be determined with this view as can bony injury to the ulnar styloid, which strongly suggest TFCC injury. Arthrography (radiocarpal and DRUJ injections) can show injury to the TFCC, and some information as to the location of the tear can be obtained (39). However, clinical correlation of arthrographic findings is crucial because there is a high incidence of age-related TFCC degeneration after age 40 (60). MRI with specialized wrist coils is becoming increasingly accurate in description of lesions of the TFCC and can also provide information about the extrinsic ligaments (Fig. 17.8) (46). Computed tomography (CT) is the best investigation for the distal radial and ulnar relationships if one is concerned about dorsal or palmar subluxation of the joint; obviously, both sides need to be scanned for comparison (61). CT is also excellent for exclusion of hamate fracture and arthritis in the pisotriquetral joint.

Treatment

Traumatic. Acute traumatic injury to the TFC complex with no associated DRUJ instability can be treated with immobilization for 6 weeks followed by rehabilitation. However, in the high-performance athlete, this may not be acceptable, and early MRI and/or arthroscopy with surgical treatment of types A, B, and D lesions for faster rehabilitation may be warranted.

Any instability of the DRUJ mandates an arthroscopic examination (62). If the TFCC injury can be reduced closed, it can be treated with immobilization for 4 weeks in ulnar deviation and flexion. The cast or brace must be above the elbow to prevent forearm rotation. If reduction is not possible with closed manipulation, then arthroscopic or open repair of the TFCC should proceed. If the lesion is in the avascular segment of the TFCC (Palmer type 1A), then the lesion can be arthroscopically debrided (63,64). It has been shown that the central two thirds of the articular disk can be removed without causing instability. Postoperatively, early motion should be encouraged. Good improvement in pain and motion should be seen by 3 to 6 weeks. If the patient has ulna-positive variance, debridement should be combined with open or arthroscopic ulnar recession to remove a potential postoperative retear (65).

Lesions in the vascular areas of the TFCC should be repaired either arthroscopically or with open techniques by passing sutures through the TFCC and tying them either to capsule or bone (49,66–68).

Degenerative. Initial treatment of degenerative lesions of the TFCC (Palmer type 2, A through E) should be conservative, using NSAIDs, a trail of immobilization, and judicious use of steroid injections. Surgical treatment of type 2 A through D lesions involves arthroscopic debridement of the TFCC with ulnar shortening osteotomy for the ulna-positive patient. In Palmer type 2D lesion, the LT dissociation should be treated with LT fusion or dorsal capsulodesis. Palmer class 2E lesions have evidence of DRUJ arthritis and may have to be treated with Bowers, Sauve-Kapandjii, or Darrach procedures that remove part or all of the distal ulna.

Distal Radial Ulnar Joint Dislocations

These are relatively uncommon injuries when seen in isolation, being much more common in association with fractures of the radius. In DRUJ dislocations, the radius moves away from the ulna, which is constant in position. However, they have conventionally been described by the position of the ulna in relation to the radius.

Ulna Dorsal

The mechanism in dorsal dislocation is believed to be forceful hyperpronation, and this lesion is seen in contact sports and in sports where the upper limbs are used for weight bearing. The DRUJ disruption is associated with a partial or complete TFCC tear. Clinically, the forearm is locked in pronation and a dorsal prominence is noted. Well-positioned lateral radiographs can confirm the diagnosis, but the best study is a CT scan.

Treatment requires closed reduction that in the acute injury can be done closed by supination of the hand with pressure dorsally on the distal ulna. Once reduction is confirmed, the arm is immobilized in supination for 4 weeks. Chronic or irreducible dislocations require open reduction through a dorsal approach over the distal ulna with repair of the TFCC. Interposition of structures such as the ECU tendon have been described.

Ulna Volar

The mechanism of ulna volar dislocations may be forced supination or a direct blow to the dorsal aspect of the distal ulna. The injury is associated with an ulnar styloid fracture or TFCC disruption. Clinically, the forearm is locked in supination with a dorsal indentation or dimple noted over the distal ulna. Well-positioned lateral radiographs can make the diagnosis, but CT is the most accurate and informative study.

In acute injuries, closed reduction can usually be obtained by pronation of the forearm with volar pressure on the distal ulna followed by immobilization of the arm in pronation for 4 weeks. Late diagnosis or irreducible dislocations should be treated by open reduction through a dorsoulnar approach.

Extensor Carpi Ulnaris Subluxation

Acute disruption or injury to the ECU sheath occurs with forced supination, ulnar deviation, and palmar flexion; it is seen in tennis players and weight lifters.

The ECU tendon has its own fibrosseous tunnel that is an important stabilizing structure of the distal radioulnar joint (69). Rupture or attenuation of this fibrosseous tunnel structure can lead to subluxation of the ECU tendon with forearm rotation, especially in ulnar deviation and flexion of the wrist. This subluxation of the ECU results in a painful snapping sensation and can cause ulnar-sided pain secondary to tenosynovitis of the tendon.

Clinically, the injury may be tender or one may feel the tendon subluxation with wrist rotation. Acute cases may be treated with immobilization of the forearm in pronation, with the wrist in slight dorsiflexion and radial deviation. Chronic subluxation requires surgical repair or reconstruction of the ECU sheath.

Triquetrohamate Impaction Syndrome

Similar to scaphoid impaction syndrome, this entity is usually caused by hyperextension in ulnar deviation; it is seen in gymnasts as a result of floor exercises and pommel horse exercises. Acute injuries can occur in football or hockey as well.

Clinically, the patient complains of dorsal wrist pain, particularly with forced wrist extension. Examination may reveal dorsoulnar swelling and point tenderness over the triquetrum and lunate. Radiographs may reveal reactive osteophytes on the dorsum of the hamate and triquetrum.

Treatment is usually nonoperative, and early return to activity may be aided by use of a soft extension block orthosis.

Tendinopathy at the Wrist

These common problems occur with repetitive resisted loading of the wrist or a sudden stress to the wrist in an athlete unaccustomed to the inciting activity (70,71). Athletes will complain of pain along the course of the tendon aggravated with resisted muscle contraction. The common course of treatment involves altering or eliminating the provocative maneuver by modification of the training program, modification of equipment, or modification of technique. Ice, splints, NSAIDs, and other modalities are frequently used. Once the initial acute inflammation subsides, a stretching, strengthening, and endurance protocol is used before return to full activity is allowed.

DeQuervain's Syndrome

This is the most common tendinopathy occurring about the wrist. It is seen often in racquet sports, golf, or baseball where repetitive forceful gripping in ulnar deviation is used. The syndrome involves inflammation within the first dorsal extensor compartment through

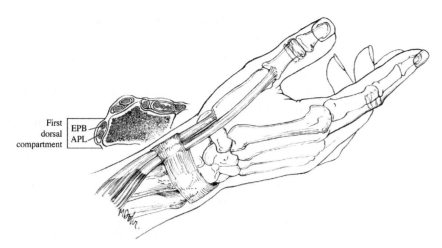

First dorsal compartment
EPB
APL

FIG. 17.9. DeQuervain's tenosynovitis occurs in the first extensor compartment that contains the abductor pollicis longus and extensor pollicis brevis tendons. Surgical release should be along the ulnar border of the first compartment so as not to cause subluxation of the tendons with thumb use.

which pass the tendons of the extensor pollicis brevis (EPB) and abductor pollicis longus (APL) (72–74). Clinically, the athlete complains of pain along the dorsal-radial side of the wrist that is aggravated with grip in ulnar deviation or with thumb use. There may also be stiffness of the thumb and weakness in opposition.

On examination, there may be swelling over the first extensor compartment and tenderness over the tendons as they pass through the sheath. Crepitus may be felt with thumb motion. The Finkelstein test (75) is very useful in diagnosis. This test is carried out by ulnar deviation of the wrist with the thumb held in the palm; this motion will reproduce the athlete's pain.

Nonoperative therapy is effective for 80% of patients with these symptoms. Therapy involves the modalities described above for all tendinopathies, but in addition the use of a thumb spica orthosis, allowing free interphalangeal joint motion, is quite helpful. Injection of a small amount of lidocaine with steroid into the sheath is diagnostic and often curative. Aggravating activities are avoided for 4 to 6 weeks.

For recalcitrant cases, operative release of the first extensor compartment has a high success rate. We prefer a longitudinal incision to minimize risk of damage to the superficial sensory branch of the radial nerve. The fibrosseous sheath is completely released along its ulnar aspect to minimize risk of tendon subluxation (Fig. 17.9). Care must be taken to inspect carefully for a separate sheath for the EPB; one must also remember that the APL can have ancillary tendons. Postoperatively, the patient is allowed to return to activities as comfort permits.

Second Compartment Tendinopathy

Tendinopathy at this location is quite common, second only to DeQuervain's in producing wrist pain. Treatment is nonoperative with release of the compartment for recalcitrant cases.

Intersection syndrome involves inflammation at the point at which the outcroppers tendons (EPL, APL, EPB) pass over the second compartment tendons (76). It is seen in athletes involved in repetitive forceful wrist flexion and extension such as rowers, weight lifters, and gymnasts. Clinical examination reveals pain, tenderness, and swelling located at the distal junction of the outcroppers and Extensor Carpi Radialis Brevis (ECRB) and Extensor Carpi Radialis Longus (ECRL) tendons. Often a palpable or audible squeak can be elicited with flexion–extension of the wrist.

Treatment is ice, NSAIDs, and rest or modification of activity. Splinting with a thumb spica splint in 15 degrees of extension is helpful. Use of local anesthetic with steroid injected in the APL bursa can help diagnosis and treatment. Splinting is continued for 2 weeks followed by therapy to recover range of motion, then strength, before return to full activity.

Surgery is rarely required but if necessary involves debridement of thickened and inflamed tissues in the area. Some release of the second compartment sheath may be required proximally, but complete sheath release should be avoided because bowstringing of the powerful wrist extensor tendons may result. Postoperatively, a thumb spica is worn for 2 weeks, and aggravating insults are avoided for 3 months. Early motion with interim splinting is started at 2 to 4 weeks followed by strengthening exercises. Return to full activity is allowed when strength is 80% to 90% of the normal side.

Extensor Pollicis Longus Tendinopathy

Inflammation at the point at which the long thumb extensor wraps around Lister's tubercle is seen in repetitive motion sports such as squash. Attritional and acute ruptures have also been reported.

Pain with thumb use and tenderness at Lister's tubercle with swelling suggest the diagnosis. Nonoperative modalities including thumb splinting are used. Rarely, transposition of the tendon over Lister's tubercle may be required.

Extensor Indicis Proprius Tendinopathy

This entity is believed to occur in patients with a musculotendon junction of the extensor indicis proprius that is distal and as such the muscle enters the sheath of the fourth extensor compartment, causing compression and then inflammation and synovitis (77,78). The pain can be reproduced with resisted extension of the index finger from the fully flexed position at the Metacarpal Phalangeal (MP) joint. The treatment involves surgical release of the proximal part of the sheath.

Extensor Carpi Ulnaris Tendinopathy

This common entity is seen in racquet sports. The ECU tendon travels below the extensor retinaculum in its own subsheath, which plays an important role in DRUJ stability. Clinically, the athlete complains of dorsoulnar wrist pain after repetitive activity. Examination reveals swelling and tenderness over the sheath. Pain can be reproduced with resisted wrist dorsiflexion with the wrist in a position of ulnar deviation and the forearm in supination. Radiologic examination may reveal calcification within the tendon, but they are usually negative. The differential diagnosis must include any cause of ulnar wrist pain or instability.

Splint immobilization for 2 weeks and steroid injection of the sheath followed by rehabilitation is often curative. Recalcitrant cases may require release of the sheath. Longitudinal incision with careful identification of the dorsal sensory branches of the ulnar nerve is followed by careful reflection of the extensor retinaculum and release of the subsheath on its radial border to avoid subluxation of the tendon. The extensor retinaculum is carefully repaired. Immobilization in a short arm or Muenster cast in neutral or pronation and slight radial deviation for 2 weeks is followed by a stretching and strengthening program. Return to full competition should be delayed until 80% of motion and strength are recovered (79).

Flexor Carpi Radialis Tendinopathy

Nerve Disorders

Nerve injury is infrequent in athletes and is usually caused by repetitive stress. The pathogenesis involves repeated vascular compression of peripheral nerves resulting in a cycle of ischemia, edema, and fibrosis that eventually leads to permanent neuronal loss. The median nerve at the wrist, the ulnar nerve at Guyon's canal, the posterior interosseous nerve, and the sensory branch of the radial nerve are susceptible in the athletic wrist.

Ulnar Nerve Compression in Guyon's Canal, or Cyclist's Palsy

This compression neuropathy is seen in cyclists, racquet sports, and handball where there is repetitive compression at the hypothenar area. Involvement can be purely sensory, purely motor, or a combination of both.

Shea and McClain (80) described compression of the ulnar nerve either just proximal to Guyon's canal or just within the canal that results in sensory and motor involvement of the ulnar nerve. Another site of compression occurs at the ulnar nerve where it exits from the canal of Guyon, near the hook of the hamate between the origins of the abductor digiti quinti and flexor digiti quinti muscles, during its passage through the substance of the opponens digiti quinti muscle, or as it crosses the palm deep to the flexor tendons and volar to the metacarpals. This second type of compression results in a pure motor palsy. Comtet et al. (81) reported a case of compression of the deep branch of the ulnar nerve by the adductor hiatus within the palm. Their patient had severe wasting in the first web space that was reversed with release of the fibrous arch. Milek and Thompson (82) reported two patients with pain in the first dorsal interosseous muscle with tenderness at the adductor hiatus but without muscle wasting.

A third type of compression involves the nerve at the distal third of the canal; this spares the motor branch and results in purely sensory findings of numbness in the ring and small fingers. Clinically, the patient usually reports pain on the ulnar volar aspect of the hand with paresthesias in the ulnar nerve sensory distribution. The patient complains of weak grip strength. Examination may reveal positive Tinel's sign over Guyon's canal. Motor involvement may result in first dorsal interosseous weakness, a positive Froment's sign, and a positive Wartenberg's sign due to unopposed extensor digiti minimi action. Late cases may involve increased two-point discrimination, a sign of neuronal loss.

The differential diagnosis includes hamate fracture, more proximal ulnar nerve compression (which might show loss of dorsal sensory branch of ulnar nerve and clawing of ulnar two digits), or hypothenar hammer syndrome (which could be excluded with Allen's test).

Treatment in cyclists involves frequent handlebar position changes to avoid pressure on the palm in the area of the hook of the hamate and the use of padded handlebars and gloves. Rest and avoidance may be required. Failure of conservative therapy or any evidence of motor involvement or pronounced sensory loss is an indication for decompression of the ulnar nerve at Guyon's canal.

Carpal Tunnel Syndrome

Compression of the median nerve at the wrist is the most common compression neuropathy found in sports.

It is seen in sports requiring repetitive grasping activity. The etiology is believed to be due to flexor tenosynovitis or lumbrical hypertrophy.

Clinically, patients complains of pain of vague and aching nature in the wrist that can radiate as far proximally as the shoulder. Weakness is described, as are distal paresthesias. Patients usually describes pain at night that awakens them and predictable occurrence of paresthesia with certain activities.

On examination, Phalen's test, the carpal tunnel compression test, and Tinel's sign are frequently found to be positive. Nerve conduction testing may reveal prolonged distal sensory latencies and decreased signal amplitude, and electromyograms may reveal muscle denervation. The differential diagnosis should include cervical radiculopathy, anterior interosseous syndrome, or pronator syndrome.

Treatment is initially nonoperative with splinting in neutral, modification of activity, and rest. Although NSAIDs may help, a steroid injection into the carpal tunnel may be both therapeutic and diagnostic. Failure of conservative therapy or severe symptoms are indications for surgical decompression.

Posterior Interosseous Nerve Symptoms, or Gymnast's Palsy

The cause of this compression neuropathy is direct compression over the nerve by repeated hyperextension of the wrist. Posterior interosseous nerve neuroma will result in pain at the extension crease of the wrist that is well localized. Nonoperative treatment involves avoidance of hyperextension and use of a soft neoprene splint. Operative treatment requires exposure of the nerve on the floor of the fourth extensor compartment with resection of a 1.5- to 2-cm section followed by careful repair of the extensor retinaculum.

Wartenberg's Syndrome

Wartenberg's syndrome involves compression of the sensory branch of the radial nerve. It can be caused by direct pressure of the nerve by equipment at the site where the nerve exits from under the edge of the brachioradialis in the distal forearm. It can also be seen as a result of a traction neuropathy resulting from repetitive forearm rotation with ulnar deviation of the wrist. This neuropathy is seen in gymnasts and weight lifters.

Clinically, the patient complains of paresthesias in the dorsoradial hand and thumb. Physical examination may reveal a Tinel's sign, reproducing symptoms over the location of the nerve as it exits from under the brachioradialis. The symptoms may be provoked with wrist flexion and ulnar deviation.

Treatment involves rest, ice, avoidance of aggravating activities, alteration of technique or equipment, and use of a palmar cock-up wrist splint. Operative treatment involves decompression of the fascia between the brachioradialis and the extensor carpi radialis tendons followed by use of a soft dressing and early motion. Dellon and MacKinnon (83) described decompression and neurolysis of the nerve. They found their best results in cases caused by an acute onset due to a single exciting episode.

VASCULAR DISORDERS

Hypothenar Hammer Syndrome or Ulnar Artery Thrombosis

Thrombosis of the ulnar artery at the wrist may be caused by an acute injury or repetitive trauma. It is seen in judo and karate athletes and also in basketball, hockey, handball, and lacrosse. The athlete complains of hypothenar pain and ulnar nerve compression symptoms. There may be variable amount of cold intolerance and vascular insufficiency. Examination may reveal a mass, tenderness over the hypothenar eminence, and a positive Tinel's sign. Allen's test will show filling only from the radial artery. Doppler or ultrasound testing may be helpful, but the definitive diagnostic test is an angiogram.

Symptoms are believed to be mediated by abnormal sympathetic function in the region of the thrombosed artery; thus, resection of the diseased section of the artery may be curative. Others have reconstructed ulnar flow with interpositional vein grafts. Nonoperative modalities such as sympathetic blocks and vasodilators have shown limited success in treating this condition.

REFERENCES

1. Howe C. Wrist injuries in sports. *Sports Med* 1994;17:163.
2. Hursh LM. Numbers and types of sports injuries. *JAMA* 1967; 199:167.
3. Simonet WT, Sim FH. Ice hockey injuries. *Am J Sports Med* 1987;15:3.
4. Strauss RH, Lanese RR. Injuries among wrestlers in school and college tournaments. *JAMA* 1982;248:2016.
5. Ellsasser JC, Stein AH. Management of hand injuries in a professional football team: review of 15 years of experience with one team. *Am J Sports Med* 1979;7:178.
6. Rettig AC, Ryan RO, Stone JA. Epidemiology of hand injuries in sports. In: Strickland JW, Rettig AC, eds. *Hand injuries in athletes.* Philadelphia: W.B. Saunders, 1992:37.
7. Rettig AC, Patel DV. Epidemiology of elbow, forearm and wrist injuries in the athlete. *Clin Sports Med* 1995;14:289.
8. Linscheid RL, Dobyns JH. Athletic injuries of the wrist. *Clin Orthop* 1985;198:141.
9. Mandelbaum BR, Bartolozzi BR, Davis CA, et al. Wrist pain syndrome in the gymnast: pathogenetic, diagnostic, and therapeutic considerations. *Am J Sports Med* 1989;17:305.
10. Dobyns JH, Linscheid RL, Chao EYS, et al. *Traumatic instability of the wrist. AAOS Instr. Course Lectures.* Vol. 24. St. Louis: Mosby, 1975.
11. Green DP. Carpal dislocations and instabilities. In: Green DP, ed. *Operative hand surgery,* 3rd ed. New York: Churchill Livingstone, 1993:861.
12. Sebald JR, Dobyns JH, Linscheid RL. The natural history of collapse deformities of the wrist. *Clin Orthop* 1974;104:140.

13. Taleisnik J. Current concepts review: carpal instability. *J Bone Joint Surg Am* 1988;70A:1262.

14. Watson HK, Ballet FL. The SLAC wrist: scapholunate advanced collapse pattern of degenerative arthritis. *J Hand Surg* 1984; 9A:358.

15. Watson HK, Jaiyoung RYU, Akelman E. Limited triscaphoid intercarpal arthrodesis for rotatory subluxation of the scaphoid. *J Bone Joint Surg Am* 1986;68A:345.

16. Berger RA. The gross and histologic anatomy of the scapholunate interosseous ligament. *J Hand Surg* 1996;21A:170.

17. Berger RA, Crowninshield RD, Flatt AE. The three dimensional behavior of the carpal bones. *Clin Orthop* 1982;167:303.

18. Dobyns JH, Berger RA. Dislocations of the carpus. In: Chapman MW, Madison M, eds. *Operative orthopedics,* 2nd ed. Philadelphia: J.B. Lippincott, 1993:1289.

19. Mayfield JK, Johnson RP, Kilcoyne RF. The ligaments of the wrist and their functional significance. *Anat Rec* 1976;186:417.

20. Mayfield JK, Williams WJ, Erdman AG, et al. Biomechanical properties of the human carpal ligaments. *Orthop Trans* 1979; 3:143.

21. Kobayashi M, Berger RA, Linscheid RL, et al. Intercarpal kinematics during wrist motion. *Hand Clin* 1997;13:143.

22. Weber ER. Concepts governing the rotational shift of the intercalated segment of the carpus. *Orthop Clin North Am* 1984;15:193.

23. Palmer AK, Werner FW. Triangular fibrocartilage complex of the wrist: anatomy and function. *J Hand Surg* 1981;6A:153.

24. Mayfield JK, Johnson RP, Kilcoyne RF. Carpal dislocations: pathomechanics and progressive perilunar instability. *J Hand Surg* 1980;5:226.

25. Short WH, Werner FW, Fortino MD, et al. A dynamic biomechanical study of scapholunate ligament sectioning. *J Hand Surg* 1995;20A:986.

26. Linscheid RL, Dobyns JH, Beabout JW, et al. Traumatic instability of the wrist: diagnosis, classification, and pathomechanics. *J Bone Joint Surg Am* 1972;54A:1612.

27. Viegas SF. The wrist. In: Gelberman R, ed. *Surgical techniques.* New York: Raven Press, 1994:88.

28. Watson HK, Ashmead D, Makhlouf MV. Examination of the scaphoid. *J Hand Surg* 1988;13A:657.

29. Easterling KJ, Wolfe SW. Scaphoid shift in the uninjured wrist. *J Hand Surg* 1994;19A:604.

30. Hardy DC, Totty WG, Reinus WR, et al. Posteroanterior wrist radiography: importance of arm positioning. *J Hand Surg* 1987; 12A:504.

31. Rockwell WB, Destouet JM, Gilula LA, et al. Radiographic approach to the painful wrist. *Orthop Rev* 1985;14:43.

32. Thompson TC, Campbell RD, et al. Primary and secondary dislocation of the scaphoid bone. *J Bone Joint Surg Br* 1964; 46B:73.

33. Linscheid A. Scapholunate ligamentous instabilities (dissociations, subdislocations, dislocations). *Ann Chir Main* 1984;3:323.

34. Meade TD, Schneider LH, Cherry K. Radiographic analysis of selective ligament sectioning at the carpal scaphoid: a cadaver study. *J Hand Surg* 1990;15A:855.

35. Gilula LA. Carpal injuries: analytic approach and case exercises. *AJR Am J Roentgenol* 1979;133:503.

36. Gilula LA, Weeks PM. Post traumatic ligamentous instability of the wrist. *Radiology* 1978;129:641.

37. Nielsen PT, Hedeboe J. Post-traumatic scapholunate dissociation by wrist cineradiography. *J Hand Surg* 1984;9A:135.

38. Jackson WT, Protas JM. Snapping scapholunate subluxation. *J Hand Surg* 1981;6A:590.

39. Levinsohn EM, Rosen ID, Palmer AK. Wrist arthrography: value of three compartment injection method. *Radiology* 1991;179:231.

40. Chung KC, Zimmerman NB, Travis MT. Wrist arthrography versus arthroscopy: a comparative study of 150 cases. *J Hand Surg* 1996;21A:591.

41. Cooney WP. Evaluation of chronic wrist pain by arthrography, arthroscopy and arthrotomy. *J Hand Surg* 1993;18A:815.

42. Cantor RM, Stern PJ, Wyrick JD, et al. The relevance of ligament tears or perforations in the diagnosis of wrist pain: an arthrographic study. *J Hand Surg* 1994;19A:945.

43. Weiss AC, Akelman E, Lambiase R. Comparison of the findings of triple injection arthrography of the wrist with those of arthroscopy. *J Bone Joint Surg Am* 1996;78A:348.

44. Eynde SV, DeSmet L, Fabry G. Diagnostic value of arthrography and arthroscopy of the radiocarpal joint. *Arthroscopy* 1994; 10:50.

45. Brown JA, Janzen DL, Adler BD, et al. Arthrography of the contralateral asymptomatic wrist in patients with unilateral wrist pain. *Can Assoc Radiol J* 1994;45:292.

46. Pederzini L, Luschetti R, Soragni O, et al. Evaluation of the triangular fibrocartilage complex tears by arthroscopy, arthrography, and magnetic resonance imaging. *Arthroscopy* 1992; 8:191.

47. Dautel G, Goudot B, Merle M. Arthroscopic diagnosis of scapholunate instability in the absence of x-ray abnormalities. *J Hand Surg* 1993;18B:213.

48. Rettig ME, Amadio PC. Wrist arthroscopy: indications and clinical applications. *J Hand Surg* 1994;19B:774.

49. Ruch DS, Poheling GG. Arthroscopic management of partial scapholunate and lunotriquetral injuries of the wrist. *J Hand Surg* 1996;21A:412.

50. Lavernia CJ, Cohen MS, Taleisnik J. Treatment of scapholunate dissociation by ligamentous repair and capsulodesis. *J Hand Surg* 1992;17A:354.

51. Blatt G. Capsulodesis in reconstructive hand surgery: dorsal capsulodesis for the unstable scaphoid and volar capsulodesis following excision of the distal ulna. *Hand Clin* 1987;3:81.

52. Wintman BI, Gelberman RH, Katz JN. Dynamic scapholunate instability: results of operative treatment with dorsal capsulodesis. *J Hand Surg* 1995;20A:971.

53. Weiss AC, Sachar K, Glowacki K. Arthroscopic debridement alone for intercarpal ligament tears. *J Hand Surg* 1997;22A:344.

54. Weiss AC. Scapholunate ligament reconstruction using a bone-retinaculum-bone autograft. *J Hand Surg* 1998;23A:205.

55. Minami A, Kaneda K. Repair and/or reconstruction of scapholunate interosseous ligament in lunate and perilunate dislocations. *J Hand Surg* 1993;18A:1099.

56. Palmer AK, Dobyns JH, Linscheid RL. Management of post traumatic ligamentous instability of the wrist secondary to ligament rupture. *J Hand Surg* 1978;3:507.

57. Pisano SM, Peimer CA, Wheeler DR, et al. Scapholunate intercarpal arthrodesis. *J Hand Surg* 1991;16A:328.

58. Weiker GG. Hand and wrist problems in the gymnast. *Clin Sports Med* 1992;11:189.

59. Palmer AK. Triangular fibrocartilage complex lesions: a classification. *J Hand Surg* 1989;14A:594.

60. Mikic ZD. Age changes in the triangular fibrocartilage of the wrist. *J Anat* 1978;126:367.

61. Weschler RJ, Wehbe MA, Rifkin MD, et al. Computed tomography diagnosis of distal radioulnar joint subluxation. *Skeletal Radiol* 1987;16:1.

62. Osterman AL, Moskow L, Low DW. Soft tissue injuries of the hand and wrist. *Clin Sports Med* 1988;7:329.

63. Minami A, Ishikawa J, Suenage N, et al. Clinical results of treatment of triangular fibrocartilage complex tears by arthroscopic debridement. *J Hand Surg* 1996;21A:406.

64. Osterman AL. Arthroscopic debridement of triangular fibrocartilage complex tears. *Arthroscopy* 1990;6:120.

65. Feldon P, Terrono AL, Belsky MR. Wafer distal ulna resection for triangular fibrocartilage tears and/or ulna impaction syndrome. *J Hand Surg* 1992;17A:731.

66. Cooney WP, Linscheid RL, Dobyns JH. Triangular fibrocartilage tears. *J Hand Surg* 1994;19A:143.

67. Trumble TE, Gilbert MA, Vedder N. Isolated tears of the triangular fibrocartilage: management by early arthroscopic repair. *J Hand Surg* 1997;22A:57.

68. Zachee B, De-Smet L, Fabry G. Arthroscopic suturing of TFCC lesions. *Arthroscopy* 1993;9:242.

69. Spinner M, Kaplan EB. Extensor carpi ulnaris: its relationship to the stability of the distal radio-ulnar joint. *Clin Orthop* 1970;68: 124.

70. Kiefhaber TR, Stern PJ. Upper extremity tendinitis and overuse syndromes in the athlete. *Clin Sports Med* 1992;11:39.

71. Stern PJ. Tendinitis, overuse syndromes, and tendon injuries. *Hand Clin* 1990;6:467.

72. Hervey FJ, Harvery PM, Horsley MW. DeQuervain's disease: surgical or non-surgical treatment. *J Hand Surg* 1990;15A:83.

73. Lacey T, Goldstein LA. Anatomic and clinical study of the variations in the insertion of the abductor pollicus longus tendon, associated with stenosing tenovaginitis. *J Bone Joint Surg Am* 1951;33A:347.

74. Wood MB, Linscheid RL. Abductor pollicus longus bursitis. *Clin Orth* 1993;93:293.

75. Finkelstein H. Stenosing tendovaginitis at the radial styloid process. *J Bone Joint Surg* 1930;12:509.

76. Grundberg AB, Reagan DS. Pathologic anatomy of the forearm: intersection syndrome. *J Hand Surg* 1985;10A:299.

77. Ritter MA, Inglis AE. The extensor indicus proprius syndrome. *J Bone Joint Surg Am* 1969;51A:1645.

78. Spinner M, Olshansky K. The extensor indicus proprius syndrome: a clinical test. *Plast Reconstr Surg* 1973;51:134.

79. Hajj AA, Wood MB. Stenosing tenosynovitis of the extensor carpi ulnaris. *J Hand Surg* 1986;11A:519.

80. Shea JD, McClain EJ. Ulnar nerve compression syndromes at and below the wrist. *J Bone Joint Surg Am* 1969;51A:1095.

81. Comtet JJ, Quieot L, Moyen B. Compression of the deep palmar branch of the ulnar nerve by the arch of the adductor pollicis. *Hand* 1978;10:176.

82. Milek M, Thompson D. Compression of the deep branch of the ulnar nerve at the adductor hiatus producing pain without muscle atrophy. *J Hand Surg* 1988;13A:283.

83. Dellon AL, Mackinnon SE. Radial sensory nerve entrapment in the forearm. *J Hand Surg* 1986;11:199.

Principles and Practice of Orthopaedic Sports Medicine,
edited by William E. Garrett, Jr., Kevin P. Speer, and Donald T. Kirkendall.
Lippincott Williams & Wilkins, Philadelphia © 2000.

CHAPTER 18

Tendinopathies about the Elbow

Jeffrey E. Budoff and Robert P. Nirschl

Tendon injuries about the elbow are usually the result of overuse from repetitive tension overload. An overuse injury occurs when tissue damage occurs over time at a rate exceeding the body's ability to heal it. As the stress tolerance of the tendon is exceeded, inflammation or tissue breakdown may occur, leading to pain and disability.

The most common example of this is lateral tennis elbow. Predisposing activities that cause repetitive eccentric loading of the lateral elbow tendons include racket sports, throwing sports, and swimming in addition to occupational activities that require stressful forearm use such as carpentry, plumbing, and textile production (1). The presenting symptoms are pain over the origin of the extensor carpi radialis brevis (ECRB) and weakness of the wrist extensors. The digital extensors may also be involved. The pain is often described as "burning" and may be noted to radiate down the forearm (2), occasionally to the long and ring fingers (3). Medial tennis elbow typically presents with pain over the flexor-pronator mass and posterior tennis elbow with pain over the triceps insertion.

Approximately 50% of tennis players can expect to get a tennis elbow at some point during their playing lifetime (4), and in one third of players this will be severe enough to interfere with activities of daily living. Once appropriately treated, up to 90% of affected players may never have a recurrence (2,5).

Throwing athletes tend to develop medial tendinosis (epicondylitis) because of the valgus stresses experienced (6). Golfers tend to develop medial tendinosis (epicondylitis) of the dominant elbow and lateral tendinosis (epicondylitis) of the nondominant elbow (7).

Tennis elbow is more frequent in patients over 35 years but may occur at a younger age in highly competitive athletes who subject their tendons to greater physiologic demands (8). The peak age of onset is between 40 and 50 years, averaging 22.6 years of prior tennis experience (5,9,10).

The onset of symptoms is usually gradual, often appearing after vigorous activity. Less commonly, acute onset may be associated with an extreme effort or direct trauma (1). In many instances no predisposing activity can be determined (11).

The patient does not have to be a competitive athlete to develop overuse injuries about the elbow. In fact, 95% of cases occur in non-tennis players (11). Musicians, carpenters, assembly-line workers, and many others subject themselves to repetitive activities on an almost daily basis, which may lead to overuse. Work or play that requires repeated pronation and supination, overuse of the wrist or finger extensors, or lifting with the hands in the palm down position are believed to be predisposing factors (12,13).

Work-related overuse syndromes often lead to lateral elbow tendinosis (epicondylitis) that is more resistant to conservative treatment and more often requires surgical management. This may be because most athletes can reduce or interrupt their participation in the aggravating activity, whereas those with work-related tendinosis do not often have that option (3). The annual incidence of non–sports-related lateral elbow tendinosis has been reported at 59 per 10,000 workers (14).

There are two types of risk factors for overuse injuries: intrinsic and extrinsic. Intrinsic risk factors relate to biomechanical abnormalities that are specific to the individual patient. These include deconditioning, weakness, inflexibility and instability, and an overall less durable collagen framework (e.g., hereditary factors). Extrinsic risk factors are related to the stresses applied to the arm and include training errors, poor technique, bad equipment, or a poor work environment. Intrinsic risk

J. E. Budoff: Department of Orthopaedic Surgery, Baylor College of Medicine, Houston, Texas 77030.

R. P. Nirschl: Department of Orthopaedic Surgery, Georgetown University, Arlington, VA 22205. McLean, Virginia 27101.

factors render the elbow more vulnerable to stress, the severity of which is increased by extrinsic risk factors.

Training errors are the number one reason for overuse injury. This includes excessive frequency or intensity of activity, inadequate rest between workouts, poor conditioning, inadequate fitness level, inadequate warm-up or warm-down, and abrupt changes in routine. Injury is most likely to occur when the athlete experiences a change in routine, known as a transition, especially if the change is so rapid that the tissue is unable to accommodate ongoing demands. Activity transitions and other training errors, such as excessively forceful gripping during weight lifting leading to medial elbow tendinosis, should be sought out in the patient's history. By correcting training errors, we may not only cure the current injury but prevent subsequent injuries.

The other side of the coin is the quality of the tissues that are being asked to absorb these repetitive stresses. Repetitive eccentric overload leads to stretching out and weakening of specific musculotendinous units, predisposing them to further injury. Injury then leads to further weakness in an ongoing cycle.

PATHOANATOMY

Lateral tennis elbow is a degenerative tendinosis of the origin of the ECRB. In addition, the anterior edge of the origin of the extensor digitorum communis (EDC) is involved in 30% of cases. Rarely, the underside of the extensor carpi radialis longus (ECRL) or the origin of the extensor carpi ulnaris is involved (1). Lateral tennis elbow is three to seven times as frequent as medial tennis elbow (3,4).

Medial tennis elbow is a degenerative tendinosis of the interface of the pronator teres and the flexor carpi radialis (56%) but has also been noted in the common flexor origin (32%), the palmaris longus, the flexor carpi ulnaris (12%), and rarely on the underside of the flexor sublimis origin (1,8,15).

Posterior tennis elbow is uncommon, accounting for only about 2% of cases (9). It represents a degenerative tendinosis of the triceps insertion and occurs in sports that require sudden elbow extension, such as overhead throwing (1,8).

The term "tendinosis" is used rather than tendinitis because it more accurately defines the histopathologic presentation of the degenerative process. The term "tendinitis" has been used to describe the theoretic chronic inflammatory changes in the overused tendon. However, histologic examination of excised pathologic tendons has consistently failed to reveal the presence of inflammatory cells. If chronic inflammatory cells are evident in the tendon, they are those of traumatic repair and include granulation tissue and scar (1,8).

The characteristic appearance of this tissue consists of invasion of immature fibroblasts and disorganized nonfunctional vascular elements (10,16). Electron microscopy has demonstrated that these vascular buds do not possess lumen (17). This granulation-like tissue has been termed angiofibroblastic hyperplasia by Nirschl (10). As tendinitis is now known to be a misnomer, it should be replaced by the term tendinosis.

Angiofibroblastic hyperplasia is intrinsically abnormal and insinuates itself through the adjacent normal-appearing tendon fibers, disrupting them. The adjacent tendon appears hypercellular, degenerated, and microfragmented (10,16). In advanced lesions, the characteristic reaction occurs in the supportive tissue and in the tendon itself. Although acute inflammatory cells are almost always absent in these supportive tissues, a mild sprinkling of chronic inflammatory cells may be noted (1,8).

It is theorized that this angiofibroblastic hyperplasia may be the result of an aborted healing response to microtears, combined with vascular deprivation in the tendon origin. Healing may not occur due to the poor vascularity of the tendon origin and the normal anatomic absence of a periosteal lining over the lateral and medial epicondyles. In addition, the normal fibroblastic repair response may be disrupted by continuing injury, and the degenerative tendinosis itself may act as a detriment to the process of tissue repair (10,16).

In general, the degree of angiofibroblastic infiltration appears to correlate generally with the duration of symptoms and the intensity of the pain (1,8). Goldie (16) believed that cases of spontaneous recovery might be explained by the replacement of this pathologic tissue by scar.

Grossly, angiofibroblastic hyperplasia characteristically appears dull, gray, friable, and edematous, as compared with the firm off-white appearance of normal tendon (1,8). Goldie (16) found free nerve endings in this tissue and believed that this explained how its presence could be painful. Although we agree that this tissue is the primary source of pathology and the patient's pain, we have been unable to identify any nerve endings within it (17).

Secondary fibrosis, tendon calcification, lateral epicondylar exostosis, and iatrogenic corticosteroid changes (cellular death and atrophy) may be associated with the primary tendinosis. At the corticosteroid injection site, nonpolarizable amorphous eosinophilic material can be identified, often without any foreign body response and usually without evidence of calcification (1,8).

Other pathologic disorders may occur in conjunction with medial elbow tendinosis, because they are also induced by repetitive valgus stress and overuse. These entities include ulnar nerve irritation and medial ulnar collateral injury and chondromalacia, synovitis, osteophytic spurring, and loose body formation of the posterior or lateral compartments (8).

There may be a subset of people particularly predisposed to the development of overuse injuries. These patients complain of multiple sites of tendon degeneration and pain, often without an impressive history of overuse. It is theorized that they may have a poorer quality of collagen, less able to tolerate stress, and more predisposed to breakdown. Nirschl (18) previously reported on this patient population and coined the term "mesenchymal syndrome" to describe them. They may encompass up to 15% of patients with overuse syndromes.

Patients with this disorder are typically, although not exclusively, female and tend to present in their late 20s or early 30s with multiple upper extremity problems such as bilateral tennis elbow, both medial and lateral; cubital tunnel syndrome; rotator cuff tendinosis; carpal tunnel syndrome; deQuervain's syndrome; or trigger finger. Osteoporosis, often from premature menopause, may also accompany the syndrome. Routine laboratory and rheumatologic screening tests are characteristically normal (8,18).

PHYSICAL EXAMINATION

Point of Maximum Tenderness

Lateral "tennis elbow," or degenerative tendinosis of the ECRB, causes tenderness over the origin of the ECRB, just anterior and distal to the tip of the lateral epicondyle. If the EDC is also involved, it will be tender just posterior and distal to the tip of the lateral epicondyle. Associated bony exostosis of the lateral epicondyle will often result in tenderness over the lateral epicondyle itself. In lateral tennis elbow, the point of maximum tenderness is invariably within 1 to 2 cm of the lateral epicondyle. If the point of maximum tenderness is distal to the level of the radial head, posterior interosseous nerve (PIN) entrapment (radial tunnel syndrome) should be suspected (4).

The lateral epicondyle, the radial head, and the radial tunnel lie in a line equidistant from each other. The point of maximum tenderness for the radial tunnel syndrome is at the proximal edge of the supinator, underneath the mobile wad of Henry, approximately 4 to 5 cm distal to the lateral epicondyle (3,19–22). Tenderness here should be compared with the other side, because this region is often a little tender to deep pressure.

The capitellum may become tender in the presence of osteochondral fractures or osteochondrosis dissecans. The capitellum is most easily palpated in flexion and is located under the most anterior aspect of the lateral soft spot, distal and anterior to the lateral epicondyle (23).

Just distal to the capitellum the radial head can be palpated; it is most easily found by passively rotating the forearm with the elbow flexed 90 degrees. It is located approximately 2 cm distal to the lateral epicondyle in a visible depression just posterior to the mobile wad of Henry. With forearm rotation, approximately three fourths of the radial head is palpable (24). Tenderness of the radial head in conjuction with an effusion is suspi-

cious for a radial head fracture, even if standard radiographs are negative.

The forearm should be rotated at varying degrees of elbow flexion. Rotation of the radial head should be smooth; any asymmetry should be suspicious for subluxation or fracture of the proximal radius. Crepitus, popping, or pain may represent radiocapitellar arthrosis, chondromalacia, osteochondritis dissecans, or a loose body.

Medial tennis elbow (or golfer's elbow) usually represents tendinosis of the pronator teres and flexor carpi radialis (13). The point of maximum tenderness usually lies within these tendons, which are distal to the medial epicondyle, on the lateral side of the flexor–pronator muscle mass. In addition, the pronator teres has an origin proximal to the medial epicondyle, which may also be tender. In medial tennis elbow, the point of maximum tenderness should be within 1 to 2 cm of the medial epicondyle. If the tenderness is more distal, other diagnoses should be considered (11).

The differential diagnosis of medial elbow pain includes injury to the medial collateral ligament (MCL), ulnar neuropathy/cubital tunnel syndrome, and a snapping medial triceps tendon (25). The anterior band of the MCL (its most significant structural component) is best palpated with the elbow gently flexed 30 to 60 degrees. It runs from the anteroinferior medial epicondyle to the medial margin of the ulna's sigmoid notch at the base of the coronoid process (26) (Fig. 18.1). Tenderness of the MCL in conjunction with pain on valgus stress is consistent with injury to this ligament.

The ulnar nerve may be palpated in the cubital tunnel, just posterior to the medial epicondyle. Percussion of an irritated ulnar nerve may lead to a positive Tinel's sign, which is pain or paresthesias radiating distally from the elbow in the distribution of the ulnar nerve (i.e., to the ulnar one and a half digits). A subluxating ulnar nerve can be palpated as it dislocates anteriorly from

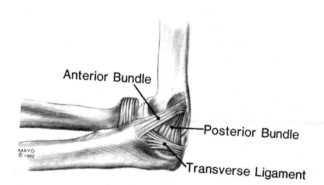

FIG. 18.1. Medial collateral ligament. Usual orientation of the ligament bundles. The transverse ligament contributes little to elbow stability. (From Morrey B, ed. *The elbow and its disorders.* Philadelphia: W.B. Saunders, 1993;566, with permission.)

its groove with elbow flexion and reduces posteriorly into its groove with elbow extension.

Posterior tennis elbow (triceps tendinosis) leads to tenderness of the insertion of the triceps tendon onto the olecranon process. The elbow should be gently flexed to deliver the olecranon from its fossa and relax the triceps muscle. This allows palpation of the olecranon, which is now covered only by the insertion of the triceps aponeurosis, its bursa, and skin (27). A gap in the substance of the tendon itself suggests frank rupture.

In patients with chronic hyperextension overload, such as throwing athletes, an exostosis may be palpable at the olecranon tip. In the presence of chronic valgus laxity, the medial margin of the olecranon may impinge on the medial wall of the olecranon fossa, often generating osteophytes. These osteophytes are a common source of loose body formation in professional throwing athletes (6,28). This area may be tender and may limit full elbow extension. Tenderness directly over the proximal ulna may suggest a stress fracture, especially in throwers (27).

The olecranon bursa, located superficial to the olecranon tip, may be inflamed, tender, or distended with fluid. Rheumatoid nodules may occur on the extensor surface of the elbow and the subcutaneous border of the ulna. These nodules are firmer to palpation than a fluid-filled bursa.

PROVOCATIVE TESTS

Lateral Tennis Elbow

If the patient has a tendinopathy, loading the injured musculotendinous units should reproduce the patient's symptoms. Test the Extensor Carp: Radialis Brevis (ECRB; a wrist extensor) by having the patient hold the elbow extended and the forearm pronated while he or she makes a fist and extends the wrist. The patient should hold this position while the examiner applies resistance (i.e., attempts to forcibly flex the wrist). Pain at the origin of the ECRB is highly suggestive of lateral tennis elbow.

The test should be repeated with the elbow flexed 90 degrees. The ECRB crosses the elbow anterior to its axis of rotation and therefore tenses with elbow extension and relaxes with elbow flexion. The amount of pain elicited by resisted wrist extension at full elbow extension and at 90 degrees of elbow flexion should be compared. The pain will usually be worse with the elbow extended and lessened with elbow flexion. If the pain is as great or worse at 90 degrees of elbow flexion (i.e., not lessened with elbow flexion), this implies a greater extent of tendon damage or degenerative tendinosis and a poorer prognosis for the success of conservative therapy.

The Exterioc Digitorum Commands (EDC) should also be checked. With the wrist in neutral, the forearm pronated, and the elbow extended, all the fingers should be extended. The patient attempts to maintain this position as the examiner applies a downward (flexing) force to the long digit or all of the digits simultaneously. Pain at the origin of the EDC (as opposed to over the radial tunnel) is positive for tendinosis of the EDC. This test should also be performed with the elbow flexed 90 degrees and the pain elicited compared with that elicited at full elbow extension. Again, pain will usually be worse with the elbow extended. Provoked pain that is not lessened by elbow flexion implies a more advanced state of pathology and a consequently poor prognosis for resolution of symptoms with conservative therapy.

The finger extension test has been previously described as provocative for radial tunnel syndrome. This test is supposed to create pain by allegedly driving the medial edge of the ECRB or a fascial extension from this muscle against the Posterior Iterosseous Nerve (PIN) (21). However, Werner (22) found that positive middle finger extension tests were related to epicondylar tenderness (and lateral tennis elbow) rather than to PIN compression. He found no evidence to support the value of this test in the diagnosis of PIN entrapment.

We also believe that pain with resisted long digit extension more commonly represents degenerative tendinosus of the origin of the EDC. It is important to note the location of the provoked pain. Provocative testing in cases of PIN entrapment should refer pain to the radial tunnel, not the lateral epicondyle. Pain referred to or about the lateral epicondyle is consistent with lateral tennis elbow (20). The finger extension test may not reliably distinguish between these two pathological entities.

Other provocative tests have been described to reproduce the symptoms of lateral tennis elbow. Passive wrist flexion with the elbow fully extended and pronated may reproduce the symptoms of lateral tennis elbow (2,20). The "coffee cup test," described by Coonrad (11), states that pain at the origin of the ECRB while picking up a full cup of coffee (or any other fluid) is almost pathognomonic for lateral tennis elbow.

The differential diagnosis of lateral tennis elbow should include PIN entrapment (i.e., supinator or radial tunnel syndrome), osteochondrosis dissecans of the capitellum, injury to the radial head, arthritis of the elbow joint, and cervical radiculopathy. Provocative supinator testing may elicit symptoms of radial tunnel syndrome. During active supination, the proximal edge of the supinator muscle may compress the PIN (22). If the patient's symptoms are reproduced by resisted active supination from the fully pronated position with the wrist (3) and elbow (20) fully extended, compression or irritation of the PIN at the arcade of Frohse is likely. Pain on supination may also be present in lateral tennis elbow (22,29) but without tenderness over the nerve. Pain on supination therefore has to be interpreted with care, not overestimating its value as an indicator of PIN entrapment (22). The symptoms of radial tunnel syndrome may also be reproduced by full passive pronation of the forearm (20,22). Placement of a pneumatic cuff over the site of nere compression and raising its pressure above venous pressure may sometimes reproduce the patient's symptoms (30).

Weakness of the finger extensors at the metacarpophalangeal joints and weakness of the extensor pollicis longus and brevis muscles is common in radial tunnel syndrome. However, weakness of the radial wrist extensors or reduced cutaneous sensation over areas innervated by the radial nerve should suggest more proximal lesions (31). It should be noted that weakness of grip is often present in the radial tunnel syndrome, probably because pain is caused by the wrist dorsiflexion of strong power grasp (20).

Electromyogram is helpful if signs of denervation are present. However, measuring radial nerve conduction velocities across the radial tunnel is not usually helpful, due to the intermittent nature of the compression. Electrodiagnostic changes may occasionally be provoked by active supination against resistance during the study (19,21,22). Therefore, although a positive electrodiagnostic study may support the diagnosis of PIN entrapment, a normal electrodiagnostic study does not exclude the diagnosis (22).

Elbow arthritis typically leads to a diffuse pain, not localized laterally, and is typically associated with decreased motion of the elbow joint (32). If there is radiocapitellar arthritis or synovitis, passive rotation of the forearm with axial compression should reproduce the symptoms. This should not produce significant pain in patients with pure lateral epicondylitis (3). Cervical radiculopathy is associated with a painful restriction of neck motion, without localized elbow tenderness (11).

Medial Tennis Elbow

Tendinosis of the flexor–pronator mass, or medial tennis elbow, usually affects the pronator teres and flexor carpi radialis (8). These symptoms may be reproduced by resisted wrist flexion and pronation.

With the elbow flexed 90 degrees and the forearm supinated, the patient makes a fist and flexes the wrist, maintaining that position as the examiner attempts to forcibly extend the wrist. If resisted wrist flexion elicits pain at the origin of the flexor carpi radialis, this tendon is involved. This test should be repeated with the elbow fully extended and the amount of pain elicited with the elbow extended and flexed compared. In contradistinction to lateral tennis elbow, medial tennis elbow usually hurts worst with the elbow flexed.

With the elbow extended and the forearm in neutral rotation, the patient should "shake hands" with the examiner. The patient should then try to forcefully pronate his or her forearm, which the examiner resists. If resisted pronation causes pain at the origin of the pronator teres, then this tendon is also involved.

It should be noted that symptoms caused by entrapment of the median nerve between the two heads of the pronator teres (the pronator syndrome) will also be reproduced by resisted forearm pronation with the elbow extended, especially if it occurs with the wrist flexed (which relaxes the flexor digitorum superficialis). However, this much rarer condition leads to irritation of the median nerve, as opposed to medial tennis elbow, which may be associated with symptoms of ulnar nerve irritation. In addition, resisted pronation with the elbow flexed should not reproduce pain caused by the pronator syndrome because only the ulnar head of the pronator teres is tense in this position and the nerve is therefore not compressed.

Posterior Tennis Elbow

In cases of triceps tendinosis, the patient's symptoms may be reproduced by resisted elbow extension. In patients with chronic hyperextension overload, with posterior exostosis formation, full extension may be limited. These patient's symptoms should be reproduced with passive elbow hyperextension. The pain may be further accentuated by applying a valgus load while hyperextending the joint, as the osteophytes are more often on the posteromedial olecranon (26).

Radiographs

Routine anteroposterior and lateral radiographs of the elbow are recommended in evaluating a patient with elbow pain. If posterior symptoms are present, we recommend an olecranon view (the reverse axial projection) taken with the elbow fully flexed. This view demonstrates osteophytes of the olecranon process or its fossa.

All radiographs should be evaluated for the presence of fracture, dislocation, subluxation, the presence of osteochondritis dissecans, loose bodies, ossification within the elbow's ligaments, heterotopic ossification, osteophyte formation, and degenerative changes.

A calcification is often noted on the lateral epicondyle of patients with lateral tennis elbow. Although of questionable prognostic significance, we usually remove these excrescences at the time of surgery. Medial tennis elbow is usually not associated with radiographic changes. Patients with posterior tennis elbow or triceps tendinosis may have an intratendinous osseous spur present, which may cause an irritative olecranon bursitis. This spur should be removed at the time of any surgical intervention.

We do not routinely obtain magnetic resonance images of the elbow in patients with tennis elbow. We believe that physical examination is the gold standard for the diagnosis of this condition, with advanced radiologic studies adding little in regard to staging, prognosis, or the determination of treatment.

Diagnostic Injection

In cases of diagnostic dilemma, a diagnostic injection can often be helpful in determining the cause of the patient's symptoms. An intraarticular injection of lidocaine, most often through the anconeus soft spot, should relieve pain due to arthritis, osteochondrosis dissecans, or other intraarticular pathology. Lidocaine injected just deep to the origin of the ECRB should relieve pain due to tendinosis of that muscle origin. The same is true with injections just deep to the flexor–pronator mass on the medial side of the elbow. Relief of symptoms after the injection of a specific area or nerve at a potential site of entrapment helps to establish the cause of the patient's complaints.

TREATMENT

General Principles

The symptoms and response to treatment have been observed to correlate with the stages of pathology. In the setting of acute tendon strain, leading to reversible inflammation without the presence of angiofibroblastic tendinosis, the symptoms are minimal (minor aching after heavy activity) and respond quickly to simple anti-inflammatory measures combined with avoidance of overuse (1).

Once angiofibroblastic invasion begins, the pathologic process is probably irreversible, but the clinical symptoms and response to treatment varies depending on the extent of involvement. Our clinical observation had been that the greater the extent of invasion, the more severe the symptoms. If less than half of the tendon is involved, the patient experiences intense activity-related pain, with only minor aching at rest. After resting, most nonstrenuous activities may be accomplished without significant discomfort. Most of these patients will respond to nonoperative therapy (1).

If greater than half of the tendon is involved with degenerative tendinosis, and especially if partial or complete rupture has occurred, significant pain will occur at rest, and activities of daily living become difficult to perform. These patients do not usually respond to nonoperative measures, and surgery is usually indicated to resolve pain (1).

In 1936 Cyriax (33) introduced an alternative possibility to structural surgery, namely a method of aggressive manipulation leading to an actual tearing of the extensor origin. He believed that it was possible for a gap left by a partial acute tear of the ECRB to be repaired by healthy granulation tissue and fibrosis. This would result in a lengthening of the tendon and a reduction of force on its insertions (33). The success of this technique has proved quite inconsistent by today's standards.

Specifics

It has been our experience that approximately 95% of patients with tennis elbow will improve with conservative therapy. Because overuse and subsequent degenerative tendinosis occurs when the repetitive forces applied to the tendon exceed its stress tolerance, there are two factors conservative therapy can address: lowering the stresses the tissue is exposed to and improving the quality of the patient's tissue by reestablishing its strength, flexibility, and endurance.

Initially, efforts may be directed toward making the patient more comfortable. This includes the standard principles of PRICEMM: protection, rest, ice, compression, elevation, medication (nonsteroidal anti-inflammatory drugs), and modalities. It is critical that the treating physician distinguish between comfort and cure. Comfort is the relief of pain but does not necessarily imply enhancement of healing or improvement in the quality of the patient's tissue. Rest and medication may result in temporary comfort, but at the expense of further deconditioning and further delay of the rehabilitative process.

Rest should be understood as the absence from abuse, not as absence from activity. Only activities that aggravate the condition should be eliminated. This does not necessarily mean abstaining from work or play if the injured tissue can be protected through a reduction in playing time or intensity. Grasping or lifting with the forearm pronated (palms down) should be avoided (2,11), and the patient should be shown how to lift with the forearm supinated (3).

Anti-inflammatory medication is helpful to control inflammation and exudation but does not provide a known specific stimulus for healing. Unless the injury is caught very early, during the reversible (inflammatory?) phase before substantial tendinosis has occurred, anti-inflammatory methods will not be sufficient to effect an ultimate cure. Likewise, cortisone injections and the comfort modalities of physical therapy (e.g., ultrasound and iontophoresis) do not specifically improve the quality of the tendon's collagen or bring in new vascularity to promote tissue healing. These measures must therefore be used only in the perspective of a larger treatment plan.

Occasionally, however, it is necessary to comfort the patient during the acute pain phase to allow him or her to proceed with curative rehabilitative exercises. We have found ice and high-voltage electrical stimulation to be the two most helpful modalities for relieving pain and inflammation. In addition, electrical stimulation may have some piezoelectric-like effect that promotes the healing process, although at this time there is no scientific certainty that a biologic stimulus to healing actually occurs. Clinical observation, however, suggests that electrical stimulation hastens the progress of rehabilitation. When used, the standard protocol is four to six sessions of high-voltage electrical stimulation over a 2- to 3-week period (1,8).

If pain is still preventing the patient from performing the prescribed exercise program, an injection of corticosteroid is appropriate. Although some have stated that steroid injections should be deferred until other conservative treatments have failed (11), we believe that the purpose of comfort-inducing measures such as steroid injections is to allow the patient to proceed with rehabilitative exercises in a comfortable and efficient manner.

When indicated, steroid injections should be placed deep to the ECRB, in the subtendinous space, just anterior and distal to the lateral epicondyle. Intratendinous injections should be avoided, because they may further damage the already injured tendon. Subdermal injection, superficial to the tendon, may lead to subcutaneous fat atrophy, leaving a permanent dimple, thinner skin, and a poorly padded vulnerable lateral epicondyle.

Steroids have been found to be somewhat helpful in approximately half the patients injected. Or, stated another way, the recurrence rate after steriod injection is as high as 50% (9,12). The repeated use of cortisone injections is inappropriate. There is no advantage, and considerable disadvantage, in administering more than two such injections (5,34). Repetitive injections may cause cellular death and potentially weaken the surrounding normal tissues, perhaps leading to attritional ruptures (1,2).

After injection, pain worsening in 50% of cases, sometimes for days, has been reported (35). Patients should be instructed to apply ice to the area of the injection for 15 to 20 minutes. This seems to minimize the painful reaction to the steroid injection in most patients (3). In our experience, the selection of cortisone type may also play a role in the frequency and intensity of postinjection pain. Depomedrol appears to have an increased propensity to produce a postinjection flare reaction and pain. Triamcinolone (Kenologg or Aristocort) tends to have a lower incidence of postinjection pain.

U.S. Food and Drug Administration studies using lithotripsy to treat recalcitrant tennis elbow in nonindustrial patients have recently begun. This noninvasive experimental treatment has shown promise in short-term follow-up.

In addition to activity limitation, other measures should be taken to reduce the stresses transmitted to the damaged tendon origins. Certain sports activities allow a variety of techniques to accomplish certain goals. Faulty techniques that place inordinately high stresses on the tendon origins should be identified and corrected.

In tennis, for example, poor swing mechanics concentrate increased force loads in the medial and lateral elbow. The tennis swing should come from the shoulder, with the use of proper body weight transfer. Proper form uses the large leg, trunk, and shoulder muscles to generate swing power. The elbow and wrist are used for control rather than force generation. Excessive use of the smaller forearm muscles for force generation places unnecessarily large stresses on these small relatively weak musculotendinous units, often leading to or exacerbating injury. For example, the inexperienced tennis player often hits the ball late, where there is rarely any body weight transfer, thereby increasing stresses on the forearm muscles.

Good tennis technique also includes ball impact in the racket's percussion center (the "sweet spot"), as the torsion of off-center hits increases the stresses the limb must absorb (1,10). Off-center impaction has been shown to cause increased electromyographic activity in the forearm extensors and may contribute to the formation of tennis elbow (7).

Many with lateral elbow pain during the forehand stroke and serve appear to overpronate the forearm during follow-through (36). Bernhang et al. (7) found that those with lateral elbow pain tended to strike the ball with the elbow ahead of the racket during their backhand strokes. A two-handed backhand stroke may decrease stresses in the injured forearm and may be recommended to those players with symptomatic tennis elbow who have not responded to other conservative measures.

Medial elbow pain may develop in the tennis serve or in the forehand stroke with the elbow leading the racket (36). Medial tennis elbow is also more common in quality players with a strong top spin forehand and a hard first flat serve (29,37).

Tennis should be avoided on wet or windy days, and players should avoid solid-core or wet tennis balls (38). Hitting a tennis ball traveling at 50 km/hr is equivalent to jerking up a weight of 25 kg (39). This force is considerably greater when the balls are wet and heavy or the velocity of the ball is increased (5). Players should therefore play with others who hit the ball at a velocity that is comfortable for the player's game.

Hitting against a backboard is often recommended by teaching tennis professionals as a practice tool or as an intermediate step before returning to the court after injury. However, this technique requires the elbow to function six times as fast as hitting on a court and requires the player to cope with the irregular bounces and angles associated with playing in an artificial environment, especially if the surface is uneven (e.g., brick walls). Consequently, this approach is not recommended to anyone with tennis elbow (5).

Each sport or activity requires individual analysis because the simple correction of faulty sports-specific mechanics may lower the stresses generated to levels the patient's tissues can withstand without discomfort (8). Athletic trainers, coaches, or tennis or golf pros are invaluable in this regard, and the patient should be encouraged to seek their input.

Improper equipment may impart greater forces than necessary onto the tendon origins. The racket grip has a significant effect on forces transmitted. There is some evidence that racket torque is best controlled using the largest comfortable grip size, possibly lessening the strain on the forearm muscles (5,7,40). In addition, the larger the grip that is used, the greater the dorsiflexion of the wrist and the less tension on the origin of the forearm extensor muscles (41).

The circumference of the handle should correspond to the working length of the hand. This is the distance from the proximal palmar crease to the tip of the ring digit, measured along the ring digit's radial border (Fig 18.2) (4,8). If grip size is uncertain, it is probably best to go to a larger grip to minimize excessive wrist wobble and torque and the tendency to grip too tightly (5,7,40). The smaller the grip, the tighter the player tends to hold the racket (42).

But although biomechanical and anecdotal evidence suggests that grip size is important, epidemiologic studies to date have not confirmed an association between grip size and the occurrence of tennis elbow. In fact, tennis elbow has been associated with both a large and a small grip (9,43). And although 84% of those with tennis elbow found changing to a larger grip helpful, 94% of those who changed to a smaller grip found this helpful. Kamien (9) found that any change of racket was generally helpful. He noted, and we agree, that no consistent pattern has emerged from the literature concerning any particular type of racket or circumference of grip. It might be noted, however, that the re-

search in this area is sparse. Grip size is probably just one of many contributing factors in the development of tennis elbow.

It is recommended that the size and weight of the equipment should match the available strength of the individual. If anything, it is preferable to use a device that is slightly lighter to ensure proper positioning of the equipment at the time of impact (1). Although epidemiologic studies have not related the incidence of tennis elbow to the type, material, or weight of the racket (9,43), a clinical observation is that a midsized (90 to 100 square inches of hitting zone) graphite composite light-weight racket offers the best protection. Good quality synthetic string at the manufacturer's low-range recommendation for string tension seems to work best (8). Looser stringing increases the dwell time of the ball on the racket, thus decreasing the shock that must be absorbed by the arm (44). Strings of smaller gauge have more "give" than thicker ones, so a player with tennis elbow may be advised not to use a string any thicker than 1.3 mm (5).

Oversized rackets have positives and negatives. Although they tend to absorb vibrations better because of their larger geometric center of percussion (sweet spot) (44), they have a greater potential for producing torque with off-center hits, and the greatest frequency and amplitude of vibrations was found in oversized rackets when the ball impacted more than 8 cm from the racket's center and especially when it struck the frame (45). Stated again, oversized rackets reduce stresses as long as the ball is struck in the racket's center. Once the ball is struck off-center, stresses are increased as compared with regular-sized rackets. Although increased torque appears to have biomechanical significance, there is little evidence that racket vibration is a cause of tennis elbow. Vibration per se may only be an aggravating factor once a player has already acquired tennis elbow (5).

Counterforce bracing has also been found to reduce the transmission of externally applied forces to the vulnerable tendon origins. It has been shown to alleviate elbow pain in 75% to 89% of players (5,9,10,43). Although the biomechanical mechanisms of this action have yet to be definitively proven, it has been theorized that counterforce bracing reduces stress in three ways.

First, the major mechanism of the brace's action is to prevent full muscular expansion, thereby not allowing a maximal contraction. This decreases intrinsic muscular forces to the muscle's injured tendinous origin. Counterforce bracing has been shown to decrease elbow angular acceleration and decrease electromyographic activity of the forearm muscles in players of all skill levels for both the serve and the one-handed backhand, without a concomitant decrease in strength output. In fact, probably due to decreased pain, counterforce bracing leads to increased grip and wrist extensor strength in symp-

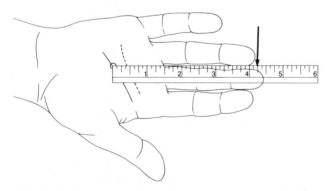

FIG. 18.2. Nirschl technique: hand size measurement. Anthropometric measurement from proximal palmar crease to tip of ring finger between long and ring finger. Measurement reflects basic working length of the hand and is especially helpful in determining implement handle size such as tennis racket.

tomatic patients (5,8,46–48). The magnitude of increase in wrist extension strength is approximately twice that seen for grip strength (48).

Second, counterforce bracing has also been demonstrated to increase wrist extensor and grip strength in asymptomatic individual (47). Stonecipher and Catlin (47) theorized that this may be due to a second mechanism of action. Deep pressure on a muscle belly may facilitate muscular contraction by activating primary afferents from the pacinian corpuscles (49). In addition, muscles are excited when the skin over the muscle is stimulated (50). The strap provides sensory stimulation to the skin overlying the extensors, possibly causing facilitation of the muscles (47).

Third, counterforce bracing may "broaden" the area of the muscle origin. Some of the forces get absorbed by the brace or by less sensitive tissues before they are transmitted proximally to the injured tissues. By acting as a secondary muscular origin, the brace effectively disseminates the concentration of forces over a wider area. It should be noted that effective counterforce bracing does not alter agonist–antagonist muscle balance, nor does it restrict joint range of motion (10,47,51). In addition, the brace probably reminds the patient that they have an elbow problem and that due caution is indicated (9).

It has been our clinical observation that counterforce brace design is more effective if the brace is wide and curvilinear (i.e., has a longer side proximally and a shorter side distally) to conform to the conical contour of the forearm. In addition, the use of two straps allows tension control over the entire width of the brace (Fig. 18.3) medial tennis elbow, an additional support just

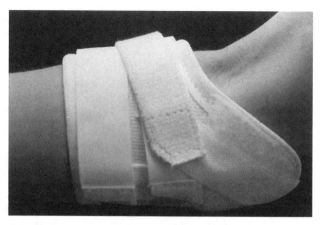

FIG. 18.4. Medial elbow counterforce brace. The same principles as noted concerning the lateral counterforce apply to the medial. It has been clinically noted that a third strap extending to the common flexor origin offers more comfort and support for medial elbow tendinosis.

distal to the medial epicondyle, over the proximal origin of the pronator teres, adds to the brace's effectiveness (1) (Fig 18.4).

Counterforce bracing controls pain, enabling the patient to better initiate each phase of the exercise program and return to sport. In most cases, a properly designed brace should be used during rehabilitative exercise, in stressful daily activities, and upon return to sport. It is usually not necessary at rest or with light activities of daily living (38).

The effect of counterforce bracing on patients with radial tunnel syndrome is, at present, unclear. Occasionally, however, bracing may exacerbate underlying ulnar neuropathy. This should be watched for, and the brace modified or discontinued if this occurs.

Wrist splints are ineffective, except in the very early acute inflammatory phase. Rigid types of immobilization, such as casting, may relieve pain but at the price of atrophy, immobility, and further deconditioning and are not recommended (1).

Although stress minimization is important, the mainstay of treatment is the improvement of the quality of the injured tissues through rehabilitative exercise. Restoration of strength, flexibility, and endurance to the appropriate musculotendinous units is necessary to allow them to safely absorb the forces imposed on them by an individual patient's life-style.

It is interesting to note that in world class tennis players, adequate power and endurance are present but flexibility is often lacking. Their exercise program should therefore be directed toward flexibility. Conversely, the average patient's muscle mass and endurance are often inadequate, and their exercise program should be designed to enhance these factors (10).

An orderly progression of graduated strength and

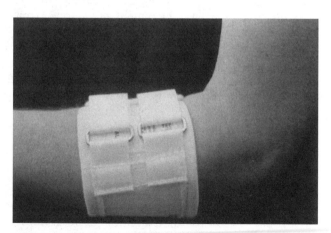

FIG. 18.3. Lateral elbow counterforce brace. The concept of counterforce bracing is to diffuse internally generated forces away from the sensitive areas of tendinosis. Wide even compression has been noted to be clinically most effective. The illustrated brace is curvilinear to best accommodate to the conical shape of the forearm and provides dual tension straps for complete counterforce control across the entire width of the brace.

endurance exercise is begun as soon as pain and inflammation have been controlled by a short rest phase and appropriate medication, as needed. The patient should be protected early with the use of an appropriate counterforce brace while performing exercises and other stressful activities. Use of the brace may be eliminated later in the program, as tolerated.

Before exercises are performed, the patient should warm up to raise body temperature a few degrees. This increases the compliance and elasticity of the body's tissues and reduces the risk of exercise-induced injury. Warm-ups should result in breaking a light sweat. This can be accomplished by 3 to 5 minutes of brisk walking, cycling, or jogging. Alternatively, the forearm may be heated with a heating pad or a hot shower.

The six key forearm exercises are wrist extension, wrist flexion, forearm pronation, forearm supination, wrist radial deviation, and wrist ulnar deviation. Each exercise should be performed at its own rate and stress tolerance; higher weights will be achieved more rapidly on some exercises than others. Each exercise should be performed slowly, with attention to proper form. The patient should be instructed not to work through pain. If pain occurs, the resistance should be decreased and the counterforce brace worn. The elbow should be flexed 90 degrees to minimize tension at the muscle origins. The forearm should be well supported on the thigh or a table.

Our program (52) begins performance of all six exercises without any weight. Using only a clenched fist, the patient performs one set of 10 to 15 repetitions of each exercise. Exercises are performed only once a day. More is not better and may exacerbate symptoms. Repetitions should be increased every few days as pain allows, until the patient is comfortably doing three sets of 10 repetitions for 2 consecutive days without increasing symptoms.

Weights are then increased in 1-pound increments. Starting with a small can of soup is a good way to begin, which may then be progressed to heavier dumbbells. Repetitions should be decreased to one set of 10 to 15 repetitions for each exercise whenever weight is added, slowly working up to three sets of 10 repetitions each for each exercise. For forearm rotation, the dumbbell is grasped on its end.

This is continued until the patient is comfortably using a 3-pound dumbbell for three sets of 10 repetitions each. When 3 pounds are reached, Isoflex or other tension tubing of graduated resistances are used on alternate days. We currently prefer this latter technique, alternating it with isotonic dumbbell exercises as rehabilitative success is enhanced.

To advance the program, the elbow is gradually straightened from 90 degrees while the forearm is still supported. Depending on symptoms, the weight may initially need to be decreased by 1 to 2 pounds and progressed until the patient is again using 3 pounds for three sets of 10 each day.

The patient should then perform the exercises with the arm straight in front of the body, the elbow straight but not locked. Again, the weight may need to be decreased and readvanced, depending on symptoms. When comfortable, the exercise frequency should be decreased to every other day to allow the muscles a day of rest to heal and prevent reinjury. The patient will then find a point where they no longer need to progress the weights and can continue with a maintenance program two to three times a week. It is important to continue the strengthening program as return to sports occurs; otherwise, the patient risks reinjury or the return of symptoms.

In addition, ball-squeezing exercises should be performed. These should be started with the elbow bent at the side and progressed as above until they are performed with the arm straight out in front. These exercises may be performed intermittently at the patient's convenience, in the car, at a desk, or while watching television. Again, these exercises should not be overdone, as overuse may cause increased pain.

If pain occurs during any exercise, the counterforce brace should be worn and the offending exercise should be modified with regards to the amount of weight used, the number of repetitions performed, or by limiting the motion performed to only the pain-free arc. If even the modified exercise is painful, the patient should stop, rest 1 to 2 days, and try again with less weight and less repetitions.

A slow steady progression has been found to be critical to the healing process. Results take time, frequently 2 to 6 months before the symptoms fully disappear. It is important to continue the exercise program and avoid painful activities, even if the patient's symptoms significantly decrease before that time (52).

Along with forearm exercises, the patient should perform elbow flexion and extension exercises and shoulder exercises. Rotator cuff tendinosis is often associated with tennis elbow. It may be frankly symptomatic, or subclinical, with signs of it elicited only on physical examination. By exercising the shoulder simultaneously with the forearm, future injuries that would be due to weakening or deconditioning may be minimized or avoided. The patient should perform rotator cuff and general shoulder strengthening exercises such as shoulder internal rotation, external rotation, forward flexion, abduction, and extension. In addition, exercises for the scapular protractors, retractors, and elevators, such as shrugs, rows, pull-downs, modified push-ups (push-up plus), and seated dips should be performed. After exercising, the patient should ice the forearm and any other sore areas for 15 to 20 minutes.

After the patient has regained near-normal strength, flexibility, and endurance, plyometrics and sport-specific activities should begin. The strength-training program should continue to even higher conditioning levels than the preinjury state. This is important, because a return to only the preinjury level still offers the potential for further force overload and reinjury. Before a final return to a sport or occupational activity, the patient should be capable of anaerobic sprint repetitions to fatigue without major activity pain (1).

Return to play should begin gradually, starting with the less stressful sport-specific activities (forehand groundstokes and volleys in the case of tennis), for short periods, interrupted by significant periods of rest. The counterforce brace should be worn. Activity may be advanced slowly, as tolerated.

In our experience, approximately 95% of patients with tennis elbow will be satisfied with the results of conservative management. That leaves about 5% of patients with tennis elbow with the choice of accepting their pain and disability, lowering their activity level to the point where their pain is tolerable, or seeking a surgical solution.

Surgery

Because tennis elbow is a quality of life issue, its operative treatment should be considered elective surgery, with the patient making the decision based on the degree of symptoms experienced, the degree of tolerable symptoms, and activity level or life-style. Usually, constant pain that interferes with activities of daily living or occurs at rest suggests the need for surgery (1).

Depending on circumstances, surgery is usually offered to patients with symptoms of long-standing duration (over 1 year), after failed conservative treatment, including at least 6 months of a concerted exercise program, temporary activity limitation, and appropriate counterforce bracing (8,11).

The principles of surgery are identification of the symptom-producing pathology, resection of the pathologic symptom-causing tissue, maintenance of normal tissues and their attachments, and quality postoperative rehabilitation (8).

Historically, surgical release, or a slide, of the extensor aponeurosis often combined with release of the orbicular ligament has been advocated (53,54). With release of the extensor aponeurosis and the orbicular ligament, the origin of the ECRB was undoubtedly released or altered as well. Garden advocated lengthening of the ECRB tendon in the distal forearm to reduce transmitted forces. All these releases have high incidences of complications, such as injury to the lateral ligament complex (occasionally even leading to posterolateral rotational elbow instability), weakness, and persistent pain. None are currently recommended (1).

Our technique involves identification and excision of any tissue involved with tendinosis. In lateral tennis elbow, the tissues involved most commonly are most, if not all, of the origin of the ECRB (100%), the anterior edge of the EDC (35%), and occasionally the underside of the Extensor Carpi Radialis Longus (ECRL). Radiographic exostosis of the lateral epicondyle occurs in 20% but has no significance regarding indications for tendon surgery (8,10). However, if prominent or tender to palpation, removal of the exostosis is recommended at the time of surgery. The surgeon should also be aware that its excision adds to the patient's postoperative pain and morbidity, because residual postoperative soreness may be extended for 1 to 2 months.

Because of the extensive origin of the ECRB (from the distal lateral humeral supracondylar ridge, the anterior ridge of the lateral epicondyle, the underside of the anterior edge of the extensor aponeurosis distal to the lateral epicondyle, the undersurface of the ECRL, the distal extensor aponeurosis, and the annular ligament), the tendon does not retract even when most of its origin is excised. It is therefore not necessary to reattach the tendon to bone. Doing so only risks the creation of a flexion contracture. Care is taken to spare the origin of the other tendons and the extensor aponeurosis. The anteromedial aspect of the lateral condyle is debrided of all tendinosis tissue and then drilled to improve the biologic environment and stimulate healing and scar formation. The normal tissues are then anatomically repaired.

Intraarticular synovitis and effusion are usually stress induced and are commonly associated with chronic and long-standing tennis elbow (11). These usually resolve after excision of the pathologic tendinosis tissue. It is unnecessary to address the joint intraarticularly in most cases.

Results of the Nirschl (1) technique of lateral tennis elbow surgery (over 750 cases) are as follows: 85% of patients experienced complete pain relief, full strength, and full return to all prior activities without pain, and 12% experienced significant pain relief and return of strength but not total normalcy. This improvement was usually enough to allow return to vigorous sports, with some pain during aggressive activities. There was a 3% failure rate, with no improvement in pain or return of strength. No patient has been observed to have had an increase in symptoms over the preoperative situation. Reasons for failure are not always clear, but possibilities include concomitant PIN entrapment and nonorganic factors. Complications have been minimal: 1% superficial infection and 1% mild (less than 5 degrees) loss of extension (1,8,22).

It might be noted that the results of tendon slide techniques are less predictable. Our observations of failure with these techniques invariably include failure to address the pathoanatomy and varying forms of iatrogenic surgical harm, including the creation of posterolateral rotatory instability.

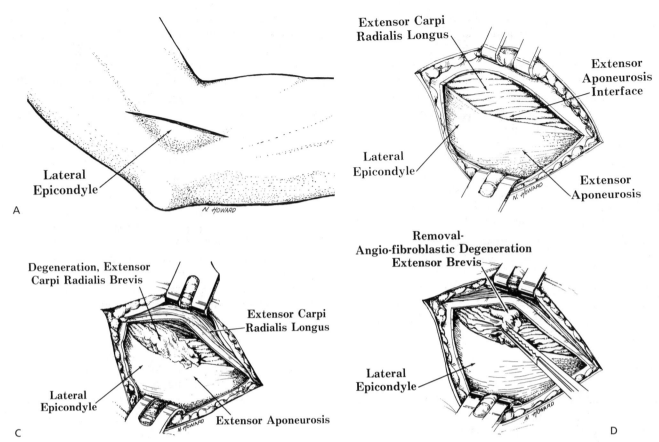

FIG. 18.5. Lateral elbow tendinosis surgery: Nirschl technique. The concept of this surgical technique is to remove all painful tendinosis tissue rather than release techniques that weaken the force generator. All normal tendon attachments are left intact. It is incumbent upon the surgeon to understand the anatomy of all tendon origins and to recognize abnormal vs. normal tendon tissue. **A:** Surgical incision. Approximately 2 inches just in length anteromedial to lateral epicondyle extending 1 inch proximal to the epicondyle to the anterolateral joint line. **B:** Exposure of extensor carpi radialis longus (ECRL) interface. The interface between the ECRL and extensor aponeurosis (extensor digitorum communis [EDC] tendon) is identified. The ECRL is soft, whereas the aponeurosis is thicker and more firm. The extensor brevis is not seen as it lies beneath the ECRL. **C:** Exposure of extensor carpi radialis brevis (ECRB). The ECRL–aponeurosis interface is incised and the ECRL is retracted anteromedially, exposing the origin of the ECRB. Note the ECRL is only 2 mm deep at this level and the dissection is primarily medial. The ECRB is distinguished 15 degrees posterolaterally. If the diagnosis is correct, the ECRB will have the characteristic gray friable tendinosis appearance. **D:** Excision of ECRB tendinosis. All tendinosis tissue is removed. This usually encompasses most of the ECRB origin. In 35% of cases, the anteromedial edge (approximately 20% of the edge) of the EDC aponeurosis can be expected to have tendinosis changes as well.

Resection and Repair of Lateral Tennis Elbow

For this technique (Fig. 18.5), the patient is positioned supine, with the arm on an arm board. A bolster or three towels are placed under to the elbow to internally rotate the shoulder and better position the elbow.

1. A straight lateral incision is made, passing just anterior to the lateral epicondyle, from 1 inch proximal to the lateral epicondyle to the level of the joint line. The incision is centered at the level of the lateral epicondyle. Care is taken not to place it too distally (a common error). It is angled approximately 30 degrees anteromedially to the axis of the humerus (A).

2. The interface between the ECRL and the extensor aponeurosis is identified and incised (B). The ECRL tendon is palpably softer and the combined origin of the extensor aponeurosis palpably firmer tissue. The interface is approximately 3 mm posterior to the posterior border of the muscle of the ECRL. The goal is to lift the ECRL off the ECRB without harming the ECRB origin. The depth of the cut should be only 2 to 3 mm (the ECRL is thin). Do not cut too deeply, because this distorts the proximal origin of the ECRB and makes it difficult to identify. Scalpel dissection proceeds horizontally (coronally) with elevation of the thin muscle of the ECRL. Retract it

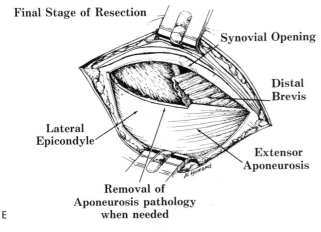

Final Stage of Resection

Synovial Opening

Distal Brevis

Lateral Epicondyle

Extensor Aponeurosis

Removal of Aponeurosis pathology when needed

E

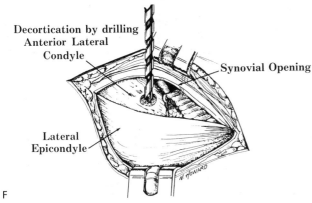

Decortication by drilling Anterior Lateral Condyle

Synovial Opening

Lateral Epicondyle

F

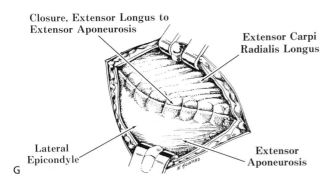

Closure, Extensor Longus to Extensor Aponeurosis

Extensor Carpi Radialis Longus

Lateral Epicondyle

Extensor Aponeurosis

G

FIG. 18.5.—*Continued* **E:** Final stage of resection. The goal of this technique is to remove pathologic tendinosis tissue. The ECRB rarely retracts as attachment points are maintained at the distal EDC aponeurosis, annular ligament, and underside of the ECRL. This illustration also depicts some resection of the anteromedial edge of the EDC aponeurosis. Under no circumstance is the aponeurosis totally released from the epicondyle because it is unnecessary and often harmful. In 20% of the Nirschl series, a bony exostosis has been noted, and if this is present, only the exostasis is removed. If this occurs, the posterior 50% of aponeurosis is left intact and the interface between the aponeurosis and ECRL is thereafter repaired in usual manner. In those instances where an intraarticular problem is suspected, a small synovial opening is made to inspect the anterolateral joint compartment. In the Nirschl series, approximately 5% of cases will demonstrate synovitis or chondromalacia. **F:** Vascular enhancement by drilling. Two to three drill holes are made through the cortical bone of the triangular recess of the lateral condyle to enhance vascular supply. The defect left by resection of the tendinosis tissue is filled in with healthy fibrotendon in the healing process. **G:** Closure of the interface. Firm closure of the ECRL to the EDC aponeurosis. Note the aponeurosis has not been disturbed from its normal attachment to the epicondyle.

anteromedially to bring the ECRB into view. The EDC (firm diagonally oriented tissue posteriorly) is untouched (C).

3. The pathologic tissue (grayish edematous tendon) often encompasses the entire origin of the ECRB to the level of the joint line. All unhealthy tendinosus tissue is excised in elliptical triangular fashion. Tendinosis is identified as degenerative, edematous, and dull tissue. Normal tendon is bright and shiny. Any questionable tissue is challenged with the "scratch test": The broad blade of the scalpel is used to scrape the tissue in question. Healthy tissue will remain firmly behind, whereas unhealthy tendinosis tissue will scratch off. This is analogous to peeling paint, where the bad paint easily scrapes off, whereas the

good paint is left behind. The bone is also scraped to be sure no tendinosis is left (D).

In 35% of cases, changes are present in the anterior underside of the extensor aponeurosis, and this area is also removed; it is unusual to have greater than 20% of its area involved. Calcific exostosis of the lateral epicondyle is present in 20%; if present, the anterior aspect of the extensor aponeurosis is partially peeled off the lateral epicondyle and the exostosis is removed with a rongeur (warn patient that this adds to postoperative pain).

4. If intraarticular pathology is suspected, a small longitudinal opening is made in the synovium anterior to the Radial Collateral Ligament (RCL) by cutting along the lateral supracondylar ridge and the lateral

compartment is inspected (E). In the standard lateral tennis elbow case, it is rare to have intraarticular pathology, and arthrotomy is not routinely performed unless clearcut intraarticular signs are noted preoperatively.

If a small rent is inadvertently made in the elbow joint's synovium, an opportunity to inspect the joint occurs. Flex the elbow to 90 degrees; if more than a drop or two of synovial fluid is expressed through this opening, examine the joint further by incising the synovium in line with the incision.

5. Two to three drill holes are placed through the exposed cortical bone of the anterior lateral condyle to cancellous depth to enhance the vascular supply (F). Because the distal attachments of the ECRB are intact and a firm attachment of the extensor aponeurosis has been maintained at all times, minimal retraction takes place. It is, therefore, unnecessary to suture the remaining ECRB to obtain proper mechanical length.

6. If an arthrotomy was made, synovial repair is performed. (Our preference is with a running 3-0 plain suture.) Firmly repair the ECRL to the anterior margin of the extensor aponeurosis with a running suture (our preference is a no. 1 PDS Structure) (G). Take care to bury the knots. The tissue quality is better in the middle of the incision; this is where the initial anchoring knot should be placed. The suture may then be run proximal then distal. Close subcutaneous tissue and then skin.

Postoperatively, splint with an elbow immobilizer at 90 degrees up to 6 days on an intermittent basis (Fig. 18.6). The patient may begin full active range of motion

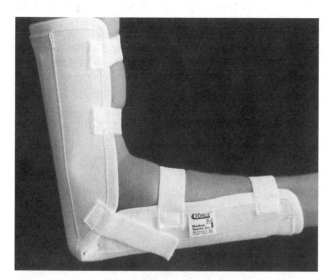

FIG. 18.6. Elbow immobilizer. An immobilizer with velcro straps is used in the immediate postoperative time period. The immobilizer is lighter, more comfortable, and more easily adaptable to wound care than a plaster splint. (Courtesy of Medical Sports, Inc., Arlington, Virginia.)

on postoperative day 3. Strength and endurance resistance exercises may be begun at 3 weeks until full strength returns (usually 4.5 months for lateral and posterior elbow resection and repairs and 5.5 months for medial resection and repairs). Light sport activities may be begun at 6 weeks postoperatively, with gradual progression. Full racket and throwing sports should be considered only after full strength returns.

Resection and Repair of Medial Tennis Elbow

The results of surgery for medial tennis elbow are less predictable than those for lateral tennis elbow. However, in a study of 50 cases of medial tennis elbow resection and repair, all patients reported significant if not complete pain relief postoperatively, and all patients had objective improvements in strength. No major complications occurred (1,15).

Medial Collateral Ligament (MCL) instability and/or ulnar nerve dysfunction may coexist with medial elbow tendinosis, and a careful preoperative evaluation should be performed to diagnose these, because their presence may modify the surgical technique. MCL instability may be addressed with MCL reconstruction using a free palmaris longus tendon graft.

Twenty-four percent to 60% of patients undergoing surgery for medial tennis elbow have some signs or symptoms of ulnar nerve irritation, usually localized to zone 3 (13,15). In addition, stretch neurapraxia of the ulnar nerve may occur in the presence of valgus laxity (1). These entities should be sought out and addressed separately.

Significant ulnar nerve compression may be addressed with an *in situ* decompression. Concomitant ulnar nerve symptoms often resolve with the elimination of the medial elbow tendinosis, which may irritate the nerve. Even in the absence of ulnar nerve symptoms, a decompression of zone 3 (for a few centimeters distal to the cubital tunnel, at the entrance of the nerve between the two heads of the Flexor Carpi Ulnaris) (FCU) should be undertaken. Failure to perform this decompression may lead to ulnar nerve compression as the flexor–pronator mass is narrowed by closing the defect left after the pathologic tissue is excised.

Indications for ulnar nerve transfer are ulnar nerve subluxation or dislocation; abnormally skeletal valgus; dynamic valgus (MCL) instability, if reconstruction is not performed; an unresolvable hostile environment in or about the cubital tunnel; and the necessity of exposing the medial elbow compartment, precluding maintenance of anatomic ulnar nerve position.

For this technique (Fig. 18.7), immediately preoperatively, mark out the patient's area of maximal tenderness in indelible marker. This locates the area of pathologic change.

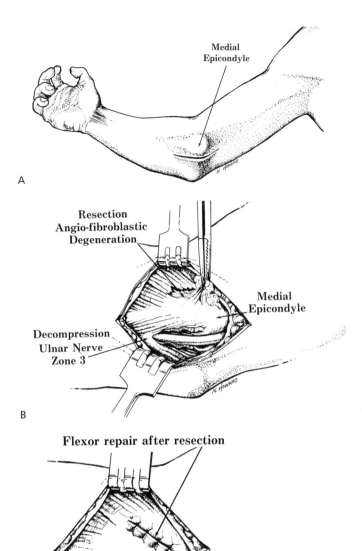

A

**Resection
Angio-fibroblastic
Degeneration**

**Medial
Epicondyle**

**Decompression
Ulnar Nerve
Zone 3**

B

Flexor repair after resection

C

FIG. 18.7. Medial elbow tendinosis surgery: Nirschl technique. The principles of medial elbow surgery are the same as the lateral elbow technique. The goal is resection of painful tendinosis tissue rather than release of the common flexor origin, which weakens. All tendon incisions are longitudinal with the excisions being longitudinal and elliptical. All normal tendon is left in normal anatomic attachment position. **A:** Medial elbow incision. The medial incision is approximately 2.5 inches in length posterior to the medial epicondyle extending from 0.5 inch proximal to the epicondyle distally. Posterior incision placement avoids interruption of the medial antebracheal cutaneous nerves, which can result in a painful neuroma or paresthesias. **B:** Excision of angiofibroblastic tendinosis. In most cases the painful tendinosis is at the interface between the pronator teres and flexor carpi radialis. The abnormal tissue may lie slightly below the surface but is identified by its grayish friable appearance. All pathologic tissue is excised longitudinally. All normal tendon attachments are not disturbed. Release of normal tissue is unnecessary and often harmful. In 40% of the Nirschl series, ulnar nerve neuropraxia has been noted. It is recommended that a decompression of the zone 3 region of the cubital tunnel be undertaken in the circumstance. **C:** Repair after resection. After elliptical resection of tendinosis tissue, the repair is completed by use of a running stitch. Note: If greater than 1 cm of elliptical excision occurs, tendon closure may tighten the cubital tunnel. Under these circumstances decompression of the cubital tunnel is recommended.

1. A 3-inch incision is made over the cubital tunnel, from 1 inch proximal to the medial epicondyle, posterior to the medial epicondyle, extending distally (A).
2. Exposure of the common flexor origin is accomplished by retraction of the skin and subcutaneous tissue anterolaterally over the medial epicondyle. Avoid branches of the medial antebrachial cutaneous nerve just distal and anterior to the epicondyle.
3. Make a longitudinal incision in the tendon origins at the area of maximal tenderness (which was marked out preoperatively), from the medial epicondyle distally for approximately 2 inches. Bluntly spread the

tendons. If the indications are correct, the lesion will come into view.

The area of pathologic tendinosis is usually found at the interface of the pronator teres and the flexor carpi radialis, close to the medial epicondyle (56%), but tendinosis has also been noted at the midcommon flexor origin (32%), in the palmaris longus, occasionally in the flexor carpi ulnaris (12%), and rarely on the underside of the flexor sublimis origin (1,15).

4. Elliptically excise all pathologic tissue (B). Resection may be carried deeply all the way to the joint, but this is rarely necessary. Do not injure the joint capsule or the MCL. All normal tissue attachments to the

medial epicondyle are left intact to avoid destabilizing the elbow.

5. Two to three drill holes (approximately 2 mm diameter) are made in the epicondyle to enhance vascular channels to the resection area. Avoid drilling the subcutaneous bone, because this leads to postoperative tenderness.
6. Close the elliptical dead space with running suture (our preference is no. 1 PDS).
7. Sixty percent of cases of (C) tennis elbow will have ulnar nerve symptoms, usually caused by zone 3 compression. Releasing the Flexor Carpi Ulnaris is usually enough to alleviate these symptoms, and ulnar nerve transfer is usually not indicated. If nerve transfer indications are present, however, our preference is subcutaneous transfer.

   Please note that it is our recommendation that the superficial fascia of the Flexor Carpi Ulnaris (zone 3 of the cubital tunnel) is released even without ulnar nerve symptoms to avoid iatrogenically creating cubital tunnel compression when the common flexor origin tightens when closed after tendinosis excision.
8. Close subcutaneous tissue and skin.

Postoperative recommendations are the same as those for the lateral procedure.

Resection and Repair of Posterior Tennis Elbow (Triceps Tendinosis)

Triceps tendinosis is commonly seen in cases of repetitive overuse of aggressive elbow extension, as occurs in pitching, football line play, track and field events (shot put, javelin throw), bowling, and heavy weight lifting. Triceps tendinosis is uncommon as an isolated entity and usually occurs in combination with other posterior pathology (olecranon osteophytes, posterior ulnotrochlear chondromalacia, etc.). These should be addressed as well, either by arthrotomy or arthroscopy. Triceps tendinosis may also be encountered in association with lateral and/or medial tennis elbow. All symptomatic pathologies are addressed at the same surgical sitting (8).

1. A longitudinal incision is made just lateral to the midline over the tricep's insertion.
2. The triceps is incised, its fibers spread, and the pathologic tissue identified.
3. Elliptically excise all pathologic tissue, including any intratendinous bony spurs, as in the medial tennis elbow resection and repair procedure. If olecranon fossa pathology is present, exposure and treatment is performed at this time.
4. Close the triceps with a running suture (our preference is no. 1 PDS), and then close the subcutaneous tissue and skin closure.

Postoperative recommendations are the same as for the lateral procedure.

SUMMARY

The understanding of all teninopathies, both for upper and lower extremities, has been widely enhanced by recent histopathologic, ummunohistologic, and electromicroscopy studies of tendon overuse abnormality. The clear evidence that degenerative rather than inflammatory failure is the core issue supports the alteration of terminology from the misnomer tendinitis to the more proper term tendinosis.

The basic concepts of the prevention and treatment of tendinosis include an enhancement and revitalization of this abnormal tissue by rehabilitative exercise. If revitalization fails, surgical excision of the tendinosis tissue is the best and most effective surgical approach. Comfort supplied by rest and medication, including cortisone injection, should not be misinterpreted as a biologic healing response. Adjunctive treatment concepts include a control of abusive overuse by equipment changes and counterforce bracing.

REFERENCES

1. Nirschl RP. Sports—and overuse injuries to the elbow. In: Morrey BF, ed. *The elbow and its disorders*, 2nd ed. Philadelphia: W.B. Saunders, 1993:537–552.
2. Burgess RC. Tennis elbow. *J Kentucky Med Assoc* 1990;88: 349–354.
3. Gellman H. Tennis elbow (lateral epicondylitis). *Orthop Clin North Am* 1992;23:75–82.
4. Nirschl RP. Tennis elbow. *Orthop Clin North Am* 1973;4:787.
5. Kamien M. A rational management of tennis elbow. *J Sports Med* 1990;9:173–191.
6. Jobe FW, Nuber G. Throwing injuries of the elbow. *Clin Sports Med* 1986;5:621–636.
7. Bernhang AM, Dehner W, Fogarty C. Tennis elbow: a biomechanical approach. *J Sports Med* 1974;2:235–260.
8. Nirschl RP. Elbow tendinosis/tennis elbow. Tendinitis II. Clinical considerations. *Clin Sports Med* 1992;11:851–870.
9. Kamien M. Tennis elbow in long-time tennis players. *Austr J Sci Med Sport* 1988;20:19–27.
10. Nirschl RP. The etiology and treatment of tennis elbow. *Am J Sports Med* 1974;2:308–319.
11. Coonrad RW. Tennis elbow. *Instr Course Lect* 1986;35:94–101.
12. Coonrad RW, Hooper WR. Tennis elbow: its course, natural history, conservative and surgical management. *J Bone Joint Surg Am* 1973;55A:1177–1182.
13. Nirschl RP. Medial tennis elbow, surgical treatment. *Orthop Trans Am Acad Orthop Surg* 1980;7:298.
14. Kivi P. The etiology and conservative treatment of humeral epicondylitis. *Scand J Rehabil Med* 1982;15:37–41.
15. Olliviere CO, Nirschl RP, Pettrone FA. Resection and repair for medial tennis elbow. *Am J Sports Med* 1995;23:214–221.
16. Goldie I. Epicondylitis lateralis. *Acta Chir Scand* 1964;339:77–113.
17. Kraushaar BS, Nirschl RP. Tendinosis of the elbow. Clinical features and findings of histological, immunohistochemical and electron microscopy studies. *J Bone Joint Surg Am* 1999;81A:259–278.
18. Nirschl RP. Mesenchymal syndrome. *VA Med Month* 1969;96:659.
19. Eversmann WW Jr. Entrapment and compression neuropathies. In: Green DP, ed. *Operative hand surgery*. New York: Churchill Livingstone, 1993:1341–1385.
20. Lister GD, Belsole RB, Kleinert HE. The radial tunnel syndrome. *J Hand Surg* 1979;4:52–59.

21. Lister G. *The hand,* 3rd ed. New York: Churchill Livingstone, 1993.
22. Werner C. Lateral elbow pain and posterior interosseous nerve entrapment. *Acta Orthop Scand* 1979;50(suppl):174.
23. Hotchkiss RN, Green DP. Fractures and dislocations of the elbow. In: Rockwood CA, Green DP, eds. *Fractures in adults.* Philadelphia: J.B. Lippincott, 1991;739–841.
24. Hoppenfeld S. *Physical examination of the spine and extremities.* Norwalk, CT: Appleton-Centure-Crofts, 1976.
25. Spinner RJ, Goldner RD. Snapping of the medial head of the triceps and recurrent dislocation of the ulnar nerve: anatomical and dynamic factors. *J Bone Joint Surg Am* 1998;80A:239–247.
26. Regan WD, Morrey BF. The physical examination of the elbow. In: Morrey BF, ed. *The elbow and its disorders,* 2nd ed. Philadelphia: W.B. Saunders, 1993;73–85.
27. Andrews JR, Wilk KE, Satterwhite YE, et al. Physical examination of the thrower's elbow. *J Sports Phys Ther* 1993;17:296–304.
28. Tullos JS, Schwab G, Benett JB, et al. Factors influencing elbow instability. *Instr Course Lect* 1981;30:185.
29. Priest JD. Tennis elbow: the syndrome and a study of average players. Minn Med 1976;59:367–371.
30. Roles NC, Maudsley RH. Radial tunnel syndrome. Resistant tennis elbow as a nerve entrapment. *J Bone Joint Surg Br* 1972; 54B:499–508.
31. Kaplan PE. Posterior interosseus neuropathies: natural history. *Arch Phys Med Rehabil* 1984;65:399–400.
32. Morrey BF. Elbow reconstructive surgery. In: Chapman MW, ed. *Operative orthopaedics.* New York: J.B. Lippincott, 1988.
33. Cyriax J. *Textbook of orthopaedic medicine,* 10th ed. Vol. 2. London: Bailliere Tindall, 1980:192.
34. Calvert PT, Allum RL, Macpherson IS, et al. Simple lateral release in treatment of tennis elbow. *J R Soc Med* 1985;78:912–915.
35. Price R, Sinclair H, Heinrich I, et al. Local injection treatment of tennis elbow—hydrocortisone, triamcinolone, and lignocaine compared. *Br J Rheumatol* 1991;30:39–44.
36. Andrews JR, Meister K. Overuse injuries of the athlete's elbow. In: Griffen LY, ed. *Orthopaedic knowledge update 5.* Rosemont, IL: American Academy of Orthopaedic Surgeons, 1994
37. Priest JD, Jones HH, Nagel DA. Elbow injuries in highly skilled tennis players. *Am J Sports Med* 1974;2:137–149.
38. Sobel J, Nirschl RP. Elbow injuries. In: Zachazewski JE, ed. *Athletic injuries and rehabilitation.* Philadelphia: W.B. Saunders, 1996: 543–583.
39. Peterson L, Renstrom P. *Sports injuries: their prevention and treatment.* Auckland: Methuen, 1986:98, 207.
40. Adelsberg S. An EMG analysis of selected muscles with racquets of increasing grip size. *Am J Sports Med* 1986;14:139.
41. Murley R. Tennis elbow: conservative, surgical and manipulative therapy [Correspondence]. *Br Med J* 1987;294:839–840.
42. Groppel J. *Tennis for advanced players and those who would like to be.* Champaign, IL: Human Kinetics, 1984.
43. Grouchow HW, Pelletier D. An epidemiologic study of tennis elbow. *Am J Sports Med* 1979;7:234–238.
44. Brody H. *Science made practical for the tennis teacher.* Vol. VI. USAQ Professional Tennis Registry, 1985.
45. Carroll R, Al-Hassani STS, Leake SF. *Vibrational characteristics of wood, metal and graphite tennis rackets.* Centre for Physical Education, University of Manchester, 1988.
46. Groppel J, Nirschl RP. A mechanical and electromyographical analysis of various joint counterforce braces on the tennis players. *Am J Sports Med* 1986;14:195–200.
47. Stonecipher DR, Catlin PA. The effect of a forearm strap on wrist extensor strength. *J Orthop Sports Phys Ther* 1984;6:184–189.
48. Wadsworth CT, Nielsen DH, Burns LT, et al. Effect of the counterforce armband on wrist extension and grip strength and pain in subjects with tennis elbow. *J Orthop Sports Phys Ther* 1989; 11:192.
49. Gowitzke BA, Milner M. *Understanding the scientific bases of human movement,* 2nd ed. Baltimore: Williams & Wilkins, 1980.
50. Hagbarth KE. Excitatory and inhibitory skin areas for flexor and extensor motoneurons. In: Payton OD, Hirt S, Newton RA, eds. *Scientific bases for neurophysiologic approaches to therapeutic exercise.* Philadelphia: F.A. Davis, 1977:125–132.
51. Nirschl RP. Tennis elbow. *Prim Care* 1977;4:367–382.
52. Nirschl RP, Sobel S. *Arm care. Virginia Sportsmedicine Institute: Tennis/Golf Elbow Program for medial and lateral tendinosis (protocol).* Arlington, VA: Medical Sport Publishing, 1996:1–88.
53. Bosworth DH. The role of the orbicular ligament in tennis elbow. *J Bone Joint Surg Am* 1955;37A:527.
54. Michele AA, Krueger FJ. Lateral epicondylitis of the elbow treated by fasciotomy. *Surgery* 1956;39:277.

Principles and Practice of Orthopaedic Sports Medicine,
edited by William E. Garrett, Jr., Kevin P. Speer, and Donald T. Kirkendall.
Lippincott Williams & Wilkins, Philadelphia © 2000.

CHAPTER 19

Elbow Injuries

Laura A. Timmerman

EPIDEMIOLOGY

Elbow injuries occur commonly in athletes. They can be a result of an acute trauma or secondary to a repetitive microtrauma. Elbow injuries are usually seen in throwing athletes, but they also occur frequently in other sports enthusiasts, such as gymnasts and golfers. To a certain extent, the nature of the elbow disorder is somewhat age dependent. The younger skeletally immature athletes are predisposed to epiphysitis, whereas the older teenager and young adult athlete develop overuse and ligamentous injuries. The older adult athlete that has been participating in the sport for several years will often present with injuries associated with degenerative changes, such as osteophytes and tendon ruptures.

Traumatic elbow injuries occur regularly in the general population and are usually the result of either a fall on an outstretched arm or a contact injury. Elbow dislocations occur regularly in both the athletic and general population. The elbow is the most common joint to dislocate in children less than 10 years of age, and after the shoulder joint, it is the second most common joint dislocation in adults (1). The incidence of elbow dislocations in the general population has been estimated to be six dislocations per 100,000 individuals, with a mean age of 30 years (2).

Several studies have attempted to quantify the incidence of injury in the adolescent pitcher (3–7). In 1965 Adams (3) first reported that 45% of pitchers participating in Little League complained of pain about the elbow and that all of 80 players in the study had radiographic abnormalities when compared with their nonthrowing side. In 1972 Torg et al. (4) reported on a group of 13-year-old pitchers, finding that 70% of them had symp-

toms about the elbow or shoulder at some time during the season. In the widely quoted Houston study on Little League, Gugenheim et al. (5) reported that of 595 pitchers (aged 8 to 12 years), approximately 17% had a history of elbow symptoms but only 1% had symptoms severe enough to prevent them from pitching. In 1980 Grana and Rashkin (6) reported on 73 pitchers with an average age of 17 years. They reported that 78% of the players complained of pain at some time but only 5% of the players had time when they could not throw secondary to pain. One of the largest series came out of Japan, where 2,574 players (aged 9 to 12 years) were followed for 3 years (7). They found that 48% of the players complained of elbow pain and 16% of the players had abnormal radiographs.

MECHANISM OF INJURY AND PATHOANATOMY

The most common mechanism of injury for the elbow in athletes is the throwing motion. For acute traumatic injuries, a fall on the outstretched arm with a hyperextension load to the elbow can result in fracture and/or dislocation. In the athletic population, overuse injuries secondary to repetitive throwing are more frequently encountered.

The throwing motion that is typically studied is the baseball pitch, but the same basic motion is used in a tennis serve or for throwing a football or javelin. The throwing motion is divided up into five basic phases: wind-up, cocking, acceleration, deceleration, and follow-through (8). In caring for throwing athletes, it is critical to understand the biomechanics of the throwing motion, because this offers a framework to sort out the athlete's symptoms to arrive at a diagnosis.

In the wind-up phase, there is little stress on the throwing elbow. The ball is taken out of the glove and the thrower positions themselves by lifting their front leg and turning their body. During the cocking phase,

Laura A. Timmerman: 112 La Casa Via # 125, Walnut Creek, California 94598.

the shoulder achieves maximum external rotation, and a large valgus torque is generated at the elbow (8); during this time the hand and ball are positioned far behind the body.

During the acceleration phase of the throwing motion, tremendous forces are generated in the elbow. The momentum that is generated in the thrower's body is transferred down the kinetic chain to the hand and then to the ball. As the thrower transfers his or her weight anteriorly and the trunk rotates, the hand and ball are left behind. The elbow is placed in an extreme valgus position, which generates tremendous tensile forces across the medial elbow and compensatory compressive forces laterally.

During the deceleration phase, there is a huge outward force on the arm, and tremendous forces are placed across the glenohumeral joint (8). During this phase the elbow comes into extension, and if the elbow extension is not decelerated properly by the biceps, brachialis, and brachioradialis, hyperextension can occur, resulting in posterior impaction injuries. During the follow-through phase, the pitcher regroups as the arm moves forward and he or she regains balance. The elbow flexes in a position of comfort, and the forces across the joint are significantly decreased as compared with the deceleration phase.

Valgus extension overload is the clinical phrase coined to explain the injuries that occur during the throwing motion. These injuries include medial tension injuries, lateral compression injuries, and posterior elbow impaction injuries (Fig. 19.1).

Medial tension injuries are a result of the valgus stress across the medial elbow during the throwing motion. These occur mainly during the arm cocking and acceleration phases, but there is also some valgus stress during the deceleration phase. The main stabilizer to valgus stress is the anterior band of the ulnar collateral ligament (UCL) (9). The demands on the UCL during throwing have been calculated to be greater than the ultimate tensile strength of the ligament (10), and it is proposed that the actual demand on the ligament is assisted with dynamic stabilization provided by the medial flexor–pronator mass muscles. With the repeated medial tension stresses, injuries can occur, including UCL laxity and tearing, ulnar nerve symptoms, flexor–pronator mass tendinitis, and medial epicondyle apophyseal injuries in the skeletally immature.

Lateral compression injuries are a result of the compressive forces the lateral elbow experiences as a result of valgus loading. In addition, during the deceleration phase the forearm pronates to also create a shearing force between the capitellum and radial head. During weight-bearing activities across the elbow such as with gymnastics, most of the axial load is transmitted through the radiocapitellar joint. Lateral injuries include osteochondritis dissecans of the capitellum in the skeletally

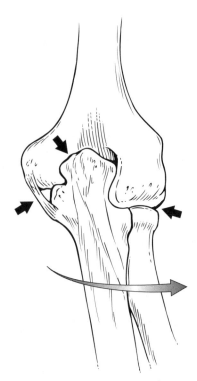

FIG. 19.1. Posterior view of the elbow, illustrating the injury sites in valgus extension overload: medial tension, lateral compression, posterior impaction.

immature and chondromalacia of the capitellum and radial head.

Posterior impaction injuries occur primarily during the deceleration phases of throwing, at which time the elbow experiences both extension and valgus forces that result in the olecranon impacting against the posteromedial humerus. This can cause inflammation, osteophyte formation on the medial olecranon with a concomitant chondral defect on the humerus, and loose body formation. In addition, stress fractures of the olecranon and ulnar nerve symptoms can develop.

CLINICAL EVALUATION

History

The most important, and often overlooked, component to the clinical evaluation of a throwing athlete is the history obtained from the patient. It is critical to carefully question the athlete regarding the onset of the pain and how the injury first occurred, at which point during the throwing motion the pain occurs, where the pain is located, and what relieves the pain.

The mechanism of injury is important information for any orthopedic history. When an acute fracture or dislocation occurs, the mechanism is often obvious, but when an athlete is complaining of pain about the elbow without apparent abnormalities, the nature of the injury is helpful. A prior history of similar pain is useful, for example, a previously injured UCL may have recurrent symptoms. Pain starting suddenly during a throwing motion, as opposed to an achy onset of pain at the end of the game, suggests an acute as opposed to a chronic type of injury. Although not common, an acute type of pain during throwing is consistent with a sudden rupture of the UCL or a medial epicondyle avulsion, bicep or tricep tendon rupture, a loose body locking in the joint, or an acute subluxation of the ulnar nerve.

It is much more common to have an athlete complain of chronic progressive pain about the elbow. To evaluate this knowledge of the location of the pain at the elbow and the timing of the pain during throwing is useful information. Medial pain is associated with UCL injuries, ulnar nerve symptoms, medial flexor mass injuries and tendinitis, olecranon stress fractures and medial epicondyle apophyseal injuries, and posteromedial olecranon osteophytes with valgus extension overload syndrome and medial subluxation of the triceps tendon. Lateral pain often suggests radiocapitellar disorders, including osteochondritis dissecans or radiocapitellar chondromalacia and lateral epicondylitis. Posterior pain is typical of valgus extension overload and less commonly triceps tendon injuries. Anterior pain is not common and is associated with biceps tendinitis, anterior capsular strain, and anterior impingement from a coronoid osteophyte.

The timing of the pain is useful: Pain that occurs during the cocking phase of throwing and ball release is often associated with medial injuries, whereas pain occurring after ball release is typical of posterior impaction or valgus extension overload type injuries. Medial pain is often difficult to sort out, and the answer to this simple question can provide helpful information regarding whether the UCL or the posterior compartment is the main source of pathology.

Other associated injuries should be taken into account. Often a thrower will injure their elbow after coming back from a shoulder injury, and it has been postulated that throwers with tight posterior shoulder capsules may develop elbow pain secondary to a change in the biomechanics of their throwing motion. The speed of the ball results from the action of a kinetic chain, and any injury along this pathway, including the legs, torso, or upper arm, can increase the likelihood of another injury. In addition, any recent changes in the mechanics of the athlete's throw, an increase or decrease in velocity or accuracy, or an increase in the amount of throwing should be noted.

Physical Examination

Physical examination of the acute traumatic injury is different than the examination for a chronic overuse disorder. The time of injury and the time of the patient's last meal should be noted, and any evidence of open injuries and distal neurovascular compromise should be immediately evaluated. Radiographs may then be obtained, and a limited physical examination is then completed, depending on the amount of discomfort that is present.

During the routine physical examination of the elbow, it is important to screen the entire upper extremity. In the older athlete, cervical disk disease can present initially as elbow pain. The range of motion of the shoulders should also be noted to detect any capsular tightness, weakness, instability, or other abnormalities on the involved side.

Initially, the patient should be examined with regard to carrying angle of the elbow. This is measured with the elbow in complete extension and the forearm maximally supinated. The normal carrying angle is approximately 13 degrees in females and 11 degrees in males. An increase in this angle, or a cubitus valgus deformity, is often noted in an older throwing athlete (11). In addition, a flexion contracture can cause the carrying angle to appear larger. This angle is also affected by previous trauma to the joint, such as a supracondylar humerus fracture resulting in cubitus varus.

The size and strength of the forearm should be noted. Girth of the maximal measurement of the forearm, approximately 5 cm below the joint line, should be recorded and compared with the other side. It is normal for the measurement to be larger on the dominant arm. Inspection for swelling within the joint is best noted in the area of the soft spot laterally.

The range of motion of the elbow in flexion and extension should then be measured with a goniometer, comparing with the normal side. Full extension should not automatically be considered normal. Often in a younger athlete, the noninjured side will have 10 to 15 degrees of hyperextension, so that a reading of zero degrees or full extension actually represents a 10- to 15-degree loss of motion. Pronation and supination measurements should also be noted, again with comparisons.

Bilateral strength testing of the biceps, triceps, wrist flexors and extensors, and pronators and supinators should be noted. Resisted strength testing of the wrist flexors and extensors should be performed to detect any evidence of tendinitis medially and laterally. Any evidence of neurologic changes or differences in reflexes should be recorded.

A careful examination of the joint should then be done with the patient both sitting and supine. With the patient supine and the arm out at the side, it is much easier to palpate and inspect the medial aspect of the joint. It is difficult to see the area of the UCL with the patient sitting, and in addition subluxation of the ulnar nerve with flexion and extension of the elbow may be missed. The anterior bundle of the UCL can be palpated along its course from the olecranon to the medial epicondyle. Injuries to the anterior bundle typically present with tenderness at the ulnar insertion. Usually this is 2 to 3 cm distal to the medial epicondyle. Tenderness over the medial epicondyle itself may indicate an epiphysitis, whereas tenderness just distal to the epicondyle is seen with medial epicondylitis or tendinitis of the pronator–flexor mass. Careful attention should be paid to the ulnar nerve because it is a frequently missed source of pathology. The nerve should be watched and palpated through the range of motion to detect any subtle subluxation of the nerve.

Laterally, the radiocapitellar joint can be palpated and then loaded with an axial force on the forearm (easier with the patient supine) to detect any grinding or pain. The lateral epicondyle and the tendon just distal should be palpated, along with the area just more distal to this over the radial nerve.

Anteriorly, the biceps tendon should be examined, and in evaluation of a possible tendon rupture, areas of ecchymosis and palpable defects should be noted, as well as the contour of the tendon.

Posteriorly, the medial and lateral humeral ridges, the olecranon, and crepitus or grind in the joint can be palpated. The insertion of the triceps should be palpated and the posterior olecranon bursa inspected.

Stress testing should then be performed. One of the most useful tests is the valgus extension overload test, which involves placing a valgus force on the forearm as the elbow is brought into extension. This test is usually positive with posterior impaction injuries of the elbow

but also may be painful with UCL injuries. Valgus stress testing is very difficult to perform because the amount of instability that one is feeling is usually less than 3 to 4 mm. A side to side comparison is necessary, and then it may not still be clear, even with later documented instability. The instability may take the force of the throwing motion to become apparent. It should be noted that the UCL can sustain plastic injury with no demonstrable valgus opening.

Testing of medial instability should be done in both the sitting and supine positions. With the athlete sitting, the elbow is flexed to 20 to 30 degrees and the forearm is then placed between the examiner's opposite arm and trunk. The examiner can then palpate the ulnohumeral joint medially while applying a valgus force to the elbow. Perhaps an easier method is to have the athlete supine, with the humerus maximally externally rotated and the arm abducted 90 degrees. This elbow is then flexed 20 to 30 degrees and a valgus force is applied to the supinated forearm.

Testing of lateral stability is evaluated, although this is a rare problem. The lateral compartment can be assessed with a simple varus force applied to the elbow, again with 20 to 30 degrees of flexion. The reverse pivot shift test of the elbow is done with the patient supine with the elbow extended with valgus stress and supination. The two forearm bones subluxate as a unit, with the radial head coming off the capitellum and the ulna externally rotating on the trochlea (Fig. 19.2) (12). This then reduces with elbow flexion and pronation. This is an unusual finding.

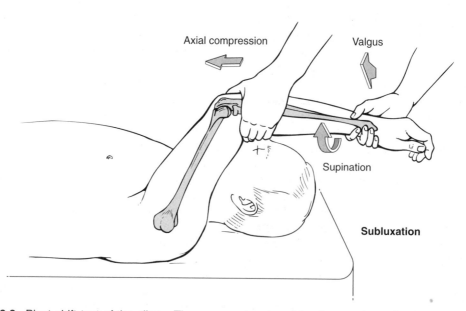

FIG. 19.2. Pivot shift test of the elbow. The arm overhead and the forearm in supination, supination and valgus moments, and axial forces are applied to the elbow, which is flexed 20 to 30 degrees. The posterolateral subluxation is visibly and palpably reduced when the elbow is flexed farther. (From O'Driscoll SW, Rell DF, Morrey BF. Posterolateral rotatory instability of the elbow. *J Bone Joint Surg Am* 1991;73A:441, 1991, with permission.)

IMAGING

A complete evaluation of any complaint of pain about the elbow should include at a minimum radiographs in the anteroposterior and lateral planes. In addition, oblique and axial views (Fig. 19.3) are often necessary to fully evaluate the joint. Stress radiography is used to evaluate the medial stability of the elbow. Commercial stressing devices have also been developed to quantify the side to side differences in medial instability (13,14). It is also useful to compare stress and nonstress views when evaluating posterolateral instability, and occasionally the radiograph will demonstrate the subluxation of the forearm bones (Fig. 19.4). Tomograms or computed tomography (CT) are useful adjuvants in evaluation of the bony structures. An arthrogram of the joint can demonstrate capsular tearing; however, this usually only is apparent acutely, and a CT arthrogram is much more useful in evaluation of subtle ligamentous injuries or the presence of loose bodies. A bone scan can demonstrate a subtle stress fracture; however, this is also seen on a magnetic resonance imaging (MRI).

MRI of the elbow has become increasingly popular over the last decade. It is very useful in evaluation of such lesions as Osteochondritis Dessicans (OCD) of the capitellum, complete tears of the UCL, and bicipital tendon injuries (15). However, the information gained from the study is only as good as the quality of the study itself, and unfortunately there is a great deal of variation in both technique and magnets with MRI studies. This is much more apparent in the elbow joint than, for example, in the knee or shoulder joint. An experienced radiologist is required to properly read the studies. An arthrogram–MRI study greatly enhances the images, as partial tears of the UCL and loose bodies may be better visualized (16). The "T sign" by MRI arthrography indicates an ulnar disinsertion of the ulnar collateral ligament on the ulna; this is the most common pathologic lesion.

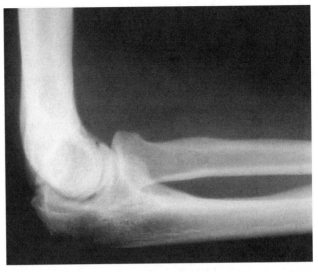

FIG. 19.4. Lateral radiograph demonstrating posterior olecranon osteophyte in a 22-year-old professional baseball player.

In the current medicoeconomic environment, plain radiographs are always indicated. They are inexpensive and will rule out serious disorders of the elbow, including the rare but regular occurrence of a tumor. It is alarming how in certain settings cost-saving measures include eliminating this important screen. The use of an MRI study is an expensive decision and should be weighed carefully. The quality of the study available locally, whether the study is going to change the course of treatment (i.e., rest vs. play), or the decision to proceed with surgery, and if a less expensive study will give the same information should all be taken into consideration.

The indicated imaging studies for specific disorders of the elbow are further reviewed in the following section.

SPECIFIC DISORDERS OF THE ELBOW

Dislocation

Pathoanatomy

The mechanism of an elbow dislocation is usually a fall on the outstretched arm, with a hyperextension load to the elbow with either a valgus or varus force, resulting in the more common posterolateral dislocation. Also seen is a straight posterior dislocation or, less commonly, a posteromedial, direct lateral, or anterior dislocation. The dislocation is classified according to the position of the forearm bones relative to the humerus. It has been demonstrated previously that a complete dislocation of the elbow is associated with tearing of both the UCL and Lateral Collateral Ligament (LCL) (17,18). In addition, a complete tear of the flexor pronator mass may

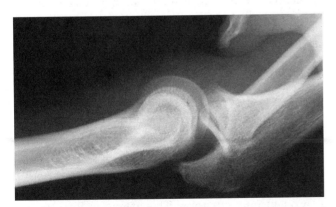

FIG. 19.3. Stress radiograph demonstrating posterolateral instability of the elbow, with subluxation of the forearm bones on the humerus, in a 15-year-old wrestler with recurrent elbow instability.

occur, and this is usually referred to as a medial elbow rupture and is grossly unstable (19).

Associated injuries with elbow dislocations include radial head fractures (10% of the dislocations), coronoid, medial and lateral epicondyle, capitellum, and trochlea fractures (20). Neurovascular injuries also occur and include brachial artery injuries, medial, ulnar, and radial nerve injuries, and acute compartment syndrome (21).

Clinical Evaluation

A careful neurovascular examination is critical before initiation of treatment. Imaging should include anteroposterior and lateral radiographs to determine the direction of the dislocation and any associated fractures. The next step should be reduction.

Treatment

Nonoperative

If a dislocation occurs at an athletic event with a trained person available to immediately reduce the elbow, this can be attempted. Ideally, the athlete should be transported to the nearest hospital so radiographs may be obtained first and intravenous sedation used, but this at times is not practical. An immediate attempt at reduction should then be attempted, with care taken to gently reduce the elbow.

Once the radiographs have been reviewed, the next step should be reduction of the joint. There are several different techniques used to reduce the elbow. The most common is the application of countertraction to the arm while a posterior force is applied to the olecranon as the elbow is extended. This will unperch the coronoid and allow it to clear the trochlea. The elbow can then be brought into flexion as the joint is reduced. Multiple attempts at closed reduction should be avoided about the elbow because of the danger of inducing a compartment syndrome or other neurovascular injury. If the joint is irreducible, the next step is open reduction.

Once the joint is reduced, repeated radiographs should be obtained to confirm the reduction and for a more careful inspection of associated fractures or loose bodies. A complete neurovascular examination should be repeated. The joint should then be gently evaluated for stability, with a stable arc of motion noted. Gross medial instability, especially in a throwing athlete, should be carefully evaluated. With evidence of a flexor–pronator mass (avulsion or tear) and a wide open valgus stress test, surgical repair is indicated (19). In the nonoverhead athlete, gross medial instability can be treated with a brace with the expectation of complete functional return. However, it is unlikely that these athletes will engage in overhead activities, even recreational activities, without pain. If the elbow is unstable at any point through the range of motion, either a hinged brace or early surgical repair should be considered.

Surgical

An irreducible elbow dislocation or a grossly unstable elbow requires early open repair. A medial approach is preferred so that the ulnar nerve can be located and protected and the flexor–pronator mass and the UCL repaired. If there is persistent instability after the medial structures are repaired, a lateral approach should be used to repair the soft tissues back to the lateral epicondyle. The lateral approach is also necessary if the radial head is buttonholed through the soft tissue.

Expected Outcome

If the complications of loss of motion and stiffness or recurrent instability are avoided, the results are generally good. A slight loss in extension is typical, and this is usually less than 10 degrees. It has been reported that only about 5% of adults have a flexion contracture greater than 30 degrees, and the incidence of recurrent instability is estimated to be between 1% and 2% of simple elbow dislocations, and this is most likely posterolateral in nature (22).

Author's Preferences

Early range of motion is critical for acceptable results after an elbow dislocation. It is also very important to verify that the elbow is stable enough to tolerate early range of motion, and if it is not, surgical repair should be done early to allow a stable range of motion. Poor results are seen after elbow dislocations for two main reasons: prolonged immobilization and an unstable elbow that redislocates after closed reduction (this may not be immediately detected) and then needs a late reduction and attempt at stabilization. Even though the current trend is toward nonoperative treatment of elbow dislocations, in athletes an early open reduction may offer superior results, especially if the UCL is disrupted in throwers.

Valgus Extension Overload

Pathoanatomy

Valgus extension overload is a term that refers to posterior impingement injuries (23). It is a result of both a valgus and extension stress at the elbow while the joint is brought into extension. This extension force results in osteophyte formation at the tip of the olecranon with fibrous tissue deposition in the olecranon fossa. Loose bodies may form, and with continued abutment of the olecranon tip against the humeral fossa with a valgus load, posteromedial osteophytes form on the olecranon, with an articular cartilage defect on the humerus as a result of the continued impingement. It is one of the most common causes of elbow pain in throwers. In a report (24) on surgery performed on a group of 72 professional baseball players, 65% of the players had posterior olecranon osteophytes removed. It was the most common operative procedure performed in this group of patients.

Clinical Evaluation

A thrower will relate that their pain occurs after ball release, as the arm is extending. They will complain of posterior or posteromedial pain or in some instances just medial pain. On physical examination a slight lack of full extension is usually apparent, and a positive valgus extension overload test is present. Other causes of medial elbow pain need to be carefully evaluated, including UCL injuries, ulnar nerve neuritis, and an olecranon stress fracture.

Imaging

Standard radiographs should be obtained, including an axial view to demonstrate the posteromedial osteophyte. The osteophyte can often be seen on a lateral radiograph (Fig. 19.4). An MRI study may demonstrate the posterior osteophyte, which is best seen on the true lateral view. Normal radiographs and MRI study do not exclude the presence of a posterior olecranon osteophyte. Imaging of the medial posterior elbow region is difficult, and the diagnosis is usually based on clinical history and physical examination findings.

Treatment

Nonoperative. Nonoperative treatment initially is focused on reducing the inflammation in the posterior elbow and regaining extension. Ice, stretching, and anti-inflammatory medications are useful. Often, a period of rest from throwing can significantly improve the symptoms. However, when the athlete resumes throwing, the symptoms usually return. Nonoperative treatment usually results in a recurrence of symptoms in the throwing athlete. Remember to rehabilitate the ipsilateral shoulder in throwing athletes.

Surgical. A posteromedial osteophyte can be removed either through an open or arthroscopic approach. In experienced hands, the arthroscopic technique offers improved visualization of the osteophyte, an opportunity to assess the valgus stability of the joint, and a more accelerated rehabilitation approach.

The open technique can either be done through a medial or lateral approach (25). If the elbow has been approached medially for a ulnar nerve transposition or a UCL procedure, the osteophyte can be removed

through a small posteromedial arthrotomy. A vertical arthrotomy is made just posterior to the bundle of the UCL. A small osteotome and rongeur are then used to remove the tip of the olecranon. The osteophyte can also be approached laterally through a small lateral arthrotomy as described previously (25).

The arthroscopic technique can be done in either the supine or prone position. The surgeon should use the position to which they are accustomed. With the arthroscope in the anterolateral portal, the medial side of the elbow joint should be inspected for any evidence of valgus instability. It has been previously described (26) that visualizing the opening medially with a valgus stress applied to the forearm with the humerus stabilized and the elbow flexed approximately 70 degrees is associated with UCL injuries, although the anterior bundle of the UCL is only partially seen at arthroscopy (Fig. 19.5). Usually, no opening between the humerus and ulna is visualized, and a gap of a few millimeters or more can be significant (Fig. 19.6).

UCL injuries commonly occur with posterior impingement injuries, and a subtle injury to the UCL that may not have been detected on clinical examination or imaging studies should be evaluated. The presence of loose bodies anteriorly should also be evaluated. The arthroscope can then be placed in the posterolateral portal under direct visualization after the soft spot portal is used, with the elbow flexed approximately 40 degrees. This portal can be difficult to make, and it is much easier if the curve of the olecranon is followed to its tip with the arthroscope and then the elbow extended slightly

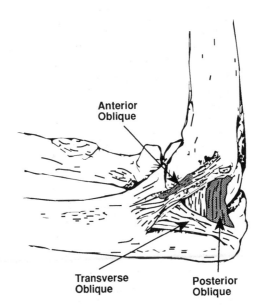

FIG. 19.5. Shaded portions of the anterior and posterior bundles of the ulnar collateral ligament demonstrate the portion of the ligament that can be viewed arthroscopically. (From Timmerman LA, Andrews JR. Histology and arthroscopic anatomy of the ulnar collateral ligament of the elbow. *Am J Sports Med* 1994;22:670, with permission.)

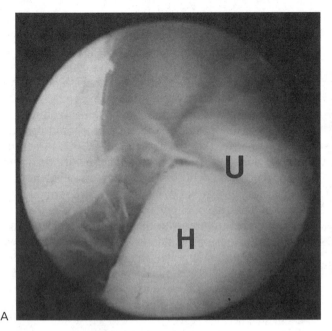

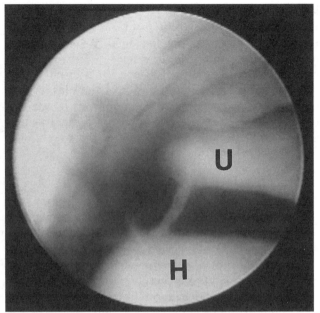

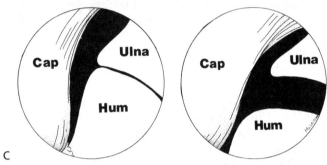

FIG. 19.6. **A:** Arthroscopic view from anterolateral portal in a right elbow of the medial elbow, humerus (*H*), and ulna (*U*). There is no opening between the humerus and ulna. **B:** With valgus stress applied, the increase in space between the ulna and humerus is demonstrated. **C:** Diagram illustrating these changes. *Cap,* capsule; *hum,* humerus; and ulna. (From Timmerman LA, Andrews JR. Undersurface tear of the ulnar collateral ligament in baseball players. *Am J Sports Med* 1994;22:34, with permission.)

to 40 to 50 degrees of flexion. If synovitis is present laterally, the shaver can clear a path for the arthroscope to enter the posterior compartment. The arthroscope is then placed in the posterolateral portal just off the humeral epicondylar ridge. A second posterior straight working portal is then made vertically through the triceps, with care taken regarding the ulnar nerve. The debrider is then brought in through the straight posterior portal, and the spur debrided (Fig. 19.7). Initially, synovitis posteriorly may make visualization difficult. Once this is debrided and the olecranon fossa is identified, the olecranon tip can be removed. Care should be taken medially because the ulnar nerve is just external to the capsule. The posteromedial corner of the olecranon tip should be addressed and the trochlea seen to rule out a chondral defect from impingement of the olecranon osteophyte (Fig. 19.8). If a full thickness chondral lesion is present, it can be debrided to stimulate bleeding and fibrocartilage formation.

Postoperatively an oral prophylactic antibiotic can be used for 3 to 4 days, as occasionally the straight posterior portal can be slow to heal because of the instrumentation in this area and can develop persistent drainage.

Once the portals are healed, a range of motion program is initiated and then a strengthening program started. An interval throwing program should then be introduced.

Expected Outcomes

The athlete should be warned of the strong tendency for posterior impingement to recur. It is important to realize that after the posterior osteophyte is removed, the stress across the UCL may be increased, because the posterior osteophyte may function as a buttress. This may result in an increased likelihood of UCL laxity or tearing. In the previously mentioned study (24) on professional baseball players, a reoperation rate of 33% was noted, most commonly involving the recurrence of posteromedial osteophytes. In addition, 25% of the players who initially underwent debridement of a posterior olecranon osteophyte went on to require a UCL reconstruction. The procedure is not curative and should instead be considered a palliative procedure. In addition, with the presence of a posterior osteophyte, the condition of the UCL should be carefully assessed, because increased ligamentous laxity may have contributed to the development of the osteophyte.

Author's Preferences

An adequate period of rest and physical therapy should precede any operative intervention, because occasionally synovitis posteriorly can present with symptoms of posterior impingement and will resolve with conservative treatment. If operative intervention is required, arthroscopic debridement is preferred, both for the advantages of improved joint visualization and a more rapid rehabilitation postoperatively. The recent trend is to debride less off the olecranon tip than previously described (25) because of the concern of increasing the stress across the UCL after excessive osteophyte debridement. Enough of the tip is removed to prevent impingement of the olecranon with extension, and any loose fragments that are still attached are removed.

Ulnar Collateral Ligament Injuries

Pathoanatomy

The UCL is composed of three bundles, the anterior, posterior, and the transverse (Fig. 19.3) (27). The anterior bundle is the main stabilizer to valgus stress (9,28). In addition, a histologic study demonstrated that the anterior bundle has a thin external layer and a thicker stout internal layer that is a part of the capsule (26)

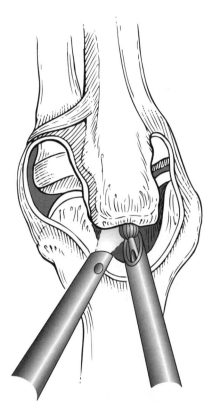

FIG. 19.7. Technique of arthroscopic debridement of a posterior olecranon spur with the arthroscopic in the posterolateral portal and the debrider in the posterior working portal with the patient in a supine position.

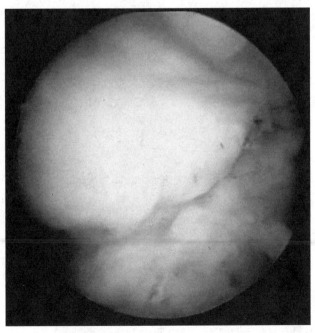
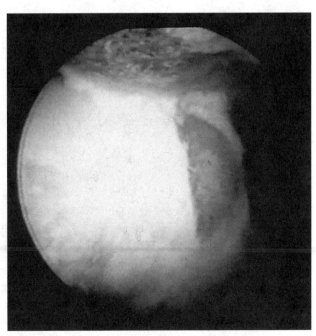

A   B

FIG. 19.8. An arthroscopic view of the posterior compartment of the elbow after arthroscopic debridement of the posterior olecranon tip (**top**) (A) with a chondral defect (or "kissing") lesion on the trochlea (B).

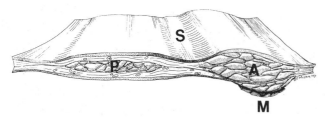

FIG. 19.9. Cross-sectional anatomy of the medial capsule of the elbow at the level of the joint line. *A,* anterior bundle; *M,* muscle, *P,* posterior bundle; *S,* synovium. (From Timmerman LA, Andrews JR. Histology and arthroscopic anatomy of the ulnar collateral ligament of the elbow. *Am J Sports Med* 22:669, 1994, with permission.)

(Fig. 19.9). This finding is important clinically because the thin outer layer may be intact (preventing contrast leakage with imaging studies), whereas the thick inner layer is torn, resulting in an undersurface tear.

Injuries to the ligament result from an excessive valgus stress across the elbow. This may result in an acute tear, as is seen with an elbow dislocation or a tagging injury suffered by a football quarterback. A chronic laxity of the ligament is more commonly seen as a result of repetitive microtrauma. An acute or chronic injury may also occur.

Clinical Evaluation

The athlete complains of medial elbow pain. Often this will only be symptomatic with the force of throwing and is most painful during the cocking portion of the throw where the maximum stress is placed across the ligament. They may have heard an audible "pop" or the injury may have happened before the athlete was warmed up or on a cold day. It is more common, however, that an acute injury is not recalled. Instead, the pain usually develops insidiously. Ulnar nerve symptoms may be present or have occurred acutely. The athlete may be unable to throw or can toss the ball but gets pain that prevents pitching. A loss of velocity or accuracy is a common complaint.

On physical examination, a slight flexion contracture is typical, with tenderness over the UCL, more commonly at the ulnar insertion. There is usually pain with valgus stress or the valgus extension overload test. It may be difficult to appreciate medial instability on examination. A Tinel's sign may be present over the ulnar nerve.

Imaging Studies

A series of plain radiographs should be taken, including anteroposterior, lateral, obliques, and axial views. Calci-

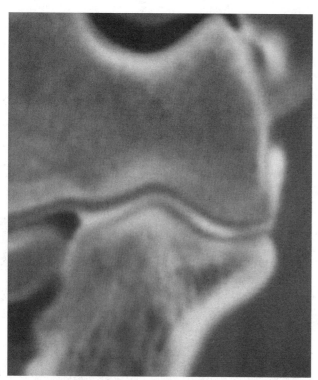
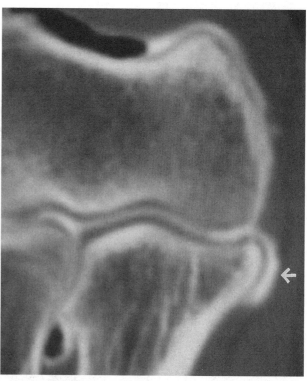

FIG. 19.10. Coronal section computed tomography arthrogram demonstrating **(A)** normal findings, with pooling of the contrast under the medial epicondyle, and **(B)** a partial tear of the ulnar collateral ligament from the ulnar insertion with the T sign, or the leaking of the contrast distally down the ulna but contained within the joint capsule. (From Timmerman LA, Schwartz ML, Andrews JR. Preoperative evaluation of the ulnar collateral ligament by magnetic resonance imaging and computed tomography arthrography. *Am J Sports Med* 1994;22:29, with permission.)

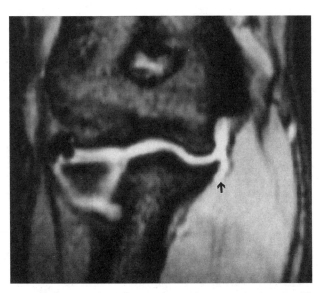

FIG. 19.11. A coronal plane magnetic resonance image with saline contrast demonstrating an ulnar collateral ligament tear with detachment from the ulna. (From Timmerman LA, Schwartz ML, Andrews JR. Preoperative evaluation of the ulnar collateral ligament by magnetic resonance imaging and computed tomography arthrography. *Am J Sports Med* 1994; 22:29, with permission.)

fications may be present in the UCL, and if the fragment is large enough, it may be symptomatic or interfere with the integrity of the ligament. The images should be carefully inspected for any sign of avulsion proximally or distally of the UCL. A CT arthrogram is useful because the contrast aids in defining the ligament. A contrast leak extracapsular is obvious for a full thickness tear, but it is important to realize that significant pathology can exist in the UCL without contrast leakage. There is an area of normal pooling under the medial epicondyle, but pooling below the level of the joint line next to the ulna is not a normal finding. Timmerman and Andrews (29) described the T sign or the presence of contrast leaking down the ulna distally as typical findings on CT arthrograms in patients with undersurface UCL tears with an intact outer layer (Fig. 19.10).

These findings can also be visualized on MRI with contrast (Fig. 19.11), with the added advantage of improved visualization of the other soft tissues about the elbow and an evaluation of the bony anatomy for evidence of OCD or other lesions (15,16). It is often difficult to fully appreciate the ligament in an MRI study without contrast, and subtle injuries to the UCL may be missed. A normal MRI study does not rule out injury to the UCL because clinically symptomatic laxity may be present in a ligament that appears normal on imaging. It is not possible to evaluate dynamic laxity with a static study.

Treatment

Nonoperative. Much is written on the operative treatment of UCL injuries (30,31), and the conservative treatment approach is generally ignored. It should be stressed that a nonoperative approach is the mainstay treatment for UCL injuries, and with rest suspected injuries to the ligament will often improve. This includes avoidance of throwing, modalities, range of motion, and then advancing to a strengthening program. Once the symptoms are resolved and the strength is normal, then an interval throwing program can be initiated. A hinged elbow brace or a removable posterior splint can be used for protection in the acute phases if necessary. Strengthening and range of motion of the shoulder should not be ignored during the rest period or the athlete may develop a shoulder injury upon return to throwing.

Surgical. The operative approach depends on the type of injury. In an acute traumatic injury, such as after an elbow dislocation or a traumatic avulsion of the flexor mass, primary surgical repair is indicated. A standard medial approach is used, with localization and transposition of the ulnar nerve. The proximal portion of the ligament can be reattached to the medial epicondyle through drill holes, and the sutures can be tied over the bony tunnel on the posterior part of the epicondyle. If the distal portion avulses off the sublime tubercle of the ulna (seen in skeletally immature), the ligament may be repaired through bony tunnels in the ulna or with the use of suture anchors. Augmentation of the ligament may be necessary. A midportion disruption may be repaired primarily with sutures; however, graft augmentation may be required.

More commonly seen is the situation of chronic laxity. Initially, the elbow should be arthroscoped from the lateral side so that the valgus stability of the elbow can be assessed (Fig. 19.6). Although there is some controversy in this area, it can be very useful in determining if valgus instability is present. It is at times easier to see the instability than to feel it on clinical examination. It is important to remember that a normal view of the medial elbow capsule does not exclude a UCL injury, because most of the anterior bundle is not visualized arthroscopically (26). An anterolateral portal introduced into the joint has minimal morbidity, and a medial portal can be evaded to avoid fluid extravasation to ease the dissection medially with the open reconstruction.

With chronic laxity, a tendon graft is required to allow stabilization of the medial side of the elbow. Palmaris longus from the ipsilateral side is generally used; however, approximately 15% of patients do not have a palmaris longus, and then a contralateral palmaris longus tendon can be used if present. Otherwise, the plantaris tendon, gracilis tendon, or a toe extensor tendon can be harvested. A length of 15 cm is desirable.

The technique involved a medial approach, with dissection and mobilization of the ulnar nerve. The small branches that supply the elbow joint usually need to be sacrificed. The proximal portion of nerve comes into contact with the intermuscular septum, and this should be excised to avoid impingement on the nerve. This septum is vascular, and careful hemostasis should be obtained.

Exposure of the anterior bundle of the UCL can be via a take-down of the flexor–pronator mass (31), a muscle fiber-splitting approach through the flexor mass (32), or by a distal exposure (33). The distal exposure involves elevating the flexor carpi ulnaris distally off its ulnar attachment. Once the interval between the ligament and flexor muscle is located, the exposure can be extended proximally to expose the entire ligament. This approach avoids taking down the flexor mass attachment from the medial epicondyle.

With the anterior bundle of the ligament exposed, the pathology of the ligament can be assessed. It often appears normal, although laxity may be detected by grasping the ligament with a pick-up. A longitudinal incision through the midportion of the anterior bundle in the line of the fibers should be done. This allows inspection of the interior of the ligament for evidence of degeneration and also for visualization of the important ulnar attachment of the deep bundle. With undersurface tears this may be detached, whereas the superficial bundle is intact (29).

The remnants of the ligament should be conserved, because the reconstruction involves an augmentation of the ligament, not a replacement. This offers more bulk of tissue medially. If a palmaris tendon graft is used, this can be harvested ipsilaterally (without an increase in morbidity) through several small transverse incisions until the musculotendinous junction is located. The muscle can be stripped off the tendon proximally to increase tendon length. A suture is then placed in each end of the tendon to allow graft passage.

The drill holes for the tendon graft are then made. Two convergent tunnels are drilled proximally to meet at the insertion of the tendon on the medial epicondyle. A 5/64-inch drill is used. Distally, right-angle drill holes are made at the sublime tubercle of the ulna, approximately 5 mm distal to the articular edge. These two drill holes can be connected with a curved very small curette initially, followed by a towel clip. Care should be taken in this step, because breakage of the bony bridge is problematic. Suture anchors have been suggested for attachment of the graft on the ulna, but the fixation appears to be inferior to that of bony tunnels. Suture loops can then be placed through each hole to ease passage of the graft. Sterile mineral oil can be placed on the graft to ease passage. The graft is then passed in a figure-8 pattern across the joint, and each end is brought out through the tunnels in the humerus (Fig. 19.12).

The graft can be tensioned over the medial epicondyle, with sutures placed through the graft to secure the ends. The elbow should be placed in about 30 degrees of flexion with a varus stress applied to the forearm.

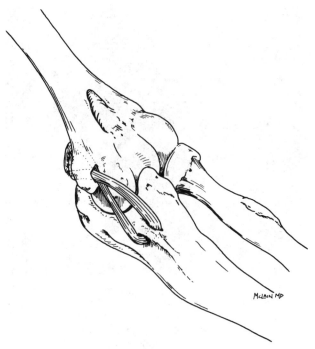

FIG. 19.12. Position of the ulnar collateral ligament graft and tunnels.

The remaining ligament is then sutured to the graft for added stability.

The ulnar nerve transposition is then completed, with the use of one or two fascial slings. The elbow should be placed through a range of motion to avoid compression over the nerve. The skin incision is then closed and the elbow is placed in a posterior splint for 10 days. The sutures are then removed and a hinged elbow braced applied with initial range of motion 30 to 90 degrees, which is increased to 10 to 110 degrees by week 4. The brace is worn for 4 to 6 weeks to provide valgus stability.

Once the athlete has regained normal range of motion of the elbow, the strengthening program can be advanced. When the athlete has full range of motion and normal strength, an interval throwing program can be initiated. This is usually after 4 to 6 months. Return to throwing generally occurs at 6 to 8 months from surgery.

Expected Outcomes

There have been two large series (31,34) addressing UCL repair and reconstruction in competitive athletes, and generally a return rate to throwing of 80% to 85% is seen. It is important to warn the athlete that the possibility of ulnar nerve paresthesias, although usually temporary, is present. In one series (31), the rate of ulnar nerve symptoms was 21% when a submuscular transposition was used. This was improved with a subcutaneous fascial sling approach (34).

Author's Preferences

Initially, a generous course of conservative treatment is indicated for UCL injuries, unless there is a severe acute traumatic disruption of the medial elbow structures. With chronic injuries, an arthroscopic examination of the elbow is done before any surgery. Typically, the athlete has undergone both a long course of rehabilitation and an arthroscopic examination of the elbow with possibly a debridement of a posterior osteophyte before a UCL reconstruction. The procedure is difficult to perform, and a trial surgery with a cadaver is strongly recommended. Postoperatively, the athlete should be warned that most high-level throwers who have undergone this procedure relate that it takes 18 to 24 months until the throw feels normal again, despite the early return to throwing at 4 to 6 months.

Little League Elbow

Pathoanatomy

Little league elbow was first described in terms of radiographic findings (35), including medial epicondylar enlargement, fragmentation, beaking, and separation of the medial epicondyle in response to excessive throwing (Fig. 19.13). It is also referred to as medial epicondylitis or a medial traction apophysitis. This disorder has been expanded by some to include the lateral compression injuries also seen in young athletes, including osteochondritis dissecans of the capitellum, but classically it should only refer to the medial disorders.

Little league elbow, or a medial traction apophysitis, most commonly occurs in throwing athletes between the ages of 9 and 12 years. The mechanism of injury is an overuse injury resulting in repeated tension stress across the epiphyseal plate of the medial epicondyle. The medial epicondyle apophysis is the last growth center about the elbow to fuse, typically around age 14 in females and up to age 17 in males.

Clinical Evaluation

The athlete complains of persistent medial elbow pain, which is worse after throwing. There is often a history of an increased amount of recent throwing. On clinical examination, there is tenderness over the medial epicondyle, with pain with resisted flexion of the wrist and with valgus stress testing of the elbow. A slight flexion contracture may also be present.

Imaging

Radiographic findings are as noted above. MRI is not usually necessary, because the diagnosis is obvious based on the history, physical examination, and radiographic findings. Occasionally, a thrower will present with an acute medial epicondyle fracture that occurred after a chronic course of medial epicondylitis (Fig. 19.14).

Treatment

Nonoperative. Nonoperative treatment is always the initial course in this injury. A period of rest from throwing, and often just from throwing a baseball with the athlete still able to play basketball or swim, is usually all that is necessary to allow the medial epicondyle to heal. Often, with mild symptoms, a pitcher can switch positions to a field position and have resolution of the pain. Usually, after 2 to 3 months of rest, the symptoms have resolved. If they are still symptomatic, a longer period of rest should be tried. If after 6 months the athlete is still symptomatic, surgical treatment is considered.

Surgical. Surgical treatment is indicated with displacement of the medial epicondyle, and only an anatomic reduction should be accepted in the throwing athlete. Care should be taken to evaluate both the anteroposterior and lateral radiographs, because significant displacement can occur on the lateral view and appear normal on the anteroposterior. If the medial epicondyle is not reduced, the tension in the UCL is affected, and also a loss in range of motion can occur.

Surgical reduction is done through a medial approach, with careful protection of the ulnar nerve. A cannulated screw with a washer can be used, with initial reduction of the fragment with a guidewire (Fig. 19.14). The elbow is then placed in a posterior splint for 7 to 10 days, with

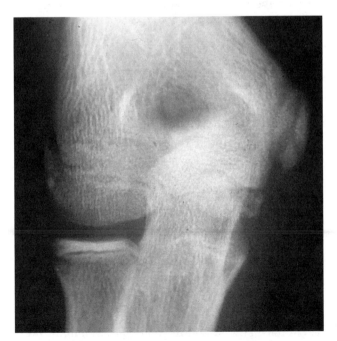

FIG. 19.13. Radiograph of Little League elbow.

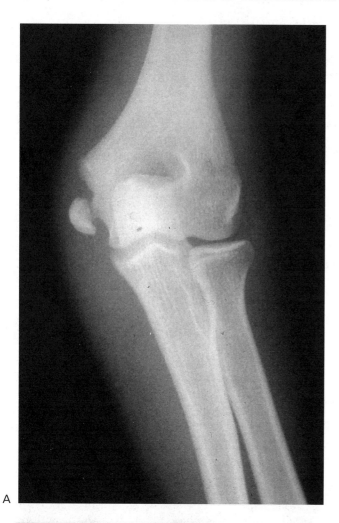

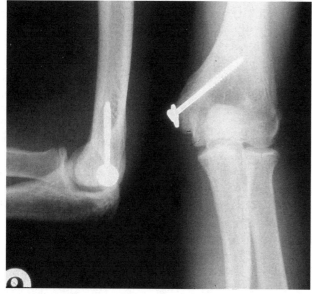

FIG. 19.14. A: Radiograph demonstrating avulsion of the medial epicondyle in a young thrower. **B:** After open reduction and internal fixation of the fragment.

early range of motion started. A removable posterior splint or hinged elbow brace is then used for an additional 2 to 3 weeks. If the screw is symptomatic, it can be removed once the fracture is healed.

Expected Outcome

Young athletes usually fully recover from this disorder with conservative treatment. If surgery is required, the key component in treatment is early range of motion. Occasionally, postoperative stiffness can be a problem.

Author's Preferences

It is important to stress to the athlete, parents, and coaches that a period of rest almost always allows this disorder to resolve. In the case of a very active athlete who is not compliant, a change in position can be offered or the opportunity to participate in different sports. If the fragment displaces, strong consideration should be given to surgical repair. This is important because it allows for early range of motion, and also it may prevent loss of motion from an improperly reduced fragment. The only poor results I have seen in this disorder are in youngsters who are immobilized for a prolonged period of time and develop arthrofibrosis and in a young athlete who had anatomic anteroposterior radiograph but had 1 cm of anterior displacement on the lateral that was initially missed. At his initial evaluation at 6 months from injury, he had a 35-degree flexion contracture. He would have been better treated with an open reduction and internal fixation of the fragment, because the anteriorly displaced ligament functions as a check to prevent extension.

Osteochondritis Dissecans

Pathoanatomy

Panner (36) first described osteochondrosis of the capitellum in 1929. This was initially described in younger athletes aged 7 to 10 years. In 1975 Woodward and Bianco (37) reported on a series of capitellar lesions in pitchers age 9 to 15 years. Irregular ossification and rarefaction with a crater formation were noted along with flattening of the capitellum and loose body formation. This was termed osteochondritis dissecans and was distinguished from osteochondrosis. Osteochondrosis occurs at an earlier age, involves the whole ossification center of the capitellum, is not associated with loose body formation, and improves with conservative treatment.

The mechanism of injury is increased lateral load across the elbow. It is most commonly seen in throwers and gymnasts. It is especially common in female gymnasts, who train extensively at a young age. The blood supply to the lateral epicondyle is from posterior vessels, and at age 8 there is no contribution from metaphyseal vessels. Once closure of the epiphysis has occurred (around age 15 in males), anastomoses have formed. Before this, however, the blood supply posteriorly is the only source to the capitellum, and with trauma to the blood supply, avascular necrosis could result. Before the introduction of arthroscopy, lateral compression injuries were proposed to be the most common pathology seen in baseball players (38), but now that the entire joint is visualized, the posterior injuries are diagnosed much more frequently.

Clinical Evaluation

The athlete most commonly presents with loss of elbow motion, and often a painless flexion contracture is the first presenting symptom of an OCD lesion. They may also complain of lateral elbow pain and occasional swelling. If loose bodies are present, symptoms such as locking or catching may be present.

Imaging

Routine radiographs should be obtained initially; however, they are often normal (39). A CT arthrogram can be used to determine if the lesion has contrast leakage behind the fragment. Tomograms alone may also outline the lesion. MRI has been shown to nicely demonstrate the lesion. Decreased signal is seen in the capitellum on T1-weighted images, with increased signal noted on T2-weighted images (15). These findings can be seen on MRI before demonstrable radiograph changes. A bone scan can also be used if an OCD lesion is suspected. In view of the improvement in MRI studies of the elbow in recent years, this study should be the second-line study ordered after radiographs are obtained. In a young athlete with a flexion contracture and otherwise normal radiographs, an MRI should be ordered early to rule out the presence of an OCD.

Treatment

Nonoperative. In the younger athlete with osteochondrosis, the symptoms will usually resolve with simple rest; in more severe cases immobilization may be necessary. Immobilization should be removable, so that the athlete can perform range of motion exercises three to four times a day. Usually, with 3 to 4 months of rest or avoidance of lateral compression activities, the pain resolves and the range of motion returns to normal. A gentle strengthening program should then be initiated, with stretching of the wrist and elbow. The strengthen-

ing program can then be advanced and an interval throwing program started before return to throwing. A gymnast should be advanced slowly back to full weight-bearing exercises.

Surgical. After failure of conservative treatment, with evidence of detachment of the fragment, or with symptoms of a loose fragment such as catching and locking, surgery should be considered. An open debridement through a lateral approach can be used, but an arthroscopic approach is preferred because it offers advantages with regards to visualization and rehabilitation (39).

At arthroscopy, the lateral compartment is best assessed from the anteromedial portal initially. With a distraction force applied to the elbow, the radiocapitellar joint can be seen. However, the OCD lesion is usually only visualized through the straight lateral or soft spot portal. Despite the small space constraints of the lateral compartment, a second portal is made. This is necessary as the working portal. It is useful for the surgeon to visualize their hands, and the instruments are handled in a parallel fashion, as opposed to the usual triangulation method with other arthroscopy. A small 2.7-mm arthroscope is helpful in the lateral compartment, as is an arthroscopic fluid system. Initially, the typically abundant synovium is debrided, and often an underlying chondral defect will be seen. Results of arthroscopic debridement of osteochondritic lesions have been previously described (40,41), and generally experience has proven that simple arthroscopic debridement of the lesion is preferred as opposed to reattachment of the lesion (39). There may be a place for mosaicoplasty types (placement of a autogenous plug of bone with articular cartilage attached) of cartilage transplants in the future, although this is still in experimental stages at this point.

Postoperatively, the patient is placed in a soft dressing, and early range of motion is encouraged. Once the swelling is resolved and motion normalized, a strengthening program is started. Usually after 8 to 12 weeks, the athlete is ready to return to an interval-throwing program or to a modified sports program. Full recovery is usually seen by 3 to 6 months.

Expected Outcomes

The results of conservative treatment of OCD lesions in the younger athlete are generally good. However, in the older thrower or athletes 10 years or older, the long-term results are far less satisfying than those seen after disorders of the medial side of the elbow. Osteochondritis dissecans involves a disruption in the articular surface of the radiocapitellar joint and can lead to long-term abnormalities with traumatic arthritis and permanent joint impairment. In a recently published series (39), 14 of 17 adolescent athletes with OCD returned to the previous sport, 2 patients required a second operation, and 1 had a poor result.

Author's Preferences

In the younger athlete, a period of rest or change in activities to avoid lateral compression of the elbow is usually enough to resolve the symptoms. If surgery is required, an arthroscopic approach is preferred, even in the smaller athletes. Simple debridement of the lesion with abrasion or microfracture of the crater offers consistently good results. The athlete often wants to resume throwing by 6 to 8 weeks, and it usually takes an effort on the physician's part to keep them from throwing for 2 to 3 months. Two lateral portals in the soft spot are required to complete the debridement arthroscopically, and it is helpful to spread these portals slightly with regards to the center of the soft spot to improve triangulation. In other words, do not place the first portal in the middle of the soft spot.

Degenerative Arthritis

Pathoanatomy

In the older athlete, degenerative arthritis of the elbow can cause limitation in motion and pain. Degenerative arthritis of the elbow without a previous history of excessive throwing or previous trauma is unusual. The presence of loose bodies in the joint with repeated locking episodes can also result in degenerative changes of the elbow. Osteophytes also form in response to repetitive stress across the joint and can result in loss of motion with the development of a flexion contracture and loss of terminal flexion.

Clinical Evaluation

The most common presenting complaint is loss of motion, resulting in difficulty participating in activities. An effusion may develop after activities. Usually, a loss in flexion and extension is noted, and occasionally a loss in pronation or supination is reported. Physical examination should focus on the measured range of motion in the passive and active range of motion. Crepitus may be present, especially over the radiocapitellar joint.

Imaging

Routine radiographs should be obtained (Fig. 19.15). A CT arthrogram is useful in outlining loose bodies and osteophytes, but it is not an absolute requirement. Although MRI will outline the degenerative changes, it is generally not worth the expense because this information can be gained from radiographs.

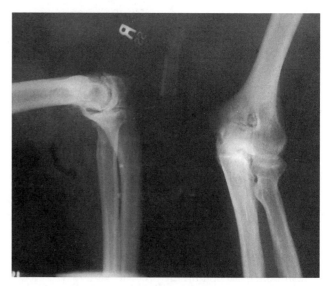

FIG. 19.15. Anteroposterior and lateral radiographs demonstrating severe degenerative changes in an elbow joint in a 46-year-old former baseball player. Note the large anterior coronoid spur, the anterior humeral osteophyte, and the multiple loose bodies posteriorly.

Treatment

Nonoperative. Nonoperative treatment should attempt to decrease pain and inflammation while working on improving range of motion and flexibility. Once these two objectives are achieved, a strengthening program can be initiated. Heat can be used to increase flexibility, with emphasis on extension, either by a dynamic splint or low-load long-duration stretching.

Surgical. Either arthroscopic or open debridement of the elbow can be performed. An arthroscopic procedure is preferred as an accelerated rehabilitation program is allowed. The arthroscopic technique for debridement of arthrofibrotic elbow joints has been previously described (42–45). The goal of surgery is to safely excise scar tissue and to restore the normal bony anatomy by debriding osteophytes and reforming the fossi about the joint that have filled in with scar tissue. Anteriorly, a large coronoid spur is usually present, and the coronoid and radial fossi are usually filled in with scar tissue. In addition, the anterior capsule is scarred and contracted. With arthroscopy performed in the supine position, the scarred capsule can be released off the humerus proximally, and this avoids directly debriding in the region of the neurovascular structures. Initially, it can be difficult to get the scope in the joint; once the arthroscope and debrider are visualized it is much easier (Fig. 19.16). The lateral compartment can be debrided by using two straight lateral portals in the soft spot. There is usually extensive scarring in the lateral compartment, and it is a relatively safe area of the elbow to debride. Once the capitellum, radial head, and olecranon are visualized,

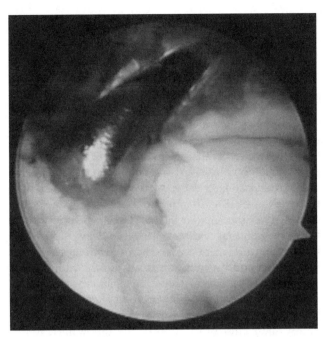

FIG. 19.16. An arthroscopic view of the anterior compartment of the elbow, demonstrating extensive anterior arthrofibrosis.

the camera can follow the debrider down the curve of the olecranon and then the posterolateral portal can be made under direct visualization. The posterior compartment is at times the most difficult part of the joint to enter, and there is usually significant scarring and osteophyte formation posteriorly. The olecranon fossa will fill in, preventing full extension. A second straight posterior portal is made to perform debridement, and once the synovitis is removed, the osteophytes on the tip of the olecranon and on the humerus are removed using a shaver, burr, or small osteotome. Extreme care must be taken posteriorly to avoid damaging the ulnar nerve. Once the scar tissue has been excised, the elbow can be gently mobilized to the limits of motion and this range noted in the operative note. However, it is the debridement itself that regains most of the motion, not the manipulation.

Postoperative rehabilitation after an arthroscopic debridement include a soft bulky dressing (a postoperative knee ice pack wrap works well) for a few days until the portals are healed and then early aggressive range of motion therapy. A dynamic splint device can occasionally be useful (46).

Surgeon's preference may dictate that an open debridement is performed. A lateral approach using the interval between the lateral border of the triceps proximally and the interval between the anconeus and extensor carpi ulnaris distally is recommended. The anconeus is released at the triceps, and if necessary the annular ligament can also be released. Using this interval, both the anterior and posterior compartments can be visual-

ized with flexion and extension of the elbow. It is less traumatic than a medial and lateral approach. The scar tissue can be released off the humerus in the same fashion as described above for the arthroscopic technique, and the osteophytes can also be removed off both the coronoid and olecranon tip. Postoperatively, the joint should be protected until the incision heals, with a posterior splint for a few days followed by a bulky dressing. Then a rehabilitation program can be initiated stressing range of motion.

Expected Outcomes

Conservative treatment offers variable results. With significant capsular contracture and osteophyte formation, therapy alone usually does not result in significant improvement in motion. With an arthroscopic release, significant improvement can be gained in function and range of motion (42).

Author's Preferences

An arthroscopic debridement is performed as described previously (42). The patient is warned that their stiffness or locking symptoms may recur and that they may eventually require a second debridement. These patients are among the most satisfied of all and generally do very well after surgery. A gain in both flexion and extension of the elbow can make a big difference in their everyday life and also in their sporting activities.

Stress Fracture of the Olecranon

Pathoanatomy

A stress fracture of the olecranon can occur in response to repetitive throwing (47,48). It is frequently misdiagnosed initially and usually presents with persistent posterior elbow pain. The proximal olecranon epiphyseal plate typically fuses at age 16 in males. In the throwing athlete, a delayed union can result, and this can persist into the throwing athlete's third decade. In the older athlete, a stress fracture may occur in this location. It is likely the result of repetitive extension stresses from the firing of the triceps muscle.

Clinical Evaluation

The athlete will usually complain of posterior or posterolateral elbow pain. This pain may be vague in nature and insidious in onset. Symptoms are similar to triceps tendinitis; however, there is usually tenderness right over the olecranon at the site of the fracture.

Imaging

Radiographs are often normally initially or the subtle findings missed at first inspection. A lateral view may

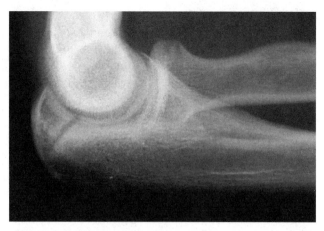

FIG. 19.17. A lateral radiograph of a stress fracture of the ulna in an 18-year-old baseball player.

demonstrate the stress fracture (Fig. 19.17). The stress fracture will be visible on MRI or CT, and a bone scan will show increased uptake at the site.

Treatment

Nonoperative. Avoidance of throwing should be tried initially, with a 6- to 8-week period of rest from throwing or aggressive strengthening activities. During this time, the patient should emphasize stretching activities and maintenance of motion. Any exercise that aggravates pain at the fracture site should be avoided. A swimming program can be started after approximately 8 weeks and then throwing started after 12 weeks. It may take 3 to 6 months to return to throwing, working through an interval throwing program.

Surgical. If conservative treatment fails, operative treatment may be necessary. Motion at the fracture site can be demonstrated at arthroscopy. Open reduction and internal fixation with either a single cancellous screw or a tension band wire technique or even a plate and screws may be necessary. Iliac crest bone graft may also be required.

Expected Outcome

Once properly diagnosed, an olecranon stress fracture will usually resolve. If operative treatment is needed, bony union can be expected in approximately 95% of cases (49).

Author's Preferences

It is important to remember this disorder and look for it on every radiograph and MRI that is ordered on throwing athletes. Also, during physical examination, remember to palpate the olecranon itself for tenderness.

It is preferable to make this diagnosis before the scope portal scars are present.

Posterior Lateral Instability

Pathoanatomy

The lateral collateral ligament complex of the lateral elbow resists varus stress, although the main stabilizer laterally is the articular surfaces (27). Morrey (50) described this complex consisting of three parts: the lateral UCL, radial collateral ligament, and the annular ligament (Fig. 19.18). The radial collateral ligament becomes lax as the annular ligament loses its tension, and it is proposed that resistance to varus stress is provided by the lateral UCL, because the attachment distally is to the ulna and it is not dependent on the radial head.

Injury to the lateral collateral ligament complex is relatively rare, and it usually presents as recurrent instability of the elbow after a dislocation. It is more commonly seen after dislocation of the elbow in children and adolescents (51). The radial head subluxates while the ulna externally rotates on the trochlea.

Clinical Evaluation

The history of recurrent locking of the elbow after a previous dislocation or traumatic injury or catching with certain movements is typical. The patient may report a loud clunk in the elbow, especially in the position of trying to push off on the elbow from a sitting position. The physical examination will be positive for the lateral

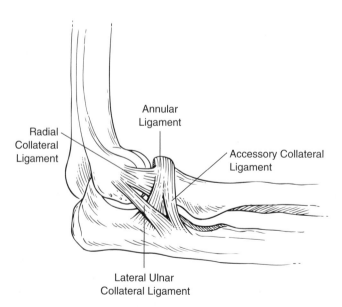

FIG. 19.18. The lateral collateral ligament complex consists of the lateral ulnar collateral ligament and the radial collateral ligament. (From Morrey BF, An KN. *The elbow*. Philadelphia: W.B. Saunders, 1985:21, with permission.)

pivot shift test of the elbow (Fig. 19.2). In addition, varus stress testing may be positive.

Imaging

A stress radiograph performed with the pivot shift maneuver is useful (Fig. 19.4). Also, an examination under fluoroscopy can be very helpful in understanding the instability.

Treatment

Nonoperative. A supportive elbow brace can be used, along with a change in activities. Symptomatic recurrent elbow instability usually requires surgical stabilization.

Surgical. Reconstruction of the lateral collateral ligament has been previously described (52). Primary repair of an acute rupture of the radial UCL has been reported (53). Specific reconstruction of the radial UCL portion of the lateral complex has been recommended, using a palmaris longus tendon graft or advancement of the existing ligament. Postoperatively, the joint is immobilized for 1 month, and then a hinged elbow brace is used for an additional month. A simple lateral collateral ligament reefing can also be performed, with advancement of the lateral capsule into the lateral epicondyle using suture anchors.

Expected Outcome

This is an unusual condition, and information on long-term results is scarce. One series (52) reported 11 patients with 7 excellent results after a lateral reconstruction. A significant report in athletes is not available, most likely due to the rare nature of the disorder.

Author's Preferences

This is an unusual disorder, and despite a large relative volume of elbow cases, only a few been treated. In cases of recurrent subluxation, a stress radiograph has been useful in detecting the presence of instability, because despite how nicely the pivot shift test of the elbow is described, it is difficult to detect. It is most likely easier once several have been done. In addition, arthroscopy has been very useful in detecting the presence of posterolateral instability, as stress can be applied with the camera in the lateral compartment and the instability directly viewed (Fig. 19.19). I have had success with simple reefing of the lateral capsule. The lateral UCL complex is detached off the lateral epicondyle (a discrete lateral UCL is not usually seen, as it is part of the capsule) and tightened with advancement of the capsule on the humerus.

Olecranon Bursitis

Pathoanatomy

Olecranon bursitis is an inflammatory process of the bursa that lies subcutaneously over the olecranon. This bursa increases in size with age and is thought to form in response to movement and friction (54). It is either septic or nonseptic (inflammatory) in nature and can

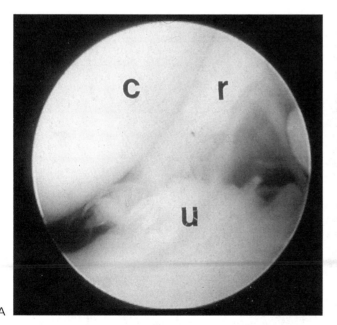
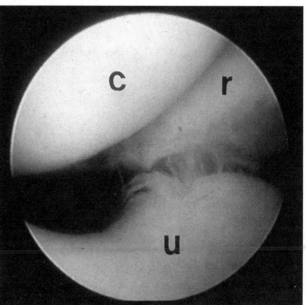

FIG. 19.19. An arthroscopic view of the lateral compartment demonstrating the posterolateral subluxation of the forearm bones on the humerus. **A:** Pre-stress, **B:** with stress. *c,* capitellum; *r,* radius; *u,* ulna.

occur acutely or chronically. Septic bursitis usually occurs after some sort of trauma to the elbow; however, penetration of the bursa is not required. Nonseptic bursitis is thought to be the result of repetitive microtrauma. It is often seen in football linemen and hockey players. It is much more common in football on artificial turf (55). It is thought that the unyielding quality of artificial turf as compared with grass results in an increased incidence of bursitis. It is also seen after repeated traumatic falls onto the elbow with swelling in the bursal sac.

Clinical Evaluation

The history may be an insidious onset of swelling, especially in the presence of a small abrasion or laceration over the bursa. In an acute traumatic onset, one blow to the elbow may lead to an immediate swelling of the bursa. With septic bursitis, the patient can appear quite ill, with the history of severe pain, swelling, tenderness, increased warmth, erythema, and pain with movement of the elbow in addition to systemis symptoms of fever, chills, and an increased white count. Examination of the elbow will show swelling and tenderness over the bursa. With acute septic bursitis, parabursal edema is seen, which may include swelling in the arm and forearm. A white count should be obtained and the temperature of the patient noted.

Imaging

Radiographs of the elbow should be obtained to evaluate for the presence of calcification in the bursal sac, to rule out the presence of a foreign body, and to evaluate the presence of osteophytes on the tip of the olecranon.

Treatment

Nonoperative. Nonoperative treatment is indicated initially, with the exception of a severe septic bursitis in a systemically ill patient. Even with a severe case, a short trial of intravenous antibiotics may significantly improve the symptoms. Aspiration is recommended initially, both to relieve the discomfort of the distended bursa and also to obtain fluid for Gram stain, culture and sensitivity, and to evaluate for the presence of gouty crystals. A compression dressing and elevation of the forearm overhead can significantly improve the swelling in the area.

For chronic nonseptic bursitis, a compressive dressing with immobilization and oral anti-inflammatory agents are indicated. If septic bursitis has been ruled out, an injection of local steroid may aid in reducing the inflammation (56). Once the athlete returns to sports, a protective elbow brace should be used.

Surgical. In acute septic bursitis that does not respond to antibiotic treatment, incision and drainage of the infected bursa are indicated. Excision of the bursa should be performed only after the septic process has resolved. With chronic recurrent nonseptic bursitis that has failed conservative treatment, excision of the bursa should be performed. This can be performed through an incision just lateral to the tip of the olecranon, with care taken to remove the entire bursa. Any osteophytes on the olecranon tip should be debrided. Closure of the defect should be carefully performed, with a compressive dressing placed and the elbow immobilized in a posterior splint. The splint should be used for the first 10 days, followed by a compressive dressing for another 2 to 3 weeks.

Expected Outcome

With appropriate treatment the expected outcome is good. It is important to remember that elbow pads are very useful as a preventive measure in contact sports and also in athletes participating in volleyball and basketball.

REFERENCES

1. Linscheid RL, O'Driscoll SW. Elbow dislocations. In: Morrey BF, ed. *The elbow and its disorders.* Philadelphia: W.B. Saunders, 1994:441–452.
2. Jossefsson PO, Nilsson BE. Incidence of elbow dislocation. *Acta Orthop Scand* 1986;47:537–538.
3. Adams JE. Injury to the throwing arm. *Cal Med* 1965;102:127–132.
4. Torg JS, Pollack H, Sweterlisch P. The effect of competitive pitching on the shoulders and elbows of preadolescent baseball players. *Pediatrics* 1972;49:267–272.
5. Gugenheim JJ, et al. Little League survey: the Houston study. *Am J Sports Med* 1976;4:189–200.
6. Grana WA, Rashkin A. Pitcher's elbow in adolescents. *Am J Sports Med* 1980;8:333–336.
7. Iwase T, Takaaki I. Baseball elbow of young players. *Tokushima J Exp Med* 1985;32:57–64.
8. Fleisig GS, Escamilla RF. Biomechanics of the elbow in the throwing athlete. *Oper Techn Sports Med* 1996;4:69–76.
9. Hotchkiss RN, Weiland AJ. Valgus stability of the elbow. *J Orthop Res* 1987;5:372–377.
10. Dillman C, Smutz P, Werner S. Valgus extension overload in baseball pitching. *Med Sci Sports Exerc* 1991;23 [Suppl]:S136.
11. King J, Brelsford HJ, Tullos HS. Analysis of the pitching arm of the professional baseball pitcher. *Clin Orthop* 1969;67:116–123.
12. O'Driscoll SW, Bell DF, Morrey BF. Posterolateral rotatory instability of the elbow. *J Bone Joint Surg Am* 1991;73A:440–446.
13. Ellenbecker TS, Mattalino AJ, Elam EA, et al. Medial elbow joint laxity in professional baseball pitchers. *Am J Sports Med* 1998;26:420–427.
14. Lee GA, Katz AD, Lazarus MD. Elbow valgus stress radiography in an uninjured population. *Am J Sports Med* 1998;26:425–427.
15. Schwartz ML, Al-Zahrani SA. Diagnostic imaging of elbow injuries in the throwing athlete. *Oper Techn Sports Med* 1996;4:84–90.
16. Timmerman LA, Schwartz ML, Andrews JR. Preoperative evaluation of the ulnar collateral ligament by magnetic resonance imaging and computed tomography arthrography. Evaluation in 25 baseball players with surgical confirmation. *Am J Sports Med* 1994;22:26–32.
17. Jossefsson PO, Johnell O, Wendeberg B. Ligamentous injuries in dislocations of the elbow joint. *Clin Orthop* 1987;221:221–225.
18. Jossefsson PO, Gentx CF, Johnell O, et al. Surgical versus nonsurgical treatment of ligamentous injuries following dislocation of the elbow joint. *J Bone Joint Surg Am* 1987;69A:605–608.

19. Norwood LA, Shook JA, Andrews JR. Acute medial elbow ruptures. *Am J Sports Med* 1981;9:16–19.
20. Timmerman LA, McBride DG. Elbow dislocations in sports. *Sports Med Arthrosc Rev* 1995;3:210–218.
21. Sadat-Ali M. Brachial artery injury in closed elbow dislocations: case report and review of the literature. *Arch Orthop Trauma Surg* 1990;109:288–290.
22. Morrey BF. Elbow dislocation in the athlete. In: DeLee JC, Drez D, eds. *Orthopaedic sports medicine*. Philadelphia: W.B. Saunders, 1994:846–843.
23. Wilson FD, Andrews JR, Blackburn TA, et al. Valgus extension overload in the pitching elbow. *Am J Sports Med* 1993;11:83–88.
24. Andrews JR, Timmerman LA. Outcome of elbow surgery in professional baseball players. *Am J Sports Med* 1995;23:404–413.
25. Andrews JR. Bony injuries about the elbow in the throwing athlete. In: *Instructional course lectures #34*. St. Louis: C.V. Mosby, 1985;323–331.
26. Timmerman LA, Andrews JR. The histologic and arthroscopic anatomy of the ulnar collateral ligament of the elbow. *Am J Sports Med* 1994;22:667–673.
27. Morrey BF, An KN. Articular and ligamentous contributions to the stability of the elbow joint. *Am J Sports Med* 1983;11:315–319.
28. Sojbjerg JO, Ovensen J, Neilsen S. Experimental elbow instability after transection of the medial collateral ligament. *Clin Orthop* 1987;218:186–190.
29. Timmerman LA, Andrews JR. Undersurface tear of the ulnar collateral ligament in baseball players. A newly recognized lesion. *Am J Sports Med* 1994;22:33–36.
30. Jobe FW, Stark A, Lombardo SJ. Reconstruction of the ulnar collateral ligament in athletes. *J Bone Joint Surg Am* 1986;68A:1158.
31. Conway JE, Jobe FW, Glousman RE, Pink M. Medial instability of the elbow in throwing athletes. *J Bone Joint Surg Am* 1992;74A:67–83.
32. Smith GR, Altchek DW, Pagnani MJ, et al. A muscle-splitting approach to the ulnar collateral ligament of the elbow. *Am J Sports Med* 1996;24:575–580.
33. Andrews JR, Timmerman LA. Surgical management of elbow problems in throwers. In: Andrews JR, Zarins B, Wilk KE, eds. *Injuries in baseball*. Philadelphia: Lippincott-Raven, 1998:233–238.
34. Azar FA, Andrews JR, Wilk KE, et al. Ulnar collateral ligament reconstruction of the elbow in athletes. Presented at American Orthopaedic Society for Sports Medicine Speciality Day Meeting, San Francisco, CA, February 1997.
35. Brogdon BG, Crowe NE. Little leaguer's elbow, USAF Hospital, Lackland Air Force Base, Texas Department of Radiology. *Am J Roentgenol* 1960;83:671–675.
36. Panner HJ. A peculiar affectation of the capitellum humeri resembling Calve-Perthes' disease of the hip. *Acta Radiol* 1929;10:234.
37. Woodward AH, Bianco AJ. Osteochondritis dissecans of the elbow. *Clin Orthop* 1975;110:35–41.
38. Indelicato PA, Jobe FW, Kerlan RK, et al. Correctable elbow lesions in professional baseball players. A review of 25 cases. *Am J Sports Med* 1979;7:72–75.
39. Baumgaraten TE, Andrews JR, Satterwhite YE. The arthroscopic classification and treatment of osteochondritis dissecans of the capitellum. *Am J Sports Med* 1998;26:520–523.
40. Jackson DW, Silvino N, Reiman P. Osteochondritis in the female gymnast's elbow. *Arthroscopy* 1989;5:129–136.
41. Ruch DS, Poehling GG. Arthroscopic treatment of Panner's disease. *Clin Sports Med* 1991;10:629–636.
42. Timmerman LA, Andrews JR. Arthroscopic treatment of posttraumatic elbow pain and stiffness. *Am J Sports Med* 1994;22:230–235.
43. Jones GS, Savoie FH III. Arthroscopic capsular release of flexion contractures (arthrofibrosis) of the elbow. *Arthroscopy* 1993;9:277–283.
44. Nowicki KD, Shall LM. Arthroscopic release of a posttraumatic flexion contracture in the elbow: a case report and review of the literature. *Arthroscopy* 1992;8:544–547.
45. Byrd JWT. Elbow arthroscopy for arthrofibrosis after type I radial head fractures. *Arthroscopy* 1994;10:162–165.
46. Hepburn GR, Crivelli KJ. Use of elbow Dynasplint for reduction of elbow flexion contractures: a case study. *J Orthop Sports Phys Ther* 1984;5:269–274.
47. Andrews JR, Schemmel SP, Whiteside JA, et al. Evaluation, treatment, and prevention of elbow injuries in throwing athletes. In: Nichols JA, Hershman EB, eds. *The upper extremity in sports medicine*, 2nd ed. St. Louis: C.V. Mosby, 1995:749–488.
48. Torg JS, Moyer RA. Nonunion of a stress fracture through the olecranon epiphyseal plate observed in an adolescent baseball pitcher. *J Bone Joint Surg Am* 1977;59A:264–265.
49. Regan WD. Acute traumatic sports injuries of the elbow in the athlete. In: Griffin LY, ed. *Sports medicine orthopaedic knowledge update*. Rosemont, IL: American Academy of Orthopaedic Surgeons, 1994:191–203.
50. Morrey BF. Biomechanics of the elbow and forearm. In: DeLee JC, Drez D, eds. *Orthopaedic sports medicine*. Philadelphia: W.B. Saunders, 1994:812–823.
51. Lansinger O, Karlsson J, Korner L, et al. Dislocation of the elbow joint. *Arch Orthop Trauma Surg* 1984;102:183–186.
52. Nestor BJ, O'Drisscoll SW, Morrey BF. Ligamentous reconstruction for posterolateral rotatory instability of the elbow. *J Bone Joint Surg Am* 1992;74A:1235–1241.
53. Imatani J, Hashizume H, Ogura T, et al. Acute posterolateral rotatory subluxation of the elbow joint: a case report. *Am J Sports Med* 1997;25:77–80.
54. Chen J, Alk D, Eventov I, et al. Development of the olecranon bursa: An anatomic cadaveric study. *Acta Orthop Scand* 1987;58:408–409.
55. Larson RL, Osternig LR. Traumatic bursitis and artificial turf. *J Sports Med* 1974;2:183–188.
56. Smith DL, et al. Treatment of nonseptic olecranon bursitis: a controlled, blinded prospective trial. *Arch Intern Med* 1989;149:2527–2530.

Principles and Practice of Orthopaedic Sports Medicine,
edited by William E. Garrett, Jr., Kevin P. Speer, and Donald T. Kirkendall.
Lippincott Williams & Wilkins, Philadelphia © 2000.

CHAPTER 20

Anatomy of the Shoulder

Jeffrey R. Dugas, Bryan T. Kelly, and Stephen J. O'Brien

Proper stability and function of the shoulder allows for directed positioning of the elbow and hand in space. During the course of evolution, articular stability of the shoulder has been exchanged for increased range of motion and greater mobility. This has left the shoulder with relatively less inherent stability when compared with other joints in the human body such as the hip. Treatment of patients with shoulder pathology, whether the result of sports-related activity or not, requires a thorough knowledge of the anatomy and function of the structures that make up the shoulder girdle. This chapter outlines in detail the gross, microscopic, functional, and surgical anatomy of the shoulder girdle.

BONES AND JOINTS

The shoulder is the most proximal joint of the upper extremity. It functions to suspend the arm from the trunk and allows for the placement of the hand in space. The unique mobility of the shoulder allows for a tremendous amount of versatility and a multitude of different hand positions for optimum function (1). The great range of motion at the shoulder is determined by four components of the shoulder complex: the glenohumeral joint, the acromioclavicular joint, the sternoclavicular joint, and the scapulothoracic gliding mechanism (2). These four joints are composed of the three major bones of the shoulder complex: the clavicle, the scapula, and the humerus. The four shoulder complex joints provide the shoulder with three degrees of freedom that permit movement of the upper limb with respect to the three planes in space and the three major axes. First, the transverse axis controls the movements of flexion and extension performed in a sagittal plane. Second, the antero-posterior axis controls the movements of abduction and of adduction, which are performed in the frontal plane. Finally, the vertical axis controls the movements of horizontal flexion and extension, which are performed in a horizontal plane with the arm abducted to 90 degrees (3). The two opposing functions of any joint are for joint mobility and to restrict joint instability and undesirable motion (4). With the high degree of shoulder mobility comes a high predisposition for shoulder instability and dislocation. A detailed understanding of the bony, ligamentous, and muscular anatomy of the shoulder and an understanding of the complex relationships between the bones and joints of the shoulder will demonstrate the delicate balance between functional shoulder mobility and pathologic shoulder instability.

Clavicle

The clavicle, the anterior member of the shoulder girdle, presents as an S-shaped tubular bone with a double curvature, convex anteriorly in the medial two thirds and concave anteriorly in the lateral one third. The major clavicular landmarks are presented in Fig. 20.1. The greater radius of curvature occurs at the medial convex curve, which is roughly triangular in cross-section. The lesser radius of curvature lying at the lateral concave curve is more flattened in a cross-sectional view. It is usually described as consisting of a body (the central two fourths), an outer end (the lateral one fourth), and an inner end (the medial one fourth) (5). The bone consists of trabecular bone within a shell of compact bone and lacks a well-defined medullary cavity (6).

The clavicle is unique in being the only long bone to ossify by the intramembranous process. It is the first bone in the body to ossify, with two primary ossification centers, which later coalesce, appearing near the center of the bone at the fifth week of fetal life. It also contains the last of the epiphyses of the body to fuse, with a third

J. R. Dugas: American Sports Medicine Institute, Birmingham, Alabama 35205.

B. T. Kelly and S. J. O'Brien: The Hospital for Special Surgery, New York, New York 10021.

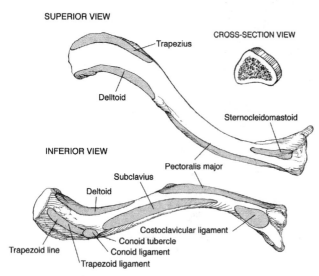

FIG. 20.1. Anteroposterior, superoinferior, and cross-sectional views of clavicle. Note the triangular shape of the mid-clavicle on cross-section. The clavicle has a dual curvature with the medial portion convex anteriorly and the lateral portion concave anteriorly.

ossification center for the sternal end appearing at about the age of 17 and fusing with the shaft at around the age of 25 (6).

There are a number of prominent bony markings on the clavicle. The medial articulation with the sternum is formed by the sternal extremity of the clavicle. This most medial aspect of the bone is triangular in shape and exhibits a slightly flared saddle-shaped articular surface that seats into the clavicular fossa of the manubrium. The costal tubercle also lies on the medial aspect of the bone. This impression represents the attachment of the costoclavicular ligament. A rhomboid fossa can be found in approximately 30% of clavicles at the medial border near the costal tubercle (4). The lateral articulation with the acromion is formed by the acromial extremity. This portion of the bone has an oval articular facet that is tilted slightly downward and lateral. The lateral aspect of the bone has two additional bony markings representing the attachment of the coracoclavicular ligament: the conoid tubercle and the trapezoid line. The coracoclavicular ligament is divided into the conoid ligament and the trapezoid ligament that insert into these two respective prominences. Between the medial and lateral bony prominences lies a long groove into which the subclavius muscle inserts: the groove for the subclavius (6,7).

The clavicle represents the origin of four muscles (the deltoid, the pectoralis major, the sternohyoid, and the sternocleidomastoid muscles) and the insertion for two muscles (the trapezius and the subclavius). Laterally, the deltoid muscle originates from the anterior inner surface and the trapezius inserts at the posterior superior surface. The subclavius muscle inserts into the groove for the subclavius at the inner surface of the

middle third of the clavicle. The pectoralis major, the sternohyoid, and the sternocleidomastoid muscles all originate from the medial clavicle. The pectoralis major muscle has its origin at the anterior surface of the medial third, whereas the sternocleidomastoid and the sternohyoid muscles have their origins from the posterior surface of the medial clavicle (Fig. 20.1).

The clavicle has several important relations to neurovascular structures with the subclavian and the axillary vessels and the nerves of the brachial plexus lying directly posterior to the middle third of the clavicle. These structures are separated from the bone only by the thin subclavius muscle and the clavipectoral fascia (8). The anterior curvature of the middle portion of the clavicle conveniently accommodates the passage of these structures. Although the most common site for fractures of the clavicle is the middle third (8), it is uncommon for clavicular trauma to cause damage to these neurovascular structures (8,9). The clavicle with the first rib together constitute the two skeletal structures defining the thoracic outlet that forms the communicating region at the root of the neck for the passage of great vessels and nerves from the mediastinum and the neck to the axilla (10).

The clavicle serves a number of important functions. Perhaps most importantly, it serves as a rigid base for muscular attachment (as noted above). Additionally, however, it forms a strut that holds the glenohumeral joint out from the trunk, thus facilitating the free movement of the arm and hand in the three planes of movement described earlier (5). This important function allows for the significantly increased motion of the human shoulder. Animals that do not require the use of their upper extremity for grasping (i.e., quadripeds) do not have clavicles (horses). The clavicle also increases the power of the arm–trunk mechanism, particularly in overhead activity (5). This function of the clavicle can be most clearly seen with the detrimental effect that the surgical removal of the clavicle has on heavy overhead activity (11,12). Conversely, excision of the medial portion of the clavicle for such conditions as neoplasms of the clavicle, nonunion of clavicular fractures, arthritis of the sternoclavicular joint, subluxation–dislocation of the sternoclavicular joint, and osteomyelitis of the clavicle has proven to result in insignificant motor weakness (13). Finally, the clavicle provides protection for the major neurovascular structures at the base of the neck described earlier and functions as one of the two major skeletal structures of the thoracic outlet.

Scapula

The scapula is a flattened triangular plate that lies on the dorsolateral aspect of the thorax, spanning the second through seventh ribs. The major scapula anatomic details are depicted in Fig. 20.2. The anterior or costal portion of the scapula is concave and is designed for

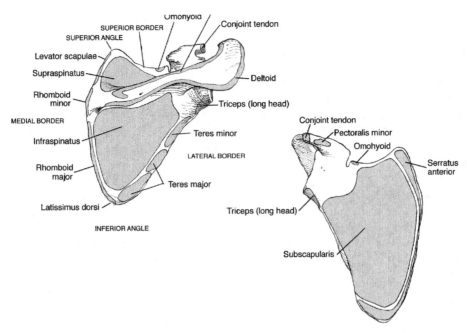

FIG. 20.2. Dorsal and ventral views of the scapula. Note muscular origins and attachments.

the smooth gliding movement across the congruent surface of the convex chest wall (14). The scapula is divided into a number of different discrete entities. The body of the scapula covers the largest surface area and is thin and translucent. The ventral surface of the body is composed of a large shallow concavity known as the subscapular fossa, which is the origin of the subscapularis muscle. The dorsal surface of the body is divided into the supraspinatus fossa (the origin of the supraspinatus muscle) and the infraspinatus fossa (the origin of the infraspinatus muscle). The three borders of the scapular body are the lateral, medial, and superior borders. In addition, the three angles of this right triangle-shaped bone are given the labels of superior, inferior, and medial angles. Four additional thickenings form discrete processes known as the coracoid process, the acromion, the spine, and the glenoid. Two different notches are created by the spine, coracoid and glenoid. The suprascapular notch is formed by the indentation of the base of the coracoid, and the greater scapular notch is formed by the coalition of the base of the spine and the neck of the glenoid. Ossification of the scapula involves at least seven different centers and begins in the eighth week of fetal life. Separate ossification centers are found for the body (one), the medial border (one), the inferior angle (one), the coracoid process (two), and the acromion (two) (6).

The thickened processes found throughout the scapula are formed by its numerous muscular attachments, 18 in all (Fig. 20.2). The thickest of these prominences lie at the superior and inferior angles and the lateral border of the body of the scapula. The lateral border exhibits thickenings at the flattened area of origin for

the teres major muscle directly above the inferior angle. The lateral border is also the site of origin for the teres minor and the long head of the triceps brachii muscle moving proximally from the inferior angle. A small slip of origin of the latissimus dorsi muscle is found directly off the inferior angle. The medial border (also known as the base) is the longest of the borders. This relatively straight border is the site of insertion for the levator scapulae and rhomboideus major and minor muscles on the dorsal side and the serratus anterior on the costal side. The superior border is the thinnest and shortest of the borders and is the site for the origin of the omohyoid muscle that lies immediately posterior to the medial side of the suprascapular notch. Additional muscular attachments are found on the coracoid: pectoralis minor, short head of the biceps brachii, and the coracobrachialis muscles; the acromion and spine of the scapula: the deltoid and trapezius muscles; and the glenoid, the long head of the biceps brachii muscle. The major ligamentous attachments of the scapula include the transverse scapular, coracoacromial, coracoglenoid, coracoclavicular, coracohumeral, acromioclavicular, and glenohumeral ligaments. These are discussed in more detail in the individual sections discussing each of the shoulder complex joints.

The coracoid process is a thick, anterior, upward projection from the neck of the glenoid (Fig. 20.2). It gives rise to the origin of two muscles (short head of the biceps brachii and the coracobrachialis), the insertion of a third muscle (pectoralis minor), and the attachment of numerous ligaments (coracoacromial, coracoglenoid, coracoclavicular, coracohumeral). Impingement of the tendinous sheath of the rotator cuff muscles beneath the coracoacromial arch is an established cause of chronic shoulder pain and disability (15–18). Because of its role in shoulder impingement, the coracoid is a much studied process. Specific attention has been placed on identifying precise radiographic and geometric measurements of the coracoid (19,20), variations in coracoacromial ligament anatomy (21–23), and anatomic relationships of the coracoid and coracoid ligaments as they relate to arthroscopy of the shoulder (24,25). Investigations on the coracoid have identified anatomic variations, including abnormal connections between the coracoid and the clavicle (26) and bony bridging of the suprascapular notch (27). The role of the coracohumeral ligament in shoulder stability and in pathologic conditions such as the frozen shoulder has also been studied (28,29).

The spine of the scapula is a bony prominence found on the dorsal aspect of the scapula that separates the supraspinatus and infraspinatus fossae. It extends from the medial border to just short of the glenoid fossa and if followed laterally ends in the acromion process. Both the spine of the scapula and the acromion serve as the origin of the deltoid muscle and the insertion for the trapezius muscle. The spine of the scapula is the least studied process as it has relatively little role in shoulder impingement syndromes or shoulder instability. However, research in the otolaryngology literature in which the scapular spine has been sacrificed for mandibular reconstruction procedures has demonstrated devastating results on subsequent shoulder function (30).

The acromion is the lateral-most projection of the spine of the scapula, forming the "roof" of the adult scapula. The acromion is roughly triangular in shape with a thick base and a thinner terminal portion. It is directed laterally at its base but curves anteriorly toward its most terminal portion. Its roughened, upper, convex portion is the site for the origin of some deltoid muscle fibers, and its concave inner margin serves as the site of insertion of a portion of the trapezius muscle. The attachment of the coracoacromial ligament is found at the apex of the acromion process anteriorly. The smooth, concave, undersurface is closely opposed by the subacromial bursa, and the medial-most portion of the process forms a smooth facet for articulation with the clavicle (6).

The acromion process has been extensively studied because of its well-established role in shoulder impingement pathology (17). Numerous studies have investigated the topographic anatomy of the acromion and provided detailed descriptions of painful shoulder motion arcs responsible for impingement-producing maneuvers (31–35). It is generally accepted that rotator cuff tendonitis and subacromial bursitis are related to soft tissue irritation and impingement of the head of the humerus underneath the coracoacromial arch in an area that is known as the supraspinatus outlet (36). It is believed that variations in acromial morphology can predispose patients to an increased risk for rotator cuff pathology (37).

In 1986 Bigliani and April (38) described three distinct acromial shapes in cadavers on the basis of lateral scapular view radiographs as depicted in Fig. 20.3. These shapes (type I, flat; type II, curved; type III, hooked) have been correlated with the incidence of rotator cuff tears (39,40). These cadaveric and patient studies demonstrated that 70% to 80% of cuff tears were associated with type III acromions, 20% to 30% of cuff tears were associated with type II acromions and only 0% to 3% associated with type I acromions. Other studies have suggested that the use of this classification system has a fair to poor level of interobserver reliability and that the diagnosis of impingement and rotator cuff tears should be based on clinical findings supplemented, when indicated, by rotator cuff imaging with less diagnostic reliance placed on the assessment of acromial morphology (41).

Significant changes in acromial morphology with age have been suggested. Wang (42) looked at the acromial morphology with respect to age in 272 patients. He concluded that the incidence of the three acromial types varies with age and that type I acromions may progress to type II acromions and then further change into type III acromions over time. Others have concluded that the variations seen in acromial morphologic condition are not acquired from age-related changes and spur formation and thus contribute to impingement disease independent of and in addition to age-related processes (43).

The acromion has two, and occasionally three, ossification centers. Liberson (44) looked at acromions with unfused epiphyses and classified them according to location as pre-acromion, meso-acromion, meta-acromion, and basi-acromion. According to Neer in 1983 (45), there is no significant increase in the number of unfused acromions associated with acromioplasties.

The glenoid cavity is formed by the broadened lateral angle of the scapula and is supported by the glenoid neck (Fig. 20.4). It is slightly pear shaped with a greater

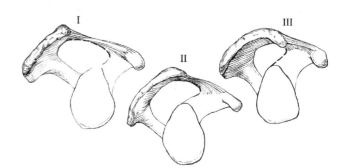

FIG. 20.3. Three types of acromion as first described by Bigliani et al. Type I is flat from anterior and posterior. Type II shows a gentle curvature from front to back. Type III has a prominent "hook" anteriorly that projects anteroinferiorly and can be a source of impingement in the subacromial space.

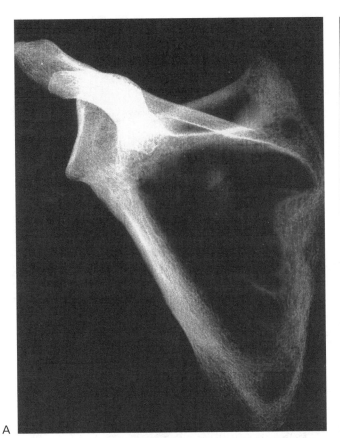

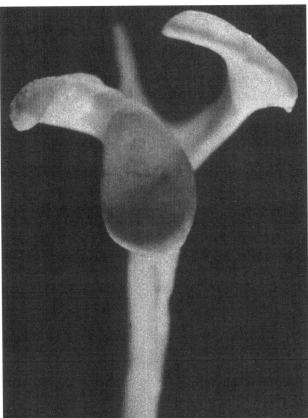

A

C

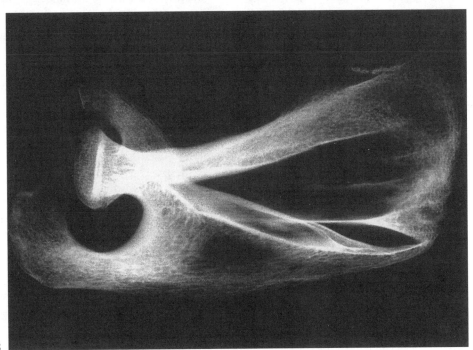

B

FIG. 20.4. (A) Anteroposterior, **(B)** superoinferior, and **(C)** lateral views of glenoid and scapula. On the lateral view **(C)**, the glenoid is shaped like an inverted "comma." The glenoid is wider superiorly than it is inferiorly. Note also the subtle lateral to medial slope of the glenoid as you look from inferior to superior. Although the glenoid is anteverted when referenced against a line perpendicular to the body axis, it is retroverted when referenced against the blade of the scapula.

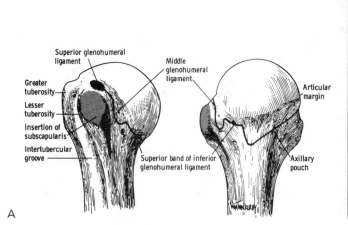
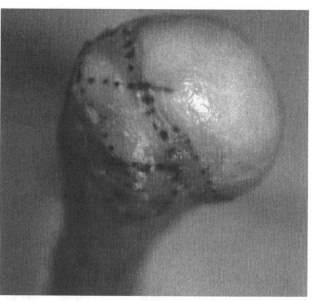

A

B

FIG. 20.5. (A) Diagrams of the proximal humerus including the insertion of the shoulder capsule and glenohumeral ligaments. **B:** Width and dimensions of the insertion of the rotator cuff musculature onto the greater tuberosity.

vertical dimension than horizontal dimension. The margin of the glenoid socket provides attachment for the fibrocartilaginous glenoid labrum. This circular, pliable, fibrous labrum contributes approximately 50% of the total depth of the socket (46). A bony prominence known as the supraglenoid tubercle represents the location for the origin of the long head of the biceps brachii tendon. The articular surface of the glenoid has an average of 6 degrees of retroversion with respect to the blade of the scapula (47). The glenoid socket and labrum combine to create a socket that is approximately 9 mm deep in the superoinferior direction and 5 mm deep in the anteroposterior direction (46). The relative contribution of the glenoid socket and labrum to shoulder stability has not been completely elucidated.

Humerus

The humerus is a long bone composed of a shaft and two articular extremities. The proximal humerus forms part of the shoulder joint and consists of the humeral head, lesser tuberosity, greater tuberosity, bicipital groove, and proximal humeral shaft (Fig. 20.5). The proximal humeral shaft can be divided into the anatomic neck and the surgical neck. The anatomic neck is the slight indentation of the head margin for the attachment of the articular capsule and lies at the junction of the head and the tuberosities. The surgical neck is the narrowed area of the shaft just distal to the greater and lesser tuberosities (48). The proximal humerus develops from three centers of ossification that coalesce between 4 and 6 years and fuse with the humeral metaphysis

between 20 and 23 years. The central articular segment epiphysis appears within 4 to 6 months of birth, the greater tuberosity epiphysis appears at approximately 3 years of age, and the lesser tuberosity epiphysis appears at approximately 5 years (49–51).

The humeral head is usually described as facing superiorly at 135 degrees to the shaft and posteriomedially such that it is retroverted 35 to 40 degrees relative to the epicondylar axis of the distal humerus (Fig. 20.6) (52–54). Numerous other important measurements defining the geometry of the humeral head have been calculated (55). The average radius of curvature of the humeral head in the coronal plane has been calculated between 2.25 (56) and 2.4 cm with a range of 1.9 to 2.8 cm (57). The average thickness of the humeral head has been calculated to be 19 ± 2.4 mm (57). There is a wide range in the size of the humeral head, and a direct correlation exists between the differences in size and

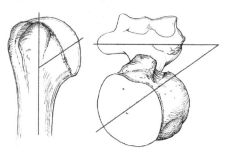

FIG. 20.6. Version of the humeral head and neck in relation to the epicondylar axis.

the heights in both men and women (57). The humeral head size strongly correlates with the lateral humeral offset, which has an average distance of 56 mm (57). The lateral humeral offset determines the position of the greater tuberosity and the rotator cuff insertions and has a significant effect on the mechanics of the rotator cuff muscles (49).

The greater tuberosity represents the most laterally projecting part of the skeleton of the shoulder. It lies just caudal to the most cephalad surface of the articular segment. It serves as the insertion site for the supraspinatus, infraspinatus, and teres minor tendons. Compression of the greater tuberosity, the supraspinatus tendon, and the biceps tendon is believed to cause impingement pain (32). Forward elevation of the humerus in the plane of the scapula results in impingement of the greater tuberosity against the anterior edge of the acromion (34).

The lesser tuberosity is separated from the greater tuberosity by the intertubercular groove. It lies directly anteriorly and is the site for the insertion of the subscapularis tendon. Both the greater tuberosity and lesser tuberosity have bony extensions distally known, respectively, as the crest of the greater tuberosity and the crest of the lesser tuberosity. The pectoralis major muscle inserts into the crest, extending from the greater tuberosity and the teres major muscle inserts into the crest extending from the lesser tuberosity.

The intertubercular groove (bicipital groove) lying approximately 1 cm lateral to the midline of the humerus lodges the long tendon of the biceps brachii muscle that traverses from its origin on the superior lip of the glenoid (47,52). Extensive anatomic studies of the course of the long head of the biceps tendon suggest a number of different anatomic variations to the origin of this structure. Vangsness et al. (58) report approximately 50% of biceps tendons arise directly from the superior glenoid labrum with the remainder attached to the supraglenoid tubercle. Bicipital tendon dislocations out of the bicipital groove have been reported for many years (59–61). The transverse humeral ligament or intertubercular ligament acts as a roof over the bicipital groove but provides minimal support in retaining the long biceps tendon in the sulcus (16,60). Some authors argue that it is the coracohumeral ligament that provides the primary restraint to dislocation of the long tendon of the biceps brachii (28,62). There are varying opinions on the incidence of biceps tendon dislocation. According to Neviaser (63), this syndrome is more common than anterior shoulder subluxation and often misdiagnosed. Others (34,64) believe that isolated biceps dislocation is extremely rare and is more commonly associated with a large tear of the rotator cuff or a fracture of the lesser tuberosity with resulting medial displacement of the tendon. The role of the long head of the biceps brachii tendon itself is not universally agreed upon. Some believe that the tendon serves as a humeral head stabilizer during elbow flexion and forearm supination (65,66). Others believe that it has an insignificant role in shoulder stabilization and functions primarily at the elbow joint (67).

The bicipital groove also receives the tendon of the latissimus dorsi muscle into its floor and the teres major muscle just medial to the groove. The pectoralis major muscle inserts into the humerus just lateral to the bicipital groove and inferior to the greater tuberosity. Distal to the bicipital groove, two additional muscles insert into the humerus approximately at the midshaft level, otherwise known as the body of the humerus. The coracobrachialis muscle inserts medially, and the prominent deltoid tuberosity is located directly laterally for the insertion of the deltoid muscle.

A slight indentation at the base of the humeral head margin represents the space between the articular cartilage of the head and the ligamentous and tendon attachments of the articular capsule (Fig. 20.5A). This region at the junction of the head and tuberosities is known as the anatomic neck of the humerus. It corresponds to the physeal line of the central articular segment. Fractures at the level of the anatomic neck of the humerus are rare and have a poor prognosis because the blood supply to the humeral head is completely disrupted. The surgical neck of the humerus is located at the level below the greater and lesser tuberosities. The line defining the surgical neck is somewhat indistinct. Surgical neck fractures are very common and have a reasonably good prognosis as the blood supply to the head is preserved (48). Codman (68) noted that most proximal humerus fractures occurred along the lines of the former physes of the proximal humerus and developed a four-segment classification system (anatomic neck, surgical neck, greater tuberosity, and lesser tuberosity). Neer (69) expanded this four-segment system to include degrees of angulation and displacement of each of the four fracture fragments. His system is based on the position of the articular segment, the greater and lesser tuberosities, and the humeral shaft and attempts to predict the effect of displacement on rotator cuff function, glenohumeral biomechanics, and articular segment vascularity (69).

Sternoclavicular Joint

The sternoclavicular joint is a diarthrodial joint that represents the only bony connection between the trunk and the upper limb (Fig. 20.7). This joint simulates in its actions a ball and socket joint, although it demonstrates less bony stability than any other joint of the body (70). It is composed of the upper end of the sternum and the proximal end of the clavicle. The two surfaces of the joint are saddle shaped and are reciprocally concavoconvex. The clavicle, which is larger than the opposing

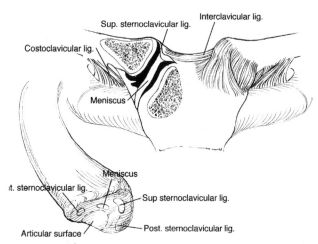

FIG. 20.7. (A) Anteroposterior and **(B)** superoinferior views of the sternoclavicular joint. Note the relative incongruence of the joint and the ligamentous attachments which provide stability in multiple planes.

sternum in both the anteroposterior and vertical dimensions, is convex in the coronal plane and concave in the transverse plane. The sternal end forms an articular fossa formed by the superolateral angle of the manubrium and the medial part of the cartilage of the first rib. The joint angles in a posteromedial direction, and its surfaces are covered with hyaline cartilage.

The two articular surfaces of the sternoclavicular joint do not have reciprocally similar radii of curvatures, which leads to significant joint incongruity. Congruence of the surfaces is improved by an intraarticular disk that separates the joint into two compartments: the discosternal and the discoclavicular (71). This fibrocartilaginous disk has a strong internal structure that buffers against joint stress and strain. Strong sinewy fibers of connective tissue are intertwined completely and interspaced with fusifom cells and true cartilage cells (71). The disk is convex–concave in configuration, with a thickened circumference and superior portion. It is attached to the upper and posterior aspect of the articular surface of the clavicle superiorly and to the cartilage of the first rib at its junction with the sternum inferiorly. Rarely, the disk is perforated, thus allowing free communication between the two compartments (71).

The intraarticular disk significantly improves joint motion and stability. Additional joint stability is provided by its surrounding extraarticular ligaments and its articular capsule that surrounds the joint and attaches to the clavicular and sternochondral articular surfaces. The capsule is weak inferiorly but is reinforced by the strong capsular ligaments known as the anterior and posterior sternoclavicular ligaments. The anterior sternoclavicular ligament may be the strongest ligament of the sternoclavicular joint and is reinforced by the tendinous origin of the sternocleidomastoid muscle (72).

The capsular ligament fibers run superiorly from their attachment to the sternum to their superior attachment on the clavicle. Together they are thought to be the most important structures in preventing upward displacement of the medial clavicle and inferior depression of the lateral clavicle (72). The interclavicular ligament passes from the superomedial aspect of each clavicle and is attached to the upper border of the sternum between. This ligament strengthens the capsule from above and tightens as the lateral end of the clavicle is depressed, assisting the capsular ligaments to hold up the shoulder. It may be absent or nonpalpable in up to 22% of the population (13).

A great deal of joint stability depends on the integrity of the costoclavicular ligament. This short, flat, rhomboid-shaped structure consists of an anterior and posterior fasciculus and runs between the cartilage of the first rib and the costal tuberosity on the undersurface of the clavicle (73). The anterior fibers arise from the anterior medial surface of the first rib and extend up laterally, whereas the posterior fibers arise from a more lateral position and extend up medially. The function of the costoclavicular ligament is principally to oppose the pull of the sternocleidomastoid muscle on the clavicle. The anterior fibers resist upward rotation and lateral displacement, whereas the posterior fibers resist downward rotation and medial displacement (72). The attachment of the costoclavicular ligament on to the clavicle has been described as one of three types. Thirty percent attach to a depression in the clavicle known as the rhomboid fossa. Sixty percent attach to a flat clavicular surface. And ten percent attach to an elevated surface off of the clavicle (73). The tendon of the subclavius muscle inserts directly lateral and anterior to the ligament.

The sternoclavicular joint receives its blood supply from the clavicular branch of the thoracoacromial artery. Additional contributions come from the internal mammary and the suprascapular arteries. The nerve to subclavius and the medial supraclavicular nerve provide neural input to the joint.

The sternoclavicular joint is the most frequently moved articulation in the body with almost all upper extremity motion being transferred proximally through the joint (74). Analysis of the movements of the joint reveal that it moves freely in almost all planes (75,76). Elevation and depression is performed about a sagittal axis, anteroposterior motion occurs about a perpendicular axis, and longitudinal rotation is executed about its length axis (74). The excursion of the joint during upward elevation is approximately 30 to 35 degrees. Anteroposterior excursion is approximately 35 degrees, and longitudinal rotation is approximately 45 to 50 degrees. Sternoclavicular joint elevation is greatest with shoulder elevation of 30 to 90 degrees, and rotation is greatest at 70 to 80 degrees of shoulder elevation (75). Fusion of the sternoclavicular joint limits shoulder abduction to 90 degrees (4). The overall mechanism of the shoulder girdle depends on a close interaction between the sternoclavicular joint and the acromioclavicular joint. As the sternal end of the clavicle moves in one direction, the acromial end moves in the opposite direction with the center of the axis of motion passing through the costoclavicular ligament (74).

Sternoclavicular dislocations are uncommon injuries and are classified as either anterior or posterior in nature. Patients that are younger than 25 years of age may present with a fracture–dislocation injury to the growth plate. The mechanism of injury is usually a direct force or blow on the point of the shoulder or on the clavicle itself. Posterior dislocations are potentially more serious than anterior dislocations because of the subjacent mediastinal and cervical structures. These patients may have resultant compression of the esophagus or trachea and compression of major vascular structures mandating careful neurovascular assessment (49). The sternohyoid, sternothyroid, and scalene muscles lie directly over a vast array of vital mediastinal structures, including the innominate artery, innominate vein, vagus nerve, phrenic nerve, internal jugular vein, anterior jugular vein, trachea, and esophagus (4). Thus, any surgical intervention around this region must be performed with extreme caution.

Acromioclavicular Joint

The acromioclavicular joint is a small synovial joint that lies between the oval articular surface of the lateral end of the clavicle and the medial border of the acromion process of the scapula (Fig. 20.8). This diarthrodial joint is the only articulation between the clavicle and the scapula with the exception of a small percentage of people who have a coracoclavicular joint (77). The ends of both the clavicle and the acromion are covered with hyaline cartilage (74), although some authors have reported degenerative changes in the late teens and early twenties, resulting in the hyaline cartilage transformation to fibrocartilage (78). The joint surfaces slope downward and medially, and there is variability with regard to the relationship of the two bony ends. Urist (79) classified anatomic variations in the articulation of the joint and reported a 49% incidence of superior overriding of the clavicle on the acromion and a 3% incidence of inferior underriding of the clavicle relative to the acromion. Only 27% of the joints examined in his study demonstrated horizontal alignment of the clavicle and the acromion in the same plane. Other authors have confirmed these anatomic variations (80,81).

As with the sternoclavicular joint, the articular surfaces of the acromioclavicular joint exhibit pronounced incongruity. Also similar to the sternoclavicular joint, a small, thin, intraarticular disk can be found between the bony articulation. This fibrocartilaginous disk can be either complete or perforated forming a meniscoid shape (74). Unlike the intraarticular disk of the sternoclavicular joint, there is a significantly higher incidence of perforated disks in the acromioclavicular joint (71,82). The acromioclavicular joint disk undergoes rapid deterioration, which first occurs in the second decade and, in most cases, results in complete obliteration by the fourth decade (74).

The acromioclavicular joint is enclosed by an articular capsule that attaches to the articular margins and is reinforced above by the superior acromioclavicular ligament and below by the inferior acromioclavicular ligament (74). Thickenings of the capsule on the anterior and posterior borders are sometimes referred to as the

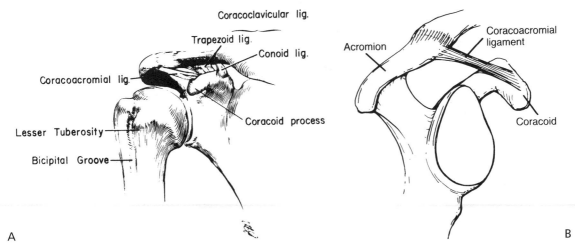

FIG. 20.8. (A and B) Two views of the acromioclavicular joint. The coracoclavicular ligaments (conoid and trapezoid) stabilize this articulation by resisting superior displacement of the clavicle, whereas the acromioclavicular (AC) joint capsule and ligament prevent anterior and posterior translation. The coracoacromial ligament is also demonstrated.

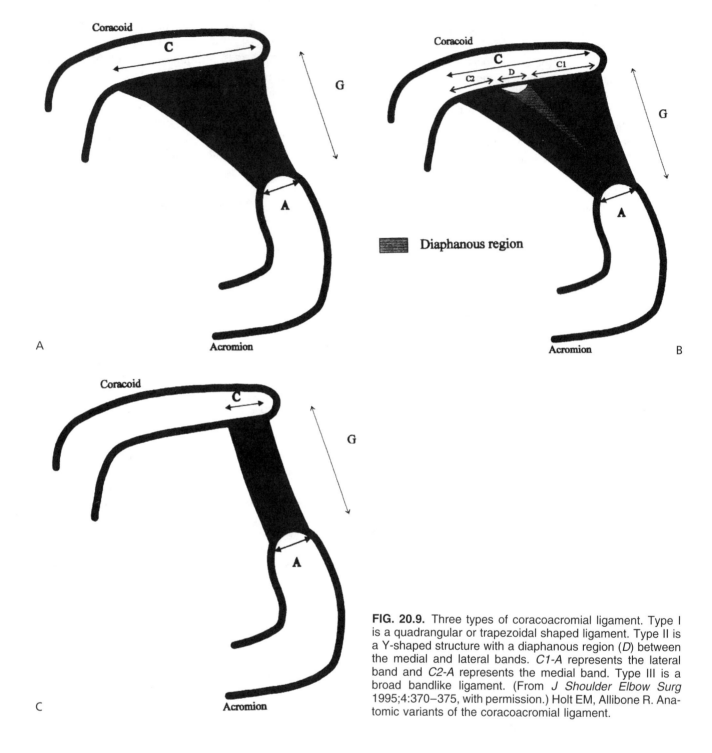

FIG. 20.9. Three types of coracoacromial ligament. Type I is a quadrangular or trapezoidal shaped ligament. Type II is a Y-shaped structure with a diaphanous region (*D*) between the medial and lateral bands. *C1-A* represents the lateral band and *C2-A* represents the medial band. Type III is a broad bandlike ligament. (From *J Shoulder Elbow Surg* 1995;4:370–375, with permission.) Holt EM, Allibone R. Anatomic variants of the coracoacromial ligament.

anterior and posterior acromioclavicular ligaments (4). Much of the integrity of this joint depends on the strong fibers of the superior acromioclavicular ligament and the insertion of the deltoid and the trapezius muscles into the clavicle and the acromion. The role of the acromioclavicular ligament in the stability of the joint was first described by Urist in 1946 (79). He demonstrated that when the anterior part of the acromioclavicular ligament and capsule was divided, posterior joint

subluxation of approximately 50% occurred. He was able to completely dislocate the joint posteriorly and subluxate the joint superiorly, when the entire capsule and the trapezius and deltoid muscle attachments were divided.

More recent serial cutting studies by Fukuda et al. (83) confirmed the role of the acromioclavicular ligament as a constraining force to posterior displacement. Fukuda et al. further demonstrated, however, that the contributions of the different ligaments in the acromioclavicular joint to joint stability varied not only with the direction of the force but also with the amount of loading and displacement. For many directions of displacement, the acromioclavicular joint contributed a greater amount to constraint at smaller degrees of displacement and lesser amounts of loading. His group found that the acromioclavicular ligament contributed an increased percentage (up to two thirds) of the constraining force to superior displacement when lesser amounts of induced load were applied (such as those experienced in daily activities) (83). Their study also demonstrated that the acromioclavicular ligament acted as a primary constraint for posterior axial rotation of the clavicle.

In addition to acromioclavicular stabilization by the capsular acromioclavicular ligament, the joint is also stabilized by the extracapsular coracoclavicular ligament. This ligament is a very strong heavy structure composed of two fasciculi called the conoid and trapezoid ligaments (Fig. 20.8). The posteromedial conoid ligament lies at the base of the coracoid process and attaches to the conoid tubercle on the posterior undersurface of the clavicle. The trapezoid ligament arises from the coracoid process anterior and lateral to the conoid origin and extends superiorly to a rough line on the undersurface of the clavicle, extending anteriorly and laterally from the conoid tubercle. The role of the coracoclavicular ligament in joint stabilization was first described by Urist (79). From his serial cutting studies he concluded that injury to the coracoclavicular ligaments allowed increased displacement of the clavicle, especially in the superior direction. Fukuda et al. (83) demonstrated more precise stabilizing roles of the conoid and trapezoid ligaments. In their study, the conoid ligament provided primary constraint to anterior and superior rotation and anterior and superior displacement of the clavicle. The trapezoid ligament, on the other hand, contributed less to clavicular movement in the horizontal and vertical planes, except when the clavicle moved in axial compression toward the acromion process. As noted earlier, Fukuda et al. demonstrated varying amounts of constraining force from each of the joint ligaments with varying amounts of loading and displacement. In general, they found the conoid ligament to contribute a greater amount of constraint with larger amounts of displacement and force.

The coracoacromial ligament has been traditionally described as a flat triangular structure with its base on the superior lateral side of the coracoid and its apex of insertion into the tip of the acromion anterior to the acromioclavicular joint (21). Holt and Allibone (22) described three main types of coracoacromial ligament shapes: quadrangular, Y-shaped, and a broad band (Fig. 20.9). This ligament does not play a significant role in acromioclavicular joint stabilization. According to Tillmann (84), the coracoacromial ligament acts as a tension band within the humeral fossa and reduces the bending movement of the coracoid process and of the acromion, thus serving to counteract the action of the pectoralis minor and of the coracobrachialis and the short head of the biceps brachii. Perhaps most significantly, it contributes to the coracoacromial arch with the coracoid process and anterior tip of the acromion and has been implicated as a source for impingement pain (32).

The acromioclavicular joint receives its blood supply from the acromial artery, a branch of the deltoid artery off the thoracoacromial axis. Additional contributions come from anastomoses between this artery, the suprascapular artery, and the posterior humeral circumflex artery. The lateral pectoral, axillary, and suprascapular nerves provide neural input to the joint.

There is variation in opinion regarding the total range of motion of the acromioclavicular joint. Original work by Inman et al. (75) reported that the total motion about the joint was approximately 20 degrees and that the motion occurred in the first 30 degrees of abduction and after 135 degrees of elevation of the arm. Inman et al. also reported acromioclavicular joint rotation of approximately 40 to 50 degrees with full elevation of the arm. Others have reported significantly less total acromioclavicular joint range of motion. Codman (68) reported only 5 degrees of motion about the joint. Rockwood and Matsen (4) reported only 5 to 8 degrees of motion detected between two pins placed in the acromioclavicular joint and measured during full range of motion of the shoulder. Further evidence for minimal range of motion at the acromioclavicular joint is suggested by nearly undetectable changes in shoulder motion after fusion of the acromioclavicular joint (48).

Scapulothoracic Joint

The concave scapula sits congruently against the ribs and smoothly glides against the convex chest wall, with its undersurface being cushioned from the ribs by the serratus anterior and subscapularis muscles (Fig. 20.2) (14). It plays an important role in arm function by stabilizing the upper extremity against the thorax and linking the upper extremity and the axial skeleton through the glenoid, acromioclavicular, clavicular, and sternoclavicular joints. The scapula sits in a resting position of approximately 30 degrees anterior rotation with respect to the frontal plane when viewed from above, 3 degrees of upward rotation with respect to the sagittal plane, and 20 degrees of forward tilt or anteflexion with respect to the frontal plane when viewed from the side (4). The motion of the shoulder joint is greater than any other joint in the body. Total shoulder complex motion consists of approximately 0 to 180 degrees of elevation, 150 degrees of internal and external rotation, and 170 degrees of flexion and extension (85). Most of this motion occurs as a composite of joint motion from the glenohumeral and scapulothoracic joints. The specific contributions of motion about these two joints during arm movement has been extensively studied and has been termed scapulohumeral rhythm (47,68,75,86,87). The relative contribution of the scapulothoracic joint to shoulder motion is described below. The basic movements of the scapulothoracic joint consist of medial and lateral displacement, elevation and depression, and tilting or rotation (sometimes referred to as protraction and retraction) (3). When the scapula moves medially, it moves progressively into the frontal plane, and when it moves laterally, it moves progressively into the sagittal plane. The total range of movement of the scapula in the horizontal plane during medial and lateral displacement forms a solid angle of 40 to 45 degrees and, in an average adult male, may translate up to 15 cm. Total range of motion of the scapula during the vertical movements of elevation and depression averages 10 to 12 cm. Total range of motion during scapula rotation is approximately 60 degrees (3).

Injury to the scapulothoracic joint is relatively rare. Dislocation of the scapula between the ribs and into the thoracic cage has been described by different authors (88–90). Some patients with preexisting conditions such as generalized laxity or locking osteochondroma may lodge the medial border of the scapula between the third and fourth ribs or in the fourth to fifth intercostal space with little violence (88,90). Other authors have reported scapula dislocation with violent trauma, which is usually associated with fracture of the scapula and ribs and tearing of the rhomboid muscles (89).

Scapulothoracic dissociation must be differentiated from scapulothoracic dislocation. This injury is caused by violent lateral or rotational displacement of the shoulder girdle with severe soft tissue injury, resulting in devastating vascular and neurologic effects. Oreck et al. (91) first described the injury as the result of severe blunt trauma or sudden forceful traction applied to the shoulder. They reported on three patients with severe blunt injury to the shoulder and an injury pattern of massive soft tissue injury to the shoulder, complete acromioclavicular joint separation, avulsion of the brachial plexus and subclavian artery, multiple open wounds, and closed fractures of the ipsilateral humerus, radius, and ulna. The injury was characterized radiographically by lateral displacement of the scapula and complete separation of the acromioclavicular joint. The displaced scapula results from disruption of the muscular attachments of the scapula, leading to impressive swelling and ecchymosis. With the skin remaining intact, this injury is essentially a closed forequarter amputation. Others have reported case series of scapulothoracic dissociations (92–94). This severe injury represents a spectrum of musculoskeletal, neurologic, and vascular injuries caused by lateral distraction or rotational displacement forces applied to the shoulder. The outcome of this injury is clearly dependent on the severity of the injury. Severe brachial plexus injury has been reported to be present in 90% of all case reports. A systematic and rational approach to clinical decision making is necessary in determining the most appropriate treatment intervention for this devastating injury.

Disruptions in the smooth articulation of the scapula on the thorax may result in scapulothoracic crepitus or "snapping scapula" (14). Often, snapping scapula is the result of abnormal anatomy, such as fracture or malunion, or pathologic processes, such as scapular exostoses (Luschka's tubercle), Sprengel's deformity, or healing rib fractures (95,96). Soft tissue abnormalities such as muscle insertion avulsions, scar formation, and bursa inflammation may also result in snapping scapula (97). Scapulothoracic crepitus, however, may not always have an anatomic source nor be the result of a pathologic condition. Often, no localized anatomic diagnosis for the snapping scapula is made, and palliative treatment including local care with heat and scapular adduction and postural shoulder shrug exercises is all that can be done (4).

Glenohumeral Joint

The glenohumeral joint is a diarthrodial joint that is formed by a unique synovial articulation resulting in a high degree of mobility balanced with stability throughout the motion range (98). The bony articulation between the glenoid and the humeral head offers very little inherent stability due to the shape and contour of the two surfaces. Glenohumeral stability is maintained, however, by a variety of factors, including both static and dynamic constraints, limited joint volume, and negative intraarticular pressure (98,99). There has been much research focusing on the articular geometry at the glenohumeral joint to provide an anatomic explanation for the inherent instability of the joint complex (47,52,57,100,101). Iannotti et al. (57) performed extensive cadaveric dissections on 140 shoulders to quantify average glenohumeral joint dimensions. In this study, the average thickness of the humeral head in both the coronal and axial planes was 20 mm. The average radius of curvature of the humeral head in the coronal plane was 24 mm and in the axial plane 22 mm. The average neck-shaft angle was 45 degrees. The glenoid demonstrated a pear-shaped configuration with the ratio of the lower half to the top half being 1:0.80. The average anterior to posterior width was found to be 29 mm at the lower half and 23 mm at the upper half. The average superior to inferior height of the glenoid was found to be 39 mm. The radius of curvature of the glenoid, measured in the coronal plane, was an average of 2.3 mm greater than the humeral head. The articular surface of the joint was found to be spherical in the central portion but slightly elliptical in the peripheral dimension. There was a strong linear correlation between the lateral humeral offset and the size of the humeral head. The average lateral humeral offset was found to be 56 mm, and it was believed that reconstruction of the lateral humeral offset was important in optimization of the moment arm of the deltoid and rotator cuff and of the normal tension of the soft tissue after shoulder reconstruction (57).

Saha performed contact studies in 20 cadaveric shoulders in which he described three variations in articular anatomy (47) (Fig. 20.10). In type A articulations, the radius of curvature of the humeral head is smaller than that of the glenoid and results in a small circular area of articulation centered in the glenoid cavity. Type B articulations are characterized by similar radii of curvature leading to a larger circular area of contact. In type C articulations, the radius of curvature of the head is greater than that of the glenoid. This configuration leads to a peripheral ring-shaped area of articulation (102). In contrast to the hip joint, the glenohumeral joint does not offer a deep stabilizing socket. The small arc of the glenoid captures very little of the humeral articular surface so that neck-rim contact and impingement is avoided throughout the wide range of shoulder motion (47,103,104). In fact, only 25% to 30% of the humeral head is covered by the glenoid throughout the range of glenohumeral motion (68,85,105). Saha described a measure of this relative uncovering as the glenohumeral index which is determined by the formula

$$\frac{\text{Maximum diameter of the glenoid}}{\text{Maximum diameter of the humeral head}} \times 100$$

The original work by Saha described average vertical and transverse glenohumeral indices. The mean value for the vertical glenohumeral index was 75%, and the mean value for the transverse index was 58%. Saha (47) believed that the transverse glenohumeral index

(smaller than the vertical) plays a more important role in the maintenance of horizontal stability.

As mentioned previously, motion of the shoulder complex is greater than any other joint in the body. This motion occurs primarily at the glenohumeral and scapulothoracic joints, although there are minor contributions from the acromioclavicular and sternoclavicular joints at extremes of the motion arc. The arm can move through an arc of motion of approximately 180-degree elevation, 150-degree internal and external rotation, and 170 degrees of flexion and extension (anterior and posterior rotation in the horizontal plane) (85).

Elevation of the shoulder is the most important movement of this joint and has been extensively studied by numerous authors (47,68,75,86,87,106–108). The relative contribution of the glenohumeral joint and the scapulothoracic joint during shoulder motion is known as scapulohumeral rhythm. Early studies by Steindler (85) reported the first 90 degrees of motion to be dependent on glenohumeral motion, followed by scapulothoracic rotation. Numerous subsequent studies have confirmed a 2:1 glenohumeral–scapulothoracic motion ratio throughout the entire motion arc (108–110). The complex movement of scapulothoracic rotation accompanies glenohumeral elevation. With upward movement of the arm, about 6 degrees of anterior rotation referable to the thorax occurs during the first 90 degrees of elevation. Beyond 90 degrees of elevation, the scapula begins approximately 16 degrees of posterior rotation, resulting in a position approximately 10 degrees posterior to the starting position. In addition to this 16 degrees of anterior–posterior rotation, the scapula rotates approximately 20 degrees of forward tilt referable to the thorax during arm elevation (111). An obligatory external rotation of the humerus accompanies maximal elevation of the humerus. The external rotation of the humerus allows the tuberosity to clear the coracoacromial arch and thus removes this mechanical constraint from full arm elevation (4). Finally, it as also been shown that external rotation of the humerus loosens the inferior ligaments of the glenohumeral joint and subsequently allows for full arm elevation by releasing the inferior checkrein effect of the inferior capsule (4).

The arterial supply of the shoulder joint includes branches of the suprascapular, anterior and posterior circumflex humeral, and circumflex scapular arteries (Fig. 20.11) (6,112,113). Extensive dissections of shoulder joints have demonstrated that the anterolateral branch of the anterior circumflex artery provides the main blood supply to the head of the humerus (112,113). The posterior circumflex artery vascularizes the posterior portion of the greater tuberosity and a small posteroinferior part of the articular segment. In addition, the posterior circumflex artery contributes an extensive web of anastomoses to the arcuate artery in the region of the greater tuberosity and joint capsule (112).

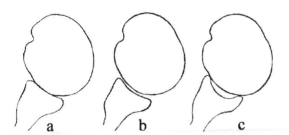

FIG. 20.10. Three types of glenohumeral articulation as first described by Saha. In type A the radius of curvature of the humeral head is less than that of the glenoid. In type B the radii of curvature are similar for both the humeral head and the glenoid. In type C the humeral head has a greater radius of curvature than the glenoid.

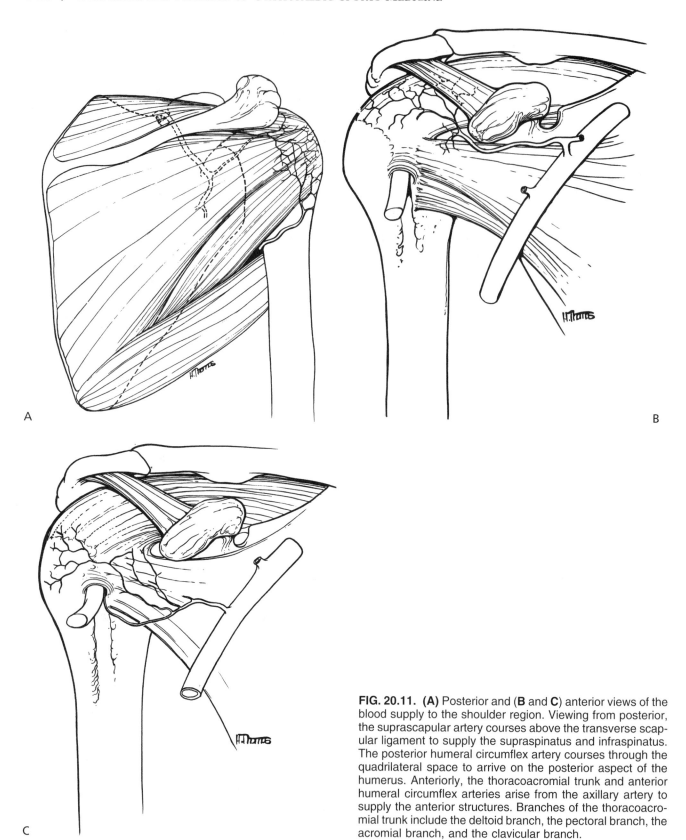

A

B

C

FIG. 20.11. (A) Posterior and **(B and C)** anterior views of the blood supply to the shoulder region. Viewing from posterior, the suprascapular artery courses above the transverse scapular ligament to supply the supraspinatus and infraspinatus. The posterior humeral circumflex artery courses through the quadrilateral space to arrive on the posterior aspect of the humerus. Anteriorly, the thoracoacromial trunk and anterior humeral circumflex arteries arise from the axillary artery to supply the anterior structures. Branches of the thoracoacromial trunk include the deltoid branch, the pectoral branch, the acromial branch, and the clavicular branch.

Most superficial and deep structures of the shoulder are innervated by a network of nerve fibers from the C-5, C-6, and C-7 nerve roots (7,114). The axillary nerve and suprascapular nerve provide most of the nerve supply to the anterior capsule and glenohumerual joint. Superiorly, two branches of the suprascapular nerve are the primary contributors to joint innervation. The suprascapular nerve and the axillary nerve provide posterior joint innervation and inferior joint innervation.

Dislocation of the glenohumeral joint is extremely common and has been described as far back as 3000 to 2500 BC (115). Shoulder dislocations account for approximately 45% of all dislocations with 85% of these in the anterior direction (116,117). Treatment of acute glenohumeral joint dislocation involves gentle and expeditious reduction, ideally after a complete set of shoulder radiographs (including anteroposterior, scapula Y lateral, and axillary view) has been obtained. Anterior dislocations are generally subcoracoid dislocations caused by abduction, extension, and external rotation producing forces that disrupt the anterior capsule and ligaments, the glenoid rim, and the rotator cuff mechanism. These dislocations are commonly associated with a Hill-Sachs defect to the posterior lateral humeral head and a Bankart tear of the anterior capsule and labrum from the glenoid lip. Anterior dislocations may also be associated with severe trauma and result in more unusual dislocation patterns. These include subglenoid (the head of the humerus lies anterior to and below the glenoid fossa), subclavicular (the head of the humerus lies medial to the coracoid process, just inferior to the lower border of the clavicle), intrathoracic (the head of the humerus lies between the ribs and the thoracic cavity), and retroperitoneal (4).

Posterior dislocations have been estimated to account for 2% of shoulder dislocations. Most commonly, posterior dislocations are subacromial but may also be found in the subglenoid and subspinous positions. Often, these dislocations are locked (118) and may result from axial loading of the adducted internally rotated arm. Inferior dislocations are extremely rare and have been described in a few series of case reports (119,120). They are thought to be produced by a hyperabduction force that causes abutment of the neck of the humerus against the acromion process, thus levering the head out inferiorly. Superior dislocations are also extremely rare and are usually caused by an extreme forward and upward force on the adducted arm (121).

Capsule and Glenohumeral Ligaments

The glenohumeral articulation is completely enclosed within its own dedicated joint capsule. The articular surface of the capsule is lined with a thin synovial membrane that also invests the path of the biceps tendon as it exits the joint capsule. In reading the material that follows, it is important to realize that the properties of human tissues change with age. The shoulder joint capsule and surrounding tissues are no exception to this rule (122). The glenohumeral capsule was noted to be a heterogeneous structure as early as Flood's description in 1829 (123). Since that time, our knowledge of the anatomy of the joint capsule and the glenohumeral ligaments has been greatly enhanced. The following paragraphs detail the gross, microscopic, and functional anatomy of the shoulder joint capsule and glenohumeral ligaments.

The humeral head is maintained in the glenoid fossa by a combination of static and dynamic restraints. Among the static restraints is the shoulder capsule. The capsule provides not only structural support and stability but also maintains the negative intraarticular pressure within the glenohumeral joint (99,124–127). Gibb et al. (124) demonstrated that venting of the shoulder capsule reduces the force necessary to translate the humeral head on the glenoid. The concept of limited joint volume has been proposed as a factor in shoulder stability. The maximum joint volume of the shoulder has been estimated at 20 mL on the basis of injection studies (128). However, a later study by Sperber and Wredmark (129) demonstrated a range of capsular volumes ranging from 18 to 52 mL in both normal and dislocating shoulders with no correlation between joint volume and body surface area. They also noted no significant difference between the normal and dislocating shoulders in the same patients.

The shoulder joint capsule is capable of resisting a tensile load of up to 2,000 N (130). This compares favorably with the elbow joint capsule, which fails at 1,500 N. Several studies have demonstrated that the weakest portion of the capsulolabral complex is the anteroinferior region (4 o'clock position in right shoulder) (122,130,131).

O'Brien et al. (132) demonstrated that the inferior capsule consists of a synovial lining and three layers of collagen fibers (Fig. 20.12). The collagen fibers are oriented from the glenoid rim to the humerus in the inner and outer layers but are circumferentially oriented in the middle layer. The inner layer of collagen fibers is thickest and the outer layer the thinnest, but the relative thickness of the layers varies depending on the region of the capsule. The capsule is made up of predominantly type I collagen, with smaller amounts of types III and V collagen present as well (130). The axillary pouch between the anterior band (AB) and posterior band (PB) of the inferior glenohumeral ligament (IGHL) is the thickest portion of the capsule, but the orientation of the collagen fibers is less organized in this region (104,132). Also noted in the axillary region is the lack of a defined outer layer of collagen fibers and an intermingling of fibers between the inner and

SAGITTAL SCHEMATIC OF HISTOLOGY

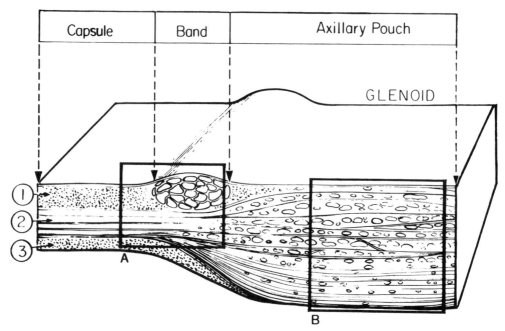

FIG. 20.12. Schematic of three layers of the glenohumeral joint capsule as originally described by O'Brien et al. Note the more organized area highlighted by the A-square that represents the anterior or posterior band. The tissue in the "hammock" region or axillary capsular tissue contains collagen in a less dense arrangement. (From O'Brien SJ, Neves MC, Rozbruck RS, et al. The anatomy and histology of the inferior glenohumeral ligament complex of the shoulder. *Am J Sports Med* 1990;18:449, with permission.)

middle layers. The capsule anterior and posterior to the inferior glenohumeral ligament complex (IGHLC) has all three layers, but the posterior capsule is thinner in total thickness than the anterior capsule, with the major difference being a thicker middle layer.

The shoulder joint capsule is innervated by a combination of nerve branches originating from the suprascapular and axillary nerves. The axillary nerve provides two branches that mainly supply the inferior capsule, whereas the branch from the suprascapular nerve supplies the superior capsule. Several studies have demonstrated that the shoulder capsule is well invested with mechanoreceptors (133,134). Vangsness et al. (134) found two types of mechanoreceptors and three types of nerve endings, whereas Bresch et al. (133) found four types of mechanoreceptors with a higher concentration at the capsulolabral junction. Jerosch et al. (135) confirmed a functional relationship to these receptors by determining that humeral translation increases after an injection of lidocaine into the joint. The proprioceptive pathway was further described by Tibone et al. (136); however, no difference was noted between stable and unstable shoulders. This study (136) and a study by Lephart et al. (137) showed that there is likely no damage to the nervous structures of the capsule with dislocation and instability but that the receptors are stimulated

abnormally in the unstable shoulder. Degeneration of the receptors and nerve fibers has been demonstrated to occur with age in nearly 100% of cadaver specimens, with endoneurial thickening and myxoid degeneration being the most common types of degeneration present (138,139). Nearly 60% of the degenerative changes in the joint capsule are found in the anteroinferior and posteroinferior regions (139).

The earliest descriptions of the glenohumeral ligaments noted them to be thickenings of the shoulder joint capsule (123,140). Beginning 50 years ago with a classic cadaveric study by DePalma et al. (82), the glenohumeral ligaments have received increasing attention, with particular emphasis on their role in shoulder stability. Based on the early studies by DePalma et al., the glenohumeral ligaments were thought to be only variably present, with the superior glenohumeral ligament the most constant. These authors also outlined six variations in the anatomy of the ligaments as they relate to periarticular spaces. In subsequent publications by Turkel et al. (104), Ferrari (141), O'Brien et al. (132), Moseley and Overgaard (142), and others (143,144), the glenohumeral ligaments have been described as varying in distinction and size but present in general. According to DePalma et al. (82), the Superior Glenohumeral Ligament (SGHL) was described as arising from the upper pole of the glenoid and the base of the coracoid process. They also noted that the ligament attached to the middle glenohumeral ligament (MGHL), the biceps tendon, and the glenoid labrum in 75% of the specimens; to the biceps tendon and labrum in 22%; to the MGHL, the IGHL, and the labrum in 2%; and to the biceps tendon only in 1%. Subsequent studies on a smaller number of specimens have noted similar variation, with the most common origin being from the glenoid labrum just anterior to the biceps tendon (143,145). The SGHL inserts in the fovea capitis of the humerus in proximity to the lesser tuberosity, along with a portion of the coracohumeral ligament. The SGHL has been noted to vary in thickness from distinct ligamentous tissue to a small region of thickening within the superior capsule. Warner et al. (144) noted that the SGHL was well developed in all but 1 of 11 specimens. They also demonstrated that in the one specimen with a poorly developed SGHL, the coracohumeral ligament was well developed. Figure 20.13 demonstrates a diagrammatic depiction of the shoulder capsule and its ligaments.

With regard to function, the SGHL has been shown to contribute little to static glenohumeral stability in the anteroposterior plane, particularly with increasing abduction (146,147). Similarly, it has been shown to minimally restrain external rotation with the arm in zero degrees of abduction (104). Basmajian et al. (148) indicated that the SGHL acts in concert with the superior tilt of the glenoid cavity and the negative intraarticular pressure to prevent downward subluxation. Based on selective cutting experiments, the SGHL is the prime static restraint to superoinferior translation of the humeral head with the arm in adduction (144,149). Warren et al. (150) discovered that for posterior dislocation to occur in the adducted flexed and internally rotated shoulder, the SGHL must be divided. In summary, the SGHL is present and functional in nearly all shoulders. Its primary function is to restrain inferior translation in the adducted shoulder. It plays a minor role in limiting external rotation and is a secondary restraint to posterior translation in the adducted flexed internally rotated shoulder.

The MGHL demonstrates the greatest variability in size and presence, being absent or poorly developed more often than the SGHL or the IGHL. DePalma et al. (82) and O'Brien et al. (132) found it to be absent in nearly 30% of specimens. When present, it most commonly arises from the anterosuperior labrum just below the SGHL. Its origin extends from just below the SGHL origin superiorly to the junction of the middle and infe-

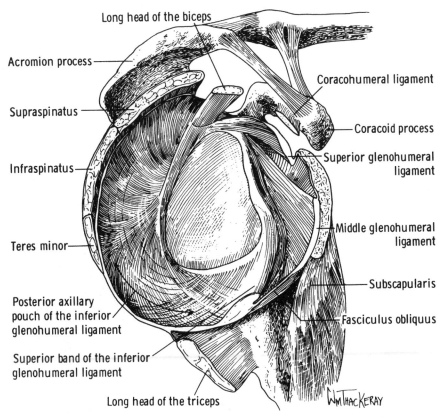

FIG. 20.13. Schematic of the glenohumeral ligaments and pericapsular tissues. (From Turkel SJ, Panio MW, Marshall JL, et al. Stabilizing mechanisms preventing anterior dislocation of the glenohumeral joint. *J Bone Joint Surg Am* 1981;63A:1208–1217, with permission.)

rior one third of the anterior glenoid rim (104). Some fibers may also arise on the neck of the glenoid. It inserts onto the medial aspect of the lesser tuberosity and is intimately associated with the deep surface of the distal 2.5 cm of the subscapularis tendon distally (141). Moseley and Overgaard (142) noted several variations in the origin of the MGHL in which all, part, or none of the ligament originates from the labrum. In most instances the MGHL is a broad fan-shaped structure greater than 2 cm in length and 3 to 4 mm in width. However, a "cordlike" MGHL has been described as part of a normal anatomic variant known as the "Buford complex" (151). Based on a retrospective review of 200 shoulder arthroscopy tapes, these authors determined that 9% had a cordlike MGHL that attached directly to the labrum near a sublabral foramen. An additional 1.5% of the patients demonstrated the three components of the Buford complex: a cordlike MGHL continuous with the anterosuperior labrum, attachment of this combined structure to the superior labrum at the base of the biceps tendon, and no additional anterosuperior labral tissue present. This constellation of findings gives the appearance of a large space posteromedial to the cordlike MGHL but should not be considered pathologic (151).

From a functional standpoint, the MGHL has been shown to limit external rotation in the lower and middle ranges of abduction but to have little effect on external rotation with the arm abducted 90 degrees (104,141,147). The MGHL has also been shown to contribute to restraint against inferior subluxation of the humeral head with the arm adducted and externally rotated (141,144). In combination with the subscapularis and IGHL, the MGHL has been shown to provide anterior stability at 45 degrees of abduction but not at zero and 90 degrees (104). The MGHL plays a secondary role in preventing anterior subluxation with the arm in 90 degrees of abduction if the AB of the IGHL is deficient (143,146,147). The MGHL parallels the SGHL as the arm is progressively abducted. It travels obliquely downward from the glenoid in zero degrees of abduction, becomes more horizontal with external rotation, and more vertical with internal rotation (143). To summarize, the MGHL is present in most shoulders with significant variability in its morphology and origin. It serves several static functions, including prevention of inferior translation and external rotation in the lower degrees of shoulder abduction and restraint against anterior subluxation in concert with other anterior structures.

The IGHLC differs from the other two glenohumeral ligaments in that there is a continuation of the anterior ligamentous tissue inferiorly and posteriorly. The IGHL was previously thought to be an individual ligament like the SGHL and MGHL extending from the labrum to the area of the triceps origin (82,142). The IGHLC is now thought to consist of an AB, a PB, and an intervening axillary segment forming a supportive "hammock" (Fig. 20.14) around the inferior aspect of the humeral head (104,132). Much of the current anatomic information about the IGHLC was described by O'Brien et al. in 1990 (132). The IGHLC originates on the anterior, inferior, and posterior margins of the labrum, the glenoid neck, and the glenoid rim. The AB generally originates between the 2 and 4 o'clock positions and has an average thickness of 2.8 mm. The PB originates between the 7 and 9 o'clock positions and has an average thickness of 1.7 mm (152). There is significant variability in the exact origin of the IGHLC within and between shoulders. The insertion of the IGHLC onto the humerus takes on one of two forms. The first is that of a "collar" around the inferior portion of the humeral head just inferior to the articular surface. The second type of insertion occurs in a "V" pattern with the AB and PB inserting adjacent to the articular surface and the axillary portion of the ligament attaching slightly distal to the inferior articular margin to form the apex of the V (132). The AB and PB are distinct structures consisting of thickened well-organized bundles of collagen. The microscopic anatomy of the inferior joint capsule is described previously in this section. In a 1992 study by Bigliani et al. (152), the tensile properties of the three portions of the IGHLC (AB, axillary pouch, PB) were shown to sustain an average strain to failure of 27%, with the AB failing at a slightly higher strain than the other two portions. These same authors also noted that failure occurred in three regions: the glenoid insertion in 40%, the midsubstance in 35%, and the humeral inser-

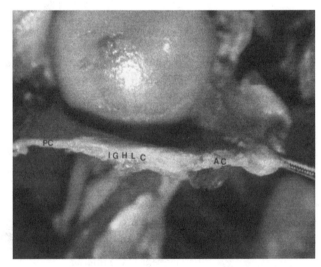

FIG. 20.14. Dissection of cadaver shoulder demonstrating the inferior glenohumeral ligament complex that includes the anterior and posterior bands and the axillary tissue between them that forms a "hammock" for the humeral head. (From Rockwood CA, Matsen FA, eds. *The shoulder,* 2nd ed. Philadelphia: W.B. Saunders, 1998, p. 21 with permission.)

tion in 25%. In a study of intact specimens, Stefko et al. (153) demonstrated that although the predominant failure at the time of dislocation is at the capsuloligamentous insertion site on the glenoid, the midsubstance undergoes an average of 2 to 3 mm of stretch, representing approximately a 7% increase in length.

Beginning in 1981 with the classic study by Turkel et al. (104), the role of the IGHLC as a stabilizing structure has received increasing attention. On the basis of selective cutting experiments, those authors determined that at 0 degrees of abduction, the subscapularis muscle provides significant stability, but with increasing abduction the IGHL prevents anterior dislocation. The IGHLC sustains increasing strain in higher degrees of abduction and external rotation when compared with other anterior structures (147). The importance of the IGHLC in shoulder stability was further confirmed by O'Brien et al. in 1995 (146) when they determined that in 90 degrees of abduction and 0 degrees of forward flexion there was maximal translation of the humeral head in the anterior–posterior direction and that the principal restraint to this motion is the IGHLC. The AB is the primary stabilizer in 0 and 30 degrees of horizontal extension, whereas the PB is the primary restraint in 30 degrees of forward flexion. Ovesen and Nielsen (154) previously demonstrated increased posterior translation with sectioning of anterior structures; however, no attempt was made to isolate specific ligaments. Warren et al. (150) demonstrated that posterior subluxation occurred in the flexed, adducted, internally rotated shoulder when, in addition to the posterior capsule, the anterior capsule was sectioned from the 12 to 3 o'clock positions. In 1992 Warner et al. (144) demonstrated that the IGHLC plays a significant role in restraining superior–inferior translation of the glenohumeral joint. With the arm adducted, the IGHLC provided little support; however, at 45 degrees of abduction the AB becomes the primary capsular restraint to inferior translation and at 90 degrees of abduction the PB provides the most restraint. Similar results were also noted in later experiments by Soslowsky et al. (155). Although the IGHLC is regarded as the structure most responsible for anterior stability, the function of the IGHLC varies with the position of the arm. Several authors have noted the "hammock" effect of the IGHLC, which is summarized here and depicted in Fig. 20.15:

In the abducted shoulder with neutral rotation, the AB and PB combine to prevent anterior–posterior translation and inferior translation. With external rotation, the AB moves superiorly along the humeral head to primarily restrain against anterior translation, whereas the PB moves further under the head, preventing inferior translation. In internal rotation the PB swings further posterior and superior, whereas the AB becomes more inferior, restricting inferior translation (127, 144–147).

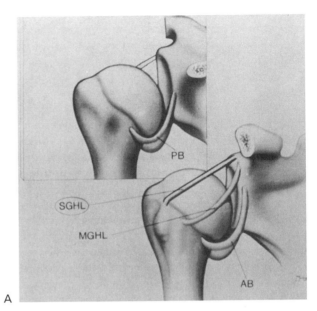

A

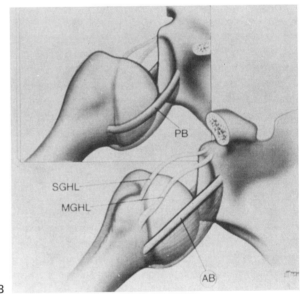

B

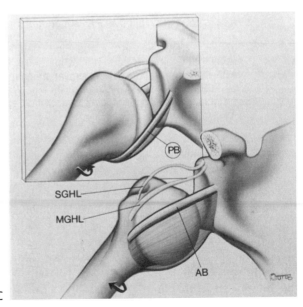

C

FIG. 20.15.—*Continued*

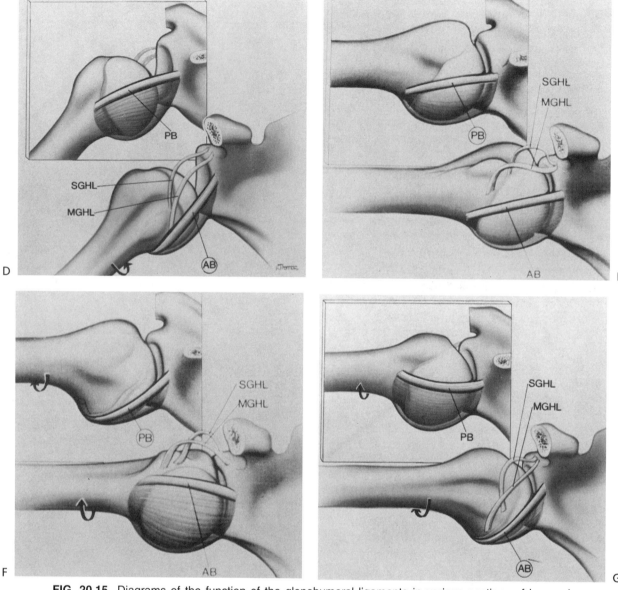

FIG. 20.15. Diagrams of the function of the glenohumeral ligaments in various postions of humeral rotation and abduction. *SGHL,* superior glenohumeral ligament; *MGHL,* middle glenohumeral ligament; *AB,* anterior band; *PB,* posterior band. The superior glenohumeral ligament is a prime restraint to inferior shoulder translation in the adducted shoulder **(A).** In 45 degrees of humeral abduction and external rotation, the anterior band moves superiorly **(B)** and the posterior band inferiorly. The opposite occurs with internal rotation **(C).** A similar mechanism takes place with 90 degrees of humeral abduction and rotation **(E, F, G).** (From Bowen MK, Warren RF. Ligamentous control of shoulder stability based on selective cutting and static translation experiment. *Clin Sports Med* 1991;10:757–782, with permission.)

Anterior translation is prevented in the adducted shoulder by a combination of structures, including the subscapularis muscle, the middle and IGHLs, and capsule (104,143,145–147,154). The capsule and glenohumeral ligament complex have also been shown to significantly restrict internal and external rotation, with the anterior structures limiting humeral external rota-

tion and the posterior structures limiting internal humeral rotation (145,156).

Labrum

There has been a gradual evolution of knowledge regarding both the structure and function of the glenoid

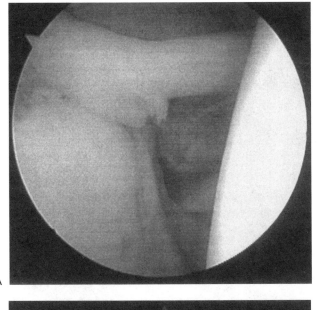

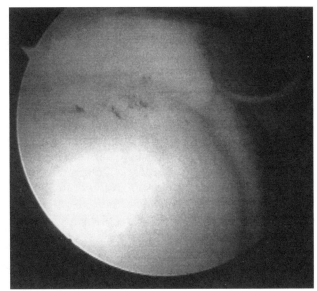

A

B

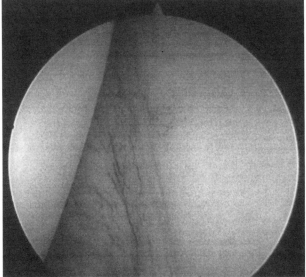

C

FIG. 20.16. Arthroscopic views of the adult labrum. The biceps tendon and anterosuperior labrum (A). The posterior labrum (B) and inferior labrum and axillary pouch (C). Note that the inferior labrum is less prominent than the superior labrum.

labrum. DePalma et al. (82) described the labrum as a triangular fibrocartilaginous structure intimately related to the biceps tendon and firmly attached to the glenoid rim. In their dissections of 45 embryos and 75 cadaver shoulders, Moseley and Overgaard (142) described the labrum as redundancy of the capsule essentially devoid of fibrocartilage. They noted a transition zone near the glenoid rim composed of fibrocartilaginous tissue. These early authors also noted that the labrum is continuous with the joint capsule at its periphery and that the articular surface of the labrum was covered with synovium. Despite these early descriptions, it was the belief of these early authors that the labrum was not a consistent structure (82,142).

More recent work has reiterated the findings that the labrum is triangular in cross-section with considerable variation in morphology but consistently present in all specimens (46,58,157,158). Prodromos et al. (158) reported that contrary to the description of Moseley and Overgaard, the labrum was not fibrous but made up of fibrocartilage. These authors also noted that although the neonatal labrum is composed of primitive mesenchymal cells with few chondrocytes, the adult labrum is distinctly fibrocartilaginous with progressive loss of chondrocytes and occasional elastin fibers (158). According to Cooper et al. (157), the adult labrum contains densely packed collagen bundles with no chondrocytes.

Although the labrum is known to be a continuous structure surrounding the glenoid rim, there are distinct differences in morphology when comparing superior and inferior regions (Fig. 20.16). The superior and anterior labrum tend to be "meniscoid-like" with loose attachments to the glenoid rim. This is in contrast to the inferior labrum, which is firmly attached to the glenoid rim and may represent a fibrous extension of the articular surface serving as an attachment site for the capsuloligamentous structures (157). Histologically, there are no differences between the superior and inferior portions of the labrum. Electron microscopy enabled Nishida et al. (159) to describe three distinct layers of collagen within the labrum. The thin outermost layer closest to the articular surface of the humeral head demonstrated a reticulated fibrilar network of fibers. The middle layer is characterized by stratification of the fibers. The deepest layer, which these authors described as the main layer, consisted of bundles of collagen fibrils densely packed and parallel to one another but oblique to the glenoid rim. On the basis of these findings, the authors postulated that the outer two layers serve as a "bumper" against the humeral head, whereas the innermost layer serves as a cushion to stabilize the joint (159).

The glenoid articular surface contributes little in the way of articular stability when compared with the bony anatomy of the hip. The presence of the glenoid labrum significantly deepens the articulation. Howell and Galinat (46) determined that the labrum nearly doubles the depth of the articular surface of the glenoid in the anterior–posterior plane. Pal et al. (160) investigated the relationship between the origin of the long head of the biceps tendon and the glenoid labrum and found that the labrum was absent or deficient at the posterior–superior aspect of the glenoid in 70% of specimens and that these specimens had a biceps tendon insertion directly onto a bony facet on the glenoid rim. Gigis et al. (161) later proposed that the origin of the biceps arises from the whole periphery of the labrum except at a deficient area near the supraglenoid tubercle. Vangsness et al. (58) determined that approximately 50% of the biceps origin is from the labrum and the other 50% is from the supraglenoid tubercle. These authors were able to demonstrate four distinct types of origin from the labrum (Fig. 20.17). The tendon originates predominantly from the posterior superior region of the labrum in types I and II (55% of specimens), takes fibers equally from the anterior and posterior superior labrum in type III (37% of specimens), and arises predominantly from anterior fibers in type IV (8% of specimens).

The vascular supply to the labrum is from branches of the suprascapular artery, the circumflex scapular artery, and the posterior humeral circumflex artery. Similar to the menisci of the knee, the vascularity of the labrum is limited to its periphery, although this is variable (157). The tributaries of the larger vessels travel to the labrum via the periosteum of the glenoid neck and the joint capsule but not from the underlying glenoid bone. Although most of the penetrating vessels are arranged in a radial pattern, few circumferentially oriented vessels are consistently found. In general, the

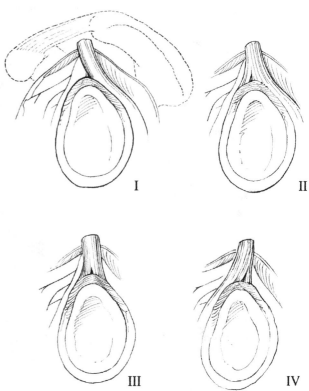

FIG. 20.17. Variations in the type of biceps tendon origin from the rim of the glenoid and superior labrum. Type I has a biceps tendon that arises entirely from the posterior labrum with no anterior contribution. In type II, most of the labral contribution is from posterior, with a small amount from anterior. Type III has equal contributions from the anterior and posterior labrum. Type IV has most of the contribution from anterior. Relative frequencies of the four types: I, 22%; II, 33%; III, 37%; and IV, 18%. (From Vangsness CT, Jr., Jorgenson SS, Watson T. The origin of the long head of the biceps from the scapula and glenoid labrum: an anatomical study of 100 shoulders. *J Bone Joint Surg Br* 1994;76B:951, with permission.)

superior and anterior portions of the labrum are less vascular than the inferior and posterior portions. Interestingly, the anterior–inferior aspect of the labrum has been shown to be the weakest in tension (131). Whether or not there is any relationship between the relative increase in vascularity in this region and the decreased strength has not been determined. According to Vangsness et al. (134), there are no mechanoreceptors within the substance of the glenoid labrum. However, free nerve endings were found in the surrounding connective tissue. Occasional free nerve endings were noted within the substance of the labrum, but only peripherally.

As noted above there is significant variability among individuals with regard to the glenoid labrum. Perhaps the most common variant is a communication with the subscapularis recess through a sublabral hole in the anterior–superior region. This sublabral foramen was noted in 4 of 11 specimens in the study by Cooper et al. (157). In another 5 of the 11 specimens there was a loose capsular attachment of the labrum to the glenoid in this area. It is important to realize that this is a normal anatomic variant and not a pathologic condition. The Buford complex is a combination of a cordlike MGHL and a sublabral foramen and is also a normal variant. An incomplete discoid variant of the labrum, similar to that seen in the knee, has been described with symptoms of painful clicking in the shoulder (162).

MUSCLES

Given the great freedom of movement enjoyed by the shoulder, it is not surprising that there are a large number of muscular attachments to the bony components of the shoulder complex. A description of the individual muscles, their bony origins and insertions, their primary roles in shoulder motion, and their vascular and nervous supplies are outlined here. The muscles of the shoulder joint can be divided into three major groups. The glenohumeral muscles attach the humerus to the scapula and include the deltoid, the rotator cuff muscles (supraspinatus, infraspinatus, subscapularis, and teres minor), the teres major, and the coracobrachialis. The scapulothoracic muscles act to anchor the scapula to the thoracic cage and include the trapezius, rhomboid major, rhomboid minor, levator scapulae, serratus anterior, pectoralis minor, and subclavius. The third group consists of muscles that connect the humerus to the axial skeleton. These muscles are also unique in the fact that they cross at least two joints. They include the pectoralis major, latissimus dorsi, biceps brachii, and triceps brachii.

Glenohumeral Muscles

Deltoid

The lateral aspect of the shoulder is surrounded by the largest and most powerful muscle of the glenohumeral group—the deltoid. This triangular, multipennate, coarsely fasciculated muscle has three major sections, the anterior, middle, and posterior deltoids. The anterior deltoid arises from the lateral third of the clavicle and the leading anterior edge of the acromion, the middle third arises from the lateral border of the acromion, and the posterior third arises from the lower lip of the crest of the spine of the scapula (163,164). The three fasciculi all converge to the insertion on the deltoid tuberosity of the humerus. The anterior and posterior thirds of the muscle are composed of long parallel fibers, whereas the middle third is composed of shorter but stronger multipennate fibers (Fig. 20.18) (6).

The deltoid is a superficial muscle overlying the greater tuberosity of the humerus and forming the broad prominence around the shoulder. The muscular fascia that surrounds the deltoid is an extension of the superfi-

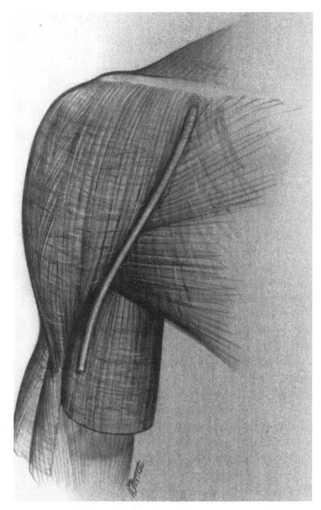

FIG. 20.18. Diagram of the deltoid muscle. The anterior, middle, and posterior components converge to insert onto the deltoid tuberosity of the humerus.

cial layer of cervical fascia from the trapezius muscle. Subcutaneous fat borders the deltoid on the external side and the subacromial or subdeltoid bursa form the deep boundary. In the floor of the bursa lies the supraspinatus tendon. The coracoid, the conjoint tendon of the coracobrachialis, and the short head of the biceps also lie deep to the anterior third of the deltoid. Anteriorly, the deltoid is adjacent to the pectoralis major muscle. The muscular fasciculi from these two muscles run parallel and together form the deltopectoral groove within which lie the cephalic vein and branches of the deltoid artery of the thoracoacromial trunk. Posteriorly, the deltoid is bounded by the infraspinatus, teres minor, and teres major muscles.

The primary roles of the deltoid in shoulder movement are elevation in the scapular plane, abduction in the coronal plane, and flexion in the saggital plane. Flexion of the shoulder is mostly the product of the anterior and middle thirds of the deltoid. The anterior third is also involved in internal rotation. The middle deltoid is most active during elevation in the scapular plane. Abduction of the shoulder increases the contribution of the posterior deltoid and decreases the contribution from the anterior deltoid. The posterior third is involved in external rotation (165–167). The activity of the deltoid increases progressively and is greatest between 90 and 180 degrees of elevation (6). The deltoid has its shortest leverage for elevation in the first 30 degrees (56), and elevation of the shoulder from 0 to 90 degrees relies heavily on the supraspinatus muscle.

The primary vascular supply to the deltoid is the posterior circumflex humeral artery (168). The deltoid branch of the thoracoacromial artery and numerous additional minor anastomosing arteries provide further vascularization of the deltoid muscle. The deltoid is innervated by the axillary nerve (C-5 and C-6), which is one of the two terminal branches of the posterior cord of the brachial plexus (169). The axillary nerve enters the posterior portion of the shoulder through the quadrilateral space where it splits into two branches.

One branch of the axillary nerve sends its fibers along the medial and inferior borders of the posterior deltoid (170), whereas the second branch ascends superiorly to supply the anterior and middle thirds.

Rotator Cuff

The rotator cuff is a sheath of tissue composed of the tendinous portions of the supraspinatus, infraspinatus, subscapularis, and teres minor muscles (Fig. 20.19). Together they surround the glenohumeral joint, humeral head, and joint capsule, forming a nearly continuous sleeve around these structures. This continuous sleeve permits the cuff muscles to provide a wide variety of movements to rotate the humerus and to oppose unwanted components of the deltoid and pectoralis muscles forces (4). The muscles and tendons of the cuff form a complex arrangement with the shoulder capsule and in the deeper regions with other neighboring structures. The fascicles of the supraspinatus tendon create a roof over the groove for the bicipital tendon, and the

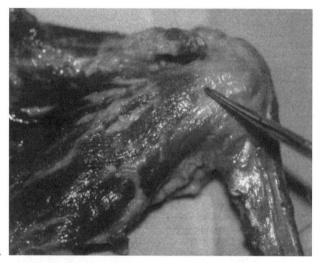

A

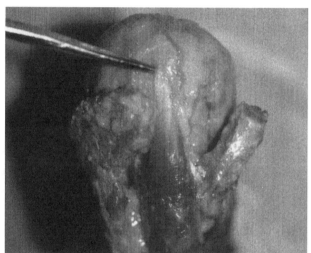

B

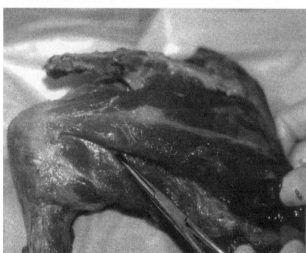

C

FIG. 20.19. Photographs of cadaveric dissections about the shoulder demonstrating the four rotator cuff muscles. Note the bipennate nature of the infraspinatus with the fat stripe separating the two heads of the muscle. **(A)** Subscapularis, **(B)** supraspinatus, and **(C)** infraspinatus and teres minor.

fascicles of the subscapularis tendon create a floor for the bicipital groove. The triangular area of tissue with its base at the coracoid process and its apex at the insertion of the coracohumeral ligament laterally on the humerus is known as the rotator interval (Fig. 20.20). This region is bordered superiorly by the anterior edge of the supraspinatus tendon and inferiorly by the superior edge of the subscapularis tendon. The interval further demonstrates the close relationship between the cuff and its neighboring structures as the coracohumeral ligament contributes fibers that envelope the supraspinatus tendon, forming a laterally based arch or suspension bridge that thickens this region of the cuff (171). A more detailed discussion on the rotator interval follows the description of the rotator cuff musculature.

The rotator cuff performs at least three major functions in the shoulder. First, the cuff muscles work to rotate the humerus with respect to the scapula. Second, they provide primary dynamic stability of the shoulder by compressing the head into the glenoid with active shoulder motion. This concept is known as concavity compression and is in contrast to the original belief that the cuff functioned primarily as a humeral head depressor. In reality, the forces of glenoid compression are significantly greater than the more minor forces of head depression (172,173). Finally, the cuff muscles provide muscular balance in the shoulder. This complex interaction of the rotator cuff and the remaining shoulder muscles requires precise timing and magnitude of the balancing forces so that detailed coordinated shoulder function can be attained and unwanted directions of humeral motion can be avoided (47,75,148,165,174,175).

In general, tendons of the rotator cuff are composed largely of water (55% wet weight) and collagen (85%

dry weight). Most collagen found in the tendon sheath is type I, but trace amounts of type III and type XII collagen are also present. The proportion of type III collagen increases with age, rotator cuff tear, and degeneration (176–178).

Six arteries provide the blood supply to the rotator cuff muscles and tendons: suprascapular artery, anterior humeral circumflex artery, posterior humeral circumflex artery, thoracoacromial artery, suprahumeral artery, and subscapular artery. Vascular flow studies by Chansky and Iannotti (179) demonstrated the frequency of contribution from each of these arteries to rotator cuff vasculature. The suprascapular, anterior humeral circumflex, and posterior humeral circumflex arteries provided blood supply 100% of the time, whereas thoracoacromial, suprahumeral, and subscapular arteries were involved in cuff blood supply 76%, 59%, and 38%, respectively. The specific functions, origins and insertions, muscular descriptions, and vascular and neural anatomy of the individual cuff muscles are detailed next.

Supraspinatus

The supraspinatus muscle occupies the entire supraspinatus fossa of the scapula, taking its origin from the medial two thirds of the dense fascia lining the bony walls of the fossa. The fibers of the muscle run from medial to lateral and terminate in a thick tendon that inserts onto the highest of three facets of the greater tuberosity of the humerus (6). This tendinous insertion has common insertions from the infraspinatus posteriorly and the coracohumeral ligament anteriorly.

The supraspinatus and infraspinatus tendons have been divided into five distinct layers based on the dissections of Clark and Harryman (180). Layer I is approximately 1 mm thick and is composed of fibers of the coracohumeral ligament that are oriented obliquely in relation to the muscle axes. The blood supply to this layer comes from large arterioles found within the muscle substance. The second layer (layer II) is approximately 3 to 5 mm thick and is composed of closely packed bundles of tendon fibers that extend directly from the muscle belly of either the supraspinatus or infraspinatus to the tuberosity. The floor of the bicipital groove is lined by fibers from this layer. The blood supply to this layer comes from the arterioles of layer I extending into the second layer between fascicles. Layer III (3 mm thick) consists of smaller tendinous bundles that lack uniform orientation with fibers and cross one another at 45-degree angles. Layer IV consists mainly of loose connective tissue in which there are thick bands of collagen. Layer V (1.5 to 2 mm thick) consists of a sheet of interwoven collagen fibrils that extend from the glenoid labrum medially to the humerus laterally (180).

Others have divided the tendon into anterior band,

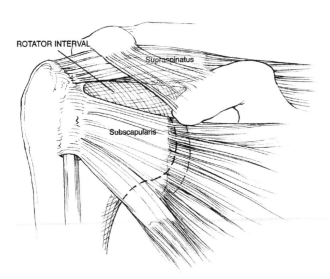

FIG. 20.20. Rotator interval. Note the triangular shape of the tissue with the base of the triangle medially at the coracoid.

middle band, and posterior band (181,182). These studies have demonstrated that the posterior portion of the supraspinatus is considerably thinner in cross-section than the anterior and middle sections (181,182). These authors conclude that the anterior portion of the tendon is the strongest and bears most of the stress.

The primary function of the supraspinatus muscle is to act concurrently with the deltoid in the first 90 degrees of abduction (6). It is, however, active with virtually any motion involving elevation, with its greatest exertion of effort at approximately 30 degrees of elevation (183,184). Several studies have demonstrated that the supraspinatus serves to reduce the required deltoid force necessary to abduct the humerus by around 30% (173,185). The absence or paralysis of the supraspinatus decreases the power of active abduction to 80% of normal at the time of take-off from the side (186). Given the muscles' circumscribed insertion around the humeral head and the orientation of its fibers directly toward the glenoid, the supraspinatus, along with the other rotator cuff muscles, plays an important role in stabilizing the glenohumeral joint by compressing the humeral head into the glenoid during active motion. It is also integral in the maintenance of muscular balance in the shoulder during arm motion.

The anatomic arrangement of the supraspinatus muscle between the subacromial bursa and acromion above and the humeral head below predisposes the muscle to compression, attrition, inflammation, and tearing. Examinations of older cadaver specimens have demonstrated that supraspinatus rotator cuff tears may be present in up to 50% of specimens (45,187,188).

The main arterial supply to the supraspinatus is from the suprascapular artery. The artery is one of three branches off of the thyrocervical trunk extending from the subclavian artery. The vessel enters the supraspinatus fossa after passing over the superior transverse scapular ligament and supplies the supraspinatus muscle from its underside (6,189). The dorsal scapular artery often supplies the medial portion of the muscle (168). A hypovascular region of the rotator cuff has been found in two thirds of specimens in the tendinous portion of the supraspinatus just medial to its insertion. This area of hypovascularity was first noted by Codman in 1934 (68) and has since been supported by other studies (189,190). Rathburn (191) noted that these hypovascular areas may be present at birth but also correspond to regions that are likely subject to increased stress and wear over time. Rathburn noted the "critical zone" of the supraspinatus tendon receives less blood flow with the arm held in adduction due to compression effect of the humeral head. The suprascapular nerve (C-5 with some C-6) provides the main innervation to the supraspinatus muscle. The suprascapular nerve extends from the superior trunk of the brachial plexus and enters the supraspinatus fossa through the scapular notch. The nerve passes under the superior transverse scapular ligament, dives deep to the muscle, and supplies muscular innervation from the underside (149,192).

Infraspinatus

The infraspinatus muscle is a thick triangular muscle that arises from the medial two thirds of the infraspinatus fossa of the scapula overlying its dense fascia and the spine of the scapula. It is in direct contact with the teres minor muscle that lies along its medial inferior border. The fibers are oriented from medial to lateral with its tendon forming within the muscle. The tendinous portion of the muscle travels over the posterior capsule and posterior aspect of the glenohumeral joint to insert onto the middle facet of the greater tuberosity of the humerus, with its deep fibers blending with the shoulder joint capsule (4,6).

The infraspinatus muscle is a primary external rotator of the humerus and accounts for as much as 60% of external rotation force (166,193,194). Additional roles of the infraspinatus muscle include humeral head depression (75,102), shoulder abduction (195), and both anterior and posterior shoulder stabilization (56,196).

The primary blood supply to the infraspinatus is from the suprascapular artery that traverses the supraspinatus fossa and passes through the notch of the scapular neck and under the inferior transverse scapular ligament to enter the upper part of the infraspinatus muscle (6,189,197). The muscle may also receive blood from the circumflex scapular branch of the subscapular artery in some patients (6,148). Similar to the supraspinatus muscle, a hypovascular region has been noted in 37% of infraspinatus tendons just medial to their insertion onto the greater tuberosity (68,189,190). The infraspinatus is supplied by the suprascapular nerve that follows the course of the suprascapular artery under the inferior transverse scapular ligament and into the upper portion of the muscle (6).

Subscapularis

The subscapularis muscle is the anterior portion of the rotator cuff that takes its origin over a broad area of the medial subscapular fossa of the scapula. Although muscle tissue occupies the entire fossa, which accounts for most of the anterior surface of the scapula, the fibers originate along ridges that are located only along the medial two thirds (6). Several fibers also arise from the lower two thirds of the groove on the axillary border of the bone. The upper 60% of the muscle fibers pass laterally and converge into the tendinous insertion onto the lesser tuberosity of the humerus. The lower 40% of the muscle fibers originating from the axillary border of the scapula insert on to the neck of the humerus for a distance of approximately 2 cm (198). The anterior humeral circumflex vessels mark the division between these upper and lower portions of the muscle (198). The tendinous portion of the muscle lies just anterior to the anterior joint capsule and becomes intimately attached to it before insertion on the humerus.

The muscle belly is multipennate in structure. The tendinous portion of the subscapularis is composed of four to six bundles of collagen fibers that extend from the myotendinous junction to the lesser tuberosity. Toward the anterior surface of the tendon, the bundles are tightly packed, whereas on the undersurface they are separated by loose connective tissue (180). Fibers from the subscapularis join some fibers from the supraspinatus to form the floor of the bicipital groove.

The subscapularis is bound anteriorly by the axillary space and the coracobrachialis bursa and superiorly by the coracoid process and the subscapularis recess. The upper portion of its deep surface is bound by the glenohumeral joint, with the MGHL lying beneath the upper portion of the tendon (6). The inferior lateral border of the muscle lies anterior to both the quadrilateral and triangular spaces (Fig. 20.20). The axillary nerve and posterior humeral circumflex artery and veins pass through the quadrilateral space, and the circumflex scapular artery passes through the more medial triangular space, all at the inferior lateral border of the muscle (6).

The subscapularis acts primarily as an internal rotator of the humerus (75,102,166,194). Additionally, because of its dense collagen internal structure, it is considered to function as one of the passive stabilizers of the shoulder joint (104,199). However, Itoi et al. (200) demonstrated that it is the least important contributor to anterior stability in the intact shoulder. As with the rest of the rotator cuff, the subscapularis plays a role in concavity compression of the humeral head into the glenoid fossa, which aids in resisting deltoid muscle shear stresses with arm elevation (75,102).

The primary blood supply to the subscapularis originates from the axillary and subscapular arteries (4,168,189). Others have suggested a large vascular supply from the anterior humeral circumflex artery and a branch off of this vessel known as the upper subscapular artery (201,202). The medial portion of the muscle may also have contributing blood supply from the dorsal or circumflex scapular artery after it penetrates the serratus anterior (203). An area of hypovascularity similar to those found in the infraspinatus and supraspinatus tendons was noted in 7% of subscapularis tendons as well (189,191). The subscapularis is innervated on its costal surface by the upper and lower subscapular nerves. The upper subscapular nerve originates from C-5 and usually contributes nerve supply to the upper 50% of the muscle, whereas the lower subscapular nerve originates from C-5 and C-6 and contributes to the lower 20% (204). A

separate middle subscapular nerve can be found in some patients and may contribute to the innervation of the remaining 30% of the muscle (205).

Teres Minor

The teres minor is a narrow elongated muscle that arises from the upper two thirds of the dorsal surface of the axillary border of the scapula and the dense fascia of the infraspinatus (6). Its fibers travel superolaterally and terminate in a tendon that inserts onto the inferior facet of the posterior portion of the greater tuberosity of the humerus. Additional fibers of the muscle insert along the proximal 2 cm of the neck of the humerus. The tendon blends deeply with the posterior capsule of the shoulder joint and is adherent to the capsule at its deep surface. The superficial surface forms a fascial plane between the deep surface of the overlying deltoid muscle. The inferior border of the muscle forms the superior margins of both the quadrilateral and triangular spaces. The teres minor is separated from the teres major muscle by the long head of the triceps brachii muscle and the axillary nerve and posterior humeral circumflex vessels as they pass through the quadrilateral space.

The teres minor muscle contracts with the infraspinatus muscle and is a primary external rotator of the humerus, providing up to 45% of external rotation force (193). The muscle is also important in humeral head compression into the glenoid with arm elevation and abduction (75,102), providing anterior shoulder stability (196).

The primary blood supply to the teres minor is from branches off the posterior humeral circumflex artery; however, several other anastomosing vessels provide important blood supply (179). The muscle is innervated by the posterior branch of the axillary nerve (6).

Rotator Interval

The rotator cuff is divided anterosuperiorly by the coracoid process between the supraspinatus and the subscapularis. The gap formed by the coracoid process medially is gradually narrowed more laterally in the space between the two cuff muscles. This gap has been termed the rotator interval and is occupied by shoulder joint capsule (Fig. 20.20). In more defining terms, the rotator interval is triangular in shape and bordered superiorly by the anterior border of the supraspinatus, inferiorly by the superior edge of the supraspinatus, and medially by the base of the coracoid process. The apex of the triangle is generally considered the transverse humeral ligament that traverses the bicipital groove. Classic anatomic descriptions of this area have stated that the coracohumeral ligament, superior glenohumeral ligament, and joint capsule tissue can be found in this interval (7,82,142). The functional role of the rotator interval tissue was demonstrated by Harryman et al. (206). These authors demonstrated that sectioning of the rotator interval tissue allowed increased external rotation of 11 degrees with the arm in 60 degrees of abduction. Shortening of the rotator interval tissue served to significantly decrease shoulder motion, including extension (18 degrees), external rotation in neutral abduction (38 degrees), and external rotation in 60 degrees of abduction (18 degrees). Internal rotation and abduction were not affected by imbrication of the interval tissue (206). Similarly, sectioning of the rotator interval tissue decreases the normal anterior and superior translation of the humeral head seen with forward flexion, whereas imbricating this tissue increases these translations. The rotator interval tissue has been proposed as a stabilizing structure of the glenohumeral joint. In sectioning studies, release of the tissue allowed for increased posterior and inferior translation of the humeral head, whereas imbrication decreased these translations (206,207). These findings were echoed in subsequent clinical studies by Field et al. (208), Rowe et al. (209), and Treacy et al. (210). The dimensions of the rotator interval can be inferred from the clinical data obtained in clinical studies on closure of the rotator interval. In the study by Field et al., the average dimensions of the rotator interval defect were 2.75 cm in width and 2.3 cm in height. We mention these numbers not as absolute dimensions but to afford the reader the image that the rotator interval is not a trivial structure.

Teres Major

The teres major muscle is a thick cylindrical muscle that arises from the posterior surface of the inferior angle of the scapula and from the intermuscular septa between it and adjacent muscles (6). It is directed superolaterally along the lateral border of the scapula toward the anterior medial humerus. It has a common tendon of insertion with the latissimus dorsi tendon, onto a crest of bone extending from the lesser tuberosity known as the medial lip of the bicipital groove. Both the teres major and latissimus dorsi fibers undergo a 180-degree spiral twist from origin to insertion such that the latissimus dorsi lies posterior to the teres major at their origin and anterior to the teres major at their insertion. The teres major forms the inferior border of both the quadrilateral and triangular spaces and the superior border of the triangular interval through which the radial nerve and the deep brachial artery can be identified (6). The muscle is also bounded by the infraspinatus and teres minor superomedially and the long head of the triceps brachii posterolaterally.

The teres major is active in adduction, extension, and internal rotation of the humerus. It acts in concert with the latissimus dorsi and pectoralis major muscles but is only recruited with resistance (6,165).

The blood supply to the muscle is derived from branches of the subscapular artery and from the thoracodorsal artery (168). Muscle innervation is from the lower subscapular nerve originating from C-5 and C-6.

Coracobrachialis

The coracobrachialis is a short bandlike muscle arising from the tip of the coracoid process, in common with and medial to the tendon of the short head of the biceps brachii. The muscle extends distally to insert on the anteromedial surface of the midportion of the humerus, near the starting point of the medial border of the bicipital groove. The muscle is bound by the short head of the biceps brachii laterally; the deltoid, deltopectoral groove, and pectoralis muscles superficially; and the coracobrachialis bursa and subscapularis to its deep surface (6).

The primary actions of the coracobrachialis include glenohumeral joint flexion and adduction (6,165). The blood supply to the muscle is usually from a single artery branching off the axillary artery but may also originate from the brachial artery (168). Innervation of the muscle comes from the lateral cord of the brachial plexus. A direct nerve branch from the lateral cord, branching off the musculocutaneous nerve (C-5 and C-6), serves the muscle. The musculocutaneous nerve penetrates the coracobrachialis at an average of 5 cm below the coracoid process. This often-described "safe zone" refers to the average position of the main trunk of the nerve 4.

Scapulothoracic Muscles

Trapezius

The trapezius muscle is the largest and most superficial muscle of the scapulothoracic muscles. The upper portion of the muscle (above C-7) takes origin from the medial third of the superior nuchal line and the external occipital protuberance of the occipital bone from the ligamentum nuchae. These upper fibers are inserted into the posterior border of the lateral third of the clavicle. The lower portion of the muscle (below C-7) takes origin from the spinous processes of the C-7 through T-12 vertebrae. The cervical and upper thoracic bundles insert onto the medial border of the acromion and the upper border of the crest of the spine of the scapula, whereas the lower thoracic muscle fibers insert into the tubercle of the crest of the scapular spine (6). Except for the thickened diamond-shaped accumulation around the lower cervical and upper thoracic fibers, the muscle is relatively thin. It is bounded by the levator scapulae and rhomboids anteriorly and by fat and skin posteriorly.

The trapezius muscle functions primarily to suspend the shoulder girdle and to act as a scapular retractor.

Muscles from the upper trapezius, levator scapulae, and upper serratus anterior muscles have a low level of activity even at rest. These muscles contract vigorously with loading of the shoulder. Different regions of the muscle contribute to different shoulder motions. The upper trapezius muscle contributes to shoulder extension and elevation of the lateral angle of the scapula, the middle fibers contribute to abduction of the arm, and the middle and lower fibers contribute most significantly to scapular retraction (165). The trapezius is not just a supporting muscle. It serves a very important role in the adjustment of the scapula during elevation of the upper limb (165). A force couple is effected between the joint actions of the upper trapezius, levator scapulae, and upper parts of the serratus anterior muscles working in conjunction with the lower part of the trapezius and the lower serratus anterior muscles. Together these muscles work to rotate the scapula on the chest wall and thus allow for the upper extremity motions of flexion, elevation, and abduction (6,185).

The trapezius muscle receives its motor innervation from the spinal accessory (cranial nerve XI) nerve, with some sensory contributions directly from the ventral rami of C-2, C-3, and C-4. The spinal accessory nerve passes through the sternocleidomastoid muscle, courses through the posterior triangle of the neck, and finally runs diagonally downward toward the underside of the trapezius (6). The nerve runs through the medial 50% of the muscle and parallel with the vertebral border of the scapula (211). The blood supply to the trapezius comes from the transverse cervical artery of the subclavian system. Its blood supply is supplemented by a muscular perforating branch of the dorsal scapular artery in the lower third of the muscle (6).

Rhomboids and Levator Scapulae

The rhomboid muscles are divided by a muscular septum into the rhomboid minor and rhomboid major. Their actions imitate the middle trapezius muscle with high levels of activity during upper extremity abduction (165). These muscles, with the levator scapulae, lie directly under the trapezius muscle. The smaller slender rhomboid minor takes origin from the lower part of the ligamentum nuchae, the spinous process of the last cervical and first thoracic vertebrae, and the associated segment of the supraspinal ligament. It is directed downward and lateral and inserts onto the medial border of the scapula at the level of the scapula spine (6). The larger rhomboid major muscle takes origin from the spinous processes of C-2 to C-5 and inserts onto the medial border of the scapula, running in a parallel direction with the rhomboid minor. The levator scapulae muscles, thicker than both the rhomboids, originate from four separate tendons off the spinous processes of C-1 through C-4. It inserts onto the medial border of the scapula above the level of the scapula spine.

In addition to assisting in shoulder abduction, the rhomboid muscles assist the serratus anterior muscle in holding the scapula depressed against the chest wall. The levator scapulae muscles are active during shoulder elevation and during scapular rotation (as mentioned earlier). All three of these muscles receive their nerve supply from the dorsal scapular nerve that arises chiefly from the C-5 nerve root off of the brachial plexus. The levator scapulae receive additional innervation from the ventral rami of C-3 and C-4 nerves (6). All three of these muscles receive their blood supply from the dorsal scapular artery that descends along the lateral border of the levator scapulae and courses toward the inferior border of the scapula.

Serratus Anterior

The serratus anterior is a muscle that is composed of three divisions, each taking origin from the ribs on the anterior lateral wall of the thoracic cage. The first division is a single slip that takes origin from the first and second ribs and the intercostal space between them. This upper slip runs superiorly and posteriorly to insert onto the superior angle of the scapula. The second division consists of three muscle slips arising from the second, third, and fourth ribs and inserting onto the anterior aspect of the medial border of the scapula. The third division consists of muscle slips arising from the fifth through ninth ribs and inserting onto the inferior angle of the scapula. The muscle is bounded anteriorly by the external oblique muscle, medially by the ribs and intercostal muscles, and laterally by the axillary space (70).

As discussed previously, the serratus anterior muscle is intimately involved in scapular rotation. The muscle is involved in a force coupling action between the upper part of the serratus and the lower part of the serratus such that the combined action rotates the scapula on the chest wall. Serratus involvement in scapular protraction and upward rotation is greater in flexion than in abduction (4).

Nerve supply to the serratus anterior is through the long thoracic nerve. The nerve has contributions from the C-5, C-6, and C-7 nerve roots off of the brachial plexus. Injury to the nerve results in paralysis of the serratus muscle and produces winging of the scapula with forward flexion. The lateral thoracic artery provides the greatest blood supply contribution to this muscle. Additional contributions come from the thoracodorsal artery, which may supply up to 50% of the muscle (4). The dorsal scapular artery and the intercostal and internal mammary arteries provide blood supply to the upper slips of the muscle (168).

Pectoralis Minor

The pectoralis minor muscle takes origin from the outer surfaces of the third, fourth, and fifth ribs and occasionally from the second rib. It runs from the origin near each rib's costal cartilage upward and laterally toward its insertion onto the medial and upper surface of the coracoid process. Muscle action results in scapular protraction and downward rotation such that the scapula is drawn forward, medially, and strongly downward with contraction (6). The medial pectoral nerve, which arises from C-8 and T-1 nerve roots, innervates the pectoralis minor as it penetrates the muscle on its way to the interpectoral space and into the pectoralis major muscle. Pectoral branches of the thoracoacromial artery provide the main blood supply to the muscle, with additional contributions from the lateral thoracic artery and short thoracic arteries off of the axillary artery (168).

Subclavius

The subclavius muscle, the smallest of the scapulothoracic muscles, arises from the junction of the first rib and its cartilage and lies parallel to the underside of the clavicle. It inserts on the underside of the clavicle between the attachments of the conoid ligament laterally and the costoclavicular ligament medially. The muscle acts to stabilize the sternoclavicular joint while in motion and draws the shoulder forward and downward (6). The muscle is innervated by the nerve to the subclavius, which branches off the superior trunk of the brachial plexus from the C-5 and C-6 nerve roots. The clavicular branch of the thoracoacromial artery provides blood supply to the muscle (6).

Multiple Joint Muscles

The next group of four muscles acting on the shoulder include the pectoralis major, the latissimus dorsi, the biceps brachii, and the triceps brachii. These muscles are unique in their action on the shoulder in that they act across two joints. Each muscle acts on the glenohumeral joint. The pectoralis muscle has additional action at the sternoclavicular joint, the latissimus dorsi acts additionally on the scapulothoracic joint, and the biceps and triceps muscles exert muscular action across the elbow joint.

Pectoralis Major

The pectoralis major muscle forms the anterior-most muscular border of the chest and consists of three discreet portions: the clavicular, sternocostal, and abdominal. The clavicular portion takes origin from the medial one half to two thirds of the clavicle. The sternocostal portion, much larger in surface area, arises from the anterior surface of the manubrium and the body of the sternum. This middle portion also has deep fascicles arising from the cartilages of the second to sixth ribs. The abdominal portion is the smallest bundle that comes off the anterior layer of the sheath of the rectus abdominis muscle. The fibers of the upper clavicular portion maintain a parallel arrangement as they course toward their insertion into the lateral lip of the bicipital groove. The middle sternocostal portion also maintains a parallel fiber arrangement and inserts directly behind the clavicular portion. The abdominal portion also inserts into the lateral lip of the bicipital groove, but these fibers are rotated 180 degrees such that they insert superiorly on the humerus. The combined tendinous insertions of these three portions thus forms a bilaminar U-shaped tendon with the fold of the tendon at the inferior portion of the bicipital groove (6).

The pectoralis muscle is invested by the pectoral fascia that extends from the clavicular and sternal origins and is continuous with both the anterior abdominal wall fascia and the axillary fascia. The muscle is bounded anteriorly by the mammary gland and the subcutaneous fat. The pectoralis minor muscle lies on the deep surface superior to the attachment to the ribs. The axillary fold forms the inferior border and the deltopectoral groove forms the superior lateral border (70). The pectoralis major muscle serves at least three different functions depending on the starting position of the humerus and on the portion of the muscle involved. The primary motions imparted upon the humerus are flexion, adduction, and internal rotation. The clavicular portion elevates the shoulder and flexes the humerus, whereas the sternocostal portion works antagonistically. The sternocostal portion is most active in internal rotation and scapular depression; however, internal rotation must be against resistance for the muscle to be called into action (165). All three portions of the muscle contribute to adduction of the glenohumeral joint and indirectly function as depressors of the lateral angle of the scapula (4).

Both the lateral and medial pectoral nerves innervate the pectoralis major muscle. These nerves are extensions of the lateral and medial cords of the brachial plexus and involve all the roots (C-5 through T-1). The lateral pectoral nerve comes from roots C-5, C-6, and C-7 and innervates the clavicular portion of the muscle. The medial pectoral nerve, carrying fibers from C-8 and T-1, innervates the remaining two portions of the muscle. The deltoid and pectoral branches of the thoracoacromial artery follow the course of the lateral and medial pectoral nerves and provide the main blood supply to the muscle. The clavicular portion is fed mainly by the deltoid branch and the sternocostal portion by the pectoral branch. Additional blood supply is received from the internal mammary artery, the fourth or fifth intercostal artery, and other anastomoses from the lateral thoracic artery (168).

Latissimus Dorsi

The latissimus dorsi is a broad triangular muscle of the lower part of the back that takes origin from the large aponeurosis from the dorsal spines of T-7 through L-5. The lower lateral most portion of the muscle has additional origin from the posterior third of the iliac crest. There are also origins from the lowest three or four ribs and the inferior angle of the scapula (201). The muscle narrows as it courses laterally past the inferior angle of the scapula and follows the spiral curve around the teres major muscle, passes around the lower edge of the posterior axillary fold, and inserts its band-like tendon into the floor of the intertubercular groove of the humerus (6).

The latissimus dorsi muscle is bound on its superficial surface only by subcutaneous fat and fascia. The inferior lateral border forms the posterior axillary fold; the anterior border forms the axillary space; and the deep surface is bound by the abdominal musculature, the posterior inferior serratus muscle, the teres major, and the posterior ribs. The primary actions of the latissimus are inward rotation and adduction of the humerus, shoulder extension, and downward rotation of the scapula (165).

The thoracodorsal nerve from the posterior cord of the brachial plexus (C-6 and C-7) innervates the latissimus dorsi. The main blood supply is from the thoracodorsal artery, which is a branch of the subscapular artery. Additional blood supply comes from the intercostal and lumbar perforators (168). The neurovascular hilum is found about 2 cm medial to the muscular border at the inferior surface of the muscle (201).

Biceps Brachii

The biceps brachii is a long fusiform muscle composed of two heads lying over the anterior aspect of the arm. The short head arises with the coracobrachialis in a broad flat tendon from the apex of the coracoid process of the scapula. The long head had been thought to arise solely from the supraglenoid tubercle, but this notion has recently been challenged. Recent studies concerning the biceps tendon have revealed that the origin of the tendon may not be solely from the supraglenoid tubercle. Pal et al. (160) demonstrated in a 1991 study that 70% of adult human cadaver specimens had a deficiency of the posterosuperior labrum where the biceps tendon crosses over it. They also showed that the major origin of the tendon of the long head of the biceps was from the supraglenoid tubercle in only 25% of specimens. The remainder took origin from a crescent ridge or accessory facet at the posterosuperior glenoid. In another study from 1995, Gigis et al. (161) stated that the origin of the biceps extends over nearly the whole periphery of the glenoid labrum except at a small area near the supraglenoid tubercle, which may be the area

of deficiency described earlier by Pal et al. In yet another large cadaveric study, Vangsness et al. (58) determined that approximately 50% of the long head of the biceps tendon arises from the supraglenoid tubercle and the remaining 50% arises directly from the labrum. From their dissections, they were able to describe four basic types of biceps tendon take-off from the labrum.

The biceps tendon is surrounded by a synovial sheath during its intraarticular course over the anterior portion of the humeral head. The tendon then passes through a special opening in the joint capsule that allows the passage of synovial fluid to the tendon. The tendon travels through the bicipital groove created by the greater and lesser tuberosities before joining the muscle belly. The bicipital groove is covered by a fibrous extension of the pectoralis major tendon, which serves to maintain the biceps tendon in the bicipital groove.

The muscular fibers of the long and short heads of the biceps converge together at about the middle of the arm to form the most prominent muscle of the anterior compartment. The fibers from the two bellies run together the remainder of their course toward the strong tendinous insertion into the biceps tuberosity of the radius. The bicipital aponeurosis is formed by the more anterior and medial tendon fibers of the muscle and arises at the bend of the elbow passing over the brachial artery and median nerve to insert over the flexor group of the forearm with the antebrachial fascia (6).

The biceps brachii functions as an elbow flexor and serves as the strongest supinator of the forearm. In addition to these roles, however, some biomechanical studies have shown that the biceps tendon provides several functions intrinsic to the shoulder joint. Pagnani et al. (212) demonstrated that the proximal tendon of the long head of the biceps contributes to anterior stability of the glenohumeral joint in the overhead position of abduction and external rotation. The same study demonstrated that the biceps tendon also helps to reduce some of the load borne by the IGHLC. A more recent biomechanical study performed by O'Brien et al., demonstrated that contraction of the tendon of the long head of the biceps resulted in significantly less translation of the humeral head in the glenoid, with a more pronounced effect in lower levels of humeral elevation (146).

Electromyogram studies of the function of the long head of the biceps at the shoulder joint have reported conflicting data. These studies have shown the role of the long head of the biceps to include shoulder flexion, shoulder abduction, shoulder internal rotation, shoulder external rotation, shoulder extension, anterior stabilization, and abduction only with resistance (165,213,214). Others have shown that bicipital activity is not associated with isolated shoulder motion but rather correlated only with motion at the elbow (215,216).

The primary innervation of the biceps brachii comes

from branches of the musculocutaneous nerve arising from the C-5 and C-6 nerve roots of the brachial plexus. The blood supply to the biceps comes from branches off the brachial artery. Studies by Salmon (168) showed that the blood supply may derive from either a single large bicipital artery (35%), multiple small arteries (40%), or a combination of both.

Triceps Brachii

The triceps brachii is a large muscle composed of three heads that occupy the entire dorsum of the arm. Of the three heads (the long head, the lateral head, and the medial head), the long head is the portion most likely to be involved in shoulder pathology. The long head of the triceps takes origin as a strong tendon off the infraglenoid tubercle of the scapula. Although it is not an intraarticular structure, it is intimately involved in the shoulder joint as its origin lies in close proximity to the glenoid labrum, and part of the tendon fibers serve as reinforcement for the IGHL portion of the shoulder capsule (4). The belly of the long head descends between the teres major and teres minor muscles, forming the medial border to the quadrangular space (containing the axillary nerve and posterior humeral circumflex artery) and the lateral border to the triangular space (containing the circumflex scapular artery) (Fig. 20.21). It runs parallel to the humerus bone and joins the medial and lateral heads for a common tendon of insertion into

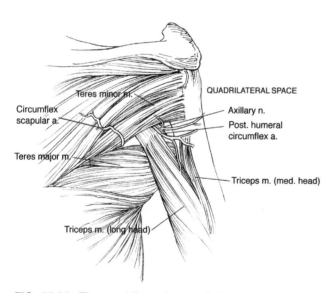

FIG. 20.21. The quadrilateral space is bordered superiorly by the teres minor, laterally by the humerus, inferiorly by the teres major, and medially by the long head of the triceps. The posterior humeral circumflex artery and the axillary nerve course through the quadrilateral space. The more medial triangular space is bordered superiorly by the teres minor, laterally by the long head of the triceps, and inferiorly by the teres major. The circumflex scapular artery coursed in this space.

the posterior part of the olecranon. The lateral head arises from the posterior surface and lateral border of the humerus. It lies lateral to the radial groove and the lateral intermuscular septum and crosses over the radial groove, covering the radial nerve and the deep brachial vessels on its course to the common tendon of insertion into the olecranon. The medial head arises from the humerus medial and inferior to the radial groove. Its origin spans most of the length of the humerus from as high as the insertion of the teres major, down the entire length of the medial intermuscular septum, and as low as the olecranon fossa of the humerus. The medial head is deep to the other heads of the triceps, and its insertion into the olecranon via the common tendon extends into the deep fascia of the forearm on either side of it (6).

The triceps brachii has its major action at the elbow as an extender. However, the long head of the triceps is believed to be involved in forced shoulder adduction and helps to offset the shear forces generated by the primary adductors (4). The primary innervation of the triceps is through the radial nerve (roots C-6 through C-8). The primary blood supply to the muscle is via the profunda brachial artery and the superior ulnar collateral artery. Additional branches from the brachial and posterior humeral circumflex arteries supply the long head near its origin (168).

BRACHIAL PLEXUS

For the hand and arm to perform the necessary fine-motor and sensory functions that are part of everyday life, an intricate network of nervous structures is required. The upper extremity receives all of its innervation via the brachial plexus, which is comprised of nerve fibers that originate in the spinal cord and exit the vertebral column as nerve roots from C-5 to T-1, with inconsistent contributions from C-4 and T-2 (Fig. 20.22). The individual motor nerve fibers of the brachial plexus originate in the ventral gray matter of the spinal cord and exit the cord as the ventral rami or roots. These roots then travel in the interval between the anterior and middle scalene muscle bellies. The C-4 through C-8 roots travel inferiorly toward the first rib, but the roots of T-1 and T-2 travel upward to reach the first rib and the rest of the roots. Although it is necessary to recognize contributions from C-4 and T-2 to the plexus, the remainder of this section is devoted to the plexus as it is most commonly composed of roots C-5 to T-1. The interwoven nature of the brachial plexus necessitate its breakdown into several anatomic regions. These regions include **R**oots, **T**runks, **D**ivisions, **C**ords, and **B**ranches. An easy mnemonic for this sequence is "**R**owdy **T**arantino **D**rinks **C**old **B**eer."

The *roots* discussed above give rise directly to several terminal nerves. These include the long thoracic nerve that is composed of fibers from C-5, C-6, and C-7. The

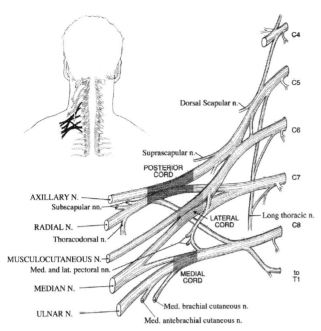

FIG. 20.22. Diagram of the brachial plexus.

the roots from C-5 to T-1. The lateral cord contains fibers originating from C-5 to C-7, and the medial cord has fibers from C-8 and T-1. The cords of the brachial plexus are named on the basis of their individual anatomic relationship to the axillary artery. Several terminal nerves arise at the cord level. The lateral pectoral nerve arises as the only terminal nerve directly from the lateral cord, whereas the medial pectoral nerve arises from the medial cord. Also from the medial cord, the medial antebrachial and medial brachial cutaneous nerves arise. From the posterior cord, the upper and lower subscapular nerves and the thoracodorsal nerve take origin.

Finally, the terminal *branches* are formed by contributions from the three cords. A large portion of the lateral and medial cords combine to form the median nerve, which also contains fibers from roots C-5 though T-1. The remainder of the medial cord goes on to form the ulnar nerve with contributions from roots C-7, C-8, and T-1, and the remainder of the lateral cord goes on to form the musculocutaneous nerve with contributions from roots C-5 through C-7. Most of the posterior cord continues laterally as the radial nerve, with a smaller amount of the cord contributing to form the axillary nerve. Interestingly, the axillary nerve receives fibers from roots C-5 and C-6 alone, whereas the radial nerve, as with the posterior cord, receives fibers from C-5 through T-1. For a complete reference on the brachial plexus and the supply to individual muscles and surface regions, please refer to Fig. 20.22.

BURSAE

A bursa is a loose connective tissue sac lined with synovium containing a small amount of fluid. There are over 50 bursae in the human body, the largest of which is the subacromial bursa in the normal human adult. Bursae in the shoulder serve to facilitate motion between relatively firm structures like bone and tendon, bone and muscle, and bone and skin. Bursae allow smooth gliding motion of one tissue plane on another by the nature of their pliability. Bursae are avascular tissues, making them ideal structures for dissection between tissue planes. The bursae of the shoulder include the subacromial bursa, the subdeltoid bursa, the subscapularis bursa; the infraspinatus bursa; and a bursal sac between the conoid and trapezoid ligaments.

The subacromial bursa and closely approximated subdeltoid bursa are often coalesced into a single structure (217). This large bursa is situated between the superior surface of the rotator cuff and the undersurface of the deltoid muscle. This bursa is consistently found extending from the musculotendinous junction of the supraspinatus, infraspinatus, and teres minor medially to the humerus beyond the tuberosities and rotator cuff

nerves to the longus coli and scalene muscles originate from the roots of C-5 through C-8. The dorsal scapular nerve is a branch off the C-5 root, as is a small branch that joins the phrenic nerve. At the lower aspect of the plexus, the first intercostal nerve is a branch from the T-1 root.

There are three *trunks* of the brachial plexus: superior, middle, and inferior. The superior trunk is composed of the C-4 and C-5 roots. The C-7 root continues distally to form the middle trunk by itself. The inferior trunk is formed by the roots of C-8 and T-1. The suprascapular nerve, which innervates the supraspinatus and infraspinatus, is a terminal branch off the superior trunk. The nerve to subclavius also is a terminal branch off of the superior trunk. No other terminal branches arise at the trunk level routinely.

The trunks each divide into anterior and posterior *divisions,* based on the relative direction of travel for each portion of the trunk. No terminal branches originate at the division level. The individual nerve fibers that form the anterior divisions supply motor and sensory function to the ventral or anterior portion of the upper extremity, whereas the fibers of the posterior divisions provide motor and sensory function to the dorsal or posterior portion of the arm.

The anterior divisions of the superior and middle trunks join to form the lateral *cord* of the plexus. The anterior division of the inferior trunk continues to form the medial cord by itself. The posterior divisions of all three trunks join to form the posterior cord. By receiving components from all the posterior divisions, the posterior cord is composed of fibers originating in all insertion. In the normal state the bursa is only 1 to 2 mm thick but may become markedly enlarged in the diseased state. The volume of the subacromial bursa has been shown to be between 5 and 10 mL in the nondiseased state (218). Pressure measurements in the subacromial bursa have been shown to increase fivefold with elevation of the arm from the side to a position of 30 degrees of abduction and 45 degrees of forward flexion (219). The subacromial bursa is the most important bursa about the shoulder in that it is frequently implicated in the etiologies of shoulder impingement and pain. The subacromial bursa has been shown to contain free nerve endings, Ruffini endings, and Pacinian corpuscles. Most nervous structures are located on the roof side of the bursa facing the acromion (220). It is believed that these nociceptors relay stimuli caused by impingement that are interpreted as pain.

The subscapularis bursa is oblong in shape and occupies the space between the glenoid neck and the upper border of the subscapularis tendon and lateral muscle belly (Fig. 20.23). There is often a communication with the glenohumeral joint between the superior and MGHLs. For this reason, this "bursa" is often thought of as a "space" instead of a bursa. Regardless, this tissue serves to protect the subscapularis as it crosses over the glenoid neck under the coracoid process. In patients with synovitis of the shoulder, it is in this area where the most intense synovial proliferation is encountered.

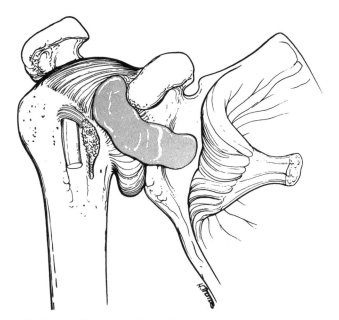

FIG. 20.23. Diagram of the subscapularis bursa. This bursa lies between the neck of the glenoid and the subscapularis muscle, allowing the muscle to glide over the bone smoothly. There is a communication between the bursa and the glenohumeral joint between the superior and middle glenohumeral ligaments. (From Rockwood CA and Matsen FA, eds. *The shoulder.* 2nd ed. Philadelphia: W.B. Saunders, 1998, p. 27 with permission.)

Other bursae that are of less clinical importance with regard to pathologic conditions are the infraspinatus bursa, situated between the insertion of the infraspinatus tendon and the joint capsule; the intermuscular bursa, between the tendons of the latissimus dorsi and the teres major; and the coracobrachialis bursa, found between the coracoid process and the subscapularis muscle belly.

SPACES

There are several soft tissue areas about the shoulder categorized as "spaces." This is a bit of a misnomer because tissues occupy these anatomic regions; they are not empty or hollow. Most of these spaces are occupied or traversed by neurovascular structures and areolar tissues. Some of the more clinically relevant areas include the axillary, subcoracoid, subacromial, quadrilateral, and triangular spaces. The subcoracoid and subacromial spaces and their contents were discussed in the sections above.

The axillary space or axilla varies in shape and size depending on the arm position. In the anatomic position (arm slightly abducted), the space is roughly pyramidal. The base of the pyramid is formed by the skin and fascia that extend from the thoracic wall to the extremity. The broad posterior wall of the space is formed by the latissimus dorsi, teres major, and subscapularis. The bicipital or intertubercular groove of the proximal humerus forms the narrow lateral wall. The anterior surface is formed by the pectoralis major and minor, and the medial wall is formed by the serratus anterior. The apex or summit of the pyramid is bounded by the first rib, the clavicle, and the upper border of the subscapularis muscle. It is through this space that the great vessels and nerves pass (197). Most of the axilla is occupied by areolar tissues and lymph nodes. The axillary fascia is fenestrated, which may explain the mobility of the tissues and overlying skin.

The quadrilateral space is an area of the posterior inferior shoulder bordered superiorly by the teres minor, laterally by the shaft of the humerus, inferiorly by the teres major, and medially by the long head of the triceps (Fig. 20.21). The key structures that traverse this space are the posterior humeral circumflex artery and the axillary nerve. Again, there is loose areolar tissue present within the space. Fibrous bands have also been noted to cross this space and may be responsible for symptoms related to compression of the neurovascular structures within the space.

The triangular space is also on the posterior inferior aspect of the shoulder (Fig. 20.21). It lies just below the quadrilateral space, separated from it by the teres major. This space is triangular in shape as its name would suggest, with the apex of the triangle pointed medially. The base (medial border) of the triangle is formed by the medial aspect of the long head of the triceps muscle. The other two borders are formed by the lower edge of the teres minor and upper edge of the teres major. Through this space passes the circumflex scapular artery.

CONCLUSION

The shoulder region of the human body contains a complex collection of structures that form the supportive and articulating attachment for the remainder of the extremity to the torso. Although the anatomy of the human shoulder is well understood, it would be unwise to consider the current knowledge final and complete. There is much to be learned, especially with regard to functional anatomy and histology of the tissues about the shoulder. We hope this chapter has furthered the reader's anatomic knowledge base and stimulated further work in this area.

REFERENCES

1. Peat M. Functional anatomy of the shoulder complex. *Phys Ther* 1986;66:1855.
2. Sarrafian SK. Gross and functional anatomy of the shoulder. *Clin Orthop* 1983;173:11.
3. Kapandji IA, Honore LH, Poileux F. *The physiology of the joints: the upper limb.* New York: Churchill Livingstone, 1982.
4. Rockwood CA, Matsen FA. *The shoulder.* Philadelphia: W.B. Saunders, 1998.
5. Moseley HF. The clavicle: its anatomy and function. *Clin Orthop* 1968;58:17.
6. Netter FH. *The CIBA collection of medical illustrations: musculoskeletal system.* Summit: CIBA-Geigy Corporation, 1987.
7. DePalma AF. *Surgery of the shoulder.* Philadelphia: J.B. Lippincott, 1983.
8. Rowe CR. An atlas of anatomy and treatment of midclavicular fractures. *Clin Orthop* 1968;58:29.
9. Howard FM, Shafer SJ. Injuries to the clavicle with neurovascular complications: a study of fourteen cases. *J Bone Joint Surg Am* 1956;47A:1335.
10. Nichols HM. Anatomic structures of the thoracic outlet. *Clin Orthop* 1967;51:17.
11. Abbott LS, Abbott LC, Lucas DB. The function of the clavicle: its surgical significance. *Ann Surg* 1954;140:583.
12. Lewis MM, Ballet FL, Kroll PG, et al. En bloc clavicular resection: operative procedure and postoperative testing of function. Case reports. *Clin Orthop* 1985;193:214.
13. Acus RW, Bell RH, Fisher CL. Proximal clavicle excision: an analysis of results. *J Shoulder Elbow Surg* 1995;4:182.
14. Ruland LJ, Ruland CM, Matthews LS. Scapulothoracic anatomy for the arthroscopist. *J Arthrosc Relat Surg* 1995;11:52.
15. Gerber C, Terrier F, Ganz R. The role of the coracoid process in the chronic impingement syndrome. *J Bone Joint Surg Br* 1985;67B:703.
16. Gerber C, Terrier F, Zehnder R, et al. The subcoracoid space: an anatomic study. *Clin Orthop* 1987;215:132.
17. Neer CS. Anterior acromioplasty for the chronic impingement syndrome in the shoulder: a preliminary report. *J Bone Joint Surg Am* 1972;54A:41.
18. Patte D. Subcoracoid impingement. *Clin Orthop* 1990;254:55.
19. Edelson JG, Taitz C. Anatomy of the coraco-acromial arch: relation to degeneration of the acromion. *J Bone Joint Surg Br* 1992;74B:589.
20. Mallon WJ, Brown HR, Vogler JB, et al. Radiographic and geometric anatomy of the scapula. *Clin Orthop* 1992;277:142.
21. Edelson JG, Luchs J. Aspects of coracoacromial ligament anat-omy of interest to the arthroscopic surgeon. *J Arthrosc Relat Surg* 1995;11:715.
22. Holt EM, Allibone RO. Anatomic variants of the coracoacromial ligament. *J Shoulder Elbow Surg* 1995;4:370.
23. Peiper HG, Radas CB, Krahl H, et al. Anatomic variation of the coracoacromial ligament: a macroscopic and microscopic cadaveric study. *J Shoulder Elbow Surg* 1997;6:291.
24. Edelson JG, Taitz C. Bony anatomy of coracoacromial arch: implications for arthroscopic portal placement in the shoulder. *J Arthrosc Relat Surg* 1993;9:201.
25. Gallino M, Battiston B, Annaratone G, et al. Coracoacromial ligament: a comparative arthroscopic and anatomic study. *J Arthrosc Relat Surg* 1995;11:564.
26. Nutter PD. Coracoclavicular articulations. *J Bone Joint Surg Am* 1941;23A:177.
27. Edelson JG. Bony bridges and other variations of the suprascapular notch. *J Bone Joint Surg Br* 1995;77B:505.
28. Edelson JG, Taitz C, Grishkan A. The coracohumeral ligament: anatomy of a substantial but neglected structure. *J Bone Joint Surg Br* 1991;73B:150.
29. Neer CS, Satterlee CC, Dalsey RM, et al. The anatomy and potential effects of contracture of the coracohumeral ligament. *Clin Orthop* 1992;280:182.
30. Panje W, Cutting C. Trapezius osteomyocutaneous island flap for reconstruction of the anterior floor of the mouth and the mandible. *Head Neck Surg* 1980;3:66.
31. Booth RE, Marvel JP. Differential diagnosis of shoulder pain. *Orthop Clin North Am* 1975;6:353.
32. Burns WC, Whipple TL. Anatomic relationships in the shoulder impingement syndrome. *Clin Orthop* 1993;294:96.
33. Hammond G. Complete acromionectomy in the treatment of chronic tendonitis of the shoulder. *J Bone Joint Surg Am* 1962;44A:494.
34. Hawkins RJ, Kennedy JC. Impingement syndrome in athletes. *Am J Sports Med* 1980;8:151.
35. Kessel L, Watson M. The painful arc syndrome. Clinical classification as a guide to management. *J Bone Joint Surg Br* 1977;59B:166.
36. Neer CS, Poppen NK. Supraspinatus outlet. *Orthop Trans* 1987;11:234.
37. Toivonen DA, Tuite MJ, Orwin JF. Acromial structure and tears of the rotator cuff. *J Shoulder Elbow Surg* 1995;4:376.
38. Bigliani LU, Morrison DS, April EW. The morphology of the acromion and its relationship to rotator cuff tears. *Orthop Trans* 1986;10:228.
39. Flatow EL, Soslowsky LV, Ticker JB, et al. Excursion of the rotator cuff under the acromion: patterns of subacromial contact. *Am J Sports Med* 1994;22:779.
40. Morrison DS, Bigliani LU. The clinical significance of variations in acromial morphology. *Orthop Trans* 1987;11:234.
41. Zuckerman JD, Kummer FJ, Cuomo F, et al. Interobserver reliability of acromial morphology classification: an anatomic study. *J Shoulder Elbow Surg* 1997;6:286.
42. Wang JC, Shapiro MS. Changes in acromial morphology with age. *J Shoulder Elbow Surg* 1997;6:55.
43. Nicholson GP, Goodman DA, Flatow EL, et al. The acromion: morphologic condition and age-related changes. A study of 420 scapulas. *J Shoulder Elbow Surg* 1996;5:1.
44. Liberson F. Os acromiale—a contested anomaly. *J Bone Joint Surg Am* 1937;19A:683–689.
45. Neer CS. Impingement lesions. *Clin Orthop* 1983;173:70.
46. Howell SM, Galinat BJ. The glenoid-labral socket: a constrained articular surface. *Clin Orthop* 1989;243:122.
47. Saha AK. Dynamic stability of the glenohumeral joint. *Acta Orthop Scand* 1971;42:491.
48. Rockwood CA, Green DP, Bucholz RW, et al. *Fractures in adults.* Philadelphia: Lippincott-Raven, 1996.
49. Browner BD, Jupiter JB, Levine AM, et al. *Skeletal trauma: fractures, dislocations, ligamentous injuries.* Philadelphia: W.B. Saunders, 1998.
50. Dameron TB, Reibel DB. Fractures involving the proximal humeral epiphyseal plate. *J Bone Joint Surg Am* 1969;51A:289.
51. Hodges PC. Development of the human skeleton. *AJR Am J Roentgenol* 1933;30:809.

52. Cyprien JM, Vasey HM, Buret A, et al. Humeral retrotorsion and glenohumeral relationship in the normal shoulder and in recurrent anterior dislocation (scapulometry). *Clin Orthop* 1983;175:8.

53. Pearl ML, Volk AG. Retroversion of the proximal humerus in relationship to prosthetic replacement arthroplasty. *J Shoulder Elbow Surg* 1995;4:286.

54. Roberts SNJ, Foley AP, Swallow HM, et al. The geometry of the humeral head and the design of prostheses. *J Bone Joint Surg Br* 1991;73B:647.

55. Boileau P, Walch G. The three-dimensional geometry of the proximal humerus: implications for surgical technique and prosthetic design. *J Bone Joint Surg Br* 1997;79B:857.

56. Perry J. Biomechanics of the shoulder. In: Rowe C, ed. *The shoulder.* New York: Churchill Livingstone, 1988.

57. Iannotti JP, Gabriel JP, Schneck SL, et al. The normal glenohumeral relationships. *J Bone Joint Surg Am* 1992;74A:491.

58. Vangsness CT, Jorgenson SS, Watson T, et al. The origin of the long head of the biceps from the scapula and glenoid labrum. *J Bone Joint Surg Br* 1994;76B:951.

59. Meyer AW. Spontaneous dislocation of the tendon of the long head of the biceps brachii. *Arch Surg* 1926;13:109.

60. Meyer AW. Spontaneous dislocation and destruction of tendon of long head of biceps brachii. *Arch Surg* 1928;17:493.

61. Petersson CJ. Spontaneous medial dislocation of the tendon of the long biceps brachii: an anatomic study of prevalence and pathomechanics. *Clin Orthop* 1986;211:224.

62. Slatis P, Aalto K. Medial dislocation of the tendon of the long head of the biceps brachii. *Acta Orthop Scand* 1979;50:73.

63. Neviaser TJ, Neviaser RJ. Lesions of the long head of biceps. *AAOS Instr Course Lect* 1981;30:250.

64. Warren RF. Lesions of the long head of the biceps tendon. *AAOS Instr Course Lect* 1985;34:204.

65. Duchenne GB. *Physiology of motion.* Philadelphia: J.B. Lippincott, 1949.

66. Kumar VP, Satku K, Balasubramaniam P. The role of the long head of biceps brachii in the stabilization of the head of the humerus. *Clin Orthop* 1989;244:172.

67. Yamaguchi K, Riew K, Galatz LM. Biceps function in normal and rotator cuff deficient shoulders: and electromyographic analysis. Annual AAOS Shoulder and Elbow Society Meeting, San Francisco, CA, 1993.

68. Codman EA. *The shoulder.* Boston: T. Todd, 1934.

69. Neer CS. Displaced proximal humeral fractures: classification and evaluation. *J Bone Joint Surg Am* 1970;52A:1077.

70. Grant JCB. *Method of anatomy.* Baltimore: Williams & Wilkins, 1965.

71. DePalma AF. Surgical anatomy of acromioclavicular and sternoclavicular joints. *Surg Clin North Am* 1963;43:1541.

72. Bearn JG. Direct observations on the function of the capsule of the sternoclavicular joint in clavicular support. *J Anat* 1967;101:159.

73. Cave AJE. The nature and morphology of the costoclavicular ligament. *J Anat* 1961;95:170.

74. DePalma AF. The role of the disks of the sternoclavicular and the acromioclavicular joints. *Clin Orthop* 1959;13:222.

75. Inman VT, Saunders M, Abbott LC. Observations on the function of the shoulder joint. *J Bone Joint Surg Am* 1944;26A:1.

76. Lucas DB. Biomechanics of the shoulder joint. *Arch Surg* 1973;107:425.

77. Lewis OJ. The coraco-clavicular joint. *J Anat* 1959;93:296.

78. Tyurina TV. Age-related characteristics of the human acromioclavicular joint. *Arkh Anat Gistol Embriol* 1985;89:75.

79. Urist MR. Complete dislocations of the acromioclavicular joint: the nature of the traumatic lesion and effective methods of treatment with an analysis of forty-one cases. *J Bone Joint Surg Am* 1946;28A:813.

80. Keats TE, Pope TL. The acromioclavicular joint: normal variation and the diagnosis of dislocation. *Skeletal Radiol* 1988;17:159.

81. Moseley HF. Athletic injuries to the shoulder region. *Am J Surg* 1959;98:401.

82. DePalma AF, Callery G, Bennett GA. Variational anatomy and degenerative lesions of the shoulder joint. In: American Academy of Orthopaedic Surgeons, eds. *Instructional Course Lectures.* Rosemont, IL: AAOS, Vol. VI. 1949:255.

83. Fukuda K, Craig EV, An KN, Cofield RH, et al. Biomechanical study of the ligamentous system of the acromioclavicular joint. *J Bone Joint Surg Am* 1986;68A:434.

84. Tillmann B. Functional anatomy of the shoulder, Fourth Congress of the European Society of Knee Surgery and Arthroscopy, Stockholm, June 25–30, 1990, 1990.

85. Steindler A. *Kinesiology of the human body under normal and pathological conditions.* Springfield: Charles C Thomas, 1955.

86. Dvir Z, Berme N. The shoulder complex in elevation of the arm: a mechanism approach. *J Biomech* 1978;11:219.

87. Freedman L, Munro RH. Abduction of the arm in scapular plane: scapular and glenohumeral movements. *J Bone Joint Surg Am* 1966;18A:1503.

88. Ainscow DA. Dislocation of the scapula. *J Coll Surg Edinb* 1982;27:56.

89. Key JA, Conwell HE. *The management of fractures, dislocations and sprains.* St. Louis: C.V. Mosby, 1964.

90. Nettrour LF, Krufty LE, Mueller RE, et al. Locked scapula: intrathoracic dislocation of the inferior angle. *J Bone Joint Surg Am* 1972;54A:413.

91. Oreck SL, Burgess A, Levine AM. Traumatic lateral displacement of the scapula: a radiologic sign of neurovascular disruption. *J Bone Joint Surg Am* 1984;66A:758.

92. Ebraheim NA, An S, Jackson WT. Scapulothoracic dissociation. *J Bone Joint Surg Am* 1988;70A:428.

93. Ebraheim NA, Pearlstein SR, Savolaine ER. Scapulothoracic dissociation (avulsion of the scapula, subclavian artery, and brachial plexus): an early recognized variant, a new classification, and a review of the literature and treatment options. *J Orthop Trauma* 1987;1:18.

94. Lange RH, Noel SH. Traumatic lateral scapular displacement: an expanded spectrum of associated neurovascular injury. *J Othop Trauma* 1993;7.

95. Cooley LH, Torg JS. Pseudowinging of the scapula secondary to subscapular osteochondroma. *Clin Orthop* 1982;162:119.

96. Milch H. Snapping scapula. *Clin Orthop* 1961;20:139–150.

97. Ciullo JV. Subscapular bursitis: treatment of "snapping scapula" or "washboard syndrome." *J Arthrosc Relat Surg* 1992;8:412.

98. Speer KP. Anatomy and pathomechanics of shoulder instability. *Clin Sports Med* 1995;14:751.

99. Kumar VP, Balasubramaniam P. The role of atmospheric pressure in stabilizing the shoulder: an experimental study. *J Bone Joint Surg Br* 1985;67B:719.

100. McPherson EJ, Friedman RJ, An YH, et al. Anthropometric study of normal glenohumeral relationships. *J Shoulder Elbow Surg* 1997;6:105.

101. Soslowsky LJ, Flatow EL, Bigliani LU, et al. Articular geometry of the glenohumeral joint. *Clin Orthop* 1992;285:181.

102. Saha AK. *Theory of shoulder mechanism: descriptive and applied.* Springfield: Charles C Thomas, 1961.

103. Matsen FA III, Lippitt SB, Sidles JA, et al. *Practical evaluation and management of the shoulder.* Philadelphia: W.B. Saunders, 1994.

104. Turkel SJ, Panio MW, Marshall JL, et al. Stabilizing mechanisms preventing anterior dislocation of the glenohumeral joint. *J Bone Joint Surg Am* 1981;63A:1208.

105. Bost FC, Inman VT. The pathological changes in recurrent dislocation of the shoulder. *J Bone Joint Surg Am* 1942;24A:595.

106. Doody SG, Freedman L, Waterland JC. Shoulder movements during abduction in the scapular plane. *Arch Phys Med Rehabil* 1970;51:595.

107. Howell SM, Galinat BJ, Renzi AJ, et al. Normal and abnormal mechanics of the glenohumeral joint in the horizontal plane. *J Bone Joint Surg Am* 1988;70A:227.

108. Poppen NK, Walker PS. Normal and abnormal motion of the shoulder. *J Bone Joint Surg Am* 1976;58A:195.

109. Bergman G. Biomechanics and pathomechanics of the shoulder joint with reference to prosthetic joint replacement. In: Koelbel R, ed. *Shoulder replacement.* Berlin: Springer-Verlag, 1987.

110. Harryman DT II, Walker ED, Harris SL. Residual motion and function after glenohumeral or scapulothoracic arthrodesis. *J Shoulder Elbow Surg* 1993;2:275.

111. Laumann U. Kinesiology of the shoulder joint. In: Koelbel R, ed. *Shoulder replacement.* Berlin: Springer-Verlag, 1987.

112. Gerber C, Schneeberger AG, Vinh TS. The arterial vascularization of the humeral head. *J Bone Joint Surg Am* 1990;72A:1486.

113. Laing PG. The arterial supply of the adult humerus. *J Bone Joint Surg Am* 1956;38A:1105.

114. Gardner E. The innervation of the shoulder joint. *Anat Rec* 1948;102:1.

115. Zimmerman LM, Veith I. *Great ideas in the history of surgery: clavicle, shoulder, shoulder amputations.* Baltimore: Williams & Wilkins, 1961.

116. Cave EF, Burke JF, Boyd RJ. *Trauma management.* Chicago: Year Book Medical Publishers, 1974.

117. Kazar B, Reloyszky E. Prognosis of primary dislocation of the shoulder. *Acta Orthop Scand* 1969;40:216.

118. Hawkins RJ, Neer CJ II, Pianta RM, et al. Locked posterior dislocation of the shoulder. *J Bone Joint Surg Am* 1987;69A:9.

119. Laskin RS, Sedlin ED. Luxatio erecta in infancy. *Clin Orthop* 1971;80:126.

120. Peiro A, Ferrandis R, Correa F. Bilateral erect dislocation of the shoulders. *Injury* 1975;6:294.

121. Speed K. *Fractures and dislocation.* Philadelphia: Lea & Febiger, 1942.

122. Reeves B. Experiments on the tensile strength of the anterior capsular structures of the shoulder in man. *J Bone Joint Surg Br* 1968;50B:858.

123. Flood V. Discovery of a new ligament of the shoulder joint. *Lancet* 1829;672–673.

124. Gibb TD, Sidles JA, Harryman DT, et al. The effect of capsular venting on glenohumeral laxity. *Clin Orthop* 1991;72:120.

125. Gray H. The articulations. In: Pickering TP, HR, eds. *Anatomy, descriptive and surgical.* New York: Bounty Books, 1977:251.

126. Habermeyer P, Schuller U, Wiedemann E. The intra-articular pressure of the shoulder: an experimental study on the role of the glenoid labrum in stabilizing the joint. *Arthroscopy* 1992;8:166.

127. Matsen FA III, Harryman DT II, Sidles JA. Mechanics of glenohumeral instability. *Clin Sports Med* 1991;10:783.

128. Reeves B. Arthrography of the shoulder. *J Bone Joint Surg Br* 1966;48B:424.

129. Sperber A, Wredmark T. Capsular elasticity and joint volume in recurrent anterior shoulder instability. *J Arthrosc Relat Surg* 1994;10:598.

130. Kaltsas DS. Comparative study of the properties of the shoulder joint capsule with those of other joint capsules. *Clin Orthop* 1983;173:20.

131. Hara H, Ito N, Iwasaki K. Strength of the glenoid labrum and adjacent shoulder capsule. *J Shoulder Elbow Surg* 1996;5:263.

132. O'Brien SJ, Neves MC, Arnoczky SP, et al. The anatomy and histology of the inferior glenohumeral ligament complex of the shoulder. *Am J Sports Med* 1990;18:449.

133. Bresch JR, Nuber G. Mechanoreceptors of the middle and inferior glenohumeral ligaments: histologic study of human cadaver shoulders. *J Shoulder Elbow Surg* 1995;4:565.

134. Vangsness CT Jr, Ennis M, Taylor JG, et al. Neural anatomy of the glenohumeral ligaments, labrum, and subacromial bursa. *J Arthrosc Relat Surg* 1995;11:180.

135. Jerosch J, Clahsen H, Hackmann-Grosse A. Effects of proprioception fibers in the capsule tissue in stabilizing the glenohumeral joint. Specialty Day: American Shoulder and Elbow Surgeons, Washington, DC, 1992.

136. Tibone JT, Fletcher J, Kao JT. Evaluation of a proprioception pathway in patients with stable and unstable shoulders with somatosensory cortical evoked potentials. *J Shoulder Elbow Surg* 1997;6:440.

137. Lephart SM, Warner JP, Borsa PA, et al. Proprioception of the shoulder joint in healthy, unstable, and surgically repaired shoulders. *J Shoulder Elbow Surg* 1994;3:371.

138. Hashimoto T, Harmada T, Sasaguri Y, et al. Immunohistochemical approach for the investigation of nerve distribution in the shoulder joint capsule. *Clin Orthop* 1994;305:273.

139. Hashimoto T, Harmada T, Nakamura T, et al. Myxoid and globular degeneration of nerves in the shoulder joint. *Clin Orthop* 1995:55.

140. Schlemm F. Veber die verstarkungsbander am schultergelerk. *Arch Anat* 1853;45–48.

141. Ferrari DA. Capsular ligaments of the shoulder: anatomical and functional study of the anterior superior capsule. *Am J Sports Med* 1990;18:20.

142. Moseley HF, Overgaard B. The anterior capsular mechanism in recurrent anterior dislocation of the shoulder: morphological and clinical studies with special reference to the glenoid labrum and the gleno-humeral ligaments. *J Bone Joint Surg Br* 1962;44B:913.

143. Warner JP, Carborn DN, Berger R, et al. Dynamic capsuloligamentous anatomy of the glenohumeral joint. *J Shoulder Elbow Surg* 1993;2:115.

144. Warner JP, Deng XH, Warren RF, et al. Static capsuloligamentous restraints to superior-inferior translation of the glenohumeral joint. *Am J Sports Med* 1992;20:675.

145. Bowen MK, Warren RF. Ligamentous control of shoulder stability based on selective cutting and static translation experiments. *Clin Sports Med* 1991;10:757.

146. O'Brien SJ, Schwartz RS, Warren RF, et al. Capsular restraints to anterior-posterior motion of the abducted shoulder: a biomechanical study. *J Shoulder Elbow Surg* 1995;4:298.

147. O'Connell PW, Nuber GW, Mileski RA, et al. The contribution of the glenohumeral ligaments to anterior stability of the shoulder joint. *Am J Sports Med* 1990;18:579.

148. Basmajian JV, Bazant FJ, Kingston CM. Factors preventing downward dislocation of the adducted shoulder. *J Bone Joint Surg Am* 1959;41A:1182.

149. Warner JP, Krushell RJ, Masquelet A, et al. Anatomy and relationships of the suprascapular nerve: anatomical constraints to mobilization of the supraspinatus and infraspinatus muscles in the management of massive rotator-cuff tears. *J Bone Joint Surg Am* 1992;74A:36.

150. Warren RF, Kornblatt IB, Marchand R. Static factors affecting posterior shoulder stability. *Orthop Trans* 1984;8:89.

151. Williams MM, Snyder SJ, Buford D. The Buford complex—the "cord-like" middle glenohumeral ligament and absent anterosuperior labrum complex: a normal anatomic capsulolabral variant. *Arthroscopy* 1994;10:241.

152. Bigliani LU, Pollock RG, Soslowsky LJ, et al. Tensile properties of the inferior glenohumeral ligament. *J Orthop Res* 1992;10:187.

153. Stefko JM, Tibone JE, Cawley PW, et al. Strain of the anterior band of the inferior glenohumeral ligament during capsule failure. *J Shoulder Elbow Surg* 1997;6:473.

154. Ovesen J, Nielsen S. Anterior and posterior instability. *Acta Orthop Scand* 1986;57:324.

155. Soslowsky LJ, Malicky DM, Blaiser RB. Active and passive factors in inferior glenohumeral stabilization: a biomechanical model. *J Shoulder Elbow Surg* 1997;6:371.

156. Branch TP, Lawton RL, Iobst CA, et al. The role of glenohumeral capsular ligaments in internal and external rotation of the humerus. *Am J Sports Med* 1995;23:632.

157. Cooper DE, Arnoczky SP, O'Brien SJ, et al. Anatomy, histology, and vascularity of the glenoid labrum: an anatomic study. *J Bone Joint Surg Am* 1992;74A:46.

158. Prodromos CC, Ferry JA, Schiller AL, et al. Histologic studies of the glenoid labrum from fetal life to old age. *J Bone Joint Surg Am* 1990;72A:1344.

159. Nishida K, Hashizume H, Toda K, et al. Histologic and scanning electron microscopic study of the glenoid labrum. *J Shoulder Elbow Surg* 1996;5:132.

160. Pal GP, Bhatt RH, Patel VS. Relationship between the tendon of the long head of the biceps brachii and the glenoidal labrum in humans. *Anat Rec* 1991;229:278.

161. Gigis P, Natsis C, Polyzonis M. New aspects on the topography of the tendon of the long head of the biceps brachii muscle. One more stabilizer factor of the shoulder joint. *Bull Assoc Anat* 1995;79:9.

162. Lee SB, Harryman DT. Superior detachment of a glenoid labrum variant resembling an incomplete discoid meniscus in a wheelchair ambulator. *J Arthrosc Relat Surg* 1997;13:511.

163. Abbott LC, Lucas DB. The tripartite deltoid and its surgical significance in exposure of the scapulohumeral joint. *Ann Surg* 1952;136:392.

164. Kumar VP, Satku K, Liu J, et al. The anatomy of the anterior origin of the deltoid. *J Bone Joint Surg Br* 1997;79B:680.

165. Basmajian JV, Deluca CJ. *Muscles alive: their functions revealed by electromyography*. Baltimore: Williams & Wilkins, 1985.

166. Kelly BT, Kadrmas WR, Kirkendall DT, et al. Optimal normalization tests for shoulder muscle activation: an electromyographic study. *J Orthop Res* 1996;14:647.

167. Shevlin MG, Lehmann JF, Lucci JA. Electromyographic study of the function of some muscles crossing the glenohumeral joint. *Arch Phys Med Rehabil* 1969;50:264.

168. Salmon M. *Anatomic studies: arteries of the muscles of the extremities and the trunk and arterial anastomotic pathways of the extremities*. St. Louis: Quality Medical Publishing, 1994.

169. Cartmill M, Hylander WL, Shafland J. *Human structure*. Cambridge: President and Fellows of Harvard College, 1987.

170. Harmon PH. Surgical reconstruction of the paralytic shoulder by multiple muscle transplantations. *J Bone Joint Surg Am* 1950;32A:583.

171. Burkhart SS, Esch JC, Jolson RS. The rotator crescent and rotator cable: an anatomic description of the shoulder's "suspension bridge." *J Arthrosc Relat Surg* 1993;9:611.

172. Sharkey NA, Marder RA, Hanson PB. The entire rotator cuff contributes to elevation of the arm. *J Orthop Res* 1994;12:699.

173. Sharkey NA, Marder RA. The rotator cuff opposes superior translation of the humeral head. *Am J Sports Med* 1995;23:270.

174. DePalma AF. Surgical anatomy of the rotator cuff and the natural history of degenerative periarthritis. *Surg Clin North Am* 1967;43:1507.

175. Speer KP, Garrett WE Jr. Muscular control of motion and stability about the pectoral girdle. In: Matsen FA III, FF, Hawkins RJ, eds. *The shoulder: a balance of mobility and stability*. Rosemont, IL: American Academy of Orthopaedic Surgeons, 1993:159.

176. Kumagai J, Sarkar K, Uhthoff HK. The collagen types in the attachment zone of rotator cuff tendons in the elderly: an immunohistochemical study. *J Rheumatol* 1994;21:2096.

177. Rodeo SA, Arnoczsky SP, Torzilli PA. Tendon healing in a bone tunnel: a biomechanical and histological study in the dog. *J Bone Joint Surg Am* 1993;75A:1795.

178. Tomonaga A, Hamada K, Gotoh M. Localization of mRNA of procollagen {alpha} 1 type III in torn supraspinatus tendons by in situ hybridization. *J Shoulder Elbow Surg* 1995;4:69.

179. Chansky HA, Ianotti JP. The vascularity of the rotator cuff. *Clin Sports Med* 1991;10:807.

180. Clark JM, Harryman DT II. Tendons, ligaments, and capsule of the rotator cuff. *J Bone Joint Surg Am* 1992;74A:713.

181. Itoi E, Berglund LS, Grabowski JJ. Tensile properties of the supraspinatus tendon. *J Orthop Res* 1995;13:578.

182. Soslowsky LJ, Carpenter JE, Bucchieri JS, et al. Biomechanics of the rotator cuff. *Orthop Clin North Am* 1997;28:17.

183. Atwater AE. Biomechanics of overarm throwing movements and of throwing injuries. *Exerc Sport Sci Rev* 1979;7:43.

184. Howell SM, Imobersteg AM, Seger DH, et al. Clarification of the role of the supraspinatus muscle in shoulder function. *J Bone Joint Surg Am* 1986;68A:398.

185. Thomson WO, Debski RE, Boardman ND III. A biomechanical analysis of rotator cuff deficiency in a cadaveric model. *Am J Sports Med* 1996;24:286.

186. Bechtol CO. Biomechanics of the shoulder. *Clin Orthop* 1980;146:37.

187. Grant JCB, Smith CG. Age incidence of rupture of the supraspinatus tendon. *Anat Rec* 1948;100:666.

188. Wilson CL, Duff GL. Pathologic study of degeneration and rupture of the supraspinatus tendon. *Arch Surg* 1943;47:121.

189. Rothman RH, Park WW. The vascular anatomy of the rotator cuff. *Clin Orthop* 1964;176–186.

190. Lohr JF, Uhthoff HK. The microvascular pattern of the supraspinatus tendon. *Clin Orthop* 1990;254:35.

191. Rathburn JB, Macnab I. The microvascular pattern of the rotator cuff. *J Bone Joint Surg Br* 1970;52B:540.

192. Bigliani LU, Dalsey RM, McCann PD, et al. An anatomical study of the suprascapular nerve. *J Arthrosc Relat Surg* 1990;6:301.

193. Colachis SC Jr, Strohm BR, Brecher VL. Effects of axillary nerve block on muscle force in the upper extremity. *Arch Phys Med Rehabil* 1969;50:645.

194. Kelly BT, Kadrmas WR, Speer KP. The manual muscle examination for rotator cuff strength: an electromyographic investigation. *Am J Sports Med* 1996;24:581.

195. Poppen NK, Walker PS. Forces at the glenohumeral joint in abduction. *Clin Orthop* 1978;135:165.

196. Cain PR, Mutschler TA, Fu FH, et al. Anterior stability of the glenohumeral joint. A dynamic model. *Am J Sports Med* 1987;15:144.

197. Hollinshead WH. *Anatomy for surgeons*. Philadelphia: Harper and Row, 1982.

198. Hinton MA, Parker AW, Drez D, et al. An anatomic study of the subscapularis tendon and myotendinous junction. *J Shoulder Elbow Surg* 1994;3:224.

199. Ovesen JO, Nielsen S. Stability of the shoulder joint. Cadaver study of stabilizing structures. *Acta Orthop Scand* 1985;56:149.

200. Itoi ES, Kuechle DK, Morrey BF, et al. Dynamic anterior stabilizers of the shoulder with the arm in abduction. *J Bone Joint Surg Br* 1994;76B:834.

201. Bartlett SP, May JW Jr., Yaremchuk MJ. The latissimus dorsi muscle: a fresh cadaver study of the primary neurovascular pedicle. *Plast Reconstr Surg* 1981;65:631.

202. Huelke DF. Variation in the origins of the branches of the axillary artery. *Anat Rec* 1959;132:233.

203. Marmor L, Bechtol CO, Hall CB. Pectoralis major muscle. *J Bone Joint Surg Am* 1961;43A.

204. McCann PD, Cardasco FA, Ticker JB. An anatomic study of the subscapular nerves: a grid for electromyographic analysis of the subscapularis muscle. *J Shoulder Elbow Surg* 1994;3:94.

205. Yung SW, Lazarus MD, Harryman DT. Practical guidelines to safe surgery about the subscapularis. *J Shoulder Elbow Surg* 1996;5:467.

206. Harryman DT, Sidles JA, Harris SL, et al. The role of the rotator interval capsule in passive motion and stability of the shoulder. *J Bone Joint Surg Am* 1992;74A:53.

207. Nobuhara K, Ikeda H. Rotator interval lesion. *Clin Orthop* 1987;223:44–50.

208. Field LD, Warren RF, O'Brien SJ, et al. Isolated closure of rotator interval defects for shoulder instability. *Am J Sports Med* 1995;23:557.

209. Rowe CR, Zarins B, Ciullo JV. Recurrent transient subluxation of the shoulder. *J Bone Joint Surg Am* 1981;63A:863.

210. Treacy SH, Field LD, Savoie FH. Rotator interval capsule closure: an arthroscopic technique. *J Arthrosc Relat Surg* 1997;13:103.

211. Jobe CM, Wood VE. The spinal accessory nerve in a trapezius splitting approach. *J Shoulder Elbow Surg* 1996;5:206.

212. Pagnani MJ, Deng XH, Warren RF, et al. Role of the long head of the biceps brachii in glenohumeral stability: a biomechanical study in cadavera. *J Shoulder Elbow Surg* 1996;5:255.

213. Basmajian JV. Integrated actions and functions of the chief flexors of the elbow: a detailed electromyographic analysis. *J Bone Joint Surg Am* 1957;39A:1106–1118.

214. Glousman R, Jobe F, Tibone J. Dynamic electromyographic analysis of the throwing shoulder with glenohumeral instability. *J Bone Joint Surg Am* 1988;70A:220.

215. Jobe FW, Moynes D, Tibone JE, et al. An EMG analysis of the shoulder in pitching: a second report. *Am J Sports Med* 1984;12:218.

216. Jobe FW, Tibone JE, Perry A, et al. An EMG analysis of the shoulder in throwing and pitching: a preliminary report. *Am J Sports Med* 1983;11:3.

217. Jobe CM. Gross anatomy of the shoulder. In: Rockwood CA MF, ed. *The shoulder*. Vol. 1. Philadelphia: W.B. Saunders, 1998:34.

218. Strizak AM, Danzig L, Jackson DW. Subacromial bursography. An anatomical and clinical study. *J Bone Joint Surg [Am]* 1982;64:196.

219. Sigholm G, Styf J, Korner L, et al. Pressure recording in the subacromial bursa. *J Orthop Res* 1988;6:123.

220. Ide K, Shirai Y, Ito H, et al. Sensory nerve supply in the human subacromial bursa. *J Shoulder Elbow Surg* 1996;5:371.

Principles and Practice of Orthopaedic Sports Medicine,
edited by William E. Garrett, Jr., Kevin P. Speer, and Donald T. Kirkendall.
Lippincott Williams & Wilkins, Philadelphia © 2000.

CHAPTER 21

Biomechanics of the Shoulder

Louis J. Soslowsky, James E. Carpenter, and John E. Kuhn

The shoulder is comprised of multiple joints all working in concert to produce the wide range of motion and activities expected of the upper limb. We present the current state of basic science, particularly of biomechanics, of several critical aspects of the shoulder. The first section reports on the biomechanics of the sternoclavicular joint, the clavicle, and the acromioclavicular joint. The second section reports on the biomechanics of the rotator cuff and the coracoacromial arch. The third section reports on the biomechanics of the glenohumeral joint, with particular emphasis on joint stability. The final section reports on the biomechanics and kinematics of the shoulder during specific sport activities.

BIOMECHANICS OF THE STERNOCLAVICULAR JOINT, CLAVICLE, AND ACROMIOCLAVICULAR JOINT

The clavicle is the sole bony connection between the upper extremity and the trunk. As such, it plays a key role in the biomechanics of the shoulder and upper extremity. It is connected by means of the sternoclavicular and acromioclavicular joints and their accompanying ligaments. It acts as a strut, maintaining the distance between the sternum and the scapula and resisting the forces that act to pull the scapula toward the chest [1,2]. This phenomena allows the trapezius and other supporting muscles to hold the scapula upward without the entire upper extremity translating toward the midline or rotating anteriorly across the front of the chest. In addition, by maintaining the scapula and humeral head

in a position away from the chest, it allows the other muscles arising from the chest that control the proximal humerus, such as the pectoralis major and latissimus dorsi, to work effectively. There are case reports of patients born without clavicles and patients who have had a complete clavicectomy for various reasons. Although these patients may be able to perform activities of daily living, their functional capacity is certainly diminished, especially with activities requiring strength with the arm out to the side. Patients who require resections of major portions of their clavicle should be warned about the functional results of losing this important support strut. The motions and stabilizers of the clavicle are best understood by separate evaluation of its joints at either end.

Sternoclavicular Joint

The mechanics of the sternoclavicular joint are best explained by evaluating its structural anatomy, normal kinematics, and restraints to abnormal forces that occur as a result of injuries. The hallmark of the sternoclavicular joint is that it is a saddle-type joint [3]. The joint surfaces are not truly congruent. The articular surface of the medial end of the clavicle is nearly twice that of the sternal side of the sternoclavicular joint. Because of this configuration, a large amount of motion is possible through the sternoclavicular joint; however, the joint itself has little bony stability. The sternal facet of the sternoclavicular faces superiorly and approximately 20 degrees posteriorly. In between the articular surfaces of the joint is an intraarticular disc [4] (Fig. 21.1). This fibrocartilagenous structure and attached ligament run from the inferior portion of the joint near the junction near the first rib in the sternum to the superior portion of the medial clavicle. As such, it is interposed in the joint and as an isolated structure has been thought to resist medial displacement of the clavicle.

L. J. Soslowsky: Departments of Orthopaedic Surgery and Bioengineering, University of Pennsylvania, Philadelphia, Pennsylvania 19104.

J. E. Carpenter and J. E. Kuhn: Section of Orthopaedic Surgery, University of Michigan, Ann Arbor, Michigan 48109.

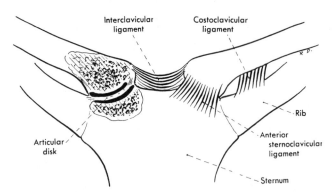

FIG. 21.1. Sternoclavicular joint anatomy depicting the intraarticular disk and associated supporting ligaments. (From Hollinshead WH, ed. *Anatomy for surgeons. Vol. 3. The back limbs.* Philadelphia: Harper & Row, 1982:262, with permission.)

The other ligamentous structures are thought to provide most of the stability to the sternoclavicular joint: the costoclavicular, interclavicular and sternoclavicular ligaments (5). The costoclavicular ligament has an anterior and posterior portion. The anterior portion primarily resists upward rotation and lateral displacement, whereas the posterior portion resists downward rotation

and medial displacement. The interclavicular ligament attaches to the superior portion of the medial clavicle, extending to the sternum and then across to the superior portion of the contralateral medial clavicle. This structure has been thought to prevent downward rotation of the distal clavicle with loading. The most structurally important restraints are the capsular or sternoclavicular ligaments. These ligaments are thickenings of the joint capsule. Of this, the anterior portion seems to be the most important. In a ligament sectioning study performed in cadavers, Bearn (6) demonstrated that the sternoclavicular ligaments are responsible for preventing the downward rotation of the distal clavicle with loading and thus attributed the "poise" of the shoulder to these structures. Only when these structures were sectioned did the distal clavicle displace inferiorly with loading (Fig. 21.2). The exact contributions of the individual ligaments toward the prevention of abnormal rotation and displacement of the medial clavicle have not been determined. It remains unclear as to why pathologic anterior dislocations of the sternoclavicular joint are much more common than posterior dislocations.

In contrast to the stabilizers of the sternoclavicular joint, its kinematics has been well studied. In describing

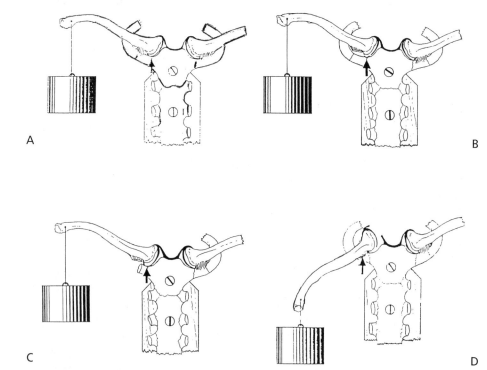

FIG. 21.2. The superior capsule of the sternoclavicular joint acts as the primary restraint to downward displacement of the lateral clavicle. *A,* Intact joint; *B,* clavicle position maintained after division of the costoclavicular ligament and intraarticular disk; *C,* clavicle position maintained after additional removal of first costicartilage; *D,* release of superior sternoclavicular joint capsule results in loss of support of the lateral clavicle. (From Bearn JG. Direct observation on the function of the capsule of the sternoclavicular joint clavicular support. *Am J Sports Med* 1967;101:159–170, with permission.)

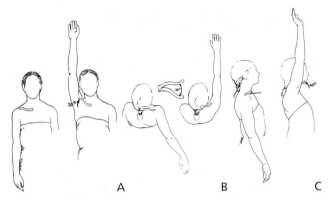

FIG. 21.3. Motions of the clavicle through the sternoclavicular joint. *A*, In full elevation, the clavicle elevates 35 degrees; *B*, with abduction and extension, the clavicle displaces anteriorly and posteriorly 35 degrees; *C*, with full elevation, the clavicle rotates on its axis 45 degrees. (From Rockwood CA. Disorders of the sternoclavicular joint. In: Rockwood CA Jr, Matsen FA III, eds. *The shoulder.* Philadelphia: W.B. Saunders, 1990:481, with permission.)

shoulder kinematics, generally the trunk (which includes the sternum) acts as the point of reference around which the motions are described. Through analysis of radiographs and the motion of pins placed in the clavicles of human volunteers, the movement of the clavicle relative to the sternum has been described (7). The range of motions as occur within a region can be depicted by a cone of approximately 35 degrees centered at the sternoclavicular joint (5). Thus, the clavicle not only rotates superiorly and inferiorly with arm elevation and abduction but also anteriorly and posteriorly with scapular protraction and retraction (Fig. 21.3). In addition, there is an axial rotation through the clavicle at the sternoclavicular joint of 45 to 50 degrees. This rotation occurs primarily with abduction and elevation of the shoulder. As the humerus is brought from the side to an overhead position, the clavicle and scapula rotate upward 45 to 50 degrees along the clavicle through the sternoclavicular joint (7). With this degree of motion at the sternoclavicular joint, it is clear why attempts at fusion of this joint are not only impractical because of the restriction of motion that would ensue but also generally unsuccessful, resulting in fixation failure and hardware migration. The effects of resection of the medial clavicle on the mechanics of the sternoclavicular articulation have not been reported. Studies of clinical outcome after resection for a variety of pathologies have generally demonstrated acceptable results. Reconstructive procedures for restoring stability at an injured sternoclavicular joint have generally relied on recreating the anterior portion of the costoclavicular ligament with biologic grafts. Results of these reconstructions have been inconsistent, and their mechanics have not been well studied.

Acromioclavicular Joint

Because of higher frequency of injury and its clinical significance, the anatomy and mechanics of the acromioclavicular joint have been better studied than those of the sternoclavicular joint. The articular anatomy of the acromioclavicular joint has been described as that of a "plane" joint (3,8). There is significant variability in the inclination of this plane from individual to individual, from almost vertical to as much as 50 degrees with the clavicle riding superior to the acromion (9). In general, this is not a perfectly congruous joint, and intraarticular disk of varying size is generally present. Rarely does a complete disk exist in the joint, but most commonly a meniscoid-type disk exists, extending from the anterior superior joint capsule (4). The typical size of the acromioclavicular joint is 9 × 19 mm (10). This articular structure has little inherent stability and is supported by the ligamentous attachments (Fig. 21.4). The acromioclavicular ligaments are thickenings of the acromioclavicular joint capsule and are not discretely defined structures. It has been found that the superior capsule is significantly thicker than the inferior capsule, thus most likely providing most of the structural support (11). In addition, Salter et al. (11) reported that the coracoacromial ligament attaches to the inferior capsule of the acromioclavicular joint and to the acromion. This attachment is

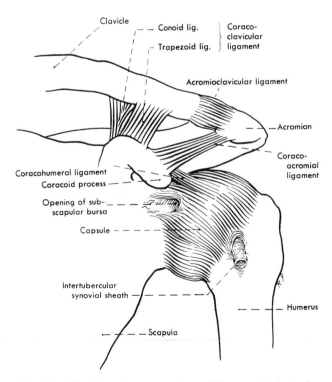

FIG. 21.4. The ligamentous anatomy of the acromioclavicular joint. (From Hollinshead WH, ed. *Anatomy for surgeons. Vol. 3. The back and limbs.* Philadelphia: Harper & Row, 1982:264, with permission.)

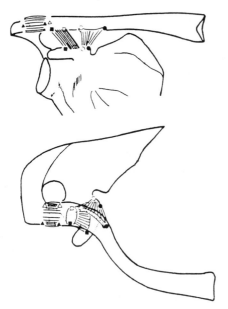

FIG. 21.5. The anatomic attachment points of the ligaments of the coracoacromial joint. The triangles indicate the acromioclavicular ligament, the squares represent the trapezoid ligament, and the circles the conoid ligament as determined by biplane radiography. (From Fukuda K, Craig EV, Kai-Nan A, et al. Biomechanical study of the ligamentous system of the acromioclavicular joint. *J Bone Joint Surg Am* 1986;68A:435, with permission.)

commonly seen during surgical release of the coracoacromial ligament, but the functional significance of this, if any, is unclear. The clavicle is further attached to the scapula through the coracoclavicular ligament. This ligament is really two separate ligaments, the conoid, which is cone shaped and slightly smaller, and the trapezoid, which is more rectangular shaped and larger (4). Using radiographic markers, Fukuda et al. (12) detailed

the anatomic attachment points of these ligaments to the coracoid and the clavicle (Fig. 21.5). Their positions help explain their relative importance in restricting displacements at the coracoclavicular joint.

Shoulder motion such as forward elevation results from coupled motions between the sternum, the clavicle, the scapula, and the humerus. The motions between the sternum and clavicle described previously have been relatively easy to determine because of the fixed nature of the sternum. However, the relative motion between the clavicle and the scapula through the acromioclavicular joint has not. This is likely because with most motions, the clavicle does not stay fixed, and thus the motion attributable to the acromioclavicular joint alone is difficult to measure, at least radiographically. In their classic study of shoulder mechanics, Inman et al. (7) determined that upward rotation of the clavicle was necessary with arm abduction (Fig. 21.6). They reported this to be 40 degrees of clavicular rotation at 180 degrees of humeral abduction. To determine this, they drilled pins into the clavicles of volunteer subjects and measured their change in rotational position as the arm was brought into abduction relative to the starting position. They concluded that this rotation occurred through the acromioclavicular joint and that preventing rotation at this joint would in fact limit the ability to abduct. By manually preventing rotation, they found that abduction was restricted to 110 degrees. These findings would suggest that any surgery or injury that prevented rotation at the acromioclavicular joint would permanently limit shoulder motion.

This concept is contrary to what other authors have reported in cases of screw fixation between the clavicle and coracoid and with coracoclavicular arthrodeses that occurred after injury to this region (13,14). Those authors reported minimal limitations of abduction and

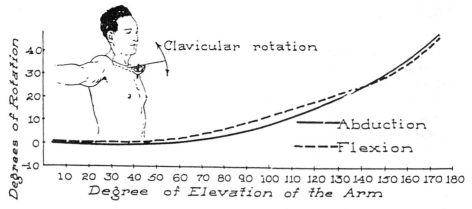

FIG. 21.6. Clavicular rotation with shoulder range of motion. This rotation was measured by observing motions of a pin placed into the clavicle percutaneously in a volunteer, whereas range of motion was performed and serial photographs obtained. (From Inman VT, Saunders JB, Abbott LC. Observations on the function of the shoulder joint. *J Bone Joint Surg* 1944;26:1–30, with permission.)

forward elevation despite this restriction of rotation at the acromioclavicular joint. Using the techniques of In-man et al., Rockwood and Young (14) placed pins in the clavicle and the acromion of volunteers, including a patient whose clavicle had been fixed to his coracoid by means of a screw. By observing the relative change in position between the two pins with arm abduction and elevation, they found that although there was a significant amount of rotation of the clavicle relative to the trunk, there was synchronous rotation of the scapula, such that the relative rotation between the two through the acromioclavicular joint was less than 10 degrees. Thus, it is most likely that little rotation occurs through the acromioclavicular joint with shoulder motion but that the scapula and clavicle rotate together as the arm is brought into a forward flexed or abducted position.

The ligamentous restraints to motion were further quantified by Fukuda et al. (12) in a biomechanical study of the acromioclavicular joint. They found that the axial rotation available through the acromioclavicular joint was small, consistent with Rockwood and Young's find-ings. In addition, they measured the amount of transla-tion available at the acromioclavicular joint. On aver-age, they found a superior/inferior displacement of 4.5 mm and anterior/posterior displacement of 17 mm. More importantly, through ligament sectioning studies, they determined the relative contributions of the acro-mioclavicular ligaments in providing joint stability. Of the directions they studied, the clinically most important are those of posterior translation and superior transla-tion. With posterior translation, they found that the acromioclavicular ligaments provided 90% of the con-straint with the conoid and trapezoid ligaments providing only a small degree of restraining force. In contrast, the relative contributions of the ligaments toward preventing superior translation of the clavicle on the acromion var-ied with the degree of displacement of the joint (Fig. 21.7). At small displacements, the acromioclavicular liga-ments provided most of the restraining force, whereas in larger displacements the conoid portion of the coracocla-vicular ligament was the most important. These quantita-tive results confirm the qualitative findings of Urist (15) in his classic observations of these ligaments. On the basis of his observations, he concluded that injury at the acromioclavicular joint capsule and its ligaments was necessary to allow for posterior subluxation or disloca-tion to occur, but that further injury to the coracoclavic-ular ligaments was necessary to allow for greater dis-placement, especially in a superior direction. Of the two coracoclavicular ligaments, the trapezoid portion has been reported to be the primary restraint to axial com-pressive loading across the acromioclavicular joint, whereas the conoid ligament plays a larger role in pro-viding stability in other directions of loading (12). As the degree of displacement increases, the role of this conoid ligament becomes even more important.

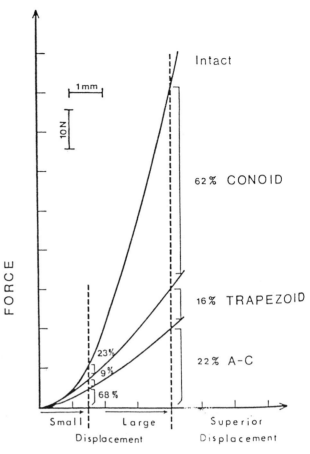

FIG. 21.7. Relative contributions of the individual ligaments to the restraint on acromioclavicular joint motion change with increasingly large displacements. At small displacements, the acromioclavicular ligament is the primarily restraint superior displacement, whereas at larger displacements, the conoid ligament becomes the dominant restraint. (From Fukuda K, Craig EV, Kai-Nan A, et al. Biomechanical study of the liga-mentous system of the acromioclavicular joint. *J Bone Joint Surg Am* 1986;68A:438, with permission.)

These biomechanical findings further support the clin-ical guidelines of preserving the acromioclavicular joint capsule and the attachments of the coracoclavicular liga-ment when resection of the distal clavicle becomes nec-essary for treatment of joint degeneration or injury. Furthermore, it is likely that rigid fixation of the clavicle to the coracoid, as is done on occasion for treatment of acromioclavicular joint injury, would not significantly limit shoulder elevation or abduction.

The biomechanics of acromioclavicular joint recon-struction have been studied with various implants in cadavers (16). These studies have suggested that the injured joint can be adequately stabilized by either fixa-tion across the acromioclavicular space with pins or plates or through loop fixation from the clavicle to the coracoid process using synthetic materials. Clinically, it has been found that prolonged fixation across the acromioclavicular joint interval will frequently lead to fatigue failure of these devices due to residual motion at the joint (17). It appears that mechanically either technique can be effective, but if fixation across the joint is prolonged, implant failure is common.

BIOMECHANICS OF THE ROTATOR CUFF AND CORACOACROMIAL ARCH

Because the rotator cuff has a central role in mechanics and function of the shoulder, its biomechanics have a predominant role in our basic science knowledge. However, the biology of aging, degenerative processes, and injury repair also play important roles. The rotator cuff is a complex musculotendinous structure comprised of four muscles, their insertions into the proximal humerus and the glenohumeral joint capsule and ligaments. The acronym SITS has been used to help remember the muscles of the rotator cuff, which are the supraspinatus (S), infraspinatus (I), teres minor (T), and subscapularis (S). These muscles work in concert with each other and with the other muscles of the trunk and shoulder girdle in a complex coordinated manner to control the shoulder and arm. The tendinous insertions of the cuff muscles merge with the joint capsule and the glenohumeral ligaments to form a continuous sleeve of tissue attaching to the humerus (18) (Fig. 21.8). In addition, structures adjacent to the cuff muscles and tendons are central to our understanding of cuff anatomy and function. The most important of these are the humeral head, coracoacromial arch, and the biceps tendon.

Rotator Cuff Vascularity

The supraspinatus tendon receives its blood supply primarily from the suprascapular artery. Near its insertion, some authors have found contributions from the posterior humeral circumflex, whereas others report blood supply from the anterior humeral circumflex and subscapular arteries. Classic studies by Codman (2) identified a "critical zone" at the supraspinatus tendon insertion as a region that had an inadequate blood supply. He believed that this was the area where damage is most often seen and inferred a causal relationship. More recently, a sparse vascular distribution at the articular side of the supraspinatus tendon and a well-vascularized bursal side has been demonstrated (19). In uninjured cuff tendons, it appears that the critical zone described by Codman is actually well vascularized with many anastomoses (20). It has been suggested that the lack of a blood supply in a certain region might be due to pressure on the tendon from the humeral head below and coracoacromial arch above (21). This pressure might "wring out the blood supply to these tendons" when the arm is at the side, thus providing an extrinsic explanation for a diminished blood supply. Thus, it appears that the normal supraspinatus tendon may be well vascularized; however injury, degeneration, tension in the cuff from muscular contraction, or compression of the cuff against the coracoacromial arch may lead to an area of inadequate blood supply.

Rotator Cuff Microstructure

Studies of the microstructure of the rotator cuff–joint capsule complex have demonstrated some important and clinically significant findings. These observations help the surgeon understand his or her findings during open or arthroscopic surgery. As the individual tendons extend toward the humerus, rather than insert as individual tendons, they intersect and blend with fibers from adjacent tendons (18) (Fig. 21.9). Through these connections, loads are transmitted transversely across the cuff, causing significant shear forces between fiber bundles. This arrangement may have importance in the initiation of cuff tears. As the cuff tendon fibers extend toward their humeral insertion, a five-layer structure to the superior cuff–capsule complex has been described (22,23). In this scheme, starting from the bursal surface, the first layer is composed of the superficial portion of the coracohumeral ligament (Fig. 21.10). Layer two is seen as closely packed parallel tendon fibers grouped in large bundles extending directly from the muscle bellies to the humeral insertions and likely is the primary load carrying portion of the cuff tendons. The third layer is

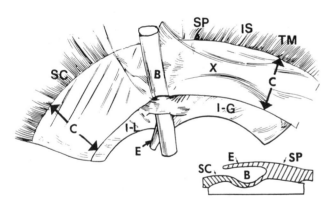

FIG. 21.8. Deep surface of the rotator cuff–capsule complex at its insertion to the humerus. *Inset:* The supraspinatus (*SP*) contributes to both the superior and inferior portions of the bicipital sheath, whereas the subscapularis (*SC*) contributes only to the floor of this sheath. Note the intricate relationship between the SC and the SP, which inserts along with the infraspinatus (*IS*) and the teres minor (*TM*) as they insert on the lesser (*I-L*) and the greater (*I-G*) tuberosities. The capsule (*C*) forms the innermost layer through which can be seen the pericapsular band (*X*) extending posteriorly from the rotator interval. Also note the biceps tendon (*B*) and its complex sheath with a slip (*E*) extending from the supraspinatus tendon. (From Clark JM, Harryman DT II. Tendons, ligaments, and capsule of the rotator cuff. *J Bone Joint Surg* 1992;5:713–725, with permission.)

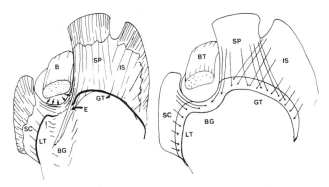

FIG. 21.9. As the subscapularis (*SC*), supraspinatus (*SP*), and the infraspinatus (*IS*) extend toward their insertion on the lesser (*LT*) and greater (*GT*) tuberosity, their fibers can blend and intermingle with the adjacent tendons. As the biceps tendon (*B* or *BT*) extends through the bicipital groove (*BG*) into the rotator interval, a sheath is formed with contributions from the supraspinatus and subscapularis tendons with a slip (*E*) superiorly extending from only the supraspinatus tendon. (From Clark JM, Harryman DT II. Tendons, ligaments, and capsule of the rotator cuff. *J Bone Joint Surg* 1992;5:713–725, with permission.)

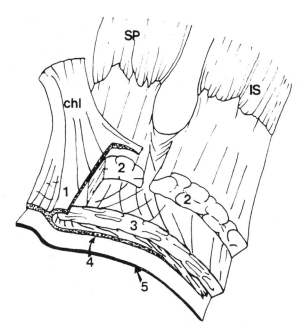

FIG. 21.10. The structure of the superior cuff capsule complex near the insertion onto the humerus is comprised of a five-layer structure. Layer one is comprised of superficial fibers that extend from the coracoid process as the coracohumeral ligament (*CHL*). Layers two and three contain the fibers of the supraspinatus (*SP*) and infraspinatus (*IS*) tendons. In layer two these fibers are oriented parallel to the axis of the cuff tendons, whereas in layer three the fibers run more obliquely and fans out to intermingle with fibers of the adjacent tendons. Layer four forms from the deep extension of the coracohumeral ligament, and layer five is the true joint capsule. (From Clark JM, Harryman DT II. Tendons, ligaments, and capsule of the rotator cuff. *J Bone Joint Surg* 1992;5:713–725, with permission.)

also a thick tendinous portion but with smaller fascicles with a less uniform orientation. Layer four is comprised of loose connective tissue in which thick bands of collagen run perpendicular to the primary fiber orientation of the cuff tendons. This is also the deep extent of the coracohumeral ligament that has been variously described as a transverse band, a pericapsular band, or a rotator cable by different authors (22,24,25). It may play a role in distributing forces between portions of the cuff. The true inner capsular layer forms a continuous layer from the glenoid to the humerus as layer five.

Coracoacromial Arch Structure and Biomechanics

A review of rotator cuff structure is incomplete without a description of the coracoacromial arch. This structure comprises the roof above the supraspinatus tendon and defines the outlet or space through which this tendon must pass (Fig. 21.11). The acromion process extends anteriorly from the scapular spine over the supraspinatus muscle and tendon. There are a number of reports on variation in the shape of the acromion, especially its anterior tip (26–28). When viewed from the lateral side, it may be relatively flat, gently curved, or have a hooked anterior edge. These variations have been labeled as type I, type II, or type III, respectively (29), and may have important implications in the pathogenesis of cuff

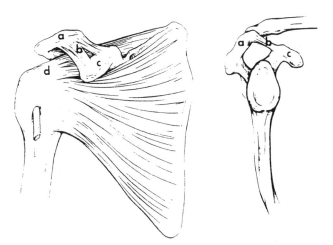

FIG. 21.11. Anterior and lateral views of the shoulder demonstrating the coracoacromial arch positioned over the supraspinatus tendon. This arch is comprised of the acromion (*a*), the coracoacromial ligament (*b*), and the coracoid (*c*). To arrive at its insertion on the greater tuberosity at the humerus, the supraspinatus tendon (*d*) must pass through this enclosed arch. Force couples about the shoulder act to maintain stability and normal kinematics. They occur in both the transverse plane as depicted by the subscapularis and infraspinatus and in the coronal plane as depicted by the rotator cuff and deltoid forces. (From Soslowsky LJ, An CH, Johnston SP, et al. Geometric and mechanical properties of the coracoacromial ligament and their relationship to rotator cuff disease. *Clin Orthop* 1994;304:10–17, with permission.)

tears and in the treatment of individuals with cuff pathology. Attached to the anterior–inferior edge of the acromion is the well-defined coracoacromial ligament. This ligament extends in two bands, a medial band and more clinically significant lateral band, to the coracoid process. The lateral band inserts primarily onto the coracoid, but the lateral-most fibers merge with fibers of the conjoined tendon and extend distally with them. Variations in the histology, geometry, and biomechanics of this ligament have been found in relation to cuff tears, suggesting that it too may play a role in cuff disease (30,31). Thus, this series of structures (acromion, coracoacromial ligament, coracoid) forms a rigid arch above the supraspinatus tendon and may compress the underlying tendon contributing to tendon injury.

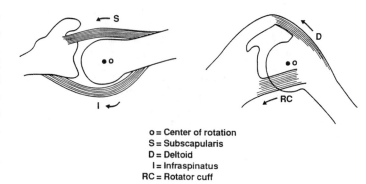

o = Center of rotation
S = Subscapularis
D = Deltoid
I = Infraspinatus
RC = Rotator cuff

FIG. 21.12. Force couples of the shoulder demonstrate the relative lines of action of the rotator cuff and the deltoid. (From Burkhart SS. Fluoroscopic comparison of kinematic patterns in massive rotator cuff tears. *Clin Orthop* 1992;284:146, with permission.)

Rotator Cuff Biomechanics

The biomechanics of the rotator cuff can be analyzed on a number of different levels. It is clear that the rotator cuff does not function in isolation. It is a part of a complex coordinated system of muscles, ligaments, and joints that affect shoulder movement. Electromyographic studies of the muscle contractions during various activities have demonstrated this complexity. Because the rotator cuff (and especially the supraspinatus) is the part of this system that is most frequently injured and dysfunctional, it has taken on special significance. For this reason, it has received much study. Inman et al. (7) were one of the early groups to measure the role of the rotator cuff in shoulder function. In finding that the cuff muscles were all active during most shoulder motions, they supported the concept of force couples around the glenohumeral joint. Using this concept, groups of muscles work together to balance each other's actions to produce the desired effect (7). For example, the cuff muscles depress and stabilize the humeral head at the same time the deltoid acts to elevate the arm (Fig. 21.12). When one of these forces is eliminated through injury or paralysis, this coupling is lost and abnormal mechanics ensue.

To investigate these concepts, a number of shoulder models have been used. Mathematical, analytic, and cadaveric models add to our understanding. Simple two-dimensional free-body models such as that presented by Inman et al. (7) including only one or two muscle forces have been used to approximate deltoid, cuff, and joint reactive forces. These studies suggest that very significant forces on the order of one's body weight can be generated at the shoulder due to the long lever arm of the upper extremity. Using radiographs to measure bony landmarks and free-body analysis, Poppen and Walker (32) predicted a joint reaction force of up to 0.9 times body weight in elevating the arm without any additional hand weights. In an effort to more realisti-

cally model the complexity of the shoulder mechanism, finite element techniques have been used to study shoulder function (33). These investigations provide a great deal of information, although validation of these models remains difficult.

Cadaveric models that use the entire glenohumeral joint while simulating muscle forces of the four cuff muscles, the three portions of the deltoid, and the long head of the biceps are very useful. By individually adjusting the tension on the tendon stumps, differing arm positions can be achieved and studied (34–36). Modifications of these forces can then be used to study pathologic conditions, most specifically cuff tears, cuff paralysis, and alterations in the coracoacromial arch. Although the techniques of simulating forces and measuring translations vary, the results found among these models are similar. There is a confirmation of the importance of the supraspinatus in initiating abduction. As shown in Fig. 21.13, when paralysis of the supraspinatus is simulated (but the cuff is still intact), the force required by the middle deltoid to abduct the arm in the scapular plane can increase by 100% at the initiation of abduction but may not be increased at all beyond 90 degrees of abduction (34). Interestingly, there is little superior translation of the humeral head with this simulated supraspinatus paralysis when compared with experimental cuff tears (36). This "spacer" effect of the superior cuff may occur because of the presence of the tendon in the subacromial space blocking translation or by allowing forces from adjacent cuff muscles to be transmitted to the superior capsule and cuff.

Actual cuff tears have been simulated by creating defects in the supraspinatus tendon and measuring the changes in kinematics. Several studies have demonstrated that small cuff tears that do not involve the infraspinatus or subscapularis have little effect on superior translation of the humeral head or on the degree of abduction achievable (24,36). This finding is particularly true if the biceps force is intact. This result helps to explain why many individuals with small or moderate tears may have normal function. In these conditions, the forces provided by the anterior and posterior portions of the intact cuff are adequate despite a defect in the superior cuff. The transverse band found in the superior capsule–cuff complex (called the rotator cable by Burkhart [24]) may provide the link necessary between the intact portions of the cuff (Fig. 21.14). However, if the tear is massive involving two or three tendons, a significant alteration in kinematics is seen. In these conditions of massive tears, there is a loss of the normal forces resulting in significant superior translation of the humeral head and limitation of abduction (36). Anatomic repair of these tears can result in normalization of kinematics. It has also been proposed that partial repair may restore function when complete repair cannot be achieved (24).

These cadaveric models have helped to define the role of the long head of the biceps tendon. The biceps functions as a humeral head stabilizer. Thus, its action depends on joint position. In cases of large or massive cuff tears, activation of biceps force reduces pathologic motion and can improve function. These findings suggest that preservation of the biceps during surgical repair of cuff tears may be important.

Recently, the effects of acromioplasty and coracoacromial ligament excision have been evaluated in cadaver models. As might be expected, if the humeral head is pushed superiorly, it will translate further if the anterior acromion and coracoacromial ligament are removed (37,38). In more detailed analysis with simu-

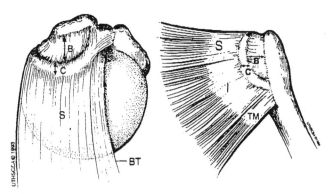

FIG. 21.14. Superior and lateral projections of the insertions of the supraspinatus (*S*), infraspinatus (*I*), teres minor (*TM*), and biceps (*BT*) at the humerus. The thickening of the cuff capsule complex just before the insertion (*C*) may act to distribute forces transversely along the cuff. Thus, small tears that incur within the region directly lateral to this band may result in no alteration of glenohumeral kinemechanics and good function clinically, and thus may not need to be repaired. Modulus of elasticity of the supraspinatus tendon. (From Brukhardt SS. Reconciling the paradox of rotator cuff repair versus debridement: a unified biomechanical rationale for the treatment of rotator cuff treas. *Arthroscopy* 1994;10:9, with permission.)

lated cuff function, significant changes in kinematics occurred after coracoacromial ligament removal only with a concomitant large or massive cuff tear (36). This effect may occur because of loss of contact with the undersurface of the acromion or from loss of tethering of the anterior tip of the acromion to the coracoid. These studies help confirm clinical observations that in some cases of massive or irreparable cuff tears or coracoacromial ligament resection results in significantly greater superior translation of the humeral head. To avoid this difficult clinical problem, preservation or reattachment of the coracoacromial ligament during surgical repair of large or massive tears has sometimes been recommended.

Although these models go a long way toward improving our understanding of rotator cuff function in normal and pathologic conditions, there are a number of limitations. Most important is the relationship of these findings to clinical symptoms. It is not known whether superior translation is related to shoulder pain. Similarly, the complex effects of pain on muscle inhibition cannot be accurately modeled.

Supraspinatus Mechanics

Although much is known about the kinematics of the rotator cuff at the whole joint level, less information is available about the mechanical properties of the individual tendons. This is true in part because it is difficult to individually isolate and functionally test significant portions of the rotator cuff with the large number of

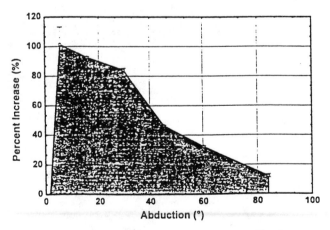

FIG. 21.13. In a biomechanical model using a cadaver, a simulated supraspinatus muscle paralysis results in significant increases in deltoid muscle force required to achieve a position of abduction. As the arm is brought into further abduction, this degree of increased force is reduced. (From Thompson WO, Debski RE, Boardman ND III, et al. A biomechanical analysis of rotator cuff deficiency in a cadaveric model. *Am J Sports Med* 1996;24:289, with permission.)

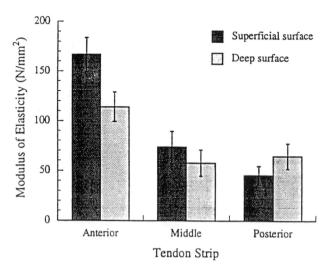

FIG. 21.15. With the tendon divided into strips, it is demonstrated that the anterior one third of the supraspinatus has the greatest modulus of elasticity and probably provides the greatest amount of force transmission from the supraspinatus muscle. (From Itoi E, Berglund LJ, Grabowski JJ, et al. Tensile properties of the supraspinatus tendon. *J Orthop Res* 1995;13:578–584, with permission.)

varying fiber orientations and interactions. Because of this predominant importance in cuff pathology and mechanics, the supraspinatus tendon has been evaluated by several techniques. It has been divided into anterior, middle, and posterior bands and studied biomechanically (39). In this study, the posterior one third of the supraspinatus tendon was found to be significantly thinner than either the anterior or middle thirds, whereas the ultimate load and stress are significantly greater for the anterior portion than the middle or posterior portion. Additionally, the modulus of elasticity is greater in the anterior one third than in the middle or posterior portions (Fig. 21.15). It appears that the anterior portion of the supraspinatus tendon is mechanically the strongest and seems to perform the primary load transmission from the supraspinatus muscle. Mechanical properties within the supraspinatus tendon have also been evaluated between the articular side and the bursal side of the tendon (40). This study demonstrated that the bursal side of the supraspinatus tendon has a lower modulus of elasticity, yet a higher ultimate strain and stress compared with the articular side of the supraspinatus before failing. On this basis, it can be suggested that the articular side of the supraspinatus tendon is more susceptible to mechanical failure in tension than is the bursal side if subjected to the same load. It is likely that differences in fiber bundle orientation and structure within these two portions of the capsule are responsible for the variations in mechanical properties. These regional variations in mechanical strength may help explain the development of partial thickness

rotator cuff tears, especially because they seem to occur more commonly on the articular surface.

Rotator Cuff Injury

Injuries to the rotator cuff are common clinical problems. The most dramatic and best studied of these injuries is that of a complete full-thickness tear. Such tears inevitably involve the supraspinatus tendon and may also involve the infraspinatus and teres minor, the subscapularis, and/or the long head of the biceps tendon. However, partial tears and tendinopathy without definable tears are also common findings. It is generally thought that these entities represent different presentations of the same disease process; however, this has not been conclusively established.

Pathology

Studies on the histopathology of rotator cuff disease have primarily relied on tissue from the subacromial bursa and the supraspinatus tendon in patients undergoing rotator cuff surgery for full-thickness cuff tears (41–

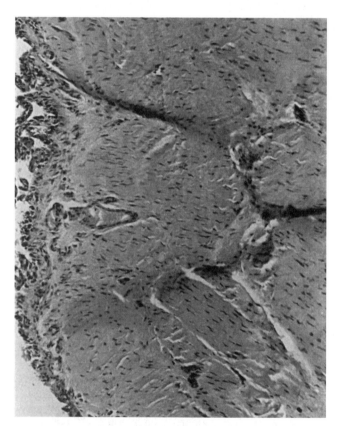

FIG. 21.16. Biopsy of a partial thickness tear near the supraspinatus insertion demonstrates extension of the tear between layers of the rotator cuff without evidence of a active repair. (From Sarkar K, Uhthoff HK. Pathophysiology of rotator cuff degeneration, calcification and repair. In: Burkhead WZ Jr, ed. *Rotator cuff disorders.* Baltimore: Williams & Wilkins, 1996:39, with permission.)

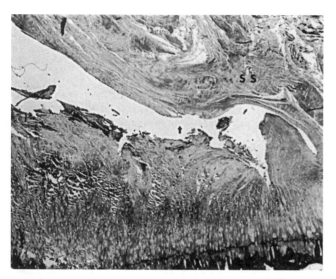

FIG. 21.17. A biopsy at the margin of a torn supraspinatus tendon demonstrates marked cellular proliferation and repair activity. (From Sarkar K, Uhthoff HK. Pathophysiology of rotator cuff degeneration, calcification and repair. In: Burkhead WZ Jr, ed. *Rotator cuff disorders.* Baltimore: Williams & Wilkins, 1996:42, with permission.)

44). A significant proliferation of reparative tissue around the edges of the tendon and in the surrounding bursal tissue with degenerative changes occurring within nearby tendon has generally been found (Fig. 21.16). True inflammatory infiltrates have not been predominate in these tissues, making the term of "tendinitis" probably not the most appropriate. However, these tissue samples have generally been taken adjacent to cuff tears and may not be characteristic of supraspinatus tendinopathy in the absence of tendon rupture.

Unfortunately, biopsies from a large number of patients with cuff disease in the absence of significant cuff tearing has not been available. In studying cadaveric tendons, less than 20% of tendons show histologic abnormalities before the age of 40, whereas this value increases to approximately 50% later in life (45). The tendon alterations found have demonstrated glycosaminoglycan infiltration, fibrocartilaginous transformation, and loss of the waviness and organization in the collagen fibers and degenerative changes. When the histologic changes are evaluated in biopsies from "rotator cuff tendinitis" patients, changes are consistent with new matrix synthesis, tissue remodeling, and wound healing. These findings are similar to those seen in biopsies from patients diagnosed with lateral epicondylitis of the elbow. Compared with normal tendon, these biopsies from supraspinatus tendons in patients with rotator cuff disease have an increased concentration of glycosaminoglycans compared with normal supraspinatus tendons (44).

Microscopic study of specimens from patients with partial-thickness rotator cuff tears may represent the earlier stages of cuff disease before a full-thickness tear develops. As such, they may provide insight to the pathogenesis of cuff disease (46). Partial tears have been found to be primarily bursal sided, articular sided, or intratendinous. They generally demonstrated a loss of the wavy fiber pattern, collagen fiber disruption, the presence of a granulation tissue response, and vascular proliferation intermixed with areas of degeneration (Fig. 21.17). The proximal stumps appear rounded and avascular with little repair response, whereas at the insertion and distal stumps, hypervascularity and granulation tissue exists. The tears extended horizontally between layers of the cuff–capsule complex, generally in the midlayer of the tendon. It is postulated that shear within the tendon is responsible for this type of tearing. Despite the proliferative tissue around these partial tears, there does not appear to be any closure of the defects.

Although there is no true consensus on what pathologic changes constitute rotator cuff disease, the most appropriate description is that of rotator cuff tendinosis. In general, a disruption of collagen fibers, a proliferation of reparative tissues, and areas of tendon degeneration can be found. Inflammatory infiltrates are not predominant, making the commonly used term tendinitis not as commonly applicable.

Etiology

Those studies that have attempted to address mechanisms of rotator cuff tendinosis can be grouped by whether they support intrinsic or extrinsic mechanisms of injury. The intrinsic mechanism states that tendon injury originates within the tendon from direct tendon overload, intrinsic degeneration, or other insult. The extrinsic mechanism states that the tendon damage is caused by injury of the tendon through compression against surrounding structures, most specifically the coracoacromial arch. Depending on which mechanism is dominant in a particular injury, different approaches toward prevention and treatment of rotator cuff disease might be appropriate.

Studies supporting intrinsic mechanisms have included vascular and anatomic investigations and evaluations of overuse syndromes. Historically, Codman (2) described a critical zone in the supraspinatus tendon near its insertion on to the humerus. This zone was thought to represent a region of poor vascularity that was at risk for injury and with little capacity for repair. Subsequent studies on the vascular supply to the supraspinatus tendon generally show an adequate blood supply in normal tendons; however aging, injury, or external compression may diminish this perfusion setting up conditions for rotator cuff disease to initiate. Histologically, regions adjacent to cuff tears have demonstrated degen-

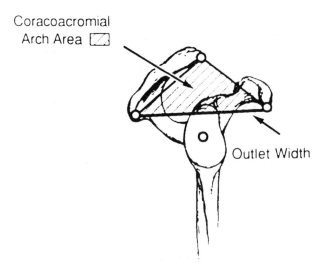

Coracoacromial
Arch Area ☐

Outlet Width

FIG. 21.18. A reduction in the coracoacromial arch area has been correlated with an increased incidence of full-thickness rotator cuff tears providing further support for an extrinsic etiology in some cases of rotator cuff disease. (From Zuckerman JD, Kummer FJ, Cuomo F, et al. The influence of coracoacromial arch anatomy on rotator cuff tears. *J Shoulder Elbow Surg* 1992;1:8, with permission.)

erative changes within the tendon (43). These changes and those of fibrocartilagenous transformation previously described may make the tendon intrinsically more susceptible to further injury and eventually tearing (44).

Studies supporting the extrinsic mechanisms of cuff tear pathogenesis have implicated impingement against the underneath surface of the acromion and the coracoacromial ligament as the primary factors for causing these tears (47). It is likely that if external compression of the rotator cuff tendons is a mechanism for rotator cuff disease as purported, then variations in the anatomy of the coracoacromial arch must be important in the disease pathogenesis. Through studying cadavers with rotator cuff tears compared with those without tears, it has been found that specimens with type III or hooked acromia (projecting further down into the subacromial space) had an increased likelihood of being associated with a full-thickness cuff tear compared with a type I or flat acromion (29). Similar findings were supported in a study of patients with symptomatic rotator cuff disease who had an increased incidence of having a hooked or type III acromion (48). Furthermore, quantitative assessment of the area of the supraspinatus outlet has demonstrated a correlation between rotator cuff tears and a reduced space for the supraspinatus (28) (Fig. 21.18).

In addition to the bony changes, changes in the coracoacromial ligament can also reduce the supraspinatus outlet area, creating an extrinsic compression on the cuff. Evaluations of shoulders with and without cuff

tears has demonstrated several significant changes in the coracoacromial ligament. Histologically, the ligament is disorganized, with a loss of normal collagen fiber orientation in shoulders with rotator cuff tears (31). There is a shortening and thickening of the coraco-

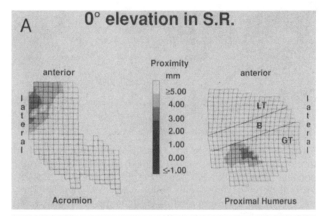

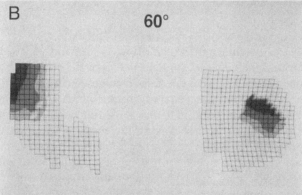

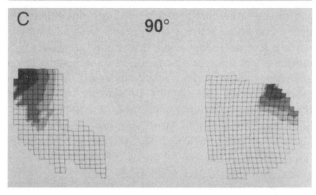

FIG. 21.19. Using stereophotogrammetery in a cadaver model, the amount and location of contact between the acromion and the rotator cuff is demonstrated. Primary contact occurs between the anterolateral portion of the acromion and the supraspinatus tendon near its insertion onto the greater tuberosity. As the degree of abduction is increased from **(A)** 0 degrees of elevation to **(B)** 60 degrees of elevation and then to **(C)** 90 degrees of elevation, the area of contact is consistent; however, the degree of contact increases. (From Flatow EL, Soslowsky LJ, Ticker JB, et al. Excursion of the rotator cuff under the acromion. *Am J Sports Med* 1994;22:784, with permission.)

acromial ligament in rotator cuff shoulders compared with shoulders without cuff tears (30). Biomechanically, there is a decrease in the modulus of the ligament, but because of a greater cross-section, there is no change in the overall structural properties. These studies clearly demonstrate alterations in the anatomy and biomechanics of the coracoacromial arch in association with rotator cuff tears, yet they are unable to determine if these changes lead to tears through compression on the supraspinatus tendon or occur as a result of altered loading after a cuff tear.

In analysis of subacromial contact, it has been demonstrated that the underneath surface of the acromion and the rotator cuff tendon are closest between 60 and 120 degrees of humeral elevation (49) (Fig. 21.19). Because this position typically represents the painful arc of motion in patients with cuff disease, it has been hypothesized that extrinsic compression of the cuff tendons against the acromion and coracoacromial ligament may be responsible for this pain. The contact occurs at the anterior–inferior portion of the acromion at the attachment of the coracoacromial ligament. This is the same area implicated as causing subacromial impingement. These areas of contact have been shown to be increased in shoulders with hooked or type III acromions. Furthermore, simulated acromioplasty can reduce the contact area. In addition, direct pressure measurements have been made on the undersurface of the acromion in cadavers, demonstrating greatest contact pressures at the anterior inferior portion of the acromion at the attachment of the coracoacromial ligament (35) (Fig. 21.20).

Thus, evidence exists for either intrinsic or extrinsic mechanisms for rotator cuff disease. It can only be stated with certainty that changes occur in both the cuff tendons and the coracoacromial arch in rotator cuff disease. Whether the tendon changes are initiated within the tendon and then through altered mechanics effect change in the arch structures or are a result of compression from primary arch abnormalities cannot be determined from these studies. Surgeons have tended to focus on the extrinsic causes because it is there where surgical corrections can be most easily entertained. Furthermore, it has been well established that acromioplasty is an effective treatment for individuals with symptomatic cuff tendinopathy without complete tears.

In an effort to more rigorously test these various hypotheses of cuff disease etiology, an animal model has been proposed (50). The advantage of using an animal model is that one can apply a known condition or injury to the shoulder and then follow and measure the response quantitatively over time. The rat has been proposed as such a model because of the anatomic similarity of the supraspinatus tendon and acromion to that of the human. Using this model, histologic changes consistent with tendinosis have been observed after either an intrinsic injury (collagenase injection), an extrinsic compression (tendon graft wrapped around the acromion), or a combination of alterations. This would suggest that injuries may occur from either mechanism or from a combination of intrinsic and extrinsic factors. Further use with this model will evaluate these effects biomechanically.

BIOMECHANICS OF THE GLENOHUMERAL JOINT AND INSTABILITY

The glenohumeral joint has evolved to allow for more motion than any other joint in the human, presumably because the human hand is so useful. With the advantages of an increased range of motion come the costs of a loss of constraint and inherent stability. As such, the human shoulder is also the most frequently dislocated major joint, and symptoms of instability in highly demanding activities, such as athletics, are common.

Many factors are important for the maintenance of shoulder stability in sports, although the relative weights of these components remain largely unknown. Although these components clearly work in concert to maintain stability, they can be divided into static and dynamic categories (Table 21.1).

Static Contributors to Glenohumeral Stability

Humeral Version

In the general population, the articular surface of the proximal humerus is inclined dorsally, with neck-shaft angles averaging between 130 and 140 degrees. In addition, the humeral head is retroverted 30 degrees relative to the transepicondylar axis of the elbow (Fig. 21.21) (7,51–59). The role that variation of these anatomic features plays in the development of instability is unclear, particularly in athletes. Although some studies have shown no differences in comparing the degree of

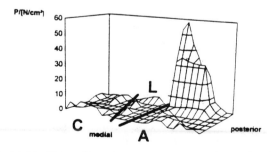

FIG. 21.20. From direct measurements on the underneath surface of the acromion made in a cadaver model, the greatest pressures occur at the anterior lateral corner of the acromion consistent with the concept of external impingement. (From Weulder N, Roetman B, Roessig S. Coracoacromial pressure recordings in a cadaveric model. *J Shoulder Elbow Surg* 1995;4:465, with permission.)

TABLE 21.1. *Static and dynamic components to shoulder stability*

Static components of shoulder stability
  Humeral version
  Glenoid version
  Articular surface area
  Articular conformity
  Glenoid labrum
  Intraarticular pressure
  Glenohumeral ligaments
Dynamic components of shoulder stability
  Rotator cuff through joint compression
  Individual components of the rotator cuff
  Rotator cuff through preloading glenohumeral ligaments
  Proprioception and reflexes
  Long head of biceps tendon
  Scapulothoracic motion

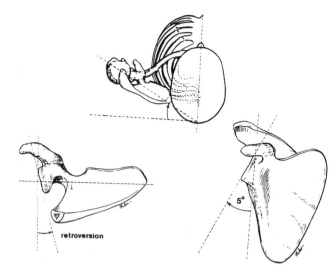

FIG. 21.22. Scapular and glenoid version. The scapula is oriented 30 to 45 degrees anterior to the coronal plane **(top)**, the glenoid fossa is oriented in approximately 7 degrees of retroversion **(left)**, approximately 5 degrees of superior tilt in most individuals. Some studies have shown more anteversion of the glenoid in patients with instability. (From Warner JJP. The gross anatomy of the joint surfaces, ligaments, labrum, and capsule. In: Matsen FA, Fu FH, Hawkins RJ, eds. *The shoulder: a balance of mobility and stability*. Rosemont, IL: American Academy of Orthopaedic Surgeons, 1993:7–28, with permission.)

retroversion in normal patients to those with anterior instability (53), others studies have shown significantly less retroversion in patients with anterior glenohumeral instability (60,61). The effect that retroversion has an instability in the athlete is unclear. In throwing athletes, retroversion may actually be increased, up to 14 degrees more than average (62). This should theoretically reduce the likelihood of developing symptoms of instability, yet current models for the development of pathology in the throwing athlete frequently invoke subtle instability as a source of symptoms (63,64). Clearly, the relationship of humeral head version in shoulder stability needs more attention, particularly in athletes.

Glenoid Version

In the resting position, the scapula is oriented 30 to 45 degrees anterior to the coronal plane (65). The glenoid fossa is oriented in 7 degrees of retroversion relative to the scapula in 75% of individuals, with a great degree of variation in the rest (51–53,66–71). Most authors agree that in the resting position, the glenoid fossa has a 5-degree superior tilt (Fig. 21.22) (53,71–73). The superior tilt of the scapula has been shown repeatedly to play a role in controlling inferior humeral head translation (72,74); however, the role of glenoid version remains unclear. Some studies have shown that patients with anterior instability have relatively more anteversion of the glenoid than normal (52), and similarly, patients with posterior instability have relatively more retroversion of the glenoid than normal (67,69,75). Other studies have failed to show these relationships (53,70). Although glenoid osteotomy for posterior instability has been advocated by many (67,69,75), the lack of reproducible reference points in assessing version and the lack of uniform conclusions make it difficult to appreciate the role of glenoid version in shoulder instability.

Surface Area and Articular Conformity

In the glenohumeral joint, the articulating surface of the humeral head is large relative to the much smaller

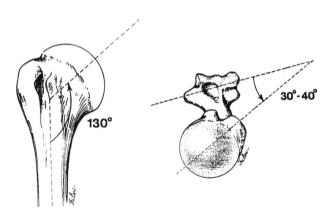

FIG. 21.21. Humeral version. The humerus neck shaft angle is dorsally inclined between 130 and 140 degrees, whereas the humeral head is retroverted between 30 and 40 degrees. Less retroversion, in some studies, has been associated with anterior glenohumeral instability. (From Warner JJP. The gross anatomy of the joint surfaces, ligaments, labrum, and capsule. In: Matsen FA, Fu FH, Hawkins RJ, eds. *The shoulder: a balance of mobility and stability*. Rosemont, IL: American Academy of Orthopaedic Surgeons, 1993:7–28, with permission.)

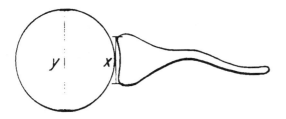

$$GHI = \frac{\text{Maximum Glenoid Diameter (x)}}{\text{Maximum Humeral Diameter (y)}}$$

FIG. 21.23. The glenohumeral index. The glenohumeral index has been calculated to be 0.75 in the transverse plane, demonstrating that only approximately 25% of the humeral head is in contact with the glenoid surface. (From Warner JJP, Caborn DNM. Overview of shoulder instability. *Crit Rev Phys Rehab Med* 1992;4:145–198, with permission.)

glenoid. This relationship has been referred to as the glenohumeral index (Fig. 21.23) and is given by the formula glenohumeral index = maximum glenoid diameter ÷ maximum humeral diameter.

This index has been calculated to be 0.75 in the sagittal plane and 0.76 in the transverse plane (51,52,76), meaning that approximately 25% of the humeral head is in contact with the glenoid surface. This has led some to describe the glenohumeral joint as analogous to a golf ball resting on a tee (77).

Although most agree that the articulating surface of the humeral head is large relative to the much smaller glenoid, there is controversy regarding the nature of that contact area. Saha (78) had described three types of humeral–glenoid articulations, based on the radius of curvature. In type A, the glenoid radius of curvature is larger than the humerus; in type B, the radii of curvatures match leading to joint conformity; and in type C, the radius of curvature of the humerus is larger than the glenoid. Other anatomic studies, and magnetic resonance imaging and computed tomography studies, tended to show matching radii of curvature, with joint conformity. Recent work by Soslowsky et al. (79,80) using stereophotogrammetry techniques accurately defined the three-dimensional articular surfaces of the glenoid and humerus and showed the articular surfaces to be nearly perfectly congruent with deviations in the radii of curvature to be less that 1% and the surfaces to be congruent within 3 mm. This results from relatively thicker articular cartilage at the periphery of the glenoid and thin cartilage in the center. The humeral articular cartilage, on the other hand, is thicker centrally and thinner at the periphery. This finding explains misconceptions about the radii of curvature when only radiographs are considered. Indeed, the glenoid bone surface (as seen on radiograph) is much flatter than the humeral head bone surface. Their findings also suggest that the humeral head maintains relative uniform contact with the glenoid surface throughout shoulder motion (79,80).

Some studies using simulated muscle forces in cadavers have demonstrated ball and socket kinematics (81). Other studies, however, have demonstrated that passive glenohumeral motion can result in translational motion of the humeral head on the glenoid and even suggest that coupled translations accompany every glenohumeral motion, particularly in the midrange to extreme ranges of motion (82–85).

Taken together, these studies suggest that the glenohumeral joint is a congruent joint, yet because the glenoid is significantly smaller than the humeral head and thus shallow and because the cartilage surfaces are deformable, translations can occur and instability can develop. Pathologic conditions that affect either the glenohumeral index or the joint conformity may lead to instability of the shoulder.

Glenoid Labrum

The glenoid labrum acts as a static stabilizer of the glenohumeral articulation by deepening the glenoid socket by 9 mm in the superior–inferior direction and by 5 mm in the anterior–posterior plane (86–88). This accounts for up to 50% of the depth of the glenoid cavity (Fig. 21.24). The labrum increases the surface

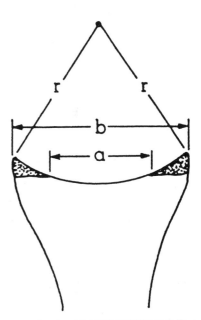

FIG. 21.24. Glenoid labrum. The glenoid labrum increases the surface area of articular contact and deepens the socket, thus improving stability. The width of the articular surface (*a*), the distance between the peripheral edges of the labrum (*b*), and the radius of the humeral head (*r*) are shown. (From Howell SM, Galinat BJ. Normal and abnormal mechanics of the glenohumeral joint in the horizontal motion plane. *Clin Orthop* 1989;243:122–125, with permission.)

area for contact with the humeral head and serves as an attachment site for the glenohumeral ligaments. Hara et al. (89) showed the weakest portion of the labrum to be in the 4 o'clock position, and when loaded to failure under tension, the labrum becomes detached in the fibrous connective tissue close to the hyaline articular cartilage. Clinically, labral lesions are often associated with traumatic glenohumeral instability, yet biomechanical studies in which an isolated Bankart lesion was created did not produce significant increases in humeral translation on the glenoid, suggesting other factors, such as plastic deformation of the glenohumeral ligaments may be required for recurrent instability (90).

Intraarticular Pressure

A number of studies have demonstrated that the force required for passive translation of the glenohumeral joint are significantly less in a vented cadaver glenohumeral joint than required for the nonvented shoulder (91–95). The normal glenohumeral joint is a closed system of finite volume. A slightly negative intraarticular pressure exists in the normal shoulder (93). Translations or distractions of the glenohumeral joint will substantially decrease the intraarticular pressure, improving glenohumeral stability. The magnitude of this effect is dependent on the position of the arm. In the abducted and externally rotated shoulder, the effect of negative intraarticular pressure is negated by the static restraints of the glenohumeral ligaments that become more effective in preventing humeral head translation (91). In summary, negative intraarticular pressure seems to have a role in centering the humeral head and may provide some restraint to pathologic translations, particularly in the neutral or early ranges of motion. However, the role of this pressure relative to other static, and dynamic restraints, is likely small.

Glenohumeral Ligaments and Capsule

Thickenings in the shoulder capsule have been identified and described for many years, yet only recently have the functional, anatomic, and material properties of these ligaments been investigated.

Histologic analysis has determined that these ligaments are comprised of collagen fiber bundles arranged in several layers of differing thickness and orientation. Although the posterior capsule has a simple pattern of radial and circular fibers, most areas of the glenohumeral capsule and ligaments demonstrate a complex pattern of cross-linking of various radial and circular fibers (23). The complex nature of the capsule suggests that the capsule should be considered cylindrical. Nevertheless, most studies have investigated the individual components of the capsule through ligament cutting studies and strain gage analysis in an effort to under-

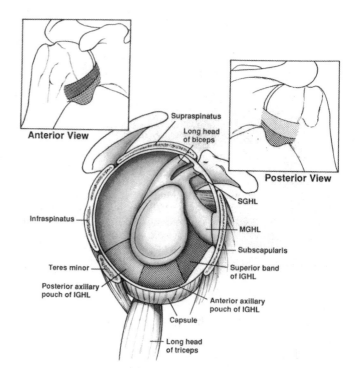

FIG. 21.25. The anatomy of the glenohumeral ligaments. The anterior aspect of the shoulder is to the right. The ligaments include the superior glenohumeral ligament (*SGHL*), the middle glenohumeral ligament (*MGHL*), and the inferior glenohumeral ligament (*IGHL*), which includes the superior band, anterior axillary pouch, and posterior axillary pouch. (From Ticker JB, Bigliani LU, Soslowsky LJ, et al. Inferior glenohumeral ligament: geometric and strain-rate dependent properties. *J Shoulder Elbow Surg* 1996;5:269–279, with permission.)

stand these static restraints. The ligaments studied most thoroughly include the superior glenohumeral ligament, the coracoacromial ligament, the middle glenohumeral ligament, and the inferior glenohumeral ligament complex (Fig. 21.25).

Superior Glenohumeral Ligament and Coracohumeral Ligament

The superior glenohumeral ligament is found in the rotator interval, parallel to the much larger extraarticular coracohumeral ligament. The superior glenohumeral ligament originates from the superior rim of the glenoid at the supraglenoid tubercle just inferior to the biceps tendon and inserts onto the lesser tuberosity of the humerus medial to the bicipital groove. It is variable in size and is found in over 90% of specimens (76,91,96–100). Unlike the coracohumeral ligament, histologic analysis of the superior glenohumeral ligament has shown it to be comprised of longitudinally arranged collagen bundles in a true ligament fashion (100).

Biomechanical studies have included strain gage analysis and ligament cutting experiments. These studies have determined that the superior glenohumeral ligament is a primary restraint to external rotation in the adducted or slightly abducted arm; is a primary restraint to inferior translation in the adducted arm; and is a secondary restraint to posterior translation in the adducted, flexed, and internally rotated shoulder (101–104).

The coracohumeral ligament has traditionally been considered a significant structure (104–110). It is an extraarticular dense fibrous structure that histologically is a thickened folding of the shoulder capsule often without the ligamentous organization of parallel bundles of collagen fibers (100). The coracohumeral ligament originates from the lateral border of the base of the coracoid process and divides into two bands. One band inserts into the greater tuberosity and tendinous anterior edge of the supraspinatus. The other band inserts on the lesser tuberosity and superior border of the subscapularis. The cross-sectional area of the coracohumeral ligament (53.7 ± 3.2 mm^2) is significantly greater than the superior glenohumeral ligament (11.3 ± 1.6 mm^2) (110).

The coracohumeral ligament is thought to be a primary restraint to inferior translation of the adducted arm and is a primary restraint to external rotation (102, 104,107). It is thought to be a secondary restraint to posterior instability with the arm in the adducted, forward flexed, and internally rotated position.

The material properties of isolated specimens of the coracohumeral ligament and the superior glenohumeral ligament demonstrate the coracohumeral ligament has greater stiffness (36.7 ± 5.9 N/mm) and ultimate load (359.8 ± 40.3 N) than the superior glenohumeral ligament (17.4 ± 1.5 N/mm and 101.9 ± 11.5 N, respectively) (110). The coracohumeral ligament, which fans out distally to converge with the rotator cuff tendons (23), fails proximally near the coracoid in bone ligament bone testing, whereas the superior glenohumeral ligament tends to fail distally as it thins near the humeral insertion. Interestingly, the coracohumeral ligament stiffness and ultimate load values were higher than those reported for the inferior glenohumeral ligament complex, and significant elongation of the coracohumeral ligament (36%) occurred before failure (110).

Middle Glenohumeral Ligament

The anatomy of the middle glenohumeral ligament is highly variable. It is poorly defined in 10% of specimens and is absent in up to 30% (76,96,98,99,103,106). Its origin may be the anterior–superior labrum, the scapular neck, or the supraglenoid tubercle, usually below the superior glenohumeral ligament and above the anterior band of the inferior glenohumeral ligament. Two morphologic variations have been described, including a cordlike structure, clearly delineated from the anterior band of the inferior glenohumeral ligament, and a sheetlike structure, blending with the anterior band of the inferior glenohumeral ligament. It may also be extremely well developed and insert onto the biceps tendon, with a portion of the underlying anterior–superior labrum absent (111). On the humerus, the middle glenohumeral ligament inserts just anterior to the lesser tuberosity with the subscapularis.

The middle glenohumeral ligament is a primary stabilizer to anterior translation with the arm abducted to 45 degrees. It is also thought to be important in limiting external rotation at 60 and 90 degrees of abduction. It may be a secondary stabilizer for inferior translation in the adducted arm (103,106,112,13).

Inferior Glenohumeral Ligament Complex

The inferior glenohumeral complex is a broad triangular structure of varying thickness that comprises the inferior shoulder capsule (96). It has been evaluated histologically and has a substantially thicker area anteriorly, called the anterior or superior band (98,112). Similarly, a thickening posteriorly has been described (98), yet others have found this structure only inconsistently (114,115). The entire structure seems to be thicker near the glenoid than the humerus (114,115).

The anterior band originates from the glenoid labrum in the 2 to 4 o'clock positions and the posterior band, when present, from the 7 to 9 o'clock positions (98). The inferior glenohumeral ligament complex runs laterally to the humeral head between the subscapularis and the triceps. O'Brien et al. (98) compared the inferior glenohumeral ligament complex with a hammock. In the abducted shoulder, external rotation will place the inferior glenohumeral ligament anteriorly, which will then restrain anterior translation of the humeral head. Correspondingly, internal rotation will direct the inferior glenohumeral ligament posteriorly, which will then restrain posterior translation of the humerus (Fig. 21.26). This effect has been demonstrated by Blasier (116), who found that the restraining effect of the inferior glenohumeral ligament in preventing posterior humeral translation of the adducted forward elevated arm was greater than that of the coracohumeral ligament when the arm was internally rotated.

The material properties of the inferior glenohumeral ligament complex have been evaluated with slow strain rates (114) and more recently with high strain rates of 10% per second (115). The anterior (or superior) band, which was the thickest region, had greater tensile strength than the inferior or posterior portions of the inferior glenohumeral ligament (115). Greater strain was observed near the bony insertion sites of the specimen than in the midsubstance of the tissue. When com-

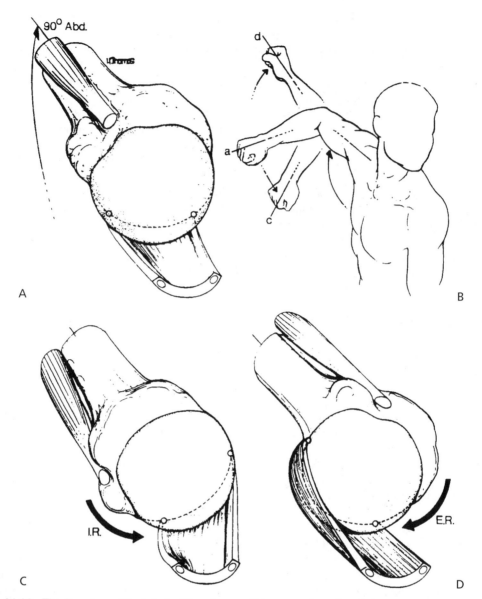

FIG. 21.26. The Function of the inferior Glenohumeral Ligament Complex. Schematic drawing showing how the IGHLC functions to support the humeral head both anteriorly and posteriorly with the arm in abduction. The arm is abducted 90 degrees and is in neutral rotation (*A*). As the arm is internally rotated (*B*), the posterior band of the IGHLC fans out to support the humeral head posteriorly (*C*). When the arm is externally rotated (*B*) the anterior band of the IGHLC fans out to support the humeral head anteriorly (*D*). (From O'Brien SJ, Neves MC, Arnoczky SJ, et al. The anatomy and histology of the inferior glenohumeral ligament complex of the shoulder. *Am J Sports Med* 1990;18:449–456, with permission.)

pared with earlier work that used slower strain rates (114), the inferior glenohumeral ligament complex responds to increased strain rates with increased strength and stiffness (115). This and numerous other studies conclude that the anterior (superior) band of the inferior glenohumeral ligament complex is a significant static restraint to anterior–inferior translation of the humeral head in the abducted externally rotated humerus (76,98,102,106,112,113) (Fig. 21.26).

Dynamic Contributors to Glenohumeral Stability

The muscles of the rotator cuff and the long head of the biceps muscle provide dynamic stability to the glenohumeral joint in a variety of ways.

Joint Compression

Numerous studies have shown that contraction of the rotator cuff and/or biceps muscles will compress the humeral head into the glenoid, resulting in an increase in the force required to translate the humeral head (86,116–119). When the rotator cuff is activated, ligament cutting studies have shown that the joint compression effect seems to be more important in stabilizing the glenohumeral joint than the capsular constraints (118).

In a series of studies by Blasier and associates (116,118,120), physiologic rotator cuff loads were simulated and shown to have a major stabilizing effect on the anterior stabilization of the glenohumeral joint. If tension on any one component of the cuff was removed, however, increased anterior humeral translation was noted regardless of which component was omitted. This suggests the entire cuff acts in concert to provide joint compression and stability. In a related experiment, these authors found the entire rotator cuff has stabilizing effects in limiting posterior translation of the humeral head as well (116). Clearly, joint compression is an essential component of glenohumeral stability.

Individual Components of the Rotator Cuff

On the other hand, individual components of the rotator cuff may have an important role in maintaining glenohumeral stability, particularly in the shoulder that is already unstable. Using electromyography, it has been shown that throwing athletes with anterior instability have demonstrable weakness in internal rotation (121,122). Because ruptures of the subscapularis have been noted in older patients with recurrent dislocations, some authors suggest that the subscapularis may have a role in preventing anterior instability, particularly in the lower ranges of abduction (123–129). Similarly, the infraspinatus and teres minor may have similar effects on posterior instability. And finally, a posterior mechanism of anterior dislocation has been described (2,124,130) in which anterior dislocation is accompanied by supraspinatus and infraspinatus tendon tears. This phenomena is seen commonly in the elderly with anterior glenohumeral dislocations and in patients with greater tuberosity fractures accompanying anterior glenohumeral dislocations (124,130). In summary, the rotator cuff is a critical component in maintaining glenohumeral stability, working as a whole to provide joint compression and as individual components that we are only now beginning to understand. Rehabilitation and strengthening of the rotator cuff is a critical component in the treatment of athletes with shoulder instability.

Preloading Glenohumeral Ligaments

The muscles of the rotator cuff may serve in a dynamic way to pretension the glenohumeral ligament complex. Histologic analysis of the shoulder capsule has demonstrated that the rotator cuff tendons insert onto and intermingle with the shoulder joint capsule at the humerus (23,131,132). Stretch receptors, Ruffini end organs, and Pacinian corpuscles have been identified in the capsuloligamentous structures (133,134). Although the capsule of the glenohumeral joint and its ligaments are relatively lax until the later ranges of shoulder motion, it has been suggested that contraction of the rotator cuff components may activate these sensors and dynamitize or preload the ligaments through complex reflex arcs (103). Similarly, these receptors may act to trigger the activation of specific cuff components through reflex arcs to protect the ligaments in which the stretch receptors are found. These reflex arcs have recently been demonstrated in a feline model (135).

Proprioception

These specialized nerve endings may also provide the glenohumeral joint with proprioception, another component of stabilization of the glenohumeral joint. Studies evaluating the proprioceptive ability in humans have determined that subjects with clinical laxity have significantly less proprioceptive skills than normal subjects (136). In addition, subjects are more sensitive to proprioception when the shoulder is near the limits of motion and during external rotation as opposed to internal rotation (137). In one clinical study, lidocaine injected into the glenohumeral joint resulted in increased passive translation in normal subjects (138). Patients with known anterior instability have less proprioceptive ability than normal subjects; however, surgical repair can restore this ability (136). These studies suggest that proprioception, through reflex mechanisms, may have an important role in glenohumeral stability, particularly in the abducted and externally rotated shoulder (139).

Biceps Tendon

Many studies have investigated the role of the long head of the biceps in shoulder stability. Like the rotator cuff, the long head of the biceps can increase joint compression and may increase the force required to translate the humeral head. In a study by Rodosky et al. (140), sectioning of the long head of the biceps tendon in the abducted externally rotated arm resulted in an increase in the strain in the inferior glenohumeral ligament. Pagnani et al. (119) demonstrated that the stabilizing role of the biceps tendon seems to be position dependent. When the arm is internally rotated, tension on the biceps diminishes anterior humeral head translation. Conversely, when the arm is externally rotated, the biceps limits posterior translation (Fig. 21.27). The biceps effect on stability is more pronounced with the arm in the lower and middle elevation angles.

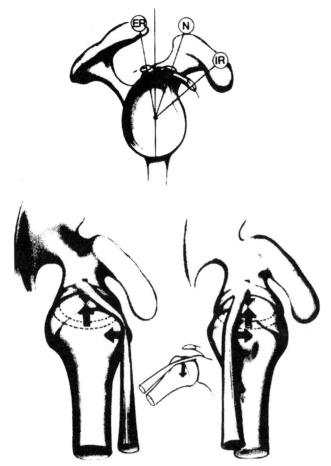

FIG. 21.27. The biceps tendon. Contraction of the biceps tendon is thought to influence glenohumeral stability by joint compression and as a static restraint. In internal rotation, the biceps moves anterior and limits anterior rotation **(bottom left)**. In external rotation, the biceps moves posterior and limits posterior translation **(bottom right)**. (From Pagnani MJ, Xiang-Hua D, Warren RF, et al. Role of the long head of the biceps brachii in glenohumeral stability: a biomechanical study in cadavers. *J Shoulder Elbow Surg* 1996;5:255–262, with permission.)

Scapular Rotators

Although the glenoid is small, it can be thought of as a platform supporting the humeral head. Its position relative to the humeral head and the forces that may create instability are critical. The position of the scapula is controlled by the scapular rotators, which are the muscles connecting the scapula to the torso, and include the trapezius, rhomboids, latissimus dorsi, serratus anterior, and levator scapulae. Abnormalities in the function of these muscles creating abnormal scapulothoracic motion may be related to glenohumeral instability (141). Scapular winging has been described as a feature of patients with anterior instability (106,142,143). Warner et al. (106) using Moire topography found scapulothoracic dysfunction was common in a population of patients

with shoulder instability. In addition, large series of patients with scapular winging, shoulder instability has been described as a related or secondary symptom (144,145). If the scapular rotators are unable to effectively position the glenoid, particularly by rotating the scapula upward during arm elevation, the glenoid may not be in position to act as a stable platform for the humeral head, and instability may result (141).

Relative Importance of the Various Components to Glenohumeral Stability

The various components of glenohumeral stability identified to date clearly have a role in maintaining shoulder stability in athletes. Yet, at this time, little work has been done to evaluate the relative roles of each different component. Nevertheless, it seems that the position of the arm is critical in determining which factors become important in stability. With the arm in a neutral position, the articular surfaces seems to have a major role. In the midrange of motion, the rotator cuff seems to have an increased role in shoulder stability, and in extremes of motion, the glenohumeral ligaments become more important (Fig. 21.28). In athletes, who are frequently using their shoulders in the mid to extreme ranges of motion, the origin of symptoms of instability may be multifactorial. As such, the approach to the athlete with instability should address all the potential factors that maintain glenohumeral joint stability.

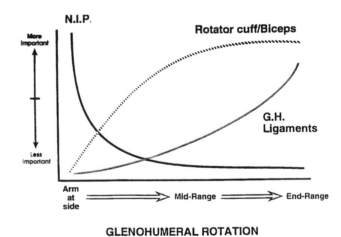

GLENOHUMERAL ROTATION

FIG. 21.28. The relative roles of the components of glenohumeral stability. The components of glenohumeral stability work in concert, yet with the arm in neutral position, negative intraarticular pressure seems to be important, with the rotator cuff becoming more important in the midrange of motion and the glenohumeral ligaments becoming more important nearer the limits of motion. (From Warner JJP, Flatow EL. Anatomy and biomechanics. In: Bigliani LU, ed. *The unstable shoulder.* Rosemont, IL: American Academy of Orthopaedic Surgeons, 1996:1–26, with permission.)

SHOULDER KINEMATICS DURING SPORTS

A variety of sporting activities has been analyzed to identify the motions and muscle activity about the shoulder. This has led to the estimation of forces about the shoulder and has provided insight into the mechanisms by which pathology develops in the athlete's shoulder. Most studies investigating glenohumeral kinematics have used high-speed cinematography, coupled with electromyographic analysis of the muscles about the athlete's shoulder. Other studies have involved biomechanical modeling using cadaver specimens. Most work has investigated the throwing shoulder; however, the shoulder kinematics of other sports have been explored as well.

Kinematics of Throwing

Pitching a baseball has been described as one of the most complex shoulder motions (146). For the purposes of study, the continuous pitching motion has been divided into five stages (Fig. 21.29). First, the *wind-up* is the initial motion, usually involving counterrotation of the body away from the target until the ball leaves the gloved hand. Second, the *stride and early cocking* stage occurs and is that period of time between the release of the ball from the gloved hand to the time when the leading stride foot makes contact with the ground. Third, *late arm cocking* occurs next and is defined as the time from stride foot contact to maximal external rotation of the throwing arm. Fourth, this is followed by *arm acceleration*, which begins with internal rotation of the humerus and continues until the ball is released. Finally, *arm deceleration and follow-through* occur after ball release and last until the motion of the throwing arm stops (146).

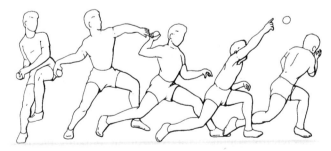

FIG. 21.29. Phases of the throwing motion. The five phases of the continuous throwing motion include wind-up, stride and early cocking, late arm cocking, arm acceleration, and arm deceleration and follow-through. (From Tibone J, Patek R, Jobe FW, et al. Functional anatomy, biomechanics, and kinesiology. In: DeLee JC, Drez D, eds. *Orthopaedic sports medicine. Principles and practice.* Philadelphia: W.B. Saunders, 1994:463–480, with permission.)

Wind-up

The wind-up motion in pitchers is one of the most variable components of the throwing motion and is not thought to be a critical component of the throwing motion. The pitcher stands facing the batter and initiates the throw by stepping backward with the stride foot. The other supporting foot is placed in front of the rubber, and weight is shifted to this supporting leg establishing a rhythm for the pitch. The body rotates 90 degrees with the throwing arm away from the batter, whereas the stride leg is elevated and flexed. The supporting leg is then flexed, lowering the body, whereas the stride leg is lowered and brought forward toward the catcher. The trunk is held back, retaining potential energy for the throw. The gloved hand, which is holding the ball, and the throwing hand move up and down, continuing the rhythm of the pitch.

Stride and Early Cocking

The stride leg moves forward and makes contact with the ground in a very predictable pattern (146). The

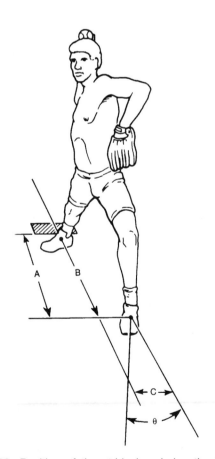

FIG. 21.30. Position of the stride leg during the baseball pitch. (From Dillman CJ, Fleisig GS, Andrews JR. Mechanics of throwing. In: Hawkins RJ, Misamore GW, eds. *Shoulder injuries in the athlete. Surgical repair and rehabilitation.* New York: Churchill Livingstone, 1996:23–30, with permission.)

length of the stride is slightly less than the pitcher's height, and the stride foot characteristically lands almost directly in front of the back foot with the toes pointed in slightly (Fig. 21.30). Appropriate positioning of the stride foot helps the pitcher use potential energy of hip rotation most efficiently. During the stride, the humerus is abducted and elevated.

Late Cocking

Once the stride leg makes contact with the ground, cocking continues by lateral motion of the trunk toward the pitcher with the initiation of hip rotation. The trunk then rotates toward the catcher and in experienced pitchers undergoes hyperextension. The arm is flexed at the elbow and the shoulder undergoes external rotation. When the trunk faces the batter, the shoulder reaches maximal external rotation. This position of maximal glenohumeral external rotation is considered a critical instant in the throwing motion (147). The position of the arm during maximal external rotation averages 94 degrees of thoracohumeral abduction, 11 degrees of

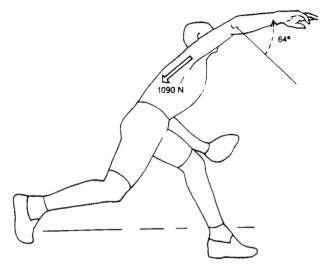

FIG. 21.32. Position of the pitcher's arm in deceleration and follow-through. At ball release the arm is adducted, the elbow is flexed, and the forearm supinates. This stage of the throwing motion is considered a critical moment and may be the time at which pathology develops in the thrower's shoulder. External rotation of the arm is 64 degrees and the elbow is flexed 25 degrees. An estimated 1,090 N of compressive force is thought to occur at the shoulder. (From Fleisig GS, Andrews JR, Dillman CJ, et al. Kinetics of baseball pitching with implications about injury mechanisms. *Am J Sports Med* 1995;23:233–239, with permission.)

horizontal adduction, and between 160 and 185 degrees of humeral external rotation (Fig. 21.31).

Acceleration

Arm acceleration begins when the humerus begins to internally rotate after the elbow begins to extend. The internal rotation torque of the humerus continues until the ball is released toward the plate. When the ball is released, the trunk is flexed, the elbow is extended, and the shoulder is internally rotating.

Deceleration and Follow-through

As the trunk moves over the stride leg, the knee is extended while the hip undergoes flexion. The shoulder is adducted, the elbow is flexed, and the forearm supinates (Fig. 21.32). The deceleration component of the baseball pitch is also considered a critical moment in the throwing cycle (147). Knowledge of the kinematics and electromyographic activity of the pitching motion has allowed the calculation of the estimated forces generated about the shoulder. In doing this, critical moments during which high forces are thought to occur. These critical moments are the point at which injury occurs in the thrower's shoulder (147). Not surprisingly, these critical moments have led to theories as to the development of pathology in the throwing shoulder.

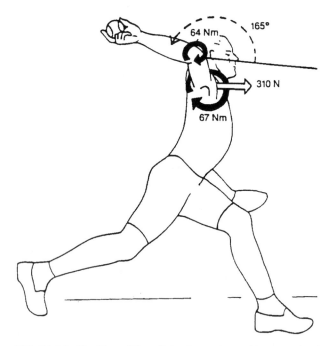

FIG. 21.31. Position of the pitcher's arm in cocking, maximal external rotation. The arm is abducted to 94 degrees and externally rotated to 165 degrees. This stage of the throwing motion is considered a critical moment and may be the time at which pathology develops in the thrower's shoulder. Forces generated during this phase of throwing include 67 N-m internal rotation torque, 310 N anterior force at the shoulder, and 64 N-m varus torque at the elbow. (From Fleisig GS, Andrews JR, Dillman CJ, et al. Kinetics of baseball pitching with implications about injury mechanisms. *Am J Sports Med* 1995;23: 233–239, with permission.)

Models for the Development of Pathology in the Thrower's Shoulder

Deceleration Model

After ball release and during deceleration of the arm, tremendous forces are thought to occur about the glenohumeral joint (Fig. 21.32). The rotator cuff and other muscles about the shoulder are responsible for a significant amount of the dissipation of these forces. As the arm is brought across the body in the deceleration and follow-through phases of pitching, the supraspinatus and infraspinatus muscles demonstrate high activity on electromyographic testing. It is important to note that these muscles are firing eccentrically. If these rotator cuff muscles are not strong enough, failure may occur, creating rotator cuff tendinopathy and possibly tearing (148,149).

With the dysfunction of the dynamic stabilizers of the glenohumeral joint, translation of the humeral head may occur in the glenoid, resulting in shearing stresses to the labrum, which may create labral tearing (149,150). In a similar fashion, lesions of the superior labrum with biceps anchor avulsions in pitchers are thought to occur as a result of traction on the tendon of the long head of the biceps during arm deceleration (151). The deceleration model, developed primarily by Andrews and colleagues, accounts for many of the findings seen in the symptomatic athlete's shoulder. It does not, however, adequately explain the increased laxity of the thrower's shoulder, which is manifested by increased external rotation and an increased sulcus sign (152,153).

Maximal External Rotation Model

The other critical moment in pitching occurs with maximal external rotation (147). At the instant of maximal external rotation, the arm is abducted to 94 degrees and externally rotated to 165 degrees (Fig. 21.31). This position is associated with high electromyographic activity of the subscapularis, pectoralis, and infraspinatus muscles, and again very high estimated forces are thought to occur about the glenohumeral joint. This, too, may be a source of pathology found in the shoulder of the throwing athlete.

Jobe et al. (63,64) presented a model for the development of pathology in the thrower's shoulder. During maximal external rotation, a phenomenon known as "hyperangulation" is thought to occur. Jobe et al. believed that pitchers with improper mechanics will horizontally abduct their arms when in maximal external rotation. This is thought to create microtrauma and stretching of the anterior structures of the glenohumeral joint capsule. This is capable of generating a vicious cycle, with more hyperangulation eventually leading to "subtle" instability and internal impingement as the greater tuberosity makes contact with the posterior–superior glenoid during arm cocking (Fig. 21.33).

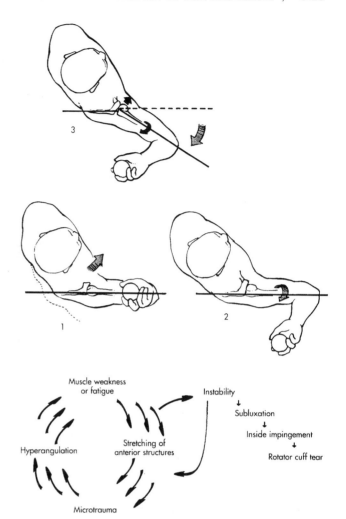

FIG. 21.33. Hyperangulation model for the development of pathology in the thrower's shoulder. In this model, improper throwing mechanics result in horizontal abduction at the glenohumeral joint, causing a stretching of the anterior capsular structures. This leads to instability and internal impingement. (From Jobe CM, Pink MM, Jobe FW, et al. Anterior shoulder instability, impingement, and rotator cuff tear: theories and concepts. In: Jobe FW, ed. *Operative techniques in upper extremity sports injuries.* St. Louis: C.V. Mosby, 1996:164–176, with permission.)

The subtle instability seen in pitchers is then thought to cause secondary anterior impingement as the rotator cuff experiences eccentric damage while trying to dynamically stabilize the lax shoulder. Jobe et al. (64) suspected that nearly all athletes with shoulder pain suffer from instability (Fig. 21.34). They called this instability subtle because throwers will often experience symptoms of pain but rarely have a sense of instability when throwing or apprehension during examination. Asymptomatic pitchers do have increased laxity when tested for external rotation or sulcus signs (152,153). However, increased laxity does not necessarily correlate with instability (85,154).

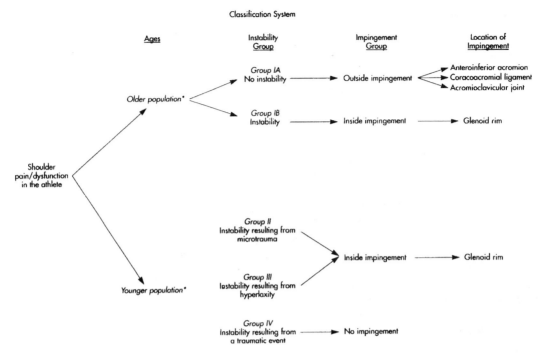

FIG. 21.34. Spectrum of instability in the overhead athlete. Note that all groups of older individuals with external impingement have instability, which is frequently difficult to detect, or "subtle." (From Jobe CM, Pink MM, Jobe FW, et al. Anterior shoulder instability, impingement, and rotator cuff tear: theories and concepts. In: Jobe FW, ed. *Operative techniques in upper extremity sports injuries.* St. Louis: C.V. Mosby, 1996:164–176, with permission.)

Another model to describe the findings in the throwing shoulder suggests that the forces generated during maximal external rotation may be responsible for the pathologic findings in the symptomatic throwing athlete. Work in our laboratory using a cadaver model identified the coracohumeral ligament and the entire inferior glenohumeral ligaments as the primary restraints to external rotation of the abducted shoulder, whereas the anterior capsule structures (superior glenohumeral ligament, middle glenohumeral ligament, and anterior band of the inferior glenohumeral ligament) were significantly less important (155). This has led to a model based on excessive external rotation to explain the findings in the symptomatic thrower's shoulder (Fig. 21.35). In this model, repeated throwing at high velocity, particularly in the presence of a weak or painful rotator cuff, leads to

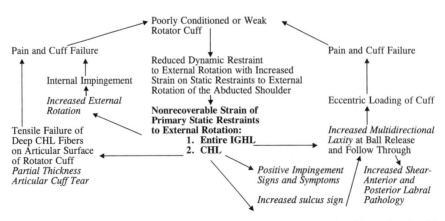

FIG. 21.35. External rotation model for the development of pathology in the thrower's shoulder. In this model, damage to the primary restraints for external rotation of the abducted shoulder are responsible for the development of pathology in the thrower's shoulder.

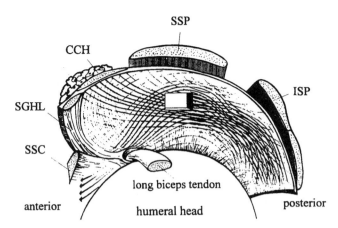

FIG. 21.36. Location of coracohumeral ligament fibers in the articular surface of the rotator cuff. (From Gohlke F, Essigkrug B, Schmitz F. The pattern of the collagen fiber bundles of the capsule of the glenohumeral joint. *J Shoulder Elbow Surg* 1994;3:111–128, with permission.)

increased strain on the primary restraints to external rotation. As the strain increases, microdamage may occur, leading to pain and nonrecoverable lengthening of the restraints.

The coracohumeral ligament is capable of significant strain before failure (110). As the coracohumeral ligament lengthens, throwers may develop pain along the coracohumeral ligament, leading to anterior impingement symptoms, with positive Neer and Hawkins impingement signs. Interestingly, the coracohumeral ligament fibers invest heavily in the articular surface of the rotator cuff (Fig. 21.36). If excessive external rotation during the throwing motion generates strain along the coracohumeral ligament, it is plausible that failure might occur along those portions of the coracohumeral ligament that invest the articular surface of the rotator cuff. This may present as an articular surface partial rotator cuff tear, a common finding in the symptomatic thrower's shoulder at arthroscopy. In addition, because the coracohumeral ligament is considered a primary stabilizer preventing inferior translation in the adducted arm, the increased sulcus sign seen in pitchers may occur as a result of nonrecoverable strain to the coracohumeral ligament during maximal external rotation of the pitching motion.

Damage to the entire inferior glenohumeral ligament would manifest as increased multidirectional laxity and may not necessarily present as anterior instability. Should this occur, increased rotator cuff strength would be required to actively and dynamically stabilize the lax shoulder during the throwing motion. In the thrower with a weak rotator cuff, this may lead to eccentric loading of the cuff that may progress to damage. Increased laxity may also produce labral shearing in multiple directions, resulting in anterior and posterior labral tears.

As the coracohumeral ligament and inferior glenohumeral ligament lengthen, increased external rotation may occur. With increased humeral external rotation, the greater tuberosity may make contact with the posterior glenoid causing internal impingement.

These models are methods of accounting for the pathologic findings seen in the symptomatic thrower's shoulder. As more is learned about throwing and the nature of the pathology seen, these models are expected to evolve. Kinetic analysis of the throwing motion has provided a great deal of information about the pathogenesis and natural history of the thrower's shoulder. Although throwing has been analyzed most, kinematic analysis of other sports has been helpful in understanding shoulder pathology in other athletes as well.

Kinematics of Swimming

The arm stroke for freestyle swimming has been analyzed kinematically and electromyographically and has been divided into four components (156,157) (Fig. 21.37): Early pull-through begins with the hand entering the water and ends when the arm is perpendicular to the torso; late pull-through continues until the hand leaves the water; early recovery begins when the hand leaves the water and continues until the arm is perpendicular to the torso; and late recovery continues until the hand enters the water again.

The fingers enter the water first, forward of and lateral to the swimmer's head, with the palm facing away from the body and the elbow flexed and above the hand. Once the hand enters the water, it reaches forward under

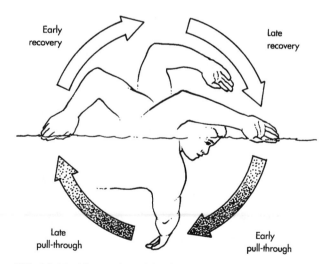

FIG. 21.37. Kinematics of the freestyle arm stroke. The four stages of the freestyle arm stroke include: early pull-through, late pull-through, early recovery, and late recovery. (From Pink MM, Perry J. Biomechanics. In: Jobe FW, ed. *Operative techniques in upper extremity sports injuries.* St. Louis: C.V. Mosby, 1996:109–123, with permission.)

the water. Once maximal reach occurs, the motion is reversed to a pulling motion, bringing the hand back toward the torso (158). At hand entry, the upper trapezius, rhomboids, supraspinatus, anterior and middle deltoids, and serratus anterior are very active (156,157). This constellation of muscle activity is retracting and rotating the scapula superiorly, which positions the glenoid as the humerus is abducted and forward flexed.

In the pull-through of the stroke, the hand follows an S-shaped curve (159), during which time the pectoralis major and teres minor are firing and acting as a force couple. The pectoralis major is internally rotating, adducting, and extending the humerus, generating the power of the stroke while the teres minor is counterbalancing the internal rotation force (156,157). Peak activity is also seen in the latissimus dorsi during the mid to late pull-through. The subscapularis demonstrated a peak activity during the late pull-through and early recovery but was active throughout the swimming stroke.

When the hand is brought out of the water at the beginning of the recovery, the middle deltoid and supraspinatus are firing to lift the arm out of the water. The scapula is retracted by the rhomboids, whereas the subscapularis continues to fire as the arm internally rotates. As the recovery continues, the infraspinatus increases its activity, which externally rotates the arm to swing the forearm and hand forward (156,157).

Throughout the swimming cycle, the supraspinatus and serratus anterior were continuously firing, which may predispose these muscles to fatigue and injury (157,160,161). Swimming injuries to the shoulder are common, with up to 67% of competitive swimmers sustaining a shoulder injury at some point in their careers (162). Swimmers with shoulder pain display a characteristic abnormal stroke in the recovery phase such that the humerus is held lower, resulting in a dropped elbow during the recovery phase. In addition, in the painful swimmer, the hand typically enters the water further laterally from the midline (157). Swimmers with painful shoulders will use the same muscle firing patterns as healthy swimmers, yet the amplitude of the muscle activity is less, particularly the serratus anterior and other periscapular muscles. These studies suggest the need for periscapular muscle training as a part of the rehabilitation of the painful shoulder in swimmers (160,161).

Kinematics of Tennis

By nature of the demands of the serve and repetitive strokes and the lever arm that a tennis racket creates, the forces on the rotator cuff in tennis are substantial. The tennis serve and the forehand and backhand strokes have been analyzed with regard to the kinematics and electromyography about the shoulder (163). The tennis serve has been divided into four stages (164) (Fig. 21.38)

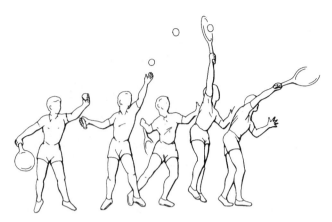

FIG. 21.38. Kinematics of the tennis serve. The tennis serve is divided into four stages: wind-up, cocking, acceleration, and follow-through. (From Tibone J, Patek R, Jobe FW, et al. Functional anatomy, biomechanics, and kinesiology. In: DeLee JC, Drez D, eds. *Orthopaedic sports medicine. Principles and practice.* Philadelphia: W.B. Saunders, 1994:463–480, with permission.)

Wind-up ends at the time of ball release and is characterized by shoulder abduction, extension, and external rotation; *cocking* begins from ball release and continues until the arm is in maximal external rotation; *acceleration* of the arm occurs next with rapid internal rotation and adduction of the arm and continues until impact with the ball; and *follow-through* continues from contact and involves adduction of the arm across the body with internal rotation of the arm. Electromyographic analysis of the tennis serve demonstrates patterns very similar to the baseball pitch. Interestingly, the serratus anterior had substantial activity during cocking and acceleration, whereas the deltoid activity is low during cocking. This pattern, which differs from pitching, is explained by the differences in trunk rotation in the tennis serve (163,164).

Forehand and backhand strokes have been divided into three stages (Fig. 21.39) (163,165). In the forehand stroke, the first stage is called racket preparation and is characterized by shoulder abduction and external rotation. This stage is relatively passive; however, trunk rotation is essential to prepare for the stroke. The second stage is called acceleration and continues until ball contact. Acceleration in the forehand is characterized by internal rotation and adduction of the shoulder with the biceps brachii, subscapularis, pectoralis major, and serratus anterior demonstrating high activity (163). Trunk rotation is also essential. The third stage is follow-through and is a deceleration of the arm as it adducts across the body. In this stage of the forehand stroke, the acceleration muscles decrease their activity, whereas the external rotators of the shoulder have increased activity to decelerate the arm.

The backhand stroke also begins with racket prepara-

Tennis—Forehand

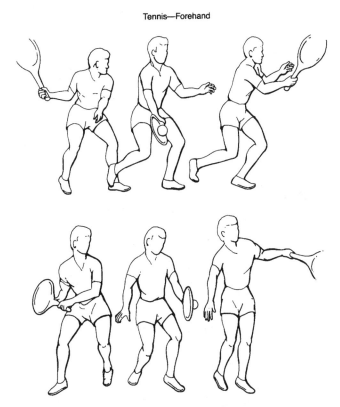

FIG. 21.39. Kinematics of the tennis forehand and backhand strokes. (From Tibone J, Patek R, Jobe FW, et al. Functional anatomy, biomechanics, and kinesiology. In: DeLee JC, Drez D, eds. *Orthopaedic sports medicine. Principles and practice.* Philadelphia: W.B. Saunders, 1994:463–480, with permission.)

tion. In the acceleration stage of the backhand, the arm is abducted and externally rotated at the shoulder. The middle deltoid, supraspinatus, and infraspinatus demonstrate high activity. The follow-through of the backhand stroke is the third stage and begins at ball strike and is characterized by decreased activity of the external rotators and increased activity of the internal rotators to decelerate the arm.

Tennis players can develop shoulder problems with improper stroke technique. If the trunk is rotated prematurely in the forehand stroke, the player loses the potential energy stored in the trunk rotation and tries to compensate for the decreased kinetic energy of the racket by overpowering the shoulder muscles. This premature trunk rotation is called "opening up too early" and can result in overloading of the internal rotators used during acceleration, leading to overuse symptoms (165). In a similar fashion, the most effective location for impact with the ball is in front of the torso. This is the location where racket velocity is maximal and is enhanced by the player stepping into the stroke. If impact is made behind the body, the arm has less time to achieve maximal velocity of the racket requiring more

rapid contraction of the rotator cuff, which can lead to overuse symptoms as well (165).

Kinematics of the Golf Swing

At this time, little information is available regarding the precise biomechanics of shoulder motion during a golf swing. Jobe et al. (166,167) investigated the function of the rotator cuff during the golf swing. The golf swing requires the use of both shoulders simultaneously, with each arm performing a different motion yet performing somewhat mirror images of each other. The left arm during the back swing is similar to the right arm during the follow-through.

Like other continuous motions of the shoulder, the golf swing has been divided into five stages (Fig. 21.40) (167): The *back swing* starts at address of the ball and continues to the end of the back swing; the *forward swing* begins at the end of the back swing to the point where the club shaft is horizontal, parallel to the ground; *acceleration* is seen from the horizontal club to impact with the ball; *early follow-through* occurs from ball impact to the point where the club shaft is horizontal again; and the *late follow-through* is the part of the swing from the horizontal club to the end of the motion. For simplicity, these stages of the golf swing are described for right-handed golfers, yet the reverse image can be applied to the left-handed swing as well.

Although the back swing is a continuous smooth motion, Cochran and Stobbs (168) divided the back swing into five segments. The first segment occurs when the shoulders are turned around the axis of the spine. Although this motion requires primarily trunk rotation, some golf professionals describe this motion as a "shoulder turn" (169). The second segment uses forward

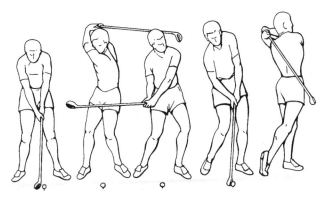

FIG. 21.40. Stages of the golf swing. The golf swing begins with the address and is followed by the back swing, forward swing, acceleration, early follow-through, and late follow-through. (From Tibone J, Patek R, Jobe FW, et al. Functional anatomy, biomechanics, and kinesiology. In: DeLee JC, Drez D, eds. *Orthopaedic sports medicine. Principles and practice.* Philadelphia: W.B. Saunders, 1994:463–480, with permission.)

flexion of the left shoulder, which raises the left arm. The third segment involves cocking the left wrist. The fourth segment of the back swing required horizontal adduction of the left arm, bringing it across the chest such that the left arm and elbow are brought closer to the right shoulder. The final segment of the back swing involves pronation of the forearm and likely some internal rotation of the glenohumeral joint, in an effort to bring the club head into the swing plane. The final position of the left arm, which is in forward flexion, internal rotation, and cross-body adduction, is thought to be responsible for the development of pathology in the left shoulder seen commonly in professional golfers with shoulder problems (169). This position may damage the posterior capsule, leading to posterior instability; and may create impingement or acromioclavicular joint loading.

Overall analysis of the motion of the golf swing demonstrates that the left shoulder is in neutral abduction/adduction and forward flexed approximately 20 degrees when the ball is addressed. During the back swing, the left shoulder will forward flex to at least 90 degrees, will horizontally adduct as much as 60 degrees, and will internally rotate slightly. The right arm meanwhile performs dissimilar motions. It is abducted slightly and externally rotated as much as 90 degrees. In general, the right arm seems to follow the grip of the club during the left arm-dominated back swing (169).

During the forward swing to impact and through the follow-through, the club is carried through the swing plane, and the right and left shoulders basically reverse their positions, such that the right shoulder is forward flexed and horizontally adducted across the chest at the end of follow-through. The left shoulder meanwhile is abducted and slightly externally rotated at the end of follow-through. During impact, with clubhead speed approaching 200 km/h in some professionals (169), the shoulders assume a position similar to the address position.

Electromyographic analysis (166,167,170) of the shoulder during the golf swing has demonstrated little deltoid activity, with a significant rotator cuff component. Interestingly, both shoulders of right-handed golfers had similar firing patterns, as the subscapularis and infraspinatus work at the extremes of shoulder motion (166). During the acceleration stage, the subscapularis reaches peak activity as the arm is internally rotating. The latissimus dorsi and pectoralis major are thought to provide power during the propulsive stage of the swing with the latissimus firing earlier, and the pectoralis contributing the most activity as the arm is powerfully rotated and adducted. Due to the fairly symmetric nature of the golf swing, we suggest strengthening the rotator cuff in both shoulders and the latissimus dorsi and pectoralis major as a part of the rehabilitation of the golfer's shoulder.

REFERENCES

1. Abbott LC, Lucas DB. The function of the clavicle: its surgical significance. *Ann Surg* 1954;140:583–597.
2. Codman EA. *The shoulder, rupture of the supraspinatus tendon and other lesions in or about the subacromial bursa.* Boston: Thomas Todd, 1934.
3. Morrey BF, An K-N. Biomechanics of the shoulder. In: Rockwood CA Jr, Matsen FA III, eds. *The shoulder.* Philadelphia: W.B. Saunders, 1990:208–245.
4. Hollinshead WH, ed. *Anatomy for surgeons. Vol. 3. The back and limbs.* Philadelphia: Harper & Row, 1982:260.
5. Rockwood CA. Disorders of the sternoclavicular joint. In: Rockwood CA Jr, Matsen FA III, eds. *The shoulder.* Philadelphia: W.B. Saunders, 1990:477.
6. Bearn JG. Direct observations on the function of the capsule of the sternoclavicular joint in clavicular support. Am J Sports Med J 1967;101:159–170.
7. Inman VT, Saunders JB, Abbott LC. Observations on the function of the shoulder joint. *J Bone Joint Surg Am* 1944;26:1–30.
8. Flatow EL. The biomechanics of the acromioclavicular, sternoclavicular, and scapulothoracic joints. In: Heckman JD, ed. *Instructional Course Lectures.* Vol. 42. Rosemont, Illinois: American Academy of Orthopaedic Surgeons, 1993:237–245.
9. DePalma AF, ed. *Surgery of the shoulder.* Philadelphia: J.B. Lippincott, 1973.
10. Bosworth BM. Complete acromioclavicular separation. *N Engl J Med* 1949;241:221–225.
11. Salter EG, Nasca RJ, Shelley BS. Anatomical observations on the acromioclavicular joint and supporting ligaments. *Am J Sports Med* 1987;15:199–206.
12. Fukuda K, Craig EV, Kai-Nan A, et al. Biomechanical study of the ligamentous system of the acromioclavicular joint. *J Bone Joint Surg Am* 1986;68A:434–440.
13. Kennedy JC, Cameron H. The acromion: complete dislocation of the acromio-clavicular joint. *J Bone Joint Surg Br* 1954;36B:202–208.
14. Rockwood CA, Young DC. Disorders of the acromioclavicular joint. In: Rockwood CA Jr, Matsen FA III, eds. *The shoulder.* Philadelphia: W.B. Saunders, 1990.
15. Urist MR. Complete dislocation of the acromioclavicular joint: the nature of the traumatic lesion and effective methods of treatment with an analysis of 41 cases. *J Bone Joint Surg* 1946;28:813–837.
16. Kiefer H, Claes L, Burri C, et al. The stabilizing effect of various implants on the torn acromioclavicular joint. *Arch Orthop Trauma Surg* 1986;106:42–46.
17. Bargren JH, Erlanger S, Dick HM. Biomechanics and comparison of two operative methods of treatment of complete acromioclavicular separation. *Clin Orthop* 1978;130:267–272.
18. Harryman DT, Clark JM. Anatomy of the rotator cuff. In: Burkhead WZ Jr, ed. *Rotator cuff disorders.* Baltimore: Williams & Wilkins, 1996:23.
19. Lohr JF, Uhthoff HK. The microvascular pattern of the supraspinatus tendon. *Clin Orthop* 1990;254:35–38.
20. Moseley HF, Goldie I. The arterial pattern of the rotator cuff of the shoulder. *J Bone Joint Surg Br* 1963;45B:780–789.
21. Rathbun JB, Macnab I. The microvascular pattern of the rotator cuff. *J Bone Joint Surg Br* 1970;52B:540–553.
22. Clark JM, Harryman DT II. Tendons, ligaments, and capsule of the rotator cuff. *J Bone Joint Surg* 1992;5:713–725.
23. Gohlke F, Essigkrug B, Schmitz F. The pattern of the collagen fiber bundles of the capsule of the glenohumeral joint. *J Shoulder Elbow Surg* 1994;3:111–128.
24. Burkhart SS. Reconciling the paradox of rotator cuff repair versus debridement: a unified biomechanical rationale for the treatment of rotator cuff tears. *Arthroscopy* 1994;10:4–19.
25. Clark J, Sidles JA, Matsen FA. The relationship of the glenohumeral joint capsule to the rotator cuff. *Clin Orthop* 1990;254:29–34.
26. Bigliani LU, Ticker JB, Flatow EL, et al. The relationship of acromial architecture to rotator cuff disease. *Clin Sports Med* 1991;10:823–838.
27. Nicholson GP, Goodman DA, Flatow EL, et al. The acromion:

morphologic condition and age-related changes. A study fo 420 scapulas. *J Shoulder Elbow Surg* 1996;5:1–11.

28. Zuckerman JD, Kummer FJ, Cuomo F, et al. The influence of coracoacromial arch anatomy on rotator cuff tears. *J Shoulder Elbow Surg* 1992;1:4–14.

29. Bigliani LU, Morrison DS, April EW. The morphology of the acromion and rotator cuff impingement. *Orthop Trans* 1986;10: 228.

30. Soslowsky LJ, An CH, Johnston SP, et al. Geometric and mechanical properties of the coracoacromial ligament and their relationship to rotator cuff disease. *Clin Orthop* 1994;304:10–17.

31. Uhthoff HK, Hammond DI, Sarkar K, et al. The role of the coracoacromial ligament in the impingement syndrome: a clinical, radiological and histological study. *Int Orthop* 1988;12: 97–104.

32. Poppen NK, Walker PS. Forces at the glenohumeral joint in abduction. *Clin Orthop* 1978;135:165–70.

33. Van Der Helm FCT. Analysis of the kinematic and dynamic behavior of the shoulder mechanism. *J Biomech* 1994;27: 527–550.

34. Thompson WO, Debski RE, Boardman, ND III, et al. A biomechanical analysis of rotator cuff deficiency in a cadaveric model. *Am J Sports Med* 1996;24:286–292.

35. Weulker N, Roetman B, Roessig S. Coracoacromial pressure recordings in a cadaveric model. *J Shoulder Elbow Surg* 1995;4: 462–467.

36. Flatow EL, Raimondo RA, Kelkar R, et al. Active and passive restraints against superior humeral translation: the biceps tendon and coracoacromial arch. *J Shoulder Elbow Surg* 1997;6:172.

37. Lazarus MD, Yung SW, Sidles JA, et al. Anterosuperior humeral displacement: limitation by the coracoacromial arch. *J Shoulder Elbow Surg* 1996;5:S7.

38. Moorman CT III, Deng XH, Warren RF, et al. The coracoacromial ligament: is it the appendix of the shoulder? *J Shoulder Elbow Surg* 1996;5:S9.

39. Itoi E, Berglund LJ, Grabowski JJ, et al. Tensile properties of the supraspinatus tendon. *J Orthop Res* 1995;13:578–584.

40. Nakajima T, Rokuuma N, Hamada K, et al. Histologic and biomechanical characteristics of the supraspinatus tendon: reference to rotator cuff tearing. *J Shoulder Elbow Surg* 1994;3:79–87.

41. McLaughlin HL, Asherman EG. Lesions of the musculotendinous cuff of the shoulder. *J Bone Joint Surg Am* 1951;33A:76–86.

42. Codman EA, Akerson IB. The pathology associated with rupture of the supraspinatus tendon. *Am J Surg* 1931;93:348–359.

43. Uhthoff HK, Sarkar K. Surgical repair of rotator cuff ruptures. The importance of the subacromial bursa. *J Bone Joint Surg Br* 1991;73B:399–401.

44. Riley GP, Harrall RL, Constant CR, et al. Glycosaminoglycans of human rotator cuff tendons: changes with age and in chronic rotator cuff tendinitis. *Ann Rheum Dis* 1994;53:367–376.

45. Chard MD, Cawston TE, Riley GP, et al. Rotator cuff degeneration and lateral epicondylitis: a comparative histological study. *Ann Rheum Dis* 1994;53:30–34.

46. Fukuda H, Hamada K, Nakajima T, et al. Pathology and pathogenesis of the intratendinous tearing of the rotator cuff viewed from en bloc histologic sections. *Clin Orthop* 1994;304:60–67.

47. Neer CS II. Anterior acromioplasty for the chronic impingement syndrome in the shoulder. *J Bone Joint Surg* Am 1972;54A:41–50.

48. Morrison DS, Bigliani LU. The clinical significance of variations in acromial morphology. *Orthop Trans* 1987;11:234.

49. Flatow EL, Soslowsky LJ, Ticker JB, et al. Excursion of the rotator cuff under the acromion. *Am J Sports Med* 1994;22: 779–788.

50. Soslowsky LJ, Carpenter JE, Debano CM, et al. Development and utilization of an animal model for investigations on rotator cuff disease. *J Shoulder Elbow Surg* 1996;5:383–392.

51. Saha AK. Mechanics of elevation of the glenohumeral joint: its application in rehabilitation of flail shoulder in upper brachial plexus injuries and in replacement of the upper humerus by prosthesis. *Acta Orthop Scand* 1973;44:668–678.

52. Saha AK. Dynamic stability of the glenohumeral joint. *Acta Orthop Scand* 1971;42:491–505.

53. Randelli M, Gambrioli PL. Glenohumeral osteometry by computed tomography in normal and unstable shoulders. *Clin Orthop* 1986;208:151–156.

54. Chaudhuri GK, Sengupta A, Saha AK. Rotation osteotomy of the shaft of the humerus for recurrent dislocation of the shoulder: anterior and posterior. *Acta Orthop Scand* 1974;45:193–198.

55. Cyprien JM, Vasey HM, Burdet A, et al. Humeral retroversion and glenohumeral relationship in the normal shoulder and in recurrent anterior dislocation (scapulometry). *Clin Orthop* 1983; 175:8–17.

56. Surin V. Blader S, Markhede G, et al. Rotational osteotomy of the humerus for posterior instability of the shoulder. *J Bone Joint Surg* 1990;72A:181–186.

57. Weber BG, Simpson LA, Hardegger F, et al. Rotational humeral osteotomy for recurrent anterior dislocation of the shoulder associated with a large Hill-Sachs lesion. *J Bone Joint Surg Am* 1984;66A:1443–1450.

58. Weber BG. Recurrent dislocation of the shoulder: treatment with subcapital rotation-osteotomy. *Acta Orthop Scand* 1974;45: 986–988.

59. Warner JJP, Flatow EL. Anatomy and biomechanics. In: Bigliani LU, ed. *The unstable shoulder.* Rosemont, IL: American Academy of Orthopaedic Surgeons, 1996:1–24.

60. Kronberg M, Brostrom L-A, Soderlund V. Retroversion of the humeral head in the normal shoulder and its relationship to the normal range of motion. *Clin Orthop* 1990;253:113–117.

61. Kronberg M, Brostrom L-A. Humeral head retroversion in patients with unstable humeroscapular joints. *Clin Orthop* 1990; 260:207–211.

62. Pieper HG. Humeral torsion in the throwing arm of handball players—an adaptation to unilateral strain. Final Program: Book of Abstracts and Outlines. 2nd World Congress on Sports Trauma, AOSSM 22nd Annual Meeting, Lake Buena Vista, Florida, 1996:769.

63. Jobe FW, Kvitne RS. Shoulder pain in the overhand or throwing athlete. *Orthop Rev* 1989;18:963–975.

64. Jobe CM, Pink MM, Jobe FW, et al. Anterior shoulder instability, impingement, and rotator cuff tears: theories and concepts. In: Jobe FW, ed. *Operative techniques in upper extremity sports injuries.* St. Louis: C.V. Mosby, 1996:164–176.

65. O'Brien SJ, Arnoczky SP, Warren RF, et al. Developmental anatomy of the shoulder and anatomy of the glenohumeral joint. In: Rockwood CA Jr, Matsen FA III, eds. *The shoulder.* Philadelphia: W.B. Saunders, 1990:1–33.

66. Doos SP, Ray GS, Saha AK. Observation of the tilt of the glenoid cavity of the scapula. *J Anat Soc India* 1966;15:114.

67. Brewer BJ, Wubben RC, Garrera GF. Excessive retroversion of the glenoid cavity: a cause of non-traumatic posterior instability of the shoulder. *J Bone Joint Surg Am* 1986;68A:724–731.

68. Hill JA, Tkach L. A study of glenohumeral orientation in patients with anterior recurrent shoulder dislocations using computed axial tomography. *Orthop Trans* 1985;9:47–48.

69. Hurley JA, Anderson TE, Dear W, et al. Posterior shoulder instability: surgical versus conservative results with evaluation of glenoid version. *Am J Sports Med* 1992;20:396–400.

70. Galinat BJ, Howell SM, Kraft TA. The glenoid-posterior acromion angle: an accurate method of evaluating glenoid version. *Orthop Trans* 1988;12:727.

71. Mallon WJ, Brown HR, Vogler JB III, et al. Radiographic and geometric anatomy of the scapula. *Clin Orthop* 1992;277: 142–154.

72. Itoi E, Motzkin NE, An KN, et al. Scapular inclination and inferior stability of the shoulder. *Trans Orthop Res Soc* 1992; 288.

73. Basmajian JB, Bazant FJ. Factors preventing downward dislocation of the adducted shoulder joint: an electromyographic and morphological study. *J Bone Joint Surg Am* 1959;41A:1182–1186.

74. Warner JJP, Deng X, Warren RF, et al. Static capsuloligamentous restraints to superior-inferior translation of the glenohumeral joint. *Am J Sports Med* 1992;20:675–685.

75. Scott DJ Jr. Treatment of recurrent posterior dislocations of the shoulder by glenoplasty: Report of three cases. *J Bone Joint Surg Am* 1967;49A:471–476.

76. Schwartz RE, O'Brien SJ, Warren RF, et al. Capsular restraints

to anterior-posterior motion of the shoulder. A biomechanical study. *Orthop Trans* 1988;12:727.

77. Rowe CR, ed. *The shoulder.* New York: Churchill Livingstone, 1988.

78. Saha AK. *Theory of shoulder mechanism: descriptive and applied.* Springfield, IL: Charles C Thomas, 1961.

79. Soslowsky LJ, Flatow EL, Bigliani LU, et al. Articular geometry of the glenohumeral joint. *Clin Orthop* 1992;285:181–190.

80. Soslowsky LJ, Flatow EL, Bigliani LU, et al. Quantification of in situ contact areas at the glenohumeral joint: a biomechanical study. *J Orthop Res* 1992;10:524–534.

81. Kelkar R, Newton PM, Armengol J, et al. Three-dimensional kinematics of the glenohumeral joint during abduction in the scapular plane. *Trans Orthop Res Soc* 1993;18:136.

82. Harryman DT II, Sidles JA, Clark JM, et al. Translation of the humeral head on the glenoid with passive glenohumeral motion. *J Bone Joint Surg Am* 1990;72A:1334–1343.

83. Harryman DT II, Sidles JA, Harris SL, et al. The role of the rotator interval capsule in passive motion and stability of the shoulder. *J Bone Joint Surg Am* 1992;74A:53–66.

84. Harryman DT II, Sidels JA, Harris SC, et al. Laxity of the normal glenohumeral joint: a quantitative in vivo assessment. *J Shoulder Elbow Surg* 1992;1:66–76.

85. Lippitt SB, Harris SL, Harryman DT II, et al. In vivo quantification of the laxity of normal and unstable glenohumeral joints. *J Shoulder Elbow Surg* 1994;3:215–223.

86. Howell SM, Galinat BJ. The glenoid-labral socket: a constrained articular surface. *Clin Orthop* 1989;243:122–125.

87. Bowen MX, Deng XH, Warner JP, et al. The effect of joint compression on stability of the glenohumeral joint. *Trans Orthop Res Soc* 1992;17:289.

88. Lippitt SB, Vanderhooft JE, Harris SL, et al. Glenohumeral stability from concavity-compression: a quantitative analysis. *J Shoulder Elbow Surg* 1993;2:27–35.

89. Hara H, Ito N, Iwasaki K. Strength of the glenoid labrum and adjacent shoulder capsule. *J Shoulder Elbow Surg* 1996;5:263–268.

90. Speer KP, Deng X, Borrero S, et al. Biomechanical evaluation of a simulated Bankart lesion. *J Bone Joint Surg Am* 1994;76A:1819–1826.

91. Warner JJP, Deng XH, Warren RF, et al. Superoinferior translation in the intact and vented glenohumeral joint. *J Shoulder Elbow Surg* 1993;2:99–105.

92. Helmig P, Sojbjerg JO, Sneppen O, et al. Glenohumeral movement patterns after puncture of the joint capsule: an experimental study. *J Shoulder Elbow Surg* 1993;2:209–215.

93. Browne AO, Hoffmeyer P, An KN, et al. The influence of atmospheric pressure on shoulder stability. *Orthop Trans* 1990;14:259.

94. Gibb TD, Sidles JA, Harryman DT II, et al. The effect of capsular venting on glenohumeral laxity. *Clin Orthop* 1991;268:120–127.

95. Kumar VP, Balasubramianiam P. The role of atmospheric pressure in stabilising the shoulder: an experimental study. *J Bone Joint Surg Br* 1985;67B:719–721.

96. DePalma AF, Callery G, Bennett GA. The shoulder joint. Part I. Variational anatomy and degenerative lesions of the shoulder bone. In: Blount WP, Banks SW, eds. *American Academy of Orthopaedic Surgeons Instructional Course Lectures XVI.* Ann Arbor, MI: JW Edwards, 1994:255–281.

97. Warner JJP, Micheli LJ, Arslanian LE, et al. Scapulothoracic motion in normal shoulders and shoulders with glenohumeral instability and impingement syndrome. A study using Moire topographic analysis. *Clin Orthop* 1992;285:191–199.

98. O'Brien SJ, Neves MC, Arnoczky SP, et al. The anatomy of the inferior glenohumeral ligament complex of the shoulder. *Am J Sports Med* 1990;18:449–456.

99. O'Brien SJ, Arnoczky SP, Warren RF, et al. Developmental anatomy of the shoulder and anatomy of the glenohumeral joint. In: Rockwood CA Jr, Matsen FA III, eds. *The shoulder.* Philadelphia: W.B. Saunders, 1990:1–33.

100. Cooper DE, O'Brien SJ, Arnoczky SP, et al. The structure and function of the coracohumeral ligament: an anatomic and microscopic study. *J Shoulder Elbow Surg* 1993;2:70–77.

101. Warren RF, Kornblatt IB, Marchand R. Static factors affecting posterior shoulder stability. *Orthop Trans* 1984;8:89.

102. Oversen J, Nielsen S. Anterior and posterior shoulder instability: a cadaver study. *Acta Orthop Scand* 1986;57:324–327.

103. Warner JJP, Caborn DNM, Berger, et al. Dynamic capsuloligamentous anatomy of the glenohumeral joint. *J Shoulder Elbow Surg* 1993;2:115–133.

104. Basmajian JV, Bazant FJ. Factors preventing downward dislocation of the adducted shoulder joint: an electromyographic and morphologic study. *J Bone Joint Surg Am* 1959;41A:1182–1186.

105. Nobuhara K, Ikeda H. Rotator interval lesion. *Clin Orthop* 1987;223:44–50.

106. Warner JJP, Deng XH, Warren RF, et al. Static capsuloligamentous restraints to superior-inferior translation of the glenohumeral joint. *Am J Sports Med* 1992;20:675–685.

107. Helmig P, Sojberg JO, Kjaersgaard-Andersen P, et al. Distal humeral migration as a component of multidirectional shoulder instability: an anatomical study in autopsy specimens. *Clin Orthop* 1990;252:139–143.

108. Neer CS II. Involuntary inferior and multidirectional instability of the shoulder: etiology, recognition and treatment. In: Stauffer ES, ed. *American Academy of Orthopaedic Surgeons Instructional Course Lectures XXXIV.* St. Louis: C.V. Mosby, 1985:232–238.

109. Edelson JG, Taitz C, Grishkan A. The coracohumeral ligament. Anatomy of a substantial but neglected structure. *J Bone Joint Surg Br* 1991;73B:150–153.

110. Boardman ND III, Debski RE, Warner JJP, et al. Tensile properties of the superior glenohumeral and coracohumeral ligaments. *J Shoulder Elbow Surg* 1996;5:249–254.

111. Snyder SJ. Diagnostic arthroscopy of the shoulder: normal anatomy and variations. In: Snyder SJ, ed. *Shoulder arthroscopy.* New York: McGraw-Hill, 1994:23–40.

112. Turkel SJ, Panio MW, Marshall JL, et al. Stabilizing mechanisms preventing anterior dislocation of the glenohumeral joint. *J Bone Joint Surg Am* 1981;63A:1208–1217.

113. O'Connell PW, Nuber GW, Mileski RA, et al. The contribution of the glenohumeral ligaments to anterior stability of the shoulder joint. *Am J Sports Med* 1990;18:579–584.

114. Bigliani LU, Pollock RG, Soslowsky LJ, et al. Tensile properties of the inferior glenohumeral ligament. *J Orthop Res* 1992;10:187–197.

115. Ticker JB, Bigliani LU, Soslowky LJ, et al. Inferior glenohumeral ligament: geometric and strain-rate dependent properties. *J Shoulder Elbow Surg* 1996;5:269–279.

116. Blasier RB, Soslowsky LJ, Malicky DM, et al. Posterior glenohumeral subluxation: active and passive stabilization in a biomechanical model. *J Bone Joint Surg* 1997;79:433–440.

117. Soslowsky LJ, Malicky DM, Blasier RB. Active and passive factors in inferior glenohumeral stabilization: a biomechanical model. *J Shoulder Elbow Surg* 1997;6:371–379.

118. Blasier BR, Goldberg RE, Rothman ED. Anterior shoulder stability: contributions of rotator cuff forces and the capsular ligaments in a cadaver model. *J Shoulder Elbow Surg* 1992;1:140–150.

119. Pagnani MJ, Xiang-Hua D, Warren RF, et al. Role of the long head of the biceps brachii in glenohumeral stability: a biomechanical study in cadavers. *J Shoulder Elbow Surg* 1996;5:255–262.

120. Malicky DM, Soslowsky LJ, Blasier RB, et al. Anterior glenohumeral stabilization factors: progressive effects in a biomechanical model. *J Orthop Res* 1996;14:282–288.

121. Glousman R, Jobe F, Tibone J, et al. Dynamic electromyographic analysis of the throwing shoulder with glenohumeral instability. *J Bone Joint Surg Am* 1988;70A:220–226.

122. Gowan ID, Jobe FW, Tibone JE, et al. A comparative electromyographic analysis of the shoulder during pitching: professional vs. amature pitchers. *Am J Sports Med* 1987;15:586–590.

123. Hawkins RJ, Koppert G. The natural history following anterior dislocation of the shoulder in the older patient. *J Bone Joint Surg Br* 1982;64B:255.

124. McLaughlin HL. Dislocation of the shoulder with tuberosity fracture. *Surg Clin North Am* 1963;43:1615–1620.

125. Pettersson G. Rupture of the tendon aponeurosis of the shoulder joint in antero-inferior dislocation: a study on the origin and occurrence of the ruptures. *Acta Chir Scand* 1942;77[Suppl]:1–187.

126. Hawkins RJ, Bell RH, Hawkins RH, et al. Anterior dislocation of the shoulder in the older patient. *Clin Orthop* 1986;206:192–195.

127. Gerber C, Krushell RJ. Isolated rupture of the tendon of the subscapularis muscle: clinical features in 16 cases. *J Bone Joint Surg Br* 1991;73B:389–394.

128. Hauser EDW. Avulsion of the tendon of the subscapularis muscle. *J Bone Joint Surg Am* 1954;36A:139–141.

129. DePalma AF, Cooke AJ, Prabhakar M. The role of the subscapularis in recurrent anterior dislocations of the shoulder. *Clin Orthop* 1967;54:35–49.

130. Craig EV. The posterior mechanism of acute anterior shoulder dislocations. *Clin Orthop* 1984;190:212–216.

131. Ferrari DA. Capsular ligaments of the shoulder: anatomical and functional study of the anterior-superior capsule. *Am J Sports Med* 1990;18:20–24.

132. Clark J, Sidles JA, Matsen FA III. The relationship of the glenohumeral joint capsule to the rotator cuff. *Clin Orthop* 1990;254:29–34.

133. Vangsness CT Jr, Ennis M, Taylor JG, et al. Neural anatomy of the glenohumeral ligaments, labrum, and subacromial bursa. *Arthroscopy* 1995;11:180–184.

134. Jerosch J, Clahsen H, Grosse-Hackman A, et al. Effects of proprioceptive fibers in the capsule tissue in stabilizing the glenohumeral joint. *Orthop Trans* 1992;16:773.

135. Guanche C, Knatt T, Solomonow M, et al. The synergistic action of the capsule and the shoulder muscles. *Am J Sports Med* 1995;23:301–311.

136. Lephart SM, Warner JJP, Borsa PA, et al. Proprioception of the shoulder in healthy, unstable and surgically repaired shoulders. *J Shoulder Elbow Surg* 1994;3:371–380.

137. Blasier RB, Carpenter JE, Huston LJ. Shoulder proprioception. Effect of joint laxity, joint position, and direction of motion. *Orthop Rev* 1994;23:45–50.

138. Jerosch J, Castro WH, Halm H, et al. Does the glenohumeral joint capsule have proprioceptive capability? *Knee Surg Sports Traumatol Arthrosc* 1993;1:80–84.

139. Carpenter JE, Blasier RB, Pellizzon GG. The effect of muscle fatigue on shoulder proprioception. *Trans Orthop Res Soc* 1993;18:3111.

140. Rodosky MW, Harner CD, Fu FH. The role of the long head of the biceps muscle and superior glenoid labrum in anterior stability of the shoulder. *Am J Sports Med* 1994;22:121–130.

141. Kibler WB. Role of the scapula in the overhead throwing motion. *Contemp Orthop* 1991;22:525–532.

142. Ozaki J. Glenohumeral movements of the involuntary inferior and multidirectional instability. *Clin Orthop* 1989;238:107–111.

143. Leffert RD, Gumley G. The relationship between dead arm syndrome and thoracic outlet syndrome. *Clin Orthop* 1987;223:20–31.

144. Fiddian NJ, King RJ. The winged scapula. *Clin Orthop* 1984;185:228–236.

145. Steinmann SP, Higgins DL, Sewell D, et al. Nonparalytic winging of the scapula (poster exhibit). Presented at the 61st Annual Meeting of the American Academy of Orthopaedic Surgeons, New Orleans, February 25, 1994.

146. Dillman CJ, Fleisig GS, Andrews JR. Mechanics of throwing. In: Hawkins RJ, Misamore GW, eds. *Shoulder injuries in the athlete. Surgical repair and rehabilitation.* New York: Churchill Livingstone, 1996:23–30.

147. Fleisig GS, Andrews JR, Dillman CJ, et al. Kinetics of baseball pitching with implications about injury mechanisms. *Am J Sports Med* 1995;23:233–239.

148. Andrews JR, Angelo RL. Shoulder arthroscopy for the throwing athlete. *Tech Orthop* 1988;3:75–81.

149. McLeod WD, Andrews JR. Mechanism of shoulder injuries. *Phys Ther* 1986;66:1901–1904.

150. Andrews JR, Kupferman SP, Dillman CJ. Labral tears in throwing and racquet sports. *Clin Sports Med* 1991;10:901–911.

151. Andrews JR, Carson WG, McLeod WD. Glenoid labrum tears related to the long head of the biceps. *Am J Sports Med* 1985;13:337–341.

152. Brown LP, Niehues SL, Harrah A, et al. Upper extremity range of motion and isokinetic strength of internal and external shoulder rotators in major league baseball players. *Am J Sports Med* 1988;16:577–585.

153. Bigliani LU, Codd TP, Connor PM, et al. Shoulder motion and laxity in the professional baseball player. *Am J Sports Med* 1997;25:609–613.

154. Warner JJP, Micheli LJ, Arslanian LE, et al. Patterns of flexibility, laxity, and strength in normal shoulders and shoulders with instability and impingement. *Am J Sports Med* 1990;18:366–375.

155. Kuhn JE, Bey MJ, Huston LJ, et al. The coracohumeral ligament and glenohumeral ligaments as restraints to external rotation: implications in the throwing athlete. 65th Annual Meeting of the American Association of Orthopaedic Surgeons, New Orleans, LA, 1997.

156. Pink M, Perry J, Browne A, et al. The normal shoulder during freestyle swimming. An electromyographic and cinematographic analysis of twelve muscles. *Am J Sports Med* 1991;19:569–576.

157. Pink MM, Perry J. Biomechanics. In: Jobe FW, ed. *Operative techniques in upper extremity sports injuries.* St. Louis: Mosby-Year Book, 1996:110–123.

158. Maglischo EW. *Swimming faster.* Mountain View, CA: Mayfield Publishing, 1982.

159. Richardson AB. The biomechanics of swimming: the shoulder and knee. *Clin Sports Med* 1986;5:103.

160. Scovazzo ML, Browne A, Pink M, et al. The painful shoulder during freestyle swimming. An electromyographic cinematographic analysis of twelve muscles. *Am J Sports Med* 1991;19:577–582.

161. Scovazzo ML, Brown A, Pink M, et al. The painful shoulder during freestyle swimming: an EMG and cinematographic analysis of twelve muscles. *Am J Sports Med* 1991;19:577–582.

162. Ruwe PA, Pink M, Jobe FW, et al. The normal and painful shoulder during breast stroke: an EMG and cinematographic analysis of 12 muscles. *Am J Sports Med* 1994;22:789–796.

163. Ryu RKN, McCormick J, Jobe FW, et al. An electromyographic analysis of shoulder function in tennis players. *Am J Sports Med* 1988;16:481–485.

164. Tibone J, Patek R, Jobe FW, et al. Functional anatomy, biomechanics, and kinesiology. In: DeLee JC, Drez D, eds. *Orthopaedic sports medicine. Principles and practice.* Philadelphia: W.B. Saunders, 1994:463–480.

165. Field LD, Altchek DW. Tennis injuries. In: Hawkins RJ, Misamore GW, eds. *Shoulder injuries in the athlete, surgical repair and rehabilitation.* New York: Churchill Livingstone, 1996:403–416.

166. Jobe FW, Moynes DR, Antonelli DJ. Rotator cuff function during a golf swing. *Am J Sports Med* 1986;14:388–392.

167. Jobe FW, Perry J, Pink M. Electromyographic shoulder activity in men and women professional golfers. *Am J Sports Med* 1989;17:782–787.

168. Cochran A, Stobbs J. *The search for the perfect swing.* Philadelphia: J.B. Lippincott, 1968.

169. Mallon WJ. Golf. In: Hawkins RJ, Misamore GW, eds. *Shoulder injuries in the athlete, surgical repair and rehabilitation.* New York: Churchill Livingstone, 1996:427–433.

170. Pink M, Jobe FW, Perry J. Electromyographic analysis of the shoulder during the golf swing. *Am J Sports Med* 1990;18:137–140.

Principles and Practice of Orthopaedic Sports Medicine,
edited by William E. Garrett, Jr., Kevin P. Speer, and Donald T. Kirkendall.
Lippincott Williams & Wilkins, Philadelphia © 2000.

CHAPTER 22

Anterior Shoulder Instability

Daniel J. Stechschulte, Jr., and Russell F. Warren

The shoulder is perhaps the most minimally constrained articulation in the body, depending on a delicate balance of stability and mobility to function effectively. Anterior glenohumeral instability is a spectrum of pathology ranging from apprehension and subluxation to frank dislocation. It is a relative term denoting "excessive" translation of the humeral head on the glenoid or the inability to maintain the humeral head centered in the glenoid. It has distinct and disparate implications in recreational, competitive, elite, and elite throwing athletes and can result from a single traumatic event or as a consequence of repetitive stress in lax individuals. Several reviews are available (1–10). Among the more commonly encountered orthopedic conditions, it can be seen at any age with age group-associated morbidity, recurrence risk, and treatment options. Many of the classic descriptions of glenohumeral anatomy and mechanisms of dislocation remain valid but have been further refined. Given the frequency of the condition, it is imperative that the orthopedic physician have a full understanding of the pathoanatomy, appropriate clinical evaluation and imaging modalities, nonoperative and operative treatments, and outcomes.

EPIDEMIOLOGY

The glenohumeral joint is the most commonly dislocated major joint. Simonet et al. (11) reported the incidence of initial traumatic anterior shoulder dislocation over a 10-year period in Olmsted County, Minnesota to be 8.2 per 100,000 person-years. Extrapolated to the

population of the United States in 1980, the authors projected 19,000 first-time traumatic anterior dislocations and greater than 25,000 total anterior dislocations, when recurrences were included. Hovelius estimated the incidence of traumatic anterior dislocations in the adult (aged 18 to 70 years) Swedish population to be 1.7% (12) and found an 8% incidence in elite ice hockey players (13). Of the 2,324 dislocations reported from the Central Outpatient Department of the Injured in Budapest from 1962 to 1964, 44.9% involved the shoulder (14). In the series of 500 shoulder dislocations reported by Rowe (15), 98% were anterior glenohumeral and only 2% were posterior.

Although frank anterior dislocation of the shoulder represents an extreme of instability that is more easily recognized, subtle instability including subluxation may be just as debilitating and more difficult to identify and manage. As such, the true incidence of anterior instability is actually unknown and certainly greater than dislocations alone.

MECHANISMS OF STABILITY

The glenohumeral joint has little intrinsic bony stability, with only 25% to 30% of the humeral head in contact with the glenoid in any one position (16–18), despite nearly congruent mating surfaces (19,20). Nonetheless, the shoulder is able to accommodate a wide range of multiplanar motions and forces with the help of a well-developed system of both passive and active soft tissue restraints (21). If intact and appropriately tensioned, this system renders the seemingly unstable glenohumeral articulation capable of limiting the excursion of the humeral head on the glenoid to less than 1.5 mm in the superoinferior plane for each 30 degrees of active motion (22). In the horizontal plane, the humeral head remains centered in all but the extremes of motion (23). With passive motions, however, significantly more translation has been shown to occur, including coupled ante-

D. J. Stechschulte, Jr.: The Kansas City Orthopaedic Institute, Leawood, Kansas 66211.

R. F. Warren: The Hospital for Special Surgery—New York Presbyterian Hospital, Weill Medical College of Cornell University, New York, New York 10021.

rior and posterior translations of the humerus on the glenoid with humeral flexion and extension, respectively (24).

Although the stability of the shoulder is certainly dependent on the area, shape, and inclination of the glenohumeral articulation and its relatively constant relationships of 30 degrees of humeral head retroversion with respect to the humeral condyles, 35 to 40 degrees of scapular anteversion relative to the coronal plane, and 7 degrees of glenoid retroversion relative to the scapular plane (25), osseous abnormalities of the glenoid or humeral head are probably rare causes of instability. In this light, Cyprien et al. (26) compared specific radiographic indices of the shoulder joint in groups of normals and recurrent anterior dislocators. They could demonstrate no significant differences in humeral retrotorsion, glenoid inclination, dimension of the glenoid, or glenoid version. However, significantly decreased glenoid diameters and contact indexes were noted when the affected and unaffected sides in unilateral recurrent dislocators were compared. A later computed tomography (CT) study using glenohumeral osteometry found no significant developmental differences in glenohumeral index, glenoid anteroposterior orientation, or humeral retrotorsion in groups of normals and recurrent anterior dislocators (27), suggesting that the side to side differences noted by the Cyprien group might be an effect and not a cause of instability.

Other passive contributors to glenohumeral joint stability include adhesion, limited joint volume, negative intraarticular pressure, the labrum, and the capsuloligamentous complex. The shoulder joint normally contains less than 1 mL of synovial fluid that forms an "adhesive seal" between the articulating surfaces (28). This seal resists distraction of the cartilaginous surfaces while allowing motion between them (29). Studies by Habermeyer et al. (30) indicate that the labrum is probably an important contributor to this effect. With an intact capsule, the joint is both closed and slightly negatively pressurized (31), resulting in significant advantages for stability. Matsen et al. (1,32) likened the relationship of the humeral head and the glenoid within a closed capsular space to a capped syringe in which attempted distraction of the plunger is resisted by an increased negative pressure within the system.

Kumar and Balasubramaniam (33) interestingly demonstrated the effect of negative intraarticular pressure in 24 cadaveric shoulders by mounting the scapula in a frame with the humerus free and monitoring for inferior translation of the humerus. No subluxation was noted until the capsule was punctured with a needle. Even in the absence of the rotator cuff musculature, the isolated intact capsule prevented any measurable subluxation until the capsule was vented, and the authors reported an audible "hissing" as the pressures equalized. Using a similar model with a standardized neutral position, Warner et al. (34) noted some inferior translation in both the intact and the vented shoulder. This effect was most significant at lower levels of abduction. Gibb et al. (35) further demonstrated that venting the capsule with an 18-gauge needle reduced the force necessary to translate the humerus anteriorly on the glenoid by an average of 15.3 N or 55%.

The glenoid labrum is a fibrous ring attached to the glenoid that serves to augment its effective depth, anchor the long head of the biceps, and serve as a transition between the glenohumeral ligaments and the glenoid. It is most firmly affixed inferiorly and can have a looser more "meniscal" attachment superiorly (36). Mobility of the labrum below the transverse equator is considered abnormal. Increasing the depth of the glenoid, the labrum also increases the force necessary to translate the humeral head off of the glenoid, serving as a "chock block" (37). Lazarus et al. (38) measured the effect of an anteroinferior chondral-labral defect on the "stability ratio" (the maximum dislocating force that can be resisted in a specific direction divided by the medially directed force compressing the head into the glenoid) for translation of the humeral head on the glenoid in the direction of the defect and found a reduction of 65%. Pagnani et al. (39) also showed no alteration in glenohumeral stability with an isolated superior labral lesion in a cadaveric model unless the insertion of the long head of the biceps was violated. As described above, the labrum probably also contributes to shoulder stability by augmenting the seal of the humerus to the glenoid.

The three anterior glenohumeral ligaments and their role in anterior instability have been the focus of much investigation. Initially identified as discrete and consistently recognizable condensations of the capsule by Flood (40) and Schlemm (41), they have been designated the superior, middle, and inferior glenohumeral ligaments (SGHL, MGHL, and IGHL, respectively). The SGHL originates at the anterosuperior margin of the glenoid and labrum and extends laterally to the most proximal aspect of the lesser tuberosity (1). The MGHL arises adjacent to the SGHL near the supraglenoid tubercle and inserts at the base of the lesser tuberosity in close association with the subscapularis tendon. Reported to be the most variable of the glenohumeral ligaments, the MGHL was nonetheless noted to be present to some degree in all 36 cadaveric shoulders examined by Turkel et al. (42). The IGHL takes origin at the anteroinferior labrum and glenoid and inserts just inferior to the MGHL on the lesser tuberosity.

Turkel et al. further subdivided the IGHL into a superior band and an axillary pouch. The latter was again divided into an anterior and posterior region. Later investigations at the same institution by O'Brien (43,44) revisited the IGHL complex and demonstrated an anterior band, a posterior band, and the interposed axillary pouch. This work combined with the observations of Ovesen and Nielsen (46), Bowen and Warren (47), O'Connell et al. (48), and Curl and Warren (49) helped to define the role of the glenohumeral ligaments in resisting specific shoulder movements. Many of these authors emphasized that capsuloligamentous structures are usually the last barrier to dislocation/instability, coming under tension only at the extremes of motion after other stabilizing structures have been defeated. In the midrange of joint motion, they are generally lax.

Based on these studies, it is apparent that the anterior band of the IGHL is the primary restraint to anterior translation of the humerus on the glenoid, particularly in the abducted externally rotated position. In addition, it limits external rotation when the arm is between 45 and 90 degrees of abduction and does play a role as an inferior stabilizer. The MGHL also contributes to a limitation of external rotation at 45 degrees of abduction and may provide a secondary restraint to anterior dislocation. Although the SGHL appears to be lax in abduction, it does play a significant role in the adducted shoulder by limiting inferior and to a lesser degree anterior translation.

Active mechanisms of glenohumeral stability are significant and include the rotator cuff muscles and the biceps. These structures compress the humeral head into the glenoid (37,50,51), effectively increasing the force necessary to dislocate (2). The rotator cuff musculature may also alter the tension of the glenohumeral ligaments and balance the humeral head on the glenoid by subtle changes in glenohumeral motion. Both the long and short heads of the biceps muscle also play a role in limiting anterior translation, particularly when the arm is abducted and externally rotated (52). Interestingly, this contribution is more significant in the presence of a Bankart lesion or some underlying instability. In further studies on the rotator cuff and biceps, these investigators also noted that the subscapularis muscle played the least significant role in anterior stability in the intact shoulder (53). In addition, the relative importance of the biceps muscle superseded that of the rotator cuff as the integrity of the capsuloligamentous structures decreased.

PATHOANATOMY

The anatomic basis for recurrent anterior instability remains a matter of some discussion. Bankart (54) proposed that the "essential lesion" was the detachment of the capsule from the anterior glenoid and labrum, and his name became associated with a surgical technique to address this defect (55). Earlier authors also recognized the significance of the problem and the efficacy of operative repair (56). Capsular deficiency or deformation

(42,57,58), subscapularis tendon injury (59–61), avulsion of the humeral IGHL insertion (62,63), and posterolateral impression fractures of the humeral head (the so-called Hill-Sachs lesion) (64,65) have also been proposed as contributors to recurrent anterior instability. Because there is some variability in the attachment of the capsule to the labrum and anterior glenoid, it is not surprising that different types of Bankart lesions have been described and classified (66).

Although a Bankart-type lesion is probably a necessary component of anterior shoulder instability, its presence alone is not sufficient to significantly increase anterior glenohumeral translation and result in dislocation in cadavers. Speer et al. (67) investigated this by creating simulated Bankart defects in cadaveric shoulders and concluded that concomitant capsular injury was necessary to produce anterior glenohumeral dislocation. Bankart (55), too, noted capsular tears to be present but believed that they healed uneventfully. Bigliani et al. (68) examined the tensile properties of the IGHL complex and found an average 27% strain to failure, demonstrating that significant plastic deformation occurs in the capsule before disruption or insertion failure.

This evidence stands in contrast to three arthroscopic studies of acute, young, first-time, traumatic anterior dislocators that show a high incidence of Bankart injuries without apparent capsular pathology. Taylor and Arciero (69) reported on 63 patients with an average age of 19.6 years who underwent arthroscopy within 10 days of an initial anterior traumatic glenohumeral dislocation and found that 97% had a Bankart defect. Only one patient had a demonstrable capsular injury and 90% had a Hill-Sachs defect of the humeral head. Baker et al. (70) studied a similar group of 45 young (average age, 21.2 years) patients and found 62% to have a Bankart lesion. However, all patients with gross instability had a Bankart defect. Interestingly, just 13% of the patients in this series demonstrated capsular pathology, and all these shoulders were stable. Norlin's (71) findings were very similar to those of Taylor and Arciero with all 24 patients in his series showing arthroscopic evidence of a Bankart lesion. The explanation for the disparity between these arthroscopic and cadaveric biomechanical studies is multifactorial. Subtle capsular injury is probably difficult to identify arthroscopically. In addition, the cadaveric specimens were elderly, whereas the patients in the clinical studies were very young. Interestingly, other arthroscopic studies by Hintermann and Gachter (72,73) on patients of a broader age range with at least one and sometimes multiple anterior dislocations showed approximately 85% to have anterior glenoid labral tears and 80% to have ventral capsular insufficiency. The authors used these findings to conclude that no single lesion defines traumatic anterior shoulder instability. Given the age-related variability in the rates of redislocation (74,75) and pathologic findings associated with shoulder instability, the age differences between the experimental groups is significant.

COMPLICATIONS

Several complications can be associated with anterior glenohumeral instability and should be familiar to the physician managing these injuries. Redislocation is the most common complication overall, with age at initial dislocation being the most important prognostic factor. Most recurrences occur within 2 years after the initial traumatic dislocation. McLaughlin and Cavallaro (77) reported a series of 573 patients in which the redislocation rate was 90% for those less than 20 years of age, 60% for those between 20 and 40, and only 10% in those patients older than 40. Other studies have supported these findings (15,78,79). Although older patients have a much lower risk of redislocation, they apparently have a higher risk of associated rotator cuff injury and avulsion, particularly after the age of 40. The Neviasers (80–82) brought this association to light and pointed out that this can easily be confused with an axillary nerve palsy.

Axillary nerve injury is also a well-known complication of shoulder dislocation, with the incidence varying with the series. In 1936, Watson-Jones (83) reported a 14% incidence, whereas Brown (84) and Blom and Dahlback (85) noted a 25% and 35% incidence, respectively. Rowe's (15) 5.4% incidence appears to be at the lower end of the range. Most axillary nerve injuries after anterior dislocation are thought to be traction neuropraxias and generally recover completely. However, a poor prognosis is associated with those injuries that do not recover by 10 weeks. Pasila et al. (86) carried out a prospective study of all shoulder dislocations presenting to the University Central Hospital of Helsinki emergency department over the 3-year period from 1973 to 1976. Twenty-six percent of the 238 patients had associated complications, including 29 brachial plexus injuries, 28 rotator cuff ruptures, and 21 axillary nerve injuries. The frequency of complications increased with the age of the patients, especially those older than 50, and in those who remained dislocated for more than 12 hours. As might be expected, no complications were observed in recurrent dislocations (87). Injuries to the axillary artery including pseudoaneurysm (88), aneurysm (89), and complete disruption (90) can occur. Open dislocation has also been reported in high energy injury (91).

Overhand or throwing athletes have unique problems associated with instability. Repetitive throwing can lead to increased anterior glenohumeral translation as the anterior stabilizing structures are stretched (92). Although active stabilizing mechanisms may compensate for this instability temporarily, overuse or fatigue can result in further anterior subluxation and produce a secondary impingement termed internal impingement (93,94). This phenomenon occurs in external rotation–abduction during the late cocking/acceleration phase of throwing when the humeral head subluxates anteriorly, allowing the deep surface of the supraspinatus to impinge into the posterosuperior glenoid. Lesions of the posterosuperior labrum and concomitant undersurface tears of the supraspinatus or infraspinatus have been identified. Because asymptomatic professional baseball pitchers have significantly increased external rotation (in abduction and at the side) and decreased internal rotation (95), it is understandable that these athletes may be predisposed to this injury.

CLINICAL EVALUATION

Anterior glenohumeral instability is a spectrum of injury with presentations ranging from locked dislocations to shoulder pain associated with minimal subluxation. A directed but detailed history should be obtained, because it is imperative to establish the mechanism of injury, the level of trauma involved, and any prior history of instability or shoulder complaints. Patients presenting after a history of dislocation should be questioned regarding the means used to accomplish reduction. In recurrent dislocation, the age at first dislocation has important prognostic implication, as noted above.

Mechanism of injury has obvious and significant implications for management. Anterior dislocation usually results from a fall onto the abducted and externally rotated extremity or rarely from a direct posterior blow. A single traumatic event or repetitive anterior strain can also lead to symptomatic subluxation. Dislocation after a high-speed fall while skiing mandates a far different approach than dislocation after reaching overhead. Thomas and Matsen (96) proposed the acronyms TUBS and AMBRII to differentiate these two clinical extremes: TUBS refers to those patients with *t*raumatic *u*nidirectional instability associated with a *B*ankart lesion and often amenable to *s*urgical stabilization, whereas AMBRII represents *a*traumatic, *m*ultidirectional, often *b*ilateral instability that should initially be managed with *r*ehabilitation but might require surgery in the form of an *i*nferior capsular shift with closure of the rotator *i*nterval. Voluntary dislocators fall into this category and should be carefully evaluated for secondary gain issues.

Physical examination should include careful inspection, palpation, and assessment of the neurovascular status of the extremity and documentation of deltoid, supraspinatus, infraspinatus, and subscapularis strength.

Range of motion and muscular atrophy should also be noted. Signs of generalized laxity including knee and elbow hyperextension, excessive dorsiflexion of the ankle, and hyperabduction of the thumb with a volar flexed wrist may be present in some patients (97). An evaluation of shoulder stability should also include an examination of inferior, posterior, and anterior translation and the apprehension and relocation tests. Traction is applied to the shoulder in the seated position and inferior translation is then graded as 1+, 2+, or 3+ (1, 2, or more than 3 cm) by the size of the subacromial "sulcus" or the distance from the inferior margin of the lateral edge of the acromion to the humeral head. A 3+ sulcus is generally indicative of multidirectional instability, but a 2+ is commonly seen in overhead athletes, particularly on the dominant side. However, a sulcus sign can occasionally result from a traumatic event in otherwise normal individuals.

The patient is then placed in the supine position with the extremity at the edge of the examining table. With the arm held in neutral rotation in the plane of the scapula, the arm is translated anteriorly and posteriorly by the examiner's hand on the proximal humerus. Simultaneously, an axial load is applied in line with the glenohumeral joint by the examiner's other hand. This force magnifies what otherwise can be subtle translations, and we refer to this as the "axial load" or "load and shift test" (Fig. 22.1). Grading is similar to that of the sulcus sign, with 1+ indicative of increased translation compared with the opposite extremity (98). A 2+ represents spontaneously reducible subluxation to the edge of the glenoid, and a 3+ indicates dislocation (99). Anterior translation of 2+ is considered pathologic. The apprehension test is positive when the patient notes a feeling

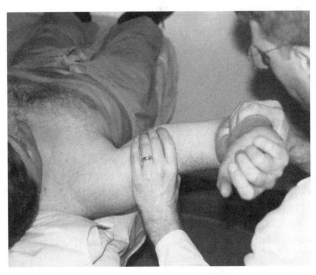

FIG. 22.2. Demonstration of the apprehension maneuver. A positive test is elicited when a feeling of impending instability is noted by the patient when the arm is brought into the abducted and externally rotated (90 degree/90 degree) position.

of impending instability as the involved extremity is brought into the 90 degree/90 degree (abduction/external rotation) position (Fig. 22.2). Significant apprehension or a combination of apprehension and pain is diagnostic of anterior instability.

The relocation test is thought to be helpful in differentiating primary impingement from secondary

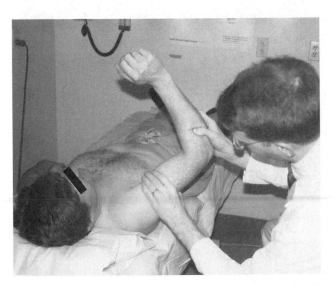

FIG. 22.1. Demonstration of the axial load or load and shift test for assessment of anterior and posterior capsular stability.

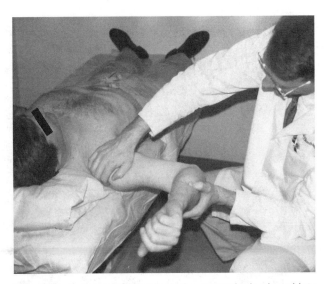

FIG. 22.3. In the relocation test, the extremity is placed into the 90 degree/90 degree position and a posterior force is applied to the anterior proximal humerus. Patients with primary impingement have no change in the character of their pain, whereas those with secondary impingement are said to note decreased pain as the humeral head is reduced.

impingement resulting from anterior instability (92, 100,101). Both present with pain in the 90 degree/ 90 degree (apprehension) position. To carry out the relocation test, the extremity is placed into the 90 degree/90 degree position and a posterior force is applied to the anterior proximal humerus (Fig. 22.3). Patients with primary impingement have no change in the character of their pain, whereas those with secondary impingement are said to note decreased pain as the humeral head is reduced. The sensitivity, specificity, and predictive value of this test have been evaluated. The relocation test failed to distinguish between patients with anterior instability and those with cuff disease when the sensation of pain alone was considered (102).

IMAGING

The radiographic features of shoulder instability have been well documented and include the Hill-Sachs lesion of the posterolateral humereal head (64) and bony abnormalities of the glenoid rim (Fig. 22.4) (103,104). Plain films should be obtained in all cases of suspected or documented anterior instability. Fractures, loose bodies, alignment, degenerative change, and calcification can be identified using a minimum of two orthogonal views. Most commonly, anteroposterior views of the glenohumeral joint with both internal and external rotation of the humerus and an axillary view (105) are sufficient. An anteroposterior view in the plane of the scapula (Grashey view) and modified axillary views such as the

West Point view (106) and the Stryker notch view (107) are preferred by some.

In patients with recurrent instability, we prefer an anteroposterior in the plane of the scapula with the humerus internally rotated, a West Point view, and the Stryker notch view. In those with acute dislocations, we obtain a shoulder trauma series. The combination of an anteroposterior view in internal rotation and a Stryker notch view have been shown to have a diagnostic yield of 92% in detecting Hill-Sachs lesions, whereas an anteroposterior view in external rotation gave only a 32% yield (103).

Other imaging modalities have been proposed as adjuncts to plain radiography in the management of anterior instability, including ultrasound (108–111), CT (112), and CT arthrography, and magnetic resonance imaging (MRI). Given the ready availability of high quality MRI at our institutions, we no longer use the other modalities in the evaluation of anterior instability. MRI provides a wealth of information regarding the state of the rotator cuff, capsuloligamentous complex, bony architecture, and the articular cartilage in a multiplanar and noninvasive fashion (Figs. 22.5 and 22.6).

MRI is more sensitive than plain radiography in detecting the early degenerative changes of osteoarthritis, has an overall accuracy exceeding 90% in the diagnosis of labral tears (113), and is accurate in assessing rotator cuff pathology (114,115). It is 100% sensitive and 95% specific for anterior labral pathology in some hands (116). Others, however, have reported a poor correla-

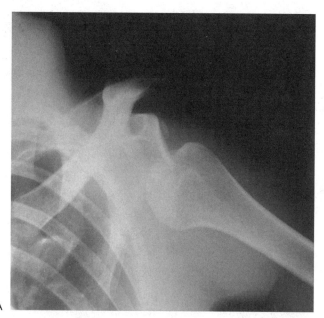

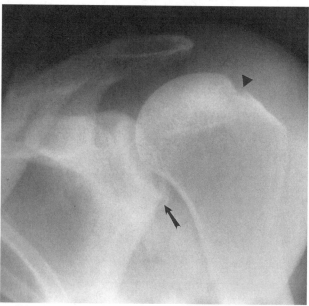

A

B

FIG. 22.4. Plain radiographs demonstrate an anterior glenohumeral dislocation before (**A**) and after (**B**) reduction. Postreduction anteroposterior (**B**) demonstrates a Hill-Sachs lesion of the posterolateral humeral head (*arrowhead*) and a typical "bony Bankart" fracture of the anteroinferior glenoid rim (*arrow*).

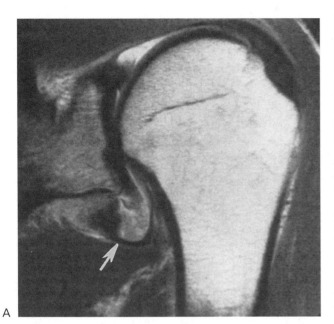 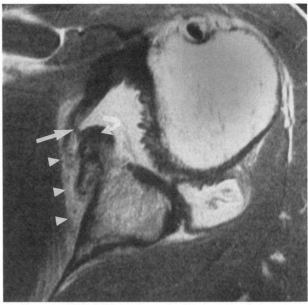

FIG. 22.5. A: Oblique coronal fast spin echo magnetic resonance (MR) image demonstrates distended axillary pouch (*arrow*), containing dependent debris, reflecting hemarthrosis. **B:** Axial fast spin echo MR image demonstrates detached anteroinferior labral fragment (*curved arrow*) that is tethered by the anterior band (*straight arrow*). Also note the presence of a true bony Bankart lesion and stripping of the anterior capsule (*arrowheads*). (MR images courtesy of Hollis G. Potter, M.D.)

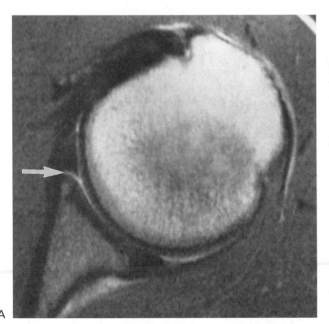 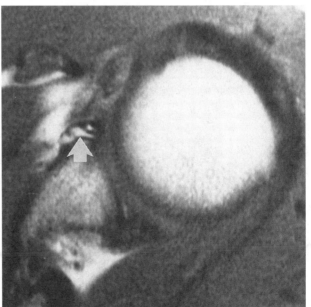

FIG. 22.6. A: Axial fast spin echo sequence demonstrates a split (*arrow*) through the midanterior labrum, centered at the equator. **B:** Axial fast spin echo MR image obtained at a more cephalad level demonstrates a ganglion cyst arising from an anterosuperior labral tear (*arrow*). (MR images courtesy of Hollis G. Potter, M.D.)

tion between MRI, histology, and gross inspection of labral injury in a cadaveric study (117).

TREATMENT

Acute anterior glenohumeral dislocations should be reduced gently but expediently using an approach familiar to the physician. Maximal muscle relaxation facilitated by intravenous administration of analgesics and a benzodiazepine is generally required. The modified Hippocratic method uses traction–countertraction and requires two individuals (Fig. 22.7). The patient lies supine with a sheet around the chest, under the involved extremity, and around the waist of an assistant on the opposite side of the table. The surgeon stands at the waist of the patient on the side of the dislocated extremity. A second sheet is passed around the waist of the surgeon and over the forearm of the dislocated extremity. With the elbow held flexed at 90 degrees, the surgeon can provide longitudinal traction through the sheet while gently rotating the humerus internally and externally. Numerous other methods of reduction have been described, including the popular method of Stimson (118) and the technique of scapular manipulation (119). Repeat radiographs and neurovascular examination should be carried out after reduction. Aspiration of hemarthrosis has been shown to relieve discomfort and can be considered, especially in older individuals (120).

Management of anterior dislocation is largely dependent on the age, occupation, and preferences of the patient. All patients should be counseled regarding their relative risk of recurrence. As noted above, most patients older than 40 will require no additional treatment except rehabilitation. Younger individuals, particularly those less than 25 years of age, have a significant risk of redislocation and may wish to consider surgery. Athletes and those whose occupations demand shoulder stability may also prefer early operative intervention.

Nonoperative Management

A short period of sling immobilization is probably appropriate after reduction of an anterior glenohumeral dislocation. Although capsular and subscapularis tendon injuries require 3 and 5 months, respectively, to heal in a primate model (76), most clinical evidence suggests that length and manner of immobilization does not have a significant impact on the rate of recurrence. McLaughlin and Cavallaro (77) found duration of immobilization after initial dislocation to be of little significance in their series of 573 dislocations. Hovelius et al. (121) prospectively compared 3 to 4 weeks of immobilization with no immobilization at all and found no difference in recurrence rate at 2-year follow-up in over 200 patients. In contrast, other investigators have reported a decreased rate of recurrence in patients immobilized for longer than 3 weeks (122).

Rehabilitation of the unstable shoulder should commence with pendulum exercises and progress to an active strengthening program for the rotator cuff, deltoid, and biceps. In patients with increased capsular laxity, these active stabilizers are of even more importance. Aronen and Regan (123) demonstrated a decreased incidence of recurrent dislocations in 20 U.S. Naval Academy midshipmen when a strengthening program was used. These authors also rigidly restricted activity until rehabilitation goals were achieved. Younger patients (less than 25 years) should generally be immobilized for 3 to 4 weeks before aggressive rehabilitation is initiated. This is less critical in older individuals who are less likely to experience a recurrence and probably more prone to lose motion as a consequence of prolonged immobilization.

In throwers and others likely to experience secondary impingement as a result of more subtle anterior instability, it is also important to strengthen the scapular stabilizers (serratus anterior, rhomboids, levator scapulae, trapezius, and pectoralis minor) and the latissimus dorsi. Anterolateral positioning of the scapula resulting from weakness or imbalance of these muscles can stress the anterior capsular structures, disrupt the normal length–tension relationships of the glenohumeral musculature, and contribute to anterior subluxation (25,124,125). Moseley et al. (126) described a core group of four exercises, including rowing, scaption (elevation of the arm in the scapular plane), push-ups with protraction, and press-ups, to address this.

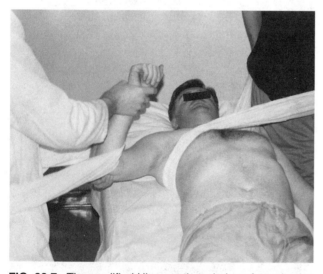

FIG. 22.7. The modified Hippocratic technique for reduction of anterior glenohumeral dislocation requires an assistant and two sheets. Gentle traction is applied to the affected extremity with one sheet as the humerus is rotated internally and externally.

Operative Management

Surgical stabilization of the glenohumeral joint is considered in patients with recurrent symptomatic instability refractory to a supervised rehabilitation program. Patients who require stability for occupational reasons or who are at very high risk for recurrence based on age at initial dislocation are also candidates. Numerous surgical procedures have been described (1) for the treatment of recurrent anterior glenohumeral instability, including the Magnuson-Stack (127), the Putti-Platt (128), the Bristow (129), the DuToit capsulorrhaphy (130), and the Bankart repair (55).

The Bankart and its modifications are anatomic reconstructions of the damaged capsulolabral structures, whereas other procedures rely on limitation of external rotation (Magnuson-Stack, Putti-Platt), interposition of a bony block (Bristow), or alteration of bony alignment by osteotomy. Although these were initially thought to be reasonable compromises to achieve stability, it has become increasingly clear that they can result in significant functional disability and can be particularly unsatisfactory for overhead athletes. Surgical limitation of external rotation is nonphysiologic at best and may lead to premature osteoarthritis at worst (131,132). Regan et al. (133) reported that half of all throwing athletes treated with a Putti-Platt procedure could not return to throwing and the other 50% significantly altered their throwing motions. Similarly, poor results were seen in throwers treated with a Magnuson-Stack procedure. Although the Bristow procedure has an acceptably low redislocation rate, most athletes cannot return to high level overhead sports. In addition, this procedure and the staple capsulorrhaphy of DuToit use hardware near the glenoid surface, which can been associated with complication (134,135) and postoperative pain (136).

The Bankart repair and its modifications remain the standard for successful open anterior stabilization, with 97% good to excellent results at 5 years in some series and a redislocation rate of 3.5% (137). A recent report has also demonstrated this procedure to offer an excellent objective long-term outcome with great patient satisfaction (138). Nonetheless, at a mean follow-up of 11.9 tears in this study, the average loss of external rotation was 12 degrees. This can be disabling for athletes, with only 33% returning to their preoperative level of competition (137) and only 50% of baseball pitchers returning to pitching (139). As should be clear from these discussions, it is relatively easy to prevent recurrent anterior dislocation but much more difficult to do so without significantly limiting function, especially in athletes.

In an effort to minimize the morbidity associated with open anterior stabilization, arthroscopic approaches have been used with variable results. A recent algorithm for arthroscopic anterior stabilization has been proposed (140). Two general techniques have evolved: suture repairs and labral tacks. Both show a recurrence rate in the range of 20%. Manta et al. (141) recently reported their 5-year results of arthroscopic transglenoid suture repairs and found only 40% of their patients to be free of instability at this extended follow-up, leading the authors to reconsider recommendation of the technique. In another recent 2- to 8-year follow-up study of the arthroscopic transglenoid suture repair, Torchia et al. (142) reported a 16.6% overall failure rate with particularly poor results in patients with a Bankart lesion and those younger than 25. The 5-year failure rate for those patients with pure capsular lesions (normal labrum and no Bankart lesion) was only 6%.

Arthroscopic stabilization with a cannulated absorbable device has also become popular but does best in patients with Bankart lesions and minimal capsular pathology (143–145). Arciero et al. (146) showed a significant decrease in the rate of recurrence of anterior instability in a prospective study comparing this technique to nonoperative management in a group of West Point cadets. As is apparent, patient selection is fundamental to success with these techniques. Contraindications to arthroscopic Bankart repair include multidirectional and volitional instability, significant capsular laxity or injury, and the absence of a true Bankart lesion. Contraindications to transglenoid suture repair include age less than 25 and the presence of anything other than a capsular injury.

Authors' Preferred Approach

Our preferred approach to recurrent traumatic anterior instability incorporates a careful examination under anesthesia followed by diagnostic arthroscopy. Even in those cases in which arthroscopic stabilization is unlikely to be indicated, diagnostic arthroscopy often supplements our understanding of the instability pattern. In those patients with a history of an acute traumatic event and arthroscopic evidence of an isolated Bankart lesion and good quality tissue, we carry out arthroscopic stabilization with a bioabsorbable tack (143). If the capsule is minimally damaged in addition to the Bankart lesion, directed capsular shrinkage with an arthroscopic radiofrequency heating device may be attempted. Although this obviates the need for an open procedure, the long-term results of this technique remain unknown.

Those patients who are not candidates for arthroscopic stabilization or who are unwilling to accept the associated increased recurrence risk (especially contact athletes) undergo open stabilization (Fig. 22.8). At our institutions, interscalene block anesthesia is used routinely. The patient is positioned supine in the modified beach chair position with the head of the bed inclined

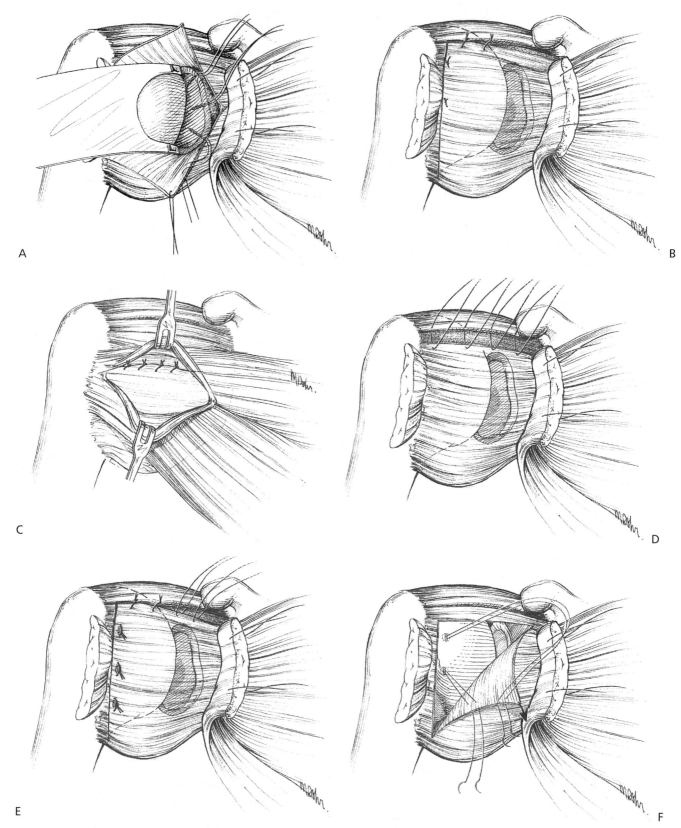

FIG. 22.8. Algorithm for approaches to anterior glenohumeral instability with selective capsular procedures. **A:** In the presence of a true Bankart lesion, lateral subscapularis tenotomy is carried out with a medial longitudinal capsulotomy. Suture anchors are placed medially along the glenoid rim. **B:** Dislocation or symptomatic subluxation without a Bankart lesion is managed operatively with a laterally based capsular shift. **C:** Symptomatic instability in throwers or overhead athletes is approached with a subscapularis split and a transverse capsulotomy. Suture anchors can then be placed medially or laterally depending on the presence of a Bankart lesion. **D:** Closure of a large rotator interval defect is the first step in the surgical management of multidirectional instability. **E:** If insufficient, this is supplemented with a laterally based capsular shift. **F:** In the presence of symptomatic instability with a large rotator interval defect and no multidirectional instability, the rotator interval is used as the transverse limb of a lateral capsular shift.

30 degrees and the operative extremity abducted approximately 45 degrees on an arm board (147). A deltopectoral approach is carried out via an incision in line with the anterior axillary fold (148). The cephalic vein is retracted laterally with the deltoid; the coracoid and clavipectoral fascia are identified. The fascia is opened lateral to the conjoined tendon, and this is extended superiorly to the coracoacromial ligament. As the conjoined tendon is gently retracted medially and the deltoid taken laterally, the subscapularis muscle is identified as the humerus is rotated back and forth. Either of two options for subscapularis take-down can be used: a subscapularis split or the more common lateral tenotomy.

A subscapularis splitting approach is used in throwers and overhead athletes to minimize the loss of external rotation. In this approach, the capsule is exposed through a transverse split in the muscle fibers. However, limited access to the superior and lateral aspects of the capsule, including the rotator interval, can be problematic. In addition, Bankart repair and capsular shift are probably more difficult with this exposure.

The more traditional lateral subscapularis tenotomy affords greater visualization and is probably appropriate for most patients. Care is taken to perform a tenotomy of the upper two thirds of the subscapularis, leaving robust tendon both medially and laterally for later anatomic repair. To avoid entering the underlying capsule, a medially angled oblique cut is used. The interval between the anterior capsule and the posterior aspect of the subscapularis is then developed.

The superolateral capsule is carefully inspected for a rotator interval defect (149). If this opening is large and extends medially to the coracoid, it should be closed with interrupted nonabsorbable sutures to tension the inferior capsule and axillary recess. In some individuals with less than gross instability, this maneuver may be sufficient to eliminate excess translation.

Once the anterior capsule has been fully exposed, a transverse incision is made above the level of the IGHL and the joint inspected. A large rotator interval defect, if present, may be used alternatively as the transverse arm of the capsulotomy. A determination is then made regarding placement of a medial or a lateral longitudinal limb. If a Bankart-type lesion is present, the transverse capsular split is extended medially onto the glenoid so that capsulolabral repair can be carried out. A longitudinal "T" off this transverse split is then made. Inferior and superior flaps are raised along the glenoid neck so that plication can be performed on the glenoid side of the joint. (If the rotator interval is used as the transverse limb, a superior flap is generally unnecessary.) The glenoid neck is prepared with a burr or sharp curettes, and suture anchors are then placed at the junction of the glenoid neck and articular surface. The capsule is then tensioned from inferior to superior with

the arm in 50 degrees abduction, 45 degrees external rotation, and neutral flexion–extension. The stability is then rechecked to ensure that the preoperative goals have been achieved. The subscapularis is repaired anatomically.

In the absence of a Bankart lesion, the transverse split in the capsule is carried laterally rather than medially. Capsular flaps are raised about the humeral neck off of a lateral T, and dissection is directed inferiorly as needed to address capsular redundancy in the axillary recess. Usually, this requires elevation of the capsule to at least the 5 o'clock position. The humeral neck is prepared similarly to the glenoid neck in a medial repair, and suture anchors are placed on the humeral side of the joint for lateral capsular tensioning in the arm position noted above. Patients with multidirectional instability, although not the focus of this chapter, also undergo a medial longitudinal capsulotomy with a modified capsular shift (99) (Fig. 22.8).

REHABILITATION

Postoperative rehabilitation begins on the first day after surgery with pendulum exercises and isometrics. The subcuticular stitch is removed at approximately 1 week postoperatively, and active assisted forward elevation and external rotation to 90 and 0 degrees, respectively, is begun. At 4 weeks the sling is discontinued, and a gradual increase in forward elevation and external rotation is initiated. Strengthening exercises using rubber tubing are also instituted at this time. Throwing athletes should achieve the "90/90" position (90 degrees of abduction and 90 degrees of external rotation) by 6 weeks after surgery, whereas nonthrowers are encouraged to reach full forward elevation by 8 to 10 weeks postoperatively. Light weight training is instituted at 6 to 8 weeks, beginning with elbow flexion exercises (curls). Bench pressing begins at 8 to 10 weeks, but military or overhead pressing is avoided at all times.

Patients with multidirectional instability are managed with a similar but more conservative protocol. Immobilization in a sling after surgery is maintained for 6 weeks, when strengthening of the rotator cuff and scapular stabilizers begins. Bench pressing is allowed at 12 weeks, but military pressing and dependent weight-lifting exercises (upright rowing, shrugs, deadlifts) are avoided permanently.

Athletes are allowed to return to full sporting activities on an individual and sport-specific basis. Contact athletes may return at 4 months, if strength equal to the nonoperated extremity is achieved. The contact athlete with multidirectional instability should be held out until at least 6 months postoperatively. Throwers generally begin a "toss program" at 3 to 4 months and gradually progress to full throwing by 5 months.

REFERENCES

1. Matsen FA, Thomas SC, Rockwood CA Jr. Glenohumeral instability. In: Rockwood CA Jr, Matsen FA, eds. *The shoulder.* Philadelphia: W.B. Saunders, 1990:526–622.
2. Matsen FA, Harryman DT, Sidles JA. Mechanics of glenohumeral instability. *Clin Sports Med* 1991;10:783–788.
3. Hawkins RJ, Mohtadi NG. Controversy in anterior shoulder instability. *Clin Orthop* 1991;272:152–161.
4. Allen AA, Warner JJ. Shoulder instability in the athlete. *Orthop Clin North Am* 1995;26:487–504.
5. Cofield RH, Kavanagh BF, Frassica FJ. Anterior shoulder instability. *Instr Course Lect* 1985;34:210–227.
6. Collins HR, Wilde AH. Shoulder instability in athletics. *Orthop Clin North Am* 1973;4:759–774.
7. Liu SH, Henry MH. Anterior shoulder instability. Current review. *Clin Orthop* 1996;323:327–337.
8. O'Brien SJ, Warren RF, Schwartz E. Anterior shoulder instability. *Orthop Clin North Am* 1987;18:395–408.
9. Pagnani MJ, Warren RF. The pathophysiology of anterior shoulder instability. *Sports Med Arthrosc Rev* 1993;1:177–189.
10. Speer KP. Anatomy and pathomechanics of shoulder instability. *Clin Sports Med* 1995;14:751–160.
11. Simonet WT, Melton LJ, Cofield RH. Incidence of anterior shoulder dislocation in Olmsted County, Minnesota. *Clin Orthop* 1984;186:186–191.
12. Hovelius L. Incidence of shoulder dislocation in Sweden. *Clin Orthop* 1982;166:127–131.
13. Hovelius L. Shoulder dislocation in Swedish ice hockey players. *Am J Sports Med* 1978;6:373–377.
14. Kazssr B, Relovszky E. Prognosis of primary dislocation of the shoulder. *Acta Orthop Scand* 1969;40:216–224.
15. Rowe CR. Prognosis in dislocations of the shoulder. *J Bone Joint Surg Am* 1956;38:957–977.
16. Bost FC, Inman VT. The pathologic changes in recurrent dislocation of the shoulder. *J Bone Joint Surg Am* 1942;24:595–613.
17. Soslowsky LJ, Flatow EL, Biglian LU, et al. Quantitation of in situ contact areas at the glenohumeral joint: a biomechanical study. *J Orthop Res* 1992;10:524–534.
18. Jobe CM, Iannotti JP. Limits imposed on glenohumeral motion by joint geometry. *J Shoulder Elbow Surg* 1995;4:281–285.
19. Soslowsky LJ, Flatow EL, Biglian LU, et al. Articular geometry of the glenohumeral joint. *Clin Orthop* 1992;285:181–190.
20. Iannotti JP, Gabriel JP, Schneck SL, et al. The normal glenohumeral relationships. An anatomical study of one hundred and forty shoulders. *J Bone Joint Surg Am* 1992;74:491–500.
21. Cooper DE, O'Brien SJ, Warren RF. Supporting layers of the glenohumeral joint. An anatomic study. *Clin Orthop* 1993;289:144–155.
22. Poppen NK, Walker PS. Normal and abnormal motion of the shoulder. *J Bone Joint Surg Am* 1976;58:195–201.
23. Howell SM, Galinat BJ, Renzi AJ, et al. Normal and abnormal mechanics of the glenohumeral joint in the horizontal plane. *J Bone Joint Surg Am* 1988;70:227–232.
24. Harryman DT, Sidles JA, Clark JM, et al. Translation of the humeral head on the glenoid with passive glenohumeral motion. *J Bone Joint Surg Am* 1990;72:1334–1343.
25. Saha AK. Dynamic stability of the glenohumeral joint. *Acta Orthop Scand* 1971;42:491–505.
26. Cyprien JM, Vasey HM, Burdet A, et al. Humeral retrotorsion and glenohumeral relationship in the normal shoulder and in recurrent anterior dislocation (scapulometry). *Clin Orthop* 1983;175:8–17.
27. Randelli M, Gambrioli PL. Glenohumeral osteometry by computed tomography in normal and unstable shoulders. *Clin Orthop* 1986;208:151–156.
28. Simkin PA. The musculoskeletal system: joints. In: Schumacher HRJ, ed. *Primer on the rheumatic diseases.* Atlanta: The Arthritis Foundation, 1993:5–8.
29. Unsworth A, Dowson D, Wright V. "Cracking joints." A bioengineering study of cavitation in the metacarpophalangeal joint. *Ann Rheum Dis* 1971;30:348–358.
30. Habermeyer P, Schuller U, Wiedemann E. The intra-articular pressure of the shoulder: an experimental study on the role of

the glenoid labrum in stabilizing the joint. *Arthroscopy* 1992;8:166–172.
31. Levick JR. Joint pressure-volume studies: their importance, design and interpretation. *J Rheumatol* 1983;10:353–357.
32. Matsen FA, Lippitt SB, Sidles DT, et al. *Practical evaluation and management of the shoulder.* Philadelphia: W.B. Saunders, 1994:242.
33. Kumar V, Balasubramaniam P. The role of atmospheric pressure in stabilising the shoulder. An experimental study. *J Bone Joint Surg Br* 1985;67:719–721.
34. Warner JJP, Deng XH, Warren RF, et al. Static capsuloligamentous restraints to superior-inferior translation of the glenohumeral joint. *Am J Sports Med* 1992;20:675–685.
35. Gibb TD, Sidles JA, Harryman DT, et al. The effect of capsular venting on glenohumeral laxity. *Clin Orthop* 1991;268:120–127.
36. Cooper DE, Arnoczky SP, O'Brien SJ, et al. Anatomy, histology, and vascularity of the glenoid labrum. An anatomical study. *J Bone Joint Surg Am* 1992;74:46–52.
37. Howell SM, Galinat BJ. The glenoid-labral socket. A constrained articular surface. *Clin Orthop* 1989;243:122–125.
38. Lazarus MD, Sidles JA, Harryman DT, et al. Effect of a chondral-labral defect on glenoid concavity and glenohumeral stability. A cadaveric model. *J Bone Joint Surg Am* 1996;78:94–102.
39. Pagnani MJ, Deng XH, Warren RF, et al. Effect of lesions of the superior portion of the glenoid labrum on glenohumeral translation. *J Bone Joint Surg Am* 1995;77:1003–1010.
40. Flood V. Discovery of a new ligament of the shoulder joint. *Lancet* 1829;1:672–673.
41. Schlemm F. Über die verstärkungsbänder am schultergelenk. *Arch Anat Physiol Wissenschaft Med* 1853;22:45–48.
42. Turkel SJ, Panlo MW, Marshall JL, et al. Stabilizing mechanisms preventing anterior dislocation of the glenohumeral joint. *J Bone Joint Surg Am* 1981;63:1208–1217.
43. O'Brien SJ, Neves MC, Arnoczky SP. The anatomy and histology of the inferior glenohumeral ligament complex of the shoulder. *Am J Sports Med* 1990;18:449–456.
44. O'Brien SJ, Neves MC, Arnoczky SP, et al. Capsular restraints to anterior-posterior motion of the abducted shoulder: a biomechanical study. *J Shoulder Elbow Surg* 1995;4:298–308.
45. Ovesen J, Nielsen S. Stability of the shoulder joint. Cadaver study of stabilizing structures. *Acta Orthop Scand* 1985;56:149–151.
46. Ovesen J, Nielsen S. Anterior and posterior shoulder instability. A cadaver study. *Acta Orthop Scand* 1986;57:324–327.
47. Bowen MK, Warren RF. Ligamentous control of shoulder stability based on selective cutting and static translation experiments. *Clin Sports Med* 1991;10:757–782.
48. O'Connell PW, Nuber GW, Mileski RA, et al. The contribution of the glenohumeral ligaments to anterior stability of the shoulder joint. *Am J Sports Med* 1990;18:579–584.
49. Curl LA, Warren RF. Glenohumeral joint stability. Selective cutting studies on the static capsular restraints. *Clin Orthop* 1996;330:54–65.
50. Cain PR, Mutschler TA, Fu FH, et al. Anterior stability of the glenohumeral joint. A dynamic model. *Am J Sports Med* 1987;15:144–148.
51. Howell SM, Kraft TA. The role of the supraspinatus and infraspinatus muscles in glenohumeral kinematics of anterior should instability. *Clin Orthop* 1991;263:128–134.
52. Itoi E, Kuechle DK, Newman SR, et al. Stabilising function of the biceps in stable and unstable shoulders. *J Bone Joint Surg Br* 1993;75:546–550.
53. Itoi E, Newman SR, Kuechle DK, et al. Dynamic anterior stabilisers of the shoulder with the arm in abduction. *J Bone Joint Surg Br* 1994;76:834–836.
54. Bankart ASB. Recurrent or habitual dislocation of the shoulder joint. *BMJ* 1923;2:1132–1133.
55. Bankart ASB. The pathology and treatment of recurrent dislocation of the shoulder joint. *Br J Surg* 1938;26:23–29.
56. Perthes G. Über Operationen bei habitueller Schulterluxation. *Deutsche Zeitschr Chir* 1906;85:199–227.
57. Townley CO. The capsular mechanism in recurrent dislocation of the shoulder. *J Bone Joint Surg Am* 1950;32:370–380.
58. Moseley HF, Övergaard B. The anterior capsular mechanism in recurrent anterior dislocation of the shoulder: Morphological

and clinical studies with special reference to the glenoid labrum and the gleno-humeral ligaments. *J Bone Joint Surg Br* 1962; 44:913–927.

59. De Palma AF, Cooke AJ, Prabhakar M. The role of the subscapularis in recurrent anterior dislocations of the shoulder. *Clin Orthop* 1967;54:35–49.

60. Symeonides PP. The significance of the subscapularis muscle in the pathogenesis of recurrent anterior dislocation of the shoulder. *J Bone Joint Surg Br* 1972;54:476–483.

61. Symeonides PP. Reconsideration of the Putti-Platt procedure and its mode of action in recurrent traumatic anterior dislocation of the shoulder. *Clin Orthop* 1989;246:8–15.

62. Nicola T. Anterior dislocation of the shoulder. The role of the articular capsule. *J Bone Joint Surg [Am]* 1942;24:614–616.

63. Bach BR, Warren RF, Fronek J. Disruption of the lateral capsule of the shoulder. A cause of recurrent dislocation. *J Bone Joint Surg Br* 1988;70:274–276.

64. Hill HA, Sachs MD. The grooved defect of the humeral head. A frequently unrecognized complication of dislocations of the shoulder joint. *Radiology* 1940;35:690–700.

65. Connolly JF. Humeral head defects associated with shoulder dislocations—their diagnostic and surgical significance. *Instr Course Lect* 1972;21:42–54.

66. Rowe CR, ed. Dislocations of the shoulder. In: *The shoulder.* New York: Churchill Livingstone, 1988:165–292.

67. Speer KP, Deng XH, Borrero S, et al. Biomechanical evaluation of a simulated Bankart lesion. *J Bone Joint Surg Am* 1994;76: 1819–1826.

68. Bigliani LU, Pollock RG, Soslowsky LJ, et al. Tensile properties of the inferior glenohumeral ligament. *J Orthop Res* 1992;10: 187–197.

69. Taylor DC, Arciero RA. Pathologic changes associated with shoulder dislocations. Arthroscopic and physical examination findings in first-time, traumatic anterior dislocations. *Am J Sports Med* 1997;25:306–311.

70. Baker CL, Uribe JW, Whitman C. Arthroscopic evaluation of acute initial anterior shoulder dislocations. *Am J Sports Med* 1990;18:25–28.

71. Norlin R. Intraarticular pathology in acute, first-time anterior shoulder dislocation: an arthroscopic study. *Arthroscopy* 1993;9: 546–549.

72. Hintermann B, Gachter A. Arthroscopic assessment of the unstable shoulder. *Knee Surg Sports Traumatol Arthrosc* 1994;2:64–69.

73. Hintermann B, Gachter A. Arthroscopic findings after shoulder dislocation. *Am J Sports Med* 1995;23:545–551.

74. Simonet WT, Cofield RH. Prognosis in anterior shoulder dislocation. *Am J Sports Med* 1984;12:19–24.

75. Hovelius L. Anterior dislocation of the shoulder in teen-agers and young adults. Five-year prognosis. *J Bone Joint Surg Am* 1987;69:393–399.

76. Reeves B. Experiments on the tensile strength of the anterior capsular structures of the shoulder in man. *J Bone Joint Surg Br* 1968;50:858–865.

77. McLaughlin HL, Cavallaro WU. Primary anterior dislocation of the shoulder. *Am J Surg* 1950;80:615–621.

78. McLaughlin HL, MacLellan DI. Recurrent anterior dislocation of the shoulder. II. A comparative study. *J Trauma* 1967;7: 191–201.

79. Hovelius L, Lind B, Thorling J. Primary dislocation of the shoulder. Factors affecting the two-year prognosis. *Clin Orthop* 1983;176:181–185.

80. Neviaser RJ, Neviaser TJ, Neviaser JS. Concurrent rupture of the rotator cuff and anterior dislocation of the shoulder in the older patient. *J Bone Joint Surg Am* 1988;70:1308–1311.

81. Neviaser RJ, Neviaser TJ, Neviaser JS. Anterior dislocation of the shoulder and rotator cuff rupture. *Clin Orthop* 1993;291: 103–106.

82. Neviaser RJ, Neviaser TJ. Recurrent instability of the shoulder after age 40. *J Shoulder Elbow Surg* 1995;4:416–418.

83. Watson-Jones R. Dislocation of the shoulder joint. *Proc R Soc Med* 1936;29:1060–1062.

84. Brown JT. Nerve injuries complicating dislocation of the shoulder. *J Bone Joint Surg Br* 1952;34:526.

85. Blom S, Dahlback LO. Nerve injuries in dislocations of the shoulder joint and fractures of the neck of the humerus. A clinical and electromyographical study. *Acta Chir Scand* 1970;136:461–466.

86. Pasila M, Jaroma H, Kiviluoto O, et al. Early complications of primary shoulder dislocations. *Acta Orthop Scand* 1978;49:260–263.

87. Pasila M, Kiviluoto O, Jaroma H, et al. Recovery from primary shoulder dislocation and its complications. *Acta Orthop Scand* 1980;51:257–262.

88. Fitzgerald JF, Keates J. False aneurysm as a late complication of anterior dislocation of the shoulder. *Ann Surg* 1975;181:785–786.

89. Waxman DL, France MP, Harryman DT. Late lateral displacement of the humeral head after closed reduction of glenohumeral dislocation: a sign of vascular injury. Report of a case. *J Bone Joint Surg Am* 1996;78:907–910.

90. Stener B. Dislocation of the shoulder complicated by complete rupture of the axillary artery. *J Bone Joint Surg Br* 1957;39: 714–717.

91. Lucas GL, Peterson MD. Open anterior dislocation of the shoulder. *J Trauma* 1977;17:883–884.

92. Kvitne RS, Jobe FW, Jobe CM. Shoulder instability in the overhand or throwing athlete. *Clin Sports Med* 1995;14:917–935.

93. Walch G, Elattrache NS, et al. Impingement of the deep surface of the supraspinatus tendon on the posterosuperior glenoid rim: an arthroscopic study. *J Shoulder Elbow Surg* 1992;1:238–245.

94. Davidson PA, Jobe CM, et al. Rotator cuff and posterior-superior glenoid labrum injury associated with increased glenohumeral motion: a new site of impingement. *J Shoulder Elbow Surg* 1995;4:384–390.

95. Bigliani LU, Codd TP, Connor PM, et al. Shoulder motion and laxity in the professional baseball player. *Am J Sports Med* 1997;25:609–613.

96. Thomas SC, Matsen FA. An approach to the repair of avulsion of the glenohumeral ligaments in the management of traumatic anterior glenohumeral instability. *J Bone Joint Surg Am* 1989; 71:506–513.

97. Marshall JL, Johanson N, Wickiewicz TL, et al. Joint looseness: a function of the person and the joint. *Med Sci Sports Exerc* 1980;12:189–194.

98. Payne LZ, Altchek DW. The surgical treatment of anterior shoulder instability. *Clin Sports Med* 1995;14:863–883.

99. Altchek DW, Warren RF, Skyhar MJ, et al. T-plasty modification of the Bankart procedure for multidirectional instability of the anterior and inferior types. *J Bone Joint Surg Am* 1991;73: 105–112.

100. Jobe FW, Kvitne RS, Giangarra CE. Shoulder pain in the overhand or throwing athlete. The relationship of anterior instability and rotator cuff impingement. *Orthop Rev* 1989;18:963–975.

101. Kvitne RS, Jobe FW. The diagnosis and treatment of anterior instability in the throwing athlete. *Clin Orthop* 1993;291:107–123.

102. Speer KP, Hannafin JA, Altchek DW, et al. An evaluation of the shoulder relocation test. *Am J Sports Med* 1994;22:177–183.

103. Pavlov H, Warren RF, Weiss CB, et al. The roentgenographic evaluation of anterior shoulder instability. *Clin Orthop* 1985;194: 153–158.

104. Engebretsen L, Craig EV. Radiologic features of shoulder instability. *Clin Orthop* 1993;291:29–44.

105. Lawrence WS. New position in radiographing the shoulder joint. *AJR Am J Roentgenol* 1915;2:728–730.

106. Rokous JR, Feagin JA, Abbott HG. Modified axillary roentgenogram. A useful adjunct in the diagnosis of recurrent instability of the shoulder. *Clin Orthop* 1972;82:84–86.

107. Hall RH, Isaac F, Booth CR. Dislocations of the shoulder with special reference to accompanying small fractures. *J Bone Joint Surg Am* 1959;41:489–494.

108. Mack LA, Matsen FA, Kilcoyne RF, et al. US evaluation of the rotator cuff. *Radiology* 1985;157:205–209.

109. Harryman DT, Mack LA, Wang KY, et al. Repairs of the rotator cuff. Correlation of functional results with integrity of the cuff. *J Bone Joint Surg Am* 1991;73:982–989.

110. Patten RM, Mack LA, Wang KY, et al. Nondisplaced fractures of the greater tuberosity of the humerus: sonographic detection. *Radiology* 1992;182:201–204.

111. Mack LA, Matsen FA. Rotator cuff. *Clin Diagn Ultrasound* 1995;30:113–133.
112. Danzig L, Resnick D, Greenway G. Evaluation of unstable shoulders by computed tomography. A preliminary study. *Am J Sports Med* 1982;10:138–141.
113. Gusmer PB, Potter HG. Imaging of shoulder instability. *Clin Sports Med* 1995;14:777–795.
114. Iannotti JP, Zlatkin MB, Esterhai JL, et al. Magnetic resonance imaging of the shoulder. Sensitivity, specificity, and predictive value. *J Bone Joint Surg Am* 1991;73:17–29.
115. Farley TE, Neumann CH, Steinbach LS, et al. Full-thickness tears of the rotator cuff of the shoulder: diagnosis with MR imaging. *AJR Am J Roentgenol* 1992;158:347–351.
116. Gusmer PB, Potter HG, Schatz JA, et al. Labral injuries: accuracy of detection with unenhanced MR imaging of the shoulder. *Radiology* 1996;200:519–524.
117. Williams GR Jr, Iannotti JR, Rosenthal A, et al. Anatomic, histologic, and magnetic resonance imaging abnormalities of the shoulder. *Clin Orthop* 1996;330:66–74.
118. Stimson LA. *A practical treatise on fractures and dislocations.* Philadelphia: Lea and Febiger, 1912.
119. Anderson D, Zvirbulis R, Ciullo J. Scapular manipulation for reduction of anterior shoulder dislocations. *Clin Orthop* 1982;164:181–183.
120. Trimmings NP. Haemarthrosis aspiration in treatment of anterior dislocation of the shoulder. *J R Soc Med* 1985;78:1023–1027.
121. Hovelius L, Eriksson K, Fredin H. Recurrences after initial dislocation of the shoulder: results of a prospective study of treatment. *J Bone Joint Surg Am* 1983;65:343–349.
122. Stromsoe K, Senn E, Simmen B. Rezidivhaufigkeit nach erstmaliger traumatischer Schulter-luxation. *Helv Chir Acta* 1980;47:85–88.
123. Aronen JG, Regan K. Decreasing the incidence of recurrence of first time anterior shoulder dislocations with rehabilitation. *Am J Sports Med* 1984;12:283–291.
124. Saha AK. Mechanics of elevation of glenohumeral joint. Its application in rehabilitation of flail shoulder in upper brachial plexus injuries and poliomyelitis and in replacement of the upper humerus by prosthesis. *Acta Orthop Scand* 1973;44:668–678.
125. Dines DM, Levinson M. The conservative management of the unstable shoulder including rehabilitation. *Clin Sports Med* 1995;14:797–816.
126. Moseley JB Jr, Jobe FW, Pink M. EMG analysis of the scapular muscles during a shoulder rehabilitation program. *Am J Sports Med* 1992;20:128–134.
127. Magnuson PB, Stack JK. Recurrent dislocation of the shoulder. *JAMA* 1943;123:889–892.
128. Osmond-Clarke H. Habitual dislocation of the shoulder. The Putti-Platt operation. *J Bone Joint Surg Br* 1948;30:19–25.
129. Helfet AJ. Coracoid transplantation for recurring dislocation of the shoulder. *J Bone Joint Surg Br* 1958;40:198–202.
130. DuToit GT, Roux D. Recurrent dislocation of the shoulder. A 24-year study of the Johannesburg stapling operation. *J Bone Joint Surg Am* 1956;38:1–12.
131. Hawkins RH, Hawkins RJ. Failed anterior reconstruction for shoulder instability. *J Bone Joint Surg Br* 1985;67:709–714.
132. Hawkins RJ, Angelo RL. Glenohumeral osteoarthrosis. A late complication of the Putti-Platt repair. *J Bone Joint Surg Am* 1990;72:1193–1197.
133. Regan WD Jr, Webster-Bogaert S, Hawkins RI. Comparative functional analysis of the Bristow, Magnuson-Stack, and Putti-Platt procedures for recurrent dislocation of the shoulder. *Am J Sports Med* 1989;17:42–48.
134. Zuckerman JD, Matsen FA. Complications about the glenohumeral joint related to the use of screws and staples. *J Bone Joint Surg Am* 1984;66:175–180.
135. Bach BR, O'Brien SJ, Leighton M. An unusual neurological complication of the Bristow procedure. *J Bone Joint Surg Am* 1988;70:458–460.
136. O'Driscoll SW, Evans DC. Long-term results of staple capsulorrhaphy for anterior instability of the shoulder. *J Bone Joint Surg Am* 1993;75:249–258.
137. Rowe CR, Patel D, Southmayd WW. The Bankart procedure: a long-term end-result study. *J Bone Joint Surg Am* 1978;60:1–16.
138. Gill TJ, Michieli LJ, Gebhard F. Bankart repair for anterior instability of the shoulder. Long-term outcome. *J Bone Joint Surg Am* 1997;79:850–857.
139. Rowe CR, Zarins B. Recurrent transient subluxation of the shoulder. *J Bone Joint Surg Am* 1981;63:863–872.
140. Lintner SA, Speer KP. Traumatic anterior glenohumeral instability: the role of arthroscopy. *J Am Acad Orthop Surg* 1997;5:233–239.
141. Manta JP, Organ S, Nirsch, RP. Arthroscopic transglenoid suture capsulolabral repair. Five-year followup. *Am J Sports Med* 1997;25:614–618.
142. Torchia ME, Caspari RB, Asselmeier MA. Arthroscopic transglenoid multiple suture repair: 2 to 8 year results in 150 shoulders. *Arthroscopy* 1997;13:609–619.
143. Warner JJP, Warren RF. Arthroscopic Bankart repair using a cannulated absorbable fixation device. *Op Tech Orthop Surg* 1991;1:192–198.
144. Speer KP, Warren RF. Arthroscopic shoulder stabilization. A role for biodegradable materials. *Clin Orthop* 1993;291:67–74.
145. Speer KP, Warren RF, Pagnani MJ. An arthroscopic technique for anterior stabilization of the shoulder with a bioabsorbable tack. *J Bone Joint Surg Am* 1996;78:1801–1807.
146. Arciero RA, Wheeler JH, Ryan JB. Arthroscopic Bankart repair versus nonoperative treatment for acute, initial anterior shoulder dislocations. *Am J Sports Med* 1994;22:589–594.
147. Skyhar MJ, Altchek DW, Warren RF. Shoulder arthroscopy with the patient in the beach-chair position. *Arthroscopy* 1988;4:256–259.
148. Leslie JT, Ryan TJ. The anterior axillary incision to approach the shoulder joint. *J Bone Joint Surg Am* 1962;44:1193–1196.
149. Harryman DT, Sidles JA, Harris SL. The role of the rotator interval capsule in passive motion and stability of the shoulder. *J Bone Joint Surg Am* 1992;74:53–66.

Principles and Practice of Orthopaedic Sports Medicine,
edited by William E. Garrett, Jr., Kevin P. Speer, and Donald T. Kirkendall.
Lippincott Williams & Wilkins, Philadelphia © 2000.

CHAPTER 23

Posterior Shoulder Instability

James P. Bradley and James E. Tibone

Posterior instability of the shoulder in athletes presents complex challenges concerning initial diagnosis and subsequent treatment. True posterior dislocations in athletes are rare; more prevalent are recurrent posterior subluxations (RPS). The diagnosis and treatment of chronic posterior instability continues to be controversial, and many treatment protocols have been advocated (1–11). Confusion exists because early authors combined chronic locked (fixed) dislocations, recurrent posterior dislocations, and RPS (12–15). McLaughlin (7) in 1962 was the first to point out that a clear demarcation should be made between fixed and recurrent shoulder instabilities. In the early 1980s, Hawkins et al. (3) made it clear and understandable.

Posterior shoulder instability can be divided into two discrete groups: true posterior traumatic dislocation and RPS (that are occasionally associated with macrotrauma but typically is precipitated by repetitive microtrauma). In other words, posterior instabilities usually present as recurrent subluxation episodes rather than frank dislocations in athletes. The classic mechanism of injury is chronic overuse leading to insidious microtrauma to the posterior capsule that subsequently becomes attenuated, thus allowing posterior subluxation (16). Rarely, a single traumatic event results in posterior subluxation, with recurrences evolving with repeated use of the shoulder. Certain athletic activities are known to force the humeral head posteriorly: the follow-through phase of throwing, the backhand stroke in tennis, the pull-through phase in swimming, certain types of weight lifting (i.e., bench press), and blocking in football offensive linemen (17).

LITERATURE REVIEW

Historically, there was a myriad of proposed treatment options for symptomatic RPS. The early literature presented small patient populations, short follow-up intervals, and a plethora of surgical alternatives. The problem emanated from the relative scarcity of clinical cases and an overall lack of understanding of the pathomechanics because of this limited exposure. In addition, a number of essential lesions have been reported as the key to recurrence. Reverse Bankart lesion (detached posterior labrum), capsular attenuation, reverse Hill-Sach's lesion (anteromedial humeral head defect), increased retrotorsion of the proximal humerus, retroversion of the glenoid, and glenoid hypoplasia have all been implied as the primary lesion responsible for recurrence. Accordingly, several surgical treatments have been designed to address one or more of the above problems. Surgical treatment options for posterior subluxations and recurrent dislocations have included biceps tendon transfers (2), reverse Bankart repair (18), subscapularis transfers (7,19,20), reverse Putti-Platt reconstruction (21,22), infraspinatus advancement (3,18), posterior staple capsulorrhaphy (16), posteroinferior capsular shifts of the glenoid or humeral sides (9,10,23), posterior bone blocks with and without capsular shifts (5,8,24,25), glenoid osteotomies (3,26–29), humeral rotational osteotomies (30,31), allograft reconstruction (32), and arthroscopic reconstruction (33). In addition, combinations of the above have been used (2,25,34–36). These surgical procedures can be divided into three types: bony, soft tissue, and combinations.

Chronologically, in 1944 Rowe and Yee (37) developed a posterior surgical approach to the shoulder and reported on two soldiers with symptomatic recurrent posterior dislocations, one having previously failed a Nicola procedure. They described a reverse Bankart procedure with the detached posterior labrum repaired to bone; both patients regained "normal function." After the report from Rowe and Yee, a posterior bone

J. P. Bradley: Department of Orthopaedic Surgery, University of Pittsburgh, Pittsburgh, Pennsylvania 15213.

J. E. Tibone: University of Southern California, Los Angeles, California 90033.

block procedure was advocated by Hindenach (4) in 1947. It entailed fixing an iliac bone graft to the posterior glenoid extracapsulary so that it projected laterally from the margin of the glenoid.

In 1949, Fried (38) described five patients who were reconstructed with an extracapsular bone block and reported good results. Similarly, Jones (5) in 1958 depicted a case report in which a posterior bone block permitted a soldier to return to full activity after having symptomatic subluxations. Subsequently, Mowery et al. (8) in 1985 reported on five patients with recurrent posterior dislocations reconstructed with an extracapsular bone block from the iliac crest. Four patients had an excellent result, and one sustained a subsequent anterior dislocation. Eventually, Fronek et al. (25) in 1989 modified this procedure and augmented their capsulorrhaphy protocol when the bony rim of the posterior glenoid was deficient or when there was significant capsular laxity with a bone block. This augmentation was needed in 5 of their 11 cases. They advocated that the humeral head should not directly impinge on the graft and the graft should be used to increase the posterior surface of the glenoid. In 1995, Murrell and Warren (9), from the same institution, further clarified the use of a posterior bone block. They considered using a tricortical block from the scapular spine to compensate for glenoid deficiency placed at the posteroinferior quadrant contiguous with its curvature to increase the articulating surface. However, they stated that this modification was used infrequently over the past 5 years to augment the open posterior capsular plication.

In 1952, McLaughlin (12) originally described a tenodesis procedure that was later modified to a concomitant bony augmentation. He reported good results on six patients stabilized with interposition of the subscapularis tendon in a "shallow vertical defect in the anterior aspect of the humeral head." In a subsequent author's note, he admitted that after submission of the above article, two cases were encountered in which it was necessary to add a posterior bone block in addition to the subscapularis transposition. A later modification described taking the subscapularis off with its underlying bony insertion to be transposed into the reverse Hill-Sach's lesion. In 1962, McLaughlin was the first to support that a sharp distinction should be made between "fixed and recurrent posterior subluxations of the shoulder." He proposed that locked posterior dislocation (LPD) with substantial anterior humeral head defects do well with subscapularis tenodesis; however, for RPS, posterior capsular plication and bone block is the procedure of choice (7).

Scott (39) was the first to report on another bony procedure, the glenoplasty (glenoid osteotomy), after having problems with bony fixation of the posterior bone blocks for recurrent dislocations. The glenoplasty is a posterior opening wedge osteotomy, followed by the introduction of a bone graft into the osteotomy site to hold the glenoid fragment in a forward-rotated position. Three soldiers were treated for RPS in which the glenoid retroversion was corrected by redirecting it anteriorly. Two patients did well and resumed their military activities, although one immediate anterior postoperative dislocation was reported and treated with closed reduction. The remaining patient still had RPS and some pain. Scott (39) believed that the glenoplasty provided a stable buttress without disruption of the shoulder mechanism, prolonged immobilization was not necessary, and a concomitant capsulorrhaphy or bone block could be performed to augment the glenoplasty. Subsequently, English and Macnab (27), reporting on four patients using this method, noted all achieved stability. Norwood and Terry (36) documented a 47% recurrence rate (9/19) and believed that the procedure yielded good results in shoulders with traumatic unidirectional posterior instability but was not indicated for those with congenitally or habitually lax shoulders. Later, Brewer et al. (26) achieved stability in four of the five shoulders, although Wilkinson and Thomas (40) demonstrated a recurrence rate of 14% (4/23). Several of these authors believed that recurrent posterior instability was secondary to excessive glenoid retroversion on axial x-rays (26,27,40).

Many salient observations of the glenoplasty procedure describe it as presently out of favor. Primarily, recent studies concerning glenoid version using axillary x-ray or computed tomography (CT) have not demonstrated glenoid version or glenohumeral index of Saha differences between normal and unstable shoulders (28,41–44). Clinically, Gerber et al. (28) reported impingement of the anterior rotator cuff between the humeral head and coracoid process after glenoplasty. Hawkins et al. (3) noted a recurrence rate of 41% (7/17) and a complication rate of 29% (5/17), including one case of avascular necrosis of the osteotomized glenoid segment. Mowery et al. (8) highlighted that it is a technically challenging procedure that necessitates considerable skill and precision to achieve success. Accurate cuts of the glenoid and constructing the bone graft are tedious, not withstanding the potential complications such as glenoid fracture, avascular necrosis of the glenoid articular fragment, nonunion or malunion of the graft, lack of correction caused by loss of the anterior cortical hinge, and graft extrusion causing loss of correction. Finally, in 1996, Hawkins (45) reported on 12 patients who underwent glenoplasty for RPS using CT to measure the change in the articular alignment. The average correction was 10.8 degrees and varied from −1 to +24 degrees. Sixteen percent (2/12) of patients had clinical instability; however, three others continued to feel "some discomfort." His conclusion, given the known risks of glenoplasty, was that this procedure should be used with caution when used for RPS.

Still other groups believe that increased proximal humeral retrotorsion is a cause of posterior instability and advocate a rotational osteotomy of the humerus to correct this deficiency (31,46). Initially, Chaudhuri et al. (46) in 1974 presented 16 cases of humeral osteotomy for instability; however, only 1 was performed to correct posterior instability. Later, surgery was required on this patient to correct recurrent anterior dislocations. Recently, rotational osteotomy for posterior instability has resurfaced. Surin et al. (31) reported on 10 cases (12 shoulders) who had RPS treated by external rotational osteotomy of the humerus. Only three patients (four shoulders) participated in overhead sports. Subjectively, 10 of the 12 shoulders were rated good to excellent; objectively, 2 shoulders were excellent, 8 good, and 2 fair. Intriguingly, many of the shoulders had significant limitations in external rotation postoperatively. However, the authors state that it did not impair their work or sports activities. Stability was accomplished in 92% of cases with one patient with multidirectional instability failing (31). They describe the osteotomy as close to the humeral head in the cancellous bone. An A.O. compression plate and screws hold the humeral head in a 30-degree externally rotated position. One complication occurred, a nonunion, which required a second procedure; also, a second operation is routinely done to remove hardware at 1-year postoperatively. They concluded that instability in more than one plane was a contraindication to humeral osteotomy (31). Nevertheless, proximal humeral osteotomy has been successful in the treatment of chronic or LPD of the shoulder when the joint is not degenerated, the humeral head defect is between 20% and 40% of the articular surface, and the patient can cooperate in a rehabilitation protocol (31). Although rarely seen in athletes, both Porteous and Miller (47) in 1990 and Keppler et al. (48) in 1993 demonstrated good results using this technique.

The second group of procedures used to treat RPS involves the reconstruction of the posterior soft tissue envelope consisting of the posterior labrum and capsule. Initially, Rowe and Yee (37) reported that on two patients with detached posteroinferior labrums, both were attached to bone using an anterior Bankart type repair. Full function and stability were restored in both shoulders. Unfortunately, reverse Bankart lesions are rare in the overall population of RPS (less than 5%) in our experience. Tibone et al. (49) reported on posterior capsulorrhaphy with a staple without detachment or advancement of the infraspinatus or teres minor in high-performance athletes. Basically, they used a Bankart repair using a staple without shifting the capsule. In the initial series of 10 athletes in 1981, no patient returned to their former throwing status, 4 had concomitant anterior instability, and 3 (30%) had recurrence of their posterior instability. It was concluded that this procedure should be supple-

mented in "ligamentously lax" individuals (49). In 1990, in a follow-up study of 20 high-performance athletes, a high failure rate was further emphasized (11). Nine patients had unsatisfactory results, six patients had recurrence of the posterior instability, three patients still had moderate or severe pain, and only one patient was able to return to further throwing status (11). Their conclusion was that posterior staple capsulorrhaphy is not acceptable treatment for posterior subluxation of the shoulder because of the high rate of failure and complications (11).

Several authors have described capsular laxity or excessive capsular redundancy as a cause of RPS (2,13,24,50). Various posterior capsulorrhaphies have subsequently been proposed to address this capsular pathology. Severin (22) in 1952 reported on two cases of a reverse Putti-Piatt procedure in which the infraspinatus tendon was divided and minimally advanced laterally over a "double-breasted" capsular plication. Later, DePalma (51) reported that advancement of the teres minor and infraspinatus laterally in three patients resulted in satisfactory results. Using a modification of this technique, Hawkins and McCormack (20) recounted good results with no recurrences in 15 cases, as did Bell and Noble (1) in 1991. Boyd and Sisk (2) used a combination of a posterior capsulorrhaphy and a posterior rerouting of the long head of the biceps in eight cases; transferring the biceps around the posterior lateral aspect of the humeral head and attaching on the posterior glenoid rim created a dynamic sling. At 2 years follow-up, all eight shoulders were stable (2).

In the late 1980, a few centers began reporting encouraging results in athletes with a posterior capsular shift (capsulorrhaphy) intended to decrease capsular redundancy and reinforce the posterior capsule and labrum. Bigliani and colleagues (10,34) believed that the "preferred operative treatment" of RPS was a posterior capsular shift as originally described by Neer and Foster (52). The posterior capsule was incised 1 cm medial to its insertion on the humerus from superior to inferior and then the capsule was split in T-fashion at the posterior midglenoid region. The superior flap is shifted inferiorly and reattached to the lateral aspect of the humeral neck, whereas the inferior flap is transferred superiorly to reduce the inferior pouch and reinforce the repair (10). Noting that in only 15% of cases is there a posterior labral detachment (reverse Bankart lesion), the authors also recommended labral repair to the glenoid rim, if present, before proceeding with the capsular shift (10). Preliminary results reported in 1989 on 25 shoulders showed an 88% good to excellent result, based on stability, pain, activity level, and range of motion (34). Importantly, these rates of success were attained, regardless of the cause (traumatic vs. atraumatic) and direction (unidirectional or multidirectional). In a follow-up evaluation in 1992 of 38 patients, the overall satisfactory results were 80%. Eleven percent had a recurrence of instability; however, of the failed procedures, all but one had prior operative attempts at stabilization. Therefore, when this group was excluded, the overall success rate was 96% (24/25 shoulders) (10,41). Fronek et al. (25), also in 1989, presented encouraging results with an overall success rate of 91% (10/11 shoulders) using a posterior capsulorrhaphy off the glenoid side sometimes supplemented with a bone block. The bone augmentation was used in cases of severely deficient posterior glenoid or when the posterior capsule or infraspinatus was attenuated (5/11 shoulders). Interestingly, 70% of the successful outcomes participated in athletics at a diminished level of competition or changed to a position that was less stressful to the affected shoulder (25). Tibone and Bradley (16) in 1993 reporting on 40 shoulders also documented a significant failure rate (40%) in predominantly elite and competitive athletes. Twenty athletes were reconstructed with a posterior staple capsulorrhaphy (early group) and 20 were stabilized with a glenoid-sided posterior capsular shift similar to Fronek et al. (25). They believed most failures were due to "ligament laxity and unrecognized multidirectional instability" (16).

Arthroscopic posterior shoulder stabilization techniques have also been developed to address the capsuloligamentous pathology associated with RPS. Papendick and Savoie (33) in 1995 initially reported on 41 cases of RPS, documenting a 95% overall satisfactory rate using the Neer-Foster scale (52). Interestingly, the patients' activity level was 16 high school athletes, six collegiate, 14 recreational, and 21 throwing athletes. Four pathology-specific arthroscopic stabilization techniques were used, including a Suretac, Mitek, suture punch, and mini-open technique (53). Their conclusions stated that capsuloligamentous structures are the primary contributor to stability and that no essential lesion is responsible for all cases of RPS; therefore, the selective procedures described are designed to anatomically repair the underlying pathology producing the instability (33). In the follow-up study, Savoie and Field (54) presented a 7-year experience on 61 patients with a mean follow-up of 34 months. They reported a 90% success rate using a combination of the UCLA and Neer scales. Wolf (55) in 1996 also used an arthroscopic suture anchor technique on 17 patients, noting an 88% successful outcome. In 1997, McIntyre et al. (56) presented 2-year results on 20 cases using an arthroscopic multiple suture technique. A suture punch was used to place multiple absorbable monofilament stitches in the posterior ligament complex and do an arthroscopic shift. Based on the athletic shoulder outcome scale (57), 17 patients were in the

excellent (15) to good (2) category; however, there was a 25% recurrence rate. Analysis of failures noted that all failures had a voluntary component to their instability.

This review emphasizes that posterior instabilities of the shoulder continue to be an orthopedic enigma. Although there has been a heightened awareness of the definition and terminology of posterior instabilities, controversy still exists concerning the best surgical treatment of these maladies.

INCIDENCE

McLaughlin's initial article in 1952 (12) noted 22 posterior dislocations or subluxations in 581 shoulder dislocations for an incidence of 4%. Most later series also demonstrated incidences of less than 5%.

PATHOANATOMY AND BIOMECHANICS

The normal biomechanics of the shoulder concerning motion and stability is extremely elaborate, involving components of both static (bony architecture, ligament complex) and dynamic (muscle tendon units) elements. A complete understanding of all these interactions in both the normal and pathologic state is still under ongoing investigation. It is agreed that a complex interaction of passive and active stabilizing forces and structures are required for clinical stability. In addition, under normal daily activities, the amount of translation of the humeral head varies significantly (58).

Bony Component

The relative sizes of the humeral head and glenoid are disproportionate. The surface area of the humeral head is two to four times that of the glenoid and the diameter of the humeral head is almost twice that of the glenoid when measured in the transverse plane (59). The small articular surface area of the glenoid is not capable of covering the much larger humeral head. Therefore, only a small portion of the humeral head is in contact with the glenoid fossa in any one position (60). This absence of articular cartilage contact adds to the inherent instability of the glenohumeral joint (61). In the uninjured state, the humeral head and glenoid are almost congruous (59). Soslowsky et al. (59) found that the joint surfaces are approximated by section of a sphere with small deviations (less than 1% of the radius), and Iannotti et al. (62) found that mating surfaces are quite congruent, with radii within 2 mm in 90% of the specimens. The apparent x-ray appearance of incongruity does not take into account the unseen humeral and glenoid cartilage. In addition, the cartilage, at the periphery of the glenoid, is thicker (63). Articular contact areas are usually greatest at the midelevation (60 to 120 degrees) rather than at the end range of total arm elevation (64). In addition, with increasing elevation, contact points on the glenoid surface tend to move posterior.

In the past, glenoid version (increased retroversion) was thought to play a greater role in posterior instabilities, but these studies now are believed to be inaccurate secondary to inconsistent reference areas. More recently, CT studies do not show significant differences between normal and unstable shoulders (28,65). However, congenital hypoplasia of the glenoid, dysplasia of the humeral neck and glenoid in Erb's palsy, and posterior glenoid fractures may be exceptions.

The humeral head and glenoid maintain a relatively constant relationship through most of the arc of motion, but at the extremes, rotation of the humeral head is coupled with translocation on the glenoid (58,66–68). External rotation of the humerus causes the humeral head to posteriorly translate on the glenoid, whereas internal rotation causes an anterior translocation. This normal pattern of anteroposterior translation does not seem to be affected when the compressive forces of the rotator cuff are eliminated by nerve blocks (69). However, when the inferior capsular structures are sectioned, the normal anteroposterior coupled translation is lost at about 45 and 90 degrees of abduction (70).

Capsuloligamentous Complex

Most work on posterior glenohumeral instabilities has concentrated on the capsuloligamentous complex of the shoulder. Initially, cadaveric and, more recently, arthroscopic evaluations have demonstrated that the shoulder capsule has specific condensations of the capsule that constitute the glenohumeral ligaments and that the capsule in the neutral position is capacious and redundant (60,71,72).

The anterior glenohumeral ligaments include the superior glenohumeral ligament (SGHL), the middle glenohumeral ligament, and the inferior glenohumeral ligament complex (IGHLC) (Fig. 23.1). The IGHLC is comprised of three discrete functional parts: the anterior band, a posterior band, and an interposed axillary pouch (73). The posterior capsule is the thinnest segment of the capsule and does not have any ligamentous thickening in its substance. The posterior capsule comprises the area posterior to the intraarticular portion of the biceps tendon down to the posterior band of the IGHLC (61). Many authors have reported that the role of the anterior glenohumeral ligament and shoulder capsule in preventing posterior instability is elaborate and varies with shoulder position and the direction of the subluxating force (53,61,73,74).

The magnitude of the work on the glenohumeral ligaments precludes discussion of all the nuances of every investigation; what is presented is a synopsis of the pre-

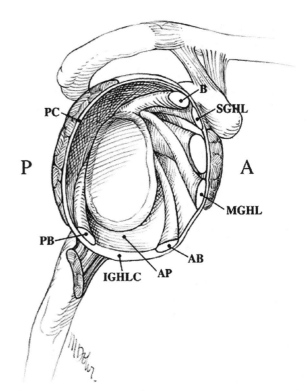

FIG. 23.1. The anatomy of the capsuloligamentous complex of the shoulder. The humeral head has been removed. *A,* Anterior; *P,* posterior; *B,* biceps tendon; *SGHL,* superior glenohumeral ligament; *MGHL,* middle glenohumeral ligament; *IGHLC,* inferior glenohumeral ligament complex; *AB,* anterior band; *AP,* axillary pouch; *PB,* posterior band; *PC,* posterior capsule.

dominant theories. Warren et al. (75) studied the static restraints to posterior translation with the arm in vulnerable position of shoulder flexion adduction and internal rotation. The infraspinatus, teres minor, and entire posterior capsule were excised; however, they were unable to demonstrate a posterior dislocation. But if the anterosuperior capsule, including the SGHL, was transected, a posterior dislocation would develop. The cadaveric studies of Warren and colleagues (61,75) led to the development the "circle concept," which states that dislocation in one direction requires capsular damage on both the same side and on the opposite side of the joint. Subsequently, O'Brien et al. (76) reported that with the shoulder in 90 degrees of glenohumeral abduction, the primary static stabilizer resisting posterior translation was the IGHLC (with the posterior inferior capsule). Additionally, the relative contribution of the components of the IGHLC changes with rotation, flexion, and extension of the arm. Specifically, if the shoulder is placed in the susceptible position of 90 degrees of abduction and is forward flexed 30 degrees, the posterior band of IGHLC becomes the prime anteroposterior stabilizer.

Similarly, Blasier et al. (77) in 1997 using a biomechanical model with a testing position of 90 degrees of forward flexion (humeral thoracic, jerk test position) with simulated muscle forces applied stated that "the single most important ligamentous or muscular factor in this study was the inferior glenohumeral ligament at large displacements in internal rotation." In agreement with O'Brien et al. (76), Blasier et al. (77) found the combination of arm internal rotation and shoulder forward flexion reoriented the IGHLC in a more anteroposterior orientation. Therefore, this orientation combined with the decrease in capsuloligamentous laxity due to internal rotation was well suited to resist translation (77). Bowen and Warren (60) helped refine the functional relationship of the three components of the IGHLC; as the shoulder is elevated and the arm internally rotated, the anterior band of the IGHLC rotates interiorly to oppose inferior translation while the posterior band of the IGHLC moves posterosuperiorly to resist anteroposterior translation. The SGHL appears to have a secondary role in opposing posterior translation when the shoulder is in a flexed adducted and internally rotated position but does not restrain posterior translation in the abducted shoulder (76). Harryman et al. (78) studied the contribution of the rotator interval in relation to shoulder stability. This rotator interval is the space between the superior border of the subscapularis and the anterior margin of the supraspinatus, both the SGHL and the coracohumeral ligament are located in this region of the capsule. They found that rotator interval opposes inferior subluxation in the adducted shoulder and functions as a secondary restraint against posterior translation.

In summary, it appears that the IGHLC is the principle static restraint opposing anterior, posterior, and inferior translation when the shoulder is abducted above 45 degrees, whereas the posterior band of the IGHLC is the primary restraint versus posterior translation with the shoulder at 45-degree elevation. The middle glenohumeral ligament assists the IGHLC in midrange elevation. In the adducted shoulder, the posterior IGHLC and the SGHL both oppose posterior translation.

Muscular Component

A complex interaction exists between the glenohumeral musculature and the capsuloligamentous structures of the shoulder (79). Presently, no model can accurately reproduce the sequential muscle activity and force generation in relation to the capsuloligamentous complex during functional activity. Efforts at understanding the dynamic muscle function are restricted by the complexity of the neuromuscular system and the limited methods to study its interaction with the static restraints. The primary method in which the glenohumeral muscles affect glenohumeral stability appears to be a dynamic one and is coupled with a coordinated system of specific

muscular contractions (79,80). Some authors believe the rotator cuff may serve a complimentary function to modify tension in the capsuloligamentous system (61). They emphasize that stretch receptors (Ruffini end organs and Pacinian corpuscles) within the capsulolabral system could be activated by tension to produce selective contraction of the glenohumeral musculature to protect the ligaments at the extremes of motion (61,81). Bowen and Warren (60) believed that activation of the rotator cuff caused the humeral head to be compressed in the glenoid, thereby increasing the load necessary to translate the humeral head.

A problem with understanding the muscular contribution to stability is that their effect depends on shoulder position. Simply stated, the resultant force a muscle produces depends on the position of the shoulder. McLaughlin et al. (7) reported that a change in position will alter the line of action of a specific muscle and consequently will alter its ability to resist a specific translation. Blasier et al. (77) cited the example of the biceps tendon and its contribution to posterior stability; with the arm in neutral rotation, the intraarticular portion of the biceps runs parallel to the supraspinatus and acts as a joint stabilizer, but with the arm in internal rotation, the biceps reorients and places a posterior directed force on the humerus, thereby aggravating the posterior translations. They also demonstrated that of all the muscles studied, the subscapularis provided the most resistance to posterior translation of the humerus.

Integrated electromyography and high-speed motion analysis of throwers has helped us understand the dynamic function of the glenohumeral muscles in relation to stability (A26,A6,A7). Jobe et al. (82) reported that deficiencies in the capsular restraints secondary to chronic microtrauma would subject the rotator cuff to fatigue, overuse, and progressive injuries. This was the so-called instability cascade. Glousman et al. (83) studied throwers with clinical anterior instability and compared electromyographic and motion analysis with a normal throwing population. They found that many of the muscles, including the supraspinatus, infraspinatus, and biceps, increased their activity during throwing, supposedly to resist the abnormal translation during late cocking and acceleration.

The understanding of the role that the glenohumeral musculature plays in shoulder stability is in its nascent stages, primarily because there is not a model that can simulate the complex neuromuscular firing patterns of normal shoulder range of motion, let alone athletic activities.

MECHANISM OF INJURY

Two distinct groups of posterior instabilities of the shoulder are apparent: true posterior traumatic dislocation and RPS. The mechanism of injury usually commonly corresponds to each separate group. Posterior dislocation is typically from a direct blow to the anterior shoulder or, more commonly, from significant indirect forces applied to the shoulder that couples shoulder flexion, adduction, and internal rotation. The most commonly cited indirect causes of this type are convulsive seizures or accidental electrical shock. The stronger internal rotators, including the latissimus dorsi, pectoralis major, and subscapularis, overpower the weaker external rotators, producing the dislocation. Yet another mechanism is a significant posterior indirect force caused by a fall onto a forward flexed shoulder on an outstretched hand.

Contrary to posterior dislocations, RPS is linked with highly repetitive forces propagated by the periscapular muscles, which develop in the follow-through phase of various athletic activities. These forces transpire as the humerus is in flexion, adduction, and internal rotation when maximal muscle forces are present in the subscapularis and deltoid muscles (80,82). Specific sports that position the glenohumeral joint in a precarious position are the follow-through of overhead throwers, tennis serve, and certain weight-lifting exercises (i.e., bench press) (17); the pull-through phase of freestyle and butterfly swimmers; and the take-away phase of the backhand stroke in tennis. The repetitive indirect forces of football linemen during blocking also aggravate posterior translation. These repetitive activities presumably cause microtrauma to the posterior static restraints that attenuate, thereby shifting the load to the dynamic muscular restraints that fatigue over time, thus allowing the RPS.

CLASSIFICATION

Recurrent posterior dislocations or LPD are extremely rare in an athletic population and are usually classified with proximal humeral fractures rather than recurrent instability. Subsequently, the classification system presented specifically relates to RPS.

Posterior subluxators are initially classified according to four parameters: frequency, direction, degree, and cause. The frequency of instability is typically recurrent. The direction is unidirectional (pure posterior), multidirectional (posterior and inferior), or global instability, in which the posterior direction is the major directional component of the instability. The degree of instability is either subluxation or dislocation. In this group by definition, it is subluxation. Cause is divided into two major groups: traumatic and atraumatic subluxations. Traumatic subluxations are subdivided into macrotrauma (single traumatic event) or microtrauma (recurrent minor trauma). Both traumatic and atraumatic subluxors can be subdivided into involuntary and voluntary subluxations. Voluntary instability can be divided into two types. The positional type occurs when the

humeral head subluxates posteriorly as the arm is forward flexed and internally rotated. When the arm is extended, the head reduces. The muscular type is caused by activation of the internal rotators to induce posterior subluxation; this type has been associated with psychiatric overlay and a poor surgical outcome. Most athletes demonstrate positional voluntary instability without psychiatric problems.

Perusing this complex classification system of a relatively rare problem, one can easily understand why accumulating large numbers of one specific classification group has been troublesome.

CLINICAL EVALUATION

History

Initially, a history of a provocative activity should be ascertained, including overhead throwers, tennis players, butterfly and freestyle swimmers, weight lifters, and football linemen. All these activities have been, due to their biomechanics, selectively associated with RPS. The athlete's chief complaint is typically pain in the shoulder without subjectively describing episodes of instability. However, the symptoms often appear or intensify when the arm is in a forward flexed, adducted, and internally rotated position (provocative position). Originally, the pain may be traced to unrecognized episodes of instability, but as the pathology temporarily develops, many patients experience persistent pain. Pollock and Bigliani (10) reported that of their patients that require surgery, fully two thirds were limited in activities outside of sports, primarily when the arm was used at or above the horizontal.

Location of the pain is variable and can be localized to the posterior shoulder, over the biceps tendon, or about the superior cuff, as in a typical impingement syndrome. It appears that the abnormal biomechanics secondary to chronic instability may also cause stress-related inflammatory changes in the rotator cuff, resulting in a secondary impingement syndrome. Neurologic and vascular symptoms are absent.

Onset of symptoms sometimes can be traced to a specific traumatic event that precipitates the initiation of the progressive pain; this is more common in football players and weight lifters. Conversely, the overhead athletes (swimmers, throwers, and tennis players) recall multiple incidents of discomfort that resolved, which becomes progressively more common and symptomatic with time.

The patient will sometimes describe crepitation and clicking when the shoulder is in a provocative position. Review by one institution showed that 90% of patients with symptomatic posterior subluxation (18/20) noted clicking or crepitation (42). Prior ligament laxity problems may become evident in a number of patients with thorough questioning. In a study at our institution, nearly 28% had a prior history of ligament laxity problems (16).

Physical Examination

Inspection of the shoulders does not usually demonstrate obvious asymmetry. Dominant arm muscular hypertrophy is common in overhead athletes and is not considered pathologic. Palpation sometimes evokes some posterior glenohumeral joint line tenderness. Pollock and Bigliani (10) reported that two thirds of their patients had posterior joint line tenderness and associated it with synovitis secondary to multiple episodes of instability. Crepitance and clicking in the same position may be attributable to posterior capsulolabral pathology. Superolateral cuff tenderness also may be apparent and usually represents inflammatory stress-related changes in the cuff secondary to the instability.

Range of motion in the dominant extremity of overhand athletes usually demonstrates excessive external rotation with concomitant loss of internal rotation secondary to adaptive changes dictated by their sport; this is considered normal. Typically, as described by Fronek et al. (25), most patients maintain normal symmetric motion, and only 3 of 20 cases showed a loss of internal rotation in their series. Strength testing is usually symmetric, unless deficiencies are noted secondary to pain from an inflamed rotator cuff. In these cases, it is not uncommon to have positive impingement signs from secondary impingement.

The position of subluxation, which is forward flexion at 90 degrees, adduction, and internal rotation, will generally reproduce the pain of subluxation. Voluntary subluxators are able to reproduce a subluxation episode without manual assistance and demonstrate the instability. This subluxation occurs between 90 and 120 degrees of forward flexion with the humeral head spontaneously reducing between 120 and 180 degrees of elevation, as the shoulder moves from forward flexion to abduction. This is sometimes termed the circumduction maneuver.

Specific tests have been designed to estimate the translocation of the humeral head on the glenoid in posterior instability. The posterior stress test is performed with the patient seated and stabilizing the medial border of the scapula with one hand while the other hand applies a posteriorly directed force to the patient's humerus, which is flexed to 90 degrees, adducted, and internally rotated. The test is positive if subluxation or dislocation occurs with pain or if an apprehensive sensation that reproduces the patient's symptoms occurs (10). Bigliani and colleagues (10,34) noted that this test was positive in most patients with posterior instability; others, however, have not found this test as reliable (3,25). Others have also described posterior stress testing with the patient in the supine position with the

arm in both 90 degrees forward flexion adduction and internal rotation and 90 degrees abduction (84). Realizing that all these tests require sensitive fingers and experience, the posterior stress test most reproducible in our hands has been a "load and shift" maneuver similar to the one described by Murrell and Warren (9). The patient is supine on a firm surface to stabilize the scapula and the humeral head free to rotate off the edge of the table. The arm is held in 90 degrees abduction neutral rotation and the humeral head is grasped between the thumb and index finger while applying a compressive load to the glenoid with the humeral head; a posterior force is then applied trying to subluxate the humeral head. Similar maneuvers are used, both anteriorly and interiorly.

Additionally, Cofield translation testing is helpful. The patient is supine with the involved shoulder off the edge of the table. The arm is held in 90 degrees of abduction and neutral rotation and the posterior translation is compared with the contralateral shoulder. Then the arm is progressively internally rotated with the shoulder in 90 degrees of abduction and compared with the uninvolved side. Typically, the normal shoulder will tighten and not subluxate between 30 and 60 degrees of internal rotation, whereas the abnormal side continues to subluxate beyond 60 degrees of internal rotation. Translation is graded as +1 if there is increased motion versus the contralateral shoulder, +2 if the head subluxes over the glenoid rim but reduces spontaneously, and +3 if there is frank dislocation without spontaneous reduction. We found that most of the 40 patients requiring surgical intervention in our study had a positive posterior stress test as described (16). This is in agreement with Fronek et al. (25) who also noted that all their patients with RPS had marked posterior translation with this test.

The Sulcus sign suggests an inferior component to the posterior instability. The sign is based on the distance between the inferior margin of the lateral acromion and the humeral head when downward traction is applied to the adducted arm. Translation is graded +1 if the distance is less than 1 cm, +2 if the distance is between 1 and 2 cm, and +3 if the distance is more than 2 cm. A Sulcus sign of +3 predicts laxity in the IGHLC and SGHL and correlates with inferior instability. Many patients with RPS will present with side to side differences in the sulcus sign; the involved side will demonstrate increased inferior translation. In patients with posterior instability, a positive finding versus the contralateral shoulder may be found in as high as three fourths of the patients (10).

Ligamentous laxity is evaluated with specific tests that include recurvatum of the knees and elbows, thumb hyperabduction with the wrist volar flexed, increased index metacarpophalangeal extension, patellar hypermobility, and the ability to touch the palms to the ground with the knees straight. Studies have documented that patients with RPS had increased laxity scores versus age- and sex-matched patients without instability (25).

IMAGING

X-rays

All athletes should be evaluated with a standard three-view roentgenographic series that includes a true anterior posterior view, an axillary view, and a supraspinatus outlet view. The x-rays are usually normal. Axillary stress x-rays are sometimes helpful in defining degree and direction of the instability if the patient can voluntarily subluxate the shoulder. The axillary view will rarely help with humeral head fractures or glenoid version. The West Point view may reveal a fracture or ectopic bone production on the anterior or posterior rim (85,86). Ferrari et al. (87) documented that extraarticular ossific lesions of the posterior glenoid (Bennett lesion) are associated with undersurface rotator cuff tears and posterior labral injuries. In rare occasions, a fracture of the lesser tuberosity will denote a posterior dislocation (88). Likewise, an impression fracture of the humeral head at the level of the lesser tuberosity (reverse Hill-Sach's lesion) is almost never seen in patients with RPS but is much more common in recurrent posterior dislocations.

CT has been used when retroversion or glenoid deficiency is suspected; however, this is uncommon. Arthroscopic CT attempts to define posterior labral and capsular pathology but has not been helpful in our experience. Bigliani et al. (41) reported that labral pathology, by CT, was over- or underread in one third of cases when compared with operative findings. In conclusion, the use of CT should be limited to patients in whom plain x-rays indicate glenoid anomalies; generally, arthroscopic CT is not recommended in the work-up of RPS.

Magnetic resonance imaging and arthroscopic magnetic resonance imaging have been useful in defining posterior labral pathology, subscapularis muscle avulsions, rotator cuff tears, and bone contusions in limited cases. Presently, their role in RPS is undefined. A fastidious history, physical examination, and routine x-rays are, at this point, more efficacious and cost effective in diagnosing RPS.

Arthroscopy and examination under anesthesia is indicated in very select difficult cases where RPS is suspected. Often, in muscular athletes or in uneasy patients, with muscle guarding, the instability is subtle and cannot be reliably documented by clinical examination or additional diagnostic tests. In such cases, a bilateral examination under anesthesia and arthroscopy of the involved shoulder is extremely useful (89,90). The examination under anesthesia will help uncover the direction and magnitude of the instability, whereas the arthroscopy permits direct visualization of posterior labral wear, capsular attenuation, and detachment.

TREATMENT

Nonoperative

The initial treatment of RPS in athletes is conservative and encompasses an intensive rehabilitation protocol. The protocol specifically encourages strengthening of the rotator cuff and posterior deltoid. Biomechanically, Blasier et al. (78) and Murrell and Warren (9) demonstrated the dynamic support of the subscapularis in assisting the IGHLC during posterior translation. In addition, the external rotators (infraspinatus, teres minor) also resist posterior subluxation (9,80). Moseley et al. (91) emphasized the importance of strong scapular rotators to position the glenoid in the most stable position to resist posterior translation. The premise is to allow the dynamic muscular stabilizers to offset the deficient static capsuloligamentous restraints. Certain exercises that place the arm in a provocative position (flexion, adduction, and internal rotation) are avoided, including bench press, incline, decline, military presses, and ergometer machines. Biofeedback, as described by Beall et al. (92), may have a place in RPS. Stimulation of the posterior deltoid muscle with surface electrodes helped to control the instability; this biofeedback allowed the patient to recognize the abnormally relaxed deltoid and to reeducate the muscle to contract in a normal manner. Rockwood et al. (43) reported that patients with RPS of either traumatic or atraumatic etiology did better with physical therapy than patients with anterior instability. Hawkins et al. (3) also documented a relatively low degree of disability with RPS after rehabilitation and recommended most patients should be treated conservatively, with rehabilitation and modification of activities. Later, Fronek et al. (25) advised that patients with moderate symptoms of RPS should be treated with rehabilitation and reserved operative management for those with severe symptoms after a failed physical therapy protocol. However, it appears that patients with a history of macrotrauma initiating the RPS do less well after rehabilitation than those who have generalized ligamentous laxity or microtrauma as their etiology (25,93). The recommendation is that the RPS physical therapy protocol is maintained for at least 6 months in an attempt to decrease the athlete's functional disability Subjectively, 70% of the athletes improve with this specific rehabilitation protocol. Objectively, the RPS is usually not eliminated, but the functional disability during athletics is improved sufficiently to allow participation in his or her sport without significant problems (16,94).

Operative treatment of athletes with RPS should only be considered when the patient is recalcitrant to conservative measures and when the pain and/or disability preclude adequate function of the shoulder. Athletes involved in overhead throwing must be advised that operative intervention may not allow them to return to their preinjury throwing status (11,16,84). Finally, all voluntary subluxators should have appropriate psychological testing before surgical intervention is recommended; however, most athletes do not have psychological disturbances and seldom use the shoulder for secondary gain.

Operative

Acute posterior dislocations (APD), which are extremely rare in athletes, are managed by reduction and immobilization of the arm in neutral rotation and slight extension for 3 weeks. A formalized posterior instability protocol is instituted similar to the rehabilitation protocol for RPS, with emphasis on regaining range of motion, strengthening of the rotator cuff, and scapular rotators. Presently, to our knowledge, the recurrence rate is unknown. Surgical management requiring open reduction is needed when closed reduction fails, if there is a risk of progressive injury to the humeral head with closed reduction, or in situations where there is a major displacement of a glenoid or humeral head fragment. A posterior approach is commonly indicated to address damage to the posterior capsule, unless a significant reverse Hill-Sach's lesion (anteriorly) would require a transfer of the lesser tuberosity (modified McLaughlin procedure) (7,12).

Neglected LPD typically require operative reduction, unless seen acutely (less than 3 weeks). Reduction from an anterior approach is preferred because of the reverse Hill-Sach's lesion. If the humeral head defect is less than 20% of the articular surface, reduce the shoulder and treat as an APD. When it is between 20% and 40%, transpose the lesser tuberosity and subscapularis into the defect, and when it is greater than 40%, proceed with a hemiarthroplasty. Another less common option when 20% to 40% of the head is involved is to perform a rotational osteotomy of the humerus. Keppler et al. (48) reported on 10 patients with LPD demonstrating between 20% and 40% head involvement by CT analysis. Using the Rowe/Zarins Scale, 80% had excellent to good results with a humeral osteotomy and two had poor results, both showing advance articular cartilage damage. A major issue is the treatment of a young athlete with a head defect larger than 40%, in which a hemiarthroplasty may have a high long-term failure rate. Recently, Gerber and Lambert (32) presented the use of an allograft reconstruction for segmental defects of the humeral head of at least 40%. Four patients with LPD were reconstructed using an allogenic segment of the femoral head. At an average follow-up of 6 to 8 months, three patients had their stability restored and maintained. One patient had mild pain and moderate

to severe dysfunction secondary to avascular necrosis after a symptomatic period of 6 years.

Historically, there has been a plethora of surgical options designed to treat RPS. The chronologic progression of these procedures is presented in the introduction of this chapter; a brief synopsis is presented below.

RPS in athletes that is symptomatic and failed a conservative rehabilitation protocol require operative intervention. Recurrence rates, after rehabilitation, vary in the literature from 30% to 96%, thus representing a significant group that may require surgery. Surgical options have focused on three types of repairs: bony, soft tissue, and a combination of both.

Bone block procedures have been used in small numbers of patients with mixed results and only address bony deficiencies, which are infrequent (4,13,38). Similarly, glenoplasty was purported to correct increased retroversion of the glenoid by osteotomizing and anteverting the glenoid surface. Recent studies concerning glenoid version documented with CT or axillary x-rays have not consistently demonstrated a glenoid version difference between normal and unstable shoulders (28,41–44). However, Hurley et al. (94) documented that the control normal patients had an average glenoid retroversion of −4 degrees, whereas the conservative and surgically treated group averages were −10.5 and −9 degrees, respectively. Similar to bone blocks, glenoplasty has been reported in small numbers, with variable results, is technically demanding, and has potentially severe complications (26,27,36,39,95). However, it may be indicated in a patient with excessive glenoid retroversion and symptomatic RPS; otherwise, glenoplasty is rarely indicated.

Rotational humeral osteotomy was used to correct increased retrotorsion of the humerus in RPS. Presently, retrotorsion of the humerus has not been well defined. Although rotation osteotomy does achieve stability (92% in one series), the significant limitations in external rotation postoperatively would not be well tolerated by athletes (31,46).

Soft tissue repairs like the "Bankart type" posterior capsular repairs, which address only the labrum, have also noted high recurrence rates. Tibone et al. (11,49), using a metal staple to repair the labrum in 20 patients, reported 45% unsatisfactory results. The authors discontinued the use of the staple in the following 20 patients, but none of these 40 athletes returned to their preinjury athletic status.

Similarly, a reverse Putti-Piatt procedure was designed to address the capsular laxity of RPS. It consisted of a capsular plication and overlapping of the infraspinatus tendon. Hawkins et al. (3) reported an 83% failure rate (five of six shoulders) secondary to recurrent instability. This recurrence rate was a small subsection computed from a large group of different operative techniques and physicians (3). Recently, Hawkins (96) reported on the reverse Putti-Platte procedure, noting that 92% (13/14 patients) of the patients were "satisfied" with their outcome. However, 28% of the patients continued to have difficulty with sporting activities. Restricted motion and damage to the infraspinatus make this procedure less desirable in athletes.

Posterior capsulorrhaphies/inferior capsular shift procedures were designed to reduce the capsular redundancy, repair the reverse Bankart Lesion, if present, and augment the posterior capsule with two layers. Fronek et al. (25) reported a significant improvement in results, 91% in 10 of 11 patients using a glenoid-based capsulorrhaphy. The authors used a bone block augmentation in 5 of 11 shoulders. Seventy percent of patients returned to athletics at a modified level. Bigliani et al. (10,34), using a posterior capsular shift described by Neer and Foster (52), documented an 80% success rate in 38 shoulders. Of the failed procedures, all but one had a prior surgical attempt at stabilization. If that group was excluded, the overall success rate was 96%. The posterior capsular shift used by Bigliani et al. (34) differed from Fronek et al. (25) in that it was a humeral-sided T-split of the capsule verses a glenoid side. Both procedures attended to the inferior capsular redundancy and a repair of a reverse Bankart lesion, if present. Brems (97) reported on a posterior/inferior capsular shift through an anterior approach at minimum 2-year follow-ups; six of seven (86%) shoulders had no prior surgery and were asymptomatic and clinically stable. Conversely, six of seven (86%) of those with prior surgery failed.

Arthroscopic posterior capsulorrhaphies using suture anchors, arthroscopic tacs, and/or thermal-assisted capsular shrinkage have been recently documented. Savoie and Field (54) presented a 7-year experience with RPS, noting a 90% success rate on 61 patients using a variety of arthroscopic techniques.

SURGICAL TECHNIQUE

We presently recommend a posterior capsulorrhaphy for RPS in athletes. The patient is placed supine on the operative table and a thorough examination under anesthesia is performed. All the specific stability tests described in the physical examination section of this text are fastidiously repeated on both shoulders and documented. The patient then is rotated on the examination table into the lateral decubitus position with the involved shoulder superior. The patient is held in position with an inflatable bean bag and kidney rests. The table is placed in a slightly reverse Trendelenburg position. Foam rests are used to protect the peroneal nerve from the pressure of the operating table where the nerve crosses the neck of the fibula on the inferior leg. Subsequently, a diagnostic shoulder arthroscopy is instituted using an anterior and posterior portal technique to eval-

uate the labrum, rotator cuff, anterior glenohumeral ligaments, posterior capsule, and glenohumeral articulation. Typical lesions include posterior labral tears and fraying, a patulous capsule, and, rarely, osteoarthrosis of the glenohumeral joint. Interestingly, reverse Bankart lesions are extremely rare in true posterior subluxators without a prior history of a significant isolated traumatic episode causing a posterior dislocation.

Once the diagnosis is confirmed by examination under anesthesia and diagnostic arthroscopy, a saber incision is initiated at the superior aspect of the shoulder, originating just posterior to the acromioclavicular joint and terminating posteriorly near the axillary fold (Fig. 23.2). The incision is generally about 10 cm in length. The deltoid muscle is exposed by undermining the subcutaneous tissue. The deltoid muscle is split in line with its fibers from the scapular spine, beginning 2 to 3 cm medial to the posterolateral corner of the acromion and extending distally approximately 5 to 6 cm (Fig. 23.3A). Care must be taken not to split the deltoid muscle distally beyond the teres minor muscle to protect the axillary nerve, which enters the deltoid muscle at the inferior border of the teres minor muscle. Typically, the deltoid muscle does not require reflection from the spine of the scapula, except in well-muscled patients. It is essential to place the split of the deltoid muscle in the correct position (medial to the posterior lateral corner of the acromion) to ensure that the glenohumeral joint is positioned just below the deltoid split.

Immediately below the deep fascia of the deltoid is the level of the external rotators of the shoulder that

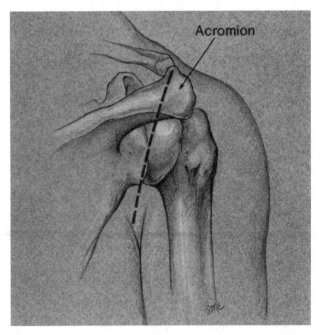

FIG. 23.2. A saber-cut incision is made from just posterior to the acromioclavicular joint toward the posterior axillary fold.

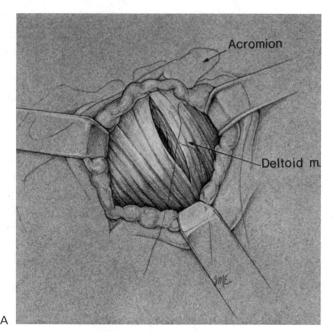 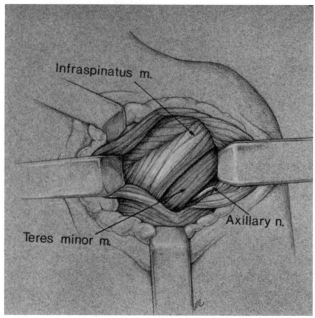

FIG. 23.3. A: The deltoid is split in line with its fibers beginning approximately 2 to 3 cm medial to the posterolateral corner of the acromion. **B:** The underlying infraspinatus and teres minor muscles are exposed.

includes the bipennate infraspinatus muscle and the teres minor (Fig. 23.3B). The interval between these two muscles is sometimes indistinct. A significant anatomic landmark is the raphe separating the two heads of the infraspinatus muscle, which is bipennate. This raphe that lies above the equator of the humeral head should not be confused with the interval separating the infraspinatus and teres minor muscles, which is usually below the equator of the humeral head. Once this hiatus between the external rotators is found, it is developed by blunt dissection; blunt retractors then are implemented to expose the posterior capsule of the shoulder (Fig. 23.4A). Currently, the interval between the bipennate heads of the infraspinatus is preferred because it is easy to locate and it places the muscular split over the midglenoid. Care must be taken not to split the infraspinatus further medially than 1.5 cm from the glenoid rim to protect the suprascapular nerve. Narrow deep Richardson retractors are ideal in this situation. The capsule needs to be freed from the overlying muscles. Because the capsule is closely associated with the tendons laterally, sharp dissection should be performed. Medially, a definite plane exists, facilitating separation with a periosteal elevator.

Once the capsule is adequately freed from the external rotators, a transverse arthrotomy is made into the posterior capsule in a lateral to medial direction up to, but not including, the labrum (Fig. 23.4A). Making a T-incision in the capsule parallel to the glenoid cavity and just adjacent to the labrum (Fig. 23.4B) then devel-

ops superior and inferior capsular flaps. These flaps are tagged with sutures to control them, and the joint is inspected. Care must be taken when developing the inferior capsular flap because of the close proximity of the axillary nerve on the undersurface of the inferior capsule.

In athletes with posterior subluxation, the pathologic findings are typically dissimilar from those athletes with anterior instability. These features include absence of a true reverse Bankart lesion, an intact labrum that is not torn away from the glenoid, a shallow labrum that may be poorly developed, and, commonly, a redundant posterior capsule. Technically, if the labrum is intact, the sutures that anchor the capsulorrhaphy are placed in the labrum. If, however, the labrum is torn, it must be reflected to permit access to the glenoid rim so that bone holes can be made and anchor sutures passed directly through the bone, as in a usual anterior Bankart repair. Suture anchors have been helpful in this circumstance.

The capsulorrhaphy is initiated by advancing the inferior flap superiorly and medially and securing it to the glenoid labrum with no. 1 nonabsorbable sutures (Fig. 23.5A). The degree of advancement of the inferior flap is tempered to correct posterior and inferior instability. The superior flap then is fastened over the inferior flap by advancing it inferiorly and medially. The arm is positioned in neutral rotation while the appropriate tension of the above capsulorrhaphy is determined. Commonly, there still may be a transverse gap in the capsule later-

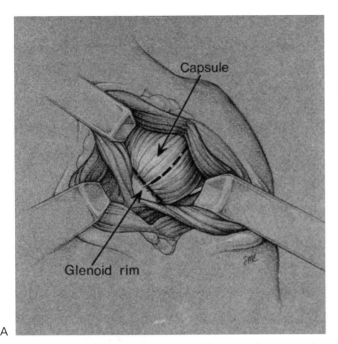

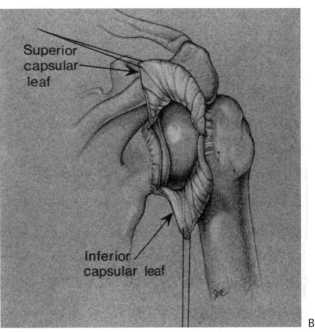

FIG. 23.4. A: The interval between the teres minor and infraspinatus muscles is developed, exposing the underlying capsule. The T-shaped incision to be made in the capsule is marked. **B:** The incision in the capsule has been made, developing inferior and superior flaps.

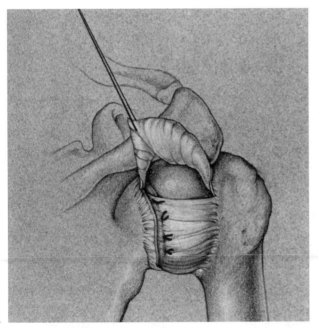

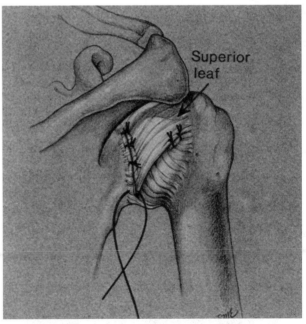

FIG. 23.5. A: The inferior capsular flap is advanced medially and superiorly and sutured to the labrum. The inset shows the split in the capsule being closed. **B:** The superior capsular flap is being sutured over the inferior capsular flap. The inset shows the split in the capsule being closed.

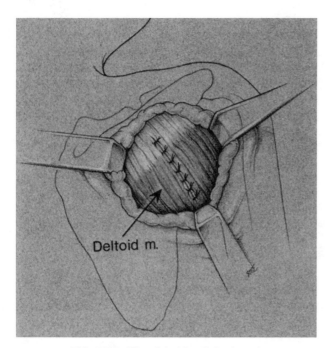

FIG. 23.6. The deltoid split is closed.

ally, with the arm in neutral. This is closed with interrupted mattress sutures (Fig. 23.5B). Augmentation of the repair with infraspinatus advancement and extraarticular bone blocks has not been necessary. The teres minor and infraspinatus muscles usually fall together without the addition of sutures. The superficial deltoid fascia then is repaired with no. 0 absorbable sutures

(Fig. 23.6). The subcutaneous tissue is approximated in routine fashion. A subcuticular stitch is used for the skin for cosmesis. Generally, no drains are necessary.

After operation, the extremity is positioned in an abduction pillow, which is commonly used for rotator cuff surgery. The shoulder is placed in slight extension and neutral rotation in the abduction pillow to take the stress off the reconstruction (Fig. 23.7 A and B). The pillow is terminated 3 weeks after operation.

POSTOPERATIVE REHABILITATION

Generally, the abduction pillow is removed 3 weeks after operation; termination is determined by the preoperative degree of ligamentous laxity. The greater the ligamentous laxity, the longer the pillow is necessary. When cessation of the pillow is deemed appropriate, active-assisted range-of-motion exercises are initiated. No resistance or passive range-of-motion exercises are attempted at this time. The emphasis is directed on elevating the arm in the scapular plane of the body and slowly regaining rotation. During the initial 3 weeks of exercise, no motion, namely, forward flexion, is attempted in the sagittal plane of the body. Forward flexion is permitted 6 weeks after operation, and active range-of-motion exercises are continued. Starting at 12 weeks, resistive exercises are initiated and progressed to increase strength and endurance. Return to sport is allowed at 6 months, except for the throwing athlete, who subsequently begins a progressive supervised

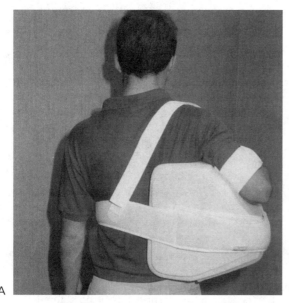
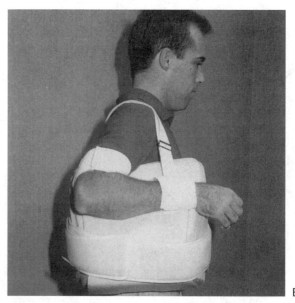

FIG. 23.7. A and B: The postoperative abduction pillow is shown with the shoulder in slight extension and neutral rotation.

throwing program. Generally, it takes the throwing athlete an additional 6 months to throw competitively.

EXPECTED OUTCOMES

Forty primarily high-performance athletes, comprising 14 elite, 15 competitive, and 11 recreational, were evaluated at a minimum 2-year follow-up. Twenty were traumatic and 20 were atraumatic; 18 were voluntary and 22 involuntary. No psychological abnormalities were documented. During surgery no true severe Bankart lesions were appreciated; rather, a redundant lax capsule was believed to be the pathology.

Range of motion was decreased in most patients, specifically in rotation. Eleven patients lost no rotation; however, external rotation was decreased in 11 patients an average of 15 degrees. Similarly, internal rotation was lost in 25 patients with an average loss of 15 degrees. Elevation was limited in three patients. Pain was significantly reduced from 75% of the patients preoperatively to 25% postoperatively. Overall, 50% of the athletes were rated excellent (12 patients) and good (8 patients). Ten percent (4) were rated fair and 40% (16) were rated poor and constituted failures.

Return to sports (at the same level) was significantly decreased with only 28% (4/14) professional or college-level athletes, 50% of the high school or competitive athletes, and 60% of the recreational athletes returning.

Failures were analyzed; 27.5% (11) had recurrent instability, whereas 12.5% (5) had no relief of their preoperative pain. Of the 11 patients with ligament laxity, 9 had recurrent instability and only 7% (2/29) without ligamentous laxity had recurrent instability.

Results from the literature are very difficult to compare because of different patient populations, specifically concerning preoperative athletic status. In addition, the lack of an accurate classification of RPS into the subgroups of traumatic, microtraumatic, and atraumatic is insufficient. In addition, some series eliminate any patients with a multidirectional component. Overall, from the literature review, successful results have varied from 50% to 90%.

AUTHORS' PREFERENCES

APD are managed by immediate reduction and immobilization of the arm in neutral rotation and slight extension for 3 weeks. A supervised posterior shoulder rehabilitation protocol is then instituted with emphasis on regaining rotator cuff and scapular rotator strength. Open reduction of APD is undertaken when closed reduction fails, if there is a risk of injury to the humeral head, or there is a major displaced fragment of the humeral head or glenoid. The approach to the glenohumeral joint is dictated by the pathology. Commonly, a posterior approach is used so that the damaged posterior capsuloligamentous structures can be repaired. However, in cases where a large reverse Hill-Sach's lesion (20% to 40% of the articular surface) is detected, an anterior approach is preferred so that transfer of the lesser tuberosity and subscapularis tendon into the defect is facilitated. The stability of the shoulder is then evaluated to determine if a posterior capsular tightening is also necessary. In most cases, this is not needed.

LPD or fixed posterior dislocations where the humeral head defect is less than 20% are treated as APD if possible, depending on the chronicity. If the head defect is between 20% and 40%, transposition of the lesser tuberosity and subscapularis tendon is recommended. When the head lesion is greater than 40% to 45% of the articular surface, a hemiarthroplasty is indicated; the exception is in a young athlete, in which case a femoral head allograft reconstruction of the anterior humeral head would be considered.

RPS in athletes that have failed conservative rehabilitation for 6 months and have functional symptomatic deficits are reconstructed using the posterior capsulorrhaphy described in the previous section. Special preoperative counseling is needed to inform the athlete concerning the decreased chances of return to sports at their preinjury status.

Future advancement in the treatment of RPS in athletes is centering on arthroscopic stabilization and thermal-assisted capsulorrhaphies. Presently, a prospective study on athletes with symptomatic RPS treated with thermal-assisted capsulorrhaphies alone, arthroscopic stabilization with suture anchors, and a combination of both is underway. In this study, the use of suture anchors has been limited to those athletes with reverse Bankart lesions; if after anchor stabilization capsular redundancy is still present, a concomitant Electro Thermal Assisted Capsulorrhapy (ETAC) is used. Temporally, the numbers are small, the follow-up is less than 1 year, and the appropriate indications are being formulated; however, the early results have been encouraging.

SUMMARY

RPS are seen in athletes predominantly secondary to repetitive macrotrauma. Approximately two thirds of the athletes with RPS respond to a proper posterior shoulder rehabilitation protocol. The primary pathology is capsuloligamentous laxity. Diagnostically, multidirectional instability must be differentiated from unidirectional posterior instability. A posterior capsulorrhaphy is the current procedure of choice for posterior unidirectional instability. Global multidirectional instability should be approached with an anterior inferior capsular shift procedure, including tightening of the rotator interval. Finally, competitive athletes with RPS can be stabilized but often still cannot compete at a high level.

REFERENCES

1. Bell RH, Noble JS. An appreciation of posterior instability of the shoulder. *Clin Sports Med* 1991;4:887.
2. Boyd HB, Sisk TD. Recurrent posterior dislocation of the shoulder. *J Bone Joint Surg Am* 1972;54A:779.
3. Hawkins RJ, Koppert G, Johnston G. Recurrent posterior instability (subluxation) of the shoulder. *J Bone Joint Surg Am* 1984;66A:169.
4. Hindenach JCR. Recurrent posterior dislocation of the shoulder. *J Bone Joint Surg Am* 1947;29A:582.
5. Jones V. Recurrent posterior dislocation of the shoulder: report of a case treated by posterior bone block. *J Bone Joint Surg Br* 1958;40B:203.
6. Matsen FA III. Glenohumeral instability. In: Evarts CM, ed. *Surgery of the musculoskeletal system.* New York: Churchill Livingstone, 1983:49.
7. McLaughlin HL. Follow-up notes on articles previously published in the journal posterior dislocation of the shoulder. *J Bone Joint Surg Am* 1962;44A:1477.
8. Mowery CA, Garfin SR, Booth RE, et al. Recurrent posterior dislocation of the shoulder: treatment using a bone block. *J Bone Joint Surg Am* 1985;67A:777.
9. Murrell GA, Warren RF. The surgical treatment of posterior shoulder instability. *Clin Sports Med* 1995;14:903.
10. Pollock RG, Bigliani LU. Recurrent posterior shoulder instability. *Clin Orthop* 1993;291:85.
11. Tibone JE, Ting A. Capsulorrhaphy with a stable for recurrent posterior subluxation of the shoulder. *J Bone Joint Surg Am* 1990;12A:999.
12. McLaughlin HL. Posterior dislocation of the shoulder. *J Bone Joint Surg Am* 1952;34A:584.
13. Nobel W. Posterior traumatic dislocation of the shoulder. *J Bone Joint Surg Am* 1962;44A:523.
14. Samilson RL, Miller E. Posterior dislocations of the shoulder. *Clin Orthop* 1964;32:69.
15. Wilson JC, McKeever FM. Traumatic posterior (retroglenoid) dislocation of the humerus. *J Bone Joint Surg Am* 1949;31A:160.
16. Tibone JE, Bradley JP. The treatment of posterior subluxation in athletes. *Clin Orthop* 1993;291:124.
17. Tullos HS, King JW. Throwing mechanisms in sport. *Orthop Clin North Am* 1973;4:709.
18. Dugas RW, Scerpella TA, Clancy WG. Surgical treatment of symptomatic posterior shoulder instability. *Orthop Trans* 1990; 14:245.
19. Hawkins RJ. Unrecognized dislocations of the shoulder. In: Stauffer ES, ed. *AAOS Instructional Course Lectures.* Vol. 34. St. Louis: C.V. Mosby, 1984:258.
20. Hawkins RJ, McCormack RG. Posterior shoulder instability. *Orthopedics* 1988;11:101.
21. Greenhill BJ. Persistent posterior shoulder dislocation: its diagnosis and its treatment by posterior Putti-Platt repair. *J Bone Joint Surg Br* 1972;54B:763.
22. Severin E. Anterior and posterior recurrent dislocation of the shoulder: the Putti-Platt operation. *Acta Orthop Scand* 1953;23: 14.
23. Goss TP, Costello G. Recurrent symptomatic posterior glenohumeral subluxation. *Orthop Rev* 1988;17:1024.
24. Ahlgreen SA, Heplund T, Nistor L. Idiopathic posterior instability of the shoulder joint: results of operation with posterior bone graft. *Acta Orthop Scand* 1978;49:600.
25. Fronek J, Warren RF, Bowen M. Posterior subluxation of the glenohumeral joint. *J Bone Joint Surg Am* 1989;71A:205.
26. Brewer BJ, Wubben RC, Carrera GF. Excessive retroversion of the glenoid cavity. *J Bone Joint Surg Am* 1986;68A:724.
27. English E, Macnab I. Recurrent posterior dislocation of the shoulder. *Can J Surg* 1974;17:147.
28. Gerber C, Ganz R, Vinh TS. Glenoplasty for recurrent posterior shoulder instability: an anatomic reappraisal. *Clin Orthop* 1987;216:70.
29. Vegter J, Marti RK. Treatment of posterior dislocation of the shoulder by osteotomy of the neck of the scapula. *J Bone Joint Surg Br* 1981;63B:288.
30. Chaudhuri GK, Sengupta A, Saha AK. Rotation osteotomy of

31. Surin V, Blader S, Markhede G, et al. Rotational osteotomy of the humerus for posterior instability of the shoulder. *J Bone Joint Surg Am* 1990;72A:181.
32. Gerber C, Lambert SM. Allograft reconstruction of segmental defects of the humeral head for the treatment of chronic locked posterior dislocation of the shoulder. *J Bone Joint Surg Am* 1996;78:376.
33. Papendick LW, Savoie FH III. Anatomy-specific repair techniques for posterior shoulder instability. *J South Orthop Assoc* 1995;4:169.
34. Bigliani LU, Endrizzi DP, McIlveon SJ. Operative management of posterior shoulder instability. *Orthop Trans* 1989;13:232.
35. Hernandez A, Drez D. Operative treatment of posterior shoulder dislocation by posterior glenoplasty, capsulorrhaphy, and infraspinatus advancement. *Am J Sports Med* 1980;14:187.
36. Norwood LA, Terry GC. Shoulder posterior subluxation. *Am J Sports Med* 1984;12:25.
37. Rowe CR, Yee LB. A posterior approach to the shoulder. *J Bone Joint Surg* 1944;26:580.
38. Fried A. Habitual posterior dislocation of the shoulder joint: a case report on 5 operated cases. *Acta Orthop Scand* 1949;18:329.
39. Scott DJ Jr. Treatment of recurrent posterior dislocations of the shoulder by glenoplasty. *J Bone Joint Surg Am* 1967;49A:471.
40. Wilkinson JA, Thomas WG. Glenoid osteotomy for recurrent posterior dislocation of the shoulder. *J Bone Joint Surg Br* 1985;67B:496.
41. Bigliani LU, Pollock RG, Endrizzi DP, et al. Surgical repair of posterior instability of the shoulder: long term results. Presented at the Ninth Combined Meeting of the Orthopaedic Associations of the English-Speaking World, Toronto, June 1992.
42. Cyprien J, Vasey HM, Burdet A, et al. Humeral retrotorsion and glenohumeral relationship in the normal shoulder and in recurrent anterior dislocation (scapulometry). *Clin Orthop* 1983;175:8.
43. Rockwood CA Jr, Burkhead WZ Jr, Brna J. Subluxation of the glenohumeral joint: response to rehabilitative exercise, traumatic vs. atraumatic instability. *Orthop Trans* 1986;10:220.
44. Saha AK. Dynamic stability of the glenohumeral joint. *Acta Orthop Scand* 1971;42:491.
45. Hawkins RJ. Glenoid osteotomy for recurrent posterior subluxation of the shoulder: assessment by computed axial tomography. *J Shoulder Elbow Surg* 1996;5:393.
46. Chaudhuri GK, Sengupta A, Saha AK. Rotation osteotomy of the shaft of the humerus for recurrent dislocation of the shoulder: anterior and posterior. *Acta Orthop Scand* 1974;45:193.
47. Porteous MJ, Miller AJ. Humeral rotation osteotomy for chronic posterior dislocation of the shoulder. *J Bone Joint Surg* 1990; 72:468.
48. Keppler P, Holz U, Thielemann FW, et al. Locked posterior dislocation of the shoulder: treatment using rotational osteotomy of the humerus. *J Orthop Trauma* 1994;8:286.
49. Tibone JE, Prietto C, Jobe FW, et al. Staple capsulorrhaphy for recurrent posterior shoulder dislocation. *Am J Sports Med* 1981;4:135.
50. Neer CS II. *Shoulder reconstruction.* Philadelphia: W.B. Saunders, 1990.
51. DePalma AF. *Surgery of the shoulder.* Philadelphia: J.B. Lippincott, 1950.
52. Neer CS II, Foster CR. Interior capsular shift for involuntary interior and multidirectional instability of the shoulder. *J Bone Joint Surg Am* 1980;62A:897.
53. Bigliani LU, Kelkar R, Flatow EL, et al. Glenohumeral stability. *Clin Orthop* 1996;330:13.
54. Savoie FH, Field LD. Arthroscopic management of posterior shoulder instability. *Oper Techn Sports Med* 1997;5:226.
55. Wolf EM. Arthroscopic shoulder stabilization using suture anchors: technique and results. Presented at AANA Annual Meeting, Washington DC, April 1996.
56. McIntyre LF, Caspari RB, Savoie FH III. The arthroscopic treatment of posterior shoulder instability: two-year results of a multiple suture technique. *Arthroscopy* 1997;13:426.
57. Tibone JE, Bradley JP. Evaluation of treatment outcomes for

the athletic shoulder. In: Matsen FA, Fu FH, Hawkins RJ, eds. *The shoulder: a balance of mobility and stability.* Rosemont, IL: American Academy of Orthopedic Surgeons, 1993:519.

58. Poppen NK, Walker PA. Normal and abnormal motion of the shoulder. *J Bone Joint Surg Am* 1976;58A:195.
59. Soslowsky LJ, Flatow EL, Bigliani LU, et al. Articular geometry of the glenohumeral joint. *Clin Orthop* 1992;285:181.
60. Bowen MK, Warren RF. Ligamentous control of shoulder stability based on selective cutting and static translation experiments. *Clin Sports Med* 1991;10:757.
61. Pagnani MJ, Warren RF. Stabilizers of the glenohumeral joint. *J Shoulder Elbow Surg* 1994;3:173.
62. Iannotti JP, Gabriel JP, Schneck SL, et al. The normal glenohumeral relationships: an anatomical study of one hundred and forty shoulders. *J Bone Joint Surg Am* 1992;74A:491.
63. Matsen FA, Harryman DT, Sidles JA. Mechanics of glenohumeral instability. *Clin Sports Med* 1991;10:783.
64. Soslowsky LJ, Flatow EL, Bigliani LU, et al. Quantitation of in situ contact areas at the glenohumeral joint: a biomechanical study. *J Orthop Res* 1992;10:524.
65. Randelli M, Gambrioli PL. Glenohumeral osteometry by computed tomography in normal and unstable shoulders. *Clin Orthop* 1986;208:151.
66. Harryman DT II, Sidles JA, Clark JM, et al. Translation of the humeral head on the glenoid with passive glenohumeral motion. *J Bone Joint Surg Am* 1990;72A:1334.
67. Howell SM, Galinat BJ. The glenoid-labral socket: a constrained articular surface. *Clin Orthop* 1989;243:122.
68. Howell SM, Galinat BJ, Renzl AJ, et al. Normal and abnormal mechanics of the glenohumeral joint in the horizontal plane. *J Bone Joint Surg Am* 1988;70A:227.
69. Howell SM, Kraft RA. The role of the supraspinatus and infraspinatus muscles in glenohumeral kinematics of anterior shoulder instability. *Clin Orthop* 1991;263:128.
70. Bowen MK, Deng XH, Warner JJP, et al. The effect of joint compression on stability of the glenohumeral joint. *Trans Orthop Res Soc* 1992;17:289.
71. Cooper DE, Arnoczky SP, O'Brien SJ, et al. Anatomy, histology, and vascularity of the glenoid labrum: an anatomical study. *J Bone Joint Surg Am* 1992;74:46.
72. Cooper DE, O'Brien SJ, Warren RF. Supporting layers of the glenohumeral joint: an anatomic study. *Clin Orthop* 1993;289:144.
73. O'Brien SJ, Neves MC, Arnoczky SP, et al. The anatomy and histology of the inferior glenohumeral ligament complex of the shoulder. *Am J Sports Med* 1990;18:449.
74. Blasier RB, Guldberg RE, Rothman ED. Anterior shoulder stability: contributions of rotator cuff forces and the capsular ligaments in a cadaver model. *J Shoulder Elbow Surg* 1992;1:140.
75. Warren RF, Kornblatt IB, Marchand R. Static factors affecting posterior shoulder stability. *Orthop Trans* 1984;8:89.
76. O'Brien SJ, Schwartz RE, Warren RF, et al. Capsular restraints to anterior/posterior motion of the shoulder. *Orthop Trans* 1988;12:143.
77. Blasier RB, Soslowsky LJ, Malicky DM, et al. Posterior glenohumeral subluxation: active and passive stabilization in a biomechanical model. *J Bone Joint Surg Am* 1997;79A:433.
78. Harryman DT II, Sidles JA, Harris SL, et al. Role of the rotator interval capsule in passive motion and stability of the shoulder. *J Bone Joint Surg Am* 1992;74A:53.
79. Bradley JP, Perry J, Jobe FW. The biomechanics of the throwing shoulder. *Perspect Orthop Surg* 1990;1:49.
80. Bradley JP, Tibone JE. Electromyographic analysis of the muscle action about the shoulder. *Clin Sports Med* 1991;10:789.
81. Terry GC, Hammon D, France P, et al. The stabilizing function of passive shoulder restraints. *Am J Sports Med* 1991;19:26.
82. Jobe FW, Moynes DR, Tibone JE, et al. An EMG analysis of the shoulder in pitching: a second report. *Am J Sports Med* 1984;12:218.
83. Glousman R, Jobe FW, Tibone JE, et al. Dynamic electromyographic analysis of the throwing shoulder with glenohumeral instability. *J Bone Joint Surg Am* 1988;70A:220.
84. Schwartz E, Warren RF, O'Brien SJ, et al. Posterior shoulder instability. *Orthop Clin North Am* 1987;18:409.
85. Engebretsen L, Craig EV. Radiologic features of shoulder instability. *Clin Orthop* 1993;291:29.
86. Pavlov H, Warren RF, Weiss C Jr, et al. The roentgenographic evaluation of anterior shoulder instability. *Clin Orthop* 1985;194:153.
87. Ferrari JD, Ferri DA, Coumas J, et al. Posterior ossification of the shoulder: the Bennett lesion. Etiology, diagnosis, and treatment. *Am J Sports Med* 1994;22:171.
88. Pagnani MJ, Warren RF. Instability of the shoulder. In: Nicholas JA, Hershman EB, eds. *The upper extremity and spine in sports medicine.* Philadelphia: J.B. Lippincott, 1994:173.
89. Cofield RH, Nessier JP, Weinstabi R. Diagnosis of shoulder instability by examination under anesthesia. *Clin Orthop* 1993;291:45.
90. Hawkins RJ, Schutte JP, Janda DH, et al. Translation of the glenohumeral joint with the patient under anesthesia. *J Shoulder Elbow Surg* 1996;5:286.
91. Moseley JP, Jobe FW, Perry J, et al. EMG analysis of the scapular rotator muscles during a baseball rehabilitation program. *Orthop Trans* 1990;14:252.
92. Beall MS Jr, Diefenbach G, Allen A. Electromyographic biofeedback in the treatment of voluntary posterior instability of the shoulder. *Am J Sports Med* 1987;15:175.
93. Bowen MK, Warren RF, Altchek DW, et al. Posterior subluxation of the glenohumeral joint treated by posterior stabilization. *Orthop Trans* 1991;15:764.
94. Hurley JA, Anderson TE, Dear W, et al. Posterior shoulder instability. Surgical versus conservative results with evaluation of glenoid version. *Am J Sports Med* 1992;20:396.
95. Bessems JH, Vegter J. Glenoplasty for recurrent posterior shoulder instability. *Acta Orthop Scand* 1995;66:535.
96. Hawkins RJ. Posterior instability of the glenohumeral joint. *Am J Sports Med* 1996;24:275.
97. Brems JJ. Anterior approach to posterior instability. *J Shoulder Elbow Surg* 1993;2[Suppl 26].

Principles and Practice of Orthopaedic Sports Medicine,
edited by William E. Garrett, Jr., Kevin P. Speer, and Donald T. Kirkendall.
Lippincott Williams & Wilkins, Philadelphia © 2000.

CHAPTER 24

Labral Injuries in Contact Sports

Anthony J. Delfico and Kevin P. Speer

Contact sports such as football, lacrosse, wrestling, and ice hockey put tremendous demands on the glenohumeral joint of the athlete. In contrast to the repetitive controlled forces that are produced in the shoulder of the overhead throwing athlete, forces exerted on the shoulder of the contact athlete are often produced by high-energy violent episodes that can generate a different spectrum of injuries than those seen in overhead athletes.

EPIDEMIOLOGY AND CLASSIFICATION

Injuries to the glenoid labrum may or may not be associated with instability of the shoulder. Whether or not instability is produced depends on the location of the labral injury and which other associated anatomic structures are injured. However, in discussing the epidemiology and classification of labral injuries, it is important to understand the basics of the classification of shoulder instability.

Instability of the glenohumeral joint may be defined in terms of its chronicity, etiology, direction, and volition. Chronicity can be described as either acute, recurrent, or chronic. The etiology of the instability is classified as traumatic, atraumatic, or the result of repetitive microtrauma. Direction is most often defined as anterior, inferior, posterior, or a combination of the three. Athletes involved in contact sports subject their shoulders to forces that most often produce acute, traumatic, anterior, involuntary instability. Such instability is associated with injury to the anterior glenoid labrum in approximately 85% of cases (1). Thus, anterior glenoid labral injury and anterior shoulder instability are closely linked

clinical entities, and injuries to the anterior glenoid labrum must be suspected and evaluated in patients presenting with signs and symptoms of instability.

Certain athletes, such as offensive linemen in football, exert unusual forces on their shoulders that produce less common patterns of labral injury as the result of very sport-specific injury mechanisms. Injuries to the posterior glenoid labrum are almost exclusively observed in contact sports and may not be associated with shoulder instability.

Anterior Labrum

The overall incidence of acute traumatic anterior glenohumeral dislocations in the general population has been estimated at 1.7% (2). Acute traumatic anterior shoulder instability is the usual cause of injury to the anterior portion of the glenoid labrum resulting from contact sports. Approximately 90% of all shoulder dislocations occur in the anterior direction (3). Types of anterior glenohumeral dislocation include subcoracoid dislocation (the most common type), subglenoid, subclavicular, intrathoracic, and retroperitoneal. The latter two types occur only very infrequently and are rarely seen as the result of sporting activities.

The natural history of injuries to the anterior glenoid labrum with associated anterior glenohumeral instability has typically been fraught with frequent recurrences of anterior dislocations. This is especially true in young active patients such as those involved in contact sports. A 90% recurrence rate in patients under 20 years of age was reported by McLaughlin and Cavallaro (4). In this study of 573 patients, the rate of recurrence was seen to decrease with the age of the patient, with a rate of 60% in patients between 20 and 40 years old and the rate decreasing to 10% in patients more than 40 years old. Multiple authors have reported similar such recurrence rates after conservative treatment of anterior shoulder dislocations (5–7).

A. J. Delfico: Department of Orthopaedic Surgery, The Valley Hospital, Ridgewood, New Jersey 07450.

K. P. Speer: Division of Orthopaedic Surgery, Section of Sports Medicine & Shoulder Surgery, Duke University Medical Center, Durham, North Carolina 27710.

The functional deficit produced by recurrent anterior shoulder instability has an even more profound effect on the athlete involved in contact sports. This is especially true if the patient's dominant arm is involved, with pain, loss of motion. and reduced strength being reported in nearly 60% of patients treated conservatively in a study by Tsai et al. (8).

Posterior Labrum

The posterior glenoid labrum may be injured as the result of a posterior dislocation of the humeral head or secondary to repetitive sheer stress applied to it by certain athletic activities. Posterior shoulder dislocations are rarely seen in athletics, but when they do occur, they may be classified by the final position of the humeral head. Subacromial dislocations are by far the most common type of posterior shoulder dislocations, followed by subglenoid and subspinous. The overall incidence of posterior shoulder dislocations is estimated at 2% of all shoulder dislocations, but this number is difficult to verify because of the high rate of missed diagnosis of this injury (9). The rate of missed diagnosis of posterior dislocations of the shoulder has been reported as more than 60% by several authors (10–12).

Although posterior dislocations of the shoulder are rarely seen in athletics, even in contact sports, the posterior labrum is frequently injured by mechanisms other than frank dislocation. Interior linemen in football appear to be the group at greatest risk for sustaining these injuries to the posterior glenoid labrum (13). Blocking techniques that place the arm in a position of forward flexion and internal rotation with the elbows locked in extension appear to be responsible for most of these injuries.

Superior Labrum

The advent of diagnostic shoulder arthroscopy has provided orthopedic surgeons with a tool capable of examining the superior labrum with new degrees of sensitivity and specificity. Lesions that were difficult to visualize through standard open approaches are now well documented. Snyder et al. (14) described a spectrum of injuries to the superior glenoid labrum beginning posteriorly and extending anteriorly and coined the term "SLAP" (superior labrum anterior to posterior) lesion. Injuries to the superior glenoid labrum are seen in both overhead throwing athletes and those involved in contact sports. Stetson et al. (15) reported that up to 17% of isolated superior labral injuries were caused by a direct blow. However, the most common mechanisms producing these injuries are traction and compression, putting both throwers and contact athletes at risk (16).

When classifying injuries to the superior glenoid labrum, Snyder et al. (14) described four distinct types of

SLAP lesions (Fig. 24.1). Type I lesions display fraying and degeneration of the superior labrum, but the labrum and biceps anchor remain firmly attached to the glenoid. Type II is described as having the labrum and biceps anchor detached from the superior glenoid. In type III lesions, a bucket-handle tear of the superior labrum exists, with the biceps anchor and remaining labrum still well attached. Type IV lesions are described as a bucket-handle tear of the superior labrum and extension of the tear into the biceps tendon. The labral flap or a portion of the tendon may displace into the glenohumeral joint with probing during arthroscopy. "Complex" type SLAP lesions were also described by Snyder et al. (14) as being a combination of two of the previously described types, with types II and IV being the most commonly

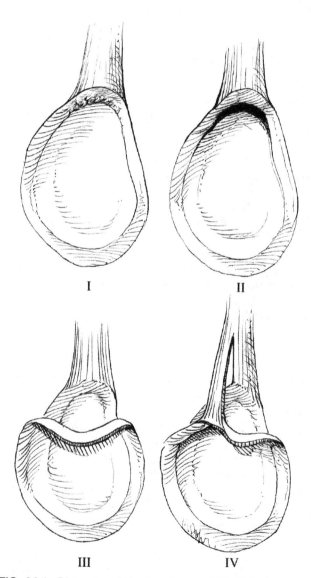

FIG. 24.1. Diagrams of the four types of SLAP lesions described by Snyder et al. (Adapted from Snyder SJ, Karzel RP, Del Pizzo W, et al. SLAP lesions of the shoulder. *Arthroscopy* 1990;6:274–278, with permission.)

involved. Maffet et al. (17) described three other patterns of complex labral tears involving the superior labrum and biceps tendon anchor. The first pattern involves a Bankart type anterior–inferior labral tear that extends into the superior labrum and is continuous with the SLAP lesion. The second complex pattern displays an avulsion of the biceps tendon with an unstable flap tear of the superior labrum. The third combination involves an extension of the separation of the superior labrum and biceps tendon into the region of the capsule beneath the middle glenohumeral ligament (MGHL).

ANATOMY

The design of the glenohumeral joint provides a tremendous range of motion at the expense of relative instability, because the shoulder is the most commonly dislocated major joint in the body (18,19). In the shoulder, a hierarchy of support mechanisms exist. This hierarchy includes passive restraint mechanisms such as the concave shape of the joint surface (which is enhanced by the glenoid labrum), the finite joint volume and negative intraarticular pressure, and the adhesion/cohesion mechanism, all of which resist displacement of the joint at minimal loads, such as the gravitational pull of the arm (9,20,21).

Dynamic Stabilizers

When larger loads are applied to the joint, active restraints are recruited to enhance stability. The rotator cuff muscles compress the humeral head into the glenoid fossa when they fire in unison and are capable of adjusting the tension of individual parts of the shoulder's capsuloligamentous complex through independent muscle contractions (22). Selective contraction of the cuff muscles helps to resist the displacing forces generated by the primary movers of the shoulder (23–25). The posteriorly directed force on the humeral head, generated by the anterior deltoid and pectoralis major, are resisted by the subscapularis, infraspinatus, and teres minor. The upward displacement of the humeral head produced by the lateral deltoid during abduction is similarly resisted by the supraspinatus.

The role of the rotator cuff in preventing anterior translation of the humeral head is less clear. Although Turkel et al. (26) proposed that the subscapularis plays a stabilizing role only in lower degrees of abduction (and adds little to shoulder stability in 90 degrees of abduction), many other authors concluded that the subscapularis is the true stabilizer resisting anterior translation (24,25,27). By compressing the humeral head into the glenolabral socket, the rotator cuff resists translation with an efficiency of approximately 40%. That is, if the compressive force exerted by the rotator cuff equals 100 units, the force resisting translation of the humeral head

will equal 40 units. By removing the glenoid labrum, the efficiency of this mechanism is reduced by 50% (1).

Capsule and Ligaments

The ligamentous and capsular restraints of the shoulder provide an essential, static component to the overall stability of the shoulder joint. The joint capsule and ligaments are normally lax through most of the range of motion of the shoulder joint—coming under tension only at extremes of motion. This laxity allows for the wide range of motion available at the shoulder. As these structures come under tension at the extremes of motion, they provide the final check reign to abnormal glenohumeral translation. Discrete thickenings within the capsule have been described as the anterior glenohumeral ligaments: the superior glenohumeral ligament (SGHL), the MGHL, and the inferior glenohumeral ligament complex (IGHLC) (Fig. 24.2). O'Brien and colleagues (28,29) defined the structures that make up the IGHLC as consisting of anterior and posterior bands separated by an intervening axillary pouch. The anterior band appears to function as the primary static stabilizer of the complex.

Cadaveric cutting studies have defined the roles played by each ligament with respect to glenohumeral stability. It appears that these ligaments take on various responsibilities depending on the shoulder position and

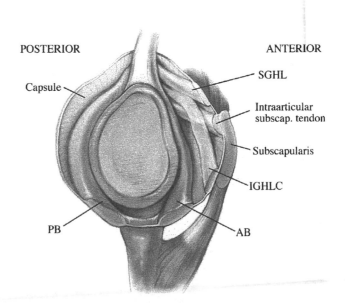

FIG. 24.2. The anterior glenohumeral ligaments. This drawing depicts the superior glenohumeral ligament (*SGHL*), and inferior glenohumeral ligament complex (*IGHLC*), including its anterior band (*AB*), and posterior band (*PB*). (Adapted from O'Brien S, Neves M, Arnoczsky SP, et al. The anatomy and histology of the inferior glenohumeral ligament complex of the shoulder. *Am J Sports Med* 1990;18:449–456, with permission.)

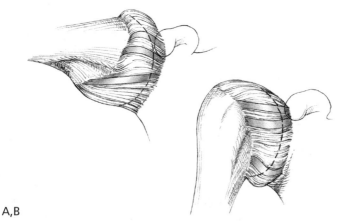

A,B

FIG. 24.3. Anterior glenohumeral ligaments **(A).** With the arm in 90 degrees of abduction, the inferior glenohumeral ligament complex (*IGHLC*) is taut and acts as the primary static stabilizer resisting anterior, posterior, and inferior glenohumeral translation. In this position the superior glenohumeral ligament (*SGHL*) is lax and acts only as a secondary static stabilizer **(B).** When the arm is in zero degrees of abduction, the SGHL becomes taut and assumes the role of the primary static stabilizer of the joint, whereas the IGHLC adopts a secondary stabilizer status. (Modified from Warner JP, Deng XH, Warren RF, et al. Static capsuloligamentous restraints to superior-inferior translation of the glenohumeral joint. *Am J Sports Med* 1992;20:675–685, with permission.)

degrees of abduction), the MGHL and the subscapularis act as secondary stabilizers, assisting the IGHLC in resisting anterior translation. The IGHLC is assisted by the SGHL in preventing inferior translation. The secondary stabilizers resisting posterior translation are infraspinatus and teres minor. With the arm at 0 degrees of abduction, the SGHL becomes the primary static stabilizer of the joint. The MGHL assists the SGHL in resisting anterior translation and the posterior capsule assists the SGHL in resisting posterior translation of the adducted humerus. Inferior translation at 0 degrees of abduction is prevented by the SGHL with assistance from the IGHLC (31).

Glenoid Labrum

The glenoid labrum is the site of the anatomic interconnection of the glenoid bone, the glenoid periosteum, the glenoid articular cartilage, the capsule, and the synovium (Fig. 24.4). The labrum serves as the site of attachment for the glenohumeral ligaments and the biceps tendon to the glenoid. The labrum is histologically composed of dense fibrous tissue with a few elastic fibers (24,32–34). This fibrocartilaginous tissue is distinct from the hyaline cartilage of the adjacent glenoid.

The inferior labrum is normally firmly attached to the underlying glenoid rim and grossly appears to be continuous with the adjacent articular cartilage. The anterosuperior labrum is more variable in its gross appearance. In up to 25% of patients, the anterosuperior labrum may appear to be detached from the underlying

the direction of the translating force being applied (Fig. 24.3) (30,31). With the arm at 45 to 90 degrees of abduction, the IGHLC takes on the role of the primary static stabilizer, resisting anterior, posterior, and inferior translation of the humeral head. In this range (45 to 90

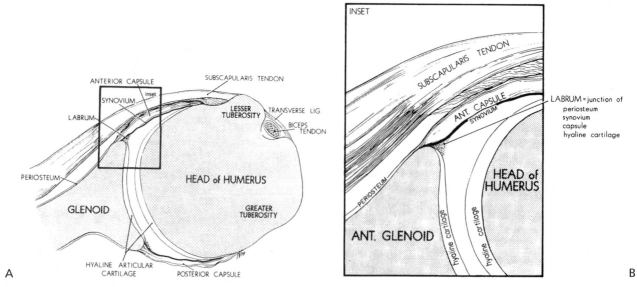

FIG. 24.4. Normal anatomy of the shoulder. **A:** A horizontal section of the glenohumeral joint. Note the close relationship of the anterior capsule and subscapularis tendon. **B:** A close-up cross-section of the anterior labrum. The labrum is made up of tissue from the adjacent hyaline cartilage, capsule, synovium, and periosteum. (From Rockwood CA, Green DP, eds. *Fractures,* 2nd ed. Vol. 1. Philadelphia: J.B. Lippincott, 1984, with permission.)

glenoid at the 1 to 3 o'clock position. This normal variant in the anterosuperior labrum is referred to as a "sublabral hole" and should not be confused with a pathologic detachment of the labrum (34). The "Buford complex" is a similar normal variant seen in approximately 1.5% of shoulders (35). When a Buford complex is present, the MGHL is present as a thickened cordlike structure that attaches to the biceps anchor, and no labral tissue is seen on the anterosuperior labrum (Fig. 24.5). The superior labrum is typically more loosely attached to the glenoid and may grossly have a more meniscal appearance than the firmly attached inferior or posterior labrum (16).

The supraglenoid tubercle lies approximately 5 mm medial to the superior rim of the glenoid. The long head of the biceps tendon inserts onto this supraglenoid tubercle and onto the superior aspect of the labrum (36). Commonly, most of the insertion appears to be into the labrum and may extend into the posterior labrum.

The blood supply of the glenoid labrum is supplied by branches of the posterior humeral circumflex artery, the suprascapular artery, and the circumflex scapular artery. The peripheral region of the labrum closest to the bone receives most of the blood supply, whereas the inner rim is relatively avascular (37). However, the nutrient vessels to the labrum do not actually arise from the underlying bone but from the surrounding capsular and periosteal vessels (37).

The glenoid labrum serves to deepen the glenoid fossa, thus adding a significant static stabilizing effect to the glenohumeral joint. Speer, Pagnani, and colleagues

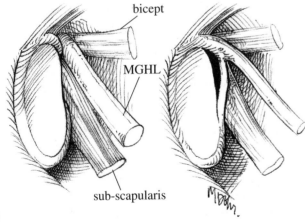

A,B

FIG. 24.5. Normal anatomic variants of the glenoid labrum. **A:** The Buford complex. The middle glenohumeral ligament (MGHL) is thickened and "cordlike" and attaches to the base of the biceps anchor. The anterosuperior labrum is absent. **B:** The sublabral hole. Present in approximately 25% of shoulders, the anterosuperior labrum is detached from the glenoid at the 1 to 3 o'clock position on the right shoulder. (Modified from Mileski RA, Snyder SJ. Superior labral lesions of the shoulder. *J Am Acad Orthop Surg* 1998;6:121–131, with permission.)

(38,39) showed that isolated labral lesions are not usually sufficient to allow glenohumeral dislocation in cadavers. However, the glenoid labrum is often seen to be injured in the athlete involved in contact sports (33,40,41). Different areas of the labrum are put at risk by different types of activities. A thorough knowledge of the anatomy of the glenohumeral joint is imperative to the understanding of the pathophysiology and treatment of these injuries.

PATHOANATOMY

Anterior Labrum

Detachment of the glenohumeral capsule and anterior labrum from the glenoid rim was proposed by Bankart (42,43) as being the essential lesion responsible for recurrent anterior glenohumeral instability. Other authors have proposed an intrasubstance tear of the anterior capsular structures is responsible for recurrent anterior instability (6,44,45). Although Bankart (43) recognized that the anterior capsule was often injured during anterior dislocation of the shoulder, he believed that the capsular injury would heal "readily and soundly." The subscapularis tendon has also been implicated as the injured structure and responsible for producing recurrent anterior instability (24–26).

The essential pathoanatomic lesion produced by anterior dislocation of the shoulder has yet to be completed elucidated. A review of the literature, performed by Lintner and Speer (1), of studies in which anterior shoulder instability was evaluated either arthroscopically or by radiologic means showed that in 400 of 472 cases a detachment of the anteroinferior capsulolabral complex (Bankart lesion) was present. Although detachment of the anterior labrum was shown to be the most common pattern of injury, it was only present in 85% of cases and cannot be considered "essential" to producing anterior instability. Furthermore, Speer et al. (39) used a cadaveric model to simulate a Bankart lesion to the anterior glenoid labrum. In this study, a 50-N anterior load was applied to the humerus and the amount of anterior translation was measured in varying degrees of shoulder abduction. An increase of 2.3 mm of anterior translation was produced at 0 degrees of abduction, and only 1.4 mm of increased anterior translation was observed with the arm in 90 degrees of abduction. The authors concluded that an isolated Bankart lesion was not capable of producing the amount of anterior glenohumeral translation necessary for an anterior dislocation to occur.

Injury to the anterior capsule and ligaments has also been implicated in producing recurrent anterior glenohumeral instability. Bigliani et al. (44) studied the ability of the IGHLC to stretch before failure. The authors were able to demonstrate that the IGHL complex failed most commonly at the glenoid insertion site (40%), followed by the midsubstance of the ligament (35%) and the humeral insertion site (25%). They also pointed out that a significant amount of stretch must occur at the ligament insertion sites, as only 35% to 45% of the overall strain was measured to occur in the ligament midsubstance.

Although detachment of the anterior labrum occurs commonly with anterior dislocation of the shoulder, it appears that this pathologic lesion alone is not capable of producing recurrent anterior instability. Stretch injury to the anterior capsular and ligamentous structures may produce plastic deformation and lengthening of these structures. Such plastic deformation obviously remains after reduction of the joint and may play a key role in producing recurrent anterior instability. Recurrent dislocations of the humeral head may produce an additive effect on the plastic lengthening of these major stabilizing structures and create even more capsular laxity and subsequent shoulder instability.

Arthroscopic assessment of the shoulder after anterior dislocation provides an excellent display of the pathoanatomy present after these injuries. As stated previously, the anterior labrum and capsule are detached from the glenoid rim approximately 85% of the time (1). At times, this anterior capsular detachment extends medially over the glenoid neck. Occasionally, an osseous or osteochondral avulsion of the anterior glenoid rim is produced.

The quality of the detached anterior labral and capsular tissues may also be observed arthroscopically. After a single traumatic anterior dislocation, these structures will often appear thick and robust. However, after chronic dislocations, the anterior capsule and labrum may acquire degenerative changes and intrasubstance injuries that cause them to appear attenuated and frayed.

The articular surface of the glenoid may also be damaged during anterior dislocation of the shoulder. Most commonly these lesions occur at the anteroinferior quadrant of the glenoid. Chronic anterior subluxation may also produce delamination injuries to the glenoid articular cartilage in this region (1).

Finally, compression fracture of the posterolateral portion of the humeral head (the Hill-Sachs lesion) should be looked for. The presence of a Hill-Sachs lesion gives the examiner an indication of the amount of force involved in producing the dislocation.

Posterior Labrum

Mair et al. (13) in reporting on nine cases of posterior glenoid labral injuries in contact athletes described detachments of the posterior glenoid labrum, which varied in size, the largest being reported as extending from the 11 o'clock position down to the 7 o'clock position on the right shoulder. In addition to being detached from the underlying glenoid, the authors reported that the posterior labrum showed signs of fraying and intrasubstance tears in all nine athletes. Articular cartilage injuries to the posterior glenoid were reported in five of the nine athletes in their study. It is important to note that all nine athletes reported in Mair's study were injured by the same mechanism of engaging an opponent with the arm in a position of forward flexion with the elbows locked in extension. Eight of the nine athletes were football lineman who repeatedly were exposed to violent contact with the arm in this provocative position. No athlete ever experienced a frank dislocation of the shoulder, and none displayed evidence of shoulder laxity in any direction (including posteriorly) on physical examination. No athlete reported in this study showed evidence of posterior capsular injury or stretch on arthroscopic examination. Similarly, no injuries were noted to the anterior labrum or inferior glenohumeral ligament.

Superior Labrum

The long head of the biceps tendon arises from the superior glenoid labrum and the supraglenoid tubercle, which lies approximately 5 mm medial to the superior apex of the glenoid rim (36). The attachment of the tendon often extends posteriorly to include a portion of the posterior labrum (36). Two distinct anatomic lesions may be seen in this area of the glenoid. The biceps anchor lesion involves avulsion of the long head of the biceps tendon from its bony anchor on the supraglenoid tubercle. The superior labrum itself may detach from the underlying glenoid, beginning posteriorly and extending anteriorly, thus creating a SLAP lesion (14). When a SLAP lesion is present, there are often signs of hemorrhage and granulation tissue beneath the biceps tendon and superior labrum. Mileski and Snyder (16) described the pathoanatomy of superior labral injuries as "the presence of a space between the articular cartilage margin of the glenoid and the attachment of the labrum and biceps anchor" (24). If traction is applied to the biceps tendon, the superior labrum may be seen to arch away from the glenoid more than 3 or 4 mm if a SLAP lesion is present (16,45). The different pathoanatomic patterns of SLAP lesions are described above under Epidemiology and Classification (Fig. 24.1).

MECHANISM OF INJURY

Anterior Labrum

Movements that produce the combination of shoulder abduction, extension, and external rotation generate forces that stress the anterior labrum and capsule, and this is the typical position seen in traumatic anterior shoulder dislocations. In anterior dislocations of the shoulder, the humeral head displaces anteriorly in relation to the glenoid. This displacement places a tensile force on the anterior capsular structures. The labrum may be pulled off the underlying glenoid. The anterior ligamentous structures and capsule sustain a sprain injury, as a result of this tensile force, which may vary in its severity. Direct impact on the proximal humerus, which may occur in contact sports, may produce an anterior subluxation of the shoulder. Such direct impact mechanisms may produce intralabral injuries or adjacent chondral injuries in the glenoid or on the humeral head at the point of contact.

Posterior Labrum

Injuries to the posterior glenoid labrum resulting from contact sports are typically produced by repetitive sheer stress applied to the posterior labrum and glenoid articular cartilage by the humeral head. These forces are created when the athlete's arm is placed in a position of forward flexion with the elbows locked in extension. Usually, the athlete (typically an offensive lineman in football) prepares him- or herself for contact with the opponent and contracts the shoulder musculature that generates compressive forces between the humeral head and glenoid. A posteriorly directed force vector is then applied to the athlete's arm by contact with the opponent, and the posterior labrum and glenoid articular cartilage are injured. Detachment of the posterior glenoid labrum that occurs as the result of contact sports appears to be a very sport-specific injury. Athletes in-

volved in violent collisions with their opponents while their arms are out in front of their bodies appear to be almost exclusively at risk. Mair et al. (13) reported on nine athletes who sustained injuries to their posterior labrums as the result of participation in contact sports in which eight were football lineman (seven offensive and one defensive). The ninth athlete was a lacrosse player who was injured when colliding with an opponent with his arm forward flexed and his elbow locked in extension while holding his stick out in front of him.

It appears that this pattern of injury to the posterior labrum is truly an "occupational hazard" of the football lineman, with a very sport-specific mechanism of injury. The National Collegiate Athletic Association produced a rule change in 1981 that allowed an offensive lineman to block with the arms fully extended and hands open while retreating. These rules were then modified in 1985 to allow this blocking technique in all situations (46). By placing the arm in this position of forward flexion and locking the elbow in extension, the posterior labrum is put at risk for injury. Muscular contraction around the shoulder in preparation for the impending contact creates compressive forces across the glenohumeral joint, and then a sheer force is applied to the posterior labrum with posteriorly directed contact to the arm.

Modified blocking techniques that place the elbow in slight flexion may help prevent these injuries. By unlocking the elbow, the triceps and pectoralis musculature may absorb some of the load applied to the arm and reduce the sheer stress being transferred to the posterior labrum (Fig. 24.6).

An acute blow to the anterior humerus is capable of

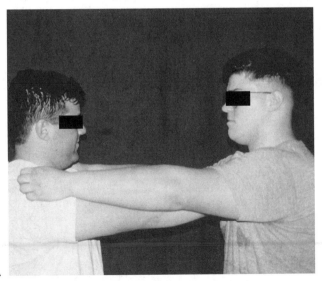
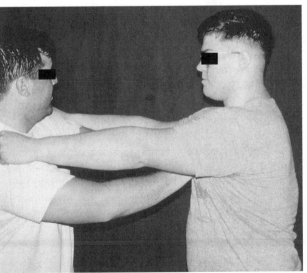

A   B

FIG. 24.6. Blocking techniques. **A:** With the player's elbows fully extended, a large shear stress is applied to the posterior labrum during contact with an opponent. **B:** By slightly flexing the elbows, the modified technique allows the player's triceps and pectoralis musculature to absorb a portion of the load and reduce the forces acting on the posterior labrum.

producing a posterior dislocation of the humeral head, along with the other well-documented mechanisms of electrocution and seizure. Although posterior dislocation of the shoulder is capable of producing an injury to the posterior glenoid labrum, these injuries are rarely seen during athletic activities, even in those sports that involve violent contact.

Superior Labrum

Most injuries to the superior glenoid labrum are produced by one of two mechanisms; traction or compression (16). Traction may be applied to the arm in either an inferior, anterior, or superior direction (17). Such traction mechanisms may occur suddenly and violently, such as during water skiing, or as the result of repetitive overhead throwing motions. The compression mechanism, which may be more common in contact sports, typically results from a fall on the outstretched arm with the arm in a position of slight abduction and forward flexion (14). Stetson et al. (15) reported that a direct blow to the shoulder was responsible for 17% of the isolated SLAP lesions seen in their series. Jones et al. (47) reported on 21 athletes with isolated SLAP lesions confirmed by diagnostic arthroscopy. Thirteen patients (62%) could recall a specific event that precipitated their injuries. Six occurred while throwing or serving (as a single event), two during a fall on the outstretched arm, two while bench pressing, two while lifting a heavy object, and one resulted from a seizure. The remaining eight patients in their study reported the insidious onset of symptoms over a period of time (between 3 months and 6 years), and the presumed mechanism of injury was thought to be repetitive microtrauma to the superior labrum in these athletic individuals.

CLINICAL EVALUATION

History

As with most musculoskeletal afflictions, diagnosis of injuries to the glenoid labrum can often be made after performing a careful history and appropriate physical examination. The history should begin with ascertaining the patient's age and chief complaint. Next, the patient's handedness, occupation, sport, and position played should be documented. Obviously, the differential diagnosis in an 18-year-old quarterback who complains of his throwing shoulder "popping out" will be different than a 35-year-old professional offensive lineman who complains of shoulder pain while bench pressing. Before focusing on the specifics of the patient's shoulder problem, it is imperative to establish whether the patient has any underlying medical conditions that may effect his or her care. It is important to document any medications the patient may be taking, along with any prior surgical

history. In addition, it is often helpful to ask if the patient has ever had any problems with the shoulder in question in the past.

Once these important details have been established in the patient's history, the examiner should begin to focus on the patient's chief complaint. The two most common chief complaints of patients with injuries of the glenoid labrum are pain and instability. Other complaints such as loss of motion, weakness, catching, or popping are typically secondary symptoms associated with either pain or instability (4). The duration of the primary complaint and its time of initial presentation must then be established. The examiner should determine whether the symptoms began after a specific single traumatic event or insidiously over an extended period of time. The onset of symptoms may be related to a change in the patient's activity level, workout program, or technique of a specific sporting activity. If the patient does associate the onset of symptoms to a specific traumatic event, it is important to document the details of this event. This includes the position of the patient's arm at the time of injury, the direction and intensity of the force applied to the arm, and how the patient was initially treated. The patient's response (or lack of response) to this initial treatment is critically important to determine.

When pain is the patient's chief complaint, it is important to characterize the nature of the pain by determining its site, time of onset, periodicity, and the presence of any radiating pain. In addition, factors that aggravate or relieve the pain should be documented. Other parameters such as the presence of night pain, the effect of analgesic medications, and an estimate of the intensity of the pain on a linear scale (e.g., "6 out of 10") should be noted. It is imperative to determine whether the patient's pain is truly originating from the shoulder or if the cervical spine is the cause of the pain. This is especially true in dealing with athletes involved in contact sports, and the examiner's history and physical examination must include a thorough evaluation of the cervical spine.

Patients with injuries to the glenoid labrum often present with pain as the chief complaint. This is especially true of patients with injuries to the superior or posterior labrum. Injuries to the anterior labrum more commonly present with instability as the chief complaint in the chronic setting. However, an acute anterior shoulder dislocation is often the cause of an anterior labral injury, and in the acute setting pain is certainly the patient's primary concern.

The most common presenting symptom in patients with injuries to the superior portion of the labrum is pain with overhead activities (14,15,17,49–52). Mechanical symptoms commonly associated with this pain include catching, popping, grinding, and locking. Mileski and Snyder (16) pointed out that the pain produced by superior labral injuries is often difficult to distinguish from impingement-type pain. SLAP-type lesions are also capable of producing symptoms such as loss of strength (17), "dead arm" symptoms (49), pain while lying on the effected shoulder (49), loss of motion, and pain with activities of daily living (52).

Injuries to the posterior labrum, occurring as the result of participation in contact sports, appear to have a very sport-specific mechanism of injury. In a report of nine athletes with posterior labral injuries by Mair et al. (13), eight athletes were football lineman (seven of these were offensive linemen). Engaging an opponent with the arm in a forward flexed position and the elbows locked in extension appears to be the common mechanism of injury in these athletes. Only two of the nine players reported by Mair et al. could recall a specific moment of injury, whereas the rest reported an insidious onset of diffuse shoulder "aching." Typically, the pain was not localized by the athletes to the posterior shoulder region. The pain was consistently described as being exacerbated by participation in contact sports and by weight lifting (specifically by the early phases of the bench-press motion). Only one of the nine athletes complained of shoulder pain with activities of daily living. The rest were symptom free when not participating in sports.

When instability is the chief complaint of the patient, it is important for the examiner to document the degree of instability (dislocation, subluxation), the direction (anterior, posterior, multidirectional), the onset (traumatic, atraumatic, overuse), and the chronicity (acute, chronic). Also, it is important to determine if the patient's instability is voluntary or involuntary in nature because a certain subgroup of voluntary dislocators may deliberately reproduce their instability and frustrate attempts at shoulder stabilization.

Although the degree of instability is usually easy to ascertain in cases of frank dislocation (the patient typically reports the shoulder "coming out" and staying out, at least for a few seconds), cases of shoulder subluxation may be more difficult for the patient to describe. Complaints of the shoulder "slipping" or feeling "loose" are common. Patients with anterior subluxation may also experience dead arm syndrome, complaining of numbness and tingling in the arm typically after throwing or when placing the arm in the provocative position of abduction and external rotation.

The direction of instability most commonly seen in athletes participating in contact sports is unidirectional anterior instability. Patients with recurrent anterior instability have been shown to have detachment of the anterior portion of the glenoid labrum in approximately 85% of cases (1). Feelings of apprehension and pain frequently are associated with complaints of instability. Apprehension may be provoked by specific activities or movements. Posterior instability may present in isola-tion or as part of a multidirectional instability pattern. However, isolated posterior instability is not common in contact athletes, even in cases of arthroscopically confirmed posterior labral injuries (13).

Physical Examination

Physical examination of the patient begins with an initial impression formulated by the examiner upon meeting the patient. Valuable information such as the patient's physiologic age, the presence or absence of generalized disease, generalized state of distress (acute or not), and overall appearance can be gained. In addition, observation of the patient's distress with shoulder motion and while performing simple tasks should be noted.

Inspection of the shoulder should then be performed. A search for muscle abnormalities (such as atrophy or winging) and the symmetry of the shoulders should be noted. On-field inspection of an injured athlete should include assessment of the integrity of the skin and soft tissues surrounding the shoulder. In an office setting, the way the arm is held or protected by the patient may provide clues about the underlying shoulder pathology.

An assessment of the active and passive range of motion of the shoulder should be performed and documented on every patient with a shoulder complaint. Inspection of the fluidity of active motion and documentation of any diskinetic or asynchronous motions (especially at the glenohumeral or scapulothoracic interface) is important. Passive motion should be tested for isolated glenohumeral elevation, external rotation with the arm in 0 and 90 degrees of abduction, and internal rotation with the arm in 90 degrees of abduction. Active internal rotation can be measured in terms of how far up the spine a patient can reach.

Next, a careful neurologic examination and muscle testing of the upper extremity should be carried out. Athletes involved in contact sports should also have a careful examination of the cervical spine performed when they present with chief complaints involving the shoulder or upper extremity.

Palpation of the shoulder and surrounding structures should then be carried out, examining for tenderness, deformity, swelling, atrophy, and temperature changes. Begin medially over the sternoclavicular joint and proceed laterally in a systematic fashion. Patients with injury to the glenoid labrum (especially the anterior and posterior labrum) may have tenderness over the joint line with deep palpation corresponding to the site of their labral injury. The nine patients reported on by Mair et al. (13) with posterior labral injuries caused by contact sports all had tenderness over the posterior joint line. Three of these athletes also were found to have tenderness over the anterior joint line.

The assessment of shoulder stability is an essential part of the physical examination in athletes with suspected injury to the glenoid labrum. This portion of the examination may be divided into two components: the assessment of the amount of passive translation of the humeral head relative to the glenoid that can be produced and the degree to which symptoms of apprehension and subluxation can be generated through provocative maneuvers.

The assessment of the degree of glenohumeral translation should begin with the patient in the sitting position and the examiner positioned beside and slightly behind the patient. Examination of the uninjured shoulder first will provide a baseline for comparison of the degree of instability present on the injured side. To assess the degree of glenohumeral translation present, it is imperative that the humeral head is in a neutral or reduced position before any displacing force is applied by the examiner. An unstable shoulder may not be concentrically reduced at the start of the examination; instead, the humeral head may lie in an anterior, posterior, or inferiorly subluxed position. Therefore, the first step in the instability examination is ensuring that the humeral head is reduced concentrically. This is accomplished by stabilizing the scapula with one hand while grasping the humeral head and applying a medially directed loading force into the glenoid fossa with the other. Once the humeral head is reduced, a displacing force may be applied (Fig. 24.7). The examiner should

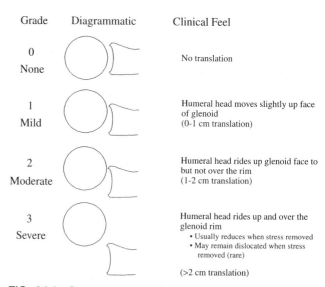

FIG. 24.8. Grading system for recording translation of the humeral head relative to the glenoid, using the load and shift test. (From Hawkins RJ, Bokor DJ. Clinical evaluation of shoulder problems. In: Rockwood CA, Matsen FA, eds. *The shoulder,* 2nd ed. Vol. 1. Philadelphia: W.B. Saunders, 1998, with permission.)

feel the humeral head gliding over the surface of the glenoid face and up the glenoid lip. As more force is applied, the humeral head may ride over the rim of the glenoid into a dislocated position.

It is most helpful to quantify the degree of translation present using a numeric grading system. The Research Committee of the American Shoulder and Elbow Surgeons published a standardized method for describing translation of the humeral head relative to the glenoid fossa (53). Using this system, instability is defined as grade 0 if completely absent, grade 1 if mild (0 to 1 cm of translation), grade 2 if moderate (1 to 2 cm of translation—up to the glenoid rim), and grade 3 if severe (more than 2 cm of translation—displacement over the glenoid rim) (Fig. 24.8).

After translating the humeral head both anteriorly and posteriorly and documenting the degree of instability present in these directions, the degree of inferior instability can then be assessed. This is accomplished by pulling inferiorly at the elbow and thus applying traction to the humerus. A "sulcus sign" may be visualized in the region just inferior to the lateral edge of the acromion if inferior instability is present (54). The space between the lateral edge of the acromion and the top of the humeral head is then palpated, and the number of centimeters between the two structures is recorded as an objective measure of inferior instability. After assessing the degree of inferior translation with the arm at the patient's side in neutral rotation, it is helpful to assess the degree of inferior translation present with the arm in 90 degrees of abduction. With the arm at the side,

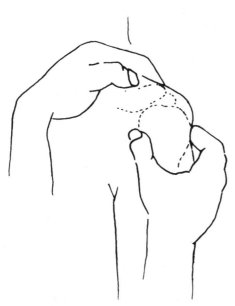

FIG. 24.7. Load and shift test. Schematic representation of the position of the examiners hands on the patient's shoulder. The examiner's left hand stabilizes the scapula, whereas the right hand initially reduces the humeral head into the glenoid and then applies a translating force to the proximal humerus. (From Hawkins RJ, Bokor DJ. Clinical evaluation of shoulder problems. In: Rockwood CA, Matsen FA, eds. *The shoulder,* 2nd ed. Vol. 1. Philadelphia: W.B. Saunders, 1998, with permission.)

in 0 degrees of abduction, the primary static restraint to inferior translation is the SGHL. However, when the arm is abducted to 90 degrees, the inferior glenohumeral ligament becomes the primary static stabilizer to inferior translation (31).

The patient should next be placed into a supine position on the examination table and the degree of anterior and posterior translation present should again be assessed. In this position the humerus is held in approximately 20 degrees of abduction and 20 degrees of forward flexion by the examiner. One hand holds the patient's elbow and applies a loading force to the humerus in the direction of the glenoid fossa and the examiner's other hand is used to grasp the patient's humeral shaft more proximally and supplies the displacing force. Again, the degree of translation is recorded using the method described above.

Other tests may be added to the stability examination that elicit apprehension of impending subluxation or dislocation with certain arm positions. The "crank test" may be used to assess the presence of anterior shoulder instability (48). This test is performed by placing the arm in a starting position of 90 degrees of abduction and neutral rotation. The arm is then externally rotated by the examiner while a gentle anterior translation force is applied to the proximal humerus. If an apprehensive feeling of impending subluxation or dislocation is elicited, the test is considered positive for anterior instability. Pain may be present, in addition to the apprehension, but the presence of pain alone without apprehension is not considered a positive test. This test may be performed in the seated or supine position.

The relocation test may add significant information to the instability examination. Initially, the crank test should be performed, and if pain or apprehension are elicited, the patient should be placed in the supine position and the test should be repeated. In this position, the edge of the examination table is used as a fulcrum and the arm is externally rotated while in a position of 90 degrees of abduction. If pain or apprehension is elicited, the amount of external rotation that produced the pain is recorded. The relocation test is then performed by applying a posterior stress to the proximal humerus with the arm in the same position of 90 degrees of abduction. The pain produced by the fulcrum test is typically relieved by this posteriorly directed force on the humerus. If a greater amount of external rotation can be achieved before symptoms are reproduced, with a posterior stress being applied to the proximal humerus, then the relocation test is considered positive for anterior instability (48,55) (Fig. 24.9). The relocation test may be quantified by the number of degrees of external rotation that are gained before symptoms are produced with the posterior force being applied to the humerus. The accuracy of the relocation test in diagnosing anterior glenohumeral instability was reported on by Speer et al. in 1994 (56), who discovered that the test was significantly more reliable when apprehension was considered as the diagnostic symptom being evaluated and less reliable when pain was used to determine instability.

The augmentation test provides similar information to the relocation test as an adjunct to the instability examination. This test is performed with the patient in the supine position, again using the examination table as a fulcrum to assist in externally rotating the arm. However, in the augmentation test, an anterior directed force is applied to the proximal humerus while the arm is being externally rotated. In cases of anterior instability, symptoms of apprehension and pain are typically elicited in fewer degrees of external rotation, when this

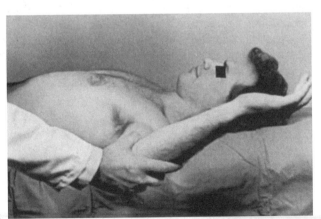
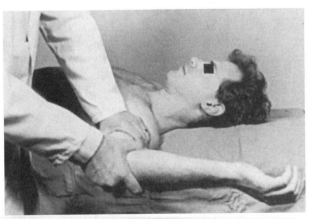

A

B

FIG. 24.9. The relocation test. **A:** The patient's abducted arm is externally rotated until pain or apprehension is felt. **B:** A posterior force is then applied to the patient's arm and the symptoms of pain and apprehension will dissipate in cases of anterior instability. Typically, the amount of external rotation attainable before pain or apprehension is produced is greater when the posterior force is being applied. (From Hawkins RJ, Bokor DJ. Clinical evaluation of shoulder problems. In: Rockwood CA, Matsen FA, eds. *The shoulder,* 2nd ed. Vol. 1. Philadelphia: W.B. Saunders, 1998, with permission.)

anterior force is applied, as compared with when no force is applied to the humerus (48).

In contrast to anterior instability, apprehension is less common and a less reliable sign when diagnosing posterior instability. Pain is the symptom that is typically elicited in patients with posterior labral injuries if the arm is forward flexed and adducted and a posterior directed force is applied to the humerus. In their study of contact athletes with injuries to the posterior labrum, Mair et al. (13) reported that all their subjects complained of pain with posterior translation of the humeral head on instability testing during the physical examination. Additionally, all patients in this study had tenderness over the posterior joint line, and they all displayed some degree of positive impingement signs on physical examination. It is important to note that despite the pain elicited by posterior translation of the humeral head, none of the patients in this study displayed increased posterior translation compared with the opposite shoulder.

Tears of the superior glenoid labrum are much more difficult to diagnose based on physical findings alone. The biceps tension test (O'Brien's test) is perhaps the best test for determining the presence of a SLAP lesion. This test is performed with the arm in a position of forward flexion, adduction, and forearm pronation. Resisted shoulder elevation is then tested in this position, and pain is usually elicited if a SLAP lesion is present. The forearm is then supinated and the test is repeated; if the pain is decreased in this position of supination, then the test is considered positive for a SLAP lesion (14).

Stetson et al. (15) reported that crepitation, snapping, or popping were present on physical examination of 43% of their patients that had isolated SLAP lesions and believed this one of the most reliable physical findings associated with injuries to the superior labrum.

The compression–rotation test may also be positive in patients with SLAP lesions (51). This test is performed with the patient in the lateral position and the arm in 90 degrees of abduction. Internal and external rotation is then applied to the humerus, and if pain is elicited, the test is considered positive for a superior labral injury.

The fact that SLAP lesions are frequently associated with injury to the rotator cuff often complicates the physical examination and creates a diagnostic dilemma (14,17,49–52). Fifty-two percent of patients with isolated SLAP lesions and no pathology of the rotator cuff visualized during arthroscopy had a positive Neer impingement sign (pain elicited by passive forward flexion of the humerus) (15). The Hawkins sign (pain elicited by forward flexion of the humerus to 90 degrees and internal rotation of the arm) is also frequently present in patients with isolated SLAP lesions and in patients with rotator cuff pathology.

Patients with damage to the superior glenoid labrum may also display signs of pain and apprehension, typically associated with anterior shoulder instability, during the crank or fulcrum test. Stetson et al. (15) reported that 39% of their patients with isolated SLAP lesions reported pain with abduction and external rotation of the humerus but only 4% displayed a decrease in their pain during the relocation test. The authors propose that this pain may be generated by traction on the torn superior labrum rather than true anterior instability.

IMAGING

Plain Radiographs

Radiographic evaluation of the shoulder with a suspected glenoid labral injury should begin with plain x-rays. The recommended views include an anteroposterior view of the glenohumeral joint, an axillary view, a West Point view, and Stryker notch view.

In cases of anterior dislocation or subluxation, there may be evidence of bony damage to the glenoid rim or calcification of the soft tissues adjacent to the anteroinferior glenoid. A true anteroposterior view of the glenohumeral joint will more reliably reveal fractures of the inferior glenoid than will an anteroposterior view taken in the plane of the thorax. The axillary view may also be useful in demonstrating bony pathology of the anterior glenoid. Rokous et al. (57) described a modified axillary roentgenogram of the shoulder (the West Point view) that provides a better look at the anteroinferior portion of the glenoid (Fig. 24.10). This portion of the glenoid is important to visualize in cases of anterior subluxation, because it may be the only area of the shoulder displaying plain radiographic evidence of pathology. The West Point view is obtained by placing the patient prone on the x-ray table with the arm abducted to 90 degrees and the involved shoulder elevated off of the table approximately 8 cm using a pad. The cassette is placed against the superior shoulder and the head is turned

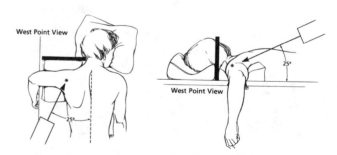

FIG. 24.10. West Point view. This view provides visualization of the anteroinferior glenoid rim. (From Rockwood CA, Jensen KL. X-ray evaluation of shoulder problems. In: Rockwood CA, Matsen FA, eds. *The shoulder,* 2nd ed. Vol. 1. Philadelphia: W.B. Saunders, 1998, with permission.)

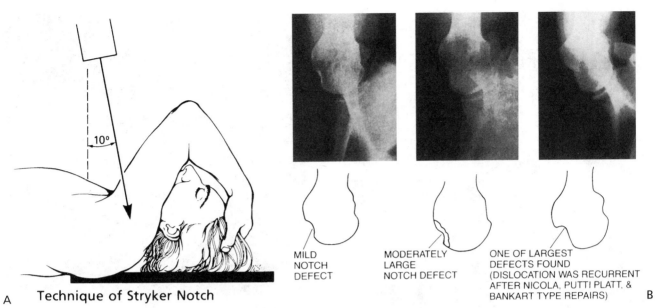

A   Technique of Stryker Notch

MILD NOTCH DEFECT

MODERATELY LARGE NOTCH DEFECT

ONE OF LARGEST DEFECTS FOUND (DISLOCATION WAS RECURRENT AFTER NICOLA, PUTTI PLATT, & BANKART TYPE REPAIRS)

B

FIG. 24.11. Stryker Notch view. **A:** Positioning of the patient to obtain a view of the posterolateral humeral head. **B:** Defects are seen in the posterolateral portion of the humeral head of three patients with recurrent anterior shoulder instability. (From Rockwood CA, Jensen KL. X-ray evaluation of shoulder problems. In: Rockwood CA, Matsen FA, eds. *The shoulder,* 2nd ed. Vol. 1. Philadelphia: W.B. Saunders, 1998, with permission.)

away from the involved side. The x-ray beam is centered on the axilla with 25 degrees of downward angulation from the horizontal and 25 degrees of medial angulation from the midline. A tangential view of the anteroinferior glenoid is obtained.

Compression fractures of the posterolateral humeral head (Hill-Sachs lesions [58]), which are frequently associated with anterior shoulder dislocations, are best viewed using the Stryker notch view (Fig 24.11) (59). The Stryker notch view is obtained by placing the palm of the hand of the affected shoulder on the top of the patients head, with the fingers pointing toward the back of the head. The cassette is place under the affected shoulder, and the x-ray beam is centered over the coracoid and directed 10 degrees cephalad. If a Hill-Sachs lesion is present, a distinct notch will be seen in the posterolateral portion of the humeral head. Hill-Sachs lesions may also be visualized on anteroposterior views with the arm in full internal rotation or occasionally on the axillary lateral view (60).

Posterior dislocations of the glenohumeral joint are frequently misdiagnosed as a result of inadequate radiographic evaluation of the shoulder. X-rays must be obtained in at least two planes, oriented 90 degrees to each other, when evaluating the injured shoulder. The two most common plain radiographic findings accompanying posterior dislocation of the glenohumeral joint include a compression fracture of the anteromedial humeral head (the ''reverse Hill-Sachs lesion'') and damage to the posterior glenoid rim. The posterior glenoid is best visualized using an axillary view. Often, computed tomography (CT) is helpful in defining posterior glenoid pathology and the extent of the compression fracture of the humeral head (60).

Injuries to the superior glenoid labrum rarely display any abnormality on plain radiographs; however, these lesion are often associated with occult instability of the shoulder, and evidence of this should be looked for (16).

Special Studies

Injuries to the glenoid labrum very often display no plain radiographic changes. Therefore, special examinations are frequently needed to help delineate the extent of labral pathology (Figs. 24.12, 24.13, 24.14, and 24.15).

An arthrogram of the shoulder joint is capable of detecting some displaced labral injuries in the shoulder. Contrast material will be seen adjacent to the glenoid rim and neck if a defect is present in the labrum. Arthrotomography has been shown, by multiple authors, to be more reliable in revealing the displaced labrum and capsular stripping associated with anterior glenohumeral instability than standard arthrography (61–64). CT arthrography has also been used to successfully diagnose glenoid labral injuries (65–68) but is generally better suited for detecting bony abnormalities than soft tissue pathology.

Magnetic resonance imaging (MRI) is currently widely used to evaluated suspected glenoid labral pathology. It provides a noninvasive alternative to arthro-

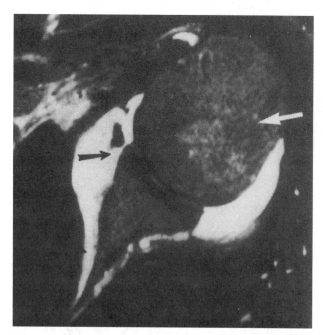

FIG. 24.12. Axial T2-weighted magnetic resonance image performed after an acute anterior dislocation of the shoulder. *Black arrow* indicates avulsion of the anterior glenoid labrum with stripping of the capsule off the glenoid neck. *White arrow* points to marrow edema in the region of a Hill-Sachs lesion. (From Linter SA, Speer KP. Traumatic anterior glenohumeral instability. *J Am Acad Orthop Surg* 1997;5:233–239, with permission.)

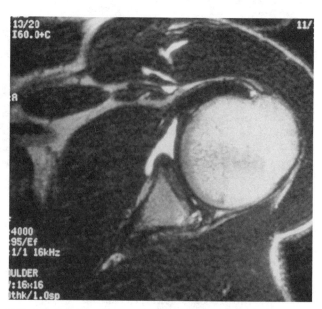

FIG. 24.14. Magnetic resonance image displaying high signal intensity in the area of the damaged posterior glenoid labrum.

graphic techniques and uses no ionizing radiation. In addition, the multiplanar views provided and the ability to evaluate other structures within the shoulder, such as the rotator cuff, make MRI extremely useful to the physician evaluating the painful shoulder. Unfortu-

nately, the reported sensitivity of MRI for detecting glenoid labral lesions has varied widely. Flannigan et al. (69) reported a 44% sensitivity and Chandnani a 46% sensitivity using conventional MRI to detect labral injury. This is in contrast to the report of Legan et al. (73) of a 95% sensitivity using MRI. Reported specificities for the use of MRI in defining labral injuries have also varied from 68% to 90% (69–73).

Gadolinium (74) or saline (75) MR arthrography has

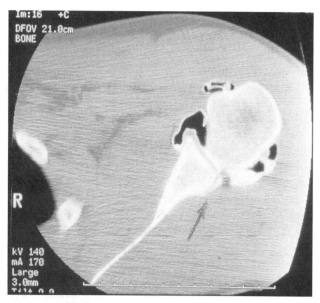

FIG. 24.13. Computed tomography demonstrating a tear of the posterior glenoid labrum (*arrow*).

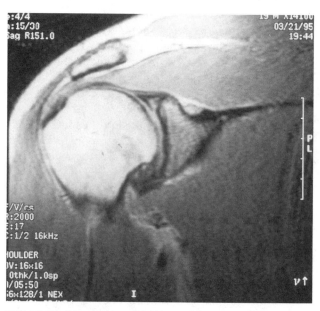

FIG. 24.15. Magnetic resonance image demonstrating a tear in the superior glenoid labrum.

been used in an attempt to increase the sensitivity and specificity of MRI in evaluating glenoid labral pathology.

Chandnani performed a prospective study demonstrating that MR arthrography provided superior results compared with CT arthrography when examining the labrum. Mileski and Snyder now recommend the use of MR arthrography in cases of suspected superior labral injury when conventional MRI fails to display pathology in this region. Radiologic findings that may indicate a labral lesion include high signal between the labrum and the glenoid rim, high signal intensity in the superior labrum–biceps anchor, displacement of the labrum, deformity, and the presence of a labral cyst (76). Despite the improved results obtained with MR arthrography, Davidson and Speer (77) showed that both MR arthrography and conventional MRI provide limited diagnostic information important to planning the patients surgical treatment. Diagnostic arthroscopy still remains the gold standard in defining glenoid labral pathology.

TREATMENT OPTIONS

Anterior Labrum

Nonoperative Treatment

Injuries to the anterior labrum produced by contact sports are typically the result of an acute traumatic anterior shoulder dislocation. Acute dislocations should be reduced as expeditiously as possible to minimize the amount of muscle spasm that must be overcome to obtain a reduction and to relieve the stretch being applied to the neurovascular structures around the shoulder. Ideally, a complete radiographic evaluation is performed before reduction to determine whether any associated bony abnormalities exist. The reduction should be performed in as gentle a manner as possible, with anesthesia used as needed.

Although many reduction techniques have been described in the literature, the authors prefer to use the traction/countertraction method (Fig. 24.16). This method of reduction is performed with the patient in the supine position. A sheet is wrapped around the patient's upper body, under the axilla of the dislocated shoulder. An assistant stands on the opposite side of the table and supplies a stabilizing countertraction force, whereas the surgeon applies traction to the dislocated arm. It is important to bend the elbow of the dislocated arm while applying traction to reduce the stretch on the neurovascular structures. Traction may be applied either directly or through a sheet wrapped around the flexed forearm. The arm is slightly flexed and abducted while the traction is applied and a gentle internal and external rotation motion may be added to facilitate reduction.

Once a reduction of the acute anterior dislocation

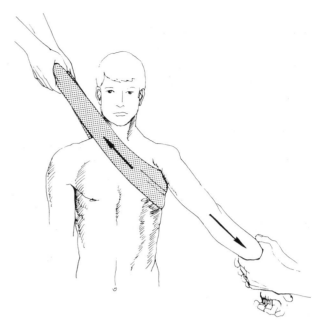

FIG. 24.16. Traction/countertraction closed reduction maneuver for anterior shoulder dislocations. (From Rockwood CA, Green DP. *Fractures,* 2nd ed. Vol. 1. Philadelphia: J.B. Lippincott, 1984, with permission.)

has been effected, a decision must be made as to how the patient will be treated. Acute traumatic anterior shoulder instability has historically been treated in a conservative manner. After obtaining a reduction of the acutely dislocated shoulder, the arm is typically placed into a sling for a variable amount of time. Multiple authors have reported unacceptably high recurrence rates with this form of treatment (Table 24.1). McLaughlin and Cavallaro (4) reporting on 573 patients treated conservatively after acute anterior shoulder dislocations found a 90% recurrence rate in patients less than 20 years old, 60% recurrence in 20 to 40 year olds, and 10% recurrence in patients over 40 year olds. Similarly, Rowe (78) reported a 94% recurrence rate in patients less than 20 years of age and a 74% recurrence rate in 20 to 40 year olds. An 88% recurrence rate after conservative management of anterior dislocations was reported by Henry and Genung (5), and Arciero et al.

TABLE 24.1. *Recurrence rates after nonoperative treatment of anterior shoulder dislocations*

Author	Journal	Year	Recurrence rate (%)
McLaughlin	*Am J Surg*	1950	90
Rowe	*Orthop Clin N Am*	1980	94
Henry	*Am J Sports Med*	1982	88
Simonet and Cofield	*Am J Sports Med*	1984	66
Arciero	*Am J Sports Med*	1994	80

(7) reported an 80% recurrence rate in 15 athletes with an average age of 20 years.

Recurrent anterior instability after closed treatment of an acute anterior shoulder dislocation must be viewed as a treatment failure. Patients with recurrent anterior shoulder instability often experience a severe functional disability. This is especially true of the athlete involved in contact sports. These athletes typically fall into the age ranges that experience the highest rates of redislocation after conservative treatment. Tsai et al. (8) reported that nearly 60% of patients with recurrent anterior instability of the shoulder complained of pain, decreased strength, and poor range of motion after closed treatment of acute dislocations. The 66% to 94% recurrence rates reported in the studies listed in Table 24.1 have led many surgeons to seek alternate forms of treatment for acute anterior shoulder dislocations.

Surgical Treatment

Operative treatment of anterior shoulder instability, regardless of the technique used, should obtain the following goals:

1. Prevent recurrent instability;
2. Maintain normal glenohumeral joint motion and mechanics;
3. Minimize postoperative morbidity;
4. Prevent complications;
5. Return the patient to the preinjury level of activity;
6. Give reproducible results (1).

Regardless of the technique used, the surgeon should strive to consistently meet all of these goals. The first decision when choosing the technique used for a given patient is whether an open or arthroscopic reconstruction will best suit the patient and his or her pathology.

Arthroscopic Treatment

Arthroscopic anterior stabilization procedures focus on reattaching the avulsed anterior labrum and anterior capsular structures back onto the glenoid rim (Fig. 24.17). Many different types of arthroscopic repair techniques have been described in the literature, and the results obtained postoperatively often vary widely between techniques, depending on the type of fixation used.

Staple fixation of the anterior labrum and capsule was initially used to treat anterior shoulder instability in open procedures. Perthes was the first to use this method of fixation in 1906 (79). The staples used for arthroscopic anterior labral repairs are smaller than those used in open repairs. During the arthroscopic reconstructions, the staples are passed into the joint with the aid of cannulas. The results obtained with techniques using staples as the mode of anterior capsulolabral fixation have been unacceptably poor regardless of whether the staples are inserted arthroscopically or using open techniques (80–83). Rates of recurrence of anterior instability as high as 46% with arthroscopic staple fixation have been reported (82). In addition, a high percentage of

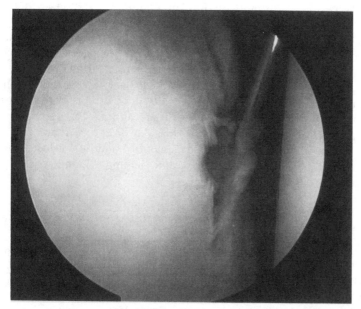
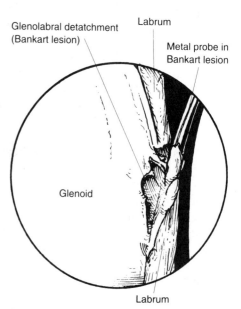

FIG. 24.17. Arthroscopic view of the anterior labrum from the posterior portal with the patient in the beach-chair position. A classic Bankart lesion (detachment of the anteroinferior labrum from the glenoid) is displayed. (From Linter SA, Speer KP. Traumatic anterior glenohumeral instability. *J Am Acad Orthop Surg* 1997;5:233–239, with permission.)

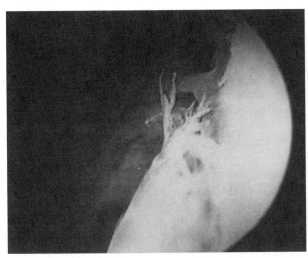
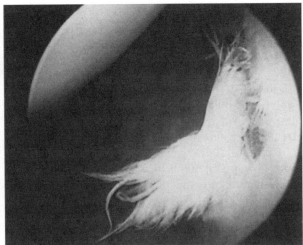

FIG. 24.18. Arthroscopic view of an anterior labrum displaying intrasubstance labral injury and poor tissue quality. Such an injury would not be considered amenable to arthroscopic labral repair. (From Linter SA, Speer KP. Traumatic anterior glenohumeral instability. *J Am Acad Orthop Surg* 1997;5:233–239, with permission.)

patients in multiple studies had complications relating directly to the staples themselves (80–83). In general, the use of staples as a means of anterior capsulolabral fixation has been abandoned.

Arthroscopic suture fixation of the avulsed anterior labrum and capsule is another alternative in the treatment of anterior shoulder instability. The technique was initially described by Morgan and Bodenstab in 1987 (84). A Beath pin was used to pass the sutures through the glenoid, from anterior to posterior, and then to reapproximate the anterior labrum and capsule. In a cohort study of 25 patients, followed for an average of 17 months, the authors reported a 100% success rate using this technique (84). A similar technique was used by McIntyre and Caspari (85), which used multiple sutures passed through the glenoid and then tied posteriorly over the infraspinatous fascia. After following this group for 33 months, the authors reported an 8% rate of recurrent anterior instability. In contrast to these good results, other groups using arthroscopic suture fixation have reported rates of recurrent instability as high as 42% and 44%, with 2- and 3-year follow-up (86,87). Factors associated with failure in these studies included shorter periods of postoperative immobilization, a history of multiple dislocations, and poor tissue quality of the anterior labrum and capsule (Fig. 24.18).

Suture anchors may be placed arthroscopically in the glenoid rim and provide the advantage of allowing the avulsed anterior structures to be repaired while avoiding having to pass a pin through the glenoid, which carries the risk of injury to the suprascapular nerve. Additionally, newer techniques using suture anchors allow patulous anterior capsular structures to be advanced and tightened with repair to the anterior glenoid. Wolf (88)

reported excellent results on 50 patients with short-term follow-up having only a 2% recurrence rate.

Bioabsorbable tack fixation, performed arthroscopically, provides the advantage of avoiding complications associated with the use of metal implants, such as staples (Fig. 24.19). Speer et al. (89) reported on a group of 52 patients, with an average follow-up of 42 months, and observed a 21% rate of recurrent instability. No complications were reported relating to the use of the bioabsorbable tacks. In the eight patients in this study who underwent open anterior reconstruction procedures for recurrent instability, all eight were found to have patulous anterior capsules that were not visualized arthroscopically. Five patients were found to have rotator cuff interval defects. Interestingly, in seven of the eight cases that underwent open anterior reconstruction, the Bank-

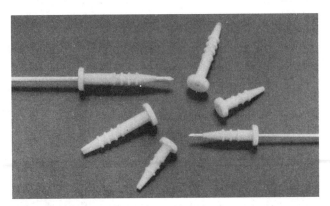

FIG. 24.19. Cannulated tack designed with a ribbed shaft and broad flat head. (From Speer KP, Warren RF. Arthroscopic shoulder stabilization—a role for biodegradable materials. *Clin Orthop* 1993;291:67–74, with permission.)

art lesion was found to be healed, and the recurrent instability was blamed on the redundancy in the anterior capsule.

Arciero et al. (7) presented a prospective study analyzing the use of nonoperative treatment versus arthroscopic Bankart suture repair for acute, traumatic, first-time, anterior shoulder dislocations in young athletes. Patients were divided into two groups. Group I patients were treated with sling immobilization for 1 month followed by physical therapy and return to full activity at 4 months. Group II patients were treated with arthroscopic Bankart repair and then underwent the same protocol as the group I patients. The authors reported an 80% rate (12/15 patients) of recurrent anterior instability in group I, with 7 of the 12 patients requiring open Bankart repairs to treat their recurrent instability. In group II, 86% (18/21 patients) had no recurrent instability at an average of 32 months follow-up. Thus, arthroscopic Bankart repair of the anterior labrum was shown to significantly reduce the rate of recurrent anterior instability in young athletes who had sustained acute, traumatic, initial dislocations.

Open Surgical Treatment

Although the rate of recurrent instability is significantly lower in patients treated with arthroscopic stabilization procedures compared with those treated conservatively, the failure rate of these arthroscopic reconstructions is still unacceptably high. A review of the world literature analyzing the results of 2,300 patients who had undergone various methods of open anterior shoulder reconstruction has shown a 3% average rate of recurrence (90). Rowe et al. (91) reported a 3.5% recurrence rate after open Bankart repair of the anterior structures. Thus, open anterior reconstruction must be considered the standard upon which we judge the success of other forms of treatment of anterior shoulder instability.

Although many methods of open anterior shoulder reconstruction have been described in the literature, currently accepted methods attempt to achieve anatomic repair of the avulsed capsule and labrum to the anterior rim of the glenoid. This is often referred to as a Bankart repair (42,43). This type of repair was actually first performed by Perthes in 1906. He recommend repair of the avulsed anterior capsule to the anterior labrum using suture passed through drill holes in the glenoid rim. Bankart (43) then popularized the procedure, and the Bankart repair performed today is based on his 1938 report. He discussed careful dissection of the subscapularis muscle in exposing the anterior capsule and reapproximation of the tendon later in the case without shortening. Sutures were passed through drill holes in the anterior glenoid neck to repair the avulsed capsule and labrum. This procedure was performed on 27 patients, and Bankart was impressed by the fact that

no recurrent dislocations were seen and that full motion was gained in each case postoperatively.

Although several changes have been made to Bankart's original method, we have come to appreciate the tremendous benefit of anatomic restoration of the anterior structures in providing stability without limiting motion.

Although arthroscopic repair of an anterior labral avulsion can produce reliable healing of the labrum (89), far lower recurrence rates have been reported using open techniques (90). Any redundancy or plastic deformation of the anterior capsule (which may be present after anterior dislocation and contribute to recurrent instability) is difficult to correct using current arthroscopic techniques but can be reliably improved with most open anterior reconstructive techniques.

Authors' Preferred Treatment

One of the primary goals in the treatment of the athlete with anterior shoulder instability is to prevent recurrent instability. With this in mind, we have adopted a treatment algorithm aimed at preventing recurrent instability and returning the athlete to his or her prior level of activity. Initially, the patient's instability must be classified as either traumatic or atraumatic. If the instability is atraumatic in origin and surgical treatment is elected, open reconstruction is the treatment of choice. Anterior shoulder instability of traumatic origin may be further broken down into unidirectional and multidirectional instability. If multidirectional instability is present, open reconstruction is, once again, the best treatment option. Cases of traumatic unidirectional instability must then be divided into acute and recurrent groups. The recurrent group is served best by open anterior shoulder reconstruction. The acute, traumatic, unidirectional instability group should undergo diagnostic arthroscopy to assess whether a Bankart lesion is present or not (Fig. 24.17). If no Bankart lesion is seen or if there is a Bankart but the quality of the detached anterior labral tissue is thought to be poor (Fig. 24.18), then the procedure should be converted to open and an anterior reconstruction should be performed. If the patient is found to have acute, traumatic, unidirectional, anterior shoulder instability with a Bankart lesion of good tissue quality, then an arthroscopic anterior labral repair can be performed (Fig. 24.20). Therefore, athletes involved in contact sports who sustain a first-time anterior shoulder dislocation are the ideal candidates for arthroscopic stabilization of their Bankart lesions. Arciero et al. (7) showed that the recurrence rate of anterior instability after arthroscopic Bankart repair is significantly lower than the rate of recurrence after conservative treatment. However, arthroscopic Bankart repair has not displayed the same success rates as open anterior reconstruction in cases involving atraumatic, multidirectional, or recur-

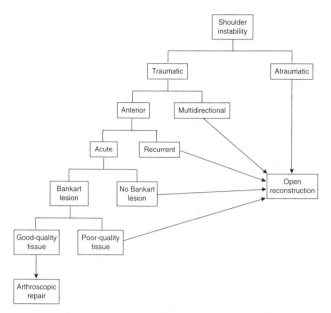

FIG. 24.20. Treatment algorithm depicting the authors' recommendations for the management of anterior glenohumeral instability. (From Lintner SA, Speer KP. Traumatic anterior glenohumeral instability. *J Am Acad Orthop Surg* 1997;5: 233–239, with permission.)

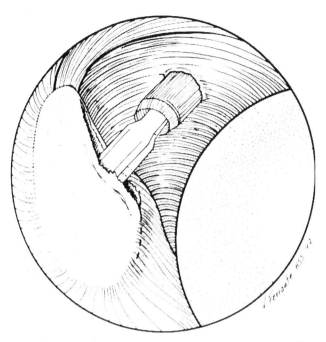

FIG. 24.21. The anterior–inferior glenoid rim is prepared by abrading it with a rasp that is introduced into the joint through an anterior portal. (From Speer KP, Warren RF. Arthroscopic shoulder stabilization—a role for biodegradable materials. *Clin Orthop* 1993;291:67–74, with permission.)

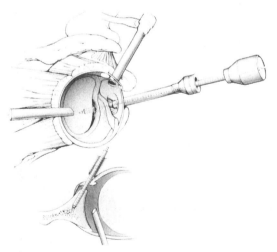

FIG. 24.22. (Top) All instruments for the insertion of the bioabsorbable tack are brought into the joint through a cannula placed in the anterior–inferior portal. **(Bottom)** This diagram displays how the cannulated drill first skewers the labrum and then creates a tunnel in the glenoid at the margin of the articular cartilage. The drill is introduced into the glenoid at an oblique angle, pointing away from the articular surface. (From Speer KP, Warren RF. Arthroscopic shoulder stabilization—a role for biodegradable materials. *Clin Orthop* 1993; 291:67–74, with permission.)

rent instability. A history of multiple dislocations, poor tissue quality (86,87), or the presence of a patulous capsule (89) have been implicated as potential causes for the increased rate of recurrent instability seen after arthroscopic repair. We believe it is imperative to strictly follow the treatment algorithm proposed when deciding whether or not a patient will benefit from an arthroscopic or open surgical procedure.

If the patient is thought to meet the criteria for arthroscopic anterior labral repair (i.e., acute, traumatic, unidirectional anterior shoulder instability with a Bankart lesion of good tissue quality), then the procedure begins with an examination under anesthesia. Diagnostic arthroscopy is then performed, and the presence or absence of a Bankart lesion is determined. The quality of the anterior capsular and labral tissue is then assessed. Initially, standard posterior and anterior–superior portals are used. If an arthroscopic repair is to be pursued, an anterior–inferior portal is established. The anterior glenoid rim is prepared using a rasp and power shaver to remove any fibrous tissue from this region and to expose an area of bleeding cancellous bone in this region (Fig. 24.21). The cannulated drill for the absorbable tack is inserted through the anterior inferior portal, and the detached anterior–inferior labrum is skewered on the drill (Fig. 24.22). A drill hole is made on the anterior glenoid rim at the chondral margin, and a guidewire is placed through the drill and into the pilot hole. The guidewire is held in place and the drill is then removed. The absorbable tack (SURETAC, Acufex Microsurgi-

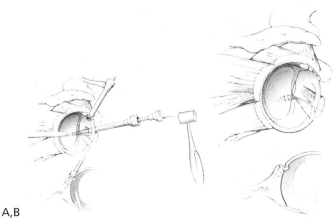

A,B

FIG. 24.23. A: The cannulated tack is driven over the guidewire with the arm in neutral rotation and 0 degrees of abduction. **B:** The final construct is examined arthroscopically to ensure adequate position of the soft tissue to the bone. (From Speer KP, Warren RF. Arthroscopic shoulder stabilization—a role for biodegradable materials. *Clin Orthop* 1993;291:67–74, with permission.)

cal, Norwood, MA) is then passed over the guidewire to secure the labrum back down to the glenoid (Fig. 24.23).

Postoperative Rehabilitation

Postoperative physical therapy after arthroscopic repair of anterior labral lesions with bioabsorbable tacks is broken down into four 4-week phases. During phase I (0 to 4 weeks) the patient is kept in a sling at all times, except when performing specific exercises to work on wrist and elbow motion and grip strength. No active or passive shoulder elevation is allowed. Phase II (4 to 8 weeks) begins to work on glenohumeral motion, beginning with passive range of motion exercises and progressing to active range of motion toward the end of phase II. Abduction and external rotation should be avoided in the early postoperative period after repair of the anterior labrum. The goal is to achieve full passive range of motion of the glenohumeral joint by 8 weeks postoperatively, but not sooner. Sling wear is discouraged (except when needed as a visible sign of vulnerability in an uncontrolled environment). Aquatic therapy is begun, and active range of motion is started with the shoulder submerged. At 6 weeks postoperatively, the patient may begin light manual periscapular and rotator cuff strengthening. Phase III (8 to 12 weeks) involves progressive strengthening of the rotator cuff and periscapular muscles and full active range of motion is sought. Phase IV (12 weeks or more) of the rehabilitation program maximizes strength of the rotator cuff, periscapular muscles, and humeral movers (deltoid, latissimus, pectoralis). Functional training to progress back to work or sports is undertaken.

Posterior Labrum

Nonoperative Treatment

Posterior labral injuries that occur as a result of contact sports typically respond poorly to conservative management. In the study by Mair et al. (13) study of nine contact athletes who sustained injuries to the posterior glenoid labrum, none of the patients displayed any significant improvement from a trial of a minimum of 6 weeks of physical therapy for rotator cuff and periscapular strengthening and nonsteroidal anti-inflammatory drugs. All nine patients complained of continued pain with bench press and inability to participate in their contact sports effectively. However, only one patient complained of pain with daily activities, whereas the rest of the patients were symptom free when not participating in their contact sports. Therefore, retirement from contact sports can be a very successful form of treatment if the athlete is inclined to pursue this option.

Surgical Treatment

Arthroscopy can play a dual role in the patient with a suspected injury to the posterior glenoid labrum. Diagnosis may be confirmed at the time of arthroscopy, and satisfactory treatment has been reported using arthroscopic techniques (13) (Fig. 24.24). Arthroscopic findings may include detachment of the labrum from the glenoid to varying degrees. The posterior capsule typically shows no sign of injury. Likewise, the anterior and inferior labrum rarely shows signs of concomitant damage. In Mair et al.'s study (13), five of nine patients displayed significant chondral damage to the posterior one third of the glenoid surface. In addition, all nine patients showed signs of intrasubstance damage to the detached

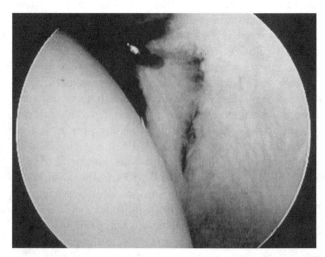

FIG. 24.24. Arthroscopic view of a posterior labral tear with the arthroscope in the anterior portal and the probe in the posterior portal.

posterior labrum, with either fraying or midsubstance tears being present.

Authors' Preferred Treatment

We prefer the beach chair position for arthroscopic treatment of posterior labral injuries. Standard posterior and anterior arthroscopy portals are established, and then a diagnostic arthroscopy is performed with the arthroscope initially in the posterior portal. The camera is then switched to the anterior portal to facilitate surgical manipulation of the posterior labrum through the posterior portal. The posterior glenoid rim is prepared in the area of the labral detachment using a rasp to expose a bleeding bony bed in this region. A cannulated drill is used to spear the posterior labrum, through the posterior portal, and then a drill hole is made at the chondral margin of the posterior glenoid rim. A guidewire is placed through the cannulated drill and left in place after the drill is removed. Then a polyglycolate bioabsorbable tack (SURETAC, Acufex Microsurgical) is impacted over this guidewire under direct arthroscopic visualization, thus securing the posterior labrum back to the glenoid. Typically, either one or two tacks are used, depending on the extent of posterior labral involvement.

Postoperative Rehabilitation

After an arthroscopic surgical repair of the posterior glenoid labrum has been performed, the patient is typically placed in a sling for 4 weeks postoperatively. At 4 weeks, active and passive range of motion exercises are begun. Motion is restricted to 40 degrees of external rotation, 140 degrees of elevation, and internal rotation to the first lumbar vertebrae. Rotator cuff and periscapular strengthening is also initiated at 4 weeks. At 8 weeks, full range of motion is allowed, and the strengthening program is continued. Formal upper body weight lifting is allowed beginning at 12 weeks with particular attention given to triceps and pectoralis strengthening. At 16 weeks, contact sports may be resumed. Before returning to play, football linemen are counseled to modify their blocking techniques and encouraged to block with their elbows slightly flexed. This position allows the upper body musculature to absorb much of the load of impact and decreases the sheer forces exerted on the posterior labrum.

Using the arthroscopic technique and postoperative rehabilitation program outlined above, Mair et al. (13) were able to return all nine of their patients back to participation in contact sports. At an average follow-up of 30 months, all nine patients had obtained full range of motion of the shoulder. All patients were able to resume bench pressing without pain, and all patients were able to return to full contact participation in their sports. There were no episodes of recurrence of symptoms reported.

Superior Labrum

Nonoperative Treatment

Conservative treatment of SLAP lesions is generally unsuccessful (16). If the athlete's symptoms are only experienced while participating in their sport, then activity modification and possible retirement from the sport may be considered in the recreational athlete. However, the mechanical symptoms and pain associated with SLAP lesions typically do not resolve over time, and most surgeons now resort to arthroscopic treatment of symptomatic injuries to the superior labrum.

Surgical Treatment

The first step in the operative treatment of SLAP lesions is an examination of the shoulder under anesthesia to search for the presence of occult instability. Occult instability of the shoulder has been cited as a potential cause of treatment failure in patients who have undergone arthroscopic debridement of SLAP lesions (16). One study of 27 patients with SLAP lesions reported a 70% rate of instability on examination under anesthesia despite the fact that none of the patients had a history of dislocation or symptoms of clinical instability (92).

After a careful examination under anesthesia has been completed, diagnostic arthroscopy should be performed, because it will allow the surgeon to accurately classify the type of SLAP lesion present. It is imperative to make an accurate classification at the time of diagnostic arthroscopy because the subsequent treatment will be entirely dependent on the type of lesion present and on the presence or absence of damage to any other structures within the shoulder. Once the lesion has been classified, a decision must be made whether to simply debride the involved labral tissue or to attempt to repair it.

Debridement of superior labral lesions has provided unreliable symptomatic relief with long-term follow-up. Cordasco et al. (92) reported on 27 patients with SLAP lesions treated with arthroscopic debridement alone. Although 78% reported excellent pain relief at 1-year follow-up, the percent of satisfactory results decreased with time, as only 63% had excellent pain relief after 2-year follow-up. In addition, only 45% of patients were able to return to their previous level of athletic activity after simple debridement of their SLAP lesions. These unsatisfactory results were attributed to the presence of occult instability associated with the superior labral injuries in 70% of these patients.

If the decision is made to proceed with a reattachment of the avulsed labrum and biceps anchor, a method of fixation must be chosen. Several types of implants have been used for this purpose, including metal screws, staples, sutures, and absorbable tacks.

Metal screws were used by Resch et al. (49) in their study of 18 patients with SLAP lesions. A 2.7-mm cannulated titanium screw with a 5-mm washer was used to stabilize six of these superior labral injuries. Eight patients were stabilized with absorbable tacks having 6.5-mm head diameters. The remaining four labral injuries were simply debrided. The patients were followed for 6 to 30 months, and 8 of 14 patients who had undergone labral repair returned to their sport and were participating at a preinjury level. Four of the 14 patients who had undergone repair of their detached labrums reported an improvement postoperatively but had not returned to their preinjury level of sports performance. Two repaired patients showed no improvement postoperatively, and only one of the four patients who had undergone debridement reported any improvement.

Staples were used by Yoneda et al. (52) to repair 10 superior labral injuries in athletes. The staples were removed at 3 to 6 months postoperatively during repeat arthroscopy, and at that time four patients showed signs of complete healing and six patients displayed superficial healing but good stability of the repaired labral tissue. The patients were followed for a minimum of 24 months postoperatively, and 80% obtained good or excellent results. No complications were attributed to the use of the staple, but the need for a second procedure to remove the staple led the authors to recommend a bioabsorbable implant in the future.

Field and Savoie (51) used a transosseous suture technique to repair 20 SLAP lesions. Fifteen were classified as type II and 5 as type IV lesions. A suture punch was used to place 2-0 PDS sutures into the avulsed superior labrum and biceps tendon, and a Beath pin was used to pass the sutures through the glenoid neck. The Beath pin was initially passed through the anterior portal, and a hole was drilled at the 1 o'clock position (for the right shoulder), through the glenoid neck, and into the infraspinatus fossa. The sutures were then tied over the infraspinatus fascia. All 20 patients received good or excellent ratings, using the Rowe scoring system, at 12- to 42-months follow-up. Six patients were throwing athletes and were able to return to their sports without limitations. No long-term complications were attributed to the subcutaneous sutures. One patient did develop adhesive capsulitis, but this was treated successfully with closed manipulation, and a good long-term result was obtained.

Snyder et al. (50) reported that 6% of their patients who underwent diagnostic glenohumeral shoulder arthroscopy between 1985 and 1993 were noted to have injuries to the superior labrum. The results of their treatment of 140 patients with SLAP lesions demonstrated the high rate of concomitant injuries within the shoulder

in these patients. Bankart lesions were noted to be present in 22% of their patients, whereas 29% had partial rotator cuff tears and 11% had full-thickness rotator cuff tears. Only 28% of the patients were diagnosed with isolated SLAP lesions. The labral injuries were treated in a variety of ways, and the high rate of associated pathologic changes within the shoulders makes interpretation of the treatment results in this report difficult. However, several important points were revealed in this large study. Type II SLAP lesions were shown to be the most common pattern encountered, with 55% of the total, followed by type I (21%), type IV (10%), type III (9%), and 5% complex patterns. Eighteen patients underwent second-look arthroscopy. When examining the type II lesions, three of five patients treated with labral debridement and glenoid abrasion were noted to have healed, compared with four of five patients who healed after absorbable tack repair of their type II injuries. Five reoperations were indicated because of fragmentation of the bioabsorbable tacks.

Stetson et al. (15) later presented a study of 23 patients with isolated SLAP lesions and an average 3.8-year follow-up. Ten patients were treated with debridement of the labral injuries (this group was composed of all four types of SLAP, including 6 type IIs.) Twelve type II lesions were treated with suture anchor labral repair, and one complex type II–III was treated with a combination of debridement and repair. Good or excellent results were reported in 82% of the patients. Snyder currently recommends repair of type II SLAP lesions using a screw type suture anchor.

Authors' Preferred Method

The treatment algorithm for injuries to the superior glenoid labrum is based on the type of SLAP lesion present. After careful physical examination under anesthesia, looking specifically for signs of glenohumeral instability, diagnostic arthroscopy is performed to classify the pattern of superior labral injury and document an concomitant pathology. Type I lesions are debrided arthroscopically. Currently, type II lesions are repaired using either suture anchors or absorbable tacks (Fig. 24.25). Type III lesions are treated with debridement and excision of the bucket-handle portion of the labral tear. The extent of involvement of the biceps tendon will dictate the treatment option chosen for type IV lesions. If less than 30% of the diameter of the biceps tendon is involved in the tear, then the torn portion of the tendon may be resected along with the damaged labrum. If the tear of the tendon involves more than 30%, then a decision must be made whether to attempt fixation of the tendon and torn labrum to the glenoid rim or to proceed with debridement of the labrum and tenodesis of the damaged biceps tendon.

Tenodesis is performed by releasing the tendon,

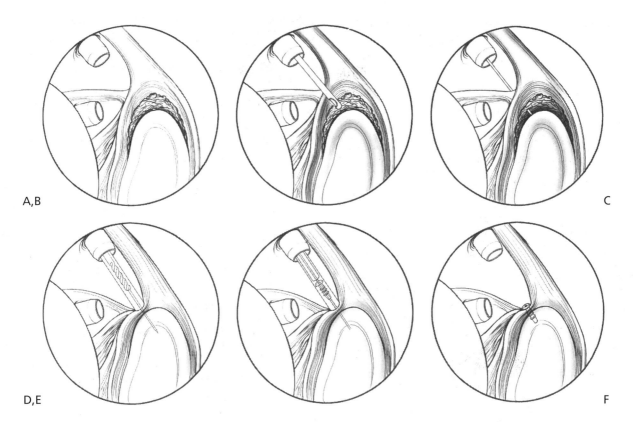

FIG. 24.25. Arthroscopic repair of a type II SLAP lesion. **A:** Avulsion of the superior labrum and biceps anchor. **B:** Shaver is used to prepare the bone along the superior rim of the glenoid. **C:** A guidewire is used to spear the superior labral tissue and biceps anchor. **D:** A cannulated drill is passed over the guidewire to create the bone tunnel for the tack. **E and F:** The tack is placed over the guidewire and impacted into position. (From Peterson CA, Altchek DW, Warren RF. Shoulder Arthroscopy. In: Rockwood CA, Matsen FA, eds. *The shoulder,* 2nd ed. Vol. 1. Philadelphia: W.B. Saunders, 1998, with permission.)

arthroscopically, at its insertion on the glenoid using an electrocautery probe brought into the shoulder through the anterior portal. Once the tendon is released, the proximal stump is debrided using the arthroscopic shaver. A mini-open incision is then made just lateral to the lateral edge of the acromion and the deltoid muscle is split in-line with its fibers. The transverse humeral ligament is incised through its midline, and the distal end of the released biceps tendon is found in the bicipital groove. A screw-in metal suture anchor is then placed in the base of the bicipital groove, and the no. 2 suture attached to the anchor is used to secure the tendon to the humeral head.

If repair of a type II SLAP lesion is elected, this is performed arthroscopically. A standard posterior arthroscopy portal is used for visualization, and a standard anterior–superior portal is used for insertion of the absorbable tack. Initially, the superior neck of the glenoid is debrided using a shaver, and the rim may be lightly decorticated using a rasp or burr. Once the bed has been prepared, the superior labrum is speared using the cannulated drill bit of the bioabsorbable tack. A guide hole is then drilled in the superior glenoid, at the chondral margin. A guidewire is placed through the cannulated drill bit, into the guide hole, and the guidewire is left in place after the drill is removed. A polyglycolate bioabsorbable tack (SURETAC, Acufex Microsurgical) is then inserted over the guidewire to secure the superior labrum and biceps tendon to the glenoid.

Postoperative Rehabilitation

Postoperative rehabilitation after arthroscopic repair of superior labral lesions using bioabsorbable tacks is very similar to arthroscopic repair of anterior labral lesions using the same fixation, and the reader is referred to the previous section on anterior labral postoperative rehabilitation for details of the protocol. Basically, the patient is kept in a sling full time for the first 4 weeks postoperatively. Passive range of motion is started at 4 weeks along with progression to active range of motion, supervised by the therapist. Light strengthening exercises are begun at 6 weeks. Full passive range of motion should be attained by 8 weeks, but not sooner. Progressive strengthening and active range of motion is then carried out over the ensuing weeks.

REFERENCES

1. Lintner SA, Speer KP. Traumatic anterior glenohumeral instability: the role of arthroscopy. *J Am Acad Orthop Surg* 1997;5: 233–239.
2. Hovelius L, Eriksson K, Fredin H, et al. Recurrences after initial dislocation of the shoulder: results of a prospective study of treatment. *J Bone Joint Surg Am* 1983;65:343–349.
3. Cave EF, Burke JF, Boyd RJ. *Trauma management.* Chicago: Year Book Medical Publishers, 1974:437.
4. McLaughlin HL, Cavallaro WU. Primary anterior dislocation of the shoulder. *Am J Surg* 1950;80:615–621.
5. Henry JH, Genung JA. Natural history of glenohumeral dislocation—revisited. *Am J Sports Med* 1982;10:135–137.
6. Simmonet WT, Cofield RH. Prognosis in anterior shoulder dislocations. *Am J Sports Med* 1984;12:19–24.
7. Arciero RA, Wheeler JH, Ryan JB, et al. Arthroscopic Bankart repair versus nonoperative treatment for acute, initial anterior shoulder dislocations. *Am J Sports Med* 1994;22:589–594.
8. Tsai L, Wredmark T, Johansson C, et al. Shoulder function in patients with unoperated anterior shoulder instability. *Am J Sports Med* 1991;19:469–473.
9. Matsen FA, Thomas SC, Rockwood CA, et al. Glenohumeral instability. In: Rockwood CA, Matsen FA, eds. *The shoulder,* 2nd ed. Philadelphia: W.B. Saunders, 1998.
10. Mestdagh H, Maynou C, Delobelle JM, et al. Traumatic posterior dislocation of the shoulder in adults. A propos of 25 cases. *Ann Chir* 1994;48:355–363.
11. Pavlov H, Warren RF, Weiss CB, et al. The roentgenographic evaluation of anterior shoulder instability. *Clin Orthop* 1985; 194:153–158.
12. Rowe CR, Zarins B. Chronic unreduced dislocations of the shoulder. *J Bone Joint Surg Am* 1982;64A:494–505.
13. Mair SD, Zarzour RH, Speer KP. Posterior labral injuries in contact athletes. *Am J Sports Med* 1998;26:753–758.
14. Snyder SJ, Karzel RP, DelPizzo W, et al. SLAP lesions of the shoulder. *Arthroscopy* 1990;6:274–279.
15. Stetson WB, Snyder SJ, Karzel RP, et al. Long term clinical follow-up of isolated SLAP lesions of the shoulder. Presented at the 65th Annual Meeting of the American Academy of Orthopaedic Surgeons.
16. Mileski RA, Snyder SJ. Superior labral lesions in the shoulder. *J Am Acad Orthop Surg* 1998;6:121–131.
17. Maffet MW, Gartsman GW, Moseley B. Superior labrum-biceps tendon complex injuries of the shoulder. *Am J Sports Med* 1995;23:93–98.
18. Kazar B, Relovsky E. Prognosis of primary dislocation of the shoulder. *Acta Orthop Scand* 1969;40:216–224.
19. Freeman BL. Recurrent dislocations. In: Crenshaw AH, ed. *Campbell's operative orthopaedics,* 8th ed. St. Louis: Mosby-Year Book, 1992:1408.
20. Simkin PA. Structure and function of joints. In: Schumacher HR, ed. *Primer on the rheumatic diseases,* 9th ed. Atlanta: Arthritis Foundation, 1988.
21. Habermeyer P, Schuller U, Wiedemann E. The intra-articular pressure of the shoulder: an experimental study on the role of the glenoid labrum in stabilizing the joint. *Arthroscopy* 1992; 8:166–172.
22. Poppen NK, Walder PS. Forces at the glenohumeral joint in abduction. *Clin Orthop* 1978;135:165–170.
23. Lippitt S, Matsen FA. Mechanisms of glenohumeral joint stability. *Clin Orthop* 1993;291:20–28.
24. Moseley HF, Overgaard B. The anterior capsular mechanism in recurrent anterior dislocation of the shoulder: morphological and clinical studies with special reference to the glenoid labrum and glenohumeral ligaments. *J Bone Joint Surg Br* 1962;44:913–927.
25. Symeonides PP. The significance of the subscapularis muscle in the pathogenesis of recurrent anterior dislocation of the shoulder. *J Bone Joint Surg Br* 1972;54:476–483.
26. Turkel SJ, Panio MW, Marshall JL, et al. Stabilizing mechanisms preventing anterior dislocation of the glenohumeral joint. *J Bone Joint Surg Am* 1981;63:1208–1217.
27. DePalma AF, Cooke AJ, Prabhakar M. The role of the subscapularis in recurrent anterior dislocations of the shoulder. *Clin Orthop* 1967;54:35–49.
28. O'Brien SJ, Neves MC, Arnoczky SP, et al. The anatomy and histology of the inferior glenohumeral ligament complex of the shoulder. *Am J Sports Med* 1990;18:449–456.
29. Schwartz RE, O'Brien SJ, Warren RF, et al. Capsular restraints to anterior-posterior motion of the shoulder [abstract]. *Orthop Trans* 1988;12:727.
30. Pagnani MJ, Warren RF. Acute injuries of the shoulder. In: Griffin LY, ed. *Orthopaedic knowledge update: sports medicine.* Rosemont, IL: American Academy of Orthopaedic Surgeons, 1994.
31. Warner JJP, Deng XH, Warren RF, et al. Static capsuloligamentous restraints to superior-inferior translation of the glenohumeral joint. *Am J Sports Med* 1992;20:675–685.
32. Gardner E. The prenatal development of the human shoulder joint. *Surg Clin North Am* 1963;43:1465–1470.
33. Townley CO. The capsular mechanism in recurrent dislocation of the shoulder. *J Bone Joint Surg Am* 1950;32:370–380.
34. Cooper DE, Arnoczky SP, O'Brien SJ, et al. Anatomy, histology, and vascularity of the glenoid labrum: an anatomical study. *J Bone Joint Surg Am* 1992;74:46–52.
35. Williams SM, Snyder SJ, Buford D Jr. The Buford complex—the "cord-like" middle glenohumeral ligament and absent anterosuperior labrum complex: a normal anatomic capsulolabral variant. *Arthroscopy* 1994;10:241–247.
36. Vangsness CT, Jorgenson SS, Watson T, et al. The origin of the long head of the biceps from the scapula and glenoid labrum. An anatomical study of 100 shoulders. *J Bone Joint Surg Br* 1994;76:951–954.
37. Arnoczky SP, Allen AA. The microvasculature of the glenoid labrum in the human shoulder. Unpublished data.
38. Pagnani MJ, Deng XH, Warren RF, et al. Effect of lesions of the superior portion of the glenoid labrum on glenohumeral translation. *J Bone Joint Surg Am* 1995;77:1003–1010.
39. Speer KP, Deng XH, Borrero S, et al. Biomechanical evaluation of a simulated Bankart lesion. *J Bone Joint Surg Am* 1994;76:1819–1826.
40. Reeves B. Arthrography in acute dislocations of the shoulder. *J Bone Joint Surg Br* 1968;48:182.
41. Reeves B. Acute anterior dislocation of the shoulder. *Ann R Coll Surg Engl* 1969;43:255.
42. Bankart ASB. Recurrent or habitual dislocation of the shoulder joint. *Br Med J* 1923;2:1132–1133.
43. Bankart ASB. The pathology and treatment of recurrent dislocation of the shoulder joint. *Br J Surg* 1938;26:23–29.
44. Bigliani LU, Pollock RG, Soslowsky LJ, et al. Tensile properties of the inferior glenohumeral ligament. *J Orthop Res* 1992;10: 187–197.
45. Snyder SJ. *Shoulder arthroscopy.* New York: McGraw-Hill, 1994:31–33, 122.
46. Atlantic Coast Conference, personal communication, Speer KP.
47. Jones CK, Speer KP, Mann C. The clinical evaluation of unstable SLAP Lesions. Submitted to *Clin J Sports Med.*
48. Hawkins RJ, Bokor DJ. Clinical evaluation of shoulder problems. In: Rockwood CA, Matsen FA, eds. *The shoulder,* 2nd ed. Philadelphia: W.B. Saunders, 1998:164–196.
49. Resch H, Goser K, Thoeni H, et al. Arthroscopic repair of superior glenoid labral detachment (the SLAP lesion). *J Shoulder Elbow Surg* 1995;4:243–248.
50. Snyder SJ, Banas MP, Karzel RP. An analysis of 140 injuries to the superior glenoid labrum. *J Shoulder Elbow Surg* 1995;4:243–248.
51. Field LD, Savoie FH III. Arthroscopic suture repair of superior labral detachment lesions of the shoulder. *Am J Sports Med* 1993;21:783–790.
52. Yoneda M, Hirooka A, Saito S, et al. Arthroscopic stapling for detached superior glenoid labrum. *J Bone Joint Surg Br* 1991;73:746–750.
53. Richard RR, et al. A standardized method for the assessment of shoulder function. *J Shoulder Elbow Surg* 1994;3:347–352.
54. Neer CS, Foster CR. Inferior capsular shift for involuntary inferior

and multidirectional instability of the shoulder: a preliminary report. *J Bone Joint Surg Am* 1980;62:897–908.

55. Boublik M, Silliman JF. History and physical examination. In: Hawkins FJ, Misamore GW, eds. *Shoulder injuries in the athlete.* New York: Churchill Livingstone, 1984:9–22.

56. Speer KP, Hannafin JA, Altchek DW, et al. An evaluation of the shoulder relocation test. *Am J Sports Med* 1994;22:177–183.

57. Rokous JR, Feagin JA, Abbott HG. Modified axillary roentgenogram. *Clin Orthop* 1972;82:84–86.

58. Hill HA, Sachs MD. The grooved defect of the humeral head: a frequently unrecognized complication of dislocations of the shoulder joint. *Radiology* 1940;35:690–700.

59. Hall RH, Isaac F, Booth CR. Dislocations of the shoulder with special reference to accompanying small fractures. *J Bone Joint Surg Am* 1959;41:489–494.

60. Rockwood CA, Jensen KL. X-ray evaluation of shoulder problems. In: Rockwood CA, Matsen FA, eds. *The shoulder,* 2nd ed. Philadelphia: W.B. Saunders, 1998.

61. Albright J, El Khoury G. Shoulder arthrotomography in the evaluation of the injured throwing arm. In: Zarins B, Andrews JR, Carson WG Jr, eds. *Injuries to the throwing arm.* Philadelphia: W.B. Saunders, 1985:66–75.

62. Braustein EM, O'Connor G. Double contrast arthrotomography of the shoulder. *J Bone Joint Surg Am* 1982;64:192–195.

63. Kleinmann PK, Kanzaria PK, Goss TP, et al. Axillary arthrotomography of the glenoid labrum. *AJR Am J Roentgenol* 1984;141:993–999.

64. Pappas AM, Goss TP, Kleinmann PK. Symptomatic shoulder instability due to lesions of the glenoid labrum. *Am J Sports Med* 1983;11:279.

65. Shuman WP, Kilcoyne RF, Matsen FA III, et al. Double-contrast computed tomography of the glenoid labrum. *AJR Am J Roentgenol* 1983;141:581–584.

66. Janke AH, Petersen SA, Neumann C, et al. A prospective comparison of computerized arthrotomography and magnetic resonance imaging of the glenohumeral joint. *Am J Sports Med* 1992;20:695–701.

67. Nottage WM, Duge WD, Fields WA. Computed arthrotomography of the glenohumeral joint to evaluate anterior instability: correlation with arthroscopic findings. *Arthroscopy* 1987;3:273–276.

68. Rafii M, Minkoff J, Bonamo J, et al. Computed tomography (CT) arthrography of shoulder instabilities in athletes. *Am J Sports Med* 1988;16:352–361.

69. Flannigan B, Kursunoglu-Brahme S, Snyder S, et al. MR arthrography of the shoulder: comparison with conventional MR imaging. *AJR Am J Roentgenol* 1990;155:829–832.

70. Kieft GJ, Bloem JL, Rozing PM, et al. MR imaging of recurrent anterior dislocation of the shoulder: comparison with CT arthrography. *AJR Am J Roentgenol* 1988;150:1083–1087.

71. Coumas JM, Waite RJ, Goss TP, et al. CT and MR evaluation of the labral capsular ligamentous complex of the shoulder. *AJR Am J Roentgenol* 1992;158:591–597.

72. Neumann CH, Petersen SA, Jahnke AH. MR imaging of the labral-capsular complex: normal variations. *AJR Am J Roentgenol* 1991;157:1015–1021.

73. Legan JM, Burkhard TK, Goff WB, et al. Tears of the glenoid labrum: MR imaging of 88 arthroscopically confirmed cases. *Radiology* 1991;179:241–246.

74. Chandnani BP, Yeager TD, Deberardino T, et al. Glenoid labral tears: prospective evaluation with MR imaging, MR arthrography, and CT arthrography. *AJR Am J Roentgenol* 1993;161:1220–1235.

75. Tirman PF, Stauffer AE, Crues JV, et al. Saline magnetic resonance arthrography in the evaluation of glenohumeral instability. *Arthroscopy* 1993;9:550–559.

76. Tirman PF, Feller JF, Janzen DL, et al. Association of glenoid labral cysts with labral tears and glenohumeral instability: radiologic findings and clinical significance. *Radiology* 1994;190:653–658.

77. Davidson JJ, Speer KP. Clinical utility of high resonance imaging and MR arthrography of the shoulder. AAOS Shoulder Meeting, Atlanta, Georgia, February 1996.

78. Rowe CR. Acute and recurrent anterior dislocations of the shoulder. *Orthop Clin North Am* 1980;11:253–270.

79. Perthes G. Uber Operationen bei habitueller Schulterluxation. *Dtsch Z Chir* 1906;85:199–227.

80. Ward WG, Bassett FH III, Garrett WE Jr. Anterior staple capsulorrhaphy for recurrent dislocation of the shoulder: a clinical and biomechanical study. *South Med J* 1990;83:510–518.

81. O'Driscoll SW, Evans DC. Long-term results of staple capsulorrhaphy for anterior instability of the shoulder. *J Bone Joint Surg Am* 1993;75:249–258.

82. Cook M, Richardson AB. Arthroscopic staple capsulorrhaphy for treatment of anterior shoulder instability [abstract]. *Orthop Trans* 1991;15:1.

83. Matthews LS, Better WL, Oweida SJ, et al. Arthroscopic staple capsulorrhaphy for recurrent anterior shoulder instability. *Arthroscopy* 1988;4:106–111.

84. Morgan CD, Bodenstab AB. Arthroscopic Bankart suture repair: technique and early results. *Arthroscopy* 1987;3:111–122.

85. McIntyre LF, Caspari RB. The rationale and technique for arthroscopic reconstruction of anterior shoulder instability using multiple sutures. *Orthop Clin North Am* 1993;24:55–58.

86. Green MR, Christensen KP. Arthroscopic Bankart procedure. Two to five year follow-up with clinical correlation to severity of glenoid labral lesion. *Am J Sports Med* 1995;23:276–281.

87. Grana WA, Buckley PD, Yates CK. Arthroscopic Bankart suture repair. *Am J Sports Med* 1993;21:348–353.

88. Wolf EM. Arthroscopic capsulolabral repair using suture anchors. *Orthop Clin North Am* 1993;24:59–69.

89. Speer KP, Warren RF, Pagnani M. An arthroscopic technique for anterior stabilization of the shoulder with a bioabsorbable tack. *J Bone Joint Surg Am* 1996;78:1801–1807.

90. Rockwood CA Jr. Part 2. Dislocations about the shoulder. In: Rockwood CA, Green DP, eds. *Fractures,* 2nd ed. Vol. 1. Philadelphia: J.B. Lippincott, 1984.

91. Rowe CR, Patel D, Southmayd WW. The Bankart procedure—a study of late results. *J Bone Joint Surg Br* 1977;59:122.

92. Cordasco FA, Steinmann S, Flatow EL, et al. Arthroscopic treatment of glenoid labral tears. *Am J Sports Med* 1993;21:425–431.

Principles and Practice of Orthopaedic Sports Medicine,
edited by William E. Garrett, Jr., Kevin P. Speer, and Donald T. Kirkendall.
Lippincott Williams & Wilkins, Philadelphia © 2000.

CHAPTER 25

Labral Tears in Throwing Sports

James R. Andrews, John H. (Russ) Fairbanks, Kevin E. Wilk,
Glenn S. Fleisig, and Martin L. Schwartz

When we examine the subjectively painful yet objectively normal shoulder in the throwing athlete, often there is functional or microinstability present that is not manifested on physical examination; consequently, a high index of suspicion should be entertained. In decreasing frequency, the pathologic conditions most commonly found in the throwing shoulder are glenoid labrum tears, partial-thickness undersurface rotator cuff tears, glenohumeral impingement, subacromial instability, biceps tendon tears, and bony abnormalities, such as a posterior glenoid exostosis (1). Anatomic instability is addressed in other chapters of this text.

EPIDEMIOLOGY

In 1941, Bennett (2) first reported on the painful throwing shoulder in professional athletes. His series demonstrated anterior lesions such as biceps tendon tears and subacromial pathology. Also mentioned was a posteroinferior exostosis of the glenoid, thought to be a secondary phenomenon due to tissue stresses during the deceleration phase of the pitch. In 1969, King et al. (3) reported increased external rotation and decreased internal rotation of the glenohumeral joint as a rather uniform finding in professional pitchers. In 1978, Barnes and Tullos (4) reported on shoulder pain in 56 pitchers of which 29 had anterior lesions, including tendonitis of the biceps, supraspinatus, pectoralis major, and latissi-

mus dorsi, and acromioclavicular joint abnormalities. Posterior lesions were found radiographically in eight patients.

In 1983, Pappas et al. (5) described "functional instability" as lesions of the glenoid labrum that allow the shoulder to click, catch, and lock secondary to partially detached fragments becoming interposed between the articular surfaces. This differs from "anatomic instability" commonly apparent as recurrent subluxation or dislocation.

In 1983, Jobe and Jobe (6) termed "microinstability" as subtle often subclinical patterns of laxity about the shoulder that lead to abnormal translation and hence accelerated wear. Jobe and Kvitne (7) also contributed to understanding of forces involved in the throwing shoulder that lead to degenerative changes in the rotator cuff.

Arthroscopy has significantly advanced understanding of the painful throwing shoulder. Andrews and Carson (8) described superior glenoid labrum tears in 1984. Their preliminary arthroscopic study of 73 throwers demonstrated anterosuperior labral tears in 83%, partial rotator cuff tears in 45%, and long head of biceps tears in 10%. Other studies have shown similar rates of correlated pathology (9,10). Indeed, single isolated lesions have proven to be uncommon.

In 1990, Snyder et al. (11) classified superior glenoid labrum injury with the term superior labrum anterior to posterior (SLAP) lesions. Thrower's exostosis has received scant attention in the literature since Bennett's report more than 55 years ago (2).

MECHANISM OF INJURY, PATHOANATOMY, AND ASSOCIATED PATHOLOGY

Normal Anatomy and Microanatomy

Moseley and Övergaard (12) described the glenoid labrum as a fibrocartilaginous transition tissue, which is

J. R. Andrews: Department of Orthopaedic Surgery, University of Alabama at Birmingham Medical School, Birmingham, Alabama 35205.
J. H. (Russ) Fairbanks: Orthopaedic Center of Natchez, Natchez, Mississippi 39120
K. E. Wilk and M. L. Schwartz: HealthSouth Medical Center, Birmingham, Alabama 35205.
G. S. Fleisig: American Sports Medicine Institute, Birmingham, Alabama 35205.

a redundant continuation of the joint capsule as it attaches to the osseous glenoid rim. Prodromos et al. (13) found decreasing labrum vascularity with age. Cooper et al. (14) described the glenoid labrum as a peripherally elevated part of the glenoid rim and also described the labrum as having much more fibrous tissue than cartilage. By definition, the superior labrum is the segment between the 10 and 2 o'clock position on the glenoid and frequently resembles a meniscus. It has a loose attachment to the superior glenoid tubercle. At the 12 o'clock position is a 5-mm extension of hyaline cartilage, which projects medially onto the superior glenoid. Beginning at the medial boundary of the hyaline articular cartilage is the supraglenoid tubercle. The biceps tendon becomes confluent with the glenoid labrum, inserting into the supraglenoid tubercle. There is a synovial reflection in that location that creates a small recess beneath the biceps tendon and the superior part of the labrum.

The anterosuperior part of the glenoid labrum has a

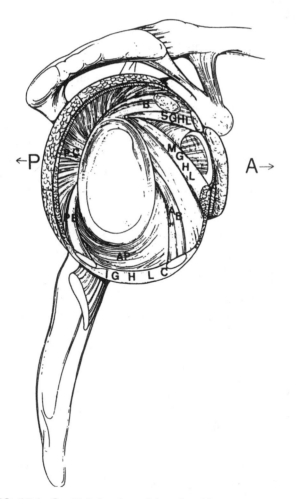

FIG. 25.1. Sagittal drawing of the glenoid, glenoid labrum, and associated capsular structures. (From Peat M, Culham E. Functional anatomy of the shoulder complex. In: Andrews JR, Wilk KE, eds. *The athlete's shoulder.* New York: Churchill Livingstone, 1994:1–13, with permission.)

meniscal shape. Its fibers insert into the middle or inferior glenohumeral ligament rather than into the actual glenoid margin in many specimens. In this area, there can be either no attachment to the glenoid rim or attachment by only a layer of thin capsular tissue. Posteriorly, the mobile superior part of the labrum is anchored and more rounded at the 10 o'clock position in half of the specimens. In the remainder, it is meniscal and more loosely attached (Fig. 25.1).

Variations on normal superior labrum anatomy should not be confused with pathologic conditions. Peripheral labrum attachment is the norm. Central labrum attachment is variable. In 12% of shoulders there is a sublabral foramen anteriorly. A Buford complex occurs in 1.5% of glenoid labrae, seen as a cordlike middle glenohumeral ligament that attaches to the labrum slightly anterior to the biceps tendon and also demonstrates a sublabral foramen (15).

Vascular supply to the superior labrum is peripheral, as in a meniscus (16). It arises from capsular and periosteal vessels rather than from the underlying bone. In the superior and anterosuperior labrum, vascularity is diminished relative to other regions of the labrum. Densely packed collagen bundles constitute the labral stroma. Mobility and a loose attachment of the labrum proximal to the glenoid equator are normal findings. Anatomic variation of the superior glenoid labrum is considered to be the rule rather than the exception.

The Normal Pitch

The pitching motion has been studied biomechanically and divided into phases (17). These phases include wind-up, stride, arm cocking, arm acceleration, arm deceleration, and follow-through. It is important to realize that pitching is a continuous activity, broken into phases only for analytical purposes. Motion analysis (18–21) and electromyographic studies (22–26) have further defined this complex phenomenon. Knowledge of a fully functioning normal shoulder provides insight into the painful throwing shoulder (Fig. 25.2).

Wind-up

Pitching is a downhill throw from a mound with a vertical height of 10 inches. Wind-up starts with a two-legged stance and ends with maximum knee lift of the lead leg. It is a phase of balance and kinetic preparation occupying nearly 60% of pitch time. As body weight is shifted posteriorly, the lead leg is flexed. Simultaneously, the hands are in front of the chest with ball in the glove. Forces about the shoulder are minimal in this preparatory phase, which ends when the ball leaves the glove.

Stride

In the stride phase, upper extremity elastic energy is stored as both arms abduct and begin to separate from

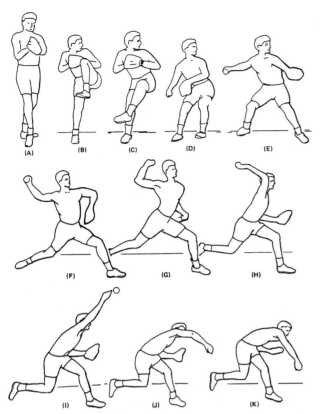

FIG. 25.2. The six phases of pitching: wind-up **(A–C)**, stride **(C–F)**, arm cocking **(F–H)**, arm acceleration **(H–I)**, arm deceleration **(I–J)**, and follow-through **(J–K)**. (From Dillman CJ, Fleisig GS, Andrews JR. Biomechanics of pitching with emphasis upon shoulder kinematics. *J Orthop Sports Phys Ther* 1993;18:402–408, with permission.)

delivery. Repetitive throwing causes increased capsular laxity with resultant increased external rotation of the shoulder. Another important variable is lever arm length as biomechanically longer limbed throwers have an advantage over shorter limbed throwers regarding pitch velocity. Therefore, genetically speaking, taller throwers with hypermobile joints are favored for pitch speed.

Motion analysis of the arm cocking phase has revealed a critical instant of forces. Average positions include elbow flexion of 95 degrees, arm external rotation of 170 degrees, and arm abduction of 94 degrees. Loads at the shoulder calculate to 67 N-m internal rotation torque, 380 N of anterior shear force, 250 N of superior shear force, and 480 N of compressive force during this critical instant (Fig. 25.3).

Electromyography of the early arm-cocking phase reveal that the trapezius and serratus anterior position the glenoid through scapular protraction and upward rotation at 60% of maximal voluntary isometric contraction (MVIC). These scapular stabilization forces also couple with the deltoids and supraspinatus to abduct the arm. The supraspinatus not only serves with the deltoid in abduction but also maintains centralization of the humeral head.

During late arm cocking when humerus external rotation reaches maximum levels, the subscapularis, pectoralis major, and latissimus dorsi greatly increase activity as "anterior wall" muscles, thus contributing to anterior joint stability. Furthermore, serratus anterior, infraspinatus, and teres minor activities reflect MVIC values of 106%, 74%, and 70%, respectively. These muscle actions

each other. External rotation is initiated in the throwing shoulder. The deltoid, supraspinatus, upper trapezius, and serratus anterior are all active during the stride phase. Kinetic energy builds as the lead leg moves toward the target. The stride phase ends when the lead foot contacts the ground.

Arm Cocking

Arm cocking begins at lead foot contact and ends with maximal shoulder external rotation. Upper extremity elastic energy accumulation continues during the arm cocking phase. With the shoulder abducted 90 degrees and the elbow flexed 90 degrees, maximal external rotation of the humerus reaches limits of between 150 and 180 degrees (arm cocking). The elbow begins to extend. The ball reaches its furthermost position behind the body; hence, elastic energy peaks. As the lead foot plants, kinetic energy is imparted into the system as the pelvis and upper torso rotate to face the target.

Shoulder motion is a prime variable in velocity development as with increasing increments of external rotation, greater amounts of elastic energy are stored for ball

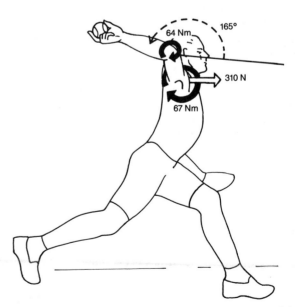

FIG. 25.3. During arm cocking, the first critical instant of the pitch occurs. (From Fleisig GS, Andrews JR, et al. Kinetics of baseball pitching with implications about injury mechanisms. *Am J Sports Med* 1995;23:233–239, with permission.)

provide external rotation and counteract humeral head anterior translation. Loading of these muscles is for the most part eccentric. During late arm cocking, biceps contraction peaks, whereas supraspinatus activity diminishes.

Arm Acceleration

The arm acceleration phase is extremely short, beginning with humerus internal rotation and ending with ball release. During arm acceleration, kinetic energy from the trunk is passed to the upper extremity. Musculature of the shoulder not only transmits this energy but also builds upon it. Extension of the elbow increases ball velocity in two ways. First, linear velocity is directly increased as a result of extension. Second, the angular velocity of shoulder internal rotation is augmented because extending the elbow reduces the amount of inertia resisting internal rotation.

Scapular muscle activity remains high during arm acceleration, acting as a stable platform for the shoulder. Posterior deltoid and supraspinatus activity is high with forces directed toward abduction. Pectoralis major and teres minor force couple with pectoralis major driving internal rotation, whereas teres minor provides a stabilizing posterior restraint. Latissimus dorsi and pectoralis major are the main upper extremity muscles that contribute to ball velocity, whereas subscapularis functions as a steering muscle to maintain optimum position of the humeral head upon the glenoid. Studies have demonstrated MVIC values for subscapularis and latissimus dorsi to be 115% and 88%, respectively, during arm acceleration.

Kinematic analysis reveals that during arm acceleration, peak angular velocity of the humerus approaches a phenomenal 7,365 degrees per second with the humerus internal rotation arc being approximately 100 degrees in 30 ms. Peak acceleration is on the order of 600,000 degrees per second. As a consequence, the humerus develops 67 N-m of internal torque just before ball release. Further, elbow extension continues and approaches an angular velocity of 2,200 degrees per second. Compressive glenohumeral load rapidly increases from 480 to over 1,000 N.

Arm Deceleration

Arm deceleration is a period of energy dissipation beginning with ball release and ending with maximal humerus internal rotation. Muscle forces during arm deceleration are eccentric. It has been shown that eccentric loading generates the greatest tensile forces. Thus, this period of rapidly decreasing angular velocity generates substantial torque about the shoulder.

During arm deceleration, scapular muscle activity continues to be maximal. Middle and posterior deltoid

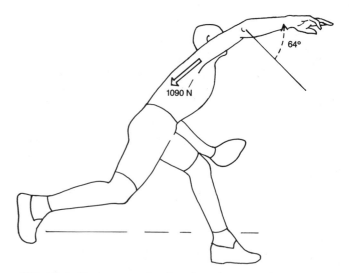

FIG. 25.4. During arm deceleration, the second critical instant of the pitch occurs. (From Fleisig GS, Andrews JR, et al: Kinetics of baseball pitching with implications about injury mechanisms. *Am J Sports Med* 1995;23:233–239, with permission.)

activity remains high in antagonism to the humeral head. Teres minor activity is foremost of all muscles with MVIC value of 84%. Latissimus dorsi continues with peak activity, whereas pectoralis major forces decline as the mechanical advantage is lost when humeral elevation drops below 90 degrees.

A second critical instant occurs during arm deceleration. While the arm is internally rotated 64 degrees and the elbow is flexed 25 degrees, a maximum distraction force of 1,090 N is generated in the shoulder (Fig. 25.4). Shoulder force in the anterior direction is 80 N, whereas it is 100 N inferiorly. Deceleration of shoulder external rotation and elbow extension is 500,000 degrees per second per second.

Follow-through

Follow-through is a phase of continued energy dissipation beginning with maximum internal rotation and ending when the thrower reaches a balanced position. Low grade noncritical eccentric loading of shoulder muscles occurs during follow-through.

In summary, each muscle group has a unique role during the pitch. Scapular muscles function to optimally position the glenoid. The deltoid functions to position the arm. The supraspinatus functions in conjunction with the deltoid and also fine tunes humeral head position relative to the glenoid. Infraspinatus and teres minor externally rotate the humerus during arm cocking. The subscapularis, pectoralis major, and latissimus dorsi provide anterior restraint during maximal humerus external rotation while also providing power during arm acceleration. During arm deceleration, teres minor maintains a high level of activity to act as posterior restraint to the humeral head.

Mechanism of Injury

Recent thought has centered on the dynamics involved in production of lesions in the throwing shoulder, such as superior labral tearing or detachment and partial tearing of the rotator cuff.

The glenohumeral joint is known to have a ball and socket character (27). In the normal throwing shoulder, translational and rotatory motion is a function of static capsular restraint and dynamic muscular action. There are linear translations and cyclic rotations of the humeral head upon the glenoid during the pitch. In the normal shoulder, these motions have physiometric limits. The repetitive forces involved in throwing can eventually alter performance of one of the soft tissue components causing dysfunction. In due course, cyclic stability is deranged, and shear forces are increased. Gradual deterioration occurs until clinically evident as a lesion-producing pain and/or loss of maximal athletic function.

Studies have been performed attempting to define normal translational behavior of the glenohumeral joint. Poppen and Walker (28) demonstrated superior—inferior translation during abduction. Howell et al. (27) demonstrated a 4-mm posterior translation with extension and external rotation. Harryman et al. (29) showed reproducible and significant translation anteriorly with flexion and adduction; moreover, there is posterior translation with both extension and external rotation.

Warner et al. (30) and Turkel et al. (31) demonstrated that at 90 degrees of abduction, the inferior glenohumeral ligament is the prime static stabilizer of the glenohumeral joint. Tightening of the anterior inferior glenohumeral ligament occurs in external rotation; conversely, the posterior inferior glenohumeral ligament tightens in internal rotation (32). It is also well known that a common physical finding in the throwing shoulder is increased external rotation and decreased internal rotation (2,33). This implies relative laxity of the anteroinferior capsular structures, thus the finding of increased external rotation. Further, there is often contracture of the posteroinferior capsule with the resultant finding of decreased internal rotation. Therefore, it can be surmised that there is indeed deviation from cyclic stability inherent in the throwing shoulder.

Jobe and Jobe (6) pointed out how repetitive microtrauma, also known as the "overuse" syndrome, in excess of normal physiologic function causes injury in soft tissue. Stresses inflicted upon the anterior capsular structures overstrain these tissues, leading to fatigue failure. After establishment of the healing response, the result is a lax attenuated ligament that allows pathologic translation and rotation during the pitching cycle.

Muscular dysfunction can detract from cyclic stability of the glenohumeral joint. It is well known that pain can inhibit muscle function at the reflex level. It is also known that malfunction of the rotator cuff can cause superior migration of the humeral head (34). These imbalances lead to translational and rotational forces exceeding physiologic norms with eventual development of pathologic lesions in the throwing shoulder (35). Analogies concerning the cruciate deficient knee with accelerated rates of meniscal and hyaline cartilage damage bring focus on the cycle of instability and secondary pathology. Interplay of the multifactorial pathologic forces is demonstrated in Fig. 25.5 (36).

Andrews and Carson (37) originally reported a tear to the superior labrum in the throwing athlete. Their study demonstrated biceps muscle activity as a possible causative agent in this anatomic derangement. Specifically, tensile forces generated by the biceps during arm deceleration tend to lift the labrum away from the glenoid.

Special attention is afforded the biceps because of its intraarticular position and role in superior glenoid labrum pathology (38,39). In stable shoulders, the primary function of the biceps is to supply elbow flexion torque. Another function of the biceps is to resist humeral distraction. Biceps activity peaks during the arm acceleration and arm deceleration phases of pitching. Its maximum value is 61 N-m shortly before ball release. It also applies compressive force to the glenohumeral joint shortly after ball release.

There is a kinetic link between anterior instability and function of the long head of biceps (40–42). An intact biceps diminishes stress placed on the inferior glenohumeral ligament. Conversely, increased laxity of the glenohumeral joint results in increased compressive force needed to resist distraction. This work load is born by the biceps. Rodosky et al. (43) showed in cadaver studies that the biceps tendon contributes to anterior shoulder stability and that rotational stability of the shoulder is decreased with biceps anchor detachment. This instability due to detachment of the superior labrum might well lead to impingement, hence the common finding of associated pathology such as undersurface tearing of the rotator cuff. These perceptions are supported by the work of Glousman et al. (22), who demonstrated that biceps activity is greater in unstable shoulders and that there are significant deviations from normal in muscles other than the biceps. For example, pectoralis major, subscapularis, latissimus dorsi, and serratus anterior all show marked decrease in activity, especially during the arm cocking phase of unstable shoulders.

Andrews et al. (44) pointed out that any force that shifts the humeral head to the glenoid rim during internal rotation causes the humeral head to be reseated off-center, thus impinging the labrum and eventually

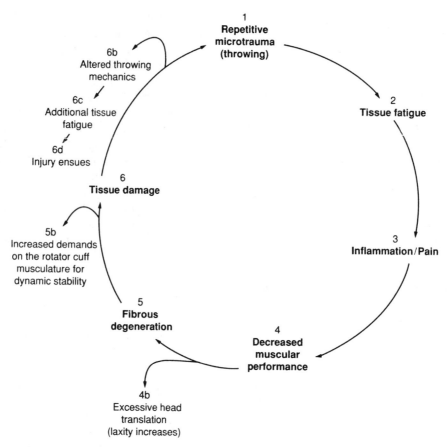

FIG. 25.5. Circular diagram of pathologic forces involved in the throwing shoulder. (From Andrews JR, Wilk KE. Shoulder injuries in baseball. In: Andrews JR, Wilk KE, eds. *The athlete's shoulder.* New York: Churchill Livingstone, 1994:369–389, with permission.)

leading to labral tearing. This repetitive injury of translation plus rotation to the anterosuperior labrum is referred to as the "shoulder grinding factor."

Jobe and Jobe (6) described internal impingement in the throwing shoulder. Often these patients present with a positive impingement sign. A painful apprehension test with a positive relocation test implies that contact between the greater tuberosity, rotator cuff, and posterosuperior labrum is relieved by posterior translation. They proposed that in a position of abduction and external rotation, slight laxity of the anterior band of the inferior glenohumeral ligament allows impingement between the posterosuperior glenoid labrum and undersurface of the rotator cuff. There could be correlation between these clinical entities and the classic combination of anterior dislocation with rotator cuff tear seen in older patients.

Many of these pathologic complexes are a problem of overrotation (45). This concept shifts reasoning from dysfunction being a static linear translational phenomenon to one which is dynamic and rotational. After all, that is the true nature of the glenohumeral joint. Overrotation occurs during the arm-cocking phase as extreme

external rotation of the glenohumeral joint takes place. With the endemic anterior capsular laxity of the thrower's shoulder, physiometric limits are exceeded. As a result, impingement develops between the undersurface infraspinatus and the posterosuperior glenoid labrum. This results in partial undersurface tearing of the infraspinatus and damage to the posterosuperior glenoid labrum. As this common pitcher's lesion propagates anteriorly, the biceps anchor is eventually involved, resulting in detachment.

A prime example is the thrower with subclinical anterior instability demonstrated by increased external rotation at 90 degrees of abduction. With these imbalances, an extremely common arthroscopic finding is partial tearing of the articular surface of the posterior supraspinatus and the anterior infraspinatus in conjunction with fraying of the posterosuperior glenoid labrum. By placing the shoulder in an athletically functional position at arthroscopy (dynamic arthroscopy), abutment of pathologic areas is noted (Fig. 25.6). This internal impingement due to overrotation is also sport specific, depending on the position of the arm while overhead.

An example of this concerns the diver's shoulder. It is

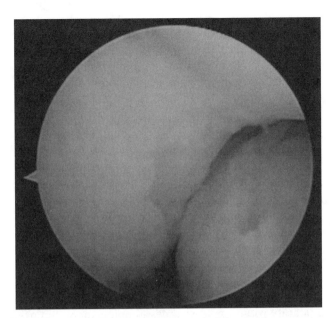

FIG. 25.6. Note pathologic abutment of the posterosuperior glenoid labrum with the undersurface of infraspinatus in this dynamic arthroscopic view of a professional pitcher's right glenohumeral joint. The upper extremity is in a position of abduction and external rotation. There is tearing of the labrum and infraspinatus.

held in a position of maximal straight overhead forward flexion plus internal rotation. At dive entry, superior loading forces are great, and subtle inferior capsular laxity develops. With dynamic arthroscopy, abutment of the superior portion of the biceps–labral complex with articular surface supraspinatus is noted, with both having pathologic tearing. We have conclusively demonstrated this phenomenon in throwers, divers, and tennis players, as Walch et al. have by using dynamic arthroscopy (Fig. 25.7). In the throwing position, impingement is seen between the posterosuperior labrum and the

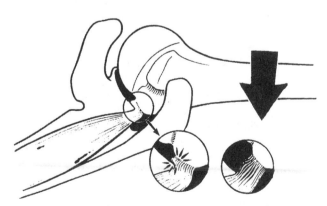

FIG. 25.7. Impingement of the superior glenoid labrum with biceps anchor against the rotator cuff undersurface in a position of abduction and eternal rotation. This process is augmented in elite throwers as a result of increased glenohumeral laxity, thus the term "overrotation."

undersurface rotator cuff (46). Other studies attest to these concepts (47,48).

Superior Glenoid Labrum Pathology

It is important to differentiate labral tearing, which involves the meniscus-like peripheral labrum, from labral detachment, which is seen as instability of the central labrum near the biceps insertion. In the Andrews et al. (44) series, the lesions were found in close proximity to the biceps tendon in 83%, with the majority being in the anterosuperior labrum. Biceps tendon fraying was seen in 10%. Glasgow et al. (49) reported that in stable shoulders, 88% of labral tears are superior and 74% are anterior when the labrum is viewed as being divided into diagonal quadrants. Snyder et al. (50) demonstrated that isolated superior labral tears were seen in only 28% of their series and that the most common concomitant pathology was of the rotator cuff with a 40% incidence. These series, though, had a low total percentage of throwers.

Flap tears (i.e., Snyder types I, III, and IV) are common superior labral lesions and are due to microtrauma. When one considers the excessive internal rotational angular velocity developed during acceleration, labral impingement can easily be surmised, especially if there is rotational dysfunction. Causative factor may include such variables as painful muscle misfiring, increased capsular laxity, or capsular contracture. Altchek et al. (51) suggested that pathologically excessive translation of the humeral head on the glenoid could be responsible for tearing of the glenoid labrum. This suggestion is consistent with the opinion of Jobe and Jobe (6), who cited microsubluxation as the cause of internal impingement and Andrews' concept of the shoulder-grinding factor.

Labral detachment (i.e., Snyder types II and complex) is accelerated by biceps contraction during late cocking as it flexes the elbow and also during deceleration as it eccentrically contracts in opposition to elbow extension. These tensile forces tend to lift the labrum off the superior glenoid. There may also be superior impingement of the biceps–labrum complex in cases of occult glenohumeral instability.

Snyder et al. (11) classified superior labrum injuries in the shoulder in 1990, calling them SLAP lesions. This series was based on lesions with traumatic etiology, not the repetitive overuse of throwers. It also implicitly differentiates between labral tearing and detachment. Classification of SLAP lesions is as follows (11):

- Type I lesion: Superior labrum appears frayed and degenerative. The (flap tear) biceps tendon anchor is normal.
- Type II lesion: Pathologic detachment of the superior labrum and biceps (detachment) anchor. The superior labrum may also be frayed.

- Type III lesion: Vertical tear through a meniscoid-like superior labrum (flap tear), producing a bucket handle lesion that may displace into the glenohumeral joint. The biceps anchor and remaining labrum stay intact.
- Type IV lesion: Vertical tear of the superior meniscoid-like labrum, which also (flap tear) extends to a variable amount into the biceps tendon. As in a type III SLAP lesion, the biceps anchor and the remainder of the superior labrum are well attached.
- Complex lesion: Combination of two or more of the other SLAP lesions. This usually consists of a type II–IV combination lesion.
- Type V lesion: A newly recognized form of a continuation of an anterior inferior labral tear into the anterior and superior labrum.

Snyder et al. demonstrated rates of SLAP lesions to be as follows; type I, 1%; type II, 55%; type III, 9%; type IV, 10%; and complex lesions, 5%. They further demonstrated that SLAP lesions were associated with the partial rotator cuff tears 29% of the time, complete rotator cuff tears 11% of the time, Bankart lesions 22% of the time, and were isolated only 28% of the time. Warner et al. (52) presented a series of shoulder arthroscopies with a 1.5% incidence of SLAP lesions, of which 10% were type II. Many superior labral detachments (Snyder II) are in fact normal anatomic variants. Also, the etiology of superior labral pathology is multifactorial.

Rotator Cuff Disease in the Throwing Athlete

Rotator cuff tears in the throwing shoulder are usually partial, spanning from the mid-supraspinatus to mid-infraspinatus. These tears tend to be centered upon the infraspinatus. They are also found predominantly on the articular side. Jobe, Perry, and colleagues have contributed a great deal to understanding of rotator cuff disease in the throwing athlete (6,7,24–26,53).

Meister and Andrews (54) proposed a classification scheme of rotator cuff disease in the overhand athlete. This system classifies lesions according to the forces involved in their etiology (compressive vs. tensile) and as a function of shoulder stability (primary vs. secondary).

Primary compressive disease (external impingement) occurs during the throwing motion as the humeral head with rotator cuff/biceps tendon rotate beneath the acromion and coracoacromial ligament. Frequently, primary compressive disease is seen in the aging overhead athlete and is uncommon at ages less than 35. A careful history will reveal the pain to occur during deceleration and follow-through when the shoulder is flexed, horizontally adducted, and internally rotated. Abnormal ac-

romial morphology, thickening of the coracoacromial ligament, rotator cuff dysfunction, degenerative spur formation, fibrosis, and cuff edema are factors that compromise the subacromial space, hence predisposing toward impingement. Mild to moderate rotator cuff weakness, stress pain, and a positive impingement sign are found on physical examination. Pain relief by subacromial lidocaine injection helps confirm the diagnosis of primary compressive disease.

Secondary compressive disease is impingement associated with other derangements. Often, the primary disease is one of occult multidirectional instability as proposed by Jobe (46). It can also be due to capsular contracture or muscle imbalance about the shoulder. With these static stabilizer abnormalities, dynamic stabilizers, such as the supraspinatus fatigue, allow abnormal rotation with resultant impingement beneath the coracoacromial arch. In younger throwing athletes, mild to moderate rotator cuff weakness, impingement findings, plus carefully sought patterns of instability indicate secondary compressive disease.

Primary tensile disease of the rotator cuff occurs during deceleration when posterior shoulder muscles contract eccentrically to counteract glenohumeral distraction forces. There is lack of subacromial impingement. Typically, these lesions begin on the articular surface of the infraspinatus. With disease progression, the tear can extend into the bursal surface and propagate into the supraspinatus and/or teres minor. Subtle cuff weakness, stress pain of infraspinatus and teres minor, posterior capsular tenderness, and a lack of instability findings are suggestive of primary tensile rotator cuff failure.

Secondary tensile disease is similar but with findings suggestive of subtle instability. Macrotraumatic failure of the rotator cuff is frequently a single event seen in an older athlete with a history of impingement symptoms for several years. It has elements of both compressive and tensile disease. It occurs with forced adduction, active abduction against resistance, or in conjunction with a traumatic dislocation. It is not uncommon for these patients to have gone through several cycles of impingement syndrome. Injectional corticosteroid therapy, although often alleviating impingement symptomatology, can in fact hasten overt cuff failure.

- Primary compressive: Impingement in throwers without other known pathology.
- Disease: Thought due to posterior capsular contracture with resultant loss of internal rotation and concomitant superior migration of humeral head. Partial tears of bursal surface associated with an abnormal subacromial space.
- Secondary compressive: Cuff disease in throwers, usually other underlying disease pathology. Most often due to anterior laxity with abnormal rotation and sec-

ondary cuff impingement. Find partial undersurface cuff tears and normal subacromial space.

- Primary tensile disease: Repetitive microtrauma failure due to eccentric overload during deceleration. Can be secondary to subtle instability. Often found isolated to infraspinatus and posterior capsule.
- Secondary tensile disease: As per primary tensile disease plus instability.
- Macrotraumatic failure: Rare catastrophic longitudinal cuff tear with or without greater tuberosity avulsion.

Bennett's Disease (Thrower's Exostosis)

Thrower's exostosis is an extracapsular ossification of the posteroinferior glenoid rarely seen except in older long-time throwers (i.e., the professional ranks). This condition was originally considered to be a traction osteophyte of the long head of the triceps (2). During open surgery, it has been demonstrated that this lesion is not located in the triceps origin. Histology has demonstrated that it is secondary ossification involving of the posterior capsule probably due to repetitive microtrauma. Indeed, this lesion is found consistently at the origin of the posterior band of the inferior glenohumeral ligament, which suggests that the microtrauma occurs during deceleration and follow-through when tensile forces associated with internal rotation are the greatest (55,56). We have recently noted by dynamic arthroscopic evaluation in very advanced prominent cases that the lesion can actually contact the posterior aspect of the humeral head and create an internal impingement phenomenon (55,56). It can actually cause an erosive defect in that area of the posterior humeral head just under the teres minor insertion associated with the overrotation phenomenon.

CLINICAL EVALUATION

History

The most important diagnostic tools for the painful throwing shoulder are a thorough history and physical examination. When evaluating the throwing shoulder, one should think in terms of the pathophysiology involved while differentiating rotator cuff disease and occult instability as part of the differential diagnosis. At the first visit it is helpful to establish what, how, when, and where so as to preemptively address concerns of insurance companies and attorneys. This documentation is particularly relevant concerning professional athletes. It is our practice to question the patient whether the problem is one of pain, weakness, loss of motion, instability, or catching (Table 25.1).

Much can be gained by a thorough history of the painful throwing shoulder, because physical findings

TABLE 25.1. *What, how, when, and where questions to patients*

- What is the frequency of the complaint?
- Is it a first occurrence problem or chronic? If chronic, how often does it happen?
- What is the mechanism of injury?
- What sport is involved?
- Did the original symptoms occur during off-season, pre-season, regular season practice, during a game, or during recreational activities?
- Is the thrower a pitcher, quarterback, or other overhead athlete?
- If disabled, how long since the thrower has been able to participate?
- How have symptoms progressed?
- How disabled is the affected shoulder?
- Are there symptoms of numbness or tingling in the extremity?
- Is there a history of muscular weakness, subluxation, or dislocation?
- Are there catches, clicks, or pops in the shoulder? How frequent are they; how long into the throwing session; and at what phase of the pitch do they occur?
- What are previously offered diagnoses?
- If the patient is a **pitcher:** What is the style of throw? Is velocity normal or decreased? Is he or she having trouble loosening up? How is accuracy affected? Is there pain at rest? Is the pain most noticed during warm-up, during the game, after the game, or the next day? Is there pain during the pitch and how severe is the pain? What phase of the throw is pain noticed? Where is the pain? What are the usual innings pitched, and how has the problem affected this variable?
- Does the athlete consider that he or she has done everything to get well with conservative treatment and rehabilitation?
- What does the athlete hope to gain from this consultation?

might tend to be sparse and ancillary testing inconclusive. Specific historical findings of functional instability (i.e., superior labral lesions, partial cuff tears, thrower's exostosis, and external and internal impingement) can be elusive. Most elite throwers can comment in detail about changes in velocity, accuracy, and innings pitched. Often these functional declines can present clues concerning the pathology. Cocking pain might indicate inflammation of the deranged anterior structures and/or rotator cuff, or more acceleration pain can point to a lesion in the posterior rotator cuff caused by eccentric overload, specifically the internal impingement phenomenon. Deceleration pain and pain throughout the pitching cycle both imply impingement. Acceleration through follow-through pain is commonly seen in pitchers with thrower's exostosis. If the location of pain is posterior and inferior during cocking, it might also represent contact pain from overrotation and extension and contact with prominent thrower's exostosis. Continuous pain, poorly localized, is suggestive of a hyaline cartilage surface defect lesion. Sharp pain may indicate an acute inflammatory process. A dull aching pain or sense of extremity heaviness is often seen in rotator cuff pathology.

Several studies report historical findings seen in athletes with superior glenoid labrum pathology. Payne and Jokl (57) reported that 100% of patients with superior glenoid labrum tears had overhead activity pain and 64% had clicking. Snyder et al. (50) reported that 49% of patients with superior labral tears had locking, catching, or popping; 19% had a history of instability. In Andrews and Carson's series (8), 95% of patients had pain during the throwing act, whereas 47% had popping or catching during throwing. Maffet et al. (58) reported 18% had locking episodes and a 16% previous dislocation rate. Resch et al. (59) reported 67% overhead snapping and 61% night pain in their SLAP lesion series. Altchek et al. (51) showed that 100% of overhead athletes having labral tears complained of overhead pain preoperatively with well-localized anterior pain reported in 60% of patients, posterior pain in 15%, and diffuse pain in 25%. Most patients with thrower's exostosis had follow-through pain in a study by Ferrari et al. (56).

Physical Examination

The first phase of physical examination is observation of the patient (6,60–62). This begins at first contact and continues throughout examination. To "read" the patient is an important part of our approach. Consistency of the physical is a hallmark of professionalism.

Inspection of the throwing shoulder usually reveals hypertrophy in the elite athlete. Atrophy or swelling should be noted. In particular, scapular position and periscapular musculature should be examined. Functional abnormalities of the scapula are evaluated by observing from posteriorly while the patient does a sitting lift-off test, along with inspection of scapulothoracic motion by active forward flexion of the glenohumeral joint, and a wall push-off test.

With the patient seated, palpation should proceed from the sternoclavicular joint, along the clavicle, AC joint, and to the lateral acromion so that point tenderness can be detected. Proceeding from anterior to lateral to posterior, the examiner also evaluates the anterior capsule, bicipital groove, coracoid, deltoid insertion, posterior capsule, and posterior soft tissues for tenderness. The examiner palpates for circumduction crepitus, which is frequently positive with subacromial disease. A painful cross arm test can suggest acromioclavicular joint disease. A load-shift test for instability is performed with the shoulder in adduction both anteriorly and posteriorly, followed by supraspinatus and teres

minor stress testing for pain or weakness. Sulcus sign testing follows evaluation for impingement. The Speed and Yergason tests are performed. They can correlate closely with strain of the long head of biceps, hence pathology in the bicipital groove. Passive internal rotation is accessed by cephalad excursion of the thumb tip along the vertebral column. Generalized ligamentous laxity of the elbow, wrist, and finger joints is also accessed.

With the patient supine, further passive range of motion testing is performed. Particular attention should be paid to differences between the upper extremities in different positions. Motion derangement is an indicator of pathology, whereas motion improvement is a sensitive index of therapeutic progress. Elite throwers often have increased passive external rotation and decreased internal rotation of the dominant glenohumeral joint. Passive glenohumeral motion testing is external rotation at 15 degrees of abduction, external and internal rotation at 90 degrees of abduction, and forward flexion.

Magnusson et al. (63) quantitated that on average, the throwing shoulder in pitchers exhibits 14 degrees more external rotation and 12 degrees less internal rotation than the nonthrowing arm. Johnson (33) showed that external rotation at 90 degrees of abduction averages 136 degrees in pitchers, whereas other players average 118 degrees in the throwing arm. These findings and those in other studies attest to the acquired laxity inherent in the throwing shoulder (2,64).

Other examination maneuvers with the patient supine include the apprehension test, relocation test, Lachman test of the shoulder, and clunk test. Lachman test of the shoulder is performed with the shoulder abducted 90 degrees and externally rotated 45 degrees. Anteriorly directed force on the humeral head is then used to compare laxity and end point firmness between the uninvolved and injured shoulders (Fig. 25.8). The clunk test is a most sensitive physical examination maneuver for

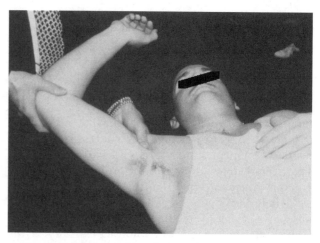

FIG. 25.8. Lachman's test of the shoulder.

detection of superior labral pathology (65). The examiner stands at the head of the bed cephalad to the affected shoulder. The hand nearest the patient's head is placed posterior to the humeral head while applying an anteriorly directed force. The hand furthest from the patient grasps the distal humerus, abducts it maximally, and applies gentle rotatory forces. Superior labral tears are trapped between the humeral head/greater tuberosity and glenoid rim, producing a palpable or audible catch (Fig. 25.9). Liu et al. (66) described the "crank" test, which is a modification of the clunk test. Their study demonstrated sensitivity, specificity, and accuracy rates of greater than 90%. The external rotation posterior impingement sign as described by Meister and Andrews (54) is very sensitive, specific, and accurate for internal impingement.

Kibler (67) described the anterior slide test that is performed by having the standing patient place hands on hips and thumbs pointing posteriorly. From posterior, the examiner places a hand atop the shoulder and with the other hand loads the humerus axially in a forward and slightly superiorly directed force. The patient is asked to push against this force. Anterior shoulder pain, a pop, or click is considered to be indicative of a superior glenoid labrum lesion. The slide test reportedly has 78.4% sensitivity and 91.5% specificity for superior labral lesions.

Finally, the patient is placed in the prone position. The posterior capsule and adjacent soft tissues are accessed for palpation tenderness. A symptomatic thrower's exostosis is suggested by posteroinferior glenoid tenderness. A posterior apprehension test can also be performed. While in the prone position, a posterior internal rotation contracture test, as described by Morgan in 1998 (*personal communication*), can be done.

A subacromial anesthetic injection is an important diagnostic maneuver to differentiate subacromial from glenohumeral pain. Great caution should be exercised in consideration of corticosteroid injection in the throwing shoulder, because it is often only a temporizing measure and can accelerate deterioration.

A literature review of physical findings accentuates what has been reported concerning these disorders. Altchek et al. (51) found that overhead athletes with labral tears demonstrated a positive impingement sign 95% of the time. None of their patients had measurable loss of motion, but all patients manifested pain during stability testing. Maffet et al. (58) found crepitus in 49%, popping in 44%, and supraspinatus tenderness in 51% of SLAP lesion patients. Impingement testing was positive in most. In a report of 18 SLAP lesions patients, Resch et al. (59) found positive examination findings of 100% for the Speed test, 67% for the Yergason test, 78% for the apprehension test, and 67% for the cross arm test. Glasgow et al. (49) corroborated 100% palpable clicks in their series of athletes with glenoid labrum tears. Andrews et al. (44) confirmed popping/catching in 79%, supraspinatus tenderness in 71%, and subluxation in 10% of patients with superior labral pathology. McGlynn and Caspari (68) showed that clicks demonstrated on physical examination corresponded with a posterolateral defect in the humeral head, which rode over the torn labrum or anterior glenoid rim at arthroscopy.

Payne et al. (69) reported on partial rotator cuff tears in young athletes. All proved to have a positive impingement test preoperatively. Limited active internal rotation was noted in 23%, and a positive apprehension test was seen in 19% of these throwers. Wright and Cofield's series (70) of partial rotator cuff tears showed mild weakness of abduction in 56%. Ferrari et al. (56) indicated that tenderness to palpation of the posteroinferior glenoid was present in 100% of patients with thrower's exostosis.

IMAGING

Diagnostic imaging of the shoulder has dramatically improved over the past 5 years. Until recently, arthrography was used to determine if a rotator cuff tear was present. Computed tomography (CT) after arthrography was also used to show labral pathology. Currently, magnetic resonance imaging (MRI) is the imaging modality of choice. MRI-arthrography has gained approval in many imaging centers because of its exceptional soft tissue contrast and ability to demonstrate subtle abnormalities.

Imaging studies serve as an adjunct to a good history, thorough physical examination, and arthroscopic evaluation. The sensitivity and specificity of MRI has increased significantly in recent years. Normal MRI studies can possibly prevent unnecessary surgery in some cases. This discussion is limited primarily to conven-

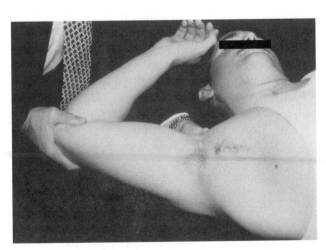

FIG. 25.9. Clunk test.

tional radiography and MRI for the evaluation of the painful shoulder in the throwing athlete.

Radiography

After thorough clinical evaluation of the shoulder, plain radiographs should be obtained. The minimum series should include anteroposterior internal rotation, anteroposterior external rotation, axillary lateral, and Stryker notch views. Optional radiographs include the West Point and acromial profile views (71).

In the throwing shoulder, anteroposterior views often reveal relative radiolucency in the greater tuberosity and surrounding proximal lateral metaphysis. Also, there may be cyst formation in those areas. We have recently noted that the so-called areas of the proximal humerus are indeed contact erosive areas secondary to internal impingement with the posterior glenoid rim from the overrotation phenomenon. Anteroposterior views can also demonstrate acromioclavicular joint arthrosis or osteophyte formation on the undersurface of the distal clavicle. Both situations can predispose the patient to impingement of the rotator cuff. Calcification in the region of the supraspinatus insertion indicates calcific tendonitis and can be seen on the anteroposterior views.

Axillary lateral or West Point views are helpful in the diagnosis of osseous Bankart lesions. Acromial profile views may reveal Bigliani type II or III acromion morphology, which indicates a tendency toward impingement syndrome. These views are also good for os-acrominales. The Stryker notch projection is helpful in demonstrating a thrower's exostosis in the posteroinferior glenoid (Fig. 25.10). This view may also show a Hill-Sachs lesion, which is pathopneumonic for a previous anterior dislocation. All plain radiographs demonstrate osseous structures only and do not show any soft tissue pathology.

Computed Tomography and Magnetic Resonance Imaging

Double-contrast CT-arthrography has proven to be a useful tool in the evaluation of soft tissue abnormalities of the shoulder. Callaghan et al. (72) demonstrated 97% accuracy in assessment of biceps–labral complex pathology. They also compared CT-arthrography of the shoulder with arthroscopy and showed that CT-arthrography was good for the delineation of glenohumeral joint pathology.

MRI demonstrates a great deal of anatomic detail in the shoulder. There is variability in the accuracy of this technique for different pathologic conditions. Legan et al. (73) showed 75% sensitivity for the detection of superior labral pathology using unenhanced MRI. Gusmer et al. (74) reported 86% sensitivity for similar cases. Rafii et al. (75) reported 89% sensitivity and 84% specificity for identifying partial rotator cuff tears using MRI. Traughber and Goodwin (76) reported only 56% sensitivity for the same type of pathology.

MRI-arthrography has been used for the evaluation of the painful throwing shoulder at our institution since 1991 (77). We believe that intraarticular contrast improves diagnostic accuracy in competitive athletes when the history and physical examination are atypical or when the physical findings are subtle. A dilute mixture of gadolinium and saline (1 mL gadoteridol in 250 mL saline) is sterilely injected into the shoulder joint under fluoroscopic guidance. The volume injected is usually 15 to 20 mL unless adhesive capsulitis is present. After injection, the glenohumeral joint is taken through a passive range of motion. The patient is positioned supine for MRI with a dedicated shoulder coil placed anteriorly.

Axial T1, sagittal T1, coronal oblique T2, and fat-suppressed coronal oblique T1-weighted images are obtained. The oblique coronal images are parallel to the supraspinatus tendon and demonstrate the rotator cuff, superior labrum, intraarticular biceps tendon, subacromial bursa, and the acromioclavicular joint. Axial images are perpendicular to the humerus, visualizing the anterior and posterior labrum, superior and middle glenohumeral ligaments, subscapularis muscle and tendon, and the biceps tendon. Sagittal images are perpendicular to the supraspinatus tendon and show the acromioclavicular joint and the rotator cuff tendons in cross-section.

It is critical to understand normal anatomic variations to distinguish them from pathologic conditions. There is variability of the anterior glenoid labrum and the anterior capsular attachment. Less variability is seen in

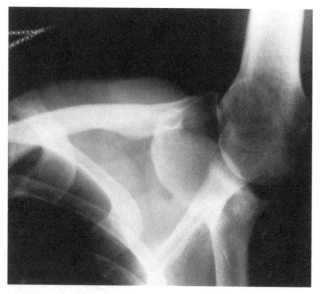

FIG. 25.10. Stryker notch view demonstrating thrower's exostosis (Bennett's lesion).

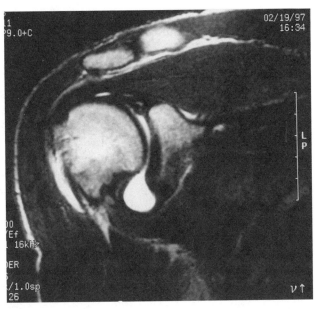

FIG. 25.11. Coronal oblique image of a right superior glenoid labrum tear. Note extravasation of contrast into the body of the labrum. (Courtesy of Martin L. Schwartz, M.D.)

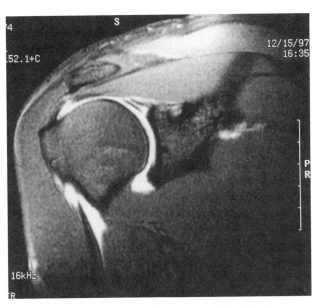

FIG. 25.13. Coronal oblique image demonstrating a partial undersurface tear of the rotator cuff. Note that the defect is filled with contrast but does not extend into the subacromial space. (Courtesy of Martin L. Schwartz, M.D.)

the posterior glenoid labrum. A normal sublabral recess is present superiorly and should not be mistaken for a tear. This recess is present at the labral–bicipital junction and is smoothly marginated, curvilinear, and fills with contrast. The Buford complex is visualized as an absent anterosuperior labrum and thickened middle glenohumeral ligament that attaches to the biceps anchor. Changes in the greater tuberosity of the humerus are

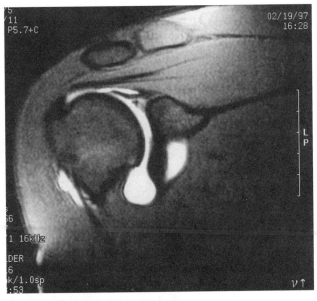

FIG. 25.12. Coronal oblique magnetic resonance image of the right shoulder demonstrating a superior labral detachment. Note the Y-shaped area of contrast that extends along the superior glenoid. (Courtesy of Martin L. Schwartz, M.D.)

seen, relating the normal stress reaction present in throwers.

Superior labral tears are best visualized on coronal oblique images as increased signal that extends to the labral surface. Contrast extends into the tear, enhancing visualization on T1-weighted images (Fig. 25.11). Superior labral detachment is seen on coronal oblique images as a T- or Y-shaped area of increased signal extending to the labral surface (Fig. 25.12).

Subacromial impingement can be demonstrated on coronal oblique or sagittal oblique images. There may be increased signal in the supraspinatus tendon, and the tendon may be distorted as it passes below the subacromial osteophyte. Iannotti et al. (78) showed a 93% positive predictive value for the detection of impingement using conventional MRI.

Partial rotator cuff tears are seen on coronal oblique images as irregularity of the undersurface of the supraspinatus tendon. There may be an associated increased signal in the substance of the tendon (Fig. 25.13). These findings are usually on the articular surface of the tendon. Contrast-enhanced MRI was shown by Karzel and Snyder (79) to improve diagnostic accuracy of partial tears as demonstrated in 81% of their patients. Rarely, partial tears will occur on the bursal surface of the supraspinatus tendon. These partial tears will go undetected with MRI unless there is fluid in the subacromial space.

TREATMENT

Nonoperative

It is important to practice preventive maintenance in off-season and during the season for the throwing shoulder

(18,80). Management programs should be individualized. Four key components of maintenance include therapeutic modalities, improving flexibility, therapeutic exercise, and conditioning. Benefits of compliance with such a program include increased power through a greater range of motion, decreased probability of injury, increased preactivity blood flow, decreased postactivity soreness, and decreased anxiety (81).

Fauls (82) first described a stretching program that has been demonstrated to greatly enhance performance. Hydrocollation and ultrasound are beneficial before warm-up activities. It has also been recommended that throwers work to maintain warmth of the pitching arm during competition, to continue muscle activity between innings, and to cool the pitching arm between innings during periods of hot weather.

Post-throwing activities should be directed toward avoidance of the inflammatory process. Elevation and cryotherapy can facilitate this aim. Between outings, high-repetition, low-resistance, rotator cuff-specific isotonic exercise should be used. Between starts, ideally a 5-day rotation, it is important to maintain shoulder function. Activities should focus on generalized and shoulder-specific exercise, stretching, and modalities with relative rest before the next start.

Nonoperative treatment of the painful throwing shoulder is individualized on a patient by patient basis. Occult instability must always be a consideration. Most injuries to the throwing shoulder do not require surgical intervention.

Rest of the painful extremity is the first consideration. It is common to see throwing athletes who are simply overthrown. Baseball is a year-round sport in some states. It is particularly easy for younger players to develop shoulder dysfunction under such circumstances. In the elite thrower, pain can develop as attrition of other throwers mount up, innings pitched per week increase, and the stresses of a long season become evident. It is helpful in these circumstances to have the player simply cease throwing for 7 to 10 days, if possible, to allow subsidence of the inflammatory response. During this period of "active rest," attention should be given to modality treatment, stretching exercise, and submaximal isometric exercise.

It is important during rehabilitative periods to limit pain reproduction. Activity that causes pain should be isolated. Often it is possible to work surrounding muscle groups maximally while relatively resting the affected group. As pain subsides in the affected group, a healing response may be assumed and activities increased accordingly.

After the rest period, progression toward throwing includes isotonic rehabilitation and an interval throwing program. Townsend et al. (83) performed neurophysiologic studies that demonstrated a combination of exercises causing a high level of activity in scapular and shoulder muscles. These include scaption in internal rotation or flexion, horizontal abduction in external rotation, and press up. Further exercises can be added to this program as needed for the individual patient. Final phases of rehabilitation include isokinetics and plyometrics.

Suspected superior labrum pathology therapy should follow the above-mentioned conventions, avoiding maneuvers that reproduce symptoms. An objective of rotator cuff disease therapy should be to maintain or increase range of motion without causing further impingement. It is best to initiate strengthening exercises only when pain has subsided. Appropriate modalities and gentle range of motion below the horizontal plane are the initial measures. Exercises above the horizontal plane should be performed later and done with the arm in external rotation so as to facilitate clearance of the greater tuberosity beneath the acromion. Repetitive stretching exercises in abduction and internal rotation should be avoided. Strengthening exercises are first started gradually, concentrating on the external rotators, the deltoid, and then the internal rotators and scapula muscles. Overly aggressive strengthening may prolong the inflammatory process. For primary tensile disease, emphasis is placed on posterior shoulder eccentric muscular strengthening. For conditions thought secondary to laxity, the appropriate dynamic stabilization program is added. Scapular strengthening is used for base stabilization in all patients. Other nonoperative options include anti-inflammatory medications and therapeutic modalities.

Surgical

Superior Labrum Pathology

Arthroscopic treatment of superior glenoid labrum lesions is strongly influenced by whether or not the biceps tendon is attached to the glenoid tubercle. Types I, III, and IV SLAP lesions (i.e., flap tears) have biceps tendon stability. These lesions respond favorably by resecting to a stable edge and appropriate rehabilitation. Because type II and complex SLAP lesions have biceps detachment, they require labral debridement plus surgical stabilization of the biceps anchor. Superior labrum surgical results are also strongly influenced by stability of the shoulder. In unstable shoulders, the prognosis for labrum resection and biceps anchor stabilization remains poor unless concomitant anterior or multidirectional instability is corrected.

Review of the literature provides interesting data from a number of studies. In 1986, Ogilvie-Harris and Wiley (84) reported that arthroscopic labrum resection yielded poor results in unstable shoulders. Altchek et al. (85) preliminarily demonstrated 85% good results in debridement of labral tears and poor results in debridement of labral detachments. In further follow-up, a high percentage of patients had clinical instability or labral lesions compatible with instability. After labral debridement, 72% of patients were better at 1 year. At 43 months, only 7% of this patient group had significant continuing pain relief. Their conclusions were that microsubluxation is causative in producing glenoid labrum pathology in the throwing shoulder. Also, long-term results of resecting torn or detached glenoid labral are poor (51).

Glasgow et al. (49) reported on 29 overhead athletes who underwent arthroscopic resection of labral tears. Their study divided patients according to stability. In stable shoulders, most labral lesions were superior or anterior. At 2-year follow-up, stable shoulders demonstrated 91% good or excellent results, whereas 75% of unstable shoulders had fair or poor results. Their conclusions were that instability should be a consideration in labrum pathology that occurs below the glenoid equator. They also concluded that a high percentage of good to excellent results can be expected for glenoid labral resection in stable shoulders.

Payne and Jokl (57) reported on 14 stable shoulders that underwent arthroscopic labral debridement. Their study demonstrated 71% good or excellent results at a 2-year follow-up. Also, large anterosuperior tears have a tendency to become unstable postoperatively, leading to unsatisfactory results.

Cordasco et al. (86) found large differences in clinical stability examination versus examination under anesthesia in patients with superior labral lesions, as pain induced guarding that seemed to hinder instability testing in awake patients. Labral debridement afforded 89% good to excellent pain relief at 1 year, which declined to 85% at 2 years. Full return to sport was 52% and 44%, respectively. Their conclusion was that an isolated labral tear without concomitant mechanical derangement is uncommon and that most superior labral tearing results from instability.

In a study with long-term follow up, Terry et al. (87) correlated labral debridement results with instability findings. Their findings indicated that a high rate of good to excellent results can be expected in patients with grade I or II laxity. In patients with grade III laxity, labral debridement with glenohumeral stabilization is indicated.

Resch et al. (59) performed arthroscopic superior glenoid labrum repair using screw fixation techniques. Their study established 86% satisfactory results. Yoneda et al. (88) treated superior labral detachment by staple fixation. At the time of staple removal 3 to 6 months later, all lesions had stabilized. After 24-months follow-up, good or excellent result rates were 80%. Poor results were seen in shoulders with anterior instability.

Snyder et al.'s (50) 1995 series is the largest concerning arthroscopic treatment of superior labrum pathol-

ogy. They concluded that suture anchor fixation of type II lesions can reliably reconstruct the normal anatomic attachment of the superior labrum. Yet bioabsorbable tacks can fragment causing the need for reoperation. Thus, they currently use suture anchor fixation.

Field and Savoie (89) reported 100% good or excellent results in treatment of types II and IV SLAP lesions with trans-glenoid suture repair. Payne et al. (69) treated 43 overhead athletes with partial rotator cuff tears arthroscopically. Their findings suggest that good to excellent results can be expected by debridement in stable shoulders. Wright and Cofield (70) demonstrated 90% satisfactory results in debridement of partial rotator cuff tears.

AUTHORS' EXPERIENCE

It is our experience that a high index of suspicion for occult instability must be maintained when evaluating the painful throwing shoulder with laxity. History taking with a focus on pathomechanics is the cornerstone of clinical evaluation. Consistent detailed physical examination further adds to clinical impressions. In the painful yet stable throwing shoulder, there are no pathopneumonic, historical, or physical findings. Indeed, there can be overlap of findings. Rotator cuff weakness, stress pain, and a positive impingement sign suggest partial undersurface tearing of the cuff. A positive clunk test tends to suggest superior labral tearing or detachment. Signs consistent with instability indicate that the problem is secondary in nature. Posteroinferior glenoid palpation pain is seen in symptomatic thrower's exostosis.

Plain radiography using the anteroposterior in internal rotation and external rotation, axillary lateral, acromial profile, and Stryker notch views are a regular part of our workup. Enhanced MRI with intraarticular gadolinium injection is performed in cases that have unclear pathology and that require arthroscopic evaluation.

Surgery is reserved for patients not responding to nonoperative care. After intubation, a careful examination under anesthesia is performed with the patient supine. Particular attention is given to comparative passive range of motion testing and evaluation for glenohumeral instability. Critical variables in the operating room are range of motion discrepancies, instability findings, location of rotator cuff lesions, and decisions as to whether superior labrum lesions are tears or detachments. Any findings suggestive of instability indicate that the pathology is a secondary phenomenon. Bursal cuff tearing implies compressive disease, whereas tensile disease is suggested by articular sided findings. Superior glenoid labrum detachment prompts the need for stabilization. It must be emphasized that glenoid labrum lesions, rotator cuff disease, and instability are usually interrelated in the throwing shoulder.

We use the lateral decubitus position for arthroscopy

within 15 pounds of suspension in a position of 70 degrees abduction and 15 degrees of forward flexion (90). A posterior arthroscopic and an anterior working portal are established for glenohumeral evaluation. The posterior portal is approximately 3 cm inferior and 1 cm medial to the posterolateral acromion. This palpable "soft spot" is between the infraspinatus and teres minor muscle bellies. The anterior portal is established under direct arthroscopic visualization from a point half way between the coracoid process and the anterior acromion. This working portal passes through the triangle bounded by the biceps tendon, subscapularis, and humeral head.

Arthroscopic evaluation begins with the biceps tendon, which should be smooth and glistening. By externally rotating the upper extremity, the biceps tendon can be followed to the bicipital groove. Synovitis surrounding the biceps tendon, cicatrix formation, or fraying of the biceps tendon are considered indicative of pathology. By rotation and sweeping of the arthroscope, the examiner can visualize the anterior capsulolabral complex. The anteroinferior labrum should be thoroughly evaluated because a Bankart lesion is often much less demonstrable arthroscopically than at open surgery. The inferior labrum is then evaluated. If it is easily visualized without additional distraction, a positive "drive-through" sign characteristic of multidirectional instability should be a consideration. By slight retraction of the arthroscope, the posterior labrum is seen. By rotating the arthroscope while advancing superiorly, the undersurface insertions of teres minor, infraspinatus, and then supraspinatus are observed. Articular cartilage is graded by the Outerbridge classification scheme.

Probing is performed along the entire labrum with particular attention to frayed areas, to the anteroinferior labrum for a Bankart lesion, and to the biceps insertion area to evaluate for superior labral detachment (Fig. 25.14). By switching the arthroscope to the anterior portal, the posterior labrum and rotator cuff are better delineated. It must be remembered that there is considerable normal variation in labral anatomy.

Often in the painful throwing shoulder without overt instability, there will be several pathologic findings in the glenohumeral joint. Any complex involving a combination of superior labral pathology with partial articular-sided cuff tearing implies instability. By removal of distraction, dynamic arthroscopy can demonstrate the pathologic process. For example, in a position of 90 degrees of abduction, extreme external rotation may reveal abutment of articular-sided infraspinatus tearing upon a posterosuperior labrum tear (Fig. 25.15). This would represent a compression internal impingement lesion due to overrotation.

Subacromial arthroscopy follows diagnostic arthroscopy of the glenohumeral joint. This is performed by removal of the arthroscope from the posterior portal

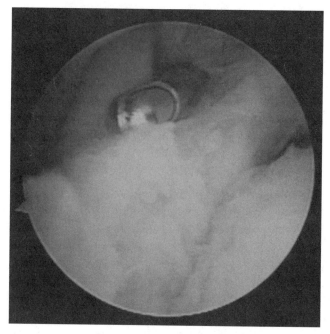

FIG. 25.14. Posterior portal arthroscopic view of superior labral detachment (Snyder type II).

followed by redirecting the cannula superiorly into the subacromial space. If a side to side sweeping motion on the undersurface of the acromion combined with advancement of the cannula to the anterolateral acromion is done, arthroscopic visualization can be en-

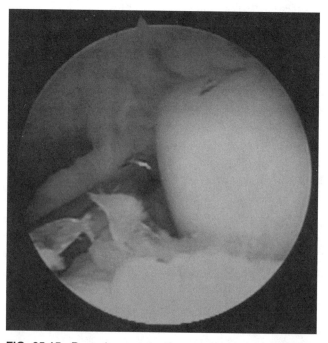

FIG. 25.15. Posterior portal arthroscopic view of partial undersurface infraspinatus tearing plus a lesion of the posterosuperior glenoid labrum in a professional pitcher. This lesion is common in elite throwers and is often due to overrotation.

hanced. A lateral portal is then established that is usually 3 cm lateral to the anterolateral acromion. An arthroscopic shaver is introduced, and the bursa is resected. Subacromial bleeding is minimized by maintaining systolic pressure less than 100 mm Hg and liberal use of electrocautery each time a bleeder is encountered. After arthroscopic subacromial bursectomy, the subacromial space is evaluated. The superior tendinous rotator cuff is evaluated for tearing. External rotation of the upper extremity facilitates visualization of the anterior fibers of the supraspinatus. The acromial undersurface periosteum and the cephalad coracoacromial ligament are examined. Finally, adequacy of subacromial space is noted.

Therapeutic arthroscopy begins with debridement of labral tears to a stable edge. Labral detachment is secured to an abraded glenoid rim with arthroscopically placed suture anchors (Fig. 25.16).

Partial rotator cuff tears are debrided to stable bleeding tissue. Acromioplasty is indicated by partial tearing of the bursal-sided rotator cuff, a hooked acromion, or surgical judgment of inadequate subacromial space. In the throwing athlete, coracoacromial ligament release or resection is usually avoided. Primary compressive disease is treated by "mini" arthroscopic acromioplasty, saving the coracoacromial ligament in most cases. Primary tensile disease is treated by arthroscopic cuff debridement to bleeding tissue without performing acromioplasty. Mini-open cuff repair in the throwing athlete is reserved for deeper penetrating tears approaching 75% thickness. It is often possible to avoid repair in

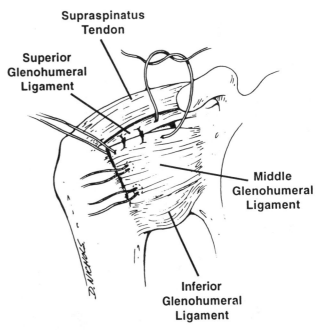

FIG. 25.17. Drawing of a mini-capsular shift. This procedure is performed by openly advancing the lateral joint capsule in a cephalad direction followed by closure of the rotator interval and anatomic repair of the subscapularis.

partial thickness lesions except when debridement has failed.

For disease secondary to acquired instability, we use the above-mentioned surgical therapy combined with either radiofrequency capsulorrhaphy or an anatomic capsular repair and/or shift. Concerning instability, we have in the past performed anatomic capsular repairs in select athletes if surgical judgment indicated the need for such a procedure. Mini-capsular shifts are carried out openly by a minimal release of the superior subscapularis, advancement of the lateral capsule in a superior direction and closure of the rotator interval (Fig. 25.17). Open stabilization in the throwing athlete as a primary procedure is avoided. In the authors' opinion, it is better to treat elite athletes arthroscopically with open procedures reserved for career salvaging and end-stage situations. For more serious anterior instability problems, we use an approach through the rotator cuff interval combined with a subscapular splint to the anterior capsule for direct repair and shift as needed.

Currently, we use a radiofrequency heat probe to perform capsular shrinkage for lower grades of acquired laxity. Early results seem encouraging, yet data are not sufficient to prognosticate what role such treatment will eventually serve in practice.

Thrower's exostosis is treated by using a full radius resector to create a capsular window at the origin of the posteroinferior glenohumeral ligament, adjacent to the glenoid labrum. An acromionizer is then used to resect the exuberant ossification (Fig. 25.18).

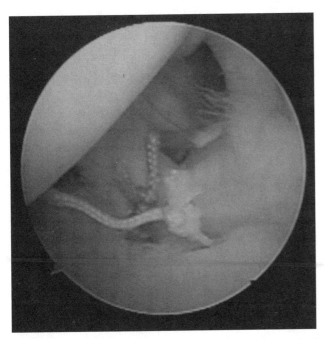

FIG. 25.16. Superior glenoid labrum detachment repaired arthroscopically with suture anchors.

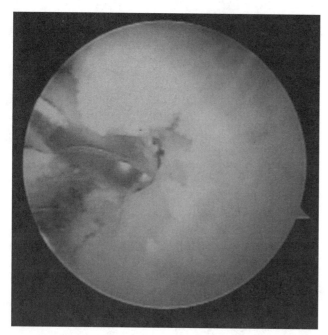

FIG. 25.18. Anterior arthroscopic view of thrower's exostosis resection in the left shoulder of a professional pitcher. A capsular window has been created and an acromionizer is being used for the resection. This lesion is consistently found subjacent to the origin of the posterior band of the inferior glenohumeral ligament.

REHABILITATION

Many patients with microtraumatic injuries respond to nonoperative rehabilitation. The key to such therapy is accurate recognition of involved tissues. For disorders not requiring surgery, such as overuse tendonitis, rotator cuff disorders, and/or superior glenoid labrum injuries, acute treatment is active rest after Biodex testing and cinemographic evaluation of the throwing motion. These studies produce information used in both improving biomechanics of the pitch and also allow monitoring of clinical progress (91,92).

Principles are similar between nonoperative and operative shoulders. We aim to restore full passive range of motion as soon as possible. Posterior capsular tightness causes the humeral head to migrate anteriorly during shoulder elevation, which may contribute to impingement of the supraspinatus.

In the painful relatively stable shoulder, most lesions are due to overuse with resultant inflammation. The first order of treatment is to calm down inflamed tissues and prevent cuff shut down. This treatment is accomplished through a 10-day period of decreasing functional stress, normalizing full passive range of motion, and strengthening. Goals of treatment are pain relief, improved function, prevention of progression, proper joint mechanics, balancing of muscle forces, strengthening of the scapular base, gradual resumption of throwing, and prevention through conditioning.

In our clinic, basic principles of shoulder rehabilitation are as follows:

1. The effects of immobility must be minimized.
2. Healing tissue should never be overstressed.
3. The patient must fulfill specific criteria to progress from one stage of rehabilitation to another.
4. The rehabilitation program must be based on current clinical and basic science research.
5. The rehabilitation program must be adaptable to each patient, allowing for the desired goals of each patient.
6. The rehabilitation process is a team effort with the physician, therapist, trainer, coach, family, and patient.

We also have developed shoulder rehabilitation cliches:

1. Structure governs function.
2. More to the shoulder complex than the shoulder.
3. Proximal stability for distal mobility.
4. Normalize arthrokinematics for normal motion.
5. Circle stability concept.
6. Classification of shoulder instability.
7. The key to the shoulder is the rotator cuff.
8. More to the shoulder than the rotator cuff.
9. More to strength training than dumbbells.
10. Treat the shoulder joint as one part of the kinetic chain.
11. Function stability results in successful outcome.
12. Isolated movement patterns strengthen weak muscles. Combined movement patterns reestablish functional activities.

Physical therapy begins postoperatively on the day of surgery. For operative patients requiring soft tissue repair, we assume that it takes 4 months to develop adequate tensile strength to tolerate physiologic loading. In our practice, all postoperative patients wear shoulder immobilizers until pain has subsided substantially. For debridement of superior labral tears and partial rotator cuff tears and acromioplasty, the immobilizer can be discontinued after several days. If superior labral detachment is stabilized, the immobilizer is continued during sleeping hours for 4 weeks postoperatively.

Phase one is the first 7–14 days after surgery when pain, inflammation, loss of motion, and muscular weakness are most prevalent. Goals are to prevent immobilization effects, regain full minimally painful range of motion, retard muscular atrophy, and reduce discomfort. These aims are accomplished by pendulum exercises plus active assisted motion with an L-bar. Internal and external rotation are improved by using both passive and active-assisted exercises at 0 to 20 degrees of abduction with progression to 90 degrees as tolerated. Anterior, inferior, and posterior capsular stretches are performed using the opposite arm to create an "overpressure." Submaximal isometrics are performed for external and internal rotators, flexors, abductors, and biceps. An important function of the rotator cuff is to dynamically stabilize and steer the humeral head during shoulder movements; thus, early isometrics for the rotator cuff are intended to reestablish voluntary humeral head control.

Phase 2 begins as pain and tenderness become minimal, range of motion approaches full, and strength nears grade 3/5. Goals are normalization of full nonpainful motion, improvement in arthrokinetics, regaining muscular strength, refining neuromuscular control, and eliminating residual inflammation. Isometrics are advanced to isotonics, emphasizing abduction and flexion to 90 degrees, scaption, internal/external rotation, and elbow flexion. The rotator cuff is unloaded by having the supine patient perform isotonic rotator cuff exercise with the shoulder in a position of 100 degrees forward flexion and 90 degrees of abduction, gradually descending to 20 degrees of abduction as pain and strength allow. As rehabilitation is advanced, the patient is switched to the lateral decubitus position to add the resistance of gravity. Scapular retraction and depression are emphasized. Late in phase 2, isokinetics in the plane of the scapula are added. Finally, the stretching routine, especially of the posterior capsule, is performed more aggressively.

Phase 3 is dynamic strengthening and begins when the patient has a full nonpainful range of motion, minimal tenderness, grade 4/5 strength, and a satisfactory clinical examination. This stage is to gain more strength and endurance, and hence power. Aggressive stretching is continued. Tubing exercises are added to the dumbbell routine to provide more constant loading with a concentric/eccentric character.

Phase 4 is return to activity beginning at 12 to 20 weeks postoperatively. It is a period of plyometrics, functional pattern emphasis, and interval sports training. Strength training is aggressive and prolonged to simulate competition demands. The Thrower's Ten Program is emphasized (93):

1. Scaption (supraspinatus)/deltoid;
2. External rotation/internal rotation (90 degrees abducted position) with exercise tubing;
3. D2 proprioceptive neuromuscular facilitation pattern flexion and extension upper extremities;
4. Shoulder horizontal abduction (prone);
5. Push-ups;
6. Press-ups;
7. Prone rowing;
8. Elbow flexion/extension;
9. Wrist extension/flexion;
10. Forearm supination/pronation: sit-ups, stretch, wall squat throws, and run.

An interval throwing program is initiated as well.

Rehabilitation should continue for 1 year postoperatively.

Most patients follow this core protocol. Labral debridement and partial rotator cuff tear patients are advanced as tolerated. It usually takes 3 to 4 months to enter phase 4. Acromioplasty patients avoid exercise in a position of greater than 90 degrees of abduction for a period of 6 weeks. Labral stabilization patients avoid isotonic shoulder and elbow flexion during phase 1 to avoid tensile stress of the biceps–labrum complex repair.

For secondary disorders involving instability, emphasis is placed on proprioceptive neuromuscular facilitation, co-contractions (rhythmic stabilization), and joint approximation as additions to the core protocol. Specifics of rehabilitation in surgically stabilized shoulders is addressed in other chapters of this text.

In summary, therapy is individualized for each patient. Nonoperative care is the mainstay in most painful throwing shoulders. Scapular stabilization provides a stable base. Correction of asymmetric capsular tightness in addition to aggressive generalized stretching is essential. Muscular balance, strengthening, and endurance should progress without undue discomfort. Advanced therapeutics, such as plyometrics, manual resistance, thrower's ten, and an interval throwing program begin only when pain is absent, motion is normal, and strength grade is 5/5. This is a team approach involving the surgeon, physical therapist, athletic trainer, throwing coach, and thrower. The most common mistake is to progress an athlete too rapidly.

SUMMARY AND CONCLUSIONS

This chapter concerns the constellation of disorders surrounding superior labral lesions in the throwing athlete. It is unusual to find isolated pathology. Often, there will be partial tearing of the rotator cuff, instability, and a symptomatic thrower's exostosis in an occasional patient.

A history should be taken with pathomechanics in mind. The physical examination can often be inconclusive. MRI-arthrography can supplement clinical impressions. Frequently, only arthroscopy fully delineates the clinical picture. Attention to detail, especially concerning the role of instability, is of great consequence.

Fortunately, many throwing athletes who present with clinical findings as discussed in this chapter can be managed nonoperatively. All treatment routines are multidisciplinary involving the thrower, surgeon, physical therapist, athletic trainer, and coach.

REFERENCES

1. Andrews JR, Angelo RL. Shoulder arthroscopy for the throwing athlete. *Techn Orthop* 1988;3:75–81.

2. Bennett GE. Shoulder and elbow lesions of the professional baseball pitcher. *JAMA* 1941;117:510–514.
3. King JW, Brelsford HJ, Tullos HS. Analysis of the pitching arm of the professional baseball pitcher. *Clin Orthop* 1969;67:116–123.
4. Barnes DA, Tullos HS. An analysis of 100 symptomatic baseball players. *Am J Sports Med* 1978;6:62–67.
5. Pappas AM, Goss TP, Kleinman PK. Symptomatic shoulder instability due to lesions of the glenoid labrum. *Am J Sports Med* 1983;11:279–288.
6. Jobe FW, Jobe CM. Painful athletic injuries of the shoulder. *Clin Orthop* 1983;173:117–124.
7. Jobe FW, Kvitne RS. Shoulder pain in the overhand or throwing athlete. The relationship of anterior instability and rotator cuff impingement. *Orthop Rev* 1989;18:963–975.
8. Andrews JR, Carson WG Jr. The arthroscopic treatment of glenoid labrum tears in the throwing athlete. *Orthop Trans* 1984;8:44.
9. Snyder SJ, Karzel RP, Del Pizzo W, et al. SLAP lesions of the shoulder. *Arthroscopy* 1990;6:274–279.
10. Tomlinson RJ Jr, Glousman RE. Arthroscopic debridement of glenoid labral tears in athletes. *Arthroscopy* 1995;11:42–51.
11. Snyder SJ, Karzel RP, Del Pizzo W, et al. SLAP lesions of the shoulder. *Arthroscopy* 1990;6:274–279.
12. Moseley HF, Overgaard B. The anterior capsular mechanism in recurrent anterior dislocation of the shoulder. Morphological and clinical studies with special reference to the glenoid labrum and the glenohumeral ligaments. *J Bone Joint Surg* 1962;4:913–927.
13. Prodromos CC, Perry JA, Schiller AL, et al. Histological studies of the glenoid labrum from fetal life to old age. *J Bone Joint Surg Br* 1990;72A:1344–1348.
14. Cooper DE, Arnoczky SP, O'Brien SJ, et al. Anatomy, histology, and vascularity of the glenoid labrum: An anatomic study. *J Bone Joint Surg Am* 1992;74A:46–52.
15. Williams MM, Snyder SJ, Buford D Jr. The Buford complex—the "cord-like middle glenohumeral ligament and absent anterosuperior labrum complex: A normal anatomic capsulolabral variant. *Arthroscopy* 1994;10:241–247.
16. Kujat R. The microangiographic pattern of the glenoid labrum of the dog. *Arch Orthop Trauma Surg* 1986;105:310–312.
17. Tullos HS, King JW. Throwing mechanism in sports. *Orthop Clin North Am* 1973;4:709–720.
18. Dillman CJ, Fleisig GS, Andrews JR. Biomechanics of pitching with emphasis upon shoulder kinematics. *J Orthop Sports Phys Ther* 1993;18:402–408.
19. Fleisig GS, Dillman CJ, Escamilla RF. Kinetics of baseball pitching with implications about injury mechanisms. *Am J Sports Med* 1995;23:233–239.
20. Gainor BJ, Piotrowski G, Puhl J, et al. The throw: biomechanics and acute injury. *Am J Sports Med* 1980;8:114–118.
21. Pappas AM, Zawacki RM, Sullivan TJ. Biomechanics of baseball pitching—a preliminary report. *Am J Sports Med* 1985;13:216–222.
22. Glousman R, Jobe FW, Tibone J, et al. Dynamic electromyographic. Analysis of the throwing shoulder with glenohumeral instability. *J Bone Joint Surg Am* 1988;70A:220–226.
23. Gowan ID, Jobe FW, Tibone JE, et al. A comparative electromyographic analysis of the shoulder during pitching. Professional versus amateur pitchers. *Am J Sports Med* 1987;15:586–590.
24. Jobe FW, Tibone JE, Perry J, et al. An EMG analysis of the shoulder in throwing and pitching. A preliminary report. *Am J Sports Med* 1983;11:3–5.
25. Jobe FW, Moynes DR, Tibone JE, et al. An EMG analysis of the shoulder in pitching. A second report. *Am J Sports Med* 1984;12:218–220.
26. Perry J. Anatomy and biomechanics of the shoulder in throwing, swimming, gymnastics, and tennis. *Clin Sports Med* 1983;2:247–270.
27. Howell SM, Galinat BJ. The glenoid-labral socket. A constrained articular surface. *Clin Orthop* 1989;243:122–125.
28. Poppen NK, Walker PS. Normal and abnormal motion of the shoulder. *J Bone Joint Surg Am* 1976;58A:195–201.
29. Harryman DT, Sidles JA, Clark JM, et al. Translation of the humeral head on the glenoid with passive glenohumeral motion. *J Bone Joint Surg Am* 1990;72A:1334–1343.
30. Warner JJP, Deng X-H, Warren RF, et al. Static capsuloligamen-

31. tous restraints to superior-inferior translation of the glenohumeral joint. *Am J Sports Med* 1992;20:675–685.
31. Turkel SP, Panio MW, Marshall JL, et al. Stabilizing mechanisms preventing anterior dislocation of the glenohumeral joint. *J Bone Joint Surg Am* 1981;63A:1208–1217.
32. Itoi E, Motzkin NE, Morrey BF, et al. Contribution of axial arm rotation to humeral head translation. *Am J Sports Med* 1994;22:499–503.
33. Johnson L. Patterns of shoulder flexibility among college baseball players. *J Athletic Training* 1992;27:44–49.
34. Weiner DS, Macnab I. Superior migration of the humeral head. A radiological aid in the diagnosis of tears of the rotator cuff. *J Bone Joint Surg Br* 1970;52B:524–527.
35. Sharkey NA, Marder RA. The rotator cuff opposes superior translation of the humeral head. *Am J Sports Med* 1995;23:270–275.
36. Andrews JR, Wilk KE. Shoulder injuries in baseball. *In The Athletes Shoulder*, New York: Churchhill Livingstone, 1994:369–389.
37. Andrews JR, Carson WG. The arthroscopic treatment of glenoid labrum tears in the throwing athlete. *Orthop Trans* 1984;8:44.
38. Rodosky MW, Rudert MJ, Harner CH, et al. The role of the biceps-superior glenoid labrum complex in anterior stability of the shoulder. *Arthroscopy* 1990;6:160.
39. Grauer JD, Paulos LE, Smutz WP. Biceps tendon and superior labral injuries. *Arthroscopy* 1992;8:488–497.
40. Itoi E, Kuechle DK, Newman SR, et al. Stabilizing function of the biceps in stable and unstable shoulders. *J Bone Joint Surg Br* 1993;75B:546–550.
41. Pagnani MJ, Deng X-H, Warren RF, et al. Role of the long head of the biceps brachii in glenohumeral stability: a biomechanical study in cadavera. *J Shoulder Elbow Surg* 1996;5:255–262.
42. Kumar VP, Satku K, Balasubramaniam P. The role of the long head of biceps brachii in the stabilization of the head of the humerus. *Clin Orthop* 1989;244:172–175.
43. Rodosky MW, Harner CD, Fu FH. The role of the long head of the biceps muscle and superior glenoid labrum in anterior stability of the shoulder. *Am J Sports Med* 1994;22:121–130.
44. Andrews JR, Carson WG, McLeod WD. Glenoid labrum tears related to the long head of the biceps. *Am J Sports Med* 1985;13:337–341.
45. Fleisig GS, Jameson GG, Dillman CJ, et al. Biomechanics of overhead sports. In: Garrett WE, Kirkendall DT, eds. *Exercise and Sport Science*. Philadelphia, PA: Lippincott Williams & Wilkins (in press).
46. Walch G, Boileau P, Noel E, et al. Impingement of the deep surface of the supraspinatus tendon on the posterosuperior glenoid rim: an arthroscopic study. *J Shoulder Elbow Surg* 1992;1:238–247.
47. Flatow EL, Soslowsky LJ, Ticker JB, et al. Excursion of the rotator cuff under the acromion. *Am J Sports Med* 1994;22:779–788.
48. Jobe CM. Posterior superior glenoid impingement: expanded spectrum. *Arthroscopy* 1995;11:530–535.
49. Glasgow SG, Bruce RA, Yacobucci GN, et al. Arthroscopic resection of glenoid labral tears in the athlete: a report of 29 cases. *Arthroscopy* 1992;8:48–54.
50. Snyder SJ, Banas MP, Karzel RP. An analysis of 140 injuries to the superior glenoid labrum. *J Shoulder Elbow Surg* 1995;4:243–248.
51. Altchek DW, Warren RF, Wickiewicz TL. Arthroscopic labral debridement. A three year follow up study. *Am J Sports Med* 1992;20:702–706.
52. Warner JP, Kann S, Marks P. Arthroscopic repair of combined Bankart and superior labral detachment anterior and posterior lesions: technique and preliminary results. *Arthroscopy* 1994;10:383–391.
53. Jobe FW, Glousman RE. Rotator cuff dysfunction and associated glenohumeral instability in the throwing shoulder. In: Paulos LE, Tibone JE, eds. Operative techniques in shoulder surgery. Maryland: Aspen Publishers, 1991:85.
54. Meister K, Andrews JR. Classification and treatment of rotator cuff injuries in the overhand athlete. *J Orthop Sports Phys Ther* 1993;18:413–421.
55. Lombardo SJ, Jobe FW, Kerlan RK. Posterior shoulder lesions in throwing athletes. *Am J Sports Med* 1977;5:106–110.
56. Ferrari JD, Ferrari DA, Coumas J, et al. Posterior ossification of

the shoulder: the Bennett lesion. Etiology, diagnosis, and treatment. *Am J Sports Med* 1994;22:171–176.

57. Payne LZ, Jokl P. The results of arthroscopic debridement of glenoid labral tears based on tear location. *Arthroscopy* 1993;9:560–565.

58. Maffet MW, Gartsman GM, Moseley B. Superior labrum-biceps tendon complex lesions of the shoulder. *Am J Sports Med* 1995;23:93–98.

59. Resch H, Golser K, Thoeni H, et al. Arthroscopic repair of superior glenoid labral detachment (the SLAP lesion). *J Shoulder Elbow Surg* 1993;2:147–155.

60. Butters KP, Rockwood CA. Office evaluation and management of the shoulder impingement syndrome. *Orthop Clin North Am* 1988;19:755–771.

61. Hawkins RJ, Hobeika P. Physical examination of the shoulder. *Orthopedics* 1983;10:1270–1279.

62. Silliman JF, Hawkins RJ. Clinical examination of the shoulder complex. In: *The Athletes Shoulder*.

63. Magnusson SP, Gleim GW, Nicholas JA. Shoulder weakness in professional baseball pitchers. *Med Sci Sports Exerc* 1994;26:5–9.

64. Brown LP, Niehues SL, Harrah A, et al. Upper extremity range of motion and isokinetic strength of the internal and external shoulder rotators in major league baseball players. *Am J Sports Med* 1988;16:577–585.

65. Andrews JR, Gillogly S. Physical examination of the shoulder in throwing athletes. In: Zarins B, Andrews JR, Carson WG, eds. *Injuries to the throwing arm*. Philadelphia: W.B. Saunders, 1985:51–65.

66. Liu SH, Henry MH, Nuccion SL. A prospective evaluation of a new physical examination in predicting glenoid labral tears. *Am J Sports Med* 1996;24:721–725.

67. Kibler WB. Specificity and sensitivity of the anterior slide test in throwing athletes with superior glenoid labrum tears. *Arthroscopy* 1995;11:296–300.

68. McGlynn FJ, Caspari RB. Arthroscopic findings in the subluxating shoulder. *Clin Orthop* 1984;183:173–178.

69. Payne LZ, Altchek DW, Craig EV, et al. Arthroscopic treatment of partial rotator cuff tears in young athletes. A preliminary report. *Am J Sports Med* 1997;25:299–305.

70. Wright SA, Cofield RH. Management of partial-thickness rotator cuff tears. *J Shoulder Elbow Surg* 1996;5:458–466.

71. Andrews JR, Byrd JWT, Kupferman SP, et al. The profile view of the acromion. *Clin Orthop* 1991;263:142–146.

72. Callaghan JJ, McNiesh LM, DeHaven JP, et al. A prospective comparison study of double contrast computed tomography (CT) arthrography and arthroscopy of the shoulder. *Am J Sports Med* 1988;16:13–20.

73. Legan JM, Burkhard TK, Goff WF, et al. Tears of the glenoid labrum: MR imaging of 88 arthroscopically confirmed cases. *Radiology* 1991;179:241–252.

74. Gusmer PB, Potter HG, Schatz JA, et al. Labral injuries: accuracy

of detection with unenhanced MR imaging of the shoulder. *Radiology* 1996;200:519–524.

75. Rafii M, Firooznia H, Sherman O, et al. Rotator cuff lesions: signal patterns at MR imaging. *Radiology* 1990;177:817–823.

76. Traughber PD, Goodwin TE. Shoulder MRI: arthroscopic correlation with emphasis on partial tears. *J Comput Assist Tomogr* 1992;16:129–133.

77. Mulligan SA, Schwartz ML, Andrews JR. MR arthrography in the evaluation of upper extremity athletic injuries. In publication.

78. Iannotti JP, Zlatkin MB, Esterhai JL, et al. Magnetic resonance imaging of the shoulder. *J Bone Joint Surg Am* 1991;73A:17–29.

79. Karzel RP, Snyder SJ. Magnetic resonance arthrography of the shoulder. A new technique of shoulder imaging. *Clin Sports Med* 1993;12:123–136.

80. Andrews JR, Wilk KE. Shoulder injuries in baseball. In: Andrews JR, Wilk KE, eds. *The athlete's shoulder*. New York: Churchill Livingstone, 1994:369–389.

81. Sain J, Andrews JR. Proper pitching techniques. In: Zarins B, Andrews JR, Carson WG, eds. *Injuries to the throwing arm*. Philadelphia: W.B. Saunders, 1985.

82. Fauls D. General training techniques to warm up and cool down the throwing arm. In: Zarins J, Andrews JR, Carson WG, eds. *Injuries to the throwing arm*. Philadelphia: W.B. Saunders, 1985.

83. Townsend H, Jobe FW, Pink M, et al. Electromyographic analysis of the glenohumeral muscles during a baseball rehabilitation program. *Am J Sports Med* 1991;19:264–272.

84. Ogilvie-Harris DJ, Wiley AM. Arthroscopic surgery of the shoulder: A general appraisal. *J Bone Joint Surg Br* 1986;68B:201–207.

85. Altchek DW, Ortiz G, Warren RF, et al. Arthroscopic labral debridement. *Orthop Trans* 1990;14:258.

86. Cordasco FA, Steinmann S, Flatow EL, et al. Arthroscopic treatment of glenoid labral tears. *Am J Sports Med* 1993;221:425–431.

87. Terry GC, Friedman SJ, Uhl TL. Arthroscopically treated tears of the glenoid labrum. Factors influencing outcome. *Am J Sports Med* 1994;22:504–512.

88. Yoneda M, Hirooka A, Saito S, et al. Arthroscopic stapling for detached superior glenoid labrum. *J Bone Joint Surg Br* 1991;73B:746–750.

89. Field LD, Savoie FH III. Arthroscopic suture repair of superior labral detachment lesions of the shoulder. *Am J Sports Med* 1993;21:783–790.

90. Andrews JR, Carson WG, Ortega K. Arthroscopy of the shoulder: technique and normal anatomy. *Am J Sports Med* 1984;12:1–7.

91. Wilk KE, Arrigo CA, Andrews JR. Standardized isokinetic testing protocol for the throwing shoulder: the thrower's series. *Isokinetics Exerc Sci* 1991;1:63–71.

92. Wilk KE, Arrigo CA. Isokinetic exercise and testing for the shoulder. In: Andrews JR, Wilk KE, eds. *The athlete's shoulder*. New York: Churchill Livingstone, 1994:523–542.

93. Arrigo CA. Arm care for the throwing athlete. In: Andrews JR, Wilk KE, eds. *The athlete's shoulder*. New York: Churchill Livingstone, 1994:653–668.

Principles and Practice of Orthopaedic Sports Medicine,
edited by William E. Garrett, Jr., Kevin P. Speer, and Donald T. Kirkendall.
Lippincott Williams & Wilkins, Philadelphia © 2000.

CHAPTER 26

Rotator Cuff Injuries

Guido Marra and Evan L. Flatow

J. G. Smith (1), an English anatomist, is credited with the first anatomic description of a rotator cuff tear, published in his report in the *London Medical Gazette* in 1834. This report described tendon rupture after shoulder trauma in a series of seven patients. Codman is credited with performing the first surgical repair of the rotator cuff. He published the results of tendon repair in two patients in 1911 (2). In 1934, he published by his classic book, *The Shoulder* (3), in which he proposed that the pathogenesis of rotator cuff tears was traumatic in nature. This was generally accepted until 1924, when Meyer (4) speculated that the pathogenesis of rotator cuff tears was due to mechanical attrition from wear caused more by the overlying acromion than by trauma. Over the next 30 years, various authors (5–7) wrote extensively about the pathogenesis and surgical management of rotator cuff tears.

Many early reports of surgical repair of the rotator cuff noted a significant number of unsatisfactory results ranging from 26% to 46% (2,3,8). In 1972, Neer advanced our understanding about rotator cuff injuries when he published his classic article on the impingement lesion (17). This landmark paper defined the clinical signs, the pathologic progression, and the treatment of this condition. For patients who failed nonoperative management of this condition, Neer advocated preservation of the deltoid along with conservative reshaping of the anteroinferior acromion (anterior acromioplasty) rather than lateral or total acromionectomy. In addition, he recommended mobilization and repair of the cuff as needed. Large series of repairs in older patients with degenerative cuff lesions using Neer's surgical principles

have reported consistent pain relief and improvement function (9–14).

Rotator cuff injuries in the young athletic population is a more complex and controversial issue. Numerous etiologies have been proposed for these conditions, including outlet impingement (15–19), impingement secondary to glenohumeral instability (20), abutment of the cuff tendon in the glenoid rim (21,22), tensile overload or shear injury to the tendon fibers (20,23–25), and avascular zones within the tendon. The introduction of shoulder arthroscopy in the evaluation and treatment of rotator cuff disease has had a profound impact (26–28). New information about glenohumeral pathology has led ato greater understanding of the pathologic lesions associated with rotator cuff injuries and has also led to increased controversy in this evolving area. The arthroscope has also revolutionized treatment options of cuff injuries with the development of arthroscopically assisted rotator cuff repair and arthroscopic rotator cuff repair.

EPIDEMIOLOGY

Numerous cadaveric studies have documented the incidence of rotator cuff tears that range from less than 5% (17) to 26.5% (29). Partial-thickness tears of the rotator cuff are more frequently encountered, with incidence reported from 13% to 37% (30). Depalma et al. (31) reported partial-thickness tears of the supraspinatus and infraspinatus in 37% of cadaveric specimens examined. The subscapularis tendon had tendon tears in 21% of specimens examined. Fukuda et al. (30) reported an overall incidence of partial-thickness tears to be 13% in a series of 249 dissections, with 3% bursal-sided tears, 7% intratendinous tears, and 3% articular-sided tears. The incidence of rotator cuff is age dependent, and frank tendon failure in patients under the age of 40 is a rare occurrence.

G. Marra: Department of Orthopaedic Surgery, Loyola University Medical Center, Maywood, Illinois 60153.

E. L. Flatow: Chief of Shoulder Surgery, The Mount Sinai Medical Center, New York, New York 10029.

MECHANISM OF INJURY AND PATHOANATOMY

Subacromial bursitis and rotator cuff tendonitis and tears have long been implicated as a cause of pain, weakness, and functional limitations about the shoulder (9,17). In the athletic population, the cause for these injuries include outlet impingement causing extrinsic tendon injury (15–19), glenohumeral instability, tendon abutment against the glenoid rim (21,22), tendon and bursal swelling in a confined space (25), tensile overload (20), intrinsic tendon injury from tendonitis (25), altered vascularity (32), or shear between different fiber bundles (23,24).

Outlet Impingement

Before Neer's classic article in 1972, impingement of the rotator cuff was thought to occur by the abutment

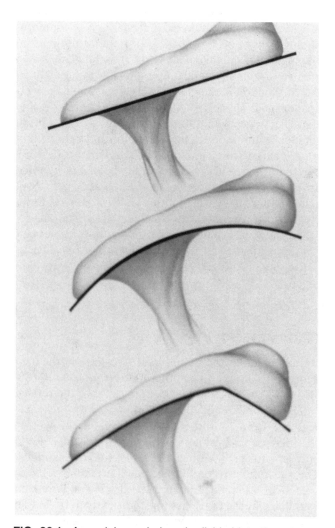

FIG. 26.1. Acromial morphology is divided into three types based on appearance on the outlet view: type I, flat; type II, smooth curve; and type III, anterior hook. (From Bigliani LU, Morrison DS, April EW. The morphology of the acromion and its relationship to rotator cuff tears. *Orthop Trans* 1986; 10:228, with permission.)

TABLE 26.1. *Neer's stages of impingement*

Stage	Age	Findings
I	<25	Edema and hemorrhage
II	Over 25	Fibrosis and tendonitis
III	Over 40	Degeneration, bony changes and tendon rupture

of the lateral edge of the acromion against the rotator cuff. Surgical treatment included complete acromionectomy and lateral acromioplasty. These surgical interventions substantially weakened the deltoid and provided mixed functional results. Neer believed that as the arm is elevated and externally rotated, the supraspinatus facet of the greater tuberosity rotated beneath the anterior inferior aspect of the acromion. Bigliani et al. (15) examined 140 shoulder in cadavers with an average age of 75 years and demonstrated a relationship between the incidence of rotator cuff tears in cadavers and acromial morphology. Acromial morphology was classified in three types (Fig. 26.1). Type I acromion (flat) was seen in 17% of the specimens, type II (curved) in 43%, and type III (hooked) in 40%. Of the specimens with full-thickness tears, 3% had a type I acromion, 24% had a type II acromion, and 73% had a type III acromion. Flatow et al. (33) demonstrated that contact of the anteroinferior acromion was centered on the supraspinatus insertion, where cuff tears are generally initiated.

Neer divided impingement into three stages, which has been subsequently modified by other authors (Table 26.1). Stage I is characterized by edema and hemorrhage and is seen in a younger population. This lesion is typically caused by overuse, has a reversible clinical course, and usually responds to conservative management. In stage II, fibrosis and tendonitis result from repetitive mechanical insults to the tendon. Patients are usually 25 to 40 years of age. Neer believed these patients should be treated conservatively for a minimum of 18 months before surgical intervention because most of these patients improved with time. In addition, he rarely performed acromioplasty in patients who were less than 30 years of age. Gartsman (34) subdivided stage II lesions into two categories: a less involved stage characterized by fibrosis and tendonitis and a more severely involved stage that included partial cuff tears. Stage III lesions included bone spur formation and tendon rupture. The typical patient in this group was over the age of 40 and required surgical intervention to improve their functional outcome.

Secondary Impingement

Jobe and Kvitne (35) popularized the theory of secondary impingement resulting from glenohumeral instability in the young athletic population. They postulated that repetitive overhead activity caused the anterior soft tissue structure deficiencies allowing for anterior subluxation of the shoulder joint. Increased anterior translation of the glenohumeral joint can result in secondary impingement. Patients with the "instability complex" are classified into four groups. Group I patients have impingement signs with no clinical evidence of instability. This groups is generally older. Group II has primary instability from anterior labral degeneration resulting in secondary instability. Patients in group III have primary instability due to hyperelastic tissue and secondary instability. Group IV patients have pure glenohumeral instability without signs impingement. Jobe and Kvitne proposed that patients with secondary impingement should have a procedure that addressed the anterior laxity and did not overly tighten the soft tissues. It was for this purpose that they developed the anterior capsulolabral reconstruction.

Posterior Superior Glenoid Impingement

Posterior superior glenoid impingement is a recently described mechanism of injury to the rotator cuff. In 1992, Walch et al. (22) reported a series of 17 overhead with shoulder pain unresponsive to conservative treatment. Pain was noted to be diffuse but tended to be worse in the posterior aspect of the shoulder. No patients exhibited any signs of glenohumeral instability. Arthroscopic examination revealed that impingement of the rotator cuff occurred between the posterior edge of the glenoid from 9 and 11 o'clock when the right arm was placed in 90 to 150 degrees of abduction. Osteochondral lesions of the humeral head were seen in eight patients. These lesion were higher than the typical Hill-Sachs defects seen in glenohumeral instability. Labral lesions included degeneration and small flap tears, but the biceps origin was never involved.

Jobe (21) reported a series of 11 patients with similar clinical finding. However, 6 patients did not have sports-related injuries, which implied that this form of impingement is not confined to the athletic population. Five structures can be involved in this process: the anterior inferior glenohumeral ligament complex and anterior glenoid labrum, the rotator cuff, the posterior superior glenoid labrum, the greater tuberosity, and the superior glenoid. If lesions are present in any one of these tructures, it is important to carefully examine the remaining structures.

Other

The vascular supply to the rotator cuff has classically been implicated as a cause of rotator cuff degeneration. Rathbun and Macnab (32) performed microinjections to define the vascular anatomy of the rotator cuff. The authors demonstrated a hypovascular zone in the leading edge of the supraspinatus tendon when the arm was adducted when compared with the abducted arm. This area corresponds to the critical zone where rotator cuff degeneration is most frequently seen. The authors postulated that in the adducted position, vessels within the supraspinatus tendon were "wrung out." Microvascular studies performed by Lohr and Unthoff (36) demonstrated that the articular surface of the supraspinatus tendon was relatively hypovascular when compared with the bursal surface. This results clinically correlate with the increased incidence of articular-sided partial-thickness cuff tears.

Fukuda et al. (23) reported a series of 17 *en bloc* specimens obtained from patients undergoing repair of partial-thickness rotator cuff tears. Bursal-sided tears were present in seven specimens, intratendinous tears were present in two, and eight specimens had articular surface tears. All specimens demonstrated intratendinous tears under microscopic observation, 15 were located in the midtendon, and 2 were eccentrically located. The authors speculated that shear forces within the tendon are responsible for the development of these tears and that the tears begin within the substance of the tendon.

CLINICAL EVALUATION

History

Patients with rotator cuff injuries will typically complain of anterior shoulder pain, most notably with activities overhead. Functional losses due to stiffness, weakness, catching, or pain are also common complaints. Often patients have nocturnal pain and difficulty sleeping on the affected arm. Pain may be localized to the coracoacromial ligament, the anterolateral acromion, or may be more diffuse due bursal inflammation.

In the young overhead athlete, complaints of pain may be nonspecific. The patient should be questioned about feelings of instability, numbness, tingling, or episodes of "dead arm" syndrome. In addition, it is important to determine the mechanics specific to the athletic activity the patients participates in. In all cases, a history of prior treatment or therapy should be elicited and its effectiveness.

Physical Examination

Physical examination in patients with suspected rotator cuff injuries should include a thorough cervical and upper extremity examination to exclude other sites of pathology. During examination, easy access to both shoulders is essential for comparison. Examination begins with visual inspection of both shoulders. Evaluation of muscle symmetry may reveal atrophy of the supraspinatus or infraspinatus (Fig. 26.2). Muscle contours should be evaluated, particularly of the deltoid and biceps. Finally, any prior surgical incisions and presence of swelling should be noted.

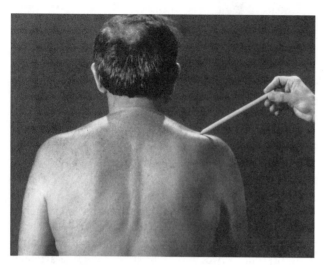

FIG. 26.2. Patient with a rotator cuff tear demonstrating atrophy of the shoulder girdle.

subacromial impingement, it is possible to elicit symptoms of impingement by maneuvering the biceps and rotator cuff under the coracoacromial arch. Neer and Hawkins (17,38) both described maneuvers to exacerbate impingement symptoms. The Neer impingement test is performed by elevating the internally rotated arm, whereas the Hawkins' impingement test is performed in forward elevation to 90 degrees, adduction across the chest, and internal rotation. Both tests bring the biceps, rotator cuff, and greater tuberosity under the coracoacromial arch. These maneuvers can be produce pain caused by other shoulder conditions such as instability, stiffness, calcium deposits, arthritis, and bone lesions. For these tests to be truly positive, the pain should be nearly completely eliminated after a subacromial injection of 10 mL of 1% xylocaine.

When evaluating the young athlete, one must be certain to exclude the diagnosis of instability as a source of anterior shoulder pain. The classic apprehension sign

Palpation is carried out to illicit exact locations of tenderness. Patients with rotator cuff injuries typically have pain over the anterior and lateral aspects of the acromion. Careful evaluation of the acromioclavicular joint is needed to ensure no concomitant acromioclavicular arthritis. Patients with subtle glenohumeral instability may also have anterior or posterior glenohumeral joint line tenderness.

Active and passive range of motion should be evaluated in elevation, internal rotation, and external rotation. Comparisons between the affected and unaffected extremity are particularly useful in the evaluation of the rotation. Patients with rotator cuff injuries will often have decreased active range of motion secondary to pain but have full passive motion. If limited active and passive range of motion is present, then adhesive capsulitis should be suspected, although shoulders with rotator cuff injuries may also develop secondary stiffness. Loss of internal rotation is common in throwing athletes and may be due to a tight posterior capsule. A tight posterior capsule is associated with rotator cuff tendonitis and instability.

Strength of the shoulder should be examined in forward elevation, abduction, internal rotation, and external rotation. Weakness is rarely seen in the small or medium-sized tears, but strength is usually reduced in the large or massive tear. This is particularly true in external rotation. Gerber et al. (37) described the lift-off test to evaluate the integrity of the subscapularis. A pathologic lift-off test is present when a patient is unable to lift the dorsum of their hand off their back (Fig. 26.3). When pain limits the examination, a xylocaine injection into the subacromial space can be used to ensure that weakness is not secondary to pain.

Because the etiology of rotator cuff tears is linked to

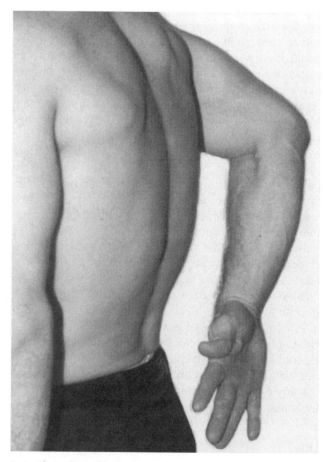

FIG. 26.3. The lift-off test evaluates the integrity of the subscapularis. The hand of the affected extremity is internally rotated and placed on the lower lumbar spine. The patient is asked to lift the dorsum of their hand off their back. If the patient is unable to lift off their hand, the test is positive, indicating compromise of the subscapularis tendon.

may be elicited when the affected arm is abducted and externally rotated. In subtle forms of instability, pain can be elicited by levering the humeral head in an abducted and externally rotated position. Disappearance of pain with anterior pressure is suggestive of subtle instability (relocation test). When uncertainty is still present, examination under anesthesia and arthroscopy may be needed.

IMAGING

Radiographs

All patients with suspected rotator cuff pathology should have plain radiographic evaluation. Standard radiographic evaluation include anteroposterior, outlet, and axillary views. Neutral, internal, and external rotation views in the anteroposterior plane of the scapula visualize the glenohumeral joint, the greater tuberosity, and the lesser tuberosity. In small cuff tears, these views are often normal, but cysts and excrescences may be visualized within the greater tuberosity. In large and massive rotator cuff tears, sclerosis may be present on the under surface of the acromion (called the sourcil sign) and the humeral head may be translated superiorly on the glenoid face (Fig. 26.4). Acromiohumeral distances that measure less than 5 mm are suggestive of large rotator cuff tears. The axillary view allows evaluation of the glenohumeral joint space, the acromioclavicular joint, the

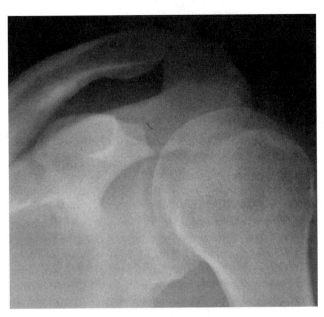

FIG. 26.5. The Zanca view is obtained by directing the x-ray beam 5 to 15 degrees cephalad, bisecting the acromioclavicular joint. This view allows clear visualization of the acromioclavicular joint by eliminating the overlap of the joint on the spine of the scapula seen on the standard anteroposterior view of the shoulder.

anterior and posterior rim of the glenoid, the presence of an os acromiale, and the tuberosities. Finally, the supraspinatus outlet view will demonstrate acromial morphology and will reveal any spurs encroaching into the subacromial space. In patients with acromioclavicular joint tenderness, a Zanca view should be obtained to evaluate this joint. This view is obtained by directing the x-ray beam 5 to 15 degrees cephalad, bisecting the acromioclavicular joint and eliminating the overlap of the joint seen on the standard anteroposterior view of the shoulder (Fig. 26.5). Rockwood also described a 30-degree caudal anteroposterior view that can reveal subacromial spurs not visible on the standard anteroposterior view (39).

Arthrograms

Shoulder arthrogram is considered to be the traditional gold standard for detecting rotator cuff tears. Lindblom described the use of radiopaque contrast for the detection of rotator cuff tears in 1939 (40). Since this description, this has evolved to become a reliable test or documenting full-thickness rotator cuff tears. Double-contrast arthrography is more frequently used than single-contrast arthrography. In this technique, 2 to 3 mL of contrast medium is introduced into the glenohumeral joint followed by 10 to 15 mL of air. Double-contrast arthrography allows accurate detection of full-thickness rotator cuff tears and visualization of the intraarticular

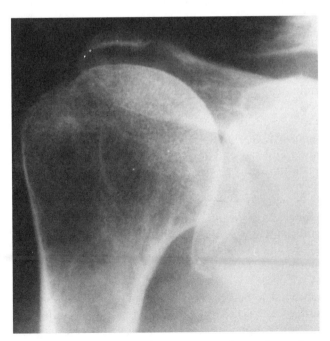

FIG. 26.4. Sclerosis may be present on the under surface of the acromion in large and massive rotator cuff tears.

portion of the biceps tendon. Reports of sensitivity of arthrography range from 85% to 100% and specificity from 85% to 95%. Arthrography is less reliable in diagnosing bursal-sided partial-thickness rotator cuff tears or intrasubstance tears. In addition, no information is provided about the condition of the muscle.

Magnetic Resonance Imaging

Magnetic resonance imaging (MRI) has emerged as the imaging study of choice in the evaluation of the rotator cuff. This study allows assessment of the quality of the rotator cuff muscles, the size of the tear, involvement of the biceps tendon, and diagnosis of partial cuff tears. Iannotti et al. (41) reported a series of 106 patients with surgically confirmed rotator cuff tears who underwent preoperatively MRI. Correlation between preoperative readings and intraoperative finding revealed a sensitivity of 100% and specificity of 95% for full-thickness rotator cuff tears (Fig. 26.6). When differentiation was made between tendonitis and partial-thickness rotator cuff tears, accuracy declined; reported sensitivity and specificity was 82% and 85%, respectively (Fig. 26.7).

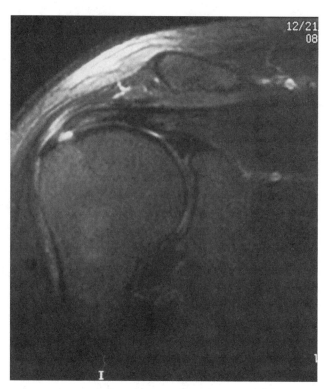

FIG. 26.7. Magnetic resonance image of the shoulder demonstrating a partial-thickness tear of the supraspinatus tendon. When partial tears constitute 50% of the tendon thickness, consideration to mini-open tendon excision and repair should be given.

TREATMENT

Nonoperative Management

Nonoperative management of rotator cuff injuries is frequently used in the competitive athlete. It is critical for the treating physician to have a clear history of disability, pain, the nature of the injury, and the athlete's training routine. The frequency and duration of the athlete's training schedule must be determined and any increase or decreases in the training cycles. When problems arise, early modification in the training technique and frequency and duration of workouts can often alleviate problems.

When training modification does not alleviate problems, then the institution of a well-structured strengthening and stretching program is necessary. If pain is sufficient, the use of a short course of nonsteroidal medicines can be beneficial. Although the use of subacromial steroid injections is widespread, its use is controversial. A double-blinded prospective trial comparing subacromial injections of steroid and placebo found no difference (42). Berry et al. (43) reported no difference in use of acupuncture, physiotherapy, subacromial injections, or anti-inflammatory medicine. Watson (44) reported a series of 89 patients undergoing rotator cuff

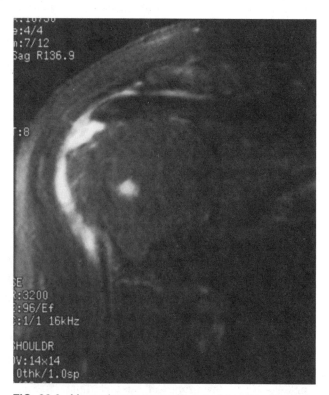

FIG. 26.6. Magnetic resonance image of the shoulder demonstrating a minimally retraction full-thickness tear of the supraspinatus tendon. These types of tears are ideal for "mini open" repair through a small extensions of the anteriolateral portal.

repair. He reported that 20 patients received more than four subacromial injections of steroid and 17 patients had poor cuff tissue at time of repair. Properly timed and judicious use of steroids can help break a chronic impingement cycle and help facilitate a proper rehabilitation program.

Rehabilitation

Initial treatment of injuries of the rotator cuff should be conservative, and its cornerstone is a comprehensive rehabilitation program with emphasis on both stretching and strengthening. The goals of the rehabilitation are threefold. First, normal passive and active range of motion must be established. Once normal range of motion is established, emphasis should be turned to reestablishing normal scapulohumeral rhythm. Finally, a program of strengthening and gradual return to competition can begin.

Stretching

It has long been recognized that capsular contracture plays a role in the pathomechanics of the impingement syndrome. Posterior tightness of the glenohumeral joint has been implicated as an causative factor in the etiology of impingement. As the arm is elevated, posterior tightness will cause superior migration of the humeral head, aggregating the impingement syndrome. Stretching of the posterior capsule is accomplished with cross-body adduction of an internally rotated arm. The use of proprioceptive neuromuscular facilitation techniques can be extremely effective in regaining motion. In the acute inflammatory phase of impingement, stretching should be performed passively in the supine position. With the scapula stabilized against the chest wall, a slow persistent arm elevation should be performed. As the arm is elevated, it is important to note the relative motion of the scapulothoracic articulation. One must be cognizant of the motion occurring at the scapulothoracic and glenohumeral joint during arm elevation. Once full passive range of motion is reached, active range of motion exercised should be instituted.

Strengthening

Strengthening programs should be directed to increase the strength of both the rotator cuff musculature and the scapular stabilizers. Rotator cuff strengthening is effectively accomplished with the use of elastic bands to provide a closed-chain kinetic strengthening. In addition, elastic bands allow concentric and eccentric muscles strengthening. In the acute phase of impingement, all exercises should be performed below the horizontal to avoid impingement of the rotator cuff.

Infraspinatus and teres minor can be isolated with

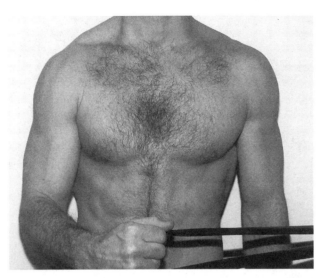

FIG. 26.8. External rotation exercises are performed with resistive elastic tube fixed across the body. With the arm held in adduction and the elbows bent at 90 degrees, concentric and eccentric exercises are performed against the resistance provided by the tubing.

the arm in an adducted position and the elbow flexed to 90 degrees. The arm is externally rotated with the elastic band brought across the chest. When full external rotation is reached, the arm is brought back to an internally rotated position, resisting the pull of the elastic band (Fig. 26.8).

The subscapularis can be exercised with the elastic band outside the body. The arm is kept adducted with the elbow flexed at 90 degrees. The arm is internally rotated against the resistance provided by the elastic band. When the arm is fully internally rotated, the arm is externally rotated slowly against the resistance provided by the elastic band (Fig. 26.9).

Jobe (45) proposed strengthening the supraspinatus tendon by elevating the arm in an internally rotated position based on electromyogram studies. Unfortunately, this also the position that maximized the impingement process by rotating the greater tuberosity under the coracoacromial arch. Speer et al. (46) found no difference in the electromyographic activity of the supraspinatus tendon with the arm internally rotated or externally rotated. Supraspinatus strengthening can be effectively accomplished with elastic band resistance exercised by elevating the externally rotated arm in the scapular plane (Fig. 26.10).

Surgical Management

Impingement

Classic treatment for the management of the impingement syndrome has been the anterior acromioplasty as described by Neer in 1972 (17). Open anterior acromio-

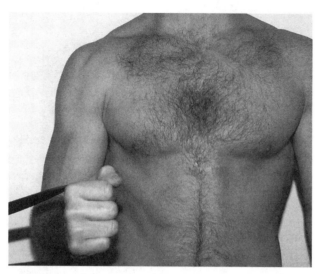

FIG. 26.9. Internal rotation exercises are performed with resistive elastic tube fixed lateral to the body. With the arm held in adduction and the elbows bent at 90 degrees, concentric and eccentric exercises are performed against the resistance provided by the tubing.

plasty has proven to be an effective treatment for impingement lesions of the rotator cuff (17,24,47,49–54). Good to excellent results have been reported from 73% to 89% with regard to pain relief and function. McShane et al. (48) modified the approach of the anterior acromioplasty by preserving the deltoid origin. This approach allowed immediate mobilization of the patient, theoreti-

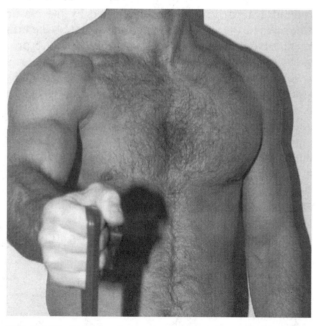

FIG. 26.10. Upper cut exercises are performed with the resistive elastic tube fixed inferior to the body. The elbow is slightly bent and the arm is against the resistance provided by the tubing.

cally decreasing the likelihood of postoperative stiffness. The natural extension of preservation of the deltoid origin is the arthroscopic acromioplasty, first described by Ellman in 1985 (55). Advantages of arthroscopic acromioplasty include the ability to evaluation the glenohumeral joint, the articular side of the rotator cuff, the ability to address intraarticular pathology, cosmesis, preservation of the deltoid origin, reduced early morbidity, and decreased hospitalization expense.

Numerous reports have validated the efficacy of arthroscopic acromioplasty with good to excellent results seen in 82% to 92% of patients (27,28,34,47,56). However, arthroscopic subacromial decompression is not without controversy. Hawkins et al. (57) reported a series of 110 patients undergoing subacromial decompression with a 2-year follow-up. Satisfactory results were seen in only 46% of patients. However, 40% of the patient were on workers' compensation, and when isolated as a group, they had only 32% satisfactory results. Hawkins et al. (50) reported a 87% satisfactory result with open decompression. Sachs et al. (58) reported a randomized prospective study comparing open with arthroscopic acromioplasty. Analysis of their results demonstrated that patients undergoing arthroscopic acromioplasty regained flexion and strength faster than patients undergoing open acromioplasty. In addition, the arthroscopic group returned to work faster, had shorter hospital stays, and used less narcotic medicine. However, at 3 months no differences were observed between the two groups.

Lazarus et al. (59) reported better results with open acromioplasty when compared with arthroscopic acromioplasty; however, the arthroscopic group demonstrated a faster recovery time. Complications of arthroscopic decompression have included injury to the deltoid origin (60), subacromial calcification and ossification (61), fracture of the acromion (60,62–64), and inadequate bone removal (60). Rockwood and Lyons (54) believed that arthroscopic decompressions may cause more weakening of the deltoid than the open approach. They believed the inferior subperiosteal exposure of the anterior acromial edge detached the deep fibers of the deltoid origin that will not heal unless this edge is reapproximated to and repaired through drill holes to the acromion.

Controversy about surgical management of impingement exists in the young athletic population. Jackson (65) reported a series of 10 athletes that underwent an open coracoacromial ligament division under local anesthesia. Six patients returned to their prior level of activity and the remaining four did not. Tibone et al. (66) reported a series of 35 cases of impingement treated by anterior acromioplasty in competitive athletes. This study reported 89% of the cases had subjective improvement in their symptoms but only 43% returned to their preinjury level of performance. However, in many early series, subtle instability patterns may have been overlooked. Jobe and Kvitne (35) proposed the anterior capsulolabral reconstruction for the unstable athletic shoulder. They reported a series of 19 athletes who underwent anterior capsulolabral reconstruction for anterior shoulder pain unresponsive to conservative treatment. Fifteen patients were able to complete one full season after rehabilitation. Proper preoperative evaluation of the athlete should distinguish the patient suffering for shoulder instability and true impingement.

Bigliani et al. (67) proposed tailoring the treatment of impingement in the younger patient to the pathology present. If diagnostic arthroscopy reveals bursal scarring, arthroscopic bursectomy and debridement of the coracoacromial ligament insertion may be performed without bone removal. When the impingement is secondary to instability, there may be subacromial scarring and inflammation that prevents adequate rehabilitation. In this setting, a soft tissue decompression of the subacromial space may allow renewed rehabilitation, avoiding the need for formal stabilization. When attritional changes are observed in the coracoacromial ligament insertion, the ligament should be excised arthroscopically. When a prominent acromion with attritional lesion is present, then an arthroscopic acromioplasty is indicated.

Partial-thickness Tears

Treatment of partial tears of the rotator cuff remains controversial. Fukuda et al. (30) advocated open excision of the involved tendon along with decompression. They reported a series of 21 cases that comprised 9 bursal-sided tears, 1 intratendous tear, and 11 articular-sided tears. Patients with bursal-sided tears were more symptomatic preoperatively. Follow-up was 15 months with 90% satisfactory results. In the older population, debridement of partial cuff tears alone does not provide satisfactory results. Ogilvie-Harris and Wiley (68) reported that of a series of 57 patients undergoing debridement of partial cuff tears, only half benefited from the procedure. Snyder et al. (69) reported 84% satisfactory results in a series of 31 patients undergoing arthroscopic debridement. In this series, decompression was performed only if there was evidence of bursal-sided attrition of the rotator cuff. Most investigators routinely include an acromioplasty in the treatment of the partial rotator cuff tear (34,53–70). Ellman (71) reported that 25% of patients undergoing an arthroscopic subacromial decompression progressed to full-thickness tears. When more than half of the tendon is torn, open tendon repair has also been advised by some authors (12,68,71). Before arthroscopy, open excision and repair of significant partial tears added little morbidity to the already open procedure (12).

Full-thickness Tears

Open rotator cuff repair remains the gold standard in the treatment of full-thickness tendon tears (10,12,72–78). The introduction of shoulder arthroscopy has led to the development of arthroscopic debridement without repair, arthroscopic subacromial decompression combined with a mini-open tendon repair, and arthroscopic tendon repair.

Debridement without Repair

Massive tears are unusual in young throwing athletes but may be seen in older athletes such as tennis players and golfers. Rockwood et al. (79) proposed open subacromial decompression and tendon debridement without repair for "irreparable" tears. Although this approach may have good results in the short run, long-term follow-up studies have shown less than optimal results. Apoil and Augereau (80) reported that over 25% of these patients developed superior migration of the humeral head and arthropathy when followed for more than 10 years. A prospective study comparing open repair versus arthroscopic cuff debridement found that open repairs had 78% satisfactory results, whereas the debridement without repair had only 39% satisfactory results (81). Ogilvie-Harris and Demaziere (82) found that over 64% of patients undergoing arthroscopic decompression and debridement had moderate functional limitations compared with 22% of patients undergoing cuff repair. Burkhart (83–85) and colleagues (86) postulated proper patient selection in using this treatment modality and a thorough understanding of the pathomechanics of rotator cuff tears. However, long-term studies of this approach are needed to validate this hypothesis.

Superior humeral dislocation has been reported after open decompression and debridement of rotator cuff tendons (87). This effect is magnified when the depressive effect of the rotator cuff on the head of the humerus is also compromised by the tendon tears. We repair the coracoacromial ligament back to the acromion after a conservative acromioplasty at the time of repair of tears where the muscles have long-standing atrophy and weakness to preserve the integrity of the coracoacromial arch.

Mini-Open Repair

The advent of arthroscopic decompression has led to the development of its combination with tendon repair through a small deltoid split (88–98). Diagnostic arthroscopy allows evaluation of the rotator cuff tear with regards to size location and degree of retraction.

Follow-up studies have reported favorable results using this approach (88–98). Baker and Liu (88) compared open repairs to arthroscopically assisted repairs and reported 80% good and excellent results with open repair group and 85% good to excellent in those treated with an arthroscopically assisted technique. Levy et al. (90) reported results of 25 patients undergoing arthroscopically assisted rotator cuff repair and found 80% good or excellent results when small to medium-sized cuff tears were fixed. Both studies also suggested that patients with small to moderate rotator cuff tears had better outcomes than those patients with larger tears. Weber and Schaefer (98) reported long-term results demonstrating that patients undergoing mini-open repair had decreased early morbidity when compared with traditional open cuff repair.

This approach is ideal for the smaller cuff tear that is easily mobilized. However, when open and arthroscopic releases are performed, it is possible to repair larger tears. Moreover, for large to massive tears, many authors prefer open repair because releases and tendon mobilization are facilitated, especially posteriorly.

Arthroscopic Repair

As arthroscopic techniques evolve in the shoulder, numerous investigator have experimented with new techniques for performing an entirely arthroscopic tendon repair. However, current techniques require some form of bone tendon anchor system. Several transfixion devices have been proposed, including staples, bioabsorbable tacs, and suture anchors. Staple fixation of the rotator cuff has been used (99,100); however, this method of fixation has a poor track record (100–103). The largest concern in the use of bioabsorbable tacs is the durability of fixation (100). Paulos et al. (104) showed that rotator cuff strength in a primate model can take up to 2 years to regain full strength. For successful rehabilitation, immediate passive motion is instituted, and as such, most authors prefer permanent fixation. Snyder and Bachner (105) and Snyder (106) developed an arthroscopic technique of tendon repair using small screw suture-anchors with encouraging early results. Concern with the use of suture anchors in cuff repair remains due to the osteopenic nature of tuberosity bone often seen in patients with cuff disease. Adequate follow-up is needed to evaluate the efficacy of this evolving technology.

Isolated Rupture of the Subscapularis Tendon

Isolated tears of the subscapularis are rare and usually are associated with other tendon tears (37,107). Most injuries of the subscapularis tendon have been in association with massive rotator cuff tears, bicipital tendon pathology, tuberosity fracture, or glenohumeral instability (107). Gerber et al. (37) reported a series of 16 patients with isolated tendon rupture of the subscapularis. All ruptures were attributed to a single traumatic

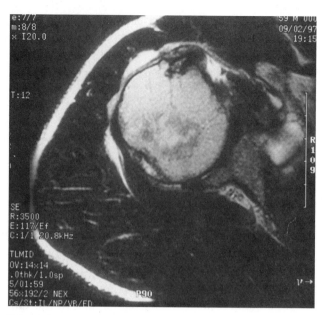

FIG. 26.11. Magnetic resonance image demonstrating a tear of the subscapularis tendon.

event, usually a high-energy injury. These patients has significant anterior shoulder pain and had difficulty performing activities above the horizontal. Patients demonstrated a "pathologic lift-off test." MRI examination was diagnostic and allowed evaluation of the long head of the biceps tendon (Fig. 26.11).

The tendon rupture was approached though an anterior deltopectoral approach. The tendon was mobilized and repaired with either bone sutures or suture anchors. When the long head of the biceps tendon was intact but medially dislocated, a soft tissue reconstruction of the transverse humeral ligament was performed. If the biceps tendon is extensively torn, a biceps tenodesis should be performed. External rotation is limited to approximately 30 degrees for 6 weeks to allow time for tendon to bone healing. The preliminary results have been favorable with regard to both pain relief and functional improvement (37).

Bennett's Lesion

In 1947, Bennett (108) reported a posterior inferior glenoid lesion in the throwing athlete with posterior shoulder pain. This lesion was thought to be a subperiosteal exostosis at the insertion of the long head of the triceps. It was found in association with labral lesions. These lesions are posterior inferior calcifications best visualized with a Bennett view of the shoulder. This view is taken in the anteroposterior plane with the arm abducted and externally rotated and the x-ray beam angle 5 degrees cephalad. Controversy exists as to the etiology of this lesion, which includes posterior capsular tears, instability, labral tears, and posterior rotator cuff injuries.

Ferrari et al. (109) reported a series of seven baseball pitchers with evidence of posterior calcification. All patients had plain radiographs, computed tomography, MRI, and arthroscopy. Radiographic evaluation revealed the calcification was extraarticular, and this was confirmed by arthroscopic evaluation. Arthroscopic findings changed in the posterior labral lesions with fibrillation of the posterior rotator cuff, and two demonstrated partial rotator cuff tears. The authors concluded that the Bennett's lesion was posterior extraarticular ossification associated with posterior labral injury and posterior rotator cuff injury and did not represent a traction injury to the long head of the triceps insertion.

Rehabilitation

Postoperative rehabilitation follows the three-phase rehabilitation program originally outlined by Neer (52). Phase I consists of exercises designed to increase the passive range of motion of the affected shoulder. Exercises include pendulum exercises, assisted supine external rotation using a stick, and assisted passive forward elevation. When applicable we use assisted extension exercises and pulley exercises. These exercises are performed five times a day with 10 repetitions of each exercise for the first 4 to 6 weeks. Phase II consists of isometric and active assistive exercises that are usually started at the 6- to 8-week period. These generally begin with active supine external rotation, elastic band exercises, and active supine forward elevation. The elastic band exercises were previously described. Finally, phase III begins active strengthening programs. This is initially performed with the weight of the extremity and hand weight ranging from 1 to 5 pounds as strength increases.

AUTHORS' PREFERENCES

Indications and Evaluation

Patients suspected of having rotator cuff injuries are started on a well-structured physical therapy program that consists of stretching to prevent stiffness that might contribute to both pain and the impingement process (52), strengthening exercises of the rotator cuff to increase humeral head depression and stability, heat, and anti-inflammatory medication. If no improvement is seen in 4 to 6 weeks, a single subacromial cortisone injection is considered. Most cases respond to nonoperative management within 4 to 6 months. However, if the patient suffers an acute injury and subsequently has profound loss of strength, early imaging of the rotator cuff is indicated. Our only indication for early cuff imaging and possible surgery is a sudden profound loss of strength, especially after an injury or dislocation, be-

cause early surgical intervention may be necessary. For chronic cases in which nonoperative management fails at 4 to 6 months, operative intervention is considered. An MRI of the shoulder is obtained to evaluated the integrity of the rotator cuff and concomitant intraarticular and extraarticular pathology. Based on the size of the tear, muscle quality, and associated pathology, an appropriate surgical intervention is determined and the patient is informed of the length of the rehabilitation process.

Impingement

In the older patient suffering from "classic" impingement patient (over 40 years old, acromial prominence, spurs or sclerosis, positive impingement sign, arc of pain, and complete but temporary relief of pain after a subacromial anesthetic injection) without evidence of a cuff tear on MRI, we generally perform an arthroscopic subacromial decompression. The patient is informed that after 1 year they can expect that pain relief will be similar to that obtained from a subacromial injection.

In the younger athletic population suffering from impingement, we perform a diagnostic arthroscopy. Any pathology found at arthroscopy is addressed at that time. In the glenohumeral joint this can include debridement or repair of glenoid labral tears or fraying, debridement of synovitis, careful debridement of articular-sided partial tears of the rotator cuff, and evaluation of the biceps tendon and insertion. In the subacromial space, evaluation of the coracoacromial ligament, bursal side of the rotator cuff, and an arthroscopic bursectomy is performed. Preoperatively, the patient is informed that these arthroscopic procedures may do little more than facilitate the postoperative rehabilitation. In patients with a type I or II acromion (67) who has bursal thickening and inflammation, a bursectomy and debridement of the coracoacromial ligament insertion is performed. This effectively increases and smooths the coracoacromial arch. When the leading edge of the coracoacromial ligament shows signs of wear, with hypertrophy and scarring, excision of the anterolateral band of the ligament is considered. Arthroscopic acromioplasty in the young population is reserved for patients with a type III acromion (67), associated with erosive changes and fibrillation of the anteroinferior acromial undersurface.

Partial Rotator Cuff Tears

When articular-sided partial rotator cuff tears are observed during arthroscopy, careful debridement with a motorized shaver is performed. After the edges of the tear are delineated, it is probed from the articular side to ensure it is not a full-thickness tear with overlying bursa. The tear is then marked with a nonabsorbable tag suture. The tag suture is identified in the subacromial space and the cuff is inspected and probed for thickness. When the partial tears are less the 50% of the thickness of the tendon, we perform an arthroscopic subacromial decompression. If the tendon tear is greater than 50%, we proceed with a mini-open repair with excision of the degenerative portion of the tendon. In our experience we rarely perform the later procedure.

Rotator Cuff Tears

When preoperative MRI demonstrates a small full-thickness tear without retraction, we inform patients that we will perform arthroscopic subacromial decompression with a mini-open tendon repair if the findings are confirmed at arthroscopy. Tendon tears that are more extensive generally require open repair.

Basic Operating Room Setup

Most shoulder cases at our institutions are performed under interscalene block. This has provided excellent intraoperative and postoperative analgesia (110). Outpatient procedures are performed under a mepivacaine block, whereas bupivacaine is used for more extensive procedures (e.g., mini-open repairs) or when an overnight stay is generally planned.

The patient is placed in a beach-chair position with the back elevated 70 degrees. Folded towels are placed beneath the medial border of the scapula and the shoulder and torso are position over the edge of the table to allow adequate room to maneuver.

After the patient is prepped and draped, the bony landmarks and arthroscopic portals are marked with a sterile pen (Fig. 26.12). This allows accurate portal placement, and later orientation when fluid distention will make palpation of these structures more difficult. We identify the anterior–lateral and posterior–lateral leading edges of the acromion, the clavicle, acromioclavicular joint, and coracoid process. The arthroscopic portals are then drawn. The standard posterior portal is placed in the "soft spot," generally located approximately 2 cm inferior and 2 cm medial to the posterior–lateral corner of the acromion. The anterior portal is marked just lateral to the tip of the coracoid. Two subacromial working portals are then marked within the skin lines of the shoulder. The anterolateral portal is marked approximately 2 cm lateral to the anterior–lateral corner of the acromion. The portals are then infiltrated with 1% lidocaine with epinephrine and the subacromial space distended with 0.25% bupivacaine with epinephrine to limit bleeding. There can be cross-innervation posteriorly, not fully covered by the block, so a few milliliters of lidocaine are injected along a path from the posterior portal to the glenohumeral capsule.

Normal saline with epinephrine is added to a concentration of 1:300,000 (10 mL of 1:1,000 solution in each 3-L bag) (62) is used for irrigation, except in the rare case of a contraindication such as a cardiac arrhythmia. This concentration of epinephrine seems more effective at limiting intraoperative bleeding than a concentration of 1:3,000,000, which others have reported (111). To date, we have not had any complications related to the

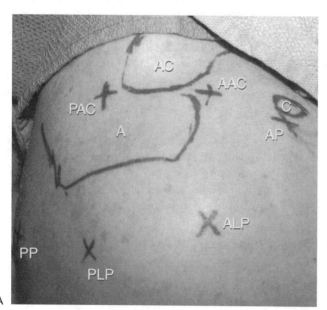
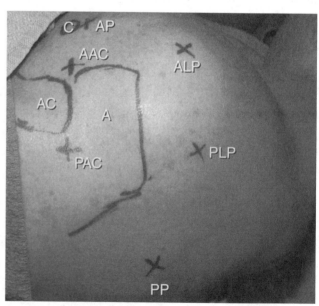

FIG. 26.12. A: Anterior view of the shoulder. **B:** Posterior view of the shoulder. *A,* acromion; *AC,* acromioclavicular joint; *C,* tip of coracoid; *AP,* anterior portal; *ALP,* anterolateral portal; *PLP,* posterolateral portal; *AAC,* anterior acromioclavicular portal; *PAC,* posterior acromioclavicular portal; *PP,* posterior portal.

use of epinephrine in the irrigation. The use of an arthroscopic pump has also been helpful in decreasing the amount of intraoperative bleeding.

Glenohumeral Arthroscopy

The arthroscope is placed through the standard posterior portal with a blunt trocar. We do not distend the joint before insertion of the sheath as this allows one to localize the glenoid rim and humeral head. If the joint appears completely normal, an anterior portal is not necessary. However, this portal is usually required and is placed under direct visualization by placing a locating needle just lateral to the coracoid into the rotator interval, followed by a plastic cannula.

The glenohumeral joint is then systematically examined. The articular surfaces of the glenoid and humerus must be carefully evaluated for chondral defects. Loss of articular cartilage is not an uncommon finding in patients whose preoperative assessment demonstrates rotator cuff disease (112). When fibrillation of the chondral surfaces is present, debridement with a motorized shaver is indicated. Attention is then turned to the biceps tendon and the superior glenoid labrum. Fraying and degeneration of the superior labrum is frequent and of uncertain significance. This area is debrided; however, we doubt this changes the clinical outcome. The stability of the biceps insertion is tested with a probe. When the biceps anchor is completely destabilized, then we generally stabilize the biceps with a biodegradable tac. Attention is then turned to the biceps tendon, and fraying of the tendon debrided. However, if more than 50% of the tendon is compromised, biceps tenodesis is considered.

Inspection of the rotator cuff is performed with the arm in the abducted position. Internal and external rotation of the arm allow inspection of the supraspinatus tendon and the posterior cuff. The insertion of the supraspinatus is at the articular margin, whereas the posterior rotator cuff has an intervening bare area. If the tendon edge is frayed, they should be debrided with a motorized shaver as this may conceal the extent of injury. The tear should be probed, and the anterior–posterior extent and medial–lateral extent of the tears should be noted (Fig. 26.13). If there is any question about whether the tear is full thickness, a colored tag suture can be placed in the area in question. The suture is used to localize the area in question on the bursal side.

Bursal Arthroscopy

We perform subacromial bursoscopy through the posterior and anterolateral portals. The arthroscopic sheath is redirected into the subacromial bursa through the posterior portal. The sheath is used to lyse bursal adhesions and to sound out the acromial morphology. The blunt trocar is next placed and bursal adhesions lysed by sliding the sheath under the acromion, coracoacromial ligament, and then out laterally underneath the deltoid.

A plastic cannula is placed into the subacromial bursal from the anterior–lateral portal under direct vision. The bursa veil is then debrided with a bipolar cautery device or a motorized shaver. After the bursal veil is removed, full visualization of the subacromial space is possible (Fig. 26.14). Arthroscopic evaluation of the subacromial space includes evaluation of the coracoacromial ligament, the undersurface of the acromion, the acromioclavicular joint, and the bursal side of the rotator cuff.

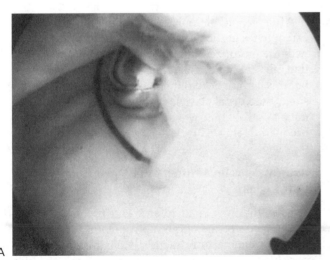
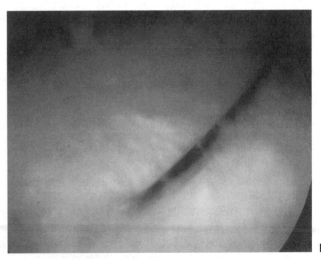

A   B

FIG. 26.13. A: Arthroscopic view of an articular-sided partial-thickness tear of the supraspinatus. A dyed absorbable suture is placed through the tear using a spinal needle introduced through the overlying anterolateral skin. The suture is grasped through the anterior portal. **B:** Suture placement allows accurate bursal-sided inspection of the partial-thickness tear. In this case, the bursal side was found intact and mini-open repair not performed.

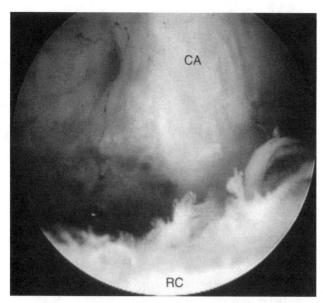

FIG. 26.14. Arthroscopic view of the subacromial space. *CA,* coracoacromial ligament; *RC,* rotator cuff.

If a suture marker was placed through, the rotator cuff should be located and inspected for wear and thickness. When dissecting toward that acromioclavicular joint, one must be careful not to shave too inferiorly as this will damage the muscle belly of the supraspinatus.

Coracoacromial Ligament Excision

The coracoacromial ligament is usually composed of anterolateral and posteromedial bands and extends posteriorly on the acromial undersurface and laterally as a "falx" beyond the anterolateral corner of the acromion (67). Often times, clinical failure of arthroscopic acromioplasty is due to incomplete release of this ligament. In the older patient we prefer to perform a complete excision of the coracoacromial ligament (113). In the young overhead athlete we excise only the anterolateral band of the coracoacromial ligament.

Anterior–Inferior Acromioplasty

Removal of the coracoacromial ligament allows adequate visualization of the anterior acromial margins and spur formation. After soft tissue debridement and when the anterolateral and anteromedial corners of the acromion are identified, accurate removal of bone is possible. We use a 6.0-mm cone-shaped burr in the anterior–lateral working portal for bone resection. Bone is remove by gently sweeping the burr from posterior toward anterior and moving lateral to medial. It is important to remove bone in a controlled fashion, taking out small amounts of bone at a time. Spurs and bony prominence are removed, and the remainder of the acromion

is sculpted so that the anterior third of the acromion is relatively flat. The acromioplasty is viewed from the anterolateral and posterior portals to ensure that is complete, and any final contouring is performed with a rasp.

When performing arthroscopic acromioplasty, one must be sure to remove an appropriate amount of bone. Clinical failure of this procedure can occur if too little or too much bone is removed (82,114). Intraoperative measurement of the subacromial space is difficult, and numerous methods of evaluation of the amount of bone resected have been proposed (97). These include removing a fixed amount of bone and using the posterior acromion as a planing guide to flatten the entire acromion (111). However, completely flattening the acromion can lead to resection of the full thickness of the anterior acromion, compromising the deltoid origin.

To investigate the effect of bone removal in the anterior acromioplasty, Flatow et al. (115) created a computer simulation of an anterior acromioplasty and looked at the effect of varying the amount of bone removal on contact on the rotator cuff. When only the anteroinferior ridges and spurs were resected, impingement was still possible. However, when the anterior third of the acromial undersurface was flattened, impingement was eliminated in all cases. Flattening of the entire acromion was unnecessary and perhaps destabilizes the head by removing the passive buffering effect of the coracoacromial arch against superior humeral subluxation. We also believe that removing a standard amount of bone in the anterior acromioplasty is ill advised. We examined 420 cadaver acromions and found an average thickness of 7.7 mm in males and 6.7 mm in females (116). A standard resection can lead to a dangerously thin acromion. The anterior acromial undersurface should be recontoured, creating a smooth surface without rough or irregular edges.

After the acromioplasty is completed, any inferior osteophytes at the acromioclavicular joint are removed with the motorized burr (51). Recent reports suggested that this can lead to late acromioclavicular joint pain, but this has not been our experience. Arthroscopic excision of the distal clavicle is only performed if the acromioclavicular joint was tender and painful on its own preoperatively (117).

Arthroscopically Assisted Mini-Open Rotator Cuff Repair

We use the mini-open rotator cuff repair for small to medium-sized tears of the supraspinatus tendon that do not have significant retraction. Repair of larger tears is possible using this technique. However, repair of large tears may be performed quicker through a standard open approach.

An arthroscopic subacromial decompression is performed as previously outlined, and the edge of the rota-

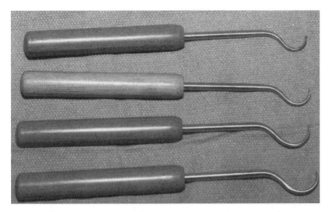

FIG. 26.15. A sharp curved awl is used to create the bone tunnel and a curved crochet hook is used to pass the sutures through the bone tunnel (Link Inc., Denville, NJ).

tor cuff tear is identified and the edge is freshened. The anterolateral working portal incision is lengthened within the skin creases to a length of 3 cm. This incision provides a more cosmetic scar than does a vertically oriented incision. Skin flaps are mobilized, and a split is made in line with the deltoid, incorporating the preexisting arthroscopic puncture hole from the anterolateral portal. Any remaining bursal tissue is resected to fully visualize the underlying rotator cuff. The arm is positioned to center the tear within the deltoid split.

Stay sutures are placed in the tendon edge, and the tear is mobilized until it reaches the greater tuberosity with the arm held in adduction. The soft tissue and bone are debrided from the greater tuberosity just lateral to the articular surface with a ronguer until a bleeding bed of bone is achieved. We secure the tendon edge to bone using bone tunnels. We find the simple two-component system from Link Inc. (Denville, NJ) very helpful. A sharp curved awl is used to create the bone tunnel, and a curved crochet hook is used to pass the sutures through the hole (Fig. 26.15). The torn edge of rotator cuff is then tied down with nonabsorbable sutures passed through bone holes that grip the tendon with a modified Mason-Allen stitch (37). The deltoid split is closed followed by a closure of the skin. Passive and assistive motion is begun immediately, but active use is avoided for 6 weeks to protect the tendon repair.

Open Rotator Cuff Repair

Large tears requiring full open repair are infrequent in young overhead athletes but may be frequent in older recreational competitors. Anesthesia and set-up is as for mini-open repair. A 6- to 7-cm incision in the skin creases is made, and flaps are elevated. The deltoid is incised in the direction of its fibers for about 4 cm from the acromial edge. The incision is taken up over the anterosuperior acromion to the front of the acromio-

clavicular joint, and the anterior acromion and coracoacromial ligament are taken down as one flap. The cuff is freed from bursal adhesions, and traction sutures are placed. It is vital to release the muscle–tendon units for gliding, motion, and to allow repair. An "interval release" may correct differential retraction between the subscapularis and supraspinatus or between the infraspinatus and supraspinatus. The capsule may need to be released under the cuff tendon to prevent tenodesis of the repair.

Repair is performed with no. 2 Ethibond with a mixture of simple and modified Mason-Allen sutures. The deltoid is repaired to bone with transosseous sutures and Mason-Allen sutures.

Rehabilitation is allowed depending on intraoperative findings. Usually, for massive tears, only passive elevation in the plane of the scapula to about 120 degrees by the surgeon, a therapist, or a trained family member is allowed. Assistive exercises, especially pulley, may place too much demand on the repaired muscles. At 6 weeks, assistive is allowed, and activity is allowed at 3 months, progressing to gentle resistive.

REFERENCES

1. Smith JG. Pathological appearances of seven cases of injury of the shoulder joint with remarks. *London Med Gaz* 1834;XIV:280.
2. Codman EA. Complete rupture of the supraspinatus tendon: operative treatment with report of two successful cases. *Boston Med Surg J* 1911;164:708.
3. Codman EA. *The shoulder. Rupture of the supraspinatus tendon and other lesions in or about the subacromial bursa.* Boston: Thomas Todd, 1934.
4. Meyer AW. Further evidence of attrition in the human body. *Am J Anat* 1924;34:241.
5. McLaughlin HL. Lesions of the musculotendinous cuff of the shoulder. 1. The exposure and treatment of tears with retraction. *J Bone Joint Surg Am* 1944;26:31.
6. McLaughlin HL. Repair of major cuff ruptures. *Surg Clin North Am* 1963;43:1535.
7. McLaughlin HL, Asherman EG. Lesions of the musculotendinous cuff of the shoulder. IV. Some observations based upon the results of surgical repair. *J Bone Joint Surg Am* 1951;33A:76.
8. Bosworth DM. An analysis of twenty-eight consecutive cases of incapacitating shoulder lesions, radically explored and repaired. *J Bone Joint Surg Am* 1940;22:369.
9. Cofield RH. Rotator cuff disease of the shoulder. *J Bone Joint Surg Am* 1985;67A:974.
10. Ellman H, Hanker G, Baer M. Repair of the rotator cuff: end-result study of factors influencing reconstruction. *J Bone Joint Surg Am* 1986;68A:1136.
11. Hawkins RJ, Missnore GW, Hobecka PE. Surgery for full-thickness rotator cuff tears. *J Bone Joint Surg Am* 1985;67A:1349.
12. Neer CS II, Flatow EL, Lech O. Tears of the rotator cuff. Long term results of anterior acromioplasty and repair. *Orthop Trans* 1988;12:735.
13. Packer NP, Calvert PT, Bayley JIL, et al. Operative treatment of chronic ruptures of the rotator cuff of the shoulder. *J Bone Joint Surg Br* 1983;65B:171.
14. Post M, Silver R, Singh M. Rotator cuff tear. Diagnosis and treatment. *Clin Orthop* 1983;173:78–91.
15. Bigliani LU, Morrison DS, April EW. The morphology of the acromion and its relationship to rotator cuff tears. *Orthop Trans* 1986;10:228.
16. Bigliani LU, Ticker JB, Flatow EL, et al. The relationship of

acromial architecture to rotator cuff disease. *Clin Sports Med* 1991;10:823.

17. Neer CS II. Anterior acromioplasty for the chronic impingement syndrome in the shoulder: a preliminary report. *J Bone Joint Surg Am* 1972;54:41.

18. Soslowsky LJ, An CH, Johnston SP, et al. Geometric and mechanical properties of the coracoacromial ligament and their relationship to rotator cuff disease. *Clin Orthop* 1994;304:10–17.

19. Zuckerman JD, Klummer FJ, Cuomo F, et al. The influence of the coracoacromial arch anatomy on rotator cuff tears. *J Shoulder Elbow Surg* 1992;1:4.

20. Jobe FW, Bradley JP. Rotator cuff injuries in baseball: prevention and rehabilitation. *Sports Med* 1988;6:378.

21. Jobe CM. Posterior superior glenoid impingement: expanded spectrum. *J Shoulder Elbow Surg* 1995;1:530.

22. Walch G, Boileau P, Noel E, et al. Impingement of the deep surface of the supraspinatus tendon on the posterosuperior glenoid rim: an arthroscopic study. *J Shoulder Elbow Surg* 1992;1:238.

23. Fukuda H, Hamada K, Nakajima T, et al. Pathology and pathogenesis of the intratendinous tearing of the rotator cuff viewed from en bloc histologic sections. *Clin Orthop* 1994;304:60–67.

24. Nakajima T, Rokuuma N, Hamada K, et al. Histologic and biomechanical characteristics of the supraspinatus tendon: reference to rotator cuff tearing. *J Shoulder Elbow Surg* 1994;3:79.

25. Uhthoff HK, Hammond DI, Sarkar K, et al. The role of the coracoacromial ligament in the impingement syndrome. A clinical, radiological and histological study. *Int Orthop* 1988;12:97.

26. Burns TP, Turba JE. Arthroscopic treatment of shoulder impingement in athletes. *Am J Sports Med* 1992;20:13.

27. Ellman H, Kay SP. Arthroscopic subacromial decompression for chronic impingement: two- to five-year results. *J Bone Joint Surg Br* 1991;73B:395.

28. Esch JC, Ozerkis LR, Helgager JA, et al. Arthroscopic subacromial decompression: results according to the degree of rotator cuff tear. *Arthroscopy* 1988;4:241.

29. Wilson PD. Complete rupture of the supraspinatus tendon. *JAMA* 1931;96:433.

30. Fukuda H, Mikasa M, Ogawa K, et al. The partial thickness tear of rotator cuff. *Ortho Trans* 1983;7:137.

31. Depalma AF, Gallery G, Bennet CA. Variational anatomy degenerative lesions of the shoulder joint. In: Blount WP, ed. *Instructional course lectures*. Ann Arbor, Michigan: JW Edwards. American Academy of Orthopaedic Surgeons, 1950:168.

32. Rathbun JB, Macnab I. The microvascular pattern of the rotator cuff. *J Bone Joint Surg Br* 1970;52B:540.

33. Flatow EL, Soslowsky LJ, Ticker JB, et al. Excursion of the rotator cuff under the acromion. Patterns of subacromial contact. *Am J Sports Med* 1994;22:779.

34. Gartsman GM. Arthroscopic acromioplasty for lesions of the rotator cuff. *J Bone Joint Surg Am* 1990;72A:169.

35. Jobe FW, Kvitne RS. Shoulder pain in the overhand or throwing athlete. The relationship of anterior instability and rotator cuff impingement. *Orthop Rev* 1989;18:963.

36. Lohr JF, Uhthoff HK. The microvascular pattern of the supraspinatous tendon. *Clin Orthop* 1990;254:35.

37. Gerber C, Schneeberger AG, Beck M, et al. Mechanical strength of repairs of the rotator cuff. *J Bone Joint Surg Br* 1994;76B:371.

38. Hawkins RJ, Bokov DJ. Clinical evaluation of shoulder problems. In: Rockwood CA, Matsen FA, eds. *The Shoulder*, 1st ed. Philadelphia: W.B. Saunders Co., 1990, p. 170.

39. Rockwood CA, Szaloy EA, Curtis RJ, et al. X-ray evaluation of shoulder problems. In: Rockwood CA, Matsen FA, eds. The Shoulder, 1st ed. Philadelphia: W.B. Saunders Co., 1990, pp. 192–197.

40. Lindblom K. Arthrography and roentgenography in ruptures of the tendon of the shoulder. *Acta Radiol* 1939;20:548–562.

41. Iannotti JP, Zlatkin MB, Esterhai JL, et al. Magnetic resonance imaging of the shoulder: sensitivity, specificity and predictive value. *J Bone Joint Surg Am* 1991;73A:17.

42. Wirthington RH, Girgis FL, Seifert MH. A placebo-controlled trial of steroid injections in the treatment of supraspinatous tendonitis. *Scand J Rheumatol* 1985;14:76.

43. Berry H, Fernandes L, Bloom B, et al. Clinical study comparing acupuncture, physiotherapy, injection and anti-inflammatory therapy in shoulder cuff lesions. *Curr Med Res Opin* 1980;7:121.

44. Watson M. Major ruptures of the rotator cuff: the results of surgical repair in 89 patients. *J Bone Joint Surg Br* 1985;67B:618.

45. Jobe FW, Moynes DR. Delineation of diagnostic criteria and a rehabilitation program for rotator cuff injuries. *Am J Sports Med* 1982;10:336–339.

46. Kelly BT, Kadrmas WR, Speer KP. The manual muscle examination for rotator cuff strength, an electromyographic investigation. *Am J Sports Med* 1996;24:581–588.

47. Altchek DW, Warren RF, Wickiewicz TL, et al. Arthroscopic acromioplasty: technique and results. *J Bone Joint Surg Am* 1990;72A:1198.

48. McShane RB, Lemberry CF, Fenlin JM. Conservative open anterior acromioplasty. *Clin Orthop* 1987;223:137–144.

49. Bigliani LU, D'Alessandro DF, Duralde XA, et al. Anterior acromioplasty for subacromial impingement in patients younger than 40 years of age. *Clin Orthop* 1989;246:111–116.

50. Hawkins RJ, Brock RM, Abrams JS, et al. Acromioplasty for impingement with an intact rotator cuff. *J Bone Joint Surg Br* 1988;70B:795.

51. Neer CS II. Impingement lesions. *Clin Orthop* 1983;173:70.

52. Neer CS II. *Shoulder reconstruction.* Philadelphia: W.B. Saunders, 1990:41.

53. Neviaser TJ, Neviaser RJ, Neviaser JS. Incomplete rotator cuff tears. A technique for diagnosis and treatment. *Clin Orthop* 1994;306:12–16.

54. Rockwood CA Jr, Lyons FR. Shoulder impingement syndrome: diagnosis, radiographic evaluation, and treatment with a modified Neer acromioplasty. *J Bone Joint Surg Am* 1993;75A:409.

55. Ellman H. Arthroscopic subacromial decompression: a preliminary report. *Orthop Trans* 1985;9:43.

56. Paulos LE, Franklin JL. Arthroscopic shoulder decompression development and application. A five year experience. *Am J Sports Med* 1990;18:235.

57. Hawkins RJ, Saddemi SR, Moor J, et al. Arthroscopic subacromial decompression. A two-year follow-up study. *J Bone Joint Surg Am* 1992;74B[Suppl III]:294.

58. Sachs RA, Stone ML, Devine S. Open vs. arthroscopic acromioplasty: a prospective, randomized study. *Arthroscopy* 1994;10:248.

59. Lazarus MD, Williams GR, Chansky HA, et al. Comparison of open and arthroscopic subacromial decompression. *Orthop Trans* 1993;17:1062.

60. Seltzer DG, Wirth MA, Rockwood CA Jr. Complications and failures of open and arthroscopic acromioplasties. *Oper Techn Sports Med* 1994;2:136.

61. Berg EE, Ciullo JV, Oglesby JW. Failure of arthroscopic decompression by subacromial heterotopic ossification causing recurrent impingement. *Arthroscopy* 1994;10:158.

62. Bigliani LU, Flatow EL, Deliz ED. Complications of shoulder arthroscopy. *Orthop Rev* 1991;20:743.

63. Marr DC, Misamore GW. Acromion nonunion after anterior acromioplasty: a case report. *J Shoulder Elbow Surg* 1992;1:317.

64. Matthews LS, Burkhead WZ, Gordon S, et al. Acromial fracture: a complication of arthroscopic subacromial decompression. *J Shoulder Elbow Surg* 1994;3:256.

65. Jackson DW. Chronic rotator cuff impingement in the throwing athlete. *Am J Sports Med* 1976;6:231.

66. Tibone JE, Jobe FW, Kerlan RK, et al. Shoulder impingement syndrome in athletes treated by an anterior acromioplasty. *Clin Orthop* 1985;198:134.

67. Bigliani LU, Rodosky MW, Newton PD, et al. Arthroscopic coracoacromial ligament resection for impingement in the overhead athlete. American Shoulder and Elbow Surgeons, Tenth Open Meeting, New Orleans, Louisiana, February 1994.

68. Ogilvie-Harris DJ, Wiley AM. Arthroscopic surgery of the shoulder. A general appraisal. *J Bone Joint Surg Br* 1986;68B:201–207.

69. Snyder SJ, Pachelli AF, Del Pizzo W, et al. Partial thickness rotator cuff tears: results of arthroscopic treatment. *Arthroscopy* 1991;7:1.

70. Ellman H. Arthroscopic treatment of impingement of the shoulder. *Instruct Course Lectures* 1989;38:177.

71. Ellman H. Diagnosis and treatment of incomplete rotator cuff tears. *Clin Orthop* 1990;254:64.

72. Bigliani LU, Cordasco FA, McIlveen SJ, et al. Operative treatment of massive rotator cuff tears: long-term results. *J Shoulder Elbow Surg* 1992;1:120.

73. Flatow EL, Fischer RA, Bigliani LU. Results of surgery. In: Ianotti JP, ed. *Rotator cuff disorders: evaluation and treatment.* Park Ridge, IL: American Academy of Orthopaedic Surgeons, 1991:53.

74. Flatow EL. Technique of rotator cuff repair. In: Kohn D, Wirth CJ, eds. *Die Schulter: Aktuelle operative Therapie.* Stuttgart: Thieme, 1992:90.

75. Grana WA, Teague B, King M, et al. An analysis of rotator cuff repair. *Am J Sports Med* 1994;22:585.

76. Harryman DT, Mack LA, Wang KY, et al. Repairs of the rotator cuff: correlation of functional results with integrity of the cuff. *J Bone Joint Surg Am* 1991;73A:982.

77. Iannotti JP. Full-thickness rotator cuff tears: factors affecting surgical outcome. *J Am Acad Orthop Surg* 1994;2:87.

78. Kirschenbaum D, Coyle MP Jr, Leddy JP, et al. Shoulder strength with rotator cuff tears: pre- and postoperative analysis. *Clin Orthop* 1993;288:174.

79. Rockwood CA Jr, Williams GR, Burkhead WZ Jr. Debridement of irreparable, degenerative lesions of the rotator cuff. *J Bone Joint Surg Br* 1992;74B[Suppl III]:294.

80. Apoil A, Augereau B. Anterosuperior arthrolysis of the shoulder for rotator cuff degenerative lesions. In: Post M, Morrey BF, Hawkins RJ, eds. *Surgery of the shoulder.* St. Louis, MO: Mosby Year Book, 1990:257–260.

81. Montgomery TJ, Savoie FH, Yerger B. A comparison of arthroscopic debridement with open surgical repair for full thickness tears of the rotator cuff. *Orthop Trans* 1992;16:742.

82. Ogilvie-Harris DJ, Demaziere A. Arthroscopic debridement versus open repair for rotator cuff tears: a prospective cohort study. *J Bone Joint Surg Br* 1993;75B:416.

83. Burkhart SS. Arthroscopic treatment of massive rotator cuff tears: clinical results and biomechanical rationale. *Clin Orthop* 1991;267:45.

84. Burkhart SS. Arthroscopic debridement and decompression for selected rotator cuff tears: clinical results, pathomechanics, and patient selection based on biomechanical parameters. *Orthop Clin North Am* 1993;24:111.

85. Burkhart SS. Reconciling the paradox of rotator cuff repair versus debridement: a unified biomechanical rationale for the treatment of rotator cuff tears. *Arthroscopy* 1994;10:4.

86. Burkhart SS, Nottage WM, Ogilvie-Harris DJ, et al. Partial repair of irreparable rotator cuff tears. *Arthroscopy* 1994;10:363.

87. Wiley AM. Superior humeral dislocation: a complication following decompression and debridement for rotator cuff tears. *Clin Orthop* 1991;263:135.

88. Baker CL, Liu SH. Comparison of open and arthroscopically assisted rotator cuff repairs. *Am J Sports Med* 1995;23:99.

89. Flynn LM, Flood SJ, Clifford S, et al. Arthroscopically assisted rotator cuff repair with the Mitek anchor. *Am J Arthroscopy* 1991;1:15.

90. Levy HJ, Uribe JW, Delaney LG. Arthroscopic assisted rotator cuff repair: preliminary results. *Arthroscopy* 1990;6:55.

91. Liu SH. Arthroscopically-assisted rotator-cuff repair. *J Bone Joint Surg Br* 1994;76B:592.

92. Paletta GA Jr, Warner JJP, Altchek DW, et al. Arthroscopic-assisted rotator cuff repair: evaluation of results and a comparison of techniques. *Orthop Trans* 1993;17:139.

93. Paulos LE, Franklin JL, Beck CL. Jr. Arthroscopic management of rotator cuff tears. In: McGinty JB, Caspari RB, Jackson RW, et al., eds. *Operative arthroscopy.* New York: Raven, 1991:529.

94. Paulos LE, Kody MH. Arthroscopically enhanced miniapproach to rotator cuff repair. *Am J Sports Med* 1994;22:19.

95. Seltzer DG, Uribe JW, Posada A, et al. Arthroscopic assisted rotator cuff repair: two year followup. *Orthop Trans* 1993;17:234.

96. Seltzer DG, Zvijac J. The technique of arthroscopy-assisted rotator cuff repair. *Techn Orthop* 1994;8:212.

97. Warner JJP, Altchek DW, Warren RF. Arthroscopic management of rotator cuff tears with emphasis on the throwing athlete. *Oper Techn Orthop* 1991;1:235.

98. Weber SC, Schaefer R. "Mini-open" versus traditional open repair in the management of small and moderate size tears of the rotator cuff. *Arthroscopy* 1993;9:365.

99. Johnson LL. *Diagnostic and surgical arthroscopy.* St. Louis, MO: Mosby, 1981.

100. Paletta GA Jr, Warner JJP, Altchek DW, et al. Arthroscopic-assisted rotator cuff repair: evaluation of results and a comparison of techniques. *Orthop Trans* 1993;17:139.

101. Bigliani LU, Steinmann SP, Flatow EL. Complications. In: Ianotti JP, ed. *Rotator cuff disorders: evaluation and treatment.* Park Ridge, IL: American Academy of Orthopaedic Surgeons, 1991:63.

102. Flatow EL, Bigliani LU. Complications of rotator cuff repair. *Comp Orthop* 1992;8:298.

103. France EP, Paulos LE, Harner CD, et al. Biomechanical evaluation of rotator cuff fixation methods. *Am J Sports Med* 1989;17:176.

104. Paulos LE, France EP, Boam GW, et al. Augmentation of rotator cuff repair: in vivo evaluation in primates. *Orthop Trans* 1990;14:404.

105. Snyder SJ, Bachner EJ. Arthroscopic fixation of rotator cuff tears: a preliminary report. *Arthroscopy* 1993;9:342.

106. Snyder SJ. *Shoulder arthroscopy.* New York: McGraw-Hill, 1994:133.

107. Mendoza Lopez M, Cardoner Parpal JC, Samso Bardes F, et al. Lesions of the subscapular tendon regarding two cases in arthroscopic surgery. *Arthroscopy* 1994;10:239.

108. Bennett GE. Shoulder and elbow lesions distinctive of baseball players. *Ann Surg* 1947;126:107–110.

109. Ferrari JD, Ferrari DA, Coumas J, et al. Posterior ossification of the shoulder: the Bennett lesion etiology, diagnosis, and treatment. *Am J Sports Med* 1994;22:171.

110. Brown AR, Weiss R, Greenberg C, et al. Interscalene block for shoulder arthroscopy: comparison with general anesthesia. *Arthroscopy* 1993;9:295.

111. Caspari RB, Thal R. A technique for arthroscopic subacromial decompression. *Arthroscopy* 1992;8:23.

112. Weinstein DM, Bucchieri JS, Pollock RG, et al. Arthroscopic debridement of the shoulder for osteoarthritis. *Arthroscopy* 1993;9:366.

113. Bigliani LU, Codd TP, Flatow EL. Arthroscopic coracoacromial ligament resection. *Techn Orthop* 1994;9:95.

114. Hawkins RJ, Chris T, Bokor D, et al. Failed anterior acromioplasty: a review of 51 cases. *Clin Orthop* 1989;243:106.

115. Flatow EL, Colman WW, Kelkar R, et al. The effect of anterior acromioplasty on rotator cuff contact: an experimental and computer simulation. American Shoulder and Elbow Surgeons, 13th Annual Closed Meeting, Manchester, Vermont, September 1994.

116. Nicholson GP, Goodman DA, Pollock RG, et al. The acromion: morphology and age related changes. A study of 420 scapulae. *Orthop Trans* 1993;17:976.

117. Flatow EL, Cordasco FA, Bigliani LU. Arthroscopic resection of the outer end of the clavicle from a superior approach: a critical, quantitative, radiographic assessment of bone removal. *Arthroscopy* 1992;8:55.

Principles and Practice of Orthopaedic Sports Medicine,
edited by William E. Garrett, Jr., Kevin P. Speer, and Donald T. Kirkendall.
Lippincott Williams & Wilkins, Philadelphia © 2000.

CHAPTER 27

Scapular Disorders

W. Ben Kibler

Disorders of scapular function are being recognized with increasing frequency. These disorders may create clinically significant symptoms localized to the scapula but may also be associated with a wide range of shoulder and arm symptoms because of the pivotal nature of the scapula as a base for the shoulder and arm. Because it is posterior and may be obscured by a large layer of muscles, the scapula has not been accurately evaluated in most shoulder and arm injury situations. This chapter addresses the anatomy of the scapula, the roles that the scapula plays in overhead throwing and serving activities, the normal biomechanics of the scapula, abnormal biomechanics and physiology of the scapula, how the scapula may function in injuries that occur around the shoulder, and treatment and rehabilitation of scapular problems.

ANATOMY

The scapula is a flat blade lying along the thoracic wall. Its wide thin configuration allows for smooth gliding of the scapula on the thoracic wall and provides a large surface area for muscle attachments both distally and proximally. Stabilization of the scapula on the thoracic wall is rather tenuous. It is attached to the axial skeleton by the strut of the clavicle and stabilized onto the chest wall by the muscle attachments to the spinous processes and the ribs. The strut configuration allows a degree of stabilization against medially directed forces but allows a large amount of scapular rotation and translation that is then controlled by the dynamic action of the muscles. Three groups of muscles attach to the scapula. The first group comprises the trapezius, rhomboids, levator scapulae, and the serratus anterior and is concerned with

stabilization and rotation of the scapula. The second group includes the extrinsic muscles of the shoulder joint—the deltoid, biceps, and triceps. They are involved in gross motor functions and movements of the arm and force generation to the hand. The final group includes the intrinsic muscles of the rotator cuff—the subscapularis, the supraspinatus, infraspinatus, and teres minor. They are responsible for fine motor movements and compression of the humerus into the shoulder joint.

ROLES OF THE SCAPULA IN OVERHEAD THROWING AND SERVING ACTIVITIES

The scapular roles in throwing and serving are concerned with achieving appropriate motions and positions to facilitate shoulder function. Optimum function occurs when normal anatomy is acted on by appropriate physiologic motor patterns, creating normal biomechanical patterns. The scapula's various roles are concerned with achieving these motions and positions to facilitate the efficient physiology and biomechanics to allow optimum shoulder function. The failure of the scapula to carry out these roles causes inefficient physiology and biomechanics and therefore inefficient shoulder function. This can cause poor performance and can cause or exacerbate shoulder injury.

The first role of the scapula is to be a stable part of the glenohumeral articulation. The glenoid is the socket of the ball and socket arrangement of the glenohumeral joint. To maintain the ball and socket configuration, the scapula must move in a coordinated relationship to the moving humerus so that the instant center of rotation, the mathematical point within the humeral head that defines the axis of rotation of the glenohumeral joint, is constrained within a physiologic pattern throughout the full range of shoulder motion in throwing or serving (1). The coordinated movements also keep the angle between the glenoid and the humerus within a physio-

W. B. Kibler: Lexington Sports Medicne Center, Lexington, Kentucky 40504.

logically tolerable range. This "safe zone" of glenohumeral activity falls roughly within 30 degrees of extension or flexion from the neutral position in the scapular plane (2). This safe zone and stable constrained center of rotation allow "'concavity/compression'" of the glenohumeral joint to be maximal. Concavity/compression is the result of intraarticular pressure, positioning of the glenoid in relationship to the humerus, and muscle activity acting in concert to maintain the ball and socket kinematics (1). Proper alignment of the glenoid allows the optimum function of the bony constraints to glenohumeral motion and allows the most efficient position of the intrinsic muscles of the rotator cuff to allow compression into the glenoid socket, thereby enhancing the muscular constraint systems around the shoulder as well (2).

The second role of the scapula is retraction and protraction along the thoracic wall. The scapula needs to retract to facilitate the position of cocking for the baseball throw, the tennis serve, or the swimming recovery. Efficient achievement of this cocking position allows for proper preloading of the anterior muscular structures and efficient change of muscle phase of contraction from eccentric to concentric on the anterior muscles and concentric to eccentric function on the posterior muscles (2,3). This position has been called the "full tank of energy" position because it allows the explosive phase of acceleration of throwing or serving. This eccentric preloading and explosive concentric contraction allows the plyometric-like activities that develop maximum power. As acceleration proceeds, the scapula must protract in a smooth fashion laterally and then anteriorly around the thoracic wall to allow the scapula to maintain a normal position in relationship to the humerus and also to dissipate some of the deceleration forces that occur in follow-through as the arm goes forward (2).

The third role that the scapula plays in the throwing and serving motion is elevation of the acromion. The acromion must be elevated during the cocking and acceleration phases to clear the acromion from the moving rotator cuff to decrease impingement and coracoacromial arch compression. In the last part of the cocking phase, through the acceleration phase, and into the early follow-through phase in pitching, the arm is abducted 85 to 100 degrees in relation to the trunk (3). In the tennis serve, the arm is progressively abducted from 85 to 104 degrees in the cocking, acceleration, and ball impact phases (WB Kibler, unpublished data). Although it is usually stated that rotator cuff fatigue may allow superior humeral head migration to cause subacromial impingement in this position (3), lower trapezius and serratus anterior muscle fatigue may also contribute to impingement if the acromion is not elevated.

The fourth role that the scapula plays is as a site for muscle attachment. The scapular stabilizers attach to the medial, superior, and inferior borders of the scapula and control the motion and position of the scapula to allow it to do all of its roles. The extrinsic muscles—the deltoid, biceps, and triceps—attach along the lateral aspect of the scapula, use the scapula as their origin to perform gross motor activities of the glenohumeral joint, and form the second cone of Saha (4). The intrinsic muscles of the rotator cuff attach along the entire surface of the scapula and are aligned in such a fashion so that their most efficient activity, working concentrically or eccentrically in a straight line of muscle pull, occurs with the arm between 70 and 100 degrees of abduction (2). In this fashion, they are biomechanically considered to be a "compressor cuff" to compress the humeral head into the socket.

The final role that the scapula plays in shoulder function is that of being a link in the proximal to distal sequencing of velocity, energy, and forces that allows the most appropriate shoulder function (3,5,6). For most shoulder activities, this sequencing starts at the ground. The individual body segments, or links, are coordinated in their movements by muscle activity and body positions to generate, summate, and transfer force through these segments to the terminal link (Fig. 27.1). This sequencing is usually termed the kinetic chain.

The largest proportion of kinetic energy and force in this sequencing is derived from the larger proximal body segments (5). Studies have shown that 51% of the total kinetic energy and 54% of the total force generated in the tennis serve are created by the lower legs, hip, and trunk (5).

The scapula is pivotal in transferring the large forces and high energy from the major source for force and energy—the legs, back, and trunk—to the actual delivery mechanism of the energy and force—the arm and the hand (5–8). Forces that are generated in the proximal segments have to be transferred efficiently and must be regulated as they go through the funnel of the shoulder. This can be accomplished most efficiently through the stable and controlled platform of the scapula. The entire arm rotates as a unit around the stable base of the glenohumeral socket. In acceleration, ball release, or ball impact, the force originally generated in the legs and trunk has been transferred distally to the arm. In this stage of the throwing or serving motion, the stable base of activity has also been transferred from the leg and trunk to the scapula. Therefore, providing stability of the scapula in relationship to the entire moving arm is the key point at this important time in the throwing sequence.

The scapula must play many diverse roles to achieve appropriate shoulder function. These roles are interrelated and are directed toward maintaining the glenohumeral instant center of rotation in the normal path and providing a stable base for muscular function.

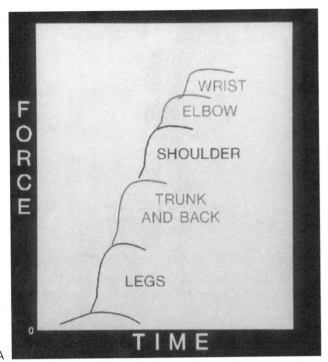

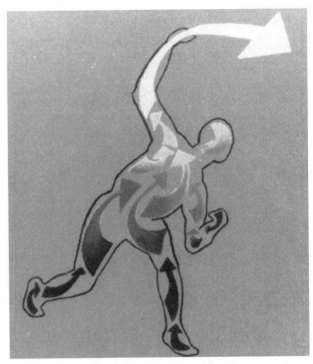

FIG. 27.1. Link sequencing allows efficient generation, summation, and transfer of kinetic energy and force from the base of support, usually the ground, to the terminal link, usually the hand. **A:** Link sequencing. **B:** Force generation.

NORMAL BIOMECHANICS AND PHYSIOLOGY OF THE SCAPULA

Large rotations and large motions occur in the scapula in the throwing and serving motions. In the normal abduction mechanism, the scapula is seen to move laterally in the first 30 to 50 degrees of glenohumeral abduction. As further abduction occurs, the scapula then rotates about a rather fixed axis through an arc of approximately 65 degrees as the shoulder reaches full elevation (9). This motion accounts for the 2:1 ratio that is observed in most throwing athletes between glenohumeral abduction and scapulothoracic rotation. Other studies have shown that this ratio varies between 1:1 and 4:1 depending on the phases of abduction; but for the entire abduction motion, the approximate 2:1 ratio holds true (6).

Translation of the scapula in retraction and protraction occurs around the curvature of the thoracic wall. Depending on the size of the individual and the vigorousness of the throwing activity, this translation may occur over distances of 15 to 18 cm (10). Retraction is mainly in a curvilinear fashion around the wall, but protraction may proceed in a slightly upward or downward position depending on the position of the arm in the throwing or serving mechanism. The motion occurs in a more superior direction with the tennis serve in which much of the acceleration is in a superior direction,

compared with the baseball throw, in which most of the acceleration is in an anterior direction (3,11).

These motions and translations occur as a result of active muscle firing, in addition to passive motion due to the angular accelerations of the trunk and arm. There is a large amount of muscle activity around the scapula in the scapular stabilizers (12–14). These muscles act mainly as force couples, which are muscles that are paired to control the movement of a joint or a body part. The appropriate force couples for scapular stabilization include the upper and lower trapezius working together with the rhomboids, paired with the serratus anterior. The appropriate force couples for acromial elevation are the lower trapezius and the serratus working together paired with the upper trapezius and rhomboids. These motor activation patterns for force couple function are specific for different desired activities. Different parts of large muscles, such as the trapezius, may be activated on different sides of the force couple, depending on the desired scapular activity. Each of these specific actions and force couples must be evaluated and rehabilitated with these different functions in mind (2,15).

ABNORMAL BIOMECHANICS AND PHYSIOLOGY

The scapular roles can be altered by many factors to create a situation for abnormal biomechanics and physi-

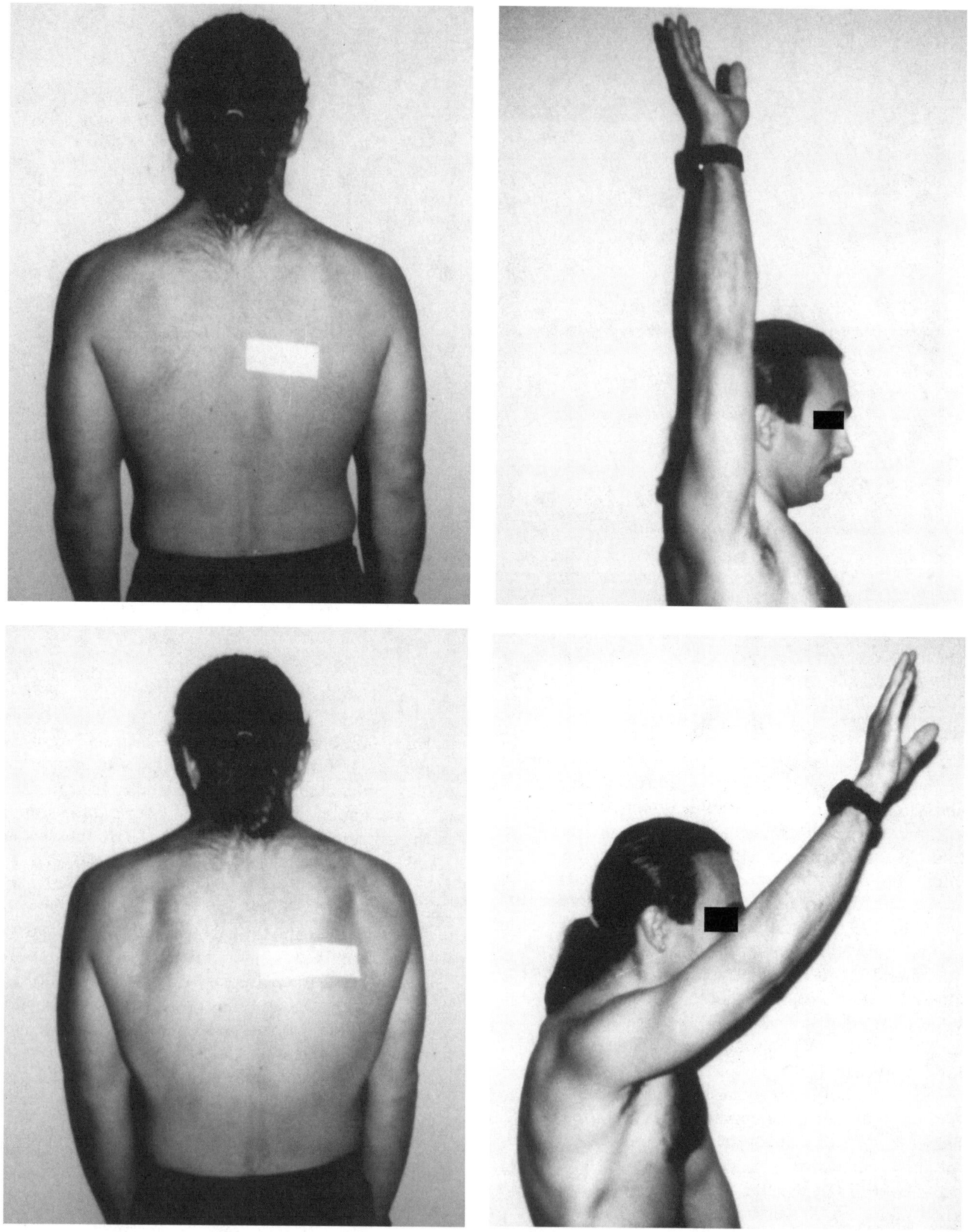

FIG. 27.2. Scapular protraction affects arm elevation before impingement. **A and B:** Normal scapular position and motion. **C and D:** Shoulder drooping, scapular protraction, and resulting early impingement.

ology. The factors may be local around the scapula or they may be distant in other parts of the kinetic chain. The factors may be directly related to an injury or may be more related to overuse, fatigue, or neuromuscular alterations.

The bony anatomy can be altered by either body posture or bony injury. A resting posture of thoracic kyphosis or neck lordosis can result in excessive protraction of the scapula so that impingement occurs early in arm elevation. In this situation, excessive muscular energy will be required to achieve the proper position of scapular retraction on the thoracic wall (Fig. 27.2). Fractures of the clavicle or scapula can alter the orientation of the scapula, the length of the clavicular strut of the scapula, or cause painful clinical situations that would inhibit muscle function. Acromioclavicular joint arthrosis or separation can also lead to abnormalities with the strut function of the clavicle and alter normal kinematics of the scapula.

Most abnormal biomechanics and physiology that occur in sports medicine injuries can be traced to alterations in the function of the muscles that control the scapula (12,16). Nerve injury either to the long thoracic nerve or the spinal accessory nerve can alter muscular function of the serratus anterior or the trapezius muscle, respectively, to give abnormal stabilization and control. This occurs in less than 5% of the problems with muscle function.

More commonly, the scapular stabilizing muscles are either directly injured from direct blow trauma; have microtrauma-induced strain in the muscles, leading to muscle weakness and force couple imbalance; become fatigued from repetitive tensile use; or are inhibited by painful conditions around the shoulder. Muscle inhibition or weakness is quite common in glenohumeral pathology, whether it be from instability, labral pathology, or arthrosis (2,12,15,16). The serratus anterior and the lower trapezius are the most susceptible to the effect of the inhibition, and they are more frequently involved in early phases of shoulder pathology (2,17). Muscle inhibition and resulting scapular instability appear to be a nonspecific response to a painful condition in the shoulder rather than a specific response to a certain glenohumeral pathologic situation. This is verified by the finding of scapular instability in as many as 68% of rotator cuff problems and 100% of glenohumeral instability problems (16,18,19). Inhibition is seen both as a decreased ability for the muscles to exert torque and stabilize the scapula and also as a disorganization of the normal muscle firing patterns of the muscles around the shoulder (16–18). The exact nature of this inhibition is not clear. The nonspecific response and the disorganization of motor patterns suggest a proprioceptively based mechanism. Pain, either from direct muscle injury or indirect sources, and fatigue or uncontrolled muscle strain have

been shown to alter proprioceptive input from Golgi tendon organs and muscle spindles.

Glenohumeral joint inflexibility can also create abnormal biomechanics of the scapula. Posterior shoulder inflexibility, due to capsular or muscular tightness, affects the smooth motion of the glenohumeral joint (19) and creates a "wind-up" effect so that the glenoid and scapula actually get pulled in a forward and inferior direction by the moving and rotating arm. This can create an excessive amount of protraction of the scapula on the thorax as the arm continues into the horizontally adducted position in follow-through. Because of the geometry of the upper aspect of the thorax, the more the scapula is protracted in follow-through, the farther it and its acromion move anteriorly and inferiorly around the thorax. The more inferiorly the scapula moves, the less it is able to elevate and avoid impingement in this phase of throwing in which the arm is still in abduction. Therefore, in the position of acceleration and follow-through, the excessive protraction may cause decreased clearance and increased risk of impingement due to the abnormal scapular biomechanics.

ROLE OF THE SCAPULA IN SHOULDER INJURIES

The abnormal biomechanics and physiology that can occur around the shoulder create abnormal scapular positions and motions that decrease normal shoulder function. This set of abnormal motions and positions has been termed scapulothoracic dyskinesis (18), floating scapula (FW Jobe, personal communication), or lateral scapular slide (20) by different authors, but basically it denotes the same phenomenon—the roles of the scapula are not being fulfilled in their normal fashion (Fig. 27.3).

Alterations in retraction and protraction will change the normal parameters of scapular motion. Lack of full retraction of the scapula on the thorax would cause loss of a stable cocking point and lack of ability to explode during acceleration out of the full tank of energy position of full cocking. This will decrease the plyometric effect to develop full power. Lack of full scapular protraction around the thoracic wall increases the deceleration forces on the shoulder (14,21) and causes alteration in the normal safe zone relationship between the glenoid and the humerus as the arm moves through the acceleration phase (1,3). Too much protraction due to tightness in the glenohumeral capsule will cause abnormalities of impingement as the scapula rotates down and forward. These cumulatively lead to abnormalities in concavity/compression due to the changes in the safe zone of the glenohumeral angle.

Loss of coordinated retraction/protraction in the throwing motion also creates a relative glenoid antetilting or functional anteversion, whereby the anterior as-

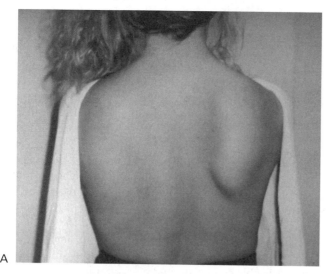 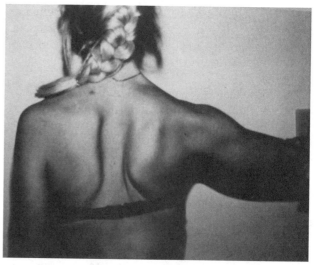

FIG. 27.3. Scapular dyskinesis. **A:** Abnormal scapular retraction (winging). **B:** Abnormal scapular elevation on arm elevation.

pect of the glenohumeral joint is more open and the normal anterior bony buttress to anterior translation is deficient. This opening up and lack of bony buttress causes increased shear stresses on the rest of the anterior stabilizing structures—the labrum and glenohumeral ligaments—causing increasing risk of shear injury or strain (22,23). This decreases the ability of the glenoid to be a stable socket for the rotating humerus as the instant center of rotation changes.

Loss of control of scapular position in the frontal plane may cause abnormal pressure between the scapula and the underlying bursae, especially at the inferior–medial and superior–medial borders. If this is present long enough, bursitis and/or scar can cause symptoms (24).

Lack of appropriate acromial elevation leads to impingement problems in cocking and in follow-through. This type of impingement is very commonly seen not only as the sole source of impingement but also as a secondary source of impingement in other shoulder problems, such as of glenohumeral instability (16,23,25). The serratus and especially the lower trapezius appear to be the first muscles involved in inhibition-based muscle dysfunction (2,17). These two muscles form a crucial part of the force couple responsible for elevating the acromion. Lack of acromial elevation and consequent secondary impingement can be seen very early in many shoulder problems such as rotator cuff tendinitis and glenohumeral instability and can play a major role in defining the clinical problems that are associated with these diagnostic entities (18,22,25).

Lack of a stable muscular anchor affects all the functions of the muscles attached to the scapula. Muscles without a stable base of origin cannot develop appropriate or maximal torque with a concentric contraction,

thereby decreasing their strength and contributing to problems not only with strength production but also in muscular imbalance. If the scapula is truly unstable on the thoracic wall, as can be seen in spinal accessory nerve palsies or in extremely inhibited muscles, then an actual reversal of the origin and insertion occurs, and the distal end of the muscle becomes the origin. When this phenomenon occurs, the scapula is actually pulled laterally by the muscle, which would be contracting from the more stable distal end on the humerus rather than from the proximal end on the scapula. This phenomenon actually increases the scapulothoracic dyskinesis and lateral scapular slide.

One of the most important abnormalities in abnormal scapular biomechanics is the loss of the link function in the kinetic chain (Fig. 27.1). The kinetic chain is the most efficient system for developing appropriate energy and force to be delivered to the hand. The scapula and shoulder are pivotal links in this chain, funneling the forces from the large segments, the legs and trunk, to the smaller rapidly moving small segments of the arm. If the scapula does become deficient in motion or position, transmission of the large generated forces from the lower extremity to the upper extremity is impaired. This creates a deficiency in resultant maximum force that can be delivered to the hand or creates a situation of "catch-up" in which the more distal links have to work at a higher level of activity to compensate for the loss of the proximally generated force. This can be very detrimental to the function of the distal links because they do not have the size, the muscle cross-section area, or the time in which to efficiently develop these larger forces. Our calculations have shown that a 20% decrease in kinetic energy delivered from the hip and trunk to the arm necessitates an 80% increase in mass or a 34%

TABLE 27.1.

	Normal	"Catch-up"	Change (%)
Shoulder velocity (m/sec)	3.3	4.43	+34
Shoulder mass (kg)	9	16.25	+80

There is a 20% decrease in trunk kinetic energy to shoulder link.

increase in rotational velocity at the shoulder to deliver the same amount of resultant force to the hand (11) (Table 27.1). This required adaptation is quite large and can cause overload problems with repeated use. In addition, the unstable scapula does not create a stable base for glenohumeral rotation as the link sequencing evolves. Therefore, the arm works off an unstable platform rather than a stable platform, decreasing the mechanical efficiency of the entire motion.

EVALUATION OF THE SCAPULA

The scapula is intimately involved with both performance and injury conditions of the shoulder. Consequently, the scapula needs to be evaluated quite closely as part of the evaluation of shoulder problems. The scapula needs to be evaluated not only locally but also distantly in relationship to its role in the kinetic chain.

Evaluation of the back and trunk is important. The degree of lumbar lordosis, any leg length asymmetry, and any hip rotational abnormalities need to be noted. Because leg and trunk muscle activity is both large (21,26) and important (8) in throwing and serving activities, it should be assessed by isokinetic dynamometers, vertical jump, or 1 or 10 repetition maximum squats. Inability to achieve normal motions or generate normal velocity in the lower extremity or trunk can affect the transfer of force to the scapula and the arm.

Thoracic and cervical posture needs to be evaluated by inspection and rotation. Thoracic kyphosis or scoliosis may have a direct relationship to the motion of the scapula by creating abnormal posturing or necessitating extra motion. Excessive cervical lordosis indicates posterior cervical muscle or fascia tightness or anterior clavicular fascia tightness, which can have an effect on scapular retraction and protraction.

The evaluation of the scapula itself should be mainly done from the posterior aspect (16,27). The examination can then proceed from posterior to anterior to allow appropriate examination of all the scapular positions and motions.

Scapular position may be evaluated in several ways. Abnormalities of winging, elevation, or rotation may first be examined in the resting position. In long-standing scapular dyskinesis, resting winging may be seen

(Fig. 27.4). Pure serratus anterior weakness due to nerve palsy will create a prominent superior medial border and depressed acromion, whereas pure trapezius weakness due to nerve palsy will create a protracted inferior border and elevated acromion. Because nerve lesions are rare and muscle dysfunction is due to fatigue or inhibition, a mixture of these two positions will be present, depending on the amount of weakness.

Motion and position should be examined both in the ascending phase and in the descending phase of the arm in both flexion and abduction. Muscle weakness and mild scapular dyskinesis will be noted more frequently in the descending phase of the arm movement. This will most commonly present as a "hitch" or a "jump" in the otherwise smooth motion of the scapula or scapular border. Sometimes the most superior aspect of the scapula will be most prominent, but more commonly the middle or inferior border becomes prominent.

Scapulothoracic bursitis ("snapping scapula") is demonstrated by painful crepitus or snapping over the superior–medial or inferior–medial borders. This usually occurs with arm abduction or scapular retraction.

A good provocative maneuver to evaluate scapular muscle strength is to do an isometric pinch of the scapulae in retraction. Scapular muscle weakness can be noted as a burning pain in less than 15 seconds. Normally, the scapula should be held in this position for 15 to 20 seconds without having the burning pain or muscle weakness. Also, wall push-ups are an effective way of evaluating serratus anterior strength. Any abnormalities of scapular winging with 5 to 10 wall push-ups may be noted.

The scapular assistance test evaluates scapular and acromial involvement in subacromial impingement. In the patient with impingement symptoms with forward elevation or abduction, assistance for scapular elevation

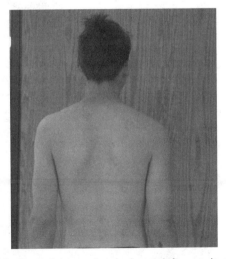

FIG. 27.4. Scapular pseudo-winging on left scapula, with medial border prominence, at resting position.

is provided by manually stabilizing the scapula and rotating the inferior border of the scapula with arm motion. This procedure simulates the force couple activity of the serratus anterior and lower trapezius. Elimination or modification of the impingement symptoms indicates that scapular dyskinesis is playing a role in the clinical symptom complex.

Quantitative measurement of scapular stabilizer strength can be achieved by the lateral slide test (Fig. 27.5). This semidynamic test evaluates the position of the scapula on the injured and noninjured sides in relationship to a fixed point on the spine as varying amounts of loads are put on the supporting musculature. Three positions are chosen for this testing procedure. The first position is with the arm relaxed at the sides (Fig. 27.5A). The second is with the hands on the hips with the fingers anterior and the thumb posterior with about 10 degrees of shoulder extension (Fig. 27.5B). The third position is with the arms at or below 90 degrees of arm elevation with maximal internal rotation at the glenohumeral joint (Fig. 27.5C). These positions offer a graded challenge to the functioning of the shoulder muscles to stabilize the scapula. The final position presents a challenge to the muscles in the position of most common function

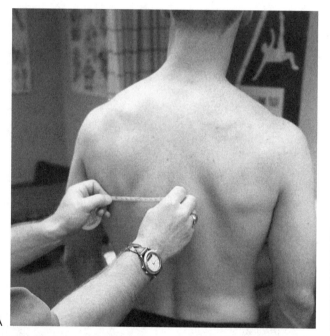

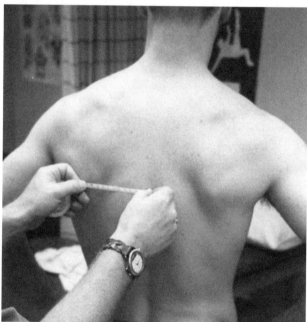

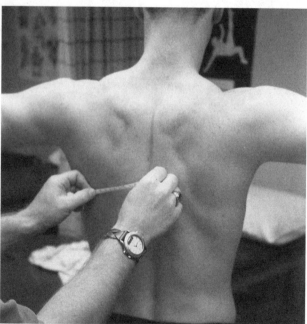

FIG. 27.5. Lateral scapular slide measurement. **A:** Position 1, with arms at side. **B:** Position 2, with hands on hips. **C:** Position 3, with arms at or below 90 degrees abduction, with glenohumeral internal rotation.

at 90 degrees of shoulder elevation. Electromyographic evaluation has shown that very few muscles are working in position 1, that the serratus and the lower trapezius are working at low levels in position 2, and that the upper trapezius, lower trapezius, serratus, and rhomboids are all working at approximately 40% of maximum in position 3. In position 1, the inferior–medial angle of the scapula is palpated and marked on both the injured and noninjured sides. The reference point on the spine is the nearest spinous process, which is then marked with an X. The measurements from the reference point on the spine to the medial border of the scapula are measured on both sides. In position 2, the new position of the inferior–medial border of the scapula is marked, and the reference point on the spine is maintained. The distances once again are calculated on both sides. The same protocol is done for position 3.

Tests for reliability and validity of this measuring system have been done. Studies on the accuracy of marking the inferior–medial border of the scapula in comparison with x-ray evaluation of the same point when marked by a lead shot have shown a correlation of 0.91 with the different positions. Therefore, it does appear that the position that is marked on the skin does correspond well with the actual position of the inferior-medial border of the scapula. Test–retest and intertest reliability has shown that the test–retest (intratester) relationship is between 0.84 and 0.88 and that the intertester reliability is between 0.77 and 0.85 depending on the position (28) (Table 27.2). Position 3 is the most difficult to measure accurately because of the muscle activity. Even so, this position achieved a test–retest and intertester reliability of greater than 0.78. Therefore, it appears that the lateral slide test does reproduce the desired scapular points and the desired measurements, is a reliable test in terms of reproducibility, and does test muscles that are actually working to stabilize the scapula.

Investigations of this testing procedure show that in asymptomatic throwing athletes, as the progression of muscle activity increases from position 1 to position 3, the amount of asymmetry of the scapular positions becomes less, indicating the increasing role of the scapu-

TABLE 27.3. *Mean asymmetry (injured side − uninjured side) measurements in cm*

Position	Symptomatic	Asymptomatic
1	0.83	0.47
2	1.41	0.39
3	1.75	0.27

lar stabilizing muscles in controlling the retraction of the scapula as the arm abducts. In a set of injured patients, this change in symmetry does not occur, and actually the degree of asymmetry increases when going from position 1 to position 3 (Table 27.3). The side-to-side differences in injured athletes are consistently greater than 0.83 cm, with a range of 0.83 to 1.75 cm. For purposes of clinical evaluation, we have established 1.5-cm asymmetry as the threshold of abnormality and accept this in any of the positions, although it is more commonly seen in position 3. Although this test does not solve all the problems about measuring scapular strength, it is a semiquantitative and reproducible test that can be used as part of evaluation and rehabilitation of these problems and does allow an objective set of criteria to determine the scapular abnormalities.

Other testing that can be done to objectify scapular position include Moire topographic analysis (18), which involves stroboscopic evaluation of the contours of the back. This shows the abnormalities of scapular position very well, but this is limited by the availability of these facilities.

Evaluation techniques for other structures that are pertinent to the scapular evaluation include evaluation of the acromioclavicular joint, the acromioclavicular angle in both retraction and protraction, and glenohumeral rotation and muscle strength (27). All these play a role in the motion and position of the scapula.

TREATMENT CONSIDERATIONS FOR SCAPULAR ABNORMALITIES

Most abnormalities that exist in scapular motion or position can be treated by treating the source of the problems (16). Very seldom is surgical treatment directed at the scapula itself; it is usually directed at the source of the underlying problems.

If there is a primary neurologic problem, such as a torn, stretched, or lacerated spinal accessory nerve or long thoracic nerve, then appropriate nerve repair or muscle transfers may be used. Scapular stabilization in serratus anterior palsy can be achieved by transfer of the pectoralis major with a fascial extension to the scapula (29) or can be achieved in trapezius palsy by rhomboid transfer and levator scapulae advancement (16,30). In advanced cases, actual stabilization of the scapula to

TABLE 27.2.

Position	Dominant	Nondominant
Intratester reliability		
1	0.85	0.87
2	0.84	0.88
3	0.86	0.85
Intertester reliability		
1	0.83	0.85
2	0.77	0.81
3	0.78	0.83

the ribs by arthrodesis can be considered. These are usually not going to be necessary in athletic populations.

Internal fixation of scapular or clavicular fractures may be necessary to restore normal anatomy or angulation of the glenoid or to restore the normal length to the strut of the clavicle (31). Acromioclavicular joint separations should be evaluated in terms of their contribution to scapular stability. If a third or fourth degree acromioclavicular separation creates a loss of the strut function and excessive scapular protraction or dyskinesis, then functional consequences may include impingement and abnormalities in strength production. Acromioclavicular joints may need to be anatomically repaired in this situation. Acromioclavicular joint arthrosis with consequent pain or acromioclavicular joint instability may need to be surgically corrected to stabilize the scapula or eliminate the pain-causing problem at the joint.

Resistant snapping scapula occasionally requires surgical attention. Rarely, true bone spurs may be identified, but the usual pathologic problem is a thickened or hypertrophic bursa. Inferior–medial bursectomies (32); superior–medial bursectomies, both open (33) and arthroscopic (34); and bony resections (32) have been reported to give good results in the small populations that do not respond to appropriate postural control, reestablishment of normal upper trapezius, lower trapezius force couples, or correction of intraarticular pathology leading to scapular dyskinesis (12,13,16,22,32).

More commonly, the underlying source of muscle inhibition or muscle imbalance needs to be addressed, whether this be the predominant glenohumeral internal derangement, such as instability, labral tears, or rotator cuff injury, or rotator cuff tendinitis with muscle weakness and inhibition. Superior glenoid labral tears and microtrauma-based glenohumeral instability are very common pain-causing contributors to scapular dyskinesis (19). Once the internal derangement is corrected, scapular muscle rehabilitation may be started.

REHABILITATION CONSIDERATIONS IN SCAPULAR DYSKINESIS

Once the complete and accurate diagnosis of all factors causing or contributing to scapular and shoulder problems is established, scapular rehabilitation should be accomplished in the context of all its roles (12,35–37).

Rehabilitation may be indicated before surgical intervention to help create more favorable postoperative rehabilitation conditions. Good preoperative scapular control can improve postoperative rehabilitation for rotator cuff repairs and glenohumeral instability reconstructions by creating a more stable neurologically coordinated base for muscle rehabilitation. In addition, preoperative scapular rehabilitation may eliminate the need for surgery. A surprisingly large percentage of "impingement" problems that are due to muscle weak-

ness or imbalance can be corrected by proper muscular reeducation and conditioning.

In the postoperative phase, kinetic chain rehabilitation may be started early, even though shoulder protection is desired. Scapular rehabilitation, especially isometric or closed chain exercises, may also be instituted before shoulder rehabilitation, within the limits imposed by the need for shoulder protection.

Because scapular dyskinesis due to altered physiology occurs early in the injury or postoperative phases, accelerated rehabilitation should be emphasized to restore normal physiologic patterns.

Rehabilitation should start at the base of the kinetic chain. This usually means correcting any strength or flexibility deficits that exist in the low back and thoracic level as a prelude to starting work on the scapular component. This phase would include exercises for flexibility in both anteroposterior and rotational directions; strengthening of the trunk in flexion, extension, and rotation; and correction of the postural abnormalities with appropriate postural exercises for the thoracic area.

Abnormalities in back alignment can be corrected with proper exercises or postural corrections (Fig. 27.6). Range of motion of the glenohumeral joint can be improved by appropriate stretching that emphasizes stretching of the posterior capsule rather than stretching of the entire upper limb. In this situation, care must be taken to ensure that the actual stretching does not occur at the scapulothoracic articulation but rather at the glenohumeral articulation. If the stretching occurs at the scapulothoracic articulation, it will actually increase the biomechanical problem, by allowing too much scapular

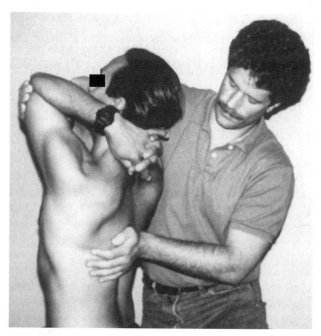

FIG. 27.6. Postural exercises should include correction of thoracic kyphosis.

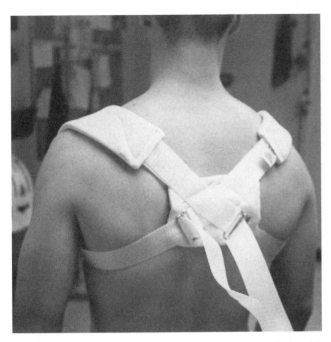

FIG. 27.7. Use of a figure of eight clavicle collar to help with scapular retraction.

protraction, rather than solving the biomechanical problem. Specific scapular rehabilitation activities should be broken down into scapular stability exercises, closed chain exercises, and open chain exercises. Scapular stability can be started early in the rehabilitation sequence. At the beginning, these exercises would involve isometric exercises, such as scapular pinch, and scapular shrug exercises for elevation. In this early stage, help with control of scapular position can be done by scapular taping in a retracted or elevated position and the use of a figure of eight collar, which is normally used for clavicle fractures (Fig. 27.7). This helps to retract and elevate the scapula and creates conditions for normalization of scapular muscle firing patterns, which are often quite disorganized and inhibited.

The most physiologic way to reorganize and reestablish normal motor firing patterns for the scapula is with the exercises that involve closed chain activities (35,36,38). Closed chain exercises simulate the normal functional patterns in that they are used with the arm at 90 degrees of glenohumeral elevation. In this fashion, they reproduce the normal physiologic patterns of co-contractions of the scapular stabilizing muscles and of the muscles of the rotator cuff. They allow normal motor

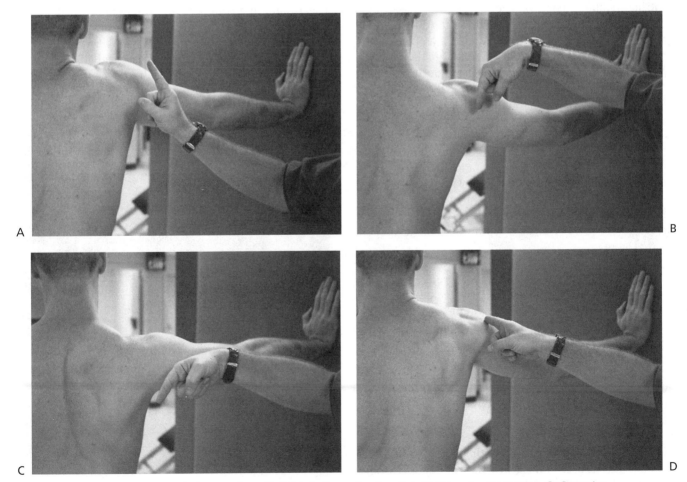

A

B

C

D

FIG. 27.8. Closed chain scapular exercises. **A:** Scapular elevation. **B:** Scapular depression. **C:** Scapular retraction. **D:** Scapular protraction.

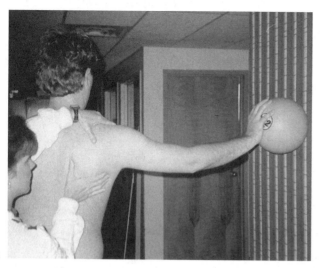
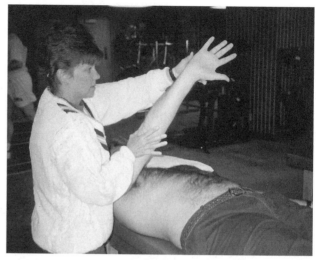

A
B

FIG. 27.9. Proprioceptive neuromuscular facilitation exercises stimulate feedback by challenging joint position and strength. **A:** Scapular stabilization. **B:** External rotation/diagonal stabilization.

patterns that create scapular elevation, depression, retraction, and protraction to occur with minimal stress and allow normal biomechanics of concavity/compression and rotation to occur. These are usually done with the hand stabilized on a wall or on a ball on the wall, and specific scapular maneuvers of elevation, depression, retraction, and protraction are carried out (Fig. 27.8).

These exercises can be done safely within the parameters set by the need for healing of the underlying injury and can be started as early as 3 weeks after surgery for glenoid labral repair or instability repair and as early as 5 weeks in rotator cuff repairs (35). These can be started at elevations of 60 degrees or less and then moved up to 90 degrees as tissue healing allows. They can be done throughout the early and middle stages of rehabilitation and can be combined with lower extremity exercises (31). Further progressions to create more load on the scapular muscles include push-ups, quadriped and biped exercises, and press-up exercises (36,37).

Open chain activities can then be initiated upon the base established by the isometric and closed chain activities. These more strenuous exercises include vigorous proprioceptive neuromuscular facilitation patterns (Fig. 27.9), diagonal patterns (Fig. 27.10), external rotation and retraction activities (Fig. 27.11), and plyometrics (Fig. 27.12), all of which create muscles ready to return to more normal physiologic function. Machines can be used in this phase to allow pull-downs, upright rows, push-ups, and push-up–plus activities to allow complete rehabilitation of the scapula.

Most scapular rehabilitation should be done before emphasis upon rotator cuff strengthening exercises. The scapula is the base from which the rotator cuff originates, and complete scapular rehabilitation allows more

normal scapular positioning and therefore more normal patterns of activation of the rotator cuff. In addition, control of elevation of the acromion decreases the chances of impingement and allows the rotator cuff muscles to pull in a compression fashion into the glenohumeral joint.

Lateral scapular slide measurements can be used as a guide for progressing through these activities. Criteria for initiating specific rotator cuff and open chain arm

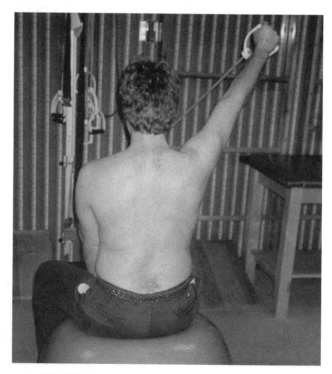

FIG. 27.10. Diagonal arm extension on plyoball.

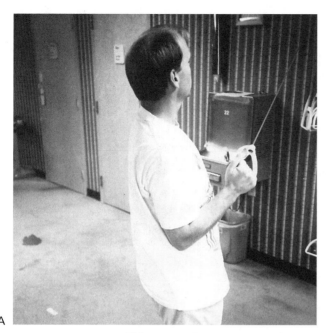 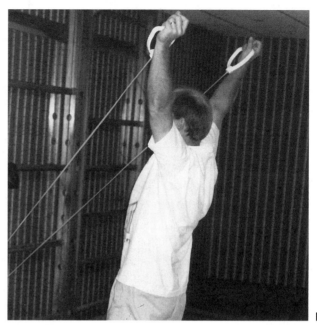

A   B

FIG. 27.11. External rotation/retraction activities. **A:** Unilateral. **B:** Bilateral.

activities would include a lateral slide asymmetry of less than 1 cm in position 3 and smooth motion of the scapula on the injured and noninjured sides with both ascent and descent.

If scapular stabilization is achieved by this strengthening program, it is often found that there are less problems in rotator cuff rehabilitation, because the rotator cuff is activated in a more physiologic fashion in the closed chain rehabilitation, and that the scapular base is much better prepared for activity of the rotator cuff muscles.

CONCLUSIONS

The scapula has a major and pivotal role in normal shoulder function. Its motion and position create the parameters to allow normal physiology and biomechanics of the shoulder to occur. Its roles include being a stable part of the glenohumeral articulation, retraction and protraction around the thoracic wall, active acromial elevation, being a base for muscle origin and insertion, and serving as a link in the kinetic chain delivering energy and force from the trunk and legs to the hand. Abnormalities in scapular position and motion can be seen in a variety of pathologic states, some intrinsic in the glenohumeral joint or scapula and some in the kinetic chain. These abnormalities alter the roles of the scapula and can decrease performance or cause or contribute to shoulder pathology. Evaluation of the scapula should be an integral part of the evaluation of shoulder pathology, and rehabilitation of the scapula should be one of the early points emphasized in shoulder rehabilitation.

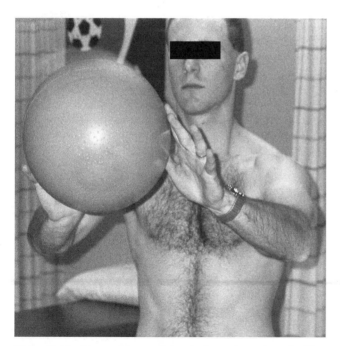

FIG. 27.12. Plyometric medicine ball catch and push. The weight of the medicine ball creates a force that is countered by the scapular stabilization and arm push-off.

REFERENCES

1. Matsen FA, Harryman DT, Sidles JA. Mechanics of glenohumeral instability. *Clin Sports Med* 1991;10:783–788.

2. Pink MM, Perry J. Biomechanics of the shoulder. In: Jobe FW, ed. *Operative techniques in upper extremity sports injuries.* St. Louis: Mosby, 1996:109–123.
3. Fleisig GS, Dillman CJ, Andrews JR. Biomechanics of the shoulder during throwing. In: Andrews JR, Wilk KE, eds. *The athlete's shoulder.* New York: Churchill Livingstone, 1994:355–368.
4. Saha AK. Dynamic stability of the glenohumeral joint. *Acta Orthop Scand* 1971;42:491–495.
5. Kibler WB. Biomechanical analysis of the shoulder during tennis activities. *Clin Sports Med* 1995;14:79–85.
6. Kennedy K. Rehabilitation of the unstable shoulder. *Oper Techn Sports Med* 1993;1:311–324.
7. Elliott BC, Marshall R, Noffal G. Contributions of upper limb segment rotations during the power serve in tennis. *J Appl Biomech* 1995;11:433–442.
8. Kraemer WJ, Triplett NT, Fry AC. An in-depth sports medicine profile of women college tennis players. *J Sports Rehabil* 1995;4:79–88.
9. Poppen NK, Walker PS. Normal and abnormal motion of the shoulder. *J Bone Joint Surg Am* 1976;58A:195–201.
10. Kibler WB. Evaluation of sports demands as a diagnostic tool in shoulder disorders. In: Matsen FA, Fu F, Hawkins RJ, eds. *The shoulder: a balance of mobility and stability.* Rosemont, IL: A.A.O.S. 1993:379–395.
11. Kibler WB, Chandler TJ. Rehabilitation for tennis and baseball. In: Griffin L, eds. *Rehabilitation of the injured knee.* St. Louis: Mosby, 1994:219–227.
12. Moseley JB, Jobe FW, Pink MM, et al. EMG analysis of the scapular muscles during a shoulder rehabilitation program. *Am J Sports Med* 1992;20:128–134.
13. Bagg SD, Forrest WJ. EMG study of the scapular rotators during arm abduction in the scapular plane. *Am J Phys Med* 1986; 65:111–124.
14. Digiovine N, Jobe FW, Pink MM, et al. An EMG analysis of the upper extremity in pitching. *J Shoulder Elbow Surg* 1992;1:15–25.
15. Speer KP, Garrett WE. Muscular control of motion and stability about the pectoral girdle. In: Matsen FA, Fu F, Hawkins RJ, eds. *The shoulder: a balance of mobility and stability.* Rosemont, IL: A.A.O.S., 1994:159–173.
16. Kuhn JE, Plancher KD, Hawkins RJ. Scapular winging. *J Am Acad Orthop Surg* 1995;3:319–325.
17. Glousman R, Jobe FW, Tibone JE. Dynamic EMG analysis of the throwing shoulder with glenohumeral instability. *J Bone Joint Surg Am* 1988;70A:220–226.
18. Warner JJP, Micheli L, Arslenian L. Scapulothoracic motion in normal shoulders and shoulders with glenohumeral instability and impingement syndrome. *Clin Orthop* 1992;285:191–199.
19. Paletta GA, Warner JJP, Warren RF, et al. Shoulder kinematics with two-plane x-ray evaluation in patients with anterior instability or rotator cuff tears. *J Shoulder Elbow Surg* 1997;6:516–527.
20. Harryman DT, Sidles JA, Clark JM. Translation of the humeral head on the glenoid with passive glenohumeral motions. *J Bone Joint Surg Am* 1990;72A:1334–1343.
21. Young JL, Herring SA, Press JM, et al. The influence of the spine on the shoulder in the throwing athlete. *J Back Musculoskel Rehab* 1996;7:5–17.
22. Kibler WB. The role of the scapula in the overhead throwing motion. *Contemp Orthop* 1991;22:525–532.
23. Jobe CM, Pink MM, Jobe FW, et al. Anterior shoulder instability, theories and concepts. In: Jobe FW, ed. *Operative techniques in upper extremity sports injuries.* St. Louis: Mosby, 1996:164–176.
24. Kuhn JE, Plancher KD, Hawkins RJ. Symptomatic scapulothoracic crepitus and bursitis. *J Am Acad Orthop Surg* 1998;6:267–274.
25. Jobe FW, Kvitne RS, Giangarra CE. Shoulder pain in the throwing athlete: the relationship of anterior instability and rotator cuff impingement. *Orthop Rev* 1989;18:963–975.
26. Watkins RG, Dennis S, Dillin WH, et al. Dynamic EMG analysis of torque transfer in professional baseball pitchers. *Spine* 1989;14:404–408.
27. Kibler WB. Clinical examination of the shoulder. In: Pettrone FA, ed. *Athletic injuries of the shoulder.* New York: McGraw-Hill, 1995:31–41.
28. Odom CJ, Hurd CE, Denegar CR, et al. Intratester and intertester reliability of the lateral scapular slide test. Master's thesis, Slippery Rock University, and presented at N.A.T.A. National Meeting, Orlando, Florida, 1996.
29. Post M. Pectoralis major transfer for winging of the scapula. *J Shoulder Elbow Surg* 1995;4:1–9.
30. Bigliani L, Perez-Sanz JR, Wolfe IN. Treatment of trapezius paralysis. *J Bone Joint Surg Am* 1985;67:871–877.
31. Fiddian NJ, King RJ. The winged scapula. *Clin Orthop* 1985;185: 228–236.
32. Sisto DJ, Jobe FW. Operative treatment of scapulothoracic bursitis in professional pitchers. *Am J Sports Med* 1986;14:192–194.
33. McCluskey GM, Biglian LU. Scapulothoracic disorders. In: Andrews JR, Wilk KE, eds. *The athlete's shoulder.* New York: Churchill Livingstone, 1994:303–316.
34. Ciullo JV, Jones E. Subscapular bursitis. Conservative and endoscopic treatment of "snapping scapula." *Orthop Trans* 1992; 16:740.
35. Kibler WB, Livingston B, Bruce R. Current concepts in shoulder rehabilitation. *Adv Operative Orthop* 1995;3:249–300.
36. Pink MM, Screnar PM, Tollefson KD. Injury prevention and rehabilitation in the upper extremity. In: Jobe FW, ed. *Operative techniques in upper extremity sports injuries.* St. Louis: Mosby, 1996:3–14.
37. Wilk KE, Arrigo C, Andrews JR. Current concepts in the rehabilitation of the athlete's shoulder. *J South Orthop Assoc* 1994;3:216–231.
38. Davies GJ, Dickoff-Hoffman S. Neuromuscular testing and rehabilitation of the shoulder complex. *J Orthop Sports Phys Ther* 1993;18:449–458.

Principles and Practice of Orthopaedic Sports Medicine,
edited by William E. Garrett, Jr., Kevin P. Speer, and Donald T. Kirkendall.
Lippincott Williams & Wilkins, Philadelphia © 2000.

CHAPTER 28

Acromioclavicular Joint Injuries in Athletes

Carl J. Basamania

Acromioclavicular joint problems in athletes are quite common (1–9). Not only is the acromioclavicular joint subject to frequent trauma in contact athletes, it is also subject to degenerative problems as a result of athletic training (10–15) or heavy labor (16,17). Acromioclavicular joint separations are second only to glenohumeral joint dislocations in their frequency of recurrence. In actuality, acromioclavicular joint separations or dislocations may occur more frequently than glenohumeral dislocations; however, patients may not seek out care for these injuries, whereas they may not have the same option with a glenohumeral joint dislocation. Most acromioclavicular joint separations tend to occur in young males (18). It is interesting to note that the first "sports medicine physician," Galen, had sustained an acromioclavicular joint separation. It is also interesting to note that he abandoned the conservative treatment of banding the injury after a short period of time because it was too uncomfortable, a problem we are often confronted with in our modern athletes (19).

There has been a great deal of controversy in regards to the treatment of these injuries. Not only has there been disagreement about whether these injuries should be treated operatively or nonoperatively, there has been an incredible number of different operations described to treat this injury. It should be pointed out, however, that there are a few other joints in the body where a complete dislocation is routinely accepted, without reduction, as the standard of care.

ANATOMY

The acromioclavicular joint is a diarthrodial joint, as is the sternoclavicular joint. These two joints make up

the only articulations between the axial skeleton in the upper extremity. The intraarticular disk of the acromioclavicular joint, which has questionable value and function (20), undergoes progressive degeneration to the point that it is rare to find "normal" joint in anyone over the age of 35 with radiographs showing progressing narrowing of the joint with age (21,22). In fact, Codman (23) stated that arthritis of the acromioclavicular joint was so common in laborers that it was "as normal as tissue as the great calluses in their hands." The articular surfaces of the joint are initially hyaline cartilage; however, it changes to fibrocartilage by 17 to 24 years of age (24). There may also be considerable variation in the inclination of the acromioclavicular joint in both the coronal and sagittal planes. In the coronal plane, it can vary from a vertical orientation to one inclined downward and medially.

Urist (25) noted that approximately half of normal acromioclavicular joints were oriented obliquely in a superior lateral to anterior medial orientation. He also found approximately one fourth of the joints were oriented vertical and the remaining one fourth were incongruent. DePalma (24) found approximately 40% of acromioclavicular joints were relatively vertical, with an average anterior medial to anterior lateral inclination of 16 degrees. Approximately half of the acromioclavicular joints were inclined approximately 25 degrees, whereas 10% had inclination of 36 degrees. He also noted that most patients with painful acromioclavicular joints had a more vertical orientation and a smaller joint surface area. Stability to the acromioclavicular joint is provided by both the acromioclavicular and coracoclavicular ligaments and the surrounding deltotrapezial fascia (Fig. 28.1). The acromioclavicular ligament complex consists of four parts: the anterior, posterior, inferior, and superior ligaments. The coracoclavicular ligament complex consists of the conoid and trapezoid ligaments. The conoid ligament originates from the posterior medial aspect of the coracoid process and inserts on the conoid

C. J. Basamania: Department of Surgery, Division of Orthopedic Surgery, Duke University Medical Center, Durham, North Carolina 27710.

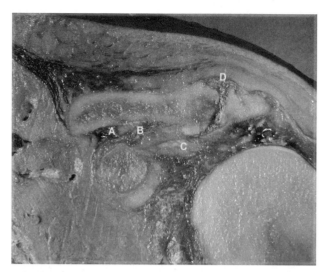

FIG. 28.1. Anatomy of the acromioclavicular joint complex. *A:* Conoid ligament. *B:* Trapezoid ligament. *C:* Acromioclavicular ligament. *D:* Superior acromioclavicular capsule.

tubercle of the clavicle. This gives the conoid ligament a slightly inferior lateral to superior medial orientation. The trapezoid ligament originates on the superior aspect of the coracoid process and inserts into the inferior lateral aspect of the clavicle. This gives it an inferior medial to superior lateral orientation. The trapazoid and conoid ligaments are oriented approximately 60 degrees to each other (Fig. 28.2). Fukuda et al. (26) showed that the function of the conoid ligament was to prevent superior translation of the clavicle relative to the coracoid. They also showed that the trapezoid ligament serves to prevent medial translation of the acromion relative to the clavicle with axial loading. The acromioclavicular ligaments act as a primary restraint to anteroposterior translation of the clavicle relative to the acromion. The deltoid and trapezius can act as dynamic stabilizers of the acromioclavicular joint. This

can actually be problematic in the acute injury setting where pain from acute separation will cause the patient to actively splint the injured shoulder by firing his or her deltoid and trapezius muscles. This may give the appearance of a normal acromioclavicular joint when in fact the patient may have a serious injury (27) (Fig. 28.3).

The amount of motion at the acromioclavicular joint has been subject to debate. Inman et al. (28) believed that there was 20 degrees of differential motion between the acromion and the clavicle. Codman, on the other hand, believed that there was only about 5 degrees of motion at the acromioclavicular joint. Rockwood (19) found by drilling pins into the clavicle and the acromion of volunteers that when the shoulder was put through a range of motion, there was only about 5 to 8 degrees of differential motion at the acromioclavicular joint. This makes intuitive sense because the distal clavicle is essentially tethered to the coracoid and the acromion by the acromioclavicular and coracoclavicular ligaments. It should be pointed out, however, that even the small amount of differential motion needs to be taken into consideration when selecting a form of fixation when treating acromioclavicular joint separations. Rockwood (19) and others (29–31) believed that coracoclavicular fixation with a screw is appropriate because there is so little differential motion. This small amount of motion, however, may be the cause of failure of coracoclavicular fixation with a screw. In what I refer to as the "stuck tent peg" phenomenon, the coracoclavicular screw can fail in much the same way as a firmly anchored tent peg can be pulled up by gently shaking it back and fourth

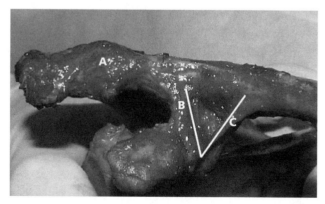

FIG. 28.2. Anatomy of the acromioclavicular joint complex. Note how the conoid ligament (*A*) and the trapezoid ligament (*B*) are angulated approximately 60 degrees to each other at their insertion on the coracoid.

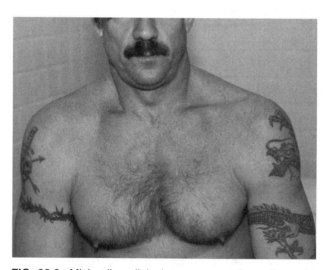

FIG. 28.3. Misleading clinical appearance of a patient who sustained a severe injury to his right acromioclavicular joint due to splinting. At the time of surgery he was found to have complete avulsion of the acromioclavicular and coracoclavicular ligaments and deltotrapezial fascia from the distal clavicle.

as one tries to pull it out of the ground. This small amount of differential motion may also be the cause of problems associated with using nonabsorbable suture in a cerclage fashion around clavicle and the coracoid. The differential motion that can be seen between the clavicle and the coracoid even with rocking the arm back and fourth with normal gait, in association with the distracted forces caused by the weight of the arm, may cause the suture to cut through the clavicle or the coracoid like a band saw (32–34).

MECHANISM OF INJURY

A fall on to the lateral aspect of the shoulder with the arm in the adducted position is probably the most common cause of injury to the acromioclavicular joint. In acromioclavicular joint separations, most authors have concluded that significant downward force on the acromion causes the acromioclavicular ligaments to rupture. If the downward force continues, the coracoclavicular ligaments may then rupture. Unfortunately, this ignores the complete mechanism of injury which, as Codman pointed out, causes the acromion to be driven downward, medially, and anteriorly relative to the clavicle. Because most of these injuries are related to a fall,

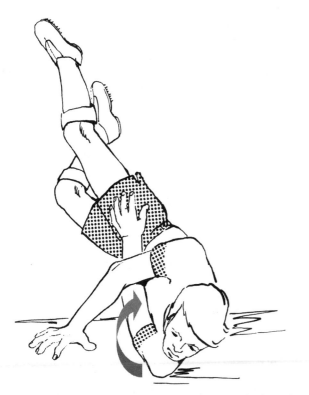

FIG. 28.4. Typical mechanism of injury for acromioclavicular separation with an anterior, medial, and interiorly directed force applied to the lateral acromion. (From Rockwood CA, Green DP, eds. *Fractures,* 2nd ed. Philadelphia: J.B. Lippincott, 1984, with permission.)

the patient either rolls their body to avoid striking the head or their head strikes the ground first, causing the body to roll toward the side that will be injured. The outer point of the shoulder then strikes the ground with the arm in an adducted position. Because of the rolling of the body toward the injured shoulder, the end result is that the acromion is driven not only inferiorly but also anteriorly and medially (Fig. 28.4).

This is probably also the same mechanism of injury as seen in distal and midshaft clavicle fractures. It is not clear what causes a fracture to occur in some patients and ligament injury to occur in others, but it may be related to the obliquity of the acromioclavicular joint with more oblique joints having a tendency to dislocate.

CLASSIFICATION OF INJURY

Rockwood pointed out that the classification of acromioclavicular joint injuries should be based on the degree of injury to the acromioclavicular and coracoclavicular ligaments in addition to the deltotrapezial fascia. The two most popular classification systems of acromioclavicular joint injuries are those popularized by Allman (35), Tossy et al. (36), and Rockwood (19). Allman (35) and Tossy et al. (36) described three degrees of severity in acromioclavicular joint separations. Type I injuries are those where the acromioclavicular ligaments are strained but intact and coracoclavicular ligaments are intact. Type II injuries are seen with higher energy and are associated with a complete tear of the acromioclavicular ligaments and a strain of the coracoclavicular ligaments. Type III injury represents the most severe injury in their classification system and is associated with even higher amounts of energy. This injury is characterized by complete rupture of both the acromioclavicular and coracoclavicular ligaments.

Rockwood believed that not all type III injuries were equivalent and that some of these represent a more severe injury and would more likely require surgical intervention. Based on this and his clinical observation that there are other forms of acromioclavicular separations, he described a more expanded modified classification system (Fig. 28.5). In his classification system, the type I injury is essentially the same as that describe by Allman and Tossy. A type II injury occurs when there is a complete disruption of the acromioclavicular ligaments and strain of the coracoclavicular ligaments with a slight increase in the coracoclavicular space. The type III injury is characterized as one where the acromioclavicular joint is dislocated and the acromioclavicular ligament is completely disrupted. The coracoclavicular ligaments are also assumed to have been disrupted and coracoclavicular interspace is approximately 25% to 100% greater than that seen in the normal shoulder. There is also disruption of the deltotrapezial fascia at

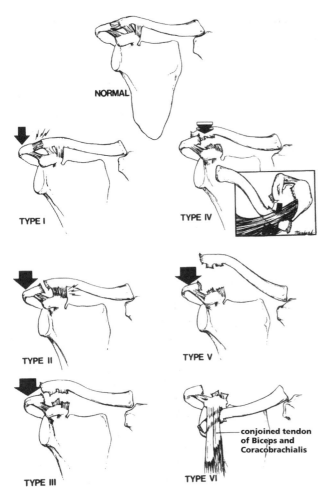

FIG. 28.5. The Rockwood classification of acromioclavicular joint ligamentous injuries. Type I: sprain of the acromioclavicular ligaments. Type II: complete disruption of the acromioclavicular joint with slight widening of the acromioclavicular joint and sprain of the coracoclavicular ligaments. Type III: complete disruption of the acromioclavicular and coracoclavicular ligaments with the coracoclavicular interspace increased by 25% to 100% more than normal shoulder. Type IV: complete disruption of the acromioclavicular and coracoclavicular ligaments of the clavicle displaced posteriorly into or through the trapezius muscle. Type V: complete disruption of the acromioclavicular and coracoclavicular ligaments with gross displacement of the acromioclavicular joint and increase in the coracoclavicular interval more than 100% greater than normal shoulder with detachment of the deltoid and trapezius fascia from the distal clavicle. Type VI: complete disruption of the acromioclavicular and coracoclavicular ligaments with detachment of the deltoid and trapezius muscle from the distal clavicle and displacement of the clavicle inferior to the acromion or the coracoid process.

its insertion into the distal clavicle. The type IV injury is essentially the same as a type III injury; however, the force on the acromion is more anteriorly directed, and hence the clavicle is displaced posteriorly into the trapezius muscle. The type V injury represents a severe form

of a type III injury, with gross displacement of the scapula relative to the clavicle and greater than 100% increase of the coracoclavicular interval. Finally, the type VI injury represents a very rare injury in which there is inferior dislocation of the clavicle beneath the coracoid. Only a handful of these cases have been reported in the literature. They are representative of severe trauma and believed to be secondary to a severe hyperadduction and external rotation of the arm (37).

I have found the Rockwood classification to be much more useful than the Allman–Tossy classification. However, I am not convinced that either classification system is representative of the mechanism of injury seen with acromioclavicular joint separations. As noted above, there is a significant inferiorly medially and anteriorly directed force on the acromion at the time of injury. Both the Rockwood and the Allman classification systems assume a force directed downward on the acromion, with the exception of the Rockwood type VI injury. Unfortunately, this is not what occurs in reality. With the exception of the situation in which a log may fall on the outside tip of the shoulder, there is almost always a medially directed force on the acromioclavicular joint. To give an example, when a person is thrown off their bicycle, their head hits the ground first, causing the body to roll onto the shoulder. When the shoulder makes contact with the ground, the vector of the forces exerted on the lateral acromion is both inferiorly and axially directed. In the classic study by Urist (25), the clavicle and the scapula were pulled apart after the acromioclavicular and coracoclavicular ligaments were sequentially divided. In both this experiment and a cadaver experiment by Rockwood (19), the assumption was made that both coracoclavicular ligaments rupture simultaneously. Because of the "V" orientation of the coracoclavicular ligaments, it is probably true that both would rupture with a direct downward force pulling apart the scapula and the clavicle (Fig. 28.6).

Fukuda et al. (26) studied the contribution of each ligament in the acromioclavicular and coracoclavicular complex to acromioclavicular stability. They found that with small displacement, the acromioclavicular ligaments were the primary restraint to both posterior and superior translation of the clavicle. With larger displacement, they found that the trapezoid ligament was a primary restraint to medial translation of the scapula with axial loading. The conoid was a primary restraint to superior translation. If one takes Fukuda et al.'s finding into account and accepts that there is a medially directed force at the time of the injury, it is entirely possible that the coracoclavicular ligaments do not rupture simultaneously. In this scenario, the person falling off their bike would land on the ground first striking their head and then their shoulder. As energy is transmitted to the acromion and hence the acromioclavicular

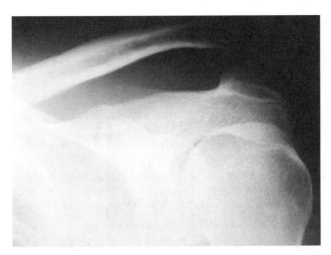

FIG. 28.6. Anterior posterior radiograph of a Rockwood type V acromioclavicular joint separation. Note the gross deformity of the coracoclavicular interval.

joint, the acromioclavicular joint ligaments would rupture first. If there was sufficient energy, the trapezoid ligament, because of its orientation, would rupture next. As the force continues to be applied to the shoulder, the scapula and acromion would be driven medially relative to the clavicle, causing the conoid ligament to assume a more vertical position. With continued displacement, the conoid ligament would become a restraint against further medial translation (Fig. 28.7). If the energy were sufficient enough, the conoid ligament would also rupture, allowing even further medial translation of the acromion and scapula relative to the clavicle.

This is actually what I have found both clinically and experimentally. With a downward and medially directed force on the shoulder, division of the acromioclavicular

ligaments causes minimal change in the coracoclavicular space distance. Sectioning of the trapezoid ligament allows an increase in the coracoclavicular interval distance of approximately 25% to 50%. However, it does not allow the medial edge of the acromion to go medial to the lateral end of the clavicle. Once the conoid ligament is divided, there is not only a significant increase in the coracoclavicular interval but also the acromion, on anteroposterior radiographs, appears to go underneath the lateral end of the clavicle. This occurs even when the deltotrapezial fascia is left completely intact. When studied with three-dimensional computed tomography, what was found was that the entire scapula actually rotated anteromedially relative to the clavicle (Fig. 28.8).

Furthermore, in many injuries that I initially classified as type IV acromioclavicular joint separations due to the relative posterior placement of the clavicle relative to the shoulder, I found that at time of surgery, the patient was placed into a supine position, and the shoulder and clavicle assumed a more normal orientation. Although situations occur in which the clavicle is actually impaled into the trapezius, this represents an unusual injury. More commonly, what I believe happens is that the instability at the acromioclavicular joint allows the shoulder to be pulled anteromedially by the pectoralis muscles. Based on these observations, I propose a classification system based on anteromedial instability of the shoulder. In anteromedially stable shoulder, the acromioclavicular and trapezoid ligaments may be injured; however, the conoid ligament remains intact. In the anteromedially unstable shoulder, the acromioclavicular trapezoid and conoid ligaments have been completely disrupted. The significance of this is that I believe the anteromedially unstable shoulders are more likely to require operative intervention.

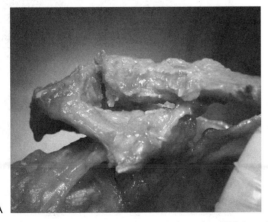

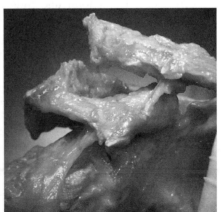

A   B

FIG. 28.7. Acromioclavicular separation after division of the acromioclavicular ligament and the trapezoid ligament. **(A)** Normal anatomic relationship **(B)** shows the acromioclavicular separation and increase in the coracoclavicular interval with medial stress applied to the scapula.

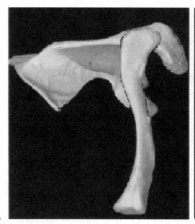
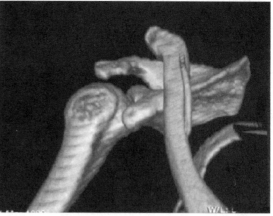

FIG. 28.8. A: Computer-generated representation of the anterior medial rotation of the scapula relative to the clavicle with complete disruption of the acromioclavicular and coracoclavicular ligaments. **B:** Three-dimensional computed tomograph of a cadaver shoulder in which the acromioclavicular and coracoclavicular ligaments have been severed but the deltotrapezial fascia left intact.

CLINICAL EXAMINATION

In the acute setting, the physical findings may range from minimal to gross deformity based on the severity of the injury and the amount of splinting by the patient. Unfortunately, it is not unusual to have a patient return for follow-up a few weeks after injury with a very obvious deformity where none was noted on the initial examination in the emergency room. Once the pain subsides from the initial injury and the patient is splinting less, the weight of the arm causes the acromioclavicular joint to subluxate. Because the early operative intervention is crucial in severe acromioclavicular joint separations, one should have a high index of suspicion in patients who have significant pain at the acromioclavicular joint and a good history for high-energy injury with minimal deformity.

In a Rockwood type I injury, there is usually minimal deformity of the acromioclavicular joint and mild to moderate tenderness to palpation. Range of motion in these patients is typically normal.

In type II injuries, there may be mild deformity due to soft tissue swelling over the acromioclavicular joint and moderate to severe tenderness to palpation of the joint. Range of motion in these patients is typically limited due to pain. Although there may not be a prominence of the distal clavicle, there may be an increase in the amount of motion in the anteroposterior plane of the distal clavicle due to injury to the acromioclavicular ligaments.

In type III and more severe injuries, the patient may present holding his or her injured arm close to the body and supporting it with the uninjured arm because of severe pain. This also helps reduce the dislocated acromioclavicular joint. Any attempted motion, even passive, in these patients is usually resisted. There may be

a significant prominence of the distal clavicle due to inferior subluxation or a drooping of the shoulder (Fig. 28.9). As noted above, these patients may have no apparent deformity due to splinting of the injury by firing of the deltoid muscle (Fig. 28.3). The distal clavicle is usually unstable in both the vertical and horizontal planes. When the injured arm is adducted across the chest, there is usually a significant prominence of the distal clavicle due to medial subluxation of the scapula relative to the clavicle.

In type IV injuries, there may be a prominence of the distal clavicle posteriorly. Although other authors

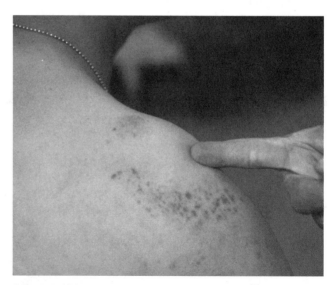

FIG. 28.9. Clinical appearance of an acute complete acromioclavicular joint separation. Note the prominence of the distal clavicle in addition to the ecchymosis and abrasions over the posterolateral aspect of the shoulder.

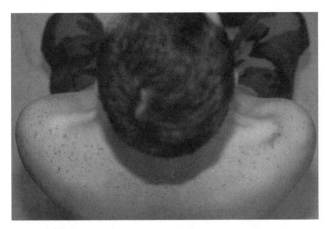

FIG. 28.10. Clinical photo of a patient initially thought to have a Rockwood type IV acromioclavicular separation. When placed in the supine position, the acromioclavicular joint self-reduced. Note how the clavicles are in normal orientation to each other; however, the right scapula is rotated anteromedially.

have suggested that this is due to posterior displacement of the distal clavicle (19,30,31), I have found that the relative prominence of the distal clavicle is due to the anterior medial displacement of the scapula that is caused by the acromioclavicular joint instability and pull of the pectoralis muscles (Fig. 28.10). It is actually almost impossible to displace the distal clavicle posteriorly because it is tethered so strongly medially. Usually, this deformity will disappear when the patient is placed into a supine position. In some of these patients, the distal clavicle may be buttonholed into the trapezius muscle, and these deformities are not easily reducible. These injuries are rare and probably represent "true" type IV injuries.

In the chronic setting, patients with type I and II injuries may have only a mild deformity at the acromioclavicular joint. Many times this deformity will actually be due to degenerative changes within the acromioclavicular joint. In type III patients and those with more severe injuries, there is usually a marked prominence of the distal clavicle due to inferior subluxation or drooping of the shoulder. Cross-body adduction in these patients will cause the distal clavicle to become markedly prominent (Fig. 28.11). These patients usually complain of chronic pain at the acromioclavicular joint. I have found that athletes may complain of decreased strength and endurance in the involved shoulder.

RADIOGRAPHIC EXAMINATION

Unfortunately, acromioclavicular joint injuries are commonly evaluated radiographically in the emergency room with standard anteroposterior and axillary views of the shoulder. The problem with this is that the acromioclavicular joint is washed out on these views of the shoulder and the acromioclavicular joint is superimposed over the acromial process (Fig. 28.12).

Because of this, subtle fractures and separations of the acromioclavicular joint may be missed. To alleviate this problem, the radiographs must be taken at "soft tissue" intensity, which uses approximately 50% less exposure than standard shoulder radiographs. If the technician is unfamiliar with this technique, a shoulder radiograph taken with chest x-ray exposure will give better visualization of the acromioclavicular joint.

Although it is important to get orthogonal radiographs on all shoulder trauma cases, additional radiographs should be obtained when an acromioclavicular joint injury is suspected.

With the standard anteroposterior views, the patient should be either seated or standing at the time of the

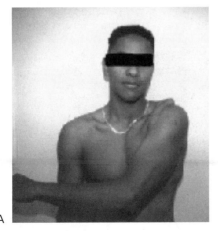

A

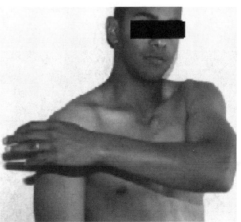

B

FIG. 28.11. A: Preoperative clinical photo of the patient with significant anteromedial instability of the shoulder. Note the significant prominence of the clavicle in the inward collapse of the shoulder relative to the clavicle. **B:** Postoperative reestablishment of the normal acromioclavicular stability.

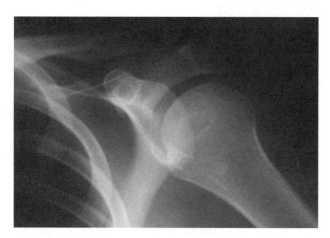

FIG. 28.12. Standard anterior posterior radiograph of the shoulder. Note the poor visualization of the acromioclavicular joint due to overpenetration.

radiographs. This may allow gravity distraction of the injured joint. Often times, however, the patient may be splinting a severely injured shoulder and this will cause the radiographs to appear normal. If possible, both acromioclavicular joints should be imaged simultaneously on the same cassette. This will allow comparison of the injury with the uninjured joint because there can be considerable variation in the orientation of the acromioclavicular joint and size of the coracoclavicular interval from patient to patient. If the patient is too large to accommodate both shoulders on the same cassette, separate cassettes can be used for each shoulder using the same radiographic techniques on each shoulder (38).

Zanca (39) found that better visualization of the acromioclavicular joint could be obtained by angling the x-ray beam 10 to 15 degrees cephalad on the anteroposterior radiographs. This provided an unobscured view of the acromioclavicular joint without superimposition of the spine of the scapula. Although this is of

limited value in acromioclavicular joint separations, it is useful in assessing patients with degenerative arthritis of the acromioclavicular joint or subtle fractures of the distal clavicle (Fig. 28.13).

Stress Views

It is not necessary to obtain stress views on clinically obvious severe acromioclavicular joint separations or in patients who have significant widening of the coracoclavicular interval on routine shoulder radiographs. Bossart et al. (40) did not believe that stress radiographs were justifiable due to their low yield in evaluation of patients without obvious injury to the acromioclavicular joint. However, I have seen numerous patients who at the time of their initial radiographic evaluation were believed to have insignificant injuries to the acromioclavicular joint and on later follow-up radiographs had complete dislocations. This is probably because the patient was trying to protect their painful injured shoulder by supporting it with the uninjured arm or by rigidly contracting the deltoid and trapezius muscles, either of which can give the appearance of the normal shoulder. This is especially common in muscular athletic patients in whom these injuries commonly occur (27). Missing a complete acromioclavicular joint dislocation on the initial examination can have significant impact on the long-term outcome of the patient. If the dislocation is detected early, a relatively easy early surgical intervention can leave the patient with a nearly normal joint. If the dislocation is not detected until later follow-up (e.g., 3 or 4 weeks later), the patient now has an injury that cannot be treated with simple surgical techniques and may require excision of the distal clavicle in addition to reconstruction of the coracoclavicular ligaments. Because of this, I believe that it is important to obtain stress x-rays on all patients suspected of having significant acromioclavicular joint injuries.

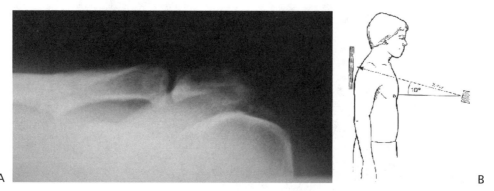

A   B

FIG. 28.13. Zanca view of the shoulder. The cephalic tilt of the x-ray allows better visualization of the acromioclavicular joint without superimposition of the spinal scapula. (From Rockwood CA, Green DP, eds. *Fractures,* 2nd ed. Philadelphia: J.B. Lippincott, 1984, with permission.)

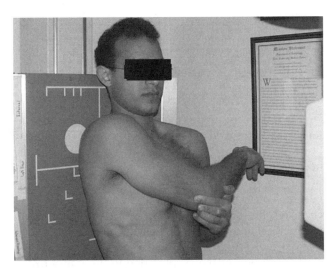

FIG. 28.14. Technique for obtaining a cross-body adduction anteroposterior radiograph of the shoulder.

The classic technique for obtaining stress radiographs is to suspend 10- to 15-pound weights from the patient's arm by tying them to the patient's wrist and then take a standard anteroposterior radiograph (27). Although some authors have suggested that the weight may be held in the hand or tied to the wrist (41) or to internally rotate the arm (42), it is preferable to have the weight tied to the wrist because it allows the patient to more completely relax the muscles about the shoulder. Unfortunately, patients with significant pain due to an acromioclavicular joint separation may still try to protect their painful shoulder by contracting the deltoid and trapezius muscles.

Alexander (43) described what he called the shoulder forward stress view to identify acromioclavicular joint dislocations. This radiograph is obtained by having the patient thrust his or her shoulders forward while a true scapular lateral radiograph is taken of the injured shoul-

der. A similar x-ray is obtained of the uninjured shoulder. In comparison with the uninjured side, the acromion will be displaced anteriorly and inferiorly relative to the distal clavicle. Although some authors have recommended this view to assess all acromioclavicular joint injuries (44), I have found this radiograph to be very difficult to interpret.

Because of the limitations with standard stress radiographs and the Alexander lateral stress view, I obtain a radiograph that I referred to as the cross-body adduction view (45). This is obtained by having the patient cross his or her injured arm across the chest while a standard anteroposterior radiograph is taken (Fig. 28.14). I have found that on patients with complete acromioclavicular joint disruptions, the acromion will appear to go medial and inferior to the distal clavicle with this view (Fig. 28.15). In laboratory studies, I have found that this only occurs when there is a complete injury to the acromioclavicular, trapezoid, and conoid ligaments. The acromion can rotate medially in the posterior band of the acromioclavicular ligament is severed; however, in laboratory studies the medial border of the acromion appeared to go inferior and medial to the lateral end of the clavicle only when the trapezoid and conoid ligaments are incompletely severed. This anterior medial subluxation of the acromion relative to the clavicle could occur when the deltotrapezial fascia was still intact. Although the acromion appears to go medial and inferior to the clavicle, three-dimensional computed tomography evaluations have shown that the acromion and scapula actually rotate anterior, medial, and inferior relative to the clavicle (Fig. 28.8). The initial idea for this radiograph came from an observation that virtually all patients with chronic, symptomatic, complete dislocations of the acromioclavicular joint all had significant medial instability of the scapular relative to the clavicle in the arm of the injured shoulder adducted across the chest (45). I have also found this study to be more reliable

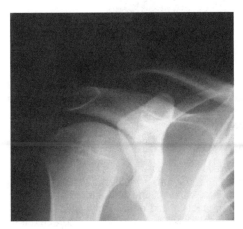
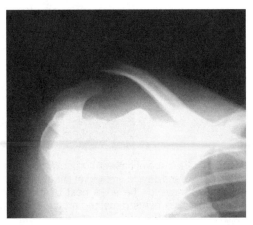

FIG. 28.15. Comparison of the standard anteroposterior radiograph of the shoulder to a cross-body adduction radiograph. Note the acromion appears to subluxate medial to the lateral aspect of the clavicle.

than routine stress x-rays and easier to interpret in the Alexander lateral stress view.

Radiographic Findings

In Rockwood type I injuries, radiographs are typically normal. Although there may be some soft tissue swelling about the acromioclavicular joint, there is no widening of the acromioclavicular or coracoclavicular interval.

In Rockwood type II injuries, there may be some widening of the acromioclavicular interval due to injury to the acromioclavicular ligaments (46). The coracoclavicular interval will be normal to slightly increased; however, the increase will be less than 25%.

In Rockwood type III injuries, the superior surface of the acromion is displaced inferior to the inferior lateral border of clavicle. The coracoclavicular interval is 25% to 100% greater than in the normal shoulder. If the superior border of acromion is inferior to the inferior lateral border of clavicle but yet the coracoclavicular interval is unchanged relative to the end injured shoulder, one should suspect a fracture of the base of the coracoid (47) (Fig. 28.16). In this situation, there is a complete disruption of the acromioclavicular ligaments; however, the coracoclavicular ligaments remain intact. It is the coracoid that displaces relative to the scapula. Fractures of the coracoid are best assessed with the Stryker notch view.

In Rockwood type IV injuries, there will be an increase in the acromioclavicular and coracoclavicular interval distances similar to that seen in type III injuries; however, the interval increases may not be dramatic because the primary deformity is posterior displacement of the distal clavicle relative to the acromion. This is best seen on an axillary view. This occurs when the distal clavicle is buttonholed posteriorly into the trapezius. A true type IV injury is very rare and must be distinguished from type III and V injuries when there is anterior medial rotation of the scapula due to the injury to the acromioclavicular and coracoclavicular ligaments and deforming forced of the pectoralis muscles. In the latter case, the axillary lateral taken in a supine position will appear normal, whereas the type IV injury will show posterior displacement.

In Rockwood type V injuries, there is dramatic increase in both the acromioclavicular and coracoclavicu-

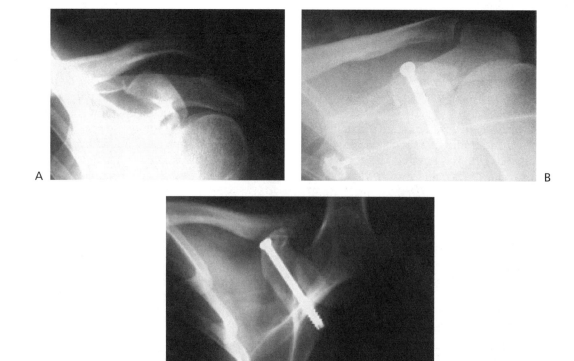

FIG. 28.16. A: Fracture of base of coracoid. Although there is significant increase in the acromioclavicular space, the coracoclavicular interval is normal. Although the fracture is well visualized on the anteroposterior view, they can be seen best of the Stryker notch view of the shoulder. **B:** Because the coracoclavicular ligaments remained intact, adequate reduction of the acromioclavicular interval was obtained through fixation of the coracoid fracture. **C:** Complete healing of the base of coracoid fracture with good position of cancellous screw.

lar intervals (Fig. 28.6). This is caused by the inferior subluxation or displacement of the scapular relative to the clavicle due to the loss of the superior suspensory mechanism of the shoulder. It should be noted that the scapula is displaced downward rather than the clavicle being displaced upward. Rockwood type VI injuries are very rare, and routine shoulder radiographs to the distal clavicle to be dislocated into the subacromial or subcoracoid space.

TREATMENT OPTIONS

Few injuries in orthopedics have had as many different treatments described as acromioclavicular joint injuries. Even within the broader categories of operative versus nonoperative treatment, numerous methods have been described, with over 35 different forms of nonoperative treatment and literally hundreds of forms of operative treatment (19,31) (Fig. 28.17B).

Few authors would suggest that anything other than nonoperative treatment is necessary for type I or II acromioclavicular joint separations. It is interesting to note that Bergfeld et al. (48) and Cox (1) have reported

these injuries may be associated with late disability. Furthermore, there are few surgeons who would recommend anything other than operative treatment for type IV, V or VI injuries. The tremendous gray area is in the treatment of type III injuries. There appears to be a current trend toward nonoperative treatment of type III injuries. A number of recent studies have shown little strength or functional differences in operatively or nonoperatively treated patients (49–60). In addition, many studies suggest a quicker returned to full function with nonoperative treatment, even in athletes (61). Unfortunately, it is difficult to draw specific conclusions about the success of either type of treatment because most studies have not controlled patient demand levels (3). In addition, it is difficult to ascertain what is meant by a "complete acromioclavicular joint dislocation" in many studies. In this climate of cost containment, one also must consider the cost of operative treatment of these injuries (62).

One particular problem in deciding operative or nonoperative treatment in athletes with type III injuries is that there are few injuries where early operative intervention can make as drastic a difference in later func-

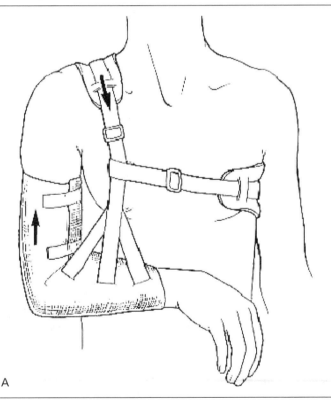

A

Nonoperative Treatment for Acromioclavicular Dislocation Reported in the Literature

Form of Treatment	Authors
Adhesive strapping	Rawlings, Thorndike and Quigley, Benson, Bakalim and Wilppula
Sling or bandage	Jones, Watson-Jones, Hawkins
Brace and harness	Giannestras, Warner, Currie, Anderson and Burgess, Anzel and Streitz
Crotch loops, stocking, garter, and strap	Darrow and associates, Spigelman, Varney and associates
Figure-of-eight bandage	Usadel
Sling and pressure dressing	Goldberg
Abduction traction and suspension in bed	Caldwell
Casts	Urist, Howard, Shaar, Hart, Trynin, Stubbins and McGaw, Dillehunt, Key and Cornwell, Gibbens

From Rockwood, C. A., and Green, D. P. (eds.), Fractures in Adults, 3rd ed. Philadelphia, J. B. Lipppincott, 1991, p 884. B

FIG. 28.17. A: Modified Kenny-Howard shoulder harness. The acromioclavicular joint is held reduced by the strap runs over the top of the shoulder and under the elbow. The additional strap around the chest prevents the harness from slipping off the shoulder. (From Rockwood CA, Green DP, eds. *Fractures,* 2nd ed. Philadelphia: J.B. Lippincott, 1984, with permission.) **B:** Table of the various nonoperative treatment techniques for acromioclavicular separations reported in the literature.

tion. To commit an athlete to a wait-and-see treatment necessitates that if they do become symptomatic at a later date, they will then require a more complicated procedure that requires resection of the distal clavicle and augmentation of the supporting ligaments, whereas early acute intervention is much easier to perform and can leave the patient with essentially a normal shoulder (4,63,64). Rockwood (19) also suggested that early operative intervention should be considered in laborers and patients involved in high demand overhead activities, such as a throwing athlete. However, he also suggested that operative intervention should not be considered in contact athletes because they are at high risk for reinjury.

In terms of pediatric patients, most can be managed nonoperatively; however, Eidman et al. (65) pointed out that patients over the age of 13 should be treated as adults.

Nonoperative Treatment

Many different techniques have been described to reduce the subluxation of the acromion relative to the clavicle in acromioclavicular joint injuries, including compressive dressings, taping, plaster casts, braces, slings, and harnesses. Generally speaking, however, the two primary treatments at this time are the use of the sling and harness or benign neglect. Use of a sling and harness device to reduce the acromioclavicular joint dates back to the time of Hippocrates, with its most current application being a device such as the Kenny-Howard shoulder harness (Fig. 28.17A). This device consists of a strap that goes around the elbow and over the top of the shoulder. This is meant to hold the dislocated acromioclavicular joint in a reduced position. To allow ligament healing, this device must be worn continuously for 3 to 6 weeks. Because of the continuous pressure applied over the distal clavicle, there can be problems of skin breakdown due to pressure necrosis. In addition, other authors have reported compression of the anterior interosseous nerve from the use of the sling and harness devise (66,67).

The current trend in nonoperative treatment is benign or skillful neglect. This entails use of the sling for comfort for approximately 1 to 2 weeks after which time the patient is allowed to return to their activities of daily living.

In type I injuries, active motion can be initiated within a day or two after the initial injury, and the athlete can return to full participation in sports when they have full strength and painless motion. This probably takes about 1 to 2 weeks.

In type II injuries, ice and analgesics, in addition to the sling, can be used for the first 2 or 3 days. The patient is told to discard the sling as symptoms permit, which is usually within the first week. The patient is

allowed to start range of motion and activities of daily living as soon as tolerated. As with the type I injuries, the patient is not allowed to return to full sports until they have full strength and painless motion. This may take up to 6 weeks. It is important that these patients are rechecked after their symptoms subside to make sure they did not sustain a more serious injury that was missed due to splinting of the injured extremity. I have seen many patients were initially diagnosed as having type I or II injuries who on later follow-up had much more severe injuries that now had to be treated as chronic separations because they were out of the time range for an acute repair.

In type III injuries, ice, analgesics, and a sling are used as in a type II injury. The sling is discontinued as the patient's symptoms allow range of motion exercises and return to activities of daily living. Most patients are essentially pain free within 2 to 3 weeks and can return to full sports participation if they have full painless motion and strength. This typically takes 6 to 8 weeks.

Operative Treatment

There has been a plethora of publications dealing with the operative treatment of acromioclavicular joint sepa-

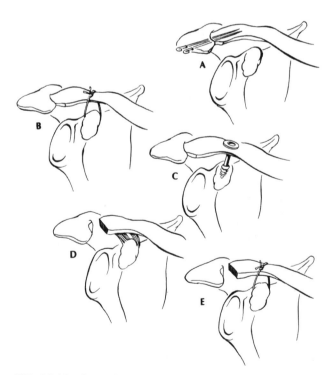

FIG. 28.18. Operative procedures of the treatment of acromioclavicular joint separations. **A:** Acromioclavicular fixation. **B:** Coracoclavicular cerclage. **C:** Coracoclavicular lag screw fixation. **D:** Distal clavicle resection. **E:** Distal clavicle resection with coracoclavicular cerclage. (From Rockwood CA, Green DP, eds. *Fractures,* 2nd ed. Philadelphia: J.B. Lippincott, 1984, with permission.)

rations. Most of these publications, however, are based on three different types of fixation—acromioclavicular, coracoclavicular, and dynamic muscle transfer—that can be combined with or without ligament augmentation and with or without resection of the distal clavicle (Fig. 28.18). Although some studies have used allograft or autograft ligament augmentation, the primary method of coracoclavicular ligament reconstruction is based on transfer of the coracoacromial ligament.

Acromioclavicular Fixation

A variety of methods of acromioclavicular fixation has been reported in the literature: use of smooth Steinmann pins, Steinmann pins augmented with tension band wires, fully threaded pins, and screws. Eskola et al. (68,69) compared screw fixation to smooth pin and threaded pin fixation and found that 15% of the patients developed symptomatic osteolysis of the distal clavicle, with most occurring in the screw fixation group.

Probably the biggest problem with pin fixation of the acromioclavicular joint is a concern for hardware migration, which has been well documented by Rockwood (19) and others (70–73). In addition to this concern, placement of transacromial pins can be quite demanding. In patients with down-sloping acromions, it can be difficult to drive the pins across the acromion and have them gain adequate purchase in the distal clavicle. There is also concern for potential damage to the lateral deltoid muscle and to the acromion, particularly in patients who have thin acromions.

Although it has not gained significant popularity in the United States, hook plate fixation has been popular in Europe. A number of authors have reported excellent results with the Balsar hook plate (74–78). Despite these reported good results, this technique requires use of a fairly expensive device, a large soft tissue dissection, and places a portion of the plate under the acromion where it may cause abrasion of the rotator cuff tendons. One study found an infection or delayed wound healing in 28% of patients (78). Furthermore, removal of the plate requires a second procedure, a large soft tissue dissection that typically must be performed in a hospital setting (75).

Coracoclavicular Fixation

A number of methods of coracoclavicular fixation have been described (19,43,79–81). This probably represents the most common type of operative fixation in United States. The two basic types of fixation consists of rigid or nonrigid constructs. Screws and wires represent a rigid form of fixation, whereas sutures, both adsorbable and nonabsorbable, and grafts, such as synthetic, allograft, and autogenous tissue, represent a nonrigid form (82). Screw fixation has the advantage of being strong

and can be placed with minimal soft tissue dissection (83); however, this type of fixation usually needs to be removed in a second procedure. Suture fixation is less rigid than screw fixation and is typically placed in a cerclage fashion around the coracoid and clavicle (84) (Fig. 28.19). This necessitates a fairly large exposure, and passing the suture beneath the coracoid can be demanding. Although unlikely, passage of instruments beneath the coracoid can potentially damage the musculocutaneous nerve or the coracohumeral ligament. One of the problems with cerclage fixation techniques is that the clavicle can be pulled anteriorly relative to its normal anatomic position, which can result in posterior acromioclavicular impingement. Some authors (85) have placed the sutures through drill holes in the clavicle (Fig. 28.20) and the coracoid to prevent this anterior migration. If absorbable sutures are used, such as PDS7 (polydioxanone), these are typically braided with a total of six to nine strands of no. 0 or no. 1 sutures. It should be pointed out that the braid must be very tight or the construct will be loose. In addition to the fact that this will provide less secure fixation, there is a risk for abrasion between the strands of the suture as it is repeatedly stretched, and this may lead to early failure. When permanent sutures, such as Mersiline or Dacron, are used in a cerclage fashion, there is a risk that this suture can erode through the clavicle or the coracoid or act as a foreign body (32–34,86,87).

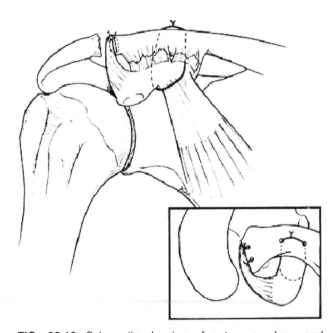

FIG. 28.19. Schematic drawing of suture cerclage and transfer of the coracoacromial ligament into the end of the clavicle. (From Weinstein DM, McCann PD, McIlveen SJ, et al. Surgical treatment of complete acromioclavicular dislocations. *Am J Sports Med* 1995;23:324.331, with permission.)

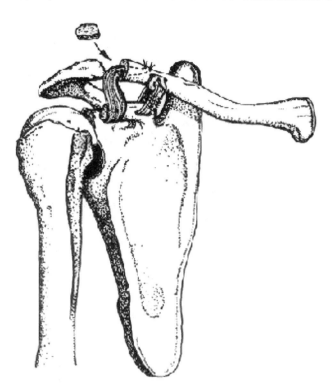

FIG. 28.20. Schematic drawing of coracoclavicular fixation using drill holes in the clavicle and coracoid. This prevents anterior subluxation of the clavicle and fracture of the clavicle or coracoid due to "sawing" motion of the suture. (From Morrison DS, Lemos MJ. Acromioclavicular separation. Reconstruction using synthetic loop augmentation. *Am J Sports Med* 1995;23:105–110, with permission.)

Dynamic Muscle Transfer

Transfer of the short of the biceps in the tip of the coracoid process has been described as treatment for both acute and chronic acromioclavicular joint separations (88,89). There appears to be little reason to recommend this procedure because it is not biomechanically sound. The basis of this operation is to pull the clavicle down to the scapula. Beside the fact that we learned long ago that dynamic transfers typically are ineffective, this procedure has a high complication rate and has been associated with musculocutaneous nerve injury and weakness (89–91).

Distal Clavicle Resection

Although Bosworth (79) believed it unnecessary to excise the distal clavicle, a number of authors have used debridement of the interarticular disk and distal clavicle excision in both acute and chronic acromioclavicular joint separations (84). Although excision of the distal clavicle may be necessary in chronic dislocations (30), it is unclear why the distal clavicle should be excised in acute injuries. Some authors have suggested that the damage to the joint and the interarticular disk will lead to later degenerative changes in the acromioclavicular joint. Although this may be so, it should be pointed out that degeneration of the acromioclavicular joint is probably natural part of aging (21,22,24) and the presence of radiographic degenerative changes does not necessarily mean the patient will be symptomatic (57). Although Fukuda et al. (26) reported that the acromioclavicular ligaments are the primary stabilizers of the acromioclavicular joint, the bony structure of the joint itself is actually an important stabilizer of the joint. Removal of the distal clavicle may not be a benign procedure (92,93) and may lead to late joint instability (94) and weakness (95). Because only some patients have symptoms related to degeneration of the acromioclavicular joint and because it can be easily treated at a later date, I prefer to resect the distal clavicle only in chronic separation cases. I have not found this compromises the later result.

If a late resection of the distal clavicle was undertaken, it is important that this procedure is not performed in patients with acromioclavicular joint instability because this may exacerbate the instability (96). It does not appear to be necessary to resect more than 10 to 15 mm of the distal clavicle. In fact, poorer results have been associated with more generous resections (97). At the time of distal clavicle resection, it is important that the surgeon check the integrity of the coracoclavicular ligaments. This can be done by palpating beneath the clavicle after the distal-most portion is removed. A trapezoid ligament can typically be felt to insert just medial to the resected end of the clavicle if 10 to 15 mm are resected. The resection of excessive amounts of the distal clavicle cannot only result in loss of the trapezoid insertion but also the insertion of the acromioclavicular ligaments. The scapula can then pivot medially about the remaining conoid ligament and impinge against the distal clavicle. Even if only 10 to 15 mm are resected off the clavicle, the surgeon should take great care to protect the acromioclavicular ligaments, especially the posterior band. If the posterior and superior portions of the acromioclavicular ligaments are damaged at the time of the resection, there can be an increase in the horizontal instability of the acromion relative to the clavicle that may result in posterior acromioclavicular impingement as the scapula rotates anteromedially (26). Additionally, care should be taken to protect the underlying suprascapular nerve because it can be injured during the resection of the distal clavicle (98).

Ligament Reconstruction

Although popularized by Weaver and Dunn (99), in 1917 Cadanet (100) described reconstruction of the coracoclavicular ligaments using transfer of the acromioclavicular ligament. Although this has been the most successful type of ligament reconstruction (31,95, 99,101), it is probably unnecessary in acute settings as the ruptured coracoclavicular ligaments have great potential for healing if reapproximated. Although the coracoacromial ligament is an excellent augmentation material, its anterior insertion on the coracoid can pull the distal clavicle into an anteriorly subluxated position when used as a ligament transfer. In addition, for this transfer to work properly, the orientation of the trapezoid ligament must be recreated for the transferred ligament to act as a tether to prevent medial translation of the scapula relative to the clavicle. Therefore, it is important that as much length of the clavicle be preserved with no more than 10 to 15 mm being resected, and placement of the transferred ligament should be into the end of the clavicle. If excessive amounts of the clavicle are resected, the transferred coracoacromial ligament will be in a vertical position. This will allow the scapula to swing as if on a pendulum and may result in acromioclavicular impingement.

OPERATIVE TECHNIQUE

Acute Injuries

The patient is placed in a beach-chair position on the operating table using a radiolucent positioner such as OSI Schlein table 7. The c-arm is positioned in such a way that its orientation is from an anterior lateral to posterior medial inclination (Fig. 28.21). This allows the coracoid to be viewed in its smallest possible diameter. The advantage of this is that it facilitates the placement of a coracoclavicular screw for fixation. When viewed in this position, a screw placed at the superior apex or midpoint of the coracoid is in the center of the coracoid from all other projections. Unfortunately, a typical mistake with the coracoclavicular screw is that it is placed either anterior or posterior to the coracoid. Because of

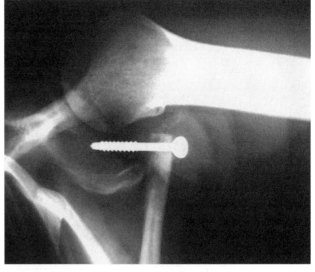

FIG. 28.22. Attempted fixation of the acromioclavicular joint using a malleolar screw. Note that the screw is lateral to the base of the coracoid.

the curve of the coracoid, it is not possible, when viewed with an anteroposterior radiograph, to tell if the screw is anterior to the coracoid, in the coracoid, or behind the coracoid. This problem is further compounded by the fact that the threads of the screw may partially engage the coracoid even when it is inserted anterior or posterior to the coracoid. This may give the surgeon a sense of false security because he or she will feel some resistance on the screwdriver as the coracoclavicular screw is being inserted and the clavicle may feel stable when it is gently stressed. Unfortunately, when the screw is placed in this fashion, it usually fails within a few days of the surgery (Fig. 28.22).

An examination under anesthesia is performed (Fig.

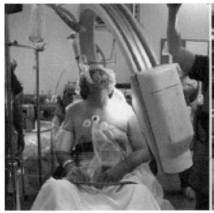
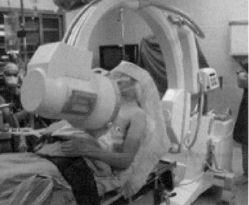

FIG. 28.21. Positioning of the patient on the operating table. The patient is placed in a radiolucent beach-chair positioner. The image intensifier is angled to posterior medial to anterolateral orientation. This allows visualization of the coracoid process in the smallest possible profile.

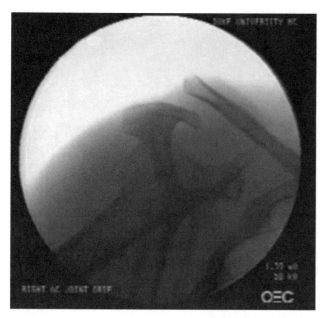

FIG. 28.23. Intraoperative demonstration of the medial instability of the shoulder due to complete disruption of the acromioclavicular and coracoclavicular ligaments.

28.23), and an attempt is then made to reduce the dislocation. If the acromioclavicular dislocation is easily reducible, I have found that it is not necessary to remove the intraarticular disk of the acromioclavicular joint (102). It also means that the distal clavicle is not buttonholed through the deltotrapezial fascia or impaled into the trapezius muscle.

The patient is then prepped and draped in the usual

sterile fashion. A saber-type incision approximately 2.5 cm long is made about 1.5 cm medial to the distal tip of the clavicle extending anteriorly from the posterior aspect of the clavicle. The subcutaneous fascia is divided down to the deltotrapezial fascia. When the deltotrapezial fascia is still intact, it is incised longitudinally in the coronal plane, extending no further laterally than the acromioclavicular joint. Although other authors have suggested that direct repair of the coracoclavicular ligaments is necessary (19,31), I have not found this to be the case (102). The acromioclavicular joint is then reduced, taking care to verify that the anterior edge of the clavicle is contiguous with the anterior edge of the acromion. If the acromioclavicular joint is not reducible, the joint is inspected and the intraarticular disk removed if necessary. It is also important to point out that the position of the clavicle relative to the acromion should be the same as that seen in the uninvolved shoulder based on preoperative radiographs. This is because there may be considerable variation from individual to individual in the orientation of the acromioclavicular joint (38).

With joint held reduced, the coracoclavicular screw is inserted in the following manner. A 3/16-inch drill bit is placed in the center of the superior cortex of the clavicle directly over the base of the coracoid. This position is verified with fluoroscopy (Fig. 28.24). A hole is then drill through the clavicle. A depth gauge can then be inserted through the drill hole in the clavicle and used as a probe to feel the anterior, medial, and

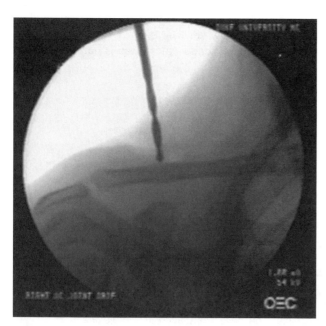

FIG. 28.24. Positioning of the first drill bit on the clavicle directly overlying the base of the coracoid.

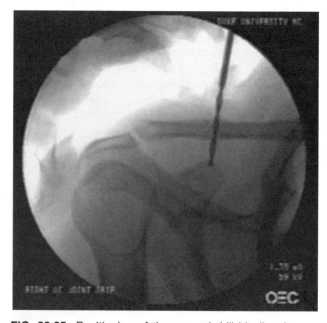

FIG. 28.25. Positioning of the second drill bit directly over the most superior aspect of the base of the coracoid. When the coracoid is viewed in its narrowest possible position, this positioning of the second drill bit ensures the drill hole will be in the center of the base of coracoid.

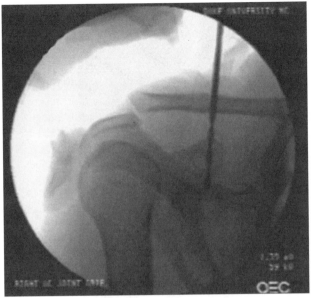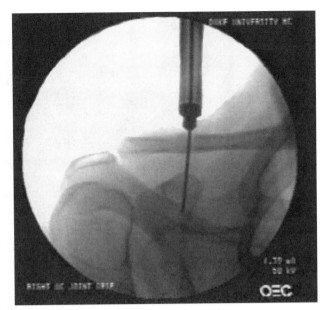

FIG. 28.26. Malposition of second drill bit relative to the coracoid due to failure to hold the acromiocla-vicular joint reduced.

lateral extent of the base of the coracoid. With the c-arm in proper position, the ideal orientation of the probe is when its tip is on the superior apex of the base of the coracoid. A 9/64-inch drill bit is inserted through the drill hole in the clavicle in the same orientation as the probe (Fig. 28.25). A hole is then drilled through the superior and inferior cortices of the base of the coracoid. The depth measurement is then made from the superior cortex of the clavicle to the inferior cortex of the coracoid (Fig. 28.26). The appropriate sized coracoclavicular lag screw and washer (Fig. 28.27) is chosen such that the distance from the base of the washer to the distal-most threads of the screw is at least equal to the depth measurement. The screw with the washer is then inserted into the

clavicle and advanced until all threads of the screw have passed through the clavicle. This will allow the screw to toggle in the clavicle and facilitate its placement of the coracoid. The smooth tip of the screw is then placed into the drill hole in the coracoid and the screw is advanced until the acromioclavicular joint is reduced and the course threads of the screw have engaged the inferior cortex of the coracoid. The reduction of the acromioclavicular joint and placement of screw is verified under fluoroscopy (Fig. 28.28).

Although the above procedure can be performed without the assistance of the c-arm, I have found that fluoroscopy greatly shortens the operative time and decreases the operative exposure and soft tissue dissection

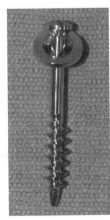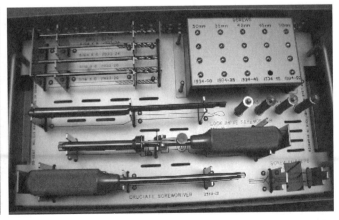

FIG. 28.27. The Depuy acromioclavicular lag screw set. The tip of the screw is blunt to allow easier placement into the coracoid drill hole. The hole in the washer is beveled to allow some angulation of the screw in the clavicle.

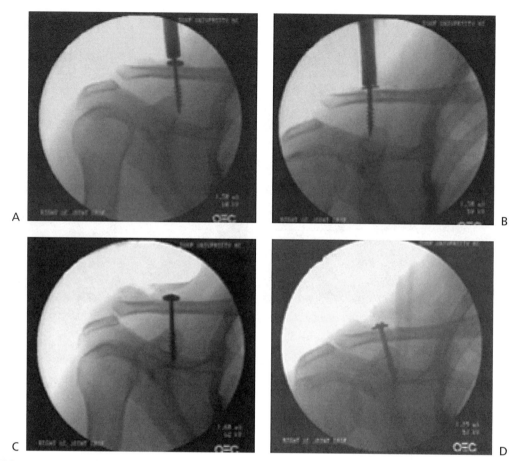

FIG. 28.28. A: Medial angulation of the lag screw. **B:** Lateral angulation of the lag screw. **C:** Malreduction of the acromioclavicular joint due to failure to hold the joint reduced during placement of the screw. **D:** Anatomic reduction of the acromioclavicular joint with placement of the lag screw in the center of the coracoid.

because the base of the coracoid does not have to be directly visualized.

Postoperative Treatment

The patient is placed in a sling before they leave the operating room and a Cryo-cuff or an ice pack is placed on the shoulder. They are typically discharged from the hospital on the same day and placed on oral pain medicines. They are told to continue to use the sling for 2 to 3 weeks, especially when they are out in public. They can come out of the sling when at home; however, they are told to limit their forward flexion to no more than 90 degrees and lift nothing heavier than a glass of water. Although the differential motion between the clavicle and the coracoid is quite small, repeated forward flexion may cause loosening of the screw due to a toggling effect.

The screw is removed under local anesthesia approximately 8 weeks postoperatively. Once the screw has been removed, the patients are told to slowly return to

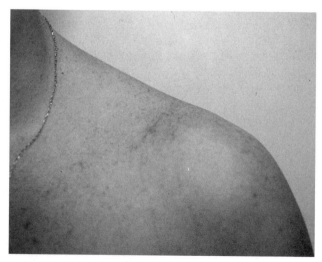

FIG. 28.29. Postoperative clinical appearance of an acromioclavicular joint separation treated acutely.

their normal activities; however, they are told to avoid heavy lifting, pushing, pulling, or contact sports for an additional 4 to 6 weeks. Full athletic participation is not allowed until the patient has full strength and full painless motion of the shoulder (Fig. 28.29).

Chronic Injuries

The positioning and preparation of the patient is essentially identical to that described above for acute injuries. The incision is essentially the same as that used in acute injuries; however, it is slightly longer to accommodate the fact that the acromioclavicular ligament is typically transferred to help stabilize the clavicle (Fig. 28.30). The incision starts at the posterior aspect of the clavicle and extends anteriorly to a point halfway between the anterior aspect of the clavicle and the palpable tip of the coracoid. The subcutaneous tissues divided carefully to avoid injury to the deltotrapezial fascia. The deltotrapezial fascia overlying the clavicle is divided coronally in a curvilinear fashion with the distal aspect of this dissection being carried laterally to about the midpoint of the acromion. Care is taken to protect the integrity

of these fascial flaps because their closure is an integral part of the surgery. The dissection is continued downward until the fascial has been completely freed from both the anterior, posterior, and superior aspects of distal clavicle.

A Crego elevator can be inserted under the distal 15 mm of the clavicle to free the deep soft tissue attachments on that surface. Once the distal clavicle has been freed from its surrounding soft tissue, a Crego elevator is placed under the distal-most portion of the clavicle to protect the underlying structures when the distal osteotomy is performed. An oscillating saw is then used to remove approximately 10 to 15 mm of the distal end of the clavicle. Although some authors have suggested removing as much as 25 mm of the clavicle, I found that recreation of a tether to prevent medial subluxation of the scapula is best obtained when as little clavicle as possible is removed. Under no circumstance should more than 15 mm be removed. If excessive amounts of the distal clavicle are removed, the transferred coracoacromial ligament may not reach the end of the clavicle. Second, even if the transferred ligament is long enough to reach the clavicle, it may be oriented too vertically.

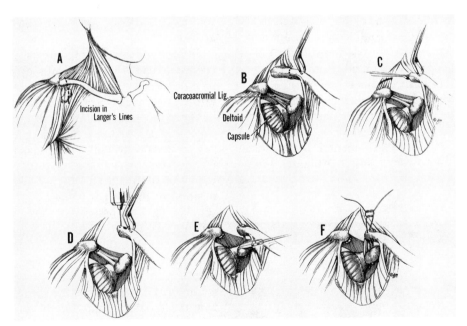

FIG. 28.30. Schematic representation of surgical technique used in chronic types III, IV, V, and VI acromioclavicular joint dislocations. **A:** Incision made in Langer's lines. **B:** Resection of the distal 10 mm of the clavicle. **C:** Curettage of the medullary canal of the distal clavicle. **D:** Detachment of the coracoacromial ligament in its insertion on the acromion and placement of dural holes and distal clavicle in the transferred ligament. **E:** Nonabsorbable suture is more when through a free end of the coracoacromial ligament and coracoclavicular lag screw is placed in the clavicle slightly over reduced. **F:** The ends of the suture in the coracoacromial ligament are passed into the medullary canal exiting through the drill holes in the superior cortex of clavicle. After the transferred ligament is secured as tightly as possible, the screw can be backed out approximately one half turn to place additional tension, transferred ligament. (From Rockwood CA, Green DP, eds. *Fractures,* 2nd ed. Philadelphia: J.B. Lippincott, 1984, with permission.)

The result is that the restraint to medial translation of the scapula will not be recreated, allowing the transferred ligament to act like a pendulum. Although the coracoclavicular interval will be reduced, some patients may experience discomfort because of persistent acromioclavicular impingement. The same situation can occur if one transfers the coracoacromial ligament into the underside of the clavicle directly overlying the coracoid. An additional problem can develop if too much clavicle is resected: The hole for the coracoclavicular lag screw may be too close to the lateral end of the clavicle and the screw may break out of the bone (Fig. 28.31).

The anterior flap of the deltotrapezial fascia is been inspected and a transverse incision is made at the level of the deep deltoid fascia. A soft tissue plane is developed with finger dissection down to the coracoacromial ligament. Once the ligament is palpated, the deep deltoid fascia can be dissected off the coracoclavicular ligament with blunt dissection. This dissection is carried laterally to the insertion of the ligament onto the underside of the anterior medial acromion. A small amount of the anterior deltoid fascia may need to be dissected off the anterior acromion to allow better exposure of the insertion of the coracoacromial ligament. Retractors are placed deep to the deep deltoid fascia to allow inspection of the coracoclavicular. A 1/4-inch Key elevator can be used to define margins of the coracoacromial ligament. There appears to be considerable variation of the width of this ligament from one individual to another. If the ligament appears broad, I prefer to take only the superior half of the ligament because this will leave the patient with a functionally intact coracoacromial ligament. If the ligament is rather narrow, the surgeon usually has to take the entire coracoacromial ligament so that the transferred ligament is substantial enough to constitute a strong transfer. Although I am

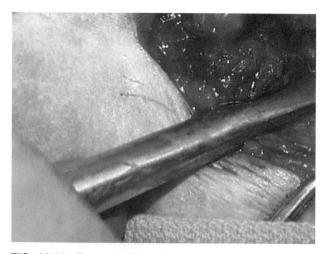

FIG. 28.31. Fracture of the distal clavicle due to excessive lateral placement of the clavicular drill hole.

somewhat concerned about disruption of the coracoclavicular arch of these patients, there has never been a study that showed any long-term detrimental effect of transferring the entire ligament. However, one only has to look at rotator cuff literature to understand the potentially detrimental effect of disrupting the coracoacromial arch.

If the entire coracoacromial ligament is transferred, I attempt to take a small portion of bone off the anterior and inferior medial aspect of the acromion where the ligament inserts. This can be accomplished by using a 1/4-inch curved osteotome. It should be pointed out that the coracoacromial ligament inserts on the medial inferior surface of the acromion rather than the anterior surface. If one attempts to remove only the anterior acromion, they may compromise the insertion of the anterior deltoid while at the same time potentially cutting fibers of the coracoacromial ligament with the osteotome.

Once the coracoclavicular ligament is freed from its surrounding soft tissue attachments, a no. 2 cottony Dacron suture is passed through the free end of the ligament in a Kessler-, Kracow-, or Bunnell-type pattern. The ligament is then pulled toward the resected end of the clavicle to check its length (Fig. 28.32). If it is not long enough, some length can be gained by freeing some of the anterior insertion of the ligament on the coracoid.

Attention is then directed to placement of the coracoclavicular screw. Under fluoroscopic guidance, a 3/16-inch drill bit is placed in the midportion of the clavicle directly over the base of the coracoid. Once the position has been ascertained, the superior inferior cortex of the clavicle is drilled. Once the drill goes through the inferior cortex, the drill bit is toggled in the clavicle to allow increased variation in the insertion of the screw into the coracoid. It should also be pointed out the when the position of the drill is being established, the shoulder should be held at reduced position. If the surgeon does not do this, the shoulder may be fixed in a laterally rotated position. Besides being a nonanatomic repair, it may also lead to non–outlet-type impingement symptoms due to the downward orientation of the lateral acromion. Furthermore, if the surgeon drills the clavicle with the shoulder in an unreduced position, he or she may find that the shoulder is then reduced, the drill hole in the clavicle will be nowhere near the base of the coracoid (Fig. 28.26). This will necessitate having to redrill the hole in the clavicle. To do so may potentially weaken the clavicle and fixation of the screw within the clavicle.

Once the initial hole is drilled in the clavicle, I prefer to take a depth gauge and use it to feel the base of the coracoid through the clavicle as described for acute injuries. Once the position has been ascertained by palpation or fluoroscopy, the base of the coracoid has been

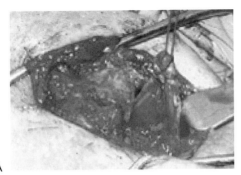
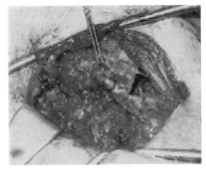

FIG. 28.32. A: Placement of sutures in the coracoacromial ligament. **B:** Testing the length of the coracoacromial ligament graft to ensure that it reaches the end of the clavicle.

drill with a 9/64-inch drill bit. The death gauge can be used to measure the distance from the superior cortex of the clavicle to the inferior cortex of the coracoid but can also be used to palpate the walls of the drill hole in the coracoid to make certain that there is bone circumferentially around the drill hole.

A curette is used to remove a small portion of cancellous bone from the medullary canal of the distal clavicle. A 2-mm drill bit is used to make two holes in the superior cortex of the distal clavicle lateral to the drill hole for the coracoclavicular screw. A trial reduction is performed to make sure that the transferred coracoacromial ligament enters the distal clavicle in the proper orientation and with the proper tension. A rasp can then be used to smooth the inferior and anterior cortex of the clavicle to prevent abrasion of the transferred ligament.

An appropriate length coracoclavicular screw is then passed through the clavicle until all the threads have passed through the hole. The threads must clear the inferior cortex of the clavicle because if they do not, it will not be possible to toggle the tip of the screw into the drill hole in the coracoid. The tip of the coracoclavicular screw can then be inserted into the drill hole in the

coracoid under either direct visualization or with the assistance of fluoroscopy. The screw is then passed into the coracoid and tightened until the clavicle is slightly overreduced relative to the acromion and coracoid. The sutures from the transferred coracoacromial ligament are then tied. The coracoclavicular screw can then be backed off approximately two turns to put more tension on the transferred ligament.

The deltotrapezial fascia is then reapproximated. In cases where there has been a long-standing dislocation of the distal clavicle, that may be considerable redundancy of the deltotrapezial fascia once the clavicle is reduced. In these cases the deltotrapezial fascia can be closed in a "pants over vest" fashion. I use nonabsorbable no. 0 sutures for this repair. This type of suture does not seem to be irritating to the patient and ensures a strong repair.

Postoperative Care

A Cryo-cuff or some other type of cold therapy wrap is placed on the patient's shoulder in the operating room. The patient's arm is supported in a sling for ap-

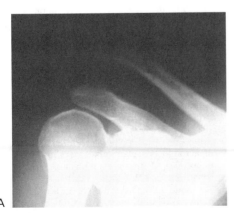
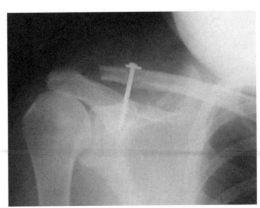

FIG. 28.33. (A) Preoperative and **(B)** postoperative radiographs of chronic type V acromioclavicular joint separation treated with transfer of the coracoacromial ligament and temporary coracoclavicular lag screw fixation.

proximately 2 to 4 weeks. The patient is given strict instructions to avoid any lifting or forward flexion of the arm passed 90 degrees. They are told to use a sling primarily when they are out in public. Sutures are removed at 7 to 10 days. Repeat radiographs are taken approximately 4 weeks postoperatively (Fig. 28.33). If the position of the screw has remained unchanged, the patient is allowed to perform activities of daily living; however, they are instructed to avoid extremes of motion and lifting. The screw is then removed under local anesthesia approximately 12 weeks postoperatively. In the next 4 to 6 weeks after screw removal, the patient is told to slowly resume their normal lifting and athletic activities. Full athletic participation, particularly overhead activities and contact sports, should be avoided until the patient has full strength and painless motion of the shoulder.

REFERENCES

1. Cox JS. The fate of the acromioclavicular joint in athletic injuries. *Am J Sports Med* 1981;9:50–53.
2. Daly PJ, Sim FH, Simonet WT. Ice hockey injuries. A review. *Sports Med* 1990;10:122–131.
3. Dias JJ, Gregg PJ. Acromioclavicular joint injuries in sport. Recommendations for treatment. *Sports Med* 1991;11:125–132.
4. McFarland EG, Blivin SJ, Doehring CB, et al. Treatment of grade III acromioclavicular separations in professional throwing athletes: results of a survey. *Am J Orthop* 1997;26:771–774.
5. Silloway KA, McLaughlin RE, Edlich RC, et al. Clavicular fractures and acromioclavicular joint dislocations in lacrosse: preventable injuries. *J Emerg Med* 1985;3:117–121.
6. Stuart MJ, Smith A. Injuries in Junior A ice hockey. A three-year prospective study. *Am J Sports Med* 1995;23:458–461.
7. Wallace WA. Sporting injuries to the shoulder. *J R Coll Surg Edinb* 1990;35:S21–S26.
8. Weaver JK. Skiing-related injuries to the shoulder. *Clin Orthop* 1987;24–28.
9. Webb J, Bannister G. Acromioclavicular disruption in first class rugby players. *Br J Sports Med* 1992;26:247–248.
10. Auge WK, Fischer RA. Arthroscopic distal clavicle resection for isolated atraumatic osteolysis in weight lifters. *Am J Sports Med* 1998;26:189–192.
11. Cahill BR. Osteolysis of the distal part of the clavicle in male athletes. *J Bone Joint Surg Am* 1982;64:1053–1058.
12. Cahill BR. Atraumatic osteolysis of the distal clavicle. A review. *Sports Med* 1992;13:214–222.
13. Mallon WJ, Colosimo AJ. Acromioclavicular joint injury in competitive golfers. *J South Orthop Assoc* 1995;4:277–282.
14. Matthews LS, Simonson BG, Wolock BS. Osteolysis of the distal clavicle in a female body builder. A case report. *Am J Sports Med* 1993;21:150–152.
15. Murphy OB, Bellamy R, Wheeler W, et al. Post-traumatic osteolysis of the distal clavicle. *Clin Orthop* 1975;108–114.
16. Stenlund B, Goldie I, Hagberg M, et al. Radiographic osteoarthrosis in the acromioclavicular joint resulting from manual work or exposure to vibration. *Br J Ind Med* 1992;49:588–593.
17. Stenlund B. Shoulder tendinitis and osteoarthrosis of the acromioclavicular joint and their relation to sports. *Br J Sports Med* 1993;27:125–130.
18. Nguyen V, Williams G, Rockwood C. Radiography of acromioclavicular dislocation and associated injuries. *Crit Rev Diagn Imag* 1991;32:191–228.
19. Rockwood CA Jr. Injuries to the acromioclavicular joint. In: *Fractures in adults*, Vol 1, 2nd ed. Philadelphia: J.B. Lippincott, 1984:860–910.
20. Salter EGJ, Nasca RJ, Shelley BS. Anatomical observations on the acromioclavicular joint and supporting ligaments. *Am J Sports Med* 1987;15:199–206.
21. Petersson CJ. Degeneration of the acromioclavicular joint. A morphological study. *Acta Orthop Scand* 1983;54:434–438.
22. Petersson CJ, Redlund-Johnell I. Radiographic joint space in normal acromioclavicular joints. *Acta Orthop Scand* 1983;54:431–433.
23. Codman EA. Rupture of the supraspinatus tendon and other lesions in or about the subacromial bursa. In: Codman EA, ed. *The shoulder.* Boston: Thomas Todd, 1934.
24. DePalma AF. *Degenerative changes in the sternoclavicular acromioclavicular joints in various decades.* Springfield: Charles C Thomas, 1957.
25. Urist MR. Complete dislocation of the acromioclavicular joint: the nature of the traumatic lesion and effective methods of treatment with an analysis of 41 cases. *J Bone Joint Surg* 1946;28:813–837.
26. Fukuda K, Craig EV, Cofield RH, et al. Biomechanical study of the ligamentous system of the acromioclavicular joint. *J Bone Joint Surg* 1986;68:434–440.
27. Harrison RB, Riddervold HO, Willett ED, et al. Acromioclavicular separation masked by muscle spasm. *Va Med* 1980;107:377–379.
28. Inman VT, McLaughlin HD, Neviaser J, et al. Treatment of complete acromioclavicular dislocation. *J Bone Joint Surg Am* 1962;44A:1008–1011.
29. Armbrecht A, Graudins J. Temporary extra-articular Bosworth' fixation in complete shoulder joint separation. Follow-up results of 41 surgically treated patients. *Aktuelle Traumatol* 1990;20:283–287.
30. Guy DK, Wirth MA, Griffin JL, et al. Reconstruction of chronic and complete dislocations of the acromioclavicular joint. *Clin Orthop* 1998;138–149.
31. Rockwood CA Jr, Williams GR Jr, Young DC. Disorders of the acromioclavicular joint. In: *The shoulder,* 2nd ed. Philadelphia: W.B. Saunders, 1998:483–553.
32. Dust WN, Lenczner EM. Stress fracture of the clavicle leading to nonunion secondary to coracoclavicular reconstruction with Dacron. *Am J Sports Med* 1989;17:128–129.
33. Martell JRJ. Clavicular nonunion. Complication with the use of mersilene tape. *Am J Sports Med* 1992;20:360–362.
34. Moneim MS, Balduini FC. Coracoid fracture as a complication of surgical treatment by coracoclavicular tape fixation. A case report. *Clin Orthop* 1982;133–135.
35. Allman FL Jr. Fractures and ligamentous injuries of the clavicle and its articulation. *J Bone Joint Surg Am* 1967;49A:774–784.
36. Tossy JD, Mead NC, Sigmond HM. Acromioclavicular separations: useful and practical classification for treatment. *Clin Orthop* 1963;28:111–119.
37. Gerber C, Rockwood CAJ. Subcoracoid dislocation of the lateral end of the clavicle. A report of three cases. *J Bone Joint Surg Am* 1987;69:924–927.
38. Keats TE, Pope TL. The acromioclavicular joint: normal variation and the diagnosis of dislocation. *Skeletal Radiol* 1988;17:159–162.
39. Zanca P. Shoulder pain. Involvement of the acromioclavicular joint: analysis of 1,000 cases. *AJR Am J Roentgenol* 1971;112:493–506.
40. Bossart PJ, Joyce SM, Manaster BJ, et al. Lack of efficacy of "weighted" radiographs in diagnosing acute acromioclavicular separation. *Ann Emerg Med* 1988;17:20–24.
41. Sluming VA. A comparison of the methods of distraction for stress examination of the acromioclavicular joint. *Br J Radiol* 1995;68:1181–1184.
42. Vanarthos WJ, Ekman EF, Bohrer SP. Radiographic diagnosis of acromioclavicular joint separation without weight bearing: importance of internal rotation of the arm. *AJR Am J Roentgenol* 1994;162:120–122.
43. Alexander OM. Dislocation of the acromioclavicular joint. *Radiography* 1948;14:139.
44. Waldrop JI, Norwood LA, Alvarez RG. Lateral roentgenographic projections of the acromioclavicular joint. *Am J Sports Med* 1981;9:337–341.
45. Basamania CJ. Medial instability of the shoulder: a new concept

of the pathomechanics acromioclavicular separations. Presented at ASES Closed Meeting, Philadelphia, November 1999.

46. Rosenorn M, Pedersen EB. The significance of the coracoclavicular ligament in experimental dislocation of the acromioclavicular joint. *Acta Orthop Scand* 1974;45:346–358.

47. Eyres KS, Brooks A, Stanley D. Fractures of the coracoid process. *J Bone Joint Surg Br* 1995;77:425–428.

48. Bergfeld JA, Andrish JT, Clancy WG. Evaluation of the acromioclavicular joint following first- and second-degree sprains. *Am J Sports Med* 1978;6:153–159.

49. Bannister GC, Wallace WA, Stableforth PG, et al. The management of acute acromioclavicular dislocation. A randomised prospective controlled trial. *J Bone Joint Surg Br* 1989;71:848–850.

50. Bjerneld H, Hovelius L, Thorling J. Acromioclavicular separations treated conservatively. A 5-year follow-up study. *Acta Orthop Scand* 1983;54:743–745.

51. Glick JM, Milburn LJ, Haggerty JF, et al. Dislocated acromioclavicular joint: follow-up study of 35 unreduced acromioclavicular dislocations. *Am J Sports Med* 1977;5:264–270.

52. Imatani RJ, Hanlon JJ, Cady GW. Acute, complete acromioclavicular separation. *J Bone Joint Surg Am* 1975;57:328–332.

53. Macdonald PB, Alexander MJ, Frejuk J, et al. Comprehensive functional analysis of shoulders following complete acromioclavicular separation. *Am J Sports Med* 1988;16:475–480.

54. Mulier T, Stuyck J, Fabry G. Conservative treatment of acromioclavicular dislocation. Evaluation of functional and radiological results after six years' follow-up. *Acta Orthop Belg* 1993;59:255–262.

55. Park JP, Arnold JA, Coker TP, et al. Treatment of acromioclavicular separations. A retrospective study. *Am J Sports Med* 1980;8:251–256.

56. Phillips AM, Smart C, Groom AF. Acromioclavicular dislocation. Conservative or surgical therapy. *Clin Orthop* 1998;10–17.

57. Smith MJ, Stewart MJ. Acute acromioclavicular separations. A 20-year study. *Am J Sports Med* 1979;7:62–71.

58. Taft TN, Wilson FC, Oglesby JW. Dislocation of the acromioclavicular joint. An end-result study. *J Bone Joint Surg Am* 1987;69:1045–1051.

59. Tibone J, Sellers R, Tonino P. Strength testing after third-degree acromioclavicular dislocations. *Am J Sports Med* 1992;20:328–331.

60. Wojtys EM, Nelson G. Conservative treatment of grade III acromioclavicular dislocations. *Clin Orthop* 1991;112–119.

61. Galpin RD, Hawkins RJ, Grainger RW. A comparative analysis of operative versus nonoperative treatment of grade III acromioclavicular separations. *Clin Orthop* 1985;150–155.

62. Schmidt A, Lill H, Lange K, et al. Acromioclavicular joint injuries: efficient therapy from the economic viewpoint. *Langenbecks Arch Chir Suppl Kongressbd* 1997;114:1262–1264.

63. Press J, Zuckerman JD, Gallagher M, et al. Treatment of grade III acromioclavicular separations. Operative versus nonoperative management. *Bull Hosp Jt Dis* 1997;56:77–83.

64. Walsh WM, Peterson DA, Shelton G, et al. Shoulder strength following acromioclavicular injury. *Am J Sports Med* 1985;13:153–158.

65. Eidman DK, Siff SJ, Tullos HS. Acromioclavicular lesions in children. *Am J Sports Med* 1981;9:150–154.

66. O'Neill DB, Zarins B, Gelberman RH, et al. Compression of the anterior interosseous nerve after use of a sling for dislocation of the acromioclavicular joint. A report of two cases [see comments]. *J Bone Joint Surg Am* 1990;72:1100–1102.

67. Vailas JC. Compression of the anterior interosseous nerve after use of a sling for dislocation of the acromioclavicular joint. A report of two cases [letter, comment]. *J Bone Joint Surg Am* 1991;73:948–949.

68. Eskola A, Vainionpaa S, Korkala O, et al. Acute complete acromioclavicular dislocation. A prospective randomized trial of fixation with smooth or threaded Kirschner wires or cortical screw. *Ann Chir Gynaecol* 1987;76:323–326.

69. Eskola A, Vainionpaa S, Korkala S, et al. Four-year outcome of operative treatment of acute acromioclavicular dislocation. *J Orthop Trauma* 1991;5:9–13.

70. Aalders GJ, Van Vroonhoven TJ, Van Der Werken C, et al. An exceptional case of pneumothorax—"a new adventure of the K wire." *Injury* 1985;16:564–565.

71. Larsen E, Bjerg-Nielsen A, Christensen P. Conservative or surgical treatment of acromioclavicular dislocation. A prospective, controlled, randomized study. *J Bone Joint Surg Am* 1986;68:552–555.

72. Lindsey RW, Gutowski WT. The migration of a broken pin following fixation of the acromioclavicular joint. A case report and review of the literature. *Orthopedics* 1986;9:413–416.

73. Oleksiuk DI, Pelipenko VP. Migration of the fixation devices into the mediastinum and spine after metallic osteosynthesis of the sternal and acromial ends of the clavicle. *Vestn Khir* 1979;123:121–122.

74. Albrecht F, Kohaus H, Stedtfeld HW. The Balser plate for acromioclavicular fixation. *Chirurg* 1982;53:732–734.

75. Eberle C, Fodor P, Metzger U. Hook plate (so-called Balser plate) or tension banding with the Bosworth screw in complete acromioclavicular dislocation and clavicular fracture. *Z Unfallchir Versicherungsmed* 1992;85:134–139.

76. Habernek H, Weinstabl R, Schmid L, et al. A crook plate for treatment of acromioclavicular joint separation: indication, technique, and results after one year. *J Trauma* 1993;35:893–901.

77. Mlasowsky B, Brenner P, Duben W, et al. Repair of complete acromioclavicular dislocation (Tossy stage III) using Balser's hook plate combined with ligament sutures. *Injury* 1988;19:227–232.

78. Sim E, Schwarz N, Hocker K, et al. Repair of complete acromioclavicular separations using the acromioclavicular-hook plate. *Clin Orthop* 1995;134–142.

79. Bosworth BM. Acromioclavicular separations: new method of repair. *Surg Gynecol Obstet* 1941;73:866–871.

80. Cox JS. Current method of treatment of acromioclavicular joint dislocations. *Orthopedics* 1992;15:1041–1044.

81. Gallay SH, Hupel TM, Beaton DE, et al. Functional outcome of acromioclavicular joint injury in polytrauma patients. *J Orthop Trauma* 1998;12:159–163.

82. Stam L, Dawson I. Complete acromioclavicular dislocations: treatment with a Dacron ligament. *Injury* 1991;22:173–176.

83. Tsou PM. Percutaneous cannulated screw coracoclavicular fixation for acute acromioclavicular dislocations. *Clin Orthop* 1989;112–121.

84. Weinstein DM, McCann PD, McIlveen SJ, et al. Surgical treatment of complete acromioclavicular dislocations. *Am J Sports Med* 1995;23:324–331.

85. Morrison DS, Lemos MJ. Acromioclavicular separation. Reconstruction using synthetic loop augmentation. *Am J Sports Med* 1995;23:105–110.

86. Colosimo AJ, Hummer CD, Heidt RSJ. Aseptic foreign body reaction to Dacron graft material used for coracoclavicular ligament reconstruction after type III acromioclavicular dislocation. *Am J Sports Med* 1996;24:561–563.

87. Neault MA, Nuber GW, Marymont JV. Infections after surgical repair of acromioclavicular separations with nonabsorbable tape or suture. *J Shoulder Elbow Surg* 1996;5:477–478.

88. Brunelli G, Brunelli F. The treatment of acromioclavicular dislocation by transfer of the short head of biceps. *Int Orthop* 1988;12:105–108.

89. Skjeldal S, Lundblad R, Dullerud R. Coracoid process transfer for acromioclavicular dislocation. *Acta Orthop Scand* 1988;59:180–182.

90. Caspi I, Ezra E, Nerubay J, et al. Musculocutaneous nerve injury after coracoid process transfer for clavicle instability. Report of three cases. *Acta Orthop Scand* 1987;58:294–295.

91. Ferris BD, Bhamra M, Paton DF. Coracoid process transfer for acromioclavicular dislocations. A report of 20 cases. *Clin Orthop* 1989;184–194.

92. Berg EE, Ciullo JV. Heterotopic ossification after acromioplasty and distal clavicle resection. *J Shoulder Elbow Surg* 1995;4:188–193.

93. Petchell JF, Sonnabend DH, Hughes JS. Distal clavicular excision: a detailed functional assessment. *Aust N Z J Surg* 1995;65:262–266.

94. Blazar PE, Iannotti JP, Williams GR. Anteroposterior instability

of the distal clavicle after distal clavicle resection. *Clin Orthop* 1998;114–120.

95. Cook FF, Tibone JE. The Mumford procedure in athletes. An objective analysis of function. *Am J Sports Med* 1988;16:97–100.
96. Mumford EB. Acromioclavicular dislocation. *J Bone Joint Surg* 1941;23:799–802.
97. Eskola A, Santavirta S, Viljakka HT, et al. The results of operative resection of the lateral end of the clavicle [see comments]. *J Bone Joint Surg Am* 1996;78:584–587.
98. Mallon WJ, Bronec PR, Spinner RJ, et al. Suprascapular neuropathy after distal clavicle excision. *Clin Orthop* 1996;207–211.
99. Weaver JK, Dunn HK. Treatment of acromioclavicular injuries, especially complete acromioclavicular separation. *J Bone Joint Surg Am* 1972;54:1187–1194.
100. Cadenat FM. The treatment of dislocations and fractures of the outer end of the clavicle. *Int Clin* 1917;1:145–169.
101. Kutschera HP, Kotz RI. Bone-ligament transfer of coracoacromial ligament for acromioclavicular dislocation. A new fixation method used in 6 cases. *Acta Orthop Scand* 1997;68:246–248.
102. Basamania CJ. Treatment of acute acromioclavicular separations utilizing coracoclavicular screw fixation. Presented at Society of Military Orthopaedic Surgeons, San Diego, 1996.

Principles and Practice of Orthopaedic Sports Medicine,
edited by William E. Garrett, Jr., Kevin P. Speer, and Donald T. Kirkendall.
Lippincott Williams & Wilkins, Philadelphia © 2000.

CHAPTER 29

Clavicular and Sternoclavicular Injuries

William N. Levine and Claude T. Moorman III

FRACTURES OF THE CLAVICLE

Epidemiology

Fractures of the clavicle are among the most frequent traumatic injuries affecting the shoulder. Although clavicular fractures account for only approximately 5% of adult fractures, they are still the most common fracture of childhood (1). They also account for nearly one half of all shoulder girdle injuries (2). Most clavicular fractures occur in the diaphysis or middle third, whereas medial third fractures are exceedingly rare. Lateral third fractures have been further classified and are discussed below.

Pathoanatomy and Mechanism of Injury

The medial ossification center of the clavicle is responsible for nearly 80% of the longitudinal growth. This ossification center typically appears between ages 12 and 18 but does not fuse until ages 22 to 25 (3). The clavicle serves as an attachment site for numerous muscles, protects underlying nerves and arteries, and is an osseous strut spanning the scapula from the chest midline.

The most common mechanism of injury to the clavicle is a direct blow to the point of the shoulder. The force is directed from the posterior aspect of the shoulder, causing buckling of the middle third of the clavicle. Neurovascular injuries have been reported but are rarely encountered in routine fractures (4–8). A fall onto an outstretched hand causes a clavicle fracture much less often than previously thought. Stanley et al. (9) showed that a fall onto the shoulder accounted for 94% of the clavicle fractures with only 6% related to a

fall onto the outstretched hand. Direct trauma in contact sports such as football, lacrosse, or rugby may also lead to this injury.

The most common location (nearly 80%) of clavicle fractures in adults and children occurs in the middle third (5). This section is biomechanically more susceptible to fracture because it is relatively devoid of muscular or ligamentous attachments. In addition, this region has the smallest cross-sectional area and is the focal point for bending, compression, and torsional stresses on the bone (10).

The Allman classification (11) was one of the early schemes introduced and divided the fractures into three groups: group I, middle third; group II, distal third; and group III, medial third. Lateral third (distal) clavicle fractures deserve special mention. These injuries have been further classified by Neer (10,12) into three types (Figs. 29.1 to 29.3). Type I fractures are interligamentous and have minimal displacement. Type II fractures are displaced secondary to a fracture medial to the coracoclavicular ligaments. The coracoclavicular ligaments are both attached to the distal fragment in type II-A lateral clavicle fractures. Neer believed that this was a stable injury due to the intact coracoclavicular ligaments. The conoid ligament is ruptured, however, in type II-B lateral clavicle fractures, whereas the trapezoid ligament remains attached to the distal segment making this a more unstable pattern. Type III lateral clavicle fractures involve the articular surface of the acromioclavicular joint alone. This injury may be missed initially, and the patient may present later with acromioclavicular joint arthrosis. We have not reliably been able to subdivide the type II fractures by clinical examination or radiographs. Therefore, we prefer to simply classify distal clavicle fractures as type I, II, or III.

Group III fractures (medial third) are the least common, comprising 5% to 6% of all clavicular fractures. These fractures are typically nondisplaced due to the sturdy costoclavicular ligaments. The articular surface

---

W. N. Levine: Department of Orthopaedic Surgery, Columbia University, New York, New York 10032.

C. T. Moorman, III: Department of Surgery, University of Maryland School of Medicine, Baltimore, Maryland 21207.

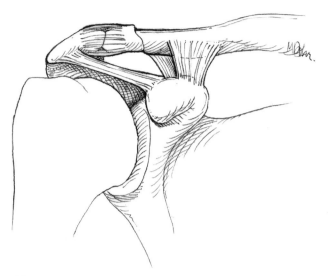

FIG. 29.1. Lateral clavicle type I fracture (Neer classification), interligamentous without displacement.

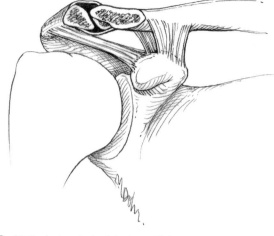

FIG. 29.3. Lateral clavicle type III fracture (Neer classification). Intraarticular fracture.

can be damaged, leading to degenerative arthritis of the sternoclavicular joint.

The medial clavicular epiphysis ossifies between the ages of 12 and 18 but does not fuse until ages 22 to 25. Therefore, most injuries involving the medial clavicle in patients under the age of 25 are growth plate injuries until proven otherwise. This is discussed in greater detail below in the section on sternoclavicular injuries.

Clinical Evaluation

The clinical presentation in adults is typically straightforward. One important aspect of the history is determination of the amount of energy absorbed by the tissue during the fracture. Pathologic fractures should be sus-

pected if the mechanism of injury does not correlate with the clavicular fracture. There will be a history of trauma, and the patient will present with pain and splinting of the involved extremity. There may be skin tenting in the moderate to severely displaced clavicle fractures.

Examination of the skin will also often reveal abrasions over the superior aspect of the shoulder, helping to clarify the mechanism of injury. Although rarely encountered, open fractures can occur, and a thorough inspection of the skin for direct bone contact should be sought. Meticulous neurovascular examination should be performed initially and followed serially. Matz et al. (8) demonstrated brachial plexus (lateral cord) neurapraxia 6 weeks after uneventful healing of midshaft clavicle fracture in a college football player. The lateral cord compression was eliminated by open excision of the

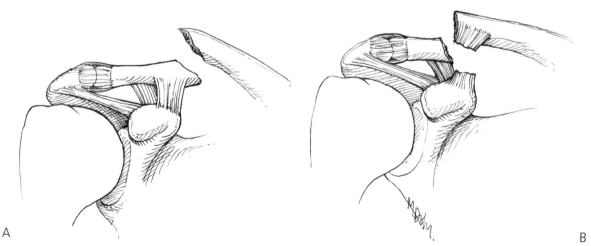

FIG. 29.2. A: Lateral clavicle type II-A fracture (Neer classification). Conoid and trapezoid ligaments attached to distal fragment. **B:** Lateral clavicle type II-B fracture (Neer classification). Conoid ligament torn, trapezoid ligament attached to distal fragment.

compressing callus spike. Nonunion of the clavicle also has a well-recognized association with neurovascular injuries (4–7,13,14).

Careful vascular examination is critical in the evaluation of patients with displaced clavicle fractures. Compression of the carotid artery, subclavian vein, subclavian artery, and traumatic aneurysms have all been described in association with clavicle fractures (6,15–17). Finally, chest auscultation should be performed to rule out associated pneumothorax or other pulmonary injury (18).

Imaging

Plain radiographs are usually all that is necessary in the diagnosis of clavicle fractures. An anteroposterior and 45-degree cephalic tilt view are recommended for fractures involving the clavicular shaft. In standard anteroposterior views, the proximal fragment is displaced upward and the distal fragment downward. The 45-degree cephalic tilt view more accurately assesses the anteroposterior relationship of the proximal and distal fragments.

For distal third fractures, anterior and posterior 45-degree oblique views should be obtained in addition to a standard anteroposterior view (12). This is especially true of the type II distal clavicle fracture that can be difficult to diagnose. The standard anteroposterior and 45-degree cephalic tilt views often do not reveal the extent of the injury. Weighted views are rarely necessary, and there is a theoretic risk of causing increased displacement of the fragments (10).

Type III fractures involve the articular surface and may be difficult to identify on plain radiographs. Computed tomography (CT) may be necessary, therefore, especially if the index of suspicion is high for this injury. Magnetic resonance imaging can also identify this injury, but CT is preferred for bony detail.

A chest radiograph should be obtained in patients with polytrauma and in patients with suspected thoracic or pulmonary injury. The chest radiograph is essential to rule out hemothorax, pneumothorax, or associated chest wall injury (rib fractures, scapulothoracic dissociation). Abnormal vascular examination should be further investigated with either Doppler ultrasound or preferably angiography.

Treatment

Nonoperative

Most clavicle fractures are successfully treated without surgery (19). In fact, most of these fractures do not require reduction. However, if severe shortening, displacement, or deformity exists, then reduction may be indicated. Reduction maneuvers are designed to bring the distal fragment up and back and then hold it in place with a figure-of-eight style bandage or spica cast. Unfortunately, this position can be uncomfortable and can lead to neurovascular complications. In addition, clavicular fracture reduction has not achieved improved results over treatment with a simple sling and swathe (5).

A sling and swathe are applied for most acute clavicle shaft fractures. Although figure-of-eight splints can be used, they are associated with an increased incidence of complications and are used less often. A recent comparison study of figure-of-eight and simple slings found no differences in healing, function, or cosmetic results (20). Clavicular shaft fractures infrequently require surgery. Indications for surgery include severely displaced fractures, neurovascular injury, open fracture or impending skin compromise, multiple trauma ("floating shoulder"), and selected type II distal clavicle fractures (21–23).

The sling and swathe is maintained until the athlete is comfortable and has painless range of motion of the extremity. This usually occurs between 2 and 4 weeks. The athlete should not return to noncontact sports until the fracture has healed and the player has regained full pain-free motion and near-normal strength. Contact athletes should be treated more conservatively, with return to collision activities between 4 and 6 months.

Operative

Although most clavicle fractures are successfully treated nonoperatively, unsatisfactory results can occur. Hill et al. (24) reported the results after closed treatment of 52 patients with middle-third clavicle fractures. Only 36 patients (69%) were satisfied with the treatment, and nonunion occurred in 15% of the reviewed patients. Initial shortening at the fracture site of more than 20 mm was significantly associated with the development of nonunion. In addition, final shortening of more than 20 mm was significantly associated with an unsatisfactory result.

Results such as in Hill et al. and a high-demand military population led Basamania to recommend operative intervention for significantly displaced clavicle fractures (Basamania, CJ unpublished data, 1998). The rationale for this approach is the faster return to full activities, the return of normal length of the shoulder girdle (loss of clavicular shortening), and the return of normal strength. This aggressive approach is not recommended universally but should be considered in those patients with high demands or in clavicle fractures with more than 20 mm shortening.

Because of the significant risk of nonunion, type II distal clavicle fractures with wide displacement are best treated with open reduction and internal fixation (10). If the acromioclavicular joint is intact and the distal fragment is of good size and bone quality, the fracture can be repaired with no. 5 permanent sutures. The repair is supplemented by stabilizing the proximal fragment to the coracoid with no. 5 sutures passed around the coracoid base. Occasionally, interfragmentary screws can be placed obliquely, obviating the need for the sutures. If the distal fragment is small, however, a modified Weaver-Dunn procedure should be performed. The small distal fragment is excised, and the coracoacromial ligament is transferred into the medial segment. Supplemental heavy sutures are placed around the base of the coracoid.

Expected Outcomes

As detailed above, most clavicle fractures heal without surgical intervention and do not cause any long-term problems. Athletes typically will return to their sport after complete healing of the fracture and return of motion and strength of the extremity. Open reduction and internal fixation of acute clavicle fractures were previously believed to be a leading cause of nonunion of the clavicle (10). However, this was most likely due to excessive periosteal stripping and inadequate fixation devices (25).

Authors' Preferences

We prefer to treat most acute clavicle fractures with a sling and swathe. The sling and swathe are used 24 hours a day for the first 2 weeks. The athlete can then begin active elbow and wrist motion and gentle pendulum exercises of the shoulder. The swathe is typically discarded at 2 weeks, whereas the sling is maintained for 4 to 6 weeks. Radiographs are obtained at 2-week intervals to document progression of healing. The sling is discarded at 6 weeks, and active shoulder motion exercises are begun without restrictions. We usually allow noncontact athletes to return to their sport as soon as they are pain free and have full range of motion and equal strength. We advise contact athletes to avoid playing for 4 to 6 months.

When operative intervention is indicated, we prefer open reduction and internal fixation with either a dynamic compression plate or preferably a limited-contact dynamic compression plate (Synthes, PA). One-third tubular plates are too weak to withstand the muscular deforming forces placed on the clavicle. Although 3.5-mm reconstruction plates have been used successfully, they are no longer recommended due to plate breakage (JB Jupiter, personal communication, 1998) (Fig. 29.4). Bone grafting is not necessary in most acute fractures. We do not have any experience with the use of the modified Hagie pin as described by Basamania, but this technique is certainly appealing because it avoids periosteal stripping and potential hardware complications. A

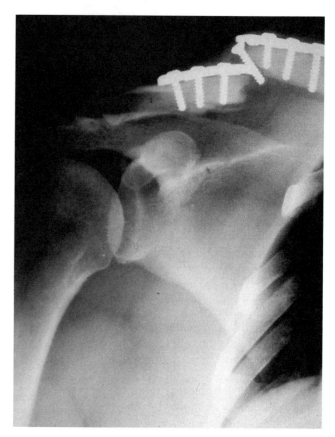

FIG. 29.4. Anteroposterior radiograph displaying fractured 3.5-mm reconstruction plate 11 weeks after open reduction/ internal fixation of a clavicle fracture. The patient denied any trauma to the extremity.

planned second procedure is necessary, however, to remove the pin.

Clavicle nonunions are treated with open reduction and internal fixation as described above. In addition, supplementation of the fixation with autologous iliac crest bone graft is recommended (5,26–34).

STERNOCLAVICULAR INJURIES

Epidemiology

The incidence of sternoclavicular dislocation is exceedingly rare, accounting for less than 1% of all joint dislocations (35). The sternoclavicular joint is the least commonly injured joint of the shoulder girdle. However, it can be difficult to make the diagnosis with routine radiographs, which can lead to a delay in diagnosis. This can be catastrophic if posterior sternoclavicular dislocation is missed, leading to compromise of the trachea, esophagus, or great vessels (35–39). Overall, anterior sternoclavicular dislocations occur three times more often than posterior dislocations.

however, for 3 months after a grade III posterior sternoclavicular dislocation.

Authors' Preferences

We prefer to treat most sternoclavicular injuries nonoperatively. A sling should be worn for comfort only in grade I injuries. Athletes with grade II injuries may require a sling for 10 to 14 days or until their symptoms dictate. We do not routinely attempt reduction of anterior grade III sternoclavicular dislocations due to their inherent instability. Patients are instructed about the natural history of this injury.

We generally treat acute posterior grade III sternoclavicular dislocations by closed reduction in the operating room. A figure-of-eight bandage is applied and maintained for 4 to 6 weeks. If an athlete is in peril on the playing field, then an attempt at closed reduction using the technique described above is performed. However, we prefer to treat these injuries in the operating room if at all possible. We will consider open reduction with the assistance of a chest surgeon only after closed reduction fails.

Finally, we do not routinely reduce either anterior or asymptomatic posterior Salter-Harris fractures of the medial clavicle epiphysis. Remodeling of these injuries is often dramatic and typically results in a painless stable joint (50).

REFERENCES

1. Tachdjiian MO. *Pediatric orthopaedics.* Philadelphia: W.B. Saunders, 1972.
2. Rowe CR. An atlas of anatomy and treatment of mid-clavicular fractures. *Clin Orthop* 1968;58:29–42.
3. Grant JCB. *Method of anatomy: by regions, descriptive and deductive,* 7th ed. Baltimore: Williams & Wilkins, 1965.
4. Connolly JF, Dehne R. Nonunion of the clavicle and thoracic outlet syndrome. *J Trauma* 1989;29:1127–1133.
5. Jupiter JB, Leffert RD. Non-union of the clavicle. Associated complications and surgical management. *J Bone Joint Surg Am* 1987;69A:753–760.
6. Kay SP, Edkardt JJ. Brachial plexus palsy secondary to clavicular nonunion. Case report and literature survey. *Clin Orthop* 1984;206:219–222.
7. Koss SD, Goitz HT, Redler MR, et al. Nonunion of a midshaft clavicle fracture associated with subclavian vein compression. *Orthop Rev* 1989;18:431–434.
8. Matz SO, Welliver PS, Welliver DI. Brachial plexus neuropraxia complicating a comminuted clavicle fracture in a college football player. Case report and review of the literature. *Am J Sports Med* 1989;17:581–583.
9. Stanley D, Trowbridge EA, Norris SH. The mechanism of clavicular fracture. *J Bone Joint Surg Br* 1988;70B:461–464.
10. Neer CS II. Fracture of the distal clavicle with detachment of the coracoclavicular ligaments in adults. *J Trauma* 1963;3:99–110.
11. Allman FL. Fractures and ligamentous injuries of the clavicle and its articulation. *J Bone Joint Surg Am* 1967;49A:774–784.
12. Neer CS II. Fractures of the distal third of the clavicle. *Clin Orthop* 1968;58:43–50.
13. Neviaser RJ. Injuries to the clavicle and acromioclavicular joint. *Orthop Clin North Am* 1987;18:433–438.
14. Ring D, Jupiter JB. Clavicular fracture, a guide to basic management. *J Musculoskel Med* 1997;14:65–73.
15. Lusskin R, Weiss CA, Winer J. The role of the subclavius muscle in the subclavian vein syndrome following fracture of the clavicle. *Clin Orthop* 1967;54:75–84.
16. Guilfoil PH, Christiansen T. An unusual vascular complication of fractured clavicle. *JAMA* 1967;200:72–73.
17. Hansky B, Murray E, Minami K, et al. Delayed brachial plexus paralysis due to subclavian pseudoaneurysm after clavicular fracture. *Eur J Cardiothorac Surg* 1993;7:497–498.
18. Dugdale TW, Fulkerson JB, Pneumothorax complicating a closed fracture of the clavicle. A case report. *Clin Orthop* 1987;221:212–214.
19. Nordqvist A, Petersson C, Redlund-Johnell I. The natural course of lateral clavicle fracture. 15 year follow-up of 110 cases. *Acta Orthop Scand* 1993;64:87–91.
20. Anderson K, Jensen P, Lauritzen J. Treatment of clavicular fractures. Figure-of-eight bandage vs a simple sling. *Acta Orthop Scand* 1987;57:71–74.
21. Bostman O, Manninen M, Pihlajamaki H. Complications of plate fixation in fresh displaced midclavicular fractures. *J Trauma* 1997;43:778–783.
22. Goldberg JA, Warwick JM, Sonnabend DH, et al. Type 2 fractures of the distal clavicle, a new surgical technique. *J Shoulder Elbow Surg* 1997;6:380–382.
23. Kona J, Bosse MJ, Staeheli JW, et al. Type II distal clavicle fractures, a retrospective review of surgical treatment. *J Orthop Trauma* 1990;4:115–120.
24. Hill JM, McGuire MH, Crosby LA. Closed treatment of displaced middle-third fractures of the clavicle gives poor results. *J Bone Joint Surg Br* 1997;79B:537–539.
25. Zenni EJ, Krieg JK, Rosen MJ. Open reduction and internal fixation of clavicular fractures. *J Bone Joint Surg Am* 1981;63A:147–151.
26. Boyer MI, Axelrod TS. Atrophic nonunion of the clavicle, treatment by compression plate, lag-screw fixation and bone graft. *J Bone Joint Surg Br* 1997;79B:301–303.
27. Bradbury N, Hutchinson J, Hahn D, et al. Clavicular nonunion. 31/32 healed after plate fixation and bone grafting. *Acta Orthop Scand* 1996;67:367–370.
28. Davids PHP, Luitse JSK, Strating RP, et al. Operative treatment for delayed union and nonunion of midshaft clavicular fractures, AO reconstruction plate fixation and early mobilization. *J Trauma* 1996;40:985–986.
29. Ebraheim NA, Mekhail AO, Darwich M. Open reduction and internal fixation with bone grafting of clavicular nonunion. *J Trauma* 1997;42:701–704.
30. Manske DJ, Szabo RM. The operative treatment of mid-shaft clavicular non-unions. *J Bone Joint Surg Am* 1985;67A:1367–1371.
31. Olsen BS, Vaesel MT, Sojbjerg JO. Treatment of midshaft clavicular nonunion with plate fixation and autologous bone grafting. *J Shoulder Elbow Surg* 1995;4:337–344.
32. Pederson M, Poulsen KA, Thomsen F, et al. Operative treatment of clavicular nonunion. *Acta Orthop Belg* 1994;60:303–306.
33. Ring D, Barrick WT, Jupiter JB. Recalcitrant nonunion. *Clin Orthop* 1997;340:181–189.
34. Seiler JG III, Jupiter JB. Intercalary tricortical iliac crest bone grafts for the treatment of chronic clavicular nonunion with bony defect. *J Orthop Techn* 1993;1:19–22.
35. Cope R, Riddervold HO, Shore JL, et al. Dislocations of the sternoclavicular joint, anatomic basis, etiologies, and radiologic diagnosis. *J Orthop Trauma* 1991;5:379–384.
36. Booth CM, Roper BA. Chronic dislocation of the sternoclavicular joint. An operative repair. *Clin Orthop* 1979;140:17–20.
37. Buckerfield CT, Castle ME. Acute traumatic retrosternal dislocation of the clavicle. *J Bone Joint Surg Am* 1984;66A:379–384.
38. Jougon JB, Lepront DJ, Dromer CE. Posterior dislocation of the sternoclavicular joint leading to mediastinal compression. *Ann Thorac Surg* 1996;61:711–713.
39. Noda M, Shiraishi H, Mizuno K. Chronic posterior sternoclavicular dislocation causing compression of a subclavian artery. *J Shoulder Elbow Surg* 1997;6:564–569.
40. Williams GR, Rockwood CA Jr. Injuries to the sternoclavicular joint. In: DeLee JC, Drez D Jr., eds. *Orthopaedic sports medicine.* Philadelphia: W.B. Saunders, 1994;512–540.
41. Rockwood CA Jr, Odor JM. Spontaneous atraumatic anterior

subluxation of the sternoclavicular joint. *J Bone Joint Surg Am* 1989;71A:1280–1288.

42. Rockwood CA Jr. Disorders of the sternoclavicular joint. In: Rockwood CA Jr, Matsen FA, eds. *The shoulder.* Philadelphia: W.B. Saunders, 1990:477–525.

43. Emery R. Acromioclavicular and sternoclavicular joints. In: Copeland S, ed. *Shoulder surgery.* Philadelphia: W.B. Saunders, 1997:84.

44. O'Donoghue DH. *Treatment of injuries to athletes,* 2nd ed. Philadelphia: W.B. Saunders, 1970:133.

45. Omer GE. Osteotomy of the clavicle in surgical reduction of anterior sternoclavicular dislocation. *J Trauma* 1967;7:584–590.

46. Wirth MA, Rockwood CA Jr. Acute and chronic traumatic injuries of the sternoclavicular joint. *J Am Acad Orthop Surg* 1996;4:268–278.

47. Lyons FA, Rockwood CA Jr. Current concepts review. Migration of pins used in operations of the shoulder. *J Bone Joint Surg Am* 1990;72A:1262–1267.

48. Rockwood CA Jr, Groh GI, Wirth MA, et al. Resection arthroplasty of the sternoclavicular joint. *J Bone Joint Surg Am* 1997;79A:387–393.

49. Acus RW 3rd, Bell RH, Fisher DL. Proximal clavicle excision, an analysis of results. *J Shoulder Elbow Surg* 1995;4:182–187.

50. Yang J, al-Etani H, Letts M. Diagnosis and treatment of posterior sternoclavicular joint dislocations in children. *Am J Orthop* 1996;25:565–569.

Principles and Practice of Orthopaedic Sports Medicine,
edited by William E. Garrett, Jr., Kevin P. Speer, and Donald T. Kirkendall.
Lippincott Williams & Wilkins, Philadelphia © 2000.

CHAPTER *30*

Nerve Injuries in the Upper Extremity

Scott Lintner

The upper extremity is a richly innervated structure with multiple motor and sensory nerve distributions. The entire nerve supply to the upper extremity originates at the cervical spine via the brachial plexus. The brachial plexus is formed by the ventral rami of the fifth through eighth cervical nerves and a portion of the first thoracic nerve. The fourth cervical nerve may contribute a small amount as may the second thoracic nerve (Fig. 30.1). The brachial plexus is organized with the five cervical roots forming three trunks that give rise to three ventral and three dorsal divisions. The divisions give rise to three cords that branch to form the five terminal nerve branches from the brachial plexus. Injuries to the brachial plexus or cervical nerve roots are not discussed in this chapter.

An injury to a nerve can be described and categorized according to Seddon's classification of nerve injuries into three types: neuropraxia, axonotmesis, and neurotomesis (1). Neuropraxic injuries occur when the nerve experiences a stretch injury but the axons and epineurium are not disrupted. This type of injury results in a local demyelination and usually resolves as the myelin is repaired. Recovery is usually complete but may take as short as a few days or as long as several months. Axonotmesis occurs when there is internal disruption of the axons but the endoneurium remains intact. With this injury, recovery requires regeneration and growth of the axons from the point of injury to the end organ. This regrowth occurs at a rate of approximately 1 mm/day. More proximal injuries carry a worse prognosis and recovery is more lengthy, but it often can be complete. Neurotomesis is characterized by complete disruption of the neural tubes along with the with endoneurium and epineurium. These injuries can be treated with surgical repair or nerve grafting procedures. The prognosis for recovery in neurotomesis injury is poor.

SHOULDER

Spinal Accessory Nerve

The spinal accessory (cranial nerve XI) nerve is a pure motor nerve providing innervation to the trapezius and sternocleidomastoid muscles. It leaves the jugular foramen at the base of the skull courses obliquely through the upper third of sternocleidomastoid muscle and then crosses the posterior triangle where it enters and terminates at the trapezius muscle. The nerve is quite superficial in its course through the cervical region, making it prone to injury, especially during surgical procedures in the neck. Direct blows to this region can also cause injury. Sports-related spinal accessory nerve injuries have reportedly occurred in wrestling and hockey (2).

Clinical Evaluation

The patient usually complains of a sagging shoulder, the inability to fully elevate the arm, and weakness. In chronic cases the patient may also complain of the cosmetic deformity caused by trapezial atrophy. Some patients may also have radicular symptoms of brachial plexus neuritis distally secondary to traction from the drooping arm. On examination, there is a sunken appearance in the supraclavicular fossa with atrophy of the trapezius. There may also be winging of the superomedial border of the scapula with resistance to arm elevation. This winging deformity can be differentiated from scapular winging due to a long thoracic nerve palsy.

Treatment

The timing of treatment should be based on the nature of the injury. Closed injuries should be followed for a

S. Lintner: Orthopaedics Indianapolis, Indianapolis, Indiana 46207.

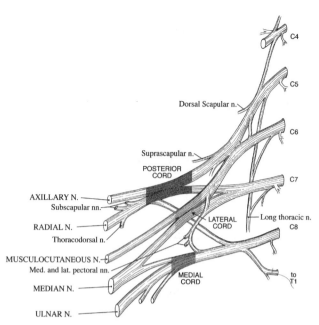

FIG. 30.1. The anatomy of the brachial plexus illustrating the roots, trunks, divisions, cords, and branches.

minimum of 6 months before exploring the nerve. More time should be given before surgical reconstruction. Open injuries that fail to respond to conservative management should be explored sooner if symptoms or electrodiagnostic studies continue to show an abnormality. Exploration between 6 and 12 weeks postinjury is an adequate amount of time for recovery after an open injury. Neurolysis, repair, or grafting could then be performed at this time.

If the nerve is in continuity and there is a failure of return of function and the patient continues to be symptomatic, then a reconstructive surgical procedure may be indicated. Bigliani et al. (3) described the surgical results of treatment for trapezius palsy. In this procedure, the levator scapulae and rhomboids are moved laterally on the scapula to help stabilize the medial scapular border. Scapular suspension procedures using fascial strips have also been described (4). This results in a static reconstruction with less motion and function postoperatively.

In those patients in whom soft tissue reconstruction has failed to provide the necessary stability or relieve the symptoms, the salvage procedure of choice is a scapulothoracic fusion (5).

Long Thoracic Nerve

The long thoracic nerve is formed from the C5-7 nerve roots. The nerve runs posterior to the brachial plexus and enters the serratus anterior. The serratus anterior covers the lateral thorax attaching to ribs I to IX. It inserts onto the deep medial surface of the scapula. It

acts in conjunction with the trapezius to stabilize the scapula for arm elevation. An open nerve injury is usually the result of a complication of a surgical procedure, such as first rib resection. Closed injuries to the nerve are usually caused by traction or may be idiopathic in nature. Brachial neuritis or Parsonage-Turner syndrome can also be a cause of serratus anterior paralysis. Other reported etiologies include postimmunizations, viral infections, surgical positioning, and prolonged bedrest (6). Most reported sports injuries have been secondary to traction type injuries (7,8).

Clinical Evaluation

Patients with a long thoracic nerve injury and paralysis of the serratus anterior often present vague symptoms of pain, but more likely due to winging of the scapula. The winging of the scapula is usually accentuated with active arm elevation and by doing a push-up–type maneuver when leaning against a wall. Electrodiagnostic studies can be used to confirm the diagnosis of long thoracic nerve palsy. Other causes of winging, such as trapezial palsy, glenohumeral instability, and painful shoulder conditions, should be ruled out. Scapular winging due to trapezial weakness secondary to an accessory nerve injury results in prominence of the medial scapula border. In long thoracic palsy, the inferior angle of the scapula moves medially and protrudes posteriorly.

Treatment

Discontinuing activities that aggravate the shoulder symptoms and that are suspected to have caused the injury is important. Recovery from a closed injury is usually spontaneous and complete. However, this may take as long as 2 to 3 years (6). Braces or external devices have not been very effective in treating this condition.

In those patients who have failed to recovery spontaneously and in whom there is no electrodiagnostic evidence of recovery, a surgical procedure may be indicated if symptoms warrant this. A transfer of the pectoralis minor to the scapula has been reported (9). Transfer of the sternal head of the pectoralis major with fascial grafting to the inferior border of the scapula has reported to provide good results (10).

Suprascapular Nerve

The suprascapular nerve is a branch off of the superior trunk and consists of nerve root C5-6. The suprascapular nerve is a pure motor nerve providing no sensory function. The nerve enters the supraspinatus fossa through the suprascapular notch deep to the superior transverse

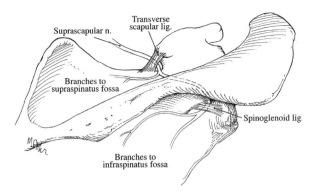

FIG. 30.2. The anatomy and potential sites of entrapment of the suprascapular nerve.

scapular ligament (Fig. 30.2). The artery and vein pass superior to the ligament. The nerve runs on the deep surface of the supraspinatus, providing innervation to this muscle. It then continues through the spinoglenoid notch, entering the infraspinatus fossa where it provides innervation to the infraspinatus muscle. The spinoglenoid ligament can be present in approximately 60% of patients, running from the glenoid neck to the spine of the scapula (11). The suprascapular notch itself may vary in its size and shape. This anatomic variety may possibly lead to an etiology for entrapment if the notch is especially narrow or shallow (12). It does appear that a larger bony notch results in a larger tunnel for the nerve to run in, decreasing the possibility of entrapment. Because of its course, the suprascapular nerve can be injured or trapped at several points along its course.

Suprascapular nerve injuries have been reported after an acute shoulder dislocation (13). Posterior glenolabral cysts from posterior labral tears may impinge upon the nerve in the spinoglenoid notch, resulting in an infraspinatus palsy. The most common cause of suprascapular nerve injury in the athlete is secondary to the throwing motion. The mechanism of injury is due to the traction produced on the nerve during the late cocking phase of the throwing motion (14). This motion causes nerve entrapment at the spinoglenoid notch that results in an isolated infraspinatus palsy (15). Electromyogram (EMG) studies reveal that less that 40% of the infraspinatus strength is necessary for throwing (15). This may allow the athlete to continue high-level participation despite the underlying pathology.

Clinical Evaluation

The patient may complain of a dull ache over the posterior aspect of the shoulder. They may also complain of weakness that may be most noticeable in movements of abduction or external rotation. As the entrapment continues, atrophy of the supraspinatus and/or infraspinatus may occur and may also cause complaints. The patient may exhibit tenderness when palpating the suprascapular notch; however, this is not always present (16). Manual muscle strength testing will usually reveal reduction in strength to abduction and external rotation. Tenderness over the spinoglenoid notch region with accompanying atrophy of the infraspinatus alone may signal entrapment at this location. Electrodiagnostic studies such as EMG and nerve conduction studies can be helpful in diagnosing and localizing this condition when such obvious findings as atrophy are not yet present. EMG studies have, however, been reported to be normal despite obvious clinical findings of a suprascapular nerve palsy (17,18). Without obvious clinical findings and normal electrodiagnostic testing, other conditions that need to be excluded would include rotator cuff tears, impingement syndrome, acromioclavicular joint degeneration, and cervical radiculopathy.

Treatment

A suprascapular nerve palsy may have a sudden onset after a specific traumatic event (13) or a somewhat insidious onset associated with chronic use. Regardless of the cause, a program of conservative treatment with follow-up is recommended as the first course of treatment.

If the pain and weakness do not improve after a minimum of 2 months of conservative management, then surgical treatment should be a consideration. Surgical decompression of the suprascapular nerve can be performed through a variety of approaches. The superior approach may be the easiest to perform and seems to cause less postoperative morbidity. After the exposure and after the identification of the suprascapular notch, the transverse scapular ligament is excised, taking care to avoid the suprascapular artery and vein. The bony notch may be enlarged if it appears abnormally narrow or shallow.

The approach to the spinoglenoid notch should be done posteriorly by releasing the deltoid muscle off the scapular spine, retracting the infraspinatus to expose the suprascapular nerve as it exits the spinoglenoid notch and enters the infraspinatus fossa. The presence of a spinoglenoid ligament should be examined and, if found, excised. If no ligament is found, a soft tissue decompression and release of the nerve is indicated. If a posterior glenolabral cyst is the cause, an intraarticular arthroscopy to address or inspect the labral lesion should also be performed. In the largest published series of patients followed for over 5 years after a suprascapular nerve release, Vastamaki and Groansson (19) reported an improvement in 81% of their patients.

Axillary Nerve Palsy

The axillary nerve is a terminal branch of the brachial plexus direct from the posterior cord. It consists primarily of nerve roots C5-6. It runs posterior to the axillary artery lying on the subscapularis muscle where it then proceeds posteriorly running immediately inferior to the glenohumeral joint and glenoid neck. It then exits the quadrangular space bordered by the teres minor, long head of the triceps, humerus and teres major, with the posterior circumflex humeral artery. At its termination, it supplies motor innervation to the teres minor and the deltoid muscles. The anterior and middle deltoid is supplied by the anterior portion of the axillary nerve. The posterior portion of the nerve supplies the posterior third of the deltoid and provides cutaneous innervation to the skin overlying the lateral aspect of the shoulder in the region of the deltoid.

Closed injuries to the axillary nerve are probably the most common. An anterior dislocation of the glenohumeral joint results in significant traction on the axillary nerve. Direct blows or a fall on the deltoid may injure the nerve along its course through the deltoid. The axillary nerve can also be injured open, especially during surgical procedures in which the deltoid fibers are split laterally. Care should be taken during the lateral surgical approach to avoid splitting the deltoid more than 4 cm distal to the lateral edge of the acromion to avoid injuring the axillary nerve as it passes through this region.

Clinical Evaluation

Patients with an axillary nerve injury will have difficulty in elevating their arm due to loss of motor function of the deltoid muscle. There will also be evidence of deltoid atrophy as the nerve lesion progresses. Some or all of the deltoid may be atrophied depending on the location of the nerve injury. Cahill and Palmer (20) described the quadrilateral space syndrome in which the axillary nerve was compressed by fibrous bands in the quadrilateral space. This is especially true in a throwing athlete with the cocking motion in throwing. In this condition, the patient presents with posterior shoulder pain in the area of the teres minor that is exacerbated by the throwing motion. In these patients, the diagnosis may need to be confirmed with an arteriogram, which will reveal an occlusion of the posterior circumflex humeral artery with abduction and external rotation.

Treatment

Treatment after a closed injury can usually consist of follow-up and repeated examinations. Rest, avoidance of aggravating activities, with or without corticosteroid injections may be helpful in treating quadrilateral space syndrome (20). If there is failure to improve using these conservative measures, a decompression of the quadrilateral space is then indicated through a posterior approach. In patients with an open injury or after a closed injury that fails to recover after 3 to 6 months of conservative management, an exploration, repair, or grafting of the nerve may be indicated. For patients with complete loss of deltoid function, larger reconstructive procedures may be indicated that are similar to those used for complete brachial plexus injuries.

Musculocutaneous Nerve

The musculocutaneous nerve is a terminal branch of the brachial plexus. It arises from a branching of the lateral cord and consists primarily of nerve roots C5, C6, and C7. The musculocutaneous nerve runs obliquely to enter the coracobrachialis approximately 5 cm below the coracoid process. The nerve then sends motor branches to the biceps brachii and brachialis muscles before continuing on to exit between the brachialis fascia and the aponeurosis of the biceps where it becomes purely sensory as the lateral cutaneous nerve of the forearm. Injury to the musculocutaneous nerve in the shoulder region is uncommon without an open wound or injury. An anterior shoulder dislocation results in a traction injury as can overzealous medial retraction during anterior surgical procedures.

Clinical Evaluation

Because of paralysis of the coracobrachialis, the brachialis, and the biceps brachii, there will be weakness of elbow flexion. If the nerve lesion is chronic, there may be atrophy as well. In more chronic situations, the patients will adapt and provide elbow flexion by use of the brachioradialis. Lesions proximal to the elbow will result in loss of sensation in the distribution of the lateral cutaneous nerve of the forearm. Davidson et al. (21) reported on 15 patients with an entrapment of the musculocutaneous nerve at the elbow by the aponeurosis of the biceps brachii. The patients reported pain in this region with burning sensations distally into the forearm. Elbow flexion strength was normal in these patients.

Treatment

If after a traumatic open wound there is obvious musculocutaneous nerve injury, an effort toward exploration and repair should be made. If there is an identifiable musculocutaneous nerve palsy after an operative procedure, a period of observation and conservative management can be tried unless there is a fear that the nerve had been transected intraoperatively. If this is the case, then immediate exploration and repair is indicated. Most intraoperative injuries are neuropraxic in nature and will recover with conservative management. If after 3 to 6 months of conservative management the nerve does not recover, then open exploration is indicated.

The distal sensory nerve entrapment as described by

Davidson et al. (21) responds well to operative decompression, with complete elimination of preoperative symptoms in 11 patients treated surgically.

ELBOW

Ulnar Nerve

The ulnar nerve is a terminal branch of the brachial plexus from the medial cord. It is composed of cervical nerve roots C8 and T1. The course is through the upper arm anterior to the medial intermuscular septum deep to the brachial artery, median nerve, and basilic vein. In the distal upper arm, the nerve passes through the intermuscular septum where it enters the posterior compartment. The fibrous tissue forming this tunnel through the septum is called the arcade of Struthers. The nerve then passes posterior to the medial epicondyle through the cubital tunnel where it emerges distally to course between the heads of the pronator teres muscle (Fig. 30.3). During its course through the upper arm, it has no significant branches. There is a branch giving sensation to the elbow joint, and distally it provides innervation to the flexor carpi ulnaris as its first branch. The ulnar nerve also supplies a portion of the flexor digitorum profundus and continues distal to the hand to provide motor innervation to the hypothenar muscle group, the ulnar two lumbricales, the adductor pollicus, and the interossei. Sensory responsibilities of the ulnar nerve consist primarily of the fifth and ulnar half of the fourth digit in the hand.

Compression of the ulnar nerve within the cubital tunnel is a common compressive neuropathy in the upper extremity. Other causes of ulnar neuropathy include subluxation of the nerve, a ganglion, anconeus epitrochlearis muscle, rheumatoid arthritis, or osteoarthritis. Ulnar nerve injury can also be caused by a direct injury to the nerve because it is subcutaneous throughout its course through the elbow.

Athletic injuries to the ulnar nerve are most common in the throwing athlete. Cross-country skiing has also been a reported cause of ulnar nerve compression. This is believed to be secondary to muscular contraction of the flexor carpi ulnaris and the triceps (22). An ulnar neuropathy may develop in the throwing athlete, especially with valgus instability of the elbow in which there is a disruption or attenuation of the ulnar collateral ligament (23). This instability results in chronic repetitive traction during the throwing motion.

Clinical Evaluation

Patients usually present with complaints of paresthesias or dysesthesias in the ulnar aspect of the hand and ulnar two digits. Throwing athletes may complain of medial elbow aching after prolonged throwing. Symptoms of numbness may occur during the throwing motion or after throwing. Weakness and/or clumsiness can also be a complaint. Examination findings include tenderness or a positive Tinel's sign over the course of the ulnar nerve, especially at the cubital tunnel. A positive elbow flexion test in which there are symptoms distally after maximal maintained elbow flexion are also indicative of ulnar neuropathy. Motor strength testing of the intrinsics of the hand and the FDP of the ring and small fingers should be tested during the examination. Radiographs should be obtained, including, anteroposterior, lateral, and cubital tunnel views. In the throwing athlete, stress testing for elbow instability should be performed. A magnetic resonance image can be used to evaluate the integrity of the ulnar collateral ligament. Electrodiagnostic testing, including EMG and nerve conduction velocities, may be helpful in evaluating this condition. In mild cases, however, these studies may be normal.

Treatment

Initial treatment should consist of nonoperative management with efforts taken to decrease the pressure at the cubital tunnel on the ulnar nerve. Extension splinting can be performed as can padding the elbow to prevent direct trauma to the ulnar nerve. In the athlete, avoidance of the throwing motion to reduce the repetitive traction on the nerve usually helps relieve the symptoms.

When conservative management fails, the surgical option is to perform a cubital tunnel release with anterior transposition of the nerve. The ulnar nerve may be placed subcutaneously, intramuscularly, or submuscularly (24). A medial epicondylectomy can be performed as well. The prognosis for return to preoperative levels of activity can be based somewhat on the severity of

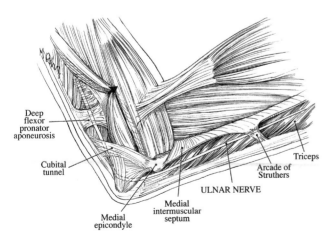

FIG. 30.3. The anatomy and potential site of entrapment of the median nerve during its course through the antecubital region.

the nerve injury. However, prognosis for return to the preoperative level of competition is good (23,25,26).

Median Nerve

The median nerve is a terminal branch of the brachial plexus formed by branches from the lateral and medial cords. It consists primarily of nerve roots C6 through T1. It courses through the upper arm medially at the level of the intramuscular septum. It passes the elbow medial to the brachial artery, proceeds distally deep to lacertus fibrosus, and then enters the pronator teres muscle (Fig. 30.4). Distal to the elbow, the anterior intraosseous nerve branches from the median nerve. The remainder of the median nerve continues distally down the forearm, running between the flexor digitorum superficialis and the flexor digitorum profundus. It enters the hand after passing through the carpal tunnel at the wrist. The median nerve provides motor innervation for the flexor carpi radialis, palmaris longus, flexor digitorum superficialis and profundus, pronator teres, flexor pollicis longus, pronator quadratus, the thenar muscles, and lumbricales I, II and III and provides sensory innervation to the radial three and a half digits. The two most common compressive neuropathies at the elbow involving the median nerve are the anterior interosseous syndrome, which is a motor neuropathy, and the pronator syndrome, which is characterized predominantly by complaints of pain.

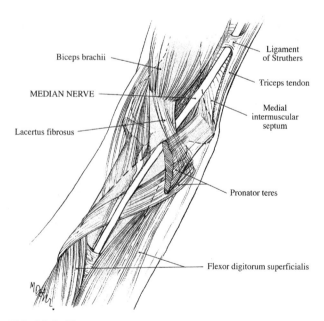

FIG. 30.4. The anatomy and potential sites of entrapment of the ulnar nerve during its course through the medial elbow region.

Pronator Syndrome

Median nerve compression in the pronator syndrome is characterized predominantly by complaints of pain. There may also be complaints of weakness, numbness, or aching in the forearm. The pathologic lesion in this case is secondary to compression of the median nerve between the ligament of Struthers and the fibrous band where the nerve runs deep to the flexor digitorum superficialis. The nerve may also be compressed at the level of the lacertus fibrosis or the intramuscular course through the pronator teres. This condition may occur in grasping sports due to repetitive stress such as weight lifting, gymnastics, or racket sports. A direct blow to the forearm may also cause this condition.

Clinical Evaluation

Positive findings include reproduction of the patient's symptoms with resistance to muscle function such as resisted pronation or supination. Direct pressure over the pronator will also reproduce symptoms. Hypertrophy of the flexor–pronator musculature may occur in athletes who use predominantly one arm for their sport. This hypertrophy can contribute to median nerve compression. Muscle weakness found in the median nerve distribution muscles is uncommon on examination (27). Electrodiagnostic studies such as EMG, nerve conduction studies, and nerve conduction velocities may not be helpful in the diagnosis but may help in excluding other possible etiologies (28).

Treatment

Conservative management should be attempted first. This would consist of rest, avoidance of aggravating activities, and splinting of the elbow in 90 degrees of flexion and neutral rotation. An anti-inflammatory agent may also be helpful.

If nonsurgical management fails to bring about an improvement, surgical decompression is indicated. This is performed through an anterior incision with the release starting at the ligament of Struther's and proceeding distally to include the lacertus fibrosus, freeing the nerve throughout its course through the pronator teres, and decompressing the fibrous band of the flexor digitorum superficialis. Good results have been achieved in surgical management. Recovery and resolution of symptoms after surgical decompression are not immediate, and recovery may take as long as several months. It should be noted that most patients respond well to nonsurgical treatment (28).

Anterior Interosseous Syndrome

This condition is a pure motor neuropathy of the muscles supplied by the anterior interosseous nerve. This consists of the flexor pollicis longus, the flexor digitorum profundus to the index finger, and the pronator quadratus. If a Martin-Grueber anastomosis is present in which the ulnar nerve combines with the anterior interosseous nerve, then the ulnar intrinsics and the flexor digitorum profundus to the other fingers may be involved. Like pronator quadratus syndrome, this condition occurs in gripping athletes and can occur after a direct blow. The onset can also be spontaneous.

Clinical Evaluation

Presenting symptoms initially are complaints of pain in the proximal forearm that gradually give rise to motor loss. Sensory examination is unremarkable. Pronator quadratus strength can be tested by fully flexing the elbow and comparing pronation strength to the uninvolved side. Elbow flexion removes the pronator teres and more fully isolates the pronator quadratus. Electrodiagnostic studies such as EMG and nerve conduction velocities will be diagnostic.

Treatment

Conservative management should be tried first. Nonsteroidal anti-inflammatory agents or oral steroids can be given. Avoidance of aggravating activities are the cornerstone of treatment. Splinting the elbow in 90 degrees of flexion and neutral rotation is also used during conservative treatment.

If conservative management fails, exploration and decompression of the nerve should be performed. Treatment outcomes from anterior interosseous nerve palsy both surgical and nonsurgical have been good (29).

Radial Nerve

The radial nerve is a terminal branch of the posterior cord. It consists primarily of nerve roots C5 through and including T1. The nerve's course is posteriorly through the spiral groove of the humerus; it then penetrates the lateral intramuscular septum in the distal third where it runs between the brachioradialis and the brachialis. In this region, motor branches arise to the brachioradialis and the extensor carpi radialis longus. At the elbow level, the radial nerve branches into the radial sensory nerve and the posterior interosseous nerve. The sensory nerve continues distally deep to the brachioradialis running between the brachioradialis and the extensor carpi radialis longus in the distal forearm to become the superficial branch of the radial nerve. The posterior interosseous nerve gives branches to the extensor carpi radialis brevis and the supinator before passing between the humeral and radial heads of the supinator. After emerging from the supinator, the nerve courses with the posterior interosseous artery. The neurovascular bundle

then runs between the superficial and deep extensor muscles of the forearm. It is here that the radial nerve gives off branches to the extensor digitorum, extensor digiti minimi, and extensor carpi ulnaris muscles. The nerve then arborizes into many branches, supplying the extensor pollicis longus, extensor indicis, abductor pollicis longus, and the extensor pollicis brevis muscles.

There are two types of radial nerve palsies in the arm. The posterior interosseous nerve syndrome is primarily a motor neuropathy and the radial tunnel syndrome is characterized predominantly by pain.

Posterior Interosseous Neuropathy

The posterior interosseous nerve may be injured by direct trauma or secondary to compression. The posterior interosseous nerve is also at risk in surgical procedures on the elbow, including elbow arthroscopy and treatment of pathology at the radial head and proximal radius. The risk of injury during elbow arthroscopy can be decreased with preinsufflation of the joint and by flexing the elbow before introduction of the instruments.

Clinical Evaluation

The patient may complain of pain in the dorsal forearm and will demonstrate weakness or paralysis of the finger and wrist extensors. Tenderness at the supinator is also common.

Treatment

Conservative management of a posterior interosseous neuropathy includes anti-inflammatory medications, avoidance of aggravating activities, and the use of a long arm splint with the arm held in supination and elbow flexion.

Failing to respond to conservative management, the posterior interosseous nerve can undergo surgical decompression. The nerve can be approached between the extensor digitorum and the extensor carpi radialis brevis, between the pronator teres and the brachial radialis, or approached through the brachioradialis muscle itself.

Most patients recover spontaneously with nonsurgical treatment. Complete recovery, however, may be quite prolonged, with wrist extensor function being the first to return (30).

Radial Tunnel Syndrome

Radial tunnel syndrome is characterized predominantly by complaints of pain. This syndrome is secondary to compression of the posterior interosseous nerve and often associated with repetitive trauma. Sites of compression include fibrous bands at the radiocapitellar joint, the vascular leash of Henry, the extensor carpi radialis brevis, the arcade of Frohse, and the distal supinator. Quite often this condition is associated with lateral epicondylitis.

Clinical Evaluation

Patients often complains of an aching in the dorsal radial aspect of the forearm. Supination will increase the symptomatology. Pain with resisted supination and resistance of the long finger extension and tenderness over the supinator are often present. The sensory examination is unremarkable and there is no motor strength deficits. Electrodiagnostic testing is not especially helpful in this condition.

Treatment

Treatment of radial tunnel syndrome includes avoidance of aggravating activities, anti-inflammatory medications, and splinting of the elbow in 90 degrees of flexion and supination. Treatment of lateral epicondylitis should also be instituted because it is often present concomitantly with radial tunnel syndrome. It should be noted that the use of a Count'R-Force brace commonly used for lateral epicondylitis may exacerbate the symptoms of radial tunnel syndrome.

If conservative management fails, a posterior interosseous nerve release and decompression can be performed in a similar fashion for posterior interosseous neuropathy. Results of surgical treatment can be somewhat unpredictable and unreliable (31). Most cases of radial tunnel syndrome respond well to conservative management.

REFERENCES

1. Seddon HJ. Three types of nerve injury. *Brain* 1943;66:237.
2. Cohn BT, Brahms MA, Cohn M. Injury to the eleventh cranial nerve in a high school wrestler. *Orthop Rev* 1986;15:59–64.
3. Bigliani LU, Perez-Sanz JR, Wolfe IN. Treatment of trapezius paralysis. *J Bone Joint Surg Am* 1985;67A:871–877.
4. Dewar FP, Harris RI. Restoration of the function of the shoulder following paralysis of the trapezius by fascial sling and transplantation of the levator scapulae. *Ann Surg* 1950;132:1111.
5. Spira E. The treatment of dropped shoulder—a new operative technique. *J Bone Joint Surg Am* 1948:30A:229.
6. Foo CL, Swam M. Isolated paralysis of the serratus anterior. A report of 20 cases. *J Bone Joint Surg Br* 1983;65B:552–556.
7. Gregg J Jr, Labosky D, Hartz M, et al. Serratus anterior paralysis in the young athlete. *J Bone Joint Surg Am* 1979;61A:825–832.
8. Johnson JTH, Kendall H. Isolated paralysis of the serratus anterior muscle. *J Bone Joint Surg Am* 1955;37A:567–574.
9. Chavezm JP. Pectoralis minor transplanted for paralysis of the serratus anterior. *J Bone Joint Surg Br* 1951;33B:2128.
10. Marmar L, Bechtal CO. Paralysis of the serratus anterior due to elective shock relieved by transplantation of the pectoralis major muscle. *J Bone Joint Surg Am* 1963;45A:156–160.
11. Demirhan M, Imhoff AB, Debski RE, et al. The spinoglenoid ligament and its relationship to the suprascapular nerve. *J Shoulder Elbow Surg* 1998;7:238–242.
12. Rengachary SS, Burr D, Lucas S, et al. Suprascapular nerve entrapment neuropathy. A clinical, anatomical, and comparative study. Part II. Anatomical study. *Neurosurgery* 1978;5:447–451.
13. Bryan WJ, Wild JJ. Isolated infraspinatus atrophy: A common cause of posterior shoulder pain and weakness in throwing athletes. *Am J Sports Med* 1989;17:130–131.
14. Ferretti A, Cerullo G, Russo G. Suprascapular neuropathy in volleyball players. *J Bone Joint Surg Am* 1987;69A:260–263.
15. Jobe FW, Tibone JE, Jobe CM, et al. The shoulder in sports. In: Rockwood CA, Matsen FA III, eds. *The shoulder.* Vol. 2. Philadelphia: W.B. Saunders, 1990:987.
16. Post M, Mayer J. Suprascapular nerve entrapment. Diagnosis and treatment. *Clin Orthop* 1987;223:126–136.
17. Clein LJ. Suprascapular entrapment neuropathy. *J Neurosurg* 1975;43:337–342.
18. Edeland HG, Zachrisson BE. Fracture of the scapular notch associated with lesion of the suprascapular nerve. *Acta Orthop Scand* 1975;46:758–763.
19. Vastamaki M, Grausson H. Suprascapular nerve entrapment. *Clin Orthop* 1993;297:135–143.
20. Cahill BR, Palmer RE. Quadrilateral space syndrome. *J Hand Surg* 1983;8:65–69.
21. Davidson JJ, Bassett FH III, Nunley IA. Musculocutaneous nerve entrapment revisited. *J Shoulder Elbow Surg* 1998;7:250–255.
22. Fulkerson J. Transient ulnar neuropathy from nardie skiing. *Clin Orthop* 1980;153:230–231.
23. Jobe FW, Fanton GS. Nerve injuries. In: Norrey BF, ed. *The elbow and its disorders.* Philadelphia: W.B. Saunders, 1985:497.
24. Eaton RR, Crowe JF, Parkes JC. Anterior transposition of the ulnar nerve using a non-compressing fasciodermal sling. *J Bone Joint Surg Am* 1980;62A:820–825.
25. Del Pizzo W, Jobe FW, Norwood L. Ulnar nerve entrapment syndrome in basketball players. *Am J Sports Med* 1977;5:182–185.
26. Rettig AC. Anterior subcutaneous transposition of the ulnar nerve in the athlete. *Am J Sports Med* 1993;21:836–839.
27. Spinner M, Linschied RL. Nerve entrapment syndromes. In: Morrey BF, ed. *The elbow and its disorders.* Philadelphia: W.B. Saunders, 1985:691.
28. Hartz CR, Linscheid RL, Gramse RR, et al. Pronator teres syndrome. Compressive neuropathy of the median nerve. *J Bone Joint Surg Am* 1981;63A:885.
29. Schantz K, Riegels-Nielsen P. The anterior interosseous nerve syndrome. *J Hand Surg* 1992;178:510–512.
30. Kaplan PE. Posterior interosseous neuropathies: natural history. *Arch Phys Med Rehabil* 1984;65:399–400.
31. Atroshi I, Johnson R, Ornstein E. Radial tunnel release: unpredictable outcome in 37 cases with a 1–5 year follow up. *Acta Orthop Scand* 1995;66:255–257.

Principles and Practice of Orthopaedic Sports Medicine,
edited by William E. Garrett, Jr., Kevin P. Speer, and Donald T. Kirkendall.
Lippincott Williams & Wilkins, Philadelphia © 2000.

CHAPTER 31

Concept of Overhead Athletic Injuries

Marilyn M. Pink and Frank W. Jobe

Have you ever heard the story of the young wife who cut the ends off the roast as she put it into the roasting pan? Her new husband asked her why that was done. She responded that she had learned it from her mother. Since he was curious, he suggested they call her mother and query her. The mother responded, "because my mother always did it." Fortunately, the grandmother was still alive, and the young man's curiosity was heightened, so they called her. This lady was able to set the record straight. She said, "because my pan was too small."

As far fetched as it may seem, this parable is related to the overhead athlete. The concept of the overhead athlete came from the overhand athlete. The baseball pitcher was one of the most prominently studied group of athletes with potential shoulder problems in the 1980s. To differentiate the overhand pitch from the underhand pitch, the baseball pitcher was dubbed the "overhand athlete." As time went on, the model that was built on the baseball pitcher began to be transferred to other groups of athletes who were also at risk for shoulder injuries. These groups included the swimmer, the golfer, the javelin thrower, the quarterback, the tennis server, and the volleyball server. Thus, the term overhand athlete (which was intended for the baseball pitcher who threw overhand) was modified to overhead athlete (to encompass all athletes whose hands went over their heads in the sporting activity). The hand over the head position inference was that the shoulder was then at 90 degrees degrees of elevation or higher. So, the very specific, accurate, and scientific model of the overhand baseball pitch evolved to be globalized to other sports. Like the roasting pan story, there was a

logic in the original model that during its evolution lost the specific relevance.

We now know that each sport has its own distinctions, own requirements, and own demands. This chapter offers an opportunity to document the historic evolution of the overhand/overhead athlete and to identify specific components of a few separate paradigms of the overhead athlete. The baseball pitcher, the freestyle swimmer, and the golfer have been chosen as three distinct models. The normal mechanics are first described and then the pathologic mechanics. The anatomy of injury is then reviewed.

OVERHAND PITCHER

Mechanics

The phases of the baseball pitch are found in Fig. 31.1. The description is that of a right-handed pitcher.

Normal Mechanics

Wind-up

During the wind-up phase, an individual can make many stylistic adaptations that will be irrelevant to the final delivery and irrelevant to any potential for injury. However, the basics of this phase are found in all successful stylistic adaptations and very much dominate the success of the delivery.

The basic components of this phase begin with the feet parallel to one another and perpendicular to the rubber on the mound. The hips are level to one another and are perpendicular to the plate. The hands are together. The body is aligned with good balance. The left leg takes a small comfortable step back, in line with home plate. The right foot is then positioned parallel to the rubber, and some coaches have the pitcher wedge the foot with the lateral half on top of the rubber.

M. M. Pink: Centinela Hospital Medical Biomechanics, Center Laboratory, Inglewood, California 90301.

F. W. Jobe: Department of Orthopaedics, University of Southern California, Los Angeles, California 90033.

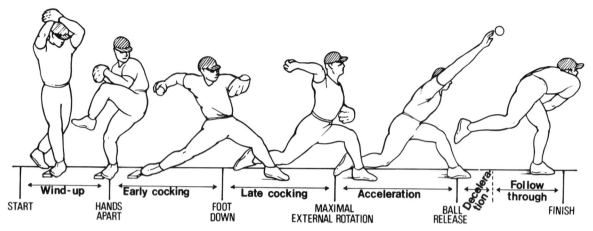

FIG. 31.1. Phases of the baseball pitch.

The left lower extremity is picked up in a controlled active fashion and the hips remain level while pointing toward home plate. As the hips begin to move forward, a "V" is formed with the hips at the apex while the torso and right leg form the two sides of the V. The hips point toward the batter. The final event of wind-up is when the hand holding the ball comes out of the glove.

Although these key points in wind-up are necessary for a successful delivery, the shoulder is relatively non-challenged. The shoulder moves slowly, the hands are together, and the muscle activity is low (1).

Early Cocking

As the hand comes out of the glove, it must stay on top of the ball. The hand on top of the ball helps the shoulder stay in more internal rotation, which is a safer position for the glenohumeral joint. The V that was initiated in wind-up becomes more pronounced in early cocking as the hips continue to advance toward home plate (Fig. 31.2). The hips stay level. Rotation of the hips is delayed as long as possible. From the perspective of the batter, the ball is hidden as the batter cannot yet determine which type of pitch will be delivered. The early cocking phase ends as the left leg slowly, easily, and comfortably comes down and the foot contacts with the mound.

The shoulder is elevated in the scapular plane to 104 degrees and externally rotated to 46 degrees (2). Two force couples are formed during early cocking: one for the scapular motion and one for glenohumeral motion. The goal of the scapular muscles is to position the glenoid for the humeral head as the arm moves into abduction. The scapula is then a stable platform upon which the humeral head can move. The upper and lower trapezius muscles upwardly rotate the scapula as they pull on the spine of the scapula. At the same time, the serratus anterior pulls the inferior angle upward, whereas the

middle trapezius, rhomboids, and levator scapulae retract the superior medial border of the scapula (1). Together these muscles tether different edges of the scapula to ensure smooth movement of this relatively large and free-floating bone (Fig. 31.3).

The three heads of the deltoid and the supraspinatus are synergistically working during early cocking to elevate the humerus (1). The supraspinatus, which inserts closer to the joint axis than does the deltoid, helps to keep the humeral head congruent with the glenoid and prevents the head from riding up the glenoid rim (Fig. 31.4). If the deltoids were to abduct the humerus without the supraspinatus, they would be able to mechanically displace the humeral head. The deltoids position the arm in space, and the supraspinatus stabilizes the head

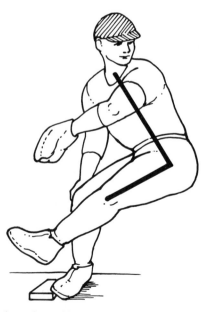

FIG. 31.2. In early cocking, the V (which was initiated in wind-up) becomes more pronounced as the hips advance toward home plate and the foot wedges into the rubber.

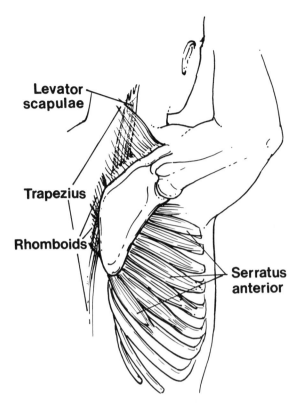

Late Cocking

As the left foot makes contact with the mound, it lands within the width of the right foot. The foot points toward home plate. The weight is evenly distributed on the two legs and the legs are firm. The torso is balanced in an upright position between the legs. The pitcher "stays closed" (delays trunk rotation) as long as possible.

The point of the late cocking phase is to move the humerus into maximal external rotation. The humerus maintains its level of elevation in the scapular plane and externally rotates from 46 to 170 degrees (2). Because the humerus maintains, rather than increases, its elevation during late cocking, the scapula does not need additional elevation. However, it does need to provide a stable base for the external rotation of the humerus. The middle trapezius, rhomboids, and levator scapulae have all been shown to be scapular retractors that function isometrically at the end of the range (4). These are key muscles in providing scapular stabilization. The serratus anterior is the key muscle opposing the retractors while stabilizing and protracting the scapula (1). In addition to forming a force couple for stabilization, these muscles may help to "tip" the scapula so that the glenoid offers maximum congruency for the humeral head.

At this time, the subscapularis, pectoralis major, and latissimus dorsi are all anterior to the glenohumeral joint. Turkel et al. (5) described the relative position of the tendons and ligaments around the glenohumeral joint in a position of 90 degrees abduction and 90 degrees external rotation (Fig. 31.5). Although this is not exactly the humeral position during late cocking, it demonstrates the relative position of the muscles. The subscapularis, teres major, pectoralis major, and latissimus

FIG. 31.3. During the early cocking phase, the scapular muscles tether different edges of the scapula to ensure smooth motion or this relatively large and free floating bone. (From Pink MM, Perry J. Biomechanics. In: Jobe FW, ed. *Operative techniques in upper extremity sports injuries.* St. Louis: Mosby-Year Book, 1996:113, with permission.)

within the glenoid. The relationship of the deltoid and supraspinatus has been noted during planar motions as well (3). This separates the supraspinatus from the rotators of the rotator cuff and functionally aligns it with the deltoids for humeral elevation.

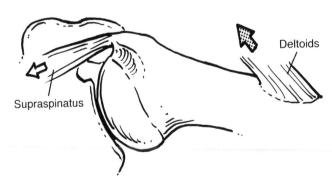

FIG. 31.4. During early cocking, the supraspinatus inserts closer to the joint axis than does the deltoid and helps to keep the humeral head congruent with the glenoid, thus preventing the head from riding up the glenoid rim. (From Pink MM, Perry J. Biomechanics. In: Jobe FW, ed. *Operative techniques in upper extremity sports injuries.* St. Louis: Mosby-Year Book, 1996:114, with permission.)

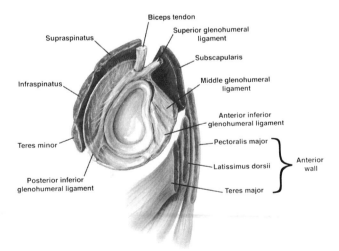

FIG. 31.5. Position of the tendons and ligaments around the glenohumeral joint in the position of 90 degrees abduction and 90 degrees external rotation (modified from Turkel et al.). (From Pink MM, Perry J. Biomechanics. In: Jobe FW, ed. *Operative techniques in upper extremity sports injuries.* St. Louis: Mosby-Year Book, 1996:114, with permission.)

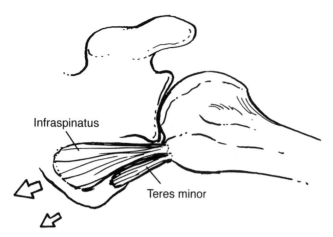

FIG. 31.6. During late cocking, the posterior position of the infraspinatus and teres minor afford a restraint to anterior subluxation as they hold the humeral head back. (From Pink MM, Perry J. Biomechanics. In: Jobe FW, ed. *Operative techniques in upper extremity sports injuries.* St. Louis: Mosby-Year Book, 1996:115, with permission.)

dorsi form the anterior wall along with the capsule and the ligaments. The anterior wall provides stability to the anterior aspect of the joint.

The posterior rotator cuff muscles are also quite active during late cocking (1). The infraspinatus and teres minor are externally rotating the humerus. In addition, their posterior placement offers a posterior restraint to the anterior subluxation as they hold the humeral head back (Fig. 31.6).

In the position of extreme external rotation, the supraspinatus is rotated posteriorly. At this point the supraspinatus is relatively ineffective as a superior compressive force. In part, this force may be provided by the subscapularis, which is now positioned superiorly. The electromyographic firing pattern supports this, be-

cause the upper portion of the subscapularis is more active than the lower portion and is more active than the supraspinatus (1). This demonstrates different functions within the subscapularis. In that this muscle has a broad origin of fibers and a narrow insertion, it is understandable how the angle of pull differs within the muscle.

The elbow increases its angle of flexion to somewhere between 55 and 90 degrees during late cocking (2). At this degree of flexion, the pronator teres and flexor carpi radialis are anterior to the ulnar collateral ligament (UCL) and thus are unable to offer any support. The flexor digitorum superficialis and flexor carpi ulnaris are in a more optimal position to contribute medial stability to the joint (Fig. 31.7).

Acceleration

Once the humerus begins to internally rotate, the acceleration phase is initiated. The ball will eventually (within 0.05 seconds) be released from the hand at over 90 miles per hour (hopefully). This motion occurs upon a very firm base provided by the lower extremities with both feet planted on the mound throughout the phase.

Very high angular velocities, torques, and joint compressive forces are reported at this time (2,6,7). A stable scapula is needed as a fulcrum for the high angular velocities and torques. In keeping with this, the scapular muscles all demonstrate relatively high activity during the acceleration phase (1).

As the humerus internally rotates, the posterior deltoid is optimally positioned to restrain the humerus with horizontal abduction as noted by its high electrical activity. The supraspinatus also is highly active as it again demonstrates its relationship to the deltoid (1) (Fig. 31.8).

The teres minor demonstrates much higher activity than the infraspinatus during acceleration (1). A subtle,

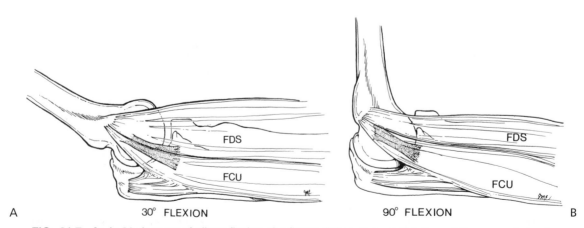

FIG. 31.7. A: At 30 degrees of elbow flexion, the flexor digitorum superficialis and flexor carpi ulnaris (FCU) are over the medial collateral ligament (MCL). **B:** At 90 degrees of elbow flexion, the FCU is over the MCL. (From Davidson PA, Pink M, Perry J, et al. Functional anatomy of the flexor pronator muscle group in relation to the medial collateral ligament of the elbow. *Am J Sports Med* 1995;23:247, with permission.)

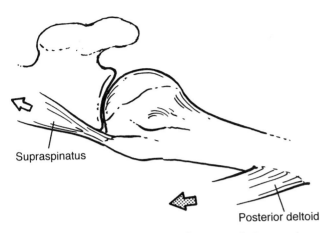

FIG. 31.8. As the humerus internally rotates during acceleration, the posterior deltoid and supraspinatus are optimally positioned to restrain the humerus with horizontal abduction. (From Pink MM, Perry J. Biomechanics. In: Jobe FW, ed. *Operative techniques in upper extremity sports injuries.* St. Louis: Mosby-Year Book, 1996:117, with permission.)

but important, point to be made here is that the teres minor and infraspinatus function differently from each other. Thus, a clinician needs to strengthen them differently.

The pectoralis major and teres minor form a force couple during acceleration. As the pectoralis major forcefully contracts at this relatively high elevation (1) for internal rotation, the teres minor holds the head back and controls the humeral internal rotation. The direction of fibers of the teres minor gives it an extension component, which may be one reason it outperforms the infraspinatus in this position.

The subscapularis, especially the upper portion, also exhibits very high activity during this phase and functions with the latissimus dorsi and the pectoralis major (1). The insertion of the subscapularis is closer to the joint axis of rotation than is the insertion of the pectoralis major and latissimus dorsi. This allows the subscapularis to function as a steering muscle as it precisely positions the humeral head in the glenoid. This is similar to the relationship of the supraspinatus with the deltoid.

A study by Bartlett et al. (8) demonstrated that the latissimus dorsi and pectoralis major may be the only upper extremity muscles to augment the force that is generated in the lower extremities and trunk. During the acceleration phase, these two muscles demonstrate a peak of muscle activity (9).

The elbow extends to −20 degrees in acceleration (2,6). Because more than 50% of pitchers have a flexion contracture (10), this −20 degrees may approach the joint extension limits.

The elbow also experiences a major valgus thrust during acceleration (11). Because advancement of the humerus precedes that of the forearm, the torque on the medial structures of the elbow are calculated to be quite high (2). The UCL is the primary stabilizer with support offered by the flexor carpi ulnaris with some assistance from the flexor digitorum superficialis (12).

Deceleration

After the ball is released, the right hip comes up and over the left leg. The right foot disengages from the mound. The excess kinetic energy that was not transferred to the ball is dissipated beginning with the arm. As in the acceleration phase, there are high calculated forces and torques to disseminate the forces (13,14). In general, all posterior muscles of the shoulder are active to control the deceleration. The teres minor demonstrates the highest level of activity of all the glenohumeral muscles (1). This is a carry-over of its activity in the acceleration phase.

Follow-through

As the arm continues to be brought down, the forces are much less to the arm. This phase appears to be fairly inconsequential. In the shoulder, the serratus anterior is the only muscle that demonstrates activity above 35% of the maximum (1). It is active as it protracts the scapula when the arm finishes its movement across the body.

Pathologic Mechanics

Wind-up

In that the stage is set during wind-up, there are numerous problems that are actually initiated in this phase, but the pathologic repercussions are not noted until later. For example, if the hips are pointing in a direction other than home plate during wind-up, the leg will later land in the faulty direction. The trunk will then exhibit compensatory rotation, and the timing of the arm will be off. Similarly, if the trunk leans back as the left leg is raised, the balance will be off throughout the pitch with excessive motion in the anterior–posterior plane (and perhaps medial–lateral motion as well). Yet, as aforementioned, the arm is at relatively low risk during wind-up because it is moving slowly, and torques are low as is the muscle activity. An astute clinician will, however, pay careful attention to the basics during the wind-up phase because any problems here will be magnified later.

Early Cocking

One of the more common faulty habits in a pitcher is the hand under the ball during early cocking. Some players will take the ball out of the glove with the hand underneath it. Others will take the ball out of the glove with the hand on top, but as they bring the arm back, they rotate the hand to beneath the ball. This erroneous technique is called "pie throwing." With the hand under the ball, the humerus moves into external rotation. As the arm is swinging back (behind the body) and up (into the throwing position), the faulty external rotation leaves the humeral head at risk to be subluxed anteriorly. Thus, there is potential for instability that can lead to anterior subluxation and subsequent injury.

Another common problem in early cocking is that of excessive early trunk rotation. During this phase, the left leg is not yet in contact with the mound. A pitcher who begins excessive rotation of the trunk obviously will not have a stable balanced base from which to rotate. In addition to a loss of balance, they will lose a lot of potential energy. Also, an individual who begins excessive rotation in early cocking opens up too soon in late cocking. ("Opening up" refers to the chest facing the batter. When the hips rotate too quickly, the trunk follows and the upper torso faces the batter too soon. To stay "closed" means that the upper torso has not rotated to face the batter. When a pitcher opens up too soon, he or she attempts to replace the lost potential energy by heaving the ball forward in acceleration.)

Late Cocking

The position of the left foot as it contacts the mound is an indicator of the earlier hip position (were they pointed toward home plate?) and of whether the pitcher will open up too soon. If the left foot lands pointing to the first base side, the pitcher will open up too soon. If it lands pointing to the third base side, the pitcher will stay closed too long, throw too far to the inside or become very off balance.

If a pitcher opens up too soon, the arm is typically left behind the scapular plane (hyperangulation) while the humerus is rotating to 170 degrees (2). This leaves the humeral head angled so that it can stretch the anterior structures and creates the potential for anterior instability and the resultant injury (Fig. 31.9). If the muscles of the anterior wall are fatigued, the probability for overstretching in the hyperangulated position is even higher.

If the arm is left behind the scapular plane, the valgus load on the elbow is increased. As stated earlier, the stress is largely borne by the UCL. Hence, this mechanical deviation can lead to medial elbow instability.

Baseball pitchers with unstable shoulders demonstrated several significant differences from pitchers with normal shoulders during the late cocking phase. First, the serratus anterior was significantly less active (9). This can be related to the clinical world because one of the most subtle signs of impending injury is scapular winging, asymmetry, or premature elevation. When the serratus anterior is no longer able to perform adequately, no other muscle can effectively substitute. Without the serratus anterior to tether down the inferior angle of the scapula, the scapula elevates early and/or wings. The serratus anterior is one of the few muscles that is constantly active. Therefore, it is more vulnerable to fatigue. A therapist would wisely put a focus on strengthening and endurance training for the serratus anterior.

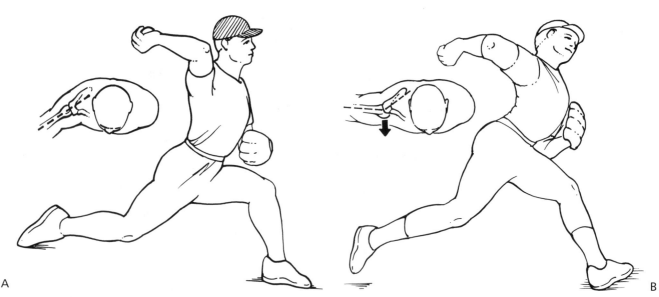

FIG. 31.9. If a pitcher opens up too soon, the arm is left behind the scapular plane, which causes potential for anterior instability and the resultant injury. **A:** Normal mechanics. **B:** Pathologic mechanics when arm is behind the scapular plane.

In the subtle stage of diminished serratus anterior activity, the astute eye of the coach or medical practitioner may note that the player tends to drop the elbow. The dropped elbow is really decreasing the degree of necessary scapular rotation and elevation. This, in turn, requires less from the serratus anterior.

In the next level of pathology, the player may begin with the aforementioned compensatory mechanics of moving the humerus into or behind the coronal plane. The player also loses some humeral external rotation, and typically the back begins to move into hyperlordosis.

Experience has shown that if the scapular asynchrony can be identified at the earliest stage, even before the athlete complains of pain or before there is a tangible consistent drop in performance, then he or she can be pulled off the field and put on a specific strengthening program to prevent anatomic damage to the static stabilizers. Chronically unstable shoulders have also demonstrated significantly less activity in the subscapularis and pectoralis major (9). The result of this is obviously a lack of support for the anterior wall.

As the subscapularis becomes less active in pitchers with unstable shoulders, the supraspinatus becomes more active (9). This could be partially related to a decrease in humeral external rotation. If the humerus is not rotated to quite the degree of the normal shoulder, the supraspinatus moves back into position to offer the superior compression to the humeral head.

It should be noted that all pathologic mechanics are not what they seem. Sometimes the pathologic mechanics are a substitution for a "downstream" problem. For example, if a pitcher has back pain, his or her arm may move into the coronal plane for reasons unrelated to the prior discussion. If the pitcher's back is sore, he or she may not be able to transmit the forces from the legs up through the trunk and out the arms. Thus, as substitution, the pitcher may attempt to regain the lost power by "heaving" the ball. The arm may move into the coronal plane to heave the ball forward. If this is done, the pitcher still ends up with anatomic damage to the shoulder. Yet the shoulder damage is really symptomatic to another problem. The athlete may attempt to rehabilitate the shoulder and return to the mound. If the core problem of a back injury was not addressed, the poor mechanics used in substitution could lead to another spate of injuries—perhaps at the shoulder, perhaps to the elbow, or perhaps at a different weak link in the chain. For this reason, the total picture of the mechanics and the effect of one body part must be considered. If an athlete presents with more than one overuse injury, it is pointing toward a mechanical deficit somewhere else in the chain. This is true not just for late cocking phase of the pitch nor for just the pitcher. The concept can be parlayed into all phases of the sport.

Acceleration

The problems mentioned in the cocking phases are also present in acceleration. The lordotic position of the back is most evident at this time. The arm behind the body is also noted, as is a dropped elbow.

A "whipping" action occurs at the elbow to substitute for the hyperangulated arm. This action brings the arm forward. The whipping in combination with the valgus forces in late cocking cause microtrauma of the UCL and in some cases an acute rupture of the ligament. In either case, medial instability of the elbow results.

Pitchers with unstable shoulders demonstrate several significant differences from pitchers with normal shoulders (9) during acceleration. First, the serratus anterior is less active. This is a carry-over from the late cocking phase with the same clinical implication. Additionally, the latissimus dorsi and subscapularis are less active. The force couple they form in the pitchers with normal shoulders is not in effect. The support for the anterior wall is also diminished. Furthermore, the augmentation of power supplied by the latissimus dorsi is no longer present. All these factors demonstrate the compound effect of the loss of the smooth gear functioning and, as a result, asynchronous motion.

Another mechanical deviation that may be noted in acceleration is the right foot may come off the ground. If this occurs, the pitcher can easily be off balance. If there is not a stable bilateral base, it is much more difficult to accumulate and transmit the large forces to throw the ball. Also, if off balance, the chances are much higher that the ball will be inaccurately placed.

Deceleration

As aforementioned, during deceleration the teres minor demonstrated the highest level of activity of all glenohumeral muscles. This has clinical relevance in that a subtle sign of injury is pain localized to the teres minor during deceleration. The rehabilitation would consist primarily of strengthening the teres minor.

Follow-through

Any faulty mechanics that are noted at this point had their genesis much earlier and the outcome (ball speed or placement) has already been determined. In baseball, there is a saying that "the game is not over until the fat lady sings." Well in terms of the pitch, by the time follow-through occurs, the fat lady is singing.

Anatomy of Injury

Shoulder

Fifty-seven percent of professional pitchers report shoulder injuries (15). This rate can be partially attrib-

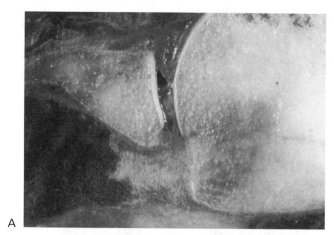
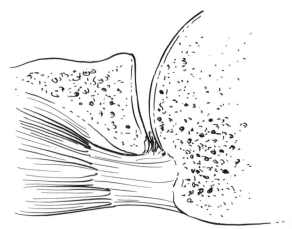

FIG. 31.10. When the arm is behind the scapular plane in the abducted and externally rotated position, the undersurface of the posterior cuff come in contact with the posterosuperior glenoid labrum. **A:** Cross-section from a cadaver. **B:** Schematic of A. (From Jobe CM, et al. Anterior shoulder instability, impingement, and rotator cuff tear: theories and concepts. In: Jobe FW, ed. *Operative techniques in upper extremity sports injuries.* St. Louis: Mosby-Year Book, 1996:170, with permission.)

uted to the repetitive nature of the sport (a professional pitcher undergoes approximately 1,000 shoulder revolutions per week) and partially to the mechanics. As the pathomechanics of the pitch have become better understood, so too has the anatomy of injury. Over the past decade, the role of instability and subluxation in injury was accepted. More recently, the link between instability and internal impingement has been defined.

When the arm is behind the scapular plane in abduction and external rotation, the undersurface of the posterior cuff comes in contact with the posterosuperior glenoid labrum (16–18) (Fig. 31.10). In the presence of anterior instability, the propensity toward injury is heightened (Fig. 31.11). This type of impingement is named posterior internal impingement to differentiate it from the classic type of impingement described by

Neer in 1972 (19) and to differentiate it from the anterior internal impingement noted in golfers and swimmers.

Thus, the continuum that leads to shoulder injury in the pitcher is multifaceted. It begins with the microtrauma from continual practice in the sport and then incorporates pathomechanics, muscular weakness and fatigue, and stretching of anterior structures. If these factors are not corrected through rehabilitation and proper coaching, anatomic damage can occur to both the skeletal and soft tissues of the joint (Fig. 31.12).

Elbow

Elbow injury in the pitcher is primarily that of medial instability caused by disruption of the UCL. The disruption can be from microtrauma or an acute tear. In the more common case of microtrauma, the repetitive wear and tear on the ligament coupled with any faulty mechanics is the culprit. Frequently, appropriate rehabilitation can return an athlete to the playing field. In the case of an acute rupture, the athlete hears a "snap" on one pitch and the ball goes wild. Surgery is the best option for this athlete.

Elbow instability along with the valgus stress leads to posterior compartment impingement and formation of osteophytes. The osteophytes can lend some stability to the elbow. However, if they break off, they not only are problematic as loose bodies, but the instability is more pronounced. For that reason, a surgeon may choose to not remove osteophytes. Also, a trainer or therapist may be wise not to forcefully stretch the typical flexion contracture (about 20 degrees) of the elbow because that could break off the osteophytes. If the osteophytes do break off, a surgeon would want to check the

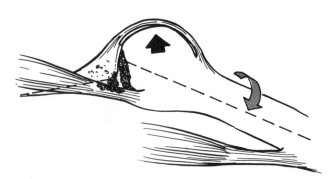

FIG. 31.11. When the arm is behind the scapular plane in the presence of anterior instability, the propensity toward injury is heightened. (From Jobe CM, et al. Anterior shoulder instability, impingement, and rotator cuff tear: theories and concepts. In: Jobe FW, ed. *Operative techniques in upper extremity sports injuries.* St. Louis: Mosby-Year Book, 1996:175, with permission.)

seen in pitching. Thus, the latissimus dorsi becomes the primary muscle of propulsion after mid–pull-through. The subscapularis forms a force couple with the latissimus dorsi. The subscapularis, which inserts closer to the axis of rotation, keeps the humeral head approximated in the joint.

Throughout the propulsive motions of the pectoralis major and latissimus dorsi, the serratus anterior is also active as it pulls the body over the arm and through the water. The serratus anterior maintains the scapula in a position of upward rotation and assists with joint congruency of the humerus and glenoid.

The posterior deltoid becomes active after the latissimus dorsi reaches its peak. The posterior deltoid is a "transition" muscle. By virtue of its extension component, it contributes to the final part of pulling while it begins to lift the humerus out of the water. (The transition is that of finishing the pull and beginning the lift.)

As the hand begins to exit the water, the group of muscles that were active at hand entry once again begin to function. The middle deltoid is active to abduct and continue lifting the arm. The supraspinatus repeats its force couple with the deltoids. The anterior deltoid abducts and begins to flex the humerus. The scapular force couple forms once more as the upper trapezius upwardly rotates the scapula, while the rhomboids retract the medial superior border and the serratus anterior assists with rotation and protraction.

Recovery

Recovery is a much shorter phase than pull-through. The purpose of recovery is simply to bring the arm into position to pull once again. The humerus is internally rotated as it is lifted out of water. It then abducts and rotates externally to a small degree (i.e., not beyond neutral rotation) order to bring the forearm around. As the hand passes the shoulder, the arm begins to move into position for hand entry once again.

The muscles that function at hand exit continue with their activity during recovery. In addition, the infraspinatus depresses and slightly rotates the humerus externally as the forearm swings around. During mid-recovery the activity in the infraspinatus is the higher than any other point in the stroke. The subscapularis is active to control the degree of humeral rotation. Of note, however, is that the activity of the infraspinatus is less than half that of the subscapularis (21). This reinforces the fact that the key rotation, here and at other points of the stroke, is internal rotation. This is in contrast to that of baseball pitchers, who go into maximal external rotation. This fact is a major argument as to the differences between these overhead sports. It mandates that each sport be acknowledged for their uniqueness rather than lumped together as one sport.

Throughout the freestyle stroke, the serratus anterior and subscapularis continually fire above 20% of their maximum. The serratus anterior is active to stabilize the scapula, which provides a stable base for the humerus. The subscapularis is continually active, again noting the predominance of internal rotation throughout the stroke (21). Monad (22) demonstrated that 15% to 20% of a muscle's maximal voluntary contraction is the highest level at which sustained activity can be performed without fatigue. Thus, these two muscles (the serratus anterior and subscapularis) appear to be susceptible to fatigue.

Another important clinical point is the different activity patterns of the teres minor and the infraspinatus. Because of their anatomic proximity and shared insertion on the humerus, one might be led to believe that they function similarly. However, this is not the case. The infraspinatus depresses and externally rotates the humerus during mid-recovery, whereas the teres minor is active during pull-through, when it forms a force couple with the pectoralis major.

Pathologic Mechanics

Early Pull-through

A swimmer with a painful shoulder may demonstrate a wider hand entry and a flatter pitch to the hand. Coaches note this position as a dropped-elbow position and remark that they can tell when swimmers are hurt, tired, or lazy because they fail to hold the elbow up. In that the hand entry position for the normal shoulder closely approximates the Neer test for impingement (23), it is understandable that the swimmer would adapt her or his mechanics to avoid the painful position. The altered hand entry position in swimmers with painful shoulders is consistent with the significant decrease in muscle activity in the anterior and middle deltoids. In addition, the scapula does not need to be upwardly rotated nor retracted as much in this position. Accordingly, there is significantly less activity in the upper trapezius and rhomboids.

Mid–Pull-through

During mid–pull-through, the most dramatic significant differences in muscle activity are noted. The serratus anterior reveals a drop in muscle activity while the rhomboids increase their activity (24). Quite likely, the serratus anterior fatigues in swimmers with painful shoulders, producing a "floating" scapula. To compensate, the rhomboids contract to stabilize the scapula. It is of interest that these two muscles are antagonists. When the serratus anterior cannot perform, there is no muscle that can assist by doing a similar action. The only way the body can stabilize the scapula is to call upon antagonistic muscles, the rhomboids, which attempt to substitute for a deficient serratus anterior. Thus, the optimum synchrony of firing seen in normal scapular rotation is disturbed at the time of propulsion.

The swimmer with shoulder pain may also exhibit excessive body roll throughout pull-through. This may be leading up to an early hand exit. Because the hand exit in the normal swimmer entails a large degree of humeral internal rotation (which is painful), the swimmer with shoulder pathology may compensate by exiting the hand before that point. One way to facilitate an early hand exit is to have excessive body roll toward the side of the hand exit. As the body rolls to that side, the hand is able to come out of the water. Usually this happens shortly after the hand passes the umbilicus. Because the most propulsive portion of the stroke is after that point, quite a bit of power can also be lost.

The altered muscle action in the swimmer with painful shoulders supports the point of decreased internal rotation at an early hand exit. The infraspinatus demonstrates significantly more activity in the painful shoulders as it externally rotates the humerus.

Recovery

As the swimmer with a painful shoulder demonstrates an early hand exit with decreased internal rotation, the elbow is also dropped. The dropped elbow (decreased internal rotation) is carried through for all of recovery. Even as the hand enters the water in a wider position, the elbow is dropped. Once again, coaches note this as dropped elbow. By keeping the arm lower and shortening the arc of motion, these swimmers avoid the painful impingement.

Likewise, the altered muscle activity in the swimmer with the painful shoulder suggests the dropped elbow.

As the hand exits the water, the anterior deltoid shows significantly less activity (24) as the lifting, abducting, and forward flexing of the humerus is blunted. There is also diminished activity in the subscapularis at mid recovery. In that the subscapularis puts the arm in the painful position of internal rotation, it is understandable that it would decrease its activity as the elbow drops and the arm avoids the extreme of internal rotation. Also, as with the serratus anterior, the subscapularis muscle activity stays above 20% of its maximum in normal shoulders throughout the stroke. This would suggest its vulnerability to fatigue. So, the diminished activity in recovery may be a response to fatigue.

A summary of the normal mechanics, pathologic mechanics, and anatomic pathology in the freestyle swimmer can be found in Fig. 31.16.

Anatomy of Pathology

Sixty-six percent of elite swimmers report shoulder pain (15). As with the pitcher, part of the blame lies with microtrauma (a distance swimmer will have approximately 16,000 shoulder revolutions per week) (15) and part with the mechanics.

Over half of the swimmers with shoulder pain report the pain during early pull-through (EF Ekman, MM Pink, FW Jobe, et al., unpublished data). More specifically, 30% of swimmers with shoulder pain report pain just before mid–pull-through (Fig. 31.17). Using the compensatory mechanics of a wider hand entry and an early hand exit diminishes the pain that is otherwise found at hand entry and hand exit. With compensation, the reported prevalence of pain at hand entry and exit is relatively low (less than 5%). Thus, it can be summarized that three points of concern in the freestyle swimmer

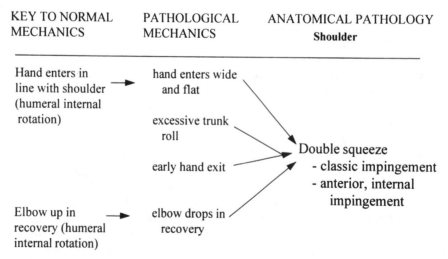

KEY TO NORMAL MECHANICS   PATHOLOGICAL MECHANICS   ANATOMICAL PATHOLOGY
                                                             Shoulder

Hand enters in line with shoulder (humeral internal rotation) → hand enters wide and flat

excessive trunk roll

early hand exit

Elbow up in recovery (humeral internal rotation) → elbow drops in recovery

Double squeeze
 - classic impingement
 - anterior, internal impingement

FIG. 31.16. Summary of the freestyle swimmer.

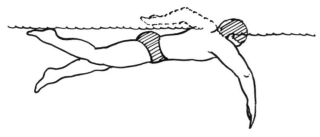

FIG. 31.17. Most painful phase of the freestyle stroke in swimmers with shoulder pain.

are hand entry, just before mid–pull-through, and hand exit. At each of these three points, the humerus is in an extreme degree of internal rotation. Once again, this is in direct contrast to the baseball pitcher whose vulnerability is at a point of maximal external rotation.

In the swimmer with a normal shoulder, the arm is in a position very similar to the Neer test at hand entry. A study was performed with cadaver limbs (AL Valadie, unpublished data) fixed in the Neer test position and cross-sections taken. All specimens demonstrated bursal surface soft tissue contact with the medial acromion and articular surface contact with the anterosuperior glenoid rim (Fig. 31.18). As the swimmer with shoulder pain widens the hand entry, this irritation is avoided.

A swimmer with a painful shoulder is not able to mechanically compensate just before mid–pull-through. A cadaver study similar to the one just mentioned was performed with the limb fixed in a position just before mid–pull-through (EF Ekman, unpublished data). The contact of the cuff tendons was similar to that demonstrated in the Neer test with both bursal articular surface contact (Fig. 31.19). At this time, there has not been a study done positioning the cadaver limb in the position

of hand exit. Thus, no conclusions can be reached as to the anatomic structures involved.

Based on available data, it appears that the swimmer's shoulder may get the "double squeeze" (i.e., both the classic impingement of the external surface and internal impingement on the anterosuperior glenoid rim). This is in contrast to the baseball pitcher who is vulnerable to impingement of the posterosuperior glenoid rim.

In a separate study, 175 competitive swimmer were examined for signs of shoulder instability (25). Less than 5% of the swimmers demonstrated anterior, inferior, or posterior instability. This also is in contrast to pitchers who tend to demonstrate anterior instability that lead to their type of injury.

GOLFER

Mechanics

The golfer is not a true overhead athlete because the shoulders are not elevated beyond 90 degrees. The club head is over the head, and the illusion of an "overhead" athlete is left. The phases of the golf swing are found in Fig. 31.20. The golfer is discussed as a right-handed golfer.

Takeaway

The takeaway phase is initiated by a sequence of movements beginning with the hands, followed by the arms, then shoulder girdle, the trunk, and finally the pelvic girdle. This sequence is subtle because the motions follow one another very quickly and can look to be almost simultaneous. The shoulder girdle is always ahead of the pelvic girdle as they turn. The pelvic girdle does not begin to rotate until the hands reach the level of the

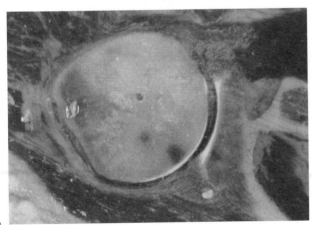
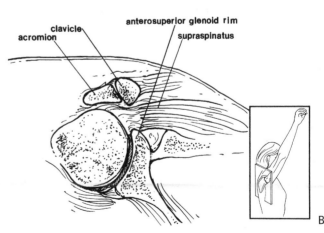

FIG. 31.18. During the Neer test for impingement there is bursal surface soft tissue contact with the medial acromion and articular surface contact with the anterosuperior glenoid. **A:** Photograph of specimen. **B:** Schematic drawing of specimen.

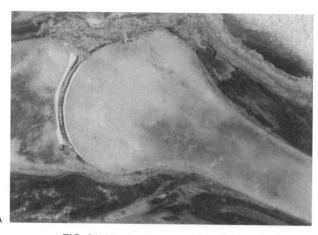

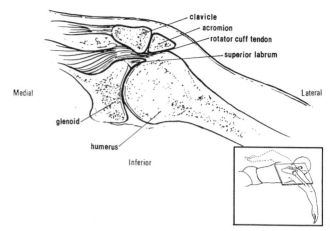

FIG. 31.19. Just before mid–pull-through, there is soft contact with both the bursal and articular surfaces. **A:** Photograph of specimen. **B:** Schematic drawing of specimen.

hips. As the pelvis begins to rotate, the left leg (the lead leg) begins to adduct and internally rotate.

Obviously, the real rotation in takeaway is in the trunk. At the top of takeaway, the golfer's back faces the direction of the flight of the ball. Very little anterior/posterior or side to side motion occurs. The head stays relatively still.

The shoulder girdle muscle activity during takeaway is that of scapular retraction and humeral external rotation in the right arm and the opposite in the left arm. In that the hands connect on the club, whatever action one arm takes, the other arm must reciprocally act. In the right arm, the three portions of the trapezius, the levator scapulae, and rhomboids are active as they retract and upwardly rotate the scapula. The infraspinatus is active as it assists with humeral external rotation. In the left arm, the primary activity is in the serratus anterior and subscapularis. These muscles are functioning to protract and upwardly rotate the scapula and internally rotate the humerus (26,27). At the end of takeaway, the left arm is in maximal horizontal adduction.

Downward Swing

Downward swing is initiated with pelvic girdle rotation. The muscle activity to start this motion is offered by the right hip extensors and adductors, along with the left adductor magnus. The left hamstrings are active as that limb accepts weight transfer on the flexed knee (28).

The pelvic girdle rotation sets up the reverse sequence from that which is present in takeaway. Trunk rotation follows that of the pelvic girdle, then the shoulder girdle, arms, and finally hands. Bilaterally, the abdominal obliques and erector spinae muscles are quite active for the trunk rotation (29). The scapular muscles are important in downward swing as they provide a stable base for the shoulder. The levator scapulae and rhomboids are quite active bilaterally at this time to stabilize the scapula. The left trapezius is also active (to retract the scapula) as is the right serratus anterior (to protract the scapula) (26). The subscapularis is active bilaterally as it holds the humerus in slight internal rotation. The pectoralis major and latissimus dorsi are also active at this time (27). This is similar to both the pitch and freestyle stroke in that they are the only upper extremity muscles that contribute power to the stroke (8).

Follow-through

Once contact is made with the ball (hopefully), the left arm begins to abduct and externally rotate while the right arm begins to horizontally adduct and internally rotate. This motion the mirror image of takeaway, and the muscle activity in the upper extremity likewise is a mirror image.

Pathologic Mechanics

If the pelvic girdle rotates too soon in takeaway, much power is lost. This is similar to the baseball pitcher who

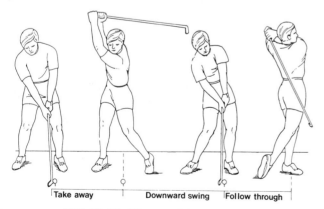

FIG. 31.20. Phases of the golf swing.

opens up too soon. If the golfer rotates the pelvic girdle too soon, the issue may simply be a bad habit, or it may be because of a limitation in trunk rotation. A trunk rotation limitation may be due to skeletal or muscular limitations or due to pain. In either case, the golfer may attempt to compensate for the lack of trunk rotation with either excessive or early pelvic or shoulder girdle motion.

It is during the top of takeaway or the top of follow-through that the shoulder is at most risk for injury. If a golfer demonstrates an excessively large arc or if there is a lack of trunk rotation with the arm compensating to give the golfer an average arc, there is potential for shoulder problems.

During downswing and follow-through, there is a risk of injury if the scapular muscles are weak. As aforementioned, the scapular muscles form a stable base from which the arms can move. If they are weak, asynchronous scapulohumeral rhythm occurs with almost certain ensuing injury.

Anatomy of Pathology

Professional golfers have a much lower incidence of injury than do professional pitchers or elite swimmers. This can be attributed to the lesser degree of humeral elevation and rotation that the sport requires (i.e., golf is not a true overhead sport). During 5 years of data collection on the Senior PGA Tour, only 98 new injuries to the shoulder were reported (Centinela Hospital Medical Center, unpublished data). These 98 injuries were less than 8% of the total reported injuries. The typical shoulder injury in the golfer is in the lead arm (the left arm in the right-handed golfer).

Overuse, however, is one of the risk factors in golf. A professional golfer may perform 2,000 or more shoulder revolutions per week. The toll that overuse takes on the shoulder is also evident in the injury database of the Senior PGA Tour. Eighty-eight percent of the injuries were classified as a "strain" and 9% as a "sprain." By definition, strain infers that the underlying problem is in the muscle and sprain infers it is in the ligament. When combining these two tissues, 97% of the shoulder injuries are thus accounted. And overuse is the etiology of most muscular and ligamentous injury.

In that the shoulder in golf is not at risk for catastrophic (macrotrauma) injury, such as that found in some overhead sports, people can play the sport well into their later years. An analogy would be to recognize that there is a Senior PGA Tour but not a senior baseball league. Because people can play the sport for life, overuse takes on an added dimension of longevity. Not only are there weekly repetitions, but the wear and tear goes on for years. Because of this longevity, factors related to aging need to be considered along with overuse.

Around the age of 35 years, the degenerative aging process can begin to be seen in the shoulder. Typically, one can find a compromise of the subacromial space, scar tissue, spur formation, cuff thinning, and probably a decreased vascular supply (30–34). In that the swing puts stress on the acromioclavicular joint, this is one of the first areas where injury occurs. The repetitious positioning of the arm across the body causes spur formation under the acromioclavicular joint, impingement of the rotator cuff on spurs, and bursal-sided partial cuff tears. Also, flexibility and resiliency of the tissue tends to decrease. Arthritic changes and degenerative breakdown begin to appear. Eventually, range of motion diminishes. Any one of these factors can cause shoulder problems in the golfer, and, unfortunately, the factors usually come in multiples.

The younger golfer (under the age of 35 years) may be more unstable. Although not a rule, some golfers do exhibit hyperlaxity. Laxity in and of itself is not pathologic; it simply notes loose ligaments (35). Yet those individuals with laxity may be at risk to develop instability (symptomatic laxity). The instability, in combination with numerous repetitions, can lead to stretched connective tissue with resultant deformation of the capsule, ligaments and labrum, and internal impingement.

The individual golfer's mechanics also give clues to potential injury. At the top of an exaggerated takeaway, a golfer may complain of anterior joint line pain in the lead (left) arm. This may be indicative of impingement of the humeral head against the anterior labrum (Fig. 31.21).

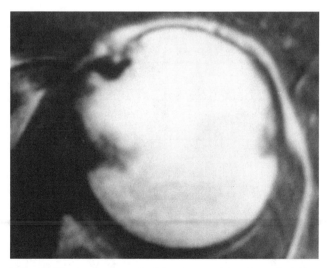

FIG. 31.21. Impingement of the humeral head against the anterior and posterior labrum. (From Jobe FW, Pink MM. Shoulder pain in golf. *Clin Sports Med* 1996;15:57, with permission.)

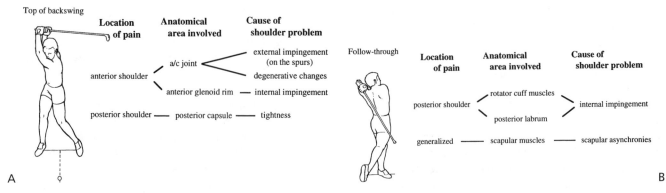

FIG. 31.22. Shoulder injuries in the lead arm during the golf swing. **A:** Top of backswing. **B:** Follow-through. (From Jobe FW, Pink MM. Shoulder pain in golf. *Clin Sports Med* 1996;15:62, with permission.)

At the top of follow-through, the humerus is abducted with some external rotation. An exaggerated follow-through can leave the golfer vulnerable to posterior labral damage in the lead arm (Fig. 31.21). The velocity and weight of the club yields high forces that could injure the joint. Also, the undersurface of the posterior rotator cuff muscles can become pinched on the labrum, which would result in undersurface fraying.

An algorithm is presented in Fig. 31.22 to summarize the potential for shoulder injuries in golfers. Although finite, this algorithm of golf mechanics gives clues to the etiology of some shoulder problems in golfers.

SUMMARY

The overhead athlete is an evolution and is in evolution. The concept of the overhead athlete began with the baseball pitcher and had been extrapolated to fit all athletes who participated in sports that require humeral elevation. We now know, though, that each sport has

Sport and Vulnerable Phase	Vulnerable Scapulohumeral Mechanics		Overhead? (humeral elevation above 90°)	Relationship of Injury and Instability?	Site of Impingement
	Elevation	Rotation			
Pitcher 1. Late Cocking	Coronal plane abduction	Maximal external	Yes	Yes	Posterosuperior, internal
Freestyle Swimmer 1. Hand entry	1. Flexion	1. Internal	1. Yes	1. No	1 & 2. Double squeeze - Anterosuperior & internal - Classic, external
2. Prior to mid pull-through	2. Flexion	2. Internal	2. No	2. No	
3. Hand exit	3. Extension	3. Internal	3. No	3. No	3. ?
Golfer (lead arm) 1. Top of takeaway	1. Horizontal adduction	1. Internal	1. No	1. No	1a. Anterior, internal b. Classic, external
2. Swing	2. Scapular asynchrony	2. Scapular asynchrony	2. No	2. No	2. Classic, external
3. Top of follow-through	3. Coronal plane abduction	3. External	3. No	3. No	3. Posterior, internal

FIG. 31.23. Summary of impingement characteristics in the pitcher, freestyle swimmer, and golfer.

unique mechanics that leave the athlete vulnerable to specific injuries (Fig. 31.23).

A clinician must understand the mechanics of the sport to acknowledge subtle symptoms of dysfunction, to accurately diagnose, and to optimally treat the injury. Our knowledge is not yet complete. With future research and a sharpening of the clinician's eye, the concept of the overhead athlete will continue to evolve.

REFERENCES

1. DiGiovine N, Jobe FW, Pink M, et al. An electromyographic analysis of the upper extremity in pitching. *J Shoulder Elbow Surg* 1992;1:15–25.
2. Feltner M, Dapena J. Dynamics of the shoulder and elbow joints of the throwing arms during a baseball pitch. *Int J Sports Biomech* 1986;2:235–259.
3. Inman VT, Saunders JBDeCM, Abbott LC. Observations on the function of the shoulder joint. *J Bone Joint Surg Am* 1944; 26A:1–30.
4. Moseley JB, Jobe FW, Pink M, et al. EMG analysis of the scapular muscles during a shoulder rehabilitation program. *Am J Sports Med* 1992;20:128–134.
5. Turkel SJ, Panio MW, Marshall JL, et al. Stabilizing mechanisms preventing anterior dislocation of the glenohumeral joint. *J Bone Joint Surg Am* 1981;63A:1208–1217.
6. Gainor BJ, Piotrowski G, Puhl J, et al. The throw: biomechanics and acute injury. *Am J Sports Med* 1980;8:114–118.
7. Pappas AM, Zawacki RM, Sullivan TJ. Biomechanics of baseball pitching: a preliminary report. *Am J Sports Med* 1985;13:216–222.
8. Bartlett LR, Storey MD, Simons BD. Measurement of upper extremity torque production and its relationship to throwing speed in the competitive athlete. *Am J Sports Med* 1989;17:89–91.
9. Glousman RE, Jobe FW, Tibone J, et al. Dynamic electromyographic analysis of the throwing shoulder with glenohumeral instability. *J Bone Joint Surg Am* 1988;70A:220–226.
10. Jobe FW, Nuber G. Throwing injuries of the elbow. *Clin Sports Med* 1986;5:621–636.
11. Tullos HS, King JW. Throwing mechanism in sports. *Orthop Clin North Am* 1973;4:709–720.
12. Davidson PA, Pink M, Perry J, et al. Functional anatomy of the flexor pronator muscle group in relation to the medial collateral ligament of the elbow. *Am J Sports Med* 1995;23:245–249.
13. Browne AO, Hoffmeyer P, Tanaka S, et al. Glenohumeral elevation studied in three dimensions. *J Bone Joint Surg Br* 1990; 72B:843–845.
14. Ferrari DA. Capsular ligaments of the shoulder: anatomical and functional study of the anterior superior capsule. *Am J Sports Med* 1990;18:20–24.
15. Johnson D. In swimming, shoulder the burden. *Sportcare Fitness* May/June 1988;24–30.
16. Walch G, Boileau P, Noel E, et al. of the deep surface of the supraspinatus tendon on the posterosuperior glenoid rim: an arthroscopic study. *J Shoulder Elbow Surg* 1992;1:238–245.
17. Jobe CM, Pink MM, Jobe FW, et al. Anterior shoulder instability, impingement, and rotator cuff tear: theories and concepts. In: Jobe FW, ed. *Operative techniques in upper extremity sports injuries.* St. Louis: Mosby-Year Book, 1996:164–176.
18. Davidson DA, Elattrache NS, Jobe CM, et al. Rotator cuff and posterior-superior glenoid labrum injury associated with increased glenohumeral motion: A new site of impingement. *J Shoulder Elbow Surg* 1995;4:384–390.
19. Neer CS II. Anterior acromioplasty for the chronic impingement syndrome in the shoulder: a preliminary report. *J Bone Joint Surg Am* 1972;54A:41–50.
20. Maglischo EW. *Swimming faster.* Mountain View, CA: Mayfield Publishing Company, 1982:53–59.
21. Pink M, Perry J, Browne A, et al. The normal freestyle swimming: An electromyographic and cinematographic analysis of twelve muscles. *Am J Sports Med* 1991;19:569–576.
22. Monad H. Contractility of muscle during prolonged static and repetitive dynamic activity. *Ergonomics* 1895;28:81–89.
23. Neer CS, Welsh RP. The shoulder in sports. *Orthop Clin North Am* 1977;8:583–591.
24. Scovazzo ML, Browne A, Pink M, et al. The painful shoulder during freestyle swimming: an electromyographic and cinematographic analysis of twelve muscles. *Am J Sports Med* 1991;19: 577–582.
25. Pink MM, Jobe FW. Biomechanics of swimming. In: Zachazewski JE, Magee DJ, Quillen WS, eds. *Athletic injuries and rehabilitation.* Philadelphia: W.B. Saunders, 1996:317–331.
26. Kao JT, Pink M, Jobe FW, et al. Electromyographic analysis of the scapular muscles during a golf swing. *Am J Sports Med* 1995;23:19–23.
27. Pink M, Jobe FW, Perry J. Electromyographic analysis of the shoulder during the golf swing. *Am J Sports Med* 1990;18:137–140.
28. Bechler JR, Jobe FW, Pink M, et al. Electromyographic analysis of the hip and knee during the golf swing. *Clin J Sport Med* 1995;5:162–166.
29. Pink M, Perry J, Jobe FW. Electromyographic analysis of the trunk in golfers. *Am J Sports Med* 1993;21:385–388.
30. Brewer BJ. Aging of the rotator cuff. *Am J Sports Med* 1979;7:102–110.
31. Kessel L. *Clinical disorders of the shoulder.* Edinburgh: Churchill Livingstone, 1982.
32. Loehr JF, Uhthoff HK. The pathogenesis of degenerative rotator cuff tears. *Orthop Trans* 1987;11:237.
33. Ogata S, Uhthoff HK. Acromial enthesopathy and rotator cuff tear: A radiologic and histologic postmortem investigation of the coracoacromial arch. *Clin Orthop* 1990;254:39–48.
34. Uhthoff HK, Sarkar K. Classification and definition of tendinopathies. *Clin Sports Med* 1991;10:707–720.
35. Pink M, Jobe FW, Kvitne RS, et al. Joint laxity, shoulder range of motion and clinical signs of shoulder pathology in swimmer. Presented to the VII International Symposium on Biomechanics and Medicine in Swimming, Atlanta, October 22, 1994.

PART IV

Lower Extremity

Principles and Practice of Orthopaedic Sports Medicine,
edited by William E. Garrett, Jr., Kevin P. Speer, and Donald T. Kirkendall.
Lippincott Williams & Wilkins, Philadelphia © 2000.

CHAPTER 32

Hip Injuries in Sports: Evaluation and Treatment of the Painful Hip

Thomas Parker Vail and Diane Beal Covington

Although injuries to the hip are most frequently minor, the spectrum of injury to the hip in sports also includes career-ending and medically devastating conditions. Thus, the early recognition and anatomic diagnosis of injury to the hip is important not only to avoid detrimental effects on sports performance, but also to minimize the long-term medical consequences of certain injuries. Injuries to the hip in sports are relatively uncommon in incidence, with most injuries self-limiting and minor, having only transient symptoms. For example, in a survey of runners, hip injuries accounted for less than 5% of the overall injuries (1). Hip injuries can present with symptoms such as recurrent or persistent pain, limitation in range of motion, or simply decreased athletic performance due to diminished hip girdle muscle strength. The goal in treating hip injuries is the early recognition and treatment of both minor problems such as bursitis and major problems such as a stress fracture, resulting in the timely return to sports without any residual long-term effect of the injury.

The mechanism of injury to the hip can depend on a variety of factors, such as the amount of repetition in the training program and the potential for high impact injury in a particular sport. Both overuse activity patterns and acute injuries can lead to symptoms attributable to the hip. For adults, overuse injuries can affect both the bony anatomy and the soft tissue structures surrounding the hip, including muscle, ligament, and cartilage structures. Occasionally, symptoms of hip pain can stem from an underlying condition such as osteoarthritis, combined with overuse. Conversely, it has been

suggested that some athletic activities are linked with an increased incidence of arthritis (2,3). Although injuries such as fractures, dislocations, and ligament tears caused by high-impact collisions or falls present distinctly, overuse injuries can present insidiously with vague complaints and nonlocalized physical findings. After consideration of the clinical history and mechanism of injury, the next important information leading to effective treatment relates to the physical condition, the age, and the specific characteristics of the individual patient.

When considering different mechanisms and presentations of hip injury, the age of the patient is crucially important. Adolescent athletes have unique problems associated with open growth plates and apophyses that must be considered in both acute and chronic conditions. Older patients may have additional considerations such as osteoporosis, calcium pyrophosphate disorder, and other underlying mild degenerative conditions. In any age group, regardless of the pathomechanism, the physician must rule out referred sources of pain when possible. For example, it is not uncommon for a child with hip pathology to present with knee pain in conditions ranging from pyarthrosis of the hip to an acutely slipped proximal capital physis. Careful physical examination will lead the physician to the hip problem. In the end, it is the anatomic diagnosis that guides the treatment plan.

The physical evaluation of the painful hip requires careful consideration of a dense collection of anatomic structures locally and distant anatomic structures that can refer pain to the hip. A differential diagnosis of conditions that can cause symptoms referred to the hip area includes degenerative conditions of the lumbar spine, such as facet arthrosis, and disk degeneration, which can cause referred pain to the buttock (Table 32.1). Stenosis of the spinal canal may present with a more symmetric pattern of radiating pain in both but-

T. Parker Vail and D. Beal Covington: Division of Orthopaedic Surgery, Duke University Medical Center, Durham, North Carolina 27710.

TABLE 32.1. *Differential diagnosis of referred hip pain*

Degenerative conditions of the lumbar spine
  Facet arthrosis
  Disk degeneration
  Stenosis
Acute disk herniation
Degenerative and inflammatory sacroiliac conditions
Peripheral nerve entrapment
  Cluneal
  Lateral femoral cutaneous
  Femoral
Intrapelvic genitourinary and gastrointestinal pathology
Lower abdominal hernias

tocks. Acute disk herniation can lead to pain in the buttock, pain radiating down the outer aspect of the thigh and leg, gluteal atrophy, and occasionally sensory changes and other neurologic findings that may be present either with or without back pain.

Degenerative and inflammatory conditions of the sacroiliac joint can also cause pain in the buttock area. Several peripheral nerve entrapment syndromes have also been implicated in hip pain. These syndromes include cluneal nerve entrapment where the cluneal nerves travel over the posterior iliac crest, penetrating the enveloping fascia, and entrapment or contusion of the lateral femoral cutaneous nerve as it pierces the fascia of the sartorius muscle and travels laterally. Intrapelvic pathology can also cause referred pain due to the developmental migration of genital organs from the inner pelvis through the inguinal canal. In males, these structures include the spermatic cord, the genitofemoral nerve, and the testes. In females, the round ligament and the genitofemoral nerve course in the inguinal canal. Ovarian cysts, inflammatory conditions, and infections of the genitourinary tract can cause pain in the groin. Lower abdominal fascial defects can lead to direct and indirect hernias, causing pain in the inguinal or pubic area.

This chapter focuses on the musculoskeletal conditions leading to a painful hip in athletic individuals. Hip pathology seen in athletes can be separated into a few general mechanistic categories: overuse injuries, including stress fractures, osteitis pubis, clicking hip (including acetabular labral injury), and bursitis; acute trauma, including fracture, hip pointer (hematoma), subluxation, dislocation, contusion, muscle avulsion; and growth-related problems caused by sports such as apophysitis, epiphyseal, and physeal injuries.

OVERUSE INJURIES

Stress Fractures

Stress fractures of the femoral neck and pubic rami are relatively well-recognized injuries that seem to have a higher incidence in women and especially in runners (4–6). Although the exact incidence is not available, femoral stress fractures are reported as the least commonly occurring stress fracture in most series (7). Nevertheless, the diagnosis and early treatment of the femoral neck stress fracture is critical to avoid the devastating complications of displacement, delayed union, and avascular necrosis that can come with delayed intervention (8). The clinical presentation of a femoral neck stress fracture can be vague. Athletic pubalgia (9), intraarticular derangement (chondral injury, labral injury, loose body), and arthritis should be considered in the differential diagnosis of unilateral anterior hip pain.

Mechanism of Injury

The mechanism of injury is debated; however, like most stress fractures it is thought to be due to trabecular fatigue failure secondary to repetitive loading. Within the broad category of stress fractures, the pathomechanism can be divided into fatigue fractures, insufficiency fractures, and fractures that may have a combined mechanism (10). In a fatigue fracture, the repetitive stress on the femoral neck exceeds the ability of the stressed bone to remodel appropriately, leading to trabecular failure. The implication is that an unfamiliar or possibly excessive and repeated load is applied to normal bone. In contrast, in an insufficiency fracture, the bone fails because of an inherent weakness in the structure of the bone, such as in osteopenia from metabolic causes. Clearly, many clinical situations include a combination of risk factors from both the fatigue and insufficiency mechanism. In athletes, particularly females, the potential for a stress fracture may be increased in the presence of the triad of osteopenia related to an improperly balanced diet or altered hormonal balance. This clinical triad has been reported in some female runners (11,12). In light of these observations, this risk of stress fracture can be minimized by shock-absorbing footwear, cross-training, and attention to general health and nutrition, including eating habits (13).

The clinical evaluation of the hip requires a high index of suspicion in a patient presenting with groin pain and possibly some limitation in the range of movement of the hip. As with all activity-related complaints, the trend over time is important to note. In particular, a pain first noted to be present during training and later is present at rest requires explanation and intervention. Initially, the patient with a developing stress fracture may not limp and may not experience symptoms when not training. Later in the progression of the fracture, the symptoms can be persistent at rest. However, rest pain may not be present until the fracture is displaced, clearly dictating that further investigation of activity-related groin or hip pain is carried out before symptoms progress to minimize the chances for fracture displacement.

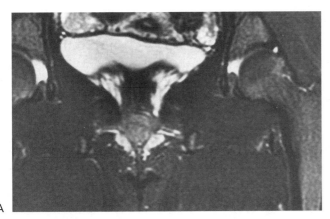 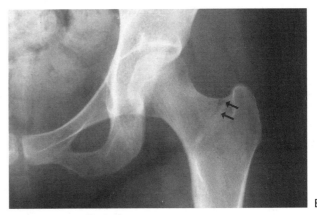

FIG. 32.1. A: Magnetic resonance image demonstrating a stress fracture of the medial femoral neck. **B:** The *arrows* indicate a stress fracture of the superior aspect of the femoral neck.

The first line of evaluation is the physical examination, which isolates the subjective and objective findings to the groin or anterior thigh area. Next, the evaluation continues with standard radiographs showing the femoral neck in two planes.

Imaging

The standard biplanar radiographs include a low anteroposterior view of the pelvis and a gentle "frog-leg" lateral, allowing scrutiny of the trabecular architecture in the femoral neck and comparison with the opposite hip. It is often difficult to diagnosis a stress fracture on radiographs because of the subtlety or nonexistence of visible findings on regular radiographs. The presence of the physeal scar and vascular channels can make interpretation of the films difficult (13–15). If the diagnosis remains unresolved after initial radiographic evaluation, regional bone scan or computed tomography (CT) can be considered. The bone scan may show increased uptake in the femoral neck, and a high-resolution CT done with thin cuts through the femoral neck may more clearly define abnormalities in the local trabecular architecture. However, the accuracy of the bone scan in identifying femoral neck stress fracture has been reported to be as low as 68% (16). A magnetic resonance imaging (MRI) study is most sensitive and specific and will allow early visualization of marrow changes in the femoral neck and head, allowing distinction to be made between injury to the femoral neck and other pathologic conditions of the femoral head such as avascular necrosis and transient regional osteoporosis (16,17) (Fig. 32.1A).

Treatment

Some attempts have been made to create algorithms for treatment of femoral neck stress fractures based on the radiographic and MRI appearance of the lesion within the femoral neck (10,18,19). The algorithm is based on distinguishing between a "tension side" and a "compression side" injury. A tension side injury occurs when there is a cortical separation or callus formation on the superior aspect of the femoral neck (Fig. 32.1B). A compression side injury presents with increased bone density on the inferior, or compression, side of the femoral neck. Compression side injuries that involve less that 50% of the femoral neck may be treated with 4 to 6 weeks of crutch walking and non-weight bearing. Compression side injuries with greater than 50% femoral neck involvement or tension side injuries are generally treated with internal fixation (10).

A displaced fracture of the femoral neck in a young active person is a true surgical emergency, with the main consideration being early minimally invasive surgical stabilization. Early stabilization is critically important to decrease the possibility of nonunion and avascular necrosis. A nondisplaced fracture can be fixed with percutaneously placed cannulated screws that travel from just above the metadiaphyseal junction of the proximal femur into the subchondral bone of the femoral head. Care must be taken to avoid penetration of the joint space with either the guide pins for the cannulated screws or the screws themselves, which can increase the chances for development of chondrolysis. Initial treatment while the diagnosis is in question should include protected ambulation with crutches.

Expected Outcome

Uncomplicated internal fixation of a nondisplaced stress fracture of the femoral neck is most frequently associated with a good result after pinning and 6 weeks of crutch ambulation. In this ideal scenario, the incidence of avascular necrosis of the hip or nonunion of the fracture are both below 10%. Completely displaced fractures can be associated with nonunion and avascular necrosis rates of up to 25% to 30%. In contrast to fatigue fracture, high-energy trauma and insufficiency fracture may predispose to the development of osteonecrosis. In a recent review of 26 patients under the age of 50 referred to a specialty clinic for treatment of symptomatic osteonecrosis of the hip, 15% had developed osteonecrosis as a complication of a stress fracture of the femoral neck (20).

In summary, a healthy patient presenting with unremitting groin or anterior thigh pain and a history of overuse will get a thorough physical examination and standard radiographic evaluation of the hip (usually a low anteroposterior radiograph of the pelvis and an orthogonal plane lateral radiograph of the affected hip and proximal femur). If the diagnosis remains unclear, we most frequently then move to an MRI evaluation to rule out stress fracture. If stress fracture is diagnosed, expeditious surgical treatment with percutaneous cannulated screws is undertaken. The patient will remain on touch-down weight-bearing restriction for 6 weeks. Rehabilitation will then begin with restoration of active and passive range of motion, followed by strengthening, and finally agility and endurance training. Regular running is not reinstituted for a minimum of 3 months.

Clicking or Snapping Hip

Confusion regarding the epidemiology of the snapping hip centers around the variety of structures in the periarticular and intraarticular anatomy that can snap, presumably causing pain. An entity called the snapping hip was first described by Binnie in 1913 (21). There were additional case reports over the following years describing the snapping hip as a periarticular process, external to the hip joint capsule. Nunziata and Blumenfeld (21) were the first to report the snapping hip as an internal or intraarticular phenomenon. The intraarticular process was described by Quirk (22) as being unique to dancers due to excessive turnout, although this problem has subsequently been noted in runners, cheerleaders, triathletes, and other recreational athletes. The reality is that the snapping hip can be caused by a variety of structures both intraarticular, such as the acetabular labrum, the chondral surface, and the osteochondral surface, and extraarticular. The most frequently cited extraarticular anatomic structures implicated in snapping include the tensor fascia, the psoas tendon, and the piriformis tendon.

Mechanism of Injury

The pathologic process leading to intraarticular injury is poorly understood. Although chondral or cartilage injury within the hip joint stemming from trauma (such as dislocation of the hip, acetabular and pelvic fracture,

femoral shaft and proximal femur fracture) can be intuitively understood, the subacute and isolated presentation of these injuries requires further study. Treatable intraarticular injuries include chondral delamination, acetabular labral tears, and chondral and osteochondral loose bodies (23,24). Chondral delamination generally results from a degenerative process or injury, leading to separation between the chondral covering and the underlying bone at the histologic tidemark. There may be a relationship between the chondral delamination and bruising of the bone that has become more easily recognized with the increasing use of MRI. Other conditions leading to chondral or osteochondral separation include developmental disorders of the hip, such as Perthes disease, and developmental dysplasia, which lead to chondral surface fragmentation.

A chondral loose body is created when the delaminated cartilage fragment becomes loose within the joint (Fig. 32.2). Osteochondral loose bodies are less common, generally related to high-energy trauma or osteonecrosis. Unstable acetabular labral tears can displace and cause mechanical symptoms of pain, catching, and locking similar to a loose body within the joint. Only recently has the clinical presentation of tears in the acetabular labrum been described (24,25). The mechanism of injury to the labrum may be much like injury to the knee joint meniscus in that it is a combination of repetitive stress and degenerative change leading to mechanical symptoms. Indeed, labral injuries can look much like meniscus injuries, with radial, circumferential (bucket-handle), and horizontal patterns.

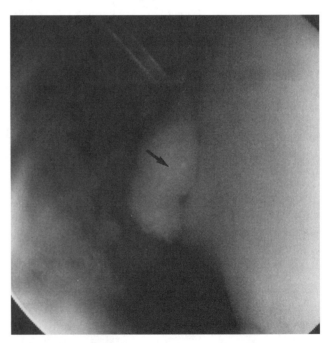

FIG. 32.2. Arthroscopic view of a chondral fragment is indicated by the *arrow.*

Certain pathoanatomy external to the hip joint can also cause clicking or snapping about the hip. Several of these entities are related to local bursal pathology, including the proximal iliotibial band and tensor fascia passing over the greater trochanteric bursa that has become thickened or inflamed from repetitive movement. Other structures that can snap include a tightened iliofemoral ligament passing over the femoral head (26) and the psoas tendon slipping over the iliopectineal eminence on the pubis (21). Other possible pathologic scenarios that have been described include anterior subluxation of the hip and stenosing tenosynovitis of the iliopsoas tendon (27).

Clinical Evaluation

Patients generally will complain of a snapping either in the anterior hip region or laterally over the greater trochanter, which may be palpable (and occasionally audible) during passive motion while supine or active movement while bearing weight. Pain, if present, is usually the result of repeated snapping (which may be voluntary and habitual), leading to local inflammation and swelling of the soft tissues (28). In the case of the numerous extraarticular entities described above, a weight-bearing examination is essential. The physician or trainer can simply place a hand over the trochanteric area while the patient walks and determine whether an external snap is present. It is also important to ask the patient to attempt to reproduce the snapping sensation. The greater trochanter may be tender to palpation when the patient is examined in the supine position if a concomitant bursitis exists.

Frequently, the symptoms of clicking or snapping are not reproducible on the examining table for either intra- or extraarticular causes of snapping. The examiner must rely on other indirect findings such as patient apprehension or positional pain. In the case of the labral tear, the pain can sometimes be provoked by flexion and internal rotation of the hip or the standing single-leg pivot test. Differential lidocaine injections, including intraarticular injection, can be very useful in separating pain eminating from one or more definable anatomic structures.

Imaging

Plain radiographs are usually unremarkable; however, further imaging may not be necessary if the physical examination reveals palpable pathology such as in the case of a snapping tensor fascia. When the diagnosis is elusive and the discomfort is persistent, an MRI can be helpful. Depending on the resolution of the MRI, some of the intraarticular pathology such as chondral lesions and labral lesions may not be visible, suspected only by the presence of a joint effusion. An MRI-arthrogram may be more sensitive in diagnosing specific intraarticular lesions. An MRI can also help to rule out osseous pathology such as osteonecrosis or early stress fracture. Increased MRI signal in the trochanteric bursa, the psoas bursa, or along the piriformis muscle can also lead to a diagnosis. Iliopsoas bursography with cineradiology, although probably no longer a first-line diagnostic modality, can show a sudden jerking motion of the iliopsoas tendon with flexion, abduction, and external rotation.

Treatment

Treatment of nearly all extraarticular inflammatory bursal conditions leading to snapping around the hip mentioned above should include a period of rest, avoidance of the habit of snapping the hip or provocative activities (if identified), and oral anti-inflammatory agents. Physical therapy may be instituted for instruction in a stretching program, particularly with the finding of a tight tensor fascia or a hip flexion contracture. If initial treatment fails, injection of corticosteroid into the trochanteric bursal area or lesser trochanteric area (depending on the source of the snapping) can alleviate symptoms in some patients. Surgical recession of a tight and painful tensor fascia, psoas tendon, or piriformis tendon is quite unusual and indicated only in the most resistant and problematic cases where the source of pain has been clearly identified.

Treatment of intraarticular pathology should also include the same initial medical management. When symptoms of pain, catching, or locking persist, minimally invasive surgery such as hip arthroscopy can be considered. Hip arthroscopy is technically demanding but frequently rewarding in the treatment of labral injury (29), chondral and osteochondral loose bodies, and other synovial conditions. Glick (30) and colleagues (31) were some of the first to describe the use of hip arthroscopy as a minimally invasive tool for hip joint assessment and intervention. Tools and techniques are being rapidly developed in this area to allow more facile access to this highly congruent and contoured joint. Presently, hip arthroscopy requires the use of some standard and some specialized arthroscopy equipment in combination with fluoroscopic imaging and joint distraction (Fig. 32.3). Surgery can be performed in the outpatient setting under regional anesthesia. Development of various joint portals has allowed access to most regions of the hip joint for chondral and articular debridement and removal of chondral debris, loose bodies, and degenerative surface lesions (32–34).

The acetabular rim, when normally developed, becomes horizontal or turns down slightly at its lateral edge. Because of this downward slope at the lateral edge, the arthroscopic cannula must take a corresponding upward course from the tip of the trochanter so that

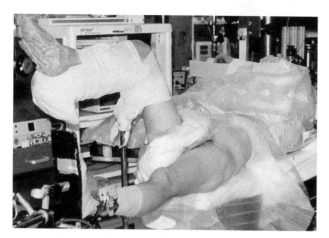

FIG. 32.3. Operative setup for hip arthroscopy.

it pierces the capsule parallel to the downward sloping acetabulum. One must keep in mind the normal anteversion of the femoral neck and acetabulum as well. The goal is to distend the joint and insert the instruments into the joint without scuffing the articular cartilage, while staying below the labrum. When inserting the arthroscopic instruments, the soft tissues at risk include the lateral femoral cutaneous nerve, femoral nerve and artery, and the sciatic nerve. The lateral femoral cutaneous nerve pierces the sartorius fascia below the inguinal ligament and lateral to the femoral vasculature. It is most at risk when creating the anterior portal. Joint distention and traction necessitate general or regional anesthesia.

Portals for hip arthroscopy have been described in anterior, posterior, and lateral positions. The most frequently used portals are the anterior and posterior lateral positions. These portals basically hug the anterior and posterior borders of the greater trochanter and aim the hip joint toward the area most frequently involved in pathology (anterolateral quadrant). The other most frequently used portal is the anterior portal that passes through the tensor–sartorius interval. Beyond these frequently used portals, others can be created around the circumference of the acetabulum depending on the location within the joint designated for access. If a low posterior portal is required, some have suggested a miniarthrotomy to avoid injury to the sciatic nerve. However, if adequate distention of the joint is achieved, a larger incision may not be required. Most work can be accomplished with the use of a standard 30-degree arthroscope, but on occasion a 70-degree scope is useful (Fig. 32.4).

Osteitis Pubis (Pubic Symphysitis)

Epidemiology

Osteitis pubis, inflammation of the symphysis pubis usually associated with erosion of one or both of the joint margins, was first described by Beer in 1924 after suprapubic surgery (35). It has also been reported to occur after prostatic, pelvic surgery, pregnancy, and trauma. Osteitis pubis has been reported as a sports-related phenomenon only in the last 25 years (36). Occurring more frequently in men than women, it has been associated

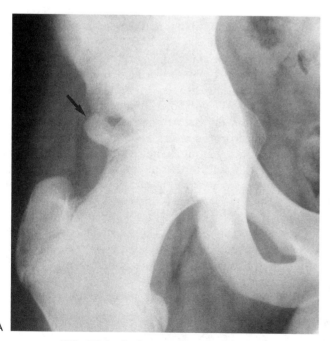

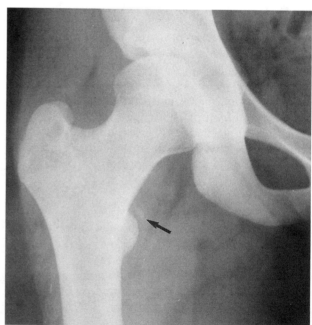

A   B

FIG. 32.4. A: An apophyseal separation of the anterior interior iliac spine is shown by the arrow.
B: The apophyseal separation of the lesser trochanter is shown by the *arrow*.

with soccer, rugby, wrestling, football, cycling, ice hockey, and tennis (37).

Clinical Evaluation

The mechanism of injury is that of repetitive minor trauma and chronic adductor and or gracilis strain, although a violent muscle contraction can result in an acute avulsion of the adductor origin and will have the same presenting symptoms (38). The presenting symptoms are commonly of pubic and adductor pain. Males may complain of scrotal pain, whereas females have perineal discomfort. There is frequently lower rectus pain as well. On physical examination, there is tenderness at the symphysis pubis, pubic rami, and pain with an adductor stretch. There may be decreased range of motion in one or both hips secondary to discomfort.

Imaging

Standard radiographic evaluation, including anteroposterior, inlet, and outlet views, may show cystic changes at one of the margins of the symphysis. Uncommonly, both sides of the pubis can be involved, and occasionally widening of the joint will be seen. Unilateral or bilateral sclerosis and symphyseal joint narrowing are sometimes features. Radiologic changes can be similar to or suggestive of tumor or infection (39). A separate bone avulsion fragment seen at the inferior aspect of the pubic symphysis can be present with adductor avulsion or enthesopathy. The presence of this fragment and associated symptoms of localized pain is referred to as the gracilis syndrome (40). Diagnosis can be confirmed by bone scan, with the finding of increased tracer uptake, particularly on the delayed views, at the inferior margin of the symphysis pubis.

Treatment

Initial treatment of pubic symphysitis consists of rest, with specific avoidance of the precipitating activity for a minimum of 6 weeks. Aerobic fitness can be maintained by alternative exercise methods. Nonsteroidal anti-inflammatory drugs (NSAIDs) are used in the early phase of treatment as well. If a satisfactory diminution of symptoms is not achieved with rest and oral medication, a local injection of corticosteroid may be considered.

Rehabilitation should be aimed at maintenance of aerobic fitness initially. Stretching and strengthening of the hip adductors should be instituted once symptoms are controlled. Specific avoidance of forceful cross-body lower extremity movement, such as lateral soccer ball movement or martial arts kicks, can hasten recovery. Referral to an orthopedic surgeon should be considered when symptoms persist despite adherence to conserva-

tive treatment for 6 weeks or if the diagnosis is in question. Surgical exploration for excision of a bony fragment and local inflammatory granulation tissue is indicated in very rare refractory cases (26). As symptoms diminish, a gradual return to preinjury activities can be expected within 6 to 12 weeks. Radiographic findings are not expected to resolve, even with successful cessation of pain.

Bursitis

Epidemiology

Inflammation of the bursa can be a chronic or acute condition resulting in significant disability for the athlete. There are several bursae located about the hip and pelvis; however, the trochanteric bursa is of most clinical significance. Nontraumatic trochanteric bursitis is most commonly seen in runners, whereas traumatic bursitis is associated with sports that involve direct contact on hard surfaces such as volleyball.

Clinical Evaluation

The development of bursitis is most commonly related to overuse, such as in runners who consistently train on the same side of the road and suffer detrimental effects of the downward camber of the road. Trochanteric bursitis can be also acute with either a fall onto the trochanter or a blow directly to the area, resulting in a hemobursa (41). Repetitive snapping of the tensor fascia over the prominent greater trochanter, with the trochanteric bursa wedged between these two structures, can lead to further inflammation of the bursa.

Patients with trochanteric bursitis usually describe fairly well-localized discomfort in the region of the greater trochanter that is made worse by lying on their affected side. Pain will sometimes be described as radiating into the lateral thigh with activity. On clinical examination there is tenderness to palpation over the greater trochanter. Symptoms are usually worsened with forced stretching of the iliotibial band. Injection of the affected bursa with marcaine is helpful as a diagnostic adjunct. In the case of inflammation of the psoas bursa, symptoms of pain in the groin are present with passive hip extension or resisted flexion. For patients with a wider pelvis or a high degree of physiologic genu valgus or varus, heel wedges can provide balance and increased normalization of pressure over the joint line at the knee.

Imaging

Routine radiographs are helpful in eliminating underlying osseous abnormalities and are usually normal. MRI is the technique of choice in evaluating bursae and other soft tissue structures but generally is not necessary when the physical examination allows anatomic localization of the complaints (17).

Treatment

Nontraumatic trochanteric bursitis is managed with rest by avoiding aggravating activities, NSAIDs, and change in running surface. If symptoms persist, injection of the bursa with a corticosteroid is indicated. Surgical excision is possible and warranted in only the most extreme situations. Physical therapy may be beneficial with modalities such as ice, ionto, or phonophoresis. Once symptoms are under control, a stretching and strengthening program should be instituted.

Traumatic hemobursa usually requires compression, icing, and rest. In the case of a large collection of blood in the bursa with palpable fluctuance or local pain attributable to soft tissue tension, aspiration may be indicated.

The expected outcome is complete return to sports after several weeks of resting, icing, stretching, and NSAIDs. Occasionally, symptoms can be more chronic and should be treated similarly to a chronic muscle strain of the associated muscle–tendon unit.

ACUTE CONDITIONS

Infection

An infection superficial to the hip joint can arise as a secondary complication of a hematoma or hip pointer. In the event of a puncture wound to the skin with an associated subcutaneous hematoma, it is wise to consider antibiotic prophylaxis with a broad-spectrum oral agent or even surgical irrigation and debridement of the hematoma if gross bacterial contamination is suspected. Other bacterial, viral, and fungal infection distally in the lower extremity, such as tinea pedis, can cause groin discomfort with associated inguinal lymphadenopathy.

Pyarthrosis of the hip and psoas abscess are two other very unusual clinical entities in healthy individuals. These entities are generally not related to athletic trauma but could be confused with minor traumatic events simply by temporal relationship. A patient with an infected joint who is otherwise healthy will generally present with rather severe pain, unwillingness to move the hip actively, or to allow the examiner to move the hip passively. The leg will be held in a slightly flexed posture, usually supported on a pillow. Classic clinical features include fever, elevated white blood cell count, increased numbers of immature cells on the peripheral white blood cell differential count, and markedly elevated erythrocyte sedimentation rate. Definitive diagnosis is made by aspiration of the hip joint with the finding of bacteria or large numbers of white blood cells on analysis of Gram stain. A pyarthrosis can be distinguished from a psoas abscess by MRI or CT. Immediate

surgical drainage is indicated in either case. Other systemic illness or immune system compromise should be ruled out for an otherwise healthy person presenting with a spontaneous deep infection.

Hip Pointer, Hematoma, or Contusion

A hip pointer is a contusion of the iliac crest that may or may not have an associated hematoma. This problem is seen most commonly in contact sports such as ice hockey but can occur in basketball, baseball, and soccer due to a hard fall. The mechanism of injury resulting in a hip pointer is a focused impact at some point between the iliac crest and the prominence of the greater trochanter caused by collision with another player, floor, or ground. The iliac wing of the pelvis is vulnerable to injury because of the relative subcutaneous position at the iliac crest. The gluteal musculature lies over the iliac wing in the externally iliac fossa. Because the iliac wing provides a relatively unforgiving support beneath the muscle, it is vulnerable to contusion in the event of a direct blow. Although in the uninjured state a space does not exist between the gluteal muscles and the external iliac fossa, an expanding hematoma can dissect between the muscular attachment and the bone surface. Additionally, the three layers of abdominal muscles attach on the superior aspect of the iliac crest. The insertion of these muscles and the thick periosteum in this area can also be the site of hematoma collection.

On physical examination of the patient with a hip pointer, there is exquisite tenderness at the anterior iliac crest. There may not be visible swelling and ecchymosis. Some patients will present with a palpable fluctuant swelling consistent with accumulation of a localized hematoma. For athletes with more subtle injury, attempts at a sit-up, particularly an oblique sit-up, will cause significant discomfort.

For most cases, the physical examination will provide enough information to make the diagnosis. In the event of high-impact injury, extreme pain, or tenderness directly over the iliac apophysis, anterior superior iliac spine, or trochanteric apophysis, radiographs can rule out a fracture of the iliac crest or apophyseal avulsion, both of which may clinically mimic a hip pointer (42,43).

Initial treatment consists of rest, short-term use of NSAIDs, and ice. Occasionally (and infrequently), aspiration or corticosteroid injection is necessary if there is an associated hematoma of sufficient size to cause pain, local inflammation, and distention of surrounding tissues (44,45).

The initial rehabilitation is directed at maintaining aerobic condition and range of motion of the hip while avoiding activities such as abdominal straining or forced hip abduction, which could exacerbate symptoms. Once comfort is achieved, the athlete can begin gluteal and abdominal muscle stretching, strengthening, and finally sports activity. Complete recovery is expected within 2 to 4 weeks.

Hip Fracture and Dislocation

Any athlete involved in high-energy contact sports or sports that involve movement at high rates of speed is at risk for a fracture of any bone in the lower extremity. Nevertheless, hip fractures are not injuries that are uniquely associated with athletes. A hip fracture is generally caused by a direct blow over the greater trochanter caused by a hard fall or tackle. Anatomically, hip fractures are divided into fractures in the region of the femoral neck and those in the intertrochanteric region (46). Femoral neck fractures are of especially great concern because of the possibility for injury to the blood supply to the femoral head, which can result in osteonecrosis (47). Femoral neck fractures are classified by the degree of displacement (48), with type I being a valgus-impacted fracture, type II nondisplaced, type III less that 50% displaced, and type IV greater than 50% displaced. The intertrochanteric fractures are classified by the number of fragments with more than 1 cm of displacement or more than 20 degrees of angulation (49). The large fragments to be counted include the femoral head and neck, the greater trochanter, the lesser trochanter, and the femoral shaft. Thus, intertrochanteric fractures are either one-, two-, three-, or four-part fractures. The treatment for all hip fractures in young individuals is anatomic reduction and internal fixation.

Dislocation of the hip in sports is rare, both in children and adults, although subluxation and dislocation have been reported to occur in football, rugby, jogging, water skiing, and snow skiing (50–56). Hip dislocation generally requires a considerable force. It is noted that the younger the child, the less force required to dislocate (57). Posterior dislocations occur far more commonly in sports than anterior dislocations of the hip (51–55,57). The two most common mechanisms of dislocation are being tackled when down on all four limbs or falling onto a flexed knee (52,55,56).

All patients with hip dislocation complain of a great deal of pain, but most are unable to rise from the ground, let alone ambulate or move the affected limb. With posterior dislocation, the leg is shortened, flexed, internally rotated, and adducted. A complete physical examination should be carried out to include neurovascular assessment, with special attention to the function of the sciatic nerve (in particular the peroneal branch), which is vulnerable in a posterior dislocation.

Standard anteroposterior and cross-table lateral radiographs should be obtained to determine the direction of the dislocation and whether there is an associated fracture of the femoral head or acetabular wall. Judet views are helpful in assessing an associated acetabular wall fracture. Postreduction films should be obtained to confirm a concentric reduction of the hip. A nonconcentric reduction may indicate a retained bone fragment or soft tissue interposition. CT can reveal the presence of fracture lines and retained femoral head and wall fragments when plane radiographs are equivocal.

Hip dislocation is considered a medical emergency because the dislocated hip compromises both its own vascular supply and potentially places adjacent neurologic structures such as the sciatic nerve at risk. A single attempt at closed reduction can be attempted by longitudinal traction with the hip slightly flexed once the patient has been stabilized in an appropriate location. An on-field reduction of a hip dislocation is generally not attempted unless a highly experienced individual is immediately at hand. If a reduction cannot be easily achieved, the patient is given appropriate pain medication and sedation and radiographs are obtained. If radiographs confirm a simple dislocation, uncomplicated by fracture, further attempts at closed reduction can be undertaken with the assistance of an anesthesiologist providing necessary levels of sedation, relaxation, and patient comfort. Indications for operative intervention to reduce the hip open include inability to reduce the hip after adequate anesthesia, a fracture fragment within the joint greater than 2 mm, neurovascular compromise, ipsilateral femoral fracture, and persistent hip instability postreduction (53,58). Loose bodies and chondral injuries can be addressed arthroscopically (59). Nearly all hip fractures in young people are treated surgically (48).

Rehabilitation is started immediately after the pain of the acute dislocation has subsided or the fracture is fixed. In general, the progression of rehabilitation starts with gently active and active assisted range of motion of the hip joint. In most cases, the weight bearing on the affected leg will be limited for 6 weeks after a fracture and 3 or 4 weeks after an uncomplicated dislocation. Once a comfortable full range of motion has been achieved and the patient has resumed bearing weight on the leg, strengthening of the hip girdle, thigh, and leg muscles can begin in earnest. Initial exercise regimens will stress low impact, isokinetic, full range strengthening. Once near equal strength has been achieved relative to the nonaffected leg, endurance and training can resume. The rehabilitation before return to training may last 3 months and the return to sports up to 6 months after a hip fracture or dislocation.

The incidence of complication of hip dislocation is less in children than in adults (55). Complications of hip subluxation and dislocation, despite appropriate and immediate care, include recurrent dislocation, avascular necrosis, sciatic nerve injury, posttraumatic arthritis, premature epiphyseal fusion in the skeletally immature patient, and myositis ossificans (53). The incidence of osteonecrosis of the femoral head after femoral neck fracture or hip dislocation ranges between 10% and 30% in the published literature (20,60). Factors that influence rate of complication include time to reduction and associated injuries.

GROWTH-RELATED PROBLEMS

Apophysitis or Apophyseal Separation

Apophyseal injuries are not uncommon in the adolescent athlete due to the relative weakness of the open physis. Avulsion may result during strenuous exercise such as in the case of disruption of the anterior superior iliac spine apophysis during sprinting. Chronic apophyseal irritation analogous to Osgood-Schlatter's disease at the tibial tubercle is also possible at the iliac and ischial apophyses. The apophyses most commonly affected about the hip are the sartorius and rectus femoris attachment to the anterior superior and inferior iliac spines, respectively; hamstrings attachment to the ischial tuberosity; and iliopsoas attachment to the lesser trochanter (61–64). The most frequently injured is the anterior superior iliac spine apophysis (Fig. 32.4A) and least commonly injured is lesser trochanteric apophysis where the iliopsoas inserts (Fig. 32.4B).

Mechanism of Injury

The mechanism of injury for an apophyseal separation in sports is most commonly a sudden stop or change in direction or a sudden and unexpected eccentric muscle contraction (as in a split). Repeated microtrauma caused by overuse or improper and unsupervised training can lead to apophyseal inflammation (apophysitis).

Clinical Evaluation

With an apophyseal avulsion, the history will usually reveal an acute onset of pain and may be accompanied by a popping sensation, whereas the presentation of apophysitis is that of gradual onset associated with activity. Typically both these conditions will present with a complaint of pain that limits their ability to participate in athletics. There will be well-localized tenderness, pain with passive stretch of the affected muscle tendon unit, and symptoms reproduced with muscle resistance. There may also be associated weakness if an avulsion has occurred.

Imaging

Plain radiographs are helpful in determining if there has been an avulsion fracture, but only if the ossification center exists. Comparison views are helpful, particularly to avoid confusion of an os acetabuli with avulsion of the anterior inferior iliac spine. Positioning of the patient is important in making the diagnosis of a lesser trochanteric avulsion. Care must be taken to externally rotate the hip to view the lesser trochanter in profile (64). Ultrasound can show changes in the absence of an ossification center (65), and further imaging is generally not necessary.

Treatment

Most apophyseal injuries respond well to nonoperative treatment to include rest, ice, NSAIDs, or other analgesic as needed. Limited weight bearing with crutches may be necessary based on symptoms. Once symptoms are controlled, a range of motion program should be instituted with a gradual progression to include instruction in proper stretching and strengthening. When full range of motion and normal strength have been achieved, a gradual return to athletic activity is possible. Surgery is not indicated for apophysitis and rarely indicated for apophyseal avulsion. However, surgery may be necessary in the case of wide displacement (more than 2 cm) of an avulsed tuberosity or iliac spine where nonunion may result in significant disability for the athlete (61,64). Because of the open growth center, the apophysis is usually sutured back into place. Anticipate return to unlimited activities is 4 to 8 weeks or longer depending on the extent of the injury.

Epiphyseal Injury

Slipped capital femoral epiphysis is the most common hip malady affecting adolescents, occurring in 0.7 to 3.4 children per 100,000 (64). Athletic injuries are not a frequent cause of slipped femoral capital epiphysis, but the diagnosis must be considered in an adolescent athlete with persistent pain in the hip and or knee. A slipped epiphysis occurs more commonly in obese males during rapid growth.

Clinical Evaluation

There is often no associated injury or only incidental trauma. Occasionally, prodromal symptoms of pain will be present. On clinical evaluation there is often a limp, and limitation in range of motion of the affected hip (internal rotation and abduction) will be present. A leg length discrepancy is sometimes noted, and the leg may be externally rotated during the stance phase of gait.

Imaging

Routine anteroposterior and lateral radiographs should be obtained. Bilateral films are recommended because bilateral involvement has been reported to occur in up to 25% to 41% of adolescents (64,66). The key is to be

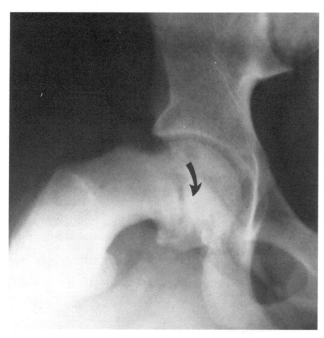

FIG. 32.5. The *arrow* indicates the direction of the slipped capital femoral epiphysis, which is in varus and retroversion.

certain of no physeal widening or metaphyseal overhang on either orthogonal view (Fig. 32.5).

Treatment

The recommended treatment of an acutely slipped epiphysis is controversial. A prompt gentle reduction and internal fixation with smooth pin or cannulated screw is appropriate. The controversy lies in whether to reduce a displaced epiphyseal separation, centering on the acuity of the injury and the degree of displacement. In general, no reduction is attempted for a chronic slip, and force should never be applied to achieve reduction in any scenario.

REFERENCES

1. Lloyd-Smith R, Clement DB, McKenzie DC, et al. A survey of overuse and traumatic hip and pelvic injuries in athletes. *Phys Sportsmed* 1985;13:131–141.
2. Lequesne MG, Dang N, Lane N. Sport practice and osteoarthritis of the limbs. *Osteoarthr Cart* 1997;5:75–86.
3. Murray RO, Duncan C. Athletic activity in adolescence as an etiological factor in degenerative hip disease. *J Bone Joint Surg Br* 1971;53B:406–419.
4. Renstrom P. Mechanism, diagnosis and treatment of running injuries. *Instruct Course Lect* 1993;42:225–234.
5. Lloyd T, Triantafyllou S, Baker E, et al. Women athletes with menstrual irregularity have increased musculoskeletal injuries. *Med Sci Sports Exerc* 1985;18:374–379.
6. Jones BH, Harris JM, Vinh TN, et al. Exercise-induced stress fractures and stress reactions of bone: epidemiology, etiology and classification. *Exerc Sports Sci Rev* 1989;17:379–422.
7. Stoneham MD, Chir MB, Morgan NV. Stress fracture of the hip in Royal Marine recruits under training: a retrospective analysis. *Br J Sports Med* 1991;25:145–148.
8. Johansson C, Ekenman I, Tornkvist H, et al. Stress fracture of the femoral neck in athletes: the consequence of a delay in diagnosis. *Am J Sports Med* 1990;18:524–528.
9. Taylor DC, Meyers WC, Moylan JA, et al. Abdominal musculature abnormalities as a cause of groin pain in athletes. Inguinal hernias and pubalgia [see comments]. *Am J Sports Med* 1991;19:239–242.
10. Shin AY, Gillingham BL. Fatigue fractures of the femoral neck in athletes. *J Am Acad Orthop Surg* 1997;5:293–302.
11. Dale E, Gerlach DH, Martin DE, et al. Menstrual dysfunction in distance runners. *Obstet Gynecol* 1979;54:47–52.
12. Russell JB, Mitchell D, Musey PL. The relationship of exercise to anovulatory cycles in female athletes: hormonal and physical characteristics. *Obstet Gynecol* 1984;63:452–456.
13. Kupke MJ, Kahler DM, Lovenzoni MH, et al. Stress fracture of the femoral neck in a long distance runner: biomechanical aspects. *J Emerg Med* 1993;11:587–591.
14. Clement DB, Ammann W, Taunton JE, et al. Exercise-induced stress injuries to the femur. *Int J Sports Med* 1993;14:347–352.
15. Lombardo SJ, Benson DW. Stress fractures of the femur in runners. *Am J Sports Med* 1982;10:219–227.
16. Shin AY, Morin WD, Gorman JD, et al. The superiority of MRI in differentiating the cause of hip pain in endurance athletes. *Am J Sports Med* 1996;25:168–176.
17. Byers GE, Berquist TH. Radiology of sports related injuries. *Curr Probl Diagn Radiol* 1996;25:1–49.
18. Blickenstaff LD, Morris JM. Fatigue fracture of the femoral neck. *J Bone Joint Surg Am* 1966;48:1031–1047.
19. Fullerton LR Jr, Snowdy HA. Femoral neck stress fractures. *Am J Sports Med* 1988;16:365–377.
20. Vail TP, Urbaniak JR. Outcomes in surgical treatment of femoral neck fracture: analysis of failures secondary to osteonecrosis. *J South Orthop Assoc* 1995;4:83–90.
21. Schaberg JE, Harper MC, Allen WC. The snapping hip syndrome. *Am J Sports Med* 1984;12:361–365.
22. Quirk R. Ballet injuries: the Australian experience. *Clin Sports Med* 1983;2:507–514.
23. Byrd JW. Hip arthroscopy for posttraumatic loose fragments in the young active adult: three case reports. *Clin J Sport Med* 1996;6:129–134.
24. Fitzgerald RH Jr. Acetabular labrum tears. Diagnosis and treatment. *Clin Orthop* 1995;311:60–68.
25. McCarthy JC, Busconi B. The role of hip arthroscopy in the diagnosis and treatment of hip disease. *Orthopedics* 1995;18:753–756.
26. Howse AJ. Orthopaedists aid ballet. *Clinical Orthopedic and Related Research* 1972;89:52–63.
27. Micheli LJ. Overuse injuries in children's sports. *Orthop Clin North Am* 1983;14:337–360.
28. Moreira FE. Anca A Scatto (snapping hip). *J Bone Joint Surg Am* 1940;22A:506.
29. Lage LA, Patel JV, Villar RN. The acetabular labral tear: an arthroscopic classification. *Arthroscopy* 1996;12:269–272.
30. Glick JM: Hip arthroscopy. In: McGinty JB, ed. *Operative arthroscopy*. New York: Raven Press, 1985:663–676.
31. Glick JM, Sampson TG, Gordon RB, et al. Hip arthroscopy by the lateral approach. *Arthroscopy* 1987;3:4–12.
32. Dvorak M, Duncan CP, Day B. Arthroscopic anatomy of the hip. *J Arthrosc Rel Res* 1990;6:264–273.
33. Hunter DM, Ruch DS. Hip arthroscopy. *J South Orthop Assoc* 1996;5:243–250.
34. Villar RN. Hip arthroscopy. *Br J Hosp Med* 1992;47:763–766.
35. Beer E. Periostitis of symphysis and descending rami of the pubes following suprapubic operations. *Int J Med Surg* 1924;37:224–225.
36. Cochrane GM. Osteitis pubis in athletes. *Br J Sports Med* 1971;5:233–235.
37. Fricker PA, Taunton JE, Ammann W. Osteitis pubis in athletes: infection, inflammation or injury? *Sports Med* 1991;12:266–279.
38. Schneider R, Kaye JJ, Ghelman B. Adductor avulsive injuries near the symphysis pubis. *Radiology* 1976;120:567–569.
39. Pavlov H. Roentgen examination of groin and hip pain in the athlete. *Clin Sports Med* 1987;6:829–843.
40. Wiley JJ. Traumatic osteitis pubis: the gracilis syndrome. *Am J Sports Med* 1983;11:360–363.

41. Peterson L, Renstrom P. *Sports injuries: their prevention and treatment.* Chicago: Year Book Medical Publishers, 1986.
42. Butler JE, Eggert AW. Fracture of the iliac crest apophysis: an unusual hip pointer. *Sports Med* 1975;3:193.
43. Godshall RW, Hansen CA. Incomplete avulsion of a portion of the iliac crest epiphysis: an injury of young athletes. *J Bone Joint Surg Am* 1973;55A:1301–1302.
44. Schneider RC, Kennedy JC, Plant ML. *Sports injuries: mechanisms, prevention and treatment.* Baltimore: Williams & Wilkins, 1985:104.
45. Fu FH, Stone DA. *Sports injuries: mechanisms, prevention and treatment.* Baltimore: Williams & Wilkins, 1994:442.
46. Vail TP, McCollum DE. Fractures of the pelvis, femur, and knee. In: Sagiston DC, ed. *Textbook of surgery: the biological basis of modern surgical practice,* 15th ed. Philadelphia: W.B. Saunders, 1997.
47. Lu-Yao GL, Keller RB, Littenberg B, et al. Outcomes after displaced fractures of the femoral neck. A meta-analysis of one hundred and six published reports. *J Bone Joint Surg Am* 1994;76A:15–25.
48. Swiontkowski M, Winquist R, Hansen S. Fractures of the femoral neck in patients between the ages of twelve and forty-nine years. *J Bone Joint Surg Am* 1984;66A:837–846.
49. Boyd HB, Griffin L. Classification and treatment of trochanteric fractures. *Arch Surg* 1949;58:858.
50. Tapper EM. Ski injuries from 1939 to 1976: the Sun Valley experience. *Am J Sports Med* 1978;6:115–121.
51. Walsh ZT, Micheli LJ. Hip dislocation in a high school football player. *Phys Sports Med* 1989;17:112–120.
52. O'Leary C, Doyle J, Fenelon G, et al. Traumatic dislocation of the hip in rugby union football. *Irish Med J* 1987;80:291–292.
53. Wolfe MW, Brinker MR, Cary GR, et al. Posterior fracture-dislocation of the hip in a jogger. *J South Ortho Assoc* 1995;4:91–95.
54. Stanisavljevic S, Irwin RB, Brown LR. Orthopedic injuries in water skiing: etiology and prevention. *Orthopedics* 1978;1:125–129.
55. Rees D, Thompson SK. Traumatic dislocation of the hip in mini rugby. *Br Med J Clin Res Ed* 1984;289:19–20.
56. Cooper DE, Warren RF, Barnes R. Traumatic subluxation of the hip resulting in aseptic necrosis and chondrolysis in a professional football player. *Am J Sports Med* 1991;19:322–324.
57. Offierski CM. Traumatic dislocation of the hip in children. *J Bone Joint Surg Br* 1981;63B:194–197.
58. DeLee JC. Fractures and dislocations of the hip. In: Rockwood CA, Green DP, eds. *Fractures in adults,* 3rd ed. Philadelphia: J.B. Lippincott, 1991:1481–1652.
59. Byrd JW. Hip arthroscopy for posttraumatic loose fragments in the young active adult: three case reports. *Clin J Sports Med* 1996;6:129–134.
60. Vail TP. The incidence of osteonecrosis. In: *The etiology, diagnosis, & management of osteonecrosis of the human skeleton.* Rosemont, IL: American Academy of Orthopaedic Surgeons, 1998.
61. Collins HR, Evarts CM. Injuries to the adolescent athlete. *Postgrad Med* 1971;49:72–78.
62. Dimon JH. Isolated fractures of the lesser trochanter of the femur. *Clin Orthop* 1972;82:144–148.
63. Peck DM. Apophyseal injuries in the young athlete. *Am Fam Physician* 1995;51:1891–1895.
64. Paletta GA, Andrish JT. Injuries about the hip and pelvis in the young athlete. *Clin Sports Med* 1995;14:591–628.
65. Lazovic D, Wegner U, Peters G, et al. Ultrasound for diagnosis of apophyseal injuries. *Knee Surg Sports Traumatol Arthrosc* 1996;3:234–237.
66. Waters PM, Millis MB. Hip and pelvic injuries in the young athlete. *Clin Sports Med* 1988;7:513–526.

Principles and Practice of Orthopaedic Sports Medicine,
edited by William E. Garrett, Jr., Kevin P. Speer, and Donald T. Kirkendall.
Lippincott Williams & Wilkins, Philadelphia © 2000.

CHAPTER 33

Injuries to the Thigh and Groin

Rolf H. Langeland and Robert J. Carangelo

Injuries to the thigh have received relatively little attention in the athletic population despite them being common and often associated with prolonged disability. Inadequate treatment of muscle contusions, muscle strains, avulsion fractures, or stress fractures will lead to delayed healing, persistent pain, and increased recurrence. Athletic activity frequently must be discontinued for several months, resulting in a discouraged athlete and frustrated physician.

The first case report of a thigh injury was described by Petit in 1722, when he reported on a quadriceps rupture (1). Stress fracture of the femur was first described by Blecker (2) in 1905. Current reports find femoral shaft stress fractures to be more common than previously expected in the athletic population, comprising up to 21% of stress fractures (3).

Soft tissue injury to the thigh and groin are known to be common in athletes. However, estimating the true incidence of thigh injuries is difficult because these injuries initially are often considered minor and therefore go unreported. Epidemiologic studies of collegiate and professional soccer teams have provided some of the best data on thigh and groin injuries. McMaster and Walter (4) found that 34% of the injuries sustained in a professional soccer season were injuries of the thigh. More recently, a Danish study (5) reported a thigh injury rate of 24% in a season, second only to ankle injury at 27%. The most recent data on thigh injuries are reported by the National Collegiate Athletic Association (NCAA) from its large ongoing study of soccer league injuries in the United States (6). The NCAA 1996–1997 soccer season found thigh injuries to account for 16% of injuries. This was second to ankle injuries, which

accounted for 21% of injuries. This study also reported injury incidence based on 1,000 hours of "athlete exposure" (AE). Injury to the thigh was at a rate of 1.51/1,000 AE. This rate is consistent with the rates reported over the last 10 years of this study.

The absolute number of thigh injuries will undoubtedly increase over the next decades because young athletes are becoming more involved in the U.S. Youth Soccer Programs (7) and as the expanding senior athletic population continues its pursuit of cardiovascular fitness.

This chapter is organized based on anatomic location of injury. The first section is an overview of the thigh anatomy. The subsequent sections are divided based on the injury location. Each section addresses epidemiology, mechanism of injury, clinical evaluation, imaging, treatment of injury, expected outcomes, and authors' preferences.

ANATOMY

The anatomy of the thigh is essentially divided into three separate compartments: posterior, medial, and anterior. These compartments surround the largest and longest bone in the body, the femur. The anterior compartment is divided from the medial and posterior compartments by a thick medial and lateral intermuscular septum. The medial and posterior compartments are divided by a thinner posterior intermuscular septum (Fig. 33.1) (8).

The posterior (hamstring, flexor) compartment is comprised primarily of the hamstring musculature (Fig. 33.2). The hamstrings include the long and short heads of the biceps femoris, the semitendinosus, and the semimembranosus. The semimembranosus muscle belly is noted to be more medial and more muscular when compared with the semitendinosus muscle. Additional structures in the posterior compartment include a portion of the adductor magnus, the sciatic nerve, the posterior femoral cutaneous nerve, and branches of the profundus

R. H. Langeland: Orthopaedic Specialty Group, Bridgeport Hospital, Fairfield, Connecticut 06430.

R. J. Carangelo: Department of Orthopaedic Surgery, University of Connecticut, Farmington, Connecticut 06032.

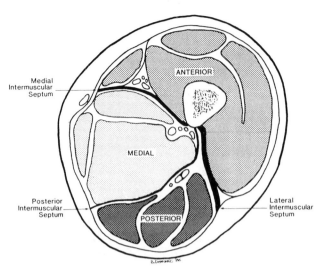

FIG. 33.1. Cross-section of the thigh outlining the three fascial compartments and the relative thickness of the intermuscular septa. (From Tarlow SD, Achterman C, Hayhurst J, et al. Acute compartment syndrome of the thigh. *J Bone Joint Surg Am* 1986;68A:1441, with permission.)

femoris artery. The long head of the biceps femoris, semimembranosus, and the semitendinosus all arise from the ischeal tuberosity, span two joints (hip and knee), and are innervated by the tibial branch of the sciatic nerve. The semimembranosus originates either from a common site on the posterolateral ischium with the semitendinosus and long head of the biceps femoris or as a separate slip anteromedial to the common origin of the other two hamstrings (9). The exception to the hamstrings is the short head of the biceps femoris, which arises from the linea aspera of the femoral shaft, crosses only the knee joint, and receives its innervation from the peroneal branch of the sciatic nerve. The biceps femoris heads form a conjoin tendon and insert onto the fibular head. The semitendinosus and the semimembranosus insert onto the proximal medial tibia, the semitendinosus forming part of the pes anserinus.

The medial (adductor, groin) compartment is comprised of the following muscles: gracilis, adductor brevis, adductor longus, adductor magnus, and obturator externus (Fig. 33.3). Additional structures in the medial compartment include the obturator nerve, the obturator artery and vein, and the profundus femoris artery. The

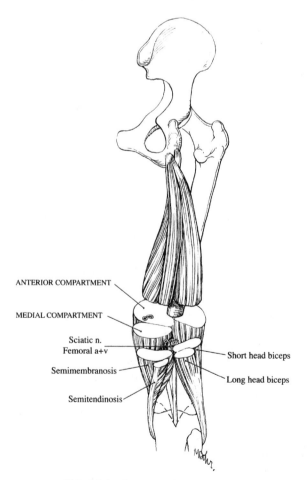

FIG. 33.2. Posterior Compartment.

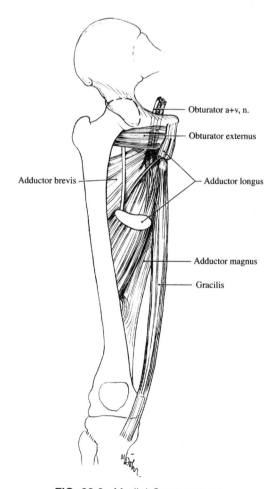

FIG. 33.3. Medial Compartment.

gracilis is the only two-joint muscle in the medial compartment, and it arises from the pubic arch and inserts on the proximal medial tibia, forming part of the pes anserinus. The adductor brevis, longus, and magnus originate from the inferior pubic ramus and insert onto the linea aspera along the femur. Innervation of most medial compartment muscles is through the anterior obturator nerve. The adductor magnus is the exception, with dual innervation from both posterior obturator nerve and the tibial portion of the sciatic nerve.

The anterior (quadriceps, extensor) compartment is formed by the following muscles: sartorius, iliacus, psoas, pectineus, vastus lateralis, vastus medialis, vastus intermedius, rectus femoris, and articularis genus (Fig. 33.4). Additional structures in the anterior compartment include femoral nerve, lateral femoral cutaneous nerve, femoral artery, and femoral vein. The rectus femoris and sartorius are the only two-joint muscles in the anterior compartment. The sartorius arises from the anterior superior iliac spine (ASIS) and inserts onto the proximal medial tibia to form part of the pes anserinus. The rectus femoris has two heads; the reflected (indirect) head, originating from the superior acetabulum, and the

straight (direct) head, originating from the anterior inferior iliac spine (AIIS). Distally, the rectus femoris fibers blend with the vastus intermedius fibers approximately 3 cm proximal to their common insertion onto the superior pole of the patella. The iliacus originates from the iliac fossa and the psoas originates from the transverse processes of L1-5; both muscles insert onto the lesser trochanter. The iliacus and psoas are innervated by the iliopsoas nerve. The pectineus arises from the pubis and inserts onto the pectineal line of the femur. The vastus lateralis arises from the vastus ridge at the greater trochanter and lateral linea aspera, inserting onto the lateral patella. The vastus intermedius originates from the anterior femur and becomes confluent with the fibers of the rectus femoris before its insertion to the superior pole of the patella. The vastus medialis arises from the medial linea aspera and inserts onto the medial patella. All the muscles of the anterior compartment, except the iliacus and psoas, receive their innervation from the femoral nerve.

The iliotibial band comprises the lateral most portion of the thigh anatomy. This structure is not located within any of the previously mentioned compartments. The iliotibial band is formed by the gluteus maximus and the tensor fascia lata. The gluteus maximus arises from the ilium and forms part of the iliotibial band, which inserts distally at Gerdy's tubercle. The tensor fascia lata originates from the anterior iliac crest and forms the other portion of the iliotibial band. Innervation of gluteus maximus is through the inferior gluteal nerve and innervation of tensor fascia lata is from the superior gluteal nerve.

MUSCLE STRAIN INJURY

"We seem to know the least of what we see the most."
William E. Garrett, Jr., MD, PhD

Muscle strain injuries are best defined as a spectrum of injury from microscopic muscle–tendon unit tears to complete ruptures or avulsions. The clinician must have a sound understanding of these injuries and their treatment because they can account for up to 30% of a typical clinical practice (10,11). In the athletic population, the most common muscle group strained in the body is the hamstrings. Specifically, the long head of the biceps femoris is most often injured, making this the most common muscle strained in the body (10,12). Muscle strain injuries frequently involve muscles that span two joints. After hamstring strains, the most common muscle groups strained, in decreasing order of frequency, are triceps surae, quadriceps, lumbar, and hip adductors (10).

Athletes at risk for muscle strain injury include "speed athletes." Track and field athletes, such as sprinters and hurdlers, and athletes of soccer, football, rugby,

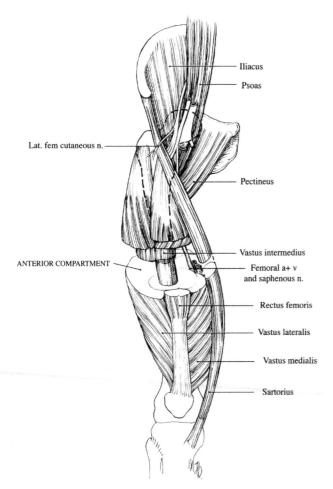

Iliacus
Psoas
Lat. fem cutaneous n.
Pectineus
ANTERIOR COMPARTMENT
Vastus intermedius
Femoral a+ v
and saphenous n.
Rectus femoris
Vastus lateralis
Vastus medialis
Sartorius

FIG. 33.4. Anterior Compartment.

gymnastics, ice hockey, and basketball are included in the group at risk for muscle injury.

These injuries represent a continuum of injury with one factor in common, eccentric muscle contraction (10–13). Eccentric muscular exercise results when a muscle develops tension while in a lengthening mode, as seen in a sprinter's hamstring tensing to slow the forward progression of the tibia in the swing phase of the running cycle. When eccentric muscle contractions occur, greater amounts of energy are absorbed and higher forces are generated using fewer motor units (14,15). This sets the stage for potential muscle injury.

In the laboratory setting, Garrett et al. (16) determined much of the pathophysiology of muscle strains. Initial findings using activated rabbit hindlimb muscles failed to show any strain injury, partial or complete. Subsequently, it was found that the forces required to cause muscle failure were several times the force normally produced during a maximal active isometric contraction (17). This suggested that passive forces, such as stretch, were required to obtain muscle strain injury (14). Maximally activated muscles were then stretched and noted to fail at the muscle–tendon junction (Fig. 33.5), thus localizing the site of the muscle strain lesion (14,16,17). The lesion occurred at the muscle–tendon junction regardless of the rate of strain or the architec-

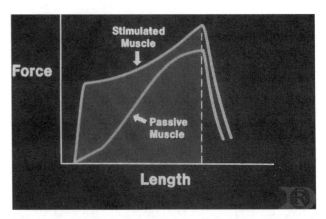

FIG. 33.6. Energy absorbed is shown as the area under each length–tension deformation curve. Relative differences in energy absorbed to failure in stimulated versus passive muscle preparations are shown. (From Garrett WE Jr. Muscle strain injuries. *Am J Sports Med* 1996;24:S3, with permission.)

ture of the muscle. In addition, it was shown that the activated muscle was protected from injury as it generated a higher force at failure and was able to absorb twice as much energy compared with the nonstimulated muscle (Fig. 33.6) (18). Therefore, any condition that results in decreased ability of the muscle to contract against stretch (eccentrically load) will predispose the muscle to strain injury (14). Conditions commonly implicated include muscle weakness, fatigue, prior muscle injury, and lack of warm-up. In a controlled laboratory study (19), fatigued muscle was found to have diminished ability to absorb energy compared with the nonfatigued muscle, thus lowering the fatigued muscle's strain threshold. Prior muscle injury has also been shown to predispose muscle to strain injury. Clinically, patients with major muscle strains usually describe a previous minor injury in the same muscle (14). Experimental muscle strain models have found that previously injured muscle will rupture at 63% of control muscle peak load (14,20). Muscle "warm-up" (increasing muscle temperature through activity) is noted to be protective against strain injury as it allows increased muscle–tendon stretch before failure (14,21).

Similarly, due to the viscoelastic properties of the muscle–tendon unit, repetitive muscle stretching is protective of strain injury as it decreases the stress on the muscle–tendon unit at any given length (14,22). NCAA soccer statistics support fatigue, lack of stretching, and lack of warm-up as major factors; as twice as many strains are found to occur in the second half of play compared with the first half (6).

At the microscopic level, typical histologic changes occur with muscle strain injuries. The injury is most commonly found at the muscle–tendon junction, with hemorrhage occurring initially. Twenty-four to 48 hours after the injury, a pronounced inflammatory response

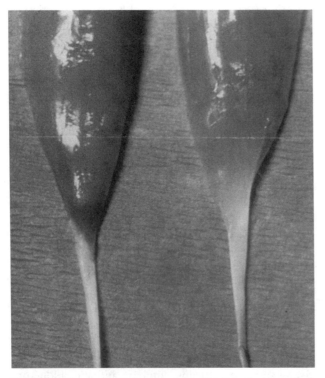

FIG. 33.5. Gross appearance of the tibialis anterior muscle of the rabbit after controlled stain injury. A small hemorrhage is evident at the distal tip of the injured (left) muscle at 24 hours. (From Garrett WE Jr. Muscle strain injuries. *Am J Sports Med* 1996;24:S3, with permission.)

is seen with fiber necrosis, capillary ingrowth, and a proliferation of disorganized fibroblasts. Collagen synthesis can be found as early as 72 hours after injury. Seven to 14 days postinjury, most inflammatory cellular response and edema have resolved. After 2 weeks, myotube and fibrous scar tissue have formed a bridge at the injury site. The collagen fibers are initially aligned perpendicular to the long axis of the injured musculotendinous unit. Secondary remodeling begins during the third and fourth weeks after injury and continues on for many months. At this stage, fibroblasts and collagen fibers begin orienting themselves along the long axis of the musculotendinous unit in a response to stress. Remodeling continues for approximately 20 weeks, at which time little histologic difference is noted at the injury site. An important factor in the healing process is that of stress. In the absence of stress, remodeling does not proceed, collagen production decreases, and the healing period is prolonged (14,18,20,23,24).

Clinically, muscle strains present with pain, swelling, erythema, and ecchymosis over the affected muscle. These findings will vary based on the severity of the strain. Pain is excentuated with passive or active stretch of the muscle. In the most severe cases (complete rupture), a palpable defect will be noted on examination.

Imaging studies of muscle strains are usually not necessary or helpful, except with suspected bony avulsions or complete ruptures. In the case of a bony avulsion, which is more commonly seen in the immature patient with open growth plates, plain radiographs may demonstrate the bony fragment and indicate the amount of retraction (25). In the adult patient, ischeal tuberosity avulsions may occur with complete rupture of the hamstrings. Complete hamstring rupture without bony avulsion is best imaged with T2-weighted magnetic resonance imaging (MRI) (26,27).

Acute muscle strain injury is treated with rest, ice, compression, and elevation (RICE) in an attempt to minimize hemorrhage and the inflammatory response. Nonsteroidal anti-inflammatory drugs (NSAIDs) are prescribed in the early stages of muscle strain to minimize the inflammatory phase. Gentle range of motion and stretching exercises are started at 3 to 5 days postinjury. Progressive stretching and strengthening exercises are continued until flexibility, strength, and balance are restored. The prognosis of the typical muscle strain is very good, and with the above treatment, most athletes return to competition within days to several weeks depending on the severity of strain. Few muscle strains require surgical repair; however, in the case of complete ischeal tuberosity hamstring rupture with distal tendon retraction, nonoperative treatment has resulted in poor functional outcome in the athlete, and surgical repair should be considered (28). (Specific muscle strain injuries and their clinical evaluation, treatment, and outcomes are discussed in depth in the following sections.)

HAMSTRINGS

Injury of the hamstring musculature is a common occurrence in the athletic population. Injuries include contusions, lacerations, strains, and complete ruptures. Hamstring strains are by far the most common injury of the posterior thigh. In comparison with all muscle strains in the body, hamstring strains are the most common, accounting for 25% of muscle strains. Hamstring strains are followed by triceps surae strains, accounting for 19% of muscle stains; quadriceps strains 17%; lumbar strains 9%; and adductor strains 8% (10).

Hamstring Strain Injury

Accurate epidemiologic estimates of hamstring injuries are difficult to obtain because most reports are sport specific and frequently do not specify the exact location of thigh injury. NCAA 1996–1997 soccer injury surveillance system data estimate muscle–tendon strain injury to occur at a rate of 2.49/1,000 hours AE. The hamstring muscle group accounts for 25% to 30% of these strain injuries. Therefore, hamstring strain injury can be estimated to occur at a rate of 0.75/1,000 hours AE (6,10). Complete rupture of the hamstring origin is a rare injury, accounting for approximately 1.5% of all hamstring injuries (6). This injury is estimated to occur at a rate of 0.08/1,000 hours AE (6,10).

By some reports, the short head of the biceps femoris has been found to be the most frequently injured muscle in the hamstring group (29,30), implicating its unique peroneal branch innervation as the etiology (30–32). More recent studies using computed tomography and MRI (12,26) demonstrated that the long head of the biceps femoris is the most frequently strained hamstring muscle. Because the hamstrings are the most common muscle group stained in the body, the long head of the biceps femoris is the most common muscle strained in the body (10,12,33).

The specific hamstring muscle strained and timing of the running gait cycle may be related. Electromyographic (EMG) evaluation of the running gait cycle has demonstrated that the semimembranosus and semitendinosus are most active during the late swing phase of the cycle, whereas the biceps femoris is most active at the take-off portion of the support phase of the cycle (34). This implies that the lateral hamstring is more at risk for injury at the take-off portion of the cycle and the medial hamstring is more at risk during the swing phase of the cycle.

Hamstring strains commonly occur in speed athletes during ballistic eccentric contraction of a tight fatigued hamstring muscle (see Muscle Strain Injury, above). The position that places the hamstring most at risk for strain injury is that of hip flexion and knee extension, because this position places the hamstring on maximum stretch.

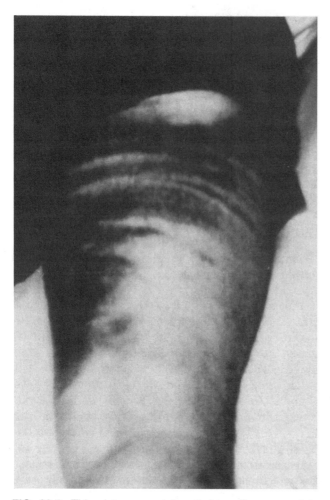

FIG. 33.7. This picture was taken 3 days after a complete hamstring muscle tear. Note the swelling and ecchymosis immediately below the buttocks and down the posterior thigh. (From Sallay PI, Friedman RL, Coogan PG, et al. Hamstring muscle injuries among water skiers. *Am J Sports Med* 1996;24:132, with permission.)

passive stretch of the posterior structures (knee extension and hip flexion). Swelling, ecchymosis, and muscle spasm are frequently associated findings but may not be present for 24 hours (Fig. 33.7).

In the most severe cases, complete hamstring rupture, a palpable defect will be noted on examination. The defect will be found just distal to the ischeal tuberosity with distal retraction of the muscle belly (Fig. 33.8). Hematoma may fill the defect after 24 hours; therefore, it is important to examine the patient early. Failure to develop tension in the distal hamstring is a consistent finding with complete rupture. This is particularly true of the medial hamstrings, because the short head of the biceps femoris may still be able to develop tension from its origin from the femoral shaft (28). In the setting of a chronic complete rupture, a palpable defect may remain and occasionally may be associated with skin dimpling when tensing the hamstrings.

Classification of a hamstring strain is based on the severity of injury. The severity of the strain is not always immediately apparent because swelling and ecchymosis frequently do not appear for 24 hours. The exception to this is the case of a complete rupture, which should be apparent immediately, with a palpable defect. Otherwise, a 24-hour delay in classification is advised to allow a more accurate assessment of severity (41).

Hamstring strains are graded as first-, second-, and third-degree strains, the third-degree strain representing a complete rupture (Table 33.1). The grade of strain is determined by the severity of pain, spasm, ecchymosis, swelling, loss of knee extension, and the presence of a defect. *Grade I strains* generally have mild pain with minimal spasm, ecchymosis, and swelling. Loss of knee extension in the prone position is less than 20 degrees and there is no defect present.

Athletes involved in kicking, punting, and hurdling are most often in a position of risk, and therefore it is not surprising that this injury is most frequently seen in soccer, football, and track and field (10).

Several other factors have been associated with hamstring injuries, including muscle fatigue, previous muscle injury, lack of adequate warm-up, poor flexibility, leg length discrepancy, electrolyte depletion, hamstring to hamstring strength imbalance, and hamstring to quadriceps strength imbalance (14,30,33,35–40).

Clinically, an athlete who sustains a hamstring strain will recall a sudden ballistic event associated with a sharp disabling posterior thigh pain occasionally associated with an audible "pop." Examination of the posterior thigh should be performed in the prone position with the knee flexed to take tension off the injury. Palpation of the hamstrings will reveal point tenderness at the site of injury, which will increase in severity with

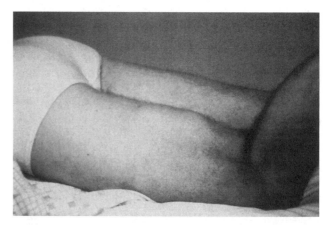

FIG. 33.8. A patient with a chronic complete hamstring muscle tear. Note the depression below the buttocks and the prominence of the retracted muscle belly distally. (From Sallay PI, Friedman RL, Coogan PG, et al. Hamstring muscle injuries among water skiers. *Am J Sports Med* 1996;24:132, with permission.)

TABLE 33-1. *Hamstring strain classification*

Grade	Pain	Ecchymosis	Spasm	Swelling	Defect	Loss of extension
I	+	+	+	+	No	<20
II	++	++	++	++	No	20–45
III	+++	+++	+++	+++	Yes	>45

From Nicholas JA, Hershman EB. *The lower extremity and spine in sports medicine,* 2nd ed. St. Louis: Mosby-Year Book Inc., 1995:45, with permission.

Grade II strains have moderate pain with moderate amounts of spasm, ecchymosis, and swelling. Loss of motion is between 20 and 45 degrees, and no palpable defect is noted. *Grade III strains* (complete ruptures) will have severe pain with significant amounts of spasm, ecchymosis, and swelling. Loss of motion will be greater than 45 degrees, and a palpable defect will be noted before hematoma formation. Distal muscle belly retraction and inability to tense the medial hamstrings may also be found.

Imaging of low-grade hamstring strains is not required. Plain radiographs will be normal, and MRI results will not change the treatment; thus, for low-grade hamstring strains, MRI is not cost effective. The exception is when evaluating a grade III strain or a controversial grade II/III strain. In these cases, plain radiographs may demonstrate a bony avulsion of the ischeal tuberosity, confirming a complete rupture. Similarly, an MRI can differentiate a complete hamstring rupture from a partial tear in the uncertain case. T2-weighted images on MRI demonstrate increased signal at the site of injury. Coronal images are most effective in evaluating partial versus complete tears at the ischium (Figs. 33.9 and 33.10). MRI of chronic complete ruptures demonstrate fatty degeneration and fibrosis of the muscle (14,26,28).

Treatment of acute hamstring strains depends on the grade of the strain; however, the initial treatment is the same regardless of severity. Initial treatment consists of RICE. The immediate goal is to minimize hemorrhage and inflammation because this will delay healing and increase scar tissue formation (10). Rest of the extremity is provided through crutch use for several days. RICE is continued throughout the acute phase, which usually lasts from 3 to 5 days.

NSAIDs have been shown to be effective in reducing pain and inflammation. Their mode of action is through direct inhibition of the enzyme cyclooxygenase that is responsible for the production of prostaglandin. Prostaglandin is a central mediator of the inflammatory process, and when inhibited the inflammatory response is minimized (43). Treatment with a NSAIDs should be implemented early in an attempt to minimize the inflammatory reaction. Once the acute inflammatory phase has passed, NSAIDs should be discontinued be-

cause of concerns regarding long-term use of NSAIDs with regard to delayed healing (14,23). In addition, the physician and athlete must be aware of the potential side effects of these medications, the most common of which is gastrointestinal distress (44).

Rehabilitation of the strain injury is implemented once the acute phase is under control, usually 3 to 5 days. The rehabilitation phase consists of a gradually

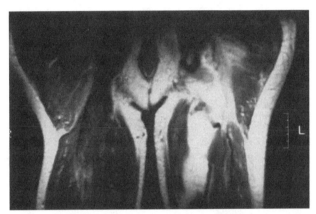

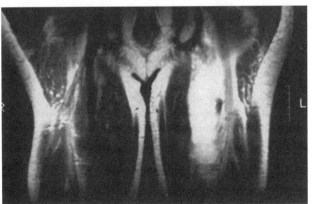

FIG. 33.9. A: T2-weighted coronal magnetic resonance image illustrating a complete tear of the left hamstring muscle complex from the ischium. The stump of the proximal tendon is clearly outlined by fluid. The contralateral side displays a normal tendon insertion onto the ischium. **B:** Note the proximity of the sciatic nerve, which is immediately adjacent to the torn tendon. (From Sallay PI, Friedman RL, Coogan PG, et al. Hamstring muscle injuries among water skiers. *Am J Sports Med* 1996;24:132, with permission.)

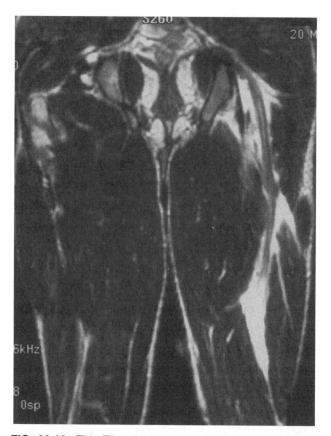

FIG. 33.10. This T2-weighted coronal magnetic resonance image of the left thigh documents a near-complete tear involving the semitendinosus and semimembranosus muscles. Most biceps femoris muscle is avulsed with the exception of a small slip laterally. (From Sallay PI, Friedman RL, Coogan PG, et al. Hamstring muscle injuries among water skiers. *Am J Sports Med* 1996;24:132, with permission.)

progressive program of stretching, strengthening, muscle balance, and restoration of hamstring function (11,30,33,36,45).

The goal of the rehabilitation phase is to reestablish muscle length, regain full range of motion, increase strength, prevent reinjury, and return the athlete to their specific sport. Muscle length is reestablished through gentle slow stretching exercises of the hamstrings. Stretching should be started as soon as symptoms allow, because it not only restores length but also provides a stress stimulus at the injury site that results in collagen proliferation, longitudinal orientation of fibers, and promotion of healing (24). Aggressive abrupt motion is avoided because this will increase bleeding and inflammation, thus increasing healing time. Once length is restored and range of motion is full, the subsequent step is to promote hamstring strength through a progressive resistance program. The resistance program should implement isometric, isotonic, and isokinetic strengthening in a sequential manner, using pain as the limiting guide for advancement. Isokinetic strengthening is used

at high speed and low resistance to stimulate the type 2 (fast-twitch) muscle fibers. Type 2 fast-twitch muscle fibers are found in a higher percentage in the hamstrings and are the fiber type most commonly affected in strain injury (40,46–49). Eccentric exercise is introduced as the final strengthening mode in the rehabilitation phase. It should be avoided initially, because it generates higher forces than concentric exercise and risks reinjury early in rehabilitation. Hamstring strengthening is continued until a 0.55 or greater hamstring-to-quadriceps strength ratio is reached. At this ratio, the hamstring has been found to be capable of protecting itself from an overpowering quadriceps that would otherwise result in reinjury (30). Once strength has been restored, the athlete may return to running and sport-specific training (Fig. 33.11).

Throughout the rehabilitation phase, modalities to decrease pain, decrease swelling, and promote muscle relaxation are used. Modalities that have had beneficial effects include ice massage, moist heat, ultrasound treatment, iontophoresis, and electric stimulation (10,11, 41,42,45). Deep massage is not recommended because this may aggravate bleeding and inflammation.

Criteria for returning to sports activity include several factors. Nicholas et al. (42) recommends equal hamstring flexibility and strength side to side, appropriate hamstring to quadriceps isokinetic ratio (more than 0.55), hip adductor/abductor strength parity, and a pain-free hamstring. DeLee and Drez (41) recommends return to sports only after isokinetic testing is within 10% of the normal side. Alternatively, functional testing (i.e., 50-yard sprints and agility box or figure-of-eight sprints) may also be used for evaluating fitness for returning to sports. If these can be accomplished pain free, the athlete is considered fit to return to sport activity.

Prevention of hamstring reinjury is of heightened importance after the first strain episode as the athlete's muscle is now predisposed to developing additional strains (14,20). Prevention strategies include endurance training of the muscle, because a fatigued muscle is more likely to strain than a nonfatigued muscle (14,19). Appropriate muscle warm-up before athletic activity is protective of strain injury (14,21). Finally, muscle stretching before and after athletic activity is a well-known strain-prevention strategy (14,22).

Grade-specific Treatment

Grade I hamstring strains are treated as described above, with RICE and NSAIDs initially, followed by additional modalities and the rehabilitation phase. Using this treatment program, prognosis is excellent, and full recovery can be expected from within days to weeks.

Grade II hamstring strains have more extensive tissue damage; however, their treatment regimen is the same

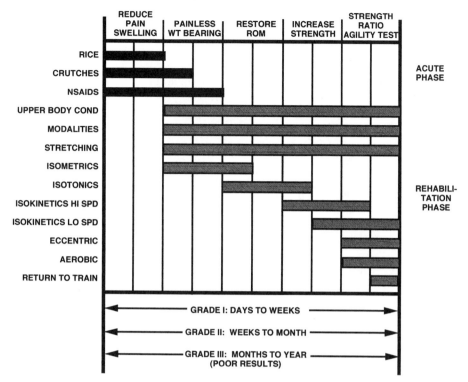

| | REDUCE PAIN SWELLING | PAINLESS WT BEARING | RESTORE ROM | INCREASE STRENGTH | STRENGTH RATIO AGILITY TEST | |

FIG. 33.11. Hamstring stain rehabilitation protocol. (From Nicholas JA, Hershman EB. *The lower extremity and spine in sports medicine,* 2nd ed. St. Louis: Mosby-Year Book, 1995:45, with permission.)

as with grade I strains. The prognosis is again excellent; however, the recovery period is prolong with full recovery expected within weeks to months. Heiser et al. (30) reported on 47 college-level football players with low-grade hamstring strains, finding an average of 14 days recovery before resuming play.

Grade III hamstring strains (complete rupture at the ischeal tuberosity) experience the greatest tissue damage of all hamstring strains. Their immediate treatment is once again with RICE to minimize hematoma formation. As with grade I and II strains, the standard regimen of NSAIDs, modalities, and rehabilitation program have been recommended (41,42); however, the results implementing this treatment protocol have been fair to poor (14,28,41,50,51). Sallay et al. (28) found an extensive recovery period from 3 to 18 months with 83% of patients reporting a pulling or cramping sensation in the posterior thigh with vigorous activity. Almost 50% of patients also reported a sense of poor leg control when attempting to run. Isokinetic muscle testing revealed an average concentric hamstring muscle strength deficit of 61% and an average quadriceps deficit of 23% compared with the opposite uninjured thigh.

Additional authors (14,41,50,51) have reported difficulties and poor results with conservative treatment of grade III complete proximal hamstring ruptures. Consequently, in the athletically active patient with a grade

III proximal hamstring rupture, several authors recommended acute surgical repair (14,28,49–51).

Authors' Preferences

Our treatment regimen for grade I and II hamstring strains is similar to most other protocols. Initial treatment consists of RICE and NSAIDs to minimize swelling and hematoma formation. Crutches are used until pain-free weight bearing is established.

Once the acute injury phase has been controlled, the rehabilitation phase is implemented. This begins with gentle stretching exercises to reestablish muscle length and range of motion. Strengthening is also initiated, in the following sequence: isometrics, isotonics, isokinetics (high speed, low resistance), isokinetics (low speed, high resistance), and eccentric strengthening. Aerobic and sport-specific training are the final steps in rehabilitation before returning to full sport activity. Pain is used as the guide for advancement throughout the rehabilitation protocol. Strengthening is continued until a hamstring-to-quadriceps strength ratio of 0.55 or greater is achieved. We also recommend agility and sprint testing as a clinical evaluation for return to sports.

Our experience in the treatment of grade III proximal hamstring ruptures using the above protocol have led to poor functional results (14,28). We therefore recommend acute repair of these injuries in the athletically active individual. In the uncertain cases, we obtain an MRI to confirm complete rupture before considering repair. Surgical repair is performed in the prone position, with a curvilinear incision centered over the ischeal tuberosity, defect, and proximal hamstring mass. The inferior boarder of the gluteus maximus and the posterior femoral cutaneous nerve are identified once the skin incision has been made. The posterior femoral cutaneous nerve is located just lateral to the ischeal tuberosity. The defect is located and the hematoma evacuated. Distal to the defect, the proximal hamstring mass is located and the individual muscles identified. The semimembranosus is found deep and medial to the semitendinosus with the long head of the biceps being most lateral of the three. The sciatic nerve can be identified deep to the biceps femoris. To expose the ischeal tuberosity, the gluteus maximus must be retracted superiorly. Care must be taken not to retract excessively on the posterior femoral cutaneous nerve or sciatic nerve, which are just lateral to the ischeal tuberosity. A bleeding bony surface is prepared on the ischeal tuberosity before reanastamosis of the proximal hamstring mass. The repair is accomplished using three to five no. 2

nonabsorbable suture anchors. The anastamosis is performed with the knee flexed to allow proximal migration of the hamstring mass. Postoperatively, the patient is maintained in a hip-knee-foot orthosis with the knee in flexion and the hip in neutral to take tension off of the repair. The knee is gradually brought into full extension over a 6-week period. At approximately 6 weeks postsurgery, the hamstring strain rehabilitation protocol is implemented (Fig. 33.11).

In the setting of chronic hamstring ruptures, chronic posterior thigh pain can eventually require surgical exploration. In these cases, we recommend a thorough exploration of the sciatic and posterior femoral cutaneous nerves, because constrictive bands of scar tissue have been noted to impinge on these nerves (Fig. 33.12). In addition, we recommend the use of an intraoperative nerve stimulator for evaluation of abnormal regions of muscle contraction secondary to scar formation. Repair of chronic ruptures usually requires distal tendon lengthening to mobilize the retracted proximal hamstrings to the ischeal tuberosity. The postoperative rehabilitation is the same as described for acute repair. Repair of chronic hamstring ruptures is technically more demanding secondary to scar formation, retraction, and muscle atrophy. We therefore recommended acute repair of proximal hamstring ruptures in the athletic population.

Avulsion Fractures

Avulsion fractures of the ischeal tuberosity are treated in the same manner as grade III hamstring strains. The diagnosis is confirmed with a palpable defect on examination and a displaced bony fragment on plain radiographs. In the case of a nondisplaced or minimally displaced ischeal tuberosity fracture with no palpable defect, we recommend protected knee flexion with a hip-knee-foot orthosis for 6 weeks. Close follow-up is required to ensure no further displacement of the bony fragment.

Displaced pediatric ischeal avulsion fractures have typically been successfully treated with nonoperative rehabilitation programs. However, when associated with severe displacement, there may be a role for acute surgical repair because troublesome bony prominences may develop and functional limitations may result (52).

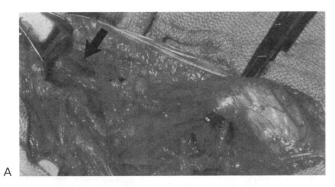

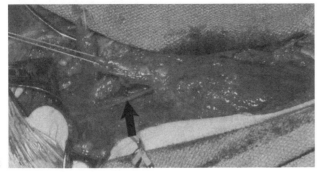

FIG. 33.12. A: The proximal hamstring tendon, identified by the clamp, is scarred and retracted distally. The *arrow* is on the ischial tuberosity. **B:** Sutures have been placed into the stump of the freed tendon ends proximally and distally. Notice the proximity of the sciatic nerve (encircled by the vessel loop) and its branches (*arrow*). (From Sallay PI, Friedman RL, Coogan PG, et al. Hamstring muscle injuries among water skiers. *Am J Sports Med* 1996;24:132, with permission.)

Ischeal Apophysitis

Pediatric ischeal apophysitis has a similar presentation to hamstring strain; however, usually there is no major traumatic event. Mean age for development of apophysitis is 14 years of age. Radiographs reveal widened and sclerotic apophysis. Prognosis is excellent with conservative treatment, including NSAIDs and stretching.

Other

For completeness we will mention less common causes of posterior thigh pain that must be considered whenever evaluating an athlete for a probable hamstring strain. Posterior thigh pain can be referred from pathology at the lumbar spine, gluteal muscles, and the sacroiliac joint. Hamstring myositis ossificans (MO), tumor, deep venous thrombosis, adductor canal syndrome, and posterior compartment syndrome can also mimic hamstring strain. These are discussed at the end of this chapter.

ADDUCTORS AND GROIN

Injury to the medial adductor compartment and groin are common to the athlete. Groin injuries are estimated to account for 2% to 5% of all sports injuries (53,54). The true incidence of groin and adductor injuries is difficult to estimate, because groin injuries are frequently grouped with pelvic and hip injuries. Recent data from the NCAA Injury Surveillance System (6) report a groin, hip, and pelvis injury rate of 0.68/1,000 hours AE.

Diagnoses that should be considered when evaluating athletes with groin pain include adductor muscle strain, iliopsoas muscle strain, adductor tubercle avulsion fracture, inferior ramus stress fracture, athletic pubalgia, and osteitis pubis. In addition, hernia, prostatitis, and hip pathology must also be considered.

Pathology in the groin region is best categorized by location of symptoms with regard to the adductor tubercle. Pain below the adductor tubercle is frequently associated with strain injury. Pain at the adductor tubercle is usually a result of avulsion fracture or inferior ramus stress fracture, and pain above the adductor tubercle is common to athletic pubalgia. Pain localized at the tubercle or just medial to the adductor tubercle is frequently found with osteitis pubis.

Chronic groin pain in the athlete is a challenging diagnostic and therapeutic problem. Symptoms are usually vague, making diagnosis difficult. The physician must have a broad knowledge of the pathoanatomy and potential diagnoses associated with chronic groin pain. Successful treatment will depend on making the correct diagnosis.

Adductor Strain Injury

Adductor strain, commonly referred to as a "groin pull," is a frequent injury found in the athletic population. Overall, adductor strains, which account for approximately 8% of strain injuries in sports, occur less frequently than hamstring and quadriceps strains (10). NCAA soccer injury surveillance data indicate an adductor strain injury rate of 0.25/1,000 hours AE (6,10). Hockey, however, has been found to have a higher rate of injury to the adductor musculature. Hockey injury data report adductor strains comprise 10% of all injuries diagnosed in hockey (49,55). Adductor strains are the most common strain injuries in hockey, with a reported injury rate as high as 0.43/1,000 hours AE (49,56). Additional sports commonly associated with adductor strain include rugby, horseback riding, tennis, track and field, karate, and gymnastics.

Adductor strains most often involve the adductor longus muscle (14,26,57,58). The adductor magnus muscle has also been implicated in groin strain injury but less frequently than the adductor longus (59). The specific injury site is the muscle–tendon junction (14,57) (see Muscle Strain Injury, above).

The mechanism of injury involves eccentric adductor muscle contraction with concurrent hip external rotation and abduction. This mechanism is typically seen in aggressively skating hockey players when shifting weight to the opposite leg. This mechanism also presents in soccer with rapid acceleration or when two soccer players kick a soccer ball at the same time (54).

Additional factors associated with adductor strain include muscle fatigue, lack of adequate warm-up, previous adductor muscle strain, poor flexibility, and adductor to adductor strength imbalance (14,36,58).

Clinically, the athlete usually presents with a history of a painful forced abduction episode resulting in immediate groin pain. Examination reveals point tenderness over the adductor longus below the adductor tubercle. Pain is accentuated with passive abduction of the hip. Complete adductor rupture will present with a palpable defect and distal muscle pain and retraction. A palpable defect with pain localized to the adductor tubercle is more likely to be associated with an avulsion fracture of the adductor tubercle.

Acute adductor strains are classified using a similar grading system as described with hamstring strains. The strain grade is based on the severity of the injury. *Grade I strains* have mild tenderness with minimal ecchymosis, spasm, and swelling. *Grade II strains* have moderate amounts of pain, ecchymosis, spasm, and swelling. *Grade III strains* (complete rupture) have severe pain with significant ecchymosis, spasm, and swelling. Distal muscle belly retraction and a palpable defect will be noted on examination before hematoma formation.

Occasionally, the athlete will present without an acute injury and without prior history of strain injury. Their groin pain will be described as being more insidious and progressive in nature. On examination, the pain is localized to the adductor muscle–tendon unit and is accentuated with hip abduction and sport-related activity. This condition is typical of a chronic overuse adductor tendonitis that results from microtears of the muscle–tendon unit secondary to repeated overload (60). In this scenario, the physician must be careful not to overlook other possible diagnoses with similar insidious onset of symptoms, such as hernia, prostatitis, and athletic pubalgia.

Imaging studies of acute low-grade adductor strains are usually not necessary. However, when there is question of the diagnosis or when considering complete adductor rupture with avulsion fracture, plain radiographs may provide insight. Radiographs of the hip and pelvis can confirm a physician's suspicion of referred pain from hip or pelvic pathology. When evaluating complete rupture or avulsion fracture plain, radiographs should always be obtained.

MRI is not indicated for acute low-grade adductor strains. However, in the uncertain case of a grade II versus grade III adductor strain, T2-weighted MRI has been shown to be most effective in confirming complete rupture (26). In addition, MRI is helpful in evaluating the etiology of groin pain in the patient with an uncertain diagnosis. MRI will differentiate muscle strain from osteitis pubis, bursitis, athletic pubalgia, and stress fractures (61).

Chronic adductor muscle strain is best evaluated using ultrasonography (62,63). Normal tendon appears fibrillar with a high-echogenic signal, whereas injured tendon is demarcated with local hypoechogenic areas and loss of fibrillar appearance (63,64). Ultrasound imaging has several advantages: rapid test time, noninvasive testing, low cost, and no radiation exposure. Ultrasonography is perhaps most useful when used to determine the exact location and extension of tendon injury before injection or surgery (62).

The treatment protocol for acute adductor strain injury is similar to that used in acute hamstring strain injury. RICE are the initial modes of treatment to minimize hemorrhage and inflammation. Crutch use allows rest of the extremity throughout the acute phase. NSAIDs are implemented early to minimize the inflammatory response. The acute phase generally lasts 3 to 5 days; however, with more severe strains the acute phase will be prolonged. Once pain-free weight bearing is obtained, a rehabilitation program is implemented. The goal of rehabilitation is to reestablish muscle length, regain full range of motion, increase strength, prevent reinjury, and return the athlete to their specific sport. Rehabilitation protocols implement a combination of stretching and progressive strengthening exercises, including isometrics, isotonics, and isokinetics (41,62). Pain reduction modalities are also used throughout the rehabilitation phase.

Criteria for return to sports activity include full pain-free range of motion with equal flexibility, isokinetic testing within 10% of uninjured side, and pain-free simu-lated sports activities (41). Recommendations for prevention of reinjury is the same as discussed under hamstring strain prevention of reinjury.

Grade-specific Treatment

Acute grade I and II adductor strain injuries are treated with the above protocol: RICE, NSAIDs, modalities, and a rehabilitation program. Prognosis is generally considered good to excellent, with the athlete returning to sports within 1 to 4 weeks. We recommend the identical rehabilitation protocol described for hamstring strains (Fig. 33.11).

Acute grade III adductor strains (complete rupture) have generally been treated with the standard nonoperative treatment protocol above. However, recent reports (41,62,65) have suggested that surgical repair of complete ruptures should be considered, because functional deficits, chronic pain, and prolonged healing periods may be experienced with nonoperative treatment. We recommend considering surgical repair of complete ruptures and displaced adductor avulsion fractures in the athletically active individual.

The initial recommended treatment for chronic adductor tendonitis is the same as the nonoperative protocol for an acute injury. Additional nonoperative intervention may include ultrasound-guided steroid injections. Martens et al. (60) found that despite 3 months of conservative management, only 38% of patients were able to return to their original activity level. This series of patients were offered subcutaneous adductor tenotomy, which produced 81% good to excellent results. Akermark and Johansson (66) also reported good results with adductor longus tenotomy for refractory cases of adductor longus tendonitis. They stressed the importance of hemostasis and avoidance of the obturator nerve branches. A final surgical approach to chronic adductor longus tendonitis involves intratendinous longitudinal split of the tendon at the site of the pathology (identified by MRI or ultrasound). Pathologic devitalized granulation tissue may be found within the tendon. The pathologic tissue is excised and the remaining normal tendon is sutured to itself (62). Postoperatively, patients are allowed weight-bearing exercise as tolerated. Return to sport activities is between 3 and 6 months.

Iliopsoas Strain

Strain injury to the iliopsoas tendon will result in groin pain that is slightly distal to the adductor tubercle. Pain is accentuated with hip extension and internal rotation. This injury has been reported in soccer and football players (49,67). The mechanism of injury is forced hyperextension of the hip against a contracting iliopsoas muscle. Hip flexion contracture and femoral nerve palsy have been associated with this injury (68). Plain radiographs and MRI will be useful when lesser trochanteric avulsion fracture or complete iliopsoas tendon disruption are suspected. Treatment of low-grade strains is conservative with RICE, NSAIDs, and a rehabilitation program. Surgical repair is considered in the skeletally mature athletic individual with avulsion fracture or complete rupture (57,69).

Adductor Tubercle Avulsion Fracture

Avulsion fracture of the adductor tubercle presents similar to an acute grade III strain of the adductor longus; however, pain may be more localized to the adductor tubercle than distally at the musculotendinous junction. There will be a palpable defect and muscle belly retraction. Plain radiographs will confirm the diagnosis in most cases. Treatment recommendation are as with grade III strain, and consideration should be given to surgical repair in the athletically active individual.

Inferior Ramus Stress Fracture

Inferior ramus stress fracture is a rare entity; however, it should be included in the differential diagnosis of groin pain localized to the adductor tubercle. As with any stress fracture, the pain is usually insidious in nature and is related to a history of overuse. Bone scan and MRI are helpful in confirming the diagnosis. Treatment is rest, avoidance of impact exercises, analgesics, and activity modification. In the female athlete with a documented stress fracture, the physician must be aware of the association with amenorrhea and anorexia. Appropriate measures must be taken to rule out this triad in any female with a stress fracture.

Osteitis Pubis

Osteitis pubis presents with insidious onset of groin pain and a history of overuse activity. Athletes who are prone to this entity include distance runners, cross-country skiers, soccer players, and hockey players. Osteitis pubis results from increased shear forces at the symphysis pubis, usually secondary to increased athletic activity. Shear forces are greatest during midstance, when the unsupported pelvis attempts to drop (69). The increased shear at the pubis results in an inflammatory reaction and pain localized to the symphysis, just medial to the adductor tubercle. Diagnosis may be difficult because these symptoms are consistent with several pathologic conditions in the groin region. Radiographs, bone scan, and MRI are helpful in confirming the diagnosis (61,69). Radiographs typically demonstrate medial symphyseal resorption, periosteal reaction, demineralization, and sclerosis. Treatment is conservative with rest, NSAIDs,

moist heat, and activity modification. Complete resolution may not occur for 3 months (70).

Athletic Pubalgia

Athletic pubalgia has been a poorly recognized and poorly understood entity. Recent literature from Europe and the United States has increased its exposure and recognition (71–74). European literature refers to this condition as "Gilmore's groin" or the "sportsman's hernia" (71–73). "Athletic pubalgia" is a descriptive term used for undiagnosed chronic groin pain in the absence of any other groin pathology (74). Specifically, inguinal hernia must be ruled out before making the diagnosis of athletic pubalgia (74) (WC Meyers, D Foley, JJ Kelly, et al., unpublished data, 1998). Because this is a diagnosis of exclusion, an extensive workup of chronic groin pain usually precedes the diagnosis and treatment.

Athletic pubalgia is not a common cause of groin pain. The true incidence is not known; however, the largest series includes 106 cases collected over an 8-year period (WC Meyers, D Foley, JJ Kelly, et al., unpublished data, 1998). This condition is found most often in veteran high-caliber athletes of soccer, football, and hockey.

The pathophysiology of athletic pubalgia is not well understood. Some have described the pathology as the earliest stage of a direct inguinal hernia (73). The pathology does appear to be related to a weakness in the abdominal wall musculature near the inguinal ligament (49,72,74). Repetitive stresses on the abdominal wall may cause microtearing or additional laxity of the abdominal wall resulting in irritation of the ilioinguinal, iliohypogastric, or genitofemoral nerves.

The pain associated with athletic pubalgia is often difficult for the athlete to describe and is usually of insidious onset, chronic in nature, and localized to the abdominal wall at the pubic tubercle. The pain can be sharp, burning, or of an aching quality lasting for hours after activity. Pain is exacerbated with kicking, running, or sit-up activity. Symptoms usually resolve with rest but return when activities are resumed. Clinically, pain is present at the pubic tubercle and is accentuated with resisted hip flexion and abdominal muscle contraction. By definition, the remainder of the groin examination is negative, including hernia and rectal examinations to rule out prostatitis.

Because athletic pubalgia is a diagnosis of exclusion, multiple imaging studies are usually obtained before making its diagnosis. Plain radiographs, bone scan, computed tomography, and MRI are obtained to exclude other possible etiologies of groin pain. Herniography has been found to be very helpful in evaluating and confirming the diagnosis of athletic pubalgia. This is the only imaging study that may be positive in an athlete with chronic groin pain and a negative examination for a hernia (75). This supports the theory that athletic pubalgia is the earliest stage of a direct inguinal hernia.

The initial treatment of athletic pubalgia includes rest and a lower abdominal wall strengthening program. However, the results with conservative treatment have not been very successful. Martens et al. (60) reported that only 30% of their patients were successfully treated nonoperatively. The remaining 70% required surgical intervention.

Operative treatment involves a pelvic floor repair. Most often, a modified Bassini-type herniorraphy has been recommended (72–74). The results with operative repair have been excellent. Several studies have demonstrated an 80% or higher success rate with pain-free return to sport activity within 3 to 4 months (72–74) (WC Meyers, D Foley, JJ Kelly, et al., unpublished data, 1998).

Although conservative treatment of athletic pubalgia has had marginal results, we do recommend a trial of physical therapy as the initial treatment for athletic pubalgia. The physical therapy protocol includes massage, stretching, and strengthening of the lower abdominal wall (Table 33.2). If a trial of physical therapy fails, we recommend general surgical consultation for modified Bassini-type herniorrhaphy.

Groin Pain: Additional Considerations

Hernia, as previously mentioned, must be evaluated in any athlete with chronic groin pain. Inguinal and femoral hernias are known to occur in the athletic population. In one series, evolving hernia was found to account for 50% of undiagnosed chronic groin pain (76). Physical examination should evaluate the inguinal canal and anterior abdominal wall for evidence of a hernia bulge. Herniography is helpful for diagnosis of uncertain cases (77,78). The treatment is surgical repair, and good results can be expected in most cases (57).

Prostatitis is frequently overlooked when evaluating chronic groin pain. Prostatitis frequently mimics adductor longus tendonitis or strain. Workup for chronic groin pain should include a rectal examination, urinalysis, and urine culture to rule out prostatitis. The recommended treatment is antibiotics and NSAIDs.

Hip pathology should always be suspected in the setting of groin pain. In the adult, osteoarthritis will refer pain to the groin. In young athletes, slipped capital femoral epiphysis and Perthes disease must be excluded. Most hip pathology will be demonstrated on radiographs. Bilateral frog-leg laterals of the hip should be obtained when evaluating for slipped capital femoral epiphysis.

Obturator nerve entrapment is not a well-recognized entity because there is only one series report of 32 patients to date (79). This condition is described as an obturator neuropathy secondary to fascial entrapment of the obturator nerve as it enters the thigh. Clinically, the athlete experiences medial thigh pain and weakness that is aggravated with exercise. The diagnosis is confirmed with an EMG and/or obturator nerve block. Definitive treatment is surgical release of the adductor longus and pectineal fascia overlying the obturator nerve. Outcome with surgical release is very good, with all patients returning to sports within 3 weeks and all EMGs returning to normal postoperatively.

TABLE 33-2. *Athletic pubalgia: physical therapy protocol*

Phase I: rest/massage
  Week 1: rest/massage.
    Deep tissue massage of muscles posterior, superior, and lateral pelvis.
    Sessions for 20–30 min focus on painful sites.
    Continue for 1 wk.
    Rest, no sport participation.

Phase II: stretching
  Week 2: begin stretching exercises.
    Stretching 2–3 times per day, hip adductors, hamstrings, hip flexors, hip rotators, and lower back (emphasize lateral bend and extension).
    Continue with massage treatment.
    Light aerobic exercise if no pain (water walking, stationary bike)
No sport participation.

Phase III: strengthening
  Week 3: begin strengthening exercises.
    Strengthen abdominal musculature, hip adductors, and hip flexors.
    Abdominal strengthening should be performed on the floor in a supine position with the back flat on the floor; legs are brought to the chest and the pelvis lifted off the floor using the abdominal muscles.
    Continue light aerobic activities.

Phase IV: functional
  Week 4: begin running—shuttle runs, agility runs, crossovers
  Continue stretching and strengthening.

Phase V: return to sport
  Gradual resumption of sport specific activities as tolerated.
  Return to competition if pain free.

From Lohnes J. *Athletic pubalgia: a cause of chronic groin pain in the athlete.* Durham, NC: Duke Univ. Med. Center, with permission.

QUADRICEPS

The four muscles of the anterior compartment include the vastus medialis, lateralis, intermedius, and rectus femoris. The latter muscle assists in hip flexion and knee extension. These muscles are mostly composed of type 2 fibers that are suited to rapid forceful activity. The primary function of the quadriceps are to contract in concert with the hamstrings to act as a decelerator during the support phase of running.

Injury to the quadriceps occurs by two mechanisms. The first is through eccentric contraction with an increase in the tensile forces beyond the threshold of the musculotendinous units, resulting in gradations of strain and rupture. The second mechanism is by forceful external compression causing contusion injury.

The incidence of quadriceps injury is difficult to ascertain. Initially, studies were performed on military personnel, but recently more studies are focusing on the athlete. Sports in which the anterior thigh is frequently injured include football, soccer, rugby, basketball, and track and field (13). McMaster and Walter (4) found that quadriceps contusions and strains accounted for 18% of the lower extremity injuries in a professional soccer team. In an evaluation of injuries in a youth soccer league, Backous et al. (80) found that 8.3% were quadriceps strains. This increased to 24% in adolescent boys near 14 years of age. Krejci and Koch (10) found that quadriceps strain ranked third behind hamstring and triceps surae, with an incidence of 17% and an injury rate of 0.5/1,000 hours AE. Lipscomb et al. (81), in a review of 42 quadriceps contusions in football players, determined that this injury occurred every 50 practices. Interestingly, quadriceps contusion in rugby players was only 2% of all injuries (82).

Quadriceps Strain Injury

Quadriceps strain is muscle injury in evolution. The spectrum encompasses delayed-onset soreness; mild, moderate, and severe strains; and frank rupture of the myotendinous complex. What each of these have in common are acute partial tears at the myotendinous junction. The severity of the strain is directly proportional to the amount of disruption of the integrity of the musculotendinous unit (20,83).

It is rare to sustain a quadriceps strain unless there is body contact that resists extension of the leg or flexion of the hip. This is in part because of the strength of the quadriceps. The normal ratio for quadriceps and hamstring strength is 3:2, but because of neglect of hamstring training, often seen in soccer, this ratio is closer to 5:1. (84). The quadriceps, save the rectus femoris, is also protected in that it does not cross two joints as does the hamstring and gastrocnemius complex, which puts these muscles at increased risk for strain. Of the quadriceps muscles, the rectus femoris is the most commonly involved muscle as it does span two joints.

The mechanism of injury is essentially a violent eccentric contraction or forceful stretching of the muscle group. The muscles are at greatest risk when the hip is extended and the knee flexed, placing them at maximal tension. Sudden resistance to knee extension and hip flexion further increases the risk of injury. Injury can also take place with sudden acceleration or an abrupt change in speed, leading to forceful muscle contraction. Other risk factors include muscle fatigue, recurrent injury, poor flexibility and conditioning, and inadequate warm-up. The amount of damage is dependent on the amount of the force and the strength of resistance. Quadriceps strains are graded as any other strain. Grade I is a mild strain and is characterized by minimal disruption of the musculotendinous complex. There is a low-grade inflammatory response with swelling, edema, and minimal loss of musculature function or restriction of motion. Grade II or a moderate strain is defined as actual damage to the myotendinous unit that compromises strength and range of motion. Grade III or severe strain represents the ultimate load to failure of the myotendinous unit (69). The structural integrity of the muscle is so compromised that rupture may occur along any part of the musculotendinous junction or muscle (59). Diagnosis depends on the recognition of the loss of function.

Often patients will present with an acute onset of anterior thigh pain with a sensation that something has torn. There is usually varying degrees of swelling, ecchymosis, muscle spasm, and loss of knee flexion depending on the severity of the strain. With a mild strain knee flexion is more than 90 degrees, for a moderate strain less than 90 degrees, and for a severe strain less than 45 degrees. Occasionally, a defect or hematoma is palpable in the anterior thigh. When contracting the quadriceps complex, a retracting palpable mass is indicative of a complete rupture (41). This finding differentiates a grade II strain from a grade III strain.

Any attempts at knee flexion will exacerbate the patients discomfort. If the rectus femoris is affected more then the vasti, the loss of knee flexion and pain will be greater with the hip extended. Conversely, if there is no increase in pain, the vastus medialis, lateralis, or intermedius may be more involved. Thigh circumference should be routinely measured and remeasured, especially when there is increasing pain and swelling in the thigh.

Plain radiographs are usually not indicated unless bony injury or avulsion fracture is suspected. The use of ultrasound for the detection of a hematoma and assisted aspiration has been suggested but is rarely practiced. MRI, specifically T2-weighted images, has the accuracy to depict the location and severity of the strain (26). Its common use is restricted, however, by the cost and actual necessity in determining the diagnosis. It is most useful in differentiating a grade II from a grade III injury.

Treatment is dependent on the severity of the quadriceps injury. The treatment protocol follows a similar pattern previously described for hamstring injury (Fig. 33.11). Briefly, the acute phase after initial assessment follows the RICE protocol. Protected weight bearing, compression, elevation, and ice will reduce the amount of hemorrhage and swelling within the thigh. The proper use of NSAIDs initially will also reduce the amount of inflammation. The rehabilitative phase includes protected range of motion, modalities, stretching, and isometric and isotonic exercises. Later, isokinetic exercise at high speeds and low resistance is incorporated in the concentric mode. Eccentric training is avoided at this stage because it generates more work per unit area of muscle then concentric work. Once isokinetics are satisfactorily completed, eccentric exercise with passive stretching is performed. Throughout the rehabilitative protocol, great care should be given to gradually advance the athlete through each step. As each step is reached, there should be less pain, more range of motion, and greater strength.

The criteria for returning to sports is similar for hamstring injuries. Suffice it to say there should be more than 90% strength compared with the contralateral limp with isokinetic testing, no pain or limitation in range of motion, normal flexibility, agility, and aerobic conditioning.

For grade I and II strains, the average time before returning to sporting activity is 2 to 3 weeks. The success for grade III strains, however, is less predictable. Rupture of the musculotendinous complex often requires surgical reconstruction to obtain a good functional result (59,83,85).

Partial Quadriceps Tendon Rupture

Partial quadriceps tendon rupture (jumper's knee) is a tendinopathy of the extensor mechanism of the knee. It most commonly affects the inferior pole of the patella at the origin of the patella tendon, but in 25% of cases the quadriceps insertion is involved (86–89). Sports that involve repetitive jumping or excessive strain on the quadriceps, such as basketball, volleyball, and weight lifting, predispose to developing partial tears of the quadriceps mechanism. A repetitive injury cascade occurs with acute and chronic inflammation secondary and eventual healing of the tendon with fibrotic tissue.

Typically, there is pain at the superior pole of the patella. This is aggravated by jumping or eccentrically contacting the quadriceps. Ultrasound and MRI may show signs of partial tears with localized areas or foci of inflammation and scar tissue (90).

Most patients will respond to conservative measures of rest, activity modification, physical therapy, and NSAIDs. Raatikainen et al. (86) reviewed 28 patients who were recalcitrant to conservative modalities and required surgery. At surgery, a palpable nodule was located in the medial or middle third of the tendon and within the posterior half. Histology characterized the nodule as dense fibrotic scar with chronic inflammation consistent with a partial rupture of the tendon. After the nodule was excised, the tendon was repaired in a side-to-side fashion with absorbable sutures. Twent-five patients had an excellent result.

Quadriceps Rupture

Historically, the writings of Galen (130–120 A.D.) described a wrestler who ruptured his patella tendon and represents the first documented extensor tendon disruption (91). Ruysch, a Dutch physician, reported on the first quadriceps injury in 1720. Until Lister in 1878 and McBurney in 1887 performed an operative repair of the quadriceps tendon, treatment was conservative with the use of splints (92,93).

Quenu and Deval in 1905 (94) reported the results on operative treatment or 26 quadriceps ruptures. Since that time, the recommended treatment for extensor tendon disruption has been surgical management. Although many authors have reported on quadriceps rupture, these have been case reports or small series. Siwek and Rao in 1981 (95) reported on the largest series of extensor tendon disruptions, which included 72 ruptures. Thirty-six were quadriceps tendon ruptures. All 30 patients operated on acutely with an end-to-end repair had an excellent or good result with knee motion 0 to 120 degrees. Similarly, Larsen and Lund (96) with 15 quadriceps tendon ruptures and Vainionpaa et al. (97) with 12 had an 83% excellent success rate with operative repair. Multiple techniques have been described to repair and reconstruct the quadriceps tendon (95–99).

In a review of 117 reported cases of extensor tendon rupture between 1880 and 1978, 88% of the quadriceps ruptures were in patients older than 40, although patella tendon disruptions were seen in patients less then 40 years old (95). Thus, there is a predisposition for an older patient population. Age-related changes in the tendon, such as fatty degeneration, tendinosclerosis, fibroid degeneration, and an attenuation of the collagen content of the fibers, decrease the strength of the musculotendinous or tendoosseous unit and increase the chance of failure under physiologic loads. Additional patients at risk include those with chronic systemic diseases like diabetes, inflammatory arthritis, chronic renal failure, collagen vascular disorders, hyperparathyroidism, and obesity (100).

Rarely, a quadriceps rupture occurs bilaterally. In fact, since Chilchester reported the first case of bilateral simultaneous rupture in 1909 (101), there has only been 39 cases documented in the English literature (102–105). They often occur exclusively in males. Chronic systemic disease or the use of anabolic steroids have been implicated in 40% to 50% of patients (100,103,104). Interestingly, there are two distinct groups of patients. In the younger patient population there is a history of chronic renal failure, gout, and hyperparathyroidism

(107,108). Those in the older group have diabetes, obesity, or no known predisposing factor (106,109). This correlation is so significant that a workup for arthritis, collagen vascular disorders, and endocrinopathies is recommended in a younger patient with bilateral quadriceps ruptures.

Most quadriceps ruptures are caused by hyperflexion of the knee while the quadriceps muscles are strongly contracting. Usually, a history of stumbling or giving way of the knee is noted. Typically, a middle-aged person has fallen on a hyperflexed knee while descending stairs. Several cases have been associated with squatting with a heavy weight (103,104,106). A history of repetitive injury and sharp or blunt trauma has also been implicated in this injury.

Patients present with acute onset pain and loss of function. There is usually a palpable gap or sulcus above the patella, hemarthrosis of the knee, and inability to extend the knee. If the patient is able to extend the knee against gravity, then the tear may be incomplete and not require operative repair (99). If there is failure to extend the knee, then both the tendon and retinaculum are ruptured and surgical repair is necessary.

Quadriceps rupture occurs 0 to 2 cm proximal to the superior pole of the patella. Rupture can occur through a portion of degenerated tendon or avulse off the superior pole of the patella. Proximal migration of the quadriceps complex, as much as 5 cm, can occur if not recognized early.

Diagnosis of the quadriceps tendon rupture is primarily by physical examination. Plain radiographs usually show loss of the quadriceps tendon shadow, suprapatellar mass, suprapatellar calcific densities, patella baja, and degenerative spurring of the patella (tooth sign) on the lateral view (110,111). Despite these radiographic findings, the diagnosis of quadriceps rupture may be elusive.

Arthrography may demonstrate extravasation of the dye into the superior defect. To avoid this invasive test and the potential complication of infection, ultrasound has been used effectively in differentiating partial from complete quadriceps tears. Bianchi et al. (112) demonstrated a high degree of sensitivity and specificity in the evaluation of tendon rupture.

MRI is a superior imaging modality (113–116). The laminated appearance of the quadriceps tendon allows distinction between partial and complete tears. T2-weighted images depict edema and hemorrhage as increased signal intensity at the site of the rupture and may demonstrate extravasation of the synovial fluid

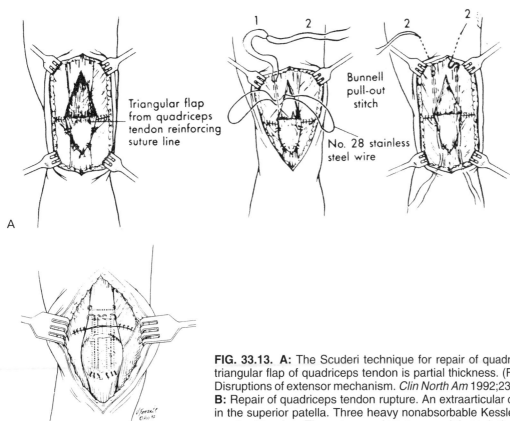

FIG. 33.13. **A:** The Scuderi technique for repair of quadriceps tendon ruptures. The triangular flap of quadriceps tendon is partial thickness. (From Haas SB, Callaway H, Disruptions of extensor mechanism. *Clin North Am* 1992;23:687–695, with permission.) **B:** Repair of quadriceps tendon rupture. An extraarticular cancellous trough is created in the superior patella. Three heavy nonabsorbable Kessler stitches are placed in the proximal tendon. The suture ends are passed through three vertical drill holes in the patella and tied at the inferior pole. The retinaculum is repaired directly. (Copyright 1992 by The Hospital for Special Surgery, with permission.)

through the defect. A corrugated appearance of the patella tendon on lateral MRI (wrinkled patella tendon) represents decreased tensile forces across it and indicates an abnormality with the extensor mechanism of the knee (115). The expense of the MRI, however, limits its usefulness and should only be applied when the diagnosis is in doubt.

Numerous surgical techniques have been described in the literature for the management of acute and chronic ruptures of quadriceps such as those advocated by Scuderi, McLaughlin, Siwek, and Miskew (95,98,99,117). Most authors agree that an end-to-end repair produces the best results (95,96,98,99,117–121).

In his study of 20 tendon repairs, Scuderi (99) used a midline approach. The tendon edges were debrided, overlapped, and then sutured together. After this a triangular flap of proximal quadriceps tendon is folded over distally and sutured to reinforce the repair. A stainless steel Bunnel pullout wire placed on either side of the patella in the retinaculum protects the repair (Fig. 33.13A).

Miskew et al. (98) described the use of Mersilene strip sutures to reinforce the end-to-end repair. This was placed through a transverse drill holes in the proximal patella and passed through the quadriceps tendon proximal to the defect.

Similarly, Levy et al. (120) used a 5.0-mm Dacron vascular reinforcement graft in a circumferential fashion around the inferior pole of the patella and proximal quadriceps (Fig. 33.14). Fujikawa et al. (121) described reconstruction of the extensor apparatus with a synthetic tubular Leeds-Keio ligament in 19 patients. The advantage of these two techniques was that no patient was immobilized postoperatively. In fact, the patients began active range of motion immediately. This is in contrast to the earlier repairs after which the patient was immobilized in a cylinder cast for 6 weeks.

When the defect occurs at the bone–tendon junction, which is often the case in patients older than 40, reapproximation of the tendon to bone is performed using no. 2 Ethibond suture placed though three longitudinal drill holes in the patella. The suture is placed through the quadriceps tendon in either a Kessler-, Krackow-, or Bunnel-type fashion. The proximal pole of the patella is debrided to create a rough bleeding cancellous bed for the tendon. The sutures are tied just distal to the inferior pole of the patella. The retinaculum is then repaired with nonabsorbable sutures (118,119) (Fig. 33.13B). Finally, a stress-relieving suture (no. 2 or no. 5 Ethibond) is placed in a circumferential purse-string fashion around the inferior pole of the patella and proximal to the quadriceps repair. The extremity is then placed in a hinged knee brace locked in extension for 6 weeks. Straight leg raising and isometric quadriceps strengthening are begun 1 week postoperatively. Weight bearing as tolerated with crutches is allowed. After 6

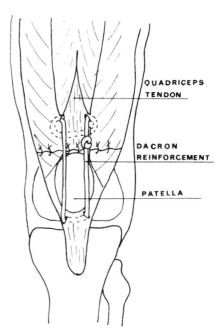

FIG. 33.14. Rupture of the quadriceps tendon. A 5-mm Dacron graft is driven transversely through the patellar ligament just below the inferior pole of the patella. The proximal lateral end of the Dacron is passed transversely through the tendon, creating two loops at the level of the musculotendinous junction. The two ends are tied together with tension. (From Levy M, Goldstein J, Rosner M. A method of repair for quadriceps tendon or patellar ligament (tendon) ruptures without cast immobilization. *Clin Orthop* 1987;218:297–301, with permission.)

weeks, intensive therapy is begun to regain knee motion and quadriceps and hamstring strength.

For chronic quadriceps rupture greater than 4 to 6 weeks, the tendon is often retracted more than 5 cm and scarred down to the underlying femur. Soft tissue releases and a quadriceps lengthening is often required. The Codivilla V-Y lengthening procedure will provide the additional length necessary for primary end-to-end repair (118).

Avulsion Fractures

Apophyseal avulsion fractures occur most commonly in children and adolescents participating in strenuous sporting activities (122–125). This is because of the unique biomechanical properties of the physeal growth plate in the skeletally immature athlete. During pubescence there is an increase in muscular strength, whereas the ultimate tensile strength of the physis decreases (126,127). This disproportionate ratio predisposes to avulsion fracture rather than ligamentous or tendon injury, which are more frequently seen in the adult (128,129).

The immature pelvis develops from 3 primary and 10 secondary centers of ossification (130,131). Of these,

ASIS and AIIS are the most commonly involved in avulsion fractures. Carp (132) and then Kohler (133) were the first to report on ASIS and AIIS, respectively, in the 1920s. The exact incidence of these fractures, however, is difficult to ascertain because there has been no large series of patients to date. Overall incidence ranged from 1.4% in Lloyd-Smith et al.'s (134) survey of hip injuries to 13.4% in a review from the Campbell Clinic (135) to 40% in Sundar and Carty's study (125).

Acute avulsion injuries occur as a result of a sudden concentric or eccentric muscular contraction. Usually there is no external trauma. Events such as sprinting, specifically at start-up or acute deceleration, have been implicated in the mechanism of avulsion fractures.

Anterior Superior Iliac Spine

The ossification center of the ASIS appears at 13 to 15 years of age and fuses to the ilium between 21 and 25 years of age (131). It is the attachment of the sartorious and some fibers of the tensor fascia lata. It is more frequently involved than the AIIS. There have been multiple reports of unilateral and a few reports on bilateral ASIS avulsion fractures (25,133,135–139,140–142). The injury most commonly occurs in runners, sprinters, or hurdlers. With the knee flexed and the hip extended, the sartorious is placed on maximal tension.

The athlete complains of acute-onset pain that is localized to the region of the ASIS. A snap or pop may be heard at the time of injury. There is often pain on palpation near the ASIS that is aggravated with passive extension or active flexion of the hip. The avulsed fragment may be palpable inferior to the ASIS.

ASIS avulsion has also presented as meralgia parasthetica with pain and numbness of the anterolateral thigh (137,143). Buch and Campbell (143) found at surgery traction on the lateral femoral cutaneous nerve by the ASIS fragment.

Radiographs show a characteristic fragment of bone measuring 1.5 to 3.0 cm displaced inferior and lateral to the pelvis. Oblique views will help differentiate ASIS from AIIS.

Treatment is primarily conservative and follows a rehabilitative protocol, as outlined by Metzmaker and Pappas (124). This is a five-phase protocol with the first stage consisting of rest, ice, analgesics, and protected gait. After the acute phase, the rest of the protocol focuses on rehabilitation with restoration of range of motion, strength, and gait. Isokinetic strength testing of the associated muscles is the preferred method for assessment of muscular strength before returning to sports (Table 33.3). Radiographs are used to observe callous formation and finally confirm healing of the avulsion fracture.

Some authors advocate open reduction internal fixation for displaced avulsion fractures greater than 2 cm. Other indications include nonunion, prolonged functional disability, and chronic pain. Veselko and Smrkolj (144) treated avulsion fractures of the ASIS with open reduction internal fixation for competitive athletes to shorten the period of recovery. Time to full recovery and return to reinjury level ranges from 3 weeks to 4 months.

Anterior Inferior Iliac Spine

The secondary center of ossification of the AIIS appears at 14 years of age and fuses at 16 years of age (131). It is the site of attachment of the straight/direct head of the rectus femoris tendon. The rectus tendon has two roles: knee extension and hip flexion. The mechanism of injury of the AIIS is similar to the ASIS in that

TABLE 33-3. *Five-stage rehabilitation program for apophyseal avulsion injuries*

Treatment phase	Days after injury	Subjective pain	Palpation subjective pain objective tissue	Range of motion	Muscle strength	Level of activity	Radiographic appearance
I	0–7	Moderate	Moderate to severe	Very limited	Poor	None, protected gait	Osseous separation
II	7 to 14–20	Minimal	Moderate	Improving with guided exercise	Fair	Protected gait, guided exercise	Osseous separation
III	14–20 to 30	Minimal with stress	Moderate	Improving with gentle stretch	Good	Guided exercise, resistance	Early callus formation
IV	30–60	None	Minimal	Normal	Good to normal	Limited athletic participation	Maturing callus
V	60 to return	None	None	Normal	Normal	Normal	Maturing callus

From Metzmaker JN, Pappas AM. Avulsion fractures of the pelvis. *Am J Sports Med* 1985;13:349–358, with permission.

forceful eccentric or concentric contraction results in avulsion of a fragment of bone. In 1935 Gallagher (145) described this injury as a "sprinters fracture." Although unilateral avulsion fractures have been reported in the literature infrequently, there have been only two reported cases of bilateral AIIS avulsions (140,146–151). AIIS fractures occur less often than injury to the ASIS.

Patients present at a younger age with a history of acute pain localized to the groin. The location of the pain is less specific than ASIS, secondary to the deep position of the AIIS within the pelvis. Hip flexion and knee extension will be painful and weak.

AIIS avulsion fracture has a characteristic appearance on radiographs. It is usually crescent or triangular shaped. Displacement is limited by the conjoined tendon and the reflected head of the rectus femoris. Comparison with the contralateral side will differentiate avulsion fracture from os acetabuli of the superior rim of the acetabulum.

Avulsion of the reflected head of the rectus femoris is extremely rare, with only one case reported in the literature (150). Radiographs revealed an avulsion fracture of the lateral acetabulum.

Treatment is conservative and follows the protocol outlined by Metzmaker and Pappas (124). Recovery time is similar to ASIS injury, with an average time to return to sports between 6 and 8 weeks.

Quadriceps Contusion

The clinical literature on quadriceps contusion is sparse. There are unique differences between a contusion and strain, and they should not be thought of as the same entity. Demographically, contusions occur in the same age group as strains. The athletes participate in more contact sports such as football or rugby. The mechanism of injury is usually a blunt force directed toward the anterior thigh. The location of the injury can be along the entire musculotendinous unit rather than at the junction. Furthermore, the muscular injury involves the deeper tissues adjacent to the bone compared with a strain, which usually involve more superficial muscle (11,152).

There are three well-known clinical studies on quadriceps contusion: Ryan et al. (153), Rothwell (154), and Jackson and Feagin (155). The study by Ryan et al. is an update of the landmark paper by Jackson and Feagin on quadriceps contusions in young athletes at West Point Academy. In the earlier study (155), 65 athletes were reviewed with quadriceps contusion and hematoma. This classified quadriceps contusions and formulated a rehabilitative protocol for treatment. The purpose of the recent update of 117 quadriceps contusions was to assess the effectiveness of a modified physical therapy protocol.

Patients present with a characteristic history of blunt trauma to the anterior thigh. There is often swelling, pain, and loss of function. Classification of quadriceps contusions is based on the amount of pain, swelling, and loss of knee flexion. Mild contusions have active flexion greater than 90 degrees, moderate contusions of 45 to 90 degrees, and severe contusions of less than 45 degrees flexion (153,155).

Walton and Rothwell (152) demonstrated a characteristic response of muscle to blunt injury using a sheep model. Initially, there is muscular tissue damage and hemorrhage followed rapidly by an acute inflammatory stage. After this, there is consolidation and resorption of the hematoma with the formation of granulation tissue. Eventually, there is maturation to dense fibrous tissue.

With a severe contusion, significant hemorrhage may occur in the quadriceps muscle and anterior compartment. It is important to measure thigh girth, compartment tension, and assess the quality of pain. Thigh compartment syndrome and/or vascular injury are extremely rare but catastrophic if not recognized early.

Ecchymosis and a sympathetic knee effusion becomes evident with 24 to 48 degrees. The knee ligaments should be tested for instability at the initial evaluation.

Plain radiographs should be obtained to rule out a fractured femur. As mentioned earlier, ultrasound or MRI may be helpful in determining the extent of soft tissue injury. Rothwell (154) used technetium scans to localize the area of muscle damage and found that intense uptake adjacent to the femur foreshadowed the development of ossification.

Ryan et al. (153) developed a treatment protocol for quadriceps contusion. This protocol had two major changes from Jackson and Feagin's study: In phase 1, the injured leg and hip rests in flexion rather than extension and there is emphasis on early flexion exercises. The results are significantly better in regard to disability and development of MO. The departure from the original protocol was based on two reasons. The position of slight hip and knee flexion increased the tension within the anterior compartment, theoretically reducing hemorrhage, swelling, and inflammation. Moreover, there has been less prolonged disability from lack of knee flexion. Interestingly, a number of studies have reported the effect of knee position on reflex inhibition of the quadriceps mechanism. When the knee is flexed 30 to 40 degrees, there is a threefold decrease in reflex inhibition with isometric quadriceps contractions (156–158).

The therapy protocol is goal oriented, individualized, and consists of three phases. Phase 1 or the immobilization phase reduces the amount of hemorrhage and swelling. Phase 2 is the restoration of motion, and phase 3 is functional rehabilitation.

In phase 1, the hip and knee are flexed to tolerance. The RICE protocol is followed until the patient is comfortable at rest and the thigh girth has stabilized. Weight bearing is as tolerated with crutch support. This phase lasts 24 to 72 degrees. The goal of phase 2 is to restore functional pain-free hours range of motion. A Continuous Passive Motion (CPM) is used, if available as an inpatient or outpatient, to assist in passive motion. Well leg gravity-assisted motion with supine and prone active flexion and isometric quadriceps exercises complete this phase. Advancement to phase 3 is contingent on painless knee flexion greater than 120 degrees, weight bearing as tolerated, and normal thigh girth. Phase 3 focuses on functional rehabilitation, flexibility, and conditioning. The patient performs isotonic and isokinetic strengthening exercises. Once full range of motion, full squat, and painless activities are achieved, then the patient is considered for return to active sports.

The criteria for participating in sports is similar to hamstring and quadriceps strains. A circular wrap and protective pad are worn to prevent recurrent trauma to the thigh. It is important to remember that during this protocol, advancement depends on pain-free functional improvement. Reinjury is a significant factor in prolonging disability.

With this protocol, Ryan et al. (153) reported that the time to recovery was 13 days for mild contusions, 19 for moderate, and 21 for severe. Other authors have shown that most athletes are able to return to sports within a 2- to 10-week period (154,155).

Myositis Ossificans

MO is a frequent complication after muscle contusion. Jackson and Feagin (155) showed a 20% incidence, Rothwell (154) 17%, and Ryan et al. (153) 9% in their series of muscular contusions. The formation of MO is a multifactorial process (159–161). Several risk factors predispose to the formation of MO: knee motion less than 120 degrees, football injury, previous quadriceps injury, delay in treatment more than 3 days, and ipsilateral knee effusion (153,159).

The pathogenesis of MO is not completely understood (162,163). In the early stages, within the first 3 weeks, there is an indurated tender mass localized to the anterior compartment (164). Osteoblastic activity is not visible radiographically but can be identified by technetium scans and ultrasound (165–167). After 3 weeks there is a "sandstorm" appearance on radiograph localized to the middle one third of the femur (154,155). As maturation proceeds, three distinct forms are identified: a stalk type with attachment to the underlying bone, a periosteal type with continuity to the underlying bone, and a broad-based type with a portion projecting into the quadriceps muscle and a radiolucent line separating it from the adjacent femur (81,155,163). At 3 to 6 months the bony mass has stabilized or diminished in size. Complete resorption is not unusual.

The differential diagnoses for MO include periosteal and parosteal osteosarcoma, synovial sarcoma, osteo-chondroma, and osteomyolytis. Histologically, MO has a zonal appearance with mature lamellar bone in the periphery and immature bone centrally.

The treatment of MO is primarily conservative, consisting of rest, NSAIDs, and active mobilization and range of motion. Despite the appearance on radiographs, there has been minimal functional disability of the quadriceps. Diphosphonates or radiation therapy are not necessary. Surgery in the early stages invites disaster. Authors have recommended waiting a minimum of 6 to 12 months before surgical intervention (41,42,81). Bone scan should show no activity. Lipscomb et al. (81) reported on 42 quadriceps contusions with a significant number of patients developing MO. Only four patients required operative intervention for functional loss of motion, pain, and quadriceps atrophy. The average time from injury to excision of the MO was 6 months. There were no recurrences.

FEMUR

Femoral Stress Fracture

Femoral stress fractures account for 5% of all stress reactions to bone (168). Involvement of the femoral shaft has varied in the literature, ranging from 1% to 43%. The early reports of Hallel et al. (169), Provost and Morris (170), Bargren et al. (171), and Giladi et al. (172) demonstrated a 20% to 43% incidence of femoral shaft stress fractures in military recruits. Former studies in athletes have suggested an incidence between 2.8% and 7.0% (168,173,174). Recently, however, Johnson et al. (3) and Clement et al. (174) demonstrated an overall incidence of 20% and 53%, respectively, in athletes. This increase in frequency may reflect an increase sensitivity for detection of the injury.

The athlete presents with vague activity-related pain poorly localized to the thigh. The athlete is usually involved in a running sport. Sullivan et al. (175), in a prospective study on runners with stress fractures, noted that the level of training exceeded 20 miles/wk. This is supported by Hershman et al. (176) and Clements et al. (174), in which athletes exceeded 56 km/wk. In addition, there is usually a change in the intensity of the workout regimen a couple weeks before the onset of symptoms.

Because of the vague symptoms, it is not uncommon for the diagnosis to be delayed 4 to 12 weeks. A high degree of suspicion, detailed history and examination, and interpretation of radiographs is essential in the diagnosis and the prevention of increased morbidity from a displaced femoral stress fracture.

The patient will describe a vague deep thigh pain localized anywhere along the length of the femur. Palpation may elicit deep thigh soreness. Sometimes there is an antalgic gait (20%) or positive Hop test (70%) (176). Johnson et al. (3) described a fulcrum test that improved the accuracy and shortened the time to 2 weeks in the diagnosis of femoral stress fractures. The fulcrum test starts with the examiners arm under the patients distal thigh as gentle pressure is placed over the dorsum of the knee. The examiner's arm is moved proximally under the thigh until a point of maximal tenderness is found.

Radiographs are the first diagnostic test ordered and rarely show classic findings of periosteal new bone formation, sclerosis, and radiolucent lines along the tension side of the bone. Seventy percent of the initial radiographs are negative. The accuracy of the radiograph depends on the grade of stress fracture. If there is a delay in diagnosis or late presentation, there is a greater chance of detection on conventional radiograph.

The bone scan is the gold standard for the diagnosis of stress fracture (177). It can detect bone changes far in advance of conventional radiographs. Changes on bone scan may be seen as early as 48 to 72 hours after injury. A stress fracture will be positive in all three phases of the bone scan. MRI can also be used to assess stress fractures with a high degree of accuracy.

Femoral stress fractures have a different distribution in the athlete compared with the military recruit. In the latter, there is an increased frequency (51%) for distal third fractures (169,170). In the athlete, the location is proximal, specifically in the posteromedial or midmedial cortex (3,176,178). The reason for this may be the stress distribution in the proximal femur. Oh and Harris (179) demonstrated that the greatest strains in the femur were localized to the medial–posteromedial cortex of the proximal femur. This is in part related to the bone morphology and the muscular forces of the thigh adductors and vastus medialis.

Early detection is the key to preventing potential displacement and increased morbidity. Conservative treatment is often adequate with modification of weight-bearing status. Cessation of all activity is required until the fracture has healed. Generally, healing occurs within 4 to 8 weeks. After this, a rehabilitative program is instituted to prepare the athlete for returning to sports. Cross-training is advocated to prevent a similar injury from recurring. Athletes can usually return to sports between 8 and 14 weeks after the onset of symptoms (3,168,176).

Traumatic Femur Fracture

Femoral fractures in the athlete are relatively uncommon. Occasionally they are seen in high-velocity sports such as alpine skiing or cross-country skiing (180–184). Sterett and Krissoff (181) reviewed 85 femur fractures sustained during alpine skiing. The incidence was 0.8 femur fractures per 100,000 skier days. The treatment of femur fractures is beyond the scope of this chapter; however, it is of paramount importance to restore alignment, rotation, and length to enable healing and return of function to a high level.

COMPARTMENT SYNDROME

Thigh contusion is a common occurrence in sports. Despite its frequency, contusion rarely results in serious injury or loss of playing time. Deep muscle contusion can occasionally lead to serious conditions of the thigh, such as compartment syndrome and MO. Most soft tissue injuries have already been addressed in previous sections. This section discusses compartment syndrome in detail.

Acute Compartment Syndrome

Acute compartment syndrome (ACS) of the thigh is an uncommon occurrence. In the trauma population, the largest series of thigh compartment syndrome includes 21 cases in 17 patients found over a 4-year period during which 6,000 trauma patients were evaluated (185). The estimated incidence of acute thigh compartment syndrome in the multitrauma population is therefore approximately 0.3%. This incidence may increase to as high as 1% when intramedullary femoral rodding has been performed in the multitrauma patient (185). In this series, ACS was found to be associated with femur fracture, systemic hypotension, use of antishock trousers, vascular injury, and prolonged mechanical compression secondary to drug overdose.

ACS of the thigh in the athletic population is extremely rare; however, case reports do exist (186–192). The true incidence of this entity in the athlete is impossible to estimate because the number of cases is too small. When ACS of the thigh does occur, it most frequently appears in the anterior compartment, followed by the posterior and medial compartments (192,193).

The mechanism of injury usually involves a direct contusion with secondary massive intracompartmental bleeding (186–188). The continuous bleeding into a closed facial space results in increased tissue pressure. Elevated pressures will eventually compromise venous outflow and arterial inflow, thus resulting in neuromuscular tissue necrosis within the compartment. Because neuromuscular tissue necrosis is a time-dependent process, immediate surgical decompression of the compartment is of the utmost importance.

Review of the sports literature reveals four cases of atraumatic ACS of the thigh secondary to exercise (190–192). One case resulted in simultaneous bilateral thigh compartment syndromes as a result of performing greater than 200 leg squats (192). The other two cases involved intensive weight training and isometric exercises of the thigh (190,191). The pathophysiology resulting in acute exercise-induced compartment syndrome has been proposed by Reneman (194) in his series of 52 patients with acute exercise-induced compartment syndrome of the lower leg. He proposed that muscular hypertrophy was the primary factor involved, resulting in a secondary obstruction of capillary venous drainage. These two factors initiated the cycle resulting in ACS.

ACS of the thigh presents clinically with the "seven Ps" of compartment syndrome: *pain* out of proportion to the severity of injury; *pain with passive stretch* of the compartment muscles in question; *pressure,* noted on examination by a tense compartment on palpation; and *pallor, paraesthesias, paralysis,* and absent *pulses,* all findings that present late in the disease process. The diagnosis should be made well before the development of these late findings.

Imaging studies should include plain radiographs to evaluate for an associated femur fracture. In the setting of a questionable arterial bleed resulting in ACS, an arteriogram can be considered; however, this must not delay the surgical treatment required to decompress the compartment. The arteriogram is, therefore, best obtained intraoperatively.

Diagnosis of ACS requires a high level of suspicion based on the history and physical examination. The diagnosis is confirmed with measurement of the intracompartmental pressures, using a handheld pressure measurement device (Stryker, Kalamazoo, MI). Each of the three compartments should be measured and recorded.

Normal intracompartmental pressure is between 0 and 8 mm Hg (195,196). The absolute pressure, requiring immediate decompression of the compartment, is controversial. Several authors have reported 30 mm Hg as their threshold (197–200), whereas others allow pressures to reach 40 mm Hg (185,201) and even 55 mm Hg (196,202) before performing decompressive fasciotomies. Taking into account all the above studies, the average of all the recommended threshold pressures is approximately 40 mm Hg. In the normotensive patient, compartment syndrome is confirmed with a pressure of 35 to 40 mm Hg. In the hypotensive patient, compartment syndrome is confirmed when the compartment pressure is within 30 to 40 mm Hg of the mean arterial pressure (49,203).

Any patient with suspected compartment syndrome should be evaluated immediately. The presence of an open injury does not exclude the possibility of ACS. The limb in question should have any restricted dressing completely removed, the limb positioned at a neutral level (not elevated), and ice avoided. Compartment pressures should be obtained and the diagnosis established early to prevent late sequellae.

Treatment for ACS of the thigh is immediate fasciotomies of the involved compartments. These are performed through a lateral incision that allows access to the anterior and posterior compartments (Fig. 33.15).

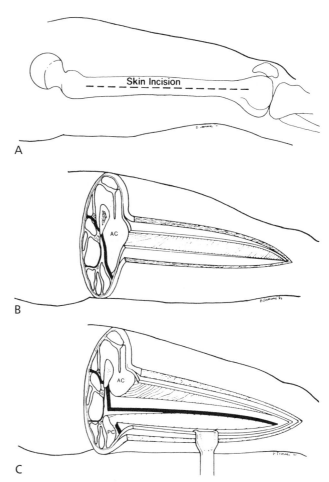

FIG. 33.15. The technique of lateral decompression of two compartments of the thigh. **A:** An incision is made from the intertrochanteric line to the lateral epicondyle. **B:** The anterior compartment (*AC*) is opened by incising the fascia lata. **C:** Retracting the vastus lateralis medially exposes the lateral intermuscular septum: that septum is then incised, decompressing the posterior compartment (*PC*). (From Tarlow SD, Achterman C, Hayhurst J, et al. Acute compartment syndrome of the thigh. *J Bone Joint Surg Am* 1986;68A:1442, with permission.)

If necessary, a separate medial incision is made for decompression of the medial compartment. In addition, myoepisiotomy may be necessary. The muscle within the compartment is examined for its color and contractility. Necrotic muscle is debrided and the wounds are packed open. The wounds undergo delayed primary closure once the swelling has subsided.

A beneficial outcome is dependent on early diagnosis and immediate treatment with the appropriate fasciotomies. Tissue damage is noted to be completely reversible at 30 minutes with pressures in the 30 mm Hg range. At 3 to 4 hours of 30 mm Hg pressure, capillary vessel damage occurs; however, full clinical recovery can be expected. Six hours' duration of a compartment syndrome will result in irreversible tissue damage with incomplete clinical recovery. Eight hours of compression leads to permanent cell death and poor functional recovery (49). These time intervals decrease when compartment pressures are greater, further supporting the urgency of diagnosis and treatment ACS of the thigh.

Chronic Exertional Compartment Syndrome

Chronic exertional compartment syndrome, also referred to as recurrent exertional compartment syndrome, has primarily been described in the lower leg (49,194,204). A review of the literature found only one case report of chronic exertional compartment syndrome of the thigh (205). This case involved the posterior compartment in a high-caliber long distance runner. Symptoms included hamstring ache, burning, tightness, and weakness that were worse with activities. Despite 6 months of conservative measures, including rest, stretching, ultrasound, whirlpool, and ice massage, there was no improvement. Preexercise and postexercise compartmental pressures revealed elevated pressures of 32 mm Hg for both. The condition was treated with a posterior compartment fasciotomy. Eight weeks postoperative, the patient was able to return to his running routine.

Chronic exertional compartment syndrome is confirmed by measuring compartment pressures pre- and postexercise. Postexercise pressures should not exceed 15 mm Hg for more than 15 minutes. An initial trial of conservative treatment is attempted. If unsuccessful, surgical fasciotomy is offered as an option.

MISCELLANEOUS

The more common injuries to the thigh and groin have been discussed in the previous sections. Despite common things being common, there are always a number of obscure entities that should be included in the differential diagnosis when the common does not present. This section presents some of the uncommon conditions of the thigh and groin.

Vascular

Adductor canal syndrome is an extremely rare condition. The etiology of this disorder is not completely understood; however, occlusion of the superficial femoral artery at Hunter's canal is usually found. Two possible mechanisms of arterial occlusion have been implicated. Verta et al. (206) described an anatomic compression of the femoral artery from an accessory band of the adductor magnus resulting in distal claudication. A traumatic compressive etiology has also been implicated, with the development of an intimal tear in the superficial femoral artery resulting in thrombosis and decreased distal blood flow (207).

The clinical presentation is that of a healthy athlete with symptoms of lower leg claudication. The athlete will experience lower leg pain that is worse with activities and better when rested. Examination will reveal diminished or absent pulses in the affected leg. It is important to remember that the saphenous nerve can also be compressed in the canal, resulting in paresthesias along the medial calf, ankle, and foot.

Diagnostic studies include ankle–brachial indices and an arteriogram. The arteriogram will indicate external compression, in which case the treatment will address the release of the accessory muscular band (206). If an intimal tear with thrombosis is found, a vascular repair will be required to reestablish normal arterial flow (41).

Hemophiliacs are known to develop intramuscular bleeds with minor trauma. These frequently occur in the iliopsoas or quadriceps and can be associated with a compressive femoral neuropathy (208,209). Initial treatment includes immediate replacement of clotting factors and splint immobilization of the affected limb. Surgical decompression should be performed only if compartment pressures reach 40 mm Hg. Hemophilic pseudotumor is a progressive cystic swelling of muscle that is a result of recurrent intramuscular hemorrhage. This occurs in only 1% of hemophiliacs and most often is associated with the quadriceps (210). Plain radiographs will demonstrate a calcific mass in proximity to the femur. Treatment consists of clotting factor replacement and immobilization. If the pseudotumor continues to enlarge resulting in compressive neuropathy and skin compromise, surgical excision may be required.

Traumatic pseudoaneurysm of the superficial femoral artery has been reported (211). A wrestler noted insidious onset of thigh swelling associated with a bruit and pulsatile mass 4 years after his initial injury. MRI and Doppler ultrasound demonstrate the aneurysm. This required surgical repair.

Bilateral muscle infarction of the thighs has been described in a case report of a 19-year-old insulin-dependent diabetic. Clinically, the patient presented with medial thigh pain. Imaging studies confirmed bilateral infarction of the medial compartments (212).

Muscular

Systemic skeletal muscle disease can frequently present primarily at the thigh. The common finding is that of thigh and hip muscle weakness. The diseases of skeletal muscle that should be considered are the muscular dystrophies and the inflammatory myopathies.

Duchenne muscular dystrophy is the most common of the muscular dystrophies. This is an X-linked recessive disorder that occurs in approximately 2.8 per 100,000 live births (213). This disease usually presents early in childhood with generalized hip and thigh muscle weakness and calf hypertrophy. The patient will often use his or her hands to climb up the legs to stand upright

(Gower's sign). Creatine phosphokinase levels are markedly elevated in this disease. Becker's muscular dystrophy is similar to Duchenne muscular dystrophy; however, its onset is at a later age. Treatment of the muscular dystrophies requires a multiteam approach in a tertiary care center (214).

Dermatomyositis and polymyositis are inflammatory and degenerative disorders of the skeletal muscle. The etiology of these disorders is unknown. They most frequently present in middle-aged women; however, they can affect patients of all ages. The initial clinical presentation is that of muscular weakness of the thighs and pelvis. Associated findings include muscle induration, contracture, and atrophy. A skin rash will also present in 40% to 60% of patients (214,215). These disorders are best treated by a rheumatologist.

Neoplasm

A final category to consider in the athletic population is that of neoplasm. Although unusual, one must always consider the possibility of tumor in the athletic individual with thigh pain. A history of night or rest pain of an aching character is a common presentation of neoplasm. Physical examination may reveal a soft tissue mass in the thigh. The workup of a suspected neoplasm includes plain radiographs, laboratory tests, and additional imaging studies. Often, a total body bone scan is obtained to rule out metastatic lesions of bone. An MRI is very useful in evaluating the consistency and extent of the lesion. Once all laboratory and imaging studies have been obtained, the working diagnosis must be confirmed with a tissue biopsy. This biopsy should be performed by an orthopedic tumor specialist, because the biopsy tract will potentially need to be excised in an additional definitive wide surgical resection. Benign tumors that are frequently found in the femur include osteoid osteoma, osteochondroma, aneurysmal bone cyst, fibrous dysplasia, and Paget's disease.

Malignant tumors of the femur include chondrosarcoma (usually in the adult or elderly population) and osteosarcoma. Osteosarcoma deserves special attention because this tumor usually occurs in the young athletic individual (second decade). Its most common location is the distal femoral metaphysis, and on plain radiograph it has a typical appearance of an ossified mass with a large soft tissue component to it (216). This requires prompt referral to an orthopedic tumor specialist. Additional malignant tumors of the femur include Ewing's sarcoma, malignant lymphoma, and malignant metastatic disease. Metastatic carcinoma to bone accounts for the greatest number of bony malignancies, and the most common long bone affected is the femur (214,216).

Benign soft tissue tumors of the thigh are relatively common. Lipoma is the most common tumor of mesenchymal origin and is frequently found in the thigh. This is usually a palpable, well-circumscribed, painless, mobile mass that has had little to no increase in size. Hemangioma is also common to the thigh. It may have a purple appearance associated with a palpable thrill.

Malignant soft tissue tumors of the thigh usually present as large, palpable, fixed, painful masses of the anterior thigh. The larger the lesion, the more likely to be malignant. Malignancies to consider include malignant fibrous histiocytoma, liposarcoma, and fibrosarcoma. Malignant fibrous histiocytoma is the most common soft tissue malignancy in adults and most often is located at the distal femur (216). These soft tissue malignancies are not common in young patients; however, malignant fibrous histiocytoma does have one peak at the second decade and a second peak at the seventh decade (216). Finally, in children, the most common soft tissue malignancy is rhabdomyosarcoma. This tumor often presents in the compartments of the thigh and is known to be very aggressive.

The details and specific treatments of these neoplasms is beyond the scope of this chapter. These neoplasms are named here as a reminder to be included in the differential diagnosis of thigh pain. When a neoplastic process has been identified, a prompt referral to an orthopedic tumor specialist and oncologist is mandatory.

ACKNOWLEDGMENTS

We thank John Lohnes and Marsha Dohrmann for their contributions to this chapter.

REFERENCES

1. Petit HL. Quoted by Loos. Ueber Subkutane Biceps Rupturen. *Beitr Klin Chir* 1901;29:410–449.
2. Blecker A. Ueber den Einfluss des Parademarsches auf die Entstehung der Fussgeshwulst. *Med Kin Berl* 1905;1:305.
3. Johnson AW, Weiss CB Jr, Wheeler DL. Stress fractures of the femoral shaft in athletes—more common than expected. *Am J Sports Med* 1994;22:248–256.
4. McMaster WC, Walter M. Injuries in soccer. *Am J Sports Med* 1978;6:354–357.
5. Yde J, Nielsen AB. Sports injuries in adolescents' ball games: soccer, handball, and basketball. *Br J Sports Med* 1990;24:51–54.
6. National Collegiate Athletic Association. *Injury surveillance system: men's and women's soccer injury/exposure summaries, 1986 to 1997.* Overland Park, KS: NCAA, 1997.
7. Soccer Industry Council of America. *National soccer participation survey.* North Palm Beach, FL: America Sports Data, 1988.
8. Tarlow SD, Achterman C, Hayhurst J, et al. Acute compartment syndrome of the thigh. *J Bone Joint Surg Am* 1986;68:1439–1443.
9. Garrett WE, Rich FR, Nikolaou PK. Computed tomography of hamstring muscle strains. *Med Sci Sports Exerc* 1989;21:506–514.
10. Krejci V, Koch P. *Muscle and tendon injuries in athletes.* Chicago: Year Book Medical Publishers, 1979.
11. Peterson L, Renstrom P. *Sports injuries: their prevention and treatment.* Chicago: Yearbook Medical Publishers, 1986.
12. Fuller, PJ. Musculotendinous leg injuries. *Aust Fam Physician* 1984;13:495–498.
13. Garrett WE Jr. Strains and sprains in athletes. *Postgrad Med* 1983;73:200–214.

14. Garrett WE Jr. Muscle strain injuries. *Am J Sports Med* 1996;24:S2–S8.
15. Stauber WT. Eccentric action of muscles: physiology, injury, and adaptation. *Exerc Sports Sci Rev* 1989;17:157–185.
16. Garrett WE Jr, Almekinders L, Seaber AV. Biomechanics of muscle tears and stretching injuries. *Trans Orthop Res Soc* 1984;9:384.
17. Garrett WE Jr, Nikolaou PK, Ribbeck BM, et al. The effect of muscle architecture on the biomechanical failure properties of skeletal muscle under passive extension. *Am J Sports Med* 1988;16:7–12.
18. Nikolaou PK, Macdonald BL, Glisson RR, et al. Biomechanical and histological evaluation of muscle after controlled strain injury. *Am J Sports Med* 1987;15:9–14.
19. Mair SD, Seaber AV, Glisson RR, et al. The role of fatigue in susceptibility to acute muscle strain injury. *Am J Sports Med* 1996;24:137–143.
20. Taylor DC, Dalton JD Jr, Seaber AV, et al. Experimental muscle strain injury. Early functional and structural deficits and the increased risk for reinjury. *Am J Sports Med* 1993;21:190–194.
21. Safran MR, Garrett WE Jr, Seaber AV, et al. The role of warm-up in muscular injury prevention. *Am J Sports Med* 1988;16:123–129.
22. Taylor DC, Dalton JD, Seaber AV, et al. Viscoelastic properties of muscle-tendon units. *Am J Sports Med* 1990;18:300–309.
23. Obremsky WT, Seaber AV, Ribbeck BM, et al. Biomechanical and histologic assessment of a controlled muscle strain injury treated with piroxicam. *Am J Sports Med* 1994;22:558–561.
24. Simon SR. *Orthopaedic basic science.* Rosemont, IL: American Academy of Orthopaedic Surgeons, 1994:47–60.
25. Fernbach SK, Wildinson RH. Avulsion injuries of the pelvis and proximal femur. *AJR Am J Roentgenol* 1981;137:581.
26. Speer KP, Lohnes J, Garrett WE Jr. Radiographic imaging of muscle strain injury. *Am J Sports Med* 1993;21:89–95.
27. Yoshioka H, Anno I, Niitsu M, et al. MRI of muscle strain injuries. *J Comput Assist Tomogr* 1994;18:454–460.
28. Sallay PI, Friedman RL, Coogan PG, et al. Hamstring muscle injuries among water skiers. *Am J Sports Med* 1996;24:130–136.
29. Roy S, Irvin R. *Sports medicine: prevention, evaluation, management, and rehabilitation.* Englewood Cliffs, NJ: Prentice-Hall, 1983:299–305.
30. Heiser TM, Weber J, Sullivan G, et al. Prophylaxis and management of hamstring muscle injuries in intercollegiate football players. *Am J Sports Med* 1984;12:368–370.
31. Agre JC. Hamstring injuries: proposed aetiological factors, prevention, and treatment. *Sports Med* 1985;2:21–33.
32. Burkett LN. Causative factors in hamstring strains. *Med Sci Sports Exerc* 1970;2:39–42.
33. Kulund DN. *The injured athlete.* Philadelphia: Lippincott, 1982:72, 85, 356–359.
34. Elliott BC, Blanksby BA. The synchronization of muscle activity and body segment movements during a running cycle. *Med Sci Sports Exerc* 1979;11:322–327.
35. Burkett LN. Causative factors in hamstring strain. *Med Sci Sports Exerc* 1970;2:39–42.
36. Casperson PC. Groin and hamstring injuries. *Athl Training* 1982;17:43–45.
37. Dornan P. A report on 140 hamstring injuries. *Aust J Sports Med* 1971;4:30–36.
38. Liemohn W. Factors related to hamstring strains. *J Sports Med* 1978;18:71–76.
39. Stafford MG, Grana WA. Hamstring/quadriceps ratios in college football players: a high velocity evaluation. *Am J Sports Med* 1984;12:209–211.
40. Sutton G. Hamstring by hamstring strains: a review of the literature. *J Orthop Sports Phys Ther* 1984;5:184–195.
41. DeLee J, Drez D. *Orthopaedic sports medicine: principles and practice.* Philadelphia: W.B. Saunders, 1994:21.
42. Nicholas JA, Hershman EB. *The lower extremity and spine in sports medicine,* 2nd ed. St. Louis: Mosby-Year Book, 1995:45.
43. Vane JR. Inhibition of prostaglandins synthesis as a mechanism of action for aspirin-like drugs. *Nature New Biol* 1971;231:232–235.
44. Knoben JE, Anderson PO. *Clinical drug data.* 6th ed. Hamilton: Hamilton Press Inc., 1988.
45. Glick JM. Muscle strains: prevention and treatment. *Phys Sports Med* 1980;8:73–77.
46. Coyle EF, Feiring DC, Rotkin TC, et al. Specificity of power improvements through slow and fast isokinetic training. *J Appl Physiol* 1981;51:1437–1442.
47. Garrett WE, Califf JC, Bassett FH. Histochemical correlates of hamstring injuries. *Am J Sports Med* 1984;12:98–103.
48. Johnson A, Polgar J, Weightman PD, et al. Data on the distribution of fiber types in thirty-six human muscles. *J Neurol Sci* 1973;18:111–129.
49. Fu FH, Stone DA. *Sports injuries: mechanisms, prevention, and treatment.* Baltimore: William & Wilkins, 1994.
50. Brewer BJ. Athletic injuries: musculotendinous unit. *Clin Orthop* 1962;23:30–38.
51. Kujala UM, Orava S, Karpakka J, et al. Ischial tuberosity apophysitis and avulsion among athletes. *Int J Sports Med* 1997;18:149–155.
52. Scholnsky J, Olix ML. Functional disability following avulsion fracture of the ischeal epiphysis. *J Bone Joint Surg* 1972;54:641.
53. Estwanik JJ, Sloane B, Rosenberg MA. Groin strain and other possible causes of groin pain. *Phys Sportsmed* 1990;18:59–65.
54. Renstrom P, Peterson L. Groin injuries in athletes. *Br J Sports Med* 1980;14:30–36.
55. NHL Injury Analysis. National Hockey League Executive Offices. 1986–1987.
56. National Collegiate Athletic Association. Injury surveillance system: men's hockey injury/exposure summaries. 1989–1990.
57. Renstrom PAHF. Tendon and muscle injuries in the groin area. *Clin Sports Med* 1992;11:815–827.
58. Merrifield HH, Cowan RFJ. Groin strain injuries in ice hockey. *J Sports Med* 1973;2:41–42.
59. Zarins B, Ciullo JV. Acute muscle and tendon injuries in athletes. *Clin Sports Med* 1983;2:167–182.
60. Martens MA, Hansen L, Mulier JC. Adductor tendinitis and musculus rectus abdominis tendonopathy. *Am J Sports Med* 1987;15:353–356.
61. Tuite MF, DeSmet AA. MRI of selected sports injuries: muscle tears, groin pain, and osteochondritis dissecans. *Semin Ultrasound CT MR* 1994;15:318–340.
62. Karlsson J, Sward L, Kalebo P, et al. Chronic groin injuries in athletes, recommendations for treatment and rehabilitation. *Sports Med* 1994;17:141–148.
63. Kalebo P, Karlsson J, Sward L, et al. Ultrasonography of chronic tendon injuries in the groin. *Am J Sports Med* 1992;20:634–639.
64. Kalebo P, Sward L, Karlsson J, et al. Ultrasonography in the detection of partial patellar ligament ruptures (jumper's knee). *Skeletal Radiol* 1991;20:378–381.
65. Sangwan SS, Aditya A, Siwach RC. Isolated traumatic rupture of the adductor longus muscle. *Indian J Med Sci* 1994;48:186–187.
66. Akermark C, Johansson C. Tenotomy of the adductor longus tendon in the treatment of chronic groin pain in athletes. *Am J Sports Med* 1992;20:640–643.
67. Mozes M, Papa M, Horoszowski H, et al. Iliopsoas injury in soccer players. *Br J Sports Med* 1985;19:168–170.
68. Takami H, Takahashi S, Ando M. Traumatic rupture of iliacus muscle with femoral nerve paralysis. *J Trauma* 1983;23:253–254.
69. Young JL, Laskowske ER, Rock MG. Thigh injuries in athletes. *Mayo Clin Proc* 1993;68:1099–1106.
70. Cochrand JM. Osteitis pubis in athletes. *Br J Sports Med* 1971;5:233.
71. Gilmore OJ. Gilmore's groin. *Sportsmed Soft Tissue Trauma* 1992;3:2–4.
72. Malycha P, Lovell G. Inguinal surgery in athletes with chronic groin pain: the "sportsman's" hernia. *Austr N Z J Surg* 1992;62:123–125.
73. Hackney RG. The sports hernia: a cause of chronic groin pain. *Br J Sports Med* 1993;27:58–62.
74. Taylor DC, Meyers WC, Moylan JA, et al. Abdominal musculature abnormalities as a cause of groin pain in athletes. Inguinal hernias and pubalgia. *Am J Sports Med* 1991;19:239–242.
75. Smedberg SG, Broome AE, Gullmo A, et al. Herniography in athletes with groin pain. *Am J Sports Med* 1985;149:378–382.

76. Lovell G. The diagnosis of chronic groin pain in athletes: a review of 189 cases. *Aust J Sci Med Sport* 1995;27:76–79.
77. Ekberg O, Blomquist P, Olsson S. Positive contrast herniography in adult patients with obscure groin pain. *Surgery* 1981;89:532–535.
78. Ekberg O, Persson MA, Abrahamsson PA. Longstanding groin pain in athletes. A multidisciplinary approach. *Sports Med* 1988;6:56–61.
79. Bradshaw C, McCrory P, Bell S, et al. Obturator nerve entrapment. A cause of groin pain in athletes. *Am J Sports Med* 1997;25:402–408.
80. Backous DD, Friedl KE, Smith NJ, et al. Soccer injuries and their relation to physical maturity. *Am J Dis Child* 1988;142:839–842.
81. Lipscomb AB Thomas E, Johnston RK. Treatment of myositis ossificans traumatica in athletes. *Am J Sports Med* 1976;4:111–120.
82. Gibbs N. Common rugby league injuries. *Sports Med* 1994;18:439–450.
83. Ryan AJ. Quadriceps strain, rupture and charlie horse. *Med Sci Sports* 1969;1:106–111.
84. Fried T, Lloyd GJ. An overview of common soccer injuries. *Sports Med* 1992;14:269–274.
85. O'Donoghue DH. Principles in the management of specific injuries. In: O'Donoghue DH, ed. *Treatment of injuries to athletes.* Philadelphia: W.B. Saunders, 1984:39–91.
86. Raatikainen T, Karpakka J, Orava S. Repair of partial quadriceps tendon rupture: observation in 28 cases. *Acta Orthop Scand* 1994;65:154–156.
87. Blazina ME, Kerlan RK, Jobe FW, et al. Jumper's knee. *Orthop Clinic North Am* 1973;4:665–678.
88. Ferritti A. Epidemiology of jumper's knee. *Sports Med* 1986;3:289–295.
89. Kelly DW, Carter VS, Jobe FW, et al. Patellar and quadriceps tendon ruptures-jumpers knee. *Am J Sports Med* 1984;12:375–380.
90. Fritschy D, de Gautard R. Jumpers knee and ultrasonography. *Am J Sports Med* 1988;16:637–640.
91. Galen. De usu partium corpus huminis librae. 1533.
92. Conway FM. Rupture of the quadriceps tendon. *Am J Surg* 1940;50:3.
93. McBurney C. Suture of the devided ends of a ruptured quadriceps extensor tendon with perfect recovery. *Ann Surg* 1887;6:170.
94. Quenu E, Duval P. Traitment operatoire des ruptures sous rotuliennes du quadriceps. *Rev Chir* 1905;31:169–194.
95. Siwek CW, Rao JP. Rupture of the extensor mechanism of the knee joint. *J Bone Joint Surg Am* 1981;63A:932–937.
96. Larsen E, Lund PM. Ruptures of the extensor mechanism of the knee joint. *Clin Orthop* 1986;213:150–153.
97. Vainionpaa S, Bostman O, et al. Rupture of the quadriceps tendon. *Acta Orthop Scand* 1985;56:433–435.
98. Miskew DBM, Pearson RL, Pankovich AM. Mersilene strip suture in repair of disruptions of the quadriceps and patella tendons. *J Trauma* 1980;20:867–872.
99. Scuderi C. Rupture of the quadriceps tendon. *Am J Surg* 1958;95:626–635.
100. De Franco P, Varghese J, Brown W, et al. Secondary hyperparathyroidism, and not beta 2 microglobulin amyloid, as a cause of spontaneous tendon rupture in patients on chronic hemodialysis. *Am J Kidney Dis* 1994;24:951–955.
101. Chilchester E. Rupture of both quadriceps extensor cruris tendons. *Br Med J* 1909;2:1343.
102. Keogh P, Shanker SJ, Burke T, et al. Bilateral simultaneous rupture of the quadriceps tendon. *Clin Orthop* 1988;234:139–141.
103. David HG, Green JT, Grant AJ, et al. Simultaneous bilateral quadriceps rupture: a complication of anabolic steroid abuse. *J Bone Joint Surg Br* 1994;77B:159–160.
104. Liow RYL, Tavarares S. Bilateral rupture of the quadriceps tendon associated with anabolic steroids. *Br J Sports Med* 1995;29:77–79.
105. Ribbens WJ, Angus PD. Simultaneous bilateral rupture of the quadriceps tendon. *British Journal of Clinical Pathology* 1989;3:122–124.
106. Munshi NI, Mbubaegbu CE. Simultaneous rupture of the quadri-

107. Lavalle C, Aprarcio LA, Moreno J, et al. Bilateral avulsion of the quadriceps tendons in primary hyperparathyroidism. *J Rheumatol* 1985;12:596–598.
108. Wilson JN. Bilateral rupture of the rectus femoris tendons in chronic nephritis. *Br Med J* 1957;4:1402–1403.
109. MacEachern AG, Plewes JL. Bilateral simultaneous spontaneous rupture of the quadriceps tendons. *J Bone Joint Surg Br* 1984;66B:81–83.
110. Kelly DW, Godfrey KD, Johanson PH, et al. Quadriceps rupture in association with the roentgenographic "tooth sign": a case report. *Orthopedics* 1980;3:1206–1208.
111. Kaneko K, et al. Radiographic diagnosis of QRT. *J Emerg Med* 1994;12:225–229.
112. Bianchi S, Zwass A, et al. Diagnosis of tears of the quadriceps tendon of the knee: value of sonography. *AJR Am J Roentgenol* 1994;162:1137–1140.
113. Spector ED, Di Marcangelo MT, Jacoby JH. The radiologic diagnosis of quadriceps tendon rupture. *N J Med* 1995;9:590–592.
114. Kuivila T, Brems J. Diagnosis of acute rupture of the quadriceps tendon by magnetic resonance imaging: a case report. *Clin Orthop* 1991;262:236–241.
115. Berlin RC, Levinsohn M, Chrisman H. The wrinkled patellar tendon: an indication of abnormality in the extensor mechanism of the knee. *Skeletal Radiol* 1991;20:181–185.
116. Zeiss J, Saddemi S, Ebraheim. MR imaging of the quadriceps tendon: normal layered configuration and its importance in cases of tendon rupture. *AJR Am J Roentgenol* 1992;159:1031–1034.
117. McLaughin HL, Francis KC, et al. Operative repair of injuries to the quadriceps extensor mechanism. *Am J Surg* 1956;91:651–653.
118. Haas SB, Callaway H. Disruptions of extensor mechanism. *Orthop Clin North Am* 1992;23:687–695.
119. Rasul A, Fischer D. Primary repair of quadriceps tendon ruptures: results of treatment. *Clin Orthop* 1993;289:205–207.
120. Levy M, Goldstein J, Rosner M. A method of repair for quadriceps tendon or patellar ligament (tendon) ruptures without cast immobilization. *Clin Orhtop* 1987;218:297–301.
121. Fujikawa K, Ohtani T, et al. Reconstruction of the extensor apparatus of the knee with the Leeds-Keio ligament. *J Bone Joint Surg Br* 1994;76B:200–203.
122. Paletta GA, Andrish JT. Injuries about the hip and pelvis in the young athlete. *Clin Sports Med* 1995;14:591–628.
123. Reed MH. Pelvic fractures in children. *J Can Assoc Radiol* 1976;27:255–261.
124. Metzmaker JN, Pappas AM. Avulsion fractures of the pelvis. *Am J Sports Med* 1985;13:349–358.
125. Sundar M, Carty H. Avulsion fractures of the pelvis in children. A report of 32 fractures and their outcome. *Skeletal Radiol* 1994;23:85–90.
126. Bright RW, Burstein AH, Elmore S. Epiphyseal plate cartilage. *J Bone Joint Surg Am* 1974;56A:688–703.
127. Morscher E. Strength and morphology of growth cartilage under hormonal influence of puberty. *Reconstr Surg Trauma* 1968;10:3–104.
128. Woo SLY, An KA, Arnoczky SP, et al. *Anatomy, biology and biomechanics of the tendon ligament and meniscus.* Chicago: Orthopaedic Basic Science, 1994.
129. Woo SLY, Ohland KJ, Weiss LA. Aging and sex related changes in the biomechanical properties of the rabbit medial collateral ligament. *Mech Ageing Dev* 1990;56:129–142.
130. Ponsetti IV. Growth and development of the acetabulum in the normal child. *J Bone Joint Surg Am* 1978;60A:575–585.
131. Watts HG. Fractures of the pelvis in children. *Orthop Clin North Am* 1976;7:615–624.
132. Carp L. Fracture of the anterior superior spine of the ilium by muscular violence. *Ann Surg* 1924;79:551–560.
133. Kohler A. *Roentgenology. The borderlands of the normal and early pathologic in the skiagram,* 1st ed. New York: William, Wood & Co., 1929:195–196.
134. Lloyd-Smith R, Clement DB, McKenzie DC, et al. A survey of overuse and traumatic hip and pelvic injuries in athletes. *Phys Sportsmed* 1985;13:131–141.
135. Canale ST, King EK. Pelvic and hip fractures. In: Rockwood

CA, Wilkins KE, King R, eds. *Fractures in children,* 3rd ed. Philadelphia: J.B. Lippincott, 1991:991–1120.

136. Draper DO, Dustman AJ. Avulsion fracture of the anterior superior iliac spine in a collegiate runner. *Arch Phys Med Rehabil* 1992;73:881–882.

137. Thanikachalam M, Petros JG, O'Donnell SO. Avulsion fracture of the anterior superior iliac spine in presenting as acute-onset meralgia paresthetica. *Ann Emerg Med* 1995;26:515–517.

138. Cleaves EN. Fracture or avulsion of the anterior superior spine of the ilium. *J Bone Joint Surg* 1938;20:490–491.

139. Robertson RC. Fracture of the anterior superior spine of the ilium. *J Bone Joint Surg* 1935;17:1045–1048.

140. Weitzner I. Fracture of the anterior superior spine of the ilium in one case and anterior inferior in another. *AJR Am J Roentgenol* 1935;39:40.

141. Hansson PG. Bilateral avulsion fractures of the anterior superior iliac spine. *Acta Chir Scand* 1970;136:85–86.

142. Khoury MB, Kirks DR, Martinez S, et al. Bilateral avulsion fractures of the anterior superior iliac spines in sprinters. *Skeletal Radiol* 1985;20:65–67.

143. Buch KA, Campbell J. Acute onset meralgia parasthetica after fracture of the anterior superior iliac spine. *Br J Accident Surg* 1993;24:569–570.

144. Veselko M, Smrkolj V. Avulsion of the anterior superior spine in athletes: case reports. *J Trauma* 1994;36:444–446.

145. Gallagher JR. Fracture of the anterior inferior spine of the ilium: "sprinter's fracture." *Ann Surg* 1935;102:86–88.

146. Crespi M. La fraturra isolata della spina iliaca anteriore inferiore. *Arch Orthop* 1961;74:438–452.

147. Lagier R, Jarret G. Apophysiolysis of the anterior inferior iliac spine. *Arch Orthop* 1975;83:81–85.

148. Gomez JE. Bilateral anterior inferior iliac spine avulsion fractures. *Med Sci Sports Exerc* 1995;161–164.

149. Bachman W. Un cas d'arrachment bilateral de i'espine iliac anteroinferiore. *Schweiz Med Wochenschr* 1941;22:721–722.

150. Deehan DJ, Beattie TF, Knight D, et al. Avulsion fracture of the straight and reflected heads of rectus femoris. *Arch Emerg Med* 1992;9:310–313.

151. Mader TJ. Avulsion of the rectus femoris tendon: an unusual type of pelvis fracture. *Pediatr Emerg Care* 1990;6:198–199.

152. Walton M, Rothwell AG. Reactions of the thigh tissues of sheep to blunt trauma. *Clin Orthop* 1983;176:273–281.

153. Ryan JB, Wheeler JH, Hopkinson WJ, et al. Quadriceps contusions: West Point update. *Am J Sports Med* 1991;19:299–304.

154. Rothwell AG. Quadriceps hematoma: a prospective and clinical study. *Clin Orthop* 1982;171:97–103.

155. Jackson DW, Feagin JA. Quadriceps contusion in young athletes. *J Bone Joint Surg Am* 1973;55A:95–105.

156. Morrissey MC. Reflex inhibition of thigh muscles in knee injury: causes and treatment. *Sports Med* 1989;7:263–276.

157. Krebs DE, Staples WH, Cutitta D, et al. Knee joint angle: its relationship tp quadriceps femoris activity in normal and post-arthrotomy limbs. *Arch Phys Rehabil* 1983;64:441–447.

158. Shakespeare DT, Stokes M, Sherman KP, et al. The effect of knee flexion on quadriceps inhibition after meniscectomy. *Clin Sci* 1983;65:64P.

159. Ellis M, Frank HG, Rad M. Myositis ossificans traumatica: with special reference to the quadriceps femoris muscle. *J Trauma* 1966;6:724–738.

160. Hiat G, Boswick JA, Stone NH. Heterotopic bone formation secondary to trauma (myositis ossificans traumatica): an unsual case and a review of current concepts. *J Trauma* 1970;10:405–411.

161. Ivey M. Myositis ossificans of the thigh following manipulation of the knee: a case report. *Clin Orthop* 1985;198:102–105.

162. Zachalini PS, Urist MR. Traumatic periosteal proliferations in rabbits. The enigma of experimental myositis ossificans traumatica. *J Trauma* 1964;4:344–357.

163. Arrington ED, Miller MD. Skeletal muscle injuries. *Orthop Clin North Am* 1995;26:411–422.

164. Norman A, Dorfman H. Juxtacortical circumscribed myositis ossificans: evolution and radiographic features. *Radiology* 1970;96:301–306.

165. Kirkpatrick JS, Koman LA, Rovere GD. The role of ultrasound in the early diagnosis of myositis ossificans. *Am J Sports Med* 1987;15:179–181.

166. Suzuki Y, Hisada K, Takeda M. Demonstration of myositis ossificans by 99m Tc pyrophosphate bone scanning. *Radiology* 1974;111:663–664.

167. Tyler JL, Derbekyan V, Lisbona R. Early diagnosis of myositis ossificans with Tc-99m diphosphonate imaging. *Clin Nucl Med* 1984;9:256–258.

168. Matheson GO, Clement DB, McKenzie DC, et al. Stress fractures in athletes: a study of 320 cases. *Am J Sports Med* 1987;15:46–58.

169. Hallel T, Amit S, Segal D. Fatigue fractures of the tibial femoral shaft in soldiers. *Clin Orthop* 1976;118:35–43.

170. Provost RA, Morris JM. Fatigue fractures of the femoral shaft. *J Bone Joint Surg Am* 1969;51A:487–498.

171. Bargren JH, Tilson DN, Bridgeford OE. Prevention of displaced fatigue fractures of the femur. *J Bone Joint Surg Am* 1971;53A:1115–1117.

172. Giladi M, Ahronson Z, Stein D, et al. Unusual distribution and onset of stress fractures in soldiers. *Clin Orthop* 1985;192:142–146.

173. Orava S. Stress fractures. *Br J Sports Med* 1980;14:40–44.

174. Clement DB, Ammann W, Taunton JE, et al. Exercise-induced stress injuires to the femur. *Int J Sports Med* 1993;14:347–352.

175. Sullivan D, Warren RF, Pavlov H, et al. Stress fractures in 51 runners. *Clin Orthop* 1984;187:188–192.

176. Hershman EB, Lombardo J, Bergfeld JA. Femoral shaft stress fractures in athletes. *Clin Sports Med* 1990;9:111–119.

177. Monteleone GP. Stress fractures in athletes. *Orthop Clin North Am* 1995;26:423–432.

178. Butler JE, Brown SL, McConnell BG. Subtrochanteric stress fractures in runners. *Am J Sports Med* 1982;10:228–232.

179. Oh L, Harris WH. Proximal strain distribution in the loaded femur. *J Bone Joint Surg Am* 1978;60A:75–85.

180. Frost A, Bauer M. Skier's hip—a new clinical entity? Proximal femur fractures sustained in cross country skiing. *J Orthop Trauma* 1991;5:47–50.

181. Sterett W, Krissoff WB. Femur fractures in alpine skiing: classification and mechanism of injury in 85 cases. *J Orthop Trauma* 1994;8:310–314.

182. Hachenbruch W. Femoral neck fractures and peritrochanteric fractures due to skiing accidents. *Fortschr Med* 1978;96:177–184.

183. Spezia P, Brennan, R, Brugman JL, et al. Femur fractures in alpine skiers. *J Orthop Trauma* 1992;6:443–447.

184. Yvars M, Kanner H. Ski fractures of the femur. *Am J Sports Med* 1984;12:386–390.

185. Schwartz JT Jr, Brumback RJ, Lakatos R, et al. Acute compartment syndrome of the thigh. *J Bone Joint Surg Am* 1989;71A:392–400.

186. Colosimo AJ, Ireland ML. Thigh compartment syndrome in a football athlete: a case report and review of the literature. *Med Sci Sports Exerc* 1992;24:958–963.

187. Klasson SC, Schilden JL. Acute anterior thigh compartment syndrome complicating quadriceps hematoma. Two case reports and review of the literature. *Orthop Rev* 1990;19:421–427.

188. Robinson D, On E, Halperin N. Anterior compartment syndrome of the thigh in athletes—indications for conservative treatment. *J Trauma* 1992;32:183–186.

189. Hutchinson MR, Ireland ML. Common compartment syndromes in athletes. Treatment and rehabilitation. *Sports Med* 1994;17:200–208.

190. Bidwell JP, Gibbons CE, Godsiff S. Acute compartment syndrome of the thigh after weight training. *Br J Sports Med* 1996;30:264–265.

191. Doube A. An acute compartment syndrome involving the anterior thighs after isometric exercise. *N Z Med J* 1995;108:413.

192. Kahan JSG, McClellan RT, Burton DS. Acute bilateral compartment syndrome to the thigh induced by exercise. *J Bone Joint Surg Am* 1994;76A:1068–1071.

193. Tarlow SD, Achterman CA, Hayhurst J, et al. Acute compartment syndrome of the thigh complicating fracture of the femur. *J Bone Joint Surg Am* 1986;68A:1439–1443.

194. Reneman RS. The anterior and the lateral compartmental syndrome of the leg due to intensive use of muscles. *Clin Orthop* 1975;113:69–80.

195. Lee BY, Berncato RF, Park IH. Management of compartmental syndrome. *Am J Surg* 1984;148:383–388.
196. Whitesides TE, Haney TC, Morimoto K, et al. Tissue pressure measurements as a determinant for the need of fasciotomy. *Clin Orthop* 1975;113:43–51.
197. Mubarak SJ, Owen CA, Hargens AR, et al. Acute compartment syndromes: diagnosis, and treatment with the aid of the Wick catheter. *J Bone Joint Surg Am* 1978;6-A:1091–1095.
198. Mubarak SJ. *Compartment syndromes and Volkmann's contracture.* Philadelphia: W.B. Saunders, 1981.
199. Mubarak SJ, Hargens AR. Acute compartment syndromes. *Surg Clin North Am* 1983;63:539–565.
200. An HS, Simpson JM, Gale S, et al. Acute anterior compartment syndrome in the thigh: a case report and review of the literature. *J Orthop Trauma* 1987;1:180–182.
201. Allen MJ, Stirling AJ, Crawshaw CV, et al. Intra-compartmental pressure monitoring of leg injuries. An aid to management. *J Bone Joint Surg Br* 1985;67B:53–57.
202. Matsen FA III, Winquist RA, Krugmire RB. Diagnosis and management of compartmental syndromes. *J Bone Joint Surg Am* 1980;62A:286–291.
203. Heppenstall RB, Scott R, Sapega A, et al. A comparative study of the tolerance of skeletal muscle to ischemia. Tourniquet application compared with acute compartment syndrome. *J Bone Joint Surg Am* 1986;68A:820–828.
204. Puranen J. The medial tibial syndrome. Exercise ischaemia in the fascial compartment of the leg. *J Bone Joint Surg Br* 1974;56B:712–715.
205. Raether PM, Lutter LD. Recurrent compartment syndrome of the posterior thigh. Report of a case. *Am J Sports Med* 1982;10:40–43.
206. Verta MJ, Vitello J, Fuller J. Adductor canal compression syndrome. *Arch Surg* 1984;119:345–346.
207. Bassett LW, Gold RH. Magnetic resonance imaging of the musculoskeletal system: an overview. *Clin Orthop* 1988;244:17–18.
208. Brower TD, Wilde AH. Femoral neuropathy in hemophilia. *J Bone Joint Surg Am* 1966;48A:487–492.
209. Hoskinson J, Duthie RB. Management of musculoskeletal problems in the hemophiliacs. *Orthop Clin North Am* 1978;9:455–480.
210. Ahlberg AK. On the natural history of hemophilic pseudotumor. *J Bone Joint Surg Am* 1975;57A:1133–1135.
211. Annenberg AJ, Vaccaro PS, Zuelzer WA. Traumatic pseudoaneurysm in a wrestler. *Ann Vasc Surg* 1990;4:69–71.
212. Barohn RJ, Bazan C III, Timmons JH, et al. Bilateral diabetic thigh muscle infarction. *J Neuroimaging* 1994;4:43–44.
213. Walton JN. *Disorders of voluntary muscle.* London: Churchill Livingstone, 1974.
214. Resnick D. *Diagnosis of bone and joint disorders,* 3rd ed. Philadelphia: W.B. Saunders, 1995.
215. Walton JN, Adams RD. *Polymyositis.* Baltimore: Williams & Wilkins, 1958.
216. Wold LE, McLeod RA, Sim FH, et al. *Atlas of orthopedic pathology.* Philadelphia: W.B. Saunders, 1990.

Principles and Practice of Orthopaedic Sports Medicine,
edited by William E. Garrett, Jr., Kevin P. Speer, and Donald T. Kirkendall.
Lippincott Williams & Wilkins, Philadelphia © 2000.

CHAPTER 34

Physical Examination of the Knee

John A. Feagin, Jr.

PHILOSOPHY OF PHYSICAL EXAMINATION

Physical examination of the knee is an art and a science. It serves as an introduction to the patient and a means of communication. The purpose of the physical examination is to arrive at the correct anatomic diagnosis. The examination should play a pivotal role in teaching the patient about the injury and treating the injury.

Examination of the well leg, as a standard for comparison, is a must. *Function* is a part of the examination and is the integration of all the anatomic parts and the symptoms that aid in diagnosis. Gait analysis is part of the functional examination for a patient with a knee injury.

The physical examination should be gentle. The patient will appreciate the art of the physician's on-hands examination and the explanations of the science involved in each part of the examination. Because the examination is administered so that it is nearly painless or that the patient indicates pain during certain parts of the examination is meaningful to the physician. The interaction between the patient and the examiner is the basis for a partnership during the treatment regimen.

Certain principles are essential to physical examination of the knee: that the unaffected side is examined first; that in the course of the examination, the examiner looks (inspection), feels (palpation), and moves both the unaffected and affected extremities; and that the result is a correct anatomic diagnosis.

The physical examination will enhance the quest for truth, which is embodied in the correct and precise diagnosis. Such truth enhances and expedites patient care, which is satisfying to the patient and, when combined with sound judgment, will decrease the cost of medical care to the patient.

CONDUCT OF THE PHYSICAL EXAMINATION

I attempt to examine the injured part in the position that I find the patient. In the office situation, I presume the patient has found a comfortable position before my arrival. I want to observe and maintain this position as long as possible. On the athletic field, the position I, as team physician, or the trainer finds the patient often speaks to the forces involved, the nature of the injury, and the diagnosis and immediate care. Certainly, examining patients in the position in which they are found is most apparent where spinal injury is a suspected component of the injury.

I always examine the well leg first and usually begin this examination gently as the patient is reciting the history. Before eliciting the history, I will confirm with the patient which leg is the "well" leg. Although this is a chapter on knee examination, "leg" is the proper term. We cannot isolate the examination solely to the knee because many diagnostic opportunities will be missed. Eliciting the history while examining the uninjured part is a way of communicating with the patient. In other words, I want to use the tactile sense in my hands to examine the knee, but I want to look at the patient as he or she is talking. For the chronic knee problem, a simple history can be "Tell me all about your knee." In the acute setting, the one-statement history simply may be "Describe what happened to your knee." The history, elicited by a simple question, is familiar and relaxing to the patient. The examiner can examine and look at both the patient–historian and the affected part. The art of eliciting the history at the same time as beginning the examination on the unaffected leg requires practice, but it is noteworthy.

I try to time the examination of the affected leg coincident with the patient's completion of the history. Rarely will the patient talk more than a few minutes in response to a single question if they are not interrupted. I never interrupt patients while they are giving their history. Sometimes, the history is not complete and the examiner

J. A. Feagin, Jr.: Department of Orthopaedics, Duke University, Durham, North Carolina 27709.

will wish for more, but this can be mentally noted and delayed until later in the physical examination. A lack of complete history will not interrupt the flow of the physical examination. A smooth flow is important to both the examiner and patient.

In the office situation, I usually find that the patient is sitting with the injured leg hanging over the examining table. I know that I want to examine the knee in the flexed position, the extended position, the prone position, and in varus–valgus. Pivot shift testing is reserved until the end of the examination because frequently it is painful. Gait also must be analyzed. The anterior cruciate ligament (ACL) and the posterior cruciate ligament (PCL) (i.e., the central pivot) must be defined first. The examination keys off these two critical components—the ACL and the PCL. My first task in examining the affected leg is to compare the conformity with the unaffected leg. Conformity deals with appearance, induration, and swelling. Temperature and tenderness are also a part of the tactile examination and are elicited with the conformity. It often amazes me the sensitivity that resides in our hands. In palpation of the knee, I wish to look for induration before eliciting tenderness or causing discomfort. Induration is an increase in tissue tension caused by swelling that may be either interstitial, intracellular, or both. Fully 50% of the time, a diagnosis can be made on just this part of the examination and the remainder of the examination is merely confirmatory. This is particularly true in meniscal lesions.

Our goal during examination is an anatomic diagnosis. Examination must be conducted in a manner that will ultimately satisfy the scientific criteria. These criteria are well outlined by the International Knee Documentation Committee based on the work initiated by Müller et al. (1). Primary and secondary restraints and the limits of motion must be defined (2–5).

Always as I am examining the knee, I remember A. Graham Apley's teachings (6) on the physical examination: Look!, Feel!, Move! This way, I will not forget anything, although I may elect to exclude some things.

Sometimes I cannot make an anatomic diagnosis on the first try with a particular patient. This usually occurs when the patient has a chronic problem or patients are at less than their best. It also may occur when I am either hurried or tired. I will then acknowledge to the patient that I cannot arrive at the requisite anatomic diagnosis and will suggest that we do an orthopaedic examination under different conditions. Perhaps just icing the knee for 15 minutes and reexamining the knee will suffice; sometimes the patient or the examiner just needs to walk about or break the encounter, or sometimes I ask the patient to aggravate the symptoms and return at a reappointed time. I will try to examine patients the second time at the time coincident with their symptoms. If the problem is overuse, I may ask them

to "overuse" the knee by 10% to 30% for a week and then reexamine them in 1 week. These opportunities to repeat the physical examination have been fruitful for me and led to more accurate anatomic diagnoses and decision making. My judgment is usually improved by the second encounter. In the fee for service practice, I do not bill the patient for the second encounter. Quite simply, I insist on an anatomic diagnosis. I achieve this approximately 85% of the time but must resort to reexamination and imaging for 100% diagnostic accuracy. I believe this simple criterion of an accurate anatomic diagnosis has made my life in orthopaedics a joy. Certainly, it has enhanced my ability to perform a physical examination because I have had to develop tests and techniques along the way to confirm diagnosis or diagnostic hypotheses. If physicians insist on an accurate and timely anatomic diagnosis, this will guarantee that we will never be "average" practitioners.

PRINCIPLES OF THE PHYSICAL EXAMINATION

Central Pivot

The ACL and the PCL form the central pivot of the knee (Fig. 34.1) (7). The ACL is defined by both the Lachman and Drawer tests and the PCL by the posterior

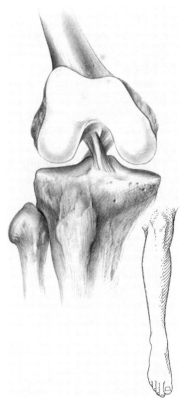

FIG. 34.1. The central pivot.

Drawer test (8). The anterior and posterior Drawer tests are not exactly the same.

The Lachman test is an active antigravity test that requires the patient's relaxation. In the hands of the skilled examiner, it can be quite accurate and is highly specific. The Lachman test, although it has been described by many in the past, was best described by Torg et al. (9) because Torg was a Lachman resident. The Drawer test may be done with the leg hanging or with the examiner stabilizing the lower leg with the knee in 90-degree flexion. The former (i.e., the lower leg unconstrained) is preferred because it enhances the displacements that can be appreciated while testing the ligaments. A sound principle is always to leave one limb segment unconstrained. This will optimize the results of the examination and is a fundamental biomechanical principle. The posterior Drawer test is a passive drop back test with the knee in 90-degree flexion and depends on gravity. Patient relaxation is rarely necessary to this test being successful. Comparison with the uninvolved side is a prerequisite for the test to be a diagnostic indicator.

In addition to straight translation, either anterior or posterior, we are also concerned with rotation as it may occur with translation. This combination will give some idea of interrelationship between the central pivot (i.e., the ACL and PCL) and the secondary restraints. For example, in the instance of a tear of the ACL and medial collateral ligament (MCL), one could expect a highly positive Lachman or Drawer test but one might also find a significant degree of external rotation in addition to the anterior translation where the MCL is also incompetent. Thus, we want to elicit the entire envelope of motion (10), be it normal or pathologic. We want to know the area under the force–displacement curve (Fig. 34.2). The physical examination elicits the area under the force–displacement curve. Translational tests with the lower limb constrained do not maximize the envelope of motion for subtle pathologies. The lower limb should be unconstrained during the ligamentous examination.

The pivot shift test, whether it is as described by Losee et al. (11) or any other version of the test (12), is aimed at combining translation with rotation and thereby eliciting the maximum area under the force–displacement curve (Fig. 34.2). Losee (13) is the master of the pivot shift (Fig. 34.3). Because a positive pivot shift is diagnostic of an incompetent ACL, he uses the test to verify to patients that he can reproduce the systems they have described and to confirm to patients that he has corrected the problem by his operation.

Few of us use the pivot shift test in such an elegant fashion, but in his hands, it is convincing to the patient both preoperatively and postoperatively. If the pivot shift is graded as described by the International Knee Documentation Committee (14), then the grades of negative, physiologic or pathologic pivot glide, pivot shift, and gross subluxation are appropriate. For gross sub-

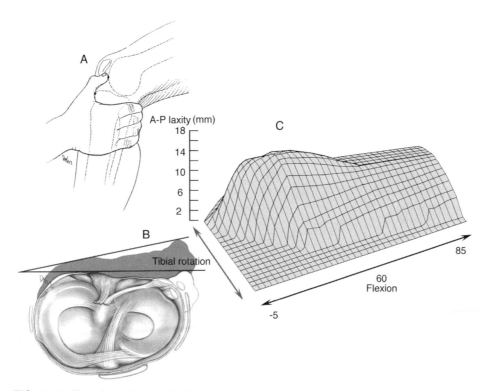

FIG. 34.2. The physical examination elicits the area under the force–displacement curve.

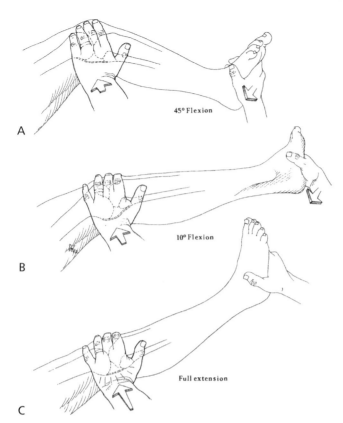

FIG. 34.3. The Losee pivot shift test.

luxation to exist, secondary restraints must also be compromised. Many adolescents and loose-jointed individuals will have a physiologic pivot glide and sometimes even a frank pivot shift, but this will cause little concern because the unaffected leg is the basis of comparison.

After the continuity or discontinuity of the central pivot (i.e., the ACL and PCL) have been determined; the secondary restraints—the MCL, lateral collateral ligament (LCL), and posterior medial and posterior lateral ligaments—are examined. The collateral ligaments are best examined at hyperextension at 0- and 30-degree knee flexion. If the foot is cradled loosely between the iliac crest and the examiner's elbow, then the lower limb will not be rigidly constrained, and the knee can be placed in these three positions (Fig. 34.4).

EXAMINATION OF THE SECONDARY RESTRAINTS

Should the examiner begin with active or passive movements? I prefer to ask the patient to move the well leg within the range of motion that is comfortable and possible. This gives a standard of comparison for the injured leg. Then I ask the patient to move the injured extremity within the bounds of comfort. This shows the range of motion available to position the leg for the ligamentous examinations.

One of the goals of movement is to place the extremity in the best position for isolating and examining the different ligamentous structures. If hyperextension can be achieved, that is a good position in which to begin. If the knee is stable in hyperextension, the medial and lateral capsuloligamentous structures and the PCL are intact. Thus, the maximum amount of information is gained quickly. The technique that Smillie (15) taught me still seems the most useful. The patient's foot is pinioned against the examiner's hip, so that both hands are free to palpate the joint lines and ligamentous structures, and the knee is then placed in hyperextension, neutral, and 30-degree flexion (Fig. 34.4).

Varus and valgus laxity in hyperextension are ominous signs that indicate disruption of key ligamentous structures. If in hyperextension the joint is lax to valgus angulation, the medial capsuloligamentous structures and the PCL are probably interrupted. If in hyperexten-

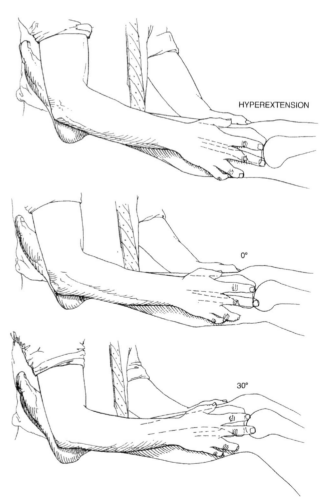

FIG. 34.4. The collateral ligaments are best examined at hyperextension, 0-, and 30-degree knee flexion.

sion the knee is lax to varus angulation, the arcuate complex, PCL, and ACL are probably disrupted. When varus angulation and valgus angulation are applied with the knee at 0-degree flexion, the ACL and PCL are less taut. Then these tests are diagnostic of medial or lateral posterior capsular injuries. At 30-degree flexion, the cruciates and posterior capsular ligaments are in their most relaxed state; then pathologic laxity indicates MCL or LCL laxity.

I believe it is important to separate the diagnosis of the posterior medial and posterior lateral capsular complexes from the MCL and LCL because they are different layers (16) and have different functions (Fig. 34.5). The posterior medial and posterior lateral capsular ligamentous complex are contiguous with the menisci and control meniscal motion. Thus, compromise of one of these complexes will affect meniscal position and function. Further, the prognosis is not the same in that the posterior medial capsular complex retracts posteriorly with injury, and although it will heal, it does not give the same stability after healing. Also, with retraction of the posterior oblique capsular ligament, there can be increased rotatory laxity that jeopardizes the meniscus and function, whereas the MCL heals quite nicely *in situ* without surgery and slight laxity does not affect

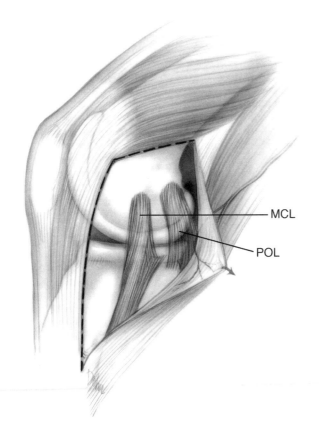

FIG. 34.5. The medial collateral ligament (*MCL*) and posterior oblique ligament (*POL*).

meniscal mechanics. In some of the literature, the MCL is not differentiated from the posterior medial capsular complex. I believe that physical examination should make this differentiation because it is important to the future function of the knee.

The Menisci

Although there are traditional meniscal tests, I prefer a meniscal examination based on the pathoanatomy. The anatomy of the medial and lateral menisci are not the same. They are tethered differently through the capsular ligaments and they have different mobility. Thus, examination of the medial meniscus is not a mirror image examination of the lateral meniscus. In both menisci, the examination is based on the integrity of the radial collagen tie fibers and the normal mobility of the menisci under load. I examine the menisci in three positions (Fig. 34.6):

1. With the knee flexed 90 degrees and the leg hanging (i.e., with gravity distracting the joint). This is optimum for palpation for tenderness. In this position, the normal menisci are not palpable (Fig. 34.6A).
2. In the figure-4 position. In the figure-4 position, the medial meniscus is compressed and the MCL has moved further posteriorly (Fig. 34.6B). This allows palpation of the injured portion of the medial meniscus and MCL and posterior oblique ligament. Because the medial meniscus is most often torn in its posterior horn, this is an especially valuable position. A torn meniscus will extrude in the flexed position, giving a positive "radial extrusion test" (Fig. 34.6C). Cystic degeneration is the basis for the radial extrusion test.
3. If I have not found tenderness, induration, or extrusion of the meniscus in either of these positions, then I will use the third position, the McMurray (17), or other displacement tests to try to see if I can compress and displace the meniscus.

In contrast to the medial meniscus, the lateral meniscus is more likely to have pathology in the mid and anterior portion, and this can be palpated better in full extension. Thus, it is important to examine both menisci through a full range of motion.

Magnetic resonance imaging (MRI) is highly sensitive and specific for meniscal pathology. I have gained increased confidence in the accuracy of physical examination of the menisci since I have adopted the radial extrusion test and made my palpatory examination discreetly over the anterior, middle, and posterior meniscal segments. MRI has helped me to define and refine my examination of the menisci.

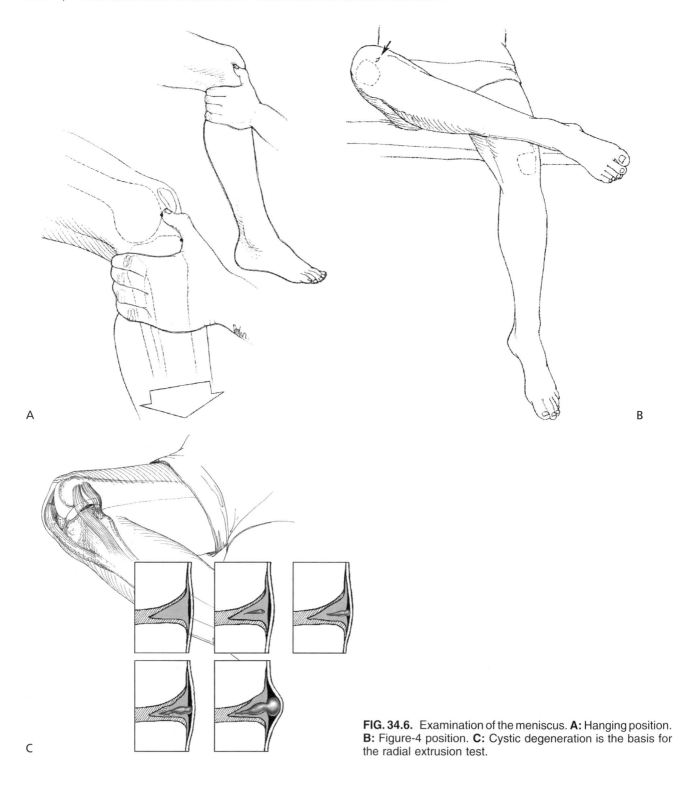

A

B

C

FIG. 34.6. Examination of the meniscus. **A:** Hanging position. **B:** Figure-4 position. **C:** Cystic degeneration is the basis for the radial extrusion test.

three positions can reveal a wealth of pathology. In addition, it is essential to examine the patellofemoral joint in a loaded condition through a range of motion because I believe that crepitus can be diagnostically revealing, and crepitus through a full range of motion is especially significant (Fig. 34.8). Also, I want to know whether the crepitus occurs when the lower pole of the patella engages the trochlear groove or, in extension,

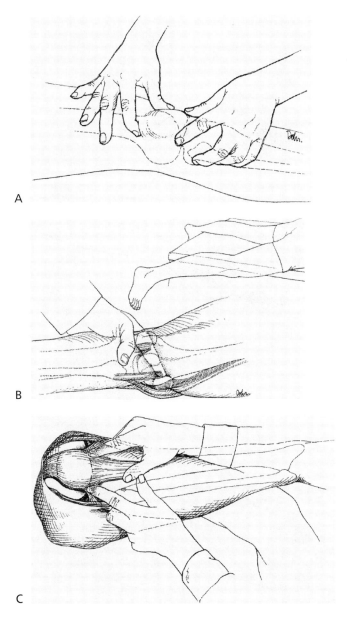

FIG. 34.7. Examination of the patellofemoral joint. **A:** The patella is examined for excursion, pain, and apprehension. **B:** With the patient in the prone position, the examiner can determine the tenderness along the capsule and the swelling and/or tenderness of the fatpad and the inferior capsular ligaments. **C:** In the position pictured, the examiner can palpate the retinacular ligaments of the patella, particularly the superior medial and lateral ligaments. The alignment of the patella with the femoral trochlear groove can also be determined.

Patellofemoral Joint

The patellofemoral joint should be examined in three positions: with the knee in extension (Fig. 34.7A), with the knee in full flexion (Fig. 34.7B), and in the prone position with the knee hyperextended (Fig. 34.7C). Physical examination of the patellofemoral joint in these

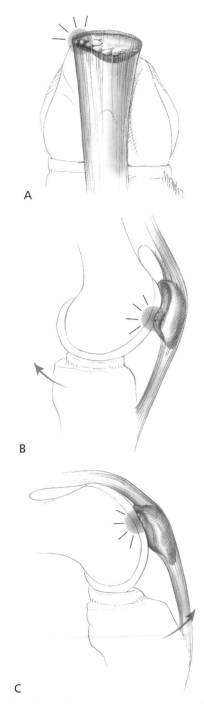

FIG. 34.8. **(A–C)** Crepitus through full range of motion is especially significant in examination of the patellofemoral joint.

when the upper pole of the patella engages the trochlear groove. Furthermore, the medial and lateral alae of the fatpad can be defined by palpation; also the size and consistency of the fatpad can be defined by palpation (Fig. 34.9). In addition, using all three positions, the infrapatella tendon can be examined in both its lax and taut positions for pathology, such as jumper's knee and Osgood-Schlatter deformity.

In examining the patella, I believe that one should use both an apprehension test and a containment test (Fig. 34.10). These define the medial and lateral patella ligaments. Frequently, in the chronic ACL-deficient knee, one will appreciate lateral tilt and lateral placement of the patella as the knee assumes increasing varus deformity. The prone position is ideal for these tests (Fig. 34.10) in that one hand can be used to manipulate the knee through a range of motion, thereby changing the tension of the supporting patella retinacular structures, whereas the other hand causes displacement or containment of the patella or palpates the fatpad, the patella tendon, and inferior capsular structures for tenderness or induration. Another reason to examine the knee and the patellofemoral joint in the prone position is to look for masses and abnormalities of the upper or lower leg. Tumors can mimic a Baker's cyst. The knee can be flexed with the hip in extension, which checks the quadriceps for contracture and the hips are easily checked for range of motion in this position. Sciatica can be detected as a contributing factor to knee pain or it can be ruled out. Thus, the prone examination of the knee and patella femoral joint is a valuable adjunct test and offers many diagnostic possibilities.

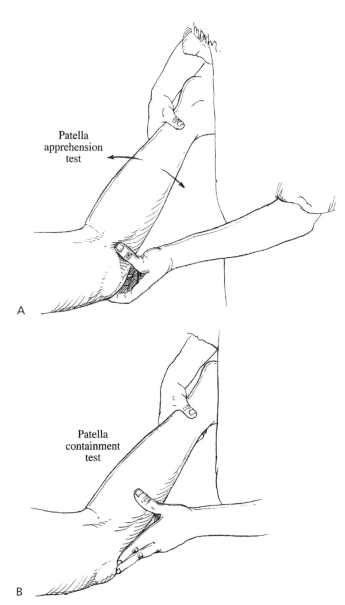

FIG. 34.10. One should use both an (**A**) apprehension test and a (**B**) containment test.

FUNCTION

The examination of the primary and secondary ligamentous structures, the menisci, patella femoral joint, and the enveloping capsular structures may be the first part of the examination, but these parts of the examination have not emphasized function. At some stage, I like to determine function by moving the knee through a range of motion, comparing this with the unaffected side. In gait examination, I watch the shoulder for antalgic sway. I also use toe walking and heel walking to define pathology. Heel walking removes some of the knee shock absorbers such as the forefoot, midfoot, and subtalar joints. If the knee is arthritic, then this will accentuate an antalgic gait or sway of the shoulders. Toe walking,

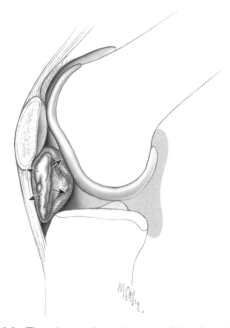

FIG. 34.9. The size and consistency of the fatpad can be defined by palpation.

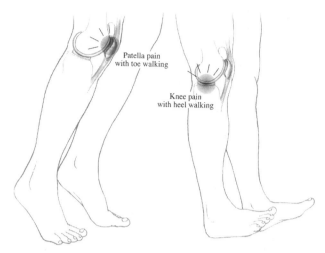

FIG. 34.11. An antalgic gait in the toe walking position indicates patella pathology.

conversely, provides excellent shock absorption for the knee joint but compresses the patella through quadriceps contraction. Thus, an antalgic gait in the toe walking position indicates patella pathology (Fig. 34.11).

IMAGING

I usually assimilate a working diagnosis from these tests. I cannot make a definitive diagnosis, but a working diagnosis allows me to contemplate the most effective imaging and to communicate a plan of action with the patient. This is the beginning of judgment. Good physical examination and good judgment makes for a "good" disposition and a happy patient.

At this stage, at the very least, I order routine radiographs or review the radiographs available to me with the patient. I believe that reviewing the radiographs with the patient is an effective teaching tool and helps the patient to understand the diagnosis and the decision-making process. On evaluating the radiographs, I am looking for a secondary trabecular pattern or spurring that suggests overload. Because radiographs reflect a long-term history of the knee mechanics, they can be quite illuminating. I prefer to review the radiographs after I have completed the physical examination so I am not tempted to shortcut the physical examination based on the radiographic diagnosis. Thus, imaging diagnosis should be used to complement physical examination and verify biomechanical abnormalities.

The choice of imaging will depend on the physical examination. Our routine radiographs include an anteroposterior, lateral, weight-bearing tunnel view (18) and Merchant (19) view of the patella. Although this combination of radiographs may be seen as excessive by some, these views are helpful to make a definitive diagnosis and a plan. How often is MRI requisite? We all agree

that MRI can be specific and sensitive for most structures of the knee. The cruciate ligaments, the secondary restraints, the menisci, the patella femoral joint, and the osseous structures are all well defined by MRI. Only two disappointments with MRI remain: the accuracy as regards chondral surfaces and the ability to obtain dynamic imaging.

Both techniques are forthcoming and will greatly enhance the value of MRI to the knee surgeon. The surgeon is the patient's advocate as regards the quality of the MRI. Less than a complete examination cannot be accepted where one is representing the patient's best interest and involved in judgments that may lead to surgery. The MRI and standard roentgenography should enhance and reinforce the physical examination.

Adjunctive imaging such as long film showing limb alignment, stress roentgenography, dynamic cinetomographic scan, and technetinum-99 scan are sometimes necessary, but these are highly selective and seldom do I consider these early in the process.

With properly selected imaging, we should move from a working anatomic diagnosis to a definitive diagnosis. It is now time to communicate completely and effectively the diagnosis with the patient, appropriate colleagues, and write the narrative in the chart. I review the imaging and the pertinent parts of the physical examination with the patient. I want to emphasis the anatomic diagnosis so that the patient also has a working diagnosis. This leads us to decision making. Sometimes it is appropriate to have the patient's family in attendance for the communicative portion of the diagnostic evaluation because decision making may involve all concerned parties. In addition, parents and spouses, coaches, the physical therapist, athletic trainers, and other team members may need to know the working diagnosis and the elements involved in decision making.

The patient must be a participant in decision making. Sometimes consultation with colleagues is necessary in decision making. This should be used as appropriate to ensure accurate diagnosis, protect the patient, allay anxiety, and ensure successful treatment. It is important to have available colleagues that can serve as effective consultants.

DECISION MAKING

After all the effort and expertise that is requisite to determining the patient's problem and a definitive diagnosis, one certainly wants to use sound judgment and effectively articulate the best solution. The best solution is seldom apparent without the patient's participating in the decision-making process. How does the patient most effectively participate in a decision-making process in which he or she has limited experience and insight?

This is the art of our profession and can be one of the most satisfying results of a well-performed physical examination and an accurate anatomic diagnosis. The performance of the physical examination gives the patient a participatory feeling. This participatory feeling initiates the shared decision-making process. The patient will be interested in the imaging and will be interested in the review and the emphasis on the positive physical findings. Frequently, the plan will be tempered by the patient's vocational and avocational needs. Thus, these needs should be elicited before decision making. I usually discuss the patient's vocational and avocational requirements during the course of the physical examination, particularly when I am in the portion of the examination that requires movement. Hopefully, the patient will focus on my query as regards to his or her activity status while I move the part through the comfortable limits of motion.

SUMMARY

Physical examination, an art and science, can be mastered by almost everyone regardless of the medical discipline. This is important because we need to communicate with the other caregivers on our team. The common denominator of communication is an anatomic diagnosis (14,20). I expect the other caregivers on my team to examine and arrive at an accurate anatomic diagnosis with the same facility and accuracy that I know. Decision making also is an art and science. Although we know the "odds" of our surgical and nonsurgical treatments, the practice of medicine and surgery is an infinite blend of circumstances. This is why the practice of medicine can be so life fulfilling. Decision making requires the integration of the science of the physical examination and anatomic diagnosis with socioeconomic factors and the patient's desires. The patient's participation in this process should be enjoyable for patient and physician alike. The best decision and the best plan for the patient is the ultimate goal of the physical examination and the physician.

REFERENCES

1. Müller W, Biedert R, Hefti F, et al. OAK knee evaluation. A new way to assess knee ligament injuries. *Clin Orthop* 1988;232:37–50.
2. Butler DL, Noyes FR, Grood ES. Ligamentous restraints to anterior-posterior Drawer in the human knee. A biomechanical study. *J Bone Joint Surg Am* 1980;62A:259–270.
3. Fukubayashi Y, Torzilli PA, Sherman MF, et al. An in vitro biomechanical evaluation of anterior-posterior motion in the knee. *J Bone Joint Surg Am* 1982;64A:258–264.
4. Grood ES, Noyes FR, Butler DL, et al. Ligamentous and capsular restraints preventing straight medial and lateral laxity in intact human knees. *J Bone Joint Surg Am* 1981;63A:1257–1269.
5. Grood ES, Stowers SF, Noyes FR. Limits of movement in the human knee. Effect of sectioning the posterior cruciate ligament and posterolateral structures. *J Bone Joint Surg Am* 1988;70A:80–97.
6. Apley AG. *A system of orthopaedics and fractures,* 4th ed. London: Butterworth Publishers, 1973:1.
7. Grood ES, Noyes FR. Diagnosis of knee ligament injuries. In: Feagin JA Jr, ed. *The crucial ligaments. Diagnosis and treatment of ligamentous injuries of the knee,* 2nd ed. New York, Edinburgh: Churchill Livingstone, 1994:371–386.
8. Noyes FR, Grood ES, Butler DL, et al. Clinical biomechanics of the knee ligament restraints and functional stability. In: Funk FJ, ed. *Symposium on the athlete's knee. Surgical repair and reconstruction.* St. Louis: C.V. Mosby, 1980.
9. Torg JS, Conrad W, Kalen V. Clinical diagnosis of anterior cruciate ligament instability of the athlete. *Am J Sports Med* 1976;4:84–93.
10. Blankevoort L, Huiskes R, deLang A. The envelope of passive knee joint motion. *J Biomech* 1988;21:705–720.
11. Losee RR, Johnson TR, Southwick WO. Anterior subluxation of the lateral tibial plateau. A diagnostic test and operative repair. *J Bone Joint Surg Am* 1978;60A:1015–1030.
12. Galway HR, MacIntosh DL. The lateral pivot shift. A symptom and sign of anterior cruciate ligament insufficiency. *Clin Orthop* 1980;147:45–50.
13. Losee RE. Pivot shift. In: Feagin JA Jr, ed. *The crucial ligaments. Diagnosis and treatment of ligamentous injuries about the knee.* New York, Edinburgh: Churchill Livingstone, 1994:407–422.
14. Daniel MD. Assessing the limits of knee motion. *Am J Sports Med* 1991;19:139–147.
15. Smillie IS. *Diseases of the knee.* Edinburgh, London: Churchill Livingstone, 1980:1–27.
16. Warren LF, Marshall JL. The supporting structures and layers of the medial side of the knee. An anatomical analysis. *J Bone Joint Surg Am* 1979;61A:56–62.
17. McMurray TP. The operative treatment of ruptured internal lateral ligament of the knee. *Br J Surg* 1918;6:377–381
18. Rosenberg TD, Paulos L, Parker RD, et al. The forty-five-degree posteroanterior flexion weight-bearing radiograph of the knee. *J Bone Joint Surg Am* 1988;70A:1479–1483.
19. Merchant AC, Mercer RL, Jacobson RH, et al. Roentgenographic analysis of patellofemoral congruence. *J Bone Joint Surg Am* 1974;56A:1391–1396.
20. Noyes FR, Grood ES, Torzilli PA. The definitions of terms for motion and position of the knee and injuries of the ligaments. *J Bone Joint Surg Am* 1989;71A:465–471.

Principles and Practice of Orthopaedic Sports Medicine,
edited by William E. Garrett, Jr., Kevin P. Speer, and Donald T. Kirkendall.
Lippincott Williams & Wilkins, Philadelphia © 2000.

CHAPTER 35

Anatomy and Biomechanics of the Knee

Bruce D. Beynnon

The knee joint is the largest and the most complex joint in the human body. The joint capsule and ligaments, which provide the structural stability to the knee, are particularly vulnerable to injury by the large moments that can be created through the forces acting along the long lever arms of the lower limb. Thus, it is not surprising that the knee is one of the most frequently injured joints. An injury to the knee, such as disruption of the anterior cruciate ligament (ACL), can result in an extensive disability because this injury may alter normal knee kinematics and therefore locomotion. An extensive background in biomechanics or mathematics is not required to understand the fundamental mechanical principles governing the knee joint. Knowledge of knee biomechanics provides an essential framework for understanding the consequences of injury and joint disorders, aids in the intelligent planning of surgical procedures, and serves as the basis for developing objective rehabilitation programs and the effect that different types of orthoses have on the knee joint.

The knee joint comprises three independent articulations: one between the patella and femur and the remaining two between the lateral and medial tibial and femoral condyles. The patellofemoral articulation consists of the patella, with a multifaceted dorsal surface, articulating with the femoral trochlear groove. The tibiofemoral articulations consist of elliptical femoral condyles with saddle-shaped tibial condyles and interposing menisci.

To the untrained observer, the knee joint may appear to function as a simple pinned hinge (ginglymus), with flexion–extension rotation the only apparent motion between the femur and tibia. However, the motion char-

acteristics of the knee joint are very complex, requiring a full 6 degrees of freedom (3 translations and 3 rotations) to completely describe the coupled, or simultaneous, joint motions. An example of coupled motion is demonstrated with flexion rotation of the knee from the extended position. With this rotation, there is a coupled posterior movement of the femoral contact regions on the tibial surface in the sagittal plane, and in the transverse plane internal rotation of the tibia relative to femur occurs. The Eularian-based coordinate system described by Hefzy and Grood (1) allow the translations and rotations to be described in anatomically referenced directions. Although there are many different types of coordinate systems used to describe three-dimensional knee motion, this system is appealing because it allows joint rotation to be expressed in terms familiar to the clinician. Grood and Noyes (2) have applied the three-dimensional coordinate system to the interpretation of various clinical examination techniques and developed a "bumper model" of the knee joint. This model is useful in describing the soft tissue restraints to anterior–posterior translation and internal–external rotation of the knee joint. In addition, the model may be applied to demonstrate the types of tibiofemoral subluxations that may result when different soft tissue structures are disrupted. Application of this approach may aid in the examination of injuries to the knee ligaments and capsular structures.

This chapter assumes a working knowledge of the biomechanical terms essential to the description of knee function. For an introduction to basic knee biomechanics, readers should consult Frankel (3), Frankel and Burstein (4), and Mow and Hayes (5) and biomechanical terminology as it applies to the knee (e.g., Noyes et al. [6] and Bonnarens and Drez [7]). A review of experimental studies and mathematical model investigations of both the tibiofemoral and the patellofemoral joints, with associated contact morphometry studies, are presented.

B. D. Beynnon: Department of Orthopaedics and Rehabilitation, McClure Musculoskeletal Research Center, University of Vermont, Burlington, Vermont 05404-0084.

DESCRIPTION OF BIOMECHANICAL TECHNIQUES

The American Society of Biomechanics has defined the term biomechanics as "the study of the structure and function of biological systems using the methods of mechanics." Specific to the knee joint, this involves modeling and experimental investigation techniques. Each is based on fundamental principles and terminology that require definition. These may be grouped into three classes of study:

1. Mathematical models of the knee joint;
2. Experimental study of the entire knee using the flexibility approach and the stiffness approach;
3. Experimental study of an individual ligament using anatomic observations, force measurement, and strain measurement.

Hefzy and Grood (1) presented a detailed review of the different modeling techniques and applications. Perhaps the most commonly described physical knee model is the crossed four-bar linkage called the "cruciate linkage" (8–12). This approach has been used to study the interaction of the cruciates with the tibiofemoral joint. The model consists of two crossed rods that represent the cruciates and two connecting bars that represent both tibial and femoral attachments of these ligaments. This approach has been used to describe the shape of both the tibial and femoral condyles, the path of the instantaneous center of knee joint rotation, and the posterior migration of the tibiofemoral contact point that occurs with knee flexion. The four-bar approach is based on rigid interconnecting cruciate linkages that are not allowed to elongate. Because the cruciates elongate during normal joint articulation (13,14), this technique may be inadequate for modeling the detailed biomechanics of the cruciates and their interactions with the tibiofemoral joint.

Crowninshield et al. (15) published one of the first theoretic investigations of the knee by means of a mathematical model. The cruciate, collateral, and capsular ligaments were represented by 13 elements. Input parameters included both *in vitro* and *in vivo* measurements of the attachment sites and dimensions of the knee ligaments. The effect of a given ligament was then investigated by eliminating an element in the model and comparing this with an actual test where the ligament was cut.

Wismans et al. (16) developed a three-dimensional tibiofemoral joint model that incorporated the nonlinear characteristics of tibiofemoral geometry and ligamentous material properties. This model was applied to investigate the biomechanics of the major knee ligaments, tibiofemoral compressive loading, and joint load–displacement response and to determine the relative position of the femur with respect to the tibia as a function of different applied joint-loading conditions. In later studies, Blankevoort and Huiskes (17) applied similar techniques to study the effects of different ACL replacement positions on tibiofemoral joint biomechanics. They also investigated the recruitment of knee ligaments (18), tibiofemoral contact in three dimensions (19), and ligament bone interaction (20).

Flexibility or Ligament Cutting Studies

This approach involves observing or measuring the displacement due to an applied joint load. A ligament is then cut and the procedure is repeated. The relative difference in displacement is then used to establish the importance of that ligament. This method is analogous to clinical laxity examinations (i.e., Lachman test), where the clinician applies a load and estimates the resulting joint displacement. Thus, this technique is useful in evaluating the sensitivity of knee laxity tests to injuries created in human cadavers. A drawback of this technique is that the difference between the behavior of a knee joint before and after excision of a ligament does not necessarily indicate that the ligament cut was responsible.

Stiffness Approach

The stiffness approach involves the application of a predetermined displacement simultaneous with measurement of the load applied to the knee joint. The structure under investigation is then cut and the test repeated. Any resultant decrease in load is recorded. This method can be used to establish the role and relative importance of a particular ligament and determines the motions resisted by that ligament.

A comparison between methodologies reveals the stiffness approach produces results that are independent of the order in which the ligaments are sectioned and therefore is a more direct approach, whereas the flexibility approach is governed by the order of ligament cutting. Thus, the results of these later studies may be difficult to interpret.

Anatomic Observation

In the clinical approach, ligament function is inferred from anatomy. Important information includes anatomic location of the ligament attachment points, orientations of major fiber bundles, and size (length and cross-sectional area). The important early observations were made by Hughston et al. (21,22), Slocum et al. (23), and Kennedy et al. (24). More recently, careful dissection techniques have been used by a number of workers to improve our understanding of the knee ligaments (25–28).

Ligament Force Measurement

Measurement of ligament or tendon force continues to be one of the biggest challenges in orthopedic biomechanics. To meet this challenge, Salmons (29) introduced the buckle transducer, a structure containing a beam over which the ligament is looped to create bending of the buckle frame. The beam is attached separately, and therefore transverse cutting of the ligament is not required. However, lengthwise incisions are required, disrupting many ligament fibers, which alters the normal function of the ligament by dissociating one group of fiber bundles from another (26,30,31). Salmons (29) and other investigators (32–34) applied this technique to various knee ligaments. This approach is limited to *in vitro* applications in cadavers or to *in vivo* studies in animals where a knee ligament is instrumented with the transducer and then the knee joint loaded. The output from the buckle transducer is then directly recorded. After testing the tissue *in situ*, the tissue is dissected free from one of its bony attachments so that a known load can be applied to the tissue-buckle system and a calibration of the gage-soft tissue system made. With this approach, the load can be determined for the tissue *in situ*.

Markolf et al. (35) presented a direct approach to the measurement of ACL force in cadaveric knees. This technique involves isolating the tibial attachment of the ACL by creating a bone plug with a coring cutter and attaching a load sensor to the external portion of the bone plug. This approach facilitates the measurement of resultant ACL force. The authors demonstrated that passive flexion–extension motion of the knee, from 10 degrees to full flexion, does not load the ACL, whereas loading of the quadriceps musculature (simulating active extension of the lower limb against gravity) developed ACL loading between the limits of 0 and 45 degrees. In addition, the authors revealed that the pressive joint load expected during common activi- of daily living acts to protect the ACL from the high forces that are developed by anterior-directed shear loads. This same protective mechanism was not demonstrated for applied internal or external tibial torque.

Strain Measurement

Several investigators have measured ligament displacement, enabling the calculation of strain pattern, to understand the effect of knee joint position and muscle activity on ligament biomechanics (36–41). Most of this work has been carried out in the *in vitro* environment with conflicting results.

Edwards et al. (38), Kennedy et al. (39), and Brown et al. (37) used mercury-filled strain gages to measure the length of ligaments at various angles of knee flexion.

Henning et al. (42) constructed a device to measure displacement in the ACL *in vivo*.

Butler et al. (43) and Woo et al. (44) developed optical techniques for the mapping of surface strains in various tissues. Butler et al. used high-speed cameras to record the movements of surface markers and measured both midsubstance and insertion site deformations of soft tissues (43,45). These techniques are an ideal method for monitoring surface strains, particularly during high rate tests, but are not useful for out-of-plane movements or for ligaments such as the cruciates that cannot be directly viewed. They also suffer from the theoretic disadvantage that the tissue of interest has to be exposed and therefore is not in a physiologic state.

Other workers have calculated strain by measuring the change of ligament attachment length under various applied joint loadings. For example, Wang et al. (41) measured the three-dimensional coordinates of pins stuck in a cadaver joint at the palpated origin and insertion points of the major knee ligaments. They recorded the relationship between torque and angular rotation between the femur and the tibia. After excision of certain ligaments, the tests were repeated to determine the contribution of these elements to torsional restraint. In the most extensive and elegant studies, Sidles et al. (46) used a three-dimensional digitizer to compute ligament length patterns. Using a slightly different approach, Trent et al. (47) measured the relative displacements of two pins embedded into the ligament attachments and located the instant centers of transverse joint rotation. Warren et al. (48) also used pins placed at ligament origins but measured displacements with a radiographic technique.

The pins or other markers used as locators of ligament origin generally estimate average ligament strain. This technique may produce confusing results because of the difficulty in choosing the center of a ligament insertion and the changes in strain from insertion site to midsubstance within a ligament.

Previous work at the University of Vermont focused on the measurement of ACL displacement in the *in vitro* environment using the Hall effect strain transducer, allowing for computing of strain (36,40,49). In recent investigations, this technique has been applied to the measurement of ACL strain *in vivo* (13,14,50).

LIGAMENT BIOMECHANICS

The primary functions of the knee ligaments are to stabilize the knee, control normal kinematics in unison with the leg muscles, and prevent abnormal displacements and rotations that may damage articular surfaces or menisci. They are the most important static stabilizers. Ligaments are primarily composed of collagen, the constituent that provides resistance to a tensile load developed along the length of the ligament, with lesser and varying amounts of elastic and reticulin fibers. Cellular elements, ground substance, vascular channels, and nerves are also present. Collagen fibers and their orientation within the tissue are responsible for the primary biomechanical behavior of each structure. The fibers of the large distinct ligaments are almost all arranged in parallel bundles, making them ideal for withstanding tensile loads, whereas capsular structures have a less consistent orientation, making them more compliant and not as strong in resisting axial loading.

The ligament insertion sites are designed to reduce the chance of failure by distributing the stresses at the bone ligament interface in a gradual fashion. This is accomplished by the collagen fibers passing from the ligament into the bone through four distinct zones: ligament morphometry, fibrocartilaginous matrix, mineralized fibrocartilage, and the bone itself (51). Despite the transitions, Noyes et al. (52) demonstrated that some strain concentration occurs near the ligamentous insertion sites. Sidles et al. (53) developed an analytic model of the ACL tibial insertion. They demonstrated that for a typical ACL insertion geometry, the transverse pressures are similar to the tensile stress along the ligament.

The knee ligaments can best control motion of the bones relative to each other if the motion takes place along the direction of the ligament fibers. For example, when the knee is loaded in valgus, the medial collateral ligament (MCL) develops a tensile stress in combination with a compressive force across the lateral compartment of the knee, creating resistance to medial joint opening. Acting alone, ligaments cannot restrain the relative rotation associated with applied torques. The ligament would simply rotate about its bony insertion sites. A second force, usually developed through bone-to-bone compression, is required. For example, as the knee is loaded with an internal torque, a transverse rotation causes the femoral condyles to ride up the tibial spines. This combination creates a compressive force across the tibiofemoral contact regions, and an oppositely directed tensile force along the cruciate and collateral ligaments. This example may help demonstrate the mechanism in which the ACL interacts with tibiofemoral bony compression to resist an applied internal rotation to the knee joint.

The ability of a ligament to resist applied tensile loading may best be described through examination of the load–elongation curve produced during tensile failure testing of an ACL. As a tensile load is applied, the ligament elongates. The slope of the measured load–displacement relationship represents the stiffness of the ligament. The steeper the slope of this curve, the stiffer the ligament. In the unloaded state, the ligament fibers are under minimal tension and the collagen fibers have a wavy pattern. As a tensile load is applied, the wavy pattern begins to straighten out. Initially, little load is required to elongate the ligament. This is characterized by the relatively flat "toe" region of the curve. The change from the toe to the linear portion of the curve represents the change in stiffness that an examiner perceives during a clinical laxity examination when a ligament's "end point" is reached.

As the tensile load continues to increase, all the collagen fibers are straightened and the curve becomes nearly linear. This region of the curve characterizes the elastic deformation of the ligament, until the yield point is reached. At this point, there is a sudden loss in the ligament's ability to transmit load. If loading continues, a maximum or ultimate failure load is reached, and a sudden drop in load is recorded, representing total failure of the ligament. The area under the load–deformation curve represents the amount of energy absorbed by a ligament during testing. Noyes et al. demonstrated that the characteristics of the ACL's load–displacement curve are dramatically affected by variables such as age (54), strain rate (55), and duration of immobilization (disuse) (56). Young adults have a yield point that can be as much as three times greater than an older person (54). Noyes et al. (55) also demonstrated the sensitivity of the ACL's load–displacement response to strain rate. Anterior cruciates that are failed rapidly (0.6 seconds) demonstrate a 20% increase in load to failure over those failed at a speed two orders of magnitude slower (60 seconds). The energy stored just before ligament failure was 30% greater in preparations tested at the high strain rate compared with those failed at the slow rate. In addition, any ligament that has been immobilized, even for short periods of time, demonstrates a reduction in strength (56).

Most orthopedic surgeons who operatively restore ACL function perform an intraarticular reconstruction with autograft material (57). Noyes et al. (52) characterized the relative strength of the various ligament replacement materials, demonstrating that a 14-mm-wide bone–patella tendon–bone preparation was 168% as strong as the normal ACL, with the strength of all other autogenous replacements less than that of a normal ACL. Woo et al. (58) demonstrated that the normal tensile strength of the ACL may be as high as 2,500 N rather than the original 1,725 N standard presented by Noyes et al. (52). This has led some surgeons to use combinations of autogenous graft material in an effort to increase the strength of the ACL replacement. Butler (59) used a primate model to demonstrate that maintaining a vascular supply to an ACL graft produces no material property differences from a similar free graft 1 year after implantation.

The Cruciates and Their Function in Joint Stability

The concept of primary and secondary knee stabilizers was introduced by Butler et al. (60), who applied the stiffness approach to human cadaver specimens. They demonstrated that the ACL is a primary restraint to anterior translation of the tibia relative to femur, providing an average restraint of 87.2% to the applied load at 30 degrees. With the knee at 90 degrees, this figure was 85.1%. After ACL transection, the remaining intact ligamentous structures provided little restraint to anterior subluxation, leading Butler et al. to describe the function of the remaining soft tissues as secondary restraints to this particular motion. The remaining ligament and capsular structures each contributed less than 3% to the total restraining force resulting from an applied anterior shear load. Butler et al. (60) also demonstrated that the posterior cruciate ligament (PCL) is the primary restraint to posterior translation of the tibia relative to femur, providing a restraining force of 94% at 90 and 30 degrees of knee flexion. None of the remaining ligamentous and capsular secondary structures contributed more than 2% of the total restraining force to an applied posterior shear load.

Fukubayashi et al. (61) used the flexibility approach to investigate the coupled behavior between anterior–posterior shear loading and internal–external tibiofemoral rotation in human cadavers. They showed that the ACL produces an internal tibial rotation with anterior shear load applied across the tibiofemoral joint, whereas the PCL produces an external tibial rotation with applied posterior shear loading. The magnitude of tibial rotation coupled with applied anterior–posterior shear loading decreased after transection of either cruciate ligament. Gollehon et al. (62) also applied the flexibility approach to human cadaver specimens in an effort to investigate the role of the cruciates, lateral collateral ligament (LCL), and deep complex (arcuate ligament and popliteus tendon) in joint stability. This investigation showed that the PCL is the principle structure resisting posterior translation of the tibia relative to femur. Isolated transection of the PCL did not affect varus angulation or external rotation of the knee. Transection of the PCL, LCL, and deep complex was then performed to investigate the effects of a combined injury. This created a significant increase in varus rotation, posterior translation, and external rotation at all angles of knee flexion, suggesting that subjects with such a combined injury may have a functionally impaired joint. Combined sectioning of the ACL and the posterolateral ligaments produced a significant increase in internal–external rotation of the tibia, indicating that patients with this combined injury may also have compromised knee function.

Grood et al. (63) applied the flexibility approach with human cadaver specimens to investigate the role of the PCL and posterolateral structures (LCL, arcuate ligament, and popliteus tendon) in joint stability. Isolated sectioning of the PCL revealed that the amount of posterior tibial translation, measured relative to the femur, was twice as much at 90 degrees than at 30 degrees of knee flexion. This occurred without abnormal axial tibial rotation and varus–valgus angulation. The concurrent increase in posterior laxity with flexion of the knee was attributed to slackening of the posterior portion of the joint capsule, which provides a secondary restraint to posterior translation. The authors concluded that clinical examination of the PCL should be performed at 90 degrees of flexion, where the secondary restraints are less effective in blocking posterior tibial translation. At this knee angle, the clinician can gain a full appreciation of the PCL contribution to joint laxity. Removal of the posterolateral complex, although leaving the PCL intact, produced an increase in both external tibial rotation and varus angulation. The increase in external rotation was greatest at 30 degrees of flexion where it was two times larger in comparison with that measured at 90 degrees.

The posterolateral complex thus provides the primary restraint to external rotation with the knee at 30 degrees. The authors (63) recommended clinical examination of the posterolateral complex with the external rotation exam while the knee is flexed between 20 and 40 degrees of flexion. A significant increase in external tibial rotation with the knee flexed to 90 degrees required transection of both the PCL and the posterolateral complex. This finding suggests that a clinical examination that demonstrates a significant increase in external tibial rotation with the knee at 90 degrees of flexion involves deficiencies in both the PCL and posterolateral complex.

Several investigators have increased our knowledge of the kinematics of the normal knee and the changes in knee kinematics as a result of ACL reconstruction. Markolf et al. (35) performed a series of studies in which they measured native ACL forces in human cadavers. They noted that although the magnitudes of the forces varied considerably from specimen to specimen, the patterns of loading with respect to direction of loading and flexion angle of the knee were consistent. Passive extension of the knee generated forces only in the last 10 degrees of extension. Adding a force through the quadriceps tendon increased the force in the ACL at all flexion angles during knee extension against resistance. Internal tibial torque generated higher ligament forces than external tibial torque. The external load applied to the knee during anterior tibial translation was approximately equal to the force in the ligament at full extension and at 20 degrees of knee flexion. Increasing tibiofemoral contact force (compressive force across the joint) decreased the force in the ligament at both full extension and at 20 degrees of flexion.

Woo et al. (64) carefully measured the forces in the ACL *in situ* using a 6 degree-of-freedom robot manipulator and universal force-moment sensor. They demonstrated that the *in situ* forces of the ACL and knee kinematics were significantly different when evaluated with a 5-degree-of-freedom unconstrained motion compared with 1-degree-of-freedom constrained motion. Anterior tibial translation increased significantly in response to an anterior tibial load in the unconstrained condition compared with the constrained condition. Constrained testing significantly altered the magnitude and direction of the *in situ* force in the ACL. They also demonstrated that the forces in the anteromedial and posterolateral bundles of the ACL changed in magnitude and distribution with knee flexion angle, suggesting that the posterolateral bundle plays an important role in resisting anterior tibial translation.

Before understanding the effects of exercises on the biomechanical behavior of an injured ACL or a healing ACL graft, it is important to understand the behavior of the normal ACL. One of our objectives has been to describe the effects of body weight, muscle forces, and knee flexion angle on ACL strain behavior (65–67). This has allowed us to understand the function of the normal ACL during exercise, and these data are now being used to study the effect of rehabilitation exercises on healing ACL grafts. Our group has measured ACL strain with the Hall effect strain transducer (Micro-Strain, Inc., Burlington, VT) and more recently with the differential variable reluctance transducer (MicroStrain, Inc.). We studied normal ACLs among patient volunteers undergoing either arthroscopic surgery for partial meniscectomy or a diagnostic procedure. The operation and study were performed under local anesthesia, which allowed the subjects full control of their musculature. After the routine surgical procedure was completed, we implanted the differential variable reluctance transducer into the ACL.

Anterior loading of the tibia at 30 degrees of flexion (the Lachman test) to the level of 150 N produced more strain within the normal anterior medial bundle (AMB) than shear testing at 90 degrees (the anterior drawer test) (14). Henning et al. (42) directly measured the displacement pattern of the anteromedial aspect of the ACL *in vivo* under anterior shear load conditions and demonstrated that the Lachman test produced greater elongation of the anteromedial band than the anterior drawer test. These data (14) agree with previously published studies that either used instrumented knee laxity testing or clinical impressions to assess the behavior of the ACL under clinical examination conditions (68). The results confirm that the Lachman test is the clinical examination of choice to evaluate the integrity of the ACL (69–73).

Isolated isometric contraction of the quadriceps musculature at 15 and 30 degrees of knee flexion produced a significant increase in ACL strain values. At 60 and 90 degrees of flexion, this activity did not change ACL strain values from those obtained when the muscles were completely relaxed. Isometric contraction of the hamstring muscles at 15, 30, 60, and 90 degrees of flexion did not strain the ACL. Simultaneous contraction of the quadriceps and hamstring muscles at 15 degrees of

knee flexion created a moderate increase in ACL strain; however, the ACL was not strained at 30, 60, and 90 degrees of flexion. Nisell et al. (74) developed a two-dimensional model of the knee that predicts that isometric quadriceps extension against a fixed resistance will produce an anterior-directed shear force on the tibia, a loading that can produce undesirable strain values on an ACL replacement, with the knee positioned between 0 and 60 degrees. According to the model, an isometric quadriceps extension effort between 60 degrees and full flexion will produce posterior-directed forces on the tibia that will strain the PCL or its replacement, but not the ACL. The model suggests that isometric quadriceps extension efforts at knee angles between 60 and 0 degrees may become unsafe for a newly reconstructed ACL, whereas this activity would be safe for a PCL reconstruction. Isometric quadriceps extension, with the knee positioned between 60 degrees and full flexion, may be unsafe for a PCL reconstruction, whereas this activity would be safe for an ACL reconstruction.

In vivo strain measured within the AMB when a seated subject performed an isotonic quadriceps contraction (active range of motion [AROM]) consistently produced a positive region of strain values between 10 and 48 degrees and an unstrained region between 48 and 110 degrees of flexion (14). AROM rehabilitation programs may now be prescribed with these two flexion angle regions adapted to the clinicians requirements. In the unstrained region, quadriceps activity associated with AROM did not produce AMB strain values different from those produced by the same knee motion without contraction of the leg musculature (knee flexion–extension motion of the subject's knee performed by an investigator and termed passive range of motion [PROM]) (14). This suggests that AROM, between the limits of 50 and 100 degrees, may be performed safely immediately after ACL reconstruction. The AROM activity may then move to the positive strain region when the reconstruction and fixation will tolerate this level of strain (at a time as yet not determined) (14). The maximum AROM strain values were greater (ranging from 4.1% to 1.5%) than the maximum PROM strain values (14). Application of a 10-pound weight boot during the AROM activity increased the AMB strain. Grood et al. (75) demonstrated, in an *in vitro* model, that leg extension exercises (in the range of 0 to 30 degrees) produce loadings potentially destructive to the repaired or reconstructed ACL. Further investigation is required to determine whether the AROM strain values between 10 and 48 degrees are large enough to produce permanent elongation of the reconstructed tissue or failure of the fixation construct. Our findings illustrate that both muscle activity and knee position determine AMB strain at rest and with joint motion (14). It appears that for AROM, the AMB is strained between the limits of full extension and 48 degrees (14). These findings are consistent with Henning et al.'s *in vivo* study (42) of two patients with injured ligaments and the findings of Markolf et al. (35).

Weight-bearing (closed-kinetic-chain) exercises have been promoted by some investigators because the compressive joint load produced by body weight forces the congruent articular surfaces together. This has been described by some as protective for a healing ACL graft. Exercises that involve contraction of the dominant quadriceps musculature in the non–weight-bearing knee (open-kinetic-chain exercises) have been characterized as antagonistic to an ACL graft and are typically prescribed once adequate healing has taken place. In an effort to provide insight into the effect of weight-bearing and non–weight-bearing exercises on an ACL graft, we investigated its strain behavior while subjects performed active flexion–extension of the leg in an open-kinetic-chain fashion, squatting (a closed-kinetic-chain exercise), and squatting with the sport cord. The maximum ACL strain values produced by squatting were not different from those produced by active flexion–extension of the knee. Squatting with the sport cord did not increase ACL strain values over squatting alone. These findings demonstrated that squatting (an exercise that involves the compressive joint load produced by body weight) does not necessarily protect the ACL any more than active flexion–extension of the knee (an exercise that is characterized primarily by contraction of the dominant quadriceps muscle group and does not include a compressive joint load produced by body weight). We also found that increasing resistance with the sport cord during squatting did not create a substantial increase in ACL strain values. This may be a benefit of closed-kinetic-chain exercises such as squatting. In contrast, our earlier work revealed that adding weight to increase resistance during open-kinetic-chain active flexion–extension of the knee produced a significant increase in ACL strain values.

We have also found a significant increase in ACL strain values when subjects move from a seated position (minimal shear and compressive loads across the knee) to a standing position (substantial compressive load and a shear force across the knee) (66). These seated and standing postures produced similar strain values when a 140 N anteriorly directed load was applied to the tibia. This finding indicates that the ACL is strained during weight bearing and the substantial compressive load produced does not reduce ligament strain (66).

Passive motion of the knee, between 110 degrees and full extension, revealed that the ACL reaches positive strain values as the joint is brought into extension and remains at or below the zero strain level between the limits of 11.5 and 110 degrees of flexion using distal leg support loading (14). Therefore, continuous passive motion of the knee within these limits should be safe for the reconstructed ACL immediately after surgery when the leg is supported throughout flexion–extension motion without applied varus–valgus loading, internal–external torques, or anterior shear forces. The limits near extension (0 to 10 degrees) can cause small magnitudes of strain (1% or less) (14). This may pose a relatively mild constraint to bracing a patient's knee in the fully extended position (0 degrees) or to the use of continuous passive motion during a rehabilitation program.

One factor critical to the long-term success of an ACL reconstruction is the location of the graft insertion sites on the femur and tibia. The locations of these bony tunnels, along with the initial tension applied to the graft, establish the new kinematic behavior of the knee. Thus, methods for locating the tunnel positions have been the subject of several investigations. Sapega et al. (31) demonstrated that none of the bundles of the ACL are of fixed length during flexion–extension of the knee, and therefore the ACL does not truly demonstrate isometric behavior. They observed the least deviations from isometry for the anteromedial sites under conditions when the gravitational dependency of the lower leg was constrained. Because the anatomic areas of the normal ACL insertion exhibit nonisometric patterns, they concluded that placement of the graft through the anteromedial portion of the anatomic attachment sites of the normal ACL will be the most isometric. One way to determine the optimal location of an ACL graft is to use an isometer. However, these instruments cannot predict the elongation behavior of the ACL graft after it is in place (76), because they are used when the knee is ACL deficient. No current commercially available isometer can mimic the material and structural properties of the selected graft, and therefore knee kinematics recorded with an isometer differ from the those with the graft in place. Using a Hall effect strain transducer to measure the elongation behavior of the patellar tendon graft *in vivo* (14,65,77–79), we demonstrated that it is possible to restore the elongation pattern of the normal ACL using an autogenous bone–patellar tendon–bone graft.

Our *in vivo* PROM investigations (13,14) and previous *in vitro* studies (26,31,36) showed that the AMB of the ACL is not "isometric." That is, the fiber length changes as the knee passes through a range of motion (14). The change in length of fibers is least in the anteromedial band (31), and thus most intraarticular reconstruction procedures now attempt to reattach an ACL graft to the attachment sites of this portion of the ligament. *In vivo* strain gage analysis immediately after the fixation of an ACL graft has allowed us to determine whether the graft strain pattern is similar to the normal ACL or unacceptable (13). Isometers have been devised to assist surgeons in identifying optimal attachment sites for an ACL reconstruction. Therefore, the *in vivo* ACL data (14) for PROM of the joint may serve as important standards by which to accept or reject isometer measurements of potential reconstruction tunnel placement sites. For PROM, the difference between mean peak and mean minimum AMB strain values was 4.2% (range, 3.0% to 7.2%) (14). If this difference is assumed to occur uniformly over the AMB length and the mean length of the AMB is equal to 36 mm (80), there would be an average change in AMB length of 1.5 mm (range, 1.1 to 2.6 mm).

The range of isometer displacement guideline should be used with two considerations when performing measurements for an ACL reconstruction tunnel placement. One, with repeated PROM of the knee, the surgeon should strive to reproduce the PROM pattern we have described (14). This would require the isometer to measure elongation (e.g., increase in length) ranging from 1.1 to 2.6 mm as the knee is brought from approximately 50 degrees (where it should be at a minimum) to extension. Two, our data represent useful criteria when used with an isometer measurement system that has load–displacement behavior similar to the normal ACL and not the highly compliant isometer systems available with present ACL reconstruction instrumentation. Care must be taken in interpreting isometer findings because the measurement is being made in an ACL-deficient knee that may have abnormal kinematics. Because the ACL is not present, a measurement system with normal ACL load–displacement behavior would restore "normal" tibiofemoral joint kinematics. Under this condition, the isometry measurement will make a potential tunnel placement prediction based on what the ACL substitute will be exposed to once implanted (81). This is not possible with current commercially available isometer systems.

Reconstruction of the ACL is performed more frequently with increasing incidence and awareness of injury to this structure. Long-term outcome studies have illustrated poor results after ACL injury without reconstruction, resulting in significant knee instability and posttraumatic arthritis (82). Several surgical techniques make use of various graft materials; however, most surgeons currently favor either the autogenous bone–patellar tendon–bone construct or the doubled or quadrupled semitendinosus–gracilis tendon graft, with an arthroscopic or arthroscopically assisted technique.

Reconstruction using the patellar tendon graft offers several advantages: a graft with superior structural properties to those of the native ACL (52,58); superior strength immediately after surgery with the interference screw fixation method; and bone-to-bone healing, offering long-term stability of the knee with decreased risk of failure. The main disadvantages have been anterior knee pain (83) and weakness of the extensor mechanism during the early phase of rehabilitation (84). Several investigators have determined the structural properties of the patellar tendon with bone blocks attached

(58,79,85–87). Noyes et al. (52) determined that a 14-mm-wide graft had 168% of the ultimate stress of the ACL. Consequently, it has been suggested that a 10-mm-wide patellar tendon graft has approximately the strength of the native ACL at the time of reconstruction. This probably decreases during healing. Woo et al. (58) demonstrated that the age of the specimen and the rate of strain applied to the specimens can affect the structural properties of the graft.

A great deal of what we know regarding the healing of ACL grafts has been learned through investigations performed in animal models (77,78). Investigations of the patellar tendon autograft in animal models have revealed that the ultimate tensile failure load values are between 11% and 57% of the control ACLs, whereas stiffness has ranged from 13% to 50% of normal ACLs after a year of healing. Adequate structural properties of an ACL graft must be accompanied by the ability of the graft to control anterior displacement of the tibia relative to the femur (e.g., prevent excessive anterior tibial translation of the tibia relative to the femur). Animal studies of healing ACL grafts have shown that anterior–posterior knee laxity increases and becomes much greater than normal after surgery.

We evaluated the effect of patellar tendon autograft elongation at the time of reconstruction on changes in anterior–posterior knee laxity at 18 months postoperatively (78) using a canine model. One group of dogs had graft elongation behavior within the 95% confidence interval of the normal ACL (group 1), whereas another group had elongation behavior more than the 95% confidence interval (group 2). At sacrifice, the anterior-posterior laxity of the knee of the dogs in group 2 was significantly greater than that of the dogs in group 1. Group 2 had significantly less linear stiffness of the graft than group 2. Anterior–posterior knee laxity values ranged from 156% to 269% of the contralateral normal knee after a year of graft healing. Investigations of healing ACL grafts that have been performed in animal models provide insight into the biomechanical behavior of the graft during healing and the biologic remodeling response of the graft. However, animals have an uncontrolled rehabilitation regimen, and the degree of similarity between animal and knees human must be carefully considered. For example, in the previously mentioned study, anterior–posterior knee laxity values ranged from 156% to 269% of the contralateral normal knee after a year of graft healing. We recently completed an investigation showing differences between healing grafts in animals and humans. We evaluated the biomechanical behavior of a matched pair of human cadaver knee specimens, one of which had an 8-month-old ACL reconstruction (88). The reconstruction had been performed with the central third of the patient's ipsilateral patellar tendon, using a tunnel–tunnel technique with interference screw fixation in the tibial and femoral bone tunnels. For the reconstructed knee, the anterior–posterior displacement values of the tibia relative to the femur were 1.85, 1.7, and 1.26 times greater than the contralateral normal knee at 10, 30, and 60 degrees of knee flexion, respectively. At all knee positions, the increase in knee laxity was produced by an increase in anterior translation of the tibia relative to the femur. The ultimate failure load of the graft was 87% of the normal ACL value, whereas the linear stiffness of the graft was 92% of normal. The energy absorbed at failure of the graft was 53% of the normal ACL value. This case study suggests that after 8 months of healing, anterior–posterior laxity of the reconstructed knee is somewhat greater than normal but that the ultimate failure load and linear stiffness values of the bone–patellar tendon–bone graft are similar to the normal ACL.

Recently, several studies have been performed to determine the patellar tendon graft harvest site morbidity. These have demonstrated little detrimental effect on the remaining patellar tendon or the strength of the extensor mechanism within 6 months after ACL reconstruction using a patellar tendon autograft (84,89–92).

There are many proponents for the use of the hamstring tendons as the source for ACL graft material. Advantages include less graft harvest site morbidity, preservation of the extensor mechanism and minimization of anterior knee pain postoperatively, and superior strength of the graft tissue when quadrupled compared with the patellar tendon and the normal ACL.

Several investigators have demonstrated that using doubled hamstring tendons for graft material yields results comparable with those with patellar tendon grafts in terms of anterior-posterior stability and functional outcome (83,93). However, both studies had short follow-up periods of 24 and 28 months, respectively. We have recently completed a prospective, randomized, double-blind trial with a minimum 3-year follow-up and have evidence that knees reconstructed with doubled semitendinosus and gracilis grafts result in a substantial increase of anterior knee laxity over time in comparison to the central one third Bone-Patellar Tendon-Bone (B-PT-B) autograft (Beynnon BD, Johnson BD, Nichols CE, et al., 2000, unpublished data). Thus, it may be important to evaluate the function of these graft tissues over longer periods of time. Tripled and quadrupled semitendinosus and gracilis tendons have increased the structural properties of the graft complex so that it is now comparable with that of the patellar tendon graft and the native ACL (64,94). In a direct comparison of patellar tendon and quadrupled semitendinosus-gracilis tendon grafts, Woo et al. (64) found that although both reconstruction techniques reduced anterior tibial translation compared with the ACL-deficient knee, the quadrupled semitendinosus–gracilis tendon graft reproduced the *in situ* forces of the intact ACL more closely—particularly with the knee in flexion.

Graft harvest site morbidity has been demonstrated to be less than that of the patellar tendon (83). The strength of the hamstring muscles after harvesting of the tendons for ACL reconstruction has been debated in the literature. Lipscomb et al. (95) reported no difference between operated and unoperated knees in hamstring strength at 26.2 months after surgery. In contrast, Marder et al. (93) reported that hamstring strength, expressed as a percentage of the unoperated knee, varied with type of graft. Patient volunteers whose ACL reconstructions involved a patellar tendon graft averaged 91% of unoperated knee strength after 26 months, whereas those whose graft consisted of a doubled hamstring tendon construct averaged 83% of unoperated knee strength.

Yasuda et al. (96) performed a randomized study to determine whether postoperative hamstring weakness was due to the harvesting technique or a result of ACL reconstruction. The strength of the hamstring muscles of patients who had the hamstring tendons harvested from the ipsilateral limb was compared with that of patients in which the hamstring tendons were taken from the contralateral limb for the ACL reconstruction. Yasuda et al. concluded that any weakness of the hamstring muscles was due to the graft harvesting procedure and not to the ACL reconstruction.

Measuring forces in the ACL and graft materials has commanded the attention of investigators in the recent literature. Most surgeons believe the initial tension applied to the graft has a significant effect on the outcome of ACL reconstruction; however, very few investigators have successfully measured graft forces accurately *in vivo*. One of the main reasons is that the patellar tendon graft uses interference screw fixation to secure the bony blocks of the graft construct. Thus, the surgeon is unable to measure tension in the midsubstance portion of the graft with accuracy, after fixation. Lewis and coworkers (97,98) reported that initial graft tension changes as early as 2 weeks after surgery, based on their work in a goat model. Their explanation is that the graft undergoes significant structural and material property changes during the healing process. Markolf et al. (99,100) demonstrated that increasing the tension applied to the graft can decrease anterior–posterior laxity of the knee significantly; this work was done in human cadavers, and no healing response could be considered in this model. They examined the biomechanical changes in the human cadaver knee joint as a result of ACL reconstruction using a patellar tendon allograft. The anterior–posterior laxity of the knee was tested with 200 N of anterior–posterior force applied to the tibia. The ACL was then resected and reconstructed. The graft tunnel positions were determined by matching the relative displacement of the graft as measured with an isometer to the measurements taken of the native ACL. The graft was then tensioned at 30 degrees of flexion to restore normal anterior–posterior laxity (laxity-matched tension condition).

Anterior–posterior laxity was also measured with a pretension that was 45 N greater than the laxity-matched tension (overtension condition). The change in anterior–posterior laxity with the tibia in neutral, internal, and external rotation was recorded at a selection of knee flexion angles. The anterior–posterior laxity of the knee was significantly less in internal and external rotation compared with the values with the tibia in neutral rotation up to 45 degrees of flexion. The isometer measurements revealed that the intact ACL changed in length by 3.1 mm between 30 degrees of flexion and full extension. At laxity-matched tension (28.2 N), the mean anterior–posterior laxities of the reconstructed knees matched that of the normal knees. Overtensioning of the graft resulted in a further decrease of 1.2 mm in anterior–posterior laxity of the reconstructed knee. During passive extension of the knee, the forces in the graft were always greater than the forces in the intact ACL using this laxity-matched tension method. At full extension, the mean force in the normal ACL was 56 N, whereas the graft force was 168 N. The overtensioned graft measured 286 N.

The mean forces in the graft were greater than those for the intact ACL over the entire range of flexion. For the overtensioned condition, graft forces produced by anterior tibial force and varus and valgus moments increased significantly. Pretensioning the patellar tendon graft required greater forces than those present in the normal ACL to restore normal anterior–posterior laxity of the knee. Forces in the graft increased significantly during certain loading conditions (external tibial torque and varus moment) that do not increase the force in the native ACL. This observation suggests that the early exposure of the knee to high-load states may place stresses on the graft that are above those seen in the normal ACL.

Yasuda et al. (101) performed a prospective randomized study of initial graft tension using autogenous doubled hamstring tendon grafts connected in series with polyester tapes fixed with the double spiked staples. Seventy patients were randomized to one of three groups based on initial graft tension: group 1, 20 N; group 2, 40 N; or group 3, 80 N. At 2-year follow-up, the average side-to-side (reconstructed minus uninjured) difference in anterior laxity was 2.2 ± 2.4 mm in group 1, 1.4 ± 1.8 mm in group 2, and 0.6 ± 1.7 mm in group 3, with a significant difference between groups 1 and 3 ($p = 0.014$). This study suggests that initial graft tension is important and that relatively high initial tension is required to reduce the postoperative anterior laxity of the knee after ACL reconstruction using a doubled hamstring tendon graft.

During the early phase of healing, the weak link of an ACL graft is its fixation. The most popular methods

of fixation have been the interference screw for the patellar tendon grafts. Currently, there appears to be no standard fixation method for hamstring tendon grafts, but the literature supports the use of a combination of screws and washers. Brown et al. (102) evaluated the effects of screw thread length, screw diameter, and screw core size on the fixation strength of patellar tendon grafts. There was no effect of screw length on pullout force, but there was a highly significant increase in pullout force for 7-mm diameter screws compared with 5.5-mm diameter screws. The minor diameter of the screw did not appear to have an effect on pullout force. Grana et al. (103) used a rabbit model to determine that the failure of the bone–patellar tendon–bone graft occurred through its intraarticular portion rather than pullout from the bone tunnel. Rodeo et al. (104) evaluated the healing of tendon directly to bone in a dog model and noted similar biomechanical and histologic findings as Grana et al., but these changes did not occur until 8 weeks after surgery. After that time, collagen fibers resembling Sharpey's fibers were observed attaching tendon to bone and graft failure was through the midsubstance.

Steiner et al. (105) evaluated several fixation techniques for both bone–patellar tendon–bone grafts and hamstring tendon grafts. The quadruple-stranded hamstring tendons secured by wrapping the graft around washers and screws exceeded the intact ACL in pullout strength but were less stiff than the normal ACL. The best fixation method for the patellar tendon graft was the interference screw technique that was not as strong (84% of the normal ACL) but much closer to the stiffness of the normal ACL. Based on our studies of soft tissue fixation, we concur with the recommendation to use screws and washers for securing hamstring tendon grafts (106). A recent study of absorbable and metal interference screws demonstrated that although in older human cadavers fixation strength may be comparable between these two types of screws, in young and middle-aged knees, the mean insertion torque and mean failure load were 500% and 150% greater, respectively, for the metal screws than for the absorbable screws (107).

Given the prevalence of ACL injuries among the athletic population, the study of knee ligament biomechanics has focused on the ACL. Recently, however, there has been an increased awareness of the functional importance of the PCL. Basic research on the anatomy and biomechanics of the PCL has augmented our understanding of role this ligament plays in providing stability to the knee (108,109). One reason for the relative lack of understanding about PCL injuries is the infrequency of their occurrence. In one long-term study of untreated isolated PCL injuries, the prognosis varied widely after 13 years, with some patients experiencing significant symptoms whereas others were able to maintain their usual knee function. This wide variation was attributed to concomitant meniscus injury (110). Articular degeneration over time was apparent on radiographs. Primary repair of the PCL has shown mixed results in one long-term study (111).

Thus, as with the ACL, surgeons are using surgical reconstruction techniques to restore normal function of this ligament. Markolf et al. (112,113) measured anterior–posterior laxity with 200 N of force applied to the tibia. The amount of force generated in the PCL during the posterior drawer test depends on the angle of flexion at which the test is performed. Near 90 degrees of flexion, all the posterior force applied to the tibia is transmitted to the ligament and the force in the ligament is not affected by internal or external tibial rotation. At smaller flexion angles, tibial rotation decreases the amount of force in the PCL during posterior drawer testing. Reconstruction of the PCL was then performed using a 10-mm-wide patellar tendon graft. Tension was applied to the graft such that anterior–posterior laxity matched that of the normal PCL before removal. The most isometric femoral tunnel position was located at a point on the proximal margin of the femoral origin of the PCL, midway between the anterior and posterior borders of the ligament. At 90 degrees of flexion, the forces in the graft were lower in the intraarticular portion of the graft compared with the force applied to the bone block in the tibial tunnel. This was due to the frictional losses from the severe bend in the graft as it passes over the posterior tibial plateau.

Additional biomechanical studies to evaluate the important factors in PCL reconstruction have concluded that the femoral attachment position of the graft is more important than the tibial attachment site in determining the posterior motion limits of the knee. There is only a small region of isometric fibers in the PCL during passive flexion–extension (114–116).

The cruciate ligaments serve as passive stabilizers of the knee and guide the joint through normal kinematics as demonstrated by the four-bar linkage model. The anterior and posterior cruciates are the primary restraints to corresponding anterior and posterior translation of the tibia relative to femur. The coupled internal–external tibial rotation that occurs with corresponding anterior–posterior shear loading is controlled in part by the cruciate ligaments and should be considered a significant aspect of a clinical examination. In addition, the cruciates act as secondary restraints to varus–valgus motion of the knee joint. Surgical reconstruction of the ACL should reproduce the *in vivo* normal ACL strain biomechanics.

Medial and Lateral Collateral Ligaments and Their Function in Joint Stability

Using the flexibility approach, Warren et al. (48) assessed the restraining action of the MCL complex in

human cadaver specimens. They demonstrated that sectioning of the superficial long fibers of the MCL complex produced a significant increase in valgus rotation of the tibiofemoral joint in experiments performed at 0 and 45 degrees of knee flexion. Sectioning the posterior oblique or deep medial portions of the MCL complex did not have a significant effect on increasing valgus knee angulation.

These findings were confirmed by Seering et al. (117), who used the stiffness approach in the study of two human cadaveric specimens. They reported that combined superficial and deep portions of the MCL provided 71% of the resistive valgus restraint in one specimen and 55% in another. Grood et al. (118) also applied the stiffness approach to investigate the medial ligament complex and presented results that supported the findings of Warren et al. (48) and Seering et al. (117). In addition, Grood et al. demonstrated that the long superficial portion of the medial ligament complex provided 57% of the valgus restraint at 5 degrees, whereas increasing to 78% at 25 degrees of flexion. The variable restraint behavior to valgus loading was attributed to the restraint provided by the posterior medial capsule, which decreased as the knee was moved from extension to flexion.

Grood et al. (118) used the stiffness approach to investigate the LCL complex. They demonstrated that in response to varus stress, this complex limits lateral opening of the joint. In response to varus loading, the LCL was found to provide 55% of the total restraint at 5 degrees, whereas 69% was provided at 25 degrees of knee flexion. There was an increase in the contribution of the LCL to the total varus restraint as the knee was moved from extension to flexion. This was attributed to a decrease in resistive support provided by the posterior portion of the lateral capsule as the knee was flexed. With the knee joint in full extension, the secondary restraints (including the cruciate ligaments and the posterior portion of the joint capsule) block opening of the knee joint after cutting the collateral ligaments (118). Simulating the forces applied by the dynamic stabilizers (iliotibial tract and biceps muscles) allowed the researchers to demonstrate the contribution to varus stability of the knee *in vivo* (118). The contribution of the dynamic stabilizers to overall stability of the knee is difficult to assess because the actual muscle force magnitudes for a specific activity are unknown. In a more recent investigation, Gollehon et al. (62) used the flexibility approach to study the contribution of the LCL and deep ligament complex (popliteus tendon and arcuate ligament) to joint stability. They reported that the LCL and deep ligament complex function together as the principal structures resisting varus and external rotation of the tibia.

There is good evidence that an isolated injury to the MCL heals satisfactorily without operative intervention

(119). Recently, attention has been drawn to the appropriate treatment of this injury in combination with rupture of the ACL. Both in an animal model and a retrospective study of human subjects, investigators have concluded that ACL reconstruction alone as treatment for combined ACL/MCL injuries results in no significant increase in valgus instability at long-term follow-up (120,121).

MENISCAL BIOMECHANICS

The Meniscus and Its Function in Load Transmission

Meniscal injuries are thought by some investigators to be the most common injury sustained by athletes (122). The menisci were originally thought to be vestigial structures that served no significant function for the tibiofemoral joint (123). As recently as 1968, Jackson (124) reported that "the exact function of the meniscus is still a matter of some conjecture." This perspective prompted many orthopedists to treat meniscal tears through complete removal (125–130). Smillie (129) recommended complete removal of the meniscus even if the posterior horn were the only structure suspected to be damaged at the time of anterior arthrotomy. It is interesting to note that as early as 1948, Fairbank (131) suggested the load-transmission function of the meniscus and postulated that complete meniscectomy frequently resulted in narrowing of the tibiofemoral joint space, flattening of the femoral condyles, and osteophyte formation. In long-term follow-up studies, performed in the late 1960s and 1970s, several investigators confirmed Fairbanks' observations, reporting a high incidence of unsatisfactory results after complete meniscectomy (132–134). It was not until the mid 1970s that several biomechanical studies confirmed the clinical observations by measuring the load-transmission function of the meniscus (135–143). These investigations predicted that between 30% and 99% of the load transmitted across the tibiofemoral joint passes through the menisci during weight-bearing activities.

Maquet et al. (137) used a contrast-injection radiography technique to measure contact area in human cadaveric specimens subjected to a physiologic compressive load. They reported a posterior translation of the medial and lateral contact areas as the knee was brought from an extended to a flexed position, along with a decrease in contact surface area with knee flexion. The contact area also decreased significantly with meniscectomy, leading Maquet et al. to postulate that the menisci transmitted a significant proportion of tibiofemoral compressive load.

Walker and Erkman (143) used a methacrylate casting technique to measure contact area in both loaded and unloaded human cadaveric specimens. They demonstrated that with no compressive joint load, tibiofemoral contact was predominately through the menisci and that a substantial increase in tibiofemoral articular cartilage contact occurred when the compressive joint load was increased to 1,500 N. The investigators also showed that the meniscal contact was primarily along the lateral and medial periphery with the knee extended, moving from an anterior to a posterior region with knee flexion.

Seedhom (138) and Hargreaves (139) reported that 70% to 99% of the tibiofemoral compressive load is transmitted through the normal menisci and that all of the load is transmitted through the posterior horns of the menisci with joint flexion past 75 degrees. These investigators also showed that partial removal of the meniscus decreased the compressive stress transmission of the joint less than did removal of the entire structure, provided the circumferential continuity of the meniscus was maintained.

Krause et al. (136) reported an increase in stress across the knee joint of approximately three times in the canine model and 2.5 times in human cadaver knees after removal of both menisci. The investigators also measured the circumferential displacement of the medial meniscus, with an applied axial compressive load, demonstrating the presence of "hoop" or tangential stress acting at the outside fibers of the meniscus. This observation led Johnson and Pope (144) to demonstrate that the meniscus absorbs energy by undergoing circumferential elongation as a load is developed across the knee joint. As the joint compresses, the wedge-shaped meniscus extrudes peripherally and its circumferentially oriented collagen fibers elongate. Thus, the meniscus absorbs energy and reduces the impulsive shock loading that would otherwise be developed across the articular cartilage and subchondral bone.

In a more recent study, Ahmed and Burke (145) directly measured the tibiofemoral pressure distribution using a microindentation transducer. Their study revealed that the medial and lateral menisci transmit at least 50% of the compressive load imposed on the tibiofemoral joint in the flexion range between 0 and 90 degrees. Removal of the medial meniscus caused a reduction in the contact area that ranged from 50% to 70%, with the latter reduction occurring at greater axial load. Because articular contact stress is inversely proportional to contact area, a 50% decrease in the contact area would cause a twofold increase in contact stress.

In a goat model, Bylski-Austrow et al. (146) demonstrated that although meniscectomy increased the knee joint contact pressure in the medial compartment by 70% over time, the pressure dropped back to 40% above normal level. They concluded that some remodeling of bone and soft tissue takes place after meniscectomy; however, this change is not sufficient to restore the normal stress distribution within the knee. Ihn et al. (147) confirmed these findings in a human cadaver model.

These mechanical investigations provide a basis for

the concept of partial meniscectomy that has been made possible by modern arthroscopic surgery. There can be no doubt that partial meniscectomy provides better results than total excision of that structure (148).

The Meniscus and Its Function in Joint Stability

Not only do the menisci provide geometric conformity to the tibiofemoral joint, optimize contact stress, and efficiently share in the transmission of the tibiofemoral compressive load, in the ACL-deficient knee they contribute to joint stability.

Johnson et al. (133) and Tapper and Hoover (135) performed postoperative clinical examinations in patients undergoing meniscectomy. Both studies revealed an increased varus–valgus and anterior–posterior laxity in 10% to 25% of patients, leading the investigators to conclude that the menisci provide some ability to stabilize the knee joint in connection with knee ligaments and bony geometry. The clinical follow-up study suggests a relationship between an increase in joint laxity after complete meniscectomy and a sequela of marginal spur formation or even degenerative changes (133).

Wang and Walker (149) evaluated the effects of transverse plane rotatory laxity before and after removal of the menisci. They specified two different types of rotatory laxity. The first, primary laxity, is joint rotation between the limits of 0.5 N-m of applied internal–external torque. This laxity represents the "looseness" of the joint before a significant resistance to the applied torque was encountered. The second, secondary laxity, is defined as joint rotation between the limits of 0.5 and 5 N-m of applied torque. The investigators measured primary and secondary rotatory laxity in human cadaver knees before and after removal of both menisci. They reported a 14% increase in primary rotatory laxity and a 2% increase in secondary laxity. Even though meniscectomy did not produce a significant increase in secondary laxity, they concluded that the menisci served as restraints to the rotation associated with primary laxity by acting as "space-filling buffers" between the tibiofemoral articular cartilage.

Hsieh and Walker (150) used an *in vitro* knee testing device to evaluate the anteroposterior load-displacement response of human cadaver knees before and after bicompartmental meniscectomy. An evaluation of one specimen, with and without a compressive load across the tibiofemoral joint, demonstrated that a dual meniscectomy produced only a minimal effect on the anteroposterior tibial displacement at 0 and 30 degrees. A similar test procedure was followed in another specimen where the cruciates were initially sectioned, followed by a dual meniscectomy. This finding demonstrated that in the absence of the cruciate ligaments, the menisci provide some resistance to tibiofemoral anteroposterior translation.

Markolf et al. (151) evaluated the effect of meniscectomy on anterior–posterior, vagus–valgus, and rotatory knee laxity in human cadavers with an instrumented laxity testing device. They observed that bicompartment removal of the menisci increased anterior–posterior joint laxity between 45 and 90 degrees of knee flexion, whereas there was only a minor increase in laxity in the rotatory and vagus–valgus planes. In a later study, Markolf et al. (152) demonstrated that although bicompartmental meniscectomy made the unloaded knee looser, in the knees with a developed tibiofemoral compressive load, laxity measurements were little affected. The same group used the instrumented laxity testing device to evaluate anteroposterior load-displacement and vagus–valgus torque-rotation responses of a subjects knee joint *in vivo* (153). They demonstrated that medial meniscectomy alone does not create a measurable increase in varus–valgus laxity, whereas a trend of increased anteroposterior laxity was observed. A significant increase in anteroposterior laxity was observed in subjects with a combined medial meniscectomy and torn ACL (153).

Levy et al. (154) used the human cadaveric model to investigate the effects of isolated medial meniscectomy and medial meniscectomy in the ACL-deficient knee. They demonstrated that an isolated medial meniscectomy did not produce a significant change in the anteroposterior load-displacement response of the knee. This finding corroborates previous work by Hsieh and Walker (150) and Bargar et al. (153). In the ACL-deficient knee without a compressive joint load, Levy et al. (154) demonstrated that resection of the meniscus caused a significant increase in the anterior displacement of the tibia relative to femur at 30, 60, and 90 degrees of knee flexion. This observation led the authors to suggest that in the ACL-deficient knee, the posterior horn of the meniscus acts as a wedge between the tibiofemoral articular surfaces, resisting anterior excursion of the tibia relative to femur. In a later study, this observation was confirmed by the same group (155). This work involved sectioning of the medial ligament structures in an ACL-deficient knee with an intact menisci and revealed an increase in anterior tibial displacement relative to femur in comparison with the knee with just the ACL cut.

In the ACL-deficient knee with an intact medial ligament complex, the mechanism of anterior tibial restraint was found to be the wedging of tibiofemoral articular surfaces apart by the meniscus, a distraction resisted by the intact medial ligament complex and capsular structures, and the development of a tibiofemoral compressive load (155). The authors hypothesized that this may be one of the mechanisms that produces posterior horn tears of the menisci in an ACL-deficient knee (155). In a more recent study, Levy et al. (156) investigated the effect of lateral meniscectomy on the motion of the human knee joint without compressive joint loading. They revealed that isolated lateral meniscectomy did not produce a significant change in the anteroposterior load-displacement behavior of the knee. In addition, the effect of the lateral meniscus on restraining anterior translation of the tibia relative to the femur was evaluated in the ACL-deficient joint. This portion of the investigation demonstrated that the lateral meniscus does not act as a restraint to anterior translation of the tibia relative to the femur, leading the authors to suggest that this structure may not behave as the medial meniscus in providing an effective posterior wedge to anterior translation (156). It is important that the results of these meniscus investigations are applied to events that occur without a compressive joint load, such as the swing phase of gait, and not to activities that include compressive joint loading.

The menisci have also been thought to assist with joint lubrication, by providing resistance to extreme joint flexion or extension, and to aid in the damping of impulsive loads transmitted across the tibiofemoral joint. However, these functions are either difficult to characterize biomechanically or to describe clinically. Despite the evidence in the literature of the detrimental biomechanical effects of total meniscectomy, a recent prospective randomized study with long-term follow-up of 200 patient volunteers with meniscal lesions demonstrated slightly higher functional scores at 1-year follow-up among those patients treated with partial meniscectomy but no significant difference in function or radiologic evidence of knee degeneration at the later follow-up (6.3 to 9.8 years) between patients treated with partial meniscectomy and those treated with complete meniscectomy (157).

PATELLOFEMORAL JOINT BIOMECHANICS

The patellofemoral joint comprises the patella, with a multifaceted dorsal surface, articulating with the femoral trochlear groove and is a key component of the extensor mechanism. In 1977, Ficat and Hungerford (158) characterized the patellofemoral joint as the "forgotten compartment of the knee." The study of patellofemoral joint biomechanics is necessary to understand its pathology, develop rational treatment regimens, and understand the effect that different rehabilitation programs have on this joint. For example, abnormally high compressive patellofemoral joint reaction (PFJR) forces produce abnormally high stress across the articular cartilage. Such stress is thought to be one of the initiating factors of chondromalacia and subsequent osteoarthritis (159–162). In addition, morphometric abnormalities in the trochlear groove or the dorsal articular surface of patella in combination with high lateral forces at the patellofemoral articulation have been thought to cause

lateral subluxation or dislocation of the patella (158, 162–164).

Patellofemoral Contact Area

In the normal knee, the patellofemoral contact area is optimally designed to respond to the increased PFJR load developed with knee flexion through a corresponding increase in contact area. This helps distribute the contact force while minimizing patellofemoral contact stress.

Goodfellow et al. (165) used the dye method to measure patellofemoral contact area with human cadaveric knees subjected to simulated weight-bearing conditions. Area measurements were made at 20, 45, 90, and 135 degrees of knee flexion. Movement of the knee from full extension to 90 degrees revealed that the contact area on the dorsal aspect of the patella moves in a continuous zone from the inferior to the superior pole of the patella. Continued flexion of the knee to 135 degrees developed two separate contact regions, one on the "odd medial facet" and the other on the lateral aspect of the patella. Huberti and Hayes (166) used pressure-sensitive film to measure the increase of patellofemoral contact area that occurs concurrently with knee flexion. At a flexion angle of 10 degrees, contact between the dorsal surface of the patella and the trochlea is initiated. The length of the patella tendon controls when the patella–trochlear contact occurs. In the case where the patella tendon is too long, patella alta may be present, and flexion of the knee greater than 10 degrees may be required to adequately seat the patella in the trochlear groove. With knee movement between extension and 90 degrees, the patella was found to be the only component of the extensor mechanism that contacts the femur, holding the quadriceps tendon away from the femur. Motion between 90 and 135 degrees produced contact of the quadriceps tendon with the femur (167). Once the quadriceps tendon contacts the femur, the compressive PFJR force is divided between the broad band of the quadriceps tendon contact with the femur and patellofemoral contact.

An example of the interaction between patellofemoral contact area and PFJR force can be demonstrated with the squatting activity. During this activity, as knee flexion increases, the PFJR force initially increases while the patellofemoral contact area available for distributing the contact force also increases, effectively distributing the articular contact stress. However, the opposite situation may occur with knee extension during weight-training programs that apply weight to the distal aspect of the tibia, with the athlete in a seated position. For this activity, the patellofemoral contact area decreases as the PFJR force increases, and therefore the PFJR stress may become high even if light weights are applied to the distal aspect of the tibia. This example may help explain why isotonic or isokinetic exercises through a full range of motion are not advised in the treatment of patellofemoral pain syndromes. Quadriceps exercises in which the knee is extended only through the last 15 to 20 degrees of extension are more likely to be tolerated, because of the decrease in PFJR force.

Patellofemoral Force Transmission

The patella transmits force from the quadriceps muscle group to the patella tendon, while developing a large PFJR force. This serves to stabilize the knee against gravity when the joint is in a flexed position and assists in the forward propulsion of the body as the knee is extended during gait. Therefore, the loads developed along the patella tendon and the PFJR force are a function of both quadriceps force and knee flexion angle. A sagittal-plane analysis can be used to demonstrate this. In a simple engineering approach, statics can be used to describe the forces and moments required to maintain the knee joint in equilibrium. For example, using this technique the quadriceps force (F_{Quads}), the PFJR force, and the patella tendon force (F_{PT}) may all be related at chosen knee flexion angles. A simplified sagittal-plane static representation of the relation between the PFJR and the quadriceps muscle forces is presented. The mass of the upper body (W), assumed to act at the hip joint, is supported by the force (F_{Quads}) developed by the quadriceps muscle groups. The vertical line below the center of mass at the subject's hip joint represents the force vector due to upper body weight, and this falls well behind the flexion axis of the knee. The distance from the center of mass force vector to the flexion axis of the knee is defined as the moment arm (c). The moment arm is relatively small, with the knee near extension. Therefore, the support mechanism provided by the quadriceps (F_{Quads}) and the developed PFJR are relatively small. The knee is in a position of greater flexion, with an associated increase in the moment arm. To maintain the knee in static equilibrium, the new force generated by the quadriceps (F_{Quads}) must increase significantly. As a result of the increased quadriceps force, the PFJR must also be larger. This model may help explain the mechanism by which both PFJR and F_{Quads} increase during squatting activities.

In the earlier analytic force analysis studies, the patella–trochlea articulation was represented as a frictionless pulley (158,159,168–174). This assumption was justified on the basis of the low coefficient of friction between the patellofemoral articular surfaces. Using this approach, the forces developed by the quadriceps muscle group were assumed to be equal to that developed along the patella tendon throughout the full range of knee motion, with the direction of the PFJR force defined as the bisector of the angle between the quadriceps and the patella tendon force vectors. Using the mechanics

principle of static equilibrium and the assumption that the patella–trochlea articulation behaves as a frictionless pulley, Reilly and Martens (173) predicted a compressive PFJR force of 0.5 times body weight for level walking. For ascending and descending stairs, the PFJR was estimated to reach 3.3 times body weight (173). Analysis of the squatting activity revealed that a maximum PFJR of 2.9 times body weight occurred at 90 degrees of flexion (173). Active extension of the lower leg with a 9-kg weight boot, while the femur was orientated in a horizontal position, produced a peak PFJR at 36 degrees of flexion (173). Maquet (175,176) questioned the frictionless pulley assumption and demonstrated with a lateral vector diagram of the patellofemoral articulation that the forces in the quadriceps mechanism and patella tendon can differ and also vary as a function of knee flexion angle (175,176). Several investigators have confirmed Maquets' findings (177–182).

In recent work performed by Huberti et al. (181), Van Eijden et al. (182), Buff et al. (179), and Ahmed et al. (177), the combined tibia, femur, and patella were evaluated using both experimental and theoretic techniques. Because the force values in the patella tendon (F_{PT}) and quadriceps muscle group (F_{Quads}) are unequal, these researchers have chosen to report results by calculating the ratio between the two force values (F_{PT}/F_{Quads}) at selected knee flexion angles. Huberti et al. (181) simulated the squatting activity in human cadaveric specimens while measuring force in the quadriceps with a tensile load cell and the patella tendon force with a buckle transducer. They revealed that for knee flexion between 0 and 45 degrees, the force developed in the patella tendon was greater than that in the quadriceps mechanism. With continued knee flexion to 120 degrees, the patella tendon force was consistently less in comparison with the quadriceps force. The authors suggested that the patella not only functions as a pulley, which changes the magnitude and direction of forces in the quadriceps and patella tendon, but in addition, the patella has two distinct mechanical functions (181). In the first and more classically described function, the anterior–posterior thickness of the patella can be attributed to increasing the effective moment arm of the quadriceps muscles and patella ligament, whereas in the second the patella acts as a lever. Therefore, the parameters that define the proximal and distal lever arms of the patella have a direct effect on the balance of forces in the quadriceps and patella tendon. The authors reasoned that the parameters were the length of the patella, location of patellofemoral contact area, and the angle between the quadriceps tendon and patella tendon (181). In a parallel experimental investigation of the squatting activity, Huberti and Hayes (166) estimated that the compressive PFJR force reached a maximum value of 6.5 times body weight. With knee flexion to

120 degrees, tendofemoral contact supported one third of the compressive PFJR force.

Van Eijden et al. (182) developed a mathematical model of the patellofemoral articulation and verified model predictions with experimental findings. Predictions of the F_{PT}/F_{Quads} ratio were similar to the experimental findings presented by Huberti et al. (181), Ahmed et al. (177), and Buff et al. (179). Van Eijden et al. demonstrated that the PFJR is approximately 50% of the quadriceps force at full extension and increases to 100% of the quadriceps force with the knee positioned between 70 and 120 degrees of flexion.

These studies have important implications for knee rehabilitation programs designed to minimize patella tendon forces, as in patellar tendinitis. In these programs, application of the large isokinetic or isometric knee moments with the knee in positions ranging between extension and 45 degrees should be avoided. In this flexion range, quadriceps activity actually produces forces of greater magnitude in the patella tendon. This has been demonstrated by Huberti et al. (181), who showed that the F_{PT}/F_{Quads} ratio is greater than 1.0 for knee positions between extension and 45 degrees. It may be advisable to restrict patellar tendinitis rehabilitation programs to flexion angles between 45 and 120 degrees, where the F_{PT}/F_{Quads} ratio is less than 1.0. This constraint will prevent an amplification of patella tendon forces. This restriction would not apply to normal gait where the bending moments and therefore quadriceps forces are not high. Because of the changing relationship between developed quadriceps force and resulting patella tendon force (F_{PT}/F_{Quads}), as the knee moves from an extended to a flexed position, the effectiveness of the quadriceps in developing an extension moment becomes substantially smaller at larger knee flexion angles, and this will also prevent the amplification of patella tendon forces.

These studies have important implications in the rehabilitation and surgical treatment of patellofemoral pain syndromes. Rehabilitation programs designed to minimize the PFJR, but not the quadriceps forces, should avoid large isokinetic, isotonic, or isometric moments with the knee positioned between 60 and 120 degrees of flexion. In this range, the predicted PFJR force is equal to the quadriceps force (182). With the requirement of minimizing the PFJR force, it may be advisable to restrict knee rehabilitation to range between the limits of extension, where the PFJR is approximately 50% of the quadriceps force, and 40 degrees, where PFJR is 90% of the quadriceps force (182). Maquet (161) investigated the surgical treatment of patellofemoral pain, demonstrating that by increasing the extensor moment arm by a 2-cm elevation of the tibial tubercle, there is a 50% reduction in the PFJR force when the knee is flexed to 45 degrees. Ferguson et al. (183) investigated the effect of anterior displacement of the tibial tubercle on patellofemoral contact stress. In this study, the patella–trochlea interface of human cadaver specimens was instrumented with miniature force sensors to monitor the patellofemoral contact stress. Anterior displacement of the tibial tubercle was found to decrease the patellofemoral contact stress between 0 and 90 degrees of flexion. The largest decrease in contact stress was achieved with a 12.5-mm elevation of the tubercle; further elevation only produced a minimal decrease in contact stress (183). This demonstrates the importance of the anterior–posterior position of the patella tendon and its role in controlling the extensor moment arm. In addition, it is equally important to realize that the proximal–distal location of the patellofemoral contact point is also critical to the function of the patella as a lever (as explained earlier).

In the frontal plane, the axis of the quadriceps force forms an angle with the patella tendon. This has been defined as the Q angle and is measured as the intersection of the center line of the patella tendon and the line from the center of patella to the anterior superior iliac spine (184). The normal Q angle is reported to range between 10 and 15 degrees with the knee in full extension (185,187). With knee flexion, the Q angle decreases because there is a coupled internal rotation of the tibia relative to the femur (158). Contraction of the quadriceps creates a bowstring effect that displaces the patella in a lateral direction, producing a contact force against the lateral margin of the femoral trochlear groove. Abnormal tracking of the patella, which allows lateral subluxation of only a few millimeters, markedly decreases the contact area, greatly increasing the local stress (force per unit area). This may contribute to patellofemoral pain and degeneration of the patella articular cartilage (chondromalacia). Other anatomic conditions can also contribute to abnormal patella tracking. These include hypoplasia of the trochlear groove, abnormal patellar articular configuration, underdevelopment of the vastus medialis, transverse plane rotational malalignment of proximal tibia relative to the distal femur, and abnormally high Q angle.

Huberti and Hayes (166) studied the effect of different Q angles by simulating the squatting activity in human cadaveric specimens while measuring patellofemoral contact pressure with pressure-sensitive film. They demonstrated that either an increase or a decrease in Q angle developed an increased peak patellofemoral pressure and associated unpredictable patterns of cartilage loading. Cox (187) presented a retrospective study of the Roux-Elmsli-Trillat procedure for realignment of the knee extensor mechanism and prevention of recurrent subluxation of the patella. An evaluation of 116 patients, followed for at least 1 year, demonstrated this procedure to be a satisfactory method for the prevention of lateral subluxation with recurrence in only 7% of the cases. Careful attention to the medial transfer of the tibial tuberosity without a posterior displacement was emphasized as the key to successful long-term results (187). Procedures that result in some posterior transfer of the tibial tuberosity, such as that described by Hauser, decrease the patellar tendon moment arm and consequently increase the patellofemoral contact stress. Fulkerson and Hungerford (188) have reviewed the clinical and radiologic outcomes of the Hauser procedure and presented evidence of progressive knee joint degeneration.

Future biomechanics research should include further *in vivo* strain measurements of the soft tissues surrounding the knee and should establish new *in vivo* measurement techniques such as force sensors. In addition, the development of an analytic model that includes both patellofemoral and tibiofemoral articulations will permit the study of injury mechanisms and the investigation of soft tissue reconstruction procedures. In turn, these will lead to better evaluation and refinement of rehabilitation strategies. Application of the *in vivo* experimental techniques and analytic models should address the relation between the biomechanical behavior of a graft or repair and resulting biologic properties. New devices, such as an implantable telemeterized load sensor, need to be designed to allow optimal matches between rehabilitation regimens and the biologic–mechanical behavior of grafts. Biomechanics research efforts should strive to establish intraoperative techniques and measurements that can accurately provide the surgeon with the ability to reestablish normal joint kinematics during a soft tissue reconstruction procedure. Future clinical biomechanical investigations of surgical procedures should include prospective, randomized, well-controlled, long-term studies that use standardized outcome evaluation techniques to assess the relative effectiveness of the many different soft tissue reconstruction techniques.

ACKNOWLEDGMENT

We acknowledge support from the National Institutes of Health (grants R01 AR39213 and R01 AR40174).

REFERENCES

1. Hefzy MS, Grood ES. Review of knee models. *Appl Mech Rev* 1988;41:1–13.
2. Grood ES, Noyes FR. Diagnosis of knee ligament injuries: biomechanical precepts. In: Fegin JA, Applewhite LB, eds. *The crucial ligaments.* New York: Churchill Livingstone, 1988: 245–260.
3. Frankel VH. Biomechanics of the knee. *Orthop Clin North Am* 1971;2:175–190.
4. Frankel VH, Burstein AH. *Orthopaedic biomechanics.* Philadelphia: Lea & Febiger, 1970.
5. Mow VC, Hayes WC. *Basic orthopaedic biomechanics.* New York: Raven Press, 1991.
6. Noyes FR, Grood ES, Torzilli PA. The definitions of terms for motion and position of the knee and injuries of the ligaments. *J Bone Joint Surg Am* 1989;71A:465–472.
7. Bonnarens FO, Drez D. Biomechanics of artificial ligaments and associated problems. In: Jackson DW, Drez D, eds. *The anterior cruciate deficient knee: new concepts in ligament repair.* St. Louis: C.V. Mosby, 1987:239–253.
8. Goodfellow J, O'Conner J. The mechanics of the knee and prosthesis design. *J Bone Joint Surg Br* 1978;60B:358–369.
9. Kapandji IA. *The physiology of the joints: annotated diagrams of the joints.* Vol. 2. Edinburgh: Churchill Livingstone, 1970.
10. Menschik A. Mechanik des kiniegelenkes. *Teil I Z Orthop* 1974;112:481–495.
11. Muller W. *The knee: form, function and ligament reconstruction.* New York: Springer-Verlag, 1983.
12. Strasser H. *Lehrbuch der Muskel und Gelenkinechanik.* Vol. 3. 1908 Berlin: Springer-Verlag.
13. Beynnon BD, Pope MH, Wertheimer CM, et al. The effect of functional knee braces on strain on the anterior cruciate ligament in vivo. *J Bone Joint Surg Am* 1992;74A:1298–1312.
14. Beynnon BD, Howe JG, Pope MH, et al. Anterior cruciate ligament strain in vivo. *Int Orthop* 1992;16:1–12.
15. Crowninshield R, Pope MH, Johnson RJ. An analytic model of the knee. *J Biomech* 1976;9:397–405.
16. Wismans J, Veldpaus F, Janssen J, et al. A three-dimensional mathematical model of the knee joint. *J Biomech* 1980;13: 677–685.
17. Blankevoort L, Huiskes R. ACL isometry is not the criterion for ACL reconstruction. *Trans Orthop Res Soc* 1991;16:203.
18. Blankevoort L, Huiskes R, de Lange A. Recruitment of the knee-joint ligaments. *J Biomech Eng* 1991;113:94–103.
19. Blankevoort L, Huiskes R, Kuiper JH, et al. Articular contact in a three-dimensional model of the knee. *J Biomech* 1991;24: 1019–1031.
20. Blankevoort L, Huiskes R. Ligament-bone interaction in a three-dimensional model of the knee. *J Biomech Eng* 1991;113: 263–269.
21. Hughston JC, Andrews JR, Cross MJ, et al. Classification of knee ligament instabilities. Part 1. The medial compartment and cruciate ligaments. *J Bone Joint Surg Am* 1976;58A:159–172.
22. Hughston JC, Eilers AF. The role of the posterior oblique ligament in repairs of the acute medial collateral ligament tears of the knee. *J Bone Joint Surg Am* 1973;55A:923–940.
23. Slocum DB, Larson RL, James SL. Late reconstruction procedures used to stabilize the knee. *Orthop Clin North Am* 1973; 4:679–689.
24. Kennedy JC, Weinberg HW, Wilson AS. The anatomy and function of the anterior cruciate ligament as determined by clinical and morphological studies. *J Bone Joint Surg Am* 1974;56A: 223–235.
25. Furman W, Marshall JL, Girgis FC. The anterior cruciate ligament—a functional analysis based on post-mortem studies. *J Bone Joint Surg Am* 1976;58A:179–185.
26. Girgis FG, Marshall JL, Monajem ARSH. The cruciate ligaments of the knee joint. *Clin Orthop* 1975;106:216–231.
27. Marshall J, Girgis FG, Zelko R. The biceps femoris tendon and its functional significance. *J Bone Joint Surg Am* 1972;54A:1444–1450.
28. Warren LF, Marshall JL. The supporting structures and layers on the medial side of the knee, an anatomical analysis. *J Bone Joint Surg Am* 1979;61A:50–62.
29. Salmons S. Meeting report from the 8th Int Conf on Medical and Biological Eng. *Bio Eng* 1969;4:467–474.
30. Hollis JM. Development and application of a method for determining the *in situ* forces in anterior cruciate ligament fiber bundles. Ph.D. dissertation, University of California, San Diego, 1988.
31. Sapega AA, Moyer RJ, Schneck C, et al. Testing for isometry during reconstruction of the anterior cruciate ligament. *J Bone Joint Surg Am* 1990;72A:259–267.
32. Barry D, Ahmed AM. Design and performance of a modified buckle transducer for the measurement of ligament tension. *J Biomech Eng* 1986;108:149–142.
33. Lewis JL, Jasti M, Schafer M, et al. Functional load directions

for the two bands of the anterior cruciate ligament. *Trans Orthop Res Soc* 1980;5:307.

34. Paulos L, Noyes FR, Grood ES, et al. Knee rehabilitation after ACL reconstruction and repair. *Am J Sports Med* 1981;9: 140–149.

35. Markolf KL, Gorek JF, Kabo M, et al. Direct measurement of resultant forces in the anterior cruciate ligament. An in vitro study performed with a new experimental technique. *J Bone Joint Surg Am* 1990;72A:557–567.

36. Arms SA, Pope MH, Johnson RJ, et al. The biomechanics of anterior cruciate ligament rehabilitation and reconstruction. *Am J Sports Med* 1984;12:8–18.

37. Brown TD, Sigal L, Njus GO, et al. Dynamic performance characteristics of the liquid metal strain gauge. *J Biomech* 1986; 19:165–173.

38. Edwards RG, Lafferty JF, Lange KD. Ligament strain in the human knee. *J Basic Eng* 1970;92:131–136.

39. Kennedy JC, Haskins RJ, Willis RB. Strain gauge analysis of knee ligaments. *Clin Orthop* 1977;129:225–229.

40. Renström P, Arms SW, Stanwyck TS, et al. Strain within the anterior cruciate ligament during hamstring and quadriceps activity. *Am J Sports Med* 1986;14:83–87.

41. Wang CJ, Walker PS, Wolf B. The effects of flexion and rotation on the length patterns of the ligaments of the knee. *J Biomech* 1973;6:587–596.

42. Henning CE, Lynch MA, Glick KR. An in vivo strain gage study of elongation of the anterior cruciate ligament. *Am J Sports Med* 1985;13:22–26.

43. Butler DL, Grood ES, Zernicke RR, et al. Non-uniform surface strains in young human tendons and fascia. *Trans Orthop Res Soc* 1983;8:8.

44. Woo SL-Y, Gomez MA, Akerson WH. Mechanical properties along the medial collateral ligament. *Trans Orthop Res Soc* 1983;8:7.

45. Butler DL, Grood ES, Noyes FR, et al. On the interpretation of our anterior cruciate ligament data. *Clin Orthop* 1985;196:26–34.

46. Sidles JA, Larson RV, Garbini JL, et al. Ligament length relationships in the moving knee. *J Orthop Res* 1988;6:593–610.

47. Trent PS, Walker PS, Wolf B. Ligament length patterns, strength and rotational axes of the knee joint. *Clin Orthop* 1976;117: 263–279.

48. Warren LF, Marshall JL, Girgis F. The prime static stabilizer of the medial side of the knee. *J Bone Joint Surg Am* 1974;56A: 665–674.

49. Fischer RA, Arms SW, Johnson RJ, et al. The functional relationship of the posterior oblique ligament to the medial collateral ligament of the human knee. *Am J Sports Med* 1985;13:390–397.

50. Howe JG, Wertheimer CM, Johnson RJ, et al. Arthroscopic strain gauge measurement of the normal anterior cruciate ligament. *Arthroscopy* 1990;6:198–204.

51. Cooper RR, Misol S. Tendon and ligament insertion: a light and electron microscopic study. *J Bone Joint Surg Am* 1970;52A:1–20.

52. Noyes FR, Butler DL, Grood ES, et al. Biomechanical analysis of human ligament grafts used in knee ligament repairs and reconstruction. *J Bone Joint Surg Am* 1984;66A:344–352.

53. Sidles JA, Clark JM, Garbini JL. Fiber anatomy and internal stresses in ligaments and tendons: a general geometric model. *Trans Orthop Res Soc* 1989;14:250.

54. Noyes FR, Grood ES. The strength of the anterior cruciate ligament in humans and rhesus monkeys age related and species related changes. *J Bone Joint Surg Am* 1976;58A:1074–1082.

55. Noyes FR, DeLucas JL, Torrik PJ. Biomechanics of ligament failure: an analysis of strain-rate sensitivity and mechanism of failure in primates. *J Bone Joint Surg Am* 1974;56A:236.

56. Noyes FR. Functional properties of knee ligaments and alterations induced by immobilization. *Clin Orthop* 1977;123:210.

57. Ameil D, Kleiner JB, Akeson WH. The natural history of the anterior cruciate ligament autograft of patellar tendon origin. *Am J Sports Med* 1986;14:449–462.

58. Woo SL-Y, Hollis JM, Adams DJ, et al. Tensile properties of the human femur anterior cruciate ligament tibia complex. The effects of specimen age and orientations. *Am J Sports Med* 1991; 19:217–225.

59. Butler DL. Anterior cruciate ligament: its response and replacement. *J Orthop Res* 1989;7:910–921.

60. Butler DL, Noyes FR, Grood ES. Ligamentous restraints to anterior-posterior drawer in the human knee. *J Bone Joint Surg Am* 1980;62A:259.

61. Fukubayashi T, Torzilli PA, Sherman MF, et al. An in vitro biomechanical evaluation of anterior-posterior motion of the knee. *J Bone Joint Surg Am* 1982;64A:258–264.

62. Gollehon DL, Torzilli PA, Warren RF. The role of the posterolateral and cruciate ligaments in the stability of the human knee. A biomechanical study. *J Bone Joint Surg Am* 1987;69A:233–242.

63. Grood ES, Stowers SF, Noyes FR. Limits of movement in the human knee effect of sectioning the posterior cruciate ligament and posterolateral structures. *J Bone Joint Surg Am* 1988;70A: 88–97.

64. Woo SL-Y, Fox RJ, Sakane M, et al. Force and force distribution in the anterior cruciate ligament and its clinical implications. *Sportorthop Sporttraumatol* 1997;13:37–48.

65. Beynnon BD, Fleming BC, Johnson RJ, et al. Anterior cruciate ligament strain behavior during rehabilitation exercises in vivo. *Am J Sports Med* 1995;23:24–34.

66. Beynnon BD, Johnson RJ, Fleming BC, et al. The effect of functional knee bracing on the anterior cruciate ligament in the weightbearing and nonweightbearing knee. *Am J Sports Med* 1997;25:353–359.

67. Beynnon BD, Johnson RJ, Fleming BC, et al. The strain behavior of the anterior cruciate ligament during squatting and active flexion-extension: a comparison of an open- and a closed-kinetic chain exercise. *Am J Sports Med* 1997;25:823–829.

68. Daniel D, Malcolm L, Losse G, et al. Instrumented measurement of anterior laxity of the knee. *J Bone Joint Surg Am* 1985;67A: 720–725.

69. Jacob RP. Observations on rotary instability of the lateral compartment of the knee. *Acta Orthop Scand* 1981;52[Suppl 1]:1–31.

70. Johnson RJ. The anterior cruciate: a dilemma in sports medicine. *Int J Sports Med* 1982;3:71–79.

71. Markolf KL, Graff-Radford A, Amstutz HC. In vivo stability—a quantitative assessment using an instrumented clinical testing apparatus. *J Bone Joint Surg Am* 1978;60A:664–674.

72. Torg J, Conrad W, Kalen V. Clinical diagnosis of ACL instability. *Am J Sports Med* 1976;4:84–92.

73. Torzilli P, Greenberg R, Hood R, et al. Measurement of anterior-posterior motion of the knee in injured patients using a biomechanical stress technique. *J Bone Joint Surg Am* 1984;66A:1438–1442.

74. Nisell R, Németh G, Ohlsén H. Joint forces in extension of the knee. *Acta Orthop Scand* 1986;57:41–46.

75. Grood ES, Suntay WJ, Noyes FR, et al. Biomechanics of the knee-extension exercise. *J Bone Joint Surg Am* 1984;66A: 725–734.

76. Fleming BC, Beynnon BD, Nichols CE, et al. An in vivo comparison between intraoperative isometric measurements and local elongation of the graft after reconstruction of the anterior cruciate ligament. *J Bone Joint Surg Am* 1994;76A:511–519.

77. Beynnon BD, Johnson RJ, Toyama H, et al. The relationship between anterior-posterior knee laxity and the structural properties of the patellar tendon graft. A study in canines. *Am J Sports Med* 1994;22:812–820.

78. Tohyama H, Beynnon BD, Johnson RJ, et al. The effect of anterior cruciate ligament graft elongation at the time of implantation on the biomechanical behavior of the graft and knee. *Am J Sports Med* 1996;24:608–614.

79. Beynnon BD, Johnson RJ, Fleming BC, et al. The measurement of elongation of anterior cruciate ligament grafts in vivo. *J Bone Joint Surg Am* 1994;76A:520–531.

80. Norwood LA, Cross MJ. Anterior cruciate ligament: functional anatomy and its bundles in rotatory instabilities. *Am J Sports Med* 1979;7:23–26.

81. Fleming BC, Beynnon BD, Johnson RJ, et al. Isometric versus tension measurements: a comparison for the reconstruction of the anterior cruciate ligament. *Am J Sports Med* 1993;21:82–88.

82. Kannus P, Jarvinen M. Conservatively treated tears of the anterior cruciate ligament. Long-term results. *J Bone Joint Surg Am* 1987;69A:1007–1012.

83. Aglietti P, Buzzi R, Zaccherotti G, et al. Patellar tendon versus doubled semitendinosus and gracilis tendons for anterior cruciate ligament reconstruction. *Am J Sports Med* 1994;22:211–218.
84. Shelbourne KD, Rubinstein RA, VanMeter CD, et al. Correlation of remaining patellar tendon width with quadriceps strength after autogenous bone-patellar tendon-bone anterior cruciate ligament reconstruction. *Am J Sports Med* 1994;22:774–778.
85. Ng GY, Oakes BW, Deacon OW, et al. Biomechanics of patellar tendon autograft for reconstruction of the anterior cruciate ligament in the goat: three-year study. *J Orthop Res* 1995;13:602–608.
86. Ng GY, Oakes BW, Deacon OW, et al. Long-term study of the biochemistry and biomechanics of anterior cruciate ligament-patellar tendon autograft in goats. *J Orthop Res* 1996;14:851–856.
87. Blevins FT, Hecker AT, Bigler GT, et al. The effects of donor age and strain rate on the biomechanical properties of bone-patellar tendon-bone allografts. *Am J Sports Med* 1994;22:328–333.
88. Beynnon BD, Risberg MA, Tjomsland O, et al. Evaluation of knee joint laxity and the structural properties of the anterior cruciate ligament graft in the human. A case report. *Am J Sports Med* 1997;25:203–206.
89. Rubinstein RA, Shelbourne KD, VanMeter CD, et al. Isolated autogenous bone-patellar tendon-bone graft site morbidity. *Am J Sports Med* 1994;22:324–327.
90. Linder LH, Sukin DL, Burks RT, et al. Biomechanical and histologic properties of the canine patellar tendon after removal of its medial third. *Am J Sports Med* 1994;22:136–142.
91. Burks RT, Haut RC, Lancaster RL. Biomechanical and histological observations of the dog patellar tendon after removal of its central one-third. *Am J Sports Med* 1990;18:146–155.
92. Beynnon BD, Proffer D, Drez DJ, et al. Biomechanical assessment of the healing response of the rabbit patellar tendon after removal of its central third. *Am J Sports Med* 1995;23:452–457.
93. Marder RA, Raskind JR, Carroll M. Prospective evaluation of arthroscopically assisted anterior cruciate ligament reconstruction. Patellar tendon versus semitendinosus and gracilis tendons. *Am J Sports Med* 1991;19:478–484.
94. Maeda A, Shino K, Horibe S, et al. Anterior cruciate ligament reconstruction with multistranded autogenous semitendinosus tendon. *Am J Sports Med* 1996;24:504–509.
95. Lipscomb AB, Johnston RK, Snyder RB, et al. Evaluation of hamstring strength following use of semitendinosus and gracilis tendons to reconstruct the anterior cruciate ligament. *Am J Sports Med* 1982;10:340–342.
96. Yasuda K, Tsujino J, Ohkoshi Y, et al. Graft site morbidity with autogenous semitendinosus and gracilis tendons. *Am J Sports Med* 1995;23:706–714.
97. Lewis JL, Poff BC, Smith JJ, et al. Method for establishing and measuring in vivo forces in an anterior cruciate ligament composite graft: response to differing levels of load sharing in a goat model. *J Orthop Res* 1994;12:780–788.
98. Smith JJ, Lewis JL, Mente PL, et al. Intraoperative force-setting did not improve the mechanical properties of an augmented bone-tendon-bone anterior cruciate ligament graft in a goat model. *J Orthop Res* 1996;14:209–215.
99. Markolf KL, Burchfield DM, Shapiro MM, et al. Biomechanical consequences of replacement of the anterior cruciate ligament with a patellar ligament allograft. Part I. Insertion of the graft and anterior-posterior testing. *J Bone Joint Surg Am* 1996;78A:1720–1727.
100. Markolf KL, Burchfield DM, Shapiro MM, et al. Biomechanical consequences of replacement of the anterior cruciate ligament with a patellar ligament. Allograft. Part II. Forces in the graft compared with forces in the intact ligament. *J Bone Joint Surg Am* 1996;78A:1728–1734.
101. Yasuda K, Tsujino J, Tanabe Y, et al. Effects of initial graft tension on clinical outcome after anterior cruciate ligament reconstruction. Autogenous doubled hamstring tendons connected in series with polyester tapes. *Am J Sports Med* 1997;25:99–106.
102. Brown CH, Hecker AT, Hipp JA, et al. The biomechanics of interference screw fixation of patellar tendon anterior cruciate ligament grafts. *Am J Sports Med* 1993;21:880–886.
103. Grana WA, Egle DM, Mahnken R, et al. An analysis of autograft fixation after anterior cruciate ligament reconstruction in a rabbit model. *Am J Sports Med* 1994;22:344–351.
104. Rodeo SA, Arnoczky SP, Torzilli PA, et al. Tendon-healing in a bone tunnel. A biomechanical and histological study in the dog. *J Bone Joint Surg Am* 1993;75A:1795–1803.
105. Steiner ME, Hecker AT, Brown CH, et al. Anterior cruciate ligament graft fixation. Comparison of hamstring and patellar tendon grafts. *Am J Sports Med* 1994;22:240–246.
106. Beynnon BD, Uh BS, Pyne JIB, et al. Semitendinosus and gracilis tendon graft fixation for ACL reconstructions. *Iowa Orthop J* 1996;16:118–121.
107. Pena F, Grontvedt T, Brown GA, et al. Comparison of failure strength between metallic and absorbable interference screws. Influence of insertion torque, tunnel-bone block gap, bone mineral density, and interference. *Am J Sports Med* 1996;24:329–334.
108. Harner CD, Xerogeanes JW, Livesay GA, et al. The human posterior cruciate ligament complex: an interdisciplinary study. Ligament morphology and biomechanical evaluation. *Am J Sports Med* 1995;23:736–745.
109. Race A, Amis AA. Loading of the two bundles of the posterior cruciate ligament: an analysis of bundle function in A-P drawer. *J Biomech* 1996;29:873–879.
110. Boynton MD, Tietjens BR. Long-term followup of the untreated isolated posterior cruciate ligament-deficient knee. *Am J Sports Med* 1996;24:306–310.
111. Richter M, Kiefer H, Hehl G, et al. Primary repair for posterior cruciate ligament injuries. An eight-year followup of fifty-three patients. *Am J Sports Med* 1996;24:298–305.
112. Markolf KL, Slauterbeck JR, Armstrong KL, et al. A biomechanical study of replacement of the posterior cruciate ligament with a graft. Part I. Isometry, pre-tension of the graft, and anterior-posterior laxity. *J Bone Joint Surg Am* 1997;79:375–380.
113. Markolf KL, Slauterbeck JR, Armstrong KL, et al. A biomechanical study of replacement of the posterior cruciate ligament with a graft. Part II. Forces in the graft compared with forces in the intact ligament. *J Bone Joint Surg Am* 1997;79:381–386.
114. Galloway MT, Grood ES, Mehalik JN, et al. Posterior cruciate ligament reconstruction. An in vitro study of femoral and tibial graft placement. *Am J Sports Med* 1996;24:437–445.
115. Covey DC, Sapega AA, Sherman GM. Testing for isometry during reconstruction of the posterior cruciate ligament. Anatomic and biomechanical considerations. *Am J Sports Med* 1996;24:740–746.
116. Stone JD, Carlin GJ, Ishibashi Y, et al. Assessment of posterior cruciate ligament graft performance using robotic technology. *Am J Sports Med* 1996;24:824–828.
117. Seering WP, Piziali RL, Nagel DA, et al. The function of the primary ligaments of the knee in varus-valgus and axial rotation. *J Biomech* 1980;13:785–794.
118. Grood ES, Noyes FR, Butler DL, et al. Ligamentous and capsular restraints preventing straight medial and lateral laxity in intact human cadaver knees. *J Bone Joint Surg Am* 1981;63A:1257–1269.
119. Lundberg M, Messner K. Long-term prognosis of isolated partial medial collateral ligament ruptures. A ten-year clinical and radiographic evaluation of a prospectively observed group of patients. *Am J Sports Med* 1996;24:160–163.
120. Yamaji T, Levine RE, Woo SL, et al. Medial collateral ligament healing one year after a concurrent medial collateral ligament and anterior cruciate ligament injury: an interdisciplinary study in rabbits. *J Orthop Res* 1996;14:223–227.
121. Hillard-Sembell D, Daniel DM, Stone ML, et al. Combine injuries of the anterior cruciate ligament and medial collateral ligaments of the knee. Effect of treatment on stability and function of the joint. *J Bone Joint Surg* 1996;78:169–176.
122. Sonne-Holm S, Fledelius I, Ahn N. Results after meniscectomy in 147 athletes. *Acta Orthop Scand* 1980;51:303–309.
123. King D. The function of semilunar cartilage. *J Bone Joint Surg Am* 1936;18A:1069–1076.
124. Jackson J.P. Degenerative changes in the knee after meniscectomy. *Br Med J* 1968;2:525.
125. Campbell WC. *Operative orthopaedics*. St. Louis: C.V. Mosby, 1939:406, 415.

126. Dandy DJ, Jackson RW. Meniscectomy and chondromalacia of the femoral condyle. *J Bone Joint Surg Am* 1975;57A:1116–1119.

127. Dandy DJ, Jackson RW. The diagnosis of problems after meniscectomy. *J Bone Joint Surg Br* 1975;57B:349–352.

128. Quigley TB. Knee injuries incurred in sports. *JAMA* 1959;171:166–170.

129. Smillie JS. *Injuries to the knee joint,* 4th ed. Edinburgh: Churchill Livingstone, 1971:68.

130. Watson-Jones OR. *Fractures and joint injuries.* Vol. 2. Edinburgh: Churchill Livingstone, 1955:769–773.

131. Fairbank TJ. Knee changes after meniscectomy. *J Bone Joint Surg Br* 1948;30B:664–670.

132. Huckell JR. Is meniscectomy a benign procedure? A long-term follow-up study. *Can J Surg* 1965;8:254–260.

133. Johnson RJ, Kettelkamp DB, Clark W, et al. Factors affecting late meniscectomy results. *J Bone Joint Surg Am* 1974;56A:719–729.

134. Tapper EM, Hoover NW. Late results after meniscectomy. *J Bone Joint Surg Am* 1969;51A:517–526.

135. Kettlekamp DB, Jacobs AW. Tibiofemoral contact areas-determination and implications. *J Bone Joint Surg Am* 1972;54A:349–356.

136. Krause WR, Pope MH, Johnson RJ, et al. Mechanical changes in the knee after meniscectomy. *J Bone Joint Surg Am* 1976;58A:599–604.

137. Maquet PG, Van De Berg AJ, Simonet JC. Femorotibial weight-bearing areas: experimental determination. *J Bone Joint Surg Am* 1975;57A:766–767.

138. Seedhom BB. Transmission of the load in the knee joint with special reference to the role of the menisci. Part I. Anatomy, analysis, and apparatus. *Eng Med* 1979;8:207–219.

139. Seedhom BB, Hargreaves DJ. Transmission of load in the knee joint with special reference to the role of the menisci. Part II. Experimental results, discussion, and conclusions. *Eng Med* 1979;8:220–228.

140. Seedhom BB, Dawson D, Wright U. Functions of the menisci—a preliminary study. *J Bone Joint Surg Br* 1974;56B:381–382.

141. Shrine N. The weight bearing role of the menisci of the knee. *J Bone Joint Surg Br* 1974;56B:381.

142. Simon. Scale affects in animal joints. *Arthritis Rheum* 1970;13:244–256.

143. Walker PS, Erkman MJ. The role of the menisci in the force transmission across the knee. *Clin Orthop* 1975;109:184–192.

144. Johnson RJ, Pope MH. Functional anatomy of the meniscus. Symposium on reconstruction of the knee. St. Louis: C.V. Mosby, 1978:3–13.

145. Ahmed AM, Burke DL. In vitro measurement of static pressure distribution in synovial joints. Part I. Tibial surface of the knee. *J Biomech Eng* 1983;105:216–225.

146. Bylski-Austrow DI, Malumed J, Meade T, et al. Knee joint contact pressure decreases after chronic meniscectomy relative to the acutely meniscectomized joint: a mechanical study in the goat. *J Orthop Res* 1993;11:796–804.

147. Ihn JC, Kim SJ, Park IH. In vitro study of contact area and pressure distribution in the human knee after partial and total meniscectomy. *Int Orthop* 1993;17:214–218.

148. Baratz ME, Fu FH, Mengato R. Meniscal tears: the effect of meniscectomy and repair in intra articular contact areas and stress in the human knee. *Am J Sports Med* 1986;14:270–275.

149. Wang CJ, Walker PS. Rotation laxity of the human knee. *J Bone Joint Surg Am* 1974;56A:161–170.

150. Hsieh HH, Walker PS. Stabilizing mechanisms of the loaded and unloaded knee joint. *J Bone Joint Surg Am* 1976;58A:87–93.

151. Markolf KL, Meusch JS, Amstutz HC. Stiffness and laxity of the knee—the contributions of the supporting structures. *J Bone Joint Surg Am* 1976;58A:583–594.

152. Markolf KL, Bargar WL, Shoemaker SC, et al. The role of joint load in knee stability. *J Bone Joint Surg Am* 1981;63A:570–585.

153. Bargar WL, Moreland JF, Markolf KL, et al. In vivo stability testing of post-meniscectomy knees. *Clin Orthop* 1980;150:247–252.

154. Levy MI, Torzilli PA, Warren RF. The effect of medial meniscectomy on anterior-posterior motion of the knee. *J Bone Joint Surg Am* 1982;64A:883–888.

155. Sullivan D, Levy IM, Shaskier S, et al. Medial restraints to anterior-posterior motion of the knee. *J Bone Joint Surg Am* 1984;66A:930–936.

156. Levy MI, Torzilli PA, Gould JD, et al. The effect of lateral meniscectomy on motion of the knee. *J Bone Joint Surg Am* 1989;71A:401–406.

157. Hede A, Larsen E. Partial versus total meniscectomy. A prospective, randomised study with long-term follow-up. *J Bone Joint Surg Br* 1992;74B:118–121.

158. Ficat RP, Hungerford DS. *Disorders of the patellofemoral joint.* Baltimore: Williams & Wilkins, 1977.

159. Bandi W. Chondromalacia patellae and femora-patellare arthrose. Atiologie Klinik and therapie. *Helv Chir Acta* 1972;11[Suppl]:3–70.

160. Insall J, Goldberg V, Salvati E. Recurrent dislocation and the high-riding patella. *Clin Orthop* 1972;88:67–69.

161. Maquet PG. Mechanics and osteoarthritis of the patellofemoral joint. *Clin Orthop* 1979;144:70–73.

162. Outerbridge RE, Dunlop JAY. The problem of chondromalacia patellae. *Clin Orthop* 1975;110:177–196.

163. Hungerford DS, Haynes D. The dynamics of patellar stabilization in knee flexion and rotation. *Trans Orthop Res Soc* 1982;7:254.

164. Insall J. "Condromalacia patellae": patellar malalignment syndrome. *Orthop Clin North Am* 1979;10:117–127.

165. Goodfellow J, Hungerford DS, Zindel M. Patellofemoral joint mechanics and pathology. *J Bone Joint Surg Br* 1976;58B:287–290.

166. Huberti HH, Hayes WC. Patellofemoral contact pressures, the influence of Q-angle and tendofemoral contact. *J Bone Joint Surg Am* 1984;66A:715–724.

167. Van Eijden TMGJ, De Boer W, Weijs WA. The orientation of the distal part of the quadriceps femoris muscle as a function of the knee flexion-extension angle. *J Biomech* 1985;18:803–809.

168. Hungerford DS, Barry M. Biomechanics of the patellofemoral joint. *Clin Orthop* 1979;144:9–15.

169. Matthews LS, Sonstegard DA, Heuke JA. Load bearing characteristics of the patellofemoral joint. *Acta Orthop Scand* 1977;48:511–516.

170. Morrison JB. The mechanics of the knee joint. *J Biomech* 1970;3:51–61.

171. Morrison JB. Function of the knee joint in various activities. *Biomed Eng* 1969;4:573–580.

172. Perry J, Antonelli P, Ford W. Analysis of knee joint forces during flexed-knee stance. *J Bone Joint Surg Am* 1975;57A:961–967.

173. Reilly DT, Martens M. Experimental analysis of the quadriceps muscle force and patellafemoral joint reaction force for various activities. *Acta Orthop Scand* 1972;43:126–137.

174. Smidt GL. Biomechanical analysis of knee flexion and extension. *J Biomech* 1973;6:79–92.

175. Maquet PG. *Biomechanics of the knee.* Berlin: Springer-Verlag, 1976.

176. Maquet PG. Biomechanics and Osteoarthritis of the knee. SICOT XI, Congress, Mexico, 1969.

177. Ahmed AM, Burke DL, Hyder A. Force analysis of the patellar mechanism. *J Orthop Res* 1987;5:69–85.

178. Bishop RED, Denham RA. A note on the ratio between tensions in the quadriceps tendon and infra-patella ligament. *Eng Med* 1977;6:53–54.

179. Buff HU, Jones LC, Hungerford DS. Experimental determination of forces transmitted through the patellofemoral joint. *J Biomech* 1988;21:17–23.

180. Ellis MI, Seedhom BB, Wright V, et al. An evaluation of the ratio between the tension along the quadriceps tendon and the patella ligament. *Eng Med* 1980;9:189–194.

181. Huberti HH, Hayes WC, Stone JL, et al. Force ratios in the quadriceps tendon and ligamentous patellae. *J Orthop Res* 1984;2:49.

182. Van Eijden TMGJ, Kouwenhoven E, Verburg J, et al. A mathematical model of the patellofemoral joint. *J Biomech* 1986;19:219–229.

183. Ferguson AB, Brown TD, Fu FH, et al. Relief of patellofemoral contact stress by anterior displacement of the tibial tubercle. *J Bone Joint Surg Am* 1979;61A:159–166.

184. Brattström H, Håken JK. Shape of the intercondylar groove normally and in recurrent dislocation of the patella. A clinical and x-ray–anatomical investigation. *Acta Orthop Scand* 1964; 68[Suppl]:1–148.

185. Insall J, Palvoka A, Wise DW. Chondromalacia patellae. A prospective study. *J Bone Joint Surg Am* 1976;58A:1–8.

186. Pevsner DN, Johnson JRG, Blazina ME. The patellofemoral joint and its implications in rehabilitation of the knee. *Phys Ther* 1979;59:869–874.

187. Cox JS. Evaluation of the Roux-Elmslie-Trillat procedure for knee extensor realignment. *Am J Sports Med* 1982;10:303.

188. Fulkerson JP, Hungerford DS. *Patellar subluxation in disorders of the patellofemoral joint.* Baltimore: Williams & Wilkins, 1990:142.

Principles and Practice of Orthopaedic Sports Medicine,
edited by William E. Garrett, Jr., Kevin P. Speer, and Donald T. Kirkendall.
Lippincott Williams & Wilkins, Philadelphia © 2000.

CHAPTER 36

Knee Meniscus

Julie A. Dodds, Douglas P. Dietzel, and Steven P. Arnoczky

The menisci are C-shaped disks of fibrocartilage interposed between the condyles of the femur and tibia. Once described as the functionless remains of leg muscle, the menisci are now realized to be integral components in the complex biomechanics of the knee joint. Knowledge of the form, function, and biology of these unique structures is an important prerequisite to applying the various clinical procedures available to treat, preserve, and replace the menisci of the knee koint.

GROSS ANATOMY

The menisci of the knee joint are actually extensions of the tibia that serve to deepen the articular surfaces of the tibial plateau to better accommodate the condyles of the femur. The peripheral border of each meniscus is thick, convex, and attached to the inside capsule of the joint; the opposite border tapers to a thin free edge (1). The proximal surfaces of the menisci are concave and in contact with the condyles of the femur; their distal surfaces are flat and rest on the plateau of the tibia (Fig. 36.1).

The medial meniscus is somewhat semicircular in form and is approximately 3.5 cm in length and considerably wider posteriorly than anteriorly (1). The anterior horn of the medial meniscus is attached to the tibial plateau in the area of the anterior intercondylar fossa in front of the anterior cruciate ligament (ACL). The posterior fibers of the anterior horn attachment merge with the transverse ligament, which connects the ante-

rior horns of the medial and lateral menisci. The posterior horn of the medial meniscus is firmly attached to the posterior intercondylar fossa of the tibia between the attachments of the lateral meniscus and the posterior cruciate ligament. The periphery of the medial meniscus is attached to the joint capsule throughout its length. The tibial portion of the capsular attachment is often referred to as the coronary ligament. At its midpoint, the medial meniscus is more firmly attached to the femur and tibia through a condensation in the joint capsule known as the deep medial collateral ligament.

The lateral meniscus is almost circular and covers a larger portion of the tibial articular surface than the medial meniscus. The anterior and posterior horns are approximately the same width. The anterior horn of the lateral meniscus is attached to the tibia in front of the intercondylar eminence and behind the attachment of the ACL, with which it partially blends. The posterior horn of the lateral meniscus is attached behind the intercondylar eminence of the tibia, in front of the posterior horn of the medial meniscus. Although there is no attachment of the lateral meniscus to the lateral collateral ligament, there is a loose peripheral attachment to the joint capsule (Fig. 36.2) (1).

Several ligaments run from the posterior horn of the lateral meniscus to the medial femoral condyle, either just in front of or behind the origin of the posterior cruciate ligament. These are known as the anterior meniscofemoral ligament (ligament of Humphrey) and the posterior meniscofemoral ligament (ligament of Wrisberg) (1,2).

J. A. Dodds: College of Human Medicine, Michigan State University, East Lansing, Michigan 48823.

D. P. Dietzel: Department of Osteopathic Surgical Specialties, Michigan State University, East Lansing, Michigan, 48824.

S. P. Arnoczky: College of Veterinary Medicine, Michigan State University, East Lansing, Michigan 48824.

ULTRASTRUCTURE AND BIOCHEMISTRY

Histologically, the meniscus is a fibrocartilaginous tissue composed primarily of an interlacing network of collagen fibers interposed with cells (Fig. 36.3). In addition, the extracellular matrix consists of proteoglycan molecules and glycoproteins (3–7).

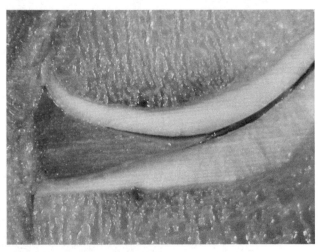

FIG. 36.1. Frontal section of the medial compartment of a human knee illustrating the articulation of the menisci with the condyles of the femur and tibia. (From Warren RF, Arnoczky SP, Wickiewicz TL. Anatomy of the knee. In: Nicholas JA, Hershman EB, eds. *The lower extremity and spine in sports medicine*. St. Louis: C.V. Mosby, 1986:657–694, with permission.)

The cells of the meniscus are responsible for synthesizing and maintaining the extracellular matrix. There is still some debate as to whether the cells of the meniscus are fibroblasts, chondrocytes, or a mixture of both and whether the tissue should be classified as fibrous tissue or fibrocartilage (8). The cells have been termed fibrochondrocytes because of their chondrocyte-like appearance and their ability to synthesize a fibrocartilage matrix. Two basic types of fibrochondrocytes have been

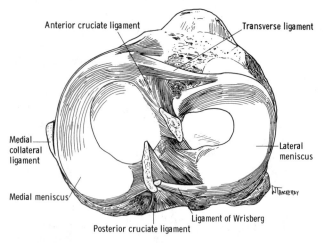

FIG. 36.2. Tibial plateau showing the shape and attachments of the medial and lateral menisci. (From Warren RF, Arnoczky SP, Wickiewicz TL. Anatomy of the knee. In: Nicholas JA, Hershman EB, eds. *The lower extremity and spine in sports medicine*. St. Louis: C.V. Mosby, 1986:657–694, with permission.)

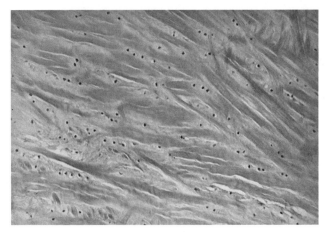

FIG. 36.3. Longitudinal section of a human meniscus (hemotoxylin and eosin, ×100).

described within the meniscus: a fusiform cell found in the superficial zone of the meniscus and an ovoid or polygonal cell found throughout the remainder of the tissue (8). Although the fusiform cells resemble fibroblasts, they are situated in well-formed lacunae and resemble the chondrocytes found in the superficial (tangential) zone of articular cartilage (8). Both cell types contain abundant endoplasmic reticulum and Golgi complexes. Mitochondria are only occasionally visualized, suggesting that, as in articular chondrocytes, the major pathway for energy production for the fibrochondrocytes in their avascular surroundings is probably anaerobic glycolysis (5,6).

The extracellular matrix of the meniscus is composed primarily of collagen (60% to 70% of the dry weight) (3–6). It is mainly type I collagen (90%) although types II, III, V, and VI have been identified within the meniscus (3–6). The circumferential orientation of these collagen fibers appears to be directly related to the function of the meniscus. In a classic study describing the orientation of the collagen fibers within the menisci, it was noted that although the principal orientation of the collagen fibers is circumferential, a few small radially disposed fibers appear on both the femoral and tibial surfaces of the menisci and within the substance of the tissue (Fig. 36.4) (9). It is theorized that these radial fibers act as "ties" to provide structural rigidity and help resist longitudinal splitting of the menisci resulting from undue compression. Subsequent light and electron microscopic examinations of the menisci have revealed three different collagen framework layers: a superficial layer composed of a network of fine fibrils woven into a meshlike matrix, a surface layer just beneath the superficial layer composed in part of irregularly aligned collagen bundles, and a middle layer in which the collagen fibers are larger and coarser and are oriented in a parallel circumferential direction (10,11). It is this mid-

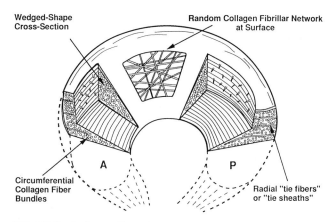

FIG. 36.4. Collagen fiber ultrastructure of the meniscus. Note the predominant circumferential orientation of the large collagen fiber bundles on the interior of the tissue. The fibers of the surface layer have no preferred orientation. Also within the interior of the meniscus are radially oriented collagen "tie" fibers. (From Mow VC, Ratcliffe A, Chern KY, et al. Structure and function relationships of the menisci of the knee. In: Mow VC, Arnoczky SP, Jackson DW, eds. *Knee meniscus: basic and clinical foundations.* New York: Raven Press, 1992:37–57, with permission.)

dle layer that allows the meniscus to resist tensile forces and function as a transmitter of load across the knee joint.

In addition to collagen, the extracellular matrix of the meniscus also consists of proteoglycans, matrix glycoproteins, and elastin (3–6). The proteoglycan content of the adult meniscus is approximately 10% of that in hyaline cartilage, although this has been shown to vary with age and location within the tissue. A study in the porcine meniscus has shown a higher (two to four times) content of hexosamine and uronic acid in the inner third of the meniscus as compared with the outer two thirds (3,4). There was also a trend toward higher concentrations in the anterior horn as compared with the posterior horn in both the medial and lateral meniscus (3,4). The glycosaminoglycan profile of the adult human meniscus has been reported to consist of chondroitin 6-sulfate (40%), chondroitin 4-sulfate (10% to 20%), dermatan sulfate (20% to 30%), and keratan sulfate (15%) (3–6).

Matrix glycoproteins, such as the link proteins that stabilize the proteoglycan–hyaluronic acid aggregates and a 116-kDa protein of unknown consequence, have also been identified within the extracellular matrix (3–6). In addition, adhesive glycoproteins such as type VI collagen, fibronectin, and thrombospondin have also been isolated from the meniscus (5,6). These macromolecules have the property to bind to other matrix macromolecules and/or cell surfaces and may play a role in the supramolecular organization of the extracellular molecules of the meniscus (5,6).

MENISCAL FUNCTION

As the knee passes through a range of motion, the menisci move with respect to the tibial articular surface. A classic study demonstrated that from 0 to 120 degrees of knee flexion, the mean meniscal excursion (defined as the average anteroposterior displacement of the anterior and posterior meniscal horns along the tibial plateau in the midcondylar, parasagittal plane) of the medial meniscus was 5.1 ± 0.96 mm, whereas that of the lateral meniscus was 11.2 ± 3.27 mm (12) (Fig. 36.5). The lack of bony opposition (i.e., convex femoral condyle and tibial plateau), an unconstrained peripheral margin, and the close approximation of its central tibial attachments appear to allow the lateral meniscus a greater degree of movement.

Rotation of the knee joint also has an effect on meniscal motion with a greater effect being observed in the lateral meniscus. The posterior oblique fibers of the medial collateral ligament appear to limit the movement of the medial meniscus in rotation, which may increase its risk of tear injury (13).

In addition to their anterior–posterior translation, the meniscus deform to remain in constant congruity to the tibial and femoral articular surfaces throughout the full range of joint motion. This allows the meniscus to provide additional joint stability (13). The anterior horn segments of the medial and lateral menisci demonstrate differing mobility compared with posterior horn segments. This differential allows the menisci to assume a decreasing radius with flexion that correlates with a decreasing radius of curvature of the posterior femoral condyle. The change in radius enables the menisci to maintain congruity with the articulating surfaces

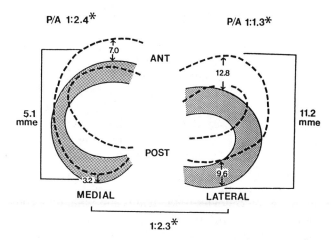

FIG. 36.5. Mean meniscal excursion (*mme*) along the tibial plateau. The ratio of posterior to anterior translation (*P/A*) was significant (*$p < 0.05$). (From Thompson WO, Thaete FL, Fu FH, et al. Tibial meniscal dynamics using three-dimensional reconstruction of magnetic resonance images. *Am J Sports Med* 1991;19:210–216, with permission.)

throughout flexion. The greatest deformation appears to occur at the anterior medial horn as it moves onto the tibial plateau with flexion and is manifested as an increase in the concavity of the superior articulating meniscal surface. This is probably due to the increasing load resulting from femoral flexion (13).

The meniscus has been shown to play a vital role in load transmission across the knee joint (14–20). Biomechanical studies have demonstrated that at least 50% of the compressive load of the knee joint is transmitted through the meniscus in extension, whereas approximately 85% of the load is transmitted in 90 degrees of flexion (14,15). In the meniscectomized knee, the contact area is reduced approximately 50% (14,15). This significantly increases the load per unit area and results in articular cartilage damage and degeneration. This evidence explains the osteophyte formation, joint space narrowing, and flattening of the femoral condyle that have been observed after total meniscectomy, as the body tries to compensate for this increased load (21).

Partial meniscectomy has also been shown to significantly increase contact pressures (22). It has been shown that resection of a little as 15% to 34% of the meniscus increased contact pressures by more than 350% (18). Thus, even a partial meniscectomy can affect the ability of the meniscus to function in load transmission across the knee (22).

Another proposed function of the meniscus is that of shock absorption. It has been suggested that the viscoelastic menisci may function to dampen the load generated during walking (18,23). Experimental studies have shown that the normal knee has a shock-absorbing capacity about 20% higher than knees that have undergone meniscectomy (23). Because the inability of a joint system to absorb shock has been strongly implicated in the development of osteoarthritis, the meniscus appears to play an important role in maintaining the health of the knee (24).

The menisci are also thought to contribute to knee joint stability. Although medial meniscectomy alone does not increase anterior–posterior joint translation significantly, it has been demonstrated that medial meniscectomy in association with ACL insufficiency significantly increases the anterior laxity of the knee (25,26). However, lateral meniscectomy, alone or in association with ACL insufficiency, has not been shown to increase knee joint laxity (25,26).

Because the menisci serve to increase the congruity between the condyles of the femur and tibia, they contribute significantly to overall joint conformity. It has been suggested that this function assists in the overall lubrication of the articular surfaces of the knee joint (13).

Finally, the menisci may serve as proprioceptive structures, providing a feedback mechanism for joint position sense. This has been inferred from the presence of type I and type II nerve endings observed in the anterior and posterior horns of the meniscus (27–30).

VASCULAR ANATOMY OF THE MENISCUS

The menisci of the knee are relatively avascular structures whose limited peripheral blood supply originates predominantly from the lateral and medial geniculate arteries (both inferior and superior) (31,32). Branches from these vessels give rise to a perimeniscal capillary plexus within the synovial and capsular tissues of the knee joint. This plexus is an arborizing network of vessels that supplies the peripheral border of the meniscus throughout its attachment to the joint capsule (Fig. 36.6) (31,32). These perimeniscal vessels are oriented in a predominantly circumferential pattern with radial branches directed toward the center of the joint. Anatomic studies have shown that the degree of vascular penetration is 10% to 30% of the width of the medial meniscus and 10% to 25% of the width of the lateral meniscus (31,32).

The middle genicular artery, along with a few terminal branches of the medial and lateral genicular arteries, also supplies vessels to the meniscus through the vascular synovial covering of the anterior and posterior horn attachments. These synovial vessels penetrate the horn attachments and give rise to endoligamentous vessels that enter the meniscal horns for a short distance and end in terminal capillary loops. A small reflection of vascular synovial tissue is also present throughout the peripheral attachment of the medial and lateral menisci on both the femoral and tibial articular surfaces. (An exception is the posterolateral portion of the lateral

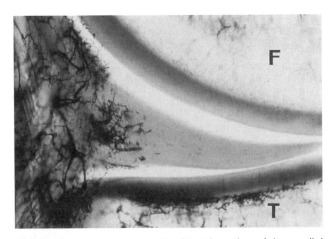

FIG. 36.6. Five-millimeter-thick frontal section of the medial compartment of the knee after vascular perfusion with India ink and tissue clearing with a modified Spalteholz technique. Branching radial vessels from the perimeniscal capillary plexus (*PCP*) can be seen penetrating the peripheral border of the medial meniscus. *F,* Femur; *T,* tibia. (From Arnoczky SP, Warren RF. Microvasculature of the human meniscus. *Am J Sports Med* 1982;10:90–95, with permission.)

meniscus adjacent to the area of the popliteal tendon.) This "synovial fringe" extends for a short distance (1 to 3 mm) over the articular surfaces of the menisci and contains small terminally looped vessels. Although this vascular synovial tissue adheres intimately to the articular surfaces of the menisci, it does not contribute vessels into the meniscal tissue (31,32).

MENISCAL HEALING

In 1885, Thomas Annandale (33) was credited with the first surgical repair of a torn meniscus, but it was not until 1936, when King (34,35) published his classic experiments on meniscus healing in dogs, that the actual biologic limitations of meniscus healing were set forth. King demonstrated that for meniscus lesions to heal, the lesion must communicate with the peripheral blood supply. Although the vascular supply of the meniscus is an essential element in determining its potential for repair, of equal importance is the ability of this blood supply to support the inflammatory response characteristic of wound repair. Clinical and experimental observations have demonstrated that the peripheral blood supply is capable of producing a reparative response similar to that observed in other connective tissues (36).

After injury within the peripheral vascular zone, a fibrin clot forms that is rich in inflammatory cells. Vessels from the perimeniscal capillary plexus proliferate through this fibrin "scaffold," accompanied by the proliferation of undifferentiated mesenchymal cells. Eventually, the lesion is filled with a cellular fibrovascular scar tissue that "glues" the wound edges together and appears continuous with the adjacent normal meniscal fibrocartilage. Vessels from the perimeniscal capillary plexus and a proliferative vascular pannus from the synovial fringe penetrate the fibrous scar to provide a marked inflammatory response (36).

Experimental studies have shown that radial lesions of the meniscus extending to the synovium are completely healed with fibrovascular scar tissue by 10 weeks (Fig. 36.7) (36). Modulation of this scar into normal-appearing fibrocartilage, however, can require several months. It should stressed that the initial strength of this repair tissue, as compared with the normal meniscus, has been found to be minimal (33% at 8 weeks, 52% at 4 months, and 62% at 6 months) (37).

The ability of meniscal lesions to heal has provided the rationale for the repair of peripheral meniscal injuries, and numerous clinical reports have demonstrated excellent results after primary repair of peripheral meniscal injuries. Postoperative examinations of these peripheral repairs have revealed a process of repair similar to that noted in the experimental models.

When examining injured menisci for potential repair, lesions are often classified by the location of the tear

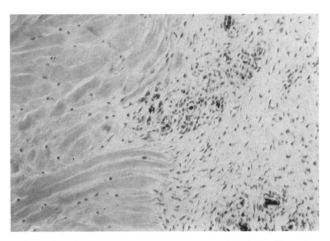

FIG. 36.7. Healing meniscus at the junction of the fibrovascular scar and the normal adjacent meniscal tissue (hemotoxylin and eosin, ×75). (From Arnoczky SP, Warren RF. The microvasculature of the meniscus and its response to injury—an experimental study in the dog. *Am J Sports Med* 1983;11:131–141, with permission.)

relative to the blood supply of the meniscus and the "vascular appearance" of the peripheral and central surfaces of the tear. The so-called *red–red* tear (peripheral capsular detachment) has a functional blood supply on the capsular and meniscal side of the lesion and obviously has the best prognosis for healing. The *red–white* tears (meniscus rim tears through the peripheral vascular zone) have an active peripheral blood supply, whereas the central (inner) surface of the lesion is devoid of functioning vessels. Theoretically, these lesions should have sufficient vascularity to heal by the aforementioned fibrovascular proliferation. The *white–white* tears (meniscus lesion completely in the avascular zone) are without blood supply and theoretically cannot heal.

Meniscus repair has generally been limited to the peripheral vascular area of the meniscus (red–red, red–white tears), but a significant number of lesions occur in the central avascular portion of the meniscus (white–white tears). Experimental and clinical observations have shown that these lesions are incapable of healing and have thereby provided the rationale for partial meniscectomy. In an effort to "extend" the level of repair into these avascular area, techniques have been developed that provide vascularity to these white–white tears. These techniques include vascular access channels (36) and synovial abrasion (38).

Initial attempts to extend the peripheral vascular response of the meniscus into the avascular zone used the creation of vascular access channels (36). This concept was based on the observation that when avascular lesions were extended into the peripheral blood supply of the meniscus, vessels would migrate into those lesions and heal them by the aforementioned process.

In an experimental study in dogs, a longitudinal lesion

in the avascular portion of the medial meniscus was connected, at its midportion, to the peripheral vasculature of the meniscus by a full-thickness vascular access channel (36). Vessels from the peripheral tissues migrated into the channel and healed the meniscal lesion by the proliferation of fibrovascular scar tissue. When using the vascular access technique, it is imperative to remember that the function of the meniscus can be destroyed through the destruction of the peripheral rim. However, because the vascularity extends into the meniscus at least 25% of its width, a vascular access channel can be created without completely disrupting the integrity of the peripheral rim of the meniscus.

Another technique of "manipulating" the vascular supply of the meniscus that has found increasing clinical utilization is the technique of synovial abrasion. In this technique, the synovial fringe is abraded in an effort to incite a more robust vascular response near the site of the meniscal lesion (38). As noted previously, the meniscal synovial fringe is a vascular synovial tissue that extends over the femoral and tibial articular surfaces of the meniscus. Although it does not contribute vessels to the meniscal stroma under normal circumstances, it plays a major role in the healing of meniscal lesions in contact with the peripheral vasculature of the meniscus. It has been theorized that by stimulating (through rasping or abrading) the synovial fringe, a proliferative vascular response could be extended over the meniscal surface to previously avascular areas of the meniscus. Although clinical results have suggested an improved healing rate when synovial abrasion is used, the exact extent and character of the repair tissue has yet to be determined.

Finally, the use of an exogenous fibrin clot has been shown to heal avascular lesions without benefit of a blood supply in a canine model (39). Previous work had suggested that white–white tears in the meniscus were incapable of repair. This was based on the belief that the meniscal cells were incapable of mounting a repair response and that a blood supply was a prerequisite for wound repair. However, in experimental studies, Webber et al. (40,41) demonstrated that meniscal fibrochondrocytes are capable of proliferation and matrix synthesis when exposed to chemotactic and mitogenic factors normally present in the wound hematoma. Using cell cultures, they demonstrated that meniscal cells exposed to platelet-derived growth factor were able to proliferate and synthesize an extracellular matrix.

In normal wound repair, hemorrhage from vascular injury gives rise to a fibrin clot that provides a scaffolding that supports a reparative response. In addition, the clot provides substances such as platelet-derived growth factor and fibronectin, which act as chemotactic and mitogenic stimuli of reparative cells. Clinical use of the fibrin clot techniques has suggested that it can improve the healing rate in meniscal tears at or near the limit of vascularity (42,43).

MENISCAL INJURIES

Epidemiology

Poehling et al. (44) reviewed 6,039 meniscal tears from 17 medical centers. From this they created a "landscape" of meniscal tears, in which 30% were complex, 26% peripheral longitudinal, 21% flap, 12% horizontal, 9.3% radial, and less than 1% discoid. The ratio of meniscal tears in males versus females was 2.5:1. The incidence of tears in females peaked at 11 to 20 years of age, whereas the incidence in males peaked between 31 and 40 years of age. The incidence of meniscal tears associated with acute ACL tears has been reported from 34% to 92%. An increased incidence of meniscal tears (as high as 98%) has been reported in chronic ACL-deficient knees (45). Lateral meniscal injury occurs more often in acute ACL tears, and medial meniscal injury occurs more often in chronic ACL-deficient knees (46,47). The instability associated with a chronic ACL tear can lead to repeated episodes of rotary subluxation and abnormal stresses on the meniscus, often causing tears. The prevention of these episodes and the preservation of the meniscus continues to be an indication for ACL reconstruction.

Mechanism of Injury

Meniscal tears most often occur with a twisting type of injury, although tears can also occur with hyperflexion. Degenerative tears often have no history of trauma, with an insidious onset of symptoms. Loss of water content secondary to meniscal degeneration is thought to cause the meniscus to become friable and susceptible to tearing.

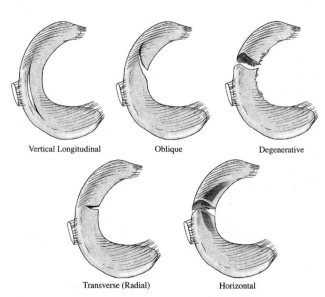

FIG. 36.8. Types of meniscal tears. (From Hoppenfeld S. *Physical examination of the spine and extremities.* Norwalk, CT: Appleton-Century-Crofts, 1976:192, with permission.)

Classification of Meniscal Tears

Five type of meniscal tears have been identified: vertical longitudinal, horizontal, flap, radial, and degenerative (44,48) (Fig. 36.8). The vertical longitudinal tear, also called the bucket-handle tear, often involves an inner mobile fragment that can sublux, limiting the range of motion of the knee. These tears are frequently found in ACL-deficient knees. The flap tear, or parrot-beak tear, may also have a mobile fragment that can displace, causing pain or "catching" symptoms. Horizontal tears begin at the inner margin of the meniscus and extend horizontally toward the capsule. This creates upper and lower flaps that may also be unstable. Meniscal cysts may be associated with these tears. Radial tears consist of a transverse fissure within the meniscus. These may propagate with weight bearing or twisting and become flap-type tears. Degenerative tears usually occur in an older population. They often consist of a complex pattern and may have associated degenerative changes on the opposing articular surfaces. Degenerative tears can also occur as a sequella to delayed treatment of simple tears, which then progress into a complex pattern.

Meniscal tears may also be associated with underlying predisposing conditions. Inflammatory diseases and metabolic conditions such as calcium pyrophosphate deposition disease may cause an accumulation of an abnormal substance within the body of the meniscus, compromising the stability and/or strength of the cartilage tissue. Discoid menisci (usually lateral) are also prone to tears due to their abnormal shape.

Clinical Evaluation

A careful history and physical evaluation should help determine approximately 75% of meniscal tears (49). Questions regarding the mechanism of injury, symptoms immediately after the injury, and residual symptoms all lead to the diagnosis. Most patients (80% to 90%) are able to recall a specific injury or mechanism that caused the tear (50). A history may be elicited of twisting, a rapid change in direction, squatting or a deep knee bend, or associated ACL deficiency (47,49,50). Symptoms may include swelling, locking, snapping, popping, inability to obtain full extension, pain with squatting or twisting, and catching. Swelling is usually delayed 1 or 2 days postinjury in isolated meniscal tears.

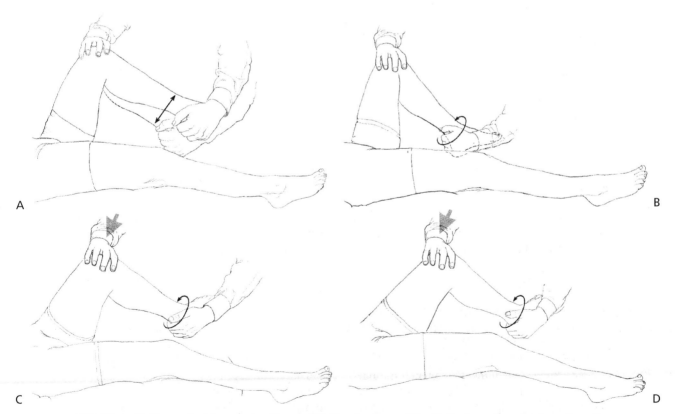

FIG. 36.9. McMurray test for meniscal tears: **(A)** Flex the knee; **(B)** with the knee flexed, internally and externally rotate the tibia on the femur; **(C)** with the leg externally rotated, place a valgus stress on the knee; **(D)** with the leg externally rotated and in valgus, slowly extend the knee. If a "click" is palpable or audible, the test is considered positive for a torn medial meniscus, usually in the posterior position. (From Hoppenfeld S. *Physical examination of the spine and extremities.* Norwalk, CT: Appleton-Century-Crofts, 1976:193, with permission.)

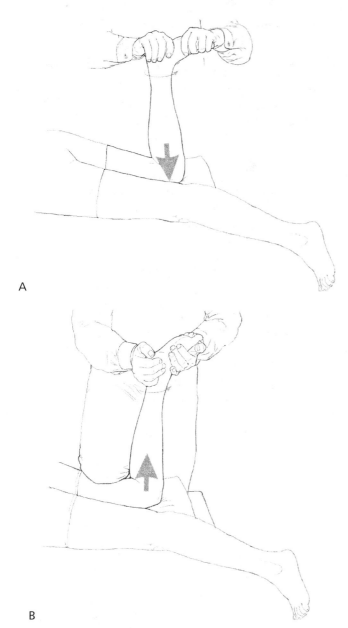

A

B

FIG. 36.10. Apley's compression **(A)** and distraction **(B)** test. (From Hoppenfeld S. *Physical examination of the spine and extremities.* Norwalk, CT: Appleton-Century-Crofts, 1976:194, with permission.)

Physical examination should include assessment of range of motion, effusion, joint line tenderness, quadriceps atrophy, McMurray's test, Apley's test, and a full flexion test (50–52). Lack of full extension (compared with the opposite knee) may indicate a bucketed longitudinal meniscal tear. Effusion may be obvious or consist of a fluid wave only. Quadriceps atrophy may occur from quad inhibition secondary to pain. McMurray's test (Fig. 36.9) is performed with the patient supine and the knee flexed. The tibia is externally rotated and the knee placed in valgus and extended. A palpable or audi-

ble click from the medial joint line or reproduction of the patient's pain suggests a medial meniscal tear. The Apley compression test (Fig. 36.10) is performed with the patient prone and the knee flexed to 90 degrees. The examiner anchors the thigh to the table (with a hand or thigh) and medially and laterally rotates the tibia. This is performed with distraction and then compression of the joint. If distraction and rotation cause pain, the problem is most likely ligamentous. If compression and rotation cause the discomfort, the problem is more likely to be meniscal. The full flexion test is performed with the patient supine and the knee flexed as far as comfort will allow. Pain at terminal flexion may indicate a lesion in the posterior horn of the meniscus.

A routine examination for meniscal tear should always include radiographs to rule out degenerative changes, loose bodies, fracture, osteochondritis dissecans, and other lesions. Double-contrast arthrography was commonly used to identify meniscal tears before the advent of magnetic resonance imaging (MRI) but has essentially fallen out of favor. The MRI has improved the ability to diagnose meniscal tears to near 90% (53). However, this accuracy is highly dependent on proper interpretation and quality of the scan. In a study of 1,014 patients, with MRI being performed at 14 centers, accuracy ranged from 64% to 95% (53). It has been shown that clinical examination can be at least as accurate as MRI in diagnosing meniscal tears (54). Arthroscopy remains the gold standard, both for diagnosing and treating meniscal tears (55).

TREATMENT OF MENISCAL TEARS

There are three options for treatment of a meniscal tear: Tears may be excised, repaired, or simply observed. Tears that are stable, short (less than 10 mm), and/or partial thickness (less than 50%) may be asymptomatic and not require treatment. This may be particularly true for lateral meniscal tears (56).

Unstable or symptomatic tears are treated with excision or repair. Meniscal excision has evolved from complete open meniscectomies to arthroscopic partial meniscectomies. The value of preserving as much meniscus as possible has been well documented in the improvement of long-term prognosis in patients with partial versus complete meniscectomies (57,58). Although preservation of the meniscus is a priority, partial meniscectomy is usually indicated for flap, complex, degenerative, and horizontal cleavage tears. Partial or complete meniscectomy is usually performed arthroscopically, using manual cutting instruments to remove most of the torn portion of the meniscus. A smooth stable rim is then created using motorized shavers.

MENISCAL REPAIR

Indication for Repair Versus Excision

When evaluating a meniscal tear for possible repair, the surgeon must consider the many factors that may affect its healing, such as location of the tear, age of the patient, chronicity of the tear, and the presence of associated injuries such as cruciate ligament insufficiency. In general, meniscal repair has proved most successful in treating longitudinal acute tears in the vascular periphery of the meniscus in young individuals with stable knees. Although other types of tears (radial, horizontal, flap, complex) have been repaired (59), the healing rate for these types of tears is significantly decreased (60). Also, healed radial tears have not shown the mechanical function and the ability to prevent articular wear seen in healed longitudinal tears.

Vascularity of the tear is the most important factor affecting healing. Longitudinal tears within 3 mm of the meniscosynovial junction are considered to be within the vascular zone of the meniscus and are most amenable to repair. Frequently, bleeding surfaces on both sides of the tear can be noted at arthroscopy. The absence of bleeding, however, does not always indicate a tear in the avascular portion of the meniscus. Tourniquet use and fluid distention pressure may be sufficient to close down small capillary circulation. Tears more than 5 mm from the meniscosynovial junction are considered avascular unless obvious signs of vascularity are noted (bleeding or partial healing) and are often candidates for partial meniscectomy. However, because of the importance of preserving the meniscus in young patients, these tears are often repaired (especially when a concomitant ACL reconstruction is performed). Vascular enhancement techniques are also recommended in these more central tears.

The condition of the meniscus is also an important factor in the ability of a torn meniscus to heal and function normally. Degenerative or severely damaged meniscal body fragments are often excised rather than repaired regardless of the location of the tear.

Finally, patient age does not appear to be a contraindication to meniscal repair. Meniscal repair of acute peripheral tears in active patients over 40 years of age is not uncommon. In fact, one study has even noted a higher healing rate in older patients (61).

Open Meniscal Repair

Initial attempts at meniscal repair were limited to peripheral detachments of the meniscus, the so-called red–red tears. These lesions were approached through a longitudinal incision in the area of the meniscal tear. This "open" technique is technically demanding and provides the surgeon very limited access to the central portion of the meniscus (62–64). Thus, only the most peripheral lesions (within 2 mm of the meniscosynovial junction) can be repaired through this approach. For open repairs, a 5- to 6-cm vertical, posterior medial, or posterolateral incision is centered at the level of the joint line. An oblique capsular incision is made to expose the underlying meniscal tear. The peripheral rim of the meniscus and the capsular bed are debrided and freshened. Double-armed sutures are used to place vertical sutures through the rim and capsular bed. Ease of preparation of the meniscal rim, the ability for "anatomic reduction" of the meniscus, and the ability to place stronger vertical mattress sutures are potential advantages (65).

Arthroscopic Meniscal Repair

The advent of arthroscopy permitted better visualization of the menisci. Through the arthroscope, the surgeon could gain access to all aspects of the meniscus, and with the development of arthroscopic surgical techniques, the repair of the more central red–white and the peripheral red–red tears was possible.

Three types of arthroscopic meniscal repair have been described; inside-out, outside-in, and all-inside. Although the specific technique used depends on meniscal tear location and surgeon preference, all have been shown to yield comparable results.

The "inside-out" meniscal suturing technique (Fig. 36.11) was proposed by Scott et al. (59) and modified by Cannon (61), Rosenberg et al. (66), and Clancy and Graf (67). In this technique, the tear is first defined arthroscopically and the edges of the meniscal lesion are debrided. A posterolateral or posteromedial exposure is then made to allow retrieval of sutures. The posteromedial incision is made just anterior to the sartorius tendon with the knee flexed and taken down to the posterior joint capsule just anterior to the semimembranosus. Care is taken to protect the sartorial branch of the saphenous nerve. The posterolateral incision dissects between the anterior border of the biceps femoris and iliotibial band at the level of the joint line. The lateral head of the gastrocnemius muscle is elevated from the posterolateral capsule to allow suture retrieval. With the knee flexed, the peroneal nerve lies posterior to the surgical dissection. After capsular exposure is gained, a single- or double-cannula system is used to pass sutures through the meniscus, across the tear, into the peripheral rim of the meniscus, and out the posterior capsule. A popliteal retractor is used to avoid piercing the popliteal neurovascular structures with needle passage. Approximately every 4 to 5 mm, sutures are placed alternately on the upper and lower surfaces of the menisci. Vertically oriented mattress sutures are preferred because of their ability to encompass more of the circumferentially oriented collagen bundles of the meniscus. If

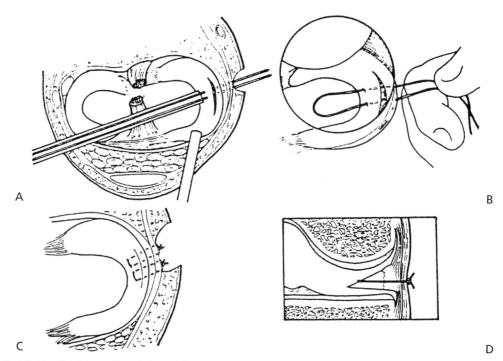

FIG. 36.11. "Inside-out" technique of meniscal repair showing **(A)** placement of needles through the lesion, **(B)** the horizontal mattress suture in place, **(C)** the sutures tied subcutaneously, and **(D)** the orientation of the sutures through the meniscal tear. (From Arnoczky SP, Dodds JA, Coper DE. Meniscal repair and replacement. In: Siliski JM, ed. *Traumatic disorders of the knee.* New York: Springer-Verlag, 1994:339, with permission.)

ACL reconstruction is performed concurrently, sutures may be tied before or after reconstruction.

The "outside-in" technique, as described by Warren (68) and Morgan and Casscells (69), was developed as an attempt to avoid the neurovascular complications originally encountered with the inside-out technique. As in the previously described technique, the meniscal tear is identified and prepared arthroscopically and the posterior medial or posterolateral capsule exposed through a small incision. An 18-gauge spinal needle is

then passed from the posterior capsule through the rim, across the tear, and into the meniscus under arthroscopic visualization (Fig. 36.12). A suture is then passed through the needle, into the joint, and brought out through an anterior portal. A large knot is tied in the end of the suture and the knot pulled back into the meniscal body by pulling the "tail" of the suture (Fig. 36.13). This process is repeated every 4 to 5 mm, alternating the knot on the upper and lower meniscal surfaces as needed to stabilize the tear. The tail ends of

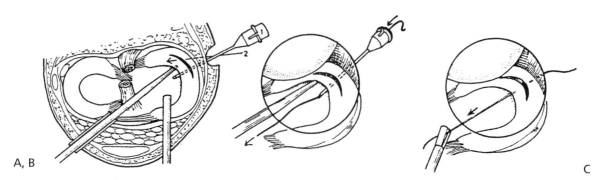

FIG. 36.12. "Outside-in" technique of meniscal repair showing **(A)** placement of an 18-gauge spinal needle across the meniscal lesion, **(B)** passage of the suture material through the needle, and **(C)** grasping of the suture to pull it out of an anterior portal. (From Arnoczky SP, Dodds JA, Coper DE. Meniscal repair and replacement. In: Siliski JM, ed. *Traumatic disorders of the knee.* New York: Springer-Verlag, 1994:339, with permission.)

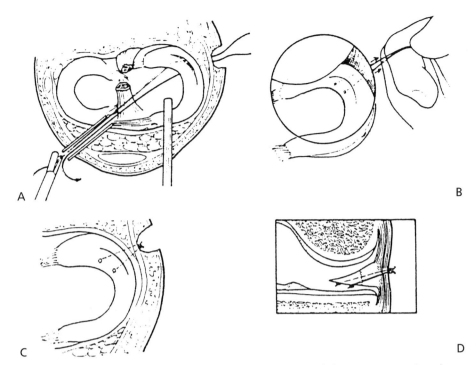

FIG. 36.13. "Outside-in" technique of meniscal repair showing **(A)** two sutures placed across the meniscal injury and exiting an anterior portal, **(B)** the sutures being pulled flush with the meniscal surface after knots have been tied in the ends of the sutures, **(C)** the free ends of the sutures being tied together subcutaneously, and **(D)** the orientation of the sutures through the meniscal tear. (From Arnoczky SP, Dodds JA, Coper DE. Meniscal repair and replacement. In: Siliski JM, ed. *Traumatic disorders of the knee.* New York: Springer-Verlag, 1994:340, with permission.)

the suture are then tied over the posterior capsule. This procedure is the preferred method for suturing peripheral anterior horn tears not accessible by other methods. For these tears, needles are passed percutaneously across the anterior horn and tied down through a small incision over the anterior capsule. An alternative technique of outside-in repair uses two needles passed across the tear, with a suture being passed through one needle and a wire snare passed through the other. The suture is passed into the joint through one needle and brought out the other needle via the snare, with the suture ends again being tied over the capsule, creating a horizontal mattress stitch.

The most recent developments in meniscal suturing have been the "all-inside" methods. These procedures allow sutures to be placed and tied entirely arthroscopically. Morgan (70) described an all-inside method applicable to peripheral (less than 3 mm rim) posterior horn tears that is a good adjunct to the other methods to allow safe access to the most central tears of the medial or lateral meniscus, near the root attachment. A posterolateral or posteromedial portal with an arthroscopic cannula is used for placement and tying of a suture that passes through the meniscal rim and body. Specialized suturing and knot-tying instruments are necessary for this type of repair.

The T-fix meniscal repair system (Smith & Nephew Endoscopy, Acufex Division, Mansfield, MA) has become increasingly used since its introduction in 1984. This system involves placing a suture that is preattached to a T-bar across the meniscal tear via a 17-gauge sheathed needle (Fig. 36.14). A small obturator pushes the "T" out of the needle (Fig. 36.15) to engage on the outer rim of the meniscus in the synovial recess. Suture tails are then tied together arthroscopically, stabilizing the tear (Fig. 36.16). This system is applicable to tears in most locations (except anterior horn tears) and has the advantage of requiring no additional incisions or portals for use.

Other all-inside repair methods involve bioabsorbable meniscal tacks or arrows that transfix the tears (Fig. 36.17). Although eliminating the need for arthroscopic knot tying required with other all-inside repairs, more conservative rehabilitation and slower return to functional activities are recommended with these devices. Pull-out strengths of these devices across meniscal tears have been shown to be similar to horizontal mattress sutures (71) but considerably less than vertical loop sutures (72).

Not infrequently, more than one repair technique may be used to repair a single meniscal tear. In unstable meniscal tears, it is helpful to first place an anchor suture

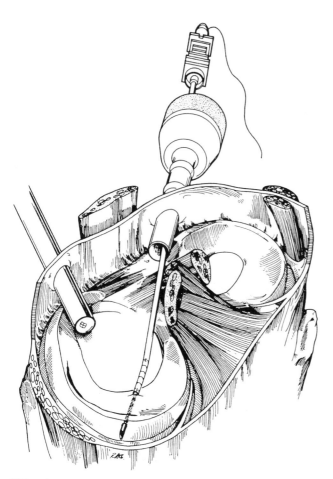

FIG. 36.14. T-fix meniscal suture being placed via sheathed cannula across meniscal tear. (From *Endoscopic meniscal repair using the T-fix (TM): instructional manual.* Technique by J. Hayhurst. Smith and Nephew, Endoscopy, Inc., Andover, MD., 1996, with permission.)

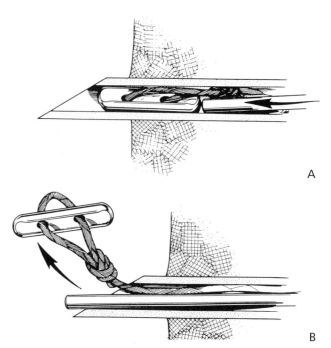

FIG. 36.15. (A) Obturator of T-fix meniscal repair system, pushing the "T" with attached suture out of the needle **(B).** (From *Endoscopic meniscal repair using the T-fix (TM): instructional manual.* Technique by J. Hayhurst. Smith and Nephew, Endoscopy, Inc. Andover, MD., 1996, with permission.)

ronment (74). This finding would suggest that nonabsorbable suture may be a more appropriate choice for meniscal repair because meniscal healing can require several months (36,37).

using an inside-out technique before placement of all-inside sutures or anchors. It is important that the surgeon is knowledgeable and skilled in several types of repair.

Type of Suture and Suture Technique

The success of meniscal repair is partially dependent on the ability of the suture fixation to maintain the initial stability of the repair under applied loads. This is dependent both on suture type and suture pattern. One study has demonstrated that vertical mattress sutures have superior pull-out strength compared with horizontal mattress or mulberry knot techniques (73). It has been shown that 1-PDS suture (Ethicon, Somerville, NJ) has better pull-out strength than 0-PDS or 2-0 Ethibond (Ethicon, Somerville, NJ) when used for vertical mattress sutures (73). However, another study has shown that PDS sutures begin to lose breaking strength at 2 weeks and retain only 40% of their original strength after 5 weeks of implantation in an intraarticular envi-

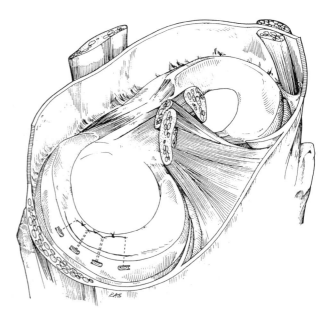

FIG. 36.16. Completed meniscal repair using T-fix meniscal repair system. (From *Endoscopic meniscal repair using the T-fix (TM): instructional manual.* Technique by J. Hayhurst. Smith and Nephew, Endoscopy, Inc. Andover, MD., 1996, with permission.)

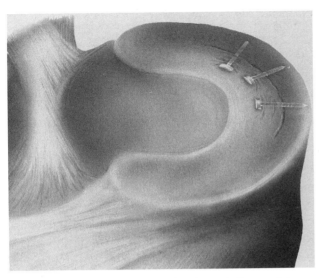

FIG. 36.17. Bioabsorbable meniscal repair "arrows" transfixing tear.

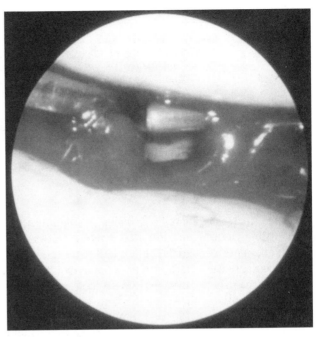

FIG. 36.19. Fibrin clot being sutured into a meniscal tear.

Vascular Enhancement

Several procedures have been proposed to improve vascularity and allow repair of some white–white tears. Fibrin clot injection (38,39) is performed by obtaining 50 to 75 mL of blood via venipuncture and precipitating a fibrin clot by stirring the whole blood in a glass vessel (Fig. 36.18). The clot is rinsed with saline to remove excess red blood cells and injected into the tear site before tensioning of the repair sutures (Fig. 36.19). Henning et al. (42) reported an improvement in healing rate of 59% to 92% with this procedure. This enhancement technique has recently been used to repair radial tears in the avascular area of the lateral meniscus adjacent to the popliteus tendon (43). Vascular access channels,

created through the peripheral meniscal rim using multiple needlesticks or trephines, have also resulted in improved healing rates (59,75). When vascular access channels are used, care must be taken to avoid complete disruption of the rim architecture because this is the key to maintaining the "hoop stresses" within the meniscus that in turn maintain the normal load-bearing status of the meniscus (19,22). Synovial abrasion is a relatively simple technique shown to enhance healing in clinical cases (59). In this technique, the synovial fringe on the femoral and tibial surfaces of the meniscus is abraded with a rasp to stimulate a proliferative vascular response. It is theorized that the vascular pannus from the synovium can be accentuated to extend into an avascular or marginally vascularized tear.

REHABILITATION

Postoperative rehabilitation after meniscal repair has varied widely among surgeons. It is probably best individualized by patient age, tear type, tear location, and stability of repair. Traditional rehabilitation guidelines are based on findings that meniscal retears occurred most frequently within the first 6 months after meniscal repair (64). Minimal weight bearing is allowed during the first 6 weeks. Although no motion is allowed for the first 2 weeks, isometric quadriceps and hamstring-setting exercises are initiated immediately. Limited motion between 30 and 70 degrees is started after 2 weeks. Further motion is allowed after 4 weeks with aggressive stretching begun at 6 weeks and crutches are discontinued 7 to 8 weeks postoperatively. Low-impact

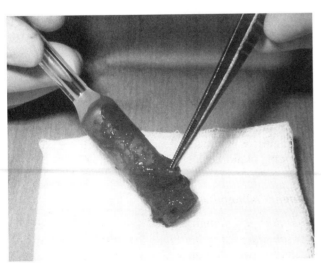

FIG. 36.18. Fibrin clot precipitated on the surface of a glass syringe barrel.

TABLE 36.1 *Accelerated rehabilitation after meniscal repair*

Time after repair	Accelerated rehabilitation physical therapy guidelines
Week 0–2	Weight bearing as tolerated; ROM exercised as tolerated; ice *Goal: full motion, no effusion, full weight bearing, normal gait*
Week 2–4	Closed kinetic chain resistance exercises; bike and swim as tolerated *Goal: full motion, no effusion, improved quadriceps strength*
Week 4–8	Strength work as needed (Cybex strength test can be used here); sports-specific functional progression *Goal: strength at least 75%; discharge from physical therapy to full activity*

ROM; range of motion.
From Shelbourne DK, Patel DV, Adsit WS, et al. Rehabilitation after meniscal repair. *Clin Sports Med* 1996;15:595–612, with permission.

activities, including bicycling, rowing, swimming, and straight-line running, are initiated 3 months after surgery if adequate strength is present and there is no pain, tenderness, or effusion. Return to full activity is allowed at 6 months. Some surgeons have recommended allowing immediate full weight bearing but immobilize the knee in full extension for 4 weeks (69). More recent "accelerated" protocols allow immediate full weight bearing and range of motion (76,77).

A typical "accelerated" rehabilitation program is shown in Table 36.1. Healing rates in patients undergoing accelerated rehabilitation have compared favorably with slower more traditional methods (76,77). However, knee flexion past 70 degrees creates posterior horn excursions of 5.1 mm medially and 11.2 mm laterally (12). To withstand this amount of motion, stability of the repair is essential. When concomitant ACL reconstruction is performed, rehabilitation normally follows the ACL protocol with minimal alteration for the repaired meniscus.

Results

Results of meniscal repair have been documented by clinical symptoms, second-look arthroscopies, arthrograms, and MRI. Lack of clinical symptoms has been shown to be a good indicator of healed or partially healed meniscal tears as noted on second-look arthroscopy (78). MRI does not appear to distinguish healed, partially healed, and unhealed meniscal tears (79).

Healing rates of open and arthroscopic repairs have been reported as 80% or higher (38,80). DeHaven et al. (81) reported an 89% success rate at 5 years after open meniscal repair. In 74 meniscal repairs using the outside-in technique, Morgan et al. (78) documented 65% healed and 19% incompletely healed tears using second-look arthroscopy and arthrograms. Success after meniscal repair has been shown to be influenced by several factors. Numerous studies have shown decreased healing rates in ACL-deficient knees (78,82). Conversely, meniscal tears repaired at the time of ACL reconstruction have shown higher healing rates (59,78). This is often attributed to eliminating patholaxity, which may stress the

repair and also to enhancing fibrin clot development. Rim width is also a significant factor, with rims of 0 to 3 mm demonstrating greater healing (59,83). Healing rates as a function of tear length have yielded inconsistent results, with increased healing noted in shorter tears by Cannon (61) but not Buseck and Noyes (83). We (J.A.D. and D.P.D.) have been very aggressive with meniscal repair, especially in younger patients and when associated with ACL reconstruction, and have noted very few patients requiring repeat arthroscopy for symptomatic nonhealed tears.

COMPLICATIONS

The complication rate of meniscal repair (1.2%) is similar to that of all arthroscopy (1.5%) (84). With the inside-out repair, injuries to the pericapsular neurovascular structures have been reported, with saphenous nerve injury being most common (69). The peroneal nerve and popliteal vessels are also at risk. Stiffness after meniscal repair has been an uncommon occurrence (85), especially with accelerated rehabilitation programs emphasizing early motion.

MENISCAL REPLACEMENT

The significance of the menisci to the overall well-being of the knee has underscored the importance of maintaining these structures whenever possible. Although techniques of meniscal repair and partial meniscectomy have limited the cases of total meniscectomy, there are instances in which total resection of the tissue is the only option. Because of the deleterious consequences to the joint as a result of meniscal loss, replacement of the meniscus through allografts or synthetic scaffolds are being explored.

Meniscal Allografts

Several experimental studies have shown that meniscal transplantation is a feasible procedure for the replacement of a severely damaged or absent meniscus (86–90). Meniscal tissue transplanted with or without viable cells has been shown to undergo a remodeling process in which host cells invade and repopulate the allograft over a 6-month period. The menisci appear to readily heal to the host tissues, and there has been no evidence of a meniscal transplant eliciting an immune response.

As clinical experience grows, the indications for meniscal transplantation are becoming more defined (91–95). At present, the best candidate for a meniscal allograft is a young individual with pain in a previously meniscectomized compartment with little or no arthritic damage. Malalignments or instabilities must be corrected in association with the transplant to avoid abnormal joint kinematics and the resulting pathologic stresses upon the meniscus. Both open and arthroscopic meniscal transplantation techniques have developed, and successful clinical outcomes (as with any surgeries) depend on the accurate placement and secure anchorage of the allograft (89,91,93,96).

Several clinical studies of meniscal allografts have been reported, and results have varied widely (92–97). Differences in surgical techniques (open vs. arthroscopic; associated surgical procedures such as ACL reconstruction), indications, and type of allografts used (cryopreserved vs. deep-frozen or irradiated vs. nonirradiated) have made direct comparisons difficult. Although most patients have reported clinical improvement, complications such as meniscal "shrinkage," peripheral extrusion of the meniscus, and failure to heal have been reported. As with most surgical techniques, long-term follow-up is required to validate meniscal transplantation as the treatment of choice for the absent or severely damaged meniscus.

Meniscal Scaffolds

A collagen scaffold created from bovine Achilles tendon has recently been used as a template for regeneration of meniscal cartilage (98). This study was undertaken with 10 patients to evaluate the safety, implantability, and ability of this scaffold to support tissue ingrowth. The collagen implants appeared to be safe with no apparent immune responses noted. The tissue was evaluated grossly, radiographically (by x-ray and MRI), and histologically. The gross appearance was similar to meniscal tissue. Radiographically, there was no evidence in change in the joint space, and the MRI showed progressive ingrowth and regeneration of tissue consistent with maturation of the collagen scaffold-meniscal tissue. The histologic appearance showed progressive new collagen and cells typical of meniscal fibrochondrocytes. Thus, this study showed that a collagen template will support human meniscal cartilage ingrowth and is apparently safely inplantable with no immediate immune response. The early results of this research are encouraging, and further research will provide more

answers in regards to the effectiveness of this and other new techniques.

REFERENCES

1. Warren R, Arnoczky SP, Wickiewicz TL. Anatomy of the knee. In: Nicholas JA, Hershman EB, eds. *The lower extremity and spine in sports medicine.* St. Louis: C.V. Mosby, 1986:657–694.
2. Heller L, Langman J. The meniscofemoral ligaments of the human knee. *J Bone Joint Surg Br* 1964;46B:307–313.
3. Adams ME, Hukins DWL. The extracellular matrix of the meniscus. In: Mow VC, Arnoczky SP, Jackson DW, eds. *Knee meniscus: basic and clinical foundations.* New York: Raven Press, 1992: 15–28.
4. Arnoczky SP, Adams ME, DeHaven K, et al. The meniscus. In: Woo SL-Y, Buckwalter J, eds. *NIAMS/AAOS workshop on the injury and repair of the musculoskeletal soft tissues.* Park Ridge, IL: Am Acad Orthop Surg, 1988:487–537.
5. McDevitt CA, Miller RR, Spindler P. The cells and cell matrix interactions of the meniscus. In: Mow VC, Arnoczky SP, Jackson DW, eds. *Knee meniscus: basic and clinical foundations.* New York: Raven Press, 1992:29–36.
6. McDevitt CA, Webber RJ. The ultrastructure and biochemistry of meniscal cartilage. *Clin Orthop* 1990;252:8–18.
7. Roughley PJ, McNicol D, Santer V, et al. The presence of a cartilage-like proteoglycan in the adult human meniscus. *Biochem J* 1981;197:77–83.
8. Ghadially FN. *Fine structure of synovial joints: a text and atlas of the ultrastructure of normal and pathological articular tissues.* London: Butterworths, 1983:103–144.
9. Bullough PG, Munuera L, Murphy J, et al. The strength of the menisci of the knee as it relates to their fine structure. *J Bone Joint Surg Br* 1970;52B:564–570.
10. Aspden RM, Hukins DWL. Structure, function, and mechanical failure of the meniscus. In: Yettram AL, ed. *Material properties and stress analysis in biomechanics.* Manchester: Manchester University Press, 1989:109–122.
11. Aspden RM, Yarker YE, Hukins DWL. Collagen orientations in the meniscus of the knee joint. *J Anat* 1985;1240:371–380.
12. Thompson WO, Thaete FL, Fu FH, et al. Tibial meniscal dynamics using three-dimensional reconstruction of magnetic resonance images. *Am J Sports Med* 1991;19:210–216.
13. Mow VC, Ratcliffe A, Chern KY, et al. Structure and function relationships of the menisci of the knee. In: Mow VC, Arnoczky SP, Jackson DW, eds. *Knee meniscus: basic and clinical foundations.* New York: Raven Press, 1992:37–57.
14. Ahmed AM. The load-bearing role of the knee menisci. In: Mow VC, Arnoczky SP, Jackson DW, eds. *Knee meniscus: basic and clinical foundations.* New York: Raven Press, 1992:59–73.
15. Ahmed AM, Burke DL. In vitro measurements of static pressure distribution in synovial joints. Part I. Tibial surface of the knee. *J Biomech Eng* 1983;105:216–225.
16. Fukubayashi T, Kurosawa H. The contact area and pressure distribution pattern of the knee. A study of normal and osteoarthritic knee joints. *Acta Orthop Scand* 1980;51:871–880.
17. Kettelcamp DB, Jacobs AW. Tibiofemoral contact. Determination and implications. *J Bone Joint Surg Am* 1972;54A:349–356.
18. Seedholm BB. Transmission of the load in the knee with special reference to the role of the menisci. Part I. *Eng Med* 1979;8:207–218.
19. Shrive NG, O'Connor JJ, Goodfellow JW. Load bearing in the knee joint. *Clin Orthop* 1978;131:279–287.
20. Walker PS, Erkman MJ. The role of the menisci in force transmission across the knee. *Clin Orthop* 1975;109:184–192.
21. Fairbank TJ. Knee joint changes after meniscectomy. *J Bone Joint Surg Br* 1948;30B:664–670.
22. Baratz ME, Fu FH, Mengato R. Meniscal tears: the effect of meniscectomy and of repair on intra-articular contact areas and stresses in the human knee. *Am J Sports Med* 1986;14:270–275.
23. Voloshin AS, Wosk J. Shock absorption of meniscectomized and painful knees. A comparative in vivo study. *J Biomed Eng* 1983; 5:157–161.

24. Burr DB, Radin EL. Meniscal function and the importance of meniscal regeneration in preventing late medial compartment osteoarthrosis. *Clin Orthop* 1982;171:121–126.

25. Levy IM, Torzilli PA, Fisch, ID. The contribution of the menisci to the stability of the knee. In: Mow VC, Arnoczky SP, Jackson DW, eds. *Knee meniscus: basic and clinical foundations.* New York: Raven Press, 1992:107–115.

26. Levy IM, Torzilli PA, Warren RF. The effect of medial meniscectomy on anterior-posterior motion of the knee. *J Bone Joint Surg Am* 1982;64A:883–888.

27. Gardner E. The innervation of the knee joint. *Anat Rec* 1948; 101:109–130.

28. Kennedy FC, Alexander IF, Hayes KL. Nerve supply of the human knee and its functional importance. *Am J Sports Med* 1982;10: 329–335.

29. Wilson AS, Legg PG, McNeur JC. Studies on the innervation of the medial meniscus in the human knee joint. *Anat Rec* 1969;165:485–492.

30. Zimny ML, Albright DL, Dabeziew E. Mechanoreceptors in the human medial meniscus. *Acta Anat* 1988;133:35–40.

31. Arnoczky SP. Gross and vascular anatomy of the meniscus and its role in meniscal healing, regeneration, and remodeling. In: Mow VC, Arnoczky SP, Jackson DW, eds. *Knee meniscus: basic and clinical foundations.* New York: Raven Press, 1992:1–14.

32. Arnoczky SP, Warren RF. Microvasculature of the human meniscus. *Am J Sports Med* 1982;10:90–95.

33. Annandale T. An operation for displaced semilunar cartilage. *Br Med J* 1885;1:779–781.

34. King D. Regeneration of the semilunar cartilage. *Surg Gynecol Obstet* 1936;62:167–170.

35. King D. The healing of the semilunar cartilages. *J Bone Joint Surg Am* 1936;18:333–342.

36. Arnoczky SP, Warren RF. The microvasculature of the meniscus and its response to injury; an experimental study in the dog. *Am J Sports Med* 1983;11:131–141.

37. Roeddecker K, Muennich U, Nagelschmidt N. Meniscal healing: a biomechanical study. *J Surg Res* 1994;56:20–27.

38. Henning CE, Lynch MA, Clark JR. Vascularity for healing of meniscus repairs. *Arthroscopy* 1987;3:13–18.

39. Arnoczky SP, Warren RF, Spivak JM. Meniscal repair using an exogenous fibrin clot. An experimental study in dogs. *J Bone Joint Surg Am* 1988;70A:1209–1217.

40. Webber RJ, Harris MG, Hough AJ Jr. Cell culture of rabbit meniscal fibrochondrocytes: proliferative and synthetic response to growth factors and ascorbate. *J Orthop Res* 1985;3:36–42.

41. Webber RJ, York L, Vander Schilden JL, et al. Fibrin clot invasion by rabbit meniscal fibrochondrocytes in organ culture. *Trans Orthop Res Soc* 1987;12:470.

42. Henning CD, Lynch M, Yearout K, et al. Arthroscopic meniscal repair using an exogenous fibrin clot. *Clin Orthop* 1990;252:64–72.

43. Van Trommel MF, Simonian PT, Potter HG, et al. Arthroscopic meniscal repair with fibrin clot of complete radial tears of the lateral meniscus in the avascular zone. *Arthroscopy* 1998;14: 360–365.

44. Poehling GG, Ruch DS, Chabon SJ. The landscape of meniscal injuries. *Clin Sports Med* 1990;9:539–549.

45. Warren RF, Marshall JL. Injuries of the anterior cruciate and medial collateral ligaments of the knee. *Clin Orthop* 1978;136: 191–197.

46. Henning CE. Current status of meniscus salvage. *Clin Sports Med* 1990;9:567–576.

47. Wickiewicz TL. Meniscal injuries in the cruciate-deficient knee. *Clin Sports Med* 1990;9:681–694.

48. Metcalf RW, Burks RT, Metcalf SM, et al. Arthroscopic meniscectomy. In: McGinty R, ed. *Operative arthroscopy.* Philadelphia: Lippincott-Raven, 1996:274–275.

49. Daniel D, Daniels E, Aronson, D. The diagnosis of meniscus pathology. *Clin Orthop* 1982;163:218–224.

50. Delee JC, Drez D. *Orthopedic sports medicine, principles and practice.* Philadelphia: W.B. Saunders, 1994:1146–1162.

51. Anderson AF, Lipscomb AB. Clinical diagnosis of meniscal tears: description of a new manipulative test. *Am J Sports Med* 1986;14:291–293.

52. Magee DJ. *Orthopedic physical assessment,* 3rd ed. Philadelphia: W.B. Saunders, 1987:506–593.

53. Fischer SP, Fox JM, Del Pizzo W, et al. Accuracy of diagnosis from magnetic resonance imaging of the knee. *J Bone Joint Surg* 1991;73:2–9.

54. Miller GK. A prospective study comparing the accuracy of the clinical diagnosis of meniscal tear with MRI and its effect on clinical outcome. *Arthroscopy* 1996;12:406–413.

55. Casscells SW. The place of arthroscopy in the diagnosis and treatment of internal derangement of the knee. *Clin Orthop* 1980; 151:135–142.

56. Fitzgibbons RE, Shellbourne KD. "Aggressive" nontreatment of lateral meniscal tears seen during anterior cruciate ligament reconstruction. *Am J Sports Med* 1995;23:156–159.

57. Jaureguito JW, Elliot JS, Lietner T, et al. Effects of arthroscopic partial lateral meniscectomy in an otherwise normal knee: a retrospective review of functional, clinical, and radiographic results. *Arthroscopy* 1995;11:29–36.

58. McGinty J, Geuss L, Marvin R. Partial or total meniscectomy. *J Bone Joint Surg Am* 1977;59:763.

59. Scott GA, Jolly BL, Henning CE. Combined posterior incision and arthroscopic intra-articular repair of the meniscus. An examination of factors affecting healing. *J Bone Joint Surg Am* 1986; 68:847–861.

60. Rubman MH, Noyes FR, Barber-Westin SD. Technical considerations in the management of complex meniscus tears. *Clin Sports Med* 1996;15:511–530.

61. Cannon WD. Arthroscopic meniscal repair. In: McGinty J, ed. *Operative arthroscopy.* New York: Raven Press, 1991:237–251.

62. DeHaven KE. Peripheral meniscal repair: An alternative to meniscectomy. *J Bone Joint Surg Br* 1981;63:463.

63. DeHaven KE. Meniscus repair: open vs. arthroscopic. *Arthroscopy* 1985;1:173–174.

64. DeHaven KE. Meniscus repair in the athlete. *Clin Orthop* 1985; 198:31–35.

65. DeHaven KE, Arnoczky SP. Meniscus repair: basic science, indications for repair and open repair. In: Schafer, M, ed. *Instructional course lectures.* St. Louis, MO: C.V. Mosby, 1994:65–75.

66. Rosenberg TD, Scott SM, Coward DB, et al. Arthroscopic meniscal repair evaluated with repeat arthroscopy. *Arthroscopy* 1986;2: 14–20.

67. Clancy WG, Graf BK. Arthroscopic meniscal repair. *Orthopaedics* 1983;6:1125–1128.

68. Warren RF. Arthroscopic meniscal repair. *Arthroscopy* 1985;1: 170–172.

69. Morgan CD, Casscells SW. Arthroscopic meniscus repair: a safe approach to the posterior horn. *Arthroscopy* 1986;2:3–12.

70. Morgan CD. The all-inside meniscus repair. *Arthroscopy* 1991;7: 120–125.

71. Albrect-Olsen P, Lind T, Kristensen G, et al. Failure strength of a new meniscus arrow repair technique: biomechanical comparison with horizontal suture. *Arthroscopy* 1997;13:183–187.

72. Dervin GF, Downing KJ, Hons BE, et al. Failure strengths of suture versus biodegradable arrow for meniscal repair: an in vitro study. *Arthroscopy* 1997;13:296–300.

73. Post WR, Akers SR, Kish V. Load to failure of common meniscal repair techniques: effects of suture technique and suture material. *Arthroscopy* 1997;13:731–736.

74. Barber FA, Gurwitz GS. Inflammatory synovial fluid and absorbable suture strength. *Arthroscopy* 1988;4:272–277.

75. Gershuni DH, Skyhar MJ, Danzig LA, et al. Experimental models to promote healing of tears in the avascular segment of canine knee menisci. *J Bone Joint Surg Am* 1989;71:1363–1370.

76. Barber FA. Accelerated rehabilitation for meniscus repairs. *Arthroscopy* 1996;10:206–210.

77. Mariani PP, Santori N, Adriani E, et al. Accelerated rehabilitation after arthroscopic meniscal repair: a clinic and magnetic resonance imaging evaluation. *Arthroscopy* 1996;12:680–686.

78. Morgan CD, Wojtys EM, Casscells CD, et al. Arthroscopic meniscal repair evaluated by second-look arthroscopy. *Am J Sports Med* 1991;19:632–637.

79. Deutsch AL, Mink JH, Fox JM, et al. Peripheral meniscal tears: MR findings after conservative treatment or arthroscopic repair. *Radiology* 1990;176:485–488.

80. Hamberg P, Gillquist J, Lysholm J. Suture of new and old peripheral meniscal tears. *J Bone Joint Surg Am* 1983;65:193–197.

81. DeHaven KE, Black KP, Griffith HJ. Open meniscus repair: technique and two to nine year results. *Am J Sports Med* 1989;17:788–795.

82. Tenuta JJ, Arciero RA. Arthroscopic evaluation of meniscal repairs: factors that effect healing. *Am J Sports Med* 1991;22:797–801.

83. Buseck M, Noyes FR. Arthroscopic evaluation of meniscal repairs after anterior cruciate ligament reconstruction and immediate motion. *Am J Sports Med* 1991;19:489–494.

84. Small N. Complications in arthroscopic surgery performed by experienced arthroscopists. *Arthroscopy* 1988;4:215–221.

85. Austin KS, Sherman OH. Complication of meniscal repair. *Sports Med* 1993;21:864–869.

86. Arnoczky SP, McDevitt CA, Schmidt MB, et al. The effect of cryopreservation in canine menisci: a biomechanical, morphologic, and biomechanical evaluation. *J Orthop Res* 1988;6:1–12.

87. Arnoczky SP, Warren RF, McDevitt CA. Meniscal replacement using a cryopreserved allograft. *Clin Orthop* 1990;252:121–128.

88. Jackson DW, McDevitt CA, Simon TM, et al. Meniscal transplantation using fresh and cryopreserved allografts. *Am J Sports Med* 1992;20:644–656.

89. Jackson DW, Simon TM. Biology of meniscal allograft. In: Mow VC, Arnoczky SP, Jackson DW, eds. *Knee meniscus: basic and clinical foundations.* New York: Raven Press, 1992:141–152.

90. Jackson DW, Whelan J, Simon TM. Cell survival after transplantation of fresh meniscal allografts. *Am J Sports Med* 1993;21:540–550.

91. Arnoczky SP, Milachowski KA. Meniscal allografts: where do we stand? In: Ewing JW, ed. *Articular cartilage and knee joint function: basic science and arthroscopy.* New York: Raven Press, 1990:129–136.

92. Garrett JC. Meniscal transplantation: a review of 43 cases with 2 to 7 year follow-up. *Sports Med Arthosc Rev* 1993;1:164–167.

93. Goble EM, Kane SM. Meniscal allografts. In: Czitrom AA, Winkler H, eds. *Orthopaedic allograft surgery.* New York: Springer-Verlag, 1996:243–252.

94. Noyes FR, Barber-Westin SD, Butler DL, et al. The role of allografts in repair and reconstruction of knee joint ligaments and menisci. *AAOS Instruct Course Lectures* 1998;47:379–396.

95. Shelton WR, Treacy SH, Dukes AD, et al. Use of allografts in knee reconstruction. II. Surgical considerations. *J Am Acad Orthop Surg* 1998;6:169–175.

96. Van Arkel ERA, deBoer HH. Human meniscal transplantation. *J Bone Joint Surg Br* 1995;77B:589–595.

97. Hamlet W, Liu SH, Yang R. Destruction of a cryopreserved meniscal allograft: a case for acute rejection. *J Arthrosc* 1997;13:517–521.

98. Stone KR, Steadman JR, Rodkey WG, et al. Regeneration of meniscal cartilage with the use of a collagen scaffold: analysis of preliminary data. *J Bone Joint Surg Am* 1997;79A:1770–1777.

99. Shelbourne DK, Patel DV, Adsit WS, et al. Rehabilitation after meniscal repair. *Clin Sports Med* 1996;15:595–612.

Principles and Practice of Orthopaedic Sports Medicine,
edited by William E. Garrett, Jr., Kevin P. Speer, and Donald T. Kirkendall.
Lippincott Williams & Wilkins, Philadelphia © 2000.

CHAPTER 37

Medial and Posteromedial Ligament Injuries of the Knee

C. Christopher Stroud and Bruce Reider

Injuries of the medial collateral ligament are common in athletes (1). Medial collateral ligament (MCL) injuries can occur in isolation or in association with other injured structures about the knee. They are most frequently seen in sports that involve the potential for direct trauma to the knee such as football, hockey, or rugby. Although it is less typical, the MCL can also be injured in activities that require cutting or twisting maneuvers such as basketball, soccer, and skiing. Most isolated injuries are benign, can be treated conservatively, and do not have long-term functional consequences to the athlete. However, combined injuries to the MCL and other knee structures are more serious and demand careful consideration and individualized treatment. It is incumbent on the treating sports-medicine physician to identify the injured structures, recognize associated injuries, and supervise a treatment program to optimize the recovery of the amateur or competitive athlete.

ANATOMY, PATHOANATOMY, AND MECHANISM OF INJURY

The anatomy of the medial aspect of the knee has been detailed by Warren and Marshall (2). The use of multiple terms to describe these structures has sometimes led to confusion. Warren and Marshall described a three-layer organization of the medial knee structures. Layer 1 is the deep investing fascia of the thigh. The MCL complex itself lies in layers 2 and 3 and is composed of two parts: a superficial part (also called the superficial

medial ligament or the tibial collateral ligament) and a deep portion (the knee joint capsular tissue) (Fig. 37.1).

The superficial MCL originates at the medial femoral epicondyle. Coursing distally and obliquely from this palpable bony landmark, these fibers insert into the proximal medial tibial metaphysis deep to the pes anserinus tendons (Fig. 37.1). Anteriorly, the fibers are subjected to increasing tension as the knee is flexed. Conversely, the posterior fibers of the superficial MCL relax slightly as the knee is flexed (3). This behavior is reversed when the knee is extended. This is due to the varying relationship of the fibers to the instant center of rotation of the knee. The superficial portion of the MCL complex has been shown to be the primary restraint to applied valgus loading of the knee, contributing 57% and 78% of medial stability at 5 and 25 degrees of knee flexion, respectively (4).

The deep portion of the MCL complex originates on the medial femoral condyle and inserts into the superior aspect of the medial meniscus. It then continues from the inferior portion of the meniscus to insert on the medial tibial metaphysis. The deep MCL consists of three parts: a thin anterior capsular portion, a midsection (consisting of the meniscofemoral and meniscotibial ligaments), and a posterior third (Fig. 37.1). Most authors recognize this third portion as the posterior oblique ligament, which consists of obliquely arranged fibers initially as part of the superficial MCL that then blend into the posteromedial capsule (5,6).

The deep MCL and posteromedial capsule act as secondary restraints at full knee extension, when this tissue is taut. The anterior and posterior cruciate ligaments have also been shown to provide secondary resistance to valgus loads (4,7,8), although much less than the medial structures. Therefore, which structures are injured depends on the position of the knee at the time of injury and the magnitude of the applied force. The

C. C. Stroud: Department of Orthopaedic Surgery, Union Memorial Hospital, Baltimore, Maryland 21218.
B. Reider: Department of Surgery (Orthopaedics), University of Chicago, Chicago, Illinois 60637.

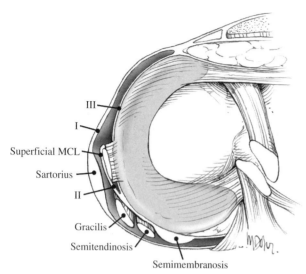

FIG. 37.1. Note the layers of the medial side of the knee and specifically the superficial medial collateral ligament as it originates from the medial femoral epicondyle to insert on the proximal medial tibial metaphysis. Cross-section at the level of the joint shows the three layers of the medial knee. Note how the deep medial collateral ligament attaches directly to the meniscal rim and how layers two and three blend together posteriorly.

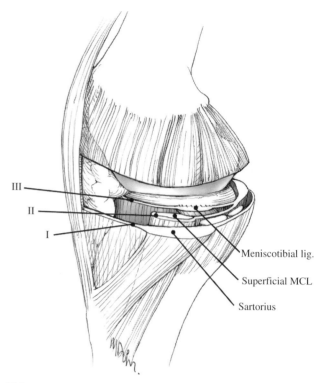

FIG. 37.2. The mechanism of most medial collateral ligament injuries involves a direct blow to the lateral aspect of the knee.

mechanism of most MCL injuries is the result of a direct blow to the lateral aspect of the knee. Distally, the tibial insertion is broad; therefore, injury most commonly occurs in the proximal portion of the ligament, at or near the femoral origin, or over the joint line. If the incident involves a rotatory component or is of severe magnitude, an associated cruciate ligament disruption may also occur.

CLINICAL EVALUATION

History

The patient with an MCL injury will usually describe receiving a blow to the lateral aspect of the knee (Fig. 37.2). He or she may describe a "rip" or a "tearing" with the sensation that the knee has "opened up." Initially, the pain is intense but may quickly diminish with time. A description of a noncontact mechanism or a feeling of rotation should increase the clinicians suspicion of a cruciate ligament injury.

Physical Examination

On initial inspection, there may be minimal or no swelling present (Fig. 37.3). As time progresses, there is usually local edema along the course of the ligament. If a large effusion is present, the clinician again must be wary of an intraarticular injury, particularly involving the cruciate ligaments. With the patient seated, the liga-

ment is then palpated as it courses obliquely from its origin on the femoral epicondyle to its insertion on the proximal medial tibia (Fig. 37.4). An area of swelling and localized tenderness often pinpoints the injured portion of the ligament. The ends of the disrupted ligament

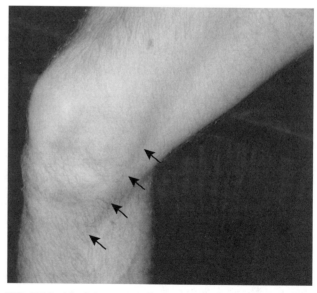

FIG. 37.3. Medial aspect of a right knee. *Arrows* denote the course of the superficial medial collateral ligament.

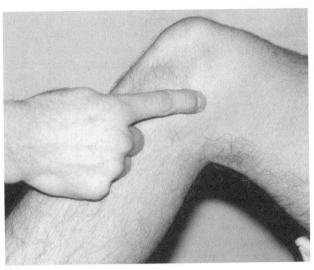

FIG. 37.4. Palpation of the course of the medial collateral ligament from its origin on the femoral epicondyle to its insertion on the proximal medial aspect of the tibia.

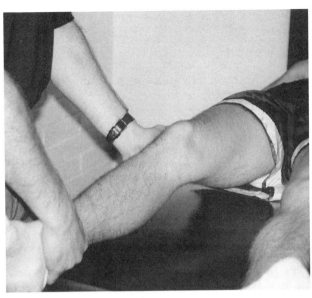

FIG. 37.6. Isolated testing of the superficial medial collateral ligament involves the same maneuver, however, with the knee in slight flexion.

can often be palpated if a lean individual is examined immediately after the injury.

The examiner then tests the stability of the medial structures with the patient in the supine position. The patient must be fully relaxed to obtain a reliable exami-

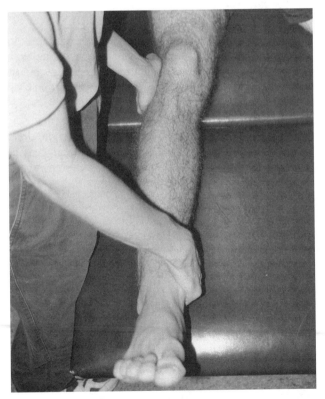

FIG. 37.5. Testing the medial collateral ligament in full extension involves applying a gentle valgus force to the relaxed patient's knee.

nation. The physician supports the injured leg, with one hand beneath the patient's heel. The outside hand is used to apply a gentle valgus force to the knee, first in full extension (Fig. 37.5). The knee is then flexed slightly to relax the posteromedial capsule, and the same gentle valgus force is applied (Fig. 37.6). This isolates the superficial MCL. The knee should not be flexed more than 10 to 15 degrees because unintended internal hip rotation will confound the examination. If the MCL is normal, the examiner will feel very little, if any, separation of the medial tibial plateau and medial femoral condyle in response to this stress. Any such separation will be met with a feeling of firm resistance or a "hard" end point. The contralateral knee is examined in a similar fashion for comparison. The testing is abnormal if excess medial opening is noted at either position. The amount of opening and quality of the end point is estimated and classified.

Classification

In the most commonly used classification system, a grade I sprain is marked by tenderness over the MCL. The ligament has been injured, but no elongation has occurred. The valgus stress test is painful but reveals no abnormal laxity and a firm end point. Grade II sprains include those in which the valgus stress test reveals an abnormal increase in laxity compared with the other side, but a firm end point is still detectable. In this situation, the ligament has been elongated but not disrupted. It can be difficult to accurately assess the character of the end point or the full amount of abnormal laxity because the valgus stress test is painful and induces protective guarding. Grade III tears are those knees with increased laxity in response to the valgus stress test with a soft or nonexistent end point. Here, the ligament has been totally disrupted, resulting in the loss of stability to the valgus test.

If abnormal laxity is noted in full extension and flexion, damage to the posteromedial capsule is present. In most of these cases there is also damage to one or both cruciate ligaments, so the examiner must evaluate the cruciates carefully when abnormal valgus laxity in full extension is noted.

Differential Diagnosis

The diagnosis of an MCL injury is usually evident with a careful history and physical examination. However, a few other conditions will present with pain localized to the medial side of the knee, including a medial bone contusion, subluxation or dislocation of the patella, or a medial meniscus tear.

A direct blow to the inner aspect of the knee may result in a contusion of the medial femoral condyle or proximal medial tibia. An exact description of the mechanism of injury and direct tenderness over the bony area will help distinguish this condition from an MCL injury. A contusion should not be associated with any abnormal laxity of the MCL.

Acute lateral patellar subluxation or dislocation may result from a direct blow to the patella or a twisting episode in which a sudden contraction of the quadriceps supplies the displacing force. The patient often experiences medial knee pain due to an avulsion of a portion of the vastus medialis obliquus origin from the adductor tubercle or intermuscular septum. Therefore, the physical examination will reveal tenderness at or near the adductor tubercle coursing proximally along the intermuscular septum. An associated medial retinacular tear, if present, will demonstrate tenderness along its insertion into the patella, rather than distally along the course of the MCL. Other physical examination findings, such as the apprehension sign, patella hypermobility, or stigmata of limb malalignment, differentiate these two conditions. Patellar subluxation and MCL sprain may sometimes occur concomitantly.

The patient with an acute medial meniscal tear will complain of medial knee pain. Examination may reveal an effusion, and tenderness is usually noted along the medial joint line. In these cases, valgus laxity should be normal. Thus, the main diagnostic difficulty arises in the face of a grade I MCL injury, in which no abnormal laxity is present. In cases in which the differentiation between a medial meniscus tear and a grade I MCL sprain is unclear, the clinician may choose to order a magnetic resonance imaging to help make the distinction. Alternatively, the patient may be followed clinically for a few weeks, because grade I MCL sprains should resolve rapidly, whereas symptoms from medial meniscus tears will usually persist.

In the skeletally immature athlete, the same forces that can produce an MCL sprain may cause a growth plate fracture. Most commonly, this would involve the distal femoral physis. Abnormal laxity associated with significant pain, swelling, and ecchymosis in an adolescent or preadolescent athlete should alert the clinician to suspect this diagnosis.

IMAGING

Routine plain radiographs of the knee, including anteroposterior, lateral, and notch views, should be obtained in all patients with a suspected knee injury. Although not helpful in the diagnosis of an isolated MCL injury, radiographs may reveal other pathology, such as a tibial plateau or growth plate fracture or an osteochondral defect.

Isolated MCL injuries rarely cause an avulsion fracture, but ectopic calcification near the medial epicondyle may subsequently develop. Radiographically, this is referred to as the Pelligrini-Stieda sign. Anterior or posterior cruciate ligament injuries may sometimes produce bony avulsions, usually involving the tibial attachment. In addition, anterior cruciate ligament (ACL) injuries are occasionally associated with the Segond fracture, a tibial flake avulsion fracture caused by the lateral capsule.

Magnetic resonance imaging provides excellent soft tissue resolution. Although rarely necessary in the evaluation of isolated collateral ligament injuries, magnetic resonance imaging provides important additional information useful to the clinician when other structures are involved. In the presence of persistent joint line tenderness, a magnetic resonance imaging will help the clinician determine whether a meniscal tear is present.

TREATMENT

Nonoperative

The treatment of an isolated MCL injury has undergone considerable change over the years. Early treatment consisted of direct surgical repair coupled with postoperative casting until the ligament healed (9–12). Flexion contractures and a loss of knee motion were common with this regime. Since then, immobilization has been shown to have deleterious effects on ligament healing and function. Woo et al. (13) noted a one-third decrease in the ultimate load to failure, compared with controls, of the MCL–bone complex after 9 weeks of immobilization in the rabbit. Not only were the mechanical properties of immobilized ligaments inferior to normals, but histologic alterations also occurred within the collagen structure, particularly at the tibial insertion site. In addition, with remobilization, the load to failure was significantly less than controls, and approximately 1 year was required for the ligament–bone junction to return to normal. Others have reported similar findings and have suggested that immobilization inhibits the maturation of healing ligaments as well (14).

Conversely, stress applied to healing MCL disruptions has been shown to have a beneficial effect on the microstructure and mechanical properties of ligaments (15–17). Gomez et al. (15) found that healing ligaments placed under tension had a higher total collagen content, more orderly arrangement of collagen fibrils, and more active remodeling than ligaments not placed under tension. The use of growth factors and gene therapy to influence healing of ligaments is also currently underway and appears to have promise (18).

Dissatisfaction with the results of surgical repair led to the popularity of nonsurgical therapy for most MCL disruptions. Subsequent clinical and animal studies have documented the satisfactory and often superior results of nonsurgical treatment coupled with an aggressive rehab program (19–30). In the laboratory, a study of MCL disruptions in mature dogs treated either nonsurgically or repaired with 3 and 6 weeks of subsequent immobilization showed that the longer period of immobilization resulted in significantly poorer mechanical properties in terms of varus–valgus laxity, load to failure, and tensile strength (28).

In a clinical study in 1983, Indelicato (24) evaluated 51 patients with an isolated complete MCL tear. Of the 36 patients available for follow-up, 16 were treated with operative repair and postoperative casting for 6 weeks, whereas 20 patients were treated nonoperatively with 2 weeks of cast immobilization followed by cast bracing for 4 weeks. A rehabilitation program followed. Equivalent good to excellent results were reported for both groups. However, the group treated with cast bracing, allowing knee motion, had a significantly quicker attainment of strength goals. The author stressed the importance of excluding associated ligamentous or meniscal injury, which ultimately affects treatment decisions and injury prognosis.

In a longitudinal study, Reider et al. (30) followed a group of recreational and competitive athletes with isolated MCL sprains for 5 years after treatment with an aggressive immediate functional rehabilitation program. They found that subjects did as well or better than historic controls treated with surgery or immobilization and continued to do well over time.

Therefore, an aggressive rehabilitation is currently favored for most isolated MCL injuries and is supported by basic science and clinical literature. This approach avoids the risks of surgery and allows the professional or recreational athlete to begin a rehabilitation program immediately after injury, thus returning the patient to competition in the shortest period of time.

Rehabilitation

Under the supervision of the physician, athletic trainer, or physical therapist, the rehabilitation of an MCL injury emphasizes the early return of motion and strength to the knee. Most programs are designed to allow the athlete to progress at his or her own pace, thus returning the patient to competition when physically and mentally ready. Player motivation is obviously a key component in the quick return to sporting activities. The primary goals to be met in any rehabilitation program include achieving full range of motion, regaining strength equal to uninjured limb, and completing an advancing series of sport-specific activities.

Once an isolated MCL injury has been identified, ice is immediately applied and the limb is elevated (Fig. 37.7). Water and ice may be placed in a plastic bag and applied directly to the medial knee for approximately 20 minutes. This is repeated every 3 to 4 hours for the first 48 hours. Ice acts as an anesthetic agent and induces local vasoconstriction, which may limit the initial hemorrhage and help contain secondary edema.

Treatment is then divided into three successive phases (Table 37.1). This goal-oriented approach allows the athlete to progress after certain basic criteria have been met in each phase. Rehabilitation time varies widely. The average time to return to sport is about 10 days for grade I injuries and 3 to 4 weeks in grade II or III injuries. Certain sports, such as soccer, place more stress on the MCL and may require a longer rehabilitation

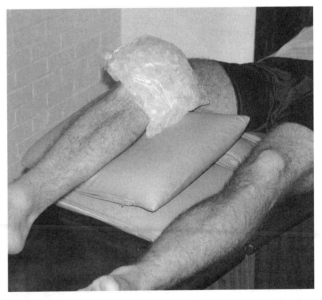

FIG. 37.7. Ice is applied to the medial knee immediately after injury and the limb is elevated.

TABLE 37.1. *Nonoperative rehabilitation program guide*

Phase I
  General
    Ice (intermittent) for 48 hr
    Elevate limb
    Electrical stimulation (E-stim)
  Weight bearing as tolerated
    Crutches may be used
  Improve range of motion
    Extension
      Towel extensions
      Prone hangs
    Flexion
      Bend over bed/table
      Wall/heel slides
Phase II
  Continue knee range of motion
  Strengthening of lower extremity
    Knee bends
    Gentle squats (no weights initially)
    Progress to resistance exercises
      Knee extensions
      Leg press
      Leg curls
  Overall conditioning
    Pool exercises
    Stationary bike (seat lowered to increase flexion)
    StairMaster
Phase III
  Continue range-of-motion/strengthening exercises
  Sport-specific activities (orderly progression)
    Walking
    Jogging
    Running
    Cutting

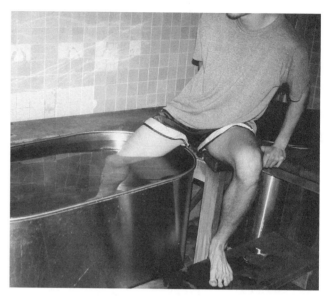

FIG. 37.8. The acutely injured knee can be immersed in a cold water bath while range of motion exercises are performed.

We recommend full-time use of the brace for the first 3 or 4 weeks, with removal permitted only for washing. Knee immobilizers or full-leg braces are excessive for this purpose and are discouraged.

The athlete strives to obtain extension or hyperexten-

time, whereas some athletes seem to progress more slowly than the norm.

Phase I

The patient is allowed to bear weight as tolerated. Crutches may be used initially and are discarded when the athlete is able to ambulate without a limp. A normal gait is usually achieved within this first week after injury. Range of motion exercises are begun as soon as possible. Initially, this can be performed in a cold whirlpool or concurrently with icing while the knee is acutely painful (Fig. 37.8).

If a grade II or III injury is present, a brace should be applied to the knee to support the MCL against valgus stresses during the healing phase. We have found the lightweight hinged braces, originally designed for prevention of bike injuries, to be optimal for this purpose because they protect the healing MCL from the low level valgus stresses that may occur during daily activities but do not limit motion or inhibit muscle function (Fig. 37.9). The athlete may subsequently wear the same brace, if desired, during the initial return to sports.

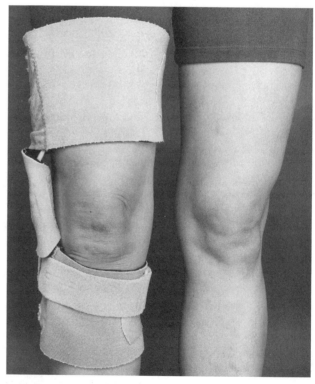

FIG. 37.9. A lightweight unilateral hinged brace is applied to the knee (McDavid, Inc., Clarendon Hills, IL).

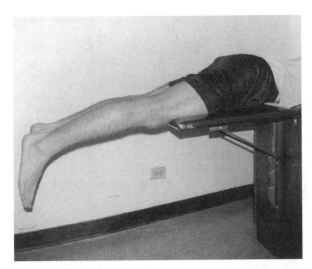

FIG. 37.10. In the prone hang exercise, both legs of the patient are suspended from the end of a table to allow full extension of the injured knee.

sion equivalent to the uninjured limb. This can be promoted through the use of towel extension exercises, in which a rolled towel or other object is placed beneath the patient's heel and the entire limb is elevated off the surface. Prone hangs, in which the patient lies prone with both limbs off the end of a table or bed, are very useful to help achieve full extension (Fig. 37.10). A heavy shoe or light ankle weight can be added to facilitate this exercise.

To improve flexion, the patient is seated on the end of a table or bed and uses gravity to attain knee flexion. The uninjured limb can be used as an assistive device for increasing flexion. Wall slides are performed with the patient supine and the legs initially extended against a wall. The contralateral limb is used for assistance as the injured leg is gradually flexed under gravity control (Fig. 37.11). Heel slides are performed with the patient sitting, grasping the ankle, and moving the knee to achieve greater than 90 degrees of flexion (Fig. 37.12).

It is not uncommon for the athlete to be unable to achieve full flexion or extension initially, because portions of the injured fibers of the MCL are stressed and may cause pain in these positions. Isometric quadriceps sets and straight leg raises help limit muscle disuse and atrophy. Electrical muscle stimulation can also be added and may act to limit reflex muscle inhibition and confuse or diminish pain input to the higher cortical centers (Fig. 37.13). This phase is completed when normal gait, minimal swelling, a full range of motion, and a baseline of quadriceps control have been achieved.

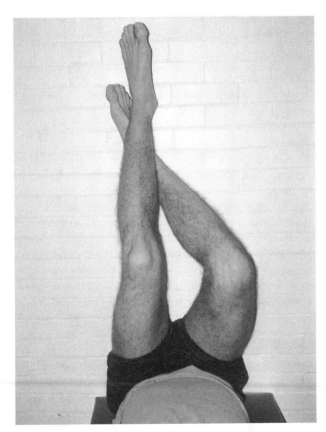

FIG. 37.11. In the wall slide exercise, the patient begins supine with both legs up against a wall. Using the uninjured limb for assistance, the knee is slowly lowered to improve knee flexion.

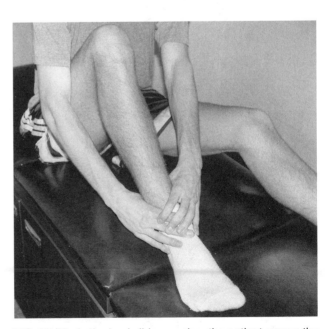

FIG. 37.12. In the heel slide exercise, the patient grasps the ankle of the extremity and slowly bends the knee to achieve increasing amounts of flexion.

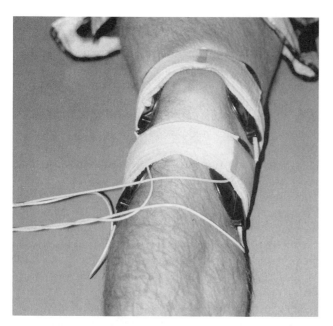

FIG. 37.13. Electrical stimulation can be applied to the injured knee to help provide a stimulus for muscular contractions in the initial phase after injury.

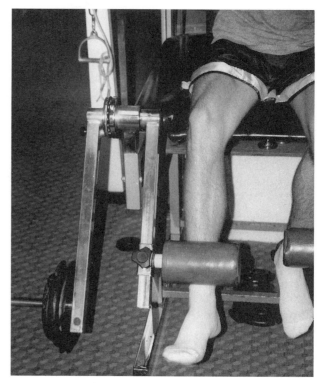

FIG. 37.15. Knee extensions and leg curls can be performed on a standard weight bench.

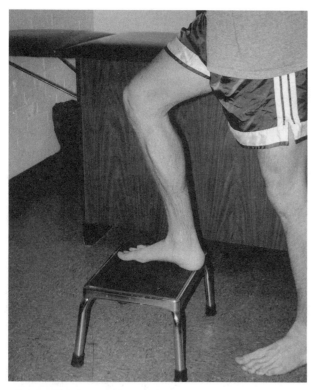

FIG. 37.14. Step-up exercises are useful in the initial rehabilitation program to promote the return of lower extremity muscular function.

Phase II

Strengthening exercises are then added while full motion is maintained. Any increase in pain or swelling is a sign that an inflammatory response is present and the athlete is progressing too quickly. Knee bends, step-ups, and squats without weights are first used (Fig. 37.14). The athlete then progresses to the use of light resistance exercises with a standard isotonic weight bench, including knee extensions, leg press, and leg curls (Fig. 37.15). Initially, light-weight high-repetition exercises are performed and are advanced to lower repetitions with higher weights. Swimming, stationary cycling, and the use of a stair climber are added to the program to maintain upper body, aerobic, and lower extremity conditioning. This phase is completed when strength of the injured extremity reaches 80% to 90% of the uninjured leg.

Phase III

The final phase focuses on a return to the athlete's previous sporting activity. The guidance of a trainer or physical therapist is particularly helpful in this phase to assess the athlete's progress and provide guidance in the proper performance of these activities.

If not already prescribed, a unilateral hinged brace is usually given to the athlete to provide some support to the healing MCL and a measure of protection against further injury. Several brace designs are available, but the applied brace should be lightweight, durable, and properly fit. Biomechanical and clinical studies have produced conflicting evidence with regards to a beneficial effect of brace use in preventing injury to the MCL (31–35). However, their use may provide the athlete with some measure of psychological support and protection to the MCL and ACL against lateral loads. Therefore, their use is currently recommended, at least in the rehabilitation process and during the remaining portion of the current season of contact sports.

A progressive running program, beginning with fast speed walking and advancing to light jogging, is performed. When comfortable, straight line running and then sprinting are introduced. Finally, cutting and pivoting exercises such as wind sprints, figure-of-eight drills, and cariocas are added. As can be seen, this orderly progression of drills and exercises allows the athlete to proceed according to his or her own level of comfort and motivation. If at any point the athlete experiences pain, increased swelling, or feels unable to accomplish any particular exercise, the program is suspended for that particular day. The athlete is able to return to competition only when he or she has successfully completed a prescribed list of functional activities.

When to Refer

The evaluation and treatment of MCL injuries requires considerable knowledge of the anatomic structures of the knee, the indications for nonoperative and operative treatment, and the complications or adverse effects that may develop. Therefore, referral may be considered when the treating primary care physician believes that an athlete may benefit from the supervision of a sports-medicine physician experienced in dealing with trainers, physical therapists, and injuries of the knee. This includes significant MCL tears that occur in isolation or are associated with other injured ligamentous or meniscal structures. If the athlete fails to progress in a reasonable amount of time, that is, when there is continued pain, swelling, or full motion is not quickly obtained, then referral is indicated.

Expected Outcome

As already mentioned, most isolated MCL tears can be successfully treated nonoperatively with minimal functional consequences. In the literature, outcomes have been assessed by evaluating medial knee stability, return to play, and reinjury rates. In 1974, Ellsasser et al. (20) found that 69 of 74 (93%) isolated grade III MCL injuries in professional football players treated with immediate motion and rehabilitation were able to return to play in less than 8 weeks. In the study by Indelicato (24), although both groups had nearly equivalent numbers of

good to excellent results and 85% of patients had less than 5 mm of increased valgus laxity compared with the uninjured limb, he noted that none of the knees "could be classified as normal in terms of stability" when compared with the contralateral side. Although this study had a relatively short follow-up (2 to 4 years), the results indicate little functional consequence of this minor degree of laxity.

In a later study, Indelicato et al. (22) found that 20 of 21 intercollegiate football players had good to excellent results after nonoperative treatment of isolated grade III MCL injuries. The rehabilitation program consisted of an initial 2-week casting period followed by mobilization in a long leg orthosis and allowed players to return to play in an average of 9.2 weeks. All players had less than 5 mm of medial laxity at follow-up examination.

In an epidemiologic study, Derscheid and Garrick (36) noted that the number of practice days lost in 51 grade I or II MCL sprains was 10.6 and 19.5 days, respectively. Interestingly, they noted that the spring season accounted for a threefold increase in the rate of these injuries and that the risk of reinjury was not statistically greater than the overall rate of injury. Jones et al. (25) noted similar findings in high school football players.

Reider et al. (30) prospectively followed 33 athletic patients with 34 grade III MCL injuries with an average follow-up of 5.2 years. Patients were treated with immediate motion and aggressive rehabilitation with use of a minimally restrictive hinged knee brace. They reported 100% good to excellent results when rated by the Hospital for Special Surgery Knee scale. Of the 29 patients with 30 injuries available for follow-up examination, 25 knees had residual increased valgus laxity of 5 mm or less compared with the contralateral side. Overall, 21 of 34 (62%) athletes returned to sports in less than 4 weeks, whereas 84% of collegiate football players did so in the same period. However, although most athletes were able to return relatively quickly, most patients did not believe that they were completely recovered until 2 to 4 months after the injuries. This did not affect the reinjury rate, because only one player was reinjured within this time frame. In regards to residual symptoms, 18 of 30 patients at the follow-up examination reported mild pain in the knee, though most listed this as occasional. Eleven of 30 patients reported the knee felt loose, but 10 of these stated this happened occasionally with stressful activities only. Swelling and crepitus were reported as occasionally present in seven and six patients, respectively, although an additional six believed crepitus occurred frequently. Upon return to athletics, only 7 of 33 patients believed that their performance was less than their preinjury level.

As can be seen, most grade I, II, and III MCL injuries are successfully treated nonoperatively. Most individuals can return to their preinjury sporting activity in a relatively short period of time, but a slightly longer time period may be required until the knee feels normal again. Residual symptoms and minor valgus laxity are relatively common but seemingly do not appear to have functional consequences.

Operative

Operative repair of an isolated MCL disruption is controversial. As mentioned, in the past, tears of this ligament were routinely repaired regardless of severity (10,12). Since then, conservative treatment has been shown to be at least equivalent to surgical repair, while returning the patients to previous activities at a faster rate. Clinicians may still consider surgical treatment of MCL injuries in cases in which there is increased valgus laxity in both flexion and full extension.

Although it is rare for such an injury to occur without disruption of one or both cruciate ligaments, cases such as this have been reported (21,27,30). These cases are so unusual, however, that it is difficult to advance beyond the level of personal opinion in recommending treatment. In 17 years of practice, the senior author has not operated on any cases of isolated MCL injuries.

A more common situation in which surgical treatment is sometimes considered is when the MCL is injured in combination with one or both cruciates ligaments. In the case of an associated ACL injury, one of two injury patterns may be seen: grade I, II, or III MCL/ACL injury when knee is stable to valgus stress in extension or MCL/ACL injury with the knee unstable to valgus stress in extension.

The literature provides some guidelines for the first situation and is unclear in the second. Shelbourne and Porter (37), in a preliminary report, discussed the results of the management of combined MCL/ACL injuries in 68 patients. Follow-up averaged 1 year. They concluded that nonoperative management of the MCL coupled with reconstruction of the ACL led to excellent subjective and objective results, including stability, strength, and range of motion of the injured limb. However, no data were given regarding residual valgus laxity and the grade of MCL tears in the study. In addition, approximately 20% of patients required either manipulation or arthroscopic scar excision to regain motion.

Noyes and Barber-Westin (38) reported on a subgroup of 34 patients with a combined MCL/ACL injury, where the knee was unstable in extension to valgus testing. These patients were treated with allograft ACL reconstruction and operative repair of the superficial and deep MCL. They noted that 82% had less than 5.5 mm of anterior displacement at follow-up and a negative pivot shift. Also, they noted that nine (36%) patients required individualized treatment for diminished range of motion, consisting of either manipulation or arthroscopic scar excision. Half of the patients were

able to return to sporting activities, albeit at a lower level of performance. They noted seven patients with moderate patellofemoral crepitus at follow-up. Concern regarding the increased prevalence of motion complications and the number of patients with patellofemoral complaints led them to recommend treating these combined injuries in a staged manner, with initial nonoperative treatment of the medial structures consisting of 3 to 4 weeks of brace protection and partial weight bearing and followed by reconstruction of the ACL in active individuals at a later date.

Animal studies have provided further support to allowing the MCL to heal with later reconstruction of the ACL in such combined injuries (39–41). Rabbits with a combined MCL/ACL injury were treated with ACL reconstruction using a flexor tendon allograft. The rabbits were divided into two groups. In one group, the MCL was repaired. In the other group, the torn ends were opposed but not sutured. The restraint to valgus testing in the repaired group was improved at 12 weeks (39) over the unrepaired animal group, but no difference in ligament stiffness or ultimate load was noted by 52 weeks (41). The anterior stability was equal in both groups. The authors concluded that primary MCL repair provided little or no long-term benefit to MCL healing after ACL reconstruction.

It should be stressed that no formal prospective randomized comparison of operatively treated versus nonoperatively treated severe MCL injuries in combination with ACL disruptions has been reported in the literature. Furthermore, if repair of the medial structures in this combined injury pattern is planned, the surgeon and patient must be prepared to accept the increased risk of stiffness and range-of-motion difficulties in return for the benefits of anatomic restoration of the injured structures. The current practice of the senior author is to perform direct repair of the MCL when abnormal valgus laxity in full extension is present in combination with disruption of one or both cruciate ligaments.

Surgical Technique

Once the decision has been made to proceed with repair of the medial structures, an examination under anesthesia is performed to confirm the diagnosis and document any addition instability. The arthroscopic examination and reconstruction of the disrupted cruciate ligament(s) is performed first. One end of each cruciate graft is fixed, usually on the femoral side, whereas the remaining end is left until the repair sutures have been placed in the MCL complex.

The exposure of the MCL depends on the concomitant surgery being performed. If only small incisions are needed for the other structures, as when allografts are used to reconstruct the cruciates, the MCL can be approached through a straight incision that begins over the medial femoral epicondyle proximally and continues longitudinally over the course of the superficial MCL to end just medial to the tibial tubercle. When the central third of the patellar tendon is used as an ACL or posterior cruciate ligament (PCL) autograft, the incision begins closer to the patella so that the MCL repair and autograft harvest can be accomplished through the same incision. A medial flap is raised to the epicondyle and joint line for exposure of the posteromedial structures.

Once the incision is made, layer 1, the sartorial fascia, is first encountered. Usually this layer is intact, although in severe injuries it will be disrupted as well. An incision is then made over the course of the superficial MCL. The site of ligament disruption is usually immediately evident. Deep to the fibers of the superficial MCL, the capsular tear is visualized. The fascia of layer 1 is retracted posteriorly to completely expose the disruption. Once adequate exposure has been obtained, nonabsorbable sutures are placed in a horizontal mattress fashion beginning at the most posterior aspect of the capsular tear and left untied. The repair then proceeds anteriorly. If the capsular tissue has been avulsed directly off the femur or tibia (a meniscofemoral or meniscotibial ligament disruption), this area is cleared of debris and suture anchors or drill holes are placed to facilitate direct reattachment to bone. If the capsular tissue has been avulsed from the peripheral rim of the medial meniscus, it is repaired directly to this structure using vertical sutures through the full thickness of the meniscal rim. Because plastic deformation of the damaged tissues has usually occurred, suture placement should be designed to imbricate the disrupted ligaments enough to restore the anatomic length.

The superficial MCL is then repaired. Disruption may occur at the femoral or tibial insertion sites or in the midsubstance of the ligament. When the ligament has been avulsed from either bony insertion, it is fixed using a screw with a spiked soft tissue washer. It is extremely important to anatomically restore the avulsed ligament to its proper attachment site.

A midsubstance disruption of the superficial MCL is repaired with a large nonabsorbable suture using a tendon repair stitch such as the Krackow technique. Care must be taken to securely reapproximate the ligament without overtightening it. The knee is taken through a range of motion to assess suture placement and the adequacy of the repair.

After all sutures have been placed to repair the deep and superficial components of the MCL, the knee is placed in a reduced position and the fixation of the cruciate graft or grafts is completed. The sutures of the deep capsular layer are then tied sequentially, beginning with the most posterior portion of the tear and progressing anteriorly. The superficial MCL is then fixed. At each stage of the closure, the knee is taken through a full range of motion to verify that motion is not restricted and that the sutures do not break or tear through the tissue.

When there is insufficient ligament tissue for a direct repair, reconstruction of the superficial MCL can be accomplished using the semitendinosus tendon (12,42,43). The tendon is mobilized proximally, leaving its distal attachment intact. The dissection is continued until the tendon can be placed up against the anatomic origin of the superficial MCL at the medial femoral epicondyle. The graft is held in place with a small Kirschner wire, and the ligament isometry is assessed. Finding the most isometric point for fixing this tendon is critical. The tendon is then fixed using a screw and spiked soft tissue washer. The tendon may also be sutured to adjacent tissue on the epicondyle for additional fixation. Once again the knee is taken through a range of motion to assess the fixation and isometry.

The sartorial fascia, subcutaneous tissue, and skin are reapproximated. A drain may be placed if necessary. A sterile dressing and a hinged knee immobilizer locked in extension are placed.

Postoperative Rehabilitation

Postoperatively, the knee is placed in a brace set to limit flexion. The range set depends on the strength of the fixation and is usually set at between 0 and 60 degrees of flexion initially. The patient is instructed to lock the brace in full extension while ambulating. Weight bearing as tolerated is allowed with crutch support. A continuous passive motion machine may be used in the initial postoperative period. After a period of 5 to 7 days, an aggressive active range-of-motion program is begun to prevent stiffness. The amount of flexion is gradually increased over the next 2 weeks. The brace is worn for the first 6 to 8 weeks after surgery and can then be discontinued. A rehabilitation program similar to the one described for nonoperative management is then begun.

Expected Outcomes

The outcomes after MCL repair is usually a function of the concomitant injuries. Significant damage to the articular cartilage will compromise the prognosis. It is common to find a few millimeters of residual valgus laxity, although this does not seem to be associated with any functional limitations.

SUMMARY

Most MCL injuries respond well to closed treatment with an aggressive rehabilitation program. This applies to most MCL injuries associated with ACL disruptions as well. Surgical repair is occasionally indicated when severely abnormal valgus laxity is encountered as part of a multiple ligament injury. Such surgery must be performed meticulously, with strict attention to the identification and anatomic repair of damaged structures.

REFERENCES

1. Wilson SA, Vigorita VJ, Scott WN. Anatomy. In: Scott WN, ed. *The knee.* St. Louis, MO: Mosby, 1994:15–54.
2. Warren LF, Marshall JL. The supporting structures and layers on the medial side of the knee. An anatomical analysis. *J Bone Joint Surg Am* 1979;61A:56–62.
3. Warren LF, Marshall JL, Gingis F. The prime static stabilizer of the medial side of the knee. *J Bone Joint Surg Am* 1974;56A:665–674.
4. Grood ES, Noyes FR, Butler DL, et al. Ligamentous and capsular restraints preventing straight medial and lateral laxity in intact human cadaver knees. *J Bone Joint Surg Am* 1981;63A:1257–1269.
5. Hughston JC, Eilers AF. The role of the POL in repairs of acute MCL tears of the knee. *J Bone Joint Surg Am* 1973;55A:923–940.
6. Hughston JC, Andres JR, Cross MF, et al. Classification of knee ligament instabilities. Part I. The medial compartment and cruciate ligaments. *J Bone Joint Surg Am* 1976;58A:159–172.
7. Haimes JL, Wroble RR, Grood ES, et al. Role of the medial structures in the intact and ACL-deficient knee—limits of motion in the human knee. *Am J Sports Med* 1994;22:402–409.
8. Inoue M, McGurk-Burleson E, Hollis JM, et al. Treatment of the medial collateral ligament injury: the importance of anterior cruciate ligament on varus-valgus knee laxity. *Am J Sports Med* 1987;15:15–21.
9. Hughston JC, Barrett GR. Acute anteromedial rotatory instability: long-term results of surgical repair. *J Bone Joint Surg Am* 1983;65A:145–153.
10. O'Donoghue DH. Surgical treatment of fresh injuries to the major ligaments of the knee. *J Bone Joint Surg Am* 1950;32:721–738.
11. Quigley TB. The treatment of avulsion of the collateral ligaments of the knee. *Am J Sports Med* 1987;15:331–341.
12. McMurray TP. The operative treatment of ruptured internal lateral ligament of the knee. *Br J Surg* 1918;6:377–381.
13. Woo SLY, Gomez MA, Sites TJ, et al. The biomechanical and morphological changes in the medial collateral ligament of the rabbit after immobilization and remobilization. *J Bone Joint Surg Am* 1987;69A:1200–1211.
14. Walsh S, Frank C, Shrive N, et al. Knee immobilization inhibits biomechanical maturation of the rabbit medial collateral ligament. *Clin Orthop* 1993;297:253–261.
15. Gomez MA, Woo SL, Amiel D. The effects of increased tension on medial collateral ligaments. *Am J Sports Med* 1991;19:347–354.
16. Hart DP, Dahners LE. Healing of the medial collateral ligament in rats. The effects of repair, motion and secondary stabilizing ligaments. *J Bone Joint Surg Am* 1987;69A:1194–1199.
17. Tipton CM, James SL, Mergner W, et al. Influence of exercise on strength of medial collateral knee ligaments of dogs. *Am J Physiol* 1970;218:894–902.
18. Woo SLY, Chan SS, Yamaji T. Biomechanics of knee ligament healing, repair and reconstruction. *J Biomech* 1997;30:431–439.
19. Ballimer PM, Jakob RP. The nonoperative treatment of isolated complete tears of the medial collateral ligament of the knee. A prospective study. *Arch Orthop Trauma Surg* 1988;107:273–276.
20. Ellsasser JC, Reynolds FC, Omohundro JR. The non-operative treatment of collateral ligament injuries of the knee in professional football players. An analysis of seventy-four injuries treated nonoperatively and twenty-four injuries treated surgically. *J Bone Joint Surg Am* 1974;56A:1185–1190.
21. Fetto J, Marshall JH. Medial collateral ligament injuries of the knee: a rationale for treatment. *Clin Orthop* 1978;132:206–218.
22. Indelicato PA, Hermansdorfer J, Huegel M. Nonoperative management of complete tears of the medial collateral ligament of the knee in intercollegiate football players. *Clin Orthop* 1990;256:174–177.
23. Indelicato PA. Isolated medial collateral ligament injuries in the knee. *J Am Acad Orthop Surg* 1995;3:9–14.
24. Indelicato PA. Nonoperative treatment of complete tears of the medial collateral ligament of the knee. *J Bone Joint Surg Am* 1983;65A:323–329.
25. Jones RE, Henley MB, Francis P. Nonoperative management of isolated grade III collateral ligament injury in high school football players. *Clin Orthop* 1986;213:137–140.
26. Kannus P. Long-term results of conservatively treated medial collateral ligament injuries of the knee joint. *Clin Orthop* 1988;226:103–112.
27. Mok DW, Good C. Nonoperative management of acute grade III medial collateral ligament injury of the knee: a prospective study. *Injury* 1989;20:277–280.
28. Woo SLY, Inoue M, McGurk-Burleson E, et al. Treatment of the medial collateral ligament injury. II. structure and function of canine knees in response to differing treatment regimens. *Am J Sports Med* 1987;15:22–29.
29. Wilk KE, Andrews JR, Clancy WG. Nonoperative and postoperative rehabilitation of the collateral ligaments of the knee. *Opin Tech Sports Med* 1996;4:192–201.
30. Reider B, Sathy MR, Talkington J, et al. Treatment of isolated medial collateral ligament injuries in athletes with early functional rehabilitation. *Am J Sports Med* 1993;22:470–476.
31. Baker BE, Van Hanswyk E, Bogosian S, et al. A biomechanical study of the static stabilizing effect on knee braces on medial stability. *Am J Sports Med* 1987;15:566–570.
32. Paulos LE, Cawley PW, France EP. Impact biomechanics of lateral knee bracing. The anterior cruciate ligament. *Am J Sports Med* 1991;19:337–342.
33. Erickson AR, Tasuda K, Beynnon B, et al. An in vitro dynamic evaluation of prophylactic knee braces during lateral impact loading. *Am J Sports Med* 1993;21:26–35.
34. Teitz CC, Hermanson BK, Kronmal RA, et al. Evaluation of the use of braces to prevent injury to the knee in collegiate football players. *J Bone Joint Surg Am* 1987;69A:2–9.
35. Sitler S, Ryan J, Hopkinson W, et al. The efficiency of a prophylactic knee brace to reduce knee injuries in football: a prospective randomized study at West Point. *Am J Sports Med* 1990;18:310–315.
36. Derscheid GL, Garrick JG. Medial collateral ligament injuries in football: nonoperative management of grade I and grade II sprains. *Am J Sports Med* 1981;9:365–368.
37. Shelbourne KD, Porter DA. Anterior cruciate ligament-medial collateral ligament injury. Nonoperative management of medial collateral ligament tears with anterior cruciate ligament reconstruction. A preliminary report. *Am J Sports Med* 1992;20:283–286.
38. Noyes FR, Barber-Westin SD. The treatment of acute combined ruptures of the anterior cruciate and medial ligaments of the knee. *Am J Sports Med* 1995;23:380–391.
39. Ohno K, Pomaybo AS, Schmidt CC, et al. Healing of the MCL after a combined MCL and ACL injury and reconstruction of the ACL: comparison of repair and nonrepair of MCL tears in rabbits. *J Orthop Res* 1995;13:442–449.
40. Woo SLY, Young EP, Ohland KJ, et al. The effects of transection of the anterior cruciate ligament on healing of the medial collateral ligament. A biomechanical study of the knee in dogs. *J Bone Joint Surg Am* 1990;72A:382–392.
41. Yamaji T, Levine RF, Woo SLY, et al. MCL healing one year after a concurrent MCL and ACL injury: an interdisciplinary study in rabbits. *J Orthop Res* 1996;14:223–227.
42. Bosworth DM. Transplantation of the semitendinosus for repair of laceration of medial collateral ligament of the knee. *J Bone Joint Surg Am* 1952;34A:196–202.
43. Helfet AJ. Injuries of the capsular and cruciate ligaments. In: Helfet AJ, ed. *Disorders of the knee,* 2nd ed. Philadelphia: J.B. Lippincott, 1982:329–342.

Principles and Practice of Orthopaedic Sports Medicine,
edited by William E. Garrett, Jr., Kevin P. Speer, and Donald T. Kirkendall.
Lippincott Williams & Wilkins, Philadelphia © 2000.

CHAPTER 38

Posterolateral Injuries of the Knee

Michael J. Maynard

The diagnosis and treatment of injuries to the structures comprising the posterolateral corner of the knee has recently entered an evolutionary phase. This is attributable to two factors: the recent appearance of important information, shedding new light on this subject, that has fostered improving awareness among orthopedic surgeons concerning the structure and function of the key elements in this zone and advancements in magnetic resonance imaging (MRI) technology that have allowed meaningful scrutiny and reinforcement of this new information.

Although isolated injuries to discrete structures of the posterolateral knee have been known to occur, the largest published series describing acute and/or chronic posterolateral knee injuries have indicated that they are much more commonly recognized in combination with associated cruciate ligament injuries.

ANATOMY AND BIOMECHANICS

Background

Historically, advancement of the practice of orthopedic surgery has required the gradual perfection of information regarding the structure and function of injured anatomic elements as foundation for the evolution of improved diagnostic logic and increasingly effective therapeutic options. Experience has demonstrated that as the quality of available information pertinent to a particular injury pattern reaches a critical level, probably closely approximating the absolute, clinical therapeutic success optimizes. Numerous examples reflect the fact that when this happens, the resulting satisfaction within the orthopedic community has often engendered the emergence of a universally accepted diagnosis and treatment rationale or "standard of care."

Thus far, no consistently satisfactory approach to the diagnosis and treatment of injuries to the posterolateral knee has emerged. In fact, several widely varying approaches to surgical reconstruction are currently advocated by several different surgeons of world-class reputation. This would appear to signify that until this time, the absolute quality of the available information concerning the structure and function of the posterolateral knee has been relatively poor.

A plausible explanation for this is that the development of anatomic information about the posterolateral corner of the knee suffered a unique setback near the middle of the 20th century. At that time, a major revision of the universally accepted anatomic nomenclature, the *Nomina Anatomica,* was published by an international congress of anatomists. The new listing of anatomic structures inadvertently omitted inclusion of a previously described and accepted connection of the popliteus tendon to the styloid of the fibula (i.e. the popliteofibular ligament (PFL). This omission was recognized by the prominent orthopedic anatomist R.J. Last. Although he explained the error in an article published in the *Journal of Bone and Joint Surgery* in 1950, his point was not fully understood either within or outside the orthopedic community. Clearly, the error was not effectively corrected with respect to the scientific community as a whole—as evidenced by the fact that since 1970, several other anatomists, ostensibly unaware of Last's work, have "rediscovered" the PFL. However, because their findings were published in that portion of the scientific literature that is most familiar to anatomists, this information did not filter through to the end users, orthopedic surgeons, until the 1990s. In fact, as a direct reflection of this error, English-language anatomy textbooks published since 1950 lack a description of any structure resembling the PFL.

Consequently, the anatomic and biomechanical studies of the posterolateral corner that have appeared over the past 40 years were founded on an incomplete knowl-

M. J. Maynard: Department of Orthopaedic Surgery, The Hospital for Special Surgery, New York, New York 10021.

edge base. Perhaps the most important and thoughtful accounts of the posterolateral anatomy that appeared in the orthopedic literature between 1950 and 1990 were published by Seebacher et al. and by Kaplan. These reports were essentially silent concerning the existence of a structurally important attachment of the popliteus tendon to the fibula. Not surprisingly, the major biomechanical investigations of the posterolateral corner published during this time period also reflected ignorance of a direct attachment of the popliteus tendon to the fibula. In retrospect, however, the results reported in these biomechanical studies ironically point to its existence. Most notably in this regard, Gollehon et al. introduced the concept of a "static function" of the popliteus—a term coined to describe the curious finding that the cadaveric popliteus muscle belly apparently developed reproducibly quantifiable tension under repeated mechanical stress testing conditions. In the light of knowledge of the PFL's existence, the mystery of this static function of the popliteus has subsequently been resolved.

Several other factors have contributed to the overall confusion in this area. For example, most anatomic reports have routinely emphasized variability in both the "robustness" and in the presence or absence of various structures in the posterolateral knee. Another factor is that all anatomic descriptions of the posterolateral knee have presented a bewildering array of "important" structures in the complete absence of any attempt to establish their relative biomechanical significance or, more germanely, their surgical relevance.

Recent Contributions

Since 1990, the PFL has reappeared in the orthopedic literature. In 1990, Sudasna et al. reported the presence of a popliteus tendon and a lateral collateral ligament (LCL) in 100% and a PFL in 98% of 50 cadaveric specimens. In this report, the next most commonly found structure was the fabellofibular ligament (FFL), which was present in 68%. In a 1993 report on the dissection of 115 knees, Watanabe et al. found a popliteus tendon and an LCL in 100% and a PFL in 94% of specimens. The next most common structure, again the febellofibular ligament, was found to be present 51% of the time. In 1996, Maynard et al. reported finding a popliteus tendon, an LCL, and a PFL in 100% of 20 knees dissected in preparation for biomechanical testing. This report did not comment on the presence of other structures.

Importantly, the anatomic reports by Kaplan and by Seebacher et al. compare closely with the reports by Sudasna et al. and Watanabe et al. regarding the relative incidence of the popliteus tendon, LCL, FFL, short lateral ligament (SLL), and arcuate ligament (AL).

Making Sense of the Posterolateral Anatomy: Structure and Function

In the course of human evolution, functional requirements (i.e., survival of the fittest) have driven the refinement of anatomic structural definition. The tremendous power of this process has endowed the association between biomechanical function and anatomic structure with such strength that it is appropriate to inductively infer function from an appraisal of structure. Applying this logic, a surgically relevant understanding of the posterolateral corner of the knee can be distilled from all the published anatomic data by conceptualizing the major posterolateral static stabilizers according to their primary mechanical functions, as intuitively defined by their architecture.

In this way, it can be appreciated that static posterolateral stability is a function of three discreet elements.

Lateral Collateral Ligament

The LCL is present essentially 100% of the time. It arises from a center of rotation of the lateral femoral condyle and provides a linkage between the femur and tibia (via the fibula) that is oriented closely perpendicular to the plane of the joint. Breaking this architectural description down into its major components allows detailed scrutiny, as follows:

1. Orientation: Perpendicular to the joint line. Preliminary implication is that the LCL functions primarily to resist force that distracts the joint surfaces.
2. Position: Lateral aspect of the knee joint. Intermediate implication is that the LCL functions primarily to resist distraction of the knee joint, particularly the lateral compartment.
3. Isometricity: Isometric. The isometric origin on the femur suggests that it functions to provide a resistive force that does not vary significantly with respect to varying angles of joint flexion.

The LCL functions primarily to resist distraction of the knee joint, particularly the lateral compartment, providing a resistive force that does not vary significantly with respect to varying angles of joint flexion. This may also be stated as follows: The LCL provides relatively constant resistance to varus rotational forces, in the coronal plane, at all positions of knee flexion.

The dynamic stabilizers most optimally positioned to support the LCL in its primary role include biceps femoris, iliotibial tract, lateral head of gastrocnemius, and popliteus. The LCL's architecture also allows it to act as a secondary static stabilizer, in resistance to anteriorly or posteriorly directed forces applied to the tibia relative to the femur and internal or external rotatory forces applied to the tibia relative to the femur, at all knee positions.

Fabellofibular Ligament, Short Lateral Ligament, and Arcuate Ligament

A summary of the anatomic reports cited above reveals that, as a group, the FFL, the SLL, and the AL are present in some combination in roughly 100% of knees. They each provide a linkage between the femur and the tibia (via the fibula) that is effectively perpendicular to the plane of the knee joint. They are positioned at the posterior edge of the lateral aspect of the knee or, if one prefers, at the lateral edge of the posterior aspect of the knee or, more succinctly, at the posterolateral corner of the knee. These structures are all nonisometric because they attach to the femur posterior to all centers of knee flexion–extension rotation. Appraisal of these structures, as a group, by their anatomic details follows:

1. Orientation: Perpendicular to the joint line. Preliminary implication is that these structures function primarily to resist force that distracts the joint surfaces.
2. Position: The posterolateral corner of the knee. Intermediate implication is that these structures function primarily to resist force that distracts the joint surfaces at the posterolateral corner of the knee.
3. Isometricity: Nonisometric.

Their nonisometric architecture indicates they provide tension that varies with joint position. They clearly provide static force resistance that is maximal at full knee extension and decreases with knee flexion. This variable contribution suggests that they "share" their primary force-resistance duties with other static or dynamic stabilizers, with a variability that is related to joint position. The dynamic stabilizer most intimately involved in this force resistance is the lateral head of the gastrocnemius because the FFL and SLL attach to the femur via the tendon of the lateral head.

These structures function primarily to resist force that distracts the joint surfaces at the posterolateral corner of the knee. They provide maximal static force at full knee extension. Their contribution to this role diminishes with increasing knee flexion, leaving the dynamic stabilizers to provide the required force resistance. This may also be stated as follows: The FFL, SLL, and AL together primarily provide static resistance to lateral knee joint hyperextension and varus/hyperextension opening of the posterolateral corner.

The dynamic stabilizers most optimally positioned to support these structures in their primary role include lateral head of the gastrocnemius, popliteus, and biceps femoris. The architecture of these structures also allows them to act as secondary static stabilizers, in resistance to anteriorly or posteriorly directed forces applied to the tibia relative to the femur and internal or external rotatory forces applied to the tibia relative to the femur at all knee positions.

Popliteofibular Ligament

As stated in the reports cited above, the popliteus tendon and the PFL are present together essentially 100% of the time. This apparatus provides a linkage between the femur and tibia (via the fibula) that is oblique to the plane of the joint. It is a nonisometric structure because it attaches to the lateral aspect of the femur off of the center of rotation established by the LCL's linkage.

1. Orientation: Oblique to the joint line, anterosuperior to posteroinferior. The PFL's obliquity with reference to the joint line enables it to efficiently provide force vectors to resist both perpendicular (joint distraction) forces and parallel (joint rotation or anteroposterior displacement) forces. Preliminary implication is that the PFL functions to resist both forces that distract the joint surfaces and external rotatory and posterior displacement forces.
2. Position: Lateral aspect of the knee joint. Compared with the LCL, the PFL is not as architecturally suited to the primary resistance of perpendicular forces and therefore must be considered a secondary stabilizer in this role. However, it is the only static structure on the lateral side with an architecture that allows it to assume resistance to forces parallel to the joint line as a primary role. Intermediate implication is that the PFL functions primarily to resist external rotation and posterior displacement of the lateral tibial plateau and secondarily to resist distraction of the lateral knee compartment (varus rotation of the knee in the coronal plane).
3. Isometricity: Nonisometric.

The PFL's nonisometric architecture indicates that it provides tension that varies with joint position. Because its attachment to the femur is anterior and distal to the center of rotation established by the LCL, the PFL is subject to a "cam effect" that causes it to develop increasing tension as the angle of knee flexion increases. As mentioned above, the logic attendant to the scrutiny of nonisometric static structures implies that there is also a significant dynamic partner, or partners, to this structure. Obviously, the most intimately associated dynamic stabilizer in this case is the popliteus muscle.

The PFL's primary function is to resist external rotation and posterior displacement of the lateral tibial plateau. It also makes a contribution to the resistance of distraction forces at the lateral knee compartment (varus rotation of the knee in the coronal plane). As knee flexion increases, the tension developed by the popliteus increases. This may also be stated as follows: The PFL's primary role is resistance to external rotational forces and posterior displacement forces applied to the lateral tibial plateau relative to the femur with increasing tension at increasing angles of knee flexion.

The dynamic stabilizers most optimally positioned to support the PFL in its primary role include the popliteus and the lateral head of the gastrocnemius. Intuitively, there is probably some degree of "balance" at all angles of knee flexion between the static tension generated in the PFL and that generated in the FFL–SLL–AL complex because one structure gains tension as the other loses it, and vice versa.

Contribution of the Proximal Tibia–Fibula Joint

Finally, it is important to realize that all the above static structures are provided a significant degree of protection against mechanical injury from the forces they resist because of their attachment to the fibula. This configuration allows excursion of the proximal tibia–fibula joint to act as a "shock absorber" in the transmission of the forces ultimately being transmitted between the femur and tibia.

This architectural detail is probably responsible for the strong association of posterolateral injury with cruciate ligament injury. Intuitively, it can be appreciated that when applied forces are of a magnitude that they are capable of causing excursion in the posterolateral knee such that the protection provided by the proximal tibia–fibula joint is surpassed—enough to actually cause damage to the posterolateral structures—the simultaneous excursion caused at the "central pivot" of the knee is probably, in most instances, enough to result in cruciate ligament injury.

The "cushioning" effect provided by the proximal tibia–fibula joint is also the reason that clinical testing of the posterolateral structures may yield relatively "sloppy" end points compared with those found in the anterior cruciate ligament, the posterior cruciate ligament (PCL), and the medial cruciate ligament, which connect the femur and tibia directly.

Biomechanical Investigations

Between 1950 and 1990, several biomechanical studies were published that described the results of coupling simulated injury to various posterolateral knee ligaments and the cruciate ligaments (selective cutting techniques) with simulation of clinical diagnostic maneuvers at various angles of knee flexion. In 1995, Veltri et al. published a study that recapitulated the classic work reported by Gollehon et al. in 1987, this time taking into account the existence of the PFL. Veltri et al. found that the PFL accounted for the "static function of the popliteus" previously reported by Gollehon et al.

The selective cutting studies mentioned above can be appropriately summarized by the following statement: "They all found that sectioning of the posterolateral ligaments resulted in increased primary posterior translation, primary varus rotation, and primary external ro-

tation." A clinically relevant summary of the specific findings reported in these studies is as follows:

Structural Deficit	Most Specific Biomechanical Effect
Isolated LCL injury	Increased varus rotation at 30 degrees of flexion
Isolated PFL injury	Increased external rotation that is greater at 30 degrees than at 90 degrees of knee flexion
Isolated PCL injury	Increased posterior translation that is maximal at 70–90 degrees of knee flexion
Combined LCL–PFL injury	Increased varus rotation, external rotation, and posterior translation that is maximal at 30 degrees of flexion
Combined LCL–PFL–PCL injury	Increased varus rotation, external rotation, and posterior translation at all angles of knee flexion

Examination of posterior translation, varus rotation (in the coronal plane), and external rotation of the tibia in relation to the femur are tests that are commonly applied by clinicians attempting to diagnose injury to the posterolateral corner, the PCL, or both. The selective cutting studies have adequately simulated all these clinical maneuvers.

Hyperextension (recurvatum) has also been clinically noted to appear in cases of posterolateral injury, as described by Hughston. Based on the structure/function discussion presented above, this clinical finding would primarily represent loss of the FFL–SLL–AL static stabilizing function. This particular issue has yet to be fully addressed in a quantitative fashion either clinically or in the biomechanics laboratory. Therefore, future biomechanical laboratory work addressing this structure–function relationship and clinical studies that include pre- and posttreatment observations of hyperextension/recurvatum could quite possibly yield important information that would significantly improve the diagnosis and treatment of posterolateral injury.

Summary

There are three important static structure–function relationships germane to posterolateral knee stability. They can be summarized as LCL, resistance to varus forces; FFL–SLL–AL, resistance to hyperextension forces; PFL, resistance to posterior displacement and external rotation forces.

Clinically significant acute or chronic injury to the posterolateral knee will always present as deficit(s) of static stability involving one or more of the above. With this understanding, the problem confronting a clinician treating injury in this zone becomes a relatively clear-cut task of first accurately identifying which instabilities exist and then surgically addressing these with appropriate repairs and/or reconstructions. One should also keep in mind that some injury patterns may additionally involve the dynamic structures (muscle–tendon units) that normally support these static stabilizers and that these should also be repaired, if possible.

MECHANISM OF INJURY

Isolated Injuries

Lateral Collateral Ligament

Isolated injury to the LCL has been reported as the direct result of a purely varus rotational stress applied to the knee. The incidence rate is apparently much less than that of isolated medial collateral ligament injury or that of combined injuries involving the LCL. This is probably attributable to the protection provided by the proximal tibia–fibula joint and other factors.

Popliteofibular Ligament

Isolated injury to the PFL has been reported in the literature as the result of the application of a sharp purely externally rotatory force to the tibia. This is also reported much less commonly than the incidence of combined injuries involving the popliteus.

Fabellofibular Ligament, Short Lateral Ligament, and Arcuate Ligament

Isolated injury to the FFL–SLL–AL group has not been addressed in the orthopedic clinical or biomechanical literature. Intuitively, it could occur as the result of a sharply applied force that distracts the posterolateral corner of the knee when the knee is at or near full extension. Such a force would tend to hyperextend the knee in the sagittal plane and simultaneously rotate the tibia into varus in the coronal plane—a varus/hyperextension force. Obviously, a varus-aligned knee would be at greatest susceptibility for injury from this type of force application. The hyperextension component of the force could tend to "protect" the PFL because it would tend to shorten the distance between the PFL's origin and insertion. Theoretically, the LCL could also be preferentially spared from the varus stress force component by the tibia–fibula joint because the FFL–SLL–AL group attaches to the fibula styloid—a point on the fibula that is superior and posterior to the LCL's attachment. During the application of a varus/hyperextension force, the styloid could act as a lever arm that would cause injury to the FFL–SLL–AL while the LCL is spared.

Combined Injuries

The most frequent mechanism of injury described in association with injuries to multiple structures in the posterolateral corner of the knee is a direct application of significant force to the medial aspect of the knee or proximal tibia with the knee at or near full extension. This type of force drives the knee into varus and hyperextension, as postulated above in the discussion of possible isolated injury to the FFL–SLL–AL. Other frequently reported mechanisms of injury have involved forces applied to the medial aspect of the leg with the knee in variable amounts of flexion and the application of violent externally rotatory forces to the knee.

Summary

The features that differentiate between the occurrence of isolated injuries and combined injuries are the magnitude and the direction of the applied forces. Smaller discreetly directed forces could lead to isolated injury, whereas larger forces are likely to result in injury to multiple posterolateral components and, as alluded to previously, injury to the cruciate ligaments.

CLINICAL EVALUATION

Acute versus Chronic Injury

The complete clinical appraisal of acute and chronic injury to the posterolateral corner of the knee involves many discreet elements. Some of these elements are more applicable to the acute setting than the chronic, and vice versa, whereas some are equally applicable to both.

Symptoms of Acute Injury: Minor or Isolated

In the setting of acute isolated posterolateral injury, the predominant symptom is usually pain in the posterolateral aspect of the knee. Complaints of dysesthesias and motor weakness in the leg and foot may also be present in some patients secondary to associated injury to the peroneal nerve. After the initial pain and swelling of an acute injury have subsided, the patient with isolated posterolateral injury may complain of instability of the knee in extension, with the knee feeling as if it "buckles" into hyperextension.

Symptoms of Acute Injury: Severe

In the setting of acute severe posterolateral injury, there is a strong likelihood of associated cruciate ligament damage. The examiner should probably approach the injury as if it were a suspected knee dislocation. Associated injuries to neurovascular structures, bone, skin, and other soft tissues may be present, a possibility that should be thoroughly evaluated.

Assessment of Knee Stability

The Lachman test should be performed to assess the integrity of the anterior cruciate ligament. The posterior drawer test, performed with the knee at 90 degrees of flexion, should be used to define the status of the PCL. Both the degree of posterior displacement of the tibia and the quality of the end point should be noted.

Clinical Tests Specific to the Diagnosis of Posterolateral Instability

The individual tests related to the three major components of static stability provided by the posterolateral knee include the varus rotation test, the external rotation recurvatum test, and the tibial external rotation test.

Varus Rotation Test

This test is performed by placing a varus stress on the knee in full extension and at 30 degrees of flexion. Increased varus laxity compared with the opposite knee is indicative of injury to the LCL.

External Rotation Recurvatum Test

The external rotation recurvatum test is performed as follows. The patient lies on the examination table in supine position with both legs resting on the table. The examiner grasps the great toe of each leg and lifts both feet while the patient is encouraged to relax the quadriceps muscles. In a patient with a posterolateral instability, the injured knee assumes a relative position of hyperextension-varus (compared with the opposite knee), whereas the tibia rotates simultaneously externally with the tibial tuberosity moving laterally. Hughston and Norwood reported that this test is specific for injury to the "AL complex" (LCL, arcuate ligament, popliteus, and lateral gastrocnemius). That conclusion agrees with the structure–function discussion, presented earlier in this text, which would lead one to expect that excessive hyperextension indicates injury to the FFL–SLL–AL structural group.

Tibial External Rotation Test

The tibial external rotation test is performed simultaneously on both knees at 30 and 90 degrees of knee flexion. This test is best performed with the patient in the prone position with the knees held together. If increased external rotation of the tibia is found at 30 degrees of knee flexion, but not at 90 degrees of knee flexion, a high probability of isolated posterolateral corner injury is

diagnosed. If increased external rotation of the tibia at both 30 and 90 degrees of knee flexion is found, a diagnosis of combined posterolateral and PCL injury is likely. A side-to-side difference of 10 degrees is significant and implies a need for treatment.

Other Considerations

In patients with acute pain, secondary muscle spasm, and guarding, it is often difficult to perform an accurate physical examination. In these patients, examination under anesthesia may be required for accurate evaluation of instability.

Some patients with chronic posterolateral instability may be able to evoke their instability pattern voluntarily. Shino et al. documented the pattern of muscle firing that enables the patient to reproduce the instability. In their study, based on electromyographic evaluation, the biceps femoris appeared to be active in the subluxation phase and the popliteus appeared to be active in the reduction phase.

The patient's gait should be informally observed. Those with a varus thrust during stance phase require valgus osteotomy of the tibia as an adjunct to definitive treatment. Formal gait analysis should be considered in cases where varus alignment or informally observed gait abnormalities raise the question of whether or not to perform an osteotomy. An abnormally high adduction moment about the knee, as quantified by formal gait analysis, provides a strong indication for the performance of a valgus high tibial osteotomy before definitive surgical stabilization.

Summary

The clinical tests specific for posterolateral instability are appropriate to both the acute and chronic setting: Varus rotation tests the LCL, external rotation recurvatum tests the FFL–SLL–AL group, and the tibial external rotation tests the PFL.

IMAGING

Radiographic Assessment

Routine plain radiographs (posteroanterior weightbearing view in full extension, posteroanterior 45-degree flexion view, and lateral view) should be obtained. They should be scrutinized for the presence of an avulsion fracture of the fibula head or Gerdy's tubercle. In some cases, posterior translation or sag of the tibia may be seen on the lateral radiograph. Alignment of the knee should also be appraised. Patients with varus malalignment should be evaluated with long leg films to accurately gauge the degree of deformity.

In cases with combined severe instabilities, it may be

difficult to determine the neutral point between anterior and posterior tibial displacements on physical examination. In these situations, some authors advocate stress radiography.

Magnetic Resonance Imaging

High-quality MRI production and interpretation is becoming widely available in assessing knee ligament injuries. MRI of the posterolateral corner should be supervised by an experienced radiologist who knows how to adjust the orientation of the imaging planes and the technical characteristics of the imaging sequences to optimize the information available concerning the soft tissues of the posterolateral corner.

TREATMENT

Nonoperative

Nonoperative treatment may be appropriate for some patients. Therapeutic components appropriate to this type of management include bracing, physical therapy, and activity modification. A program involving these options should be tailored to the symptoms presented by each patient.

Operative

A reasoned surgical approach to posterolateral instability should be predicated on the chronicity of the injury and an accurate appraisal of the specific structures involved.

Over time, various approaches to the surgical treatment of posterolateral instability have been advocated. The earliest schemes, such as those described by Slocum and by Hughston, basically involved advancement and/or "reefing" of the injured posterior and lateral soft tissues. More recently developed techniques, such as those described by Warren, by Jacob, and by Noyes, incorporate grafting into the treatment of injured posterolateral structures.

The details of the reconstructive techniques advocated by Warren, Jacob, and Noyes are published in the orthopedic literature. Description and comparison of them is beyond the scope of this discourse. It is, however, appropriate to note here that they differ significantly from each other and that they have produced variable results, even in the best hands. Yet together they currently represent the standard of care for the treatment of posterolateral injuries.

It is important for the surgeon contemplating operative treatment of injuries in this zone to realize that successful performance of these procedures, and those described below, demands advanced skill in the appraisal of the native posterolateral tissue integrity and in the selection, preparation, and utilization of the grafts required for the restoration of posterolateral knee stability.

AUTHOR'S APPROACH

Basic Considerations

Aside from the constellation of skin, neurovascular, other soft tissue, or bony injuries that might complicate the clinical picture in posterolateral knee injury, the main factors to be considered in the planning for surgical correction of acute or chronic posterolateral instability are consideration of whether a tibial osteotomy is required for ultimate success and consideration of the options for restoration, as necessary, of each of the three primary static elements of posterolateral stability: resistance to varus opening (LCL), resistance to hyperextension (FFL–SLL–AL), and resistance to lateral tibial external rotation or posterior displacement (PFL).

Tibial Osteotomy

Valgus high tibial osteotomy should probably be performed before soft tissue repair of the posterolateral corner if the knee alignment is in mechanical varus (at or beyond neutral anatomic alignment), an abnormally high adduction moment about the knee is found upon formal gait analysis, or an obvious varus thrust is present in the stance phase of gait. Persistence of any of the above circumstances would apply repetitive distraction force to the posterolateral corner, leading to ultimate failure of any restorative effort.

Proximal Tibia–Fibula Joint

As previously explained, the proximal tibia–fibula joint plays an important role in the normal functioning of the posterolateral stabilizers. It is therefore important to avoid violation of this joint in the performance of a tibial osteotomy. Obviously, this necessitates that a fibula osteotomy is performed distal to the joint, instead.

Restoration of Stability

In the worst case scenario, the surgeon should be prepared to perform complete autograft or allograft reconstruction of the LCL, the PFL, and the FFL–SLL–AL. Therefore, it is the author's preference to have an Achilles tendon allograft available, on standby, at every procedure, because this single graft source can be applied to the global reconstruction of any or all ligaments, if necessary.

Surgical Approach

A standard lateral incision is used, centered over the lateral joint line. It is extended distally to allow exposure of the fibula head and the peroneal nerve as it crosses the fibula neck and proximally to allow access to the attachment site of the lateral head of the gastrocnemius.

The interval between the posterior edge of the iliotibial band and the biceps tendon sheath is identified and developed. The iliotibial band is then mobilized anteriorly by progressively dissecting it from all of its undersurface attachments and its attachment to Gerdy's tubercle (which is later repaired), starting at its posterior edge and working anteriorly. This maneuver allows easy access to all structures important to posterolateral stability.

The peroneal nerve is next addressed. It should first be identified proximally as it proceeds posterior to the biceps tendon. It is then inspected, and an epineurolysis is performed if hematoma is present within the neural sheath. The nerve is completely mobilized, from proximal to the biceps tendon to beyond the fibula neck, and then carefully protected, in all cases where drilling, or other instrumentation, of the fibula head is to be performed.

Proximal Tibia–Fibula Joint

Once the iliotibial band has been adequately mobilized and the peroneal nerve has been addressed, the integrity of the proximal tibia–fibula joint should be examined. If the joint is found to be unstable and/or subluxed, this must be corrected. In cases of proximal fibula head subluxation, the fibula head is restored to its normal anatomic position relative to the tibial plateau via a shortening osteotomy of the fibula neck or shaft, which is fixed with either an intramedullary screw or a plate and screws. If gross instability of the joint is present, arthrodesis may be performed by obliterating the joint articular surfaces and firmly apposing the newly exposed bony surfaces with one or more screws. In some cases of clear-cut posterolateral instability, primary treatment of a deranged proximal tibia–fibula joint may prove to be the definitive remedy.

After the proximal tibia–fibula joint has been addressed, the integrity of the major posterolateral static stabilizers is assessed. All three elements (LCL, PFL, and FFL–SLL–AL) should be examined before correction of damage to any of them is undertaken. This is because the correction of significant deficits in two or three elements may be most appropriately accomplished using a unified grafting approach.

Lateral Collateral Ligament

If the LCL is damaged, options for restoration include advancement of the LCL into its femoral origin, reconstruction or augmentation using local biceps tendon autograft, and reconstruction or augmentation using distant autograft or allograft.

Advancement of the LCL into its femoral origin is used only if careful examination reveals that ligament damage is restricted to the femoral attachment site and no more that 3 to 5 mm of adjacent ligament. If more than 3 to 5 mm is damaged, augmentation or reconstruction should be performed. Advancement is achieved by detaching the ligament from its femoral attachment, debriding the injured tissue, gaining control of the remaining ligament with sutures both at its free end and along its length, and then using these sutures to draw the end of the ligament into a bony bed prepared at the isometric femoral attachment point. The sutures are passed across the width of the femur, through bone tunnels originating in the bony bed, and are tied down on the medial side of the femur with tensioning of the ligament performed at full knee extension, in neutral rotation, while a valgus force is applied to the knee to close the lateral compartment.

The biceps tendon is the optimal choice if graft reconstruction (or augmentation) of the LCL is appropriate. This is because its fibula attachment is anatomically identical to the LCL's; it actually encircles the LCL's fibula attachment. The graft is harvested by carefully protecting the tendon's fibula attachment while elevating a proximally contiguous piece of tendon, approximately 2 to 3 cm wide by 6 to 8 cm long, from the underlying muscle. This flat piece of tendon is manually "tubularized" and then controlled by weaving sutures from its fibula attachment to its free end. Separate sutures are placed at the free end to allow proper tensioning. The graft is then advanced into a bony tunnel prepared at the isometric point on the lateral femoral condyle by drawing the sutures through bone tunnels drilled across the femur. The graft should be tensioned and secured with the knee positioned at full extension and neutral rotation, while a valgus moment is applied to the knee to close the lateral joint compartment.

Reconstruction of the LCL using allograft or distant autograft is the procedure of choice if the LCL is unusable, biceps tendon autograft is not available, and/or if injury to other elements of posterolateral stability makes a unified graft reconstruction approach desirable.

Popliteofibular Ligament

If the PFL/popliteus tendon is damaged, the options for restoration include advancement of the popliteus tendon into its femoral attachment, tenodesis of the popliteus tendon to the fibula, and allograft or autograft augmentation or reconstruction.

Advancement of the popliteus tendon into its femoral attachment site is used if careful examination reveals that the structural integrity of the popliteus tendon itself is maintained but the femoral attachment site is disrupted. This is accomplished, in a manner that is completely analogous to the similar procedure described for the LCL, by detaching the tendon from its femoral attachment, debriding the injured tissue, gaining control of the remaining tendon with sutures both at its free end and along its length, and then using these sutures to draw the end of the tendon into a bony bed prepared at the anatomic femoral attachment point, just distal and anterior to the attachment site of the LCL. The sutures are passed across the width of the femur, through bone tunnels originating in the bony bed, and are tied down on the medial side of the femur. The tendon must be tensioned with the knee at approximately 70 degrees of flexion.

Tenodesis of the popliteus tendon to the posterior portion of the fibula head is appropriate if the normal attachment of the popliteus tendon to the fibula has been disrupted while the popliteus tendon, from its femoral attachment to the point where it crosses the fibula, is otherwise intact. This is accomplished by preparing a bony bed on the medial surface of the most posterior and superior projection of the fibula styloid and then placing sutures through the tendon that secure it to this bony bed. This fixation should be performed such that the tendon begins to develop significant tension at approximately 70 degrees of knee flexion. This is accomplished using sutures placed into the appropriate zone of tendon and then brought through the fibula head where they are tied down over a bony bridge. Alternatively, one may use suture anchors, placed in the prepared bony bed, for tenodesis fixation.

Allograft or autograft augmentation or reconstruction of the PFL, from the femur to the fibula, is undertaken if the popliteus tendon has intrasubstance damage, is completely unusable, and/or if injury to other elements of posterolateral stability makes a unified graft reconstruction approach desirable.

Fabellofibular Ligament, Short Lateral Ligament, and Arcuate Ligament

If inspection reveals damage to the FFL–SLL–AL group, the options for restoration include advancement of the ligaments into the femoral attachment site, repair of the fibula styloid attachment, and reconstruction of a restraint to hyperextension, from the femur to the fibula, using allograft or autograft.

Advancement of the FFL–SLL–AL into their femoral attachment site (at the under surface of the attachment of the lateral head of the gastrocnemius to the femur) is the procedure of choice if examination of these tissues reveals that their fibula attachment is intact and that the integrity of these ligamentous tissues is otherwise acceptable. This advancement is accomplished, in a manner that is completely analogous to the similar procedure described for the LCL and popliteus tendon, by detaching the ligaments from their femoral attachment, debriding the injured tissue, gaining control of the remaining ligament with sutures both at its free end and along its length, and then using these sutures to draw the end of the tendon into a bony bed prepared at the anatomic attachment point, at the distal portion of the lateral head of the gastrocnemius insertion. The sutures are passed anteriorly or diagonally, through bone tunnels originating at the anatomic attachment site, and are tied down over a bony bridge on the femur. Tensioning of these tissues should be performed at approximately 20 to 30 degrees of knee flexion such that strong tension is developed when the knee is brought toward full extension.

Repair of the fibula styloid attachment of the FFL–SLL–AL group may be appropriate if this attachment has been avulsed, leaving the integrity of the remaining tissue and their femoral attachment relatively intact. This is accomplished, in a manner analogous to that described for tenodesis of the popliteus tendon to the fibula, by preparing a bony bed on the tip and posterior surface of the fibula styloid. The tissues are reattached under tension at 20 to 30 degrees of knee flexion. This may be accomplished using sutures through the ligaments and bone or via the use of suture anchors placed in the prepared bony bed.

Allograft or autograft reconstruction of the FFL–SLL–AL group (from the femur to the fibula) is undertaken if the native tissues are unusable and/or if injury to other elements of posterolateral stability makes a unified graft reconstruction approach desirable.

Graft Reconstructions

Graft Selection

Factors to be considered in graft selection include the effective length of the structure(s) to be reconstructed, the number of structures to be reconstructed, and the availability or desirability of autograft versus allograft tissues. Autografts to be considered include middle-third patella tendon (bone–tendon–bone), quadriceps tendon (bone–tendon), and hamstring tendon (semitendinosus and gracilis tendons). Allografts to be considered include patella tendon (bone–tendon–bone) and Achilles tendon (bone–tendon or tendon alone).

Because of their larger available size, both in width and length, allografts generally posses a versatility advantage with respect to autografts in posterolateral reconstruction. For example, a whole patella tendon allograft may be fashioned into an implant with two or three ligament–bone arms attached to a single bone plug on one end or into multiple bone–tendon–bone constructs. Likewise, an Achilles tendon allograft may be fashioned into an implant with two or three long ligaments attached to a single bone plug. Alternatively, an Achilles tendon graft may be divided into several separate long ligament grafts with or without bone plugs. Obviously, this versatility allows the performance of numerous possible applications in posterolateral reconstruction, only a few of which are discussed below.

Autograft tissues are preferred by the author, if available, in the circumstance of an acute injury. In the acute setting, every attempt is made to preserve and use as much native posterolateral tissue as possible because it is expected that the acute healing process will have a beneficial effect on native tissue with respect to ultimate repair and remodeling. Autograft tissue is favored, under these conditions, for use as less-bulky "augmenting" tissue. These autografts are generally smaller than the comparable allografts used in the chronic setting, but they are routed and secured in exactly the same fashion.

Single Element Reconstruction

If only one of the three elements of posterolateral stability requires graft reconstruction, a patella tendon (bone–tendon–bone) construct of autograft or allograft origin is the optimal choice. This type of graft offers the best combination of strength, stiffness, and options for fixation. Before graft preparation, however, available tendon length of this type of graft should be appraised with respect to the distance, from femur to fibula, required for the element to be reconstructed, for obvious reasons. If the available bone–tendon–bone graft source is too short, the next choice is a bone–tendon construct such as quadriceps tendon or Achilles tendon.

Because the fibula head is small and fragile, it can safely accommodate bone tunnel fixation of only one graft bone plug. Furthermore, interference screw fixation is not often satisfactory in the fragile bone of the fibula head and is not routinely recommended. Therefore, if a bone–tendon construct is used, the bone plug end should be placed in a femoral bone tunnel, because an interference screw may be safely used, whereas fixation of the soft tissue end in the fibula should be via sutures tied over a bony bridge or ligament button.

Lateral Collateral Ligament

For isolated LCL reconstruction, a 6- to 8-mm graft should be fashioned, depending on the size of the patient. The fibula bone tunnel should be placed at the anterolateral corner of the fibula head at the anatomic LCL origin. The graft's fibula end is drawn into the tunnel first and is fixed in place, with sutures drawn through two holes, placed through the bottom of the bone tunnel, that emerge from the fibula cortex distally. These sutures are tied down over a cortical bone bridge and/or ligament button to provide graft fixation. On the femoral side, the graft is drawn into a bone tunnel placed at the isometric point on the lateral femur relative to the fibula origin of the graft. This point is found using

the trial-and-error technique described by Warren. Fixation of this end of the graft is achieved by tying the draw sutures down on the medial side of the knee. Additionally, interference screw fixation may also be safely achieved on a bone plug in the femoral bone tunnel. The graft should be tensioned in the femoral tunnel and secured with the knee positioned at full extension and neutral rotation, while a valgus moment is applied to the knee to close the lateral joint compartment.

Popliteofibular Ligament

For isolated PFL reconstruction, an 8- to 10-mm graft should be fashioned, depending on the size of the patient. The fibula bone tunnel should be placed at the medial surface of the fibula styloid, with care taken to avoid injury to the styloid attachment of the FFL–SLL–AL group. The graft's fibula end is drawn into the tunnel first and is fixed in place, with sutures drawn through two holes, placed through the bottom of the bone tunnel, that emerge from the fibula cortex distally. These sutures are tied down over a cortical bone bridge and/or ligament button to provide graft fixation. On the femoral side, the graft is drawn into a bone tunnel placed at the usual position of the popliteus tendon on the lateral femur, just anterior and distal to the LCL attachment site. Fixation of this end of the graft is achieved by tying the draw sutures down on the medial side of the knee. Additionally, interference screw fixation may also be used on a bone plug in the femoral bone tunnel. The PFL is a nonisometric structure. As previously explained, the cam effect inherent in its architecture causes it to develop increasing tension with increasing knee flexion. Therefore, the graft should be tensioned and secured in the femoral tunnel, with the knee positioned at 70 to 80 degrees of flexion and neutral rotation.

Fabellofibular Ligament, Short Lateral Ligament, and Arcuate Ligament

For isolated FFL–SLL–AL reconstruction, an 8- to 10-mm graft should be fashioned, depending on the size of the patient. The fibula bone tunnel should be placed at the fibula styloid with care to avoid injury to the PFL's fibula attachment. The graft's fibula end is drawn into the tunnel first and is fixed in place, with sutures drawn through two holes, placed through the bottom of the bone tunnel, that emerge from the fibula cortex distally. These sutures are tied down over a cortical bone bridge and/or ligament button to provide graft fixation. On the femoral side, the graft is drawn into a bone tunnel placed at the attachment site of the lateral head of the gastrocnemius. Fixation of this end of the graft is achieved by tying the draw sutures down on the medial side of the knee. Again, additional interference screw fixation may be achieved on the bone plug in this femoral bone tunnel. The FFL–SLL–AL group is nonisometric. As previously explained, the architecture of this group of structures causes them to develop increasing tension with increasing knee extension. Therefore, the graft should be tensioned and secured in the femoral bone tunnel with the knee positioned at 20 to 30 degrees of flexion and neutral rotation.

A Unified Approach to Graft Reconstruction of Two or Three Elements of Posterolateral Stability

If more than one of the elements of posterolateral stability requires reconstruction, I prefer to use a "unified" approach that reconstructs or augments all three elements. The main advantages of this technique are that a single graft is used and a single bone tunnel is placed in the fibula. The procedure combines features of the approaches advocated by Warren, Jacob, and Noyes.

The graft may be either an autogenous semitendinosus and gracilis composite or an allograft Achilles tendon, 7 to 8 mm in width, with a bone plug at one end. Minimum tendon length required is approximately 25 cm. The fibula bone tunnel is placed transversely, anterior to posterior, across the widest portion of the fibula head.

Graft implantation begins with placement of one end of the graft into a bone tunnel at, or near, the femoral insertion of the popliteus. Fixation is achieved in this femoral tunnel with sutures tied down on the medial side of the femur. If an Achilles tendon graft is used, the bone plug is placed at this site and secondary interference screw fixation is also placed.

The graft is then routed through the fibula bone tunnel from posterior to anterior. At this point, the graft recapitulates the popliteus connection from femur to fibula. This portion of the graft should now be tensioned with the knee at approximately 70 degrees of flexion at neutral rotation. Fixation is achieved by placing heavy sutures through the tendon and the adjacent fibula bone.

The graft is next drawn superiorly. Using the trial-and-error technique, described by Warren, the isometric point for attachment of this graft to the femur is identified. It should be noted that because the graft origin from the anterior surface of the fibula is different from the LCL origin, the isometric point on the femur for the graft may not coincide with the LCL's attachment site. Once the appropriate isometric point is identified, a bone tunnel can be placed in the femoral condyle. The tunnel entrance should be placed such that the isometric point is at its posteroinferior edge. The tunnel emerges at, or just above, the insertion site of the lateral head of the gastrocnemius.

Once the femoral bone tunnel has been constructed, the graft is drawn through it from anterior to posterior.

At this point, the graft recapitulates the course of the LCL. This limb of the graft is tensioned with the knee at 0 to 20 degrees of flexion and neutral rotation, while valgus stress is placed on the knee to close the lateral joint. Fixation is achieved by placing heavy sutures through the graft and the bone at the mouth of the femoral tunnel.

Finally, the graft is again routed through the fibula bone tunnel from posterior to anterior. If necessary, the fibula tunnel may be carefully enlarged with a small sharp curette. Use of a graft leader may reduce the need for this maneuver. The graft now recapitulates the course of the FFL–SLL–AL. This limb of the graft is tensioned with the knee at approximately 20 degrees of flexion. Final graft fixation is again secured with sutures placed through the graft and the bone. If the graft has significant residual length emerging from the fibula tunnel, additional fixation with a screw and ligament washer may be possible on the fibula, distal to the tunnel opening, or on the nearby tibia.

Other Surgical Considerations

Once the static stabilizers have been addressed, attention should be given to repair of the dynamic stabilizers and other supporting structures. In the acute setting, all obvious or suspected damage to the posterior and lateral joint capsule, the biceps tendon, the iliotibial band, the lateral head of the gastrocnemius, and the popliteus muscle–tendon junction should be repaired as appropriate. In the chronic setting, imbrication of the joint capsule and advancement of the dynamic stabilizers, including the biceps, the lateral head of the gastrocnemius, the iliotibial band, and the popliteus muscle belly, should be considered.

Postoperative Care

In general, posterolateral reconstructions should be protected with limited weight bearing and bracing for an extended period. Passive range of motion may begin immediately. Hyperextension is avoided at all times. Flexion past 90 degrees is delayed until after 6 weeks postoperatively and is limited to 135 degrees until 1 year postoperatively. Ambulation is allowed, with toe-touch weight bearing, in a long leg brace locked in full extension during the first 8 weeks. After 8 weeks, progressive weight bearing as tolerated is initiated in a valgus-unloader type of brace that allows a 0 to 90-degree range of motion. This bracing is continued until 6 months postoperatively. Closed kinetic chain exercises, such as bicycling and squats, are allowed at 6 weeks postoperatively. Open kinetic chain quadriceps and hamstring exercises are delayed until 3 months postoperatively.

Principles and Practice of Orthopaedic Sports Medicine,
edited by William E. Garrett, Jr., Kevin P. Speer, and Donald T. Kirkendall.
Lippincott Williams & Wilkins, Philadelphia © 2000.

CHAPTER 39

Diagnosis and Treatment of Knee Tendon Injury

Scott A. Rodeo and Kazutaka Izawa

BASIC ASPECTS

Tendon Structure and Function

A knowledge of basic tendon structure and function is important for understanding the principles of tendon healing and repair. Chapter 35 provides a detailed review of basic tendon structure. Like other fibrous connective tissues, tendon is composed primarily of type I collagen. The other principal constituents of tendon include water, proteoglycan, elastin, and other noncollagenous proteins. The material properties (strength) of tendon are determined principally by collagen. Tissue strength is positively correlated with total collagen content, density of stable (pyridinoline) cross-links, collagen organization, collagen fibril diameter, and elastin content. Many of these factors change as the tendon ages. The ability of tendon to resist plastic deformation (creep) is related to the content of small-diameter collagen fibrils, whereas the ability to resist high tensile loads is related to the content of large diameter fibrils (1).

Recent studies have focused on proteoglycans in tendon (2). The principal proteoglycan of tendon is decorin; biglycan, lumican, and fibromodulin are also found. Tendons that experience compressive loads contain an elevated content of glycosaminoglycan, which probably represents a functional adaptation to the mechanical environment (3). Proteoglycans in tendon probably play an important role in regulation of collagen fibril diameter and may serve to separate individual fiber bundles and to minimize shear stress as fiber bundles move relative to each other. Elastic fibers within the tendon may contribute to the shock-absorbing capacity of tendon

and may contribute to the maintenance of the collagen crimp pattern.

Age-related Changes in Tendon

Age has a significant influence on the properties of tendons around the knee and thereby may affect the susceptibility to injury. Aging results in an increased amount of insoluble collagen, increased maturation of collagen cross-links, increased collagen fibril diameter, reduced collagen turnover, decreased proteoglycan and water content, and a reduction in cellularity and vascularity (4–8). These age-related changes, which can occur by the third decade of life, may result in a stiffer, less compliant, and weaker tendon, causing increased susceptibility to injury. The susceptibility to injury may be especially increased if there are concomitant pathologic alterations, such as calcification, mucoid degeneration, or hypoxic degeneration. Age-related tendon alterations result in a diminished healing capacity. It has been hypothesized that age-related changes are due to decreased physical activity, and experimental data suggest that exercise can slow the decline in biochemical properties of a tendon with aging (8).

Effect of Mechanical Load on Tendon

Mechanical load has a significant affect on connective tissues such as tendon. The effect of mechanical load is relevant to the design of rehabilitation programs after tendon injury and repair (9–11). Recent *in vivo* and *in vitro* experiments demonstrate that immobilization of tendon decreases its tensile strength, stiffness, and total weight (12). Microscopically, there is a decrease in cellularity, overall collagen organization, collagen fibril diameter, and collagen cross-links. The proteoglycan and water content are also altered. Subsequent tendon remobilization results in recovery of normal biochemical and biomechanical properties, but recovery takes longer

S. A. Rodeo: Department of Surgery, Cornell University Medical College, New York, New York 10021.

K. Izawa: Departmemt of Orthopaedic Surgery, Taneyama National Hospital, Osaka 5605552, Japan.

than the period of immobilization (12–17). Remobilization of tendon results in an acceleration of collagen synthesis and cross-link formation (18). The three-dimensional orientation of tendon fibers becomes more organized in response to tensile load. During the remobilization process, the tendon collagen fibers may still be deficient in content, quality, and orientation, with a concomitant risk for reinjury during postimmobilization activities. Early tendon mobilization is important to minimize the adverse effects of immobilization.

Adaptive differences to the types of applied load are also observed. In areas subjected primarily to tensile forces, tendons show linearly arranged dense collagen fibrils, higher rates of collagen synthesis, and lower proteoglycan content (predominantly smaller proteoglycans such as decorin). In contrast, in regions where tendons are subjected primarily to compression and friction, there is an increased amount of both small and large proteoglycans and thinner collagen fibrils organized in a network with fewer cross-links (19). Although the mechanism of response to exercise is unclear, it is hypothesized that intermittent stress and relaxation produces a direct cellular response. Alterations in a number of basic mechanisms appear to be involved in signal transduction in tendon cells: protein phosphorylation, cytosolic Ca^{2+}, and inositol-triphosphate concentration; interstitial fluid flow-induced electrical potentials; cell-surface molecules (integrins); and gap junctions through which tendon cells communicate are all influenced by mechanical loading.

Metabolic Disorders Affecting Tendon

A number of local and systemic metabolic abnormalities have been found to affect the biochemical composition and biomechanical properties of tendon and tendon insertions, and many of these conditions will present with tendon pathology around the knee (most commonly the patellar tendon). These conditions can affect the tendon substance or the tendon insertion site. Normal healthy tendon rarely fails within its substance; ruptures usually occur at the muscle–tendon junction or at the tendon–bone junction (20). The occurrence of midsubstance rupture of the patellar or quadriceps tendon should prompt consideration of the presence of an underlying tendon disorder.

One of the most common causes of intrinsic tendon weakening in sports medicine is the use of local or systemic corticosteroids. Experimental studies have demonstrated that local corticosteroid injections can impair healing of ligament, probably by inhibition of the inflammatory phase of healing (21). Bilateral patellar tendon rupture has been reported after local steroid injections (22). Fluoroquinolone antibiotics (e.g., ciprofloxacin) have also been associated with tendon ruptures, possibly due to pathologic alterations in tendon

extracellular matrix (23). Tendons may also be weakened by abnormal deposition of metabolic products in the tendon. For example, deposition of calcium pyrophosphate occurs commonly in the gastrocnemius and quadriceps tendons in chondrocalcinosis of the knee and may contribute to knee pain (24). Patellar tendon rupture has been reported in hyperparathyroidism and systemic lupus erythematosus (25). Dystrophic calcification occurs in hyperparathyroidism with deposition of calcium hydroxyapatite and urate crystals in tendon, which may weaken the tendon. Pathologic alterations in tendon matrix with resultant tendon weakening also may occur in gout, renal failure, rheumatoid arthritis, and systemic lupus erythematosus (25–27). In these conditions, tendon weakening probably occurs due to the basic disease process and the frequent associated use of corticosteroid treatment. Bilateral quadriceps tendon ruptures have been reported in association with gout and renal failure (26,27). Abnormal deposition of proteoglycan and hyaluronic acid in tendon has been reported in hypothyroidism (28,29).

Pathologic changes also occur at tendon entheses or the underlying bone in several metabolic conditions. Monosodium urate deposits (tophi) often occur at the patellar tendon insertion in gout, resulting in pain and swelling (30). A similar enthesopathy has been described in calcium pyrophosphate deposition disease (chondrocalcinosis) (24). Pathologic changes at the patellar tendon insertion has been reported in association with isotretinoin (a retinoid used to treat severe cystic acne) treatment (31). Retinoids have been found to result in skeletal hyperostoses and proliferation of new bone at tendon insertions, such as the patella tendon.

Conditions that affect bone strength may affect tendon insertions, causing activity-related pain. Avulsion of the patellar tendon from its tibial insertion has been reported in Paget's disease, in which there is rapid bone turnover and remodeling (32). Renal disease and primary or secondary hyperparathyroidism weaken bone due to resorption. Ruptures of the patellar tendon insertion have been reported in these conditions. Similarly, synovial proliferation in rheumatoid arthritis can cause bone erosions and weaken tendon insertions. All these conditions may increase the susceptibility of knee tendons to injury, and recognition of such underlying abnormalities is important to provide proper treatment and to properly advise the patient to prevent recurrent injury.

Pathophysiology of Tendon Injury

Acute tendon injury may be direct, occurring due to contusion or laceration, or indirect, occurring due to acute tensile overload. Acute tensile overload usually results in injury to the muscle–tendon junction or avulsion fracture, because the healthy tendon can withstand higher tensile loads than the muscle. The most common site of failure in an acute muscle–tendon unit injury is at the musculotendinous junction (16). The hamstrings, rectus femoris, and gastrocnemius seem to be predisposed to acute strain injury, perhaps because they cross two joints, and as a result tension can be developed within the muscle by passive joint positioning. Strain injury to the musculotendinous junction usually occurs due to lengthening of the muscle while it is simultaneously contracting (eccentric contraction).

Overuse tendon injuries around the knee, occurring due to repetitive microtrauma, most commonly involve the patellar tendon. The adaptive and reparative ability of tendon can be exceeded when the tendon is strained repeatedly to 4% to 8% of its original length. Such repetitive strain can result in microscopic and/or macroscopic injury to collagen fibrils, noncollagenous matrix, and the microvasculature, resulting in inflammation, edema, and pain. It is currently believed that the earliest pathophysiologic alteration occurs in the paratenon that surrounds the tendon, resulting in peritendinitis (also called paratenonitis). There is inflammatory cell infiltration, tissue edema, and fibrin exudation in the paratenon. If the basal reparative ability of the tendon is overwhelmed by continued overload, the inflammation can become chronic with resulting proliferation of synovial cells, fibroblasts, and capillaries, which eventually leads to fibrosis and thickening of the paratenon.

It is believed that continued tendon overload and chronic peritendinitis leads to tendinosis (intrinsic tendon degeneration). It appears that tendons go through acute, recurrent, subchronic, and chronic phases of peritendinitis before actual degeneration develops. The cellular mechanism(s) by which acute or chronic inflammation lead to tendon degeneration is poorly understood. An experimental model in rabbits demonstrated that chronic inflammation of paratenon results in tendinosis (33). It must be noted, however, that a causal link between chronic peritendinitis and tendinosis has not been conclusively established. A popular model is that tendon degeneration occurs due to failure of the cell matrix to adapt to excessive load (34). Repetitive tendon overload may result in altered cellular function and impaired metabolic activity due to release of inflammatory mediators and cytokines, leading to an ineffectual healing response.

Tendinosis involves histopathologic alterations to cells, collagen fibers, and noncollagenous matrix components. There is angiofibroblastic hyperplasia, consisting of proliferation of fibroblasts and new capillaries. Various histologic abnormalities are found, with the most common being collagen fragmentation and mucoid degeneration with glycosaminoglycan deposition (principally chondroitin sulfate). Inflammation is notably absent in tendinosis (35). The result of such pathologic alterations is decreased tensile strength of the tendon.

Furthermore, degenerative tendon with diminished vascularity cannot heal subclinical injury with microfailure of tendon fibers. The result is progressive loss of functional tendon fibers, which increases the load on the remaining tendon, thus increasing its susceptibility to progressive failure.

Pathologic changes can also occur at the site of tendon attachment to bone. In the skeletally immature child, tensile overload often results in pathologic alterations at the apophysis, resulting in apophysitis. The most common site of apophysitis around the knee occurs at the tibial tuberosity (Osgood-Schlatter disease). Histologically, avulsion of small areas of the ossification center are found. Insertion tendinopathy can also occur in adults in which the pathologic alterations include collagen fragmentation with disorganization and thickening of the fibrocartilage zone of the insertion. A recent study has demonstrated a significant negative correlation between degenerative changes and tensile strength at the supraspinatus insertion (36).

Recent studies have identified several factors that are probably important in the development of tendon degeneration. Tissue hypoxia due to poor vascularity (which may be intrinsic and/or a result on overuse-induced injury to the microvasculature) results in impaired metabolic activity. Other factors that may affect the ability of tendon to adapt to repetitive loading include age, immobilization, hormones (such as estrogen), and drugs (corticosteroid injections and fluoroquinolone antibiotics can lead to pathologic matrix alterations). Extrinsic factors that may contribute to tendon overuse injury include joint instability, malalignments (such as excessive hindfoot pronation, genu valgum, increased femoral anteversion), decreased flexibility, muscle weakness and imbalance, and excessive body weight. The type of loading (tension, compression, or shear), pattern of load (concentric or eccentric), and magnitude of force also affect the response of the tendon to repetitive loading.

Tendon Healing and Repair

Previous studies have focused on the different healing mechanism between intrasynovial (e.g., the popliteus tendon) and extrasynovial tendons (e.g., the patellar tendon). It is likely that tendons heal by both intrinsic and extrinsic mechanisms. Although extrasynovial tendons often heal by infiltration of extrinsic cells derived from paratenon (including inflammatory cells, which result in adhesion formation), intrasynovial tendons can heal via intrinsic cells (epitenon and endotenon cells). An intrinsic healing capacity has been conclusively demonstrated by the presence of αI procollagen mRNA in epitenon and endotenon cells in healing tendon (37). Experimental studies suggest genetically predetermined structural and metabolic properties accounting for the differential cellular activity between these tendon types.

There are three phases during the tendon healing process: inflammatory, proliferative, and remodeling. Healing of extrasynovial tendon after injury or repair begins with formation of a hematoma, which contains inflammatory cells, blood cells, fibrin clot, and cellular and matrix debris. Cells derived from the paratenon proliferate and migrate into the wound site. Phagocytic cells phagocytose the necrotic debris at the wound site. Granulation tissue and new capillary buds are formed. New collagen synthesis can be detected by the third day. During the proliferative phase (starting at days 4 through 7), there is significant fibroblast proliferation and collagen production. Early matrix synthesis is disorganized and is oriented perpendicular to the axis of the tendon. Cells from the endotenon and epitenon proliferate and migrate into the wound site. During the third and fourth weeks, the newly formed matrix in the repair site begins to become organized and becomes oriented along the long axis of the tendon. This reorganization of the matrix occurs in response to stress on the tendon. The third phase of tendon healing is the remodeling phase. During this phase, the amount of scar tissue decreases but the biomechanical properties of the healed tendon increase. This is due to organization of the newly formed matrix and collagen cross-linking and other post-translational modifications of matrix proteins. Gradual remodeling continues for at least 6 months. During the remodeling phase, tendon vascularity and cellularity gradually return to normal.

Healing of intrasynovial tendon after injury or repair is predominantly via an intrinsic repair process. The healing process begins with migration of cells from the epitenon into the wound. These cells remove necrotic debris from the early granulation tissue that forms at the injury site. Proliferation of cells from the endotenon follows the phagocytosis by the epitenon cells, and these endotenon cells then produce new matrix to heal the tendon defect. The intrinsic repair response predominates during controlled motion, whereas tendons heal by ingrowth of connective tissue from the tendon sheath during immobilization.

Recent studies have begun to elucidate the histologic and biomechanical characteristics of tendon-to-bone healing, such as is required after patellar tendon and quadriceps tendon repair in the knee. Tendons attach to bone via direct or indirect types of insertions. The direct insertion contains an intermediate zone of fibrocartilage between the tendon and bone, whereas in indirect insertions the collagen fibers of the tendon become continuous with bone (Sharpey's fibers). No studies have directly examined healing of quadriceps or patellar tendon to bone; however, experimental studies have examined the histologic and biomechanical characteristics of healing of a tendon graft in a bone tunnel and

healing of a tendon to the surface of bone (38,39). Tendon-to-bone healing begins with formation of a fibrovascular interface tissue between the tendon and bone. The healing process appears to begin with mesenchymal cells derived from bone marrow. There is progressive bone ingrowth into this interface tissue, with gradual reestablishment of a tendon insertion by either endochondral or intramembranous bone formation, resulting in formation of a direct or indirect insertion, respectively. The gradual increase in strength of the healing tendon-to-bone attachment correlates well with the progressive bone ingrowth and maturation of the interface. The type of insertion that forms (direct or indirect) probably depends on multiple factors, including anatomic location, mechanical load, and species-specific factors. In a larger animal model (goats), an indirect insertion formed, whereas studies in lower animals demonstrate formation of a direct insertion (40). Further study is required to determine the basic cellular mechanism of tendon-to-bone healing.

New Methods to Improve Tendon Healing

There has been a great deal of research on the ability to influence the basic biology of tendon healing using pharmacologic and physical modalities. Various growth factors have been found to affect cell proliferation, matrix synthesis, and cell migration in intrasynovial and extrasynovial tendons. The most promising growth factors are transforming growth factor-β, insulin-like growth factor type 1, and platelet-derived growth factor (41–44). Transforming growth factor-β is a potent stimulator of matrix synthesis, whereas platelet-derived growth factor and insulin-like growth factor type 1 are powerful mitogenic agents. There are differences in sensitivity and response to some growth factors between intrasynovial and extrasynovial tendons, possibly due to a difference in growth factor receptor density. Gene transfer into cells of tendon and tendon sheath has been demonstrated using a recombinant adenovirus, raising the possibility of using gene therapy to deliver genes that code for cytokines that are important in tendon healing (45). Improvement in patellar tendon healing using gene therapy has been demonstrated in animal models. New research into tissue regeneration has demonstrated the possibility of using absorbable polymers, collagen gels, and mesenchymal stem cells to augment tendon healing. Novel physical modalities have also been found to augment tendon healing. Ultrasound has been reported to improve scar maturation and to decrease inflammatory cell infiltration into healing flexor tendon (46–48). A combination of ultrasound, electrical stimulation, and laser stimulation were found to increase collagen synthesis, tensile strength, and Young's modulus in healing rabbit Achilles tendon. These novel approaches and emerging technologies will hopefully be useful for improving the results of patellar tendon and quadriceps tendon repair in the future.

CLINICAL ASPECTS

Injury to tendons around the knee are common injuries that can occur due to both acute macrotrauma and repetitive microtrauma. Such injuries often cause disbling symptoms and require treatment. Approximately one third of sports injuries seen at outpatient clinics involve the knee (49). The highest incidences of injury are in soccer, basketball, volleyball, and long-distance running. The most common knee tendon injuries are quadriceps tendon ruptures, patellar tendinitis, Osgood-Schlatter disease, iliotibial band (ITB) friction syndrome, and hamstring strains.

Quadriceps Tendon Injury

Epidemiology

Quadriceps tendon ruptures tend to occur in patients over 40 years of age and with three times the frequency of patellar tendon ruptures. These injuries are seldom seen in younger patients. Unilateral quadriceps tendon ruptures occur approximately 15 to 20 times more frequently than do bilateral ruptures (50). Most ruptures occur transversely within 2 cm of the superior pole of the patella and often progress in a horizontal direction into the medial and lateral retinacula. Ruptures of the extensor mechanism, including patellar tendon rupture, occur most often in male patients (51).

Mechanism of Injury

Failure of the tendon most frequently occurs during an eccentric contraction. The usual mechanism is a violent reflex contraction of the muscle that is initiated against body weight with the knee in a partially flexed position. The knee may be going into flexion, despite quadriceps contraction, due to high external loads. However, it has been shown that the normal tendon is able to tolerate very high tensile loads (20). In addition, quadriceps tendon fibers interdigitate among separate bone lamellar systems (osteons or bone marrow spaces) of the patella, which suggests that the tendon insertion is very strong (52). Thus, it appears that tears often occur through a degenerative area within the tendon in patients older than 40 years of age. Tendon degeneration due to a systemic disease tends to occur bilaterally and may precipitate bilateral tendon rupture (53). Systemic conditions such as lupus erythematosus, diabetes mellitus, gout, hyperparathyroidism, uremia, rheumatoid arthritis, and osteomalacia (26,54) can affect the material properties of the tendon. Direct steroid injection can also weaken tendon (55). In healthy younger individu-

als, although rare, the rupture is usually due to direct trauma. DeLee and Craviotto (56) reported rupture of the quadriceps tendon after harvest of a central third patellar tendon graft for anterior cruciate ligament reconstruction.

Clinical Evaluation

Acute quadriceps tendon rupture causes immediate onset of pain and moderate swelling. A "pop" is sometimes felt or heard. Pain before the rupture is sometimes present. The patient is usually unable to extend the knee against resistance in a complete rupture. In a chronic partial rupture, the patient may complain of difficulty climbing stairs and giving way during walking. The patient may be able to walk with the knee in full extension. A palpable defect may be found just above the proximal pole of the patella with subcutaneous hematoma in a complete tear. There is usually inability to actively extend the knee; however, an ability to partially extend the knee may remain due to an intact medial and lateral retinaculum.

At the time of surgery, a careful examination under anesthesia should be performed to rule out concomitant ligamentous injury. An incomplete tear without a distinct episode of direct trauma may initially be misdiagnosed. Careful examination is required to diagnose an incomplete tear because there may not be a palpable tendon defect and full knee extension may still be possible. It is very important to take an accurate medical history of past and present medical problems and medications, including injections or surgery, because quadriceps tendon rupture may be associated with systemic disease. Occasionally, tears in patients with systemic diseases are first seen by nonorthopedic surgeons and physicians, and the injury may be mistaken for a neurologic paralysis (57).

Imaging

Plain radiographs may show a patella baja, avulsion of small bone fragments from the superior pole of the patella, calcification within the quadriceps tendon, or a suprapatellar bony spur. The "tooth sign," which is a degenerative bony spur at the superior pole of the patella seen on a tangential view, has been reported in association with quadriceps tendon degeneration (58). Lateral radiographs of the uninjured knee may be obtained to evaluate patellar height.

Arthrography may be useful for the diagnosis of a complete tear, in which there will be extravasation of dye from the suprapatellar pouch (59). Ultrasonography has been shown to demonstrate focal tendon degeneration or partial tears of the tendon. Bianchi et al. (60) studied 29 cases of quadriceps rupture diagnosed with ultrasonography and demonstrated a high degree of sensitivity and specificity. Because it is simple and cost effective, ultrasonography may also be useful for serial examinations to follow tendon healing. The principal drawback with ultrasonography is that it is highly operator dependent and requires an experienced technician.

Magnetic resonance imaging (MRI) is the most sensitive, specific, and accurate modality for evaluation of tendon injuries due to its superior soft tissue resolution. In the setting of a quadriceps tendon rupture, MRI demonstrates focal tendon discontinuity, increased signal intensity within the tendon, altered tendon morphology, and evidence of patella baja (61). The patellar tendon may appear lax due to loss of tension in the extensor mechanism. Because it is tomographic, MRI can accurately depict the exact width and thickness of the tear and preexisting pathologic changes within the tendon, such as underlying chondromucoid degeneration. MRI also allows visualization of all other intraarticular and extraarticular structures around the knee. Zeiss et al. (62) used MRI to evaluate normal and ruptured quadriceps tendons and reported that the normal quadriceps tendon has a laminated appearance with either two (30%), three (56%), or four (6%) layers. Incomplete ruptures were seen as focal discontinuities of individual layers with other layers remaining intact.

Nonoperative Treatment

For an incomplete tear, conservative treatment may be indicated; however, there is little information in the literature to guide in patient selection and expected outcomes. If MRI demonstrates a small partial thickness tear and knee extension strength is well preserved compared with the uninjured side, nonoperative treatment may be recommended. After acute injury, ice, compression, elevation, and anti-inflammatory medication are prescribed. The leg should be placed in a long leg splint with the knee fully extended. Aseptic aspiration of the hematoma may be helpful for both diagnostic and therapeutic purposes. After the initial swelling has resolved, the leg is placed in a cylinder cast or a removable double-upright hinged brace in full extension for 4 to 6 weeks. Straight leg raising isometric exercises may be started immediately. Partial weight bearing is recommended during the initial 4 weeks, followed by progression to full weight bearing in extension. Between 4 and 6 weeks (based on the size of the tear), the hinges on the brace are opened to allow restoration of normal gait. The brace is discontinued after 2 weeks of ambulation with the hinges open, as long as active leg control, strength, and gait are adequate.

After 4 to 6 weeks in full extension in the cast or brace, protected active flexion exercises begin with a gradual restoration of full flexion over the next 2 to 4 weeks. Aggressive attempts to rapidly increase knee flexion should be avoided, because the healing tendon is still remodeling and may stretch excessively. A recommended goal is to achieve 90 degrees of flexion within 2 weeks of cost removal. Progressive resistance exercises for the quadriceps are then begun, starting with closed chain isotonics and progressing to isokinetic exercises. Full sports activities should be avoided for at least 4 months after the injury. Healing should be carefully monitored if conservative treatment of an incomplete tear is elected to detect development of a complete rupture. If there is evidence of delayed healing or progressive rupture, early surgical intervention is recommended because delayed repair may be associated with inferior results.

Operative Treatment

Immediate repair of complete ruptures appears to yield improved overall results. Multiple surgical techniques for repairing the ruptured tendon have been described. The particular repair technique chosen may be guided by surgeon preference, the extent of retraction of the torn tendon, and the length of the residual tendon attached to the patella. Direct repair is possible for most acute tears. A midline longitudinal incision is used to expose the torn tendon. The tendon stumps are debrided of any necrotic, degenerative, and inflammatory tissue. If there is sufficient tendon proximally and distally, an end-to-end repair is performed with multiple no. 2 and no. 5 nonabsorbable mattress sutures. A tendon grasping suture, such as a Kessler or Bunnell suture configuration, is used to ensure a secure repair. The retinaculum is also carefully repaired with multiple interrupted nonabsorbable sutures. After the repair is complete, knee range of motion, tension on the repaired tendon, patellar position and tracking are carefully evaluated. The position of flexion at which there begins to be significant tension on the repair is carefully noted; this degree of flexion will be used to determine the limits of active flexion in the early postoperative period.

Most quadriceps tendon ruptures occur within 1 to 2 cm of the tendon–bone junction, with or without avulsion fragments of the patella. Often, a small amount of vastus intermedius tendon will remain attached to the superior pole of the patella. In such a case, the tendon stump is debrided of any necrotic, degenerative, and inflammatory tissue. A small horizontal trough is made at the proximal pole of the patella with a rongeur or high-speed bur. If a small stump of tendon remains on the patella, the trough should be made deep to the stump and the stump can then be used for augmentation of the repair. Anterior placement of the trough should be avoided because this may induce superior patellar tilt. Several sets of heavy nonabsorbable sutures are passed through the tendon in a Kessler or Bunnell suture configuration. Two parallel longitudinal drill holes are made in the patella. These drill holes enter into the trough and exit over the inferior pole of the patella (Fig. 39.1). The sutures from the tendon are then passed through these holes. The tendon is then reduced to the superior pole of the patella, and the sutures are tied with the knee in full extension. A careful retinacular repair is performed using nonabsorbable suture.

Chronic ruptures may be difficult to treat due to contraction of the tendon, degeneration of the residual tendon, and muscle atrophy from prolonged disuse. The tendon is mobilized by releasing adhesions to the surrounding soft tissues, skin, and underlying femur. Rarely, to mobilize the central tendon, it may be necessary to detach the vastus medialis and/or vastus lateralis muscles from the tendon. The muscles are then repaired back to the tendon after the tendon has been repaired to the patella. Quadriceps tendon lengthening using a Z-plasty or V-Y technique may be required to aid in tendon mobilization.

Several techniques are available to aid in repair of a retracted tendon. Techniques described by Scuderi and Codivilla can be used to close the gap. In the Scuderi technique, a partial-thickness triangular flap is fashioned from the anterior surface of the proximal tendon stump (63). This triangle is usually 7.5 cm long on each side and 5 cm wide at the base. The base of the triangle is made 5 cm proximal to the rupture. The apex of the triangle is turned distally and sutured across the rupture. The Scuderi technique may be modified such that the apex of the triangular flap is sutured to the distal stump at the proximal pole (64).

Another repair technique to bridge a large tendon gap is the Codivilla technique (65). An inverted V is cut through the full thickness of the proximal segment of the quadriceps tendon. This flap is split into an anterior part of one third of its thickness and a posterior part of two thirds. The anterior part of the flap is turned distally and sutured as in the Scuderi technique. The upper part of the V is then closed with sutures.

Augmentation materials such as strips of fascia lata autograft or allograft, semitendinosus and gracilis tendon, or synthetic materials can be used as well. Levy et al. (66) reported favorable results of four cases of quadriceps tendon repair with a Dacron vascular graft. A circumferential suturing or wiring may also be used for protection of the repair. A heavy no. 5 nonabsorbable suture or 5-mm Mersilene tape is passed through the proximal aspect of the patellar tendon along the inferior pole of patella and then through the quadriceps tendon above the repair site. In this way a circumferential loop is created that will serve to stress relieve the repair site. An 18-gauge wire may also be used, with placement through a drill hole in the tibial tubercle. The wire should be removed after 8 weeks.

Postoperative Rehabilitation

Postoperative rehabilitation includes protection of the repair during the early healing phase. The limb is placed into a hinged double-upright brace. Partial weight bearing in full extension is allowed immediately in most cases. If the repair is tenuous, non-weight bearing may be prescribed initially. If the patient is believed to be potentially noncompliant, consideration may be made for immobilization in a long leg cast for the first 3 weeks with the knee in full extension. Generally, however, a hinged brace is used so that protected early motion may begin. Full weight bearing is allowed once the patient has regained adequate motor control of the limb. Ambulation out of the brace is allowed when sufficient muscle strength and greater than 90 degrees of flexion have been achieved. The brace is usually worn for 6 to 8 weeks.

Early active flexion is allowed within a range that does not place high stress on the repair (this is determined intraoperatively). Up to 90 degrees of flexion may be possible after immediate repair of acute quadriceps tendon ruptures. Early limited motion will provide some mechanical load to the tendon. There is extensive basic and clinical evidence that load can enhance tendon healing (9,11–13). Motion will also prevent immobilization-induced articular cartilage degeneration. Continuous

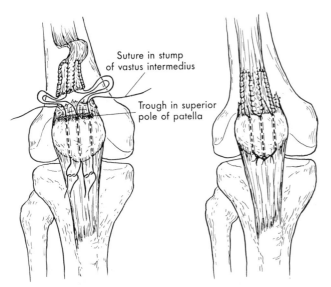

Suture in stump
of vastus intermedius

Trough in superior
pole of patella

FIG. 39.1. Quadriceps tendon repair is performed by placing several sets of heavy nonabsorbable sutures through the tendon in a Kessler or Bunnell suture configuration. Two parallel longitudinal drill holes are made in the patella, entering into the trough on the superior aspect of the patella and exiting over the inferior pole of the patella. The sutures from the tendon are then passed through these holes, the tendon is reduced to the superior pole of the patella, and the sutures are tied with the knee in full extension. (From Philips B. Disorders of muscles, tendons and associated structures: traumatic disorders. In: Crenshaw AH, ed. *Campbell's operative orthopaedics,* 8th ed. St. Louis: Mosby Year Book, 1992:1919, with permission.)

passive motion may be used in the first 3 to 4 weeks to aid in early motion. Only passive extension is allowed during the initial 6 weeks. Isometric quadriceps contractions and straight leg raising exercises may begin immediately for acute repairs. After 6 weeks, active extension exercises are begun. Initially, only the weight of the leg is used for quadriceps exercises. A progressive strengthening program is then followed, with progression to isotonic and isokinetic exercises. Electrical stimulation for the quadriceps may be useful. Active, active-assisted, and passive range-of-motion exercises are also progressed after the 6-week point. Strenuous sports or occupational activities may not be allowed until 6 months after surgery.

If a delayed repair has been performed or if the repair is believed to be tenuous, the postoperative rehabilitation must be modified appropriately. Straight leg raising exercises may be delayed until 2 to 3 weeks postoperatively and limited weight bearing may be followed for the first 6 weeks. Restoration of range of motion will also be slower in this setting.

Expected Outcomes

Overall, the results after quadriceps tendon rupture are superior to those after patellar tendon rupture (51,67). After acute repairs and appropriate rehabilitation, most patients achieve normal gait, full quadriceps strength, and satisfactory flexion (120 to 130 degrees). Secondary ruptures are rare after the repair. The principal factor in determining outcome is the length of time between injury and surgery. Chronic quadriceps tendon rupture is associated with disuse atrophy of the muscles of the injured leg, retraction of the quadriceps, and knee joint contracture. Age is also a factor, with better overall results reported in younger patients (67). Delayed quadriceps tendon repair is often associated with persistent quadriceps weakness and extensor lag.

Authors' Preferred Treatment

Repair of quadriceps tendon rupture within the first 2 to 4 weeks allows anatomic end-to-end repair. A vertical midline incision is used. The tendon ends are identified, freed from any early adhesions, and the torn end of the tendon is debrided back to healthy tendon. Retinacular tears should also be exposed and debrided, if necessary, in preparation for suture repair. Heavy nonabsorbable sutures (no. 2 or no. 5) are then woven through the proximal tendon with a tendon-gripping configuration (such as Kessler, Bunnell, or Mason-Allen stitch). A trough is made at the superior pole of the patella at the tendon attachment site using a burr or rongeur. Two parallel longitudinal drill holes are made in the patella, and the sutures are passed through these holes so that they exit over the inferior pole of the patella. The tendon

is reduced to the trough, and the sutures are tied over the inferior pole. Care must be taken to not excessively shorten the tendon. Patellar position and tracking should be evaluated before securing the repair sutures. The knot may be brought to one side so that it is not prominent over the front of the knee. The retinaculum is repaired using no. 0 absorbable sutures. After the repair is secured, the knee is brought through a range of motion and the position of flexion where there is significant tension on the repair is carefully noted; this degree of flexion will be used to determine the limits of active flexion in the early postoperative period.

Delayed quadriceps tendon repair may require the use of augmentation techniques and extensive mobilization, or even lengthening, of the retracted tendon. Adhesions between the tendon and the surrounding soft tissues are released. The Scuderi technique, as described above, is recommended for delayed repairs. A V-Y or Z-plasty lengthening may be necessary in cases with marked tendon retraction. A significant defect at the repair site may also be augmented with semitendinosus and gracilis tendons. The repair may be protected with a circumferential suture passed proximal and distal to the repair site. This circumferential loop serves to stress relieve the repair site.

Complications

Residual weakness of the extensor mechanism and inability to achieve full knee flexion are the most common complications after surgery. A residual extensor lag may occur after delayed repair. Infection and wound problems can occur, especially if there is poor soft tissue coverage over the tibial tubercle or if the wound closure is under tension, which may occur if augmentation materials are prominent at the repair site. Pull-out wires, which have been used in the past, are not recommended due to the risk for infection. Lateral patellar tilt may be induced if the retinacular repair is not balanced, and excessive patellofemoral contact stress may result from excessive shortening of the extensor mechanism. Excessive tightness of the retinacular repair may even induce patella infera, which can have detrimental consequences (67). Superior patellar tilt may be induced if the trough at the superior pole of the patella is placed anteriorly. These complications can be avoided by careful assessment of patellar position during the repair. Rerupture of the repair appears to be rare.

Iliotibial Band Friction Syndrome

Epidemiology

This condition was first described in young men in vigorous military training (68). Iliotibial band (ITB) friction syndrome occurs most commonly in long-distance runners and cyclists. It is especially common in athletes who engage in downhill running, such as cross-country runners.

Mechanism of Injury and Pathoanatomy

ITB friction syndrome is an overuse tendon injury caused by repetitive rubbing of the ITB over the lateral femoral epicondyle during flexion and extension of the knee. Pain and inflammation are produced by impingement of the posterior edge of the ITB over the lateral femoral epicondyle. This usually occurs just after footstrike in the gait cycle, at approximately 30 degrees of knee flexion. Downhill running seems to predispose to this problem because knee flexion angle at footstrike is reduced. Extrinsic factors related to this problem include excessive training mileage, downhill running, and running on a banked track. Intrinsic factors that have been identified include varus knee alignment, hindfoot pronation, leg length discrepancy (the shorter leg is affected), and ITB inflexibility.

Clinical Evaluation

The most common symptom is lateral knee pain which is worst at approximately 30 degrees of flexion and relieved in full extension. The pain is exacerbated by downhill running. Physical examination demonstrates tenderness in the region of the lateral femoral condyle with occasional crepitus. There is usually no effusion, and tests for meniscal or ligament injury are negative. Ober's test may demonstrate inflexibility of the ITB. There may occasionally be a palpable thickening of the band. The differential diagnosis includes lateral meniscus injury, patellofemoral syndrome, biceps tendinitis, and stress fracture.

Imaging

Plain radiographs of the knee are usually negative, but MRI may demonstrate increased thickness of the ITB and fluid collection, consistent with a bursa, deep to the ITB (69). Increased uptake over the lateral femoral epicondyle has been described on bone scan (70). Plain radiographs are recommended routinely, but MRI or bone scan are not part of the routine evaluation of this problem. MRI is recommended only if symptoms fail to respond to extensive conservative treatment.

Nonoperative Treatment

Conservative treatment modalities include rest, ice, flexibility exercises, anti-inflammatory medications, and modalities such as ultrasound or massage therapy. Steroid injection may be considered in recalcitrant cases. Foot orthoses may be considered if there is abnormal hindfoot alignment. Suggested alterations in the running regimen include avoiding downhill running, running faster (because there is higher knee flexion angle at footstrike when running faster), and running on the opposite side of the road or track if running on a banked surface.

Operative Treatment

Surgical treatment is reserved for those cases that do not respond to 3 to 6 months of conservative management. Preoperative MRI may be helpful in determining the size and location of ITB thickening and any associated bursa. Surgery consists of removal of the fibrotic thickened bursa between the ITB and the lateral femoral epicondyle and incision of the posterior edge of the ITB to remove the site of impingement. Any excessive prominence of the lateral femoral epicondyle should also be removed, if present. Arthroscopic inspection of the knee should be performed to rule out any other cause of the knee pain. Arthroscopic resection of the bursa between the ITB and the lateral femoral epicondyle and removal of a prominent epicondyle may also be considered. Arthroscopic localization may be aided by using a needle placed from the outside into the thickened region of the band.

Postoperative rehabilitation includes progressive range of motion and strengthening exercises. Immediate full weight bearing without a brace is allowed. ITB flexibility work is important. Strengthening is performed with isotonic and isokinetic exercises. Quadriceps strengthening and hamstring stretching exercises are important to prevent patellofemoral pain. Progression to sport-specific exercises and return to activity are based on range of motion and strength. Return to running may begin at approximately 4 weeks, but care should be taken to progress gradually to prevent patellofemoral pain.

Expected Outcomes

With early diagnosis and appropriate rehabilitation, return to full activity may be expected. However, because this is an overuse injury, there is always a chance for recurrence, especially if the athlete resumes the activities that initiated the problem. The most important factor in preventing recurrence is elimination of predisposing factors such as ITB inflexibility. The risk of recurrence may also be decreased by altering the running regimen and perhaps the running surface.

Authors' Preferences

With early diagnosis and a well-designed treatment program, most patients with ITB friction syndrome will improve with nonoperative treatment. Identification and correction of predisposing factors is important. For runners, the frequency, intensity, and duration of running must be carefully determined. The relationship between the onset of symptoms and any changes in the training regimen should be determined. The important aspects of nonoperative treatment are rest, ice, flexibility exercises, anti-inflammatory medications, and, possibly, modalities such as ultrasound, electrical stimulation, or massage therapy. Steroid injection would only be considered for recalcitrant symptoms (longer than 3 months) that have not responded to conservative treatment and if imaging studies clearly demonstrate a fibrotic thickened bursa between the ITB and the lateral femoral epicondyle. The steroid should not be directly injected into the ITB to avoid the potential adverse effects of corticosteroid on collagenous tissues.

Hamstring Tendon, Popliteus Tendon, and Gastrocnemius Tendon Injury

Epidemiology

Hamstring muscle strains are very common injuries in runners (especially sprinters), hurdlers, and jumpers. These injuries are also common in soccer and football players. Acute disruption of the medial gastrocnemius at the musculotendinous junction can occur in middle-aged recreational athletes.

Mechanism of Injury and Pathoanatomy

Most hamstring muscle strains occur at the proximal muscle–tendon junction of the biceps femoris muscle and usually do not present with knee pain. Rarely, tendinitis or strain injury will occur in the distal aspect of the muscle–tendon unit and result in knee pain. These injuries may be due to repetitive overuse and present as a tendinosis/peritendinitis. Alternatively, there may be a single injury that results in a strain or tear at the muscle–tendon junction. This type of injury usually occurs in a poorly flexible muscle–tendon unit that is fatigued from exercise. Complete disruption of the biceps muscle at the distal muscle–tendon junction has been reported in a runner (71). Such injuries may prove debilitating because the biceps is the most powerful knee flexor (72).

Recent anatomic studies have demonstrated the complex anatomy of the biceps femoris muscle complex at the lateral side of the knee (17). This study demonstrated expansions from the biceps tendon to the iliotibial tract and the lateral collateral ligament and reported an association between anterior knee instability (positive Lachman test) and injury to the expansion from the biceps to the iliotibial tract, demonstrating the relationship between biceps femoris complex injury and anterior instability.

Injury to the gastrocnemius tendons at the knee is uncommon. Repetitive overload of the gastrocnemius–soleus complex usually results in peritendinitis/tendinosis of the Achilles tendon rather than at the proximal tendon at the knee. Because the gastrocnemius muscle crosses two joints, the combination of knee hyperextension and ankle dorsiflexion can lead to failure at the muscle–tendon junction during eccentric contraction. The medial head of the gastrocnemius is more prone to injury than the lateral head because of its larger size and more oblique fiber orientation.

Overuse injury of the pes anserinus tendons (sartorius, gracilis, and semitendinosis) may also occur. A case of medial knee pain due to friction between the anterior edge of the pes anserinus and the medial femoral condyle, analogous to ITB friction syndrome, has been reported (73). Histologic analysis of tissue over the medial femoral condyle in this case showed proliferation of periosteal cells, formation of fibrocartilage, and endochondral ossification.

Isolated acute or chronic injury of the popliteus tendon is uncommon. Lateral knee pain due to popliteus tenosynovitis, ganglion cyst of the tendon, and calcium deposition have been reported (74–76). Overuse injury of the popliteus tendon has been described as a cause of lateral knee pain, especially in persons performing downhill running (77). This condition is associated with lateral knee pain when weight bearing on the knee at 15 to 30 degrees of flexion. This condition may occur due to repetitive high loads on the popliteus tendon as it resists anterior femoral displacement relative to the tibia as the knee is increasingly flexed during downhill running. Acute rupture of the popliteus tendon from its femoral insertion with associated mildly increased posterolateral rotatory laxity has also been reported (78).

Clinical Evaluation

Diagnosis of acute or chronic injury involving the biceps femoris, pes anserinus, popliteus, or gastrocnemius tendons is made principally by the location and pattern of pain, mechanism of injury, and a careful physical examination. Tenderness, pain with resisted contraction, pain with passive stretch, and occasional swelling over the involved structure verify the diagnosis. Intraarticular knee effusion is uncommon, and signs for meniscal and ligament injury will be negative.

Most hamstring muscle strains occur at the proximal muscle–tendon junction of the biceps femoris muscle and thus do not present with knee pain. However, strain injury or tendinitis may occur in the distal aspect of the muscle–tendon unit and results in knee pain. The pain is usually well localized to the back of the knee. Examination may reveal tenderness at the site of the hamstring strain. Rarely, ecchymosis or even a palpable defect will be present. Detection of a defect in the muscle/tendon may be facilitated by having the patient contract the muscle while the examiner palpates. Decreased flexibility of the hamstrings is often present. Passive stretch and active contraction of the hamstrings usually reproduce pain.

Gastrocnemius muscle–tendon injury usually presents as calf pain but may occasionally be associated with knee pain. The medial head of the gastrocnemius is more commonly injured than the lateral head. Overuse injury of the pes anserinus tendons presents as activity-related pain along the anteromedial aspect of the knee, which may be exacerbated by repetitive flexion and extension. Resisted knee flexion or passive stretch may reproduce the pain. Popliteus tendon injury presents as lateral-sided knee pain, which may be exacerbated during downhill running. Examination may reveal tenderness at the femoral insertion of the popliteus tendon, and pain may be elicited by passive external rotation of the tibia.

Imaging

Plain radiographs should be obtained routinely in the evaluation of the knee. Plain radiographs are usually negative but may rarely reveal foci of calcification in the involved tendon. For most tendon injuries, advanced imaging is not indicated during the initial evaluation. Imaging may be indicated if symptoms persist despite comprehensive treatment. MRI is the most accurate modality for imaging tendon injuries due to its superior soft tissue contrast. Ultrasound has also been used for tendon imaging, but this modality is highly operator dependent, and the overall resolution, sensitivity, and specificity are inferior to MRI. A case of pes anserinus tendinitis due to friction between the anterior edge of the pes anserinus and the medial femoral condyle, analogous to ITB friction syndrome, has been reported in which bone scan revealed increased uptake over the medial femoral condyle (73).

Nonoperative Treatment

Recommended treatment of these overuse tendon injuries is similar to treatment of other tendon injuries. Conservative treatment with rest, ice, anti-inflammatory medications, flexibility exercises, modalities such as ultrasound, and, occasionally, steroid injection are usually curative. A compression wrap is recommended to decrease bleeding in an acute strain injury at a muscle–tendon junction.

Identification of specific intrinsic (specific muscle weakness or inflexibility, knee or ankle malalignment) or extrinsic factors (training errors, excessive training) is important in preventing recurrent injury. Muscle strengthening is important for prevention of recurrent

injury. Because these injuries often occur during eccentric muscle contraction, muscle strengthening may help to prevent injury by increasing the ability of muscle to absorb and dissipate force. Before return to sports, there must be no tenderness over the injured tendon, full knee range of motion and muscle flexibility, and muscle strength and endurance equal to at least 90% of the normal side with isokinetic testing.

Operative Treatment

Surgical treatment is rarely required. Surgery should be considered if symptoms persist after 3 to 6 months of well-structured conservative management. Surgical treatment should be based on a distinct anatomic abnormality identified on imaging studies. For example, a discrete focus of high-signal intensity within a tendon has been found to correlate with histologically demonstrated tendon degeneration. Excision of such a focus of abnormal tendon with repair of the remaining normal tendon would be recommended in this setting if conservative treatment failed to relieve symptoms. A chronically thickened fibrotic tendon sheath may also be identified on imaging studies, and surgical release of this pathologic tendon sheath may also be effective. Rupture of the popliteus tendon, although uncommon, should be repaired to restore normal posterolateral knee stability.

Expected Outcomes

Most overuse tendon injuries will resolve with appropriate treatment. Time missed from practice and competition is quite variable, ranging from 1 to 2 days to as long as 6 weeks, depending on the severity of the injury and the underlying cause of the injury. Identification and correction of any specific predisposing factors will aid in preventing recurrence. Hamstring strain injuries commonly recur, most likely because the athlete returns to the offending activity. There is always a risk of recurrence of tendon overuse injuries if the athlete returns to the activity that caused the injury.

Authors' Preferences

With early diagnosis and a well-designed treatment program, most patients with overuse tendon injury will improve with nonoperative treatment. Identification and correction of predisposing factors is important. The important aspects of nonoperative treatment are rest, ice, flexibility exercises, anti-inflammatory medications, and modalities such as ultrasound, electrical stimulation, or massage therapy. Attention should especially be paid to improving flexibility to prevent recurrent hamstring strain injury. Steroid injection would only be considered for recalcitrant symptoms (longer than 3 months) that have not responded to conservative treatment and if imaging studies clearly demonstrate a pathologic abnormality in the tendon. Steroids should not be directly injected into tendons.

Patellar Tendinitis ("Jumper's Knee")

Epidemiology

The clinical entity of "jumper's knee" was first described by Blazina et al. (79). Patellar tendinitis is a common condition affecting the proximal attachment of the patellar tendon to the distal pole of the patella and is found particularly in those engaged in sporting activities such as basketball, volleyball, and soccer. Activities with repetitive jumping predispose to patellar tendinitis, which is why this condition is often called jumper's knee. However, patellar tendinitis does not occur only in jumping athletes. It can occur in any activities in which repeated extension of the knee is required.

The most common age is from the late teens to the thirties, although this condition may occur in older individuals. Martens et al. (80) reported that volleyball and soccer were the most common sports involved. Blazina et al. reported that patellar tendinitis usually occurred in tall individuals, and Lian et al. (81) found a significant difference in body weight between patient and control groups in their study of volleyball players with jumper's knee. This condition has also been reported in association with several pathologic conditions (e.g., rheumatoid arthritis and gout). Sinding-Larsen-Johannsson disease is sometimes described in association with patellar tendinitis; however, the former condition is more accurately termed an apophysitis and is described in another section of this chapter.

Mechanism of Injury

Although it is basically a chronic overuse injury of the patellar tendon, the precise pathomechanics that lead to injury have not been well described. Repetitive microtrauma or a single macrotraumatic event may initiate the underlying pathologic process. Johnson et al. (82) suggested that patellar tendinitis may represent an impingement of the distal patellar pole on the middle third of the patellar tendon in flexion because the fibers of the tendon do not all insert directly at the patellar apex but continue over the anterior surface of the patellar apex. These authors supported their hypothesis with MRI evaluations of patellar tendinitis and believed that such a mechanism would explain the characteristic site of the lesion and explain why surgical release of the tendon at the patellar apex is often beneficial. Laduron et al. (83) advocated another type of impingement that occurred between the deep fibers of the patellar tendon and the lateral part of the femoral trochlea when the knee is fully extended.

Several anatomic factors have been related to patellar tendinitis, including patella alta, abnormal patellofemoral tracking, patellar instability, chondromalacia, Osgood-Schlatter disease, and mechanical malalignment or leg length inequality (84). The relationship of such factors to patellar tendinitis remains to be clarified. Other studies have characterized factors during the jumping motion associated with patellar tendinitis. Lian et al. (81) found that volleyball players with jumper's knee demonstrated better performance in jump tests than uninjured athletes, particularly in jumps involving eccentric force generation, presumably resulting in greater stress on the patellar tendon. Richards et al. (85) studied lower extremity movement biomechanics for 10 elite volleyball players and concluded that the likelihood of patellar tendon pain was related to high forces and rates of loading in the knee extensor mechanism, combined with large external tibial torsional moments and deep knee flexion angles.

The pathologic abnormality in this condition appears to be an area of tendon degeneration (tendinosis) within the proximal patellar tendon. Histologically, the tissue is characterized as "angiofibroblastic hyperplasia" with fibroblast proliferation, new blood vessel formation, chondromucoid deposition, and collagen fragmentation. The gross and microscopic appearance is similar to that seen in chronic lateral epicondylitis. Notably, inflammatory cells are usually absent in surgical biopsies. However, in the early phases of the condition, there may be inflammation in the paratenon ("peritendinitis"), but very little histologic confirmation is available from early cases because surgery is rarely indicated at this stage. This abnormal tissue may represent the result of an ineffectual healing response to repetitive microtears within the tendon. Once this abnormal tissue develops, the natural healing response may not be capable of healing the lesion, resulting in chronic symptoms.

Clinical Evaluation

In the acute phase, the patient experiences anterior knee pain focused on the distal patellar pole and the proximal part of the patellar tendon. There is usually tenderness to palpation over this region. The tendon itself may become swollen. Active knee extension against resistance causes pain. These symptoms usually disappear after a period of rest, despite pathologic change in the tendon or its attachment site. Blazina et al. (79) described four stages of jumper's knee based on symptoms. In stage 1 there is pain only after activity, whereas in stage 2 there is pain at the beginning of activity that disappears after a warm-up but may reappear with fatigue. In stage 3 there is constant pain at rest and with activity. In stage 4 there is complete rupture of the patellar tendon.

Imaging

The diagnosis of patellar tendinitis is made based on the clinical presentation. However, plain radiographs should be obtained in the initial evaluation of all patients with patellar tendinitis. Plain radiographs may show decreased bone mineral density at the distal pole of the patella. With prolonged symptoms, osteophyte may form at the distal pole, the tooth sign (which represents periosteal reaction of the anterior patellar surface) may be present, and tendon calcification may be evident.

MRI is the most accurate modality for imaging the patellar tendon due to the excellent soft tissue contrast. MRI is recommended for evaluation of chronic symptoms and in planning surgical intervention. MRI may demonstrate significant thickening of the proximal one third of the tendon, especially on the posterior and central or medial aspect (82,86). Focal enlargement of the tendon may exceed 7 mm in the anteroposterior dimension (86). In chronic cases, MRI will demonstrate a focus of abnormal signal intensity in the posterior aspect of the proximal tendon. The abnormal signal may extend to the distal pole of the patella. Yu et al. (86) correlated MRI findings with pathologic findings in athletes with chronic patellar tendinitis. Pathologically, the areas of abnormal signal intensity on MRI corresponded to tissue containing hyaline degeneration, tendon fibroblast proliferation, prominent angiogenesis with endothelial hyperplasia, loss of longitudinal collagen architecture, and microtears with collagen fiber separation. The presence of a focus of abnormal signal in the tendon usually indicates irreversible changes within the tendon, and these cases may require surgical intervention. Conversely, the absence of a tendon abnormality on MRI may suggest that conservative treatment will most likely be effective. MRI can thus be very helpful in planning treatment.

Ultrasound may demonstrate a focal hypoechoic region at the deep portion of the tendon adjacent to the lower pole of the patella (87). Ultrasound may be useful in the outpatient or emergency room setting for its real-time imaging; however, the quality of the images is highly operator dependent, and ultrasound is therefore not widely used at this time in the United States. Bone scintigraphy may show abnormally increased uptake at the distal pole of the patella, although it is not suitable for the routine diagnosis because of its low sensitivity (88).

Nonoperative Treatment

In the acute phase of patellar tendinitis, ice, rest, and avoidance of the offending activity are recommended. Nonsteroidal anti-inflammatory drugs can be used for several weeks. Physiotherapy may be started after the acute pain has resolved. Quadriceps and hamstring muscle stretching and isometric exercise in a limited range of motion are started. Modalities such as ultrasound and massage may be helpful. Errors in jumping or running technique should be identified and corrected. Physical therapy should be continued, including progressive eccentric muscle strengthening, until there is complete remission of the symptoms (89). Restoration of full flexibility of the extensor mechanism is the most important factor in preventing recurrence. An elastic knee support or a patellar brace may be useful to protect the tendon if abnormal patellofemoral tracking or patellar instability is present. Some cases of patellar tendinitis may require a prolonged period of conservative treatment.

Operative Treatment

Surgical intervention is recommended if prolonged conservative management fails to resolve symptoms. In chronic cases there is usually a focus of abnormal degenerative tendon in the proximal patellar tendon at the attachment site to the patella. MRI will demonstrate the precise location and extent of abnormality within the tendon and is thus very helpful in planning surgery. Surgery consists of resection of the degenerated tendon and bone at the apex of the patella. The paratenon is opened and preserved. Careful surgical exploration demonstrates a focus of abnormal tissue. This area is usually gray in appearance and may have a somewhat gelatinous or gritty consistency. The appearance of the abnormal tissue is similar to that seen in chronic lateral epicondylitis. The focus of degenerate tendon is often on the deep aspect of the patellar tendon and so may only be evident after the proximal tendon is opened longitudinally in line with its fibers. This abnormal focus of degenerate tendon is thoroughly excised. The excision also includes a small amount of bone at the insertion site on the patella. Small drill holes may be made in the inferior pole of the patella to promote healing. The defect in the tendon is closed with side-to-side interrupted absorbable sutures without tension. The paratenon is carefully closed over the tendon repair site. After the repair is complete, the knee is brought through a range of motion, and tension on the repaired tendon, patellar position, and patellar tracking are carefully evaluated. The position of flexion at which there begins to be significant tension on the repair is carefully noted; this degree of flexion will be used to determine the limits of motion in the early postoperative period.

Postoperative Rehabilitation

The leg is placed in a knee immobilizer or hinged knee brace for 4 to 6 weeks, and partial weight bearing in full extension is permitted initially. Isometric quadriceps muscle exercise can be started immediately after surgery. Active flexion to the limits determined intraoperatively is begun immediately. Flexion of at least 90 degrees should be safe immediately postoperatively because no significant tendon shortening should be created by the surgery. Active extension exercises against gravity are delayed for 4 weeks to allow full tendon healing. A progressive program of quadriceps strengthening and flexibility is then initiated. The load on the patellar tendon is progressively increased, and activity-specific exercises are gradually added. Criteria for return to sports include absence of tenderness at the repair site, full range of motion, and isokinetic quadriceps strength equal to at least 90% of the normal side. Return to full activity is allowed at approximately 4 months after surgery. Residual pain during activity is sometimes observed for several months after return to sports. During the healing phase, the patellar tendon is probably at some increased risk of rupture and thus care is taken to carefully follow symptoms during return to vigorous activity.

Expected Outcomes

The results of surgery, including a full return to sports, are generally favorable (80,90). Successful return to sports has been reported in approximately 80% to 90% of patients. However, some residual activity-related discomfort at the tendon repair site is not uncommon during the first 6 months after return to sports. Patients must be informed of this possibility.

Authors' Preferred Treatment

Most cases of patellar tendinitis can be successfully treated with a well-designed rehabilitation program. Careful examination of running and/or jumping technique and training regimen will be helpful in identifying etiologic factors. Flexibility training is an especially important component of the rehabilitation program. If symptoms persist, MRI is recommended to determine if there is a structural abnormality in the tendon. If there is a focus of degenerate tendon on MRI and symptoms persist, surgical intervention is recommended. Our experience has been that the presence of an abnormal focus of degeneration within the tendon as seen on MRI indicates an irreversible lesion that most likely will not resolve with conservative management. Resection of the degenerative tendon and bone at the insertion site with careful tendon repair, as described above, is recommended for such cases.

Complications

Recurrence rates are low after surgical intervention. However, as noted above, activity-related discomfort may persist for up to 6 months after return to activities.

Excessive shortening of the tendon may increase patellofemoral contact stress and result in patellar pain and should thus be avoided. Even with normal tendon length and patellofemoral mechanics, extensor mechanism dysfunction may occur from quadriceps inhibition and result in anterior knee pain. This should resolve with careful physical therapy. Rupture of the tendon is a possibility during the early healing period, and thus the healing tendon is protected postoperatively and return to activity must be gradual.

Patellar Tendon Rupture

Epidemiology

Patellar tendon rupture is an uncommon condition compared with quadriceps tendon rupture. In a series from the Mayo Clinic, patellar tendon rupture occurred one third as often as quadriceps tendon rupture (91). Most patellar tendon ruptures occur in patients who are less than 40 years of age. Most ruptures occur at the tendon–bone junction at the distal pole of the patella. This injury is frequently associated with sports that place high loads on the knee, such as football, basketball, and soccer. Patellar tendinitis also occurs commonly in these sports. Bilateral simultaneous rupture is quite rare but has been reported in a young athlete without any history of predisposing conditions (92).

Mechanism of Injury

Histologic examination of torn patellar tendon often demonstrates underlying microscopic tendon degeneration preceding spontaneous tendon rupture. It is likely that such pathologic alterations predispose the tendon to rupture, because normal tendon rarely fails during ultimate tensile testing. However, dynamic loading during sports activities can generate very high tendon forces and may lead to rupture (93). Patellar tendon ruptures can also occur in association with systemic conditions, as described above for quadriceps tendon injuries. Local steroid injection can also weaken tendon and predispose to rupture (94,95). Aging may lead to degenerative change of the tendon and deterioration of biomechanical properties of the tendon, although one study reported minimal differences in tensile and viscoelastic properties between younger and older age groups (96). Previous surgery such as anterior cruciate ligament reconstruction using the central third of the patellar tendon as a graft, intramedullary nailing of the tibia, and total knee arthroplasty have also been related to early and late postoperative patellar tendon ruptures (97). Previous surgery may affect the vascularity of the patellar tendon, resulting in tendon weakening. In younger patients, patellar tendon injury may occur with direct trauma (such as laceration) or as a result of chronic overuse injury (such as jumper's knee or Osgood-Schlatter disease).

Clinical Evaluation

The most common location of patellar tendon rupture is at the inferior pole of the patella. Disruption of the patellar tendon causes similar findings to quadriceps tendon rupture in that the patient is usually unable to generate or maintain full extension of the knee against gravity. A palpable discontinuity of the tendon may be easily appreciated just below the distal pole of the patella. Significant hematoma is usually present. The patella migrates proximally, and there may be abnormal medial and lateral patellar mobility. Chronic ruptures may present with a persistent extensor lag, decreased quadriceps strength, and decreased range of motion.

Imaging

Plain radiographs should be obtained in the evaluation of all suspected patellar tendon ruptures. Plain radiographs often demonstrate patella alta, with or without a bony fragment at the inferior pole of the patella. Calcification within the tendon and a bone spur over the distal pole of the patella may be present. A lateral radiograph at 30 degrees of flexion will demonstrate patella alta based on an Insall-Salvati ratio of less than 0.80 (98). Comparison lateral radiographs of the contralateral knee are also helpful to evaluate patellar height.

MRI accurately demonstrates the site of tendon disruption, underlying tendon degeneration (based on increased intratendon signal), patellar position, and any other associated injuries. MRI may also be very helpful in the detection of quadriceps atrophy in chronic cases, which will be demonstrated as abnormal signal within the muscle. MRI is not routinely recommended in the evaluation of suspected patellar tendon injury because this diagnosis can usually be made based on clinical evaluation. MRI is recommended, however, if there is a suspicion of partial rupture, significant muscle atrophy, or other associated pathology. If MRI is unavailable, arthrography may demonstrate extravasation of dye if there is disruption of the medial and lateral extensor retinaculum and the capsule. Arthrography is no longer routinely used.

Nonoperative Treatment

Partial tears can be treated conservatively by immobilization of the leg in full extension. Partial weight bearing in full extension is allowed for the first 2 to 3 weeks, after which full weight bearing in extension is allowed. Straight leg raising exercises may begin immediately. After 4 to 6 weeks of immobilization, based on the size of the tear, active flexion and passive extension is begun.

Knee flexion is limited to 30 degrees for the first 2 weeks, after which flexion is progressed by 30 degrees every 2 weeks. Active-assisted extension exercises may begin at the 6-week point. At 8 weeks, a progressive quadriceps stengthening program, using isotonic and isokinetic exercises, is started (99). Quadriceps flexibility is also gradually increased. Return to sports is allowed when there is no tenderness over the patellar tendon, full range of knee motion, and isokinetic quadriceps strength equal to at least 90% of the normal side.

Operative Treatment

Complete tears should be treated surgically as soon as possible to avoid contracture of the extensor mechanism. Acute ruptures may be directly repaired. A careful examination under anesthesia is first performed to rule out concomitant ligament instability. A straight vertical midline incision is used to expose the torn tendon and the retinaculum. The tendon stumps are debrided of all degenerated and inflammatory tissue and mobilized to oppose the torn ends easily. Care should be taken to avoid injury to the infrapatellar fat pad because it may provide blood supply to the healing patellar tendon.

The most common site of rupture is at the attachment to the inferior pole of the patella, with or without an avulsion fragment of bone. A small horizontal trough is made at the distal pole of the patella with a rongeur or burr. Nonabsorbable no. 2 or no. 5 sutures are placed into the tendon using a locking suture configuration, such as a Kessler, Mason-Allen, or Bunnell stitch. Two or three longitudinal drill holes are made in the patella, taking care to avoid violating the articular surface. The sutures are passed from the tendon into the drill holes, exiting over the superior pole of the patella. The tendon is reduced to the trough in the inferior pole of the patella and are then tied with the knee in full extension. Any retinacular tears are repaired with multiple interrupted no. 0 absorbable sutures. If the rupture occurs in the middle of the tendon with sufficient remaining tendon proximally and distally, an end-to-end repair is performed with multiple no. 2 or no. 5 nonabsorbable mattress sutures. If the repair site is close to the patella or tibial tuberosity, one set of sutures may be passed through drill holes in the patella or tibial tuberosity, respectively. If possible, the paratenon is closed as a separate layer over the repaired tendon. When the repair is complete, knee range of motion, tension on the repaired tendon, patellar position, and patellar tracking should be carefully evaluated. The knee should be able to flex at least to 90 degrees. Correct patellar tendon length and patellar height can be judged by using an intraoperative radiograph or by prepping the contralateral limb to allow for direct comparison during surgery.

The repair may be protected with a circumferential loop of 18-gauge wire, Mersilene tape, Dacron graft, heavy suture, or semitendinosus and gracilis tendon (100–102). Bioabsorbable suture materials or tendon grafts have the advantage of possibly decreasing stress shielding, hardware problems such as infection, and the necessity for removal. These materials are placed through the distal quadriceps tendon or, less commonly, a drill hole in the superior aspect of the patella, and through a drill hole in the tibial tuberosity. McLaughlin and Francis (103) described a technique in which a circumferential wire is secured to the tibia with a bolt. The circumferential wire or suture should be secured with the knee between 45 and 90 degrees of flexion to avoid overconstraining the extensor mechanism. These reinforcing materials allow early mobilization. If a wire is used, it should be removed at 8 to 10 weeks after repair. When the semitendinosus and gracilis tendons are used for augmentation of the repair, they are placed through a transverse drill hole in the patella and through a drill hole in the tibial tuberosity (Fig. 39.2) (100,101). These tendons are then sutured to the patellar tendon. Other options for augmentation include distal reflection of a strip of the central third of the quadriceps tendon or use of fascia lata.

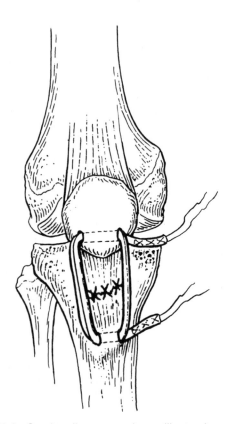

FIG. 39.2. Semitendinosus and gracilis tendons can be placed through drill holes in the proximal tibia and through the proximal pole of the patella to augment the patellar tendon repair. (From Larson RV, Simonian PT. Semitendinosus augmentation of acute patellar tendon repair with immediate mobilization. *Am J Sports Med* 1995;23:82–86, with permission.)

Chronic ruptures are more difficult to treat due to proximal retraction of the extensor mechanism and muscle atrophy. The quadriceps tendon is mobilized by releasing any adhesions to the surrounding soft tissues. The vastus intermedius tendon may need to be mobilized from adhesions to the underlying femur. Preoperative traction may be useful in cases with severe proximal retraction. A Steinman pin is placed transversely through the patella, and then traction is applied with progressively increasing weight over 2 to 4 weeks. Traction should be continued until normal patellar height is restored and there is at least 90 degrees of flexion. Once the patella has been restored to its anatomic position, the patellar tendon repair or reconstruction is carried out as the second stage. Patellar traction has also been described using an Ilizarov fixator in which olive wires are placed vertically in the patella and then connected to a tibial frame. The wires are tensioned 1 mm/day to pull the patella distally (104). Advantages of this technique are that it allows knee motion and weight bearing of the injured leg during the period of traction, and the tendon repair site can also be protected by the Ilizarov frame postoperatively, with gradual stress transfer to the healing tendon by removing the traction. In cases of severe patellar retraction, a Z lengthening or V-Y lengthening of the quadriceps tendon may be required to correct patellar height.

Because the tissue quality of the remaining tendon in chronic cases is often inferior, augmentation or the repair and/or patellar tendon reconstruction are often indicated. There are several options for augmentation and reconstruction. As described above, semitendinosus and gracilis tendons can be used. These tendons are useful for augmentation if there is some remaining patellar tendon; however, they are insufficient for use as a sole replacement for an irreparable tendon. An Achilles tendon allograft with a calcaneal bone block has been used for patellar tendon reconstruction (105). A trough is made at the tibial tubercle to receive the calcaneal bone block, which is then secured with two cancellous screws. Care is taken to recreate a normal Q-angle when choosing the site for attachment of the bone block to the tibial tuberosity. The tendinous portion of the allograft is divided into three strips, the central third of which is passed through a 9-mm-wide longitudinal tunnel in the patella. This central slip of tendon then emerges proximally through a small slit in the quadriceps tendon and is sutured to the quadriceps tendon with no. 2 nonabsorbable sutures. The medial and lateral thirds of the allograft tendon are passed proximally and sutured to the medial and lateral retinaculum with no. 2 nonabsorbable sutures. Care is taken to avoid producing an imbalance in the tension in the medial versus lateral retinaculum when suturing the allograft to the retinaculum. The allograft is also sutured to any remaining native patellar tendon. Appropriate graft length is determined by ensuring that the knee will flex to 90 degrees and by evaluation of the Insall-Salvati ratio. Intraoperative radiographs may be helpful to confirm appropriate patellar height.

Reconstruction can also be performed using a patella–quadriceps tendon autograft (Fig. 39.3) (106). The graft is taken from the central third of the quadriceps tendon with an attached bone block from the proximal patella. The length of tendon harvested is determined by the length of the normal patella tendon. The bone block is fixed to a bony trough at the tibial tubercle with a 4-mm cancellous screw. A small horizontal trough is made at the distal pole of the patella with a rongeur or burr. Heavy nonabsorbable (no. 5) sutures are placed into the tendon using a locking suture configuration, such as a Kessler, Mason-Allen, or Bunnell stitch. Two longitudinal drill holes are made in the patella, taking care to avoid entering the graft donor site in the proxi-

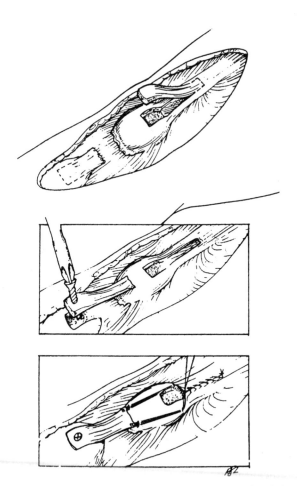

FIG. 39.3. The central third of the quadriceps tendon is harvested with an attached bone plug. This bone plug is then placed into a trough in the tibial tuberosity and the tendon is secured to the patella with heavy sutures passed through drill holes in the patella. (From Williams RJ, Brooks DD, Wickiewicz TL. Reconstruction of the patellar tendon using a patella-quadriceps tendon autograft. *Orthopedics* 1997;20:554–558, with permission.)

mal patella. The sutures are passed from the tendon into the drill holes, exiting over the superior pole of the patella. The tendon is reduced to the trough in the inferior pole of the patella and are then tied with the knee in full extension. The tendon graft is then sutured to the patellar tendon remnant. The bone that was removed to create the trough in the tibial tuberosity is used to graft the defect in the superior pole of the patella, and the quadriceps tendon donor site is sutured.

Patellar tendon reconstruction can also be performed using a bone–patellar tendon–bone autograft from the contralateral knee, as is used for anterior cruciate ligament reconstruction. The graft is fixed in a trough made at the tibial tuberosity with a cancellous screw. The patellar side is fixed by modifying the bone plug to make it wedge shaped. This bone plug is then attached to a matching trough on the patella, which is made with an obliquely oriented surface. A screw can then be oriented 45 degrees to the axis of the patella, thus avoiding violation of the articular surface of the patella. Alternatively, the graft can be harvested with a bone plug from only the tibial side, creating a bone–patellar tendon graft. This graft is then used as described above for a patella-quadriceps tendon autograft. Reconstruction using a bone–patellar tendon–bone allograft has also been reported and represents another option for reconstruction after chronic ruptures (105).

There are several other special circumstances in which repair or reconstruction of the patellar tendon may be required. Use of the central third of the patellar tendon for anterior cruciate ligament reconstruction has been associated with postoperative rupture of the remaining patellar tendon. This injury can usually be treated by direct repair. Direct repair may be difficult if rupture occurs at the tibial attachment, and in this setting reconstruction may be required. Sleeve fracture of the patella is an injury that occurs in skeletally immature children and involves avulsion of a small portion of the bony inferior pole of the patella with a large attached piece of articular surface. If not recognized and reduced early, these injuries can result in formation of ectopic bone between the inferior patella and the patellar tendon with a resultant extensor lag. Treatment at that point requires excision of the ectopic bone and repair of the patellar tendon to the patella.

Another special circumstance that may require patellar tendon reconstruction is infrapatellar contracture syndrome. Paulos et al. (107) described this complication after anterior cruciate ligament reconstruction. There is fibrosis in the infrapatellar fat pad and anterior knee capsule resulting in patellar tendon contracture and patellar entrapment. This condition can result in significant motion loss and anterior knee pain. Early treatment includes arthroscopic lysis of adhesions, removal of the fibrotic infrapatellar tissue, manipulation, and aggressive range of motion exercises. Often, however, open capsular and retinacular releases are required to restore full range of motion. In advanced cases, complete reconstruction of the patellar tendon may even be required. The procedures and principles described above for treatment of chronic patellar tendon rupture apply in this setting. Shortening of the quadriceps tendon and Z lengthening of the contracted patellar tendon may also be required in this setting.

If the patient has a history of previous infection and has failed all attempts at repair and reconstruction, the final salvage for chronic extensor mechanism disruption is knee arthrodesis. There are several techniques available for knee arthrodesis, including plate fixation, external fixation, and intramedullary implants. The recommended position is 0 to 5 degrees valgus and 10 to 15 degrees of flexion. The patella may be left intact or the patellar articular surface may be resected.

Postoperative Rehabilitation

Postoperative rehabilitation is influenced by the perceived strength of the repair site. For acute repairs, weight bearing as tolerated is allowed in a double-upright hinged brace with the knee in full extension. The brace is worn for 6 to 8 weeks after surgery. When a secure repair is achieved, the affected leg can be mobilized immediately after surgery using a continuous passive motion machine, which is continued for approximately 2 weeks until an arc of motion of at least 90 degrees is achieved. Active flexion and passive extension exercises are begun by the second week. Flexion is limited to the point at which there is tension on the repair, as determined intraoperatively. Straight leg raising exercises are allowed immediately after surgery. At 6 weeks postoperatively, active assisted extension exercises are initiated. Range-of-motion exercises and progressive resistance exercises for the quadriceps are performed with a physical therapist.

Postoperative rehabilitation will be more gradual after repair or reconstruction for a chronic rupture. Weight bearing and flexion exercises are delayed for 2 weeks. Partial weight bearing is prescribed for the first 4 weeks, after which the patient may progress to weight bearing as tolerated. Straight leg raises may be delayed for 2 weeks. Active extension exercises are allowed at 6 weeks, but resistance exercises are delayed until 12 weeks postoperatively.

Expected Outcomes

Generally, good results have been reported after surgical treatment. There are a few reports on the long-term outcome of patellar tendon repair in athletes (108,109). Kuechle and Stuart (110) reported on six patients, all of whom were able to achieve their preinjury levels of sports at an average of 18 months after injury. One important factor that influences functional recovery appears to be restoration of normal patellofemoral tracking. Care should be taken to appropriately balance the patella and to avoid shortening the patellar tendon to avoid late patellofemoral pain. Inferior results have been reported after delayed surgery due to muscle atrophy, proximal retraction of the extensor mechanism, and knee joint contracture.

Authors' Preferred Treatment

Acute ruptures should be repaired within the first 2 weeks of injury. Repair is performed with heavy sutures placed through drill holes in the patella, as described. Midsubstance ruptures are directly repaired with heavy sutures and are augmented with semitendinosus tendon passed through the distal quadriceps tendon or a transverse drill hole in the patella and through a drill hole in the tibial tuberosity. Ruptures at the tendon attachment site on the tibial tuberosity, which are uncommon, are repaired with sutures through drill holes and are also augmented with semitendinosus tendon.

Our first choice for patellar tendon reconstruction of a chronic rupture is to use a patella–quadriceps tendon autograft (106) as described above. If this tissue is unsuitable for use as a graft, we would recommend use of allograft Achilles tendon. Use of tissue from the contralateral knee would be recommended if allograft was not available or if the patient refused use of allograft tissue. Augmentation with both semitendinosus and gracilis tendons together is recommended for reconstructions performed for chronic rupture.

Complications

The complication rate and the need for reoperation after patellar tendon repairs appear to be higher than that after quadriceps tendon repair. Secondary ruptures, although uncommon, are more frequent after patellar tendon repair compared with quadriceps tendon repair. Patellar malalignment with abnormal patellar kinematics appears to be the most frequent complication after patellar tendon repair. Lateral patellar tilt may be induced if the retinacular repair is not balanced, and excessive patellofemoral contact stress may result from excessive shortening of the extensor mechanism. Patella infera may occur due to entrapment of the patellar tendon by fibrosis in the infrapatellar fat pad and can cause significant pain and loss of flexion (107).

Residual weakness of the extensor mechanism and inability to achieve full knee flexion are also common complications after surgery. A residual extensor lag may occur after delayed repair. Infection and wound problems can occur, especially if there is poor soft tissue coverage over the tibial tubercle or if the wound closure is under tension, which may occur if augmentation materials are prominent at the repair site. Pull-out wires, which have been used in the past, are not recommended due to the risk of infection.

Injuries in the Skeletally Immature

Epidemiology

Several overuse injuries are unique to the skeletally immature patient. Osgood-Shlatter disease is one of the most frequent lesions in the knee in active young patients. Pain is usually localized around the tibial tubercle. Sinding-Larsen-Johansson disease occurs in a similar population as Osgood-Shlatter disease. The pathologic lesion in Sinding-Larsen-Johansson disease is located in the distal pole of the patella. Typically, the patient is in the preteenage or early teenage years, and boys are more commonly affected than girls. Sinding-Larsen-Johansson disease usually occurs in girls at an earlier age (10 to 13 years) than in boys, which is probably related to earlier skeletal maturity. Jarvinen (49) studied 890 athletes with knee disorders and reported that the most common knee disorders were patellar tendinitis (20%) and Osgood-Shlatter disease (10%). Kujala et al. (111) found a 21% prevalance of Osgood-Shlatter disease in a group of athletic adolescents but only a 4.5% prevalance in a group of similar age who were nonathletic. The condition occurs bilaterally in 20% to 30% of patients.

Mechanism of Injury

Several etiologic factors are related to these conditions. The most important factor is repetitive microtrauma. A subsequent single episode of macrotrauma, such as landing from a high jump, may aggravate these conditions. Repeated direct contact to the knee is another form of repetitive microtrauma that can result in these conditions. Another essential factor is the growth process itself. During periods of rapid growth, there may be a decrease in flexibility of the muscle–tendon unit due to imbalance of growth between bone and muscle, which may render the apophysis susceptible to overuse injury (112). The role of anatomic factors, such as patella alta in Osgood-Schlatter disease (111), has also been studied by several authors. Sen et al. (113) reported a smaller patellar angle (which is formed by lines drawn along the articular surface and the inferior patellar apex) in patients with Osgood-Schlatter disease. These authors speculated that with a smaller patellar angle, a greater quadriceps muscle force is required to perform the same function (113).

Clinical Evaluation

Patients with Osgood-Schlatter disease present with activity-related pain around the tibial tubercle. Physical examination demonstrates local tenderness, swelling, and the formation of a bump over the tibial tubercle. Tenderness may also be noted around the patella and patellar tendon, and quadriceps atrophy may be present. An extensor lag may be present if there is significant pain. There may be tightness of the quadriceps, hamstrings, gastrocnemius, and ITB. A positive Ely test due to quadriceps tightness is also a common finding. Resisted knee extension reproduces pain, whereas straight leg raising is usually painless. The presentation of Sinding-Larsen-Johansonn disease is similar to that of Osgood-Schlatter disease, but the involved site is at the inferior patellar pole in Sinding-Larsen-Johansonn disease. Similar symptoms can occur proximally at the junction of the quadriceps tendon and the patella.

Imaging

A discrete ossicle at the tibial tubercle on plain radiographs has been reported in 32% to 50% of cases of Osgood-Schlatter disease. A bony prominence of variable shape at the tibial tubercle may also be observed. Plain radiographs are important to exclude other pathologic entities such as neoplasm and infection. MRI is often recommended as well to image the soft tissues. Rosenberg et al. (114) studied 28 cases of Osgood-Schlatter disease using multiple imaging modalities and stressed the importance of soft tissue abnormalities, such as tendinitis and bursitis, as detected by computed tomography and MRI. In addition, they speculated that Osgood-Schlatter disease might not be produced by an avulsion fracture of the patellar tendon because the ossicle was seen in only 32% of the cases and it seldom united despite symptomatic relief. Plain radiographs in Sinding-Larsen-Johansson disease may reveal a bony avulsion, soft tissue calcification, or an elongation of the inferior pole of the patella. MRI is an effective modality for diagnosis and follow-up in Sinding-Larsen- Johansson disease. De Flaviis et al. (115) reported on the efficacy of ultrasonographic diagnosis of Osgood-Schlatter and Sinding-Larsen-Johansson diseases and concluded that ultrasound is simple and reliable for the evaluation of these conditions. However, ultrasonography has been found to be highly operator dependent.

Nonoperative Treatment

Because Sinding-Larsen-Johansson disease and Osgood-Schlatter disease have a common mechanism of injury, similar nonoperative treatment regimens can be followed. These conditions usually resolve with conservative measures. The initial treatment includes a period of rest, ice, and anti-inflammatory medication. The use of steroid or xylocaine injections into peritendinous tissue is still controversial. Lower extremity stretching and muscle strengthening exercises are recommended. Sports activity should be based on the severity of the symptoms. Knee braces may also be useful to control symptoms, especially when muscle strength and flexibility are not fully recovered. Orthotics or shoe inserts to decrease impact loads on the extremity may also be helpful. A simple protective pad or a knee protector should be used when kneeling or if direct knee contact occurs in sports or daily activities. If symptoms progress during daily activities, brace or cast immobilization or crutch support may be required in rare cases. The use of such measures should be limited to a maximum of 3 weeks.

Surgical Treatment

A small percentage of patients with these conditions will have persistent symptoms and will be significantly disabled after a trial of comprehensive conservative treatment. In patients with Osgood-Schlatter disease, excision of free ossicles and debridement of the degenerative tendon will usually relieve the symptoms completely. Similarly, surgical debridement of the degenerative tendon provides relief of the symptom of Sinding-Larsen-Johansson disease when conservative measures fail. Any loose bony fragments are carefully excised. A hinged double-upright knee brace or cylinder walking cast is applied and worn for 2 to 3 weeks. Full weight bearing in extension is allowed immediately with avoidance of active extension for up to 4 to 6 weeks if the procedure involved repair of the tendon to bone. Early knee motion in a range that does not result in high strain on the repair will be guided by the limits determined intraoperatively. Straight leg raising exercises may begin immediately. After the tendon repair has healed (4 to 6 weeks), range of motion and strengthening are progressed.

Expected Outcomes

Krause et al. (116) reviewed the natural history of untreated Osgood-Schlatter disease in 69 knees in 50 patients and found that 76% of patients had no limitation of activity, although only 60% could kneel without discomfort. They concluded that bony abnormalities such as ossicles or prominence of the tibial tubercle were related to persistent symptoms that did not resolve with conservative treatment. Hogh and Lund (117) reported on a group of patients with Osgood-Schlatter disease who had symptoms for an average of 8 years. Excision of bony abnormalities produced good results in all these patients.

Authors' Preferred Treatment

Conservative treatment is usually successful. Vigorous flexibility exercises and avoidance of the offending activity are the mainstays of treatment. If the symptoms do not respond to conservative treatment, MRI is used for evaluation of the tendon attachment. If MRI demonstrates an abnormal focus within the tendon, surgical treatment is recommended.

Complications

Persistent anterior knee pain with associated quadriceps weakness may occur with or without surgical treatment. Nonunion of the free ossicle, patella alta, patellar subluxation, and premature fusion of the anterior part of the proximal tibial physis with resulting genu recurvatum have been reported as complications of Osgood-Schlatter disease after both conservative and surgical treatment. It is currently controversial whether surgery should be delayed to allow for physeal closure.

REFERENCES

1. Parry DAD, Barnes GRG, Craig AS. A comparison of the size distribution of collagen fibrils in connective tissues as a function of age and a possible relation between fibril size distribution and mechanical properties. *Proc R Soc Lond B* 1978;203:305.
2. Berenson MC, Blevins FT, Plaas AHK, et al. Proteoglycans of human rotator cuff tendons. *J Orthop Res* 1996;14:518.
3. Flatow EL, Djurasovic M, Bigliani LU, et al. Variation in proteoglycan gene expression in human rotator cuff tendons. *Trans Orthop Res Soc* 1997;22:27.
4. Hamlin CR, Kohn RR, Luschin JH. Apparent accelerated ageing of human collagen fibers. *Diabetes* 1975;24:902.
5. Ippolito E, Natali PG, Postacchini F. Morphological, immunological, and biochemical study of rabbit Achilles tendon at various ages. *J Bone Joint Surg Am* 1980;62A:583.
6. Shadwick RE. Elastic energy storage in tendons: mechanical differences related to function and age. *J Appl Phys* 1990;68:1033.
7. Shadwick RE. The role of the collagen crosslinks in the age related changes in mechanical properties of digital tendons. *Proc North Am Congr Biomech* 1986;1:137.
8. Vailas AC, Perrini VA, Pedrini-Mille A, et al. Patellar tendon matrix changes associated with ageing and voluntary exercise. *J Appl Phys* 1985;58:1572.
9. Attia E, Bhargava MM, Warren RF, et al. The effect of cyclic load on growth, matrix production and migration of tendon fibroblasts is cell density dependent. *Trans Orthop Res Soc* 1996; 21:2.
10. Houglum P. Soft tissue healing and its impact on rehabilitation. *J Sports Rehabil* 1992;1:19.
11. Tanaka H, Manske PR, Pruitt Dl, et al. Effect of cyclic tension on lacerated flexor tendons in vitro. *J Hand Surg Am* 1995;20:467.
12. Hannafin JA, Arnoczky SP, Hoonjan A, et al. Effect of stress deprivation and cyclic tensile loading on the material and morphologic properties of canine flexor digitorum profundus tendon: an in vitro study. *J Orthop Res* 1995;13:907.
13. Aoki M, Kubota H, Pruitt DL, et al. Biomechanical and histologic characteristics of canine flexor tendon repair using early postoperative mobilization. *J Hand Surg Am* 1997;22:107.
14. Enwemeka CS. Functional loading augments the initial tensile strength and energy absorption capacity of regenerating rabbit Achilles tendons. *Am J Phys Med Rehabil* 1992;71:31.
15. Loitz BJ, Zernicke RF, Vailas AC, et al. Effects of short-term immobilization versus continuous passive motion on the biomechanical and biochemical properties of the rabbit tendon. *Clin Orthop* 1989;244:265.
16. Taylor DC, Dalton JD Jr, Seaber AV, et al. Experimental muscle strain injury. Early functional and structural deficits and the increased risk for reinjury. *Am J Sports Med* 1993;21:190.

17. Terry GC, LaPrade RF. The posterolateral aspect of the knee. Anatomy and surgical approach. *Am J Sports Med* 1996;24:732.
18. Karpakka J, Väänänen K, Orava S, et al. The effects of preimmobilization training and immobilization on collagen synthesis in rat skeletal muscle. *Int J Sports Med* 1990;11:484.
19. Vogel KG, Ordog A, Pogany G, et al. Proteoglycans in the compressed region of human tibialis posterior tendon and in ligaments. *J Orthop Res* 1993;11:68.
20. McMaster PE. Tendon and muscle ruptures: clinical and experimental studies on the causes and location of subcutaneous ruptures. *J Bone Joint Surg Am* 1933;15:705.
21. Wiggins ME, Fadale PD, Barrach H, et al. Healing characteristics of a type I collagenous structure treated with corticosteroids. *Am J Sports Med* 1994;22:279.
22. Clark SC, Jones MW, Choudhury RR, et al. Bilateral patellar tendon rupture secondary to repeated local steroid injections. *J Accident Emerg Med* 1995;12:300.
23. McGarvey WC, Singh D, Trevino SG. Partial Achilles tendon ruptures associated with fluoroquinolone antibiotics: a case report and literature review. *Foot Ankle Int* 1996;17:496.
24. Yang BY, Sartoris DJ, Resnik D, et al. Calcium pyrophosphate dihydrate crystal deposition disease: frequency of tendon calcification about the knee. *J Rheumatol* 1996;23:883.
25. Babini SM, Arturi A, Marcos JC. Laxity and rupture of the patellar tendon in systemic lupus erythematosus. Association with secondary hypoparathyroidism. *J Rheumatol* 1988;15:1162.
26. Bhole R, Flynn JC, Marbury TC. Quadriceps tendon ruptures in uremia. *Clin Orthop* 1985;195:200.
27. Levy M, Seelenfreund P, Fried A, et al. Bilateral spontaneous and simultaneous rupture of the quadriceps tendons in gout. *J Bone Joint Surg Br* 1971;53B:510.
28. Josza L, Szederkenyi G. Mucopolysaccharide content of the human aorta in hypothyroidism. *Endokrinologie* 1966;50:116.
29. Likar IN, Robinson RW, Likar LJ. Glycosaminoglycans and hormones: mesenchymal response in endocrinopathies. In: Varna RS, et al., eds. *Glycosaminoglycans and proteoglycans in physiological and pathological processes of body systems.* Basel: Karger, 1982:412.
30. Gerster JC, Landry M, Rappoport G, et al. Enthesopathy and tendinopathy in gout: computed tomographic assessment. *Ann Rheum Dis* 1996;55:921.
31. Scuderi AJ, Datz FL, Valdivia S, et al. Enthesopathy of the patellar tendon insertion associated with isotretinoin therapy. *J Nucl Med Mar* 1993;34:455.
32. Lapinsky AS, Padgett DE, Hall FW. Disruption of the extensor mechanism in Paget's disease. *Am J Orthop* 1995;24:165.
33. Backman C, Boquist L, Friden J, et al. Chronic achilles paratenonitis with tendinosis: an experimental model in the rabbit. *J Orthop Res* 1990;8:541.
34. Leadbetter WB, Mooar PA, Lane GJ, et al. The surgical treatment of tendinitis. Clinical rationale and biologic basis. *Clin Sports Med* 1992;11:679.
35. Kannus P, Jozsa L. Histopathological changes preceding spontaneous rupture of a tendon. A controlled study of 891 patients. *J Bone Joint Surg Am* 1991;73A:1507.
36. Sano H, Ishii H, Yeadon A, et al. Degeneration at the insertion weakens the tensile strength of the supraspinatus tendon. *Trans Orthop Res Soc* 1997;22:860.
37. Hamada K, Tomonaga A, Gotoh M, et al. Intrinsic healing capacity and tearing process of torn supraspinatous tendons: in situ hybridization study of (1(I) Procollagen mRNA. *J Orthop Res* 1997;15:24.
38. Rodeo SA, Arnoczky SP, Torzilli PA, et al. Tendon-healing in a bone tunnel. *J Bone Joint Surg Am* 1993;75A:1795.
39. St. Pierre P, Olson EJ, Elliot JJ, et al. Tendon-healing to cortical bone compared with healing to a cancellous trough. *J Bone Joint Surg Am* 1995;77A:1858.
40. Hattersley G, Cox K, Soslowsky LI, et al. Bone morphogenetic proteins 2 and 12 alter the attachment of tendon to bone in a rat model: a histological and biomechanical investigation. *Trans Orthop Res Soc* 1998;23:96.
41. Duffy FJ, Seiler JG, Hergrueter CA, et al. Intrinsic mitogenic potential of canine flexor tendons. *J Hand Surg Br* 1992;17:275.
42. Hart DA, Frank CB, Murphy PG. Potential clinical applications

43. of growth factors and unique cell populations to promote anterior cruciate ligament healing. In: Jackson DW, ed. *The anterior cruciate ligament: current and future concepts.* New York: Raven Press, 1993:401.
43. Lee J, Green MH, Amiel D. Synergistic effect of growth factors on cell outgrowth from explants of rabbit anterior cruciate and medial collateral ligaments. *J Orthop Res* 1995;13:435.
44. Letson AK, Dahners LE. The effect of combinations of growth factors on ligament healing. *Clin Orthop* 1994;308:207.
45. Lou J, Manske PR, Aoki M, et al. Adenovirus-mediated gene transfer into tendon and tendon sheath. *J Orthop Res* 1996;14:513.
46. Gum SL, Reddy GK, Stehno-Bittel L, et al. Combined ultrasound, electrical stimulation, and laser promote collagen synthesis with moderate changes in tendon biomechanics. *Am J Phys Med Rehabil* 1997;76:288.
47. Jackson BA, Schwane JA, Starcher BC. Effect of ultrasound therapy on the repair of Achilles tendon injuries in rats. *Med Sci Sports Exerc* 1991;23:171.
48. Turner SM, Powell ES, Ng CS. The effect of ultrasound on the healing of repaired cockerel tendon: is collagen cross-linkage a factor? *J Hand Surg* 1989;14:428.
49. Jarvinen M. Epidemiology of tendon injuries in sports. *Clin Sports Med* 1992;11:493.
50. Caborn DNM, Boyd DW. Tendon ruptures. In: Fu F, ed. *Knee surgery.* Baltimore: Williams & Wilkins, 1994:911.
51. Siwek CW, Rao JP. Ruptures of the extensor mechanism of the knee joint. *J Bone Joint Surg Am* 1981;63A:932.
52. Clark JM, Stechschulte DJ. The interface between bone and tendon at an insertion site: a study of the quadriceps tendon insertion. *J Anat* 1990;192:605–616.
53. Lauerman WC, Smith BG, Kenmore PI. Spontaneous bilateral rupture of the extensor mechanism of the knee in two patients on chronic ambulatory peritoneal dialysis. *Orthopedics* 1987;10:589.
54. Costigan PS, Innes A. Spontaneous bilateral rupture of the quadriceps mechanism in chronic renal failure. *J R Coll Surg Edinb* 1992;37:343.
55. Unverferth LJ, Olix ML. The effect of local steroid injections on tendon. *J Sports Med* 1973;1:31.
56. DeLee JC, Craviotto DF. Rupture of the quadriceps tendon after a central third patellar tendon anterior cruciate ligament reconstruction. *Am J Sports Med* 1991;19:415.
57. MacEachern AG, Plewes JL. Bilateral simultaneous spontaneous rupture of the quadriceps tendons. *J Bone Joint Surg Br* 1984;66B:81.
58. Nance EP, Kaye JJ. Injuries of the quadriceps mechanism. *Diagn Radiol* 1982;142:301.
59. Aprin H, Broukhim B. Early diagnosis of acute rupture of the quadriceps tendon by arthrography. *Clin Orthop* 1985;195:185.
60. Bianchi S, Zwass A, Abdelwahab IF, et al. Diagnosis of tears of the quadriceps tendon of the knee: value of sonography. *AJR Am J Roentgenol* 1994;162:1137.
61. Kuivilla TE, Brems JJ. Diagnosis of acute rupture of the quadriceps tendon by magnetic resonance imaging. *Clin Orthop* 1991;262:236.
62. Zeiss J, Saddemi SR, Ebraheim NA. MR imaging of the quadriceps tendon: normal layered configuration and its importance in cases of tendon rupture. *AJR Am J Roentgenol* 1992;159:1031.
63. Scuderi C. Ruptures of the quadriceps tendon: study of twenty tendon ruptures. *Am J Surg* 1958;95:626.
64. Katzman BM, Silberberg S, Caligiuri D, et al. Delayed repair of a quadriceps tendon. *Orthopedics* 1997;20:553.
65. Scuderi C, Schrey EL. Quadriceps tendon ruptures. *Arch Surg* 1950;61:42.
66. Levy M, Goldstein J, Rosner M. A method of repair for quadriceps tendon or patellar ligament (tendon) ruptures without cast immobilization. *Clin Orthop* 1987;218:297.
67. Larsen E, Lund PM. Ruptures of the extensor mechanism of the knee joint. *Clin Orthop* 1986;213:150.
68. Renne JW. The iliotibial band friction syndrome. *J Bone Joint Surg Am* 1975;57:1110.
69. Ekman EF, Pope T, Martin DF, et al. Magnetic resonance imaging of iliotibial band syndrome. *Am J Sports Med* 1994;22:851.

70. De Geeter F, De Neve J, Van Steelandt H. Bone scan in iliotibial band syndrome. *Clin Nucl Med* 1995;20:550.
71. David A, Buchholz J, Muhr G. Tear of the biceps femoris tendon. *Arch Orthop Trauma Surg* 1994;113:351.
72. Brunet ME, Kester MA, Cook SD, et al. Biomechanical evaluation of superficial transfer of the biceps femoris tendon. *Am J Sports Med* 1987;15:103.
73. Fornasier VL, Czitrom AA, Evans JA, et al. Case report 398: friction by pes anserinus. *Skeletal Radiol* 1987;16:57.
74. Holden NT. Deposition of calcium salts in the popliteus tendon. *J Bone Joint Surg Br* 1955;37B:446.
75. Howard CB, Bonneh DY, Nyska M. Diagnosis of popliteus tenosynovitis by ultrasound. *J Orthop Sports Phys Ther* 1992;16:58.
76. Scapinelli R. A synovial ganglion of the popliteus tendon simulating a para meniscal cyst. Two case reports. *J Bone Joint Surg Am* 1988;70A:1085.
77. Mayfield GW. Popliteus tendon tenosynovitis. *Am J Sports Med* 1977;5:31.
78. Westrich GH, Hannafin JA, Potter HG. Isolated rupture and repair of the popliteus tendon. *Arthroscopy* 1995;11:628.
79. Blazina ME, Kerlan RK, Jobe FW, et al. Jumper's knee. *Orthop Clin North Am* 1973;4:665.
80. Martens M, Wouters P, Burssens A, et al. Patellar tendinitis: pathology and results of treatment. *Acta Orthop Scand* 1982; 53:445.
81. Lian O, Engebretsen L, Ovrebo RV, et al. Characteristics of the leg extensors in male volleyball players with jumper's knee. *Am J Sports Med* 1996;24:380.
82. Johnson DP, Wakeley CJ, Watt I. Magnetic resonance imaging of patellar tendonitis. *J Bone Joint Surg Br* 1996;78B:452.
83. Laduron J, Shahabpour M Anneert JM, et al. Use of dynamic US and MR imaging in the assessment of trochleotendinous knee impingement syndrome. RSNA 79th Scientific Assembly and Annual Meeting, 1993:208.
84. Kujala UM, Osterman K, Kvist M, et al. Factors predisposing to patellar chondropathy and patellar apicitis in athletes. *Int Orthop* 1986;10:195.
85. Richards DP, Ajemian SV, Wiley JP, et al. Knee joint dynamic predict patellar tendinitis in elite volleyball players. *Am J Sports Med* 1996;24:676.
86. Yu JS, Popp JE, Kaeding CC, et al. Correlation of MR imaging and pathologic findings in athletes undergoing surgery for chronic patellar tendinitis. *AJR Am J Roentgenol* 1995;165:115.
87. Khan KM, Bonar F, Desmond PM, et al. Patellar tendinosis (jumper's knee): findings at histopathologic examination, US, and MR imaging. *Radiology* 1996;200:821.
88. Green JS, Morgan B, Lauder I, et al. The correlation of bone scintigraphy and histological findings in patellar tendinitis. *Nucl Med Com* 1996;17:231.
89. Stanish WD, Rubinovich RM, Curwin S. Eccentric exercise in chronic tendinitis. *Clin Orthop* 1986;208:65.
90. King JB, Perry DJ, Mourad K, et al. Lesion of the patellar ligament. *J Bone Joint Surg Br* 1990;72B:46.
91. Anzel SH, Covey KW, Weiner AD, et al. Disruption of muscles and tendons: an analysis of 1014 cases. *Surgery* 1959;45:406.
92. Podesta L, Sherman MF, Bonamo JR. Bilateral simultaneous rupture of the infra patellar tendon in a recreational athlete. A case report. *Am J Sports Med* 1991;19:325.
93. Scott SH, Winter DA. Internal forces at chronic running injury sites. *Med Sci Sports* 1990;22:357.
94. Kennedy JC, Willis RB. The effects of local steroid injections on tendons: a biomechanical and microscopic correlative study. *Am J Sports Med* 1976;4:11.
95. Noyes F, Nussbaum N, Torvilk P, et al. Biomechanical and ultrastructural changes in ligaments and tendons after local corticosteroid injections. *J Bone Joint Surg Am* 1975;57A:876.
96. Johnson GA, Tramaglini DM, Levine RE, et al. Tensile and viscoelastic properties of human patellar tendon. *J Orthop Res* 1994;12:796.
97. Kretzler JE, Curtin SL, Wegner DA, et al. Patellar tendon rupture: a late complication of a tibial nail. *Orthopedics* 1995;18:1109.
98. Aglietti P, Buzzi R, Insall J. Disorders of the patellofemoral joint. In: Insall J, ed. *Surgery of the knee.* New York: Churchill Livingstone, 1992:241.
99. Karlsson J, Kalebo P, Goksor LA, et al. Partial rupture of the patellar ligament. *Am J Sports Med* 1992;20:390.
100. Kelikian H, Riashi E, Gleason J. Restoration of quadriceps tendon function in neglected tear of the patella tendon. *Surg Gynecol Obstet* 1957;104:200.
101. Larson RV, Simonian PT. Semitendinosus augmentation of acute patellar tendon repair with immediate mobilization. *Am J Sports Med* 1995;23:82.
102. Lindy PB, Boyton MD, Fadale PD. Repair of patellar tendon disruptions without hardware. *J Orthop Trauma* 1995;9:238.
103. McLaughlin HL, Francis KC. Operative repair of injuries to the quadriceps extensor mechanism. *Am J Surg* 1956;91:651.
104. Isiklar ZU, Varner KE, Lindsey RW, et al. Late reconstruction of patellar ligament ruptures using Ilizarov external fixation. *Clin Orthop* 1996;322:174.
105. Burks RT, Edelson RH. Allograft reconstruction of the patellar ligament. *J Bone Joint Surg Am* 1994;76A:1077.
106. Williams RJ, Brooks DD, Wickiewicz TL. Reconstruction of the patellar tendon using a patella-quadriceps tendon autograft. *Orthopedics* 1997;20:554.
107. Paulos LE, Wnorowski DC, Greenwald AE. Infrapatellar contracture syndrome: diagnosis, treatment, and long-term followup. *Am J Sports Med* 1994;22:440.
108. Donati RB, Cox S, Echo BS, et al. Bilateral simultaneous patellar tendon rupture in a female collegiate gymnast. A case report. *Am J Sports Med* 1986;14:237.
109. Kelly DW, Carter VS, Jobe FW, et al. Patellar and quadriceps tendon ruptures—jumper's knee. *Am J Sports Med* 1984;12:375.
110. Kuechle DK, Stuart MJ. Isolated rupture of the patellar tendon in athletes. *Am J Sports Med* 1994;22:692.
111. Kujala UM, Kvist M, Heinonen O. Osgood-Shlatter's disease in adolescent athletes: retrospective study of incidence and duration. *Am J Sports Med* 1985;13:236.
112. Micheli LJ, Starter JA, Woods E, et al. Patella alta and the adolescent growth spurt. *Clin Orthop* 1986;213:159.
113. Sen RK, Sharma LR, Thakur SR, et al. Patellar angle in Osgood-Schlatter disease. *Acta Orthop Scand* 1989;60:26.
114. Rosenberg ZS, Kawelbulum M, Cheung YY, et al. Osgood-Schlatter lesion: fracture of tendinitis? Scintigraphic, CT, and MR imaging features. *Radiology* 1992;185:853.
115. De Flaviis L, Nessi R, Scaglione P, et al. Ultrasonic diagnosis of Osgood-Schlatter and Sinding-Larsen-Johansonn disease of the knee. *Skeletal Radiol* 1989;18:193.
116. Krause BL, Williams JPR, Catterall A. Natural history of Osgood-Schlatter disease. *J Pediatr Orthop* 1990;10:65.
117. Hogh J, Lund B. The sequelae of Osgood-Schlatter's disease in adults. *Int Orthop* 1988;12:213.

Principles and Practice of Orthopaedic Sports Medicine,
edited by William E. Garrett, Jr., Kevin P. Speer, and Donald T. Kirkendall.
Lippincott Williams & Wilkins, Philadelphia © 2000.

CHAPTER 40

Acute and Chronic Injuries to the Patellofemoral Joint

Nader Q. Kasim and John P. Fulkerson

ANATOMY AND PATHOGENESIS

The patella is an integral part of the extensor mechanism of the knee. It is the largest sesamoid bone in the body, lying in and surrounded by the quadriceps tendon. The ossification center generally appears at the age of 2 to 3 years but can be delayed as late as 6 years (1).

The patella is essentially triangular in shape with a distally directed apex. It is composed of a proximal and distal pole, with a medial and lateral margin. The transverse diameter is slightly larger than the longitudinal diameter. The proximal pole is relatively thick, receiving the insertion of the vastus muscles and rectus femoris. The patellar ligament originates from the distal pole of the patella and inserts into the tibial tubercle. Its relative inelasticity keeps a reasonably fixed distance between the pole and the tibial tubercle throughout motion of the knee. Fibers from the vastus medialis and vastus lateralis insert into the medial and lateral margins of the patella, respectively (2).

The four passive soft tissue stabilizers of the patella are shown in Fig. 40.1. They help guide the patella during knee flexion and extension. The patellar tendon is slightly wider proximally than distally. Its distal and lateral obliquity contributes to overall valgus alignment of the extensor mechanism. Increased obliquity may contribute to recurrent patellar instability. The quadriceps tendon is composed of three layers. The superficial layer is derived from the rectus femoris, with the deep layer formed by the vastus intermedius. The middle layer of the quadriceps tendon is formed by the vastus medialis and vastus lateralis.

The vastus muscles send longitudinal fibers adjacent to the patella that compose the medial and lateral retinaculae. They insert into the upper tibia and the medial and lateral borders of the patella. The lateral retinaculum is composed of a superficial and deep layer (3). The superficial layer consists of oblique fibers running distally and anteriorly, with the deep fibers being oriented more transversely (Fig. 40.2). The bulk of the fibers of the lateral retinaculum run between the iliotibial band and the lateral margin of the patella and patellar tendon. Increasing knee flexion displaces the iliotibial band posteriorly, which increases the lateral pull on the patella and may lead to patellar tilt or subluxation (4). The medial retinaculum inserts into the upper two thirds of the medial patellar margin. It is also composed of two layers. The medial patellofemoral ligament inserts into the medial femoral epicondyle, and the medial patellotibial ligament inserts into the tibia and medial meniscus. Two of the main functions of the medial and lateral retinaculae are to maintain the alignment of the patella in its articulation with the femur throughout the range of motion of the knee and to aid in active extension of the knee.

The quadriceps muscle is also considered an active stabilizer of the patella. The vastus medialis consists of an obliquus and longus portion. The vastus medialis obliquus (VMO) is more obliquely oriented, sending fibers distally and laterally at an angle ranging from 55 to 70 degrees in relation to the long axis of the quadriceps tendon (5). It is thus better suited to limit the lateral displacement of the patella. The vastus lateralis inserts onto the patella with a more acute angle than the VMO. The angle with respect to the long axis of the quadriceps tendon ranges from 22 to 45 degrees. The most distal part of the vastus lateralis is anatomically distinct and is named the vastus lateralis obliquus. It is better suited to apply a lateral pull on the patella (6).

N. Q. Kasim and J. P. Fulkerson: Department of Orthopaedic Surgery, University of Connecticut Medical School, Farmington, Connecticut 06032.

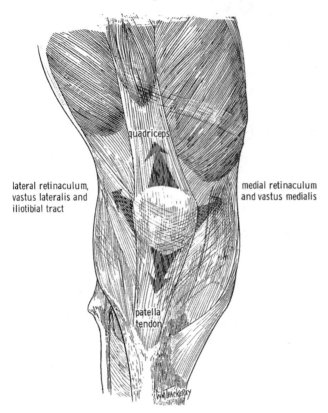

FIG. 40.1. Soft tissue stabilizers of the patella. (From Insall JN, Windsor RE, Scott WN, et al. *Surgery of the knee.* New York: Churchill Livingstone, 1993:243, with permission.)

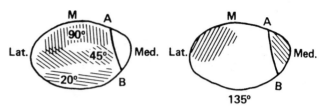

FIG. 40.3. Areas of contact on the articular surface of the patella with increasing knee flexion. (From Fulkerson JP. *Disorders of the patellofemoral joint.* Baltimore: Williams & Wilkins, 1997:29, with permission.)

The articular surface of the patella is the thickest in the human body. The thickest region (up to 5 mm) is on the central ridge. Its articulation with the anterior surface of the femoral condyle varies according to the position of the knee. The contact area starts in the lower portion of the patella with the knee in extension and moves proximally as the knee is flexed (Fig. 40.3). The vertical ridge of the patella, which corresponds to the distal femoral articular groove, divides the articular surface into a medial and lateral facet. Goodfellow et al. (7) described the presence of an "odd" facet near the medial patellar border delineated by a secondary ridge on the medial facet (Fig. 40.4). This tends to contact the femoral trochlea with the knee in full extension. The superior three fourths of the posterior surface of the patella is articular, with the inferior fourth being nonarticular.

The femoral trochlea consists of a sulcus and medial and lateral facets. The sulcus is continuous with the

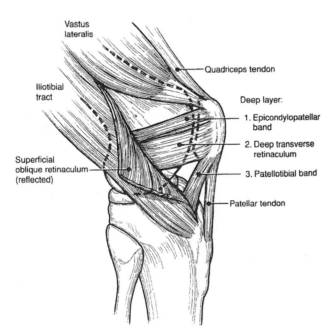

FIG. 40.2. Superficial and deep layers of the lateral retinaculum. (From Insall JN, Windsor RE, Scott WN, et al. *Surgery of the knee.* New York: Churchill Livingstone, 1993:244, with permission.)

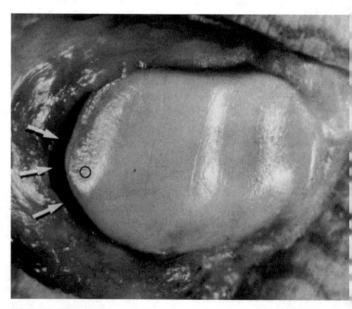

FIG. 40.4. Articular surface of the patella with odd facet (*arrows and circle*). (From Fulkerson JP. *Disorders of the patellofemoral joint.* Baltimore: Williams & Wilkins, 1997:5, with permission.)

intercondylar notch, and the facets are in continuity with their corresponding femoral condyles. The lateral facet is typically a few millimeters more prominent than the medial facet. This asymmetry along with the congruence between the central ridge of the patella and the trochlear sulcus contributes to the osseous stabilization of the patella. This stabilizing function of the osseous surfaces may be lost to a certain extent in knees with a flatter sulcus (4).

BIOMECHANICS

It is important to understand the biomechanics of the patellofemoral joint to understand the pathogenesis. Clinical studies have supported the idea of the patella as an important contributor to knee extension power (8–10). The product of the extensor muscle force with its moment arm defines the knee extensor moment (11). The patella functions to displace the extensor mechanism anteriorly, thereby significantly increasing the extensor moment arm (12). This increase leads to less muscle force necessary to produce a given level of extension power, ultimately decreasing the patellofemoral contact loads (13).

The patellofemoral joint reaction force defines the compressive forces experienced by the patella during different activities. It results from the tension developing in the quadriceps and patellar tendons with contraction of the quadriceps muscle. As shown in Fig. 40.5, the patellofemoral joint reaction force is the resultant vector of the quadriceps tendon force (M1) and the patellar tendon force (M2). As the knee flexes and the angle between M1 and M2 decreases, the resultant vector of the patellofemoral joint reaction force increases. Therefore, as a person performs a squat, increased quadriceps force is required to maintain a position with increased knee flexion (4). However, other factors can also affect the patellofemoral joint reaction force, including displacement of the body center of gravity and the dynamic acceleration and deceleration of knee flexion. Reilly and Martens (14) reported high values of the patellofemoral joint reaction force during different activities. They calculated the force to be 0.5 × body weight with level walking at minimal knee flexion, 3.3 × body weight at up to 60 degrees of knee flexion with stair climbing, and up to 7.8 × body weight with deep knee bends of 130 degrees.

The patellofemoral contact pressures is the ratio of the joint reaction force to the contact area. These values are very important when discussing the biomechanics if the patellofemoral joint. The contact area of the patella moves proximally with increasing knee flexion with a corresponding increase in the surface area. The contact area increases steadily up to 90 degrees. Afterward, the quadriceps tendon contacts the anterior femur and helps resist the increasing patellofemoral joint reaction force

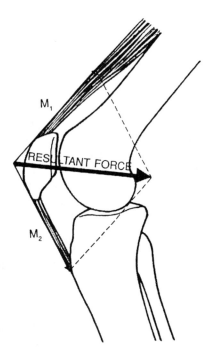

FIG. 40.5. Biomechanics of the patellofemoral joint. Resultant force of quadriceps tension (M1) and patellar tendon tension (M2) acting perpendicular to the articular surface. (From Fulkerson JP. *Disorders of the patellofemoral joint.* Baltimore: Williams & Wilkins, 1997:25, with permission.)

and lowers the pressures. As mentioned earlier, the contact force increases with flexion and squatting, which is partially compensated for by a corresponding increase in the contact area. The contact pressures are highest between 60 and 90 degrees of knee flexion. These observations help explain why patients with patellofemoral symptoms do not tolerate deep knee bends or resisted knee extension exercises. More suitable exercises for quadriceps rehabilitation include straight leg raises or short arc isotonic exercises (4).

CLINICAL EVALUATION

A complete evaluation of the patellofemoral joint should always start with a thorough history. Complaints of pain with climbing or descending stairs and squatting often relate to the extensor mechanism. Strong eccentric or concentric quadriceps contractions required for these activities cause pain in patients with patellofemoral disorders. A history of patellar dislocation or the sense of shifting of the patella leads to the suspicion of patellar instability. The sense of "giving way" is not always due to instability because quadriceps weakness alone may cause these symptoms.

The onset of patellofemoral symptoms may help in making a diagnosis. Acute high-energy or blunt trauma can disrupt the soft tissue restraints or cause bony injury. Acute patellar dislocations or subluxations can result from indirect forces in athletes. They are often caused by high-energy valgus/external rotation injuries. Pain of an insidious nature may often be due to an underlying deficit of strength or flexibility. Patients with this history are especially likely to have some underlying patellar malalignment (15).

A history of overuse can often lead to activity-related anterior knee pain. The overuse can produce tissue overload within the patella or the surrounding soft tissue restraints. This typically depends on the type of activity and whether there is any weakness of inflexibility. Patients with patellar malalignment may be predisposed to overload, but normally aligned knees can also have overuse pain syndromes.

A thorough examination of the patellofemoral joint involves a visual assessment and a clinical evaluation. The patient should always be barefoot and in shorts when being examined. Observing the patient's lower extremity alignment while standing is important. Any pelvic obliquity or limb length discrepancy and any gross abnormalities in the gait pattern should be noted.

Quadriceps muscle atrophy may result from the patellofemoral syndrome and may also contribute to its cause. Bilateral thigh circumference should be measured at a standard distance from the superior pole of the patella. Any quadriceps weakness related to atrophy may affect the dynamic control of the patella and its stability. Lateral patellar tilt and subluxation is resisted by the VMO. The quadriceps also resists collapse of the knee into flexion during weight bearing. Eccentric contraction of the quadriceps controls the knee flexion as the body is lowered while descending stairs. Failure of this shock absorption may result from weak quadriceps, which can increase the loads on the patellofemoral joint. A deficient VMO may also result in malalignment that can lead to asymmetric loads on the joint. Therefore, many patients with weak quadriceps have pain when descending stairs (15).

Pronation of the foot can affect patellar tracking (16). Evaluating heel position during standing is a good measure of foot pronation. An obligatory internal rotation of the tibia results from prolonged and excessive foot pronation during walking. This internal rotation is translated to the femur rotating the lateral femoral trochlea against the lateral patellar facet during weight bearing. This may lead to or aggravate the patellofemoral syndrome. Custom-made orthotics can help control the hindfoot and relieve the patellofemoral symptoms (17).

The Q angle is believed to be important in estimating the lateral moment acting on the patella. It is the angle formed by a line connecting the anterior iliac spine to the center of the patella with a line from the center of the patella to the tibial tubercle (Fig. 40.6) (15). However, studies by Aglietti et al. (18) did not show a significant difference between the Q angles in patients with patellofemoral syndrome and control subjects. Despite its im-

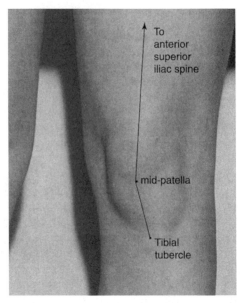

FIG. 40.6. Measurement of the quadriceps (Q) angle with patient standing. (From Fulkerson JP. *Disorders of the patellofemoral joint.* Baltimore: Williams & Wilkins, 1997:45, with permission.)

portance in measuring the valgus extensor moment on the knee, the Q angle has not been proven to directly correlate with the incidence of patellofemoral symptoms through scientific evidence (15).

As the knee is brought into flexion, the patella engages in the trochlea at a flexion angle of 30 to 40 degrees. Observing passive patellar tracking can shed light on the contribution of the soft tissue restraints to patellar alignment. A patella that is positioned too far medially or laterally will tend to suddenly shift into the trochlea during flexion. Also, contracting the quadriceps while the leg is extended will shift the patella if it is malpositioned. The bayonet sign (J sign) as described by Ficat is an abrupt lateral translation of the patella just before full extension of the knee is achieved.

Tilting of the patella can often be seen on clinical inspection. Attempts at inverting a laterally tilted patella by elevating the lateral facet and depressing the medial facet will reveal tightness in the lateral retinaculum (19). Normally, the lateral facet can be elevated between 0 and 15 degrees above horizontal. A neutral or negative angle can be obtained with a tight lateral retinaculum. The test should be done with the knee in full extension to relax the quadriceps muscles. The results should always be compared with the patients' contralateral knee.

Decreased medial or lateral glide of the patella signifies a tight lateral or medial retinaculum, respectively. Firm pressure is applied to the medial and lateral borders of the patella to test for translation (Fig. 40.7). Excessive glide or play of the patella can be determined

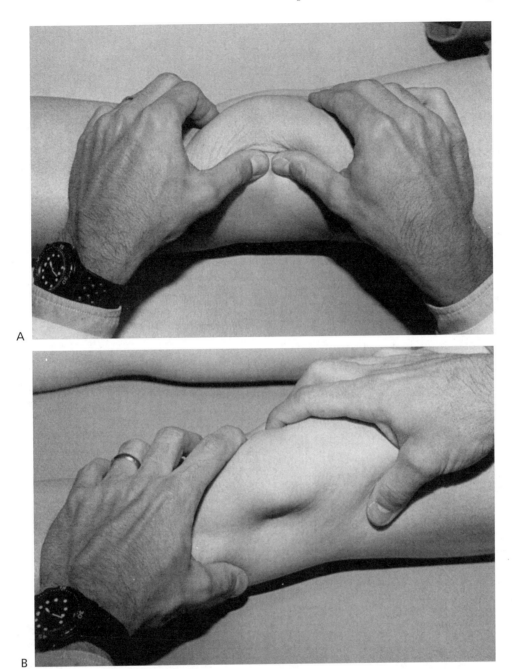

FIG. 40.7. Medial (**A**) and lateral (**B**) glide tests performed with knee in extension. (From Fulkerson JP. *Disorders of the patellofemoral joint.* Baltimore: Williams & Wilkins, 1997:51, with permission.)

by manually subluxating it in the medial–lateral direction. The apprehension sign is caused by a lateral force to the patella that elicits the sense of subluxation or dislocation and patient apprehension (20). When applying a medial force on the patella, excessive tilt must be controlled to prevent the patella from externally rotating. This may lead to the sense of increased medial displacement of the patella. The patellar glide test assesses the static factors that affect patellar alignment. An estimate of the amount of translation can be determined by dividing the patella into longitudinal quad-

rants and noting how many quadrants can be translated with the glide test.

Medial subluxation of the patella, although not as common as lateral subluxation, may be determined by the Fulkerson relocation test. The test involves holding the patient's knee in full extension with the patella pushed medially and actively or passively flexing the knee rapidly while letting go of the patella. The sensation of pain with this maneuver, which re-creates the patient's symptoms, can confirm the diagnosis of medial instability. To further confirm the diagnosis, the Fulker-

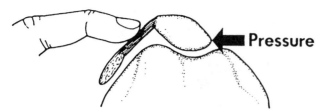

FIG. 40.8. Palpation of soft tissue around the patella. Soft tissue is placed under tension before palpation. (From Fulkerson JP. *Disorders of the patellofemoral joint*. Baltimore: Williams & Wilkins, 1997:54, with permission.)

son test applies a Trupull brace such that a medial to lateral pull is applied. Relief of symptoms confirms a diagnosis of medial patella subluxation.

Parapatellar tenderness should be carefully evaluated. Palpation of all soft tissue restraints of the patella should be performed. This includes the medial and lateral retinaculum, the patellar tendon, all quadriceps tendon insertions, and the medial femoral condyle for the medial parapatellar plica. It is important to place each structure under tension before palpation to avoid transmitting pressure to any underlying structures (Fig. 40.8). All scars need to be palpated for neuromata and the adductor hiatus for signs of saphenous nerve entrapment. The patellar retinaculae and tendon are highly innervated regions and are often the source of anterior knee pain. Kasim and Fulkerson (21) showed neuromatous degeneration of small nerves and neovascularization within resected regions of painful retinaculum in patients with anterior knee pain. This neuromatous degeneration has been previously found by Fulkerson et al. (22) from retinacular tissue excised after lateral release.

Palpation around the medial femoral condyle is important to discover a painful parapatellar plica and an injured medial patellofemoral ligament due to lateral patellar dislocation. Focal tenderness in the peripatellar retinaculum, muscle, and tendon may be associated with patellar malalignment. Recurrent stretching of a tight retinaculum during knee motion can give rise to pain and tenderness in this region (16). Tenderness within the patellar tendon often denotes tendinitis or tendinosis. The quadriceps muscle and tendon may be tender due to overuse syndromes.

Retropatellar tenderness is a characteristic finding in patients with chondromalacia. Direct patellofemoral compression can elicit tenderness in these patients. Insall et al. (23) described applying direct compression with the knee slightly flexed to ensure contact of the articular surface with the femoral groove. This method may avoid trapping the synovium in the suprapatellar pouch that can elicit pain in a normal knee. The patella should be compressed against the femur at all angles of knee flexion. Care should be taken to avoid applying pressure to the retinacular tissue. The pain elicited is

often due to articular lesions, causing irritation of the subchondral bone. It is important to note the flexion angle that gives the most pain because it may help determine what region is damaged on the patellar articular surface. Any crepitus with active and passive knee flexion should be noted. Although normal knees often have crepitus, a discreet catch or click that recreates the patient's symptoms is important for making the diagnosis.

A knee effusion may be determined by milking the suprapatellar pouch with one hand and checking if the patella is ballotable with the other hand (15). An effusion may be caused by many intraarticular lesions that include patellofemoral arthrosis and osteochondral lesions. Reflex quadriceps inhibition may be caused by a joint effusion, where as little as 20 to 30 mL of fluid can inhibit the VMO (24). Such inhibition can cause dynamic malalignment and lead to patellofemoral pain.

Direct palpation of the medial or lateral facet may

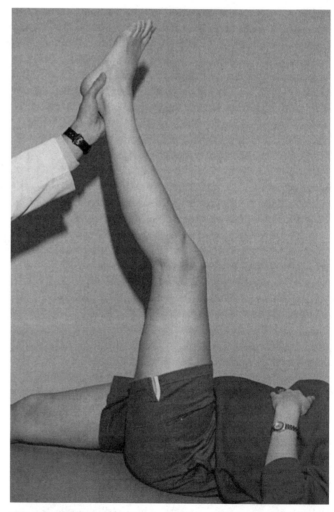

FIG. 40.9. Measuring the popliteal angle to evaluate hamstring tightness while patient is supine. (From Fulkerson JP. *Disorders of the patellofemoral joint*. Baltimore: Williams & Wilkins, 1997:59, with permission.)

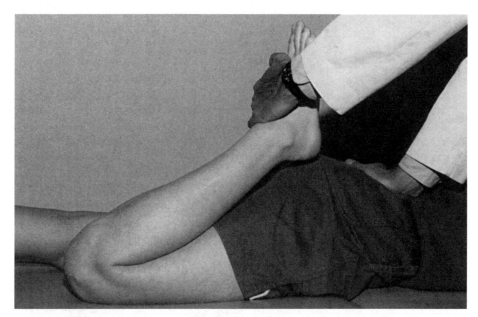

FIG. 40.10. Examination for quadriceps flexibility while patient is prone. (From Fulkerson JP. *Disorders of the patellofemoral joint.* Baltimore: Williams & Wilkins, 1997:61, with permission.)

be accomplished in a patella that is easily subluxable. Inversion or eversion of the patella can allow for direct facet palpation. Any tenderness noted needs to be differentiated from retinacular tenderness because the palpation is performed through the retinaculum.

Examination for flexibility is important in patients with patellofemoral injury. Evaluation for hamstring tightness is done with the patient supine. Flex each hip separately to 90 degrees and determine the popliteal angle (Fig. 40.9). A comparison with the contralateral side is necessary. An excessively tight hamstring can lead to a relative knee flexion contracture that increases the quadriceps forces required for knee extension. This can cause an increase in the patellofemoral joint reaction force.

Quadriceps flexibility is determined with the patient in the prone position. The pelvis is stabilized as each knee is flexed (Fig. 40.10). The heel to buttock distance is recorded for both legs. A tight quadriceps muscle can increase patellofemoral joint reaction forces during knee flexion because greater resistance needs to be overcome. Inflexibility can also lead to overload injuries to other regions such as the patellar or quadriceps tendons.

Ober's test is used to evaluate iliotibial band flexibility (Fig. 40.11). With the patient in the lateral position, the lower hip is maximally flexed while the pelvis is stabilized. The upper hip is extended to neutral with the knee flexed to 90 degrees. Allow the upper leg to drop while maintaining the knee flexion and hip extension. The iliotibial band is placed on stretch with this maneuver and thus allows observation of its flexibility. The leg should drop to a position at least parallel to the table, but a comparison with the contralateral leg needs to be performed. Pain in the distal aspect of the iliotibial band can also signify excessive tightness. Inflexibility of the iliotibial band can lead to patellar malalignment and a tight lateral retinaculum.

A thorough history and physical examination is invaluable in helping diagnose and treat patients with patellofemoral injuries. Only after this is completed should other tests such as imaging studies be obtained to corroborate the clinical suspicions.

RADIOGRAPHIC EVALUATION

Despite the importance of a thorough history and physical examination for patients with anterior knee pain, imaging studies are often required to help corroborate the diagnosis. Standard radiographs are often enough to evaluate patients with injuries to the patellofemoral joint. Standing anteroposterior and lateral radiographs may show sclerosis or fractures of the patella and other pathologic processes but are poor tools for evaluating alignment. The lateral x-ray taken in 30 degrees of flexion can demonstrate patella alta or baha and the functional relationship of the patellar facets to the femur. The Insall-Salvati ratio (25) is derived from a lateral x-ray with the knee in 20 to 70 degrees flexion (Fig. 40.12). It is the ratio of the patellar tendon length to the height of the patella. The value is normally $1.03 \pm 20\%$. Values out of this range may signify patella alta or baha. However, variations in the morphology of the patella that cause differences in lengths of the articulating and nonarticulating portions of the patella decrease

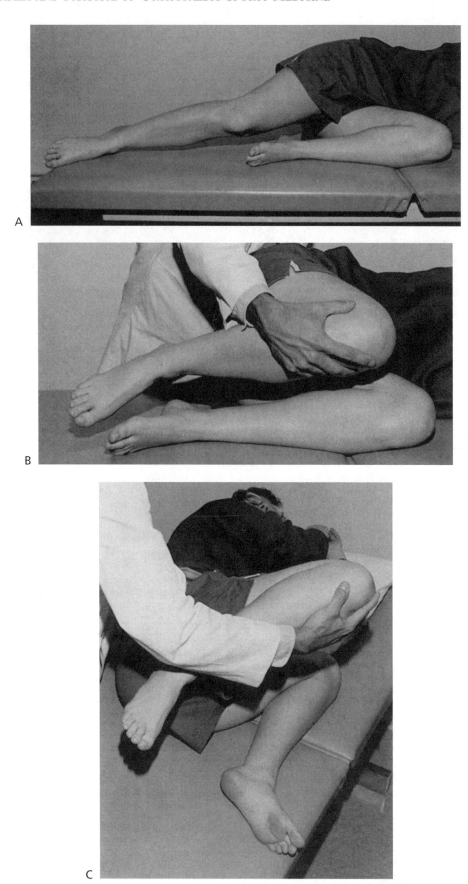

FIG. 40.11. *Continued*

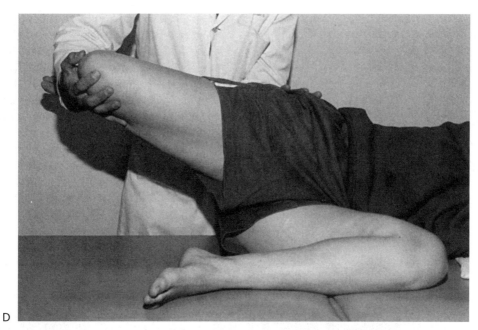

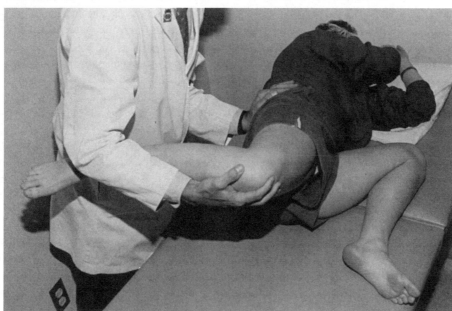

FIG. 40.11. *Continued* (**A–E**) Ober's test to evaluate iliotibial band tightness. With patient in lateral position, the pelvis is stabilized while the lower hip is fully flexed. The upper hip is extended with the knee flexed. The leg is allowed to drop with gravity while the femur is controlled for rotation. (From Fulkerson JP. *Disorders of the patellofemoral joint.* Baltimore: Williams & Wilkins, 1997:65, with permission.)

the sensitivity of the Insall-Salvati ratio. Caton et al. (26) described the ratio between the patellar articular length and the distance between the distal pole of the patella and the tibial tubercle (Fig. 40.12). The ratio is 0.8 in normal knees with 30 degrees of flexion.

A lateral view of the patellofemoral joint can also provide information regarding rotation of the patella. Maldague and Malghem (27) described the use of a precise lateral radiograph of the knee to determine pa-

tellar alignment. The precise lateral radiograph, however, requires the posterior and distal femoral condyles to be overlapped. A normally aligned patella has the central ridge posterior to the lateral facet (Fig. 40.13A). A patella that is laterally tilted shows overlap of the lateral facet and central ridge, with extreme rotation showing the lateral ridge posterior to the central ridge (Fig. 40.13B). This view helps determine patellar tilt but provides little help in evaluating translation.

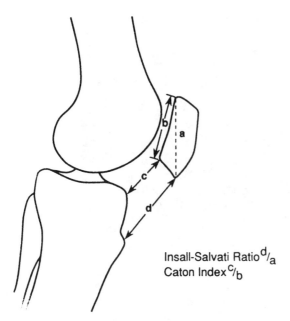

FIG. 40.12. Measurement of the Insall-Salvati ratio (*d/a*) and the Caton index (*c/b*). (From Fulkerson JP. *Disorders of the patellofemoral joint.* Baltimore: Williams & Wilkins, 1997: 81, with permission.)

Axial views of the knee have become critical in evaluating patellofemoral disorders. Maquet (28) examined tangential or "sunrise" views and suggested that reorientation of the osseous trabeculae of the lateral facet may signify excess pressure on the facet. Laurin et al. (29) evaluated axial x-rays with the knee at 20 degrees of flexion to study patellar alignment (Fig. 40.14). This view is often difficult to obtain but can provide helpful information in detecting subtle alignment abnormalities. They described the lateral patellofemoral angle as an index of patellar tilt (Fig. 40.15). The angle is formed by a line along the lateral facet and a line drawn across the anterior portions of the femoral trochlea. The normal patellofemoral joint has an angle that opens laterally. This angle is appropriate for measuring patellar tilt and has little use in assessing subluxation.

Merchant et al. (30) used a tangential radiograph to describe the congruence angle. Figure 40.16 shows the technique of obtaining a Merchant view. The knee is flexed to 45 degrees with the x-ray beam projected at 30 degrees above the horizontal. The angle formed by the femoral trochlea (sulcus angle) is bisected. This sul-

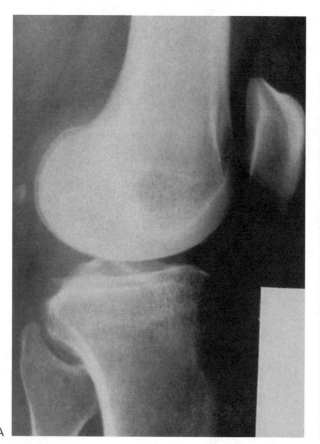

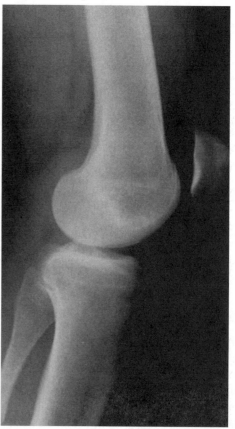

FIG. 40.13. A: Normal rotation of the patella on true lateral view with central ridge posterior to lateral facet line. **B:** Tilt of the patella with overlap of central ridge and lateral facet line. (From Fulkerson JP. *Disorders of the patellofemoral joint.* Baltimore: Williams & Wilkins, 1997:76–77, with permission.)

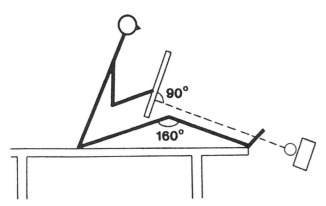

FIG. 40.14. Tangential x-ray of the patellofemoral joint. The knee is at 160 degrees, and the x-ray beam is directed cephalad, parallel to the anterior border of the tibia. (From Laurin CA, Dussault R, Levesque HP. The tangential x-ray investigation of the patellofemoral joint. *Clin Orthop* 1979;144:17, with permission.)

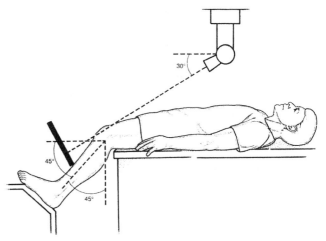

FIG. 40.16. Technique of obtaining a Merchant's axial view of the knee. The knee is flexed to 45 degrees and the beam is directed caudad, 30 degrees down from the horizontal. (From Insall JN, Windsor RE, Scott WN, et al. *Surgery of the knee.* New York: Churchill Livingstone, 1993:268, with permission.)

cus angle normally measures 138 degrees. An angle greater than 150 degrees may predispose to patellar subluxation or dislocation. The congruence angle is formed by the bisector of the trochlea with a line drawn from the apex of the sulcus to the apex of the patella (Fig. 40.17). An angle that opens medially is negative and that which opens laterally is positive. Values less than 16 degrees are considered normal by Merchant et al. However, Aglietti et al. (31) defined the upper limit of normal as 4 degrees. They stated that patients with

angles greater than 23 degrees often had patellar dislocations. This angle assesses subluxation as apposed to the lateral patellofemoral angle that assesses tilt. The congruence angle can be determined at angles other than the 45-degree angle described by Merchant et al. Smaller angles, however, usually require computed tomography (CT) to evaluate because they are technically difficult to obtain accurately with plain radiography.

Malghem and Maldague (32) used the axial x-rays to describe patellar "subluxability." This denotes the tendency of the patella to subluxate when stress is applied to it or the knee is rotated. Subluxation describes

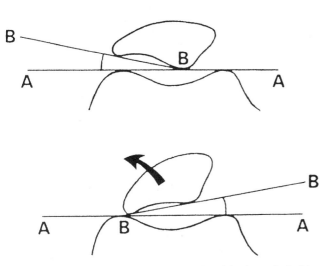

FIG. 40.15. Lateral patellofemoral angle of the knee (left side is lateral). *Line AA* joins the top of the femoral condyles, and line *BB* joins the limits of the lateral facet. The angle is formed by *lines AA and BB*, which open laterally when normal (*upper diagram*). The angle opens medially or the lines are parallel in instances of patellar tilt (*lower diagram*). (From Laurin CA, Dussault R, Levesque HP. The tangential x-ray investigation of the patellofemoral joint. *Clin Orthop* 1979;144:18, with permission.)

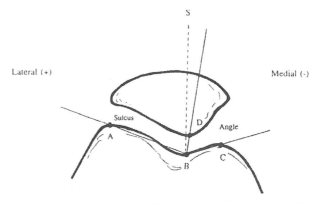

FIG. 40.17. Diagram of the Merchant congruence angle. The sulcus angle (*ABC*) is bisected by the reference line (*BS*). A line (*BD*) is drawn from the sulcus (*B*) to the lowest aspect of the patella (*D*). The congruence angle (*DBS*) is negative if *D* is medial to line *BS* and positive if *D* is lateral to line *BS*. (From Larsen B, Andreasen E, Urfer A, et al. Patellar taping: a radiographic examination of the medial glide technique. *Am J Sports Med* 1995;23:468, with permission.)

displacement without stress or knee rotation. The x-rays are 30-degree axial views with external tibial rotation. A patella that displaces is considered subluxable.

More recently, CT has been used as an effective tool to evaluate the patellofemoral relationship. It is often useful when the patient has clinically suspected patellofemoral problems with negative axial x-rays. Laurin et al. (29) recognized the importance of evaluating the joint with the knee in the least possible flexion to demonstrate true pathology and malalignment. Sunrise views in the range of maximum instability (0 to 30 degrees of flexion) are often technically difficult and are not consistently helpful in evaluating the malalignment syndrome.

The CT is well suited to evaluate the patellofemoral joint because it avoids the problems of overlapping images and variable reference points. Schutzer et al. (33) used midpatellar transverse tomographic cuts from 0 to 30 degrees to describe normal patellar alignment. The normally aligned patella enters the femoral trochlea early in flexion, has no tilt beyond 10 degrees of flexion, and has a congruence angle of 0 at 10 to 20 degrees of flexion. Congruence angles greater than 0 at 10 degrees of knee flexion are considered abnormal. Schutzer et al. (33) also showed that some patients with patellofemoral symptoms and abnormal congruence angles at 10 to 20 degrees had correction of this abnormality with further knee flexion. Patients who have abnormal congruence at angles greater than 20 degrees as well may be considered to have more severe malalignment.

CT is also helpful in measuring the patellar tilt angle. This angle is formed by a line along the lateral facet and one along the posterior femoral condyles (Fig. 40.18). Normal values are greater than 8 degrees. This angle measures patellar tilt, whereas the congruence angle is more useful for measuring subluxation. Finally,

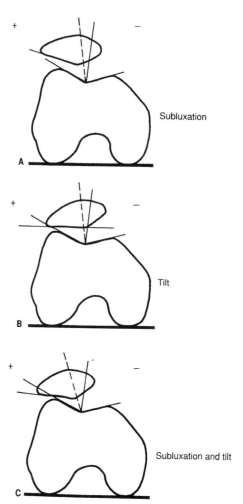

FIG. 40.19. The position of the patella on computed tomography images. The position of the patella may show subluxation alone (A), tilt alone (B), or subluxation and tilt together (C). (From Insall JN, Windsor RE, Scott WN, et al. *Surgery of the knee.* New York: Churchill Livingstone, 1993:275, with permission.)

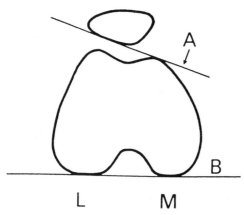

FIG. 40.18. The patellar tilt angle formed by a line along the posterior femoral condyles and another one along the lateral facet. (From Fulkerson JP. *Disorders of the patellofemoral joint.* Baltimore: Williams & Wilkins, 1997:92, with permission.)

Schutzer et al. (33) developed a classification including four patterns of malalignment using axial CTs (Fig. 40.19): type 1, subluxation alone; type 2, subluxation with tilt; type 3, tilt alone; type 4, no malalignment. The types were subdivided further depending on the presence of no articular lesion, minor chondromalacia, and osteoarthrosis.

Other radiographic modalities have been used less frequently. Magnetic resonance imaging (MRI) can assess patellar tracking at low flexion angles but is more useful to detect lesions of the articular cartilage and other knee pathology. In the current medicoeconomic environment, the expense of MRI should limit its use to situations where the other less expensive modalities are unable to detect any abnormalities within the patellofemoral joint. CT is less expensive than MRI and offers greater ability to obtain axial slices at varying knee flexion angles. CT arthrography can also be used to study the patellofemoral articulation (34). A thorough history and physical examination with good quality plain radiographs is usually enough to diagnose and treat injuries to the patellofemoral joint. Bone scans can aid in detecting other lesions within the patella and RSD.

SOFT TISSUE INJURY

Many patients with anterior knee pain have tenderness localized to the patellar tendon. This patellar tendinitis, or jumper's knee, is often found in athletes who jump frequently, such as basketball or tennis players. The tenderness is often localized to the origin of the patellar tendon on the distal pole of the patella. The patient will usually complain of pain in the anterior knee with activities that stress the extensor mechanism, such as squatting or jumping.

Bursitis is a common disorder, with many bursae localized around the anterior knee (Fig. 40.20). Prolonged kneeling and blunt trauma to the anterior knee can lead to bursitis. Retropatellar bursitis, localized behind the distal patellar tendon, gives symptoms that can mimic patellofemoral arthritis. Examination with a relaxed quadriceps muscle in the fully extended knee will often reveal pain within the bursa itself.

Direct trauma to the anterior knee can traumatize the infrapatellar fat pad. Fat pad syndrome may also arise from pinching of the pad between the femoral condyles and the tibial plateau with knee extension. Patients with genu recurvatum may be more at risk because the area for the fat pad is reduced (35). Direct palpation of the fat pad will reveal tenderness, which should be differentiated from generalized synovitis of the knee.

Nonoperative Management

The mainstay of treatment for most soft tissue injuries is nonoperative. Stretching exercises for the extensor mechanism in the prone position and eccentric quadriceps muscle strengthening is important. High-impact loading activities during early rehabilitation should be avoided. This includes isokinetic exercises that may greatly increase the loads in the patellofemoral joint. Stationary cycling, swimming, and isometric exercises provide good nonimpact exercises.

Simple elastic sleeves may provide relief because they can vary the soft tissue tensions around the anterior knee without altering patellar tracking. Nonsteroidal anti-inflammatory medication and modalities such as hydrocortisone iontophoresis may be helpful in many

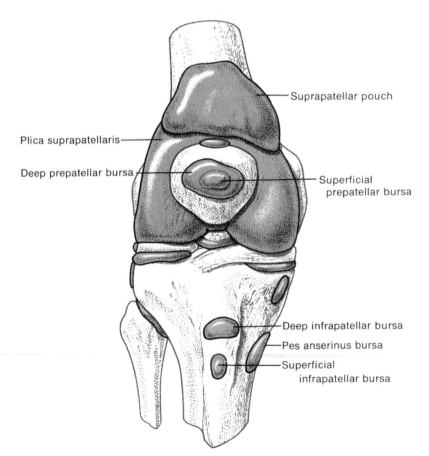

FIG. 40.20. Bursae in the front of the knee. (From Fulkerson JP. *Disorders of the patellofemoral joint.* Baltimore: Williams & Wilkins, 1997:145, with permission.)

cases. Direct corticosteroid injections into an inflamed bursa or fat pad can be curative in combination with rehabilitation. Care must be taken to avoid injecting the patellar tendon directly because this may cause weakening of the tendon, predisposing it to rupture.

Operative Management

In the rare case that conservative treatment is not successful with these injuries, operative management is used. Patients with refractory patellar tendinitis infrequently require open exploration of the tendon. Limited resection of localized chronic granulation tissue may treat the problem. Arthroscopic excision of any impinging fat pad may cure the fat pad syndrome.

LATERAL PATELLAR PRESSURE SYNDROME

Natural History

Anterior knee pain brought on by physical activity may present in the early teens in patients with lateral patellar tilt. Typically, this problem is present since childhood but not clinically apparent. The stress on a chronically tilted patella can increase substantially with longitudinal bone growth. Despite this finding of lateral patellar tilt syndrome in young patients, it remains more common in older female patients with chronic anterior knee pain. The onset of the symptoms can often follow direct trauma or a twisting injury to the knee.

A chronically tilted patella can lead to adaptive shortening of the lateral retinaculum. A tight retinaculum, however, can also lead to patellar tilt and lateral compression syndrome. Ficat et al. (36) theorized that excessive tightness in the lateral retinaculum can tilt the patella, leading to increased pressure on the lateral facet and subsequent degeneration and pain. The vector of posterior pull on a tight lateral retinaculum during knee flexion is high and may lead to stretching and overload within the retinaculum. Results may include pain with lateral facet compression and irritation of the small sensory nerves within the retinaculum (22). Chronic lateral patellar tilt can lead to lateral facet overload and deficient medial facet contact pressure. Articular cartilage degeneration on either facet may result. The lateral compression syndrome thus often starts with soft tissue pain and eventually leads to articular cartilage degeneration.

Evaluation

Examination of the patient often reveals crepitus within the patellofemoral joint with flexion and extension of the knee. Comparison with the contralateral leg is important to determine if any of the catching or clicking recreates their pain. Patellar tracking should be evaluated with passive flexion and extension of the knee to rule out lateral subluxation.

Lateral retinacular tightness needs to be assessed. Attempts at depressing the medial facet and elevating the lateral facet past neutral is performed, and restrictions to medial displacement of the patella is noted. Systematic palpation of all soft tissue restraints of the patella is done with careful attention to the lateral retinaculum. Fulkerson (37) prospectively examined 78 knees in patients with patellofemoral pain and found tenderness within the lateral retinaculum in 90% of the cases.

Radiographic evaluation starts with standard anteroposterior, lateral, and axial views. The anteroposterior view provides little information for lateral patellar tilt, but a true lateral view may reveal rotation and tilt of the patella as demonstrated by Maldague and Malghem

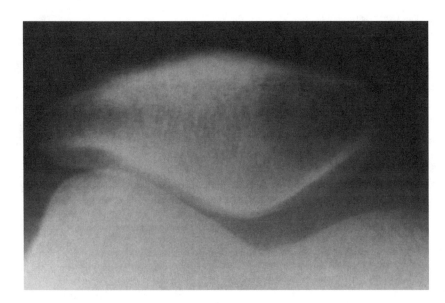

FIG. 40.21. Axial view of the patellofemoral joint. Cartilage loss and lateral patellofemoral joint space narrowing giving appearance of "false subluxation." (From Fulkerson JP. *Disorders of the patellofemoral joint.* Baltimore: Williams & Wilkins, 1997:157, with permission.)

(27). The axial view provides the most information for the lateral compression syndrome. The lateral patellofemoral angle should be determined (Fig. 40.15). A normal angle opens laterally, whereby a medially opening angle denotes lateral patellar tilt. In chronic cases, a loss of cartilage joint space in the lateral patellofemoral joint denotes significant cartilage degeneration and can often be mistaken for "false subluxation" (Fig. 40.21).

CT is also helpful because it is the only method where the posterior condyle reference line is reproducible to measure the patellar tilt angle (Fig. 40.18). Control studies of asymptomatic patients (38) showed that the patellar tilt angle is greater than 7 degrees at any flexion angle. CT can also be used to determine whether the patient has progressive tilt with increasing knee flexion because serial images can be taken with the knee in increasing flexion.

Nonoperative Management

The initial treatment for most orthopaedic problems, including patellofemoral pain syndrome, is conservative. Nonoperative measures include activity modification, rehabilitation programs, knee supports, patellar taping, anti-inflammatory medications, orthotics, and reassurance. Perhaps the most important aspect of a nonoperative program is patient education. Success will often depend on a cooperative and compliant patient who is well informed. Patient education provides reassurance that life- or limb-threatening pathology does not exist and helps relieve any excess anxiety.

An important focus of rehabilitation in patients with patellar tilt is stretching and mobilization of tight quadriceps and lateral retinacular tissue. Tight quadriceps can be stretched in the prone position, and a tight lateral retinaculum can be manually stretched with passive medial displacement of the patella with the knee fully extended. A tight iliotibial band needs to also be addressed because this may increase the posterior pull of the lateral retinaculum during knee flexion and accentuate the lateral tilt syndrome.

Strengthening of the quadriceps, especially the VMO, can provide significant improvement. Isometric quadriceps exercises such as progressive resistive straight leg raises are very effective and rarely painful. Resistive knee extension exercises from 90 degrees to full extension are often painful and contraindicated because they impart high loads on the patellofemoral joint (39). Short-arc isotonic exercises in the last 30 degrees of extension may be of benefit in some patients.

Activity modification is useful in the conservative approach to treatment but is often difficult for some patients to follow. Many patients are young athletes who want to continue their sports, and others have more severe symptoms that arise with simple activities of daily living. Whitelaw et al. (40) treated 85 patients with anterior knee pain with conservative measures and found a higher success rate in patients who also restricted their activities. Improved knee function was also found in those patients who maintained a home exercise program.

Nonoperative treatment should include at least 6 months of conservative measures, including supervised physical therapy. Surgical intervention for the lateral patellar compression syndrome is used only when there is failure of improvement and disabling symptoms persist.

Operative Management

The mainstay of treatment for patients with a tight lateral retinaculum is a lateral release. This includes those who have radiographic evidence of lateral tilt. Patients with advanced degeneration of the patellofemoral joint and subluxation do less well with this procedure. A lateral release may also be successful when there is tenderness within the retinaculum that may be due to neuromatous degeneration of the small nerves. The release may decompress and dennervate this region and the neuroma, providing pain relief (22).

The lateral release can be performed arthroscopically or open. An arthroscopic examination of the knee joint to rule out any other intraarticular pathology should be performed before either technique. Meniscal pathology and the articular surface of the patella should be examined. The entire lateral retinaculum and synovium is released under direct vision, including the proximal epicondylopatellar band and the distal patellotibial band. Partial release of any tight retropatellar tendon fat may also be helpful (15). Distally, the release should continue to the level of the tibial tubercle with extreme care taken to avoid injuring the lateral meniscus. Proximally, the vastus lateralis obliquus tendon is released along the plane between it and the main tendon of the vastus lateralis (Fig. 40.22). This allows complete release of both the static and dynamic lateral patellar support structures.

An open lateral release can safely be performed through a 3- to 5-cm incision. The subcutaneous tissue is undermined to allow complete visualization of the entire retinaculum and safe release. Once the release is done, the patella should be everted to 90 degrees to ensure a complete release and to examine the articular surface of the patella. If a tourniquet is used, it should be let down at this point to allow thorough hemostasis, including the superior lateral geniculate vessel. The knee is then flexed and extended multiple times to evaluate tracking. Continued abnormal tracking may signify lateral subluxation of the patella. At this point, the skin and subcutaneous tissues are closed and a pressure dressing is placed over the lateral patellofemoral joint to prevent hematoma formation.

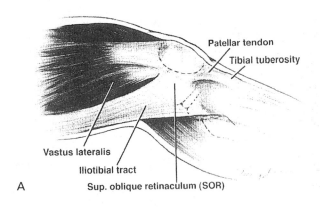

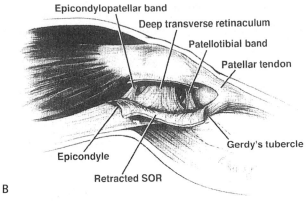

FIG. 40.22. A: Lateral retinaculum. **B:** Incision in superficial lateral retinaculum for lateral release revealing deep transverse retinaculum. (From Banas MP, Ferkel RD, Friedman MJ. Arthroscopic lateral retinacular release of the patellofemoral joint. *Opin Tech Sports Med* 1994;2:292, with permission.)

The main advantage of the arthroscopic lateral release is cosmetic due to the avoidance of an incision. The disadvantage is that hemostasis is more difficult to perform. Electrosurgery has been used more frequently with arthroscopy recently that can decrease hematoma formation. Caution must be taken when using electrocautery to avoid cauterizing the skin.

Postoperative Rehabilitation

Range-of-motion exercises and weight bearing are usually started in the immediate postoperative period. Early flexion is obtained to prevent scar formation across the release as it is opened widely with knee flexion. Quadriceps strengthening is also important to obtain good results. Straight leg raising exercises need to be started as early as possible to help rehabilitate the quadriceps muscles. Once the patient is comfortable, the patella can be manipulated with medial glides and lift-up of the lateral patellar border to prevent adhesions (4). Eventually, short-arc resistive extension exercises are performed in the last 10 to 20 degrees of extension. An exercise bicycle is also helpful during rehabilitation with

the seat raised high and minimal resistance. This rehabilitation should continue indefinitely with a well-developed home exercise program.

Outcomes

Comparison of the results in the literature on lateral release is difficult because no true standardized method of rating the outcomes have been universally accepted. Some factors, however, have been associated with successful or unsatisfactory results. Gecha and Torg (41) defined some prognosticators for success in a series of patients undergoing lateral release. Better results were obtained when there was no malalignment, tilt, or laxity present. Other negative factors include genu varum, valgum or recurvatum, increased femoral anteversion, external tibial torsion, and abnormal foot pronation. Significant lateral facet degeneration also can negatively affect the results of surgery.

Postoperatively, failure to appropriately rehabilitate the quadriceps muscles, including the VMO, can lead to poor results. Adequate muscular training can also help to centralize the patella postoperatively. It is evident that successful results depend on preoperative, intraoperative, and postoperative factors.

ACUTE DISLOCATIONS OF THE PATELLA

Etiology

Patellar dislocation may occur due to direct trauma in patients with or without preexisting patellar malalignment. Patients who have subluxation of the patella may predispose them to dislocation. Indirect trauma causing twisting of the knee with a laterally directed vector of stress on the patella can cause dislocation. The patella has a tendency to displace laterally in the normal knee due to the Q angle. The bony architecture of the lateral trochlea as a buttress helps to balance this tendency (15). The patella is also balanced functionally by the VMO and passively by the medial ligaments. An acute or recurrent dislocation often involves some form of breakdown in this equilibrium.

The bony architecture of the patellofemoral joint may play a role in dislocation. Brattstrom (42) measured the sulcus angles in 131 patients with recurrent dislocations and determined that the angle was 10 degrees greater in these patients than in control group (200 subjects). Accurate assessment of the sulcus angle can be made using CT or MRI. Abnormal patellar morphology may have an effect on dislocation. A chronically malaligned patella may lead to secondary morphologic changes that can increase the chances of complete patellar dislocation. However, direct or indirect trauma to the knee can cause patellar dislocation without the presence of preexisting malalignment or bony abnormalities.

Clinical Evaluation

Patients often report a giving way of their knee after an injury has occurred. They sometimes describe that their knee has "dislocated" and then subsequently relocated. The knee is usually swollen on presentation, making it difficult to assess the bony architecture. Aspiration of the knee can help in the examination. A limitation of range of motion is seen due to the swelling and tenderness. The patient also often resists knee flexion because it may pull the patella laterally and give them the sense or redislocation. The patella should be stabilized in the trochlear groove when attempting to flex the knee. The patella often relocates before the patient is seen by the physician when the patient extends the knee after the injury. On occasion, the patella remains dislocated, requiring acute management.

A careful examination of the entire knee must be performed to rule out other injury. Testing for cruciate injury, joint line tenderness, and quadriceps or patellar tendon rupture is important. A defect near the proximal or distal pole of the patella and an inability to perform a straight leg raise confirms the diagnosis of tendon rupture. A systematic examination should then be done for the supporting structures of the patella. Tenderness is found in the medial retinaculum with apprehension at any attempts at lateral patellar displacement. Swelling may also be noted near the insertion of the VMO. The lateral retinaculum may or may not be tender. Other tests requiring flexion and extension of the knee are difficult secondary to the pain and swelling.

Radiographic Evaluation

Routine anteroposterior, lateral, and Merchant axial views should always be taken after an acute patellar dislocation. The radiographs are often unremarkable, but some findings may be indicative of patellar dislocation. Osteochondral fragments or bony avulsions are often seen in the parapatellar region. The osteochondral fractures are usually from the medial patellar facet or lateral femoral condyle (43). They are usually produced when the medial patellar facet strikes the lateral femoral condyle during relocation. Loose osteochondral fragments can often be seen in the lateral gutter on an axial view. The articular damage to the medial facet is frequently seen during arthroscopy (Fig. 40.23).

Lateral displacement of the patella within the sulcus can also be seen on the Merchant view secondary to disruption of the medial stabilizers of the patella. Evidence of a high riding patella or a shallow femoral sulcus should be noted. CT and MRI are rarely necessary after a patellar dislocation. CT may help diagnose malalignment, and MRI can reveal other intraarticular pathology including bony contusions.

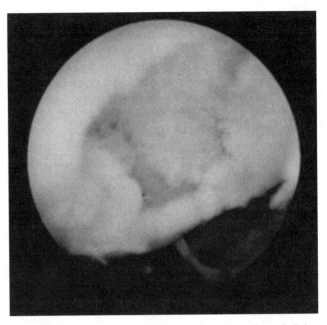

FIG. 40.23. Injury to medial facet after relocation of dislocated patella. (From Fulkerson JP. *Disorders of the patellofemoral joint.* Baltimore: Williams & Wilkins, 1997:205, with permission.)

Treatment

Infrequently, patients will be seen with an unreduced patella. These cases need to be treated as an orthopaedic emergency. Closed reduction of the patella should be performed. Patients with an unreduced dislocation often have significant pain and muscle spasms. Aspiration of the joints with large effusions can provide some relief of these symptoms. Relaxation of the quadriceps muscles by placing the leg in full knee extension can be achieved. Intravenous pain medicine and muscle relaxants may also be of benefit. Allowing the patient's leg to rest in full extension will frequently lead to spontaneous relocation. On occasion, medially directed pressure on the patella is required to achieve relocation. Rarely, unreducible dislocations need to be openly reduced.

Rest and activity restriction are essential in the management of patients with acute dislocation. Activities that increase patellofemoral pressure should be avoided. These include any weight-bearing activities with a flexed knee such as squatting, jumping, climbing, and kneeling. Aspiration of large effusions may help alleviate pain and allow for earlier rehabilitation. In general, the level of pain should dictate the amount of activity restriction, and any activity causing knee pain should be avoided.

Immobilization of the knee after an acute dislocation is commonly used to allow healing of the medial retinaculum. Larsen and Lauridsen (44) confirmed that first-time dislocators should be treated conservatively. Nonoperative measures should be used only if the surgeon is sure that there is no major articular fragment displacement. The knee is immobilized for 4 to 6 weeks to allow restoration of stability. Quadriceps strengthening with straight leg raises is started as soon as the patient is comfortable. The patient begins partial weight bearing in the brace and advances to full weight bearing as tolerated. Once the brace is removed, quadriceps strengthening continues for prolonged periods.

The presence of an osteochondral fragment on x-ray should warrant surgical intervention. Small fragments may be excised with open or arthroscopic techniques. Larger fragments should be replaced to help restore articular congruence and prevent future problems. Articular injury may be substantial even in the face of normal radiographs, and the acute period is the best time to restore the displaced fragments.

Hawkins et al. (45) believed that immediate arthroscopic intervention would benefit those patients with a history of underlying malalignment. A tight lateral retinaculum should be released at the time of surgery to help restore proper tracking. A medial plication can also be performed initially, but most surgeons believe that major reconstructive procedures should be avoided in the acute setting.

Fulkerson's Preference

Immobilization is the treatment of choice when there is no evidence of a major osteochondral fragment or underlying malalignment. The patient works on progressive quadriceps strengthening exercises emphasizing the VMO. A large fragment creating a significant defect in the lateral trochlea should be pinned through a limited arthrotomy. Smaller fragments (<1 cm) can be removed arthroscopically. A lateral release is also done at the time of surgery when there is evidence of significant lateral tilt with a tight lateral retinaculum. Major reconstructive procedures should generally be avoided after an acute patellar dislocation.

Outcomes

The outcomes for conservative and surgical treatment of acute patellar dislocations have been studied by several authors (Tables 40.1 and 40.2). There is a trend for higher redislocation rates in younger patients who typically have more predisposing factors. Cofield and Bryan (46) reported redislocation rates of up to 44% in 50 patients treated conservatively and suggested surgical repair for patients with underlying malalignment and displaced intraarticular fragments. Hawkins et al. (45) also noted improved outcomes with surgical treatment when there is evidence of predisposing signs such as increased Q angle, patella alta, and abnormal patellar alignment. Cash and Hughston (47) found redislocation rates with conservative management of 20% when there was no predisposing signs and 43% with anatomic abnor-

TABLE 40.1. *Outcomes for conservative treatment of acute patella dislocations*

Author/reference	Year	No. of knees	Treatment	Average follow-up (mo)	Redislocation (%)	Remarks
Cofield and Bryan (46)	1977	50	Conservative		44	High redislocation rate; 52% of the knees were considered unsatisfactory; 27% required further surgery.
McManus et al. (103)	1979	26	Cast 6 wk	31	19	Dislocations in children; 42% complained of instability without dislocation and 38% were asymptomatic.
Larsen and Lauridsen (44)	1982	79	Cast or bandage	71	NA	Unable to define factors that may predispose to redislocation except age of less than 20 yr.
Hawkins et al. (45)	1986	20	Arthroscopy (9) Cast (11)	40	15	All patients that experienced redislocation had obvious lower limb malalignment; some degree of pain was present in 75% of the cases.
Cash and Hughston (47)	1988	74	Cast	96	36	Recurrence rate is higher in presence of signs of patellofemoral dysplasia of the opposite knee (43%) than when these are absent (20%); higher redislocation rate in younger patients.

NA, not available.

TABLE 40.2. *Outcomes for surgical treatment of acute patellar dislocations*

Author/reference	Year	No. of knees	Treatment		Average follow-up (mo)	Redislocation (%)	Remarks
Boring and O'Donoghue (104)	1978	17	Modified Hauser	9	98	0	There were no redislocations, but 2 knees had subluxation (12%); 12 knees (70%) were painful, although 8 were so only rarely; all had moderate retropatellar crepitation.
			Medial reefing	8			
Jensen and Roosen (105)	1985	23	Medial reefing	23	39	9	Pain with motion was present in 39%, retropatellar crepitus and signs of chondromalacia in 35%; the addition of lateral release did not improve the results.
			Lateral release	8			
Cash and Hughston (47)	1988	16	Medial reefing		97	0	Satisfactory results were obtained in 87%.
Dainer et al. (106)	1988	29	Arthroscopy and cast	14	25	14	All the recurrences were in the group treated with lateral release, which had a lower incidence of satisfactory results (73%) than those treated without lateral release (93%).
			Arthroscopy and lateral release	15			
Vainionpää et al. (107)	1990	55	Medial reefing	55	24	9	Satisfactory results in 80%; snapping was reported by 66% and giving way by 20%.
			Lateral release	37			

malities. They had a 0% redislocation rate in 16 patients treated operatively. The trend in the literature for outcomes after acute patellar dislocation seems to show better results after surgical intervention when there are predisposing factors (as described by Hawkins et al.). Despite a decrease in recurrence rate, there was a significant incidence of pain and crepitus. The outcome is therefore best optimized by thoroughly evaluating each case to determine if there are any indications for operative treatment.

RECURRENT SUBLUXATION AND DISLOCATION

Recurrent patellar subluxations and dislocations is a disabling disorder and has had many procedures developed for its treatment. Multiple studies have shown a predominance of this disorder in the second decade. Ficat (48) found a peak at 15 years, and Baum and Bensahal (49) found one at 14 years. Crosby and Insall (50) noted a decrease in frequency with age in a study of 26 patients treated nonoperatively. The literature also reveals a female predominance, with most patients presenting with multiple events of subluxations or dislocations. These frequent injuries have been associated

with damage to the patellar articular cartilage (51). The initial episode often occurs as a result of a twisting injury or from an external rotation and valgus stress applied to the knee during an athletic event.

Clinical Evaluation

The patient should be observed standing for any signs of excessive foot pronation or knee angular deformities. The Q angle of the injured and contralateral side is important to determine. Insall (52) believed that an excessive quadriceps (Q) angle and patella alta can lead to recurrent subluxations and dislocations. After an acute episode, the patient may have a hemarthrosis and pain along the medial border of the patella. More commonly, the patient does not complain of pain but may describe the feeling of insecurity with the involved knee.

A thorough examination of patellar tracking should be done in all cases. The knee is flexed and extended both actively and passively to test for subluxation. A positive J sign (abrupt lateral translation of the patella just before full extension) is often noted. The medial and lateral mobility of the patella is checked with the knee in full extension. With the quadriceps relaxed, lateral hypermobility is frequently observed. A patella that can be laterally subluxated more than half of its width signifies laxity. Comparison with the opposite side is required. Decreased medial displacement of the patella indicates a tight lateral retinaculum. This can be determined as well by attempting to lift the lateral edge of the patella past the horizontal.

A significant physical finding in patients with recurrent subluxations and dislocations is a positive apprehension sign described by Fairbank (53). With the knee fully extended and the quadriceps relaxed, the patella is subluxated laterally with firm pressure on its medial border. Passive flexion of the knee at this point may cause discomfort or the feeling of pending dislocation. The patient will often contract the quadriceps to recenter the patella and may attempt to displace the examiners hands.

Signs of patellofemoral crepitus and quadriceps weakness need to be evaluated. Crepitus with active and passive knee motion may denote articular damage. Associated discomfort should be determined, and comparison with the contralateral side is always checked. Quadriceps atrophy can be seen as the patient contracts the quadriceps muscle. The VMO is especially important, because weakness can lead to functional malalignment. Electromyographic studies (54) have shown decreased activity in the VMO as compared with the vastus lateralis in seven of eight patients with patellar subluxation. This was particularly evident in the last 30 degrees of extension.

Evaluation for systemic hypermobility should always be performed. Ehlers-Danlos or Marfan's syndrome is suspected when there is marked hypermobility. Appropriate referrals need to be made for these patients. The knees and elbows are checked for hyperextension, and the thumb to forearm distance is measured. Runow (55) showed that patellar dislocation was six times more common in patients with signs of systemic hypermobility.

Radiographic Evaluation

Standard radiographs are used to check for predisposing factors of patellar subluxation and dislocation. Patella

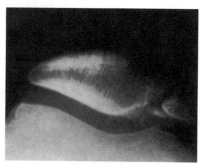

FIG. 40.25. Osteochondral fracture of medial facet after patellar dislocation. (From Fulkerson JP. *Disorders of the patellofemoral joint.* Baltimore: Williams & Wilkins, 1997:210, with permission.)

alta as determined by the Insall-Salvati ratio (25) has been associated with recurrent patellar subluxation (18). Values for patellar tendon length to patellar height averaged 1.23 in patients with subluxation and 1.04 in controls.

The Merchant view (30) can be used to determine the congruence angle (Fig. 40.17). Aglietti et al. (31) stated that angles greater than 23 degrees predispose the knee to dislocation. The femoral sulcus is also best viewed on axial radiographs. Larger angles were found in patients with recurrent instability (18). Calcification within the medial retinaculum can be seen due to recurrent dislocations (Fig. 40.24) and osteochondral fractures (Fig. 40.25).

CT or MRI is used when malalignment is less evident. They allow axial views in lower flexion angles without overlapping bony contours. The congruence angle can be accurately measured at various knee flexion angles. The height of the lateral femoral condyle should also be determined. Schutzer et al. (33) reported that the height of the condyle with respect to the deepest point of the sulcus is less in patients with patellar subluxation.

Nonoperative Treatment

Conservative therapy should initially be attempted in patients with recurrent patellar instability. The initial goals are aimed at stretching tight lateral structures and strengthening the quadriceps muscles. Wasting and weakness of the quadriceps muscles is a common finding associated with patellar subluxation. Most rehabilitation programs stress strengthening of the quadriceps muscles. Strengthening of the VMO is emphasized because an imbalance between the vastus medialis and vastus lateralis can contribute to lateral patellar tracking. The exercise programs usually involve isometric resistive quadriceps strengthening with the knee in extension. Straight leg raising with ankle weights may be used. Resisted exercises with the knee in flexion

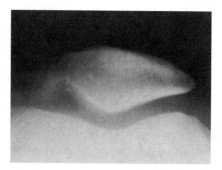

FIG. 40.24. Calcification within the medial retinaculum in a patient with recurrent patellar dislocations. (From Fulkerson JP. *Disorders of the patellofemoral joint.* Baltimore: Williams & Wilkins, 1997:209, with permission.)

should be avoided because it can exacerbate the symptoms.

Multiple braces have been designed to prevent patellar subluxation and alleviate patellofemoral pain. Varying degrees of success have been reported with these braces (56,57). The Trupull brace (Depuy-Orthotech, Tracy, CA) was recently introduced by one of the authors (J.P.F.). It applies consistent support for the patella by using a unique concept of pull strap fixation to separate fixation straps. In the middle 1980s, McConnell (58) introduced her technique and program of patellar taping, which is still widely used today. The taping is intended to reduce pain, control patellar maltracking, and allow enhanced quadriceps muscle rehabilitation. McConnell (58) reported success rates of up to 96% in the athletic population. Larsen et al. (59) radiographically determined that the taping was effective in medializing the patella but was ineffective in maintaining this after exercise.

Stretching plays a significant role in the treatment of patellar subluxation. Tightness of the lateral retinaculum, hamstring muscles, and iliotibial band are all contributing factors for lateral patellar tracking. A well-structured rehabilitation program must therefore include stretching protocols for these regions. A tight lateral retinaculum may be stretched and mobilized with passive medial displacement of the patella with the knee in extension.

The appropriate combination of nonoperative measures can result in a high rate of success with cooperative patients. Many return to their desired activity level with a substantial decrease in their pain and avoid the need for surgical intervention.

Operative Treatment

Conservative therapy has been shown to be successful in most young patients with patellar subluxation and dislocation. However, a subset of patients has persistent anterior knee pain and recurrent instability despite appropriate nonoperative measures. Most orthopedists believe that surgical intervention should be considered only after a minimum of 4 to 6 months of adequate conservative treatment has been tried. At this point, the precise etiology must be established. The back and hips should be examined to rule out the possibility of referred pain. Abnormal foot and ankle mechanics should be treated when necessary. Finally, the patient should demonstrate flexibility of the hamstrings and iliotibial band and objective increases in quadriceps strength.

Before proceeding with surgical intervention, the following questions should be answered (60): Is there evidence of referred pain? Is there parapatellar soft tissue pain? Is there x-ray or CT evidence of patellar tilt, subluxation, or both at 10 and 20 degrees flexion? Is there evidence of joint deterioration and is the pain

clearly associated with it? Is the problem structural or related to psychiatric problems and secondary gain? Have other causes of anterior knee pain not related to malalignment been eliminated? Is there evidence of RSD.

A surgical approach to malalignment should be undertaken only after these questions are answered.

Proximal Realignment

Proximal realignment procedures are aimed at altering the line of pull of the quadriceps muscles to help correct patellofemoral incongruence. Insall et al. (4) described their procedure using a rearrangement of the muscular attachments to the patella (Fig. 40.26). A midline incision is made to expose the patella and quadriceps expansions. Proximally, the vastus medialis, vastus lateralis, and the quadriceps tendon must be exposed.

After appropriate exposure is obtained, an arthrotomy is performed starting within the quadriceps tendon near its apex and extending distally within the tendon near the border of the vastus medialis. The incision is continued distally across the medial border of the patella and medial to the patellar tendon. The quadriceps expansion is then dissected free from the bone medially, with care taken to avoid tearing the thin layer that is elevated off the patella. The synovial lining medial to the patella is divided, and the fat pad is incised in line with the arthrotomy. The patella at this point can be everted for inspection.

A lateral arthrotomy is then made starting in the muscle fibers of the vastus lateralis and extending distally to the level of the tibial tubercle. Unlike the medial arthrotomy, this incision is made lateral to the patella and attempts are made to maintain the integrity of the synovium. Multiple vessels may need to be coagulated to avoid hematoma formation. The tourniquet if used is usually released at this point to allow for appropriate hemostasis.

Reconstruction of the quadriceps is then performed to alter the line of pull of this muscle in a more medially directed manner. The distal portion of the vastus medialis is brought laterally and distally to overlap the upper pole of the patella and quadriceps tendon and sutured in place. The typical overlap is 10 to 15 mm depending on the amount of preoperative laxity. The medial flap is then brought across the lower pole of the patella and sutured there. The remainder of the closure is then performed distally and proximally where the flaps lie, and the knee must be able to be flexed to 90 degrees without suture rupture. Also, the patella must be centrally aligned in the trochlea even in varus and valgus, without medial tilt.

One of the most common technical errors comes from not extending the lateral incision proximally enough

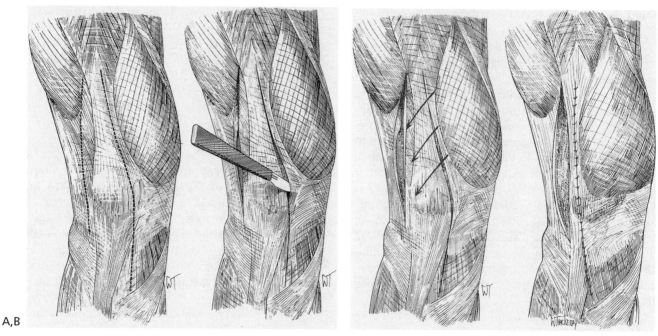

A,B

C,D

FIG. 40.26. Insall's proximal patellar realignment. **A:** Medial arthrotomy along medial border of quadriceps tendon, over medial border of the patella, and medial to patellar tendon. Lateral release incision. **B:** Quadriceps expansion elevated carefully off the patella. **C:** Medial flap is advanced distally and laterally in line with the fibers of the vastus medialis obliquus fibers. **D:** Advanced margin is sutured in place. (From Insall JN, Windsor RE, Scott WN, et al. *Surgery of the knee.* New York: Churchill Livingstone, 1993:330–331, with permission.)

into the vastus lateralis to allow for appropriate quadriceps rearrangement. A second error comes from overtightening the distal closure that may affect patellar tracking during knee flexion.

Postoperatively, the patient is allowed full weight bearing as tolerated with straight leg raises done as soon as possible. Flexion is also permitted early, with progression to 90 degrees by 4 weeks. Straight leg raises are done each day, and resistive quadriceps extension exercises are avoided.

TABLE 40.3. *Results of Insall's proximal realignment procedure*

Author/reference	Year	No. of knees	Diagnosis	Average follow-up (mo)	Satisfactory results (%)	Remarks
Insall et al. (108)	1983	75	Pain and subluxation	48	91	Better results when the patella was centered in the sulcus after the operation; no correlation with the severity of chondromalacia.
Scuderi et al. (62)	1988	60	Subluxation and dislocation	42	81	Only one redislocation (1.7%); females and older patients had inferior results; better results with patella centralization.
Abraham et al. (109)	1989	35	Pain and dislocation	76	62	Less satisfactory results in knees with patellofemoral pain (53%) than in knees with recurrent dislocation (78%).
Aglietti et al. (110)	1991	11	Dislocation	102	91	Only one case was unsatisfactory due to insufficient quadriceps rehabilitation.

Outcomes

The results of Insall's proximal realignment procedure have been reported in the literature (Table 40.3). Insall (61) reviewed his results for 75 knees at an average follow-up of 4 years. All patients had chronic symptoms that interfered with everyday activities, and all had failed extensive conservative measures. Forty patients had complaints of patellar pain, 29 had complaints of instability, and 6 had both. There was a 91% satisfactory rate, with better results correlating with improved centering of the patella postoperatively. No obvious correlation was made with the degree of chondromalacia found at surgery.

Scuderi et al. (62) described a satisfactory rate of 81% in 42 patients, with a redislocation rate of 1.7% (1 patient). Improved patellar centralization had a positive affect on the outcome, and better results were also obtained in males and younger patients. Abraham et al. (63) had a satisfactory rate of 62% in 76 patients, with better results obtained in knees with recurrent dislocations as compared with patellofemoral pain.

As is usually the case, appropriate patient selection is important for obtaining good results. The patient must understand their problem and must be well motivated for postoperative rehabilitation. The degree of patellofemoral arthritis is also important to determine because it can influence the surgical outcome.

Distal Realignment

Distal realignment procedures, including medialization and anteriorization of the tibial tubercle, play a major role in the treatment of patellar subluxation and dislocation. The indications typically include the presence of significant malalignment, patellar subluxation with or without dislocation, and varying degrees of patellar arthrosis. The following is a description of some of the more commonly used distal realignment procedures.

Procedures

Soft tissue realignments are typically performed on the skeletally immature patient. Various procedures have been described, including a combined lateral release with a medial soft tissue plication, semitendinosus tenodesis, and pes anserinus transfer. The Roux-Goldthwait procedure (Fig. 40.27) has remained popular over the years, first described by Roux in 1888 (64) and later by Goldthwait in 1895 (65).

The approach for the Roux-Goldthwait procedure has historically started with a transverse skin incision made between the inferior pole of the patella and the tibial tubercle. The skin flaps are mobilized proximally and distally to expose the tibial tubercle and the medial and lateral retinaculae. A lateral release is performed

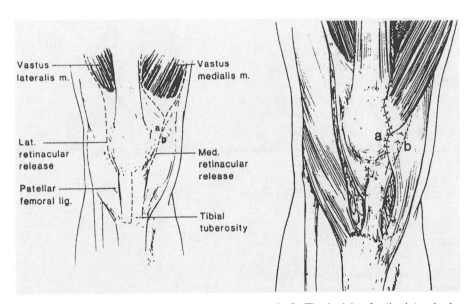

FIG. 40.27. The Roux-Goldthwait realignment procedure. **Left:** The incision for the lateral release and the medial plication. The patellar tendon is split longitudinally and the lateral half is released distally. **Right:** The completion of the realignment. The lateral half of the patellar tendon is advanced medially beneath the remaining tendon and sutured under a periosteal flap. The lateral release is completed, and the vastus medialis obliquus is advanced to the superomedial border of the patella. (From Fondren FB, Goldner JL, Bassett FH. Recurrent dislocation of the patella treated by the modified Roux-Goldthwait procedure. A perspective study in forty-seven knees. *J Bone Joint Surg Am* 1985;67A:993–1005, with permission.)

starting at the level of the tibial tubercle and extending proximally to the level of the vastus lateralis muscle (66).

A second incision is made in the medial retinaculum extending proximally to the musculotendinous junction of the VMO. The VMO is advanced and sutured to the superomedial margin of the patella after it is realigned and its medial edge depressed. This step is a modification of the original description. The retinacular flaps created are overlapped and sutured to properly align the patella (66).

The final step includes releasing the lateral half of the patellar tendon from the tibial tubercle, which is freed from the remaining tendon up to the level of the inferior patellar pole. The freed half is passed medially under the remaining tendon and sutured to a periosteal flap in the proximal medial tibia. Care again must be taken to ensure appropriate tension to realign and centralize the patella (66).

Common technical errors with the Roux-Goldthwait procedure include incomplete lateral release and/or insufficient transfer of the tendon, leading to recurrent dislocations. Medial overcorrection, although less common, may result from excessive overlap of the medial retinacular flaps and an excessive medial transfer of the tendon. Finally, distal advancement of the tendon may lead to increased patellar tilt and pressure in the lateral patellofemoral joint.

Patients were initially placed in a cylinder cast for 6 weeks followed by gentle flexion exercises. More recently, a cast or splint is used for 2 weeks followed by extension bracing with gentle assisted flexion exercises. Cautious extension exercises against gravity are implemented at 6 weeks, with heavy resistance avoided for a minimum of 3 months. The patient uses crutches with partial weight bearing for 4 to 6 weeks, slowly weaning off the crutches after this period.

Once skeletal maturity is reached, multiple procedures involving moving of the tibial tubercle have been performed. One of the earliest ones described is the Hauser procedure reported in 1938 (67). The Hauser repair also involves a complete lateral release with a medial capsular reefing. The entire patellar tendon with a block of tibial tubercle is transferred medially and posteriorly into a new bed cut in the tibia. It is held in place with a screw or staple (68) (Fig. 40.28).

The Hauser procedure has not enjoyed as successful a track record as some of the other realignment procedures. Some of the more common pitfalls include excessive distal and posterior displacement of the tuberosity leading to increasing compressive forces of the patellofemoral joint and potential patellar baha. Multiple authors have associated osteoarthritis of the joint with this procedure. Undercorrection of the malaligned patella is a frequent error leading to recurrent dislocations. Finally, overcorrection can also occur due to excessive medial displacement of the tuberosity. The Hauser pro-

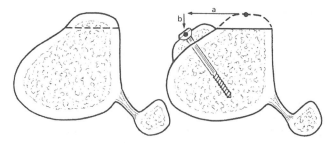

FIG. 40.28. Hauser procedure for transfer of the tibial tubercle. The tubercle is transferred medially and posteriorly due to the triangular shape of the proximal tibia. (From Insall JN, Windsor RE, Scott WN, et al. *Surgery of the knee.* New York: Churchill Livingstone, 1993:337, with permission.)

cedure is presently used infrequently due to its relatively poor long-term results.

The Elmslie-Trillat procedure (69) has been performed for patients with chronic subluxation and/or dislocation with minimal patellofemoral chondrosis. The technique involves a lateral release with a medial rotation of the tuberosity on a periosteal hinge (Fig. 40.29). The approach involves a curvilinear lateral parapatellar incision extending slightly distal to the tibial tubercle. A complete lateral release is then performed. A small osteotome is used to outline the tibial tubercle proximally and to cut the cortical bone along the borders of the patellar ligament distally. A curved osteotome is then placed under the patellar ligament proximally and driven distally 6 to 8 cm, creating a layer of bone that is 5 to 10 mm thick. The tubercle is not freed distally

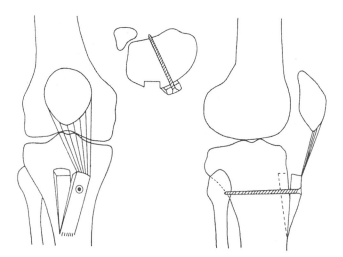

FIG. 40.29. Medial rotation of the tibial tubercle. An osteotomy is performed creating a long tuberosity shingle that is rotated medially and held in place with a bicortical screw. (From Miller BJ, LaRochelle PJ. The treatment of patellofemoral pain by combined rotation and elevation of the tibial tubercle. *J Bone Joint Surg Am* 1986;68A:419–423, with permission.)

but tapered to allow it to hinge as the proximal part is rotated medially. It is then fixed in a position that demonstrates the best patellar tracking without medial or lateral tethering during knee flexion.

The common technical errors are the same as with any tubercle transfer procedures. Over- or undercorrection of the patellar malalignment can lead to medial subluxation or recurrent dislocation, respectively.

The postoperative rehabilitation regimen includes isometric quadriceps exercises as soon as the patient is able. The leg is placed in a cast or a brace and the patient is allowed partial weight bearing with crutches. Full weight bearing is allowed in a cylinder cast at 2 weeks. The cast is removed by the fifth postoperative week, and full weight bearing is continued. Active and passive quadriceps exercises are started with a physiotherapist, with weight resistant exercises begun at 6 weeks (70).

Patients who demonstrate varying degrees of patellofemoral arthritis along with patellar malalignment require some form of anteriorization of the tibial tubercle and the distal realignment to reduce patellofemoral contact pressure. One of the more common procedures used today is anteromedialization (AMZ), described by Fulkerson (71) in 1983, and is used primarily when patellofemoral arthritis is present along with malalignment. The approach consists of a lateral incision starting at the level of the distal pole of the patella, midway between the tibial tuberosity and Gerdy's tubercle, and extending distally 10 to 12 cm to the anterior tibial ridge. A complete lateral release is then performed, extending through the vastus lateralis obliquus tendon without incising the main vastus lateralis tendon. Once the release is completed, the patella is lifted to examine the articular surface. The extent and pattern of the articular damage is important to note, which may also be corroborated with arthroscopic examination.

A drill guide (Depuy-Orthotech) is used just medial to the tibial tubercle to make parallel drill holes at an oblique angle aiming posterolaterally across the tibia. The obliquity of the angle is varied according to how much anteriorization and medialization is desired (Fig. 40.30). An osteotome or saw is used to connect the drill holes, adding an oblique cut from the proximal hole to a point just proximal to the lateral patellar tendon insertion. Care must be taken to fully complete the osteotomy proximally to avoid extension of the cut into the proximal tibial articular surface. The cut is completed distally to a level 5 to 8 cm distal to the tuberosity. The bony pedicle is then medialized until appropriate patellofemoral alignment is obtained with knee flexion and extension and anteriorized according to the obliquity of the osteotomy (71). Two cortical lag screws are used to fix the osteotomy.

Patients use a knee immobilizer and partially bear weight with crutches. Isometric quadriceps setting exer-

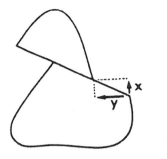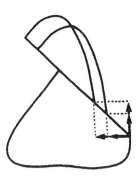

FIG. 40.30. Anteromedialization of the tibial tubercle. The relative amount of anteriorization and medialization depends on the obliquity of the osteotomy. (From Post WR, Fulkerson JP. Arthritis of the patellofemoral joint. In: Fu FH, Harner CD, Vince KG, eds. *Knee Surgery*. Baltimore: Williams & Wilkins, 1994:195–225, with permission.)

cises are started immediately. Weight bearing is increased as quadriceps strength is improved. The immobilizer is worn for 4 weeks during ambulation. Gentle active flexion exercises are started early as long as rigid fixation of the osteotomy is achieved. Resisted extension exercises are typically not used but may be started at 6 to 8 weeks postoperative when full healing of the osteotomy is demonstrated. These resistive exercises should be gentle to avoid a significant increase in the patellofemoral contact pressure.

A major pitfall of the AMZ procedure involves inappropriate "mapping" of the patellar articular degeneration. The procedure tends to load the proximal and medial region of the patella and requires a preserved articular surface in this area. An arthroscopy should always be performed before the procedure to examine the patellofemoral joint. Undercorrection of the malalignment, with associated patellar subluxation, may also occur. Finally, two bicortical screws are typically used to ensure rigid internal fixation. The two drill holes for the screws should not be placed in the same line to help avoid splitting the bony pedicle.

Outcomes

The surgical results for distal realignment procedures are better when there is minimal to no arthritis present. Early series on the Hauser procedure have shown success in preventing recurrent dislocations but poor outcomes with regards to patellofemoral symptoms. Barberi et al. (72) found that less than 50% of patients were free of pain at long-term follow-up after the Hauser procedure. Juliusson and Markhede (73) noted a 12% objective satisfactory rate in 40 patients who underwent this procedure. Goutallier and Debeyre (74) observed a detrimental biomechanical effect of a posteromedial transfer of the tibial tubercle, which may help explain the poor long-term results with the Hauser procedure.

The Goldthwait procedure (65) has also never gained widespread popularity because it pulls down on the lateral facet, which may adversely affect patellar contact pressures. The Elmslie-Trillat procedure (69) is preferred for distal realignment. Cox (75) reported that only 7% of his patients experienced subluxation after this procedure. Its benefit lies in the fact that it allows pure medial transfer of the tibial tubercle without posteriorization that can lead to increased patellofemoral contact pressures.

Buuck has reviewed the long-term result (average 8 years) of Fulkerson's anteromedial tibial tubercle transfers (15). The long-term satisfaction rate was 91% with poorer results in patients with worker's compensation and crush type injuries. Pidoriano also studied Fulkerson's results with respect to the severity and location of articular damage found at the time of operation (15). He found that patients with central or distal lesions and lateral facet pathology had better results than those with proximal damage. The Fulkerson AMZ procedure has become the treatment of choice by many surgeons for patients with malalignment and mild patellofemoral arthritis. The key to improving the results lies in the appropriate mapping of the articular damage to ensure the proper indications for the procedure.

PATELLOFEMORAL ARTHRITIS

History

Articular degeneration within the patellofemoral joint can result from inflammatory or mechanical insults. Acute high-energy trauma or chronic malalignment are the common mechanical causes for articular degeneration. Malalignment and recurrent instability lead to elevations in the joint contact forces, which has a deleterious effect on the joint surfaces. Determining whether there is a history of prior injury or instability is therefore important to help direct treatment. A patient with pain after blunt trauma has a different problem than one who has had an insidious onset of symptoms that have progressed without significant trauma.

Activity-related anterior knee pain is a common complaint in the presence of patellofemoral disorders. The typical aggravating activities include stair climbing, squatting, or prolonged sitting, which involve resisted knee extension or prolonged knee flexion. Constant pain not increased by activity is usually caused by nonmechanical or referred symptoms. Evidence of neuromas or hip and back problems should be sought.

Patellofemoral pain is often accompanied by instability. The instability may be secondary to malalignment or quadriceps muscle weakness. Instability leading to recurrent patellar dislocations can cause significant damage to the articular surface. Each event may cause compressive or shear trauma to the patella or femoral trochlea that can lead to significant degeneration. A careful history is necessary to reveal if instability exists so as to include surgical realignment in the treatment plan (76).

Chondromalacia Patellae

Traditionally, the term chondromalacia has been used to denote pathologic changes in the patellar articular surface. Various stages involving gross and microscopic findings have been described (77). Outerbridge classified chondromalacia into four different grades (78):

- Grade 1, Swelling and softening of the articular cartilage;
- Grade 2, Fragmentation and fissuring (less than one-half inch);
- Grade 3, Area greater than one-half inch;
- Grade 4, Cartilage erosion down to bone.

Closed chondromalacia shows a continuous articular surface and falls into grade 1. Open chondromalacia shows obvious fibrillations within the surface. Osteoarthritis, involving narrowing of the joint space, osteophyte formation, and subchondral sclerosis, is thought to be a different stage of the same process (23).

Localization of the chondromalacia is important to determine the pathophysiology and potential solutions of patellofemoral disorders. Lesions on the lateral patellar facet are often due to an imbalance of the "tension" in the medial and lateral retinacula. A tight lateral retinaculum that tilts the patella will adaptively shorten to perpetuate the increased lateral pressure. Pain may often be localized to the lateral retinaculum (79). Fulkerson et al. (22) demonstrated neuromatous degeneration of the small nerves within the lateral retinaculum of patients undergoing a lateral release. Hypertrophy of the lateral capsule and abnormal insertion of the iliotibial tract can also lead to lateral tilt or subluxation (36).

Chondromalacia of the central portion of the patella is often caused by an increase in the resultant of flexion due to excessive tension in the extensor mechanism. This may be related to excessive tightness in the soft tissue restraints of the extensor mechanism or other anatomic problems such as hypertrophy of the patella, hypoplasia of the tibial tubercle, and abnormal convexity of the trochlea (36).

Medial facet pathology has multiple etiologies, including excessive medial pressure and incongruity of the medial patellofemoral compartment. This may result from medial capsulitis, excessive genu varum, or rotational abnormalities (36). Medial facet chondromalacia may also be caused by its impingement on the lateral trochlea after repetitive relocations of a subluxating patella (16).

Direct trauma to the patella remains a significant cause of proximal pole chondromalacia. A direct blow, usually with the knee flexed, to the anterior knee can contuse the proximal patellar articular cartilage, ultimately leading to its degeneration. This has historically caused many cases of chondromalacia of the patella and must be kept in mind during the workup of patellofemoral disorders. Anteriorizing procedures can also actually shift contact pressure onto a proximal pole lesion.

Clinical Evaluation

A complete evaluation starts with observation of the lower extremity. Torsional deformities, foot pronation, angular knee deformities, and gait patterns should be noted. Patellar tracking and quadriceps muscle atrophy is evaluated. The quadriceps circumference is measured at a fixed distance from the superior pole of the patella and is compared with the contralateral side. The Q angle and tubercle sulcus angle is measured to determine any underlying predisposition to malalignment. The tubercle sulcus angle describes the position of the tibial tubercle with respect to the inferior pole of the patella with the knee at 90 degrees (80). Any evidence of a positive J sign is also noted. These observations will help one decide whether malalignment is a significant part of the underlying problem.

Provocative tests are useful to determine the origin of the symptoms. Direct compression of the patella while flexing the knee will typically produce pain in the presence of patellofemoral arthritis. Resisted isometric extension exercises will also produce pain in most patients. These maneuvers should be done at different flexion angles to help determine which region of the patellofemoral joint is involved.

It is important to determine whether the knee pain is originating from the parapatellar soft tissue or the joint surfaces. Fulkerson (19) described systematic palpation of the soft tissue around the knee. Structures that are palpated should be placed on stretch to avoid compression of underlying tissue. Special attention is paid to regions where there are points of intersection. Patients often have tenderness at the junction of the medial retinaculum with the patellar tendon and inferior pole of the patella. Direct palpation of the patellar facet may be performed by tilting the patella but is difficult due to the interposition of the retinaculum. Painful crepitus should be checked because it may signify a chondral flap or inflamed plica.

Lower extremity flexibility can significantly affect the patellofemoral joint. The quadriceps, hamstrings, iliotibial band, and gastrocnemius–soleus complex should all be examined for excessive tightness. A tight quadriceps can directly increase the forces within the patellofemoral joint. Hamstring tightness can cause a functional knee flexion contracture that can also increase these forces. A tight iliotibial band, through its attachments with the lateral retinaculum, can directly increase

the lateral joint forces with knee flexion. Finally, gastrocnemius–soleus muscle contracture can lead to excessive foot pronation and subsequent patellar malalignment. All these abnormalities may result in anterior knee pain and need to be evaluated to help direct treatment.

Radiographic Evaluation

Standard anteroposterior, lateral, and axial views are obtained for all patients with anterior knee pain. Degenerative arthritis of the tibiofemoral joint should be noted along with other associated abnormalities. Axial views may reveal asymmetry in the subchondral sclerosis of the patellar facets. Increased regions of local sclerosis may indicate unbalanced stress within the patellofemoral joint (76). Joint space narrowing may also be noted on the axial view as a result of articular degeneration.

Patellar malalignment can be measured with the Merchant's congruence angle and the Laurin's lateral patellofemoral angle. They denote lateral subluxation and tilt, respectively. CT has been used as well to determine these values because it can be performed at lower flexion angles and avoids the problem of bony overlap. Accurate measurements of patellar alignment is important to obtain whenever surgery is considered.

Bone scans are helpful in cases where the source of pain is unclear. Increased activity reflects a bony rather than a soft tissue problem. Increased blood flow or bone remodeling can result from various pathologic processes such as tumor, trauma, or metabolic diseases (76). The information obtained from a bone scan can confirm the presence of reflex sympathetic dystrophy in chronic cases of anterior knee pain (81).

Nonoperative Treatment

The treatment for patellofemoral arthritis should be geared toward decreasing the joint reaction forces within the patellofemoral joint. Avoiding activities that result in high joint reaction forces or prolonged knee flexion is recommended. Physical therapy is used to increase flexibility and balanced muscle strength. Tight structures such as the iliotibial band or lateral retinaculum are stretched. Prone stretching of the quadriceps will help reduce stiffness in the anterior knee structures. Strengthening exercises are important and should emphasize the quadriceps and VMO. Regaining appropriate strength will help improve the functional level of many patients. Isometric exercises in a nonpainful range of motion are performed to prevent worsening of symptoms. Taping or bracing may be of benefit to allow more aggressive rehabilitation with less pain. DeHaven et al. (82) showed an 82% success rate for nonoperative measures in a prospective study of 100 athletes with chondromalacia patellae. Only 8% of these patients required surgery, whereas two thirds were able to return to unrestricted activities.

The inflammatory component of the arthrosis can be treated with nonsteroidal anti-inflammatory medication. Aspirin has been frequently used as the medication of choice for patients with patellofemoral pain. Typically a dosage of 0.6 g four times a day has been used for severe pain. Besides its analgesic qualities, aspirin has been clinically shown to protect the articular cartilage after recurrent patellar dislocations and inhibit its degradation by cathepsin enzymes (83). However, it has not been shown to promote healing of the cartilage matrix in the presence of established defects (84). Other anti-inflammatory agents can be used in patients not tolerating aspirin. Intraarticular steroids have an adverse effect on articular cartilage and are not recommended (85).

Operative Treatment

Operative intervention for patellofemoral arthritis is performed only after an appropriate conservative regimen is completed. Multiple procedures have been developed to treat patellar arthrosis. These procedures are aimed at directly addressing the articular damage or improving alignment to relieve the excess stresses within the patellofemoral joint. The former category includes procedures such as patellar shaving, drilling, resurfacing, and abrasion of the subchondral bone. The latter includes realignment procedures aimed at stopping the underlying abnormality to slow the progression of degeneration. Proximal and distal realignment, tibial tubercle elevation, and lateral retinacular release are included in this group (7).

Realignment procedures are used in cases where chondromalacia or arthritis is considered as secondary to biomechanical abnormalities. Correcting these abnormalities can reduce the asymmetric and excessive loads on the patellofemoral joint.

The Maquet procedure as described in 1963 (28,86) is a direct anteriorization of the tibial tubercle (Fig. 40.31). In his study, Maquet discussed two means by which the patellofemoral contact forces decreased. An anteriorly displaced patellar tendon works at the end of a longer lever arm, thus increasing the efficiency of the quadriceps muscle. The muscle requires less effort to produce the same work, ultimately reducing the force transmitted by the patella to the femur. Also, the anterior displacement of the patellar tendon increases the angle formed by the vector of force of the quadriceps and patellar tendons. Widening this angle will also decrease the resultant force that represents patellofemoral compression. Maquet (28) used knee models to calculate that a 2-cm advancement of the patellar tendon reduces the compressive forces during weight bearing by 50%.

The approach of the Maquet technique includes an incision that is medial and parallel to the tibial crest

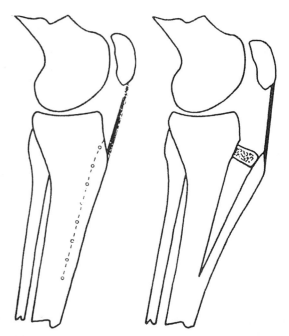

FIG. 40.31. Anteriorization of the tibial tubercle (Maquet procedure). The tuberosity is osteotomized creating a long shingle that is elevated and held in place with a piece of iliac crest bone graft. (From Maquet P. Advancement of the tibial tuberosity. *Clin Orthop* 1976;115:225–230, with permission.)

below the tuberosity. A Kirschner wire is used to drill parallel holes across the tibial crest, creating a wedge of bone 7 to 8 mm thick that includes the tubercle. This is continued distally, and an osteotome is used to create a shingling of the anterior tibial cortex ending 12 cm distal to the tubercle. The proximal margin, which includes the tuberosity and patellar tendon, is wedged open and held elevated by a piece of iliac crest bone graft. The remaining gap is filled in with more bone graft (28).

These patients do not require immobilization and immediately start active knee motion. They ambulate with support as soon as comfortable and discard the crutches after 2 weeks. Full range of motion is usually achieved by 3 months. One pitfall of the Maquet procedure comes from releasing the cortex at the distal extent of the osteotomy, thus destabilizing the osteotomy. Excessive anteriorization can also increase tension on the skin, leading to anterior skin slough.

The AMZ procedure as described by Fulkerson (71) in 1982 is used to manage patients with arthritis associated with malalignment. The outline of the procedure has been discussed earlier. Similar to the Maquet procedure, AMZ allows for varying degrees of anteriorization of the tibial tubercle. At the same time, the patellar tracking may be improved with medialization. The relative amount of medialization versus anteriorization depends on the obliquity of the osteotomy and can be varied according to the major underlying abnormality.

Arthroscopic mapping of the articular degeneration is done first to make sure that the appropriate indications are met to improve outcomes. The proximal medial surface of the patella should be free from significant degeneration because this area receives increased loads after surgery.

Excessive pressure on the lateral patellar facet may lead to articular degeneration in this region. A shortened tight lateral retinaculum creates lateral tilt of the patella that leads to excessive lateral pressure. A complete lateral retinacular release should relieve the tethering of the patella and decrease the pressure on the lateral facet. Fulkerson et al. (87) showed with CT studies an improvement of the lateral tilt after retinacular release. The increased strain in the lateral retinaculum has also been shown to lead to neuromatous degeneration of the small nerves within the tissue (22). A complete release will often treat the soft tissue pain that is frequently present in patients with anterior knee pain.

Abrasion arthroplasty has been frequently used to treat damaged articular cartilage. Injured articular cartilage heals with fibrocartilage, which has inferior mechanical properties compared with hyaline cartilage. Debridement of diseased cartilage down to subchondral bone can induce the formation of the fibrocartilage. Superficial debridement will not result in this same healing response. However, it still may be of benefit because it removes loose flaps of cartilage and debris that cause inflammation within the joint. Despite its inferior properties, fibrocartilage still may represent an improvement in regions where hyaline cartilage is absent or fibrillated (76).

Ficat et al. (88) described spongialization as a treatment for diseased patellae. The procedure is essentially an extension of the commonly performed abrasion arthroplasty. The abrasion is usually carried down to the subchondral plate to allow fibrocartilage regeneration. With spongialization, the entire region of diseased cartilage is resected, including the subchondral bone, to leave an exposed bed of cancellous bone. Ficat et al. explained that the subchondral bone is removed because it is often abnormal and a source of pain in these cases. The regenerated tissue comes from the underlying marrow of the cancellous bone.

Cases of severe patellofemoral arthritis often require resection arthroplasty or patellar resurfacing. The importance of the patella for the function of the extensor mechanism has been explained in the biomechanical section. Studies have shown a decrease in quadriceps strength after patellectomy (89). Resection arthroplasty has been performed less frequently recently and is saved for patients who have failed all other treatment options and continue to have disabling pain.

The use of the patellar prosthesis was first reported in 1955 by McKeever (90). The purpose of patellar resurfacing is to treat significantly diseased articular carti-lage without losing the quadriceps mechanical lever arm. The typical prosthesis is a cobalt–chromium alloy that approximates the anatomic shape of the normal patella (Fig. 40.32). This shape allows improved tracking and decreased liklihood of dislocation (91).

A midline or medial parapatellar incision is used to expose the patella. A medial arthrotomy is performed to allow inspection of the patellar articular surface. The greatest thickness of the patella is determined in the region of the ridge between the medial and lateral facets. An oscillating saw is then used to remove the articular surface of the patella. The amount of surface removed should approximate the thickness of the prosthesis, taking into account the fact that the patella may be thinner than normal secondary to articular degeneration. A template is used to mark the cut surface for the anchoring system of the particular prosthesis being used. Trial prostheses are used to ensure appropriate tracking of the patella, and the patellar prosthesis is then cemented in place. The thickness of the patella at this point should be within 1 to 2 mm of the original size (91).

Patellar hemiarthroplasty has not gained widespread acceptance, and patellectomy is still used for severe patellofemoral arthritis. A wide variety of techniques has been used to remove the patella. A midline incision is made to expose the patella, and then the patella is removed through either a longitudinal incision through

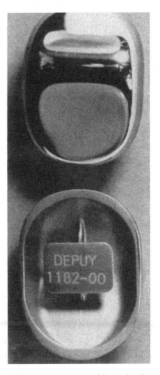

FIG. 40.32. Patellar prosthesis with articular surface on the left and anchoring surface on the right. (From Worrell RV. Prosthetic resurfacing of the patella. *Clin Orthop* 1979;144:92, with permission.)

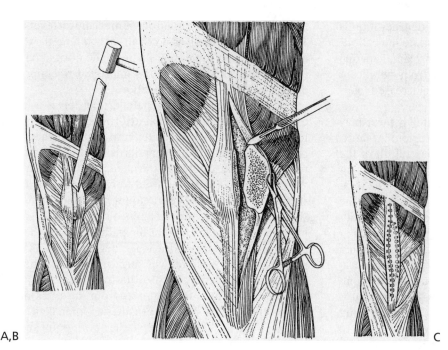

A,B

C

FIG. 40.33. Boyd and Hawkins technique for patellectomy. A longitudinal incision is made down the central portion of the quadriceps tendon, over the center of the patella, and down the center of the patellar tendon. The patella is split in half and carefully freed from the overlying quadriceps expansion. The wound is closed by imbricating one side over the other. (From Fulkerson JP. *Disorders of the patellofemoral joint.* Baltimore: Williams & Wilkins, 1997:325, with permission.)

the extensor mechanism or a transverse incision. Care is taken to preserve the integrity of the tissue that is elevated off the patella to allow secure closure. Kaufer (12) recommended a transverse incision and repair for patellectomy. He showed that less force was required to extend the knee after a transverse repair when compared with a longitudinal one. The flaps may also be imbricated, which can affect the transmission of tensile forces to the tibia during active knee extension.

Boyd and Hawkins (92) described using a longitudinal incision through the extensor mechanism for excision of the patella (Fig. 40.33). The incision is extended into the quadriceps and patellar tendons, and the patella is divided in half before excision. Each half of the patella is removed with care to preserve the fibers for later closure. The longitudinal split in the extensor mechanism is then closed after imbricating the two sides. The knee is flexed to 90 degrees to ensure that the repair is stable. This is the approach recommended by the senior author (J.P.F.).

Compere et al. (93) described a procedure that removes the patella and creates a tube that will support any regenerated bone (Fig. 40.34). Reports suggesting that calcification can cause pain after patellectomy have led to the development of this technique. A medial and lateral parapatellar incision is made, and the patella is removed without disruption of the dorsal fibers of the quadriceps expansion. The medial border of the fibers is then brought underneath and sutured to the lateral border, creating a "tube." The vastus medialis is then advanced laterally and distally and sutured to the created tube. Regardless of the technique used, careful

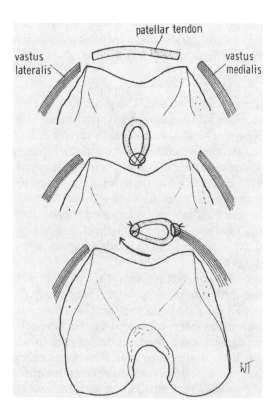

FIG. 40.34. Compere's technique for patellectomy with creation of a tube to contain any bone regeneration. (From Kelly MA, Insall JN. Patellectomy. *Orthop Clin North Am* 1986; 17:291, with permission.)

attention must be paid to ensure a secure closure and appropriate tracking with knee flexion.

Outcomes

The key to successful outcome after surgery for patellofemoral arthritis lies in correctly diagnosing the underlying cause of the articular degeneration. Any associated malalignment should be corrected during surgery to improve articular congruency. One common finding, however, is that severe arthritis decreases the liklihood of success with simple realignment procedures.

The lateral retinacular release has been the treatment of choice for patients with anterior knee pain associated with lateral patellar tilt. The degree of articular degeneration has shown a correlation to success rates in many studies. Osborne and Fulford (94) showed poor long-term results in patients with grade 3 or 4 Outerbridge changes. Christensen et al. (95) revealed a success rate of only 17% at long-term follow-up for similar patients. More recently, Shea and Fulkerson (96) reported 92% success rate for lateral release with patellar tilt and minimal articular degeneration, with only 22% success in the presence of grade 3 or 4 Outerbridge changes. Determining the extent of articular damage can therefore have a significant effect on results after lateral retinacular release.

Anteriorization is performed to relieve some of the pressure within the patellofemoral joint. Maquet (28) reported a satisfactory rate of 97% after 4.7 years in 37 patients undergoing his procedure. He advanced the tuberosity 2 to 3 cm and had one patient develop skin necrosis. Ferguson (97) elevated the tubercle only 1.25 cm and noted a success rate after 2 years of 86%. The success rate was 92% in patients whose primary diagnosis was osteoarthrosis. In general, the best reported results have been in knees with osteoarthrosis and minimal malalignment. The amount of elevation necessary has not been clearly defined, but more elevation may be required in the face of more severe degeneration.

Patients with malalignment associated with chondromalacia require realignment and tubercle elevation. Fulkerson et al. (98) reported a success rate after 2 years of 89% in patients undergoing AMZ for severe patellofemoral arthritis. No patients had excellent results, however, in this series. The average tubercle elevation was 10.6 mm. Morshuis et al. (99) reported satisfactory results in 70% of their patients undergoing the AMZ for patellofemoral pain. The results were better in those with less severe arthritis. Fulkerson (98) later determined better results for patients who had sparing of the proximal medial articular surface with distal central or lateral lesions.

Abrasion arthroplasty, drilling, and spongialization have had varying degrees of success in the treatment of patellofemoral arthritis. The goal of shaving is to remove any loose pieces of cartilage that may irritate the joint. The results of shaving alone have not been shown to be uniformly satisfactory in the literature. Bentley (100) compared his results of four different procedures for chondromalacia and found the worst results with shaving alone (25% satisfactory rate). The other procedures included patellectomy, distal realignment with lateral release, and cartilage excision with drilling of subchondral bone. Patellar abrasion alone provides poor outcomes in the presence of malalignment and should be an adjunct to realignment procedures. It has been shown to provide relief when loose flaps of cartilage are discovered and removed.

The outcomes after drilling or spongialization have also been unpredictable. They are typically used with advanced chondromalacia to expose the subchondral bone and allow for fibrocartilage ingrowth. Ficat et al. (88) reported a satisfactory rate of 79% after spongialization in 85 patients. The average follow-up was 6 months to 3 years. Bentley (100) reported only 35% satisfactory rate after 7 years in 20 patients undergoing cartilage excision and drilling. The outcome after these procedures have been inconsistent, and they may be better suited as adjuncts to tubercle elevation or realignment procedures.

Patellar resurfacing procedures and patellectomies are considered salvage procedures for end-stage arthritis of the patellofemoral joint. The advantage of resurfacing over patellectomy is that the lever arm of the quadriceps mechanism is preserved. De Palma et al. (101) reported good to excellent results in 15 of 17 patients using the McKeever prosthesis. Longer follow-up of these patients, however, revealed a decline in the satisfaction rate. Insall et al. (4) used a different prosthesis with a dome shape to its articulating facet for 29 patients and noted good to excellent results in 16 knees with poor results in 10 knees. Worse outcomes have been shown in the presence of tibiofemoral arthritis and persistent malalignment.

Patellectomy is considered as the last resort for patients with severe patellofemoral arthritis. The outcome for 100 patients from the Hospital for Special Surgery (102) at an average follow-up of 5 years was reviewed for patients over and under 40 years old. Good or excellent results were noted in 76% of the younger patients and 71% of the older patients. Arthritis of the tibiofemoral joint has been associated with worse results. There is also a trend toward better results for patients with comminuted fractures or severe arthrosis confined to the patellofemoral joint. Despite many reports of good results after patellectomy, the patella should be preserved whenever possible. It should be performed in the presence of severe patellofemoral arthritis without maltracking or when realignment procedures have failed. Another indication is the severe comminuted patella fracture where adequate reduction cannot be obtained.

TABLE 40.4. *Indications for operative treatment for patellofemoral pain*

Lateral release
  Consistent tenderness and tightness in the lateral retinaculum, usually associated with patellar tilt or subluxation.
  Painful arthrosis in the patellofemoral joint with radiographically documented lateral patellar tilt and minimal or no subluxation.
  In association with a realignment procedure of the patella for chronic subluxation or dislocation.
Soft tissue realignment
  Skeletally immature with a history of recurrent patellar dislocation.
  Realignment of the patella without diminishing overall patellar contact stress (minimal or no arthrosis).
Medial tibial tubercle transfer
  Skeletally mature patient with chronic subluxation/dislocation and minimal chondrosis.
Anterior tibial tubercle elevation
  Skeletally mature patient with distal patella chondrosis and little or no malalignment present.
Anteromedial tibial tubercle transfer (closed epiphysis a prerequisite)
  Persistent patellofemoral pain related to malalignment with excessive patellar tilt or elevated congruence angle, with a need for relief of patellar contact stress due to distal and/or lateral patellar arthrosis.
  Lateral facet arthrosis and elevated quadriceps angle > 22 degrees (patella centered in the trochlea).
  Failed lateral release without evidence of lateral retinacular reattachment and with significant residual lateral tilt.
Patellar resurfacing
  Severe patellofemoral arthritis without malalignment that has not responded to all other treatment modalities.
Patellectomy
  Salvage procedure for cases of unreducible comminuted patella fractures.
  Severe arthritis without malalignment that has failed all other treatment methods.

SUMMARY

Most patients with injuries to the patellofemoral joint fortunately improve with conservative measures. However, a subset of patients requires surgical intervention. It is important to rule out other causes of knee pain first and then determine the precise etiology to choose the appropriate surgical option (60). Table 40.4 can be used when planning operative treatment for patellofemoral pain (60). Despite the tremendous advancements made in the treatment options for patellofemoral joint injuries, it remains one of the more challenging areas to treat in orthopaedics.

REFERENCES

1. Johnson EE. *Fractures of the patella. Rockwood and Green's fractures in adults,* 3rd ed. Philadelphia: Lippincott Williams & Wilkins 1991:1762.
2. Goss CM, ed. *Gray's anatomy of the human body,* 28th ed. Philadelphia: Lea and Febiger, 1966.
3. Fulkerson JP, Gossling HR. Anatomy of the knee joint lateral retinaculum. *Clin Orthop* 1980;153:183–188.
4. Insall JN, Windsor RE, Scott WN, et al. *Surgery of the knee,* 2nd ed. New York: Churchill Livingstone, 1993:241–385.
5. Reider B, Marshall JL, Koslin B, et al. The anterior aspect of the knee joint—an anatomical study. *J Bone Joint Surg Am* 1981;63A:351–356.
6. Hallisey M, Doherty N, Bennet W, et al. Anatomy of the junction of the vastus lateralis tendon and the patella. *J Bone Joint Surg Am* 1987;69A:545–549.
7. Goodfellow J, Hungerford DS, Zindel M. Patellofemoral joint mechanics and pathology. 1. Functional anatomy of the patellofemoral joint. *J Bone Joint Surg Br* 1976;58B:287.
8. Insall JN. Intra-articular surgery for degenerative arthritis of the knee. A report of the work of the late K.H. Pridie. *J Bone Joint Surg Br* 1967;49B:211–228.
9. Steurer PA, Gradisar IA, Hoyt WA, et al. Patellectomy: a clinical study and biomechanical evaluation. *J Bone Joint Surg Am* 1976;58A:736.
10. Sutton FS, Thompson CH, Lipke J, et al. The effect of patellectomy on knee function. *J Bone Joint Surg Am* 1976;58A:537–540.
11. Frankel VH, Burstein AH. Orthopaedic biomechanics. Philadelphia: Lea and Febiger, 1970.
12. Kaufer H. Mechanical function of the patella. *J Bone Joint Surg Am* 1971;53A:1551–1560.
13. Kaufer H. Patellar biomechanics. *Clin Orthop* 1979;144:51–54.
14. Reilly DT, Martens M. Experimental analysis of the quadriceps muscle force and patellofemoral joint reaction force for various activities. *Acta Orthop Scand* 1972;43:126.
15. Fulkerson JP. *Disorders of the patellofemoral joint.* Baltimore: Williams & Wilkins, 1997.
16. Fulkerson JP, Shea KP. Current concepts review: disorders of patellofemoral alignment. *J Bone Joint Surg Am* 1990;72A:1424–1429.
17. Tiberio D. The effect of excessive subtalar joint pronation on patellofemoral mechanics: a theoretical model. *JOSPT* 1987;:160–165.
18. Aglietti P, Insall JH, Cerulli G. Patellar pain and incongruence. *Clin Orthop* 1983;122:217–224.
19. Fulkerson JP. Awareness of the retinaculum in evaluating patellofemoral pain. *Am J Sports Med* 1982;10:147–149.
20. Fulkerson JP, Hungerford DS. *Disorders of the patellofemoral joint.* Baltimore: Williams & Wilkins, 1990.
21. Kasim NQ, Fulkerson JP. Resection of clinically localized segments of painful retinaculum as the treatment of selected patients with anterior knee pain. AANA, San Diego, CA, April 1997.
22. Fulkerson JP, Tennant R, Jaivin J, et al. Histologic evidence of retinacular nerve injury associated with patellofemoral malalignment. *Clin Orthop* 1985;197:196.
23. Insall JN, Falvo KA, Wise DW. Chondromalacia patellae: a prospective study. *J Bone Joint Surg Am* 1976;58A:1–8.
24. Spencer JD, Hayes KC, Alexander IJ. Knee joint effusion and quadriceps inhibition in man. *Arch Phys Med Rehabil* 1984;65:171–177.
25. Insall JN, Goldberg W, Salvati E. Recurrent dislocation of the high-riding patella. *Clin Orthop* 1972;88:67.
26. Caton J, Deschamps G, Chambat P, et al. Les rotules basses. A propos de 128 observations. *Rev Chir Orthop* 1982;68:317–325.
27. Maldague B, Malghem J. Imagerie du Genou en 1987. In: *Cahiers d*Enseignement de la SO.F.C.O.T.* Paris: Expansion Scietifique Francaise, 1987:347–370.
28. Maquet P. Advancement of the tibial tuberosity. *Clin Orthop* 1976;115:225–230.
29. Laurin CA, Dussault R, Levesque HP. The tangential x-ray investigation of the patellofemoral joint: x-ray technique, diagnostic criteria and their interpretation. *Clin Orthop* 1979;144:16–26.
30. Merchant AC, Mercer RL, Jacobsen RH, et al. Roentgenographic analysis of patellofemoral congruence. *J Bone Joint Surg Am* 1974;56A:1391–1396.
31. Aglietti P, Insall JN, Cerulli G. Patellar pain and incongruence. I. Measurements of incongruence. *Clin Orthop* 1983;176:217–224.

32. Malghem J, Maldague B. Patellofemoral joint: 30 degree axial radiograph with lateral rotation of the leg. *Radiology* 1989; 170:566–657.

33. Schutzer SF, Ramsby GR, Fulkerson JP. Computed tomographic classification of patellofemoral pain patients. *Orthop Clin North Am* 1986;17:235–248.

34. Boven F, Bellemans M, Geurts J, et al. A comparative study of the patellofemoral joint on axial roentgenogram, axial arthrogram, and computed tomography following arthrography. *Skeletal Radiol* 1982;8:179–181.

35. Smillie IS. *Injuries of the knee joint.* Baltimore: Williams & Wilkins, 1962.

36. Ficat RP, Philippe J, Hungerford DS. Chondromalacia patellae: a system of classification. *Clin Orthop* 1979;144:55–62.

37. Fulkerson JP. The etiology of patellofemoral pain in young active patients: a prospective study. *Clin Orthop* 1983;179:129.

38. Fulkerson JP, Kalenak A, Rosenberg T, et al. Patellofemoral pain. *AAOS Instruct Course Lecture* 1992;XLI.

39. Kaufman KR, An K, Litchy WJ, et al. Dynamic joint forces during knee isokinetic exercises. *Am J Sports Med* 1991;19: 305–316.

40. Whitelaw GP, Rulla DJ, Markowitz HD, et al. A conservative approach to anterior knee pain. *Clin Orthop* 1989;246:234–237.

41. Gecha SR, Torg JS. Clinical prognosticators for the efficacy of retinacular release surgery to treat patellofemoral pain. *Clin Orthop* 1990;253:203–208.

42. Brattstrom H. Shape of the intercondylar groove normally and in recurrent dislocation of the patella. *Acta Orthop Scand* 1964;68[Suppl]:134–148.

43. Ashtrom JP. Osteochondral fracture in the knee joint associated with hypermobility and dislocation of the patella: report of eighteen cases. *J Bone Joint Surg Am* 1965;47A:1491.

44. Larsen E, Lauridsen F. Conservative treatment of patellar dislocations. *Clin Orthop* 1982;171:131–136.

45. Hawkins R, Bell R, Anisette G. Acute patellar dislocations. The natural history. *Am J Sports Med* 1986;14:117–120.

46. Cofield R, Bryan R. Acute dislocation of the patella: results of conservative treatment. *J Trauma* 1977;17:526–531.

47. Cash JD, Hughston JC. Treatment of acute patellar dislocation. *Am J Sports Med* 1988;16:244–249.

48. Ficat P. *Pathologie femeoro-patellaire.* Paris: Masson et Cie, 1970.

49. Baum C, Bensahal H. Luxation recidivante de la rotule chez l'enfant. *Rev Chir Orthop* 1973;59:583–592.

50. Crosby EB, Insall J. Recurrent dislocation of the patella. *J Bone Joint Surg Am* 1976;58A:9–13.

51. Macnab I. Recurrent dislocation of the patella. *J Bone Joint Surg Am* 1952;34A:957–976.

52. Insall JN. "Chondromalacia patellae." Patellar malalignment syndrome. *Orthop Clin North Am* 1979;10:117–127.

53. Fairbank HAT. Internal derangement of the knee in children. *Proc R Soc* 1937;3:11.

54. Mariani PP, Caruso C. An electromyographic investigation of subluxation of the patella. *J Bone Joint Surg Br* 1979;61B: 169–171.

55. Runow A. The dislocating patella: etiology and prognosis in relation to generalized joint laxity and anatomy of the patellar articulation. *Acta Orthop Scand* 1983;54[Suppl]:201.

56. Levine J, Splain SH. Use of infrapatellar strap in the treatment of patellofemoral pain. *Clin Orthop* 1979;139:179–181.

57. Palumbo PM. Dynamic patellar brace: a new orthosis in the management of patellofemoral disorders. *Am J Sports Med* 1981;9:45–49.

58. McConnell JS. The management of chondromalacia patellae: a long-term solution. *Aust J Physiother* 1986;32:215–223.

59. Larsen B, Andreasen E, Urfer A, et al. Patellar taping: a radiographic examination of the medial glide technique. *Am J Sports Med* 1995;23:465–471.

60. Fulkerson JP, Schutzer SF. After failure of conservative treatment for painful patellofemoral malalignment: lateral release or realignment? *Orthop Clin North Am* 1986;17:283–288.

61. Insall JN. Disorders of the patella. In: *Surgery of the knee.* New York: Churchill Livingstone, 1984:191.

62. Scuderi G, Cuomo F, Scott NW. Lateral release and proximal realignment for patellar subluxation and dislocation: a long-term follow-up. *J Bone Joint Surg Am* 1988;70A:856–861.

63. Aglietti P, Pisaneschi A, De Biase P. Lussazione recidivante di rotula: tre tipi di trattamento chirurgico. *G Ital Orthop Traumat* 1992;XIII:25.

64. Roux C. Luxation habituelle de la rotule: traitement operatoire. *Rev Chir Paris* 1888;8:682.

65. Goldthwait JE. Dislocation of the patella. *Trans Am Orthop Assoc* 1895;8:237.

66. Fondren FB, Goldner JL, Bassett FH. Recurrent dislocation of the patella treated by the modified Roux-Goldthwait procedure. A prospective study of forty-seven knees. *J Bone Joint Surg Am* 1985;67A:993–1005.

67. Hauser EDW. Total tendon transplant for slipping patella. *Surg Gynecol Obstet* 1938;66:199.

68. Chrisman OD, Snook GA, Wilson TC. A long-term prospective study of the Hauser and Roux-Goldthwait procedures for recurrent patellar dislocation. *Clin Orthop* 1979;144:27–30.

69. Trillat A, Dejour H, Couette A. Diagnostic et traitement des subluxations recidivantes de la rotule. *Rev Chir Orthop* 1964; 50:813–824.

70. Miller BJ, LaRochelle PJ. The treatment of patellofemoral pain by combined rotation and elevation of the tibial tubercle. *J Bone Joint Surg Am* 1986;68A:419–423.

71. Fulkerson JP. Anteromedialization of the tibial tuberosity for patellofemoral malalignment. *Clin Orthop* 1983;177:176–181.

72. Barbari S, Raugstad TS, Lichtenberg N, et al. The Hauser operation for patellar dislocation: 3–32 year results in 63 knees. *Acta Orthop Scand* 1990;61:32–35.

73. Juliusson R, Markhede G. A modified Hauser procedure for recurrent dislocation of the patella. A long-term follow-up study with special reference to osteoarthritis. *Arch Orthop Trauma Surg* 1984;103:42–46.

74. Goutallier D, Debeyre J. Le recentrage rotulien dans les arthroses femero-patellaires lateralisees. *Rev Chir Orthop* 1974;60: 377–386.

75. Cox JS. Evaluation of the Roux-Elmslie-Trillat procedure for knee extensor realignment. *Am J Sports Med* 1982;10:303–310.

76. Post WR, Fulkerson JP. Arthritis of the patellofemoral joint. In: Fu FH, Harner CD, Vince KG, eds. *Knee surgery.* Baltimore: Williams & Wilkins, 1994:195–225.

77. Wiles P, Andrews PS, Bremner RA. Chondromalacia of the patella. A study of later results of excision of articular cartilage. *J Bone Joint Surg Br* 1960;42B:65–70.

78. Outerbridge RE. The etiology of chondromalacia patellae. *J Bone Joint Surg Br* 1961;43B:752.

79. Fulkerson JP, Shea KP. Mechanical basis for patellofemoral pain and cartilage breakdown. In: Ewing JW, ed. *Articular cartilage and knee joint function: basic science and arthroscopy.* New York: Raven Press, 1990:93–101.

80. Kolowich PA, Paulos LE, Rosenberg TD, et al. Lateral release of the patella: indications and contraindications. *Am J Sports Med* 1990;18:359–365.

81. MacKinnon S, Holder L. The use of three phase radionuclide bone scanning in the diagnosis of RSD. *J Hand Surg* 1984;9A: 556–563.

82. DeHaven DE, Dolan WA, Mayer PJ. Chondromalacia patellae in athletes. Clinical presentation and conservative management. *Am J Sports Med* 1979;7:5–11.

83. Chrisman OD, Snook GA, Wilson TC. The protective effect of aspirin against degradation of human articular cartilage. *Clin Orthop* 1972;84:193–196.

84. Chrisman OD. Symposium: early degenerative arthritis of the knee. *J Bone Joint Surg Am* 1969;51A:1027.

85. Roach JE, Tomblin W, Eyring EJ. Comparison of the effects of steroid, aspirin and sodium salicylate on articular cartilage. *Clin Orthop* 1975;106:350–356.

86. Maquet P. Consideration biomechanique sur l'arthrose du genou. Un traitement biomechanique de l'arthrose femoropatellaire. L'advancement du tendon rotulien. *Rev Rheum* 1963; 30:779.

87. Fulkerson JP, Schutzer SF, Ramsby GR, et al. Computerized tomography of the patellofemoral joint before and after lateral release or realignment. *Arthroscopy* 1987;3:19–24.

88. Ficat RP, Ficat C, Gedeon P, et al. Spongialization: a new treatment for diseased patellae. *Clin Orthop* 1979;144:74–83.
89. Watkins MP, Harris BA, Wender S, et al. Effect of patellectomy on the function of the quadriceps and hamstrings. *J Bone Joint Surg Am* 1983;65A:390–395.
90. McKeever DC. Patellar prosthesis. *J Bone Joint Surg Am* 1955; 37A:1074–1084.
91. Worrell RV. Prosthetic resurfacing of the patella. *Clin Orthop* 1979;144:91.
92. Boyd HB, Hawkins BL. Patellectomy: a simplified technique. *Surg Gynecol Obstet* 1948;86:357.
93. Compere CL, Hill JA, Levinnek GE, et al. A new method of patellectomy for patellofemoral arthritis. *J Bone Joint Surg Am* 1979;61A:714–718.
94. Osborne AH, Fulford PC. Lateral release for chondromalacia patellae. *J Bone Joint Surg Br* 1982;64B:202–205.
95. Christensen F, Soballe K, Snerum L. Treatment of chondromalacia patellae by lateral retinacular release of the patella. *Clin Orthop* 1988;234:145.
96. Shea KP, Fulkerson JP. Preoperative computed tomography scanning and arthroscopy in predicting outcome after lateral retinacular release. *Arthroscopy* 1992;8:327–334.
97. Ferguson AB. Elevation of the insertion of the patellar ligament for patellofemoral pain. *J Bone Joint Surg Am* 1982;64A: 766–771.
98. Fulkerson JP, Becker GJ, Meaney JA, et al. Anteromedial tibial tubercle transfer without bone graft. *Am J Sports Med* 1990;18: 490–496.
99. Morshuis WJ, Pavlov PW, DeRooy KP. Anteromedialization of the tibial tuberosity in the treatment of patellofemoral pain and malalignment. *Clin Orthop* 1990;255:242–250.
100. Bentley G. The surgical treatment of chondromalacia patellae. *J Bone Joint Surg Br* 1978;60B:74–81.
101. De Palma AF, Sawier B, Hoffman JD. Reconsideration of lesions affecting the patellofemoral joint. *Clin Orthop* 1960;18:63.
102. Kelley MA, Insall JN. Patellectomy. *Orthop Clin North Am* 1986;17:289.
103. McManus F, Rang M, Heslin DJ. Acute dislocation of the patella in children: the natural history. *Clin Orthop* 1979;139;88.
104. Boring TH, O'Donoghue DH. Acute patellar dislocation: results of immediate surgery repair. *Clin Orthop* 1978;136;182.
105. Jensen CM, Roosen JV. Acute traumatic dislocation of the patella. *J Trauma* 1985;25(2);160.
106. Dainer RD, Barrack RL, Buckley SL, et al. Arthroscopic treatment of acute patellar dislocation. *Arthroscopy* 1988;4 (4);267.
107. Vainionpaa S, Laasonen E, Silvennoinen T, et al. Acute dislocation of the patella: a prospective review of operative treatment. *J Bone Joint Surg [Br]* 1990;72B;366.
108. Insall JN, Aglietti, P, Tria AJ. Patellar pain and incongruence. II. Clinical application. *Clin Orthop* 1983:176;225.
109. Abraham E, Washington E, Huang TL. Insall proximal realignment for disorders of the patella. *Clin Orthop* 1989:248;61.
110. Aglietti P, Pisaneschi A, De Biase P. Lussazione recidivante di rotula: tre tipi di trattamento chirurgico. *Cr Ital Ortop Traumat* 1992:XIII(1);25.

Principles and Practice of Orthopaedic Sports Medicine,
edited by William E. Garrett, Jr., Kevin P. Speer, and Donald T. Kirkendall.
Lippincott Williams & Wilkins, Philadelphia © 2000.

CHAPTER 41

Treatment of Anterior Cruciate Ligament Injuries

K. Donald Shelbourne and Douglas A. Foulk

The anterior cruciate ligament (ACL) has become the most extensively studied ligament in the body. Since 1980 and the birth of the ACL Study Group, more than 1,000 basic science and clinical studies have been published describing the anatomy, biomechanical properties, mechanism of injury, diagnosis, and treatment of the ACL. Reconstruction of the ACL after injury has become the preferred form of treatment despite an unclear understanding of the natural history of a knee without a functioning ACL. Rehabilitation after ACL reconstruction has changed dramatically in the past 10 years based primarily on clinical observations. Recent subjective and objective results after reconstruction far exceed those of the past. Unfortunately, we still do not know if restoring normal stability and full mobility changes the long-term destiny of this injury. Long-term follow-up studies of modern treatment hopefully will help to answer this question. In this chapter, we present what is currently known about ACL injuries and treatment. We also share our experience in treating over 5,000 ACL injuries in the past decade and a half at the Methodist Sports Medicine Center in Indianapolis, Indiana.

EPIDEMIOLOGY

Population-based studies in the United States and Denmark found injury rates of 0.30 and 0.38 per 1,000 people per year, respectively (1,2). Sports, including football, basketball, soccer, and skiing, account for most ACL injuries. Feagin et al. (3) estimated as many as 100,000

ACL injuries per year are the result of skiing accidents. Hewson et al. (4) estimated that a college football player, over a 4-year career, may have as high as a 16% chance of an ACL injury.

Many factors have been recognized that increase one's risk for ACL injury. Age appears to be one of those factors. Stanitski et al. (5) found that greater than 60% of children presenting with an acute hemarthrosis will have an ACL tear. Daniel et al. (6) found the incidence of ACL injury to be greater than twice the general population for those individuals 15 to 44 years of age. Miyaska et al. (1) and Nielsen et al. (2) found that within this age group, those younger than 19 years of age are at even greater risk. Historically, adolescent ACL injuries were believed to be rare, explained by the relative weakness of the physeal plate compared with the ligament. McCarroll et al. (7) and Lipscomb and Anderson (8) more recently reported that of the ACL-injured patients seen, the overall incidence of midsubstance ACL tears was 3% to 4% in the skeletally immature adolescent. Why we are seeing this injury more often now is unknown, but it probably can be attributed to an increase in sports participation within this age group and a greater awareness of and improved diagnostic techniques for all sports injuries in the younger athlete.

Overall, the absolute number of ACL injuries in men is greater than in women. Recently, however, great attention has been given to the relative increase in the number of female ACL injuries. Arendt and Dick (9) reviewed data gathered between 1989 and 1993 by the National Collegiate Athletic Association Injury Surveillance System. ACL injury rates in comparable men and women's sports, specifically soccer and basketball, were analyzed. Noncontact ACL tear rates for women were 2.5 and 4 times higher in those sports, respectively. High injury rates for women have been documented in other sports as well (10). The explanation for these observed

D. Shelbourne: Methodist Sports Medicine Center, Indianapolis, Indiana 46202.

D. A. Foulk: Department of Orthopaedics, University of Colorado Health Science Center, Denver, Colorado 80222.

differences is unknown, although many theories have been proposed, including muscle function and strength, sport-specific skill, anatomic differences, and hormones (11–14).

Recently, there has been great interest in the anatomy of the femoral intercondylar notch and its relationship to ACL injuries. A stenotic or narrowed notch has been suggested as increasing one's risk for ACL injury (15,16). Shelbourne et al. (17) found that, on average, women have narrower notch widths than men even when the men and women are of equal size. In addition, when men and women have equal size notch widths, their tear rates are equal. After ACL reconstruction, when the ligament (graft) size is the same (10 mm) in all patients, there does not appear to be a gender difference in graft tear rate.

MECHANISM OF INJURY AND PATHOANATOMY

The mechanisms by which the ACL can be injured are numerous. Sports that involve cutting, twisting, jumping, and landing in conjunction with velocity changes expose the ACL to injury. Noncontact mechanisms, when all high-risk sports are included, account for more ACL tears than those injuries that involve contact. Fetto and Marshall (18) described two basic mechanisms of injury: a valgus force applied, either with contact or more often with no contact, to a flexed knee with the leg in external rotation and hyperextension of the knee with the leg internally rotated. A more unusual mechanism most often seen in skiing is that of knee hyperflexion while attempting to prevent a fall backward. Paletta et al. (19) found that in alpine skiing, beginners typically injure the ACL by a valgus/external rotation (ski tip out) mechanism and those with more advanced skills by varus/internal rotation (ski tip in) or by a third mechanism, flexion with quadriceps loading.

Johnson et al. (20) analyzed thousands of ski-related ACL tears by history and video tape and described the "phantom foot" ACL injury. The tail of the downhill ski along with the high stiff-backed boot produces a lever that applies twisting and bending loads to the knee. A "boot-induced" ACL tear can also occur when a skier lands off balance after a jump. Pressure from the boot against the back of leg combined with quadriceps muscle contraction to keep the knee extended can produce an ACL injury.

When injury to the ACL occurs, more often than not it is isolated. Hirshman et al. (21) found that of 500 significant knee ligament injuries, 48% were isolated ACL tears. Thirteen percent of the injuries in this study were combined injuries to the ACL and medial collateral ligament (MCL). Other combinations occurred in 2% or less of the cases. O'Donoghue (22) described the "terrible triad" that involves injury to the ACL, MCL,

and medial meniscus. To the contrary, Shelbourne and Nitz (23) found that the lateral meniscus is more frequently damaged in combined ACL–MCL injuries, particularly when the MCL is partially torn. A complete discussion of combined ligament injuries and their management is covered elsewhere in this text.

Injury to the medial and/or lateral meniscus is common when the ACL is torn. We have found that the overall incidence of meniscal injury after an acute ACL tear is approximately 69% (Table 41.1). Acutely, lateral meniscus tears outnumber medial meniscus tears. Fortunately, many of these tears can heal or remain asymptomatic, particularly those that are lateral, peripheral, and posterior to the popliteus tendon (24). In the chronic ACL-deficient knee, medial meniscus tears are present more often, and overall, these tears tend to be more complex and less amenable to repair (25).

Occult injuries to the chondral and subchondral regions of the femur and tibia, though not historically recognized, have been given considerable attention since the advent of magnetic resonance imaging (MRI). Speer et al. (26) found that more than 90% of acute ACL-injured knees have femoral and/or tibial contusions present on MRI. These lesions are most often seen on the weight-bearing surface of the lateral femoral condyle and posterolateral tibial plateau and may represent a microfracture. Graf et al. (27) found that femoral lesions are usually in the middle third of the condyle and tibial lesions in the posterior third, demonstrating the degree of subluxation that occurs when the ACL is torn (Fig. 41.1). Correlation between the MRI findings and changes in the articular surface when examined arthroscopically was present in about two thirds of the cases. Some studies suggest that these lesions resolve quickly, within 6 to 10 weeks (27). Stein et al. (28) found that about one third of the lesions persisted 2 years after injury, particularly those within the lateral tibial plateau. At the present time, the prognosis of these injuries remains unknown.

In our experience, injury to the articular surface (grade III or IV) seen at arthroscopy is present in both acute and chronic ACL tears but is more common with

TABLE 41.1. *Injuries associated with ACL tears*

	ACL reconstructions	
	Chronic	Acute
Number of reconstructions	1,304 (56)	1,042 (44)
Neither menisci torn	204 (16)	314 (30)
Only lateral menisci torn	261 (20)	302 (29)
Only medial menisci torn	390 (30)	167 (16)
Both menisci torn	449 (34)	259 (25)
Grade III or IV chondromalacia	430 (33)	125 (12)

Values are number of instances, with percents in parentheses.
ACL, anterior cruciate ligament.

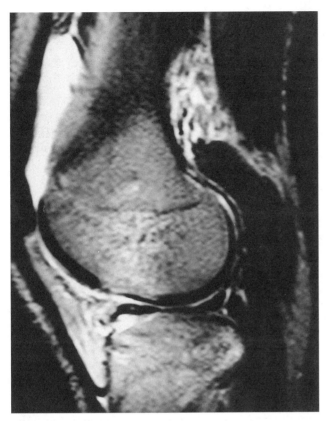

FIG. 41.1. Magnetic resonance imaging shows a bone bruise on the lateral femoral condyle and the posterior lateral tibial plateau.

chronic injuries (Table 41.1). Lateral femoral and tibial damage again appears most frequently. At the present time, no one knows the long-term impact these injuries will have on knee function, although it is logical to believe that they do contribute to earlier degeneration even if knee stability has been restored.

CLINICAL EVALUATION

Evaluation of all musculoskeletal injuries, including an athletic knee injury, begins by obtaining a good history. This includes not only the events surrounding the injury, but information such as the athlete's year in school, sport and position played, other sports played, and future athletic plans. Knowing as much about the athlete as possible will facilitate making treatment decisions.

Injury to ACL in most situations is a major traumatic event with a characteristic history. The athlete will usually describe the knee as "coming apart." An audible "pop" heard or felt by the athlete will occur in 35% to 65% of ACL tears (18,29). In our experience, few athletes (5%) will be able to continue participation and most will require assistance getting off the playing field. An effusion secondary to bleeding will occur within 6 to 12 hours after injury unless significant capsular dam-

age is present, allowing blood to leak from the joint. Full weight bearing will be difficult, as will full extension of the knee. Noyes et al. (29) found that 60% to 70% of knees that have a traumatic hemarthrosis will have an ACL injury. Sometimes, the ACL can be torn by what sounds to be insignificant trauma. The examiner must not be misled by this history and a minimally swollen knee.

Athletes with a history of prior knee injury and chronic ACL deficiency may describe one or many additional giving-way episodes since their initial injury. They may also describe intermittent locking secondary to an unstable meniscus tear or recurrent swelling and pain indicative of early arthrosis.

It is important to determine if the presenting injury is acute or recurrent because it is rare to sustain a displaced bucket-handle meniscus tear at the time of an acute ACL injury. Lack of full extension after an acute injury is usually secondary to pain with extension from a mismatch between the ACL stump and the intercondylar notch. In the chronically unstable knee, extension loss after a giving-way episode may be secondary to a locked displaced meniscus tear, usually on the medial side. Understanding the difference between the acute and chronic ACL injury will assist in knowing when it is and is not appropriate to prescribe aggressive physical therapy exercises to regain extension. If you suspect a bucket-handle meniscal tear with a chronic ACL-deficient knee and extension does not return easily with physical therapy exercises, an MRI is warranted to determine if the loss of extension is from a displaced meniscus or a bone bruise.

Physical examination of an acute knee injury is history based. In other words, examining the ACL first when the injury is suspected avoids performing potentially painful and unnecessary components of a full knee examination. Whether the knee is examined in the office or on a sideline, a comfortable and relaxed patient is essential. If possible, observe the patient's gait and ability to lift the injured leg. After an ACL injury, a bent knee limp is common as is weakness of the quadriceps muscles. Both lower extremities must be entirely exposed and well supported beyond the heel to allow an accurate examination. We recommend a complete examination of the uninjured knee first to gain patient confidence and obtain a baseline for comparison.

Historically, the anterior drawer test, translation of the tibia forward relative to the femur with the knee in 90 degrees of flexion, was thought to be the best clinical test for ACL injury. Torg et al. (30) found this test to be positive in only 50% of ACL injuries if the posterior horn of the medial meniscus and/or posterior capsule are intact. Torg et al. believed in 1976, as most do today, that the Lachman test was the most reliable and reproducible examination method to confirm ACL injury. In the acute setting, and when performed correctly, the

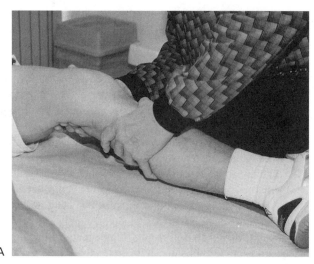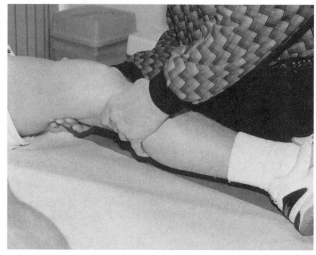

A   B

FIG. 41.2. The Lachman test. **A:** The patient's leg, including the heel, is supported by the table and is relaxed. The examiner's right hand is holding the femur and can feel if the patient has relaxed the hamstrings. The examiner's left hand grips the tibia firmly. **B:** The examiner pulls forward with the left hand to determine anterior laxity and the presence or absence of an end point.

Lachman test has a sensitivity of 87% to 98% for detecting an ACL tear (31). Though the test is named after John W. Lachman, Noulis in 1875 was the first to describe the test (32).

A relaxed patient is mandatory to conduct an accurate Lachman test. Supine positioning with the hip external rotated and the knee supported in slight flexion facilitates relaxation. The hand on the lateral side of the knee grasps the femur, whereas the other inside hand grasps the tibia. A quick firm motion pulling the tibia forward while pushing the femur posteriorly will allow one to feel for an end point and quantitate the amount of translation (Fig 41.2). Increased translation and a soft or absent end point compared with the uninjured knee can confirm the ACL injury. It is more important to interpret the Lachman test as positive or negative than it is to quantify the amount of laxity. To date, no study has shown a correlation between the grade of laxity appreciated and the resultant functional instability.

Galway and MacIntosh (33) in addition described the lateral pivot shift phenomena. Creating this after an acute ACL injury can be difficult secondary to patient guarding. Chronically, this test can provide

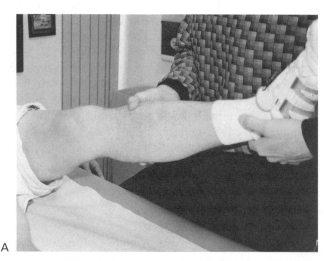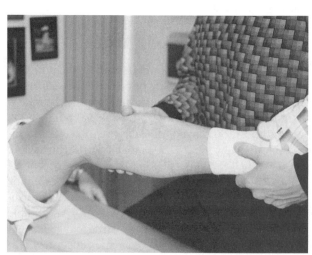

A   B

FIG. 41.3. Modified flexion rotation drawer. **A:** The examiner cradles the patient's calf, ankle, and foot so the patient can relax the leg totally with the knee in slight flexion. **B:** The examiner gently flexes the knee, which causes a reduction of the tibia while applying a slight valgus force to the knee and external rotation of the foot.

additional confirmation of ACL injury. However, the flexion rotation drawer test, a variation of the pivot shift, can be performed painlessly, on an acutely injured knee. While cradling the calf and flexing the knee, a posteriorly directed force on the tibia will cause reduction of the tibia as the femur rotates from an externally rotated position (Fig. 41.3). A comparison with the uninjured knee again will prevent the examiner from misinterpreting this test in a patient with a mild physiologic laxity.

After the ACL has been evaluated, the MCL, the lateral collateral ligament (LCL), and the posterior cruciate ligament (PCL) need to be assessed for injury. The reader is referred to other chapters for a detailed review of these ligaments and their evaluation. Joint line tenderness, though present frequently after ACL injury, is not predictive of meniscal injury and is usually secondary to the adjacent capsular damage (34). The major nerve and blood vessels around the knee must also be evaluated after any ligamentous injury. To our knowledge, significant neurovascular injury has not been reported to be associated with an isolated ACL tear; however, in combination ligament injuries involving the ACL, neurovascular structures are at greater risk for injury.

In some cases, the status of the ACL may remain in question at the conclusion of a detailed history and examination. The most cost-effective approach at this point is to reduce pain and swelling and to reevaluate the knee several days later. MRI and certainly diagnostic arthroscopy can be avoided in almost all cases with no significant time lost or risk of additional injury.

IMAGING

Imaging of the acute knee injury, as with any musculoskeletal problem, begins with plain radiographs. Routine examination should include a posteroanterior weight-bearing view (35), lateral view with 60 degrees of knee flexion, and bilateral patellofemoral views as described by Merchant et al. (36). The Rosenberg view (35) is more accurate in assessing joint space narrowing than the traditional anteroposterior view. The posteroanterior view also allows measurement of the intercondylar notch. Most often plain x-rays are normal; however, an avulsion or osteochondral fracture may be seen. A Segond fracture or lateral capsule avulsion may be seen on the posteroanterior or anteroposterior view and is thought to be highly predictive of ACL injury (37,38). When the ACL is injured in combination with a collateral ligament, an avulsion of the femoral attachment of the MCL or fibular attachment of the LCL may be seen infrequently on the radiograph.

Fracture of the tibial spine may occur in both children and adults. Meyers and McKeever (39,40) classified this fracture according to the degree of displacement. Type I fractures are nondisplaced, type II demonstrate slight elevation, and type III are completely displaced.

Stäubli (41) described a reproducible technique to obtain stress radiographs of the ligamentous injured knee using a modified Telos machine. This allows objective measurement of the direction and magnitude of the instability after an injury. Unfortunately, the complexity and time involved in obtaining these views makes the routine use of them impractical for the most part.

MRI usually is not needed to evaluate an acute knee injury because of the accuracy of the history and physical examination. Unfortunately, many patients want an MRI examination to be done despite the expense. More important than confirming ACL injury is the additional information that can be obtained with regard to the menisci, subchondral bone, and other ligamentous structures. Rarely is the acute management altered because of these findings. They may, however, be of prognostic value and in certain situations help the physician and patient make treatment decisions. For example, in the skeletally immature athlete or the athlete who desires to return to play in a brace after ACL injury, evaluation of the menisci by MRI can detect, in the former case, a meniscal injury that may require repair and, in the latter case, help predict further meniscal injury if play is allowed. In the chronic ACL-deficient setting, an MRI can differentiate extension loss secondary to a displaced meniscus tear or extension loss secondary to a new bone bruise from a recent giving-way episode.

When uninjured, the ACL appears on MRI as an uninterrupted signalless band that may display several distinct fiber bundles (42). Damage to the ligament may be seen as increased signal within the ligament on T2-weighted image, waviness of the fibers, or a complete absence. The accuracy of detecting an ACL tear by MRI is high (43). One study found that the accuracy depends on the imaging center in which it is performed (43). Vahey et al. (44) reported on the MRI findings in both acute and chronic ACL-deficient knees. They found that edematous soft tissue as opposed to fluid in the intercondylar notch is most characteristic of an acute ACL tear. In the chronic setting, as others have suggested, visualization of variable-sized fragments without edema is most indicative of ACL damage. This is in contrast to a report by Mink et al. (45), who found nonvisualization of the ACL to be most common. In addition to increased signal within the ACL and/or discontinuity of the ligament on the sagittal image, many other secondary findings of ACL damage have also been reported. Mink and Deutsch (46) described occult osseous lesions (low signal on T1-weighted image and high signal on T2-weighted image) in the epiphyseal and metaphyseal regions of the tibia and femur. These so-called bone bruises are most common in the lateral

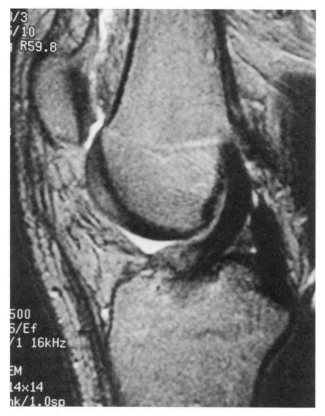

FIG. 41.4. Magnetic resonance imaging shows an anterior cruciate ligament graft at 3 months after reconstruction. The graft was placed parallel and posterior to Blumensaat's line.

tibia and femur when the ACL has been torn. Anterior translocation of the tibia measured in the midsagittal plane of the lateral femoral condyle (47), posterior displacement of the lateral menisci (48), and PCL buckling (49) have been reported to be associated with an ACL tear. Tung et al. (48) found that these signs were specific (90% to 100%) but not particularly sensitive (18% to 73%).

Finally, use of MRI after reconstruction of the ACL can provide information about graft position and integrity. Howell et al. (50) reported on graft appearance in the impinged and unimpinged knee. High signal in the graft near the tibial tunnel when associated with anterior tibial tunnel placement indicates graft impingement and the potential for failure of the graft in the future. An unimpinged ACL graft that is parallel and posterior to Blumensaat's line on MRI is key to a successful long-term result (Fig. 41.4).

TREATMENT OF THE INJURY

A unified treatment approach to ACL injuries is yet to be defined. Though most individuals who sustain an ACL tear are active in some type of sports, their expectations after injury are different based on their stage of life. Children, adolescents, and younger adults most often desire a return to their preinjury sport and are unable to do so with an unstable knee. Many older adults, however, may be willing to modify their activity to avoid giving-way episodes and the need for surgical intervention, although age itself is not a criteria for being a candidate for an ACL reconstruction.

Unfortunately, the ideal natural history study of the ACL-deficient knee does not exist at this time. Presently, we are working on a long-term follow-up study of greater than 800 patients who are at least 5 years post-ACL reconstruction to determine if the reconstruction prevents early joint degeneration. It is apparent now that a knee that continues to give way recurrently over time has a high incidence of additional meniscal and chondral damage that will lead to accelerated joint degeneration. Thus, at the present time, counseling patients as to the most appropriate treatment for them can only be based on factors that are known to place the knee at risk for further injury and relating those factors to the individual patient.

Nonoperative Treatment

Many patients who tear the ACL will elect not to undergo reconstruction. For the skeletally immature athlete, this decision is only a temporary one. The adult, however, may have minimal limitations with activities of daily living and low-risk sports and may feel no need to undergo surgical treatment. The main key to counseling the patient is to determine the patient's desire to participate in twisting and pivoting activities and the likelihood of suffering recurrent giving-way episodes. Regardless of the situation, the initial management of an acute ACL tear involves decreasing the patient's discomfort and swelling, followed by restoring full range of motion (phase I). The rehabilitation mainly emphasizes regaining full extension, because it is the torn ACL stump in the notch that prevents obtaining extension easily. The Cryo/Cuff (Aircast, Inc., Summit, NJ) applies cold and compression in a safe and effective manner, facilitating rapid achievement of these goals (51). Some patients will have poor leg control because of pain and swelling. The use of a knee immobilizer and crutches for several days will encourage early weight bearing and prevent the development of a disabling limp.

As pain and swelling decrease, emphasis shifts to restoring range of motion, especially extension. Patients with an acutely torn ACL feel unstable as the knee extends secondary to both instability and pain from the torn ACL, causing pain as the knee extends. Passive methods such as prone hangs and heel props are used to achieve full hyperextension. Isometric quadriceps muscle exercise assists with maintaining extension and preventing quadriceps muscle shutdown. A hyperextension device (Fig. 41.5) can be used in short duration several times per day to accelerate regaining full hyperextension or assist in cases where it is difficult to achieve. If achieving full hyperextension is painful or difficult in the first week after injury despite these methods, one should consider an MRI evaluation, particularly in chronic ACL-deficient cases to rule out extension block secondary to a displaced bucket-handle meniscus tear. In our experience, only 1% to 2% of patients with acute ACL tears have a displaced bucket-handle meniscus tear. These patients usually have more of a flexion contracture that is painful to the patient when working on extension exercises. Flexion, on the other hand, typically returns with less effort. As swelling subsides, wall slides and active flexion exercises are usually all that is necessary.

Strengthening can begin once extension is restored and flexion exceeds 115 to 120 degrees (phase II). Many strengthening protocols have been advocated after an ACL tear. Recently, more emphasis has been placed on functional retraining. DeCarlo et al. (52) and Palmitier et al. (53) recommend closed kinetic chain rehabilitation programs, including single leg knee bends, step-ups, leg press, hip sled, and a stair-stepper machine to lessen joint sheer stress via joint compression and muscle cocontraction.

Phase III of the rehabilitation program emphasizes a functional return to activities that are believed to be safe based on knee stability and patient confidence. Both isokinetic and functional strength testing can be performed at this point to guide decision making. Athletes with full range of motion and strength at least 85% to 90% of the contralateral lower extremity can return to

TABLE 41.2. *International Knee Documentation Committee activity levels*

Level	Activity
I	Jumping, pivoting, hard cutting (basketball, football, soccer)
II	Lateral motion; less jumping and hard cutting (baseball, racket sports, skiing)
III	Jogging, running, swimming

low-risk activities, including running, bicycling, and swimming with minimal risk of reinjury.

Return to high-risk cutting and pivot activities with an ACL-deficient knee, in our experience, usually is not possible without sustaining additional giving-way episodes. Even when a battery of functional tests, including strength and knee laxity testing (KT-1000 arthrometer), are performed, we have been unable to predict which nonoperatively treated knees will be stable in these high-risk situations. The International Knee Documentation Committee (IKDC) has divided sports into three separate categories based on perceived risk of injury to the knee (Table 41.2) (54). Daniel et al. (6) found athletes who participate greater than 50 hr/yr in level I or II sports and have arthrometer measurements 5 mm or greater than the normal contralateral knee (55) to be at greatest risk for additional injury and the need for subsequent surgical intervention.

The usefulness of braces in the nonoperatively treated ACL-deficient patient remains questionable. No study to date has shown that bracing an ACL-deficient knee will prevent episodes of instability if one returns to high-risk activities. In fact, Beynnon et al. (56) found no stress shielding of the native ACL with custom or off-the-shelf braces when the high anterior sheer loads seen in sports were applied to the knee. Bracing may, however, provide some benefit to the patient in lower risk activities by enhancing proprioception.

Finally, when a patient chooses nonoperative treatment after an ACL tear, evaluation of the menisci should be performed, especially if he or she wants to return to high-risk sports. MRI is an excellent way to do this because it is noninvasive and does not require radiation. If repairable meniscal tears are seen (mainly in the medial meniscus), it is best to advise against returning to level I or II activities and to recommend ACL reconstruction combined with meniscal repair. If no meniscal damage can be documented, returning to a low-risk sport or low-risk position in a high-risk sport may be allowed with the agreement that if further instability episodes occur, participation will cease.

Surgical Treatment

In 1885, Mayo Robson (57) performed the first reported cruciate ligament repair. He sutured both the ACL and

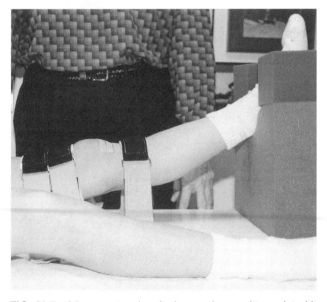

FIG. 41.5. A hyperextension device can be used to assist with obtaining full hyperextension equal to the contralateral knee.

PCL back to their femoral attachments with a reported excellent functional result. Thirty years later, Hey-Groves (58) substituted the ACL with a proximally based strip of the iliotibial band, routing it through the femur and tibia, again yielding an excellent result. Others during this time were attempting artificial ligament reconstruction with wire and suture (59). Since those early times, many other procedures have been described, attempted, and subsequently abandoned. Primary repair, though reported to be successful in elite skiers (60), is no longer performed because the long-term failure rates are high (61). Extraarticular procedures, most often using the iliotibial band in isolation (62,63) or in combination with an intraarticular reconstruction, appear to fail in the former and provide no additional stability in the latter (64,65). Prosthetic reconstructions that use material such as Dacron or Goretex (W.L. Gore and Associates, Inc., Flagstaff, AZ) predictably fail in the long term and have been associated with complications secondary to the generation of wear debris (66–68). Ligament augmentation devices have not been shown to improve stability results when used with autogenous or allograft tissues (69,70). Thus, at the present time, most surgeons perform an intraarticular reconstruction of the ACL primarily using an autograft tendon and less often an allograft tendon.

Historically, reconstruction of the acutely torn ACL was performed immediately or as soon as possible after injury. Subacute reconstruction, defined as the patient regaining full range of motion and not having subsequent giving-way episodes, is now favored by most surgeons because of studies that demonstrate a high rate of knee stiffness if surgery is done acutely (71,72). However, it is the condition of the knee (full range of motion including hyperextension, minimal swelling, and good strength) that should determine when reconstruction is performed rather than a defined interval of time after injury. This preoperative time period, whether 1 or 12 weeks or more, allows the clinician adequate time to educate the patient and his or her family about the injury, treatment, and rehabilitation. This purposeful delay also allows psychological preparation because most patients with an acute ACL tear undergo a series of steps after the injury that include anger, depression, denial, and acceptance. The surgery can be scheduled around school or work activities. The delay in surgery allows a predictable and easier return of full range of motion with a very low incidence (<1%) of postoperative procedures to treat symptomatic extension deficits and flexion contractures (73).

The goals of ACL reconstruction are to reestablish a normal knee with full range of motion, good stability, and strength and to prevent additional meniscal and/or chondral damage. The procedure that a surgeon selects to meet these goals must satisfy the following criteria. The success rate in restoring normal stability and full mobility (including hyperextension) must be high. The graft used should have an initial strength equal to or greater than the native ACL, allow secure fixation, and have minimal long-term donor site morbidity. The placement of the graft needs to be anatomic so that fixation of the graft can be secure enough to allow an accelerated rehabilitation program followed by a return to preinjury activities as the patient desires.

Since 1963 when Jones (74) first used the central one third of the patellar tendon for ACL reconstruction, this graft has become the graft of choice by most surgeons. The patellar tendon graft is preferred because of its ease in harvest, predictable width (average 29 mm; range, 22 to 35 mm) and length (minimum 34 mm; KD Shelbourne, unpublished data, 1998), initial strength approximating the native ACL, and the advantage of bone-to-bone healing within the tibial and femoral tunnels. The patellar tendon graft allows a 9 to 10 mm wide graft for all patients. The length has always been greater than the original ACL length (range, 20 to 32 mm). The patellar and tibial bone plugs can be customized in width and length to fit appropriately in the tibial and femoral tunnels. Even in situations where a tibial tubercle ossicle is present, a patellar tendon autograft can be harvested and the ossicle excised (75).

A wide variety of fixation methods can be used with a patellar tendon graft. Laboratory testing suggests that large interference screw fixation in the tibia and femur has the greatest pullout strength (76). Screws placed in a divergent manner, however, may weaken this form of fixation (77). The demand for great amounts of pullout strength needs to be questioned, however, as properly placed anatomic grafts should have very little need to be securely fixed. Other techniques using suture tied through a button or over a screw post on both the femoral and tibial sides have been shown to be successful in properly placed grafts. Rigidly fixed grafts placed improperly may cause range of motion deficits or may be prone to graft failure when or if full range of motion is achieved.

Historically, graft site morbidity was thought to be the major disadvantage of the patellar tendon autograft. It appears now that graft-site morbidity, including patellofemoral pain and crepitus, do not occur more frequently than in the general population if postoperative rehabilitation emphasizes restoration of full knee hyperextension followed by restoration of the knee extensor mechanism (78). Activity-related patellar tendinitis does occur, although rarely restrictive, and can be minimized if quadriceps muscle strength is restored before returning to a higher level of activities. Patellar contracture and or baja occurred frequently in the past after patellar tendon harvest (79,80). Postoperative rehabilitation programs currently do not involve immobilization or restrict quadriceps muscle activity associated with patellar contractures or baja in the past. Shelbourne et al. (81) found insignificant patellar tendon shortening in patients who had preoperative and postoperative rehabilitation programs to regain full range of motion. Finally, catastrophic extensor mechanism injuries, including patellar tendon rupture (82,83) and fracture (84), have been reported after graft harvest. Shelbourne et al. (85) showed that harvesting a 10-mm-wide patellar tendon graft in patients regardless of the width of the native ACL (range, 22 to 36 mm) can result in a return to equal extensor mechanism strength by 6 months postoperatively without a risk of patellar tendon rupture or patella fracture. Patellar fracture may be prevented by harvesting a shorter (<25 mm) bone plug and bone grafting the patellar defect.

Howell (86) showed that the gracilis and semitendinosis tendons when used in combination and double looped have an initial load-to-failure strength greater than the native ACL and a 10-mm patellar tendon autograft. In addition, the stiffness of this graft more closely approximates that of the native ACL, believed by some to be important. Newer fixation techniques appear to be as strong as those used with patellar tendon reconstruction. Tendon healing in the bone tunnels, however, may be slower than the bone-to-bone healing with patellar tendon grafts, creating some concern about subjecting the graft to an accelerated rehabilitation program. Hamstring tendon grafts do not disrupt the extensor mechanism, theoretically decreasing or eliminating the morbidity associated with patellar tendon harvest. Strength deficit after hamstring tendon(s) harvest does not appear to be a significant functional problem. Marder et al. (87) did, however, find a greater peak torque deficit within a group of patients reconstructed with hamstring tendons compared with a group reconstructed with patellar tendon. Graft harvest of the hamstring tendons can be difficult, and if care is not exercised, premature amputation can occur, resulting in a shortened graft. It appears that both the patellar tendon and hamstring tendon grafts, if properly placed, can give an equal long-term success rate. At the present time, however, it is not known if the decrease in donor site morbidity with the hamstring tendons outweighs the advantage of patients being able to return to sports competition sooner when they receive a patellar tendon graft for ACL reconstruction.

Using allograft tissue to reconstruct the ACL is attractive to some surgeons because of the absence of donor site morbidity and ability to vary graft size. Of the tissues reported to be usable in ACL reconstruction, bone–patellar tendon–bone is used most often. Graft tissue is procured under sterile conditions, and donors are screened for infectious diseases (88). Storage of the tissue is performed by deep freezing at −70 to −80° C or by freeze drying. Gamma irradiation (2.5 Mrad) may prevent viral transmission and avoid graft damage that has been associated with higher radiation dosages (89,90). Concern about disease transmission is real, although only one reported case of HIV infection has occurred after allograft ACL reconstruction (91,92). Buck et al. (92) calculated viral transmission risk at 1:1,700,000. Immunogenicity of an allograft used in ACL reconstruction appears to be of minimal significance (93). Although graft strength at the time of implantation is equivalent to autogenous tissue, it appears that incorporation and remodeling proceed more slowly than seen with autograft tissue in laboratory studies (94). With this in mind, exposing an allograft to an accelerated rehabilitation program may lead to graft elongation and inferior stability results.

The technique a surgeon selects to perform an ACL reconstruction (arthroscopically assisted or open) is not as important as precise tibial and femoral tunnel placement. Anterior tibial tunnel placement has been shown to cause graft impingement, leading to a loss of full knee extension and possibly graft failure (95). Anterior femoral tunnel placement may prevent restoration of full knee flexion unless the graft elongates when full range of motion is obtained. This position also may result in graft laxity when the knee is in extension. Most surgeons prefer using a guide to create the tibial and femoral tunnels. These guides key off the notch roof or PCL for the tibial tunnel and the over-the-top position for the femoral tunnel. It is common to perform a notchplasty of the lateral femoral condyle. A notchplasty needs to be performed only if the ACL graft is larger than the native ACL because the native ACL fits into the intercondylar notch in full extension. When using a 10-mm patellar tendon graft, we make sure the width of the notch from the lateral border of the PCL to the lateral femoral condyle is at least 10 mm to accommodate the new ligament (Fig. 41.6).

The amount of tension that should be applied to an ACL graft at the time of implantation is currently unknown. The tension must be great enough to restore stability to the joint but not great enough to capture it. Full range of motion (full hyperextension to full flexion) must be confirmed in the operating room by the surgeon to avoid potential joint capture.

Postoperative rehabilitation is covered in detail below (see Authors' Preference). We continue to believe that a successful result after ACL reconstruction depends primarily on placement, fixation, and tensioning of the graft so that the knee can be placed through full range of motion while the patient is still on the operating room table. Many times, a failure after surgery is blamed on the rehabilitation program or the patient's noncompliance with the rehabilitation program. We believe that

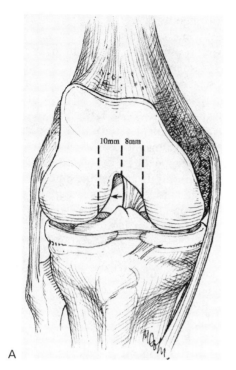

A

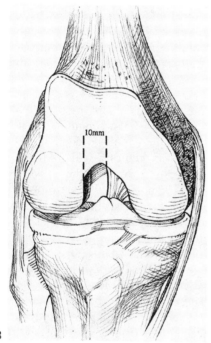

B

FIG. 41.6. A: *Arrow* shows the space between the posterior collateral ligament and the lateral femoral condyle. **B:** A lateral notchplasty is performed to allow 10 mm of space for the 10-mm-wide anterior cruciate ligament graft.

most failures are due to improper surgical technique and not rehabilitation activities.

Expected Outcomes

The outcome after the treatment of any injury is both objective and subjective. There is also a short-term and long-term component to the assessment. Studies carried out in the past have shown that objective evaluation can differ significantly from a patient's subjective assessment (96). The IKDC knee evaluation form is an attempt to bring together the objective and subjective components of the evaluation (97). It is also designed to allow a more universal comparison of treatment results. Surgeons performing ACL reconstructions should evaluate their results with a tool such as the IKDC form to validate their intervention. Follow-up must be long term, although during the early postoperative period, follow-up visits need to be frequent enough to detect graft failure and assess the outcome of meniscal treatment.

We perform weight-bearing radiographs as described by Rosenberg (35) preoperatively and at 2, 5, 10, and 15 years after reconstruction. Objective knee stability testing (KT-1000 arthrometer manual maximum difference between knees) is performed preoperatively and postoperatively at 4 to 5 weeks, 3 and 6 months, and 1, 2, 5, 10, and 15 years after surgery. Quadriceps muscle strength is measured with the Cybex II dynamometer, leg press test, and the single leg hop test at similar times. Subjective evaluation includes the modified Noyes questionnaire (98) and the current IKDC form.

Despite the significant bias that exists in all natural history studies of ACL-deficient knees, most physicians treating this injury believe that the prognosis after an ACL tear is poor if the patient develops recurrent instability. Unfortunately, meniscal and chondral damage sustained at the time of the acute injury may significantly influence the outcome despite treatment, operative or nonoperative, that provides the patient with functional stability. Successful treatment in the short term means eliminating giving-way episodes that, hopefully, will minimize the premature degeneration of the joint and guarantee long-term success.

Nonoperative treatment of an ACL injury can be successful if the patient is willing to modify his or her life-style appropriately to avoid additional giving-way episodes. For many patients, this is difficult to accomplish. Bonamo et al. (99) found that despite a regimented strengthening program, including sport-specific exercises, 40% of the 79 recreational athletes who sustained an ACL tear and elected nonoperative treatment had to significantly modify their athletic activity to avoid giving-way episodes. Only 11% demonstrated excellent results. Hawkins et al. (100) and Andersson et al. (101) similarly found that 75% to 80% of prospectively followed ACL-deficient patients treated nonoperatively could not return to level I or II sports activities, although most could participate in some lower risk sport. In fact, Daniel et al. (6) found that it is one's inability to return to sports because of instability that brings them to surgical treatment. Others have found that even when a mild grade of instability is present or the patient is relatively sedentary, half will fare poorly with nonoperative treatment (102). Both Warren (103) and Daniel et al. (6) found that the outcome of nonoperative treatment is worse as the severity of laxity increases, particularly in those who continue to participate in high-risk sports. Finally, studies do confirm that patients with chronic anterior instability develop meniscal tears (usually medial) with greater frequency and, in addition, are more likely to have chondral injuries than those with acute ACL injury (104,105). Despite a successful ACL reconstruction that restores stability, patients with preexisting meniscal tears or chondral injuries may have more long-term problems.

Many retrospective studies have been performed to evaluate the results of intraarticular reconstruction of the ACL. It is difficult to compare these studies because there are differences in patient groups, reconstruction methods, and postoperative rehabilitation programs. In addition, most studies have not used a uniform evaluation system. A study by Shelbourne et al. (98) of patients who had an ACL reconstruction with an autogenous patellar tendon graft showed that at least 87% of patients were able to return to their preinjury level of activity. There does not appear to be any difference in outcome related to the technique used for reconstruction. A recent study by O'Neill (106) and the previous study by Marder et al. (87) found no significant difference in functional outcome or objective stability when patellar tendon autograft was compared with semitendinosus/gracilis autograft in a prospective randomized fashion.

It is not known whether an allograft reconstruction of the ACL yields clinical results similar to reconstruction with autogenous tissue. Olson et al. (107) found that only 74% of patients undergoing allograft ACL reconstruction could return to their preinjury level of activity. Seventy percent of the patients had objective stability with KT-1000 arthrometer testing compared with studies of autogenous graft tissue in which greater than 80% demonstrate near normal stability.

Shelbourne and Gray (73) recently reported results of a long-term follow-up study of autogenous patellar tendon reconstructions followed by an accelerated rehabilitation program during which the return to activities was dictated by the condition of the knee and not a time from surgery. Objectively, the mean manual maximum KT-1000 arthrometer difference between the reconstructed knee and the normal contralateral knee was 2.0 ± 1.5 mm. Quadriceps muscle strength tested isokinetically was greater than 90%. The IKDC knee evaluation rating revealed that 42% of the knees were normal, 47% were near normal, 10% were abnormal, and 1% were severely abnormal. Radiographically, greater than 90% of the knees had no joint space narrowing. The mean time to return to sports-specific activities was 6.2 weeks. The patients reported that they returned to competition at full capability at a mean of 6.2 months after surgery.

AUTHORS' PREFERENCES

At the Methodist Sports Medicine Center in Indianapolis, Indiana, we have more than 15 years of experience treating ACL injuries and more than 5,000 ACL reconstructions have been performed. Consistent data collection, while analyzing the results of both our successful and failed reconstructions, has allowed us to develop a treatment approach to ACL injuries. Since 1982, this approach has undergone and continues to undergo significant evaluation and subsequent change based on our observations and results of treatment. This section describes our approach to ACL injuries and how it has become what it is today.

The treatment goal for all ACL injuries is restoration of functional stability and full motion while minimizing morbidity. Most patients who tear the ACL have high expectations and desire a rapid return to their preinjury state. With this in mind, it is not surprising that most ACL tears are treated by reconstruction. We recommend surgical reconstruction to all school-aged athletes and to those individuals who want to return to high-risk activities.

After the diagnosis of an ACL tear, treatment should begin immediately (phase I). Proper education that includes a description of the injury, anatomy, treatment options, and expected outcome facilitates early rehabilitation. Having patients talk with other ACL-injured or ACL-reconstructed patients who are in various stages of their rehabilitation helps to extinguish anxiety and fear. We agree with Smith et al. (108), who found that competitive athletes in particular have significant depression, anger, and decreased vigor after major injury. These psychological changes can last for several weeks. Recognition of this process and assistance with resolution of the injury will improve communication with both the athlete and the family and will expedite preoperative rehabilitation.

Since 1990, we have not performed ACL reconstruction on an acute basis before full range of motion was restored, and this approach decreased our incidence of symptomatic extension loss to less than 1%. Unfortunately, athletes and their families want to proceed with reconstruction immediately after injury because they believe it will lead to an earlier return to participation. We have found that waiting to perform surgery until the patient has regained full range of motion, including hyperextension, not only minimizes the potential for postoperative stiffness but allows a faster return of strength postoperatively, thus allowing an earlier return to sports (109,110). During this preoperative rehabilitation period, the patient must be aware that the ACL does not heal and, despite decreased swelling and return of full motion and strength, the knee remains unstable and at risk for additional injury if high-risk sports are resumed.

After preoperative rehabilitation and before surgical treatment of the ACL tear, patients undergo preoperative isokinetic and isometric (leg press force plate) strength testing along with KT-1000 arthrometer measurements. We do emphasize preoperative strengthening after restoration of full motion. Closed kinetic chain exercises (knee bends, step-ups, leg press, bike, and stair-stepper) are well tolerated and safe.

When a young skeletally immature athlete tears the ACL, several unique situations may arise. They may not be able to undergo an ACL reconstruction because of the fear of growth disturbance. Although no study has demonstrated the effect of drilling across an open physes, Lipscomb and Anderson (8) did document one physeal injury in 24 athletes with open physes undergoing ACL reconstruction with hamstring tendons and staple fixation. Others have shown that nonanatomic reconstructions or repair of the ACL, although potentially safer with regard to growth disturbance, does not restore knee stability in a predictable fashion (111). Thus, we believe it is best to wait and perform one anatomic procedure when the risk of growth disturbance is minimal. We use Tanner staging (patient self-comparison with a chart), menstrual history, growth history, parental height, and serial radiographs to determine when the reconstruction is safe (112). Tanner stage 3 to 4, beginning of menses, completion of the preadolescent growth spurt, and physeal blurring on radiographs lend support to proceeding with an anatomic reconstruction with an autogenous patellar tendon graft. Our results with using these criteria and an autogenous patellar tendon graft reconstruction have resulted in no growth disturbance and excellent clinical results.

While waiting for the patient to obtain adequate physical maturity, education about the potential for significant reinjury during this period, activity modification, and use of a brace most often will prevent additional injury. The athlete, however, may miss one or two seasons of participation. An athlete occasionally may want to continue participation in a lower risk sport after an ACL tear. We use MRI to evaluate the menisci before allowing the athlete to return to sports. More specifically, our purpose is to evaluate the medial meniscus because peripheral medial meniscus tears have been found to be a greater problem than lateral tears, which can heal without repair. If repairable medial meniscal tear is seen on MRI, a meniscal repair is performed. If no medial meniscal tear is seen or after the patient has completed the rehabilitation after meniscal repair, the patient may be allowed to participate in a low-risk sport. Usually, a brace is recommended. The risk, however, must be discussed with the athlete and his or her family in detail. Additional giving-way episodes preclude continued participation.

Our approach to combined ACL–MCL injuries has been described in detail (113). It is important to determine the site of MCL injury (proximal, midsubstance, or distal). Proximal injuries tend to heal with greater knee stiffness, necessitating a delay of the ACL reconstruction until full range of motion is restored. Distal injuries, on the other hand, usually require a period of immobilization (2 to 4 weeks) to reestablish acceptable medial stability. Knowing that all grades of isolated MCL injuries can heal with excellent stability when treated nonoperatively allows us to convert this combined injury into an isolated ACL tear. Third-degree MCL tears are treated with weekly cylinder casts until the MCL begins to heal and has an end point upon physical examination. Second-degree MCL tears are immobilized in a splint for comfort until the patient can walk with a normal gait. While the MCL heals and once full restoration of motion is achieved, ACL reconstruction alone can be performed in those patients who require knee stability for high-risk activities (114).

Injury to the ACL and lateral side of the knee, in our opinion, requires prompt identification and surgical treatment. MRI can be helpful in delineating the extent and location of the lateral side injury. Frequently, the lateral structures of the lateral capsule off the tibia, the lateral cruciate ligament, and the biceps tendon are avulsed from their distal attachments and retracted proximally, making direct repair difficult if delayed beyond 7 to 10 days. We perform an ACL reconstruction and a direct repair of the injured lateral structures by stapling the lateral capsule and its associated soft tissue attachments back to the bare spot on the tibia.

Chronic ACL-deficient patients who present with a recent giving-way episode and a "stuck" bent and swollen knee in many cases have a displaced bucket-handle tear of the meniscus. Since 1989, we have staged the management of this problem first by repairing the meniscus, if possible, and then by restoring full knee motion before proceeding with an ACL reconstruction (115). This approach was developed as a result of observing significant motion problems in this subgroup of chronic ACL-deficient patients when we simultaneously repaired or removed the locked meniscus and performed an ACL reconstruction. By staging the procedures, we were aggressive with preserving more menisci because we knew we would be able to observe the meniscus again at the time of ACL reconstruction and have found that many meniscus tears that we were previously excising would actually heal well by the time of the ACL reconstruction. This approach has helped us appreciate the ability of the repaired menisci to heal despite weight bearing and rehabilitation exercises. In addition, the problem of regaining full range of motion was eliminated by the two-staged procedure.

Our operative procedure has been described in detail. We continue to use exclusively a 10-mm autogenous patellar tendon graft both for primary and revision reconstructions. Correct placement of the tibial and femoral tunnels is the key to a successful result. Our technique emphasizes direct visualization of the tibia and femur and tunnel creation independent of each other. We do not use interference screw fixation in either the tibia or femur. Although the polyethylene button is a weaker form of fixation when tested *in vitro,* we have not seen a fixation failure and are able to maximize the surface area for bone healing within the tunnels. The buttons allow flexible fixation, easy tensioning, no radiographic change, and easier revision surgery if needed later as no bone holes are still present. The buttons have been strong enough to not cause graft failure despite our rehabilitation program.

We do not believe that immediate arthroscopic intervention is necessary to treat meniscal damage that has been identified after injury. The tears can be treated with equal success at the time of delayed reconstruction if giving-way episodes are avoided. We have found that many meniscal tears are healed or are healing by the time of ACL reconstruction, which has allowed us to better understand the natural history of these tears. Stable meniscal tears seen at the time of reconstruction are not removed but rather abraded and trephinated to facilitate healing. Those tears that do require repair are sutured by an inside-out technique, tying over the capsule via a small medial or lateral incisions. The success rate of this treatment has been followed and reevaluated over time. In general, we are leaving more lateral tears and partially removing more degenerative medial tears.

Postoperative rehabilitation (phase II) begins in the operating room when the surgeon confirms that full range of motion, including hyperextension, can be achieved. This ensures that the graft has not been over-tensioned. Patients remain in the hospital for one night after surgery. This allows the use of continuous IV ketorolac that in most cases eliminates the need for supplemental narcotics (116). An alert patient who does not need supplement narcotics for pain control can begin extension exercises immediately and regain quadriceps muscle control quickly. We have continued to use the Cryo/Cuff because of its ability to compress the knee joint and prevent a postoperative hemarthrosis while providing analgesia (117).

A continuous passive motion (CPM) machine is used immediately after surgery. This device, although not shown to improve ultimate outcome in some studies, predictably elevates the extremity above the level of the heart, keeps the patient at bedrest, initiates early range of motion, and minimizes postoperative swelling. In the past, the CPM machine moved the knee from 0 to 90 degrees, but many patients had significant swelling. Once we realized that it was the extremes of motion that were our main goals, we set the CPM machine to move from 0 to 30 degrees. The exercises to achieve the extremes of motion were performed at specific times during the day. The day after surgery, patients increase their flexion within the machine to a maximum of 110 degrees (flexion limited by the machine) four to five times per day, holding the knee in the flexed position for 10 minutes each time. Three to four times a day while the leg was out of the CPM machine, patients increase knee flexion to 120 degrees and hold it there for 5 minutes without developing increased swelling afterward.

Actively lifting the extremity from the CPM for extension exercises, isometric quadriceps contraction, and

TABLE 41.3. *Summary of clinic visits and goals during rehabilitation*

Time	Clinic goals
Before surgery	Purposeful delay in surgery to prepare the patient for reconstruction
	Isokinetic/isometric testing
	Full passive extension (hyper)
	Minimize swelling
	Normal gait and good leg strength
	KT-1000 testing[a]
1 wk after surgery	Full passive knee extension (normal hyperextension) to 110-degree flexion
	Good leg control
	Soft tissue healing
2 wk after surgery	Full passive extension
	120-degree flexion
	Normal gait
	Begin quadriceps strengthening (bicycle, leg press, Stairmaster)
5 wk after surgery	Full knee extension (hyper)
	Full flexion
	60–65% isokinetic quadriceps strength
	KT-1000 testing[a]
	Begin sport-specific activities/agility drills to regain proprioception; progress to competition as able
10 wk after surgery	Full active ROM
	70–75% isokinetic quadriceps strength
	KT-1000 testing[a]
	Competition or full athletic activity as desired
4 mo after surgery	Follow-up strength and functional testing
	KT-1000 testing[a]
	80–85% isokinetic quadriceps strength
	Consistent participation in athletic activity
6 mo after surgery	Follow-up strength and functional testing
	KT-1000 testing[a]
	90% isokinetic quadriceps strength
	Full participation in athletic activity

[a] KT-1000 Knee Arthrometer, MEDmetric, San Diego, California.
ROM; range of motion.

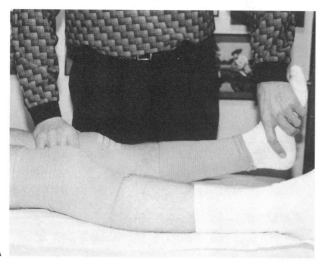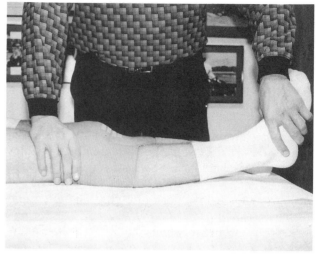

FIG. 41.7. A: To confirm symmetric hyperextension, the examiner holds the thigh securely down on the table while using the other hand to lift the patient's foot. The amount of hyperextension and the ease of which the knee extends is compared with the contralateral normal knee **(B).**

short-arc quadriceps exercises are all used immediately after surgery to restore leg control. Early quadriceps activation and the flexion exercises will place tension on the patellar tendon and will aid in the prevention of a patellar tendon contracture.

Although our rehabilitation has been termed "accelerated" as far as allowing an early return to activities, patients must understand the importance of minimizing swelling in the immediate postoperative period. We encourage patients to get up only to use the bathroom and for meals during the first postoperative week. Full weight bearing is allowed immediately after surgery, but the amount of time is limited. Patients are discharged the morning after surgery when they have minimal swelling, full hyperextension, flexion to 100 degrees, and good quadriceps muscle control.

The scheduled clinic visits and goals for the first year after surgery are summarized in Table 41.3. Rapid restoration of full knee hyperextension in the postoperative period is critical to avoid the potential problem of graft/ notch mismatch. Despite previous opinions that restoration of full hyperextension would lead to instability, we have found evidence to the contrary. Postoperative stability demonstrated by both objective and subjective measures has improved with this more aggressive approach to knee extension (118). We have also found that the incidence of anterior knee pain 1 year after ACL reconstruction in patients who achieve full hyperextension to be equal to a normal control population (78). In our clinic we evaluate hyperextension by the method shown in Fig. 41.7. Comparison should be carried out with the contralateral knee. Loss of any extension should be addressed early in the rehabilitation because it much easier to restore at this time. Use of

an hyperextension device, as mentioned earlier in this chapter, can be helpful when patients are having difficulty.

Leg strengthening (phase III) cannot be accomplished well until swelling is minimal, hyperextension has been restored, and flexion is at least 120 degrees. Attempting to strengthen the leg before achieving these goals can result in increased swelling and pain along with difficulty maintaining the achieved range of motion. Using closed kinetic chain exercises (step-ups, quarter squats, leg press, hip sled, stair-stepper), leg strength is improved while minimizing soreness.

Returning to sports (phase IV) after an ACL reconstruction depends on many factors with significant variability in the duration of time from surgery. We do not use strict criteria of strength return to allow athletes to resume sports. Quadriceps strength of at least 65% of the contralateral leg, tested isokinetically at 180 degrees/s, is sufficient to allow more aggressive sporting activities with little fear of initiating patellar tendon soreness and swelling. Patients will need 2 to 3 months of performing their sport before they will feel like they are competing at 100% capability. The athlete's sport, position, and preinjury ability will dictate to a significant degree the rate and level to which they can return. No patient is pushed to return sooner than desired. Rather, the physician's role is to encourage and monitor progress, prevent complications, and allow a return to activities as quickly as desired as long as the specific rehabilitation goals have been achieved.

Fortunately, complications after ACL reconstruction are now infrequent. Infection has been reported to occur in less than 1% of cases (119). Deep venous thrombosis appears to occur no more frequently than seen with

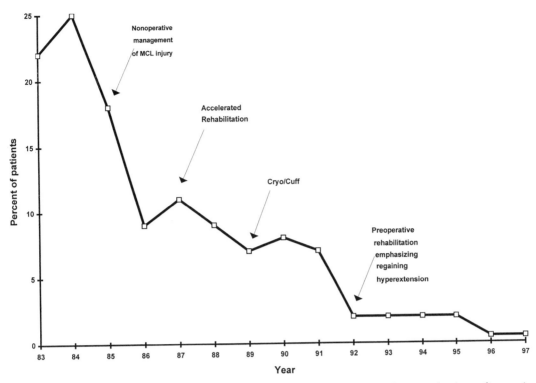

FIG. 41.8. The percent of patients requiring a scar resection for symptomatic extension loss after acute and semiacute anterior cruciate ligament reconstruction.

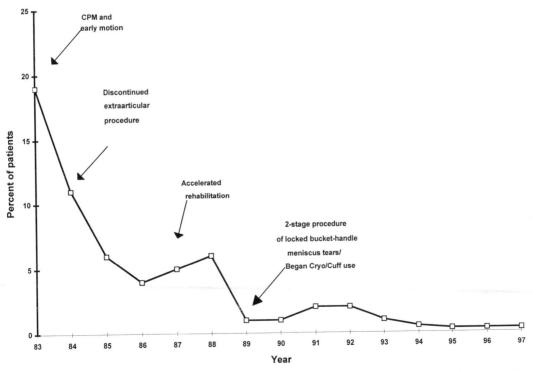

FIG. 41.9. The percent of patients requiring a scar resection for symptomatic extension loss after chronic anterior cruciate ligament reconstruction.

TABLE 41.4. *Classification of arthrofibrosis of the knee*

Type	Description
1	Extension loss of (10) compared with contralateral knee
	Normal flexion
2	Extension loss of >10 compared with contralateral knee
	Normal flexion
3	Extension loss of >10 compared with contralateral knee
	Flexion loss of >25
	Decreased medial and lateral movement of the patella
	No patellar infera
4	Extension loss of >10
	Flexion loss of 30
	Marked patellar tightness

knee arthroscopy alone. Fracture of the femur and neurovascular injuries are extremely rare (120). What does remain a problem, however, is the symptomatic loss of full range of motion. In the past, this was the result of immediate surgery after an acute ACL tear without regaining full range of motion before surgery or by prolonged immobilization postoperatively. Knees were stable after this treatment approach, but stiffness resulted in many patient complaints, including quadriceps weakness, anterior knee pain, and patellar tendinitis. Many changes in our management of ACL injuries have occurred since 1982 in an effort to decrease the incidence of postoperative stiffness. These changes in both the acute and chronic ACL-deficient knee are summarized in Figs. 41.8 and 41.9.

When difficulty regaining full range of motion does occur, conservative treatment with techniques already described in the postoperative rehabilitation are usually successful. We have found it helpful to classify range of motion loss after ACL surgery (Table 41.4). This scheme, in our opinion, predicts the amount of scarring present and the type of intervention needed. In cases where conservative methods fail, we perform arthroscopic scar excision followed by serial extension casting. Although this postoperative regimen is very labor intensive, our patients have been very pleased with the outcome (121–123).

SUMMARY

The goals of an ACL reconstruction and rehabilitation are to restore stability, full range of motion, and full function in all patients. With an understanding of precise surgical technique and advances in perioperative rehabilitation, the more recent results obtained after surgery have been encouraging. It is always the patient's desire that the knee feel normal again after surgery. The patient's concept of how the knee feels after surgery depends on the difficulty or lack of difficulty the patient has with rehabilitation and with return to activities. It is possible for the rehabilitative course after surgery to be smooth and predictable when the patient has a thorough understanding of the goals of each phase of rehabilitation. We believe that the future for an athlete suffering an ACL tear is bright and that most patients can look forward to returning to athletic activities safely with a long-term excellent result.

REFERENCES

1. Miyaska KC, Daniel DM, Stone ML, et al. The incidence of knee ligament injuries in the general population. *Am J Knee Surg* 1991;4:3–8.
2. Nielsen AF, Yde J. Epidemiology of acute knee injuries: a prospective hospital investigation. *J Trauma* 1991;31:1644–1648.
3. Feagin JA Jr, Lambert KL, Cunningham RR, et al. Consideration of the anterior cruciate ligament injury in skiing. *Clin Orthop* 1987;216:13–18.
4. Hewson GF Jr, Mendini RA, Wang JB. Prophylactic knee bracing in college football. *Am J Sports Med* 1986;14:262–266.
5. Stanitski CL, Harrell JC, Fu F. Observations on acute knee hemarthrosis in children and adolescents. *J Pediatr Orthop* 1993;13:506–510.
6. Daniel DM, Stone ML, Dobson BE, et al. Fate of the ACL injured patient: a prospective outcome study. *Am J Sports Med* 1994;22:632–644.
7. McCarroll JR, Rettig AC, Shelbourne KD. Anterior cruciate ligament injuries in the young athlete with open physes. *Am J Sports Med* 1988;16:44–47.
8. Lipscomb AB, Anderson AF. Tears of the anterior cruciate ligament in adolescents. *J Bone Joint Surg Am* 1986;68A:19–28.
9. Arendt E, Dick R. Knee injury patterns among men and women in collegiate basketball and soccer. *Am J Sports Med* 1995;23:694–701.
10. Jackson DS, Furman WK, Berson BL. Patterns of injuries in college athletes. A retrospective study of injuries sustained in intercollegiate athletes in two colleges over a two-year period. *Mt Sinai J Med* 1980;47:423–426.
11. Haycock CE, Gillette JV. Susceptibility of women athletes to injury: myth vs. reality. *JAMA* 1976;236:163–165.
12. Huston LJ, Wojtys EM. Neuromuscular performance characteristics in elite female athletes. *Am J Sports Med* 1996;24:427–436.
13. Knapik JJ, Bauman CL, Jones BH, et al. Preseason strength and flexibility imbalances associated with athletic injuries in female collegiate athletes. *Am J Sports Med* 1991;19:76–81.
14. Zilsko JA, Noble HB, Porter M. A comparison of men's and women's professional basketball injuries. *Am J Sports Med* 1982;10:297–299.
15. LaPrade RF, Burnett QM. Femoral intercondylar notch stenosis and correlation to anterior cruciate ligament injuries. A prospective study. *Am J Sports Med* 1994;22:198–203.
16. Souryal TO, Freeman TR. Intercondylar notch size and anterior cruciate ligament injuries in athletes. A prospective study. *Am J Sports Med* 1993;21:535–539.
17. Shelbourne KD, Davis TJ, Klootwyk TE. The relationship of the intercondylar notch width of the femur and the incidence of anterior cruciate ligament tears. *Am J Sports Med* 1998;26:402–408.
18. Fetto JF, Marshall JL. The natural history and diagnosis of anterior cruciate ligament insufficiency. *Clin Orthop* 1980;147:29–38.
19. Paletta GA, Levine DS, O'Brien SJ, et al. Patterns of meniscal injury associated with acute anterior cruciate ligament injury in skiers. *Am J Sports Med* 1992;20:542–547.
20. Johnson R, Shealy J, Ettlinger C. *Training tips for knee-friendly skiing.* Burlington, VT: Vermont Safety Research, 1996.
21. Hirshman HP, Daniel DM, Miyaska K. The fate of unoperated knee ligament injuries. In: Daniel DM, Akeson WH, O'Connor

JJ, eds. *Knee ligaments: structure, function, injury and repair.* New York: Raven Press, 1990:481–503.

22. O'Donoghue DH. Surgical treatment of fresh injuries to the major ligaments of the knee. *J Bone Joint Surg Am* 1950;32A:721–738.

23. Shelbourne KD, Nitz PA. The O'Donoghue triad revisited. Combine knee injuries involving anterior cruciate and medial collateral ligament tears. *Am J Sports Med* 1991;19:474–477.

24. Fitzgibbons RE, Shelbourne KD. "Aggressive" non-treatment of lateral meniscal tears seen during anterior cruciate ligament reconstruction. *Am J Sports Med* 1995;23:156–159.

25. Keene GC, Bickerstaff D, Rae PJ, et al. The natural history of meniscal tears in anterior cruciate ligament insufficiency. *Am J Sports Med* 1993;21:672–679.

26. Speer KP, Spritzer CE, Bassett FH III, et al. Osseous injury associated with acute tears of the anterior cruciate ligament. *Am J Sports Med* 1992;20:382–389.

27. Graf BK, Cook DA, DeSmet AA, et al. "Bone bruises" on magnetic resonance imaging evaluation of anterior cruciate ligament injuries. *Am J Sports Med* 1993;21:220–223.

28. Stein LN, Fischer DA, Fritts HM, et al. Occult osseous lesions associated with anterior cruciate ligament tears. *Clin Orthop* 1995;313:187–193.

29. Noyes FR, Bassett RW, Grood ES, et al. Arthroscopy in acute traumatic hemarthrosis of the knee: incidence of anterior cruciate tears and other injuries. *J Bone Joint Surg Am* 1980;62A:687–695.

30. Torg JS, Conrad W, Kalen V. Clinical diagnosis of anterior cruciate ligament instability in the athlete. *Am J Sports Med* 1976;4:84–93.

31. DeHaven KE. Diagnosis of acute knee injuries with hemarthrosis. *Am J Sports Med* 1980;8:9–14.

32. Paessler HH, Michel D. How new is the Lachman test? *Am J Sports Med* 1992;20:95–98.

33. Galway HR, MacIntosh DL. The lateral pivot shift: a symptom and sign of anterior cruciate ligament insufficiency. *Clin Orthop* 1980;147:45–50.

34. Shelbourne KD, Martini DJ, McCarroll JR, et al. Correlation of joint line tenderness and meniscal lesions in patients with acute anterior cruciate ligament tears. *Am J Sports Med* 1995;23:166–169.

35. Rosenberg TD, Paulos LE, Parker RD, et al. The forty-five degree posteroanterior flexion weight-bearing radiograph of the knee. *J Bone Joint Surg Am* 1988;70A:1479–1483.

36. Merchant AC, Mercer RL, Jacobsen RH, et al. Radiographic analysis of patellofemoral congruence. *J Bone Joint Surg Am* 1974;56A:1391–1396.

37. Milch H. Cortical avulsion fracture of the lateral tibial condyle. *J Bone Joint Surg [Am]* 1936;18:159–164.

38. Woods GW, Stanley RF Jr, Tulles HS. Lateral capsular sign: x-ray clue to a significant knee instability. *Am J Sports Med* 1979;7:27–33.

39. Meyers MH, McKeever FM. Fracture of the intercondylar eminence of the tibia. *J Bone Joint Surg Am* 1959;41A:209–222.

40. Meyers MH, McKeever FM. Fracture of the intercondylar eminence of the tibia. *J Bone Joint Surg Am* 1970;52A:1677–1684.

41. Stäubli HU. Stress radiography to document cruciate ligament function. *Sports Med Arthros Rev* 1997;5:1–10.

42. Mink JH, Reichen MA, Crues JVIII, eds. *Magnetic resonance imaging of the knee.* New York: Raven Press, 1987.

43. Fischer SP, Fox JM, Del Pizzo W, et al. Accuracy of diagnosis from magnetic resonance imaging of the knee. A multi-center analysis of one thousand and fourteen patients. *J Bone Joint Surg Am* 1991;73A:2–10.

44. Vahey TN, Broome DR, Kayes KJ, et al. Acute and chronic tears of the anterior cruciate ligament: differential features at MR imaging. *Radiology* 1991;181:251–253.

45. Mink JH, Levy T, Crues JV. Tears of the anterior cruciate ligament and menisci of the knee: MR imaging evaluation. *Radiology* 1988;167:769–774.

46. Mink JH, Deutsch AL. Occult cartilage and bone injuries of the knee: detection, classification, and assessment with MR imaging. *Radiology* 1989;170:823–829.

47. Vahey TN, Hunt JE, Shelbourne KD. Anterior translation of the tibia at MR imaging: a secondary sign of anterior cruciate ligament tears. *Radiology* 1993;187:817–819.

48. Tung GA, Davis LM, Wiggins ME, et al. Tears of the anterior cruciate ligament: primary and secondary sign at MR imaging. *Radiology* 1993;188:661–667.

49. Boeree NR, Ackroyd CE. Magnetic resonance imaging of anterior cruciate ligament rupture. A new diagnostic sign. *J Bone Joint Surg Br* 1992;74B:614–616.

50. Howell SM, Berns GS, Farley TE. Unimpinged and impinged anterior cruciate ligament grafts: MR signal intensity measurements. *Radiology* 1991;179:639–643.

51. Mindrebo N, Shelbourne KD. Knee pressure dressings and their effects on lower extremity venous capacitance and venous outflow. *Orthop Int* 1994;2:273–280.

52. DeCarlo MS, Porter DA, Gehlson G, et al. Electromyographic and cinematographic analysis of the lower extremity during closed and open kinetic chain exercise. *Isokinet Exerc Sci* 1992;2:24–29.

53. Palmitier RA, An KN, Scott SG, et al. Kinetic chain exercise in knee rehabilitation. *Sports Med* 1991;11:402–413.

54. Fithian DC, Luetzow WF. Natural history of the ACL deficient patient. *Sports Med Arthros Rev* 1996;4:319–327.

55. Daniel DM, Malcom LL, Losse G, et al. Instrumented measurement of anterior laxity of the knee. *J Bone Joint Surg Am* 1985;67A:720–726.

56. Beynnon BD, Pope MH, Wertheimer CM, et al. The effect of functional knee braces on strain on the anterior cruciate ligament in vivo. *J Bone Joint Surg Am* 1992;74A:1298–1312.

57. Mayo Robson AW. Ruptured cruciate ligaments and their repair by operation. *Ann Surg* 1903;37:716–718.

58. Hey-Groves EW. Operation for the repair of the crucial ligaments. *Lancet* 1917;2:674–675.

59. Smith A. The diagnosis and treatment of injuries of the crucial ligaments. *Br J Surg* 1918;6:176–189.

60. Higgins RW, Steadman JR. Anterior cruciate ligament repairs in world class skiers. *Am J Sports Med* 1987;15:439–447.

61. Engebretsen L, Svenningson S, Benum P. Poor results of anterior cruciate ligament repair in adolescence. *Acta Orthop Scand* 1989;59:684–686.

62. Reid JS, Hanks GA, Kalenak A, et al. The Ellison iliotibial-band transfer for a torn anterior cruciate ligament of the knee: a long term follow-up. *J Bone Joint Surg Am* 1992;74A:1392–1402.

63. Vail TP, Malone TR, Bassett FH III. Long-term functional results in patients with anterolateral rotatory instability treated by iliotibial band transfer. *Am J Sports Med* 1992;20:274–282.

64. O'Brien SJ, Warren RF, Pavlov H, et al. Reconstruction of the chronically insufficient anterior cruciate ligament with the central third of the patellar ligament. *J Bone Joint Surg Am* 1991;73A:278–286.

65. Strum GM, Fox JM, Ferkel RD, et al. Intraarticular versus intraarticular and extraarticular reconstruction for chronic anterior cruciate ligament instability. *Clin Orthop* 1989;245:188–198.

66. Barrett GR, Line LL, Shelton WR, et al. The Dacron ligament prosthesis in anterior cruciate ligament reconstruction. A four year review. *Am J Sports Med* 1993;21:367–373.

67. Paulos LE, Rosenberg TD, Grewe SR, et al. The Gore-Tex anterior cruciate ligament prosthesis. A long term follow-up. *Am J Sports Med* 1992;20:246–252.

68. Woods GA, Indelicato PA, Prevof TJ. The Gore-Tex anterior cruciate ligament prosthesis: two versus three year results. *Am J Sports Med* 1991;19:48–55.

69. Moyen BJ, Jenny JY, Mandrino AH, et al. Comparison of reconstruction of the anterior cruciate ligament with and without a Kennedy ligament-augmentation device. A randomized, prospective study. *J Bone Joint Surg Am* 1992;74A:1313–1319.

70. Noyes FR, Barber SD. The effect of a ligament augmentation device on allograft reconstructions for chronic ruptures of the anterior cruciate ligament. *J Bone Joint Surg Am* 1992;74A:960–973.

71. Shelbourne KD, Wilckens JH, Mollabashy A, et al. Arthrofibrosis in acute anterior cruciate ligament reconstruction. The effect of timing of reconstruction and rehabilitation. *Am J Sports Med* 1991;19:332–336.

72. Mohtadi NGH, Webster-Bogaert S, Fowler PJ. Limitation of

motion following anterior cruciate ligament reconstruction. A case-control study. *Am J Sports Med* 1991;19:620–625.

73. Shelbourne KD, Gray T. Anterior cruciate ligament reconstruction with autogenous patellar tendon graft followed by accelerated rehabilitation. A two- to nine-year followup. *Am J Sports Med* 1997;25:786–795.

74. Jones KG. Reconstruction of the anterior cruciate ligament: a technique using the central one-third of the patellar ligament. *J Bone Joint Surg Am* 1963;45A:925–932.

75. McCarroll JR, Shelbourne KD, Patel DV. Anterior cruciate ligament reconstruction in athletes with an ossicle associated with Osgood-Schlatter's disease. *Arthroscopy* 1996;12:556–560.

76. Kurosaka M, Yoshiya S, Andrish JT. A biomechanical comparison of different surgical techniques of graft fixation in anterior cruciate ligament reconstruction. *Am J Sports Med* 1987;15: 225–229.

77. Lemos MJ, Jackson DW, Lee TQ, et al. Assessment of initial fixation of endoscopic interference femoral screws with divergent and parallel placement. *Arthroscopy* 1995;11:37–41.

78. Shelbourne KD, Trumper RV. Preventing anterior knee pain after anterior cruciate ligament reconstruction. *Am J Sports Med* 1997;25:41–47.

79. Rosenberg TD, Franklin JL, Baldwin GH, et al. Extensor mechanism function after patellar tendon graft harvest for anterior cruciate ligament reconstruction. *Am J Sports Med* 1992;20: 519–526.

80. Sachs RA, Daniel DM, Stone ML, et al. Patellofemoral problems after anterior cruciate ligament reconstruction. *Am J Sports Med* 1989;17:760–765.

81. Shelbourne KD, Rubinstein RA Jr, Braeckel CJ, et al. Assessment of patellar height after autogenous patellar tendon anterior cruciate ligament reconstruction. *Orthopaedics* 1995;18:1073–1077.

82. Hardin GT, Bach BR Jr. Distal rupture of the infrapatellar tendon after use of its central third for anterior cruciate ligament reconstruction: case report. *Am J Knee Surg* 1992;5:140–143.

83. Marumoto JM, Mitsunaga MM, Richardson AB, et al. Late patellar tendon ruptures after removal of the central third for anterior cruciate ligament reconstruction. A report of two cases. *Am J Sports Med* 1996;24:698–701.

84. Bonatus TJ, Alexander AH. Patellar fracture and avulsion of the patellar ligament complicating arthroscopic anterior cruciate ligament reconstruction. *Orthop Rev* 1991;20:770–774.

85. Shelbourne KD, Rubinstein RA, VanMeter, CD, et al. Correlation of remaining patellar tendon width with quadriceps strength after autogenous bone-patellar tendon-bone anterior cruciate ligament reconstruction. *Am J Sports Med* 1994;22:774–777.

86. Howell SM. Arthroscopically assisted technique for preventing roof impingement of an anterior cruciate ligament graft illustrated by the use of an autogenous double-looped semitendinosus and gracilis graft. *Opin Tech Sports Med* 1993;1:58–65.

87. Marder RA, Raskind JR, Carroll M. Prospective evaluation of arthroscopically assisted anterior cruciate ligament reconstruction. Patellar tendon versus semitendinosus and gracilis tendons. *Am J Sports Med* 1991;19:478–484.

88. Bright R, Friedlander G, Snell K. Tissue banking. The United States Navy Tissue Bank. *Mil Med* 1977;142:503–510.

89. Fideler BM, Vangsness CT, Moore T, et al. Effects of gamma irradiation on the human immunodeficiency virus: A study in frozen human bone-patellar ligament-bone grafts obtained from infected cadavers. *J Bone Joint Surg Am* 1994;76A:1032–1035.

90. Gibbons MJ, Butler DL, Grood ES, et al. Effects of gamma irradiation on the initial mechanical and material properties of goat bone-patellar tendon bone allografts. *J Orthop Res* 1991; 9:209–218.

91. Asselmejer MA, Caspari RB, Bottenfield S. A review of allograft processing and sterilization techniques and their role in transmission of the human immunodeficiency virus. *Am J Sports Med* 1993;21:170–175.

92. Buck BE, Malium TI, Brown MO. Bone transplantation and human immunodeficiency virus. An estimate of risk of acquired immunodeficiency syndrome (AIDS). *Clin Orthop* 1989;240: 129–136.

93. Shino K, Kimura T, Hirose H, et al. Reconstruction of the ante-

rior cruciate ligament by an allograft tendon graft. An operation for chronic ligamentous insufficiency. *J Bone Joint Surg Br* 1986;68B:739–746.

94. Jackson DW, Grood EW, Goldstein J, et al. A comparison of patellar tendon autograft and allograft used for anterior cruciate ligament reconstruction in the goat model. *Am J Sports Med* 1993;21:176–185.

95. Howell SM, Clark JA. Tibial tunnel placement in anterior cruciate ligament reconstructions and graft impingement. *Clin Orthop* 1992;238:187–195.

96. O'Donoghue DH. An analysis of and results of surgical treatment of major injuries of the ligaments of the knee. *J Bone Joint Surg Am* 1955:37A:1–13.

97. Wojtys EM, ed. *The ACL deficient knee.* Rosemont, IL: American Academy of Orthopaedic Surgeons Monograph Series, 1993:122.

98. Shelbourne KD, Whitaker JH, McCarroll JR, et al. Anterior cruciate ligament injury: evaluation of intra-articular reconstruction of acute tears without repair. Two to seven year followup of 155 athletes. *Am J Sports Med* 1990;18:484–489.

99. Bonamo JJ, Fay C, Firestone T. The conservative treatment of the anterior cruciate ligament-deficient knee. *Am J Sports Med* 1990;18:1618–1623.

100. Hawkins RJ, Misamore GW, Merritt TR. Follow-up of the acute nonoperated isolated anterior cruciate ligament tear. *Am J Sports Med* 1986;14:205–210.

101. Andersson C, Odensten M, Gillquist J. Knee function after surgical or nonsurgical treatment of acute rupture of the anterior cruciate ligament: A randomized study with a long-term follow-up period. *Clin Orthop* 1991;264:255–263.

102. Clancy WG, Ray JM, Zoltan DJ. Acute tears of the anterior cruciate ligament. Surgical versus conservative treatment. *J Bone Joint Surg Am* 1988;70A:1483–1488.

103. Warren RF. Meniscectomy and repair of the anterior cruciate ligament-deficient patient. *Clin Orthop* 1990;252:55–63.

104. Giove TP, Miller SJ, Kent BE, et al. Non-operative treatment of the torn anterior cruciate ligament. *J Bone Joint Surg Am* 1983;65A:184–192.

105. McDaniel WJ, Dameron TB. Untreated ruptures of the anterior cruciate ligament. *J Bone Joint Surg Am* 1980;62A:696–705.

106. O'Neill DB. Arthroscopically assisted reconstruction of the anterior cruciate ligament. *J Bone Joint Surg Am* 1996;78A:803–813.

107. Olson EJ, Harner CD, Fu FH, et al. Clinical use of fresh frozen soft tissue allografts. *Orthopaedics* 1992;15:1225–1232.

108. Smith AM, Scott SG, O'Fallon WM, et al. Emotional responses of athletes to injury. *Mayo Clin Proc* 1990;65:38–50.

109. Shelbourne KD, Foulk DA. Timing of surgery in acute ACL tears on the return of quadriceps muscle strength following reconstruction using autogenous patellar tendon graft. *Am J Sports Med* 1995;23:686–689.

110. Wasilewski SA, Covall DJ, Cohen S. Effect of surgical timing on recovery and associated injuries after anterior cruciate ligament reconstruction. *Am J Sports Med* 1993;21:338–342.

111. Andrews M, Noyes FR. Anterior cruciate ligament allograft reconstruction in the skeletal immature athlete. *Am J Sports Med* 1994;22:48–54.

112. Tanner JM. *Growth of adolescence,* 2nd ed. Oxford, England: Blackwell Scientific, 1962.

113. Shelbourne KD, Patel DV. Management of combined injures of the anterior cruciate ligament and medial collateral ligament. *J Bone Joint Surg Am* 1995;77A:800–806.

114. Shelbourne KD, Porter DA. Anterior cruciate ligament-medial collateral ligament injury: nonoperative management of medial collateral ligament tears with anterior cruciate ligament reconstruction. *Am J Sports Med* 1992;20:283–286.

115. Shelbourne KD, Johnson GE. Locked bucket-handle meniscal tears in knees with chronic anterior cruciate ligament deficiency. *Am J Sports Med* 1993;21:779–782.

116. Shelbourne KD, Liotta FJ. Preemptive program. Pain management for anterior cruciate ligament reconstruction. *Am J Knee Surg* 1998;11:116–119.

117. Shelbourne KD, Rubinstein RA, McCarroll JR, et al. Postoperative cryotherapy for the knee in ACL reconstructive surgery. *Orthop Int* 1994;2:165–170.

118. Rubinstein RA, Shelbourne KD, VanMeter CD, et al. Effect on

knee stability if full hyperextension is restored immediately after autogenous bone-patellar tendon-bone anterior cruciate ligament reconstruction. *Am J Sports Med* 1995;23:365–368.

119. Graf B, Uhr F. Complications of the intraarticular anterior cruciate reconstruction. *Clin Sports Med* 1988;7:835–848.

120. Noah J, Sherman OH, Roberts C. Fracture of the supracondylar femur after anterior cruciate ligament reconstruction using patellar tendon and iliotibial band tenodesis: a case report. *Am J Sports Med* 1992;20:615–618.

121. Fisher SE, Shelbourne KD. Arthroscopic treatment of symptomatic extension block complicating anterior cruciate ligament reconstruction. *Am J Sports Med* 1993;21:558–564.

122. Shelbourne KD, Johnson GE. Outpatient surgical management of arthrofibrosis after anterior cruciate ligament surgery. *Am J Sports Med* 1994;22:192–197.

123. Shelbourne KD, Patel DV, Martini DJ. Classification and management of arthrofibrosis of the knee after anterior cruciate ligament reconstruction. *Am J Sports Med* 1996;24:857–862.

Principles and Practice of Orthopaedic Sports Medicine,
edited by William E. Garrett, Jr., Kevin P. Speer, and Donald T. Kirkendall.
Lippincott Williams & Wilkins, Philadelphia © 2000.

CHAPTER 42

Posterior Cruciate Ligament

Leslie J. Bisson and William G. Clancy, Jr.

The posterior cruciate ligament (PCL) is the strongest of the two cruciate ligaments and is the primary restraint to posterior tibial translation at 90 degrees of knee flexion. The recent emphasis on reconstructive surgery in cases of anterior cruciate ligament (ACL) injury has stimulated an increased interest in the PCL, and investigators have begun to study the anatomy, biomechanics, and function of the PCL in greater detail. Additionally, there have been attempts to better document the natural history of the PCL-deficient knee and to define the optimum time and method of reconstruction in cases in which surgery is deemed necessary. Despite the large numbers of articles published recently on these topics, the management of injury to the PCL continues to be controversial, because support for both surgical and nonsurgical management can be found in the orthopedic literature.

In this chapter, we provide a summary of what is known about the epidemiology, mechanism of injury, biomechanics and pathoanatomy, clinical evaluation, imaging, treatment, and results of treatment of injuries to the PCL. A section at the end of the chapter outlines the preferences of the senior author (W.G.C.), who has reconstructed over 400 knees with PCL insufficiency.

EPIDEMIOLOGY

Injuries to the PCL are much less frequent than those to the ACL (1–3). Indeed, it is thought that the PCL is injured about one tenth to one twentieth as often as the ACL (4). The incidence of both isolated and combined PCL injuries in series of surgically treated knee injuries ranges from 3.49% (5) to 20% (6,7). How-

ever, the symptoms and clinical signs of isolated PCL injury may be subtle both to the patient and the physician, and the injury may often be missed (8–10). When diagnosed, the isolated PCL injury is often treated nonoperatively. These factors suggest that the true incidence of PCL injury is higher than that quoted in the literature. It is interesting to note that approximately 2% to 5% of the players participating in the National Football League's predraft physical examinations have evidence of isolated PCL laxity and that most of these players are unaware of having had a significant ligamentous injury (11). In a study that analyzed 500 knee ligament injuries with pathologic motion as measured by a KT-1000 arthrometer, 63% were found to be ACL injuries, whereas 7% were PCL injuries (12). Seventy-five percent of the ACL injuries were isolated, as compared with 49% of the PCL injuries. It is not uncommon for PCL injuries to have associated injury to the ACL, medial collateral ligament (MCL), and the posterolateral corner (PLC) (13–15).

ANATOMY

Gross Anatomy

The PCL originates from the lateral portion of the medial femoral condyle at the point where the roof of the intercondylar notch meets the wall of the medial femoral condyle, approximately 1 cm proximal to the articular cartilage (16). The most distal fibers, however, are within 3 mm of the articular surface (17,18). The origin is in the shape of a semicircle, with the horizontal portion facing proximally and having an average length of 32 mm (Fig. 42.1). The overall length of the ligament from origin to insertion averages 38 mm, and the average thickness of the PCL is 13 mm (17). The cross-sectional shape of the PCL is irregular along the length of the ligament and changes with the angle of knee flexion, with the most marked changes occurring near the femo-

L. J. Bisson: American Sports Medicine Institute, Birmingham, Alabama 35205.

W. G. Clancy: Department of Orthopaedic Surgery, University of Alabama at Birmingham, Birmingham, Alabama 35205.

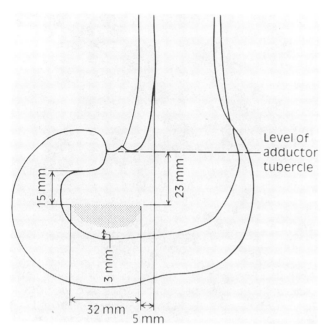

FIG. 42.1. Dimensions of the femoral origin of the posterior cruciate ligament. (From Girgis FG, Marshall JL, Al Monajem ARS. The cruciate ligaments of the knee joint: anatomical, functional and experimental analysis. *Clin Orthop* 1975;106: 216–231, with permission.)

ral origin (19). The ligament inserts on the fovea of the proximal tibia, which is located in a depression between the tibial plateaus 1 cm distal to the articular surface (Fig. 42.2). The average width of this attachment site is 13 mm (17,18).

The tibial footprint is rectangular, but viewed in three

dimensions it is seen to bend across the posterior aspect of the tibial plateau (19). The PCL is narrowest in its midsubstance, fanning out both proximally and distally (17). The PCL is about 50% larger than the ACL at its femoral origin and about 20% larger than the ACL at its tibial insertion (19). It has often been divided into two functional bundles named for their femoral origin followed by their tibial insertion (Fig. 42.3). The bulk of the ligament consists of the anterolateral or antero-central portion, which arises from the anterior part of the site of origin of the PCL on the femur and inserts on the lateral portion of the insertion site on the tibia. These fibers are nonisometric and tighten with flexion of the knee. A smaller portion of the ligament consists of a posteromedial/posterior oblique bundle, which arises from the posterior part of the origin of the PCL on the femur and inserts on the medial part of the tibial insertion site. These fibers tighten with extension of the knee (20). The posteromedial/posterior oblique bundle of the ligament contains some fibers that are isometric throughout the range of motion of the knee.

The PCL is located near the longitudinal axis of rotation of the knee and is slightly medial to the center of the knee (17). It is directed vertically in the frontal plane and at an angle of 30 to 35 degrees in the sagittal plane. The angle of the PCL in the sagittal plane becomes more horizontal with increasing angles of knee flexion (17) (Fig. 42.4).

The PCL is covered anteriorly, medially, and laterally with synovium. which is reflected from the posterior capsule (8). Distally, the insertion of the PCL blends with the proximal tibial periosteum and the posterior capsule.

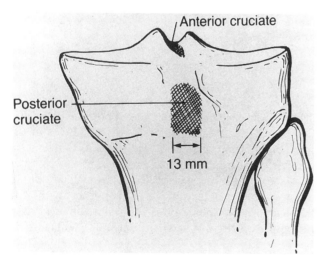

FIG. 42.2. Dimensions of the tibial insertion of the posterior cruciate ligament. (From DeLee JC, Bergfeld JA, Drez D, Jr, et al. The posterior cruciate ligament. In: DeLee JC, Drez D Jr, eds. *Orthopaedic sports medicine. Principles and practice.* Philadelphia: W.B. Saunders, 1994, with permission.)

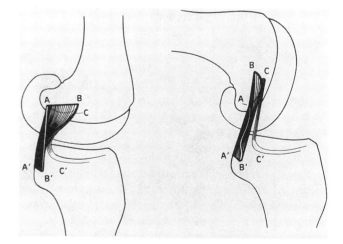

FIG. 42.3. Changes in fiber tension in the posterior cruciate ligament as the knee moves from extension to flexion. **A–A′:** Posteromedial bundle; **B–B′:** anterolateral bundle; **C–C′:** ligament of Humphrey. (From Girgis FG, Marshall JL, Al Mona-jem ARS. The cruciate ligaments of the knee joint: anatomical, functional and experimental analysis. *Clin Orthop* 1975;106: 216–231, with permission.)

Harner et al. (19) used quantitative electron microscopy to compare collagen fibril distribution and area within different portions of the PCL. Ultrastructurally, the PCL begins proximally with a bimodal distribution of large collagen fibrils. This changes to a unimodal distribution of relatively smaller fibrils by the distal midsubstance. This change in fibril size, which corresponds to a gross change in ligament size, was suggested by these investigators to serve a role in the smooth transition of tensile force.

Vascular Supply

Most of the vascular supply of the PCL is from the middle geniculate artery, which is a branch of the popliteal artery that arises just posterior to the popliteal surface of the femur and penetrates the posterior capsule of the knee joint (21). The synovium surrounding the PCL also contributes a large portion of the blood supply of the ligament (21,22), and the base of the PCL is supplied in part by capsular vessels from the inferior geniculate arteries and the popliteal artery (21). Also, several small vessels arising directly from the popliteal artery penetrate the PCL at various portions of its course and send branches both proximally and distally in the ligament.

Innervation

The knee is innervated by an anterior and posterior group of nerves (23). The anterior group is comprised of the femoral, peroneal, and saphenous nerves, and the posterior group consists of the obturator and posterior articular nerves. The posterior articular nerve is the largest nerve supplying the joint and is a branch of the posterior tibial nerve. Fibers from this nerve were noted to penetrate the posterior capsule and synovial lining of the cruciate ligaments (23). Golgi–tendon-like organs have been seen in the cruciate ligaments, particularly near the insertion sites of the ligaments (24,25). These structures are thought to have a proprioceptive function in the knee.

Meniscofemoral Ligaments

Most knees have meniscofemoral ligaments that are present in addition to the PCL. These ligaments originate from the medial femoral condyle, pass anterior and posterior to the PCL, and insert on the lateral meniscus (Fig. 42.4). The anterior meniscofemoral ligament is also known as the ligament of Humphrey, and the posterior meniscofemoral ligament is also known as the ligament of Wrisberg. The incidence of these ligaments in cadaver dissections has ranged from 71% to 100% (26–29). The posterior meniscofemoral ligament originates from the femur at the posterior portion of the

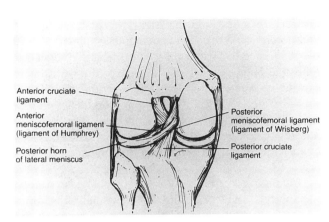

FIG. 42.4. Relationship of the meniscofemoral ligaments to the posterior cruciate ligament. (From DeLee JC, Bergfeld JA, Drez D, Jr, et al. The posterior cruciate ligament. In: DeLee JC, Drez D Jr, eds. *Orthopaedic sports medicine. Principles and practice.* Philadelphia: W.B. Saunders, 1994, with permission.)

site of origin of the PCL and runs obliquely behind the PCL to attach to the posterior horn of the lateral meniscus (28). Fibers of this ligament may also attach to the posterior tibia or posterior capsule. In this case the ligament's attachments to the lateral meniscus are via the posterior capsule and popliteus (18,28,30). This ligament may be nearly 50% as large as the PCL (28). The anterior meniscofemoral ligament fibers originate within the anterior portion of the footprint of the PCL on the medial femoral condyle, pass anterior to the PCL, and insert on the posterior horn of the lateral meniscus. This ligament is usually less than one third the size of the PCL (28).

BIOMECHANICS AND PATHOANATOMY

The major biomechanical function of the PCL is to provide resistance to posterior tibial translation. Secondary functions include providing resistance to hyperextension (after injury to the ACL) (17,31), limiting external rotation, and preventing varus–valgus rotation.

The biomechanics of the PCL have been well studied by Butler et al. (32), who used cutting studies to define the contribution of the PCL to stability of the knee. They found the PCL to be the primary restraint to posterior tibial translation with the knee in 90 degrees of flexion. They reported that the PCL contributes 95% of the restraining force to posterior translation at this degree of knee flexion. Similar results were found when the knee was studied at 30 degrees of flexion. The absolute amount of posterior translation after isolated section of the PCL increased as the flexion angle of the knee increased. The investigators also evaluated the role of the secondary restraints in resisting the posterior drawer test and found that the posterolateral capsule and popliteus muscle–tendon complex supplied 59% of the resistance to further posterior translation, once the PCL had been cut. Sixteen percent of the restraint to further posterior translation after section of the PCL was provided by the MCL. The authors believed that secondary restraints were used only when the PCL was absent but pointed out that the secondary restraints may confuse the finding of clinical laxity when manual forces are used.

Gollehon et al. (33) and Grood et al. (34) also studied the ability of the PCL to prevent abnormal translations of the knee and explored the interplay between the PCL and the lateral collateral ligament (LCL) and deep lateral ligament complex (which is composed of the arcuate ligament, popliteus tendon, fabellofibular ligament, and posterolateral capsule). The findings of Gollehon et al. are summarized below.

Anterior–Posterior Translation

Gollehon et al. (33) also concluded that the PCL was the primary structure preventing posterior tibial translation at all angles of knee flexion. They found the PCL to be most functional at higher angles of knee flexion. Therefore, patients with isolated PCL injuries have more normal function at angles closer to full extension. Isolated section of the LCL or the deep lateral ligament complex produced no increase in posterior translation at any angle of knee flexion, whereas combined section of the lateral collateral and deep lateral ligament complex resulted in small increases in posterior translation at all angles of knee flexion. At 0 and 30 degrees of flexion, section of either the PCL or the lateral collateral and deep lateral ligament complex resulted in similar increases in posterior translation. Combined cutting of the PCL, LCL, and deep lateral ligament complex caused large (i.e., 20 to 25 mm) increases in posterior translation at all flexion angles when compared with either the intact knee or knees in which isolated sectionings of either ligament or ligament complex had been performed.

Varus–Valgus Rotation

Gollehon et al. (33) also found that the LCL and the deep lateral ligament complex act together to provide the primary restraint to varus rotation of the tibia. When the LCL and deep lateral ligament complex are intact, section of the PCL does not lead to any increase in varus rotation. However, section of the PCL after section of the LCL and the deep lateral ligament complex leads to increases in varus rotation. This allowed greater than 30 degrees of varus angulation at 60 degrees of knee flexion. Knees with injury to the PCL and the posterolat-

eral structures were unstable in extension and at 30 degrees of flexion.

Internal–External Rotation of the Tibia

Section of the deep lateral ligament complex alone leads to a small (approximately 6 degrees) increase in external rotation at 90 degrees of flexion. Isolated cutting of the LCL causes small (approximately 2 to 3 degrees) increases in external rotation at 0, 30, and 90 degrees of flexion. Cutting both the lateral collateral and deep lateral ligament complex results in further increased external rotation at all flexion angles. Section of the PCL alone leads to no increase in external rotation. However, section of the PCL after section of the LCL and the deep lateral ligament complex causes further increased external rotation at 60 and 90 degrees of knee flexion but no increase in external rotation at 30 degrees of flexion. The authors concluded that increased external rotation at 30 degrees of flexion is a sign of PLC injury, whereas increased external rotation at 30 degrees, which is even greater at 90 degrees, is a sign of injury to both the PCL and the posterolateral structures.

Articular Contact Pressures

It has been shown experimentally that injury to the PCL leads to increased contact pressures in the medial and patellofemoral compartments of the knee (35). However, the incidence of degenerative arthritis after PCL injury and the degree to which each compartment is involved remains controversial (1,36–40).

Tensile Strength

Kennedy et al. (41) measured the tensile strength of the PCL in excised ligament specimens and showed that it was approximately twice as strong as the ACL. Prieto et al. (42) tested the femur–PCL–tibia complex in young cadaveric knees and reported a linear stiffness of approximately 200 N/mm and an ultimate load of approximately 1,600 N. In a related study, Race and Amis (43) tested the anterolateral and posteromedial components of the PCL separately and concluded that the anterolateral component was significantly stiffer and stronger than the posteromedial component.

Recently, Harner et al. (19) reported the tensile properties of the anterolateral, posteromedial, and meniscofemoral portions of the PCL and characterized their relative stiffnesses and strengths within the same knee. They found that when compared with the posteromedial and meniscofemoral portions, the anterolateral component of the PCL had the highest stiffness by a factor of 2.3 and 2.9, respectively; the highest ultimate load by a factor of 2.9 and 3.4, respectively; and the highest failure energy by a factor of 4.1 and 11.1, respectively. The mean stiffnesses were as follows: anterolateral component, 120 N/mm; posteromedial component, 57 N/mm; and meniscofemoral component, 49 N/mm. The mean ultimate loads were as follows: anterolateral component, 1,120 N; posteromedial component, 419 N; and meniscofemoral component, 297 N.

Meniscofemoral Ligaments

Boyd and Bergfeld carried out studies of the meniscofemoral ligaments and their function in preventing posterior tibial translation (J. Boyd and J.A. Bergfeld, personal communication, 1991). When isolated from the PCL, the meniscofemoral ligaments were found to provide 10% of the resistance to the posterior drawer test, whereas the PCL provided 85% of the resistance.

MECHANISM OF INJURY

When discussing the mechanism of injury to the PCL, it is helpful for the examiner to differentiate between low-energy (i.e., athletic) and high-energy (i.e., motor vehicle accident) etiologies because of the higher incidence of combined ligamentous injuries and associated

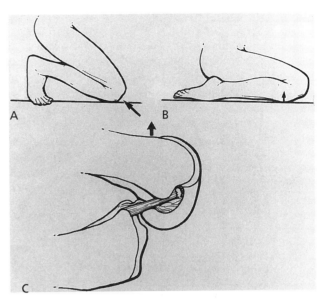

FIG. 42.6. Mechanisms of injury to the posterior cruciate ligament (PCL). (From DeLee JC, Bergfeld JA, Drez D, Jr, et al. The posterior cruciate ligament. In: DeLee JC, Drez D Jr, eds. *Orthopaedic sports medicine. Principles and practice.* Philadelphia: W.B. Saunders, 1994, with permission.) **A:** A fall onto the flexed knee with the foot in dorsiflexion results in force being transmitted through the patellofemoral joint. **B:** A fall onto the flexed knee with the foot in plantarflexion results in force being transmitted to the tibial tubercle and hence to the PCL. **C:** A hyperflexion injury can result in an avulsion of the origin of the PCL from the femur.

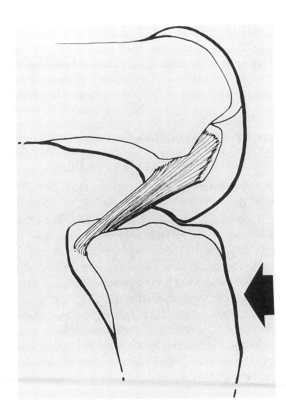

FIG. 42.5. Mechanism of injury to the posterior cruciate ligament: a posterior force applied to the proximal tibia with the knee in 90 degrees of flexion. (From DeLee JC, Bergfeld JA, Drez D, Jr, et al. The posterior cruciate ligament. In: DeLee JC, Drez D Jr, eds. *Orthopaedic sports medicine. Principles and practice.* Philadelphia: W.B. Saunders, 1994, with permission.)

injuries in the latter (44). Injury to the PCL has been described as occurring in one of four classical ways (Figs. 42.5 to 42.7): a posterior force applied to the tibia with the knee in flexion, a fall onto the flexed knee with the foot in plantarflexion, hyperflexion, and hyperextension. Two other less-common means of injury have been recently described, including a noncontact external rotation/posterior translation injury (45) and an external rotation/valgus injury (46).

A posterior force applied to the proximal tibia with the knee in flexion is a common mechanism of PCL injury (Fig. 42.5), and this often accounts for the injury seen after a motor vehicle accident. In this case the flexed knee is struck by the posteriorly moving dashboard. This is thought to often result in an isolated midsubstance injury to the PCL (47), but the magnitude of the forces involved in a motor vehicle accident can also result in fractures or injuries to other ligaments.

The most common cause of PCL injury in sports was initially described by the senior author (W.G.C.). The mechanism consists of a fall onto a flexed knee while the foot is in plantar flexion (1,48) (Fig. 42.6A and B). This position of the foot allows the blow to be delivered to the tibial tubercle and therefore to be transmitted to the PCL. It should be noted that this injury, like that of the first mechanism, occurs with the knee joint in 90

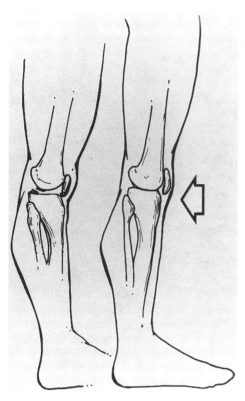

FIG. 42.7. Mechanism of injury to the posterior cruciate ligament: hyperextension. (From DeLee JC, Bergfeld JA, Drez D, Jr, et al. The posterior cruciate ligament. In: DeLee JC, Drez D Jr, eds. *Orthopaedic sports medicine. Principles and practice.* Philadelphia: W.B. Saunders, 1994, with permission.)

degrees of flexion. If the foot is in dorsiflexion, the flexion of the knee joint is greater than 90 degrees when the tibia strikes the ground. In this case it is thought that the force is transmitted to the patellofemoral joint rather than to the PCL and thus may cause a patellar fracture but spares the PCL.

Fowler and Messieh (9) reported that hyperflexion alone can result in PCL injury (Fig. 42.6C). This mechanism may often result in avulsion of the origin of the PCL from the medial femoral condyle with a portion of the periosteum remaining attached. This periosteal fragment may allow anatomic repair of the avulsed ligament back to its origin, resulting in a stable knee. It is our experience that a hyperflexion injury more often produces an interstitial PCL failure. With hyperflexion the amount of tibial/femoral displacement is somewhat limited, producing failure in the zone of plasticity. There is not sufficient displacement to produce ultimate yield of the ligament. A number of these patients will tighten up one grade over a 3-month period. A grade II posterior drawer (femoral condyles flush with the anterior tibia) will become a grade I posterior drawer.

The three mechanisms of injury listed above will often result in injury that is limited to the PCL. The knee

may exhibit minimal swelling, and the patient may be unaware of the significance of the injury. These injuries can occur in the midsubstance of the ligament and allow the ligament to remain in continuity but to functionally exhibit laxity. The posterior drawer test may be positive, but ligament continuity can be demonstrated on magnetic resonance imaging (MRI). It has been the experience of the senior author that these injuries in continuity may often undergo contraction as they heal, resulting in diminished posterior translation on posterior drawer testing as the time from injury increases.

The final classic mechanism of PCL injury occurs when a posteriorly directed force is applied to a hyperextended knee with the foot fixed on the ground (Fig. 42.7). In this case, ACL failure happens first, followed by capsular and PCL injury at 30 degrees of hyperextension, and finally by popliteal artery failure at 50 degrees of hyperextension (41). A variant of this injury pattern common to contact sports involves a blow to the anteromedial tibia with the foot planted. This forces the knee into hyperextension and varus and often results in combined injury to the PCL and PLC.

In addition to these commonly observed mechanisms of injury, Shelbourne and Rubenstein (45) described three cases of PCL injury that occurred due to a noncontact external rotation force coupled with posterior translation that took place while the athlete changed direction with the foot planted but unloaded. Shelbourne et al. (46) also described a combined PCL–MCL injury caused by a valgus and external rotation force applied to a flexed knee with the foot fixed but unloaded.

CLINICAL EVALUATION

Isolated Posterior Cruciate Ligament Injury

It has been stated by many authors that diagnosis of injury to the PCL can often be confusing, particularly when it occurs acutely and is isolated. The presence of quadriceps muscle spasm may mask some of the findings on physical examination, and the isolated injury to the PCL may be dismissed by the athlete as insignificant (11). The presence of a tense effusion such as occurs with an acute ACL injury is usually absent. For this reason the history and physical examination are of paramount importance, not only to diagnose the injury itself but also to determine the site of the injury and therefore to determine the appropriate treatment plan.

History

Knowledge of the mechanism of injury in cases of suspected PCL injury can help determine the likelihood of injury to the ligament and suggest the potential site of involvement along the length of the PCL. Injury to the midsubstance of the PCL often occurs after a direct blow to the anterior proximal tibia with the knee flexed (9,49). Midsubstance injuries also may occur after a fall onto the flexed knee with the foot in plantarflexion, which concentrates the bulk of the force on the tibial tubercle (48). A blow to the anteromedial aspect of the proximal tibia with the knee in extension is a common mechanism in sport-related injuries and also results in midsubstance injury to the PCL and injury to the PLC structures. A pure hyperflexion injury without a force being applied directly to the proximal tibia often results in avulsion of the origin of the ligament from the medial femoral condyle, offering a chance for primary repair (48).

In cases of chronic PCL injury, a common complaint is discomfort in the knee while weight bearing in a semiflexed position, such as ascending or descending stairs or squatting down to pick something up (50). Aching in the knee when walking long distances was also found to be a common complaint (50). Approximately 50% of patients with symptomatic PCL insufficiency will complain of instability in the knee when walking on uneven ground (50). Approximately half of the patients reported by Cross and Powell (8) complained of retropatellar pain in the knee that was not present initially but developed at some point after the injury. Swelling and stiffness may vary and may depend on the degree of associated chondral damage. These authors also reported that some patients would complain of instability while walking on uneven ground.

Physical Examination

An acute injury to the PCL may often be missed for several reasons. Often the athlete is unaware of significant injury, because most patients have a full range of motion with very little hemarthrosis (1,11,50,51). Often it is only the posterior drawer test that causes any pain. The presence of a contusion over the proximal anterior tibia may be very helpful in suggesting injury to the PCL in this setting.

The importance of noting the relationship of the proximal tibia to the femur when the knee is flexed to 90 degrees cannot be overemphasized. When the PCL is intact, flexion of the knee to 90 degrees results in the anterior proximal tibia being positioned approximately 1 cm anterior to the distal femoral condyles (Fig. 42.8). This is referred to as a normal anterior step-off. Loss of this normal anterior step-off signifies injury to the PCL. The importance of detecting this posterior subluxation has been emphasized by Clancy et al. (1), which they state is best noted from the side with the knee flexed to 90 degrees. This posterior subluxation of the proximal tibia with the knee flexed to 90 degrees is also known as the posterior sag sign (of Godfrey).

The posterior drawer test performed at 70 to 90 degrees of flexion has been regarded as the most reliable

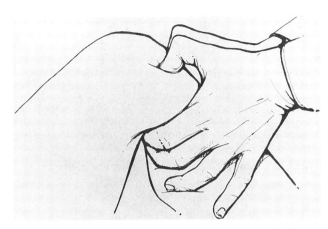

FIG. 42.8. When the posterior cruciate ligament is intact, flexion of the knee to 90 degrees should result in the proximal tibial emminence being anterior to the distal femoral condyles by approximately 1 cm. (From DeLee JC, Bergfeld JA, Drez D, Jr, et al. The posterior cruciate ligament. In: DeLee JC, Drez D Jr, eds. *Orthopaedic sports medicine. Principles and practice.* Philadelphia: W.B. Saunders, 1994, with permission.)

sign of PCL disruption (52,53) (Fig. 42.9). This test is graded with respect to the opposite knee. Loss of the normal anterior tibial step-off when compared with the opposite side, but with the proximal tibial eminence remaining anterior to the distal femur, is considered to

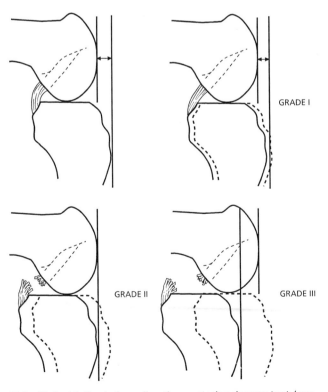

FIG. 42.9. Method of grading the posterior drawer test (see text for explanation).

be a 1+ posterior drawer. When the proximal tibial emmience can be translated posteriorly to the point where it is flush with the distal femoral condyles, the posterior drawer is graded 2+. This is thought to signify complete disruption of the PCL. Translation of the proximal tibial emmience posterior to the distal femoral condyles is considered to be grade 3+ and is thought to signify complete PCL and posterolateral ligament injury. This test, however, has been reported to be positive in as few as 10% to 76% of patients with acute PCL disruptions (13,29,31,52). Hughston et al. (13) found that only 31% of their patients with an acute PCL injury had a positive posterior drawer, whereas Loos et al. (54) found a positive posterior drawer in 51% of their acute PCL disruptions. Kennedy and Grainger (31), Moore and Larson (52), and Savatsky et al. (53) reported a positive posterior drawer in 51%, 67%, and 76%, respectively, of their acute injuries. Clancy et al. (1) stated that a 2+ posterior drawer, with the tibia held first in neutral and then in external rotation, is diagnostic of a complete disruption of the PCL. They also emphasized that 80% of patients with complete disruption of the PCL would have a normal posterior drawer sign with the tibia held in internal rotation. This loss of the posterior drawer with the tibia held in internal rotation is explained by the fact that internal tibial rotation tightens the meniscofemoral ligaments, which are usually intact after injury to the PCL. These ligaments are then able to resist attempted posterior tibial translation during the posterior drawer maneuver. The authors also found meniscal injury to be uncommon both clinically and at arthroscopy when the PCL was injured. Finally, these investigators also stated that muscle spasm and pain could significantly limit the utility of the posterior drawer test.

The accuracy of the posterior drawer test in the chronic setting has been documented by Rubinstein et al. (55). These examiners found that the posterior drawer test, including palpation of the tibial step-off, was the most sensitive and specific clinical test of PCL insufficiency. Clinical examination for chronic PCL injury was 96% accurate, 90% sensitive, and 99% specific. The interobserver agreement for the grade of the injury was 81%.

Because the presence of muscle spasm has been shown to limit the effectiveness of the posterior drawer test in the acute setting, Daniel et al. (56) introduced the quadriceps active drawer test to detect PCL injury (Fig. 42.10). This test is based on the biomechanical relationship between the line of action of the patellar tendon and the resultant quadriceps muscle force. In an intact knee, the line of action of the patellar tendon tends to pull the proximal tibia anterior at low knee flexion angles. At high knee flexion angles, the PCL causes the femur to roll back on the proximal tibia, and the line of action of the patellar tendon therefore tends

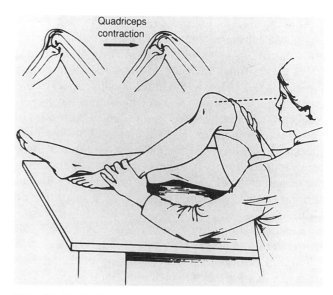

FIG. 42.10. Performance of the quadriceps active drawer test. See text for explanation. (From Daniel DM, Stone ML, Barnett P, et al. Use of the quadriceps active test to diagnose posterior cruciate ligament disruption and measure posterior laxity of the knee. *J Bone Joint Surg Am* 1988;70A:386–391, with permission.)

to pull the proximal tibia posterior. The angle of knee flexion at which the line of action of the patellar tendon is directly perpendicular to the surface of the tibial plateau is called the quadriceps neutral angle and occurs at 60 to 90 degrees of flexion in the intact knee. In a knee with the PCL injured or absent, roll-back of the femur on the tibia does not occur with increasing knee flexion. Therefore, the line of action of the patellar tendon is always directed anteriorly.

The quadriceps active drawer is performed with the subject relaxed in the supine position with the knee flexed 70 to 90 degrees. The examiner stabilizes the patients foot on the table and then asks the patient to slide the foot distally on the table. In the normal knee, the patellar tendon line of action will be directed posteriorly, and this quadriceps contraction will not cause any anterior translation of the proximal tibia. However, in the patient with deficiency of the PCL, the posterior sag of the proximal tibia will result in the line of action of the patellar tendon being directed anteriorly, and this quadriceps contraction will result in a notable anterior translation of the proximal tibia. Daniel et al. (56) found the quadriceps active drawer test to be positive in 41 of 42 knees with documented disruption of the PCL. Anterior translation did not occur in the contralateral normal knee of these patients nor did it occur in 25 knees with known disruption of the ACL. These authors found this test to be useful in both acute and chronic cases.

Combined Posterior Cruciate Ligament and Collateral Ligament Injury

History

Combined injuries to the PCL and PLC structures are often caused by a blow to the anteromedial tibia with the knee in extension. This mechanism of injury is not uncommon in sport-related injuries to the PCL. A blow delivered to the lateral aspect of the knee causes a valgus force at the knee joint and first injures the MCL and the posteromedial capsule. Once these structures have been injured, the cruciate ligaments are the next restraints to valgus rotation. This mechanism of injury may cause combined ACL–MCL or PCL–MCL injuries. Finally, impact to the medial aspect of the knee first causes disruption of the LCL and the PLC structures. If the injury is severe enough, the central pivot ligaments are next to fail. This mechanism results in combined injury to the ACL and posterolateral structures or the PCL and posterolateral structures.

The patient with combined PCL and collateral ligament injury often has a significant amount of pain when compared with the patient with an isolated PCL injury. Disruption of the capsule that occurs in conjunction with collateral ligament injury may allow dissection of the hemarthrosis into the thigh and leg and therefore limit the amount of effusion present. The primary concern in the knee with multiple ligament injuries is the possibility of neurovascular injury. It has been reported that approximately 50% of knee dislocations reduce spontaneously at the time of injury and are consequently not evident at the time of initial evaluation (57). For this reason, any patient with disruption of multiple knee ligaments must be suspected of having had a knee dislocation, and careful attention must be paid to the vascular and neurologic status of the extremity. Consultation of a vascular surgeon to determine the need for anteriography or exploration is mandatory in cases with any change in the vascular status of the injured extremity. Arteriography to rule out intimal injury is recommended for known instances of dislocation, even in the presence of normal pulses. It also should be kept in mind that patients with combined PCL and lateral ligamentous injury have an incidence of peroneal nerve injury that approaches 30% (57).

An individual with chronic PCL and posterolateral laxity will often complain of instability of the knee that is particularly bothersome when walking on uneven ground. The knee is felt to give way at the posterolateral aspect, and pain is felt medially and posterolaterally. The medial pain is due to increased medial joint loads that are a result of both the increased medial compartment loads secondary to PCL insufficiency (35) and to the varus thrust present during gait. The posterolateral pain is a result of stretching of those structures during the varus thrust component of gait.

Physical Examination

The patient with suspected combined PCL and posterolateral ligament complex injury is first examined using the above-mentioned tests to assess the integrity of the PCL. Varus laxity with the knee held in 30 degrees of flexion indicates injury to the fibular collateral ligament and possible injury to the posterolateral structures. Placing the leg in the figure-of-four position allows palpation of the LCL and enables one to confirm its integrity. The external rotation recurvatum test can help to determine the presence of injury to the posterolateral structures and is performed by grasping the great toes of each leg with the knees in extension and lifting each leg off of the examining table. Hyperextension and increased external rotation of the involved leg suggests significant injury to the posterolateral structures (Fig. 42.11). The posterolateral drawer test, which is positive when the lateral tibial plateau rotates externally and posteriorly at the end of the posterior drawer test, is another helpful test in determining the presence of injury to the posterolateral structures. However, it should be noted that these test have a relatively low sensitivity, being present in only 25% and 33% of patients, respectively (58).

Gollehon et al. (33) showed that a 15-degree increase in tibial external rotation at 30 degrees of knee flexion

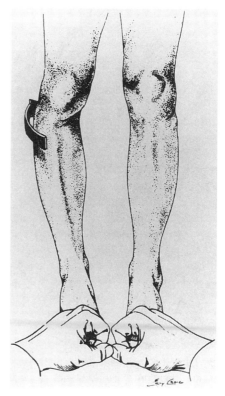

FIG. 42.11. The external rotation recurvatum test. (From Hughston and Norwood. *Clin Orthop* 1980;147:82, with permission.)

is indicative of significant injury to the posterolateral structures. Increased external rotation of the tibia at 90 degrees of flexion indicates injury to both the PCL and posterolateral ligament complex. The reverse pivot shift test, introduced by Jakob et al. (16), is another test that is used to assess the posterolateral ligaments. In the reverse pivot shift test, the knee is reduced in full extension. As the examiner applies a valgus and external rotation force while flexing the knee, the lateral tibial plateau can be felt to subluxate posteriorly. This creates a shifting sensation similar to that felt during the classic pivot shift in patients with ACL laxity. All the above tests are more profoundly positive in the presence of associated PCL insufficiency.

Injury to the MCL in combination with PCL injury is detected by increased valgus laxity at both full extension and 30 degrees of flexion. The above-mentioned tests for PCL injury are also positive. There will also be a greater posterior translation of the medial tibial plateau during the posterior drawer test at 90 degrees of knee flexion. It should be noted that PCL/MCL injury is less common than PCL/PLC injury. Finally, patients with injury to the PCL and both the medial and lateral sides of the knee will exhibit symmetric posterior displacement of both tibial plateaus during the posterior drawer test.

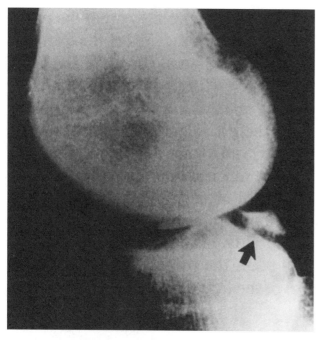

FIG. 42.12. Lateral radiograph of the knee demonstrating avulsion of the insertion of the posterior cruciate ligament from the tibia. (From Cooper DE, Warren RF, Warner JJP. The posterior cruciate ligament and posterolateral structures of the knee: anatomy, function and patterns of injury. *Instr Course Lect* 1991;40:249–270, with permission.)

IMAGING

Routine Radiographs

Standard anteroposterior, lateral, tunnel, and axial patellofemoral views are usually taken in patients with acute PCL injury but often are not diagnostic. The lateral radiograph may show an avulsion of the PCL from its tibial insertion, but this is a relatively uncommon injury (10,59–61) (Fig. 42.12). In cases of chronic PCL insufficiency, radiographs may show evidence of arthrosis of the medial and patellofemoral articulations.

Plumb-line weight-bearing radiographs are essential in the preoperative patient to allow determination of the mechanical alignment of the limb (5). If the patient with posterolateral laxity and varus alignment has a ligamentous reconstruction without correction of the mechanical axis by osteotomy, the abnormal stresses imposed on the reconstruction by the varus alignment would be expected to result in failure of the reconstruction.

Stress Radiographs

We have found stress lateral radiographs to be helpful in documenting the presence of injury to the PCL. Comparison radiographs taken at 70 to 90 degrees of flexion with first an anterior and then a posterior stress are helpful both for diagnosis of PCL insufficiency and for comparing with postoperative stress radiographs to allow objective comparison of results among investigators. Correction of the total anteroposterior translation to that present in the normal opposite knee is one objective way of suggesting that the restoration of normal biomechanics of the knee has been achieved.

The utility of stress radiographs in the documentation of complete PCL injury and in the differentiation between complete and partial tears of the PCL has been recently studied by Hewett et al. (62). These investigators found that 8 mm or more of increased posterior translation occurring with the application of an 89-N posterior load at 70 degrees of flexion was indicative of a complete rupture of the PCL. They also found that stress radiographs were superior to both KT-1000 arthrometry and clinical examination in assessing the status of the PCL.

Magnetic Resonance Imaging

MRI has greatly increased the accuracy with which acute ligamentous injuries of the knee may be detected and correctly diagnosed and has allowed the detection of other associated injuries to the menisci, cartilage, and subchondral bone (63). MRI in patients with suspected injury to the PCL cannot only confirm the injury but can also determine the site of injury to the ligament

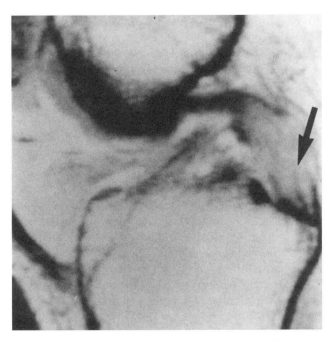

FIG. 42.13. Lateral magnetic resonance image of the knee demonstrating midsubstance disruption of the posterior cruciate ligament. (From DeLee JC, Bergfeld JA, Drez D, Jr, et al. The posterior cruciate ligament. In: DeLee JC, Drez D Jr, eds. *Orthopaedic sports medicine. Principles and practice.* Philadelphia: W.B. Saunders, 1994, with permission.)

(Fig. 42.13). It has also been noted by the senior author (W.G.C.) that MRI may show a lesion in continuity of the PCL. This injury is characterized by increased signal in the midsubstance of the ligament without evidence of complete disruption and is characterized by laxity of the PCL on clinical examination. Clancy has found that this injury may heal with a decrease in the initial laxity.

Bone Scan

A bone scan may be helpful in following the patient with pain and isolated PCL insufficiency. Isolated chronic PCL insufficiency rarely leads to instability, and the disability from this injury is more often due to pain secondary to articular cartilage changes. For this reason, it has been suggested that serial bone scanning may allow early diagnosis of changes of the articular cartilage in the patient who is being treated nonoperatively. Early recognition of increased joint contact pressures secondary to the abnormal knee biomechanics present in the knee with PCL insufficiency may allow a reconstruction to arrest these changes before irreversible progression takes place. This argument, however, assumes that reconstruction of the PCL restores the knee biomechanics to normal and prevents further deterioration of the articular cartilage. To date, this has not been shown in any scientific study.

TREATMENT

The treatment of the knee with a PCL injury is controversial, and recommendations have been made for both operative and nonoperative management. A large part of the controversy is because very few studies in the orthopedic literature document the long-term results of any form of treatment. Many studies do not differentiate between results obtained for knees with isolated PCL injury versus combined injury patterns or between results obtained in cases of chronic versus acute PCL insufficiency. The relative infrequency of PCL injury combined with the conventionally narrow indications for operative treatment also make it difficult for one surgeon to gain a large experience in the treatment of the PCL-insufficient knee. The following section reviews the current literature with respect to the treatment of the PCL-injured knee, dividing the results into those obtained for avulsion injuries, isolated PCL injuries, combined instability patterns, and chronic PCL insufficiency. A section at the end of the chapter outlines the preferences of the senior author (W.G.C.) in his experience of over 400 operative cases of PCL reconstruction.

Nonoperative

Several authorities have recommended nonoperative management for isolated PCL injuries (9,31,36,40,50, 64,65). Short-term follow-up studies of patients treated without surgery indicated that these individuals generally did well (9,64,65), but more recent long-term follow-up reports have documented worse results and radiographic deterioration with increasing time from the injury (38,66). When the PCL is torn, the patella and patellar tendon take on a more prominent role in the prevention of posterior tibial translation (8,67). Also, the increased posterior tibial sag that occurs in the PCL-deficient knee shortens the moment arm of the quadriceps, decreasing its mechanical advantage (68). Therefore, the nonoperative management of PCL injuries should emphasize quadriceps strengthening as a key component of the rehabilitation program (64). However, restoration of satisfactory quadriceps strength does not necessarily ensure a good long-term clinical result (38).

Rehabilitation

The goal of physical therapy is to strengthen the muscles that act to prevent posterior tibial translation, particularly the quadriceps, while minimizing gravity-induced posterior tibial sag (69). Open kinetic chain hamstring exercises (which are performed with the foot free, in contrast to closed kinetic chain exercises, which are performed with the foot fixed), which cause posterior tibial translation in the PCL-deficient knee, are avoided (70). Closed kinetic chain exercises, such as the squat, cause less shear force at the tibiofemoral joint (70) and are the preferred method for strengthening. However, properly performed open kinetic chain exercises, such as the leg extension, may be used if certain precautions are followed. Green et al. (71) found that open kinetic chain extension exercises in the range from 70 to 0 degrees of flexion minimized posterior tibial translation. Placement of the resistance pad distally on the leg during the exercise routine lessens articular contact pressures in the medial compartment and diminishes the posterior stresses on the secondary restraints (36,72).

The rehabilitation program used for the patient with PCL injury involves three phases: a maximum protection phase, which is used during the first 2 weeks after injury; a moderate protection phase, used from weeks 4 to 6 after injury; and a minimal protection phase, used 6 to 8 weeks after injury.

The maximum protection phase is initiated after the diagnosis of an acute PCL injury and is progressed over the first 2 to 3 weeks. Weight bearing as tolerated is encouraged using two crutches, and a brace permitting range of motion from 0 to 60 degrees is prescribed according to the preferences and comfort of the patient. When the individual is comfortable, he or she begins straight leg raises; knee extension from 60 to 0 degrees; quad isometrics at 60, 40, and 20 degrees; and mini-squats and leg presses from 0 to 45 degrees. Over the next 2 to 3 weeks, full weight bearing is achieved, the patient begins cycling for range of motion, and leg press range of motion increases up to 60 degrees of flexion.

The moderate protection phase takes place from weeks 3 to 6 after the injury. Range of motion is increased to normal as the individual tolerates, and bracing (if used) is discontinued. Resistance exercises are increased, and the patient may begin activities such as rowing and stairmaster machines. Running may be initiated in the pool during this phase. Light resistance hamstring curls and step-ups are also introduced.

The minimal protection phase begins at weeks 6 to 8. All strengthening exercises are continued, a running program is used, and the patient may gradually return to sporting activities. Criteria to be met before returning to sport include the absence of pain, tenderness, and swelling and isokinetic testing documenting at least 85% strength on the injured compared with the normal side.

When to Refer

We believe that patients initially diagnosed with either acute or chronic isolated injury to the PCL may be initially managed with the above rehabilitation program. Patients with injury to another major knee ligament in addition to the PCL should be referred for

surgical consultation, as should individuals with isolated PCL injury who continue to have pain or instability despite use of the above rehab program for at least 3 months.

Operative

Avulsion Fractures of the Tibial Insertion of the Posterior Cruciate Ligament

Most authors have recommended operative repair of a displaced bony avulsion of the tibial insertion of the PCL (10,36,59,60,73) (Figs. 42.14 and 42.15). Undisplaced fractures are treated with immobilization of the knee in extension, using the intact collateral ligaments to help prevent posterior sag (74,75).

Lee (76) in 1937 reported on one patient with an avulsion fracture treated with repair. McMaster (73) described obtaining a functional range of motion and no instability in two patients treated with operative repair, but the follow-up was limited to only 3 months in both patients.

Trickey (10) reported the results of treatment of bony avulsion fractures of the tibial insertion of the PCL in 13 patients. Eight avulsions were treated operatively

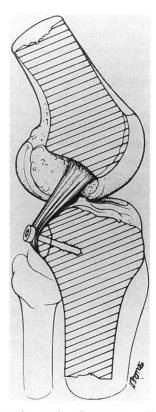

FIG. 42.14. Posterior cruciate ligament avulsion from the tibia fixed with a screw. (From Bowen MK, Warren RF, Cooper DE. Posterior cruciate ligament and related injuries. In: Insall et al., eds. *Surgery of the Knee.* New York: Churchill Livingstone, with permission.)

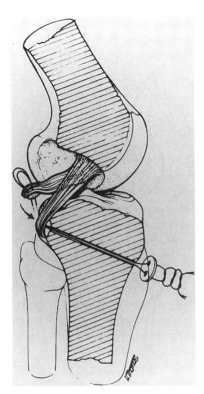

FIG. 42.15. Tibial avulsion of the posterior cruciate ligament reattached with sutures placed through the bony fragment and secured over a button. (From Bowen MK, Warren RF, Cooper DE. Posterior cruciate ligament and related injuries. In: Insall et al., eds. *Surgery of the Knee.* New York: Churchill Livingstone, with permission.)

and five nonoperatively. Two operatively treated patients had a residual flexion contracture but were said to have a stable knee. Three nonoperatively treated patients had residual instability, and one lost flexion. Only one nonoperatively treated patient regained a full range of motion and had a stable knee.

Torisu (59) summarized the results of treatment of 21 patients with avulsion fractures of the tibial insertion of the PCL. Small or nondisplaced fractures were treated with immobilization in a cast, whereas large or displaced fragments were fixed with staples. All patients had an excellent or good result at an average of 4 years of follow-up. Torisu (60) also noted that it was possible to obtain satisfactory results in fractures treated with repair if the fracture was less than 7 weeks old but that repairs delayed beyond 11 weeks from the time of injury resulted in less satisfactory results.

Isolated Posterior Cruciate Ligament Injury

Most authors have recommended a nonoperative approach to the treatment of isolated PCL injuries. Dandy and Pusey (50) described 20 patients with isolated PCL injuries who were treated nonoperatively. Patients were treated with either cast immobilization or early range of motion and followed for an average of 7.2 years. All patients were referred due to symptoms arising from the knee and therefore do not represent a true example of the natural history of the injury. Despite the presence of symptoms, the authors did not believe that the patients' disabilities warranted operative reconstruction of the PCL. It should be noted, however, that radiographs to evaluate the presence of degenerative joint disease were not performed in this study.

Teitjens (77) reported the results of nonoperative treatment in 50 patients with isolated PCL tears. Eighty percent of the patients achieved a good or excellent functional result. Twenty percent complained of either disabling instability (10%) or meniscal tears (10%). Teitjens concluded that reconstruction was not warranted in most patients with isolated rupture.

Cross and Powell (8) summarized the results of treatment of 116 patients with PCL injury, 67 of whom were treated without surgery. These authors also did not use radiographic criteria to define their results and did not divide patients into groups with combined versus isolated PCL injuries. Fifty-four patients had good or excellent results, 4 had fair results, and 9 had poor results. There was a slight correlation between the result and quadriceps function.

Parolie and Bergfeld (64) reported the results of nonoperative management of PCL injury in 25 patients followed for an average of 6.2 years. Eighty percent of their patients were satisfied with their knee function, and 68% had returned to their previous level of sporting activity. Quadriceps strength as measured by Cybex testing was the most important prognostic factor for a good result. All patients who were satisfied had higher values for quadriceps strength in the involved leg, and all patients who were dissatisfied had lower values for quadriceps strength in the involved leg.

Torg et al. (40) followed 14 isolated and 29 combined PCL injuries for an average of 6.3 years and concluded that the patients with isolated injuries remained asymptomatic and did not require reconstruction. It is significant to note, however, that 60% of the patients with isolated injuries and radiographic follow-up had evidence of medial compartment degeneration on x-ray.

Fowler and Messieh (9) reported on 13 patients with isolated PCL injuries treated nonoperatively and followed for an average of 2.6 years. All individuals returned to their previous level of sporting activity. The authors noted these good subjective results despite the fact that only three knees were rated as good using objective stability criteria and the remainder were rated as only fair. These authors believed that good functional results did not depend on obtaining objective stability and that nonoperative treatment of the isolated PCL injury was a reasonable option.

Dejour et al. (66) noted that although the instability that occurs secondary to an isolated PCL injury is well tolerated, degenerative changes inevitably appear with longer term follow-up.

Keller et al. (38) summarized the results of nonoperative management in 40 of 54 individuals with isolated PCL injury who were followed for an average of 6 years. They noted that 90% of patients still complained of knee pain, 65% believed that the knee limited their activity, and 43% had difficulty in walking. These subjective complaints were related to the degree of laxity of the PCL noted on objective testing. Radiographic changes were correlated with the amount of time since the injury. These authors did not find a correlation between quadriceps strength and functional or objective results.

Geissler and Whipple (78) used arthroscopy to study the intraarticular abnormalities associated with isolated PCL insufficiency. After a mean interval of 2.2 years from the time of injury, they found articular cartilage lesion of grade II or higher in 49% of their patients and meniscal lesions in 36%.

Boynton and Tietjens (79) reported the natural history of isolated PCL insufficiency in 38 patients at average follow-up of 13.4 years. Eighty-one percent of their patients had at least occasional pain in their knee, and 56% of their patients had at least occasional swelling. An increase in the time from injury was associated with increased degenerative changes as seen on radiographs. However, several patients remained essentially asymptomatic, even at long-term follow-up.

Several general conclusions can be made from the above studies. First, the subjective results of nonoperative treatment of the isolated PCL injury are not excellent. Even the most optimistic of the above studies demonstrate a 20% to 25% failure rate of nonoperative management, and the study by Keller et al. (38) noted that most patients continue to complain of knee pain and activity limitations. Second, there may be some degree of correlation between quadriceps strength and outcome. Third, there does not appear to be a strong association between subjective results and ligamentous stability. Finally, a substantial number of knees with isolated PCL injury will go on to develop degenerative changes, particularly in the medial compartment, with time.

To recommend reconstructive surgery to the patient with isolated injury to the PCL, one must show that the results of reconstruction are superior to those of nonoperative management and that the risks of surgery are outweighed by the benefits of ligamentous reconstruction. It needs to be shown that surgery offers a higher success rate than nonoperative management and that the long-term results of surgery result in a lower incidence of degenerative arthritis than occurs in the knees treated without surgery. There are currently no prospective randomized studies of operative versus non-operative treatment of the knee with PCL injury to guide us in our analysis of this issue. Very few reports of the operative management of PCL injury divide the patients into groups with isolated PCL versus combined PCL and other ligamentous injury. Studies by Bianchi (6) and by Loos et al. (54) noted mixed results in the patients with surgically treated isolated PCL insufficiency. Most patients rated their results as good or fair, but the operative procedures commonly failed to restore objective stability. Despite this, the patients rarely complained of functional instability. A more recent study by Richter et al. (80) reported 8-year follow-up results in 53 patients with acute isolated and combined PCL instabilities treated with operative repair. Although the posterior drawer test was normal to 1+ in 46 patients, no patient had a normal result according to the International Knee Documentation Committee scoring system and only 13% were graded as nearly normal. In contrast to these reports, Clancy et al. (1) reported excellent subjective and objective results in 15 patients treated operatively for acute PCL insufficiency. The authors used a technique of ligament repair supplemented with a central third patellar tendon autograft passed through bony tunnels. Ten patients were evaluated at a 2-year follow-up (8 of whom had had isolated PCL injuries), and all 8 had excellent (7) or good (1) results. Seven patients had trace and one patient had 1+ posterior laxity at follow-up. This study offers promising objective and subjective results for the patient with acute isolated PCL laxity. It remains to be seen whether reconstruction of the isolated PCL injury will result in a decrease in the long-term incidence of degenerative arthritis.

Acute Posterior Cruciate Ligament Combined with Other Ligaments

Disruption of the PCL and other major ligaments, including the MCL, LCL, arcuate ligament complex, popliteus muscle–tendon unit, or other structures alone or in combination, is usually due to higher energy mechanisms of injury but may also occur in sport-related injuries. The diagnosis of the structures injured is key to the decision-making process and the plan for operative reconstruction, as discussed above. Because injury to the PCL combined with injury to one or more other major knee ligaments results in gross derangement of the normal biomechanics of the knee, most authorities have advocated operative treatment for the combination of PCL disruption along with injury to other major knee ligaments. For this reason, there are no large long-term studies of the results of nonoperative treatment of these injuries. This makes it impossible to determine objectively whether or not surgical management improves upon the natural history of these combined injuries. A wide variety of surgical approaches and tissues for augmentation and/or reconstruction has been suggested as useful for treatment.

Kennedy and Grainger (31) believed that repair of an injured PCL was superior to reconstruction and found few indications for a major reconstruction. When a reconstruction was believed to be necessary, they recommended use of the hamstring tendons passed through drill holes in the tibia and medial femoral condyle, a procedure originally proposed by Hey-Grooves.

McCormick et al. (81) described a patient with disruption of the PCL and LCL, and they reconstructed the PCL by passing the tendon of the popliteus through drill holes in the medial femoral condyle at the anatomic origin of the PCL. They did not describe how the injury to the LCL was treated.

Soughmayd and Rubin (82) reported a case in which the semimembranosus tendon was used to reconstruct the PCL by preserving its distal attachment and passing the proximal end of the tendon through the medial femoral condyle. This patient had persistent 1+ posterior laxity after the surgery but returned to his previous level of activity.

Moore and Larson (52) summarized the results of 18 patients operated on an average of 2.6 days after their injury and followed for 30.8 months. Avulsion injuries were repaired using sutures passed through drill holes, whereas nonrepairable tears were reconstructed using the medial head of the gastrocnemius tendon and reattaching it to the medial femoral condyle using a bone block and drill holes. The associated ligamentous injuries were repaired, and patients were casted postoperatively. Seven patients had an excellent result, seven results were good, three fair, and one poor.

Hughston et al. (13) reviewed 32 individuals with acute combined injuries involving the PCL. Twenty-two patients had ACL tears, 21 had medial meniscus tears, and 3 had lateral meniscus tears. The PCL was repaired in each case, but in nine cases this failed to restore knee stability. In these cases the medial meniscus was used for the reconstruction, with six of the nine harvested menisci having had peripheral tears, whereas the other three menisci were normal. The authors evaluated 20 of the knees 5 to 6 years after surgery. Thirteen knees were rated as good, 4 as fair, and 3 as poor. No knee was believed to be normal after this injury.

Loos et al. (54) reported their experience in a mixed series of 102 PCL injuries, 46 of which were combined with other ligamentous injury and which were repaired acutely. The authors did not divide the patients into groups according to the injury pattern and did not differentiate between isolated and combined injuries. They had 32% poor results, and 4 of the 46 patients underwent reoperation.

Bianchi (6) summarized his experience in 19 patients with combined PCL injuries (16 MCL, 3 LCL, 8 ACL, 10 medial meniscal, 3 lateral meniscal, and 2 medial and lateral meniscal tears) that were treated operatively. Midsubstance ruptures were reconstructed using hamstring tendons, whereas avulsion injuries were repaired with sutures passed through bone. The treatment of the associated injuries was not specifically addressed. Forty-eight percent of the results were good, 44% fair, and 8% poor.

DeLee et al. (57) treated 10 patients with complete disruption of the PCL, ACL, and LCL. All patients initially had a 3+ posterior drawer. All injuries were repaired primarily, with avulsions being repaired to bone and midsubstance tears repaired with sutures. No patient had a reconstruction or ligament augmentation. Five of seven patients available for follow-up at an average of 7.5 years had good results, whereas two had poor results. Six of the seven patients had negative posterior drawer testing, whereas one had a 3+ posterior drawer.

Baker et al. (83) reviewed 13 surgically treated patients with acute PCL and PLC instability at an average of 56 months. Midsubstance tears were sutured end to end, avulsions were repaired back to bone, and one midsubstance tear was reconstructed with the lateral meniscus as a graft. ACL avulsions were repaired, whereas midsubstance tears were treated with excision of the ACL. Tears of the arcuate ligament complex were repaired primarily. Eight individuals had good objective results and three had poor results, and all 11 patients returning for follow-up evaluation had good functional results.

Pournaras and Symeonides (84) also used suture repair of the ligament in a series of 20 patients treated for isolated and combined ligament injuries. This procedure did not eliminate posterior instability, and all patients had evidence of a positive posterior drawer sign on follow-up examination. Despite the objective results, 15 patients had good subjective results.

Many of the above reports did not divide the patients into groups according to the specific injury pattern, and the materials used for repair or reconstruction in these studies are considered to be inferior to the central third patellar tendon or Achilles tendon autograft or allografts used today. Despite these shortcomings, it can be concluded from these studies that the results of treatment of combined PCL and other major ligament injuries lead to a satisfactory functional outcome in most patients. What is disturbing is that the objective results demonstrate that the stability of the knee is far from normal. If the goals of surgery are to recreate the stability and kinematics of the knee in the situation in which the PCL is intact, it appears that these goals have not been met by any reconstructive method described to date. Newer methods of PCL reconstruction that attempt to reproduce the anatomy of the PCL using more than one graft and multiple femoral tunnels appear promising both biomechanically and clinically, but results using these methods are still considered preliminary.

Chronic Posterior Cruciate Ligament Insufficiency

Chronic PCL insufficiency usually results in symptoms either from degenerative changes in the medial and patellofemoral compartments or from instability due to injury or subsequent stretching of the secondary restraints, particularly the PLC. There are few reports of successful nonoperative management of these injuries. However, a report by Hughston and Degenhardt (14) demonstrated that nearly half of their patients with chronic PCL insufficiency obtained functional stability with the aid of an aggressive rehabilitation program. The characteristics of that group were not specifically defined, and it has been suggested that perhaps the individuals responding to nonoperative management had a lesser degree of instability present initially (47).

Several authors have advocated surgical management of the patient with symptomatic chronic insufficiency of the PCL, and a number of procedures and ligament substitutes have been proposed. Tellberg (85) summarized the results of PCL reconstruction using lateral meniscus as a graft. Seven of his 45 knees had chronic PCL insufficiency, and his results were mixed. He believed that meniscus was an excellent graft source for several reasons, including its length and size, because it was not dependent on restoration of a blood supply, and because it was the only graft material normally found in the intraarticular environment.

Hughston and Degenhardt (14) reviewed 94 knees with chronic PCL injury. Thirty-nine knees failed to obtain functional stability using an aggressive exercise program and required surgery. Most patients (29) had reconstruction using the medial head of the gastrocnemius tendon; other materials included medial meniscus (4), artificial ligament (6), and meniscus and tendon of the medial head of the gastrocnemius (1). The investigators found a high incidence of associated instability of the PLC in these patients, which they contrasted with the small number found in their series of acute PCL injuries. They believed that this difference could be attributed to a gradual stretching of the arcuate complex with time. Twenty-six knees were available for follow-up at an average of 45 months. Functional results included 20 knees rated as good, 4 as fair, and 2 as poor. Objectively, there were 9 good, 15 fair, and 2 poor results. Forty percent of the patients had at least a 2+ posterior drawer sign after reconstruction. As in several other studies, there was minimal correlation between objective and functional results.

Kennedy and Galpin (86) used the tendon of the medial head of the gastrocnemius to address chronic PCL insufficiency in 21 patients. Eighteen of these indi-

viduals were followed for at least 8 months, and 80% had good or excellent results. These authors also noted persistence of the posterior drawer sign after surgery. The operation also failed to correct preoperative patellofemoral complaints.

Insall and Hood (87) also used the tendon of the medial gastrocnemius to reconstruct the PCL-insufficient knee but removed a block of bone with the tendon before reattaching it to the medial femoral condyle. Six of eight patients had good or excellent results, and all eight had improved stability after surgery. These authors believed that the additional stability afforded by bony fixation allowed earlier mobilization.

Tibone et al. (68) compared transfer of the medial head of the gastrocnemius tendon for functional PCL insufficiency with nonoperative treatment. All patients had posterior drawer signs of 2+ to 3+ preoperatively. Nine of 10 surgically treated patients continued to have a positive posterior drawer sign in external rotation after the surgery, and the posterior drawer sign in internal rotation was positive after surgery in 5 of 10. No comment was made regarding the treatment of associated combined ligamentous instabilities, and the authors did not mention the presence of any associated malalignments. Six of 10 surgically treated patients had medial compartment changes, with 3 of these 6 also having lateral compartment changes. Only one patient in the operative group had degenerative changes, and these were rated as minimal.

More recently, surgeons have been using other graft materials to substitute for the PCL, including central third of the patellar tendon and hamstring autografts and patellar tendon and Achilles tendon allografts. Autografts provide strong readily available tissue without the risk of disease transmission, whereas allografts have the advantage of no donor site morbidity. Reconstructions using these materials emphasize placement of bony tunnels at the sites of origin and insertion of the PCL, followed by insertion of strong graft tissue to substitute for the ligament. Paulos (88) described an arthroscopically assisted technique and recommended use of an Achilles tendon allograft, believing that the tendon offers excellent strength, allows bony fixation in the femur, passes easily through bone tunnels, and may minimize postoperative patellofemoral problems.

Clancy et al. (1) summarized their experience in 33 patients with chronic PCL insufficiency in whom reconstruction was done using a central third of the patellar tendon autograft. Twenty-three of 33 patients had evidence of degenerative changes on preoperative radiographs. The number of patients with radiographic changes increased as the time from injury to surgery increased, and there was a poor correlation between preoperative radiographs and articular damage noted at surgery. Thirteen patients were available for evaluation at a minimum of 2 years. Four patient had associated ACL repairs, one had repair of the PLC, and one had repair of the MCL. Preoperative complaints were of disabling pain and of instability. All had at least a 2+ posterior drawer, and all but five patients had radiographic evidence of degenerative changes. All but two patients had good or excellent results. Of the six patients with combined instabilities, five believed their knee was improved. Five patients had a 1+ posterior drawer, and one was graded as trace. All these patients were satisfied with their results. There was one excellent, four good, and one fair result.

Importantly, although the above studies included patients with associated laxity of the posterolateral structures, none specifically mentioned the preoperative alignment of the limb. The significance of varus alignment of the limb and, more importantly, of a varus thrust during gait has recently been stressed by several authors (36,89,90). Soft tissue procedures performed on the PLC in a limb that has a varus thrust during gait will tend to stretch out and fail over time. Despite the lack of studies demonstrating a long-term benefit, many authors (89,90) believe that the most reliable procedure in such a setting is a high tibial osteotomy.

Postoperative Rehabilitation

We divide postoperative rehabilitation after PCL reconstruction into five phases: immediate postoperative phase (first 2 weeks after surgery), maximum protection phase (weeks 2 to 6), controlled ambulation phase (weeks 6 to 12), light activity phase (weeks 12 to 16), and return to activity phase (weeks 16 to 24).

In the immediate postoperative phase, the patient is encouraged to bear 50% of weight as tolerated using two crutches, to do ankle and hip exercises, and to perform knee extensions from 60 to 0 degrees.

During the maximum protection phase, full weight bearing is allowed; multiangle quad isometrics at 60, 40, and 20 degrees are done; leg press and squats from 0 to 60 degrees are introduced; and well-leg bicycling is performed. By week 4, range of motion should be to 90 degrees and bicycling can be encouraged for range of motion and endurance. Exercises in the pool are initiated at week 5.

The controlled ambulation phase aims to increase quad strength by initiating swimming, closed kinetic chain rehabilitation, and a stretching program. By week 12 the patient may begin lateral step-ups, cycling for endurance (30 minutes), hamstring curls from 0 to 60 degrees with low weight, and a walking program.

The light activity phase continues with the above exercises and allows a light running program. By 5 to 6 months after the surgery, the patient should be performing plyometric exercises and agility and balance drills and may return to sport when KT-2000, isokinetic testing, and functional testing yield satisfactory results according to the surgeon.

Expected Outcomes

It can be concluded from the above series that most properly selected individuals who undergo PCL reconstruction for either isolated or combined injuries will obtain a satisfactory subjective result. The goals of surgery should be to return the individual to his or her preinjury activity level, to provide normal subjective and objective stability, to restore the biomechanics of the knee to normal, and to prevent the onset or progression of degenerative changes, while avoiding operative complications. It appears that at the current time, we can return most individuals with isolated PCL insufficiency to their preinjury activity level and to restore subjective (but not objective) stability. The results of surgery in the setting of combined PCL and other major knee ligament injuries are less predictable but still offer satisfactory subjective results in most patients. However, we are still searching for an operation that reliably restores objective stability, recreates normal biomechanics, and prevents or delays the onset of degenerative disease. Although newer methods of reconstruction using multiple grafts to recreate both anatomic bundles of the PCL appear promising both biomechanically and clinically, long-term clinical studies using these methods are currently unavailable.

AUTHORS' PREFERENCES

The senior author (W.G.C.) has surgically treated more than 400 patients for symptomatic isolated or combined PCL insufficiency. The following section summarizes his preferences in the management of these demanding injuries.

Acute Posterior Cruciate Ligament Injury

Most patients with acute injury limited to the PCL are treated nonoperatively. The major exception to this is the patient with the displaced fracture of the origin or insertion of the PCL, which is treated with anatomic open reduction and internal fixation, followed by early motion. We believe that the grade of the posterior drawer test is very important in defining the extent of ligamentous injury. A posterior drawer test graded as 1+ usually signifies incomplete injury to the PCL, which is often manifest anatomically as an interstitial lengthening of the ligament. This is considered to be a tear in continuity and may be seen as such on the MRI. It has been our experience that these degrees of injury often tighten as healing progresses, and the amount of laxity on posterior drawer testing often diminishes to trace with appropriate nonoperative management. Laxity on posterior drawer testing graded as 2+ is consistent with a complete disruption of the PCL. In the absence of other major ligamentous injury, we continue to prefer to treat this injury without surgery. An aggressive rehab program that focuses on maximizing the ability of the quadriceps muscle to substitute for the PCL is prescribed, and surgery is recommended only if the patient exhibits continued instability or medial joint pain secondary to increased contact pressures in the medial compartment. In the patient with medial joint line pain, normal radiographs, and a history of PCL insufficiency, we have found the bone scan to be useful in defining the source of the pain. Theoretically, reconstruction of the PCL before radiographic changes become evident may correct the increased medial joint pressures by restoring the normal kinematics of the knee and therefore prevent or delay the onset of osteoarthritis. This, however, has not been shown clinically. The patient with 3+ laxity on posterior drawer testing has injury not only to the PCL but also to the secondary restraints to posterior translation, most commonly the PLC structures. The treatment of these combined PCL and other major ligamentous injuries is discussed below.

Posterior Cruciate Ligament Injury Combined with Other Ligaments

Ligamentous injury of the knee not limited to the PCL usually includes injury to the PLC, ACL, MCL, or some combination thereof. These injuries are due to higher energies, and result in combined instabilities that are usually inadequately compensated for by other ligaments or surrounding muscles. In most cases, we prefer to treat these injuries surgically, with repair or reconstruction of the injured structures being done as the situation dictates. We discuss these on a case-by-case basis below.

PCL Combined with Posterolateral Corner Injury

When these injuries are recognized in the acute setting, we prefer early (i.e., within 3 weeks) surgery to allow satisfactory repair of the injured PLC structures rather than having to perform a secondary reconstruction. The knee is splinted until the acute pain subsides, and active and active-assisted range of motion is encouraged. Allowing 5 to 7 days to elapse from the time of injury until the time of surgery permits the joint capsule to seal and avoids extravasation of arthroscopy fluid into the leg from the injured posterolateral structures during the arthroscopic part of the procedure. The PCL is first reconstructed using the procedure outlined below, and the PLC structures that are injured are then repaired through a standard lateral approach.

Posterior Cruciate Ligament Combined with Anterior Cruciate Ligament Injury

As recalled from the section on evaluation, these injuries are often unrecognized knee dislocations, and appropriate attention must be paid to the neurovascular structures, with vascular consultation being obtained as necessary. Once the knee is reduced, it is splinted until the acute pain of the injury subsides, which is usually a few days. Active range of motion is begun within the limits of pain, and once a satisfactory range of motion is obtained (i.e., full extension and approximately 120 degrees of flexion), elective reconstruction of the ACL and PCL are performed. The ACL is reconstructed using an endoscopic technique that places the patellar tendon graft at the anatomic sites of origin and insertion of the ACL, and the PCL is reconstructed using the technique described below. Early postoperative range of motion and weight bearing is begun, and an accelerated rehab program is prescribed.

Posterior Cruciate Ligament Combined with Medial Collateral Ligament Injury

Injury to the PCL combined with MCL injury is somewhat unusual but certainly does occur. Grade I or II MCL injuries combined with PCL disruption can usually be treated without surgery, and the emphasis is on early range of motion and quadriceps strengthening. Grade III MCL injuries, which are defined by laxity to valgus stress applied at full extension, are characterized by injury to the posterior oblique portion of the MCL and the anterior longitudinal portion. We prefer to treat these injuries with splinting until range of motion exercises can be initiated, followed by early repair of the MCL and posterior oblique ligament and reconstruction of the PCL. It is important to ensure isometric repair of the MCL and posterior oblique ligament to avoid creating a flexion contracture in the postoperative period. The PCL is reconstructed using the procedure described below.

Chronic Posterior Cruciate Ligament Insufficiency

The patient with chronic insufficiency of the PCL may or may not have concomitant injury to the posterolateral structures. If the PCL injury is isolated, a rehab program to strengthen the quadriceps is first prescribed. Failure of this program to result in improvement of symptoms over a period of 3 or more months results in our offering the patient the option of a PCL reconstruction. More commonly, the symptomatic patient with chronic PCL insufficiency also has some laxity of their secondary restraints, particularly the posterolateral structures. In this setting we offer the patient a PCL reconstruction, and we also reconstruct the posterolateral structures using a tenodesis of a portion of the biceps tendon, as previously described (91).

Authors' Technique for Two-band and Two Femoral Tunnel Reconstruction of the Posterior Cruciate Ligament

We believe that there is excellent biomechanical evidence to support the theory that the PCL acts primarily as two separate functional bundles, with the anterolateral or anterocentral portion of the ligament acting predominantly in flexion and the posteromedial or posterior oblique portion of the ligament acting predominantly in extension (92). Because of the size of the sites of origin and insertion of the PCL, reconstruction of the ligament using a single graft necessitates that only one of these two bundles is reconstructed. Most researchers to date have preferred to reconstruct the anterolateral or anterocentral portion of the ligament and have recommended tensioning the graft at 90 degrees of flexion (93,94). This method reduces the posterior drawer as measured at the time of surgery, but it the objective results of this method seem to deteriorate as the interval from surgery increases. We believe that the increase in laxity that occurs in the interval from the immediate postoperative period until the time of further follow-up is because this portion of the PCL tightens with flexion and loosens with extension. Because most functional activities are performed at less than 70 degrees of flexion, the graft is subjected to posterior stresses at flexion angles that are significantly less than those at which it was tensioned. This allows subsequent cyclic fatigue and lengthening of the graft. The posteromedial and posterior oblique portions of the PCL contain some fibers that exhibit isometric behavior under certain conditions, but placement of a 10- to 11-mm graft at the sites of origin and insertion of these fibers results in a large portion of the graft being outside of the anatomic boundaries of the PCL. We therefore prefer to reconstruct both bundles of the PCL and pass two separate grafts through two separate femoral tunnels. These grafts are then passed through a single tibial tunnel, with the anterolateral/anterocentral graft being tensioned at 90 degrees of flexion and the posteromedial/posterior oblique graft being tensioned at 30 degrees of flexion. This technique is fully described below.

The technique of PCL reconstruction developed and refined by the senior author involves 11 steps: examination of the knee under anesthesia, arthroscopic inspection of the knee joint, harvest of a patellar tendon graft (used to reconstruct the anterolateral/anterocentral bundle), debridement of the PCL remnant from the femur, debridement of the tibial insertion site of the PCL, creation of the tibial tunnel, creation of the femoral tunnels, harvest of the hamstring or quadriceps tendon graft (used to reconstruct the posteromedial/

posterior oblique bundle), passage of the grafts into the femur, passage of the grafts into the tibia, and fixation of the grafts. Attention to detail and satisfactory performance of each step in the proper order is necessary to ensure a satisfactory result.

Step 1: Examination of the Knee under Anesthesia

Every ligamentous reconstructive procedure should begin with a complete examination under anesthesia. This is necessary both to document the presence and degree of insufficiency of the PCL and to determine the presence or absence of injury to other major ligaments, particularly the PLC structures. The technique for performing and grading the posterior drawer and the method for examining the PLC structures are described above.

Step 2: Arthroscopic Inspection of the Knee Joint

After the examination under anesthesia, the 30-degree arthroscope is introduced into the knee joint via a medial peripatellar portal. This portal is created vertically along the medial border of the patellar tendon at the level of the inferior pole of the patella, with the knee in approximately 30 degrees of flexion. It should be noted that we do not use a tourniquet during any of our reconstructive procedures of the knee. The senior author believes that avoidance of a tourniquet allows better hemostasis during the procedure and also decreases postoperative quadriceps inhibition. The knee is inspected in a systematic fashion, with particular attention being paid to the medial and patellofemoral compartments. Substantial involvement of these compartments with degenerative changes may be considered a relative contraindication to PCL reconstruction. The contents of the intracondylar notch are inspected, and the site of injury to the PCL is identified. It should be noted that chronic cases of PCL injury often show only laxity of the ligament, which may be most evident as diminished tension of the ligament at its insertion site into the tibia. There may also appear to be abnormal laxity of the ACL, which is usually due to the abnormal posterior position of the tibia and which is reduced with placement of the proximal tibia into its normal position with respect to the distal femur.

Step 3: Harvest of the Patellar Tendon Graft

Once the site and degree of injury to the PCL has been confirmed arthroscopically, a graft from the central third of the patellar tendon is harvested. Harvest of the graft at this point in the procedure allows subsequent creation of a central portal through the fat pad at the site of the defect in the patellar tendon, and this portal will be used both to debride the remnant of the PCL from the femur and to position the tibial guide for the tibial tunnel. The incision along the medial border of the patellar tendon is extended both proximally and distally, and the medial and lateral borders of the patellar tendon are defined. We prefer to harvest a 10-mm-wide graft from the central third of the patellar tendon and take 10-mm-wide by 20-mm-long grafts from both the patella and the tibial tubercle. The graft is prepared by an assistant to allow easy passage through 10-mm tunnels, and three no. 5 Ethibond sutures are placed through each end of the graft.

Step 4: Debridement of the Posterior Cruciate Ligament Remnant from the Femur

The arthroscope is now reinserted into the knee through the medial peripatellar portal, and the motorized shaver is introduced through a central fat pad portal that is created in the defect left by harvest of the patellar tendon graft. The origin of the PCL from the medial femoral condyle is then debrided. Care is taken to preserve a portion of these fibers during the debridement, because they serve as a valuable landmark for later tunnel placement. We have noted that there is a curved ridge on the medial femoral condyle (which is somewhat analogous to the "resident's ridge" on the lateral femoral condyle) posterior to which there are no fibers of origin of the PCL. Preservation of this landmark is also quite helpful during femoral tunnel placement.

Step 5: Debridement of the Tibial Insertion Site of the Posterior Cruciate Ligament

Debridement of the tibial insertion site of the PCL is accomplished through a posteromedial portal, which is created at the level of the junction of the proximal medial tibia with the posterior portion of the medial femoral condyle. The arthroscope is advanced into the intracondylar notch, and the motorized shaver is inserted through the posteromedial portal. Debridement is carried out with the shaver always facing toward the tibia order to avoid inadvertent damage to the posterior capsule or neurovascular structures. Placement of the arthroscope into the posteromedial portal allows identification of the tibial fovea. This area is then defined using first a curved shaver placed through the central fat pad portal and then by use of an angled curette. It is important to fully visualize the insertion site of the PCL to ensure proper placement of the tibial guide pin and to avoid popliteal artery or tibial nerve damage during subsequent drilling.

Step 6: Creation of the Tibial Tunnel

Once the site of insertion of the PCL has been fully identified, a guide pin is driven from the anterior tibia

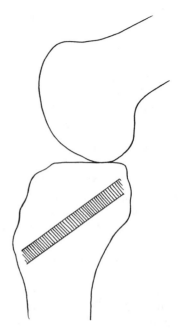

FIG. 42.16. Ideal site for the tibial tunnel, which enters the tibia distal to the site of graft harvest from the tibial tubercle and exits the proximal tibia in the center of the insertion site of the posterior cruciate ligament.

(approximately 12 to 15 mm distal to the site of graft harvest from the tibial tubercle) into the center of the insertion of the PCL (Fig. 42.16). We believe that the entry point of the guide pin into the tibia is quite important, because it creates a rather vertical tunnel (which eases graft passage into the tibia and also facilitates tensioning of the graft) and also because it avoids creating an oblique hole at the exit site of the tunnel in the fovea. Drilling a hole that enters medial or lateral to the tibial tubercle creates an oblique exit hole in the tibial fovea and may result in excessive medial or lateral placement of the graft. A 10-mm reamer is then driven over the guidewire, followed by a 12-mm reamer. The arthroscope remains in the posteromedial portal during reaming to ensure that neither the guide pin nor the reamers penetrate the knee joint during reaming. Once the tibial tunnel has been reamed, the foveal site is debrided of any remaining tissue. A no. 5 Ethibond suture is next passed through the tibial drill hole and out the central fat pad portal. This suture will be used during passage of the graft into the tibial tunnel.

Step 7: Creation of the Femoral Tunnels

The femoral tunnels are now created using the remaining fibers of the PCL on the medial femoral condyle as a guide (Figs. 42.17 and 42.18). We drill a 10-mm anterior/proximal tunnel and an 8-mm posterior/distal tunnel, keeping the tunnels separated by a 3- to 4-mm bony bridge. A 00 curette is used to make marks in the

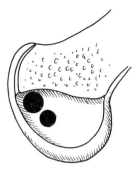

FIG. 42.17. Ideal sites for the positions of the femoral tunnels, as viewed from the side of a left knee with the lateral femoral condyle removed.

medial femoral condyle at the desired tunnel sites. The anterior/proximal tunnel guide pin should enter the intracondylar notch at the 10:30 position in a left knee (the 1:30 position in a right knee) and be approximately 6 mm posterior to the articular surface of the medial femoral condyle. The posterior/distal tunnel is placed approximately 5 mm posterior and 5 mm distal to the anterior/proximal tunnel, taking care to ascertain that the tunnel sites remain within the anatomic site of origin of the PCL and that both tunnels will be entirely anterior to the ridge in the medial femoral condyle (see step 4, above). An incision is made over the vastus medialis muscle at the level of the adductor tubercle, and the fibers of the vastus medialis are elevated anteriorly. A vector guide is then used to place a pin from the region of the adductor tubercle into the desired position of the anterior/proximal tunnel, and a 10-mm reamer is driven over this guide. A second guide pin is driven from a

separate site in the medial femoral condyle into the desired site of the posterior/distal tunnel, and an 8-mm reamer is driven over this guide pin. Care is taken to ensure that an adequate bony bridge separates these two tunnels. Two separate no. 5 Ethibond sutures (which will be used later for graft passage) are passed through these tunnels and exit out the central fat pad portal.

It should be noted that we have had recent success with placement of the above femoral tunnels using an endoscopic technique. Using this method, the femoral tunnel sites are marked with the 00 curette as described above. We then use a specially designed custom guide and flexible guide pins and reamers to ream the two tunnels from the inside of the notch. Each tunnel is reamed to a depth of 25 to 30 mm with the appropriately sized reamer, and a 4.5-mm drill is used to drill out the medial femoral cortex. The grafts are then fixed using an Endobutton device, allowing an entirely endoscopic reconstruction.

Step 8: Harvest of the Hamstring or Quadriceps Tendon Graft

At this point we harvest the graft that will be used to reconstruct the posteromedial/posterior oblique portion of the PCL. Depending on the preference of the surgeon, either the quadriceps tendon or the semitendinosis tendon may be used. If the quadriceps tendon is used, we make a separate incision centered over the superior pole of the patella. The quadriceps insertion into the patella is identified, and an 8-mm-wide by 15- to 20-mm-long bone plug is harvested from the patella. An 8-mm-wide strip of quadriceps tendon is taken that runs the length of the tendon. If the quadriceps tendon is excessively thick, only the superficial lamina of the tendon is harvested. A no. 5 nonabsorbable braided suture is placed through the tendon, which will be used to fix the tendon in the tibia.

If the surgeon prefers, the semitendinosis tendon may be used instead of the quadriceps tendon. The semitendinosis tendon is harvested in standard fashion, using the distal end of the original incision. The tendon is doubled over itself to form a double-stranded graft and can be fixed in the femur using either a standard button or an Endobutton (if an endoscopic technique is chosen).

Step 9: Passage of the Grafts into the Femur

The grafts are passed into the femoral tunnels using the previously placed sutures through the central fat pad portal and the femoral tunnels (Fig. 42.19). The quadriceps or semitendinosis graft is placed first and is then fixed at the medial femoral condyle using either a simple button (open technique) or an Endobutton (endoscopic technique). After femoral fixation of this graft, the patel-

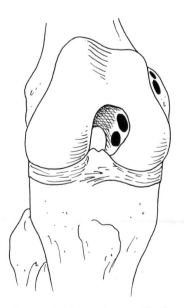

FIG. 42.18. Ideal sites for the positions of the femoral tunnels, as viewed in a right knee.

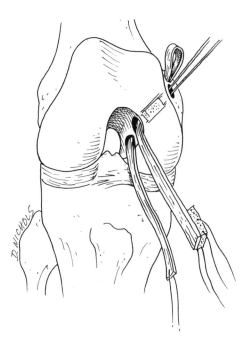

FIG. 42.19. Passage of the hamstring and patellar tendon grafts into the femur in a right knee (see text for explanation).

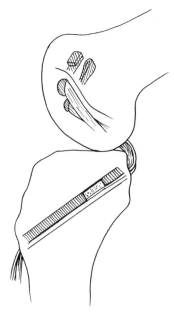

FIG. 42.21. Final view of a two-bundle posterior cruciate ligament reconstruction as it would appear in a left knee, seen from the lateral side with the lateral femoral condyle removed.

lar tendon graft is passed into the femur and fixed in similar fashion.

Step 10: Passage of the Grafts into the Tibia

Once both grafts have been fixed at the medial femoral condyle, they are passed through the central fat pad portal and into the tibia (Figs. 42.20 and 42.21). This is

done using the previously placed suture through the tibial tunnel and can be facilitated with the used of a specialized graft passer (Depuy), which encloses the grafts and provides a smooth surface to slide through the tibial tunnel. We have found that application of an anterior drawer at the time of graft passage into the tibia helps the graft to turn the corner at the proximal part of the tibial tunnel.

Step 11: Fixation of the Grafts

The final step in the procedure is fixation of the grafts to the tibia. The patellar tendon graft is fixed first and is tensioned at 90 degrees of flexion with an anterior drawer test. The sutures from the patellar bone plug are tied over a screw and washer, which is tightened at the end of the procedure. The quadriceps or hamstring graft is tightened at 30 degrees of flexion, and these sutures are tied over the same screw as those from the patellar tendon graft. The wounds are then irrigated and closed in routine fashion. A standardized rehab protocol begins on the first postoperative day, and the patient is usually discharged from the hospital on the second postoperative day.

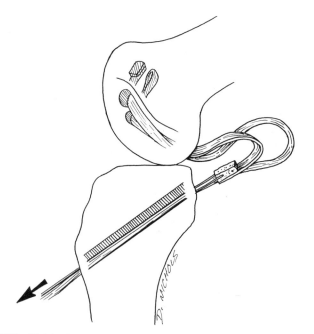

FIG. 42.20. Passage of the hamstring and patellar grafts into the tibia in a left knee (see text for explanation).

REFERENCES

1. Clancy WG, Shelbourne KD, Zoellner GB. Treatment of knee joint instability secondary to rupture of the posterior cruciate ligament. *J Bone Joint Surg Am* 1983;65A:310–332.
2. Johnson JC, Bach BR. Current concepts review: posterior cruciate ligament. *Am J Knee Surg* 1990;3:143–153.

3. Kannus P, Bergfeld J, Jarvinen M, et al. Injuries to the posterior cruciate ligament of the knee. *Sports Med* 1991;12:110–131.
4. Bach BR. Graft selection for posterior cruciate ligament surgery. *Op Tech Sports Med* 1993;2:104–109.
5. O'Donoghue DH. Surgical treatment of injuries to ligaments of the knee. *JAMA* 1959;169:1423–1431.
6. Bianchi M. Acute tears of the posterior cruciate ligament: clinical study and results of operative treatment in 27 cases. *Am J Sports Med* 1983;11:308–314.
7. Clendenin MB, DeLee JC, Heckman JD. Interstitial tears of the posterior cruciate ligament of the knee. *Orthopaedics* 1980; 3:764–772.
8. Cross MJ, Powell JF. Long-term followup of posterior cruciate ligament rupture: a study of 116 cases. *Am J Sports Med* 1984;12:292–297.
9. Fowler PJ, Messieh SS. Isolated posterior cruciate ligament injuries in athletes. *Am J Sports Med* 1987;15:553–557.
10. Trickey EL. Rupture of the posterior cruciate ligament of the knee. *J Bone Joint Surg Br* 1968;50B:334–341.
11. Bergfeld JA. Diagnosis and nonoperative treatment of acute posterior cruciate ligament injury. *Instr Course Lect* 1990;208.
12. Daniel C. Knee ligament injuries. *AAOS postgraduate course "the knee–current concepts."* St. Thomas, VI, June, 1992.
13. Hughston JC, Bowden JA, Andrews JR, et al. Acute tears of the posterior cruciate ligament. Results of operative treatment. *J Bone Joint Surg Am* 1980;62A:438–450.
14. Hughston JC, Degenhardt TC. Reconstruction of the posterior cruciate ligament. *Clin Orthop* 1982;154:59–77.
15. Lipscomb AB, Johnston RK, Snyder RB. The technique of cruciate ligament reconstruction. *Am J Sports Med* 1981;9:77–81.
16. Jakob RP, Hassler H, Staeubli HU. Observations on rotatory instability of the lateral compartment of the knee. *Acta Orthop Scand* 1981; [Suppl]:191.
17. Girgis FG, Marshall JL, Al Monajem ARS. The cruciate ligaments of the knee joint: anatomical, functional and experimental analysis. *Clin Orthop* 1975;106:216–231.
18. Warren RF, Arnoczky SP, Wickiewicz TL. Anatomy of the knee. In: Nicholas JA, Hershman EB, eds. *The lower extremity and spine in sports medicine.* St. Louis, MO: Mosby, 1986:657–694.
19. Harner CD, Xerogeanes JW, Livesay GA, et al. The human posterior cruciate ligament complex: an interdisciplinary study. Ligament morphology and biomechanical evaluation. *Am J Sports Med* 1995;23:736–745.
20. Kennedy JC, Roth JH, Walker DM. Posterior cruciate ligament injuries. *Orthop Digest* 1979;7:19–32.
21. Scapinelli R. Studies on the vasculature of the human knee joint. *Acta Anat* 1968;70:305.
22. Arnoczky SP, Rubin RM, Marshall JL. The microvasculature of the cruciate ligaments and its response to injury. An experimental study in dogs. *J Bone Joint Surg Am* 1979;61A:1221–1229.
23. Kennedy JC, Alexander IJ, Hayes KC. Nerve supply of the human knee and its functional importance. *Am J Sports Med* 1982; 10:329–335.
24. Schultz RA, Miller DC, Kerr CS, et al. Mechanoreceptors in human cruciate ligaments. *J Bone Joint Surg Am* 1984;66A:1072–1076.
25. Schutte MJ, Diabezies EJ, Zimny ML, et al. Neural anatomy of the human anterior cruciate ligament. *J Bone Joint Surg Am* 1987;69A:243–247.
26. Brantigan OC, Voshell AF. The mechanics of the ligaments and menisci of the knee joint. *J Bone Joint Surg Am* 1941;23A:44–66.
27. Candiollo L, Gautero D. Morphologie et fonction des ligaments menisco-femoraux de l'articulation du genori chez l'homme. *Acta Anat* 1959;38:304.
28. Heller L, Langman J. The menisco-femoral ligaments of the human knee. *J Bone Joint Surg Br* 1964;46B:303–313.
29. Radoievitch S. Les ligaments des menisques interarticulaires du genou. *Ann Anat Pathol* 1931;8:400.
30. Kaplan EB. Some aspects of functional anatomy of the human knee joint. *Clin Orthop* 1960;23:18–28.
31. Kennedy JC, Grainger RW. The posterior cruciate ligament. *J Trauma* 1967;7:367–376.
32. Butler DL, Noyes FR, Grood ES. Ligamentous restraints to ante-rior-posterior drawer in the human knee. A biomechanical study. *J Bone Joint Surg Am* 1980;62A:259–270.
33. Gollehon DL, Torzilli PA, Warren RJ. The role of the posterolateral and cruciate ligaments in the stability of the human knee: a biomechanical study. *J Bone Joint Surg Am* 1987;69A:233–242.
34. Grood ES, Stowers SF, Noyes FR. Limits of movement in the human knee. The effects of sectioning the PCL and posterolateral structures. *J Bone Joint Surg Am* 1988;70A:88–97.
35. Skyhar MJ, Warren RF, Ortiz GJ, et al. The effects of sectioning of the posterior cruciate ligament and the posterolateral complex on the articular contact pressures within the knee. *J Bone Joint Surg Am* 1993;75A:694–699.
36. Cooper DE, Warren RF, Warner JJP. The posterior cruciate ligament and posterolateral structures of the knee: anatomy, function and patterns of injury. *Instr Course Lect* 1991;40:249–270.
37. Hughston JC, Andrews JR, Cross MJ, et al. Classification of knee ligament instabilities. Part 1. The medial compartment and cruciate ligaments. *J Bone Joint Surg Am* 1976;58A:159–172.
38. Keller PM, Shelborne KD, McCarroll JR, et al. Nonoperatively treated isolated posterior cruciate ligament injury. *Am J Sport Med* 1993;21:132–136.
39. Pournaras J, Symeonides P, Karkavelas G. The significance of the posterior cruciate ligament in the stability of the knee. *J Bone Joint Surg Br* 1983;65B:204–209.
40. Torg JS, Barton TM, Pavlov H, et al. Natural history of the posterior cruciate ligament-deficient knee. *Clin Orthop* 1989; 246:208–216.
41. Kennedy JC, Hawkins RJ, Willis RB, et al. Tension studies of human knee ligaments. Yield point, ultimate failure, and disruption of the cruciate and tibial collateral ligaments. *J Bone Joint Surg Am* 1976;58A:350–355.
42. Prietto MP, Bain JR, Stonebrook SN, et al. Tensile strength of the human posterior cruciate ligament (PCL). *Trans Orthop Res Soc* 1988;13:195.
43. Race A, Amis AA. Mechanical properties of the two bundles of the humal posterior cruciate ligament. *Trans Orthop Res Soc* 1992;17:124.
44. Rubinstein RA Jr, Shelbourne KD. Diagnosis of posterior cruciate ligament injuries and indications for nonoperative and operative treatment. *Op Tech Sports Med* 1993;2:99–103.
45. Shelbourne KD, Rubinstein RA. Isolated posterior cruciate ligament rupture: An unusual mechanism of injury. A report of 3 cases. *Am J Knee Surg.*
46. Shelbourne KD, Mesko JW, McCarroll JR, et al. Combined medial collateral ligament-posterior cruciate rupture. Mechanism of injury. *Am J Knee Surg* 1990;3:41–44.
47. DeLee JC, Bergfeld JA, Drez D, Jr, et al. The posterior cruciate ligament. In: DeLee JC, Drez D Jr, eds. *Orthopaedic sports medicine. Principles and practice.* Philadelphia: W.B. Saunders, 1994.
48. Donovan TL, Behling F, Nagel D. Posterior cruciate injury on artificial turf. *Orthop Trans* 1977;1:20.
49. Fowler PJ. The classification and early diagnosis of knee joint instability. *Clin Orthop* 1980;147:15–21.
50. Dandy DJ, Pusey RJ. The long-term results of unrepaired tears of the posterior cruciate ligament. *J Bone Joint Surg Br* 1982;64B:92–94.
51. Cross MJ. Conservative surgery in posterior cruciate ligament disruption. *J Bone Joint Surg Br* 1983;65B:99.
52. Moore HA, Larson RL. Posterior cruciate ligament injuries. Results of early surgical repair. *Am J Sports Med* 1980;8:68–78.
53. Savatsky GH, Marshall JL, Warren RF, et al. Posterior cruciate ligament injury. *Orthop Trans* 1980;4:293.
54. Loos WC, Fox JM, Blazina ME, et al. Acute posterior cruciate ligament injuries. *Am J Sports Med* 1981;9:86–92.
55. Rubinstein RA Jr, Shelbourne KD, McCarroll JR, et al. The accuracy of the clinical examination in the setting of posterior cruciate ligament injuries. *Am J Sports Med* 1994;22:550–557.
56. Daniel DM, Stone ML, Barnett P, et al. Use of the quadriceps active test to diagnose posterior cruciate ligament disruption and measure posterior laxity of the knee. *J Bone Joint Surg Am* 1988;70A:386–391.
57. DeLee JC, Riley MB, Rockwood CA. Acute straight lateral instability of the knee. *Am J Sports Med* 1983;11:404–411.

58. DeLee JC, Riley MB, Rockwood CA. Acute posterolateral rotatory instability of the knee. *Am J Sports Med* 1983;11:199–205.
59. Torisu T. Isolated avulsion fracture of the tibial attachment of the posterior cruciate ligament. *J Bone Joint Surg Am* 1977;59A: 68–72.
60. Torisu T. Avulsion fracture of the tibial attachment of the posterior cruciate ligament. Indications and results of delayed repair. *Clin Orthop* 1979;143:107–114.
61. Trickey EL. Injuries to the posterior cruciate ligament. Diagnosis and treatment of early injuries and reconstruction of late instability. *Clin Orthop* 1980;147:76–81.
62. Hewett TE, Noyes FR, Lee MD. Diagnosis of complete and partial posterior cruciate ligament ruptures. Stress radiography compared with KT-1000 arthrometer and posterior drawer testing. *Am J Sports Med* 1997;25:648–655.
63. Vellet AD, Marks PH, Fowler PJ, et al. Occult post-traumatic osteochondral lesions of the knee: Prevalence, classification, and short term sequelae evaluated with MR imaging. *Radiology* 1991;178:271–276.
64. Parolie JM, Bergfeld JA. Long-term results of nonoperative treatment of isolated posterior cruciate ligament injuries in the athlete. *Am J Sports Med* 1986;14:35–38.
65. Satku K, Chew CN, Seow H. Posterior cruciate ligament injuries. *Acta Orthop Scand* 1984;55:26–29.
66. Dejour H, Walch G, Peyrot J, et al. The natural history of rupture of the posterior cruciate ligament. *Rev Chir Orthop* 1988;74:35–43.
67. Cain TE, Schwab GH. Performance of an athlete with straight posterior knee instability. *Am J Sports Med* 1981;9:203–208.
68. Tibone JE, Antich TJ, Perry J, et al. Functional analysis of untreated and reconstructed posterior cruciate ligament injuries. *Am J Sports Med* 1988;16:217–222.
69. Maday M, Fu FH, Harner CD, et al. Posterior cruciate ligament reconstruction using fresh frozen allograft tissue: indications, techniques, results and controversies. Presented as a Scientific Exhibit at the Annual Meeting of The American Academy of Orthopaedic Surgeons, San Francisco, California, Feb. 18–23, 1993.
70. Lutz GE, Palmitier RA, An KN, et al. Comparison of tibiofemoral joint forces during open-kinetic-chain and closed-kinetic-chain exercises. *J Bone Joint Surg Am* 1993;75A:732–739.
71. Green RB, Noble PC, Woods GW, et al. Rehabilitation of the posterior cruciate deficient knee: a biomechanical simulation. *Orthop Trans* 1989;13:319.
72. Jurist KA, Otis JC. Anteroposterior tibiofemoral displacements during isometric extension efforts. The roles of external load and knee flexion angle. *Am J Sports Med* 1985;13:254–258.
73. McMaster WC. Isolated posterior cruciate ligament injury: literature review and case reports. *J Trauma* 1975;15:1025–1029.
74. Ogata K, McCarthy JA. Measurement of length and tension patterns during reconstruction of the posterior cruciate ligament. *Am J Sports Med* 1992;20:351–355.
75. Ogata K, McCarthy JA, Dunlap J, et al. Pathomechanics of posterior sag of the tibia in posterior cruciate deficient knees. *Am J Sports Med* 1988;16:630–636.
76. Lee HG. Avulsion fracture of the tibial attachments of the cruciate ligaments. Treatment by operative reduction. *J Bone Joint Surg Am* 1937;29:460.
77. Tietjens BB. Posterior cruciate ligament injuries. *J Bone Joint Surg Br* 1985;67B:674.
78. Geissler WB, Whipple TL. Intraarticular abnormalities in association with posterior cruciate ligament injuries. *Am J Sports Med* 1993;21:846–849.
79. Boynton MD, Tietjens MB. Long-term followup of the untreated isolated posterior cruciate ligament-deficient knee. *Am J Sports Med* 1996;24:306–310.
80. Richter M, Kiefer H, Hehl G, et al. Primary repair for posterior cruciate ligament injuries. An eight-year followup of fifty-three patients. *Am J Sports Med* 1996;24:298–305.
81. McCormick WC, Bagg RJ, Kennedy CW Jr, et al. Reconstruction of the posterior cruciate ligament. Preliminary report of a new procedure. *Clin Orthop* 1976;118:30.
82. Southmayd WW, Rubin BD. Reconstruction of the posterior cruciate ligament using the semimembranosus tendon. *Clin Orthop* 1980;150:196–197.
83. Baker CL, Norwood LA, Hughston JC. Acute combined posterior cruciate and posterolateral instability of the knee. *Am J Sports Med* 1984;12:204–208.
84. Pournaras J, Symeonides P. The results of surgical repair of acute tears of the posterior cruciated ligament. *Clin Orthop* 1991; 267:103–107.
85. Tillberg B. The late repair of torn cruciate ligaments using menisci. *J Bone Joint Surg Br* 1977;59B:15–19.
86. Kennedy JC, Galpin RD. The use of the medial head of the gastrocnemius muscle in the posterior cruciate deficient knee. *Am J Sports Med* 1982;10:63–74.
87. Insall JN, Hood RW. Bone-block transfer of the medial head of the gastrocnemius for posterior cruciate insufficiency. *J Bone Joint Surg Am* 1982;64A:691–699.
88. Paulos L. Posterior cruciate and associated ligament injuries. *Instr Course Lect* 1992.
89. Drez DJ Jr. Nonoperative treatment of PCL injuries. *AAOS course "the knee—current concepts."* St. Thomas, VI, May 1992.
90. Jackson DF. Posterior cruciate and associated ligament instabilities. Instructional Course Lectures, AAOS Annual Meeting, Washington, DC, 1992.
91. Clancy WG. Repair and reconstruction of the posterior cruciate ligament. In: Chapman MW, ed. *Operative orthopaedics.* Vol. 3. Philadelphia, PA: J.B. Lippincott, 1988:1651–1655.
92. Covey DC, Sapega AA, Sherman GM. Testing for isometry during reconstruction of the posterior cruciate ligament. *Am J Sports Med* 1996;24:740–746.
93. Burns WC, Draganich LF, Pyevich M, et al. The effect of femoral tunnel position and graft tensioning technique on posterior laxity of the posterior cruciate ligament-reconstructed knee. *Am J Sports Med* 1995;23:424–430.
94. Stone JD, Carlin GJ, Ishibashi Y, et al. Assessment of posterior cruciate ligament graft performance using robotic technology. *Am J Sports Med* 1996;24:824–828.

Principles and Practice of Orthopaedic Sports Medicine,
edited by William E. Garrett, Jr., Kevin P. Speer, and Donald T. Kirkendall.
Lippincott Williams & Wilkins, Philadelphia © 2000.

CHAPTER 43

Articular Cartilage

Andrew S. Levy and David H. Goltz

ARTICULAR CARTILAGE INJURY

Integral to human athletic performance is the smooth function of our articulations. Proper joint function requires adequate strength and stability and a smooth gliding articular surface to allow an effortless range of motion. It has long been known that dysfunction of this natural bearing surface results in pain and limitation of function (1). It has also been known that injury to this structure may result in progressive degeneration into osteoarthritis (2). However, better understanding of the mechanics and anatomy of cartilage injury has only started to come into focus over the last 10 years. We now have a better understanding of articular cartilage as a composite tissue with specific mechanical and physiologic properties.

The junction of calcified from noncalcified tissues has increasingly become implicated as the site of the essential lesion in articular cartilage injury. The limitations of articular cartilage to repair itself to have come under increased scientific scrutiny. These limitations have led to extensive investigation into various revolutionary techniques for treating articular cartilage lesions. However, tremendous controversy surrounds many of these techniques. Although the understanding of the mechanics and physiology of cartilage injury have begun to be understood, much is left to be learned about the natural history of these injuries and how the natural history can be altered by the physician.

STRUCTURE

Articular cartilage consists of a highly specialized extracellular matrix surrounding a sparse population of chondrocytes. Chondrocytes are derived from mesenchymal

cells, and it has been demonstrated that perivascular mesenchymal cells in cell culture can be recruited to form chondrocytes or osteocytes under the influence of certain morphogenetic factors (3). The chondrocytes are responsible for the production and maintenance of the extracellular matrix. Cartilage is aneural and avascular, leaving chondrocyte viability dependent on diffusion of metabolites from the synovial fluid.

The extracellular matrix in articular cartilage is responsible for its smooth gliding properties. The extracellular matrix consists of primarily type II collagen, proteoglycans, and water. Other components, such as types V, VI, IX, X, and XI collagen, lipids, and inorganic substances, are present in smaller amounts.

Type II collagen, which makes up 90% to 95% of the collagen present in articular cartilage, is largely responsible for the ability of cartilage to resist shear stress (4,5) (Fig. 43.1). The collagen fibrils of type II collagen are wound into a consistent triple helix. However, the substitution of glycine residues with other amino acids results in breaks in the triple helix such as in type IX collagen. This may allow for important cross-linking to occur between types II and IX collagen, thereby stabilizing the entire collagen network and decreasing solubility of the collagen (4,6). Although the function of type X collagen is not known, it has been identified in its highest concentrations in the zone of calcified cartilage and may play an important role in this deepest layer (4).

The proteoglycans present in cartilage consist of glycosaminoglycans, including chondroitin sulfate and keratin sulfate side chains bound to a protein core to form the aggrecan macromolecule (Fig. 43.2). The protein core is bound noncovalently to hyaluronate via link protein to form large aggregates of aggrecan–hyaluronate complexes. Glycosaminoglycans in cartilage contain both carboxy-terminal and sulfated ends, which are ionized in solution. These ionized groups result in aggrecan molecules being highly hydrophilic and

A. S. Levy and D. H. Goltz: Center for Advanced Sports Medicine, Knee and Shoulder, Summit, New Jersey 07901.

Pure Shear

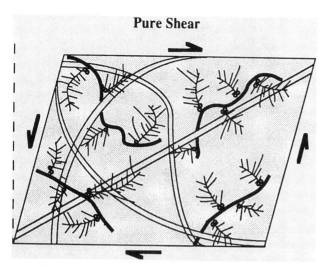

FIG. 43.1. Cartilage in pure shear. The tension of the type II collagen provides shear stiffness. (From Langer F, Gross AE, Greaves MF. The auto-immunogenicity of articular cartilage. *Clin Exp Immunol* 1972;12:31–37, with permission.)

account for the swelling pressure of cartilage. As a pressurized proteoglycan gel with collagen fiber reenforcement, cartilage is highly resistant to compressive loads.

Articular cartilage is organized into four distinct layers: superficial, middle, deep, and the calcified cartilage (4,7) (Fig. 43.3). In the superficial layer, cells and collagen are arranged in a plane parallel to the joint surface and proteoglycans are at their lowest concentration. This surface is especially well suited to facilitate the gliding motion of joints and the large sheer forces acting at the articular surface. The middle layer has more rounded cells and an oblique orientation to the collagen fibers. In the deepest layer, the cell population is at its largest concentration as is the proteoglycan concentration. The collagen fibers in the deepest layer are oriented perpendicular to the joint surface. Deepest and adjacent to bone is the calcified cartilage. The calcified cartilage is separated from the noncalcified deep cartilage layer by an eosinophilic staining wavy line referred to as the tidemark. This junction of calcified from noncalcified tissue has been shown in recent cadaver, animal, and mathematical models to be a likely source for

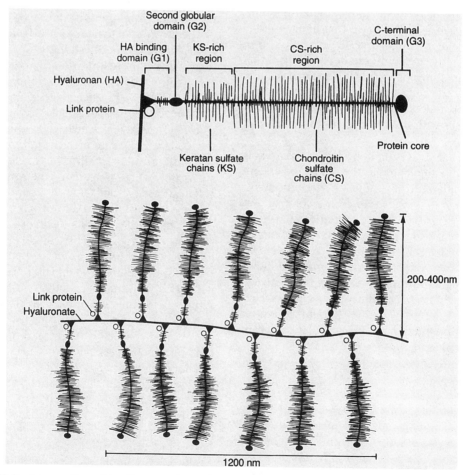

FIG. 43.2. Aggregating proteoglycan molecule in cartilage composed of keratin sulfate and chondroitin sulfate chains bound to a protein core molecule. (From Buckwalter JA, Mow VC, Ratcliffe A. Restoration of injured or degenerated articular cartilage. *J Am Acad Orthop Surg* 1994;2:192–201, with permission.

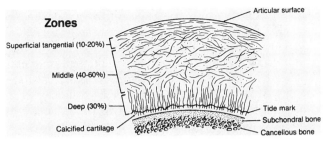

FIG. 43.3. Layered structure of cartilage collagen network showing three noncalcified zones: the calcified cartilage zone, subchondral bone, and tidemark. (From Langer F, Gross AE, Greaves MF. The auto-immunogenicity of articular cartilage. *Clin Exp Immunol* 1972;12:31–37, with permission.)

the initial injury in cartilage injuries due to sheer stress (8). Indeed, the level of the tidemark is the junction between hard and soft tissues, and with its vertically oriented collagen, it is poorly suited to resist sheer stresses.

FUNCTION

The function of articular cartilage is to allow a smooth resilient bearing surface for the articulations. The requirements of the ideal bearing surface are a low coefficient of friction, high resistance to stress, and the capacity for self-repair.

Through a combination of factors, articular cartilage maintains a low coefficient of friction. Water molecules are delivered on the surface of the articular cartilage when a load is applied. The water is "squeezed" through pores present in the collagen and proteoglycan network. These water molecules add to the already-present synovial fluid surface film. The fluid-phase portion of cartilage thus adds to the low friction surface layer between the two articular surfaces. The tangential orientation of the superficial layer also contributes to the natural low-friction surface, and under normal conditions, cartilage functions smoothly for decades.

Cartilage demonstrates time-dependent deformation under a constant load, the viscoelastic property of creep. It is most likely the result of the water molecules being slowly squeezed out of the proteoglycan gel. To some extent, deformation depends on resistance to stress in the solid components. However, water molecules experience drag as they are squeezed through the porous collagen fiber network toward the articular surface, thereby resulting in cartilage's excellent ability to resist compression.

INJURY

Under most physiologic stresses, articular cartilage is able to maintain its highly specialized function without injury. Consequently, the mechanism of articular degen-

eration has long been postulated to represent an abrasive wear phenomenon. Unfortunately, little evidence supports the concept of abrasive wear, resulting in articular cartilage lesions.

Analytical studies by Ateshian et al. (8) demonstrated that articular cartilage behaves as a bi- or perhaps triphasic material. Consequently, shear and blunt forces are manifested at the junction of the uncalcified and calcified cartilage. Using this mathematical model, the authors were unable to derive a situation whereby shearing forces would produce surface failure (abrasion) without first causing damage at the tidemark.

This has been demonstrated in a cadaver model in which loads with variable speed and force were applied to porcine femoral condyles (9). Interestingly, the low-speed low-energy injuries resulted in injuries below the articular surface, at the junction of the calcified and noncalcified tissues. Another cadaver model used blunt injury to articular cartilage and analyzed the zone of injury found microscopically in relation to the size of the injury device (10). This study demonstrated that the zone of injury is larger than the footprint of any given blunt impact. A zone of sheer forces radiates from the impact site, producing injury to the junction of calcified and noncalcified tissues.

Animal studies have supported the concept of sheer forces producing injury to the junction between the calcified and noncalcified cartilage zones. Additionally, it is known that low-speed low-energy blows produce selective injury to the deep structures (9–11) while leaving the articular surface intact (Fig. 43.4). These data

FIG. 43.4. Light micrograph of rabbit chondral delamination after shear compressive impaction by 700-g weight. Note separation at tidemark (*arrow*).

infer that the junction between calcified and noncalcified tissues may represent the "weak link" in articular cartilage's ability to resist shear forces. Transarticular loading of canine metacarpal–phalangeal joints has resulted in cracks appearing in the calcified cartilage (11) that went on to osteoarthritis, thereby strengthening the argument that injury to the deeper layers may ultimately lead to articular degeneration. However, this study used primarily compressive forces to selectively injure the calcified layer.

Recently, this phenomenon has been demonstrated in athletes (12) and in patients with a history of mechanical symptoms (1,13,14). Many of these patients demonstrate arthroscopic evidence of lesions that appeared to have a significantly larger deep component than the immediately evident surface lesion. Upon probing, the uncalcified tissue appeared to have "pealed" off the calcified layers (Fig. 43.5).

The correlation between an acute shear force injury such as during disruption of the anterior cruciate ligament and cartilage lesions is not definite, but increasing evidence of the poor prognosis of predominantly shear force injuries is mounting (11,12). Indeed, a reconstructed ligament may restore stability to the knee, but the prognosis of the articular surface may depend on factors other than stability (15). Although an unstable knee is functionally limiting, it has also been correlated with meniscal pathology. Meniscal pathology resulting in meniscectomy is known to correlate with joint degeneration, but initially stable or stable reconstructed knees with intact menisci have also gone on to joint degeneration (15). The origin of this pathology may be the initial silent insult to the articular cartilage at the time of anterior cruciate ligament disruption. Additionally, athletes involved in pivoting sports have developed cartilage lesions without ligament or meniscal pathology (12). The high sheer forces at the level of the tidemark in aggressive pivoting athletes may be sufficient in some situations to induce injury to the cartilage.

In contrast, large high-speed forces acting primarily in compression result in surface cracks in articular cartilage (9,16,17). Although any blunt injury results in a combination of shear and compressive forces, direct high-energy blows to the cartilage will result in primarily compressive forces. Examples of these types of injuries would include a motor vehicle accident where the femoral condyle directly strikes the dashboard or a direct blow to the anterior surface of the patella. Animal studies have demonstrated that softening of the articular surface occurs after appearance of these linear cracks in the cartilage (18).

Progression of occult articular cartilage injuries is an area of active scientific investigation in which much is yet to be learned. One possible explanation focuses on the potential space created between the calcified and noncalcified cartilage at the time of injury. As the joint is loaded, water molecules may be delivered to this potential space as the cartilage undergoes viscoelastic creep (8). Thus pressurized, the potential space may expand at the level of the tidemark with each loading of the joint. Eventually, the enlarged potential space may communicate with the joint surface and a surface lesion will become evident. When probed, this small lesion will appear to have delaminated from the calcified tissue, revealing a much more extensive deep lesion.

Another theory postulates that the biologic response to injury may result in a construct more poorly suited to tolerate physiologic loads. A well-designed animal study found that impulsive loading of rabbit knees resulted in subchondral plate fractures that healed into a mechanically stiffer construct (via tidemark advancement) than the normal joint (19). These joints degenerated with time.

Although different mechanisms of injury account for damage to the articular surface, it is becoming increasingly evident that the essential lesion responsible for articular degeneration after injury may be damage at the level of the calcifed–noncalcified cartilage tidemark. The understanding of occult articular injury is a new area of scientific study, and an appreciation for the destructive effects of acute shear forces is growing.

Although abrasive and third body wear does not appear to cause chondral lesions, it will certainly result in progression of articular injury and degeneration and eventually osteoarthritis. Acute injury, progression of injury, multiple small insults, absent menisci, alignment,

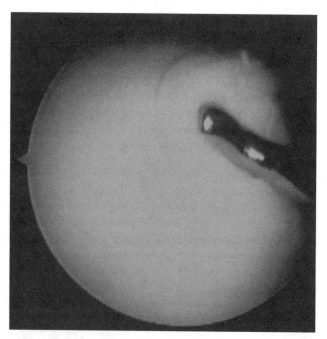

FIG. 43.5. Arthroscopic photo of probing of articular cartilage demonstrating chondral delamination without crater formation.

and instability are among the multitude of variables that may eventually result in osteoarthritis. It is unlikely that abrasive wear could result in an acute articular lesion. However, an articular lesion that progresses or does not heal could certainly result in a roughened articular surface, which could abrade the surface with which it articulates.

HEALING

Injury to the cartilage at either the surface or the deep layers would not be significant if cartilage had a strong ability to heal. Unfortunately, cartilage has a limited ability for self-repair (20–30). Numerous studies have demonstrated that acutely injured chondrocytes respond with the production of collagen and proteoglycans. This increased matrix production, however, is insufficient to fill the injured region and does not result in hyaline cartilage. Furthermore, chondrocytes lack the ability to migrate into the adjacent lesion and produce minimal mitotic activity after adolescence (31).

The primary factor related to cartilage's poor healing response is the lack of blood supply to the chondrocytes. This precludes the formation of fibrin clot and inhibits the inflammatory cascade that most tissues use in healing. Consequently, chondral injuries that do not penetrate the subchondral bone remain for up to 2 years after injury (31).

Violation of the subchondral bone, however, can elicit a vigorous healing response. The lesion first fills with blood, creating a hematoma and resulting in the production of a fibrin clot (23,24). This allows migration of mesenchymal precursor cells and results in primary fibrous repair tissue formation (22). This is followed by a variable hyaline-like phase with variable deterioration with time due to the failure of the repair tissue to develop tangential superficial layers (32).

CLINICAL EVALUATION

The isolated chondral lesion was not reported in the literature until 1987 (14). We now know that an estimated that 900,000 Americans suffer cartilage injuries each year (33). In a recent attempt to delineate the prevalence of chondral lesions, Curl et al. (34) reviewed 31,516 arthroscopies over a 4-year period. They noted 53,569 hyaline cartilage lesions in 19,827 patients. Of these, in patients under age 40 years, grade IV lesions of the femur accounted for 5% of all arthroscopies.

Patients with articular cartilage lesions may present with a myriad of confusing signs and symptoms, but the most common complaint is knee pain. The pain is generally intermittent and may or may not have been related to an acute injury. The pain may be reproducible with certain activities or within a specific arc of motion (12). Mechanical symptoms of popping, locking, and catching may occur if a fragment has broken loose or a flap of delaminated cartilage is present. Intermittent effusions occur in approximately 70% of patients with articular lesions. Care should be taken to elicit any history of prior knee injury. Approximately 50% of patients will recall some precipitating event whether it is ligament or meniscal injury, problems with patellar instability, or blunt trauma, which was initially dismissed as a contusion. No matter how far in the remote past, these injuries may have resulted in an occult articular injury, which may now manifest with pain and mechanical symptoms.

Physical examination should proceed with thorough inspection of the knee and alignment, palpation of structures, range of motion testing, and evaluation of joint stability. Special attention should be paid to the joint line and femoral condyles as tenderness may be present if a lesion is located far enough anteriorly to permit palpation. Clinically evident joint effusion is present in only about 30% of patients, although swelling is a common complaint. Joint crepitation may be present but in only 25% of patients (12). Lesions in the patellofemoral joint are more difficult to identify. The patellofemoral grind and quadriceps resistance tests are sometimes helpful. However, these lesions can easily be mistaken for anterior knee pain syndrome, patellar instability, chronic chondromalacea, or early patellofemoral osteoarthritis. In the more acute setting with mechanical symptoms and joint line tenderness, the differential should include meniscal pathology and loose body (1).

Although history and physical examination can reveal some cartilage lesions, they are sometimes difficult to identify. The key to making the diagnosis is to maintain a high index of suspicion, especially in aggressive pivoting athletes. However, imaging studies can assist in narrowing the differential diagnosis.

IMAGING

Plain radiographs are of limited value in the diagnosis of articular cartilage injury. However, due to the difficulty of making the diagnosis of a chondral lesion, x-rays are frequently obtained in the process of eliminating other possibilities from the differential diagnosis. Standard anteroposterior, lateral, and sunrise views can readily rule out both tibiofemoral and patellofemoral osteoarthritis. In the acute setting, x-rays are frequently needed to rule out fractures. If osteochondritis is strongly suspected and is not evident on standard views, a tunnel view film may reveal the lesion with sclerosis of the subchondral bone.

Although magnetic resonance imaging (MRI) has been well established in the diagnosis of meniscal and ligament pathology (35,36), it is controversial in the diagnosis of chondral lesions. With its superb ability to demonstrate soft tissue anatomy, it has become a commonly used diagnostic tool. Cartilage lesions greater than 3 mm have been reported to be imaged well in patients, especially if a joint effusion is present (37). Because of the penetration of synovial fluid or blood into the interstices of these lesions, they may appear as defects or linear delaminations with increased signal intensity on T2 imaging. However, if the lesion is not contiguous with the articular surface, imaging will be very difficult. Lesions 2 mm or greater have been identified on MRI with the introduction of intraarticular gadolinium (38). Despite the Increased sensitivity with gadolinium, the cost and invasive nature of this adjunct have resulted in infrequent use in clinical practice. Still others have dismissed MRI as being highly unreliable in diagnosing chondral lesions, with a sensitivity of as low as 21% (12). The flaw of MRI in identifying cartilage lesions relates to the nature of the studies investigating them; MRI is useful for identifying lesions if it is already known that one exists (39). New cartilage imaging sequencing is promising and may increase the efficiency of MRI in identifying chondral lesions.

The true utility of MRI in the evaluation of chondral lesions is in the modality's ability to image the subchondral structures. MRI may reveal an occult lesion not seen on x-ray or at arthroscopy (40). In the acute setting, subchondral injury has been referred to as a bone bruise (41) or a bone contusion. Increased signal on T2 and decreased signal on T1 in a geographic nonlinear pattern characterizes these familiar MRI findings. They are found in 47% to 83% of acute anterior cruciate ligament disruptions (42–46), most frequently involving the lateral femoral condyle and lateral tibial plateau. They have also been found in the talus (47), proximal humerus (48), medial malleolus (49), and distal radius (50,51). One study (52) observed dimpling or softening of the cartilage over bone bruises. However, acute bone

bruises have not been highly associated with acute cartilage lesions seen at arthroscopy (45). Long thought to represent a microtrabecular fracture, recent animal studies revealed this MRI finding to represent either a fracture of the subchondral plate or a separation of the calcified from noncalcified cartilage tidemark (53).

The natural history has been followed to resolution in the short term (43), but the long-term prognosis is not known. Preliminary work has identified thinning of the cartilage on MRI at 5 years after injury. However, because no histologic data have accompanied this finding, it is not known what pathologic process is occurring. Perhaps the cartilage is thinning or perhaps the calcified cartilage tidemark is advancing. Indeed, if a bone bruise on MRI is found after a significant subluxation of a joint, this may suggest a more severe occult articular lesion than initially suspected. The long-term natural history of these lesions is yet to be reported; however, evidence is increasingly implicating subchondral injuries in the development of frank articular surface lesions.

Technetium-99 bone scan has been reported in the diagnosis of occult osseous lesions, which may represent occult subchondral injury. Bone scans have identified subchondral lesions in the calcaneus (54). However, scintography does not demonstrate soft tissue structures, thus limiting its utility.

Arthroscopic imaging and careful probing are the gold standard in the diagnosis of articular cartilage lesions. Numerous classifications have been published describing the appearance of chondral lesions (1,13,14,55–58). However, it is critical to note that most of these classifications involve not only visualizing the articular surface but also noting the consistency of the cartilage when arthroscopically probed (Fig. 43.5). Essentially, most classification schemes describe lesions, either open or closed. Closed lesions are simply softening of the

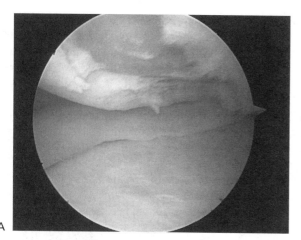
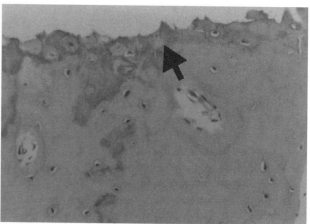

FIG. 43.6. A: Arthroscopic photo of "full-thickness" chondral lesion on the femoral condyle. **B:** Light micrograph of biopsy from same lesion however reveals that calcified cartilage (*arrow*) is still present at base of lesion.

cartilage on probing, with or without surface changes. Open lesions are classified according to size and depth of involvement. Full-thickness lesions involve true exposed subchondral bone, whereas partial-thickness lesions may only involve the layers superficial to the calcified cartilage (Fig. 43.6). Larger and deeper lesions obviously have a worse prognosis. It is also useful to classify the lesions for purposes of clear communication; however, one must state which classification is being used.

Arthroscopy is invaluable in the evaluation of articular cartilage lesions. Arthroscopy allows direct visualization and classification of the lesion. Coincident meniscal or ligament pathology can be addressed, and if amenable, the chondral lesion can be treated at the same operative sitting. If a more extensive lesion is found, accurate assessment of the pathology can be attained, thus permitting the patient and physician to pursue an objective evaluation of the various more complicated treatment options.

TREATMENT OPTIONS

The presentation of chondral injuries is quite variable, and a specific inciting event is only determinable in 25% of cases (12). Consequently, the duration and nature of nonoperative treatment will vary as well. In most cases a course of nonoperative treatment should be instituted for at least 12 weeks before surgical intervention is contemplated. Closed chain muscle strengthening combined with cryotherapy and oral anti-inflammatories are the mainstay of this treatment. Supportive braces (i.e., elastic or neoprene often assist in controlling effusions and are believed to be beneficial by many individuals with chondral lesions). Open chain strengthening may be used in some cases when the work can be performed outside the painful arc of motion. Intraarticular cortisone injections are contraindicated in athletes due to the direct deleterious effect on the articular chondrocytes and the potential for additional knee injury. No data exist concerning the success of nonoperative treatment in patients with chondral lesions.

The ultimate goal in the surgical treatment of articular cartilage lesions is the reproduction of viable hyaline cartilage bound to a restored subchondral bone plate and the surrounding hyaline cartilage. The achievement of this goal implies that arthritic deterioration is prevented and reversed with resumption of full asymptomatic function. At present these goals remain elusive, and success of treatment has been directed toward reduction of pain and swelling and improved function. Additional difficulties exist in comparing animal studies of articular cartilage. The animal models used often have articular cartilage properties extremely different from human cartilage, and the lesions created rarely resemble the human condition. Furthermore, the outcomes of these studies have been based on the ability of filling the cartilage holes or the production of hyaline-like tissue. No evidence exists to suggest that tissue that is more hyaline-like will diminish pain, improve function, and prevent deterioration of the joint.

Despite these fundamental problems in cartilage treatment, the central phenomenon of persistent cartilage defects progressing eventually to diffuse arthritis mandates continued research into treatment options (2,59). Furthermore, the frequency of patients presenting with painful swollen knees that limit function necessitates that we continue to treat these injuries despite the knowledge that our current treatment methods may prove inadequate in preventing eventual joint deterioration.

The operative treatment of chondral injuries of the articular surface can be divided into four basic principles. In advanced articular cartilage destruction, the altering of joint forces may be used to decrease pain and improve function. In isolated chondral lesions, treatment includes stabilization of loose or worn articular cartilage, stimulation of a repair process derived from the subchondral bone, and regeneration of an articular surface (via transplantation of a cell line or a precursor tissue into the defect). In many cases, a treatment option will include a combination of different techniques.

The anatomic location of the lesion must be taken into account when treating chondral lesions. This is most true of the patellofemoral joint where most lesions are the result of lateral patellofemoral compressive forces such as tilt and subluxation. In these cases, all surgical cartilage treatment options are likely to fail if the underlying mechanical problem is not addressed. Furthermore, different areas within the joint are not easily accessible for many treatment options.

ALTERATION OF JOINT FORCES

Alteration of joint forces is usually reserved for chondral injuries that have progressed to fulminate unicompartmental arthritis. Options include osteotomy, unloading braces, and shoe inserts. Although these techniques offer short time efficacy in advanced cases of arthritis, they are not frequently used in definitive treatment of chondral lesions. Consideration for osteotomy is, however, strongly recommended after failed initial cartilage repair. It is important to remember that prolonged unloading of articular cartilage will make it more susceptible to accelerated degeneration when it is remobilized (2). However, the short time use of an unloading brace may be used in cartilage repair and regeneration during the postoperative rehabilitation. These braces diminish approximately 15% (60) of the forces in the medial compartment and may thus protect a healing cartilage region while still allowing some forces to propagate through the tissue.

CARTILAGE STABILIZATION AND DEBRIDEMENT

The pain associated with chondral lesions is attributed to the free nerve endings found in the subchondral bone and the effects of cartilage debris mitigated effusions (1,59). Consequently, the removal of debris from the joint is performed to diminish its irritative effects on the synovium. This may be done either through lavage or direct particulate removal. The exact mechanisms whereby isolated chondral lesions irritate free nerve endings in subchondral bone are unknown. This may be attributed, however, to unstable chondral flaps producing mechanical irritation of the subchondral plate. Stabilization of the walls of the chondral lesion is thus performed. Unfortunately, the term stable has not been well defined, and one must be careful to avoid completely "peeling the orange." Several authors (12,14) have demonstrated that the visible chondral lesion averages approximately one third of the final lesion once debridement is concluded. Additional data exist to suggest that tapering chondral edges is less mechanically advantageous than maintaining vertical chondral lesion walls (58). Isolated cartilage stabilization and debridement is more common in the early arthritis phase of chondral lesions and in extensive or multiple lesions to diminish pain. In the isolated chondral lesion, stabilization and debridement are the initial preparatory phase in the treatment. Cartilage stabilization and debridement are easily accomplished arthroscopically and may be expedited through the use of bent curettes and osteotomes.

CARTILAGE REPAIR

Cartilage repair is based on the utilization of the subchondral bone as a source of the necessary ingredients to fill the defect, diminish pain, and improve function. At the heart of chondral repair techniques is the inability of hyaline cartilage to repair itself due to the poor blood supply and minimal cellular replicative capacity of its chondrocytes. Consequently, chondral repair involves penetration of the subchondral bone to access vascular channels to promote bleeding into the lesion (24) (Fig. 43.7). This results in fibrin clot formation and delivery of bone matrix growth factors and mesenchymal precursor cells into the defect (2).

Early on, hyaline-like cartilage with a high proportion of type II collagen may be found in the repair matrix (32). Over time, however, type I collagen becomes more prevalent, resulting in a fibrocartilage fill of the lesion (25). No evidence exists to suggest that the fibrocartilage binds to the surrounding normal hyaline cartilage. It is theorized that the fibrocartilage's beneficial effect is due to its ability to seal over the lesion, thus diminishing mechanical stress on the subchondral bone (Fig. 43.8).

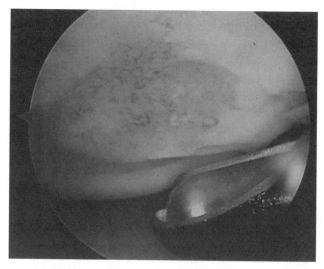

FIG. 43.7. Arthroscopic photo after debridement of chondral lesion and stimulation of punctate bleeding via controlled abrasion.

This same sealant effect may also reduce joint effusions by diminishing cartilage debris from floating free into the joint (61).

Biomechanically, fibrocartilage is markedly inferior to normal hyaline cartilage in response to shear and compressive stress (59). This combined with the stress riser between the fibro- and hyaline cartilage makes survivability questionable over long periods of time. The predictability of a successful outcome of fibrocartilage producing treatments may be quite variable in different patients.

Techniques of cartilage repair include abrasion, drilling, and "microfracture." These techniques vary mainly

FIG. 43.8. Light micrograph of biopsy from clinically successful fibrocartilage repair tissue 2 years postoperative.

on their method of achieving subchondral penetration. All these techniques first use chondral stabilization and debridement as part of the procedure. A significant advantage of these techniques is that they can all be performed arthroscopically on an outpatient basis with minimal morbidity to the patient. Despite the apparent prevalence of these techniques, little data exist on the outcome of these treatments, and no comparative studies have been published.

Cartilage lesion abrasion is differentiated from abrasion arthroplasty in that in chondral lesion abrasion, only the base of an isolated chondral lesion is abraded to penetrate the subchondral bone and stimulate punctate bleeding. Abrasion arthroplasty has been described in arthritic patients as a diffuse deep abrasion of entire joint surfaces to produce a massive bleeding bone surface. In contrast, abrasion of a chondral lesion often uses a shaver rather than a burr to minimize deep penetration of the subchondral bone. Short-term data (1 to 2 years) demonstrated that this technique is effective in athletes in diminishing symptomatology and permitting a return to competitive sports at approximately 10 to 12 weeks (12). Most athletes did note persistence of dull aching pain after strenuous activity. The overall relief of symptoms in this athletic population was comparable with the preliminary data published on the results of cartilage cell transplant in nonathletes (62).

Another common way of penetrating the subchondral bone at the base of a chondral lesion is through drilling. Theoretically, this technique preserves part of the calcified cartilage layer while creating vascular channels to allow bleeding from the subchondral bone. The exact depth of penetration via drilling has not been determined. There are two basic concerns with this technique. The first is that the speed of the drill may generate excessive heat and produce localized osteonecrosis. The second is that the vascular channels themselves result in columns of fibrocartilage that adversely effects later treatment options (63). In a single report of this technique via open arthrotomy, patients returned to full activity at 6 months with 69% rated as good, 3% as fair, and 28% as poor (58).

Another alternative technique for cartilage repair involves the use of specially designed "awls" to make perforations in the subchondral bone. Light arthroscopic shaving to remove debris follows this. The theoretic advantage of this microfracture technique is that access to undifferentiated mesenchymal cells is provided without the drawbacks of drilling. The inventors have described a 70% to 80% success rate in reducing symptoms for lesions less than 2 cm in diameter. In horses, microfracture technique generated 50% more type II collagen than controls and demonstrated 60% to 90% fill of full-thickness lesions (64). The inventors have also compared this technique to deep abrasion in horses. Six weeks after treatment, the microfracture group lesions

were noted to have a more hybrid cartilage fill that was believed to be more hyaline like than that of the deep abrasion group (64).

LASER CHONDROPLASTY

Lasers (light amplification by stimulated emission of radiation) are used in orthopedics to produce an intense beam for cutting, coagulating, and ablating of tissue. This occurs due to the absorption of laser energy and its subsequent conversion to heat based on the water content of a given tissue. In the late 1980s, surgeons began applying the thermodestructive effects of the laser to damaged articular cartilage. The use on articular cartilage lesions achieved prominence in 1989 when some investigators claimed that the holmium laser could be used to stimulate hyaline cartilage formation (65).

Further research has questioned these findings and also suggested that the penetration of laser energy is deeper than once thought and that there is a delayed zone of cartilage destruction that occurs after the initial lasing (Fig. 43.9). This area is more extensive than the initial zone of visible damage (66). Immediately after 0.5-J per pulse laser treatment of full (five pulses) and partial (one to two pulses) thickness defects in sheep, a zone of damage was noted extending up to 500 μm below the crater. Two to 4 weeks after laser surgery, hyperchromatic nuclei were seen up to 800 to 900 μm distal to the ablation crater and loss of osteocytes was

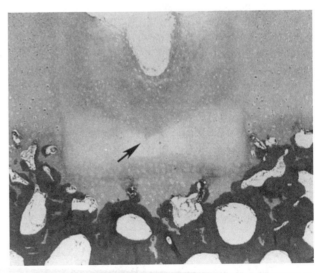

FIG. 43.9. Light micrograph of laser ablation of articular cartilage. Four weeks after partial ablation, the crater persists and damage extends more than 900 μm from crater edge. The damage zone (*arrow*) is characterized by loss of nuclei and destroyed extracellular matrix. (From Trauner KB, Nishioka NS, Flotte T, et al. Acute and chronic response of articular cartilage to homium: YAG laser irradiation. *Clin Orthop* 1995;310:52–57, with permission.)

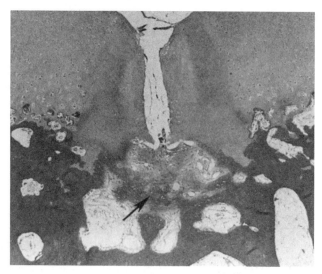

FIG. 43.10. Light micrograph of laser ablation of articular cartilage. Ten weeks after full-thickness ablation, the crater persists and damage extends more than 900 μm from crater edge. The damage zone now includes disruption of the subchondral bone (*arrow*). (From Trauner KB, Nishioka NS, Flotte T, et al. Acute and chronic response of articular cartilage to homium: YAG laser irradiation. *Clin Orthop* 1995;310:52–57, with permission.)

noted in the subchondral bone (Fig. 43.10). There was no healing of partial-thickness lesions, and some fibrocartilaginous healing was noted in the full-thickness defects. Ten weeks after laser treatment, no repair tissue was left in the full-thickness lesions and no repair response had occurred in the partial-thickness lesions. Granulation tissue was present in the damaged subchondral bone but not in the chondral ablation crater. This increased damage with time is attributed to a photoacoustic effect. At present, there is little evidence to suggest that laser use will produce significant hyaline repair. The nature and quantity of fibrocartilage repair also remains questionable given the animal data.

Recently, monopolar and bipolar radiofrequency probes have been utilized in the treatment of degenerative chondral lesions. Despite the creation of descriptive terms such as coblation (cold ablation) these devices all operate above 45° centigrade (the threshold for cell death). Further research is required before radiofrequency can be recommended in the treatment of focal chondral lesions.

CARTILAGE REGENERATION

Cartilage regeneration is the major alternative to the stimulation of the host repair response. Regeneration implies the transplantation of functional cells or precursor cells into the defect. Regenerative techniques include autogenous perichondral transplant, autogenous periosteal transplant, autogenous chondrocyte trans-

plant, autogenous osteochondral grafting, and allograft osteochondral transplant.

Rib perichondrium has been used in an attempt to fill osteochondral lesions in young patients. Its use has not been documented in isolated chondral lesions. Early success in osteochondral lesions did not persist due to the high propensity for perichondrium to calcify. Its use is not recommended in chondral lesions.

Periostium is plentiful throughout the body, although its thickness diminishes with age. Several studies have demonstrated that the cambium layer of periosteum can differentiate into chondrocytes and form hyaline cartilage (2). When sutured to the base of a lesion, a hyaline-like repair tissue was formed with similar histologic characteristics (87% type II collagen) and biomechanical characteristics as normal hyaline cartilage. The use of continuous passive motion has been found to be advantageous in increasing the success rate of periosteal transplantation in animals (67). Preliminary data demonstrated the efficacy of this technique in reducing pain in lesions of the patella and the femoral condyle (68). Controversy exists as to whether the periostium is best placed cambium layer facing into the joint (67–69) or into the lesion (62,70).

The advantages of periosteal transplant are that the supply is virtually unlimited and that minimal instrumentation and commercial supplies (cell culturing) are not required. Unfortunately, the promising early results of periosteal transplant to the femur appear to diminish with time (Fig. 43.11) (71). The patient morbidity is fairly high, because this requires a formal arthrotomy and continuous passive motion. Additional concerns exist because the cellularity of the periosteal

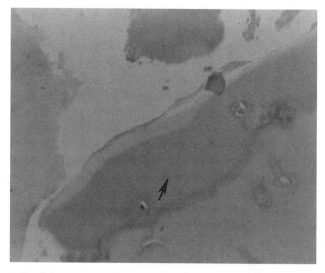

FIG. 43.11. Light micrograph of tidemark advancement (*arrow*) at base of chondral lesion 1 year after failed periosteal grafting.

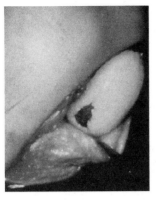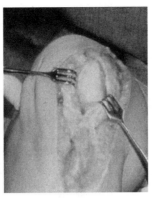

FIG. 43.12. Human femoral condyle lesion before and after combined periosteal and autogenous chondrocyte transplantation. (From Genzyme. Articular Cartilage Study Group. AAOS Annual Meeting, San Francisco, California, 1995.)

harvest appears to be closely related to the experience of the harvester (71).

To augment the periosteal transplantation, in 1989 Grande et al. (72) reported placing cultured autogenous chondrocytes under periostium sutured directly to the surrounding hyaline cartilage. In rabbit defects, this was found to produce greater filling of the defects than in controls (periostium alone sutured to cartilage). Histologically, this repair tissue was believed to be significantly more hyaline-like than the controls. In 1994, Brittberg et al. (62) reported on the results of this technique in 23 human subjects. They reported eight good (occasional pain and swelling), six excellent, and two fair and poor results on femoral lesions 1 year after transplantation (Fig. 43.12). Patellar lesion treatment yielded three fair, two poor, and two good results. Arthroscopic second looks revealed soft repair tissue in the defects without incorporation into the surrounding hyaline cartilage. This conflicted with the data from previous studies that showed early degeneration at 12

weeks after transplantation (73). These improved results were attributed to changes in postoperative regimen.

Minas et al. (74) also reported on 16 cases of chondrocyte transplants in humans. Fifty percent of patients reported decreased pain at 3 months, with an improvement to 80% at 6 months with only one patient requiring revision. Subsequently, Breinan et al. (75) reported on a long-term canine study using cultured autologous chondrocytes. In this study, the authors compared unfilled defects to the calcified cartilage to those covered with periostium flap sewn to the cartilage surface to those filled with cultured autogenous chondrocytes. The 6-week, 3-month, and 6-month results showed a more complete fill with hyaline-like cartilage in the autogenous cell transplanted group (Fig. 43.13). At 12 and 18 months, however, no significant differences were noted in the three groups (Fig. 43.14).

This extended time frame of improvement is correlated with the three-phase progression of this technique (76). The proliferative phase accounts for the first 4 weeks after transplantation and is characterized by rapid increase of the total chondrocyte population. The maturation phase occurs from weeks 4 to 8 and includes differentiation of the transplanted chondrocytes into hyaline-like chondrocytes. During this phase, extracellular matrix production increases and a smooth articular surface appears. The transformation phase occurs from 2 to 6 months after transplantation and involves multilayer organization into hyaline-like cartilage. The most marked changes occur at the deep zones where chondrocytes nourished by subchondral blood vessels transform into a calcified layer to reconstitute the subchondral plate. Although these phases have been demonstrated in animal models, the occurrence of the transformation phase and its time frame have yet to be documented in human studies. Little information exists as to what occurs in humans after the 6-month point.

Enthusiasm for this technique in the United States

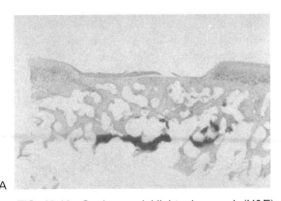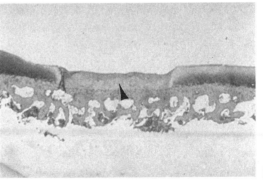

A   B

FIG. 43.13. Canine model light micrograph (H&E) of periosteal patch alone **(A)** vs. chondrocyte transplant **(B)** at 6 weeks after operative. Note apparent restoration of chondral layer (*arrow*) in chondrocyte treated site. (From Breinan HA, Minas T, Hsu HP, et al. Effect of cultured chondrocytes on repair of chondral defects in a canine model. *J Bone Joint Surg Am* 1997;79-A:1439–1451.)

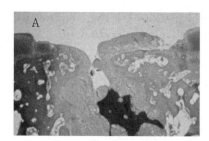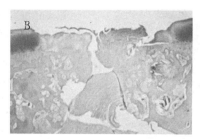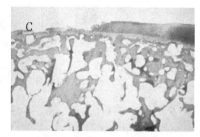

FIG. 43.14. Canine model light micrograph (Safranin O) of no treatment **(A)** vs. periosteal patch alone **(B)** vs. chondrocyte transplant **(C)** at 1 year after operative. Note lack of restoration of chondral layer in all cases. (From Breinan HA, Minas T, Hsu HP, et al. Effect of cultured chondrocytes on repair of chondral defects in a canine model. *J Bone Joint Surg Am* 1997;79-A:1439–1451, with permission.)

has been hampered by theoretic and economic concerns. It is well known that cultured chondrocytes frequently dedifferentiate into fibrochondrocytes. This occurs primarily in monolayer cultures and is accompanied by a loss of phenotype, increased type I collagen production, and decreased type II collagen and aggrecan production (77). Furthermore, if they manage to survive the transplant back into the knee joint, little data exist as to whether the hyaline-like cartilage will truly function like and bind to the surrounding hyaline cartilage.

Economically, the cost of the cells alone is $10,000, and third-party payers are extremely unwilling to approve its use except in rare salvage cases. Despite these difficulties, 1,810 chondrocyte harvests have been performed, resulting in 808 implantations by 583 surgeons as of February 1999 (78). In the 240 cases with 24-month follow-up, 85% reported a reduction in pain and swelling, with 8% noting an increase in these symptoms. Overall patient evaluated improvement averaged 3.1 (on a 10-point scale) from preoperative evaluation.

Autogenous Osteochondral Grafting

The rational behind osteochondral grafting is the vast array of analytic, cadaver, animal, and, recently, human data that demonstrate the common essential lesion in the development of chondral lesions occurs at or near the tidemark where the subchondral plate (subchondral bone and calcified cartilage) interfaces with the uncalcified cartilage. By replacing the entire osteochondral unit, one could theoretically address and remove the actual site of damage that has led to the visible lesion.

The first known report of transplanting articular cartilage bone fragments is by Judet and Henri in 1908 for the treatment of osteochondritis dissecans (79). In 1959, Campbell et al. (80) reported using fresh osteochondral autografts with little or no destruction occurring over the first year. In 1961, Pap and Krompecher (81) reported the transplantation of articular cartilage fragments and their associated less than 5 mm of subchondral bone in 51 dogs. They noted survival of the articular cartilage of up to 2 years provided normal physiologic

loads were applied. In 1962, Entin et al. (82) performed autogenous osteochondral transplantation from the foot to the hand and found that the cartilage was not replaced.

In 1963, Campbell et al. (83) again reported on the use of osteochondral grafting on 42 dog knees. In this study, grafts were limited to 1 × 2 cm in width and length, with subchondral bone depth limited to less than 5 mm. They noted that the osseous portion healed by 14 days via creeping substitution and that the articular cartilage appeared grossly and histologically normal at 500 days after grafting. They did, however, note that the articular cartilage of the grafts did not bind to the surrounding cartilage. They also speculated that increasing the depth of the subchondral bone might lead to increased necrosis of deep bone.

The healing of osteochondral autografts has been further studied by McDermott et al. (84). It appears that the surface osteocytes in the subchondral bone survive, whereas those deeper than 3 mm are replaced within the first 4 weeks.

Limited biomechanical studies have also been performed to evaluate the effects of graft size on function. It has been shown that a 15% increase in diameter results in a 50% increase in torsional strength of the grafts (85). The potential unknown effects of radius mismatch must, however, temper this.

In 1994, Hangody and Karpati (86) reported on a technique termed "mosaicplasty." Mosaicplasty uses multiple plugs of autogenous osteochondral graft to fill chondral lesions. Based on unpublished work on dogs (36 surgeries on 18 dogs), this procedure was performed on 122 humans. There were 57 medial femoral condyle lesions, 48 lateral femoral condyle lesions, and 17 patella lesions with greater than 1 year follow-up. The lesions ranged from 1 to 8 cm², and grafts varying from 2.7 to 4.5 mm diameter were obtained from the lateral and medial edge of the condyles to fill the defect via an open arthrotomy. At 1 year follow-up, there were no cases of loosening or backing out of the grafts, and the average HSS score was 88.4 (range, 61 to 100). Second-look arthroscopy was performed in many cases and showed good congruency.

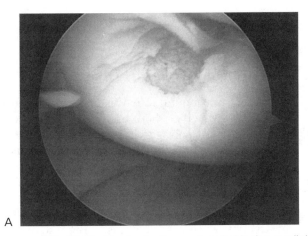
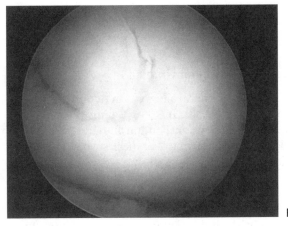

A   B

FIG. 43.15. Twelve by 7-mm chondral lesion medial femoral condyle **(A)** treated by arthroscopic placement of osteochondral plugs **(B)**.

The use of osteochondral autografts has also been described in conjunction with anterior cruciate reconstruction. In 29 cases, 1- to 1.5-cm defects of the femoral condyles were filled with osteochondral plugs (5 mm wide and 10 to 15 mm long) harvested from the intercondylar notch. At 2 to 3 years after transplantation, the articular cartilage on the transplants appears (via MRI and probing) to have survived. The surrounding area is filled with fibrocartilage. Clinically, this has correlated with 19 excellent outcomes in 22 cases (87).

The resurgence in enthusiasm for osteochondral grafting is associated with the increased development of techniques that permit more predictable arthroscopic harvesting and delivery of the plugs. This, however, applies only to limited areas of the femoral condyles (Fig. 43.15). The use of this technique on the patella, trochlea, posterior femoral condyles, and talus requires open arthrotomy (Fig. 43.16). Additionally, the treatment of defects greater than 12 mm in diameter often requires open arthrotomy to ensure perpendicular graft placement.

Difficulties with osteochondral grafting include those associated with perpendicular graft placement, graft impaction forces, cartilage thickness mismatch, and radius of curvature differences. Further concerns arise due to the continued necessity for fibrocartilaginous fill around

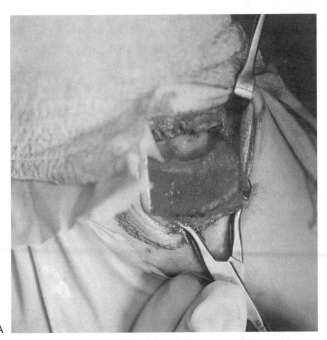
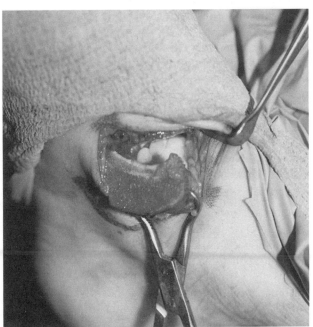

A   B

FIG. 43.16. Twenty-millimeter chondral lesion of talus **(A)** treated by medial maleolar osteotoma and open osteochondral grafting **(B)**. Plugs harvested from ipsilateral knee.

the plugs and potential remaining stress riser production between the two nonbinding cartilages.

Allograft Osteochondral Grafting

The use of osteochondral allografts in tumor treatments dates back to the 1950s. In 1959, Campbell et al. (80) reported using fresh osteochondral autografts with little or no destruction occurring over the first year. However, when fresh and frozen allografts were used, they became fibrillated and degenerated within a few months. This deterioration of the articular cartilage in allografts has also been documented in cryopreserved cases. It appears that the subchondral collapse produced by bone turnover in the metaphysis produces the cartilage destruction (84,88). Thus, the fate of the transplanted articular cartilage in allografts is related to the fate of the subchondral bone.

It appears that the proteoglycans in the cartilage matrix act as a barrier to prevent recognition of the foreign antigens on the transplanted chondrocytes (89). This protects the transplanted chondrocytes from humeral and cell-mediated immune reactions (83,90,91). Several authors have subsequently shown that immune responses do not occur to osteochondral allograft chondrocytes surrounded by intact matrices (92,93).

Cellular survival of chondrocytes has been improved with two-stage cryopreservation techniques. Cryoprotectant use has subsequently produced 85% to 95% chondrocyte survival rates with maintenance of chondrocyte phenotype (94). For allograft cartilage transplant to be successful, the allograft must heal to the surrounding bone incompletely so that extensive revascularization and resorption does not result in cartilage collapse.

To date, no studies exist that address the use of modern osteochondral grafting techniques for allograft. Theoretically, if successful, this would improve graft thickness and radius of curvature mismatch concerns in autograft techniques.

CARTILAGE STIMULATION VIA GROWTH FACTORS

An exciting area of cartilage repair and regeneration involves the use of growth factors. These polypeptides attach to chondrocyte cell surface receptors (integrins) and influence matrix production, proliferation, migration, and replication (2). The two most promising factors at present are insulin-like growth factor type 1 and transforming growth factor-β. These have been shown to enhance matrix synthesis in animal studies. Unfortunately, these growth factors are not specific for chondrocytes and can effect an entire joint adversely. Further research is needed into delivery, regulation, and modu-

lation of these factors before they are used in human joints.

AUTHORS' PREFERRED TREATMENT

Treatment of chondral lesions is first and foremost determined by whether there has been a previous treatment rendered (salvage situation) or if the planned treatment is the initial intervention (primary situation). Secondarily come the size and location of the lesion. The third consideration is the patient-specific factors, including limb alignment, morphology, and life issues.

Patient preparation and preoperative discussion is paramount for success in all cases. Because of the frequent overlap in symptoms with meniscal pathology, we inform all arthroscopy patients of a likelihood that an articular cartilage procedure may be required at surgery. One must explain the potential divergence in surgical technique and postoperative treatment regimen should a cartilage lesion be identified.

For primary lesions of the trochea, tibia, talus, and posterior femoral condyles, debridement of unstable borders and stimulation of fibrocartilage is our preferred option (Fig. 43.17). Debridement is best accomplished by controlled "scooping" of unstable chondral borders using bent curettes and osteotomes. Scraping the calcified cartilage to stimulate punctate bleeding via these same bent curettes and osteotomes follows this. Alternatively, this can be accomplished using microfracture awls. The debris is then removed using a rotatory shaver on suction. Successful penetration of the subchondral bone can be confirmed by placing the shaver near the lesion with suction wide open and inflow closed. Diffuse punctate bleeding necessary for fibrin clot formation is thus confirmed. Postoperatively, the patients are started on range of motion exercises, and cryotherapy is used for control of pain and swelling. Anti-inflammatory medicines are avoided for 6 weeks to avoid disrupting the repair response. The basic science data on the effect of early weight bearing and fibrocartilage

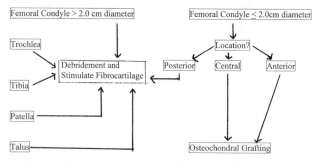

FIG. 43.17. Algorithm for authors' preferred initial treatment of symptomatic chondral lesions.

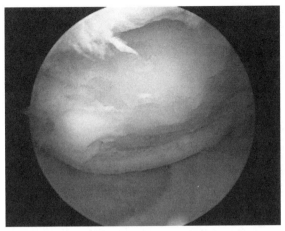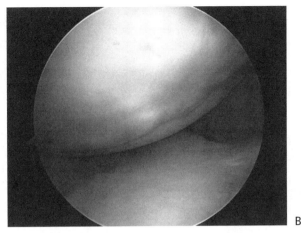

A   B

FIG. 43.18. Large (25-mm diameter) chondral lesion of medial femoral condyle **(A)** treated by open osteochondral grafting. Four months later, repeat arthroscopy **(B)** reveals plug integrity and fibrocartilage fill.

fill is conflicting. Although many surgeons prefer to keep these patients non-weight bearing, we have not seen a problem with early weight bearing and routinely encourage it as the patient regains quadriceps control. The stationary bicycle is a mainstay of early rehabilitation and closed chain exercises are instituted as range of motion increases. Return to running and sports are patient specific and achieved in a goal-oriented program of progression. This averages 10 to 12 weeks in most cases.

We prefer to use osteochondral grafting in the primary treatment of lesions in the central and anterior third of the femoral condyles (Fig. 43.18). We do not hesitate to perform a miniarthrotomy for lesions greater than 12 mm in diameter and in any situation where perpendicular placement may be jeopardized by the arthroscopic technique. The 6-mm-diameter 8-mm-deep plug is our mainstay, but this may be supplemented by 4- and 8-mm-diameter plugs. Care must be taken to gently tap the graft into place to avoid delaminating its surface.

Postoperatively, early active range of motion, bicycle, and isometric quadriceps exercises are initiated while the limb is kept non-weight bearing for 3 weeks. From 3 to 6 weeks, partial weight bearing is initiated. After 6 weeks, the patient is advanced to full weight bearing and strengthening exercises are instituted. Sports-specific rehabilitation is initiated at 10 to 12 weeks with full return to activities based on a functional assessment.

The primary treatment of a chondral lesion should not be termed a failure until at least 6 months after operation. If pain and/or swelling persist and function is diminished, consideration can be given to a salvage procedure (Fig. 43.19). In salvage situations, it is important to allow the subchondral plate to recover from the initial surgery. Once a patient has failed a less aggressive treatment option, our preference is to perform a carticel technique for lesions of the femoral condyle and trochlea (Fig. 43.20). It is important to begin preparing the patient for this procedure and its implications before harvesting the chondrocytes for culture. If this is unachievable due to socioeconomic reasons, consideration is given toward osteochondral grafting via a formal open arthrotomy. For lesions of the talus, open osteochondral grafting via a malleolar osteotomy has produced relief for many patients who have failed debridement of osteochondral lesions.

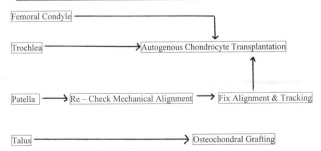

FIG. 43.19. Algorithm for authors' preferred salvage treatment after failed initial treatment of symptomatic chondral lesions.

SUMMARY

The treatment of articular cartilage lesions remains one of the great challenges facing orthopedic surgeons today. The technique of chondrocyte transplantation has opened the door for the application of biologic solutions to difficult problems. These techniques will prove the keystone of further advances into biologic joint repair and replacement. Enthusiasm, however, must be tempered by the numerous gaps in cartilage science and the overwhelming need for further long-term data to demonstrate the efficacy of these techniques in thwart-

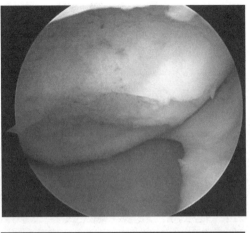

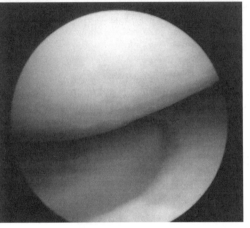

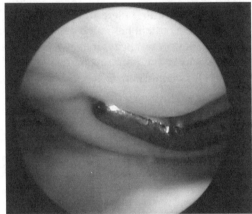

FIG. 43.20. A: Arthroscopic photo of a patient who presented with an isolated chondral lesion of the medial femoral condyle after failing simple debridement. **B:** Arthroscopic photo of same patient after further debridement and stimulation of punctate bleeding via controlled abrasion. **C:** Arthroscopic photo during chondrocyte biopsy of same patient 6 months after the controlled abrasion. Despite fibrocartilage fill, the patient remained extremely symptomatic. **D:** Arthroscopic photo of a patient 6 months status after chondrocyte transplantation. **E:** Arthroscopic photo of a patient 6 months after chondrocyte transplantation. Despite visual appearance, probing reveals sacklike consistency of repair tissue.

ing the presumed eventual progression of these lesions toward osteoarthritis. The orthopedic surgeon must increase his or her knowledge of the basic science of articular cartilage to best choose from the various cartilage treatments.

REFERENCES

1. Zamber RW, Teitz CC, McGuire DA, et al. Articular cartilage lesions of the knee. *Arthroscopy* 1989;5:258–268.
2. Buckwalter JA, Mow VC, Ratcliffe A. Restoration of injured or degenerated articular cartilage. *J Am Acad Orthop Surg* 1994;2: 192–201.
3. Takahashi S, Urist MR. Differentiation of cartilage on three substrata under the influence of an aggregate of morphogenetic protein and other bone tissue noncollagenous proteins. *Clin Orthop* 1986;207:227–238.
4. Mankin HJ, Mow VC, Buckwalter JA, et al. Form and function of articular cartilage. In: Simon SR, ed. *Orthopaedic basic science.* Rosemont, IL: AAOS, 1994:1–44.
5. Mow VC, Ratcliffe A. Structure and function of articular cartilage and meniscus. In: Mow VC, Hayes WC, eds. *Basic orthopaedic biomechanics.* Philadelphia: Lippincott-Raven, 1997: 113–177.
6. Mayne R, Irwin MH. Collagen types in cartilage. In: Kuettner KE,

Schleyerbach R, Hascall VC, eds. *Articular cartilage biochemistry.* New York: Raven Press, 1986:23–38.

7. Buckwalter JA, Hunziker EB. Articular cartilage biology and morphology. In: Mow VC, Ratcliffe A, eds. *Structure and function of articular cartilage.* Boca Raton, FL: CRC Press, 1993.

8. Ateshian GA, Lai WM, Zhu WB, et al. An asymptotic solution for the contact of two biphasic cartilage layers. *J Biomech* 1994;27:1347–1360.

9. Tomatsu T, Imai N, Takewuchi N, et al. Experimentally produced fractures of articular cartilage and bone. *J Bone Joint Surg Br* 1992;74-B:457–462.

10. Borrelli J Jr, Torzilla PA, Grigiene R, et al. Effect of impact load on articular cartilage: development of an intra-articular fracture model. *J Orthop Trauma* 1997;11:319–326.

11. Vener MJ, Thompson RC, Lewis JL, et al. Subchondral damage after transarticular loading: an in vitro model of joint injury. *J Orthop Res* 1992;10:759–765.

12. Levy AS, Lohnes J, Sculley S, et al. Chondral delamination of the knee is soccer players. *Am J Sports Med* 1995;24:634–639.

13. Imai N, Tomatsu T. Cartilage lesions in the knee of adolescents and young adults: arthroscopic analysis. *Arthroscopy* 1991;7:198–203.

14. Terry GC, Flandry F, Van Mansen JW, et al. Isolated chondral fractures of the knee. *Clin Orthop* 1988;234:170–177.

15. Daniel DM, Stone ML, Dobson BE, et al. Fate of the ACL injured knee. *Am J Sports Med* 1994;22:632–644.

16. Haut RC. Contact pressures in the patellofemoral joint during impact loading on the human flexed knee. *J Orthop Res* 1989;7:272–280.

17. Xiaowel L, Haut RC, Altiero NJ. An analytical model to study blunt impact response of the rabbit P-F joint. *J Biomech Eng* 1995;117:485–491.

18. Haut RC, Ide TM, De Camp CE. Mechanical response of the rabbit patellofemoral joint to blunt impact. *J Biomech Eng* 1995;117:402–408.

19. Radin EL, Parker HG, Pugh JW, et al. Response of joint to impact loading. III. Relationship between trabecular microfractures on cartilage degeneration. *J Biomech* 1973;6:51–57.

20. Hunter W. On the structure and diseases of articulating cartilages. *Phil Trans R Soc* 1743;42(B):514–521.

21. Bennett GA, Baur W. Further studies concerning the repair of articular cartilage in dog joints. *J Bone Joint Surg* 1935;17:141–150.

22. Bennett GA, Baur W, Maddock SJ. A study of the repair of articular cartilage and the reaction of normal joints of adult dogs to surgically created defects of articular cartilage, "joint mice," and patellar displacement. *Am J Pathol* 1932;8:499–524.

23. Calandruccio RA, Gilmer WS. Proliferation, regeneration, and repair of articular cartilage of immature animals. *J Bone Joint Surg Am* 1962;44-A:431–455.

24. Campbell CJ. The healing of cartilage defects. *Clin Orthop* 1969;64:45–62.

25. DePalma AF, McKeever CD, Subin SK. Process of repair of articular cartilage demonstrated by histology and autoradiography with tritiated thymidine. *Clin Orthop* 1966;48:229–242.

26. Fuller JA, Ghadially FN. Ultrastructural observations on surgically produced partial thickness defects in articular cartilage. *Clin Orthop* 1972;86:193–205.

27. Ito LK. The nutrition of articular cartilage and its method of repair. *Br J Surg* 1924;12:31–42.

28. Mankin HJ. Localization of tritiated thymidine in articular cartilage of rabbits. II. Repair in immature cartilage. *J Bone Joint Surg Am* 1962;44-A:688–698.

29. Mankin HJ. The reaction of articular cartilage to injury an osteoarthritis. Parts 1 and 2. *N Engl J Med* 1974;291:1285–1292, 1335–1340.

30. Paget J. Healing of cartilage. *Clin Orthop* 1969;64:7–8.

31. Mankin HJ. The response of articular cartilage to mechanical injury. *J Bone Joint Surg Am* 1982;64-A:460–466.

32. Mitchell N, Shepard N. The resurfacing of adult rabbit articular cartilage by multiple perforations through the subchondral bone. *J Bone Joint Surg Am* 1976;58-A:230–233.

33. Genzyme. Presented at AAOS 1995 annual meeting: Cartilage repair symposium, San Francisco, CA.

34. Curl WW, Krome J, Gordon ES, et al. Cartilage injuries: a review of 31,516 knee arthroscopies. *Arthroscopy* 1997;13:456–460.

35. Rangger C, Klestil T, Kathrein A, et al. Influence of magnetic resonance imaging on indications for arthroscopy of the knee. *Clin Orthop* 1996;330:133–142.

36. Jackson DW, Jennings LD, Maywood RM, et al. Magnetic resonance imaging of the knee. *Am J Sports Med* 1988;6:29–38.

37. Wojtys E, Wilson M, Buckwalter K, et al. Magnetic resonance imaging of knee hyaline cartilage and intraarticular pathology. *Am J Sports Med* 1987;15:455–463.

38. Gylys-Morin VM, Hajek PC, Sartoris DJ, et al. Articular cartilage defects: detectability in cadaver knees with MR. *Am J Radiol* 1987;148:1153–1157.

39. Speer KP, Spritzer CE, Goldner L, et al. Magnetic resonance imaging of traumatic knee articular cartilage injuries. *Am J Sports Med* 1991;19:396–402.

40. Handelberg F, Shahabpour M, Casteleyn P. Chondral lesions of the patella evaluated with computed tomography, magnetic resonance imaging and arthroscopy. *Arthroscopy* 1990;6:24–29.

41. Mink JH, Deutsch AL. Occult cartilage and bone injuries of the knee: detection, classification, and assessment with MR imaging. *Radiology* 1989;170:823–829.

42. Speer KP, Spritzer CE, Bassett FH, et al. Osseous injury associated with acute tears of the anterior cruciate ligament. *Am J Sports Med* 1992;20:382–389.

43. Speer KP, Warren RF, Wickiewicz TL, et al. Observations on the injury mechanism of anterior cruciate ligament tears in skiers. *Am J Sports Med* 1995;23:77–81.

44. Vellet AD, Marks PH, Fowler PJ, et al. Occult post-traumatic osteochondral lesions off the knee: prevalence, classification, and short-term sequelae evaluated with MR imaging. *Radiology* 1991;178:271–276.

45. Graf BK, Cook DA, De Smet AA, et al. "Bone bruise" on magnetic resonance imaging evaluation of anterior cruciate ligament injuries. *Am J Sports Med* 1993;21:220–223.

46. Spindler KP, Schils JP, Bergfeld JA, et al. Prospective study of osseous, articular and meniscal lesions in anterior cruciate ligament tears by magnetic resonance imaging and arthroscopy. *Am J Sports Med* 1993;21:551–557.

47. Zanetti M, De Simoni C, Wetz HH, et al. Magnetic resonance imaging of injuries to the ankle joint: can it predict clinical outcome? *Skeletal Radiol* 1997;26:82–88.

48. Anzilotti KF Jr, Schweitzer ME, Oliveri M, et al. Skeletal radiology, rotator cuff strain: a post-traumatic mimicker of tendonitis on MRI. *Skeletal Radiol* 1996;25:555–558.

49. Nishimura G, Yamato M, Togawa M. Trabecular trauma of the talus and medial malleoulus concurrent with lateral collateral ligamentous injuries of the ankle: evaluation with MRI. *Skeletal Radiol* 1996;25:49–54.

50. Kettner NW, Pierre-Jerome C. Magnetic resonance imaging of the wrist: occult osseus lesions. *J Manipulative Physiol Ther* 1992;15:599–603.

51. Shih C, Chang CY, Penn IW, et al. Chronically stressed wrists in adolescent gymnasts: MR imaging appearance. *Radiology* 1995;195:855–859.

52. Coen MJ, Caborn DN, Johnson DL. The dimpling phenomenon: articular cartilage injury overlying an occult osteochondral lesion at the time of anterior cruciate ligament reconstruction. *Arthroscopy* 1996;12:502–505.

53. Goltz DH, Levy AS, Parsons R. The MRI bone bruise: what is it, really? Proceedings of the AAOS annual meeting, New Orleans, LA 1998.

54. Soudry G, Mannting F. Hot calcaneus on three-phase bone scan due to bone bruise. *Clin Nucl Med* 1995;20:832–934.

55. Jackson RW. Meniscal and articular cartilage injury in sport. *J R Coll Surg Edinb* 1989;34[Suppl]:s15–s17.

56. Baur M, Jackson RW. Chondral lesions of the femoral condyles: a system of arthroscopic classification. *Arthroscopy* 1988;4:97–102.

57. Noyes FR, Stabler CL. A system for grading articular cartilage lesions at arthroscopy. *Am J Sports Med* 1989;17:505–513.

58. Dzioba RB. The classification and treatment of acute articular cartilage lesions. *Arthroscopy* 1988;4:72–80.

59. Mayer G, Seidlein H. Chondral and osteochondral fractures of

the knee joint—treatment and results. *Arch Orthop Trauma Surg* 1988;107:154–157.

60. Wickiewicz TL. Presented at the AOSSM annual meeting, Sun Valley, ID, 1997.

61. Farkas T, Lippiello L, Mitrovic D, et al. Papain induced healing of superficial lacerations in articular cartilage of adult rabbits. *Trans Orthop Res Soc* 1977;2:204.

62. Brittberg M, Lindahl A, Nilsson A, et al. Treatment of deep cartilage defects in the knee with autologous chondrocyte transplantation. *N Engl J Med* 1994;331:889–895.

63. Genzyme. Articular cartilage study group, AAOS annual meeting, New Orleans, LA, 1998.

64. Steadman R. Biological resurfacing of large articular cartilage defects. Presented at AAOS annual meeting: Meniscus and articular cartilage study group, San Francisco, CA, 1997.

65. Miller DV, O'Brien SJ, Arnoczky SS, et al. The use of the contact Nd:YAG laser in arthroscopic surgery: effects on articular cartilage and meniscal tissue. *Arthroscopy* 1989;5:245–253.

66. Trauner KB, Nishioka NS, Flotte T, et al. Acute and chronic response of articular cartilage to homium:YAG laser irradiation. *Clin Orthop* 1995;310:52–57.

67. Delaney-JP, O'Driscoll SW, Salter RB. Neochondrogenesis in free intraarticular periosteal autografts in an immobilized and paralyzed limb. An experimental investigation in the rabbit. *Clin Orthop* 1989;248:278–282.

68. O'Driscoll SW, Kelley FW, Salter RB. Durability of regenerated articular cartilage produced by free autogenous periosteal grafts in major full-thickness defects in joint surfaces under the influence of continuous passive motion. A follow-up report at one year. *J Bone Joint Surg Am* 1988;70-A:595–606.

69. O'Driscoll S, Salter R, Kelley F. The chondrogenic potential of free autogenous periosteal grafts for biological resurfacing of major full-thickness defects in joint surfaces under the influence of continuous passive motion: an experimental investigation in the rabbit. *J Bone Joint Surg Am* 1986;68-A:1017–1035.

70. Lorentzen R. Chondral lesions of the patella treated with periosteal grafts. Presented at Sports Medicine 2000, Stockholm, Sweden, 1995.

71. O'Driscoll S. Presented at the AAOS annual meeting, San Francisco, CA, 1997.

72. Grande DA, Pitman MI, Peterson L, et al. The repair of experimentally produced defects in rabbit articular cartilage by autologous chondrocyte transplantation. *J Orthop Res* 1989;7:208–218.

73. Shapiro F, Koide S, Glimcher MJ. Cell origin and differentiation in the repair of full-thickness defects of articular cartilage. *J Bone Joint Surg Am* 1993;75-A:532–553.

74. Minas T, Spector M, Shortroff S, et al. New animal, human data reported for autologous chondrocyte transplants [as reported by J. Fischer]. *Orthop Today* 1996;16:18–19.

75. Breinan HA, Minas T, Hsu HP, et al. Effect of cultured chondro-cytes on repair of chondral defects in a canine model. *J Bone Joint Surg Am* 1997;79-A:1439–1451.

76. Itay S, Abramovici A, Nevo Z. Use of cultured embryonal chick epiphyseal chondrocytes as grafts for defects in chick articular cartilage. *Clin Orthop* 1987;220:284–303.

77. Green W. Articular cartilage repair. Behavior of rabbit chondro-cytes during tissue culture and subsequent allografting. *Clin Orthop* 1977;124:237–250.

78. Genzyme Cartilage Repair Registry, Vol. 5, Feb. 1999.

79. Judet, Henri. Essai sur la greffe des tissues articulares. *Comp Rend Acad D Sci* 1908;146:193–196, 600–603.

80. Campbell CJ, Grisolia A, Zanconato G. The effects produced in the cartilaginous epiphyseal plate of immature dogs by experimental surgical traumata. *J Bone Joint Surg Am* 1959;45-A:1221–1242.

81. Pap K, Krompecher S. Arthroplasty of the knee- experimental and clinical experiences. *J Bone Joint Surg Am* 1961;43-A:523–537.

82. Entin MA, Alger JR, Baird RM. Experimental and clinical transplantation of autogenous whole joints. *J Bone Joint Surg Am* 1962;44-A:1518–1536.

83. Campbell CJ, Ishida H, Takahashi H, et al. The transplantation of articular cartilage: an experimental study in dogs. *J Bone Joint Surg Am* 1963;45-A:1579–1592.

84. McDermott AG, Langer F, Pritzker KP, et al. Fresh small-fragment osteochondral allografts: long-term follow-up study on first 100 cases. *Clin Orthop* 1985;197:96–102.

85. Pelker RR, Friedlaender GE. Boimechanical considerations in osteochondral grafts. In: Friedlaender GE, Goldberg VM, eds. *Bone and cartilage allografts.* Rosemont, IL: American Academy of Orthopaedic Surgeons, 1991:155–162.

86. Hangody L, Karpati Z. A new surgical treatment of localized cartilagenous defects of the knee. *Hung J Orthop Trauma* 1994;37:237–242.

87. Bobic V. Arthroscopic osteochondral autograft transplantation in anterior cruciate ligament reconstruction: a preliminary clinical study. *Knee Surg Sports Traumatol Arthrosc* 1996;3:262–264.

88. Mankin HJ, Fogelson FS, Thrasher AZ, et al. Massive resection and allograft transplantation in the treatment of malignant bone tumors. *N Engl J Med* 1976;294:1247–1255.

89. Chen FS, Frenkel SR, Di Cesare PE. Chondrocyte transplantation and experimental treatment options for articular cartilage defects. *Am J Orthop* 1997;26:396–406.

90. Brown KL, Cruess RL. Bone and cartilage transplantation in orthopaedic surgery: a review. *J Bone Joint Surg Am* 1982;64-A:270–279.

91. Sengupta S. The fate of transplants of articular cartilage in the rabbit. *J Bone Joint Surg Br* 1974;56-B:167–177.

92. Langer F, Gross AE, Greaves MF. The auto-immunogenicity of articular cartilage. *Clin Exp Immunol* 1972;12:31–37.

93. McKibbon B, Ralis ZA. The site dependence of the articular cartilage transplant reaction. *J Bone Joint Surg Br* 1978;60-B:561–566.

94. Tomford W, Mankin H. Investigational approaches to articular cartilage preservation. *Clin Orthop* 1983;174:22–27.

Principles and Practice of Orthopaedic Sports Medicine,
edited by William E. Garrett, Jr., Kevin P. Speer, and Donald T. Kirkendall.
Lippincott Williams & Wilkins, Philadelphia © 2000.

CHAPTER 44

Multiligament Injuries of the Knee

Laurence D. Higgins, Mark Clatworthy, and Christopher D. Harner

The multiple-ligament knee injury is an infrequent injury, and significant controversy regarding its treatment continues to exist. The early evaluation of such knee injuries, due to the high rate of associated vascular and nerve injury, has received significant and appropriate study. Failure of early diagnosis of vascular injuries has led to alarmingly high amputation rates, approaching 90% in some series (1). As a more precise acute evaluation of such injuries has evolved, attention has now shifted toward the outcome of these injuries and algorithms for their treatment. Early nonoperative treatment failures have yielded to more aggressive operative repair or reconstruction to maximize the patient's functional outcome. Despite the relative rarity of these injuries, a thorough understanding of these complex injuries is mandatory to appropriately manage patients with multiple-ligament injuries.

DEFINITION

Most knee dislocations involve injury to both the anterior (ACL) and posterior cruciate ligaments (PCL). However, case reports of such injuries with an intact cruciate ligament exist (2–4). Additionally, involvement of collateral ligaments is common, as is the posterolateral corner (particularly when the PCL has been injured). Concomitant injury to the meniscus and the articular cartilage is often found, and although fractures may exist, their occurrence is usually limited to those injuries

resulting from high-energy trauma (i.e., motor vehicle injuries).

ANATOMY

The anatomy of the anterior and PCLs has been well covered in the preceding chapters. In this chapter we address the anatomy of the posterolateral structures (PLS) and posteromedial structures (PMS) of the knee.

Posterolateral Structures

The principal anatomic structures of the posterolateral corner of the knee are the lateral collateral ligament (LCL), the popliteus tendon, the popliteofibular ligament, the arcuate ligament, the short lateral ligament, the fabellofibular ligament, the biceps tendon, and the iliotibial tract. The anatomy of these structures is complex. This is thought to be due in part to the evolutionary changes that have taken place in this area. The fibula head initially articulated with the femur (5,6). With distal fibula migration, the popliteus gained a femoral attachment while still maintaining its fibula insertion. This evolutionary development explains the complexities of the popliteus hiatus and the intraarticular course of the popliteus tendon. In addition, the biceps femoris insertion moved from the proximal tibia to the fibula.

Seebacher et al. (7) defined three layers of the posterolateral corner to aid our understanding of this area. Layer I is the most superficial layer. It is comprised of the iliotibial tract, its anterior expansion, the superficial portion of the biceps tendon, and its expansion posteriorly. The iliotibial band (ITB) inserts into Gerdy's tubercle. The peroneal nerve lies deep to this layer, posterior to the biceps tendon. The biceps femoris muscle is comprised of the long and short head. The long head is divided into two tendinosus insertions, a direct and an anterior arm and three fascial components—a reflected arm and lateral and anterior aponeurotic insertions (8).

L. D. Higgins: Department of Surgery, Division of Orthopaedics, Duke University Medical Center, Durham, North Carolina 27710.

M. Clatworthy: Department of Sports Medicine, University of Pittsburgh, Pittsburgh, Pennsylvania 15232.

C. D. Harner: Division of Sports Medicine, Department of Orthopaedics, University of Pittsburgh, Pittsburgh, Pennsylvania 15232.

The direct arm is inserted into the posterolateral aspect of the fibula head, whereas the anterior arm is attached to the lateral edge of the fibula passing superficial to the LCL. A bursa lies between them. The reflected arm is attached to the posterior aspect of the ITB just proximal to the fibula head. The insertions of the short head are sixfold (9,10). There are two tendinous components, a direct inserting into the medial aspect of the fibula deep to the LCL and an anterior passing deep to this and inserting into the posterior aspect of the tibial tuberosity. Three muscular attachments insert into the long head, the posterolateral capsule and the ITB and an aponeurotic expansion attaches to the posteromedial aspect of the LCL.

Layer II consists of the lateral quadriceps retinaculum lying anteriorly, whereas the two patellofemoral ligaments lie posteriorly. The proximal ligament is attached to the terminal fibers of the lateral intermuscular septum, whereas the distal ligament ends posteriorly in the fabella when present or when absent at the femoral insertion of the posterolateral capsule and the lateral head of gastrocnemius. This layer is incomplete.

Layer III is the deepest layer that forms the posterolateral capsule of the knee joint. Posteriorly to the overlying ITB, the capsule divides into two laminae. The superficial lamina encompasses the LCL. This arises in a fanlike fashion from a saddle between the lateral epicondyle and supracondylar process. As it courses distally, its deep fibers insert into the lateral aspect of the fibula, whereas the lateral fibers blend with the superficial fascia of the anterior compartment of the leg. The superficial lamina ends posteriorly at the fabellofibular ligament or short lateral ligament. If the fabella is present, the fabellofibular ligament courses parallel to the LCL from the fibula to the fabella, inserting posterior to direct arm of the long head of biceps. The short lateral ligament if present is found adjacent to the lateral limb of the arcuate ligament running from the femoral origin of the lateral head of gastrocnemius to the fibula. The lateral inferior geniculate vessels lie between the superficial and deep lamina. The deep lamina passes along the edge of the lateral meniscus to form the coronary ligament and the hiatus for the popliteus tendon. Thus, the popliteus tendon courses through layer III before its intraarticular course. The deep lamina terminates posteriorly at the Y-shaped arcuate ligament. This is arcuate ligament composed of medial and lateral limbs that cross over at the popliteus musculotendinosus junction. The medial limb (oblique popliteal ligament) is a coalescence of the oblique popliteal expansion of the semimembranous and the capsular arm of the posterior oblique ligament arising from the medial side of the knee. This limb crosses the midpoint of the knee at the level of the tibial insertion of the PCL and courses superolaterally to insert into the inferiomedial edge of the fabella if present. If not, it inserts into the

posterior capsule overlying the lateral femoral condyle. The lateral limb arises from the posterior capsule and inserts into the posterior aspect of the fibula. The final and most important structure of the deep lamina is the popliteofibular ligament (11–13). This ligament provides a fibula fixation point for the popliteal tendon. It arises just anterior to the fibula styloid, thus anterior and deep to the lateral limb of the arcuate and fabellofibular ligament. It joins the popliteus tendon just proximal to the musculotendinosus junction.

The popliteus muscle arises from the posteromedial aspect of the tibia and courses superomedially. The musculotendinous junction lies at the level of the fibula head. The tendon then courses laterally through the popliteal hiatus into the posterolateral aspect of the knee joint. It is inserted into the popliteal fossa, which lies anterior and inferior to the lateral epicondyle of the femur. Medial to the popliteal tendon, the muscle attaches to the posterior capsule, the medial limb of the arcuate, and the inferior surface of the posterior horn of the lateral meniscus. This is the meniscal aponeurosis described by Last (14). It begins just lateral to the fovea of the PCL and extends laterally to the musculotendinous junction. This substitutes for the absent coronary ligament to the posterior horn of the lateral meniscus.

There is great variability in the anatomy of this region. The LCL and popliteus are consistently present, whereas the popliteofibular ligament is present 94% (15) to 98% (16) of the time. Seebacher et al. (7) showed that the arcuate ligament alone reinforced the capsule in 13%, the fabellofibular alone in 20%, and both in the remaining 67%. Susanna and Harnsiriwattanagit (16) dissected the posterolateral corner of 50 knees and demonstrated that the fabellofibular ligament was present in 68%, the short lateral ligament in 4%, and the arcuate was only a thin membranous structure in 24%.

Posteromedial Structures

The medial structures of the knee form a complex static and dynamic stabilizing mechanism. Static support is provided by the superficial medial collateral ligament (MCL), the posterior oblique ligament, and the deep MCL. Dynamic support is afforded by the semimembranosis, pes anserine, and the vastus medialis. Both these stabilizing mechanisms provide control for both valgus and rotatory stresses across the knee. Warren et al. (17) popularized the three-layer concept of the medial aspect of the knee. Although a detailed anatomic description is beyond the scope of this chapter, a detailed description of the pertinent anatomy and biomechanics may be found in Chapter 37.

Biomechanics

Our understanding of the relative importance of the structures of the posterolateral complex as they relate to the stability of the knee and their relationship with the cruciate ligaments has been determined by a number of serial sectional studies.

Gollehon et al. (18) demonstrated that sectioning of the PCL alone does not increase varus or external rotation. However, if the LCL and PLS are also divided, there is a greater increase in posterior translation and varus instability. External rotation increased when the knee is flexed greater than 30 degrees. Grood et al. (19) reported that isolated sectioning of the PLS alone resulted in increased external rotation at 30 and 90 degrees of flexion. However, external rotation is greater at 30 degrees (13 vs. 5.3 degrees for 90 degrees). If the PCL is then sectioned, greater increases are then noted at 90 degrees (20.9 vs. 18.9 degrees for 30 degrees). Noyes et al. (20) confirmed increased external rotation with sectioning of the PLS and noted further rotation with concomitant sectioning of the PCL. Veltri et al. (13) assessed the importance of sectioning the PCL and ACL in conjunction with a posterolateral injury. They showed that with isolated sectioning of the PLS, there is increased posterior translation, coupled external rotation with a posterior force, external rotation, and varus. All increases are maximal at 30 to 45 degrees of flexion. When the ACL is also sectioned, they found maximal increases of anterior and posterior translation at 30 degrees of flexion. Varus and internal rotation also increased and was maximal at 30 degrees. Combined sectioning of the PCL and PLS has resulted in increased posterior translation, varus, and external rotation at all angles of knee flexion. They concluded that because no increase is seen of the external rotation test at 30 degrees of flexion, the diagnosis of a combined ACL–PLS injury may be difficult to determine because the standard external rotation test at 30 degrees may not be reliable.

The structural properties of the popliteofibular and LCL were recently measured under tensile loading conditions (11). The mean load to failure of the popliteofibular ligament is 425 ± 165 N, whereas the LCL is 750 ± 433 N.

Our comprehension of the interplay of these ligaments has been further enlightened with studies using a robotic/universal force-moment sensor. Preliminary studies in our research center have investigated the biomechanical interaction between the PCL and PLS in response to posterior tibial loads and external tibial torque. We observed that in situ forces in the intact PCL were significantly higher in the PLS-deficient knee in response to these loading conditions (21). Likewise, the in situ forces of the PLS increased up to six times after sectioning of the PCL (22). We have also investigated the effects of a 44-N popliteus muscle load to the knee. This load resulted in a significant decrease in the in situ force in the PCL and a decrease in posterior tibial translation in the PCL-deficient knee (23). These

preliminary studies demonstrate a significant interaction between the PCL and PLS in restraining both posterior tibial translation and external rotation.

We recently evaluated the ability of a PCL graft to effectively restore normal knee kinematics and in situ forces of the intact PCL in both the isolated PCL and combined PCL–PLS injuries in cadaver knees. In the isolated PCL injury model, the PCL reconstruction reduced posterior laxity to within 1 to 2.5 mm of the intact knee at 30 and 90 degrees in response to a 134-N posterior load. The resulting knee kinematics and in situ forces in the PCL graft were not significantly different from the intact knee. In the combined PCL–PLS injury model, PLS deficiency resulted in an average increase in posterior laxity of the reconstructed knee of 5.7 mm at 30 degrees and 4.8 mm at 90 degrees of flexion. External rotation increased up to 14 degrees, whereas varus rotation increased up to 7 degrees.

Biomechanical studies focusing on the PMS demonstrate that the deep MCL is the first ligament disrupted with a valgus load is applied (24). The next structure to be injured is the posterior oblique ligament followed by the superficial MCL (25). Warren et al. (17) showed that the superficial MCL is the primary restraint to abduction and external rotation loads on the medial side of the knee. Grood et al. (26) also found that the superficial MCL is the primary restraint to pure valgus loads and the posterior oblique ligament and cruciates are secondary restraints. Ritchie et al. (27) evaluated the role of the medial structures in the PCL-deficient knee. They showed that the superficial MCL rather than the meniscofemoral ligaments is the primary restraint to posterior translation in the PCL-deficient knee when the tibia is internally rotated.

Clinical Relevance of Biomechanical Testing

Selective cutting studies determine the angle of knee flexion at which particular ligaments function primarily. This enables us to determine the correct position for examining these ligaments.

The results of these studies demonstrate that increases in posterior translation, varus, and external rotation occur with injury to the PLS (11–13,18–20). An isolated PCL results in increased posterior translation at all angles; however, it is maximal at 70 to 90 degrees. Thus, this is the angle of knee flexion for the posterior drawer test. Conversely, varus and external rotation have been shown to be maximal at 30 degrees for an isolated posterolateral corner injury; thus, we test at this angle of flexion for the isolated injury. With a combined injury, posterior translation, varus, and external rotation increase at all ranges; thus, we also test at 90 degrees to differentiate between an isolated and a combined injury.

Our robotic studies show that it is imperative to repair the PLS in a combined injury. Failure to perform this may at least partly explain the inconsistent results that have been reported for PCL reconstruction.

INCIDENCE

The true incidence of these injuries is unknown, and reported rates have been derived from hospital admission data. Of two million admissions to the Mayo Clinic, Hoover (1) documented only 14 knee dislocations in a 50-year period, whereas Meyers and Harvey (28) reported on 53 cases in Los Angeles County Hospital over a 10-year period. Recently, Wascher et al. (29) presented 50 knee dislocations over a 7-year period at a busy level 1 trauma center in New Mexico, which is similar to the rate at the University of Pittsburgh (30). These latter two articles illustrate the referral nature of these injuries to centers familiar with their management. Although still a rare injury, the incidence of these injuries is likely increasing due in part to improved recognition, increased use and sensitivity of noninvasive radiographic studies, the growth of the population involved in sports, and increased speed and utilization of vehicles.

CLASSIFICATION

There is no widely accepted classification system for knee dislocations. Although direction of the dislocation is critically important, other variables of significance include timing, degree of dislocation (subluxation vs. dislocation), mechanism (including magnitude of energy), and vascular status. Each criterion has prognostic value for outcome, and because no universally agreed upon system exists, one should include all the above information when discussing such an injury.

The direction of dislocation is routinely classified as the position of the tibia with respect to the femur. Not only may the tibia displace anteriorly, posteriorly, medially, or laterally with respect to the femur, combinations of the above may occur. Although anterior dislocations are widely regarded as the most common, posterior dislocations are often observed. If the medial femoral condyle has created a "button-hole" through the anteromedial capsule, an irreducible posterolateral dislocation occurs that is the most common of the combination directions. Attempts at reduction of this posterolateral dislocation may cause a "dimple sign" as the skin furrows at the level of the medial joint line caused by an invagination of a portion of the medial capsule (31). A classification system by Kennedy is the most widely used and is expounded on in the following section on mechanism.

It is generally accepted that spontaneous reduction of knee dislocations may occur, and therefore the position of dislocation is difficult to determine. Furthermore, not all multiple-ligament–injured knees sustained a frank dislocation, and therefore for the purpose of no-menclature, any patient that has torn three or more ligaments should be regarded as having sustained a knee dislocation (32,33). The purpose of this definition is to alert the physician of the seriousness of the injury manifested by a high incidence of vascular and/or nerve injury observed when three or more ligaments are disrupted.

Low-energy dislocations occur most commonly from sporting activity and may portend a better prognosis for vascular injuries (32). However, it is incumbent upon the treating physician to evaluate meticulously the vascular status of any knee dislocation regardless of mechanism, direction, or amount of energy imparted. Further evaluation of the incidence of associated injuries (as a function of the energy of the injury) is needed before definitive recommendations can be made regarding treatment.

MECHANISM

In 1963, Kennedy (34) published his experiments on the mechanism of knee dislocations and created a classifications system. Anterior dislocations were created with extreme hyperextension and were reliably reproduced in the laboratory. Posterior dislocations required significant torque and are now believed to occur as a result of a posteriorly directed blow to the proximal tibia (35).

Medial and lateral dislocations are less frequent and, in Kennedy's experiments, required a large force to reproduce. These injuries are likely to result from angular and rotatory moments and are often reduced at presentation or easily reduced. The irreducible posterolateral dislocation may be caused by an adduction internal rotation mechanism on a flexed unweighted extremity (36). It must be emphasized that the pattern of ligamentous instability is highly variable and may not be discernible based on the direction of dislocation.

ASSOCIATED INJURIES

Vascular Injuries

Injuries to the popliteal artery are potentially catastrophic. Although the anatomic configuration of popliteal artery predisposes it to injury as it courses posterior to the midaspect of the knee, the rate of dislocation may be directly related to the energy of the injury. Low-energy injuries, often occurring with sports participation, are reported to have an incidence as low as 5%; high-energy injuries have a reported incidence of 20% to 50% (1,34,35,37–43). Green and Allen (38) documented a 32% vascular injury rate after a thorough review of the literature with a slightly higher rate (40%) in anterior and posterior dislocations. Although it is generally accepted that low-energy injuries have a slightly lower vascular injury rate, hyperextension injuries, by their very nature, have high injury rate to the popliteal vessels due to the tethering at the adductor hiatus proximally and the soleal arch distally (30).

Nerve Injuries

The reported incidence of nerve injuries in documented knee dislocations has varied between 9 and 49% (40–42,44–46). Although most cases involve the common peroneal nerve with posterolateral and medial knee dislocations, tibial nerve involvement has also been documented (47). Complete nerve transections may occur; however, interstitial stretch, even at sites well proximal to the fibula, have been documented. Because of the variable nature and site of the injury, over 50% of the injuries fail to improve (28,30,45).

Bony Injuries

Because of the high energy of many of these injuries and their association with multiple trauma, fractures may be encountered in up to 60% of knee dislocations. Cole and Harner (30) reported that an associated tibial plateau fracture rate of 10% to 20% is often associated with inferior outcomes. In addition to plateau fractures, small avulsions and proximal fibula fractures are frequently encountered with an overall incidence as high as 60%, predominately with medial or lateral dislocations (28,44,46). Furthermore, open dislocation have been reported by both Shields et al. (40) and Meyers and Harvey (28) in up to 35% of cases, particularly with anterior and posterior dislocations. Moore (48) coined the phrase "fracture–dislocations" of the knee and proposed early bony and soft tissue stabilization to achieve satisfactory results.

EVALUATION AND MANAGEMENT

Initial Evaluation

The initial evaluation of any potential multiligamentous-injured knee begins with both a high index of suspicion and a thorough history. The acutely traumatized knee is often extremely painful and therefore difficult to examine. When the knee is dislocated, the diagnosis is often straightforward and apparent on the initial examination. The presence of any ligamentous instability warrants thorough radiographic evaluation, and clinical suspicion of a knee dislocation when two ligaments are injured must be maintained. It is critical to understand the mechanism of injury, because one surmise what associated structures may potentially be compromised. If the examination is limited by pain or if associated injuries prevent adequate evaluation, alternative methods (i.e., magnetic resonance imaging) should be used.

Many knee dislocations are missed at the index emergency room evaluation when attention is appropriately directed to other life-threatening injuries. However, it is incumbent upon the orthopedic surgeon and emergency room staffs to evaluate fully these patients to document knee reduction and neurovascular status to appropriately care for these injuries. Furthermore, specific clinical signs that may herald a knee dislocation should be sought. For example, the presence of a dimple sign, pathognomonic for unreduced posterolateral dislocation, must be noted.

Adequate documentation of pedal pulses and contralateral limb pedal pulses, in addition to ankle–brachial indexes bilaterally is of the highest priority for these complex injuries. The presence of diminished pulses may occur (as is witnessed with intimal tears), and an arteriogram should be ordered. If there is doubt regarding the presence of diminished pulses, ankle–brachial ratios should be made. If the ankle–brachial ratio is less than 0.8, an arteriogram should be obtained to exclude serious vascular insult (31). It must be emphasized that meticulous attention should be paid to the vascular status because complete vascular disruption may not be immediately apparent due to adequate collateral circulation (38).

Emergency Surgery

Currently, the authors have three indications for emergent surgical treatment of knee dislocations. Vascular injury leading a compromised blood supply to the leg is an absolute surgical indications. Second, all open dislocations require a minimum of an acute irrigation and debridement to reduce the risk of infection. Finally, an irreducible dislocation must be addressed acutely due to the potential for skin and muscle necrosis and subsequent vascular compromise.

Although it is not mandatory to address the ligamentous pathology for those cases with an indication for emergency surgery, thoughtful repair during surgical exposure is encouraged. In those patients with irreducible dislocations, substantial dissection may be required to obtain stable reduction. Some authors recommend concomitant ligamentous reconstruction during these cases. Currently, no data support emergent repair or reconstruction, and we prefer to schedule these cases within 2 weeks of the injury.

Reduction

Unreduced knee dislocations should be immediately reduced, ideally in the emergency room to diminish the potential damage to the neurovascular structures. With specific traction and reduction maneuvers with conscious sedation, successful reduction is often easily achieved. For anterior dislocations, traction with distal femoral elevation is often successful; posterior dislocations are addressed with proximal tibial extension. The physician must be cognizant of the mechanism and direction of dislocation for a successful reduction and must avoid excessive traction or hyperextension forces that may create further neurovascular injury. As noted earlier, the presence of a dimple sign signifies an irreducible posterolateral dislocation that must be addressed in the operating room (30,49).

Once reduction is maintained, a knee immobilizer is used until definitive treatment occurs. If necessary, a spanning external fixator is applied until ligament reconstruction is performed. If vascular repair occurred at the initial presentation, the request by the vascular surgeon to place the knee in flexion should be followed with extreme caution. The predilection for posterior subluxation of the tibia with knee flexion may create an irreducible dislocation if maintained in this position for even brief periods. Ideally, the knee is maintained near full extension or in full extension to confirm reduction. Orthogonal radiographs must be performed (anteroposterior and lateral views of the knee) to document reduction and should be followed closely until ligament reconstruction. Furthermore, if the patient returns to the operating room for further management, repeat radiographs are recommended.

Vascular Injuries

If the pedal pulses are absent upon reduction, disappear after the reduction maneuver, or evidence of ischemia is present, emergent vascular consultation is mandatory. With amputation rates approaching 85% in one large series if revascularization was not performed within 8 hours, time is obviously critical (38). If the reduction was accomplished in the operating room, consultation should occur in this setting, and a "one-shot" arteriogram may be obtained in the operating room before vascular exploration begins to aid in surgical planning. Vascular exploration should occur with close consultation between the vascular and orthopedic surgeons to ensure appropriate surgical incisions for later ligament reconstruction. Typically, reverse saphenous venous grafts are used for bypass. If the popliteal vein is injured, the simultaneous reconstruction of the popliteal vein is strongly advocated to prevent venous outflow obstruction, insufficiency, or thrombosis and to minimize postphlebotic syndromes. Furthermore, long-term arterial patency may be improved with popliteal vein repair and possible avoidance of chronic venous insufficiency (30,47,50,51). As with any revascularization procedure, prophylactic fasciotomies are required to prevent reperfusion injuries to the lower extremity. It is our preference to limit orthopedic intervention at this time to ensure a well-reduced knee with a healthy vascular status. However, obvious injuries that are easily managed during the course of vascular exploration may be addressed at this time.

In addition to the absence of pulses, other signs of vascular compromise must be sought. Ischemia may present as pallor, poor capillary refill, cyanosis, and diminished temperature; one must caution against reliance on palpable pulses only. In fact, numerous cases of severe vascular injury have been reported in the presence of pedal pulses (52–54). Furthermore, a complete vascular evaluation may require formal arteriography to elucidate the presence of intimal tears, occasionally missed by one-shot arteriograms (51,53). Arteriograms obtained in formal vascular laboratories often include digitally subtracted images with multiple planes and sequences. One should never attribute any significant abnormalities of vascular flow to self-limiting arterial spasm. The presence of a small intimal tear may progress rapidly to arterial thrombosis and may occur with symmetrically palpable pulses. Adequate documentation does exist that important vascular compromise requiring operative treatment may be sufficiently managed by serial examination by a vascular surgeon (43). With the publication of case reports accounting significant vascular trauma occurring with normal Doppler examination, many authors recommend arteriography for all suspected knee dislocations in their treatment algorithms (33,37,41,44,55).

Although the focus on vascular injuries and their management has been emphasized in the acute evaluation, vigilance must be maintained. The development of compartment syndrome, loss of pulse due to thrombosis, or further vascular compromise may occur well after presentation. Regular neurovascular monitoring and documentation is critical for the care of these patients. The use of anticoagulation is controversial in this population for those without a defined vascular injury. Because of the potential for prolonged immobilization and concomitant injuries, we use chemical prophylaxis. Low-molecular-weight heparin (Lovenox, Rhone-Poulenc Rorer Pharmaceuticals Inc., Collegeville, PA) is used in the immediate postinjury setting and discontinued before reconstructive surgery. Other regimens include enteric-coated aspirin, subcutaneous heparin, or mechanical means (sequential compression devices); if vascular repair is performed, the vascular surgeon may require short-term systemic heparinization.

Nerve Injury

Although nerve injuries are not uncommon, the lack of a large series in the literature makes reliable prognostication impossible. In a meta-analysis published by Good and Johnson (31), 50 cases were reported in 195 patients with knee dislocation (26%). Sixty percent experienced no improvement (30/50 cases), with only 16 cases recovering completely (32%). Although varying degrees of nerve injury may have been present, these results demonstrate the severe nature of these injuries. Furthermore, only three of seven patients who underwent nerve decompression experienced any benefit.

Although some authors recommend an "expectancy period" of 3 months to allow spontaneous improvement (56), Lundborg (57) proposed a more aggressive approach. By using sural nerve cable grafts and acute microsurgical nerve repair, the repair is technically easier to perform at the time of injury. Currently, most authors recommend observation of such injuries with temporary orthotic management.

In a grossly intact nerve with a preoperative deficit, we recommend a release of the fascial bands overlying the peroneal nerve as it enters the lateral compartment. This may protect the nerve from further injury associated with postoperative swelling. Currently, we do not advocate immediate nerve grafting if the nerve is in continuity while neurolysis is performed judiciously, because some evidence supports enhanced nerve recovery (28). If a transected nerve is encountered during ligamentous repair, the nerve ends are tagged if microsurgical repair is not feasible and cable grafting is performed later.

The loss of active dorsiflexion may rapidly create plantar flexion contractures and prevention is the simplest treatment. Ankle–foot orthosis should be placed early in the management of peroneal nerve injuries. Management of persistent nerve injuries includes dynamic or fixed orthosis, tendon transfers, or arthrodesis.

DEFINITIVE MANAGEMENT

Currently, most authors recommend operative management of multiligament knee injuries to provide a stable knee with full range of motion. Exceptions to this approach include those patients who are sedentary or elderly, stable after reduction, or who will likely be noncompliant in the postoperative state. With new repair and reconstruction techniques, subjective instability is less likely than a loss of motion after surgical treatment (30,31,35,37,41,42,45,58–63). It must be emphasized that successful results require a meticulous examination and preoperative planning to address the pathology.

Critical to the successful management of these injuries is a thorough understanding of the injury pattern. Although acute evaluation is often limited due to significant pain or distracting injury, a delay of several days after injury may provide ample opportunity to obtain a full thorough examination and order appropriate diagnostic tests. Furthermore, we prefer to perform reconstruction and/or repair on a semielective basis. With these complex cases, it is imperative that the surgical team is familiar with these techniques to prevent delays and to maximize patient outcome. A limited treatment of bony avulsions or ligament repair may be considered at the time of a vascular approach on an acute basis, with reconstruction to follow after the surgeon and operative team has appropriately planned.

As a general rule, all grade III laxity patterns must be addressed surgically to obtain good results. Although we believe that the PCL, if injured and clinically confirmed to be a grade III laxity pattern, must be reconstructed, lesser laxity patterns are not routinely reconstructed. For example, a multiligamentous knee injury with a grade I PCL laxity pattern will have its associated injured ligaments repaired or reconstructed, and the PCL will be carefully observed and not reconstructed. If the PCL is determined to have a grade II laxity pattern, reconstruction will be considered only in those patients with high functional demands. Current techniques do not return PCL reconstruction to normal laxity patterns, and therefore only grade III injuries and their associated posterolateral corner injuries are surgically addressed (30).

Surgical management of these injuries is rarely performed acutely, as we to delay operative treatment for 1 to 2 weeks after the index injury. Currently, irreducibility of the knee serves as one of the few acute surgical indications. A period of operative delay serves several functions. This allows a period of observation for vascular injury and an opportunity for a complete evaluation of the injury pattern. Currently, the exact period of high risk for arterial thrombosis is unknown, and therefore close observation is necessary to prevent catastrophic complications.

Furthermore, this operative delay allows capsular healing to occur that will facilitate the arthroscopic repair or reconstruction of the cruciate ligaments. During this period, if the knee is not grossly unstable, a gentle range of motion is permitted (while appropriately braced), which may reduce swelling. We prefer to schedule these cases semielectively, which allows the appropriate surgical team to be present (those familiar with complex knee reconstruction) and to obtain necessary equipment or allograft tissue if needed.

Another advantage of delaying surgery is to diminish the risk of arthrofibrosis. Shelbourne et al. (32) proposed a treatment algorithm for knee dislocations to reduce the incidence of knee stiffness. Patients with combined cruciate ligament injuries involving either the MCL or LCL underwent surgical repair without ACL reconstruction. A delayed ACL reconstruction was advocated to reduce the likelihood of arthrofibrosis often witnessed with combined cruciate ligament reconstruction and/or repair if the injured MCL. Although arthrofibrosis requiring manipulation is not uncommon, surgeons vary markedly in their approach regarding timing of repair and reconstruction (30,32,35,41,58,64–66). We currently favor repair and/or reconstruction of all injured structures at the time of surgery.

Preoperative Evaluation

The analysis of ligament injury is facilitated by a thorough examination and diagnostic studies. Plain radiographs including anteroposterior, lateral, and oblique views will frequently demonstrate bony avulsions and persistent subluxation and must be obtained. Furthermore, fractures about the knee, particularly of the tibial plateau and supracondylar femur, will need operative stabilization. If treatment of these fractures is facilitated by computed tomography, we recommend obtaining these studies. For those patients without fractures, magnetic resonance imaging is routinely obtained to aid in preoperative planning and diminish operative time. Furthermore, detailed discussions with the patient are aided if a complete understanding of the pathology is available.

Examination under anesthesia is critical. This confirms all laxity patterns and determines which incisions are to be used. During examination, particular attention should be directed to the collateral ligaments and the posterolateral corner. A meticulous arthroscopic evaluation of the meniscus, articular cartilage, cruciate ligaments, popliteal tendon, and the posterior capsule follows to further direct operative repair.

TIMING OF SURGERY

Acute repairs of ligaments may be performed within the first 2 weeks after injury, without compromise to the ultimate results. Therefore, the surgeon has this opportunity to adequately monitor and evaluate the injury without compromise to the result. The most critical component of this period is the close vascular observation. Delayed vascular injury, either in the form of clot formation, intimal tear, or arterial occlusion, is uncommon but a potentially devastating complication. Only when the vascular status of the leg is optimized should repair or reconstruction follow (45). If vascular repair has been performed, the use of a tourniquet may be contraindicated. The vascular surgeon should be consulted preoperatively to discuss antithrombotic management in the perioperative setting.

Operative delay longer than 14 days may compromise the surgeons ability to repair both the collateral ligaments and the posterolateral corner (12,45,63). The proliferative scar formation that occurs after knee dislocations obscures operative planes and makes surgical repair more difficult. Several authors (12,45) have recommended that if surgical delay is inevitable (perhaps due to other injuries), it is preferable to regain full range of motion to diminish the risk of arthrofibrosis. If subsequent instability occurs, delayed reconstruction is then indicated.

Ligament Avulsions

The routine evaluation of certain knee dislocations may demonstrate bony avulsions of the ligaments from their origin or insertion. Rather than formally reconstruct these injuries, anatomic repair of these avulsions often yields excellent results, often surpassing the results with reconstruction. Avulsion of the PCL from its tibial insertion is not uncommonly seen, and the avulsed bony–ligament complex should be secured with suture or screw fixation. For tibial eminence fractures with an adequate bony avulsion attached to the ACL, small drill holes tied over a bony bridge yield excellent ligament repair and results.

Midsubstance ligament injuries to the ACL, PCL, and LCL are typically not amenable to surgical repair. For these injuries, the formal reconstruction as described in earlier chapters is recommended. For injuries to the midsubstance of the MCL, however, primary repair is an option if residual laxity is a concern. For these MCL injuries, careful inspection of the meniscus often demonstrates a tear or detachment of the overlying MCL; this must be simultaneously addressed. As with all repairs and reconstructions, anatomic placement of the ligament is crucial. Careful note of which ligaments are repaired must be noted to direct postoperative physical therapy. It is generally accepted that reconstructions are stronger than ligament repairs, and postoperative rehabilitation should reflect this.

Graft Choice

Multiligamentous knee injuries requiring reconstruction pose problems for graft selection. Surgeon preference is the most critical factor in determining the ideal graft for reconstruction. Although autograft options are available, the addition of donor site morbidity to a previously compromised knee may be unfavorable. If several ligaments are in need of reconstruction, autograft shortage may occur, driving the surgeon to consider either contralateral graft options or the use of allograft. Although autograft choices may heal faster, we prefer to use allograft for reconstruction to avoid donor sit morbidity, iatrogenic trauma, and to decrease operative time.

The use of allograft has several other advantages and risks. Surgical incisions for autograft harvest are avoided, which may be advantageous in a recently traumatized knee. Second, tourniquet time is reduced, an important consideration for multiligament reconstruction, particularly if neurovascular injury has occurred. Knee stiffness and postoperative pain may also be diminished by using allograft tissue (67). The risk of disease transmission is the greatest disadvantage to the use of allograft. In 1989, the purported risk of procuring tissue from a donor with human immunodeficiency virus transmission was stated to be 1:1.667,000 (68) if all screening measures were used. With the advent of polymerase chain reaction technologies, the risk is certainly smaller; quantification is difficult. There have been no reported cases of transmission of the human immunodeficiency virus in over 500,000 musculoskeletal allografts from a 10-year period ending in 1995 (69). A more thorough discourse on the risks of allograft is beyond the scope of this chapter.

Operative Approach

Examination Under Anesthesia

The successful treatment of all combined ligament-injured knees begins with is accurate diagnosis. Although preoperative planning and review of radiographic studies are critical steps, the examination under anesthesia will ultimately determine the surgical approach and finalize which ligaments need to be addressed. The examination of the contralateral extremity to serve as a control (if it is uninjured) is routinely used. Particular attention must be directed to the collateral ligaments, PCL, and the posterolateral corner. The pattern of instability will determine which incisions will be used and to direct the step-by-step approaches to the reconstruction.

Patient Position

For all multiligament injuries, we prefer the patient to be supine with a tourniquet as high as possible on the thigh. The addition of a sandbag taped to the bed to assist in maintaining the leg in a flexed position is similarly recommended. The use of a lateral post is routine to aid in visualization for the arthroscopic portion of the procedure. If the medial side is uninjured and does not need to be surgically addressed, the addition of a "bump" under the hip to assist in exposure of the lateral side may also be considered. The tourniquet is not inflated unless necessary, and its use is avoided entirely if concomitant neurovascular injuries have occurred.

Lateral Side Injuries

A complete understanding of the anatomy of the lateral side of the knee is mandatory for repair and reconstruction of these injures. Furthermore, wide exposure is mandatory for the successful treatment of all lateral side injuries. No attempt is made, particularly for injuries to the LCL and posterolateral corner, to treat these injuries with small incisions or with inadequate exposure. Each injured structure must be meticulously identified and anatomic repair is essential.

A 15-cm incision begins at the posterior aspect of the ITB, courses over the lateral epicondyle, and ends between Gerdy's tubercle and the fibular head. The extent of the injury is often apparent with disruption of the ITB, biceps tendon, LCL, arcuate ligament, popliteus tendon, peroneal nerve, and lateral meniscus all potentially involved. In delayed cases, exuberant scarring may make dissection difficult and time consuming. Attention is initially directed to isolating the peroneal nerve to prevent inadvertent injury.

The peroneal nerve is isolated proximally, just deep and posterior to the biceps tendon, and inspected for evidence of injury. Evidence of injury is documented; however, no attempt should be made to perform cable grafting if the nerve is grossly in continuity. The nerve is thereafter protected for the entire duration of the procedure. Distal dissection of the nerve continues until it is seen entering the anterolateral musculature. The fascial bands in this area are released, and neurolysis is performed if hematoma warrants.

The biceps tendon is inspected and is often injured. A common location is avulsion off the fibular head. The plane on the posterior aspect of the ITB is developed and inspection completed. At this point, the decision whether to reflect the portion of the ITB off Gerdy's tubercle or to use "windows" in the ITB should be made. To reflect the posterior aspect of the ITB, subperiosteal dissection of the ITB must be made starting at the posterior aspect. Stay sutures placed into the posterior margin retracting anteriorly will provide adequate exposure. Repair with suture anchors at the end of the procedure will complete closure of the deep layer for this exposure.

The use of several windows through the ITB also provides adequate exposure while preserving the intact ITB. Although this approach is somewhat more difficult, we prefer this when the ITB is intact to preserve any structures that are not disrupted from the index injury. Three windows as described by Terry and LaPrade (9) are created to completely visualize the lateral side of the knee. By using three fascial incisions and one lateral midcapsular incision, visualization of all the lateral and PLS was possible. It should be noted that not all incisions are necessary, and the exposure should be directed by the injury pattern. This technique serves to maintain the ITB's integrity if it is not injured during the index injury. Although no data exist supporting the importance of maintaining the continuity of the ITB, preservation of normal anatomy seems optimal.

The first fascial incision splits the ITB at the midpoint of Gerdy's tubercle and continues proximally and allows inspection of the biceps, LCL, and the ITB. A vertical lateral capsular incision allows examination of the popliteus attachment to the femur, the lateral meniscus, and the remainder of the midthird capsular ligament. The second fascial incision is made in the interval between the long head of the biceps and the ITB. This window permits exposure of the biceps attachments and, if injured, to the fabellofibular ligament. The third fascial incision, along the posterior border of the long head of the biceps, allows inspection when the biceps is retracted anteriorly and the peroneal nerve (after neurolysis) is retracted posteriorly. The fabellofibular ligament, posterior popliteofibular ligament, and the arcuate ligament are visualized in this interval.

Medial Side Injuries

Medial side injuries are common with multiligament knee injuries, particularly when there is PCL involvement. The loss of cruciate ligament stability to valgus stress has been implicated in poor MCL healing (26) and has been invoked as the justification for acute medial side repair. Currently, we recommend acute repair of grade III MCL injuries with marked medial instability. Lesser instability patterns are treated nonoperatively, and persistent instability has not been problematic. Ideally, if other ligament injuries do not mandate early operative intervention (i.e., posterolateral corner injury), low-grade injuries to the MCL are treated nonoperatively with surgical delay and primary healing. This approach allows the patient to regain knee motion and reduce the risk of knee stiffness (70). The risk of knee stiffness with medial and cruciate repair is three to four time higher, and therefore such risk is acceptable only in grade III injuries with poor potential to heal (71). Therefore, patients with combined ligament insufficiencies in conjunction with a grade III MCL undergo a more aggressive approach with cruciate reconstruction and MCL repair on an acute basis.

The Hughston technique for anatomic repair is used. A medial "hockey stick" incision is made beginning at the vastus medialis, coursing over the medial epicondyle, and ending on the anteromedial tibia. Cruciate reconstruction is typically performed before addressing the medial side, although a medial parapatellar arthrotomy is readily available through this approach to reconstruct the cruciate ligaments. Once the sartorial fascia is divided and retracted, the medial structures are meticulously inspected.

The critical step in repairing the medial structures is assessing the injured structures. The MCL may be avulsed from the medial epicondyle, and repair here is made primarily. The use of a soft tissue washer and screw or suture anchors provides excellent fixation if the reattachment site is anatomic. Finding the isometric point of fixation is critical because failure to reattach the ligament in this fashion will either fail or lead to permanent restriction of knee motion. If the ligament is torn distal to its insertion, no attempt to repair this to the side of the femur with a screw is made because this will create a nonanatomic origin. Rather, the use of sutures to repair the ligament is encouraged after superficial and deep MCL are

isolated. The sutures are passed individually, and the knee is ranged after each stitch is placed to ensure that it is not captured from inadvertent suture placement. The meniscus, capsule, and posterior oblique ligament are inspected and repaired as necessary.

Cruciate Reconstruction

The technical details of cruciate ligament reconstruction are covered in separate chapters and are not discussed. However, because of the complex nature of these injuries, several practical considerations are discussed, particularly when combined cruciate ligament reconstruction is considered.

Posterior Cruciate Ligament Reconstruction

PCL reconstruction is accomplished with an arthroscopic-assisted technique using a doubled bundle approach. Because of residual laxity with reconstruction of the anterolateral bundle only and compelling biomechanical data supporting the use of a double bundle technique, this is our preferred method. The addition of the posteromedial bundle reconstruction reduced posterior translation by a mean of 3.5 mm with reproduction of more normal PCL kinematics (72).

The tibial tunnel is drilled with the arthroscope in the posteromedial portal after adequate visualization of the tibial footprint is obtained. With the PCL guide in the medial portal, the guide pin should ideally enter the inferolateral aspect of the PCL footprint. Intraoperative fluoroscopy or plain radiographs are routinely used to confirm guide pin placement. The tibial tunnel is drilled with the last few millimeters completed by hand to prevent inadvertent injury to the posterior structures.

The femoral tunnels are created via an enlarged lateral portal. With the arthroscope in the medial portal, the anterior/proximal tunnel is placed at the 10:30 position in the left knee, approximately 6 to 7 mm off the articular surface. An allograft Achilles tendon is our graft of choice, and the bone plug is fashioned to be 10 mm in diameter and 25 mm in length. A 10-mm tunnel is drilled approximately 25 mm deep. Bone debris are removed and the tunnel impacted with an appropriately sized dilator. The posterior/distal tunnel is placed within the PCL footprint, leaving a bone bridge between the two tunnels. The size of the tunnel depends on the graft available. Currently, we favor doubled semitendinosis yielding a 6- to 7-mm graft. The tunnels are similarly drilled and dilated.

Fixation of the Achilles grafts on the femur may be accomplished with the use of interference screws, Endobutton (Acufex, Boston, MA) device, or with a polypropylene button secured on the medial femoral condyle. We prefer to secure the semitendinosis with a bioabsorbable screw placed through the lateral portal. Tibial

Step 1:
    Tibial tunnels
        PCL
        ACL
Step 2:
    Femoral tunnels
        ACL
        PCL (anterior / proximal)
        PCL (posterior/ distal)
Step 3:
    PCL Graft passage
        Pass PCL (Achilles tendon allograft) into tibial tunnel through lateral
        portal via antegrade approach
        Pass PCL (semitendinosis graft) into tibial tunnel through lateral portal via
        antegrade approach
Step 4:
    Secure PCL grafts in femur
Step 5:
    ACL graft passage
        Pass ACL into femoral tunnel via retrograde approach
Step 6:
    Secure ACL graft in femur
Step 7:
    Collateral ligament repair
        Secure collateral ligament repairs or reconstructions
Step 8:
    Cycle PCL and ACL grafts
Step 9:
    Secure PCL tibial fixation
        Secure anterolateral bundle (anterior / proximal) with knee at 90°
        Secure posteromedial bundle (posterior / distal) with knee at 30°
Step 10:
    Secure ACL tibial fixation
        Secure ACL in full extension

FIG. 44.1. Ten step order for ACL/PCL and collateral ligament repair.

fixation is routinely accomplished with AO cortical screws with soft tissue washers.

Before tibial graft fixation, the grafts are cycled to remove any laxity in the graft. With distal traction, the knee is cycled a minimum of 20 times from 0 to 90 degrees. The anterolateral bundle is first secured in 90 degrees of flexion with the hamstring graft tensioned at 30 degrees of flexion (73). The sequence of graft fixation and tensioning is critical and depends on the nature of the injury (Fig. 44.1).

Anterior Cruciate Ligament Reconstruction

The specifics of ACL reconstruction are well covered in Chapter 00. However, with the absence of a PCL for ACL tibial tunnel position, the anterior horn of the lateral meniscus may serve as a reference. By using the posterior aspect of the anterior horn of the lateral meniscus and confirming tunnel location radiographically, accurate tunnel position is possible (30). One must be cognizant of the PCL tunnel when placing the ACL tibial tunnel. The femoral tunnel is routinely placed for ACL reconstruction in multiligament knee injuries. Ideally, tunnel placement will not result in impingement, and a thorough investigation after all grafts have been passed is mandatory.

REHABILITATION

There are few article in the literature investigating rehabilitation for multiligament knee injuries. Although some advocate early motion, the risk of injury to the graft and residual laxity have been prime concerns. Currently, we recommend that the leg is immobilized in full extension for a period of 4 weeks. This generally ensures knee reduction and prevents excessive hamstring moments from stretching the PCL or PLS structures. Similarly, weight bearing is prohibited in the first 6 postoperative weeks. The patient is encouraged to perform straight leg raises and quad sets while immobilized. Active hamstring exercises begin at least 3 months postoperatively.

After the first postoperative week, gentle passive range of motion in the prone position with the assistance of a physical therapist is begun. The motion is performed with a slight anterior drawer to protect the PCL and PLS. At 6 weeks, the patient begins active knee motion. Weight bearing advances from week 6 to full weight bearing at 3 months.

REFERENCES

1. Hoover NW. Injuries of the popliteal artery associated with fractures and dislocations. *Surg Clin North Am* 1961;41:1099–1124.
2. Bellabarba C, Bush-Joseph CA, Bach BRJ. Knee dislocation without anterior cruciate ligament disruption. A report of three cases. *Am J Knee Surg* 1996;9:167–170.
3. Cooper DE, Speer KP, Wickiewicz TL, et al. Complete knee dislocation without posterior cruciate ligament disruption. A report of four cases and review of the literature. *Clin Orthop* 1992;284:228–233.
4. Shelbourne KD, Pritchard J, Rettig AC, et al. Knee dislocations with intact PCL. *Orthop Rev* 1992;21:607–608.
5. Haines RJ. The tetrapod knee joint [abstract]. *J Anat* 1942;76: 270–301.
6. Herzmark MH. The evolution of the knee joint [abstract]. *J Bone Joint Surg Am* 1938;20:77–84.
7. Seebacher JR, Inglis AE, Marshall JL, et al. The structure of the posterolateral aspect of the knee. *J Bone Joint Surg Am* 1982; 64:536–541.
8. Terry GC, Hughston JC, Norwood LA. The anatomy of the iliopatellar band and iliotibial tract. *Am J Sports Med* 1986;14:39–45.
9. Terry GC, LaPrade RF. The posterolateral aspect of the knee. Anatomy and surgical approach. *Am J Sports Med* 1996;24: 732–739.
10. Terry GC, LaPrade RF. The biceps femoris muscle complex at the knee. Its anatomy and injury patterns associated with acute anterolateral-anteromedial rotatory instability. *Am J Sports Med* 1996;24:2–8.
11. Maynard MJ, Deng X, Wickiewicz TL, et al. The popliteofibular ligament. Rediscovery of a key element in posterolateral stability. *Am J Sports Med* 1996;24:311–316.
12. Veltri DM, Warren RF. Posterolateral instability of the knee. *Instr Course Lect* 1995;44:441–453.
13. Veltri DM, Deng XH, Torzilli PA, et al. The role of the cruciate and posterolateral ligaments in stability of the knee. A biomechanical study. *Am J Sports Med* 1995;23:436–443.
14. Last RJ. Anatomical details of the knee joint [abstract]. *J Bone Joint Surg Br* 1950;32B:93–99.
15. Watanabe Y, Moriya H, Takahashi K, et al. Functional anatomy of the posterolateral structures of the knee [abstract]. *Arthroscopy* 1993;9:57–62.
16. Sudsana S, Harnsiriwattanagit K. The ligamentous structures of

the posterolateral aspect of the knee [abstract]. *Bull Hosp Joint Dis* 1990;50:35–40.

17. Warren LA, Marshall JL, Girgis F. The prime static stabilizer of the medial side of the knee. *J Bone Joint Surg Am* 1974;56:665–674.

18. Gollehon DL, Torzilli PA, Warren RF. The role of the posterolateral and cruciate ligaments in the stability of the human knee. A biomechanical study. *J Bone Joint Surg Am* 1987;69:233–242.

19. Grood ES, Stowers SF, Noyes FR. Limits of movement in the human knee. Effect of sectioning the posterior cruciate ligament and posterolateral structures. *J Bone Joint Surg Am* 1988;70:88–97.

20. Noyes FR, Stowers SF, Grood ES, et al. Posterior subluxations of the medial and lateral tibiofemoral compartments. An in vitro ligament sectioning study in cadaveric knees. *Am J Sports Med* 1993;21:407–414.

21. Harner CD, Vogrin T, Höher J, et al. Injury to the posterolateral structures has profound effects on the function of the posterior cruciate ligament [abstract]. *Trans Orthop Res Soc* 1998;23:47.

22. Hoher J, Harner CD, Vogrin TM, et al. In situ forces in the posterolateral structures of the knee under posterior tibial loading in the intact and posterior cruciate ligament-deficient knee. *J Orthop Res* 1998;16:675–681.

23. Harner CD, Hoher J, Vogrin TM, et al. The effects of a popliteus muscle load on in situ forces in the posterior cruciate ligament and on knee kinematics. A human cadaveric study. *Am J Sports Med* 1998;26:669–673.

24. Kennedy JC, Fowler PJ. Medial and anterior instability of the knee. An anatomical and clinical study using stress machines. *J Bone Joint Surg Am* 1971;53:1257–1270.

25. Mueller W. *The knee: form, function and ligament reconstruction.* Berlin: Springer-Verlag, 1983.

26. Grood ES, Noyes FR, Butler DL, et al. Ligamentous and capsular restraints preventing straight medial and lateral laxity in intact human cadaver knees. *J Bone Joint Surg Am* 1981;63:1257–1269.

27. Ritchie JR, Bergfeld JA, Kambic H, et al. Isolated sectioning of the medial and posteromedial capsular ligaments in the posterior cruciate ligament-deficient knee [In Process Citation]. *Am J Sports Med* 1998;26:389–394.

28. Meyers MH, Harvey JPJ. Traumatic dislocation of the knee joint. A study of eighteen cases. *J Bone Joint Surg Am* 1971;53:16–29.

29. Wascher DC, Dvirnak PC, DeCoster TA. Knee dislocation: initial assessment and implications for treatment. *J Orthop Trauma* 1997;11:525–529.

30. Cole BJ, Harner CD. The multiple ligament injured knee. *Clin Sports Med* 1999;18:241–262.

31. Good L, Johnson RJ. The dislocated knee. *J Am Acad Orthop Surg* 1995;3:284–292.

32. Shelbourne KD, Porter DA, Clingman JA, et al. Low-velocity knee dislocation. *Orthop Rev* 1991;20:995–1004.

33. Varnell RM, Coldwell DM, Sangeorzan BJ, et al. Arterial injury complicating knee disruption. *Am Surg* 1989;55:699–704.

34. Kennedy JC. Complete dislocation of the knee joint. *J Bone Joint Surg Am* 1963;45:889–904.

35. Roman PD, Hopson CN, Zenni EJJ. Traumatic dislocation of the knee: a report of 30 cases and literature review. *Orthop Rev* 1987;16:917–924.

36. Quinlan AG. Irreducible posterolateral dislocation of the knee with button-holing of the medial femoral condyle. *J Bone Joint Surg Am* 1966;48:1619–1621.

37. Frassica FJ, Sim FH, Staeheli JW, et al. Dislocation of the knee. *Clin Orthop* 1991;263:200–205.

38. Green NE, Allen BL. Vascular injuries associated with dislocation of the knee. *J Bone Joint Surg Am* 1977;59:236–239.

39. Kendall RW, Taylor DC, Salvian AJ, et al. The role of arteriography in assessing vascular injuries associated with dislocations of the knee. *J Trauma* 1993;35:875–878.

40. Shields L, Mital M, Cave EF. Complete dislocation of the knee: experience at the Massachusetts General Hospital. *J Trauma* 1969;9:192–215.

41. Sisto DJ, Warren RF. Complete knee dislocation. A follow-up study of operative treatment. *Clin Orthop* 1985;198:94–101.

42. Taylor AR, Arden GP, Rainey HA. Traumatic dislocation of

the knee. A report of forty-three cases with special reference to conservative treatment. *J Bone Joint Surg Br* 1972;54:96–102.

43. Treiman GS, Yellin AE, Weaver FA, et al. Examination of the patient with a knee dislocation. The case for selective arteriography. *Arch Surg* 1992;127:1056–1062.

44. McCoy GF, Hannon DG, Barr RJ, et al. Vascular injury associated with low-velocity dislocations of the knee. *J Bone Joint Surg Br* 1987;69:285–287.

45. Taft T, Almekinders LC. The dislocated knee. In: Fu FH, Harner CD, Vince K, eds. *Knee surgery.* Baltimore: Williams & Wilkins, 1994:837–858.

46. Thomsen PB, Rud B, Jensen UH. Stability and motion after traumatic dislocation of the knee. *Acta Orthop Scand* 1984;55:278–283.

47. Welling RE, Kakkasseril J, Cranley JJ Complete dislocations of the knee with popliteal vascular injury. *J Trauma* 1981;21:450–453.

48. Moore TM. Fracture–dislocation of the knee. *Clin Orthop* 1981;156:128–140.

49. Hill JA, Rana NA. Complications of posterolateral dislocation of the knee: case report and literature review. *Clin Orthop* 1981;212–215.

50. Bishara RA, Pasch AR, Lim LT, et al. Improved results in the treatment of civilian vascular injuries associated with fractures and dislocations. *J Vasc Surg* 1986;3:707–711.

51. O'Donnell TFJ, Brewster DC, Darling RC, et al. Arterial injuries associated with fractures and/or dislocations of the knee. *J Trauma* 1977;17:775–784.

52. Grimley RP, Ashton F, Slaney G, et al. Popliteal arterial injuries associated with civilian knee trauma. *Injury* 1981;13:1–6.

53. Ottolenghi CE. Vascular complications in injuries about the knee joint. *Clin Orthop* 1982;165:148–156.

54. Savage R. Popliteal artery injury associated with knee dislocation: improved outlook? *Am Surg* 1980;46:627–632.

55. Chapman JA. Popliteal artery damage in closed injuries of the knee. *J Bone Joint Surg Br* 1985;67:420–423.

56. White J. The results of traction injuries to the common peroneal nerve. *J Bone Joint Surg Br* 1968;50:346–350.

57. Lundborg G. Peripheral nerve injuries: pathophysiology and strategies for treatment [editorial]. *J Hand Ther* 1993;6:179–188.

58. Fanelli GC, Giannotti BF, Edson CJ. Arthroscopically assisted combined anterior and posterior cruciate ligament reconstruction. *Arthroscopy* 1996;12:5–14.

59. Malizos KN, Xenakis T, Mavrodontidis AN, et al. Knee dislocations and their management. A report of 16 cases. *Acta Orthop Scand* 1997;275[Suppl]:80–83.

60. Marks PH, Harner CD. The anterior cruciate ligament in the multiple ligament-injured knee. *Clin Sports Med* 1993;12:825–838.

61. Montgomery JB. Dislocation of the knee. *Orthop Clin North Am* 1987;18:149–156.

62. Shapiro MS, Freedman EL. Allograft reconstruction of the anterior and posterior cruciate ligaments after traumatic knee dislocation. *Am J Sports Med* 1995;23:580–587.

63. Veltri DM, Warren RF. Operative treatment of posterolateral instability of the knee. *Clin Sports Med* 1994;13:615–627.

64. Almekinders LC, Logan TC. Results following treatment of traumatic dislocations of the knee joint. *Clin Orthop* 1992;284 203–207.

65. Noyes FR, Barber-Westin SD. Reconstruction of the anterior and posterior cruciate ligaments after knee dislocation. Use of early protected postoperative motion to decrease arthrofibrosis. *Am J Sports Med* 1997;25:769–778.

66. Simonian PT, Wickiewicz TL, Hotchkiss RN, et al. Chronic knee dislocation: reduction, reconstruction, and application of a skeletally fixed knee hinge. A report of two cases. *Am J Sports Med* 1998;26:591–596.

67. Harner CD, Olsen E, Fu FH. The use of fresh frozen allograft in knee ligament reconstruction: indications, techniques, results and controversies. In: Wojtys EM, ed. *The ACL-deficient knee.* Washington, DC: The American Academy of Orthopaedic Surgeons, 1994:28–46.

68. Buck BE, Malinin TI, Brown MD. Bone transplantation and human immunodeficiency virus. An estimate of risk of acquired

immunodeficiency syndrome (AIDS). *Clin Orthop* 1989;240: 129–136.

69. Tomford WW. Transmission of disease through transplantation of musculoskeletal allografts. *J Bone Joint Surg Am* 1995;77:1742–1754.

70. Hillard-Sembell D, Daniel DM, Stone ML, et al. Combined injuries of the anterior cruciate and medial collateral ligaments of the knee. Effect of treatment on stability and function of the joint. *J Bone Joint Surg Am* 1996;78:169–176.

71. Shelbourne KD, Baele JR. Treatment of combined anterior cruciate ligament and medial collateral ligament injures. *Am J Knee Surg* 1988;1:56–58.

72. Harner CD, Janaushek MA, Kanamori A, et al. Biomechanical analysis of a double bundle posterior cruciate ligament reconstruction. *Am J Sports Med* 2000;28:144–151.

73. Petrie RS, Harner CD. Double bundle PCL reconstruction technique: University of Pittsburgh approach. *Op Techn Sports Med* 1999;7:118–126.

Principles and Practice of Orthopaedic Sports Medicine,
edited by William E. Garrett, Jr., Kevin P. Speer, and Donald T. Kirkendall.
Lippincott Williams & Wilkins, Philadelphia © 2000.

CHAPTER 45

Ankle Impingement Syndromes

Thomas P. Knapp, William M. Hayes, and Bert R. Mandelbaum

Acute ankle sprains and chronic pain/instability syndromes are a common and disabling spectrum of disorders in athletes. Relatively "minor" ankle sprains are common with the athlete returning to competition and training with minimal downtime. It is the moderate/severe sprains that can cause significant morbidity, leading to long downtime, chronic recalcitrant pain, functional instability, weakness, loss of proprioception, and consequent athletic disability. Management goals for ankle sprains for the sports medicine professional should include prevention, minimization of morbidity, and performance facilitation.

In sports, despite the best rehabilitation programs, there is a subgroup of athletes with residual ankle symptoms. These symptoms include pain, weakness, functional instability, gross instability, and inability to participate in sports. Smith and Reischl (1) in their description of young athletes reported that in basketball players who had ankle sprains, 50% had residual symptoms. More importantly, 15% continued with symptoms that compromised their performance. Freeman et al. (2), on the other hand, found 40% of their patients with ankle sprains had residual symptoms. In this subpopulation, the "acute ankle sprain" was not "just a sprain." The descriptive terms for these residual symptoms included chronic ankle sprains, meniscoid lesions, or an unstable ankle. It is imperative to view this syndrome spectrum as an overlapping of pain, instability, and impingement (Fig. 45.1) Allowing the clinician to define, classify, diagnose, and treat this subgroup of disorders is the focus of this chapter.

EPIDEMIOLOGY OF ANKLE SPRAINS

Epidemiologically, lateral ligamentous sprains represent the most frequent injury sustained by an athlete

(3). In fact, 85% of all ankle injuries are sprains (3). Garrick (4) reported that 31% of soccer injuries are acute ankle sprains, whereas 45% of basketball and 25% of volleyball injuries are acute ankle sprains. Therefore, ankle sprains are the most common athletic injury.

MECHANISM OF INJURY AND PATHOANATOMY

The cornerstone for understanding the pathoanatomic spectrum is defining normal anatomy. The ankle is bounded by the tibial plafond superiorly, fibula laterally, medial malleolus, and talus inferiorly. All these surfaces are covered by hyaline cartilage. This bony framework is held together by a complex ligamentous complex, including the anterior talofibular (ATFL), calcaneofibular, posterior talofibular, deltoid, and the distal tibiofibular syndesmosis (ligamentous mass that joins the tibia to the fibula). The ankle is also surrounded on all sides by numerous tendons.

Plantar–flexion/inversion is the most common mechanism of injury of acute ankle sprains (5). The ATFL tears first, followed by the calcaneofibular and posterior talofibular ligaments. There are far more lateral ligament injuries than medial ligament injuries. The longer lateral malleolus obstructs eversion of the ankle, whereas the shorter medial malleolus offers little obstruction to inversion. Further, there is a natural tendency for inversion. Studies have shown the ATFL sustains the least maximal load to failure of all the components of the lateral complex (6). Hence, it is the most frequently injured. Additionally, the deltoid ligament (superficial and deep) is stronger than the lateral complex ligaments and therefore more difficult to tear. Eversion, or syndesmotic sprains, are less frequent but may have a greater morbidity.

In 1950, Wolin et al. (7) were the first to define the term "chronic ankle sprains" in nine patients after ankle sprains with intractable anterolateral pain, no instabil-

T. P. Knapp, W. M. Hayes, and B. R. Mandelbaum: Santa Monica Orthopaedic and Sports Medicine Group, Santa Monica, California 90404.

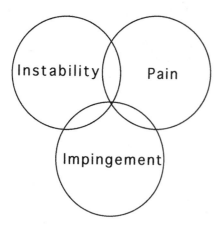

FIG. 45.1. Ankle Impingement Syndrome Spectrum.

ity, and a palpable mass in the anterolateral ankle joint. They theorized the mass to be hyalinized connective tissue from the talofibular joint capsule. Wolin et al. believed repeated pinching of the tissue led to pain and swelling. These patients underwent arthrotomy and exploration because of the chronicity of the symptoms. Surgical findings included a "meniscoid" mass between the fibula and talus in the lateral gutter. Histologic sections revealed a combination of ligamentous, fibrous, fibrocartilaginous, and inflammatory tissue and hypertrophic synovium. This has been confirmed in subsequent arthroscopic studies (8–10). These studies have discovered at arthroscopy that the mass of tissue involved with dynamic impingement is more extensive and is not uniquely localized in the lateral gutter. What is found is a dense mass of hypertrophic tissue in the anterolateral tibiotalar joint space extending from the anterior capsule posteriorly into the lateral gutter. Histologically, these studies have corroborated the findings of Wolin et al. and have clearly improved our understanding of the pathoanatomic changes leading to anterior capsular impingement.

More recently, McCarroll et al. (11) described an identical lesion in four soccer players. Waller (12), in 1982, described a repetitive inversion injury leading to chronic pain anterolaterally. He thus coined the term "anterolateral corner compression syndrome."

In 1990, Bassett et al. (9) reported impingement from a separate distal fasciae of anterior tibiofibular ligament. They theorized that tear of the ATFL causes increased laxity, allowing the talar dome to extrude anteriorly in dorsiflexion causing impingement. "Bassett's ligament" is present in most human ankles and may be a cause of talar impingement, abrasion of the articular cartilage, and pain in the anterior aspect of the ankle. It is of interest that resection of this ligament usually will alleviate the pain caused by the impingement.

What then is the cause of anterolateral pain seen with "chronic ankle sprains"? Healing of ligament sprains is invariably accompanied by scarring. Recurrent sprains

lead to an abundant scar mass in the area of the ATFL and in the anterolateral capsule. This mass may be a combination of scarified capsule and ligamentous tissue. A pedunculated mass of scar tissue and/or hypertrophic synovium may actually protrude intraarticularly. The hypertrophic tissue is an impediment to normal healing and to complete symptomatic resolution. With significant impingement, patients invariably fail to improve with conservative means. Sprains may cause ankle ligament laxity and attenuation and therefore become dysfunctional as a check rein. As a consequence, the ankle becomes relatively unstable. The combination of this occult instability with the pathologic "scar mass" results in clinical and subjective complaints of pain, functional instability, and loss of function.

CLINICAL EVALUATION

The diagnosis and treatment of acute ankle sprains is relatively straightforward and has been well elucidated previously (13).

What are the diagnostic clues that can accurately lead the sports medicine specialist to the correct diagnosis of an ankle impingement syndrome? The diagnosis is made by using a systematic approach and by maintaining a high level of suspicion. The clinician must specifically inquire about past ankle injuries and treatments. The characteristic presentation of ankle impingement syndrome is an athlete with repetitive sprains and intractable anterolateral ankle pain despite an intensive program of physical therapy, pharmacologic intervention, and rehabilitation. Subjective symptoms include pain with exertional activities such as pivoting and pushing off. Pain is only present with activities and exercise. Often the symptoms are absent before or after such exertion. Physical examination reveals anterolateral tenderness, bogginess, and occasionally erythema and diffuse swelling.

IMAGING STUDIES

Radiographic evaluation includes anteroposterior, lateral, and mortise views of the ankle. Additionally, if clinically indicated, anteroposterior, lateral, and oblique views of the foot are obtained. When dealing with athletes, it is important to not overread x-rays. Many have been fooled into believing they have discovered the source of the acute symptoms when in actual fact it is simply the "acute discovery of chronic disease." This was shown by Massada (14). In a study of 88 professional soccer players, he found a high prevalance of radiographic changes in asymptomatic ankles. Interestingly, 59.1% were found in the right ankle and 52.3% in the left. He theorized that these radiographic images seem to indicate the existence of an osseous remodeling phenomena in response to overuse and overstress of the ankle. He coined the phrase "radiographic arthrosis of sportsman" to describe these radiographic findings in the asymptomatic athlete. Described were changes in the neck of the talus ("squatting facet") and/or the anterior articular border of the distal epiphysis of the tibia (talotibial exostosis).

Stress views are obtained to corroborate the absence of pathologic ligamentous laxity. Stress views are reserved for the fully rehabilitated athlete with continued instability symptoms. Key to the diagnosis of instability is demonstration of abnormal radiographic stress views. However, stress views can give contradictory information. Seligson et al. (15) casted doubt on the validity of ankle stress views in a study published in 1980. In this study, bilateral ankle stress testing was performed on 25 subjects in a device that controlled position of the foot and the amount of force applied during the examination. Both inversion testing in the anteroposterior plane and anterior drawer testing in the lateral plane were performed in the same group of symptom-free patients. The reproducibility of the test was demonstrated. Previous history of injury, left versus right handedness, side, and arthropometric measurements did not affect the test. There was no difference in the inversion test between ankles tested in neutral and plantar flexion. In functionally normal ankles, the range of inversion "talar tilt" was 0 to 18 degrees, whereas the maximum of anterior displacement on drawer testing was 3 mm. Their conclusion was that anterior drawer testing appears to evaluate lateral ligamentous integrity of the ankle more critically than the talar tilt test. The usefulness of stress views was also called into question recently by Cardone et al. (16), who performed a retrospective review of 43 patients. They were able to diagnose 30 ATFL, 20 calcaneofibular ligament, and no posterior talofibular ligament injuries. An important finding from this study was ligamentous injuries were found in 12 of 23 with normal stress x-rays.

Secondary diagnostic techniques (e.g., bone scan, computed tomography, magnetic resonance imaging [MRI]) can facilitate interpretation and aid in the proper diagnosis but primarily by exclusion. MRI is a sensitive indicator of osteochondral defects but is insensitive in confirming the diagnosis of anterolateral impingement. Liu et al. (17) showed that physical examination was

TABLE 45.1. *Differential diagnosis of ankle impingement pain*

1. Osteochondral lesions of the talus
2. Calcific densities beneath the medial or lateral malleoli
3. Peroneal subluxation or dislocation
4. Tarsal coalition
5. Subtalar joint dysfunction
6. Degenerative joint disease
7. Soft tissue impingement

TABLE 45.2. *Ankle impingement syndrome classification*

Grade I:	Normal x-rays, anterolateral capsular thickening seen on MRI and verified arthroscopically.
Grade II:	Extraarticular or intraarticular osteophytes with articular surfaces entirely normal.
Grade III:	Bony abnormalities involving articular surface (i.e., osteochondritis dissecans).
Grade IV:	Previous intraarticular fracture.

MRI, magnetic resonance imaging.

94% sensitive and 75% specific in making the diagnosis, whereas MRI was 39% sensitive and 50% specific. This was confirmed by Farooki et al. (18), who demonstrated 42% sensitivity, 85% specificity, and 69% accuracy of MRI.

Table 45.1 lists the differential diagnoses to ankle impingement pain. Also, Bartolozzi et al. (8) proposed a classification system for stable ankles with impingement symptoms (Table 45.2).

ANKLE IMPINGEMENT TREATMENT

Literature is scarce on the treatment of this important pathologic entity. Fortunately, arthroscopic intervention has expanded our spectrum of therapeutic alternatives. It should be emphasized, however, that anterior capsular impingement requiring arthroscopic surgical intervention represents a very small percentage of the total group. A word of warning must be heeded. During arthroscopic debridement, it is imperative that the surgeon not excise the ATFL in his or her zeal to debride the pathologic mass.

What should the approach be to the ankle with chronic instability but no impingement? The first step is to differentiate the entity from the incompletely rehabilitated ankle, which can also be present with chronic anterolateral pain and functional instability. An exhaustive systematic therapy program incorporating strengthening and mobilization, modalities, nonsteroidal antiinflammatory agents, and occasional steroid injections is pursued. In step 1, the rehabilitation program involves an initial baseline assessment of range of motion and baseline isokinetic testing. The physical therapy protocol incorporates modalities (ice, phonophoresis, electrical and muscle stimulation), exercise and strengthening (isometrics, isokinetics, and isotonics), range of motion activities (stretching, joint mobilization), and functional progression as indicated with multidirectional exercises, proprioceptive training, and sport simulation. In step 2, if step 1 is unsuccessful, then it is necessary to proceed to diagnostic arthroscopy and modified Brostrom lateral ligament reconstruction. The success rate from this protocol is 85% to 90%.

EXPECTED OUTCOMES

Most athletes with impingement will respond to systematic nonoperative management. This is predicated, however, on the proper diagnosis and carefully monitored rehabilitation.

The success rate with a properly diagnosed and skillful arthroscopically treated ankle is excellent. Bartolozzi et al. (8) found 77% of their patients with excellent or good results after arthroscopic debridement. Ferkel et al. (10) reported in a similar study an 84% success rate with a 6-week return to sports.

What is the ultimate outcome of the nonoperated ankle with chronic lateral instability? Lofvenberg et al. (19) recently answered this question when they detailed the outcome of nonoperated patients with chronic lateral instability of the ankle in a 20-year follow-up study. They reported on 37 patients studied 18 to 23 years after their index visit who were conservatively treated because of chronic lateral instability of the ankle; 32 of 49 ankles still suffered from instability. Degenerative changes were observed in only 6 of 46 radiographically examined ankles. The key finding of this study was no correlation to age or persistent instability. Therefore, although instability may persist, it appears that there is no increased incidence of degenerative changes.

AUTHORS' PREFERRED TREATMENT

Most patients referred to our facility have undergone previous diagnostic studies, rest, rehabilitation, and frequently arthroscopic surgery. It is important to not take previous workup for granted. In a sports medicine professional's desire to make the diagnosis and institute treatment, the correct diagnosis is frequently overlooked. This is avoided by systematically following the basics: "When in doubt, examine the patient." The patient's history and physical examination will yield the correct diagnosis over 90% of the time.

We do believe stress views have a place in the evaluation on chronic instability, but we always obtain comparison views. Moreover, we have found lateral radiographs with an anterior drawer test to be much more helpful than talar tilt comparison. Despite this, an anterior drawer of greater than 3 mm or a talar tilt greater than

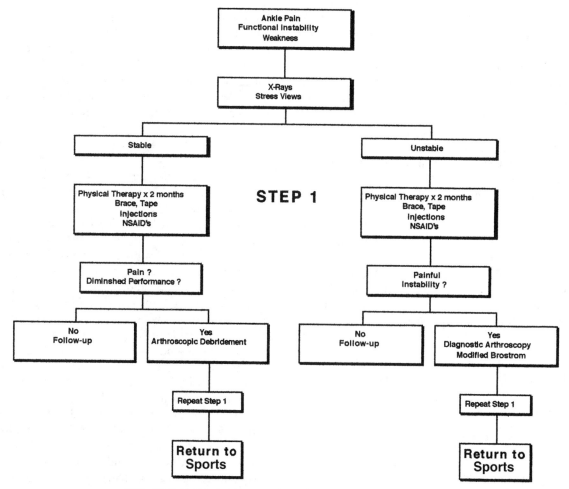

FIG. 45.2. Ankle impingement syndrome treatment algorithm.

5 degrees when compared with the contralateral ankle is considered diagnostic of instability.

As stated earlier, there are many entities that cause anterolateral ankle pain. Subjective functional instability may be present secondary to pain, but laxity is specifically not a component of the syndrome. We have found it helpful to divide ankles into two groups: unstable with or without impingement and stable with or without impingement.

A systematic and organized approach to diagnosis and appropriate therapeutic intervention for chronic recurrent ankle sprains is presented in the algorithm in Fig. 45.2 (8). Note that MRI does not appear in the algorithm. We use MRI when our physical examination does not suggest instability or impingement to search for osteochondral lesions or occult tendinosis. The use of differential lidocaine injections to separate out coexistent pathology should be used liberally. Frequently, the actual diagnosis is multifactorial. Remember the old adage "What has four wings and flies?" The answer: two birds.

SUMMARY

In summary, acute ankle sprains must be recognized and rehabilitated aggressively. Nonoperative management with functional bracing is as effective as surgical intervention with an earlier return to sports. Chronic lateral ankle pain has many causes, one of which is the anterior capsular impingement syndrome. This is an entity that develops in a subgroup of athletes' ankles after recurrent sprains. It is characterized by the formation of hypertrophic scar tissue, synovium, and fibrocartilage in the anterolateral aspect of the ankle joint. A constellation of symptoms refractory to conservative management, including pain, weakness, and functional instability, and diminution in performance is the result. To date, surgical management via arthroscopic debridement has yielded uniformly good and excellent results, especially in grade I or grade II injuries (8).

REFERENCES

1. Smith RW, Reischl SF. Treatment of ankle sprains in young athletes. *Am J Sports Med* 1986;14:465–471.
2. Freeman MAR, Dean MRE, Hanham IWF. The etiology and prevention of functional instability of the foot. *J Bone Joint Surg Br* 1965;47B:676–677.
3. Attarian DE, McCracken HJ, DeVito DP, et al. A biochemical study of human lateral ankle ligaments and autogenous reconstructive grafts. *Am J Sports Med* 1985;13:377–381.
4. Garrick JM. The frequency of injury, mechanism of injury, and epidemiology of ankle sprains. *Am J Sports Med* 1977;5:241–242.
5. Balduini FC, Tetzlaff J. Historical perspectives on injuries of the ligaments of the ankle. *Clin Sports Med* 1982;1:3–12.
6. Cox JS. Surgical and nonsurgical treatment of acute ankle sprains. *Clin Orthop* 1985;198:118–126.
7. Wolin I, Glassman F, Sideman S, et al. Internal derangement of the talofibular component of the ankle. *Surg Gynecol Obstet* 1950; 91:193–200.
8. Bartolozzi AR, Mandelbaum BR, Finerman GAM, et al. The anterior capsular impingement syndrome of the ankle. Presented at the 13th Annual Meeting of the American Orthopaedic Society for Sports Medicine, Orlando, 1987.
9. Bassett FH, Gates HS, Billys JB, et al. Talar impingement by the anteroinferior tibiofibular ligament. *J Bone Joint Surg Am* 1990;72A:55–59.
10. Ferkel RD, Karzel RP, Del Pizzo W, et al. Arthroscopic treatment of anterolateral impingement of the ankle. *Am J Sports Med* 1991; 19:440–446.
11. McCarroll JR, Schrader JW, Shelbourne RD, et al. Meniscoid lesions of the ankle in soccer players. *Am J Sports Med* 1987;15:255–257.
12. Waller JF. Hindfoot and midfoot problems in the runner. In: Mack RP, ed. *Symposium on the foot and leg in running.* St. Louis: Mosby, 1982:64–71.
13. Knapp TP, Mandelbaum BR. Ankle sprains and impingement syndromes. In: Garrett WE, ed. *The U.S. soccer sports medicine book.* Baltimore: Williams & Wilkins, 1996:360–368.
14. Massada JL. Ankle overuse injuries in soccer players. *J Sports Med Phys Fitness* 1991;31:447–451.
15. Seligson D, Gassman J, Pope M. Ankle instability: evaluation of the lateral ligaments. *Am J Sports Med* 1980;8:39–41.
16. Cardone BW, Erickson SJ, Den Hartog BD, et al. MRI of injury to the lateral collateral ligamentous complex of the ankle. *J Comput Assist Tomogr* 1993;17:102–107.
17. Liu SH, Nuccion SL, Finerman G. Diagnosis of anterolateral ankle impingement. Comparison between magnetic resonance imaging and clinical examination. *Am J Sports Med* 1997;25:389–393.
18. Farooki S, Yao L, Seeger LL. Anterolateral impingement of the ankle: effectiveness of MR imaging. *Radiology* 1998;207:357–360.
19. Lofvenberg R, Karrholm J, Lund B. The outcome of nonoperated patients with chronic lateral instability of the ankle: a 20-year follow-up study. *Foot Ankle* 1994;15:165–169.

Principles and Practice of Orthopaedic Sports Medicine,
edited by William E. Garrett, Jr., Kevin P. Speer, and Donald T. Kirkendall.
Lippincott Williams & Wilkins, Philadelphia © 2000.

CHAPTER 46

Surgical Complications of the Knee

Herb O. Boté and Lonnie E. Paulos

LIGAMENT RECONSTRUCTION

Significant advances have been made in the reconstruction of ligament insufficiency during the last 15 years. The focus of research has been mainly on anterior cruciate ligament (ACL) reconstruction. Posterior cruciate ligament (PCL) and multiple-ligament injuries have been getting increased attention secondary to an increasingly active patient population and increased incidence of traumatic injuries. The publicity of injuries and treatment of professional athletes have also heightened the awareness of patients dealing with similar situations. There has also been a trend in ligament injuries in the older population (1). This would approximate to 95,000 new injuries each year. Complications have focused mainly on the choice and preparation of the graft, tunnel placement, and arthrofibrosis.

Complications Arising from the Graft

The choices of which type of graft to use for ligament reconstruction are many. There are advantages and disadvantages for each type. The two most popular types are the bone–patellar tendon–bone (PTB) and the hamstring (HS) autogenous grafts. Proponents of PTB grafts cite studies that demonstrate comparable tensile strength of the graft compared with native ACL (2–4). The study by McKernan et al. (5) and the review by Brown and Steiner (6), however, have shown the strength of doubled semitendinosus/gracilis grafts to approach that of the native ACL. Brown and Steiner (6) demonstrated that the ultimate tensile strength of a doubled semitendinosus/gracilis graft to be 3,879 N, exceeding the value obtained for the strength of the ACL by Woo et al. (4) (2,160 N) and the tensile strength of PTB (2,977 N) obtained by Cooper et al. (2).

Another reason for preference for PTB grafts is the belief that bone to bone healing occurs at a much faster rate than tendon to bone healing. Recent studies using a canine model (7) and rabbit model (8) have demonstrated that HS grafts undergo similar healing and ligamentization processes as PTB grafts. Johnson (9) showed that the semitendinosus graft in humans was histologically normal by 3 months with evidence of revascularization and maturation patterns of normal ACL. Complications from utilization of PTB grafts have been due mainly to donor site morbidity. Numerous reports have documented quadriceps weakness, patellar irritability, and flexion contracture (10–14). In a prospective study, Sachs et al. (14) demonstrated a 65% rate of quadriceps weakness below 80% of the contralateral limb in patients in which PTB were used. O'Brien et al. (13) reported a 37% rate of patellar pain after harvest of PTB grafts. There are studies, however, that demonstrate patellofemoral pain and arthrosis without the use of PTB grafts (15,16). Patellar ligament ruptures and quadriceps tendon ruptures have been noted after use of PTB grafts (17–20). Bonamo et al. (17) reported on two cases in which the patellar tendon ruptured 4 and 8 months after ACL reconstruction. Both ruptures occurred at the inferior pole of the patella. The ligament defects were noted to be well healed. Marumoto et al. (19) described two patellar ligament ruptures occurring 3 and 6 years after the index reconstruction. Patellar fractures are also noted to occur after PTB graft harvest (21,22). Simonian et al. (22) described two cases of stellate patella fractures after an indirect mechanism of injury. Patella baja after closure of the patellar ligament defect has been reported in the literature (23,24). Tria et al. (23) studied 29 consecutive ACL reconstructions using PTB grafts. All defects were closed. They found a 76% incidence of patella baja postoperatively. This finding, however, did not have a direct correlation with patellofemoral pain or arthrosis. Because of this finding, we do not recommend closure of the tendon defect or limit the closure to the peritenon.

H. O. Boté and L. E. Paulos: The Orthopedic Specialty Hospital, Salt Lake City, Utah 84107.

Allogeneic tissue for use as ACL graft has enjoyed limited success in the literature. Their use has been advocated mainly as a secondary source of graft for use in revision reconstruction and for multiple ligament reconstruction (25–28). There are few long-term data on the results of allograft reconstruction. Most have been 1- to 2-year follow-up studies (29–36). There have been very few long-term follow-up studies with allografts. Malek and DeLuca (37) showed a deterioration of average knee scores from 84 to 72 and good to excellent results from 80% to 48% comparing 2- and 5-year follow-up. Ethylene oxide sterilization has been shown to have deleterious effects on soft tissue allografts (38,39). Jackson et al. (39) showed a 6.4% incidence of intraarticular reaction resulting in an effusion. Synovial biopsies revealed a chronic inflammatory response characterized by fibrin, collagen, and phagocytic cells. Gas chromatography revealed ethylene chlorohydrin, a toxic byproduct of ethylene oxide. Removal of the graft resulted in resolution of the effusion and inflammation. In a 2-year follow-up study, Roberts et al. (38) showed a 22% rate of graft dissolution on repeat arthroscopy. Large femoral cysts were also noted in these cases. Only 17 of the 36 patients studied were considered to have functional knees. Ethylene oxide sterilized grafts are currently not recommended for use in allograft reconstruction.

Transmission of viral disease has been the main public fear of allograft tissue. Transmission of human immunodeficiency virus type I (HIV) has been documented in two cases (40,41). The first case in 1988 was due to a femoral bone allograft from a donor that was HIV positive that eventually developed acquired immunodeficiency syndrome (AIDS) complex. The recipient received the allograft for elective spinal fusion for idiopathic scoliosis 4 months before U.S. Food and Drug Administration approval of antibody testing of donor and donor tissue for HIV. Donor screening for HIV risk had not yet been instituted at the time of transplant. The donor had a history of intravenous drug abuse and a lymph node biopsy that was not elicited before the donation. Both donor and recipient eventually succumbed to complications from AIDS. The second case was reported in 1992. The recipient had undergone a revision total hip arthroplasty using a femoral head allograft. The donor was a 22-year-old man who died of a gunshot wound to the head. Serum from the donor was tested negative for HIV at two different institutions. Recipients of both kidneys, the liver, and the heart eventually tested positive for HIV. Recipients of unprocessed femoral heads and bone–patellar ligament–bone also tested positive for the virus. Recipients of freeze-dried bone chips and heat treated femoral head, however, tested negative for the virus. It was thought that the process of freeze

drying removed the medullary contents of the bone and thus the virus.

Transmission of hepatitis B and C in musculoskeletal allografts has also been documented in the literature (42–46). Similar donor screening and tissue processing protocols have evolved from information obtained from these studies. Fresh frozen allografts have been shown to produce slightly better results than freeze-dried specimens (29,47). There is, however, an increased risk of transmission of bloodborne pathogens with its use (40–43).

Gamma irradiation of allograft tissue is an alternative to ethylene oxide sterilization. Alteration of collagen structure has been shown in a number of studies (48–50). Gibbons et al. (48) demonstrated significant decreases in the maximum stress, maximum strain, and strain energy density to maximum stress when frozen PTB specimens were subjected to 3 Mrad of gamma radiation. Two megarads of radiation did not show significant change in the parameters measured. Fideler et al. (50), however, showed that even 2 Mrad of radiation will significantly decrease maximum force, strain energy, modulus, and maximum stress of the specimens tested. The International Atomic Energy Agency has recommended a dose of 2.5 Mrad for the sterilization of medical products (51). Tissue banks commonly use between 1.5 and 2.5 Mrad for sterilization of allografts (52). Fideler et al. (53) showed that irradiation with 2.5 Mrad did not eradicate the presence of HIV DNA in confirmed infected PTB specimens. The ability of the irradiated HIV DNA to infect the host is still under investigation. To date, the jury is still out on the effectiveness and deleterious effects of gamma irradiation of soft tissue allografts. Artificial allografts are only of historical note

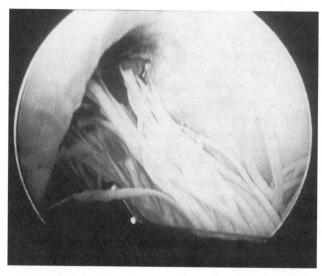

FIG. 46.1. Failed Gortex anterior cruciate ligament graft.

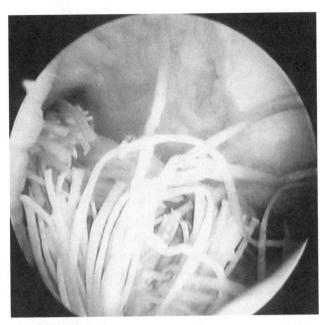

FIG. 46.2. Failed Gortex anterior cruciate ligament graft at 3 years.

subject the graft to increased strain as the knee is flexed. This in turn will lead to overconstraint and loss of flexion or graft elongation.

Positioning of the femoral attachment in the over the top position will cause excessive laxity in the graft as the knee is flexed and increased tension as the knee is extended (56,58,81). Tibial tunnel placement has less direct influence on graft length changes than the femoral tunnel attachment site. Inadvertent anterior tibial tunnel placement, however, has been shown to increase the incidence of graft impingement in the intercondylar notch (65–69,75). Howell and Taylor (69) studied tibial tunnel placement and graft impingement using cadaveric, clinical, and magnetic resonance imaging (MRI) data. They showed that an ACL graft placed anterior to a line drawn from the femur to the tibial plateau along Blumensaat's line, with the knee in full hyperextension, will result in intercondylar roof impingement (Fig. 46.4). MRI will show increased signal intensity of the ACL graft at the area of notch impingement. This has led surgeons to perform a notchplasty to ensure that the ACL graft will have adequate clearance under the

at this time. We observed a 50% complication rate at 3 to 5 years in our series of patients (Figs. 46.1 and 46.2).

Tunnel Placement Complications

Tunnel placement is the most critical and the most technically dependent portion of ACL reconstruction. Errors in tunnel placement can lead to graft stretching, graft failure, and overconstraint of the knee, resulting in loss of motion. An extensive review of this subject was published by Jauregito and Paulos in 1996 (54). Attention in the past has been focused mainly in the femoral tunnel placement and its isometric position (55–64). Recently, however, increased attention has been given to the accurate placement of tibial tunnels (65–77). Functionally, the ACL has been divided into two bundles: anteromedial and posterolateral (78,79). Although ACL reconstruction is designed to recreate the isometric attachment of the ACL in the knee, this has been difficult to achieve perfectly in the clinical setting (62,80). Most current techniques attempt to recreate the anteromedial bundle during reconstruction (63,81). The goal of reconstruction is to eliminate knee instability without creating excessive graft tension. Increase graft tension will lead to loss of motion or permanent elongation leading to recurrent instability. Anterior femoral tunnel placement will lead to an increase in distance between the femoral and tibial attachment sites as the knee is flexed (55,56,58–60,63,64) (Fig. 46.3). This will

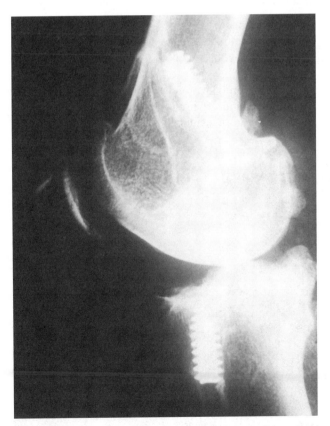

FIG. 46.3. Anterior femoral tunnel placement in this patient led to graft stretching with continued knee flexion and eventual graft failure.

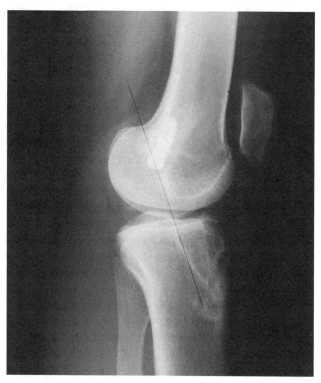

FIG. 46.4. A 20-year-old woman presents to our office with persistent knee pain with extension and instability 4 years after her anterior cruciate ligament reconstruction.

intercondylar roof even with the knee in hyperextension.

The intercondylar notch has taken a central role in the subject of graft impingement. In addition to the issue of tunnel placement just described, the morphol-

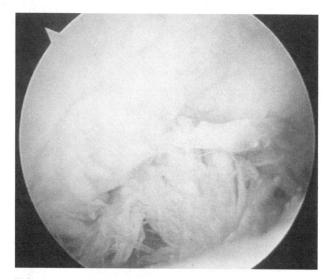

FIG. 46.5. Notch regrowth led to impingement and graft failure in this patient.

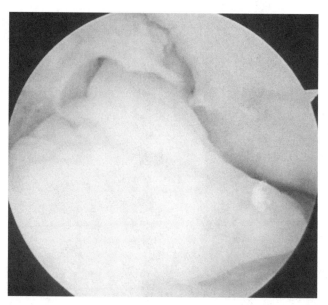

FIG. 46.6. Intercondylar notch view of left knee with "cyclops" lesion formation on the anterior cruciate ligament graft.

ogy of the intercondylar notch has been shown to contribute to ACL tears and to graft failure (67,71,82–86). Inadequate notchplasty and notch regrowth have also been implicated in graft failure (Fig. 46.5). The formation of a lump of scarlike tissue, commonly known as a "cyclops lesion" has been attributed to anterior graft impingement (87–90) (Fig. 46.6). Watanabe and Howell (89) reported on 19 patients that complained of persistent effusion, extension deficit, recurrent instability, and knee pain. Second-look arthroscopy revealed fragmentation and extrusion of graft material into the outlet of the notch. A fibrous nodule was also noted on repeat arthroscopy. Jackson and Schaefer (87) reported on 13 patients who complained of loss of full extension and an audible and palpable clunk with terminal extension. The symptoms and range of motion improved with manipulation and arthroscopic debridement. Preoperative MRI studies of these lesions reveal abnormal increased signal characteristics consistent with fibrous tissue anterior to the ACL graft (90). Histologic analysis reveals dense disorganized fibroconnective tissue that undergoes conversion to fibrocartilagenous tissue (88).

Common Complications and Authors' Preferred Treatment

Patellofemoral Pain

In our institution we prefer to use doubled semitendinosus and gracilis autografts for primary ACL reconstructions to minimize the risk of postoperative patellofemoral pain. Femoral fixation is achieved by anchorage of the looped graft into the anterior femoral cortex. The femoral fixation device is directly linked to the graft without use of a suture that could invariably deform. The use of allograft tissue is reserved mainly for multiple ligament reconstructions and/or revision reconstructions. We also use the contralateral HS for isolated revision ACL reconstructions. Because of our high success rates with use of HS grafts, PTB grafts have only rarely been used in revision situations and in athletes who demand a rapid return to sports and show no clinical evidence of patellofemoral pathology.

Anterior Femoral and Tibial Tunnel Placement

We prefer to treat errors in tunnel placement in two stages. During the first stage we debride the graft and the original femoral and tibial tunnels. Both the femoral and tibial tunnels are packed with bone graft from a femoral head allograft. The second stage is performed after 3 months of healing. This consists of the revision reconstruction with the appropriate choice of graft. Most errors in tunnel placement occur in the femoral side. In some situations the femoral tunnel is so far anterior, we are able to perform the revision in one stage using the original tibial tunnel and a more posterior femoral tunnel. Use of a soft tissue graft and avoidance of interference screw femoral fixation is advantageous in this situation. Special attention should be used in tunnel bone grafting so that all soft tissue is removed from within the bony tunnel because this would prevent healing of the graft to host bone. To prevent anterior femoral tunnel placement, we routinely identify the over-the-top position and place the femoral guide pin 2 to 3 mm anterior to this spot.

Notch Impingement

Notch impingement is related to tibial tunnel placement. We prefer to place the tibial guide pin in the posterior portion of the footprint of the native ACL just anterior to the PCL. The angle subtended by the guide pin and the tibial plateau surface is predetermined at 50 degrees. Most errors in tibial tunnel placement have been anterior and medial deviation. Anterior deviation will result in graft impingement in the intercondylar notch during extension. Our solution to this problem is to resect additional bone from the superior and lateral intercondylar notch. After the notchplasty, we routinely use the 0-degree arthroscope inserted into the tibial tunnel as a gauge to the adequacy of the notchplasty (Fig. 46.7). At full extension there should be no encroachment of any portion of the intercondylar notch as seen from the arthroscope within the tibial tunnel (Fig. 46.8).

Chronic notch impingement results in loss of extension and formation of scarring anteriorly on the graft,

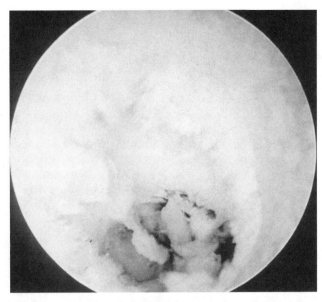

FIG. 46.7. Arthroscopic view using a 0-degree arthroscope through the tibial tunnel with the knee in full extension. There is a potential impingement of the anterior cruciate ligament graft by the superior portion of the intercondylar roof.

termed a cyclops lesion. Treatment is by arthroscopic debridement of the lesion and resumption of range of motion exercises. Notch regrowth, despite adequate initial notchplasty, in another problem that is receiving increased attention as a cause of notch impingement (Fig. 46.9). We are currently conducting a clinical study as to the association of notch regrowth to graft rerupture. Arthrofibrosis and patellar entrapment is a disas-

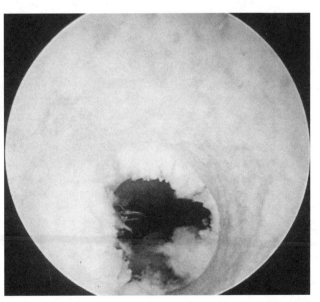

FIG. 46.8. Same view and patient as in Fig. 46.7 after superior notchplasty.

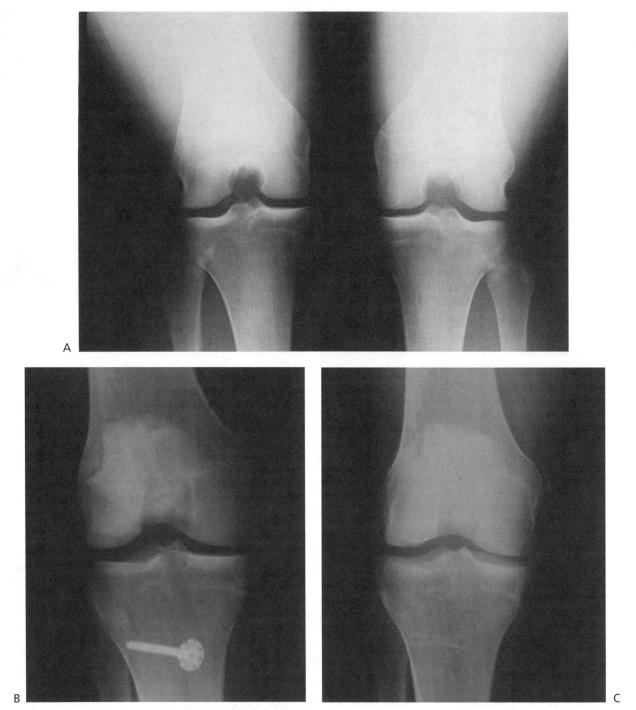

FIG. 46.9. A: Notch radiograph before anterior cruciate ligament (ACL) reconstruction. **B:** Notch radiograph of the same patient 1 week after ACL reconstruction. **C:** Notch radiograph 21 months after ACL reconstruction showing evidence of regrowth of the lateral intercondylar notch.

trous complication that is discussed in detail in the last section of this chapter.

MENISCAL SURGERY

King (91), in his now classic study, demonstrated that canine menisci will heal as long as there was a viable vascular network to supply the healing wound. Fairbank (92) would later show that removal of the meniscus would place the knee at risk of degenerative joint disease. Since then, an attempt has been made to preserve as much of the meniscus as possible in hopes of preventing this sequela. Arnoczky and Warren (93,94) have been instrumental in demonstrating the vascular anatomy of the meniscus. With this foundation, meniscal repair is now the standard of care in the treatment of meniscal tears within the vascularized zone. Meniscectomy continues to be a viable option in the face of degenerative or complex tears. Meniscal transplantation is a burgeoning new field that is just recently gaining acceptance. We deal mainly with the complications of these three procedures.

Complications in Meniscal Repair

Arthroscopically assisted meniscal repair is the current standard of care in treatment of meniscal tears within the vascularized zone of the meniscus. The technique described have ranged from outside-to-inside, inside-to-outside, and all-inside. This wide variability makes it difficult to compare the different results that have been published. Added to this are the different leg positioning, suture material, suturing techniques, and instrumentation.

Small (95), in a survey of 8,791 knee arthroscopies, documented a 1.52% complication rate in medial meniscal repairs. The nature of the complications was not given in the study. The author qualified his results by the fact that the surgeons reporting in his survey had an average of 14 years of knee arthroscopic experience. It might be inferred that a higher rate will be obtained by less experienced arthroscopists. Austin and Sherman (96) reported on 101 consecutive meniscal repair. They found an overall complication rate of 18%. They had a 13% complication rate in lateral meniscal repair compared with a 19% rate with medial meniscal repair. Females had a higher likelihood of complication. There was a 10% rate of arthrofibrosis with concomitant ACL reconstruction.

Studies using second-look arthroscopies reported reoccurrence of tears. It is unclear, however, if the pathology is actually a recurrence or a failure to heal. Eggli et al. (97) reported 14 reruptures in 52 patients followed for an average of 7.5 years, giving a 27% failure rate. Two patients were treated with repairs and 12 were treated with partial meniscectomies. The average time to rerupture was 11.2 months. None of their failures occurred after 44 months. Sixty-four percent of the failures occurred within 6 months after the repair. None of the patients in this study required an ACL reconstruction. DeHaven et al. (98), on a minimum 10-year follow-up study, reported a 21% incidence of retears on 33 open repairs. All failures occurred in knees that were unstable by arthrometer testing. Horibe et al. (99) reported on 31 patients evaluated by second-look arthroscopy. Five patients (14%) had no evidence of healing. Seven patients had evidence of tears in a different location from the original tear. Jensen et al. (100) reported 10 retears in 49 patients. None of the retears occurred

in patients who had meniscal repair in conjunction with an ACL reconstruction.

Several factors have been associated with meniscal repair healing. Most authors agree that concomitant meniscal repair and ACL reconstruction has a high likelihood of a satisfactory outcome (101–104). It is postulated that ACL reconstruction results in increased intraarticular bleeding and clot formation. This in turn brings in the cytokines necessary to promote accelerated healing. It is also postulated that patients with meniscal and ACL ruptures present more acutely. Stone et al. (103) reported a 100% healing rate if the meniscal repair was performed within 8 weeks from the time of the injury. Those repaired after 8 weeks showed only a 64% healing rate. Hamberg et al. (105) demonstrated an 11% rerupture rate if tears were repaired more than 12 months from the time of the original injury. Only 1 of 15 repairs reruptured if performed acutely. Eggli et al. (97) found a 9% increase in failure if the repairs were delayed more than 8 weeks from the time of the injury. They also found that repairs done on tears with more than 3 mm of rim width had a 40% retear rate as compared with 13% if the rim width of the residual meniscus was less than 3 mm.

Arthrofibrosis is another commonly reported complication associated with meniscal repair. Ryu and Dunbar (106) reported a 10% incidence of arthrofibrosis in 31 meniscal repairs. Austin and Sherman (107) also reported a 10% incidence in their report, but most of these were associated with combined ACL reconstruction. Rokito et al. (108) presented follow-up data on 243 meniscal repairs and found that 14 of the 15 documented cases of arthrofibrosis were in patients that had concomitant meniscal repair and ACL reconstruction. A more detailed discussion of arthrofibrosis and patellar entrapment syndrome (PES) is discussed at a later part of this chapter.

Saphenous neuropathy is another commonly reported complication (96,101,106,109,110). Barber (101) reported a 22% incidence in their series. They used an inside-out technique, tying their sutures over subcutaneous tissue. All symptoms resolved with time. Stone and Miller (109) reported a 38% incidence in their 51 meniscal repairs using an inside-out technique. Symptoms resolved with conservative treatment within 3 to 12 months. Morgan and Casscells (110) also reported a transient saphenous neuropathy that resolved within 4 months. Partial peroneal nerve palsy have also been reported (102,107,111,112). They are not as frequent, but the injury is potentially more disastrous to the patient. Jurist et al. (111) reported on a case in which the peroneal nerve was tethered and wrapped around two sutures that had been placed from inside-out. Miller (112) also reported on a case in which the nerve was entrapped by a suture by an inside-out technique also. Both cases resolved after reoperation and release. The one case reported by Cannon and Vittori (102) completely resolved except for hypoesthesia in the first web space. All authors reached the consensus that a well-placed posterior incision is vital to the protection of the neurovascular structures. Specifically designed retractors are also available to assist with direct visualization of needles and sutures being passed. Leg positioning has also been shown to be important. Most authors (106,110) recommend 20 to 30 degrees of knee flexion for medial meniscal repairs and 90 degrees of flexion in lateral repairs.

Other complications associated with meniscal repairs are superficial cellulitis (109), thrombophlebitis (102,109), and reflex sympathetic dystrophy (101). Septic arthritis has also been associated with meniscal repairs (113). Symptoms presented 7 to 10 days after surgery. Large effusion and fever were the most common complaints. The organism isolated was *Staphylococcus* in all cases. Definitive treatment consisted of resection of the bucket-handle tear. This report illustrates the point that the clinician must be aware of complications no matter how unlikely. Most complications, however, can be avoided with careful placement of incisions and retractors and optimal leg positioning.

Complications with Meniscectomy

Degeneration of the knee after total meniscectomy is well documented in the literature (92,114–117). Every effort has been made to try to preserve as much meniscal tissue as possible in the face of a tear. Small (95) in his survey found a 1.78% complication rate with medial meniscectomy and a 1.48% rate in lateral meniscectomies out of a total of 8,791 knee arthroscopies. The most common complication is continued degeneration despite adequate debridement of the pathology. Friedman et al. (118) reported on 44 patients who had recurrent symptoms of knee pain after arthroscopic partial meniscectomy. They found that medial sided procedures correlated with poorer results. They also found that a history of reinjury and mechanical symptoms had a direct correlation with good and excellent results. In a follow-up study averaging 8.5 years, Fauno and Nielsen (119) found 53% of patients had Fairbanks changes in the operated knee as opposed to the nonoperative contralateral knee. They also found an increased incidence of reoperation in patients that had flap tears of the meniscus. Ferkel et al. (120) found poor results with patients who had advanced chondromalacia changes, aged more than 40 years, prior knee surgeries, and symptoms greater than 2 months. They also found that bucket-handle, longitudinal, and flap tears were associated with good to excellent results. By contrast, horizontal cleavage, degenerative, and complex tears had a higher rate of poor results.

Osteonecrosis has also been known to follow arthroscopic meniscectomies (121,122). With the advent of laser as an adjunct to meniscectomy, there are now increasing reports of osteonecrosis after these procedures (123–125). Muscolo (122) reported on eight patients who had preoperative MRI that showed no evidence of osteonecrosis. After arthroscopic meniscectomy, however, all eight patients complained of continued knee pain. Repeat MRI revealed changes consistent with osteonecrosis of the medial femoral condyle. They could not isolate a definite cause for the phenomenon. They postulated that there could have been osteonecrosis before the arthroscopy, but this was not evident on the preoperative MRI. Another hypothesis was the inducement of osteonecrosis by the procedure itself.

A third hypothesis was attributed to additional procedures performed during the arthroscopy. Rozbruch et al. (123) reported on a case of osteonecrosis after use of a 60-W contact neodymium:YAG laser. The osteonecrosis was present on both the medial femoral and tibial subchondral bone. The patient was treated with an osteoarticular allograft. Janzen et al. (124) reported on two patients diagnosed with osteonecrosis after arthroscopic partial meniscectomies using neodymium:YAG laser. They also had femoral and tibial changes at the site of the meniscectomy. One patient required a total knee arthroplasty and the other a high tibial osteotomy. Holmium:YAG lasers have also been implicated in cartilage sloughs (125). Both patients studied showed changes in the lateral femoral condyles on second-look arthroscopy. The jury is still out on the benefits of laser meniscectomy as opposed to standard means. The advantage of quicker recovery time and less risk of instrument breakage have not been shown in the literature. The Holmium:YAG laser seems to be the safest choice in the market. It avoids the gas insufflation needed with CO_2 lasers and allows pulsed energy transmission, avoiding the thermal effect and wide zone of necrosis caused by neodymium:YAG lasers (126).

Pseudoaneurysm of the popliteal artery has also been reported after arthroscopic meniscectomy (127–131). Potter and Morris-Jones (127) reported on two patients that had undergone arthroscopic meniscectomy. There was documented difficulty in removing the damaged meniscus in both cases. One case noted a small amount of bleeding after meniscus removal. Tourniquets were used in both cases. In both cases, deflation of the tourniquet demonstrated a slowed reperfusion of the extremity. One case had a pale pulseless leg postoperatively. Both were diagnosed with arteriograms, and both were treated with urgent reverse saphenous vein bypass grafting. Vincent and Stanish (130) reported on two cases of pseudoaneurysm of the medial and lateral geniculate arteries. Both cases resolved with surgical ablation. Peroneal nerve injury has also been reported in the literature (132). A neuroma in continuity was found on second-look surgery. Despite sural nerve grafting, functional motor and sensory activity did not return. There was a 7-month delay from the time of injury to the time of presentation.

Complications of Meniscal Transplantation

To date there have been few long-term follow-up studies of the results of allograft meniscal transplantations. Milachowski et al. (133) reported on 22 patients receiving either lyophilized or deep frozen meniscal allograft replacement. They found graft shrinkage to be the major complicating factor, especially in the lyophilized group. More episodes of postoperative effusions also occurred in the lyophilized group. Deep frozen allograft were noted to have fewer complications. In a report of three failures, de Boer and Koudstaal (134) showed loosening of the graft attachment in all three cases. All transplants were soft tissue only without bone blocks as a source of attachment. One of the failures was associated with a varus knee alignment. All three eventually required removal for pain relief. In a report of 63 patients and 67 knees, Cameron and Saha (135) found six posterior horn tears in the allograft. All six were treated with partial meniscectomy. The morphology of the graft was not described in the study. Two patients had infections that resolved with antibiotic treatment.

Common Complications and Authors' Preferred Treatment

Retears

Complications such as retears and failure to heal are relatively straightforward problems. Most likely, a certain percentage of meniscal repairs fail to heal and yet remain asymptomatic. Those patients that become symptomatic should be treated according to the viability of the tear. Partial meniscectomy is the solution when it appears that the vascularity within the pathologic area is nonexistent. Repair should be reserved for young individuals with adequate blood supply to the area in question. Augmentation with a clot should be considered at the time of repair. Allograft meniscal transplantation should be considered in young individuals in whom meniscectomy has been performed. Knee malalignment should also be corrected at the time of surgery.

Neuropathy

Saphenous nerve neuroma after medial meniscal repair should be excised if modalities do not relieve the pain.

Paresthesias in the absence of nerve entrapment should be observed. Motor involvement of the common peroneal nerve should be treated with emergent exploration to prevent permanent damage. We prefer to repair all posterior horn tears with combined open and arthroscopic suturing techniques with direct visualization of the knee capsule and sutures.

Persistent Pain

Pain after meniscectomy can be referred pain from weak quadriceps and HS muscles. It can also be a result of patellofemoral pathology that was unmasked by surgery. Misdiagnosis of patellofemoral symptoms can be a cause of continued pain. Progressive joint degeneration is highly likely with subtotal meniscectomy. Initial treatment should consist of quadriceps and HS strengthening in a supervised rehabilitation program. Surgical consideration should not be discussed until conservative treatments fail and a specific anatomic pathology is identified.

PATELLOFEMORAL SURGERY

The discussion in this section focuses mainly on the complications of patellofemoral surgery for lateral patellar compression syndrome, malalignment, and trauma. More specifically, complications related to lateral releases, proximal and distal realignments, and salvage surgeries are discussed. The reader is referred to other studies for more detailed discussions of patellofemoral pathology (136–138).

Complications of Lateral Release

Merchant and Mercer (139) were the first to discuss the release of the lateral retinaculum to the superior pole of the patella. Small (140) reviewed 10,262 arthroscopic procedures and found 32 complications in 446 lateral retinacular releases for a complication rate of 7.2%. Hemarthrosis accounted for approximately 65% of the complications. This was directly related to tourniquet use, a subcutaneous technique, and the use of a drain for 24 hours. He recommended release of the tourniquet and cauterization of bleeding before closure and perioperative drainage for 2 to 3 hours with removal before discharge.

Other authors have reported quadriceps tendon rupture and weakness, medial patellar subluxation, and patellar hypermobility (141–146) associated with failed lateral retinacular release. Hughston and Deese (143) reported on 60 knees who failed to improve. There was evidence of vastus lateralis atrophy and retraction as shown by computed tomography. They also documented a 50% incidence of medial subluxation on examination. Using kinematic MRI, Shellock et al. (146) showed 60% incidence of medial subluxation in 40 patients with persistent symptoms after lateral release. Isolated lateral release should be avoided in patients with evidence of hypermobile patellae due to the increased risk of postoperative medial and lateral instability (143–146). Proximal realignment should be considered in these situations or a distal realignment if the tubercle sulcus angle is excessive. Kolowich et al. (144) demonstrated that patellar glides of less than two quadrants in the medial and lateral direction, lateral patellar tilt of less than 5 degrees, and a tubercle sulcus angle of less than 5 degrees led to a more predictable and consistent result. They recommended dividing both the retinaculum and the synovium up to but not beyond the level of the vastus lateralis.

Complications of Proximal Realignment

Proximal realignment comprises a lateral release and a medial imbrication. Complications include recurrent instability, medial subluxation, patellar malrotation, and loss of motion (144,147,148). Recurrence rates of between 20% and 25% have been reported (147,149,150). Medial subluxation can result if the medial side is over-tightened in the presence of a hypermobile patella and an incompetent lateral restraint (144,147). Patellar malrotation and increased patellofemoral contact stresses have been reported (147,148). In our institution we place a suture anchor into a bony trough along the superomedial patella to which we pull the medial patellofemoral ligament if it is torn from the patella. We avoid anterior placement of the vastus medialis obliquus to avoid medial patellar tilt. We also avoid advancement below the equator of the patella to avoid malalignment in the medial/lateral plane.

Complications of Combined Proximal and Distal Realignment

Combined proximal and distal realignment procedures are indicated for individuals with a history of patellar subluxation/dislocation and a tubercle sulcus angle greater than 5 degrees (144). Complications include loss of range of motion, premature epiphyseal closure, bony block displacement, neurovascular injury, infrapatellar tendon rupture, medial patellar subluxation, persistent lateral patellar subluxation, patella baja, and accelerated osteoarthritis. An open epiphyses is a contraindication to distal bony realignment procedures. Premature closure can occur, resulting in distal migration of the patellar tendon insertion, recurvatum deformity, external tibial torsion, and proximal axial tibial deformity (147,149,151,152).

Displacement of the bone block usually occurs with attempts at early mobilization without rigid fixation (149,151,153). When recognized, reoperation with internal fixation and bone grafting is recommended. Rupture of the patellar tendon has been described as a complication of the Roux-Goldthwait procedure (147,154). This is thought to be due to scarring of the transferred half of the tendon with a resultant increased force on the remaining tendon. Isolated peroneal nerve palsy has been reported in the literature (155). Because it was reported as an isolated nerve injury, it was thought to be due to direct pressure by an expanding hematoma and not from vascular compromise. The complications occurred only in patients who did not have the tourniquet released before closure. Compartment syndrome has been reported after the Hauser procedure (156,157). Deficits ranged from mild weakness to above knee amputations. Studies revealed that a leash of recurrent anterior tibial vessels were cut, resulting in continued bleeding after retracting into the depth of the wound. The crucial error was failing to consider the possibility of a compartment syndrome.

Overcorrection or undercorrection has also been reported to cause medial subluxation and persistent lateral subluxation (144,158). Correction to achieve a tubercle sulcus angle of 0 degrees helps avoid this complication (144). The Hauser procedure is commonly associated with patella baja and patellofemoral osteoarthritis (147,149,151,152,159,160,161). Patients will usually complain of retropatellar pain, crepitance, and limitation of motion. Physical examination and radiographs will reveal distal displacement of the patella. Infrapatellar contracture syndrome (IPCS) is a complication of patella baja and is discussed in detail later in this chapter. Studies have reported moderate to severe patellofemoral osteoarthrosis in 60% to 70% patients followed (149,161). It has been postulated that the posteromedial bevel of the proximal tibia will result in posterior displacement of the tibial tuberosity, leading to increased patellofemoral contact forces (151,152).

Complications of Salvage Procedures

The Maquet procedure, patellofemoral arthroplasty, and patellectomy are three salvage procedures used in patients with patellofemoral pain and arthrosis.

Maquet (162) is credited for the procedure that anteriorizes the patella to unload the patellofemoral joint. He recommended a minimum of 2 cm of anteriorization to maximize the benefit of the procedure. This amount of displacement, however, gave him a 9.7% complication rate due to skin necrosis. Other authors have similar complications (163–167). Mendes et al. (165) recommended testing the skin for extensibility. Both he and Radin (167,168) recommended avoiding the procedure in patients with multiple scars near the operative site. They also reported using tissue expanders and multiple relaxing incisions to relieve tension. Ferguson et al. (164) recommended avoiding elevation beyond 1.5 cm because they had no evidence of added benefit. Graft displacement, osteotomy displacement, and nonunion have also been reported in the literature (163–165). Some authors have recommended avoidance of hardware fixation to prevent wound complications. Wedging the graft has caused reports of tuberosity fracture and displacement. Radin and Labosky (167) recommended wedging the graft well proximal of the attached end of the tubercle. Graft displacement can be avoided by careful attention to fitting the graft and placing the knee through a full range of motion. We prefer to use 6.5-mm cancellous Aesculaps screws with a flat head to avoid prominence. Scar tenderness over the donor site has been reported as high as 24% by Mendes (165).

Patellofemoral arthroplasty is not a popular option for the treatment of patellofemoral pathology due to its unpredictable results (169,170). Arciero and Toomey (171) reported that tibiofemoral osteoarthritis, persistent patellofemoral malalignment, and component malposition were associated with unsatisfactory outcomes in their series. Cartier et al. (172) reported 50% of their complications due to component malposition. Blazina et al. (169) reported 101 secondary procedures out of 85 patellofemoral replacements. These were due to lateral subluxation, prosthesis toggling, patellar clunking, component malposition, and loss of motion. Insall et al. (170) reported a 45% failure rate in 28 patients secondary to persistent pain.

Patellectomy is indicated for intractable pain from chondromalacia patella and severely comminuted patellar fractures (173–175). The most commonly reported complication is quadriceps weakness with an extensor lag (176–178). Lennox et al. (176) reported a 60% loss of strength when they compared strength with the contralateral unoperated side. A decrease in quadriceps efficiency of as much as 30% was reported by Kaufer (179). This was most noted in the terminal 60 degrees of extension. Rupture of the extensor mechanism has been attributed to the increased force requirement on these patients.

It has also been postulated that this decrease in efficiency makes it difficult to support the loaded limb in the stance phase of gait (177). An increase in tibiofemoral compressive forces due to altered forces has also been reported (178,180). Evidence of tricompartmental knee osteoarthritis is, therefore, regarded as a relative contraindication to patellectomy. Subluxation of the quadriceps mechanism has also been described after patellectomy (181,182). Careful attention should be paid at the time of the operation so that the quadriceps mechanism and medial and lateral retinaculum are properly balanced. Calcification of the quadriceps tendon can inter-

fere with the postoperative rehabilitation after patellectomy. Compere et al. (175) described a technique of tubing the tendon to limit the calcification and protect the patellofemoral articulation. Results of total knee arthroplasty after patellectomy have been unsatisfactory. This is due mainly to instability and weak extensor mechanism (183). Those authors also reported an increased incidence of component failure as well. Buechel (184) reported using a 2.5 by 1-cm bone graft in the anatomic location of the patella, resulting in increased function for his patients.

Common Complication and Authors' Preferred Treatment

Hemarthrosis

This complication is a common cause of residual stiffness after knee arthroscopy. We perform our lateral release under tactile guidance. We then reinsert the arthroscope with the tourniquet deflated and cauterize the superior and inferior lateral geniculate vessels. We then insert a drain that is removed after 24 hours. We have also started using a pain pump that delivers a constant amount of local anesthetic to reduce the immediate postoperative pain.

Over/Undercorrection

This complication is related more to accurate diagnosis than to intraoperative complications. Overcorrection in a lateral release occurs from a release that extends into the muscle belly, causing a weakened lateral quadriceps and medial subluxation. Initial treatment should consist of quadriceps strengthening. Lateral retinacular reconstruction with the use of fascia lata allograft has been used in our institution in recalcitrant cases.

Undercorrection usually occurs in isolated lateral release and/or proximal realignment. This usually occurs from a missed diagnosis of increased tibial tubercle–femoral sulcus angle. Treatment will invariably be distal realignment consisting of a tubercle osteotomy.

Patella Baja

This complication can have idiopathic or iatrogenic etiology. Idiopathic causes usually occur from fibrosis of the infrapatellar fat pad. Iatrogenic etiology usually occur from performance of a Maquet osteotomy in the face of a low lying patella (Fig. 46.10). Initial treatment should consist of patellar mobilization, anti-inflammatory medications, and quadriceps strengthening. Surgical treatment includes infrapatellar fat pad debridement with placement of a retropatellar tendon gortex graft and proximal tibial tubercle osteotomy.

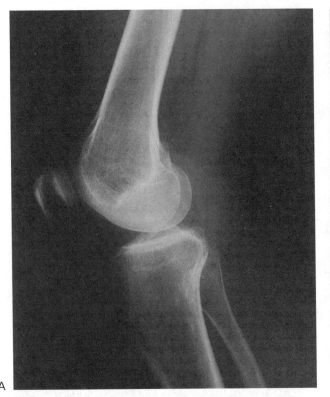

A

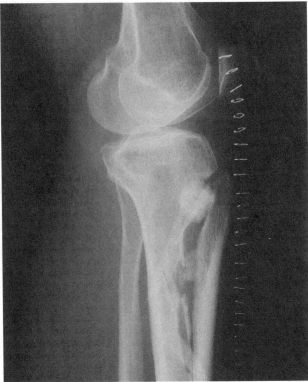

B

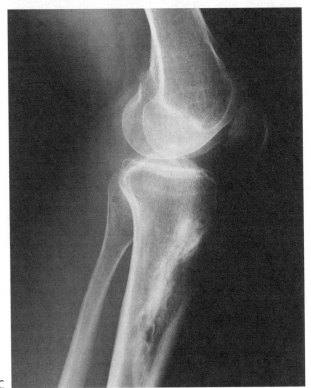

C

FIG. 46.10. A: Lateral radiograph of left knee before Maquet osteotomy. **B:** Immediate postoperative lateral radiograph of the same patient after a Maquet osteotomy. **C:** Nine months postoperatively of the same patient after presenting to our office with patella infera and severe knee pain and weakness.

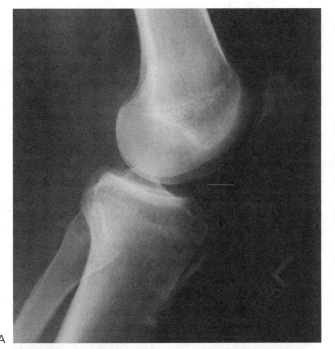

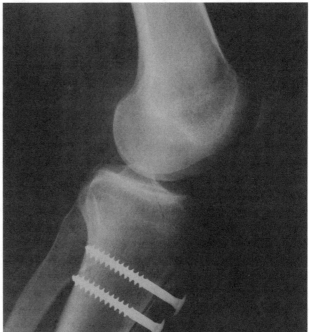

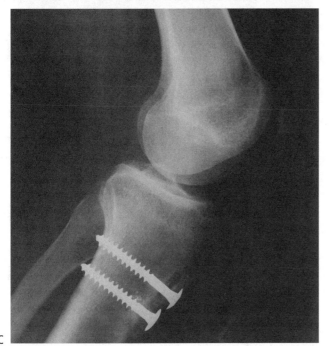

FIG. 46.11. A: Lateral radiograph of the left knee of a patient who presented to our office complaining of persistent tibial tubercle pain 2 years after tibial tubercle osteotomy, internal fixation, bone grafting, and hardware removal. **B:** Lateral radiograph of same patient 7 months after revision tibial tubercle osteotomy and internal fixation. The patient complains of persistent pain and weakness in the knee. **C:** The same patient 2 months after revision osteotomy and iliac crest bone grafting. He had complete resolution of pain.

Nonunion

Although uncommon, there is a high risk of this complication in distal realignment surgery (Fig. 46.11). At the time of the initial realignment, we are attentive in attaining rigid fixation in the osteotomy site. We will pack cancellous bone graft in the defect created from the realignment. We treat nonunions with extensive debridement of the osteotomy site and autogenous iliac crest bone grafting.

PATELLAR ENTRAPMENT

PES is a major cause of reduced range of motion after knee surgery. PES is defined as a loss of knee extension of at least 10 degrees or at least 25-degree loss of knee flexion with significantly reduced patellar mobility associated with peripatellar surgery (185). Isolated IPCS is a subset of PES. It is associated with reduced patellar mobility secondary to contracture of the infrapatellar tissues as demonstrated by reduced superior patellar glide with the knee in maximum extension (186). Paulos et al. (187) in 1987 published the results of 28 consecutive patients with IPCS. They divided the etiology as primary or secondary. They postulated that the primary cause was due to "exaggerated pathologic fibrous hyperplasia" of the anterior knee structures. Secondary causes included nonisometric graft placement, prolonged immobilization, and quadriceps weakness. ACL reconstruction is commonly associated with IPCS and arthrofibrosis (186–191). Reflex sympathetic dystrophy is differentiated from PES by the quality and degree of pain and by the presence of autonomic symptoms. Skin changes are also seen in reflex sympathetic dystrophy but not PES.

Three stages have been described to classify IPCS (186,187). Stage I is the prodromal stage. Patients usually present with periarticular swelling and inflammation. They have failed to progress in rehabilitation with a significant inability to gain extension. Examination will reveal periarticular edema, particularly near the patellar tendon and fat pad. Painful and tender active range of motion is present. A quadriceps lag (i.e., passive range of motion greater than active range of motion) is apparent. Patellar tilt and patellar glide are decreased. Although most patients present within 2 to 8 weeks from the index procedure, patients can present with this stage months after the initial surgery.

Stage II is the active stage. These are usually patients who had unrecognized prodromal symptoms. Patients present with decreased patellar mobility. Secondary procedures such as manipulations and arthroscopic lysis of adhesions have been performed before this stage. The "shelf sign" is usually present at this time (Fig. 46.12). This sign appears when induration in the anterior tissues extends to the distal attachment of the patellar tendon and creates and abrupt step-off or "shelf" from the patellar tendon to the tibial tubercle. Patellar mobility is decreased in all directions with a zero or negative patellar tilt test. Quadriceps lag is no longer present secondary to restrictions in active and passive flexion and extension. There is patellofemoral crepitation with significant quadriceps atrophy. The patient will demonstrate a bent knee or "short leg" gait.

Stage III is the residual or "burned out" stage. There is continued quadriceps atrophy. Peripatellar and retinacular tissues demonstrate increased suppleness. Patellar mobility is still decreased but not as severely as in stage II. Residual patella infera and patellofemoral arthrosis may be the only symptoms present. The diagnosis of patella infera requires the use of lateral knee radiographs. The inferior pole of the patella should lie at the roof of the intercondylar notch (Blumensaat's line) on a 30-degree flexion lateral radiograph. Numerous methods have been described to quantify the degree of patellar tendon contraction. The principle has been to determine the ratio of the patellar articular surface to the length of the patellar tendon (192–194). We prefer to use the method described by Blackburne and Peel (192) because it shows the least amount of variability. This ratio is obtained by comparing the distance from the distal pole of the patellar articular cartilage with a perpendicular line drawn at the level of the tibial plateau and the length of the patellar articular surface (TA). Patella infera is considered when the ratio is less than 0.54.

Prevention is the key to the approach to PES and IPCS. Fu et al. (195) presented data that demonstrated poorer outcome and increased incidence of patella infera predominantly in male and older patients. Numerous studies have also documented that surgery in the acutely injured knee predisposes the patient to

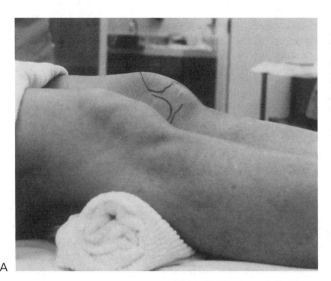
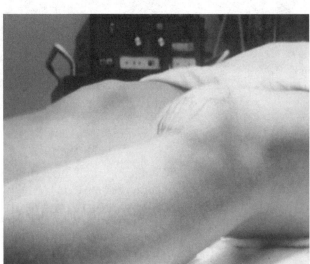

A   B

FIG. 46.12. A and B: Two cases of shelf sign of left knee.

arthrofibrosis (189–191,196). Paulos et al. (186) found that 10 of 12 (83%) patients with poor outcomes had surgery during the acute stage of injury. Fifteen of 19 (79%) patients diagnosed with patella infera were also operated on during the acute phase of injury. They stated that in their series "it is apparent that index surgery performed acutely may lead to a more refractory type of IPCS." They stated, however, that it is more prudent to wait for inflammation to subside and for the patient's range of motion to return rather than arbitrarily designate a period of time at which it is safe to operate. Associated ligamentous injuries have also been implicated as contributing to postoperative knee stiffness (196). Other studies (186,189), however, have not been able to demonstrate this association with any significance. The type of ACL graft has also been mentioned as contributing to arthrofibrosis after reconstructive procedures. Numerous reports have implicated the use of central third patellar tendon autograft as a risk to development of arthrofibrosis (186,188,197–199). Paulos et al. (186) showed that 17 of 19 patients who were diagnosed with patella infera had central third patellar tendon autografts. Firm conclusions could not be made, however, because most of their patients were referred from outside institutions.

Authors' Preferred Treatment Approach

Treatment of PES and IPCS is dependent on early recognition (186,187). If the patient shows no progress despite early range of motion and patellar mobilization, a trial of nonsteroidal anti-inflammatory drugs, corticosteroid dose packs, and transcutaneous electrical nerve stimulation units should be given. Forceful manipulation of the knee should be avoided, but range of motion should be maintained with a leg press program and low-impact exercises such as swimming and cycling. Regaining an active quadriceps contraction is mandatory before any surgical considerations. Extension boards may be used briefly during the course of treatment but should be discontinued until after surgery if ineffective. Patients that progress to stage II often require surgery. Continued manipulation and forceful physical therapy may only worsen the symptoms. Our surgical protocol (186) requires an open arthrotomy to achieve lateral or medial retinacular release and debridement of all adhesions, including medial and suprapatellar plicae and scarified fat pad. All fibrotic tissue between the inferior pole of the patella and anterior tibia should be resected. The patellar tendon should be released from the anterior tibia but not from the tibial tubercle. In addition, an interposition Gortex graft is usually sutured to the posterior patellar ligament to prevent recurrent adhesion. The retropatellar tendon bursa should be released.

If an ACL reconstruction has been performed, graft placement and impingement should be checked. An anterior tibial tunnel placement will result in graft impingement in the intercondylar notch. Howell et al. (200) demonstrated that tibial tunnels placed 5 mm anteromedial from the center of the ACL footprint will require an additional 5- to 6-mm resection of bone from the intercondylar roof compared with 2- to 3-mm resection when the tunnel is placed within the center. A nonisometric and overtensioned graft may require lengthening or removal. Revision of the notchplasty should be performed as necessary. If patella infera of 8 mm or more is present, a proximal displacement tibial tubercle osteotomy should be performed. Normal patellar mobility must be achieved along with a patellar tilt of 45 degrees.

For patients who have progressed to stage III, the options are limited. Surgical debridement requires both intraarticular and extraarticular debridement as previously described. If advanced patellofemoral arthrosis is present, however, debridement and release by themselves will not be enough. Consideration should be given to proximal displacement osteotomy, Maquet osteotomy, patellectomy, and even total knee arthroplasty.

Postoperatively, continuous passive motion machines and night extension splints should be instituted immediately. Drains should be left in place for 24 to 48 hours. Daily physical therapy with judicious use of transcutaneous electrical nerve stimulation units should be ordered. An epidural analgesic should be used for pain control whenever possible. Oral steroids should be avoided until complete wound healing has occurred. It is paramount that extension is gained immediately even if flexion is sacrificed. Extension contractures can be successfully treated with manipulation or arthroscopic lysis of adhesions. According to Paulos et al. (186), they obtained extension gains of 14 degrees and flexion gains of 33 degrees with this protocol. Mean patellar tilt increase was 6 degrees and patellar glide increased by one quadrant. Lysholm scores averaged 72.2 of 100. At final follow-up, the mean Tegner score was 4.3 as compared with preinjury Tegner scores of 6. Despite the lack of significant improvements demonstrated by the activity scores, 85% of the respondents would repeat their original decision in favor of the index surgery.

There has been increased awareness of PES (and IPCS) since the publication of the study by Paulos et al. (187). Prevention and early recognition is the key to a successful outcome. Once diagnosed, forceful manipulation should be avoided and judicious use of anti-inflammatories should be instituted. Voluntary quadriceps contraction is mandatory, and reestablishment of extension is paramount. Surgery should include extensive open intraarticular and extraarticular debridement. Salvage procedures should be reserved for those with advanced patellofemoral arthrosis.

REFERENCES

1. Miyasaka KC, Daniel DM, Stone ML. The incidence of knee ligament injuries in the general population. *Am J Knee Surg* 1991;3:43–48.
2. Cooper DE, Deng XH, Burnstein AL, et al. The strength of the central third patellar tendon graft: a biomechanical study. *Am J Sports Med* 1991;21:818–824.
3. Noyes FR, Butler DL, Grood ES, et al. Biomechanical analysis of human ligament grafts used in knee ligament repairs and reconstructions. *J Bone Joint Surg Am* 1986;66(A):348–360.
4. Woo SLY, Hollis JM, Adams DJ, et al. Tensile properties of the human femur anterior cruciate ligament tibia complex. The effects of specimen age and orientation. *Am J Sports Med* 1991; 19:217–225.
5. McKernan DJ, Wiss JA, Deffner KT, et al. Tensile properties of gracilis, semitendinosus and patellar tendons from the same donor. *Trans Orthop Res Soc* 1995;20:39–37.
6. Brown CH, Steiner ME. Anterior cruciate ligament Injuries. In: Siliski JM, ed. *Traumatic disorders of the knee.* New York: Springer-Verlag, 1994.
7. Rodeo SA, Arnoczky SP, Torzilli PA, et al. Tendon healing in a bone tunnel. A biomechanical and histological study in the dog. *J Bone Joint Surg Am* 1993;75(A):1795–1803.
8. Kohn D, Rose C. Primary stability of interference screw fixation. Influence of screw diameter and insertion torque. *Am J Sports Med* 1994;22:334–338.
9. Johnson LL. The outcome of a free autogenous semitendinosus tendon graft in human anterior cruciate ligament reconstruction surgery. A histological study. *Arthroscopy* 1993;9:131–142.
10. Rubenstein RA Jr, Shelbourne KD, VanMeter CD, et al. Isolated autogenous bone-patellar tendon-bone graft site morbidity. *Am J Sports Med* 1994;22:324–327.
11. Clancy WG Jr, Nelson DA, Reider B, et al. Anterior cruciate ligament reconstruction using one third of the patellar ligament, augmented by extra-articular tendon transfers. *J Bone Joint Surg Am* 1982;64(A):352–359.
12. Johnson RJ, Eriksson E, Haggmark T, et al. Five to ten year follow-up evaluation after reconstruction of the anterior cruciate ligament. *Clin Orthop* 1994;183:122–140.
13. O'Brien SJ, Warren RF, Pavlov H, et al. Reconstruction of the chronically insufficient anterior cruciate ligament with the central third of the patellar ligament. *J Bone Joint Surg Am* 1991;73(A): 278–286.
14. Sachs RA, Daniel DM, Stone ML, et al. Patellofemoral problems after anterior cruciate ligament reconstruction. *Am J Sports Med* 1989;17:760–765.
15. Engebretsen L, Benum P, Fasting O, et al. A prospective, randomized study of three surgical techniques for treatment of acute ruptures of the anterior cruciate ligament. *Am J Sports Med* 1990;18:585–590.
16. Marder RA, Raskind JR, Carroll M. Prospective evaluation of arthroscopically assisted anterior cruciate ligament reconstruction. Patellar tendon versus semitendinosus and gracilis tendons. *Am J Sports Med* 1991;19:478–484.
17. Bonamo J, Krinick RM, Sporn AA. Rupture of the patellar ligament after use of its central third for anterior cruciate reconstruction. *J Bone Joint Surg Am* 1984;66(A):194–1297.
18. DeLee JC, Craviotto DF. Rupture of the quadriceps tendon after a central third patellar tendon anterior cruciate ligament reconstruction. *Am J Sports Med* 1991;10:415–416.
19. Marumoto JM, Mitsunaga MM, Richardson AB, et al. Late patellar tendon ruptures after removal of the central third for anterior cruciate ligament reconstruction. A report of two cases. *Am J Sports Med* 1996;24:698–701.
20. Hardin GT, Bach BR. Distal rupture of the infrapatellar tendon after use of its central third for anterior cruciate ligament reconstruction. Case report. *Am J Knee Surg* 1992;5:140–143.
21. Christen B, Jakob RP. Fractures associated with patellar ligament grafts in cruciate ligament surgery. *J Bone Joint Surg Br* 1992;74(B):617–619.
22. Simonian PT, Mann FA, Mandt PR. Indirect forces and patella fracture after anterior cruciate ligament reconstruction with the patellar ligament. Case report. *Am J Knee Surg* 1995;8:60–64.
23. Tria AJ Jr, Alicea JA, Cody RP. Patella baja in anterior cruciate ligament reconstruction of the knee. *Clin Orthop* 1994;299: 229–234.
24. Dandy DJ, Desai SS. Patellar tendon length after anterior cruciate ligament reconstruction. *J Bone Joint Surg Br* 1994;76(B): 198–199.
25. Noyes FR, Barber-Westin SD. Reconstruction of the anterior cruciate ligament with human allograft. Comparison of early and later result. *J Bone Joint Surg Am* 1996;78(A):524–537.
26. Noyes FR, Barber-Westin SD, Roberts CS. Use of allograft after failed treatment of rupture of the anterior cruciate ligament. *J Bone Joint Surg Am* 1994;76(A):1019–1031.
27. Safran MR, Harner CD. Revision ACL surgery: techniques and results utilizing allografts. *Instruct Course Lect* 1995;44:407–415.
28. Bullis DW, Paulos LE. Reconstruction of the posterior cruciate ligament with allograft. *Clin Sports Med* 1994;13:581–597.
29. Indelicato PA, Bittar ES, Prevot TJ, et al. Clinical comparison of freeze-dried and fresh frozen patellar tendon allografts for anterior cruciate ligament reconstruction of the knee. *Am J Sports Med* 1990;18:335–342.
30. Shino K, Inoue M, Nakamura H, et al. Arthroscopic follow-up of anterior cruciate ligament reconstruction using allogeneic tendon. *Arthroscopy* 1989;5:165–171.
31. Meyers JF, Caspari RB, Cash JD, et al. Arthroscopic evaluation of allograft anterior cruciate ligament reconstruction. *Arthroscopy* 1992;8:157–161.
32. Shelton WR, Papendick L, Dukes AD. Autograft versus allograft anterior cruciate ligament reconstruction. *Arthroscopy* 1997;13: 446–449.
33. Victor J, Bellemans J, Witvrouw E, et al. Graft selection in anterior cruciate ligament reconstruction-prospective analysis of patellar tendon autografts compared with allografts. *Int Orthop* 1997;21:93–97.
34. Horstman JK, Ahmadu-Suka F, Norrdin RW. Anterior cruciate ligament fascia lata allograft reconstruction: Progressive histologic changes toward maturity. *Arthroscopy* 1993;9:509–518.
35. Indelicato PA, Linton RC, Huegel M. The results of fresh frozen patellar tendon allografts for chronic anterior cruciate ligament deficiency of the knee. *Am J Sports Med* 1992;20:118–121.
36. Wainer RA, Clarke TJ, Poehling GG. Arthroscopic reconstruction of the anterior cruciate ligament using allograft tendon. *Arthroscopy* 1988;4:199–205.
37. Malek MM, DeLuca JV. Freeze dried achilles tendon allograft in anterior cruciate ligament reconstruction: two and five year follow-up comparison. Presented at AAOS 60th Annual Meeting, San Francisco, 1993.
38. Roberts TS, Drez D Jr, McCarthy W, et al. Anterior cruciate ligament reconstruction using freeze dried, ethylene oxide sterilized, bone-patellar tendon-bone allografts. Two year results in thirty-six patients. *Am J Sports Med* 1991;19:35–41.
39. Jackson DW, Windler GE, Simon TM. Intraarticular reaction associated with the use of freeze dried, ethylene oxide sterilized bone-patellar tendon-bone allografts in the reconstruction of the anterior cruciate ligament. *Am J Sports Med* 1990;18:1–10.
40. Simonds RJ, Holmberg SD, Hurwitz RL, et al. Transmission of human immunodeficiency virus type 1 from a seronegative organ and tissue donor. *N Engl J Med* 1992;326:726–732.
41. Centers for Disease Control. Transmission of HIV through bone transplantation: case report and public health recommendations. *MMWR Morb Mortal Wkly Rep* 1988;37:597–599.
42. Shutkin NM. Homologous serum hepatitis following the use of refrigerated bone-bank bone. *J Bone Joint Surg Am* 1954;36(A): 160–162.
43. Eggen BM, Nordbo SA. Transmission of HCV by organ transplantation [letter]. *N Engl J Med* 1992;326:411.
44. Pereira BJ, Milford EL, Kirkman RL, et al. Transmission of hepatitis C virus by organ transplantation. *N Engl J Med* 1991; 325:454–460.
45. Pereira BJ, Milford EL, Kirkman RL, et al. Low risk of liver disease after tissue transplantation from donors with HCV [letter]. *Lancet* 1993;341:903–904.
46. Conrad EU, Gretch DR, Obermeyer KR, et al. Transmission of the hepatitis C virus by tissue transplantation. *J Bone Joint Surg Am* 1995;77(A):214–224.

47. Levitt RL, Malinin T. Allograft reconstruction of the anterior cruciate ligament—a six year experience with 300 allografts [abstract]. *Arthroscopy* 1991;7:318–319.

48. Gibbons MJ, Butler DL, Grood ES, et al. Effects of gamma irradiation on the initial mechanical and material properties of goat bone-patellar tendon-bone allografts. *J Orthop Res* 1991;9:209–218.

49. De Deyne P, Haut RC. Some effects of gamma irradiation on patellar tendon allografts. *Connect Tissue Res* 1991;27:51–62.

50. Fideler BM, Vangsness CT Jr, Lu B, et al. Gamma irradiation: effects on biomechanical properties of human bone-patellar tendon-bone allografts. *Am J Sports Med* 1995;23:643–646.

51. Van Winkle W Jr, Borick PM, Fogarty M. Destruction of radiation resistant microorganisms on surgical sutures by ⁶⁰Co irradiation under manufacturing conditions. In radiosterilization of medical products. Proceedings of a symposium, Budapest, June 1967 and Recommended Code of Practice, Vienna, International Atomic Energy Agency, 169–180, 1967.

52. Jackson DW. Use of allografts for anterior cruciate ligament reconstruction. *Am Acad Orthop Surg Bull* 1992;40:10–11.

53. Fideler BM, Vangsness CT Jr, Moore T, et al. Effects of gamma irradiation on the human immunodeficiency virus. A study in frozen human bone-patellar tendon-bone grafts obtained from infected cadavera. *J Bone Joint Surg Am* 1994;76(A):1032–1035.

54. Jauregito JW, Paulos LE. Why grafts fail. *Clin Orthop* 1996; 325:25–41.

55. Good L, Odensten M, Gillquist J. Sagittal knee stability after anterior cruciate ligament reconstruction with a patellar tendon strip: a two year follow-up study. *Am J Sports Med* 1994;22: 518–523.

56. Hefzy MS, Grood ES, Noyes FR. Factors affecting the region of most isometric femoral attachments. Part II. The anterior cruciate ligament. *Am J Sports Med* 1989;17:208–216.

57. Sidles JA, Larson RV, Garbini JL, et al. Ligament length relationships in the moving knee. *J Orthop Res* 1988;6:593–610.

58. O'Brien WR. Isometric placement of anterior cruciate ligament substitutes. *Op Tech Orthop* 1992;2:49–54.

59. Melhorn JM, Henning CE. The relationship of the femoral attachment site to the isometric tracking of the anterior cruciate ligament graft. *Am J Sports Med* 1987;15:539–542.

60. Muneta T, Yamamoto H, Sakai H, et al. Relationship between changes in length and force in vitro reconstructed anterior cruciate ligament. *Am J Sports Med* 1993;21:299–304.

61. Good L, Gillquist J. The value of intraoperative isometry measurements in anterior cruciate ligament reconstruction: an in vivo correlation between substitute tension and length change. *J Arthrosc Rel Surg* 1993;9:525–532.

62. Colville MR, Bowman RR. The significance of isometer measurements and graft position during anterior cruciate ligament reconstruction. *Am J Sports Med* 1993;21:832–835.

63. Brand MG, Daniel DM. Considerations in the placement of intraarticular anterior cruciate ligament graft. *Op Tech Orthop* 1992;2:55–62.

64. Acker JH, Drez D. Analysis of isometric placement of grafts in ACL reconstruction procedures. *Am J Knee Surg* 1989;2:65–70.

65. Howell SM. Arthroscopically assisted technique for preventing roof impingement of an anterior cruciate ligament graft illustrated by the use of an autogenous double looped semitendinosus and gracilis graft. *Op Tech Sports Med* 1993;1:58–65.

66. Howell SM, Barad SJ. Knee extension and its relationship to the slope of the intercondylar roof. Implications for positioning the tibial tunnel in anterior cruciate ligament reconstructions. *Am J Sports Med* 1995;23:288–294.

67. Howell SM, Clark JA. Tibial tunnel placement in anterior cruciate ligament reconstructions and graft impingement. *Clin Orthop* 1992;283:187–195.

68. Howell SM, Clark JA, Farley TE. Serial magnetic resonance study assessing the effects of impingement on the MR image of the patellar tendon graft. *Arthroscopy* 1992;8:350–358.

69. Howell SM, Taylor MA. Failure of reconstruction of the anterior cruciate ligament due to impingement by the intercondylar roof. *J Bone Joint Surg Am* 1993;75(A):1044–1055.

70. Muneta T, Yamamoto H, Ishibashi T, et al. The effects of tibial tunnel placement and roofplasty on reconstructed anterior cruciate ligament knees. *Arthroscopy* 1995;11:57–62.

71. Tanzer M, Lenczner E. The relationship of intercondylar notch size and content to notchplasty requirement in anterior cruciate ligament surgery. *Arthroscopy* 1990;6:89–93.

72. Goble EM, Downey DJ, Wilcox TR. Positioning of the tibial tunnel for anterior cruciate ligament reconstruction. *Arthroscopy* 1995;11:688–695.

73. Miller MD, Olszewski AD. Posterior tibial tunnel placement to avoid anterior cruciate ligament graft impingement by the intercondylar roof. An in vitro and in vivo study. *Am J Sports Med* 1997;25:818–822.

74. McGuire DA, Hendricks SD, Sanders HM. The relationship between anterior cruciate ligament reconstruction tibial tunnel location and the anterior aspect of the posterior cruciate ligament insertion. *Arthroscopy* 1997;13:465–473.

75. Yaru NC, Daniel DM, Penner D. The effect of tibial attachment site on graft impingement in an anterior cruciate ligament reconstruction. *Am J Sports Med* 1922;20:217–220.

76. Romano VM, Graf BK, Keene JS, et al. Anterior cruciate ligament reconstruction. The effect of tibial tunnel placement on range of motion. *Am J Sports Med* 1993;21:415–418.

77. Morgan CD, Kalman VR, Grawl DM. Definitive landmarks for reproducible tibial tunnel placement in anterior cruciate ligament reconstruction. *Arthroscopy* 1995;11:275–288.

78. Girgis FG, Marshall JL, Al Monajem ARS. The cruciate ligaments of the knee joint: Anatomical function and experimental analysis. *Clin Orthop* 1975;106:216–231.

79. Odensten M, Gillquist J. Functional anatomy of the anterior cruciate ligament and a rationale for reconstruction. *J Bone Joint Surg Am* 1985;67(A):257–262.

80. Barrett GR, Treacy SH. The effect of intraoperative isometric measurement on the outcome of anterior cruciate ligament reconstruction: a clinical analysis. *Arthroscopy* 1996;12:645–651.

81. Sapega AA, Moyer RA, Schneck C, et al. Testing for ismetry during reconstruction of the anterior cruciate ligament: anatomical and biomechanical considerations. *J Bone Joint Surg Am* 1990;72(A):259–267.

82. Harner CD, Paulos LE, Greenwald AE, et al. Detailed analysis of patients with bilateral anterior cruciate ligament injuries. *Am J Sports Med* 1994;22:37–43.

83. Houseworth SW, Mauro VJ, Mellon BA, et al. The intercondylar notch in acute tears of the anterior cruciate ligament: a computer graphics study. *Am J Sports Med* 1987;15:221–224.

84. Souryal TO, Moore HA, Evans JP. Bilaterality in anterior cruciate ligament injuries. *Am J Sports Med* 1988;16:449–454.

85. Howell SM. Arthroscopic roofplasty: a method for correcting an extension deficit caused by roof impingement of an anterior cruciate ligament graft. *Arthroscopy* 1992;8:375–379.

86. Good L, Odensten M, Gillquist J. Intercondylar notch measurement with special reference to anterior cruciate ligament surgery. *Clin Orthop* 1991;263:185–189.

87. Jackson DW, Schaefer RK. Cyclops syndrome: loss of extension following intraarticular anterior cruciate ligament reconstruction. *Arthroscopy* 1990;6:171–178.

88. Marzo JM, Bowen MK, Warren RF, et al. Intraarticular fibrous nodule as a cause of loss of extension following anterior cruciate ligament reconstruction. *Arthroscopy* 1992;8:10–18.

89. Watanabe BM, Howell SM. Arthroscopic findings associated with roof impingement of an anterior cruciate ligament graft. *Am J Sports Med* 1995;23:616–625.

90. Recht MP, Piraino DW, Cohen MA, et al. Localized anterior arthrofibrosis (cyclops lesion) after reconstruction of the anterior cruciate ligament: MR imaging findings. *AJR Am J Roentgenol* 1995;165:383–385.

91. King D. The healing of semilunar cartilages. *J Bone Joint Surg Am* 1936;18(A):333–342.

92. Fairbank TJ. Knee joint changes after meniscectomy. *J Bone Joint Surg Br* 1948;30(B):664–670.

93. Arnoczky SP, Warren RF. Microvasculature of the human meniscus. *Am J Sports Med* 1982;10:90–95.

94. Arnoczky SP, Warren RF. The microvasculature of the meniscus and its response to injury, An experimental study in the dog. *Am J Sports Med* 1983;11:131–141.

95. Small NC. Complications in arthroscopic surgery performed by experienced arthroscopists. *Arthroscopy* 1988;4:215–221.

96. Austin KS, Sherman OH. Complications of arthroscopic meniscal repair. *Am J Sports Med* 1993;21:864–868.

97. Eggli S, Wegmuller H, Kosina J, et al. Long term results of arthroscopic meniscal repairs. An analysis of isolated tears. *Am J Sports Med* 1995;23:715–720.

98. DeHaven KE, Lohrer WA, Lovelock JE. Long term results of open meniscal repair. *Am J Sports Med* 1995;23:524–530.

99. Horibe S, Shino K, Maeda A, et al. Results of meniscal repair evaluated by second-look arthroscopy. *Arthroscopy* 1996;12: 150–155.

100. Jensen NC, Riis J, Robertsen K, et al. Arthroscopic repair of the ruptured meniscus: one to 6.3 year follow-up. *Arthroscopy* 1994;10:211–214.

101. Barber FA. Meniscus repair. Results of an arthroscopic technique. *Arthroscopy* 1987;3:25–30.

102. Cannon WD Jr, Vittori JM. The incidence of healing in arthroscopic meniscal repairs in anterior cruciate ligament reconstructed knees versus stable knees. *Am J Sports Med* 1992;20:176–181.

103. Stone RG, Frewin PR, Gonzales S. Long term assessment of arthroscopic meniscus repair. A 2 to 6 year follow-up study. *Arthroscopy* 1990;6:73–78.

104. Rosenberg TD, Scott SM, Coward DB, et al. Arthroscopic meniscal repair evaluated with repeat arthroscopy. *Arthroscopy* 1986; 2:14–20.

105. Hamberg P, Gillquist J, Lysholm J. Suture of new and old peripheral meniscus tears. *J Bone Joint Surg Am* 1983;65(A):193–197.

106. Ryu RK, Dunbar WH. Arthroscopic meniscal repair with two year follow-up. *Arthroscopy* 1988;4:168–173.

107. Austin KS, Sherman OH. Complications of arthroscopic meniscal repair. *Am J Sports Med* 1993;21:864–868.

108. Rokito AS, Kvitne RS, Lee MR, et al. Long term results following meniscal repair. Book of Abstracts and Outline. Presented at Specialty Day, American Orthopaedic Society for Sports Medicine, Orlando, Florida, 1995:45–46.

109. Stone RG, Miller GA. A technique of arthroscopic suture of torn menisci. *Arthroscopy* 1985;1:226–232.

110. Morgan CK, Casscells SW. Arthroscopic meniscus repair. A safe approach to the posterior horns. *Arthroscopy* 1986;2:3–12.

111. Jurist KA, Green PW III, Shirkoda A. Peroneal nerve dysfunction as a complication of lateral meniscal repair. A case report and dissection. *Arthroscopy* 1989;5:141–147.

112. Miller DB. Arthroscopic meniscus repair. *Am J Sports Med* 1988;16:315–320.

113. Myerthall S, Ogilvie-Harris DJ. Failure of arthroscopic meniscal repair following septic arthritis. *Arthroscopy* 1996;6:746–748.

114. Dandy DJ, Jackson RW. The diagnosis of problems after meniscectomy. *J Bone Joint Surg Br* 1975;57(B):349–352.

115. Jackson JP. Degenerative changes in the knee after meniscectomy. *Br Med J* 1968;2:525–527.

116. Johnson RJ, Kettlekamp DB, Clark W, et al. Factors affecting late results after meniscectomy. *J Bone Joint Surg Am* 1974; 56(A):719–729.

117. Tapper EM, Hoover NW. Late results after meniscectomy. *J Bone Joint Surg Am* 1969;51(A):517–526.

118. Friedman MJ, Brna JA, Gallick GS, et al. Failed arthroscopic meniscectomy: prognostic factors for repeat arthroscopic examination. *Arthroscopy* 1987;3:99–105.

119. Fauno P, Nielsen AB. Arthroscopic partial meniscectomy: a long term follow-up. *Arthroscopy* 1992;8:345–349.

120. Ferkel RD, Davis JR, Friedman MJ, et al. Arthroscopic partial medial meniscectomy: an analysis of unsatisfactory results. *Arthroscopy* 1985;1:44–52.

121. Santori N, Condello V, Adriani E, et al. Osteonecrosis after arthroscopic medial meniscectomy. *Arthroscopy* 1995;11:220–224.

122. Muscolo DL, Costa-Paz M, Makino A, et al. Osteonecrosis of the knee following arthroscopic meniscectomy in patients over 50 years old. *Arthroscopy* 1996;12:273–279.

123. Rozbruch SR, Wickiewicz TL, DiCarlo EF, et al. Osteonecrosis of the knee following arthroscopic laser meniscectomy. *Arthroscopy* 1996;12:245–250.

124. Janzen DL, Kosarek FJ, Helms CA, et al. Osteonecrosis after contact neodymium:yttrium aluminum garnet arthroscopic laser meniscectomy. *AJR Am J Roentgenol* 1997;169:855–858.

125. Thal R, Danziger MB, Kelly A. Delayed articular cartilage slough: two cases resulting from holmium: YAG laser damage to normal articular cartilage and a review of the literature. *Arthroscopy* 1996;12:92–94.

126. Dillingham MF, Price JM, Fanton GS. Holmium laser surgery. *Orthopedics* 1993;16:551–555.

127. Potter D, Morris-Jones W. Popliteal artery injury complicating arthroscopic meniscectomy. *Arthroscopy* 1995;11:723–726.

128. Jimenez F, Utrilla A, Cuesta C, et al. Popliteal artery and venous aneurysm as a complication of arthroscopic meniscectomy. *J Trauma* 1988;28:1404–1405.

129. Guermazi A, Zagdanski AM, de Kerviler E, et al. Popliteal artery pseudoaneurysm revealed by deep vein thrombosis after arthroscopic meniscectomy. *Eur Radiol* 1996;6:217–219.

130. Vincent GM, Stanish WD. False aneurysm after arthroscopic meniscectomy. A report of two cases. *J Bone Joint Surg Am* 1990;72(A):770–772.

131. Vassallo P, Reiser MF, Strobel M, et al. Popliteal pseudoaneurysm and arteriovenous shunt following arthroscopic meniscectomy: case report. *Cardiovasc Intervent Radiol* 1989;12:142–144.

132. Rodeo SA, Sobel M, Weiland AJ. Deep peroneal nerve injury as a result of arthroscopic meniscectomy. A case report and review of the literature. *J Bone Joint Surg Am* 1993;75(A):1221–1224.

133. Milachowski KA, Weismeier K, Wirth CJ. Homologous meniscus transplantation. Experimental and clinical results. *Int Orthop* 1989;13:1–11.

134. de Boer HH, Koudstaal J. Failed Meniscus Transplantation. A report of three cases. *Clin Orthop* 1994;306:155–162.

135. Cameron JC, Saha S. Meniscal allograft transplantation for unicompartmental arthritis of the knee. *Clin Orthop* 1997;337: 164–171.

136. Evans IK, Paulos LE. Complications of patellofemoral joint surgery. *Orthop Clin North Am* 1992;23(4):697–709.

137. Insall JN, Aglietti P, Tria AJ. Patellar pain and incongruence. II. Clinical applications. *Clin Orthop* 1983;176:225–232.

138. Merchant AC. Classification of patellofemoral disorders. *Arthroscopy* 1988;4:2355–240.

139. Merchant AC, Mercer RL. Lateral release of the patella: a preliminary report. *Clin Orthop* 1974;103:40–45.

140. Small NC. An analysis of complications in lateral retinacular release procedures. *Arthroscopy* 1989;5:282–286.

141. Betz RR, MaGill JT, Lonergan RP. The percutaneous lateral retinacular release. *Am J Sports Med* 1987;15:477–482.

142. Blasier RB, Ciullo JV. Rupture of the quadriceps tendon after arthroscopic lateral release: a case report. *Arthroscopy* 1986;2: 262–263.

143. Hughston JC, Deese M. Medial subluxation of the patella as a complication of lateral retinacular release. *Am J Sports Med* 1988;16:383–388.

144. Kolowich PA, Paulos LE, Rosenberg TD, et al. Lateral release of the patella: indications and contraindications. *Am J Sports Med* 1990;18:359–365.

145. Langeland N. Recurrent dislocation of the patella following lateral retinacular release: a case report. *Arch Orthop Trauma Surg* 1983;102:65–66.

146. Shellock FG, Mink JH, Dutsch A, et al. Evaluation of patients with persistent symptoms after lateral retinacular release by kinematic magnetic resonance imaging of the patellofemoral joint. *Arthroscopy* 1990;6:226–234.

147. Hughston JC, Walsh WMM. Proximal and distal reconstruction of the extensor mechanism for patella subluxation. *Clin Orthop* 1979;144:36–42.

148. Huberti HH, Hayes WC. Contact pressure in chondromalacia patellae and the effects of capsular reconstructive procedures. *J Orthop Res* 1988;6:499–508.

149. Crosby EB, Insall J. Recurrent dislocation of the patella. *J Bone Joint Surg Am* 1976;58(A):9–13.

150. Scuderi G, Cuomo F, Scott WM. Lateral release and proximal realignment for patellar subluxation and dislocation: a long term follow-up. *J Bone Joint Surg Am* 1988;70(A):856–861.

151. Barbari S, Raugstad TS, Lichtenberg N. The Hauser operation for patellar dislocation: 3–32 year results in 63 knees. *Acta Orthop Scand* 1990;61:32–35.

152. Cox JS. Evaluation of the Roux-Elmsie-Trillat procedure for the knee extensor realignment. *Am J Sports Med* 1982;10:303–310.

153. Fulkerson JP, Becker GJ, Meaney JA, et al. Anteromedial tibial tubercle transfer without bone graft. *Am J Sports Med* 1990; 18:490–497.

154. Slocum DB, Larson RL, James SL. Late reconstruction of ligamentous injuries of the medial compartment of the knee. *Clin Orthop* 1974;100:23–55.

155. Garland DE, Hughston JC. Peroneal nerve paralysis: complications of extensor reconstruction of the knee. *Clin Orthop* 1979;140:169–171.

156. Wall JJ. Compartment syndrome as a complication of the Hauser procedure. *J Bone Joint Surg Am* 1979;61(A):185–191.

157. Wiggins HW. The anterior tibial compartment syndrome: a complication of the Hauser procedure. *Clin Orthop* 1975;113:90–94.

158. Chrisman OD, Snook GA, Wilson TC. A long term prospective study of the Hauser and Roux-Goldthwait procedures for recurrent patellar dislocation. *Clin Orthop* 1979;144:27–30.

159. Blazina ME, Fox JM, Carlson GJ, et al. Patella baja: a technical consideration in evaluating results of tibial tubercle transplantation. *J Bone Joint Surg Am* 1975;57(A):1027.

160. Linclau L, Dokter G. Iatrogenic patella baja. *J Bone Joint Surg Am* 1976;58(A):9–13.

161. Hampson WGJ, Hill P. Late results of transfer of the tibial tubercle for recurrent dislocation of the patella. *J Bone Joint Surg Br* 1975;57(B):209–213.

162. Maquet PGJ. Consideration biomechanique sur, l'arthrose du genou. Un traitement biomechanique de l arthrose femoropatellaire. L'Advancement du tendon routulien. *Rev Rheum* 1963; 30:779.

163. Bessette GC, Hunter RE. The Maquet procedure: a retrospective review. *Clin Orthop* 1988;232:159–167.

164. Ferguson AB, Brown TD, Fu FH, et al. Relief of patellofemoral contact stress by anterior displacement of the tibial tubercle. *J Bone Joint Surg Am* 1979;61(A):159–166.

165. Mendes DG, Soudry M, lusim M. Clinical assessment of Maquet tuberosity advancement. *Clin Orthop* 1987;222:228–238.

166. Radin EL. Anterior tibial tubercle elevation in the young adult. *Orthop Clin North Am* 1986;17:297–302.

167. Radin EL, Labosky DA. Avoiding complications associated with the Maquet procedure. *Comp Orthop* 1989;2:48–53.

168. Radin EL. The Maquet procedure-anterior displacement of the tibial tubercle: Indications, contraindications, and precautions. *Clin Orthop* 1986;213:241–248.

169. Blazina ME, Fox JM, Del Pizzo, et al. Patellofemoral replacement. *Clin Orthop* 1979;144:98–103.

170. Insall J, Tria AJ, Aglietti P. Resurfacing of the patella. *J Bone Joint Surg Am* 1980;62(A):933–936.

171. Arciero RA, Toomey HE. Patellofemoral arthroplasty. A 3 to 9 year follow-up study. *Clin Orthop* 1988;236:60–71.

172. Cartier P, Sanouiller JL, Grelasamer R. Patellofemoral arthroplasty. 2–12 year follow-up study. *J Arthroplasty* 1990; 5(1):49–55.

173. Baker CL, Hughston JC. Miyakawa patellectomy. *J Bone Joint Surg Am* 1988;70(A):1489–1494.

174. Bentley G, Dowd G. Current concepts in etiology and treatment of chondromalacia patellae. *Clin Orthop* 1984;189:209–228.

175. Compere CL, Hill JA, Lewinek GE, et al. A new method of patellectomy for patellofemoral arthritis. *J Bone Joint Surg Am* 1979;61(A):712–719.

176. Lennox IA, Cobb AG, Knowles J, et al. Knee function after patellectomy. A 12 to 48 year follow-up. *J Bone Joint Surg Br* 1994;76(B):485–487.

177. Sutton FS, Thompson CH, Lipke J, et al. Effect of patellectomy on knee function. *J Bone Joint Surg Am* 1976;58(A):537–540.

178. Watkins MP, Harris BA, Wender S, et al. Effect of patellectomy on the function of the quadriceps and hamstrings. *J Bone Joint Surg Am* 1983;65(A):390–395.

179. Kaufer H. Mechanical function of the patella. *J Bone Joint Surg Am* 1971;53(A):1551–1560.

180. Steurer PA, Gradisar IA, Hoyt WA, et al. Patellectomy: a clinical study and biomechanical evaluation. *Clin Orthop* 1979;144: 84–90.

181. Kelly MA, Insall JN. Patellectomy. *Orthop Clin North Am* 1986;17:289–295.

182. Kettelkamp DB. Current concepts review: management of patellar malalignment. *J Bone Joint Surg Am* 1987;63(A):1344–1348.

183. Larson KR, Cracchiolo A, Dorey FJ, et al. Total knee arthroplasty in patients after patellectomy. *Clin Orthop* 1991;264:243–254.

184. Buechel FF. Patellar tendon bone grafting for patellectomized patients having total knee arthroplasty. *Clin Orthop* 1991; 271:72–78.

185. Paulos LE, Meislin R. Patellar entrapment following anterior cruciate ligament surgery. In: Jackson DW, ed. *The anterior cruciate ligament: current and future concepts*, 1st ed. New York: Raven Press, 1993:440–510.

186. Paulos LE, Wnorowski DC, Greenwald AE. Infrapatellar contracture syndrome. Diagnosis, treatment and long-term follow-up. *Am J Sports Med* 1994;22:550–449.

187. Paulos LE, Rosenberg TD, Drawbert J, et al. Infrapatellar contracture syndrome. An unrecognized cause of knee stiffness with patella entrapment and patella infera. *Am J Sports Med* 1987;15:331–341.

188. Harner CD, Irrgand JJ, Paul J, et al. Loss of knee motion after anterior cruciate ligament reconstruction. *Am J Sports Med* 1992;20:499–506.

189. Mohtadi NG, Webster-Bogaert S, Fowler PJ. Limitation of motion following anterior cruciate ligament reconstruction: a case control study. *Am J Sports Med* 1991;19:620–625.

190. Shelbourne KD, Wilckens J, Molabashy A, et al. Arthrofibrosis in acute anterior cruciate ligament reconstruction: the effect of timing of the reconstruction and rehabilitation. *Am J Sports Med* 1991;19:332–336.

191. Strum GM, Friedman MJ, Fox JM, et al. Acute anterior cruciate ligament reconstruction: analysis of complications. *Clin Orthop* 1990;253:184–189.

192. Blackburne J, Peel T. A new method of measuring patellar height. *J Bone Joint Surg Br* 1977;58(B):241.

193. Insall J, Salvati E. Patella position in the normal knee joint. *Radiology* 1971;101:101–104.

194. Noyes FR, Wojtys EM, Marshall MT. The early diagnosis and treatment of developmental patella infera syndrome. *Clin Orthop* 1991;265:241–252.

195. Fu F, Paul JP, Harner C, et al. The development of flexion contractures following arthroscopic anterior cruciate ligament reconstruction. *Am J Sports Med* 1991;19:560.

196. Graf B, Uhr F. Complications of intra-articular anterior cruciate ligament reconstruction. *Clin Sports Med* 1988;7:835–848.

197. Bonamo JJ, Krinick RM, Sporn AA. Rupture of the patellar ligament after use of its central third for anterior cruciate reconstruction. A report of two cases. *J Bone Joint Surg Am* 1984; 66(A):1294–1297.

198. DeLee JC. Complications of arthroscopy and arthroscopic surgery. Results of a national survey. *Arthroscopy* 1990;1:214–220.

199. Shino K, Nakagawa S, Inoue M, et al. Deterioration of patellofemoral articular surfaces after anterior cruciate ligament reconstruction. *Am J Sports Med* 1993;21:206–211.

200. Howell SM, Clark JA, Farley TE. A rationale for predicting anterior cruciate graft impingement by the intercondylar roof. A magnetic resonance imaging study. *Am J Sports Med* 1991; 19:276–281.

Principles and Practice of Orthopaedic Sports Medicine,
edited by William E. Garrett, Jr., Kevin P. Speer, and Donald T. Kirkendall.
Lippincott Williams & Wilkins, Philadelphia © 2000.

CHAPTER 47

The Degenerative Knee

Garron G. Weiker and James DeVellis

Keeping athletes healthy enough to participate in their chosen activities at a level they find acceptable without undo pain or risk is generally a challenge. The athlete who already has degenerative disease in his or her knee presents a special aspect of that overall challenge. It is generally accepted now that even those athletes with arthritis have a right and probably an obligation to continue participating in activities. We have transitioned from benign neglect to aggressive conservative treatment and surgical intervention for the knee with limiting pain and no mechanical symptoms. We have recently seen the development and implementation of many new injectable and oral treatments for arthritis and new surgical techniques to replace and improve articular surface. In this chapter we review the underlying disease process, discuss evaluation capabilities, and present the tried and true forms of surgical intervention and the newer and presently developmental techniques.

EPIDEMIOLOGY

Degenerative joint disease, or osteoarthritis, is the most common form of progressive joint disease seen in adults. It affects nearly 6% or 60 million American adults. The incidence increases with age and is quoted as being 0.1% in the 25- to 34-year-old range and between 10% and 30% in the 65- to 75-year-old range (1). Osteoarthritis is a major cause of disability in the United States, with approximately 68 million work loss days and 4 million hospitalizations per year. Felson et al. and others have reviewed the pattern and incidence of osteoarthritis in a community-based model and documented the occurrence of new cases related to aging and the higher incidence in females (4–7).

Multiple studies have sought to identify those things specifically related to an increased incidence of this problem. Identification of risk factors is significant not only for the athlete and his or her competition desires but also to American society. Once the factors are defined, we can attempt to develop ways to avoid the onset and/or progression of degenerative joint disease.

Age and Gender

As earlier noted, several reviews have shown a higher incidence of osteoarthritis among women than among men. In the Framingham Cohort Study there were three factors of osteoarthritis directly related to age and gender. There definitely was an increased incidence in the disease in women at all ages with an approximate ratio of 1.7:1. The rate of disease progression was also higher in women with 1.4:1. They also noted that in each age group, the onset of new cases of osteoarthritis of the knee was more frequent in women than in men. These conclusions were based on a review of radiographic criteria using a modified Kellgren-Lawrence scale. The scale is rated 0 through 4: 0, no evidence of arthritis; 1, questionable osteophytes and/or questionable joint space narrowing; 2, definite osteophytes with possible joint space narrowing or definite mild joint space narrowing with or without osteophytes; 3, definite joint space narrowing of at least 50% with or without cysts and/or sclerosis; and 4, severe joint space narrowing. Osteophytes were usually present in types 3 and 4. The patients were also evaluated on the basis of their subjective pain symptoms and their perceived functional capacity (11).

Manninen et al. (10) performed a 10-year study of farmers in Finland using radiographic techniques and subjective evaluations. They also demonstrated a significantly increased incidence of osteoarthritis of the knee in female patients and a progressive increase in incidence in both genders with progressive age.

G. G. Weiker and J. DeVellis: Department of Orthopaedic Surgery, Cleveland Clinic Foundation, Cleveland, Ohio 44195.

Weight

Body weight, both absolute and relative to overall size, has been studied in relationship to the incidence and development of osteoarthritis (10,12,13). There is a definite positive association between relative weight and the incidence of knee osteoarthritis as observed both in longitudinal and cross-sectional studies (12–17). When the incidence of advanced osteoarthritis of the knee is analyzed in reference to the body mass index (weight divided by height squared), the relationship seems to be linear in nature. The risk factors increase by 1.4 per standard deviation above the index body mass (3.8 kg/m^2). Obesity was also identified as the dominant factor in bilateral osteoarthritis of the knees. This study by Manninen did not take into consideration other risk factors such as previous trauma, level of activity, or type of occupation and occupational exposure.

Hochberg et al. (20) looked at the relationship between body fat and body weight and osteoarthritis of the knee. They concluded that increased percent body fat was definitely associated with increased osteoarthritis in a dose-response relationship. They also noted bilateral osteoarthritis of the knees related to obesity in women but not in men. The measure of body fat distribution with a waist-to-hip ratio variance was associated with bilateral osteoarthritis in men. These correlations between measurements of body fat distribution and body fat percentage with the fatty mass index may explain the apparent paradox. Whereas osteoarthritis is more related to percent body fat in women and waist-to-hip ratio in men, both entities are related to increased body mass index and the associated increased load.

Although obesity does effect both the weight-bearing tibial femoral joint and the patellofemoral joint of the knee, there are some variations. Cicuttini et al. (21) noted that those patients who also demonstrate osteoarthritis changes in the distal interphalangeal joints had much more significant osteoarthritis in the tibial femoral joint than in the patellofemoral joint.

Injury

Primary osteoarthritis is, by definition, idiopathic and is less prevalent than secondary osteoarthritis. Secondary osteoarthritis may be the result of previous trauma, congenital deformity, metabolic disease, endocrinopathies, neuropathies, or infection. In the general practice of orthopedic surgery, the most common form of secondary osteoarthritis we see is related to previous trauma. The onset of posttraumatic osteoarthritis may be related to direct damage to the articular surfaces, intraarticular fractures with a residual step-off, or angulation causing asymmetric loading. Damage to the articular surface

itself fills in primarily with a fibrocartilaginous matrix that does not possess the same biomechanical properties as normal articular surface (18). This fibrocartilage does not have the long-lasting biomechanical capability to sustain load bearing in many cases and therefore breaks down, causing additional problems. The ability to repair articular cartilage is age dependent, and skeletally immature individuals may, on occasion, produce a repair patch that functions very adequately.

The history, evaluation, and treatment of osteoarthritis of the knee requires close attention to any biomechanical abnormalities produced by previous trauma. As previously noted, although weight is a more significant factor in the development of osteoarthritis of the knee in women than it is in men, the history of previous trauma to the knee is more prevalent and more directly related in men than it is in women (19).

Occupational Exposure

Although there has been a general conception that specific occupations have an increased risk of the development of osteoarthritis of the knee, we have no studies that conclusively demonstrate this relationship. The literature, at present, is somewhat difficult to understand and interpret because of the many variations and failures in study design and data collection. Recently, Maetzel et al. (22) reviewed the literature on this subject from the past 28 years. Their study was designed to examine the data and summarize the odds in those studies that provided moderate to strong evidence. They found nine studies with particular attention directed to osteoarthritis of the knee and reviewed those for study design and analysis.

In four of the nine studies, there was moderate or strong evidence that supported the association of occupational exposure and osteoarthritis of the knee. Men were shown to have a consistently positive relationship between osteoarthritis of the knee and work that involved repetitive knee bending. This was best demonstrated in a prospective review (24). The evidence for a similar association was not well demonstrated in female workers. This correlation between work that required repetitive knee bending was not as strong or conclusive as the correlation between osteoarthritis and previous trauma or obesity (14).

Sports Participation

Buckwalter and Lane (25) reviewed the literature regarding sports participation and the development of osteoarthritis of the knee. As in the case of occupational exposure, it is difficult to analyze the data in this group without including confounding variables of genetic background, trauma, weight, and occupational exposure (28). There are conflicting data in regard to long-term sports participation and its relationship to osteoarthritis of the knee. There is another problem in that many of the past studies have used radiographic joint space measurements and the presence or absence of osteophytes as the basis for their definition of osteoarthritis. Those radiographic findings may not always correlate directly with degeneration of the articular surface and so-called osteoarthritis in the early stages (26).

People who participate in sports that subject their joints to intense impact and torsional loading seem to have an increased prevalence of osteoarthritis (28,29). Chronic low-impact repetitive exercise does not appear to cause the same level of damage as that seen with high impact. Long distance running, which is rated as relatively low impact and torsion, shows no higher risk of developing knee osteoarthritis than age-matched control subjects (30,31). These studies are lacking in that the time necessary to complete them is somewhat limited and therefore the studies usually result in primarily retrospective evaluation.

Recent animal studies have failed to demonstrate any long-term affect on the articular surface or increased rate of osteoarthritis in lifelong running exercise protocols (33). Dogs were placed on a long distance running program with physiologic loads and supraphysiologic loads (130% body weight); they demonstrated no significant ligament, meniscal, or articular surface damage. Mechanical testing also showed no significant difference in the articular cartilage from the running group versus the control group. Definite conclusions are difficult to establish, but there appears to be a strong general trend. It appears that there is a risk of articular cartilage degeneration in athletes who participate in activities that require repetitive high levels of impact and torsion and that this is exacerbated by history of previous joint injury (26,32). Moderate habitual exercise does not appear to increase the risk of developing osteoarthritis of the knee.

Genetic Predisposition

Most orthopedic surgeons we know believe that they see a consistent pattern of familial vulnerability to osteoarthritis. Some of this may be related to environmental factors such as weight and activity level. Spector et al. (34) looked at genetic influence related to osteoarthritis in women by reviewing 130 pairs of identical twins and 120 pairs of fraternal twins. The participants were screened both radiographically and by clinical evaluation. Results showed a strong genetic influence on the rate of osteoarthritis of the knee with a range between 39% and 65%. This percentage was independent of any recognizable or known environmental or demographic confounders. Similar conclusions have been reached in other studies, and one showed a definite predisposition

for development of osteoarthritis of both the hip and the knee (35).

PATHOANATOMY

Osteoarthritis is the progressive degradation and loss of articular cartilage. It is followed by the body's attempts at repair, remodeling, sclerosis of the subchondral bone, and eventually the development of osteophytes (36,37). The presence of pain, loss of joint motion, recurrent effusions, and deformity are all factors that must be included when diagnosing the clinical syndrome of osteoarthritis. The finding of osteophytes, whether palpated or seen radiographically, does not in and of itself make the diagnosis. On the microscopic level, localized fibrillation and disruption of the surface layer is the first visible sign related to osteoarthritis. As the disease progresses, these surface irregularities become full-blown clefts. At the same time, the articular surface becomes increasingly more and more irregular and the clefts penetrate deeper until there are fissures that actually reach the subchondral bone. Fragmentation of this irregular roughened articular surface takes place initially in a small fine pattern and then eventually progresses to larger and larger fragments that break loose. This breakdown and loss of the surface layers results in a reduction of cartilage volume and thickness (36,37). At the same time, these microscopic changes start the cartilage loses water content and breakdown and simultaneous synthesis. In osteoarthritis this balance is disrupted, and homeostasis is lost as the breakdown progresses ahead of regenerative capability (18). It is unlikely any single factor is causative in this process. More likely, the degradation represents a series of events and the coming together of multiple factors.

Review of the literature fails to show any conclusive evidence of a direct relationship between metabolic factors such as hypertension, glucose intolerance, or hypercholesterolemia and the development of osteoarthritis (14,38). Consistently, the literature does reflect an association between those factors that are mechanical in nature, such as obesity, previous trauma, joint surface irregularity, and the genetic vulnerability to osteoarthritis (19).

Mechanical Factors

We can generalize and describe osteoarthritis as a progressive loss of articular cartilage that proceeds at a rate beyond the body's capability of simultaneous repair (37). Many mechanisms have been proposed as the cause of this imbalance. They can be summarized as factors that cause the joint surface to see increased forces that are beyond tolerance. This may be as a result of abnormal tracking and abnormal sheer forces, loss of some of the normal protective structures, or simply a dramatically increased load such as obesity.

The literature clearly reflects the effect of total meniscectomy on the human knee. There is definitely an increased rate of progressive degenerative change both clinically and radiographically in those people who have had complete meniscectomies (39–44). The load-bearing function of the meniscus has been repeatedly studied (45–47), and these studies have increased our awareness of the importance of the meniscus. The knowledge led to the concept of partial meniscectomy for treatment of meniscal tears. It has also become generally accepted now that repair of the meniscus, when possible, is preferential to any form of resection. Recent long-term studies of partial meniscectomies performed arthroscopically have demonstrated improvement in both radiographic and clinical result as compared with total meniscectomy (48–52). These studies have shown that partial meniscectomy can give good results as far as pain relief and have minimal long-term effect on the development of radiographically evidenced arthritic changes. If there is visible articular cartilage surface change or damage at the time of meniscectomy, the rate of degradation and development of osteoarthritis is faster and pain relief is less certain. It should be noted that there is significant effort across the country to perfect techniques to replace diseased menisci before the development of arthritic change. The two predominant schools of thought at present are allograft meniscal implants and modified collagen scaffolds to stimulate meniscal regrowth. Both approaches show promise but are not yet perfected and ready for general use.

Rangger et al. (49) reported on the follow-up of 284 patients 5 years after arthroscopic partial meniscectomy. This study showed the anticipated progression of radiographic signs related to arthritic change. They found the patients who were over 40 years of age at the time of partial meniscectomy had a higher rate of arthritic degeneration than did younger patients. Rangger et al. noted that chondral damage existing at the time of arthroscopy was a likely indicator of a more rapid progression of subsequent osteoarthritic change. Burks et al. (50) also looked at the long-term affects of arthroscopic meniscectomy. Radiographic evaluation was done on 146 patients an average of 15 years after arthroscopic meniscectomy. Based on the weight-bearing AP of the knee, their results did not demonstrate a significant difference related to age of the patient at the time of surgery. They did find that isolated medial meniscal tear patients had less progressive osteoarthritis change than did isolated lateral meniscal tear patients. They also found that knees that had a valgus inclination had less progressive change in the medial compartment than did those who were neutral or varus (44,53–56). Multiple studies, including Rangger et al.'s, demonstrated that knees with anterior cruciate ligament (ACL) deficiency

and partial meniscectomy had a more rapid progressive arthritis than stable knees with the same type of meniscectomies.

The long-term history of the ACL-deficient knee has been studied extensively (56–67). Patients who elected nonoperative treatment showed increased radiographic evidence of osteoarthritic change. Those patients with ACL injury and meniscal pathology that required excision had an even more rapid progression and increase in severity of osteoarthritis. Daniel et al. (67) did point out that many of these natural history studies have been retrospective and are likely to contain a built-in bias. Patients who come in to be evaluated with long-standing ACL insufficiency are likely to be those who have symptoms, and therefore the studies automatically, by design, exclude those asymptomatic patients who have not sought medical care. In Daniel et al.'s own prospective study (67) of ACL-deficient patients, there was a lower incidence of posttraumatic arthritis than in other studies but still a definite increased tendency toward arthritic degeneration than seen in the general population. The only other factor of significance was that those patients who modify their activity levels to the point that they are no longer symptomatic are less likely to develop arthritis than are those who insist on continuing all activities despite symptoms (57).

In keeping with earlier comments, it is noted that the ACL-deficient knee with meniscal and/or articular surface damage at the time of initial evaluation is likely to develop degenerative arthritis changes. Multiple reports have demonstrated that meniscus injury, articular surface injury, and subchondral bone injury are all frequently associated with ACL rupture (69–72). Any of the aforementioned associated injuries can and will influence the statistical probability of the early of osteoarthritis (68). Roos et al. (73) examined 1,012 patient with previous arthroscopy and radiographs in an effort to correlate the onset of arthritis in relationship to age at the time of injury and time since the reported injury. They found that radiographic changes were identified at approximately 40 years of age after ACL injury either isolated or with meniscus and/or collateral ligament injury. Most of their patients were under the age of 25 at the time of the designated injury event. In the group of meniscal injury patients followed in the same fashion, the average age of radiographic evidence of arthritis onset was 50 years. Those patients also sustained most of these injuries between the ages of 20 and 30. In both groups, the average time of onset for the radiographic change was 10 years after the original injury. For those patients who had meniscal injury between the ages of 17 and 30, there was an average time of 15 years to the point of radiographically recognized change. Those over the age of 30 at the time of meniscal injury had only 5 years, on the average, before the onset of radiographic changes. They concluded that osteoarthritis of the knee does indeed show progression and progresses more rapidly as time passes. They also concluded that osteoarthritis changes appear sooner after injury in the older group of patients.

Articular Cartilage Damage

Direct damage to the articular surface may be either the result of a blunt force or from indirect trauma transmitted through the joint. In experimental studies, disruption of normal articular cartilage requires contact stresses of approximately 25 MPa or more (74). Other studies have shown that intact loading of bone can generate 25 MPa in the articular surface without causing fracture of the bone (75). Theoretically, this load could result in chondrocyte death and cartilage fissuring. These loads may actually represent the so-called bone bruise of magnetic resonance imaging (MRI) (74–76). Although there is no full long-term follow-up, studies of bone bruises in correlation with eventual osteoarthritis show that it is probable this entity is significant. It is entirely possible that irreversible damage to the articular cartilage occurs at the time of a single high-energy impact load that results in the MRI bone bruise (77). This irreversible damage to the articular surface may well serve to be the focal point that leads to progressive degenerative changes within the joint (78). At present we cannot directly correlate the bone bruise with eventual osteoarthritis, but there is strong suspicion that will be the result as time goes on and the studies are extended.

Curl et al. (79) in a review of 31,516 arthroscopies looked specifically for chondral injury documented at the time of arthroscopy. In 19,827 of these patients they identified 53,569 articular surface lesions. Most of these lesions involved either the patella or the medial femoral condyle, and most were graded as III or IV. Five percent of these lesions were grade IV lesions in patients under the age of 40. Although there was no proof, it was suspected that these lesions were largely the result of specific focal impact loads at the time of the injury that resulted in arthroscopic intervention. Again, at present, we have no long-term documentation of the outcome of these lesions.

CLINICAL EVALUATION

History

It is easy to overlook or underemphasize history as a part of the evaluation in these patients. The history is critical in that it determines, to a large extent, the recommendations concerning treatment. We all know, but often forget, that we are not treating a knee. We are treating a patient. The initial history should include not only the typical primary complaint of dull aching arthritic type pain but a much more complete picture of the patient's problems and subsequent disabilities.

We need to determine the duration of the symptoms and the character of the onset. It is important to know whether the patient went abruptly from asymptomatic to significantly symptomatic or had gradual progression. Was there a point in time when there was a dramatic or significant increase in symptom intensity? Was that related to any specific event or activity? It is important to know whether or not there are any mechanical symptoms as a component of the overall picture. In other words, does the patient have any locking, popping, catching, snapping, buckling, partial buckling, or any of the other mechanical descriptions they may give? Generally speaking, the patient who has aching arthritic pain with no mechanical symptoms is unlikely to benefit from a simple arthroscopic clean-out.

The history needs to incorporate any underlying disease processes, family history of arthritis, involvement of other joints, or any other associated symptoms. We need to know the types of activity in which they have participated and to what extent they were involved. This should include not only their sports activity but also their employment and hobby histories that may affect the knee. The classic example is the older person who participates in general activities but really has a fascination with gardening and tends to "duck walk" along the rows of the garden as they work. It is important to know the time of day when the pain is greatest and its relationship to activity. The activity history should include the type of activities that cause the greatest problems and the duration of activity and the temporal relationship between that activity and the pain. Activity history should also find out if the individual has given up any activities because of knee symptoms and when they gave those up.

The final aspects of the general history determines prior history of significant previous injury and/or physician intervention. Has the patient previously had a documented meniscal tear treated? Was it partially resected? What was the postoperative rehabilitation? When did they stop doing the rehabilitation and does that correlate with the onset of present symptoms? After completing the generalized history evaluation, ask the patient to pinpoint as closely as possible the point of maximum discomfort. With true generalized osteoarthritis they will have difficulty doing this. The patient will describe it as globally about the knee or perhaps medially or laterally. With a true mechanical component they are often able to place one finger on the medial joint line or on the lateral joint line and say "that is where I feel most of my pain." If they have a history of recurrent effusions, we need to find out what seems to precipitate those, how fast they go away, and if the patient has found anything that seems to increase the rate of resolution. All these components of the history and anything else that the patient may volunteer must be assembled to form a picture to guide the rest of the evaluation.

Physical Examination

The sequence and exact method of physical examination will vary among clinicians. Regardless of the exact method, the most important thing is consistency. The examination should always be performed with the patient in shorts and with shoes and socks off. The initial observation of the patient standing should be done both from in front and behind, observing the general body habitus, lower extremity alignment, and any deformities. Dynamic evaluation should follow with observation of the patient's gait and gentle partial knee bends. In the arthritic knee, special attention should be paid to patellofemoral tracking, evidence of thrust, or appearance of instability.

The seated examination is generally next. Observe skin quality, extremity symmetry, and muscle mass. The patient is then asked to actively extend and flex the knee while the examiner observes the tracking and palpates lightly for crepitation. Supine examination follows the seated position with initial attention to evidence of deformity and/or effusions. Passive and active range of motion is assessed, and the knee is palpated for localization of tenderness. A dramatic response to palpation that is greater than seems appropriate for this situation should call to mind the possibility of reflex sympathetic dystrophy or hysteria. Any evidence of previous surgical incisions should cause a review of the history to be certain that previous surgical intervention has been adequately documented and defined. Undoubtedly, the best information on previous surgery is to request, or have the patient request, copies of the previous operative reports and any intraoperative photos or videos available. Palpable marginal spurring and crepitance is again noted and points of focal tenderness are identified.

Joint line tenderness in this group of patients with arthritic knees is very likely to be degenerative meniscal pathology but may also represent marginal spurs that are sensitive. Variations on the classic McMurray's examination, Apley compression test, or Steinmann rotation test all have their place and are of value (80–82). Typically, the degenerative meniscus tear does not result in a dramatic McMurray type clunk or any locking of the joint but rather as pain caused by attempting these various provocative maneuvers.

Although the ligamentous status of the knee is less often of major importance in this particular population of patients, it should be evaluated. The examiner needs to remember that collapse of the medial compartment, which is often seen in the form of a varus knee, will examine much like a medial collateral ligament laxity due to the increased space in the medial joint. It is not at all rare to find increased excursion on the Lachman

exam and even occasionally a positive lateral pivot shift. This may reflect a remote injury to the ACL. With careful questioning, it is frequently possible to determine a causative event in high school, college, or sandlot sports that the patient had essentially forgotten. Often, these ACL-deficient knees are stable to examination because they have already developed enough marginal arthritic spurring to cause a secondary stabilization affect (83–86).

The examination then should finalize on the patellofemoral joint. This has already been initially evaluated with observation both walking and seated and by palpating for crepitus. The lateral apprehension sign and medial facet tenderness is checked, and a Clark patellar compression test or some other form of patellofemoral compression test is done. During the seated observation, watch for an abrupt lateral deviation of the patella as the knee reaches extension. When present it represents the so-called J sign, with inherent maltracking of the patella.

Finally, the examination should include evaluation of the peripheral neurovascular and hip status to rule out referred knee pain.

IMAGING STUDIES

Radiography

Radiographic evaluation has become a standard and fundamental portion of the workup for most knee problems. Radiographs not only confirm the existing problem but also give ancillary information as far as possible underlying advanced aseptic necrosis, calcified loose bodies, cystic areas, or bony tumors. We use a standard series of four views for the initial examination of the knee. The first view is a standing anteroposterior done in full extension. That view gives some idea of overall knee alignment, evidence of chondrocalcinosis, evidence of marginal osteophytes, and evidence of loss of medial or lateral joint space if it is significantly advanced (93). The second view is a 45-degree posterior anterior flexed weight-bearing view. This view, as described by Rosenberg et al., is excellent for showing any evidence of significant joint surface cartilage loss in the primary weight-bearing zone. The combination of the anteroposterior and partially flexed PA gives a good overall evaluation of the amount of articular cartilage loss that may be present. Third is a lateral taken with the knee in 30 degrees of flexion. This allows us to look at the contour of the condyles, the evidence for loose bodies or chondrocalcinosis, and evidence of spurs or ectopic calcification. If the view is taken at 30 degrees, it can also be used in conjunction with the Insall-Salvati, Blumenstat, or Blackberne and Peele measurements for patellar position (91,92,94). Each of these methods of measuring is used to determine the presence of patella alta or baja. The final view we routinely take is the Merchant patellofemoral view (87). On occasion this will be augmented in the younger patient with early disease with views taken in 30 and 60 degrees and the primary 45-degree Merchant. This allows analysis of the articular space within the patellofemoral joint and positioning of the patella. It allows us to look for evidence of abnormal patellar tilt or abnormal displacement out of the trochlear groove.

This combination of views allows a relatively complete radiographic assessment of the human knee and addresses the primary areas of concern related to osteoarthritis. On the anteroposterior view, the Fairbanks system is used. The rating of arthritic changes is based on the osteophytes, subchondral sclerosis, and squaring off of the femoral condyles as seen of this series (39). When it is necessary to have an accurate assessment of the limb alignment such as in considering high tibial osteotomy or some other form of realignment procedure, it is best to have a full-length standing anteroposterior view. If the patient has demonstrated a significant thrust on ambulation, it is wise to take this view standing one legged on the involved leg to demonstrate the position of the knee in weight-bearing posture (95).

Magnetic Resonance Imaging

MRI technology is still evolving. Initially it was believed to be too costly, and the machines were tied up performing life-saving evaluations. As the machines became more readily available in the community, the shift was to perform MRIs basically on every patient who walked in the door and who was willing to submit to the study. The MRI offers a distinct advantage in its ability to evaluate soft tissue structures within and around the knee and the bone marrow. Although the MRI is capable of giving us a high percentage of accuracy and sensitivity for meniscal pathology, it is seldom necessary in this group of patients. A good history and physical examination is likely to give us 97% to 99% accuracy in identifying the common posterior horn degenerative tear of the medial meniscus. In our practice, we limit the MRI to that occasional patient where we are uncomfortable with the working diagnosis after history and physical or to the patient who is so apprehensive they need the study to psychologically accept the findings and recommendations. I certainly would not recommend getting an MRI in people with early degenerative joint disease changes and mild to moderate symptomatology. The study often will show significant signal changes within the meniscal substance that is probably related to aging and can be very confusing as far as future planning if it is actually read as representing a tear (96,97).

In those cases where the examination does not ring true and obvious, the MRI has the potential for demonstrating the early changes of osteonecrosis, bone marrow-related diseases, and occult fractures. Until recently, the MRI has been of minimal to moderate value in visualizing articular cartilage lesions. A study of 28 patients by Speer et al. (99) concluded that the MRI could not reliably exclude articular cartilage damage. Since that time, newer imaging techniques and machines have evolved. Using a volumetric, fat-suppressed, spoiled gradient-recalled, signal acquisition in the steady state, it is possible to accurately record the volume of articular cartilage. The use of this equipment by properly trained radiologists can offer a very high degree of consistency and sensitivity in evaluating articular surface changes not visualized on plain radiographs.

NONOPERATIVE TREATMENT

Unless the patient is experiencing mechanical symptoms of locking or true buckling, there is little place for consideration of surgical intervention at the time of initial diagnosis. Most patients will respond to conservative management in the early and moderate stages of the disease. There is no specific algorithm or exact pattern to the nonoperative management of degenerative arthritis in the knee even though there are some general principles and patterns to keep in mind. Early treatment should routinely include any necessary activity modification, appropriate weight loss, physical therapy for motion and strengthening, and pharmacologic aides as appropriate.

Weight Loss, Activity Modification, and Exercise

As described earlier, it has been clearly shown that articular cartilage degeneration of the knee is directly related to obesity, especially in women. Although there is a paucity of literature that demonstrates any positive correlation between weight loss and decreasing symptoms, studies have indirectly demonstrated a causal relationship (19,100,102,103). Felson et al. (102) noted an affect on reviewing the information from the Framingham Study and interval radiographs taken over a 10-year period. For every 10-pound weight loss or weight gain, there was a corresponding decrease or increase in the likelihood of the study group developing osteoarthritis (102). In another uncontrolled study of obese patients who had undergone gastric stapling for weight loss, McGoey et al. (100) found that 57% of patients with knee pain who lost 100 pounds experienced relief of their symptoms. In addition to the direct possibility of decreasing symptoms by weight loss, the patients need to be counseled regarding appropriate weight for total knee replacement if their disease process continues.

It is generally accepted that weight loss alone is not the complete answer. Weight loss coupled with activity modification is recommended. The activity modification should include decreasing high impact and torsion loading while increasing activities beneficial for weight loss, conditioning, and strengthening of the lower extremity. The literature does demonstrate improvement in strength and decreasing symptoms for osteoarthritis of the knee with appropriate rehabilitation exercise (103,104). The pain also seems to be improved by a rehabilitation program that prevents flexion contractures and the associated unhealthy gait. A fitness walking program has been shown to improve functional status without increasing knee pain in the osteoarthritic knee (105). Once initial muscle rehabilitation strengthening has been accomplished, the patients are able to improve their gait pattern by increasing velocity, cadence, and stride length without significantly increasing pain (106,107).

In those patients who are already actively involved in running, tennis, fitness walking, or golf, the actual rehabilitation effort should avoid repetition of those same activities. They should participate in activities such as closed chain kinetic conditioning, exercise cycling, swimming, or other low-impact low-torsional stress-type activities. This allows them to maintain their cardiovascular fitness and improve their functional gait without adding to the impact and torsional loading that they are receiving in their normal daily activities.

Nonprescription Medications

Patients are presently bombarded by a plethora of media advertising efforts directed at convincing them to use both prescription and nonprescription treatments for osteoarthritis. A large number of "natural" medications have flooded the market. The emphasis in advertising and patient response seems to be directed toward the glucosaminoglycan-like products, chondroitin sulfates, and shark cartilage. The advertisers claim that these substances can restore natural glucosaminoglycan levels to the knee joint and therefore restore a more homeopathic state in the arthritic joint.

In reviewing the rheumatologic literature, glucosamine seems to be the one item in this group that is clearly of some benefit. Glucosamine is an amino monosaccharide that functions in the body as a precursor of a disaccharide unit in glycosaminoglycans. Glucosamine is normally produced by the chondrocytes but appears to be decreased in the osteoarthritic state. The advertisers claim that taken orally it can add the additional raw materials for cartilage matrix production and have a specific anti-inflammatory role and a role in stimulating chondrocyte metabolism (119). In several randomized controlled studies, the efficacy of glucosamine sulfate was compared with placebo (108–114). In all these studies, the short-term effects of glucosamine taken in a dosage of 500 mg three times per day were superior to

the placebo from the fourth to the eighth week. There were no reported adverse side effects in comparison with the placebo group. Glucosamine was then compared with ibuprofen in randomized clinical trials (115,116). Vaz found that ibuprofen 1,200 mg/day in three divided doses was superior to glucosamine sulfate initially but that the pattern reversed by 8 weeks. By the 8-week point, the benefits from glucosamine significantly outweighed the benefits of ibuprofen. Tolerance was high in both study groups, but the ibuprofen group did have a higher rate of adverse side affects. These studies seemed to show a definite place in the overall armamentarium for the use of glucosamine 500 mg three times a day in the management of early to moderately advanced arthritis of the knee.

Acetaminophen has generally been ignored as a treatment for osteoarthritis by the orthopedic community even though commercial advertising strongly indicates that it is beneficial. In controlled studies, the use of acetaminophen was compared with nonsteroidal anti-inflammatory drugs (NSAIDs) and found to be equal in efficacy. In randomized control studies comparing the use of ibuprofen and naproxen to acetaminophen, there was no statistically significant differences in the outcomes between the groups (117,118). Williams et al. (117) found that withdrawal due to lack of efficacy was slightly higher in the acetaminophen group than in the naproxen group over a 2-year period. The withdrawal due to adverse side affects was higher in the naproxen group. At this time, based on the literature, we recommend acetaminophen as the initial line of analgesia control for early to moderately severe degenerative joint disease.

Nonsteroidal Anti-inflammatory Medications

Over the last two decades, the use of NSAIDs has generally become the primary and initial approach for early osteoarthritis of the knee. With current knowledge it is debatable whether this is wise. Perhaps analgesic medications with lesser potential side effects such as acetaminophen should be initially considered (120). NSAIDs accomplish their anti-inflammatory functions specifically by preventing the enzyme cyclooxygenase (COX) from converting arachidonic acid into prostaglandin. Because the prostaglandin causes the primary inflammatory response, chemical blockage of their formation decreases the inflammatory process. Unfortunately, NSAIDs are not specific in blocking this primary inflammatory COX pathway. They also block the COX pathway involved in the maintenance of homeostasis in both the renal and gastrointestinal systems. Because of this secondary undesirable COX pathway blockage, side effects are relatively common. The most common is gastrointestinal irritation and potential ulceration. In addition to the gastrointestinal side effects, there have been reported problems with renal impairment, platelet inhibition, hepatotoxicity, central nervous system toxicity, and increased potassium levels.

Of the multiple NSAIDs on the market today, each manufacturer claims to demonstrate superior efficacy, and many of them claim to have fewer side effects. No one NSAID has truly been proven to be vastly superior to the others. Although individuals do respond to certain drugs more dramatically than to others, the overall populous has been shown to have roughly the same response to the different NSAIDs. In the average orthopedic practice, it is probably wise to use NSAIDs on a short-term basis after ruling out preexisting renal disease, gastric disease, or other contraindications. Patients on long-term therapy should be monitored periodically with routine analysis of complete blood count, urinalysis, serum creatinine, and liver enzymes (121). This is probably best managed by their family physician or general internist. If and when the pharmaceutical companies are able to develop a newer NSAID package that selectively blocks the COX-1 pathway and prevents inflammation without blocking the other more beneficial affects, the general usage of NSAIDs will be safer and more appropriate.

Intraarticular Injections

Corticosteroids

Intraarticular cortical steroids have been used for many years as a primary treatment modality for osteoarthritis of the knee. Over time they have shown little evidence of morbidity (123,124). Despite this, we have some hesitancy concerning the random and frequent use of intraarticular steroids. It is well documented that corticosteroids initially cause some collagen linkage changes with a mechanical weakening of the chondral surface. Although this is reversible, it does coincide with the maximum anti-inflammatory effect of the injection. That gives the patient a false sense of well-being when the articular surface is at its weakest. Extreme activity during that period of time, when the chondral surface is transiently weakened, may cause accelerated wear and tear. The indication for intraarticular corticosteroid injection should be advanced osteoarthritis unresponsive to routine treatment modalities and medications. Injections should not be given if there is any evidence of infection, cellulitis, or other overlying skin problems and probably should not be given to people with a history of bleeding coagulopathies or to those on anticoagulant therapy. The injections may be soluble or microcrystalline preparations. The soluble preparations are absorbed quickly, reach their maximum efficacy quickly, and lose efficacy quickly. The microcrystalline preparations are more slowly absorbed and therefore have a slower onset, lower peak affect, and a much longer action.

Double-blinded placebo-controlled studies looking at the efficacy of intraarticular corticosteroids have demonstrated mixed success (125–128). These studies indicate that the injections are more effective than placebo treatment for short-term relief during the first 2 to 3 weeks postinjection. Beyond 2 to 3 weeks, the steroids were not shown to be more effective than the placebo control. In 1996, Jones and Doherty (128) specifically looked at patients receiving intraarticular steroid injection in an effort to establish clinical predictors of response to the injection. They were unable to find any specific predictor or group of predictors that would allow them to identify better responders. Although the clinical effects of intraarticular corticosteroids are short lived, they do have dramatic initial effects and may well offer an interim solution in those patients with very advanced disease and a need for specific temporary relief.

Hyaluronic Acid

Synovial fluid in osteoarthritic joints has been demonstrated to have lower elasticity and viscosity than synovial fluid from normal joints. This is thought to be the result of a decreased concentration and molecular size of hyaluronan in that fluid (129). Based on that finding, an effort has been made to restore the elasticity and viscosity of the synovial fluid in arthritic joints by the instillation of intraarticular hyaluronan. This approach has been used extensively abroad and in Canada but has only recently been allowed into the U.S. marketplace (130). There are currently two U.S. Food and Drug Administration-approved forms of hyaluronan available for usage in the United States: Hylan G-F20 (Synvisc), administered in three weekly intervals, and sodium hyaluronate (Hyalgan), given in five weekly injections.

Review of the available literature shows that a Canadian multicenter randomized trial of Hylan G-F20 was compared with NSAIDs alone and with NSAIDs combined with Hylan G-F20. At 26 weeks into the study, both groups receiving the Hylan G-F20 showed improved status as compared with NSAIDs alone (131). Earlier results at 12 weeks for the three groups showed little differential between them. Sodium hyaluronate has been tested in several randomized, double-blind, placebo-controlled trials (132–137). Little effect was seen during the series of five weekly intraarticular injections, but there was a definite statistical improvement after the 5-week period. These benefits lasted from 3 to 12 months, and the best results were identified in patients over the age of 60 years. Hyaluronan has also been compared with intraarticular methylprednisolone (138,139). After 60 days the hyaluronan group had a greater clinical response and fewer symptoms than the methylprednisolone group. There does appear to be a role for the use of intraarticular injections in osteoarthritic knees. Studies are still sparse in this area, but it appears that patients over the age of 60 years and patients who can have the injections in conjunction with the use of oral NSAIDs have the greatest likelihood of a positive response.

Bracing and Pedorthotics

Osteoarthritis (or degenerative joint disease) of the knee involves the medial compartment approximately 10 times as often as it does the lateral compartment (140). This is likely related to the knee alignment and subsequent increased load bearing through the medial compartment during weight-bearing activities (142). The Japanese were reportedly the first to make an effort at redistributing the forces across the knee. They attempted to instill wedge insole orthoses in patients with unicompartmental medial arthritis in an effort to shift the forces into the lateral compartment (141,142). This promise of altering the mechanical alignment of the knee was studied by Sasaki and Yasuda (142), who followed 105 patients. They placed a 5-degree heel wedge on the lateral side of the heel in 105 patients with medial compartment osteoarthritis. These patients were followed for a period of 1 to 5 years. They did show some significantly valid results with the best of those being obtained in patients who demonstrated mild osteoarthritis rather than advanced disease. In 1993, Keating et al. (144) found similar results in 85 patients using a lateral heel wedge in a 1-year follow-up. Their patients demonstrated a significant improvement, and even those with advanced osteoarthritis demonstrated recognizable improvement.

Following the same concept of attempting to unload the medial compartment but shifting to the knee itself, the orthotics companies have now developed varus or valgus unloading knee braces. These braces function on a three-point bending principle with pressure at the joint line or epicondylar area of the knee countered by pressure midcalf and midthigh on the opposite side. By placing the center pad over the lateral side of the knee and the proximal distal pads on the medial side, it is possible to create valgus (145). Some braces require custom fitting and others are designed for off-the-shelf utilization. Those that come off the shelf are generally designed with adjustable increasing or decreasing pad pressure. This is done by changing the thickness of the pads themselves or by using an inflatable bladder.

Various biomechanical or gait analysis studies have demonstrated conclusive evidence that the adductor moment seen in the physiologically varus knee is decreased by application of a valgus unloader brace (146,147). The use of valgus unloader braces in patients with medial compartment osteoarthritis has demonstrated improvement in pain scores. Function scores improve the most in those activities related to daily life (148–151). In a prospective review with 1-year patient follow-up in 1998, Hewett et al. (151) found improved function and decreased pain after the patients wore a valgus unloader brace for an average of 7 hours per day for 5 days a week. They concluded that the goal of bracing should be to buy a short amount of time for patients who wished to avoid or delay having definitive surgery. In addition to relieving pain and buying time, the brace is also a relatively effective way of testing to see if a patient will benefit from high tibial osteotomy. Personal experience has been that the braces are most effective in those patients who can wear them for specific activities that cause difficulty rather than wearing them for a specific time period of the day.

OPERATIVE INTERVENTION ARTHROSCOPY

As the arthroscope has evolved from a diagnostic tool in the early 1970s to a surgical tool in the 1990s, the selection of patients benefited by the use of the arthroscope has also evolved. The arthroscope is no longer used for only young athletes. Early practitioners noticed significant improvement in osteoarthritic symptoms after arthroscopic lavage of the joint (152,153). Subsequently, as the arthroscope made its dramatic entrance into clinical practice in the 1970s, the value of debridement for arthritic knees became generally recognized. Unfortunately, there is still some controversy regarding the usefulness of this tool in the management of osteoarthritis. Evolution of arthroscopic techniques for osteoarthritis of the knee has resulted in a general picture of the most appropriate candidate but not necessarily a rigid pattern. The general rule of thumb indicates that the arthroscope is appropriate only after conservative approaches fail or when knee symptoms are largely mechanical in nature. Those patients who report mechanical symptoms that we have come to equate with the presence of loose bodies or fragments of articular surface or meniscus are more likely to respond beneficially to arthroscopy (154,155). If the presentation is that of a deep aching pain, especially night pain or rest pain with little mechanical component, the arthroscopic clean-out and debridement is less likely to offer significant benefit (154,155).

There is still some debate as to the value of arthroscopy or arthroscopic surgery versus arthroplasty because there is no definite answer (156). There is a confusion in terms associated with the definition of joint debridement, and there is also an obvious difference in surgical ability and aggressiveness among various arthroscopists. The literature is replete with articles identifying everything from excellent results to poor results. There is no simple way to separate and clear up the confusion between quality of procedure versus quality of the surgeon. The thing that remains abundantly clear is that the arthroscope allows us to perform procedures in a minimally invasive fashion with low morbidity and no interference with more definitive procedures in the future (157). To put it another way, the arthroscope offers us an opportunity to give patients with arthritic knees significant relief with minimal risk and without burning any bridges for future treatment.

Several reports do support the effectiveness of simple joint lavage for relieving the pain of arthritic knees (158–160). Explanation of this success includes the possibilities that the lavage removes cartilaginous debris or crystals or rinses out degradative metalloproteases and/ or other inflammatory factors (157). When a direct comparison is done, arthroscopic lavage has a better success rate at 1-year follow-up than does simple needle lavage (160). Although there is some possible debate concerning placebo affect in these studies, they are the only preliminarily randomized trials available at this time (161).

The arthroscope also gives us the opportunity for a cameo look at the joint surfaces and the ability to identify, classify, and define the amount of arthritis present at the time of surgery. Although there have been several different classification schemes for grading arthritic changes, no system has been universally accepted. The most generally accepted and extensively used is that proposed by Outerbridge (184), who defines the appearance of articular cartilage damage in four grades:

- Grade I: softening and swelling.
- Grade II: fragmentation and fissuring less than 0.5 inches.
- Grade III: fragmentation and fissuring greater than 0.5 inches.
- Grade IV: erosion down to subchondral bone.

Though the system is easy to memorize and work with, it does lack description of lesion size or depth unless the depth reaches subchondral bone. Other systems designed to improve on this classification have been described but not generally accepted (185,186). Noyes and Stabler (187) published another classification scheme that takes into account surface description and extent of involvement, diameter of lesion, and site of lesion. Although this system is the most precise classification system presently available, it is cumbersome to use and difficult to accurately remember. Much of the confusion will continue to remain concerning evaluation and treatment of chondral lesions until a generally acceptable and effective classification system is in place.

Formal joint debridement has been extensively reported in the literature (155,162–167). Magnusen (162) reported an open arthrotomy technique to remove painful marginal spurs and mechanical irritants from the knee. That procedure did improve function and de-

crease pain, but it also required a wide surgical exposure and extensive physical therapy. The formal Magnusen-type procedure has fallen out of favor with many surgeons since the advent of the motorized arthroscope instrumentation. (It is our personal preference to revert to the open Magnusen-type debridement when there are large palpable marginal spurs about the entire joint.) Although it is possible to do a full debridement with the arthroscopic instrumentation, the duration and magnitude of the procedure is far greater with the arthroscope than it is with open arthrotomy. The ideal combination seems to be to clean out the weight-bearing area and the intercondylar notch arthroscopically and then convert to simple arthrotomy and open debridement of the major spurs. The arthroscopic debridement, as noted, does allow the advantage of removing degenerative meniscal tissue, loose cartilaginous articular fragments, and inflamed or impinging synovium (157). General review of debridement techniques has shown good to excellent results in approximately 70%. The success rate gradually declines as time goes on and the arthritic changes progress.

Abrasion arthroplasty and aggressive early motion combine to form a smooth surface of reparative fibrocartilage. Histologic studies show that this material is indeed a fibrocartilage rather than hyalin cartilage and generally has poor long-term wear characteristics (168). Abrasion arthroplasty was shown to have limited success rates in several studies (1,3,71,155,164,166,169). The result after abrasion arthroplasty seemed to degrade quite rapidly. Because of this rather limited and unpredictable success rate, the process has presently fallen out of favor.

Similar in concept to the abrasion arthroplasty is a process of drilling multiple holes through the subchondral bone as described by Pridie in 1959 (172). In addition is the so-called picking or microfracture technique as described by Rodrigo et al. in 1994 (173). Both techniques rely on the bleeding from the subchondral bone to create a fibrin clot and then motion to stimulate transformation to fibrocartilage. It was emphasized that existing cartilage should be debrided back to a stable rim. Postoperative patients were to be restricted from weight bearing, and it was recommended that continuous passive motion should be used postoperatively. In that first study, 46 of the 77 patients did have continuous passive motion for 8 weeks, and that group had an 85% improvement rate versus only 55% in the non-continuous passive motion group. Second-look arthroscopy in this group of patients with the picking procedure did show reparative cartilage with mechanical wear properties closer to hyalin cartilage (174). Long-term result of this technique is still pending, and modern restrictions on cost of care and general fiscal responsibility makes 8 weeks of continuous passive motion difficult to establish.

CARTILAGE REPAIR AND REGENERATION

Osteochondral Transplant

Osteochondral autografting is a more recent innovation in the series of efforts to reestablish functional chondral surface on weight-bearing areas. This involves harvesting osteochondral plugs of apparently normal articular cartilage that are not from primarily weight-bearing areas and transplanting them into chondral or osteochondral defects in the weight-bearing zone. Donor sites are typically taken around the inner edge of the intercondylar notch or from the periphery of the femoral condyles along the areas of the trochlea. There have been limited long-term follow-up studies, but the results have been promising. Outerbridge et al. (175) reported on 10 patients with a 6.5-year average follow-up and all showing excellent results. Other reports have shown similar excellent short-term results using this osteochondral autografting technique (176–178). Because the plugs are osteochondral in nature, they offer structural support for the transposed cartilage surface and heal by osseus ingrowth of the bony portion of the plug. Larger defects have required numerous plugs to fill them, and larger plugs result in more space between the plugs. Approximately 40% of the defect is filled with actual transplanted articular hyalin cartilage and the remaining 60% of the area that is the intervening space between plugs heal with reparative fibrocartilage. It is generally recommended that patients remain non-weight bearing for 6 to 8 weeks after the implantation of the osteochondral plugs.

Some authors have recommended the use of fresh osteochondral allograft tissue from precisely matched donors (179,180). In 5- to 7-year follow-up studies of those patients, 90% have been rated as good to excellent. The procedure does require precise tissue matching, and there is still the potential risk of disease transmission with the use of any allograft tissue.

Chondrocyte Transplantation

Implantation of autologous chondrocytes grown *in vitro* has been studied in the Scandinavian countries and more recently imported into this country. The treatment requires two procedures. The initial procedure is to identify and define the defect area, debride it, and take living cartilage cells for culture. These cells are then cultured *in vitro* to create a paste of living chondrocytes that is subsequently reimplanted under a periosteal patch during the second procedure (181). Animal studies by Brittberg et al. (182) showed excellent results that in turn led to the initiation of human trials. A 2-year follow-up did show 14 of 16 patients with good to excellent results. The longest follow-up now present is 9 years, and again results have been good to excellent with no demonstrable graft failure or evidence of enchondral

ossification (183). The major stumbling blocks to this are that the treatment does require two separate operative interventions, the recovery and maturation of the pouch takes up to 30 months, and the cost of *in vitro* culturing remains high. Although multiple surgeons in the United States have been approved for use of this technique, none of them has enough cases with a long enough follow-up to offer any conclusive data.

OSTEOTOMIES OF THE KNEE

In line with the same principle as previously discussed under varus and valgus unloading braces, it is possible to do a bony realignment of the knee to unload a specific compartment. By shifting the weight from a primarily diseased compartment into a healthier compartment, one can theoretically decrease the symptoms. Although both varus and valgus osteotomies have been described, most unicompartmental knee disease is medial and most high tibial osteotomies are valgus to unload the medial side. Experience has shown that lateral compartment arthritis requiring varus osteotomy of more than 3 to 5 degrees is likely to be more effectively treated by distal femoral osteotomy than by proximal tibial. Although there are multiple studies that describe the efficacy of this procedure, criteria for the procedure, and the possible problems related to it, there are no firm and fast guidelines as yet.

There is no specific age limit for valgus high tibial osteotomy or varus distal femoral osteotomy. Some may say 55 years of age is the upper limit and recommend total knee replacement after that. We have to be aware that the aging population we deal with is also redefining activity levels in the 50s, 60s, and 70s. Those patients who are in good health except for degenerative changes in the knee should be considered as potential osteotomy candidates. Total knee replacement is unacceptable if the patient's desired level of activity would be excluded by following the appropriate postoperative protocol for that operation. Those who desire to be active in jumping, running, twisting, or impact loading activities should be offered a procedure that gives them some chance to get back to that activity level. Those patients who have no significant high-level activity desires but wish to be comfortable with a standard sedentary life-style should seriously consider total knee replacement.

Weight reduction continues to play a major role in patient evaluation and treatment planning. However, obesity has been clearly demonstrated to represent a negative prognostic factor for total knee replacements. It does not seem to have a dramatic impact on the outcome of osteotomies. Patients who are willing to follow a weight-reduction protocol may find that their knee symptoms decrease enough with the loss of weight that they can either delay or permanently avoid any form of major operative intervention (188).

Most authors do include range of motion as a significant factor in preoperative planning. It is generally accepted that a flexion contracture of greater than 15 degrees or flexion of less than 90 degrees make the likelihood of success with osteotomy unacceptably low (189). Rarely, it may be necessary to combine ligament reconstruction and osteotomy in the same patient to relieve arthritic symptoms and instability problems simultaneously (190,191).

If the decision is made to consider distal femoral or high tibial osteotomy, the preoperative planning should include full-length weight-bearing anteroposterior radiographs of the extremity. This allows measurement of the mechanical axis from the center of the femoral head to the center of the tibiotalar joint (192). Using that measurement, it is possible to anticipate the amount of varus or valgus required to bring the knee into the correct alignment position. If the patient demonstrates a dynamic thrust on ambulation, the long x-ray should be taken weight bearing on one limb with the knee in the thrust position for preoperative planning. As noted earlier, a trial of one of the varus or valgus unloader braces also may be beneficial in helping the surgeon decide whether or not this procedure will offer significant benefit.

Proximal Tibial Osteotomy

The proximal or high tibial valgus producing osteotomy, classically described by Coventry (193), is a lateral closing wedge osteotomy. It continues to be the most popular method of high tibial osteotomy today. The procedure involves removing a wedge of bone from the lateral side of the tibial metaphysis with the apex of the wedge all the way at the medial cortex. The medial cortex is weakened by several drill holes but left intact. The space where the wedge was removed is mechanically closed by breaking the tibia over into its new position. The amount of correction is determined by preoperative radiographic planning and is approximately 1 degree per 1 mm of wedge taken. This technique is simple and straightforward. It has a high rate of union because there is a large cancellous surface area (194,195). Multiple different forms of fixation have been used over the years, including casts (196), staples (193), plates and screws (197), and external fixation (198). All forms of fixation do require a postoperative period of limited weight bearing and observation to allow the osteotomy site adequate healing. It has been generally accepted that the postoperative mechanical axis of the limb should run through the middle third of the lateral knee compartment. Adequate correction should be planned to achieve that goal (197). Both undercorrection and overcorrection have been demonstrated to cause less than ideal results (188).

Other than excessive or inadequate correction, the problems most commonly related to high tibial osteotomy are injury of major blood vessels. Reports have implicated the popliteal artery, the posterior tibial artery, and the anterior tibial artery (199). Injuries to the common peroneal nerve, deep peroneal nerve, and superficial peroneal nerve have also been reported (199). Other reports have reflected problems with malunion, nonunion, infection, deep venous thrombosis, stiffness, postoperative knee instability, and continued pain. Most of these problems are related to poor preoperative planning, poor patient selection, or limited technical capability.

The success rate with high tibial osteotomies has varied widely throughout the literature and generally shows a decrease in success rate over a progressive time span. Good to excellent results have been routinely reported for up to 5 years in most patients (200–202). More recent reports have shown results that have remained good to excellent in 63% of patients at 10 to 15 years of follow-up. Although some adult reconstruction surgeons have complained that the closing wedge high tibial osteotomy makes total knee replacement more difficult, those who are accomplished surgeons find that it does not prohibit a good result.

Distal Varus Osteotomy

Although lateral compartment arthritis is less common than medial, it is often more rapidly progressive and can present a difficult surgical challenge. Results with the proximal tibial varus osteotomy have not been as good as valgus osteotomies (204). The recommendation at present is for distal femoral osteotomy to establish varus position as treatment of unicompartmental lateral osteoarthritis of the knee. Two recent studies have demonstrated a favorable result of varus distal femoral osteotomies in more than 90% of patients after a 4-year follow-up (204,205). As with the valgus high tibial osteotomy, there is no specific formula for determining the amount of osteotomy correction. The standing long film should be analyzed to allow enough correction to bring the mechanical axis through the midportion of the medial tibial plateau (206). The literature reflects use of a blade plate as the most effective stabilization technique for distal femoral osteotomy (207). Complications are similar to those reported with high tibial osteotomy with both undercorrection and overcorrection being the most frequent and causing significant problems. A recent report described 57% of 21 patients who underwent distal femoral varus osteotomy as having a significant complication (208).

TOTAL KNEE ARTHROPLASTY

Since the total knee arthroplasty became a common procedure, it has been generally recognized that long-term success rises dramatically if patients are deferred until at least the age of 60. These patients are then counseled postoperatively not to participate in any high-impact loading or torsion-loading activities. They are advised that this would cause premature wear of the polyethylene and/or aseptic loosening of the components. More recent reports demonstrate excellent long-term results in younger patients (209–212). These studies are limited in that they have small numbers and only intermediate duration follow-up. They also include a mixture of patients with inflammatory arthropathies and osteoarthritis. This younger group has demonstrated little regard for recommendations concerning activity status, and many of them have continued to be active in tennis, skiing, and other activities. Although they are cautioned against high-level activities, history has shown that the younger group is less compliant.

Recently, Diduch et al. (213) presented a series of 88 patients with 103 total knee replacements all under the age of 55. This group underwent total knee replacement with a cemented posteriorly stabilized prosthesis and were followed long term. They demonstrated a 94% knee survival rate. Definition of failure was the need to replace one or both components. The patients were also evaluated with an activity score rating. It was noted that 60% of the patients participated in activities requiring high impact such as tennis or downhill skiing. All these patients had failed previous types of treatment and had an average of two surgical procedures before having a total knee arthroplasty. The authors believed that the cemented posteriorly stabilized total knee arthroplasty is a viable option for this younger more active group of patients. Although they recognized that this group would have a more active life-style, they still recommended that patients are counseled against participation in high-impact activities.

REFERENCES

1. Felson DT, Naimark A, Anderson JJ, et al. The prevalence of knee osteoarthritis in the elderly: The Framingham Osteoarthritis Study. *Arthritis Rheum* 1987;30:914–918.
2. Farrell AJ, Blake DR, Balmer RM, et al. Increased concentration of nitrite in synovial fluid and serum samples suggest increased nitric oxide synthesis in rheumatic diseases. *Ann Rheum Dis* 1992;51:1219–1222.
3. Kramer JS, Yelin EH, Epstein WV. Social and economic impacts of four musculoskeletal condition: a study using national community-based data. *J Rheumatol* 1983;26:901–907.
4. Felson DT, Zhang Y, Hanna MT, et al. The incidence and natural history of knee osteoarthritis in the elderly. *Arthritis Rheum* 1995;38:1500–1505.
5. Olivieri Sa, Felson DT, Reed Ji, et al. Incidence of symptomatic hand, hip, and knee osteoarthritis among patients in a health maintenance organization. *Arthritis Rheum* 1995;38:1134–1141.
6. Bagge E, Bjelle A, Valkkenburg HA, et al. Prevalence of radiographic osteoarthritis in two elderly populations. *Rheumatol Int* 1992;12:33–38.
7. Wilson MG, Michet CJ, Ilstrup DM, et al. Idiopathic symptomatic osteoarthritis of the hip and knee: a population-based incidence study. *Mayo Clin Proc* 1990;65:1214–1221.
8. Felson DT. Epidemiology of hip and knee osteoarthritis. *Epidemiol Rev* 1988;10:1–28.
9. Schouten JSAG, van den Ouweland FA, Valkenburg HA. A 12-year follow-up study in the general population on prognostic factors of cartilage loss in osteoarthritis of the knee. *Ann Rheum Dis* 1992;51:932–937.
10. Manninien P, Riihimaki H, Heliovaara M, et al. Overweight, gender and knee osteoarthritis. *Int J Obesity* 1996;20:595–597.
11. Kellegren JR, Lawrence JS. The epidemiology of chronic rheumatism. In: *Atlas of standard radiographs.* Oxford: Blackwell Scientific, 1963.
12. Felson DT, Anderson JJ, Naimark A, et al. Obesity and knee osteoarthritis: the Framingham Study. *Ann Intern Med* 1988;109:18–24.
13. Hart DJ, Spector TD. The relationship of obesity, fat distribution and osteoarthritis in the general population: the Chingford Study. *J Rheumatol* 1993;20:331–335.
14. Hart DJ, Doyle DV, Spector TD. Association between metabolic factors and knee osteoarthritis in women: the Chingford Study. *J Rheumatol* 1995;22:118–1123.
15. Spector TD, Hart DJ, Doyle DV. Incidence and progression of osteoarthritis in women with unilateral knee disease in the general population: the effect of obesity. *Ann Rheum Dis* 1994;53:565–568.
16. Harts AJ, Fischer ME, Bril G, et al. The association of obesity with joint pain and osteoarthritis in the HANES data. *J Chronic Dis* 1986;39:311–319.
17. Davis MA, Ettinger WH, Neuhaus JM, et al. The association of knee injury and obesity with unilateral and bilateral osteoarthritis of the knee. *Am J Epidemiol* 1989;130:278–288.
18. Mankin HJ, Mow VC, Buckwalter JA, et al. Form and function of articular cartilage. In: *Orthopaedic basic science.* Rosemont, IL: American Academy of Orthopaedic Surgeons, 1991.
19. Felson DT, Chaisson CE. Understanding the relationship between body weight and osteoarthritis. *Bailliere's Clin Rheumatol* 1997;11:671–681.
20. Hochberg MC, Letherbridge-Cejku M, Scott WW, et al. The association of body weight, body fatness and body fat distribution with osteoarthritis of the knee: data from the Baltimore longitudinal study of aging. *J Rheumatol* 1995;22:488–493.
21. Cicuttini FM, Spector T, Baker J. Risk factors for osteoarthritis in the tibiofemoral and patellofemoral joints of the knee. *J Rheumatol* 1997;24:1164–1167.
22. Maetzel A, Makela M, Hawker G, et al. Osteoarthritis of the hip and knee and mechanical occupational exposure: a systematic overview of the evidence. *J Rheumatol* 1997;24:1599–1607.
23. Sahlstrom A, Montgomery F. Risk analysis of occupational factors influencing the development of arthrosis of the knee. *Eur J Epidemiol* 1997;13:675–679.
24. Felson DT, Hannan MT, Naimark A, et al. Occupational physical demands, knee bending, and knee osteoarthritis: results form the Framingham study. *J Rheumatol* 1991;128:170–189.
25. Buckwalter JA, Lane NE. Athletics and osteoarthritis. *Am J Sports Med* 1997;25:873–881.
26. Spector TD, Harris PA, Hart DJ, et al. Risk of osteoarthritis associated with long-term weight-bearing sports. *Arthritis Rheum* 1996;39:988–995.
27. Deacon A, Bennell K, Kiss ZS, et al. Osteoarthritis of the knee in retired, elite Australian rules footballers. *Med J Austr* 1997;166:187–190.
28. Buckwalter JA, Lane NE, Gordon SL. Exercise as a cause of osteoarthritis. In: Kuetter KE, Goldberg VM, eds. *Osteoarthritic disorders.* Rosemont, IL: American Academy of Orthopaedic Surgeons, 1995:405–417.
29. Licensee MG, Dang N, Lane NE. Sport practice and osteoarthritis of the limbs. *Osteoarthr Cart* 1997;5:75–86.
30. Lane NE, Bloch DA, Jones HH, et al. Long-distance running, bone density, and osteoarthritis. *JAMA* 1986;255:1147–1151.
31. Lane NE, Michel B, Bjorkengren A, et al. The risk of osteoarthritis with running and aging: a five year longitudinal study. *J Rheumatol* 1993;20:461–468.
32. Rall K, McElroy G, Keats TE. A study of the long term effects of football injury in the knee. *Miss Med* 1984;61:435–438.
33. Newton PM, Mow VC, Gardner TR, et al. The effect of lifelong

exercise on canine articular cartilage. *Am J Sports Med* 1997;
25:282–287.

34. Spector TD, Cicuttini F, Baker J, et al. Genetic influences on osteoarthritis in women: a twin study. *Br J Med* 1996;312:940–943.

35. Chitnavis J, Sinsheimer JS, Clipsham K, et al. Genetic influences in end-stage osteoarthritis. Sibling risks of hip and knee replacements for idiopathic osteoarthritis. *J Bone Joint Surg Br* 1997;79:660–664.

36. Buckwalter JA, Mankin HJ. Articular cartilage. Part I. Tissue design and chondrocyte-matrix interactions. *J Bone Joint Surg Am* 1997;79A:600–611.

37. Buckwalter JA, Mankin HJ. Articular cartilage. Part II. Degeneration and osteoarthrosis, repair, regeneration, and transplantation. *J Bone Joint Surg Am* 1997;79A:612–632.

38. Martin K, Letherbridge-Cejku M, Muller D, et al. Metabolic correlates of obesity and radiographic features of knee osteoarthritis: data from the Baltimore Longitudinal Study of Aging. *J Rheumatol* 1997;24:702–707.

39. Fairbanks TJ. Knee joint changes after meniscectomy. *J Bone Joint Surg Br* 1948;30B:664–670.

40. Cox JS, Nye CE, Schaefer WW, et al. The degenerative effects of partial and total resection of the medial meniscus in dog's knees. *Clin Orthop* 1975;109:178–183.

41. Tapper EM, Hoover NW. Late results after meniscectomy. *J Bone Joint Surg Am* 1969;51A:517–526.

42. Johnson RJ, Kettlekamp DB, Clark W, et al. Factors affecting late results after meniscectomy. *J Bone Joint Surg Am* 1974;56A:719–729.

43. Jackson JP. Degenerative changes in the knee after meniscectomy. *Br Med J* 1968;2:525–527.

44. Allen PR, Denham RA, Swan AV. Late degenerative changes after meniscectomy. *J Bone Joint Surg Br* 1984;66B:666–671.

45. Kurosawa H, Fukubayashi T, Nakajima H. Load-bearing mode of the knee joint. Physical behavior of the knee with or without menisci. *Clin Orthop* 1980;149:283–290.

46. Seedhom BB, Hargreaves DJ. Transmission of load in the knee joint with special reference to the role of the menisci. II. Experimental results, discussion and conclusions. *Eng Med* 1979;8:220–228.

47. Walker PS, Erkman MJ. The role of the meniscal force transmission across the knee. *Clin Orthop* 1975;109:184–192.

48. Bolano LE, Grana WA. Isolated arthroscopic partial meniscectomy. Functional radiographic evaluation at five years. *Am J Sports Med* 1993;21:432–437.

49. Rangger C, Klestil T, Gloetzer, et al. Osteoarthritis after arthroscopic partial meniscectomy. *Am J Sports Med* 1995;23:240–244.

50. Burks RT, Metcalf MH, Metcalf RW. Fifteen-year follow-up of arthroscopic partial meniscectomy. *Arthroscopy* 1997;13:673–679.

51. Maletius W, Messner K. The effect of partial meniscectomy on the long-term prognosis of knees with localized, severe chondral damage. A twelve- to fifteen-year follow-up. *Am J Sports Med* 1996;24:258–262.

52. Matsusue Y, Thomson NL. Arthroscopic partial medial meniscectomy in patients over 40 years old: a 5- to 11-year follow-up study.

53. Covall DJ, Wasilewski SA. Roentgenographic changes after partial meniscectomy: % year follow-up in patients more than 45 years old. *Arthroscopy* 1992;8:242–246.

54. Gillquist J, Oretorp N. Arthroscopic partial meniscectomy. *Clin Orthop* 1982;167:29–33.

55. Fauno P, Neilson AB. Arthroscopic partial meniscectomy: a long-term follow-up. *Arthroscopy* 1992;8:345–349.

56. Funk FJ. Osteoarthritis of the knee following ligamentous injury. *Clin Orthop* 1983;172:154–157.

57. Noyes FR, Mooar PA, Matthews DA, et al. The symptomatic anterior cruciate-deficient knee. Part I. The long-term functional disability in athletically active individuals. *J Bone Joint Surg Am* 1983;65A:154–62.

58. Fetto JF, Marshall JL. The natural history and diagnosis of anterior cruciate ligament insufficiency. *Clin Orthop* 1980;147:29–38.

59. Feagin JA, Lambert KL, Cunningham RR, et al. Consideration of the anterior cruciate ligament injury in skiing. *Clin Orthop* 1987;216:13–18.

60. Arnold JA, Coker TP, Heaton LM, et al. Natural history of anterior cruciate tears. *Am J Sports Med* 1979;7:305–313.

61. McDaniel WJ, Dameron TB. The untreated anterior cruciate ligament rupture. *Clin Orthop* 1983;172:158–163.

62. Pattee GA, Fox JM, Delpizzo W, et al. Four- to Ten-year follow-up of untreated anterior cruciate ligament tears. *Am J Sports Med* 1989;17:430–435.

63. Kannus P, Jarvinen M. Conservatively treated tears of the anterior cruciate ligament. Long-term results. *J Bone Joint Surg Am* 1987;69A:1007–1012.

64. Clancy WG, Ray JM, Zoltan DJ. Acute tears of the anterior cruciate ligament. Surgical versus conservative treatment. *J Bone Joint Surg Am* 1988;70A:1483–1488.

65. Hawkins RJ, Misamore GW, Merritt TR. Follow-up of the acute non-operated isolated anterior cruciate ligament tear. *Am J Sports Med* 1986;14:205–210.

66. Andersson C, Odensten M, Good L, et al. Surgical or non-surgical treatment of the acute rupture of the anterior cruciate ligament. A randomized study with long-term follow-up. *Joint Bone Joint Surg Am* 1989;71A:965–974.

67. Daniel DM, Stone ML, Dobson BE, et al. Fate of the ACL-injured: A prospective outcome study. *Am J Sports Med* 1994;22:632–644.

68. Fithian DC, Luetzow WF. Natural history of the ACL-deficient patient. *Sports Med Arthrosc Rev* 1996;4:319–327.

69. Dehaven KE. Diagnosis of acute knee injuries with hemarthrosis. *Am J Sports Med* 1980;8:9–14.

70. Noyes FR, Bassett RW, Grood ES, et al. Arthroscopy in acute traumatic hemarthrosis of the knee. Incidence of anterior cruciate tears and other injuries. *J Bone Joint Surg Am* 1980;62A:687–695.

71. Rosen MA, Jackson DW, Berger PE. Occult osseous lesions documented by magnetic resonance imaging associated with ACL rupture. *Arthroscopy* 1991;7:45–51.

72. Gillquist J, Hapberg G, Oretorp N. Arthroscopy in acute injuries of the knee joint. *Acta Orthop Scand* 1977;48:190–196.

73. Roos H, Adalberth T, Dahlberg L, et al. Osteoarthritis of the knee after injury to the anterior cruciate ligament or meniscus: the influence of time and age. *Osteoarthr Cart* 1995;3:261–267.

74. Repo RU, Finlay JB. Survival of articular cartilage after controlled impact. *J Bone Joint Surg Am* 1977;59A:1068–1076.

75. Thompson RC, Oegema TR, Lewis JL, et al. Osteoarthritic changes after acute transarticular load: an animal model. *J Bone Joint Surg Am* 1991;73A:990–1001.

76. Spindler KP, Schils JP, Bergfeld JA, et al. Prospective study of osseous, articular, and meniscal lesions in recent anterior cruciate ligament tears by magnetic resonance imaging and arthroscopy. *Am J Sports Med* 1993;21:551–557.

77. Borrelli J, Torzilli PA, Grigiene R, et al. Effect of impact load on articular cartilage: development of an intra-articular fracture model. *J Orthop Trauma* 1997;11:319–326.

78. Newberry WN, Zulkowsky DK, Haut RC. Subfracture insult to a knee joint causes alterations in the bone and in the functional stiffness of the overlying cartilage. *J Orthop Res* 1997;15:450–455.

79. Curl WW, Krome J, Gordon S, et al. Cartilage injuries: a review of 31,516 knee arthroscopies. *Arthroscopy* 1997;13:456–460.

80. McMurray TP. The semilunar cartilages. *Br J Surg* 1941;29:407.

81. Apley AG. The diagnosis of meniscus injuries: some new clinical methods. *J Bone Joint Surg Br* 1929;29B:78.

82. Ricklin P, Ruttiman A, del Buono MS. Meniscal lesions. In: *Practical problems of clinical diagnosis.* New York: Grune & Stratton, 1973.

83. Torg JS, Conrad W, Kalen V. Clinical diagnosis of anterior cruciate ligament instability in the athlete. *Am J Sports Med* 1976;4:84–93.

84. Galway RD, Beaupre A, MacIntosh DL. Pivot shift. *J Bone Joint Surg Br* 1972;54B:763.

85. Losee RE, Johnson TR, Southwick WO. Anterior subluxation of the lateral tibial plateau: a diagnostic test an operative repair. *J Bone Joint Surg Am* 1978;60A:1015–1130.

86. Grood ES, Stowers SF, Noyes FR. Limits of movement in the human knee: effects of sectioning the posterior cruciate ligament

and posterolateral structures. *J Bone Joint Surg Am* 1988;70A:88–97.

87. Greenfield MA, Scott WN. Arthroscopic evaluation and treatment of the patellofemoral joint. *Orthop Clin North Am* 1992;23:587–600.

88. Merchant AC, Mercer RL, Jacobsen RH, et al. Roentgenographic analysis of patellofemoral congruence. *J Bone Joint Surg Am* 1972;56A:1391–1396.

89. Rosenberg TD, Paulos LE, Parker RD, et al. The forty-five degree posteroanterior flexion weight-bearing radiograph of the knee. *J Bone Joint Surg Am* 1988;70A:1479–1483.

90. Aglietti P, Insall JN, Cerulli G. Patellar pain and incongruence. *Clin Orthop* 1983;176:217–224.

91. Blackburne JS, Peel TE. A new method of measuring patella height. *J Bone Joint Surg Br* 1977;59B:241.

92. Insall J, Salvati E. Patella position in the normal knee joint. *Radiology* 1971;101:101–104.

93. Newhouse KE, Rosenberg TD. Basic radiographic examination of the knee. In: Fu F, Harner C, Vince K, eds. *Knee surgery.* Vol. I. Baltimore: Williams & Wilkins, 1994.

94. Blumensatt C. Die Lageabweichungen and Verrenkungen der Kniescheibe. *Ergebn Chir Orthop* 1938;31:149–223.

95. Insall J, Shoji H, Mayer V. High tibial osteotomy. *J Bone Joint Surg Am* 1974;56A:1397–1405.

96. Kornick J, Trefelner E, McCarthy S, et al. Meniscal abnormalities in the asymptomatic population at MR imaging. *Radiology* 1990;177:463–465.

97. Hodler J, Haghighi P, Pathria NM, et al. Meniscal changes in the elderly: correlation of MR imaging. *Radiology* 1992;184:221–225.

98. Chan WP, Lang P, Stevens MP, et al. Osteoarthritis of the knee: comparison of radiography, CT and MR imaging to assess extent and severity. *AJR Am J Roentgenol* 1991;157:799–806.

99. Speer KP, Spritzer CE, Goldner JL, et al. Magnetic resonance imaging of traumatic knee articular cartilage injuries. *Am J Sports Med* 1991;19:396–402.

100. McGoey BV, Deitel M, Saplys RFJ, et al. Effect of weight loss on musculoskeletal pain in the morbidly obese. *J Bone Joint Surg Br* 1990;72B:322–323.

101. Williams RA, Foulsham BM. Weight reduction in osteoarthritis using phentermine. *Practitioner* 1981;225:231–232.

102. Felson DT, Zhang Y, Hannan MT, et al. Risk factors for incident radiographic knee osteoarthritis in the elderly: the Framingham study. *Arthritis Rheum* 1997;40:728–733.

103. Doucett SA, Goble EM. The effect of exercise on patellar tracking in lateral patellar compression syndrome. *Am J Sports Med* 1992;20:434–440.

104. O'Neill DB, Micheli LJ, Warner JP. Patellofemoral stress: a prospective analysis of exercise treatment in adolescents and adults. *Am J Sports Med* 1992;20:151–156.

105. Kovar PA, Allegrante JP, Mackenzie CR, et al. Supervised fitness walking in patients osteoarthritis of the knee. A randomized, controlled trial. *Ann Intern Med* 1992;116:529–534.

106. Fransen M, Margiotta E, Crosbie J, et al. A revised group exercise program for osteoarthritis of the knee. *Physiother Res Int* 1997;2:30–41.

107. Fisher NM, White SC, Yack HJ, et al. Muscle function and gait in patients with knee osteoarthritis before and after muscle rehabilitation. *Disabil Rehabil* 1997;19:47–55.

108. Pujalte JM, Llavore EP, Ylescupidez. Double-blind clinical evaluation of oral glucosamine sulphate in the basic treatment of osteoarthrosis. *Curr Med Res Opin* 1980;7:110–114.

109. D'Ambrosio E, Casa B, Bompani R, et al. Glucosamine sulphate: a controlled clinical investigation in arthrosis. *Pharmatherapeutica* 1981;2:504–508.

110. Vajaradul Y. Double-blind clinical evaluation of intra-articular glucosamine in outpatients with gonarthrosis. *Clin Therap* 1981;3:336–343.

111. Reichelt A, Forster KK, Fischer M, et al. Efficacy and safety of intramuscular glucosamine sulfate in osteoarthritis of the knee. A randomized, placebo-controlled double-blind study. *Arzneimittelforschung* 1994;44:75–80.

112. Crolle G, D'Este E. Glucosamine sulphate for the management of arthrosis: a controlled clinical investigation. *Curr Med Res Opin* 1980;7:104–109.

113. Tapadinhas MJ, Rivera IC, Bignamini AA. Oral glucosamine sulphate in the management of arthrosis: report on a multi-centre open investigation in Portugal. *Pharmatherapeutica* 1982;3:157–168.

114. Noack Osteoarthritis Cartilage 1994.

115. Lopes-Vas A. Double-blind clinical evaluation of the relative efficacy of ibuprofen and glucosamine sulphate in the management of osteoarthrosis of the knee in outpatients. *Curr Med Res Opin* 1982;8:145–149.

116. Müller-Fassbender H, et al. Glucosamine sulphate compared to ibuprofen in osteoarthritis of the knee. *Osteoarthr Cart* 1994;2:61–69.

117. Williams HJ, Ward JR, Egger MJ, et al. Comparison of naproxen and acetaminophen in a two-year study of treatment of osteoarthritis of the knee. *Arthritis Rheum* 1993;36:1196–1206.

118. Bradley JD, Brandt KD, Katz BP, et al. Comparison of an anti-inflammatory dose of ibuprofen, an analgesic dose of ibuprofen, and acetaminophen in the treatment of patients with osteoarthritis of the knee. *N Engl J Med* 1991;325:87–91.

119. Jimenez SA. *The effects of glucosamine on human chondrocyte gene expression.* Madrid, Spain: The Ninth Eular Symposium, 1996:8–10.

120. Hochberg MC, Altman RD, Brandt KD, et al. Guidelines for the medical management of osteoarthritis. Part II. Osteoarthritis of the knee. *Arthritis Rheum* 1995;38:1541–1546.

121. Moskowitz R. The appropriate use of NSAID's in arthritic conditions. *Am J Orthop* 1996;[Suppl]:4–6.

122. Dupuy DE, Spillane RM, Rosol MS, et al. Quantification of articular cartilage in the knee with three-dimensional MR imaging. *Acta Radiol* 1996;3:919–924.

123. Hollander JL. Intra-articular hydrocortisone in arthritis and allied conditions. *J Bone Joint Surg Am* 1953;35A:983–990.

124. Hollander JL, Jesser RA, Brown RR. Intrasynovial corticosteroid therapy: a decade of use. *Bull Rheumatol Dis* 1961;11:239–240.

125. Dieppe P, Sathapatayavongs B, Jones H, et al. Intra-articular steroids in osteoarthritis. *Rheumatol Rehabil* 1980;19:212–217.

126. Friedman D, Moore M. The efficacy of intra-articular steroids in osteoarthritis: a double-blind study. *J Rheumatol* 1980;7:850–856.

127. Gaffney IC, et al. Intra-articular triamcinolone hexacetonide in knee osteoarthritis: factors influencing the clinical response. *Ann Rheumatol Dis* 1995;54:379–381.

128. Jones A, Doherty M. Intra-articular corticosteroids are effective in osteoarthritis but there are no clinical predictors of response. *Ann Rheumatol Dis* 1996;55:829–832.

129. Balazs EA, Watson D, Duff IF, et al. Hyaluronic acid in synovial fluid. Molecular parameters of hyaluronic acid in normal and arthritic human synovial fluid. *Arthritis Rheum* 1967;10:357–376.

130. Peyron JG. Intra-articular hyaluronan injections in the treatment of osteoarthritis: state-of-the-art review. *J Rheumatol* 1993;20[Suppl 39]:10–15.

131. Adams ME, Atkinson MH, Lussier AJ, et al. The role of viscosupplementation with hylan G-F 20 (Synvisc) in the treatment of osteoarthritis of the knee: a Canadian multicenter trial comparing hylan G-F 20 alone, hylan G-F 20 with nonsteroidal anti-inflammatory drugs (NSAID's) and NSAID's alone. *Osteoarthr Cart* 1995;3:213–225.

132. Dixon A, Jacoby R, Berry H, et al. Clinical trial of intra-articular injection of sodium hyaluronate in patients with osteoarthritis of the knee. *Curr Med Res Opin* 1988;11:205–213.

133. Grecomoro G, Martorana U, Di Marco C. Intra-articular injection with sodium hyaluronate in gonarthrosis; a controlled clinical trial versus placebo. *Pharmatherapeutica* 1987;5:137–141.

134. Dahlberg L, Lohmander LS, Ryd L. Intra-articular injections of hyaluronan in patients with cartilage abnormalities and knee pain. *Arthritis Rheum* 1994;37:521–528.

135. Henderson EB, Smith EC, Pegley F, Blake DR. Intra-articular injections of 750 KD hyaluronan in the treatment of osteoarthritis: a randomized single centre double-blind placebo-controlled trial of 91 Patients demonstrating lack of efficacy. *Ann Rheumatol Dis* 1994;53:529–534.

136. Lohmander LS, Dalen N, Englund G, et al. Intra-articular injections in the treatment of osteoarthritis of the knee: a randomized,

double blind, placebo controlled multicentre trial. *Hyaluronan Multicentre Trial Group. Ann Rheumatol Dis* 1996;55:424–431.

137. Wu JJ, Shih LY, Hsu HC, et al. The double-blind test of sodium hyaluronate (ARTZ) on osteoarthritis of the knee. *Chin Med J* 1997;59:99–106.

138. Pietrogrande V, Melanotte P, D'Angelo B, et al. Hyaluronic acid versus methylprednisolone intra-articularly injected for treatment of osteoarthritis of the knee. *Curr Therap Res* 1991;50:691–700.

139. Leardini G, Mattara L, Franceschini M, et al. Intra-articular treatment of knee arthritis: a comparative study between hyaluronic acid and 6-methylprednisolone acetate. *Clin Exp Rheumatol* 1991;9:375–381.

140. Albach S. Osteoarthosis of the knee: a radiographic investigation. *Acta Radiol* 1968;277[Suppl]:7–72.

141. Prodromas CC, Andiacchi TP, Galante JO. A relationship between gait and clinical changes following high tibial osteotomy. *J Bone Joint Surg Am* 1985;67A:1188–1194.

142. Sasaki T, Yasuda K. Clinical evaluation of the treatment of osteoarthritic knees using a newly designed wedged insole. *Clin Orthop* 1987;221:181–187.

143. Yasuda K, Sasaki T. The mechanics of treatment of the osteoarthritic knee with a wedged insole. *Clin Orthop* 1987;221:181–187.

144. Keating EM, Faris PM, Ritter MA, et al. Use of a lateral heel and sole wedges in the treatment of medial osteoarthritis of the knee. *Orthop Rev* 1993;921–924.

145. Pollo FE. Bracing and heel wedging for unicompartmental osteoarthritis of the knee. *Am J Knee Surg* 1998;11:47–50.

146. Pollo FE, Otis JC, Wickiewicz TL, et al. Biomechanical analysis of valgus bracing for the osteoarthritic knee. *Gait Posture* 1994;2:63.

147. Lindenfeld TN, Hewett TE, Andriachhi TP. Joint loading with valgus bracing in patients with varus gonarthrosis.

148. Bowton EJ, Hoffinger SA, Larson RV, et al. Kinetic analysis of medial hinge knee brace for medial compartment gonarthrosis. *Orthop Trans* 1994;18:910–911.

149. Matsuno H, Kadowaki KM, Tsuji H. Generation II knee bracing for severe medial compartment osteoarthritis of the knee. *Arch Phys Med Rehabil* 1997;78:745–749.

150. Horlick SG, Loomer RL. Valgus knee bracing for the osteoarthritic knee. *Clin J Sports Med* 1993;3:251–255.

151. Hewett TE, Noyes FR, Barber-Westin SD, et al. Decrease in knee joint pain and increase in function in patients with medial compartment arthrosis: a prospective analysis of valgus bracing. *Orthopaedics* 1998;21:131–138.

152. Burman MS, Finkelstein H, Mayer L. Arthroscopy of the knee joint. *J Bone Joint Surg* 1934;16:25–32.

153. Watanabe M, Takeda S, Ikeuchi H. *Atlas of arthroscopy.* Tokyo, Japan: Igaku Shoin, 1957.

154. Baumgaertener MR, Cannon WD, Vittori JM, et al. Arthroscopic debridement of the arthritic knee. *Clin Orthop* 1990;253:197–202.

155. Ogilvie-Harris DJ, Fitsialos DP. Arthroscopic management of the degenerative knee. *J Arthroscopy* 1991;7:151–157.

156. Jackson RW, Gilbert JE, Sharkey PF. Arthroscopic debridement versus arthroplasty in the osteoarthritic knee. *J Arthroplasty* 1997;12:465–470.

157. Goldman RT, Scuderi GR, Kelly MA. Arthroscopic treatment of the degenerative knee in older athletes. *Clin Sports Med* 1997;16:51–68.

158. Jackson RW, Rouse DW. The results of partial arthroscopic meniscectomy in patients over 40 years of age. *J Bone Joint Surg Br* 1982;64B:481–485.

159. Edelson R, Burks RT, Bloebaum RD. Short-term effects of knee washout for osteoarthritis *Am J Sports Med* 1995;23:345–349.

160. Livesley PJ, Doherty M, Needorf M, et al. Arthroscopic lavage of osteoarthritic knee. *J Bone Joint Surg Br* 1991;73:922–926.

161. Moseley JB, Wray NP, Kuykendall D, et al. Arthroscopic treatment of osteoarthritis of the knee: a prospective, randomized, placebo-controlled trial. *Am J Sports Med* 1996;24:28–34.

162. Magnuson PB. Joint debridement: surgical treatment of degenerative arthritis. *Surg Gynecol Obstet* 1941;73:1–9.

163. Sprague NF. Arthroscopic debridement for degenerative knee joint disease. *Clin Orthop* 1981;160:118–123.

164. Bert JM, Maschka K. The arthroscopic treatment of unicompart-

mental gonarthrosis: a five-year follow-up study of abrasion arthroplasty plus arthroscopic debridement and arthroscopic debridement alone. *J Arthroscopy* 1989;5:25–32.

165. Gross DE, Brenner SL, Esformes I, et al. Arthroscopic treatment of degenerative joint disease of the knee. *Orthopedics* 1991;14:1317–1321.

166. Rand JA. Role of arthroscopy in osteoarthritis of the knee. *J Arthroscopy* 1991;7:358–363.

167. Jackson RW, Silver R, Marans H. Arthroscopic treatment of degenerative joint disease. *J Arthroscopy* 1986;2:114.

168. Mankin HJ. The response of articular cartilage to mechanical injury. *J Bone Joint Surg* 1982;64:460–466.

169. Chandler EJ. Abrasion arthroplasty of the knee. *Contemp Orthop* 1985;11:21–29.

170. Friedman MJ, Berasi CC, Fox JM, et al. Preliminary results with abrasion arthroplasty in the osteoarthritic knee. *Clin Orthop* 1984;182:200–205.

171. Johnson LL. Arthroscopic abrasion arthroplasty. Historical and pathological perspective: present status. *J Arthroscopy* 1986;2:54–69.

172. Pridie AH. A method of resurfacing osteoarthritic knee joints. *J Bone Joint Surg Br* 1959;41:618.

173. Rodrigo JJ, Steadman JR, Silliman JF, et al. Improvement of full thickness chondral defect healing in the human knee after debridement and microfracture using continuous passive motion. *Am J Knee Surg* 1994;7:109–116.

174. Rodkey WG, McIlwraith CW, Frisbie JT, et al. Microfracture technique to treat chondral defects in a large animal model: histology, biochemistry and molecular biology. Steadman-Hawkins Sports Medicine Fellows conference, 1997.

175. Outerbridge HK, Outerbridge AR, Outerbridge RE. The use of lateral patellar autologous graft for the repair of a large osteochondral defect in the bone. *J Bone Joint Surg Am* 1995;77A:595–606.

176. Bobic V. Arthroscopic osteochondral autograft transplantation in anterior cruciate ligament reconstruction. A preliminary clinical study. *Knee Surg Sports Traumatol Arthrosc* 1996;3:262–264.

177. Hangody L, Sukosd L, Szigeti I, et al. Arthroscopic autogenous osteochondral mosaicplasty. *Hung J Orthop Trauma* 1996;39:49–54.

178. Matsusue Y, Yamamuro T, Hama H. Case report: arthroscopic multiple osteochondral transplantation to the chondral defect in the knee associated with anterior cruciate ligament disruption. *Arthroscopy* 1993;9:214–216.

179. Garrett JC, Kress KJ, Mudano M. Osteochondritis dissecans of the lateral femoral condyle in the adult. *Arthroscopy* 1992;8:474–481.

180. Convery Fr, Meyers MH, Akeson WH. Fresh osteochondral allografting of the femoral condyle. *Clin Orthop* 1991;273:139–145.

181. Mankin HJ. Chondrocyte transplantation-one answer to an old question. *N Engl J Med* 1994;331:940–941.

182. Brittberg M, Lindahl A, Nilsson A, et al. Treatment of deep cartilage defects in the knee with autologous chondrocyte implantation. *N Engl J Med* 1994;331:889–895.

183. Minas T, Nehre S. Current concepts in the treatment of articular cartilage defects. *Orthopaedics* 1997;20:525–538.

184. Outerbridge RE. The etiology of chondromalacia patellae. *J Bone Joint Surg Br* 1961;43B:752–757.

185. Casscells SW. Gross pathological changes in the knee joint of the aged individual: a study of 300 cases. *Clin Orthop* 1978;132:225–232.

186. Insall J. The Pridie debridement operation for osteoarthritis of the knee. *Clin Orthop* 1974;101:61–67.

187. Noyes FR, Stabler CL. A system for grading articular cartilage lesions at arthroscopy. *Am J Sports Med* 1989;17:505–513.

188. Matthew LS, Goldstein SA, Malvitz TA, et al. Proximal tibial osteotomy: factors that influence the duration of satisfactory function. *Clin Orthop* 1988;229:193–200.

189. Phillips MJ, Krakow KA. High tibial osteotomy and distal femoral osteotomy for valgus or varus deformity around the knee. *AAOS Instruct Course Lect* 1998;47:429–436.

190. Noyes FR, Barber SD, Simon R. High tibial osteotomy and ligament reconstruction in varus angulated, anterior cruciate liga-

ment-deficient knees. A two-to seven-year follow-up study. *Am J Sports Med* 1993;21:2–12.

191. Neuschwander DC, Drez D Jr, Paine RM. Simultaneous high tibial osteotomy and ACL reconstruction for combined genu varum and symptomatic ACL tear. *Orthopaedics* 1993;16: 679–684.

192. Hsu RWW, Himeno S, Coventry MB, et al. Normal axial alignment of the lower extremity and load-bearing distribution at the knee. *Clin Orthop* 1990;255:215–227.

193. Coventry MB. Osteotomy of the upper tibia for degenerative arthritis of the knee: a preliminary report. *J Bone Joint Surg Am* 1965;47A:984–990.

194. Murphy SB. Tibial osteotomy for genu varum: indications, preoperative planning, and technique. *Orthop Clin North Am* 1994; 25:477–482.

195. Paley D, Maar DC, Herzenberg JE. New concepts in high tibial osteotomy for medial compartment osteoarthritis. *Orthop Clin North Am* 1994;25:483–498.

196. Insall J, Shoji H, Mayer V. High tibial osteotomy. *J Bone Joint Surg Am* 1974;56A:1397–1405.

197. Miniacci A, et al. Proximal tibial osteotomy. A new fixation device. *Clin Orthop* 1989;246:250–259.

198. Grill F. Correction of complicated extremity deformities by external fixation. *Clin Orthop* 1989;241:166–176.

199. Handal EG, Morawski DR, Santore RF. Complications of high tibial osteotomy. In: Fu F, Harner CD, Vance KG, eds. *Knee surgery*. Vol. II. Baltimore: Williams & Wilkins, 1994.

200. Coventry MB. Osteotomy about the knee for degenerative and rheumatoid arthritis: indications, operative technique, and results. *J Bone Joint Surg Am* 1973;55A:23–48.

201. Insall JN, Joseph DM, Msiak C. High tibial osteotomy for varus gonarthrosis: a long-term follow-up study. *J Bone Joint Surg Am* 1984;66A:1040–1048.

202. Healy WL, Riley LH Jr. High tibial valgus osteotomy: a clinical review. *Clin Orthop* 1986;209:227–233.

203. Yasuda K, Majima T, Tsuchida T, et al. A ten- to fifteen-year follow-up observation of high tibial osteotomy in medial compartment osteoarthrosis. *Clin Orthop* 1992;282:186–195.

204. Healy WL, Anglen JO, Wasilewski SA, et al. Distal femoral varus osteotomy. *J Bone Joint Surg Am* 1988;70A:102–109.

205. McDermott AG, Finklestein JA, Farine, et al. Distal femoral varus osteotomy for valgus deformity of the knee. *J Bone Joint Surg Am* 1988;70A:110–116.

206. Morrey BF, Edgerton BC. Distal femoral osteotomy for lateral gonarthrosis. In: Eilbert E, ed. *Instructional course lectures XLI.* Rosemont, IL: American Academy of Orthopaedic Surgeons, 1992:77–85.

207. Healy WL, Wasilewski SA, Krakow KA. Distal femoral varus osteotomy for the painful valgus knee. *Techn Orthop* 1989; 4:47–52.

208. Mathews J, Cobb AG, Richardson S, et al. Distal femoral osteotomy for lateral compartment osteoarthritis of the knee. *Orthopaedics* 1998;21:437–438.

209. Dalury DE, Ewald FC, Christie MJ, et al. Total knee arthroplasty in a group of patients less than 45 years of age. *J Arthroplasty* 1995;10:598–602.

210. Ewald FC, Christie MJ. Results of cemented total knee replacement in young patients. *Orthop Trans* 1987;11:442.

211. Hungerford DS, Krackow KA, Kenna RV. Cementless total knee replacement in patients 50 years old and under. *Orthop Clin North Am* 1989;20:131–145.

212. Stuart MJ, Rand JA. Total knee arthroplasty in the young adult. *Orthop Trans* 1987;11:441–442.

213. Diduch DR, Insall JN, Scott WN, et al. Total knee replacement in young, active patients: long-term follow-up and functional results. *J Bone Joint Surg Am* 1997;79A:575–582.

Principles and Practice of Orthopaedic Sports Medicine,
edited by William E. Garrett, Jr., Kevin P. Speer, and Donald T. Kirkendall.
Lippincott Williams & Wilkins, Philadelphia © 2000.

CHAPTER 48

Anterior Cruciate Ligament Functional Bracing

Edward M. Wojtys

The use of braces to protect the anterior cruciate ligament (ACL)-deficient or -reconstructed knee has changed substantially over the past 30 years. Initially, the goal of an ACL brace was to replace the function of the injured ligament. As reconstructive procedures improved through the 1980s and 1990s, the role of the ACL brace has evolved. ACL braces are now more often used to provide protection for ACL grafts or partially torn ligaments. Replacing the function of the ACL and protecting an ACL substitute are variants of the same goal: decreasing ACL strain by controlling tibial–femoral motion. To replace the function of an ACL, a brace must limit anterior tibial translation (ATT) and internal/external tibial rotation. Protection of an ACL graft might be accomplished by the same motion-limiting mechanisms, but the degree of needed "brace effect" may be less. ACL graft protection might be accomplished by partially limiting tibial–femoral motion and thus simply dampening the forces transmitted to the ACL. ACL graft protection might also be accomplished by augmenting other protective mechanisms such as the neuromuscular response to impact forces or tibial torques. Completely replacing the function of an ACL with a brace appears to be a much more formidable task, probably an unattainable one. All these factors and limitations deserve consideration in defining the role of the functional knee brace today.

In light of this dual role for ACL functional bracing (replacement or protection), it is helpful to initially discuss why brace an ACL-injured or -reconstructed knee in the first place. The most common response is usually to maintain tibiofemoral stability. Part of the stability goal is to prevent giving-way episodes of the tibial–femoral joint by limiting abnormal ATT and/or rotation. The short-term goal of preventing increased ATT and

giving-way episodes should keep the patient from falling or sustaining further damage to menisci and hyaline cartilage. The long-term goal of these efforts to maintain tibial–femoral stability is preventing further or accelerated degenerative change.

An obstacle to accomplishing these bracing goals that manufacturers still confront in 1998 is the fact that we still do not know what forces an ACL experiences *in vivo,* either for activities of daily living or sports. This factor makes it difficult to judge what level of function a brace must provide in replacing or protecting an injured ACL. Although we are slowly gaining information about strain values and force levels during basic rehabilitation exercises (1), no doubt those seen during contact sports and peak athletic performance will be much higher. This information is desperately needed by the brace industry to confirm the efficacy of bracing.

To achieve the goals of ACL replacement or ACL graft protection, brace testing today must be performed under conditions similar to those found *in vivo.* We must consider the specific situation under which a brace will be asked to perform, keeping in mind the demands of the ACL-deficient knee will be different than those of a partially injured cruciate and those will also be different than a reconstructed ligament. Chronic injuries with secondary restraint laxity will also pose more of a challenge than the acutely injured isolated ligament tear. Also, biomechanical and physiologic factors can and do change over time, meaning the role of the brace may need to change. The acute injury situation, the postoperative scenario, and the return to full activity can all present different challenges. The level of activity in which the brace will be used must also be kept in mind. Will the brace be used in the rehabilitation setting under low or high forces? Will there be full weight bearing or protected weight bearing? Is the brace for activities of daily living or for sports competition? All these factors have implications in terms of the stresses and strains placed on the ligament, menisci, and joint surfaces. Finally, to be effective, the performance of the brace must

E. M. Wojtys: MedSport, Department of Surgery, University of Michigan, Ann Arbor, Michigan 48106.

accelerate with the function of the patient. Therefore, researchers need to be very specific when approaching these activity and sport-specific problems. Manufacturers need to identify which activities braces are produced for. With these parameters in focus, the role of ACL functional bracing can be more clearly defined.

All through these efforts to redefine the role of ACL functional use, care must be taken to identify potential problems with brace use (2). We must look for signs of muscle inhibition, increased strain on ligaments, and so on to make sure these devices do not place brace users at increased risk for other problems.

Unfortunately in some situations, the brace may provide a false sense of security for both patient and the physician. Caution should be exercised in athletic participation in cutting and jumping sports. Currently, there is little science available to justify a return to vigorous sports participation with a braced unstable knee.

Finally, what physicians, therapists, trainers, and patients need is proof that braces actually do work. In a time of increased competition for the health care dollar, brace efficacy must be well documented. Manufacturers need to provide evidence for their claims of function. Brace prescribers and purchasers should demand high-quality proof of function and not settle for anecdotal testimonials from professional athletes.

HOW CAN A BRACE WORK?

Initially, most braces were designed to limit tibial–femoral motion. The hope was that the brace could serve as a mechanical restraint to the increased ATT and rotation experienced after ACL rupture. Unfortunately, this has become a very difficult task for bracing. It is complicated by the fact that the femur, and to a lesser extent the tibia, is encompassed in a soft tissue envelope containing primarily muscle. Depending on the level of activity of the muscle and the physical abilities of the patient, the musculature may or may not be able to respond and stiffen itself and the knee joint when needed. Because muscle sits in the interface between the bony tibia and femur and the brace, its stiffness is critically important to the performance of a brace designed to limit tibial–femoral motion. The best way for a brace to control tibial–femoral motion would be by direct attachment to both the femur and tibia. Because this is not feasible, the soft tissue envelope that encompasses the femur and tibia must be dealt with. Unfortunately, this envelope is dynamic, changing with training and various activities. It can also be drastically altered by injury and/or surgery. This soft tissue envelope frequently atrophies with disuse and then hypertrophies with training and conditioning. Knee joint pain and swelling will also alter muscle response and performance. Because of these factors and others, it is important to recognize that this soft tissue envelope, which is

usually primarily muscle, provides a varying interface for the brace. Consequently, brace performance is directly related to soft tissue stiffness and to muscle performance. Conversely, the opposite may also be true: Muscle performance may be dependent on brace performance (2).

A second brace function mechanism that is often discussed is the augmentation of proprioception (3–5). The ACL is not merely a static restraint, but it also provides mechanoreceptor afferent input to the central nervous system necessary for muscle protection of the knee joint (6). When the ACL is torn, this function is lost, and other systems may be recruited to perform the same function (7). This proprioceptive function is mentioned in the brace literature and is the target of some bracing efforts. Unfortunately, proprioception is for the most part a static phenomenon. It is very difficult to change individual proprioceptive abilities. Although training and conditioning may very well improve the awareness of afferent input, it is unlikely the afferent impulse expands or multiplies with "proprioceptive training." The afferent portion of this system is not capable of expansion for the most part. Although some evidence shows that one portion of the afferent system (muscle spindles) can be modulated, the rest of the afferent receptor system does not appear to change with training and conditioning. The motor (efferent) portion of this system does have the capacity to change; however, most studies of muscle performance with brace use are mixed in their results at best (2,8–10). Most studies that examine isokinetic performance indicate little, if any, improvement with brace use (2,10,11). Because the afferent limb of the proprioceptive loop is very limited in its capacity to expand its function and because the efferent or motor segment has not shown significant improvement with brace use (2), it is unlikely that bracing can augment proprioception. Although some functional activities may benefit from brace use, it is difficult to assign that positive change to augmented proprioception.

BRACE DESIGN

Several research studies indicate that the shell bilateral postdesign probably functions the best on the ACL-deficient knee (2,12–16). The shell design provides the most brace limb contact thought to improve function and comfort. Despite all the attention given to the hinge configuration (14), it is questionable whether these make a real difference in brace function (17). In fact, hinge position is probably more important than hinge design (16,17). This fact is due primarily to the compliant nature of the thigh and leg compartments. If these were solid composites, then the hinge design would be more important and would probably need to closely mimic knee motion (a combination of sliding and gliding). Because of the soft tissue compliance of those compartments, the hinge design probably has little effect on tibial translation and rotation control. However, hinges may play a role in the level of comfort by affecting the amount of pistoning that occurs with rigorous brace use.

For a brace to function effectively, it must be fit well. Obviously, some body types and shapes are more difficult to brace due to their configuration and frequently present bracing challenges. Many times, if the brace is going to provide some function, multiple adjustments and possibly refabrications are needed to achieve optimal fit. The need for readjustment and fine tuning should be discussed with the patient from the start of brace use. Otherwise, the patient may become frustrated with the effort needed to get a brace to fit and subsequently work. This frustration may lead to a failure to realize the benefits of brace use.

Even if the brace fits well statically, it must stay in good proximal–distal orientation during activities to function properly. If a brace easily migrates proximally or distally, it may piston and become uncomfortable with activities. When this happens, patients are likely to discard the device. Research work that monitored brace position with exercise has shown a disturbing amount of migration with some braces (2). Interestingly, the custom braces tested did not outperform off-the-shelf braces in proximal–distal migration with exercise, making the extra cost of the custom brace difficult to justify (2,17). When a brace migrates and its rotation axis moves farther away from that of the knee, it most likely will become ineffective and uncomfortable.

Another factor to consider in brace design is the ability of the ACL brace to produce a posterior tibial force (8). Braces that produce a posterior tibial load are frequently described as "dynamic," the thought being that this should lead to added benefit in resisting ATT with posterior tibial loading. Cadaver work supports these contentions (18). Interestingly, *in vivo* work on some braces does not seem to agree. Beynnon's work used posterior loads of 45 and 22 N to investigate this effect. In all testing conditions used in that study (anterior loading with and without weight bearing and internal and external rotation testing), there were no differences in ACL strain between the two strap tensions (45 and 22 N) used to produce a posterior tibial load. These results raise the question of whether a counteractive posterior tibial load can produce a beneficial effect *in vivo* in an ACL-reconstructed or -deficient knee.

SUBJECTIVE REPORTS

The most positive area of the brace literature is the subjective reports of function. How much emphasis should be placed on these reports is open to debate. A positive approach by the brace user is helpful, but it

may not be enough to justify the cost of bracing today. In reality, the positive subjective feeling experienced while wearing a brace should be buoyed by objective proof of brace function. When this proof of function is not present, the brace prescriber must consider the possibility that a false sense of security may be given to the patient, possibly leading to an increased chance of further injury. Most clinicians would agree that an ACL functional brace should never be used as a substitute for adequate muscle rehabilitation after injury and/or surgery. Unfortunately, this scenario is all too frequent. A less than adequately rehabilitated patient after injury and/or surgery believes he or she can return to rigorous sports with a brace. Reinjury is often the result. When reinjury does not occur, the brace is often given credit for the successful result without consideration of other factors such as the level of neuromuscular protection the patient is able to provide. Although it is obvious to most that many patients feel much more confident about their abilities in the brace, it is also clear that no brace can replace adequate rehabilitation in terms of strength, power, speed, and agility. This particular clinical situation is all too frequent in this day of aggressive rehabilitation and early attempts to return to sports after ACL reconstruction. Unfortunately, the price paid for such judgment errors can be formidable and long lasting.

After the introduction of the Lenox-Hill knee brace in the early 1970s, Nicholas (19) was one of the first to report the positive subjective findings using the Lenox-Hill brace, stating that "many patients did not wish to have surgical treatment after their instability was controlled by the brace." Bassett and Fleming (20) and Colville et al. (21) echoed the same positive reports of Nicholas. Mishra et al. (22), however, was the most enthusiastic, reporting that 85% of brace users eliminated their episodes of giving away.

A close look at the report by Bassett and Fleming (20) showed that 81% of the patients had an improved anterior drawer and all had an improved Lachman test. Unfortunately, 70% of these patients continued to complain of subluxation episodes in the brace.

The review by Colville et al. (21) of 45 patients showed that 70% reported improved athletic performance in the brace, whereas 91% thought that it was beneficial to them. The most important finding in this study was that the absolute laxity of the ACL-deficient knee was unchanged by the brace but that the relative resistance to anterior displacement was increased. This finding offers insight into how some knee braces may improve function today. Although the braces are incapable of eliminating all abnormal ATT and tibial rotation, they may be able to increase the overall stiffness of the limb. This overall increase in the stiffness across the knee joint may represent the best explanation of brace function.

From these subjective reports, it is clear that some individuals do find braces helpful. The most important question becomes, by what mechanism is this positive influence provided? This positive effect is especially prevalent when the activities performed do not require jumping, pivoting, or deceleration. Knee bracing will undoubtedly be more successful with "in-line" activities that do not include pivoting or jumping because the risks of tibial subluxation are not as high.

Patients frequently look at braces as an insurance policy against recurrent injury. Many feel "protected" in the brace and refuse to participate in vigorous activities without their brace. In today's liability-minded society, the brace prescriber is frequently placed in a hazardous position regardless of his or her view of brace function. The treating physician may even be pressured into prescribing braces despite the lack of adequate proof of function in many situations. However, refusing to brace a patient that requests bracing is probably an unwise course to follow. Educating the patient about knee protection and the limitations of brace function is a good first step. After that, the patient may be in the best position to help decide whether or not to brace. If a patient is still convinced that a brace is important for protection, it is probably unwise to refuse such treatment. Essential to such discussions are the facts about knee injury rates with and without bracing. Relevant to those discussions may be the work of Tegner and Lorentzon (23), who reviewed the knee injury rates of 600 elite Swedish hockey players. They concluded that there was no difference in knee injury rates with or without knee brace use.

The possibility that a brace may give an athlete a false sense of security that could create hazardous situations must be kept in mind in discussions with parents, coaches, and agents. Discussing these factors with athletes who are attempting to return to play after injury and/or operation should be routine. Failure to do so may create an uncomfortable situation if injury occurs. Providing the athlete with the limitations of brace function and what must be present in terms of muscle function to protect a knee is essential in decision making about braces.

Along these lines, there are several well-known professional athletes who are inseparable from their knee orthoses on the field of play, a fact that we and our patients are constantly bombarded with by the brace-marketing features. Keep in mind that it is unknown by most what problem is being treated with the brace in these situations. Frequently, it is unclear what degree or severity of injury is present. Many athletes wear braces prophylactically, giving the injured patient a false sense of what bracing can do. Second, most professionals have tremendous neuromuscular abilities, making comparisons with injured normal patients unrealistic. Just because elite athletes are seen using a particular device does not mean that that device is the explanation for their success.

OBJECTIVE TESTING

Research on ACL knee braces has used knee arthrometers (4,9,12,24), radiographic techniques (25), and direct measurements of strain in the ACL (17,26). The problem with all these techniques is that they are static or at best quasistatic. Most frequently, testing occurs on a nonaxially loaded limb. Unfortunately, many testing models do not reflect the *in vivo* situation at the knee, and in fact, some models for testing may induce knee joint positions and kinematics that are nonphysiologic.

Initially, most brace research was done with cadavers (27,28). This model obviously has limitations because there is little opportunity to adequately maintain the tension in the soft tissue envelope over the femur and tibia. On the other hand, cadaver research does offer a view of what the brace will do when soft tissue is not tensioned. In the injury situation, this may in fact be the case and may be part of the dysfunction equation that allows injury to occur in some individuals. There may not be an adequate muscle response to deforming forces, and that may actually be why some knee injuries occur. Poor muscle function after injury and/or surgery may also explain continuing problems with knee control. Therefore, assuming adequate muscle response and good soft tissue tension in brace research may be assuming too much.

Recognizing some of the shortcomings with cadaver testing, surrogate knee models were developed (15,29). Unfortunately, their stiffness characteristics did not mimic that of the human knee *in vivo*, whereas their ranges of tibial translation and rotation were limited in direction and degree. In fact, most surrogate knee models only allowed for anterior–posterior tibial translation, which is only one of the 6 degrees of freedom seen in the human knee.

Complicating the choice of the best model for brace testing is the fact that displacement testing is fraught with the problem of measuring relatively small amounts of tibial–femoral motion at the knee that is covered with a soft tissue envelope. Radiographic measurements, arthrometers, linear potentiometers, and robotic systems have all contributed to our understanding of ATT and tibial rotations in the unstable knee. Regardless of the technique used, tibial laxity measurements are best made under displacement loads greater than 200 N, whereas knee stiffness characteristics are best determined at loads less than 100 N (30). These relative guidelines apply to tests with no axial load applied across the knee by either muscle contraction or weight bearing. When joint compression loads are applied across the tibial–femoral joint, the loads required for displacement testing will escalate.

Recently, some impressive brace research has been performed *in vivo* (26). These studies benefit from the addition of active muscle to the brace equation. Undoubtedly, the timing, amplitude, and coordination of muscle activity will affect the stiffness of the knee and soft tissue envelope on which the brace performs. Desperately needed in these studies is the separation of the effects of joint compression produced by muscle contractions and weight bearing and the effects of bracing (26). Ideally, these factors would be additive in the bracing equation of function. At present we are unsure if they are.

Most helpful in the struggle to identify and characterize brace function is a study by Beynnon et al. (17) that investigated the effect of bracing on the strain in the ACL under various conditions. Their studies used a Hall-effect strain transducer in knees with a normal ACL. Under low anterior shear loads (100 N) at 30 degrees of flexion and without joint compression forces from weight bearing or muscle contractions, the DonJoy (4 pt. Sport ACL brace) and Townsend (Townsend Industries) braces did reduce the strain in the ACL by a statistically significant degree. Under low internal rotation torques (5 N-m), the DonJoy, Townsend, C.T.i (Innovation Sports), and Lenox-Hill (Lenox-Hill Brace Shop) braces all produced statistically significant reductions in ACL strain. Unfortunately, because of our lack of knowledge of *in vivo* forces in the ACL, we do not know if these are clinically significant reductions in strain. Furthermore, when the anterior tibial shear load was raised to 180 N (45 pounds), none of the braces tested (previously mentioned braces plus the Bledsoe Sports rehab brace [Medical Technology], 3D Dynamic functional rehab brace [3D Orthopedics], and Leiman Multi-Leg II brace [U.S. Manufacturing]) provided a strain-shielding effect on the ACL. When the internal rotation torques reached 10 N-m, all strain-shielding effect was lost. Also, important were the findings that none of the braces produced a strain-shielding effect during active tibial–femoral motion between 10 and 120 degrees or during isometric contraction of the quadriceps. These findings certainly raise questions about the use of braces during routine rehabilitation after ACL surgery, yet alone for a return to athletics. On the positive side, possibly the most significant finding in this study (17) is that there was no increase in ACL strain while bracing the knee, suggesting that at least braces do not increase the risk of ACL injury.

In the area of rehabilitation from ACL surgery, where functional braces are most commonly used today, recent work by Beynnon et al. (26) showed that the ACL is strained during weight bearing and that the compressive load produced across the knee joint during weight bearing does not significantly reduce ACL strain values compared with the non–weight-bearing knee. The protective strain-shielding effect of the ACL brace in the non–weight-bearing knee decreased as the anterior load or internal rotation torque applied to the tibia increased. Weight-bearing forces can be stabilizing or destabilizing to the tibial–femoral joint depending on the direction of forces applied and the position of the joint. The problem with the addition of compressive forces in these models is that testing becomes more difficult. For instance, the displacement forces needed to produce ATT during weight bearing are much higher than in the unweighted joint. Non–weight-bearing conditions are frequently used for safety's sake because smaller displacement forces are needed. Yet these conditions usually do not mimic *in vivo* athletic activities.

Several groups (17,18,21,26) have shown that some knee braces can control tibiofemoral motion for low level anterior tibial directed forces and low levels of internal and external tibial rotation torque. Unfortunately, as forces begin to approach the levels of force expected during ADL, ACL strain values were not affected by bracing. Nevertheless, these objective reports are encouraging and suggest that further research is needed.

SUMMARY

The time has come for brace manufacturers to supply activity- and condition-specific data concerning brace function. Brace consumers should not rely on the anecdotal claims of brace function from high-level athletes. Although the objective data available on brace function do not match the subjective reports from brace users and manufacturers, researchers must keep an open mind and continue to identify devices that may be capable of augmenting knee function and protecting injured or reconstructed knee ligaments.

REFERENCES

1. Beynnon BD, Fleming BC, Johnson RJ, et al. Anterior cruciate ligament strain behavior during rehabilitation exercises in vivo. *Am J Sports Med* 1995;23:24–34.
2. Wojtys EM, Kothari SU, Huston LJ. Anterior cruciate ligament functional brace use in sports. *Am J Sports Med* 1996;24:539–546.
3. Blackburn T. The effect of bracing on knee proprioception and single leg stance in an ACL deficient population. Presented at the 22nd Annual AOSSM Meeting, Orlando, Florida, June 16–20, 1996.
4. Branch TP, Hunter R, Donath M. Dynamic EMG analysis of anterior cruciate deficient legs with and without bracing during cutting. *Am J Sports Med* 1989;17:35–41.
5. Voight ML, Blackburn TA, Nashner L. Neuromuscular function changes with ACL functional brace use. Presented at the 24th Annual AOSSM Meeting, Vancouver, British Columbia, Canada, July 12–15, 1998.
6. Tsuda E, Harata S, Okamura Y, et al. The direct evidence of ACL-hamstring reflex in humans. Presented at the 24th Annual AOSSM Meeting, Vancouver, British Columbia, Canada, July 12–15, 1998.
7. Solomonow M, Baratta R, Zhou BH, et al. The synergistic action of the anterior cruciate ligament and thigh muscles in maintaining joint stability. *Am J Sports Med* 1987;15:207–213.

8. Acierno SP, D'Ambrosia C, Solomonow M. Electromyography and biomechanics of a dynamic knee brace for anterior cruciate ligament deficiency. *Orthopedics* 1995;18:1101–1107.

9. Cawley PW, France EP, Paulos LE. The current state of functional knee bracing research: a review of the literature. *Am J Sports Med* 1991;19:226–233.

10. Houston ME, Goemans PH. Leg muscle performance of athletes with and without knee support braces. *Arch Phys Med Rehabil* 1982;63:431–432.

11. Knutzen KM, Bates BT, Hamill J. Electrogoniometry of post-surgical knee bracing in running. *Am J Phys Med* 1983;62:172–181.

12. Beck C, Drez D, Young J, et al. Instrumented testing of functional knee braces. *Am J Sports Med* 1986;14:253–256.

13. Beynnon BD, Howe JG, Pope MH, et al. Anterior cruciate ligament strain in-vivo. *Int Orthop* 1992;16:1–12.

14. France EP, Cawley PW, Paulos LE. Choosing functional knee braces. *Clin Sports Med* 1990;9:743–750.

15. Liu SH, Lunsford T, Gude S, et al. Comparison of functional knee braces for control of anterior tibial displacement. *Clin Orthop* 1994;303:203–210.

16. Vailas JC, Pink M. Biomechanical effects of functional knee bracing: Practical implications. *Sports Med* 1993;15:210–218.

17. Beynnon BD, Pope MH, Wertheimer CM. The effect of functional knee-braces on strain on the anterior cruciate ligament in vivo. *J Bone Joint Surg Am* 1992;74-A:1298–1312.

18. Wojtys EM, Loubert PV, Samson SY, et al. Use of a knee brace for control of tibial translation and rotation: a comparison, in cadavers, of available models. *J Bone Joint Surg Am* 1990;72-A:1323–1329.

19. Nicholas JA. The five-one reconstruction for anteromedial instability of the knee: indications, technique, and the results in fifty-two patients. *J Bone Joint Surg Am* 1973;55-A:899–922.

20. Bassett GS, Fleming BW. The Lenox Hill brace in anterolateral rotatory instability. *Am J Sports Med* 1983;11:345–348.

21. Colville MR, Lee CL, Ciullo JV. The Lenox Hill brace: an evaluation of effectiveness in treating knee instability. *Am J Sports Med* 1986;14:257–261.

22. Mishra DK, Daniel DM, Stone ML. The use of functional knee braces in the control of pathologic anterior knee laxity. *Clin Orthop* 1989;241:213–220.

23. Tegner Y, Lorentzon R. Evaluation of knee braces in Swedish ice hockey players. *Br J Sports Med* 1991;25:159–161.

24. Bagger J, Ravn J, Lavard P, et al. Effect of functional bracing, quadriceps and hamstrings on anterior tibial translation in anterior cruciate ligament insufficiency: a preliminary report. *J Rehabil Res Dev* 1992;29:9–12.

25. Jonsson H, Kärrholm J. Brace effects on the unstable knee in 21 cases: a roentgen stereophotogrammetric comparison of three design. *Acta Orthop Scand* 1990;61:313–318.

26. Beynnon BD, Johnson RJ, Fleming BC, et al. The effect of functional knee bracing on the anterior cruciate ligament in the weight-bearing and nonweightbearing knee. *Am J Sports Med* 1997;25:353–359.

27. Hoffman AA, Wyatt RW, Bourne MH, et al. Knee stability in orthotic knee braces. *Am J Sports Med* 1984;12:371–374.

28. Wojtys EM, Goldstein SA, Redfern MS, et al. A biomechanical evaluation of the Lenox Hill knee brace. *Clin Orthop* 1987;220:179–184.

29. Cawley PW, France EP, Paulos LE. Comparison of rehabilitative knee braces: a biomechanical investigation. *Am J Sports Med* 1989;17:141–146.

30. Markolf KL, Kochan A, Amstutz HC. Measurement of knee stiffness and laxity in patients with documented absence of the anterior cruciate ligament. *J Bone Joint Surg Am* 1984;66-A:242–252.

Principles and Practice of Orthopaedic Sports Medicine,
edited by William E. Garrett, Jr., Kevin P. Speer, and Donald T. Kirkendall.
Lippincott Williams & Wilkins, Philadelphia © 2000.

CHAPTER 49

The Leg

Barry P. Boden

STRESS FRACTURES

Epidemiology

Stress fractures are most commonly seen in athletes and military recruits. Although the reported incidence of stress fractures in the general athletic population is less than 1%, the incidence in runners may be as high as 15% (1). In a review of 370 athletes with stress fractures, the tibia was the most commonly involved bone (49.1%), and the fibula was the fifth most common site of injury (6.6%) (2). Bilateral stress fractures occurred in 16.6% of cases (2). Stress fractures of the tibia and fibula are especially common in long distance runners (3). The physician should not overlook the diagnosis of stress fractures in the growing population of active elderly citizens (4).

Pathogenesis

Stress fractures result from excessive repetitive loads on the bone that cause an imbalance between bone resorption and formation. An abrupt increase in the duration, intensity, or frequency of physical activity without adequate periods of rest may lead to an escalation in osteoclast activity. The exact mechanism responsible for initiating stress fractures remains unclear. One theory holds that excessive forces are transmitted to bone when the surrounding muscles become fatigued (5,6). Alternatively, muscles may contribute to stress fractures by concentrating forces across a localized area of bone, thus causing mechanical insults above the stress-bearing capacity of the bone (7).

In addition to local mechanical influences, systemic factors, including nutritional deficiencies, hormonal im-

balances, sleep deprivation, collagen abnormalities, and metabolic bone disorders, may contribute to the development of stress fractures (8). A high incidence of stress fractures has been reported in women (9). Therefore, it is especially important to investigate intrinsic factors in female athletes. The "female athlete triad" refers to a female athlete with an eating disorder, amenorrhea, and osteoporosis. Women participating in high-level figure skating, gymnastics, and cross-country running are particularly prone to this triad. In an effort to minimize body fat and maintain high athletic performance, many develop eating disorders during puberty. A high incidence of amenorrhea and oligomenorrhea has been described in competitive female distance runners (9). The prevalence of menstrual irregularities may reach as high as 50% in elite distance runners and ballet dancers. The resultant estrogen-deficient state leads to decreased bone mineral density and an increased risk of stress fractures. Treatment with oral contraceptives may help to reverse this condition.

Anthropomorphic risk factors for the development of stress fractures have been analyzed in several reports by Giladi and colleagues (10–13). Three risk factors for stress fractures were identified: a narrow tibial width, higher degree of external rotation of the hip, and a cavus foot. The authors postulated that narrow tibias have less resistance to bending forces, thereby predisposing them to stress fractures (10). The cavus foot may precipitate stress fractures because of inferior shock-absorbing characteristics (12).

Clinical Evaluation

Early diagnosis is essential for avoiding complications and returning the athlete to play as soon as possible. The onset of pain is insidious over a period of days to weeks. Symptoms are aggravated by activity and relieved with rest. Examination reveals localized pain to

B. P. Boden: Uniformed Services University of the Health Sciences, The Orthopedic Center, Rockville, Maryland 20850.

palpation over a confined area of the tibia or fibula. Hopping on the affected leg may elicit pain.

Imaging

Radiographs are initially normal for the first 2 to 3 weeks of symptoms. Periosteal reaction and cortical lucency may be appreciated on later films. Radionuclide imaging has traditionally been the gold standard for confirming clinically suspected stress fractures. In the early stages of a stress fracture, before any changes on plain films, bone scans are highly sensitive for detecting stress injuries (14–16).

Nuclear imaging is particularly helpful in distinguishing medial tibial stress syndrome (MTSS) from stress fractures. MTSS shows linear increased uptake on delayed images (phase III) along the posteromedial aspect of the middle and distal tibia. In contrast, stress fractures characteristically reveal discrete localized areas of increased uptake on all three phases of a technetium-99 diphosphonate bone scan (Fig. 49.1, Table 49.1). As healing of the stress fracture occurs, radionuclide images (phase I) and blood pool images (phase II) of the nuclear scans may revert to normal (17). The intensity of activity on delayed images decreases over 3 to 12 months. Occasionally, minor abnormalities may persist for 18 months.

Although nuclear imaging has a high sensitivity in detecting stress fractures, this imaging modality lacks specificity. Several reports have documented that 40% to 50% of scintigraphic findings occur at asymptomatic sites (16,18). These areas of increased uptake may represent subclinical sites of bone remodeling as a result of stress. The clinical significance of these lesions is controversial. Although many progress to stress fractures if untreated, other lesions resolve despite continuous training (19). A brief rest period is appropriate for these lesions.

In the future, magnetic resonance imaging (MRI) may replace scintigraphy as the imaging modality of choice (Fig. 49.2). One advantage of MRI over scintigraphy is the ability to more precisely define the anatomic location and extent of stress fractures. Fredericson et al. (20) found that the degree of bone involvement can be correlated with clinical symptoms using MRI. This allows a more accurate assessment of the severity of injury and the recovery time. In addition, MRI avoids radiation exposure and requires less imaging time than three-phase bone scintigraphy (21). The major disadvantage of MRI is the cost.

A spectrum of stress-related bone changes has been documented using MRI. An MRI grading scheme using T1 inversion recovery times has been proposed (20–22)

TABLE 49.1. *Nuclear imaging features of tibial stress fractures and MTSS*

	Stress fractures	MTSS
Three phase	Any phase or all phases can be positive	Positive on delayed phase
Shape	Round, localized	Linear/vertical
Location	Any location	Posteromedial one third of middle-to-distal tibia

MTSS, medial tibial stress syndrome.

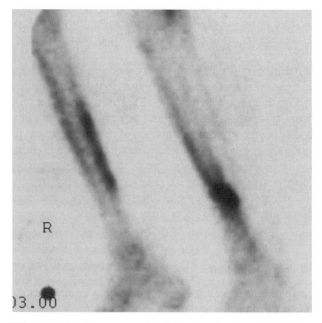

FIG. 49.1. Nuclear scan of athlete who developed MTSS on right leg (linear uptake along one third of tibia) and stress fracture of left leg (focal uptake).

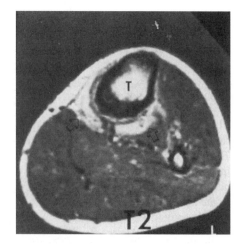

FIG. 49.2. Axial magnetic resonance image at level of tibial stress fracture reveals periosteal edema and ring of cortical bone elevated from the cortex. (From Gersten K. Lower leg. In: Martire JR, Levinsohn EM, eds. *Imaging of athletic injuries: a multimodality approach,* 1st ed. New York: McGraw-Hill, 1992:57, with permission.)

TABLE 49.2. *Radiologic grading system of tibial stress fractures*

Grade	Radiograph	MRI	Treatment
1	Normal	Periosteal edema (T2)	3 wk rest
2	Normal	Periosteal edema (T2) Marrow edema (T2)	4–6 wk rest
3	Discrete line (+/−) Periosteal reaction (+/−)	No definite cortical break Periosteal edema (T2) Marrow edema (T1, T2)	6–9 wk rest
4	Fracture or periosteal reaction	Fracture line Periosteal edema (T2) Marrow edema (T1, T2)	12–16 wk rest

MRI, magnetic resonance imaging.

(Table 49.2). Grade 1 injuries, which represent an early stress phenomenon, demonstrate periosteal edema on T2-weighted images with no focal bone marrow abnormality. Grade 2 lesions reveal severe periosteal and bone marrow edema on T2-weighted images. Grade 3 changes include periosteal edema on T2 images and bone marrow edema on T1- and T2-weighted images. Grade 4 lesions demonstrate a definite fracture line, severe periosteal edema on T2 images, and marrow edema on T1- and T2-weighted images. The classification scheme may be simplified by grouping grades 1 and 2 injuries as low-grade stress fractures and grades 3 and 4 lesions as high-grade stress fractures (21). Radiographs are normal for grade 1 and 2 lesions, often show a linear periosteal reaction for grade 3 injuries, and reveal a clear stress fracture for grade 4 lesions. Based on the MRI grading of tibial stress fractures, the recovery time can be estimated as follows: 3 weeks for grade 1; 4 to 6 weeks for grade 2; 6 to 9 weeks for grade 3; and 12 to 16 weeks for grade 4 injuries (10,21). Indications for obtaining an MRI have not been clearly defined.

Treatment

Management of stress fractures varies depending on the underlying etiology. Training errors are the most common cause of stress fractures. Intrinsic factors such as nutritional, hormonal, and medical abnormalities need to be assessed. Medical evaluation is considered for any patient with increased risk factors such as female athletes, athletes with recurrent or multiple stress fractures, and stress fractures with delayed healing times.

Most tibia and fibula stress fractures can be treated by rest followed by a gradual resumption of activity. Surgery may be necessary for problematic stress fractures such as those located at the anterior cortex of the tibia or the medial malleolus. Ideally, stress fractures are best managed through prevention. Athletes, coaches, and parents should be educated about the deleterious effects of overtraining and the importance of periodic rest days. In addition, coaches should be alerted to the high incidence of stress fractures in female athletes. The effectiveness of shock-absorbing orthotics on the incidence of tibial stress fractures remains controversial (23–25).

Tibial Shaft Stress Fractures

In athletes, the tibial shaft is the most common site of stress fractures (2). Tibial stress fractures may occur at any site along the shaft of the bone (Fig. 49.3) but are most frequently encountered in the posteromedial cortex or compression side. The onset of pain is insidious and usually occurs at the end of running activities. If the exercise is continued, symptoms may develop during activity and persist for several hours after the event.

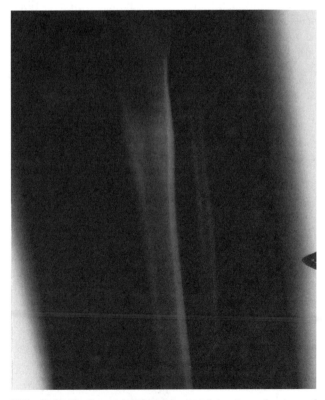

FIG. 49.3. Radiograph demonstrating late stress fracture of the proximal tibia with cortical thickening.

Tenderness is usually present at the site of the stress fracture. Occasionally swelling is noted, and in the later stages callus formation may be palpable.

Tibial stress fractures on the posteromedial cortex respond favorably to discontinuation of the inciting activity. During this time the athlete can maintain aerobic fitness with low-impact exercises such as stationary bicycling, swimming, and stair-climbing machines. Upon resolution of pain, a gradual resumption of impact exercises is initiated.

Supplemental use of a pneumatic brace may allow athletes to return to activity sooner than traditional treatment alone (26). The pneumatic brace has been proposed to work similarly to a functional weight-bearing cast (27,28). By unloading the tibia at the site of the stress fracture, the brace theoretically hastens the healing time. Alternatively, the pneumatic brace may act as a venous tourniquet, shifting electrolytes into the interstitial fluid space. This creates an electronegative charge that stimulates osteoblastic bone formation (28). In a randomized prospective study comparing treatment modalities, Swenson et al. (26) found that patients in the brace group returned to full unrestricted activity at an average of 21 days. This was significantly better than the average of 77 days for the group treated with rest alone.

Anterior Cortex Tibial Stress Fractures

A less common, but more problematic, location of tibial stress fractures is the anterior cortex of the middle third of the tibia (Fig. 49.4). Stress fractures at this tension side of the bone have been reported to exhibit poor healing properties. In addition to constant tension on the anterior aspect of the tibia, limited blood supply may predispose this site to nonunion or delayed union. In 1985, Green et al. (29) reported six stress fractures of the middle third of the tibia that failed to heal with simple immobilization. Since then, numerous authors have presented different treatment modalities to achieve union of these recalcitrant lesions (30–32).

In contrast to compression tibial stress fractures, which usually occur in distance runners, tension tibial stress injuries occur in athletes performing repetitive jumping and leaping activities. Patients present with point tenderness over the anterior aspect of the central third of the tibia. These problematic tibial stress fractures have the potential to progress to a complete fracture (29). Radiographs are often initially normal but subsequently develop a characteristic V- or wedge-shaped defect in the anterior cortex with the open end of the V being directed anteriorly (32). The radiographic appearance has also been referred to as the "dreaded black line" because of its prolonged healing time. Radionuclide imaging may demonstrate minimal activity, indicating nonunion of the stress fracture (30). The dif-

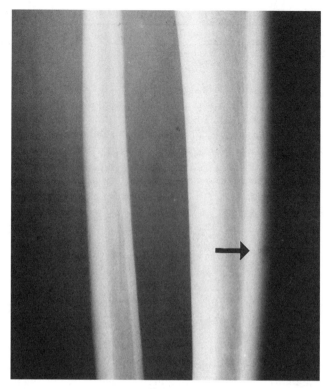

FIG. 49.4. Radiograph of subtle anterior tibial stress fracture (*arrow*) in athlete participating in gymnastics and cheerleading. The stress fracture appearance has been referred to as the "dreaded black line."

ferential diagnosis should include infection, tumors, MTSS, and exertional compartment syndrome.

Initial treatment of anterior midtibial stress fractures is generally a trial of rest, with or without immobilization, for a minimum of 4 to 6 months. For stress fractures with delayed healing, numerous treatments have been proposed. Prompt healing has been reported in patients after excision and bone grafting of the lesion (29). Rettig et al. (32) evaluated a treatment regimen of rest and external electrical stimulation. In their series, seven of eight patients showed complete healing after an average of 8.7 months of treatment. Other authors have described less favorable results with electromagnetic stimulation (29). Chang and Harris (31) reported good to excellent results in five patients with recalcitrant stress fractures who were treated with reamed unlocked tibial nails. The author prefers treatment with a reamed tibial intramedullary rod for anterior cortex tibial stress fractures that fail to heal after 4 to 6 months of immobilization with external stimulation.

Medial Malleolus Stress Fractures

The medial malleolus is an uncommon location for stress fractures to occur. In 1988, the first series of medial malleolar stress fractures was reported in six athletes

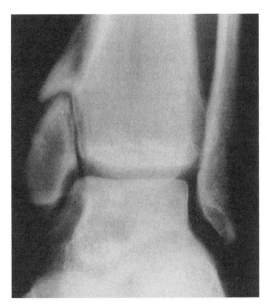

FIG. 49.5. Mortise radiography reveals nonunion of medial malleolus. (From Reider B, Falroniero R, Yurkufsky J. Nonunion of a medial malleolus stress fracture. A case report. *Am J Sports Med* 1993;21:478–481, with permission.)

(33). The following characteristics defined these fractures: tenderness over the medial malleolus with an ankle effusion, pain during athletic activities for several weeks before an acute episode, and a vertical or oblique fracture line on radiographs originating from the tibial plafond and the medial malleolar junction. The clinical course is characterized by pain of gradual onset that increases with activity and is relieved by rest. The authors hypothesized that these stress fractures are caused by repeated ankle dorsiflexion and tibial rotation during running. These maneuvers place increased stress at the junction of the medial malleolus and the tibial plafond (33).

Shelbourne et al. (33) advocated internal fixation with malleolar screws for patients with a fracture line present on radiographs. For individuals with a positive bone scan and negative radiographs, treatment was individualized based on the level of athletic activity. Athletes desiring early return to competition were treated with internal fixation, whereas the remaining subjects were treated with ankle bracing. Both treatments resulted in a full return to activity in all patients by 6 to 8 weeks. Because of the high shear forces placed at the fracture site, improper management early in the clinical course may promote a nonunion (Fig. 49.5) (34). In this circumstance, open reduction and internal fixation with two cancellous screws is required. Bone grafting may also be necessary.

Distal Fibula Stress Fractures

Although stress fractures may occur at any site in the fibula (Fig. 49.6), the most common location is the distal third of the bone. The usual site of fibular stress fractures is just proximal to the inferior tibiofibular ligaments at the junction of cortical and cancellous bone (6). This injury predominantly occurs in distance runners who train on hard surfaces (35). Devas and Sweetnam (36) postulated that rhythmic contraction of the long toe flexors causes micromotion of the fibula, leading to stress fractures.

Patients present with pain over the distal fibula and ankle. Symptoms usually develop insidiously over several days to weeks. Onset may be abrupt when a cortical fracture occurs (36–38). The symptoms are relieved by rest and aggravated by physical activity. Pain is elicited by pressing the fibula toward the tibia. Occasionally, callus formation is palpable.

In the early stages, radiographic findings are subtle or absent. The earliest change is a hazy patch of new bone in the fibula just proximal to the ankle joint (Fig. 49.7). With progression of the lesion, callus or a fracture line may be visualized (36).

Stress fractures of the distal fibula have an excellent prognosis when diagnosed early and treated with a 3-

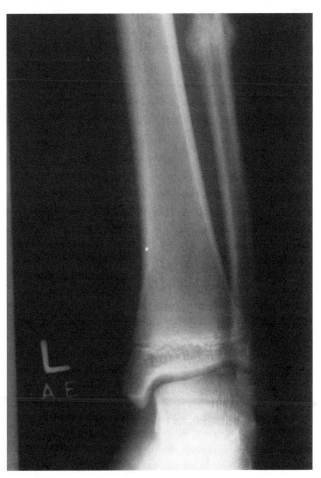

FIG. 49.6. Radiograph demonstrating healing fibula stress fracture.

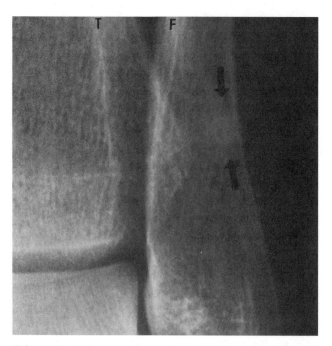

FIG. 49.7. Anteroposterior radiograph demonstrates distal fibula stress fractures (*arrows*) just proximal to tibiofibular ligaments. (From Gersten K. Lower leg. In: Martire JR, Levinsohn EM, eds. *Imaging of athletic injuries: a multimodality approach,* 1st ed. New York: McGraw-Hill, 1992:63, with permission.)

to 6-week period of rest. Without treatment, symptoms may persist for 3 to 6 months (36).

Proximal Fibula Stress Fractures

Although fibular stress fractures are usually in the distal two thirds of the bone, proximal fibular stress fractures have also been reported (39–41). These stress fractures occur in sedentary individuals who abruptly begin a vigorous exercise program. The exact etiology of proximal fibular stress fractures is unknown but may be related to a combination of muscle forces and compression loading. Symeonides (41) reported several military recruits who developed proximal fibular stress fractures after performing intense jumping exercises from a squatting position.

Affected patients present with diffuse proximal and lateral leg pain that is often exacerbated by exercise or knee range of motion. Tenderness to palpation is frequently noted over the proximal fibula. Instability of the proximal tibiofibular joint should be excluded on examination. Plain films may reveal periosteal new bone formation at the neck of the proximal fibula. Radionuclide imaging is a useful diagnostic tool in uncertain cases. Resolution of symptoms occurs with cessation of the offending activity. Supportive care with crutches is occasionally required for a short duration.

TIBIA AND FIBULA FRACTURES

Fractures of the tibia and fibula are uncommon injuries in athletes. Although these injuries can occur in any sport, soccer players are at high risk due to the high energy associated with the kicking maneuver. Shin guards, the only standard protective equipment in soccer, are effective in decreasing the number of minor injuries to the lower extremity but are less protective against forces that can result in fractures. In one study, soccer players who sustained 31 fractures of both the tibia and fibula, the tibia only, or the fibula only were retrospectively reviewed (42). Most fractures occurred at or near the junction of the middle and distal thirds of the lower leg (Fig. 49.8). The mechanisms of injury typically involved contact during a slide tackle, two opposing players swinging for a loose ball, or a collision during a fast break with a goalie. In over half of the injuries, the point of impact was with the shin guard before the fracture. The authors concluded that currently available shin guards are inadequate at protecting against fractures (42).

In the limited number of reports on leg fractures in athletes, there appears to be a relatively high incidence of complications. In a report of tibia and fibula fractures in soccer players, a 41% incidence of major complications of 31 fractures was documented (42). Because of the tremendous forces necessary to fracture both the tibia and fibula, these fractures may be associated with

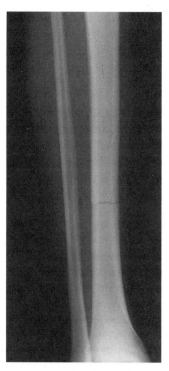

FIG. 49.8. Tibial fracture at the junction of the middle and distal third of the bone in a young soccer player who was kicked while wearing shin guards.

soft tissue injuries, compartment syndromes, and/or healing problems. Delayed union, varus malunions, or nonunions are known complications of isolated tibia fractures with an intact fibula (43). Conversely, it is possible that an isolated fibula fracture may not receive adequate stress transfer at the fracture site when the tibia is intact. Slauterbeck et al. (44) reviewed three athletes who sustained isolated fibula fractures from a direct blow. Because each case was associated with a refracture, the ultimate healing time was prolonged at an average of 23 weeks. These reports suggest that leg fractures in athletes are associated with high forces and high complication rates. Caution should be exercised at attempting to return athletes to sports activities after a leg fracture before the standard healing time in the general population (42,45).

MEDIAL TIBIAL STRESS SYNDROME (SHIN SPLINTS)

Numerous terms such as shin splints, shin soreness, soleus syndrome, and MTSS have been used to describe activity-related pain along the middle to distal aspect of the posteromedial tibia. Because the shin refers to the anterior aspect of the tibia, MTSS is a more appropriate descriptive term for this condition. MTSS was originally used as a nonspecific term referring to overuse syndromes of the leg. This confusion over leg syndromes can be attributed to an initial lack of understanding of the pathomechanics of MTSS, stress fractures, and compartment syndromes. In an attempt to more clearly define the syndrome, the American Medical Association suggested that the diagnosis is limited to musculotendinous inflammation, excluding stress fractures and ischemic disorders (46).

Epidemiology

Epidemiologic studies on MTSS reveal that most cases occur in runners and military recruits with the incidence ranging between 4% and 13% (47,48). However, the syndrome may occur in any sport or activity in which the athlete repetitively places weight-bearing impact forces on the leg. James et al. (48) reviewed 180 runners with 232 conditions and found a 13% incidence of MTSS, with most injuries occurring in distance runners. Andrish et al. (47) performed a perspective study on MTSS at the U.S. Naval Academy. They followed 2,777 first-year midshipmen during two consecutive summer training sessions. Ninety-seven cases of MTSS were diagnosed for an incidence of 4.07%. In another perspective study, Watson (49) followed 324 athletes participating in a variety of sports over a 12-month period. He reported 32 cases of MTSS, or an incidence of 9.9%. Wadley and Albright (50) conducted a prospective study of a women's college gymnastics team over a 4-year period.

They identified six cases of MTSS from a total of 106 injuries for an incidence of 5.7%.

Pathogenesis

Although MTSS has been shown to be a distinct entity from stress fractures and compartment syndrome, little data are available regarding the exact pathophysiology. Stress fractures and MTSS have been shown to have different pathologic processes based on the scintigraphic images. In 1972, it was hypothesized that MTSS represented a deep posterior compartment syndrome (51). Since this initial report, several studies have demonstrated normal compartment pressures in patients with MTSS (52,53).

Biopsies of the periosteum at the site of tenderness have revealed conflicting results. In two reports, the specimens demonstrated an inflammatory picture consistent with periostitis (53,54). Detmer (55) reported the largest series of patients, 18, with chronic MTSS who were treated operatively. Biopsies of the fascia and periosteum in 10 of these chronic cases revealed no inflammation or vasculitis. The author proposed that the pathogenesis of MTSS is related to stress at the periosteum of the tibia (55). In the acute phase, the periosteum may reveal inflammatory changes with the fascial tissue still firmly attached to the tibia. An adequate period of rest during this early phase may allow the inflammation to resolve. However, in chronic cases the periosteum may become disengaged from the bone either by a ballistic avulsion or subperiosteal hemorrhage. It is unclear whether the periosteum is able to heal back to the tibia in these chronic cases. Continuing stress on the innervated, but disengaged, periosteum may be responsible for the persistent pain noted with normal exercise. Therefore, the acute phase may represent a periostitis, whereas the chronic phase is referred to as periostalgia. Confirmation of this theory requires further study.

Anatomy

There has been much conjecture regarding the exact anatomic structures responsible for this traction-induced syndrome. The muscles that have been implicated in this condition are the soleus (54–56), the flexor digitorum longus (57), and the tibialis posterior (52, 58,59). The tibialis posterior muscle is an unlikely culprit because of its more proximal and lateral attachment to the tibia.

Based on two cadaver studies, the soleus origin appears to be the most likely anatomic structure that contributes to MTSS. In one study, the authors performed anatomic dissections of human cadavers and correlated clinical findings with electromyography and nuclear images (60). The site of increased tenderness on clinical palpation and the site of increased activity on bone scans

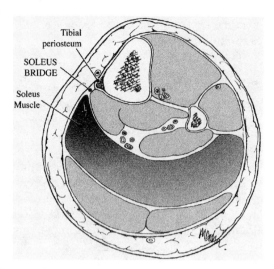

FIG. 49.9. Cross-section of leg reveals anterior and posterior fascia of soleus converging to form soleus bridge.

corresponded to the medial origin of the soleus muscle in the cadaveric dissections. The authors found that the soleus muscle has an aponeurotic covering both anteriorly and posteriorly that enveloped the muscle. These aponeurotic coverings fuse to form a strong facial layer referred to as the "soleus bridge" that attaches directly to the posteromedial border of the tibia for three fourths of its length (Fig. 49.9) (60,61). In another comprehensive cadaveric study, Beck and Osternig (62) dissected 50 cadaver legs to identify the structures that attach to the tibia at the site of MTSS symptoms. They found that the soleus, the flexor digitorum longus, and the deep crural fascia attached most frequently at the site of pain in MTSS. In no specimen was the tibialis posterior attached in the vicinity of the clinical symptoms. Based on the strength and location of the soleus bridge, the authors concluded that the soleus is the major contributor to the development of MTSS. The flexor digitorum longus periosteum may play a less important role in the genesis of MTSS.

Biomechanics

The runner with excessively pronated feet has been shown to be predisposed to the development of overuse syndromes (63). As the leg is loaded during running, the tibia internally rotates, resulting in a compensatory eversion of the subtalar joint. This foot motion, referred to as pronation, is a normal occurrence during gait and functions as a shock absorber of the initial contact forces.

The association of excessive pronation of the foot with the development of MTSS has been described by several authors (50,64–66). Viitasalo and Kvist (66) compared 35 male athletes with MTSS to 13 male long distance runners with no symptoms. The authors mea-

sured several biomechanical aspects of the foot and ankle while standing and running on a treadmill. They found that in standing and at heel strike the Achilles tendon angle (the angle between the calcaneus midline and the lower leg midline) was greater (more pronation) in the MTSS group than in the control group. In addition, the MTSS group had higher angular displacement values in eversion than the control group. This indicates more pronounced pronation in MTSS patients, leading to increased tension on the soleus and flexor digitorum longus fascial attachments to the tibia.

Messier and Pittala (64) analyzed selected biomechanical, anthroprometric, and training variables in 17 runners with MTSS and 19 asymptomatic runners. Data on hindfoot movement was obtained using high-speed cinematography. Their results revealed that maximum pronation is a significant discriminator between runners with and without MTSS. Furthermore, they showed a significantly greater maximum pronation velocity in the runners with MTSS. There was also a trend toward less dorsiflexion range of motion in the MTSS group. The velocity of pronation may be an important factor in placing strain on the fascia of the soleus during an eccentric contraction.

Using a static model to assess foot posture, Sommer and Vallentyne (65) also found a relationship between foot pronation and the incidence of MTSS. Both hindfoot and forefoot varus alignment occurred more often in subjects with a history of MTSS than in controls. The authors proposed that a standing foot angle (angle between medial malleolar–navicular prominence and navicular prominence–first metacarpal head segment) of less than 140 degrees serves as a threshold for assessing the risk of MTSS.

Clinical Evaluation

Similar to stress fractures, MTSS is common in runners, especially distance runners, sprinters, hurdlers, or athletes involved in ballistic sports such as gymnastics or basketball. MTSS typically occurs in individuals who substantially increase the intensity or duration of their activity. In addition, changes in footwear or hard running surfaces may be related to the onset of MTSS (48).

Patients with MTSS present with recurrent pain along the middle and distal thirds of the tibia (67,68). The pain is usually present at the beginning of the workout and can vary in intensity from a dull ache to severe pain with prolonged activity. The symptoms often disappear while exercising only to return during the cool-down period. Bilaterality may occur in 50% of subjects (55). Rest alleviates the symptoms in the early phase of the syndrome; however, in more advanced cases, the pain may persist during and after the workout. Some athletes are able to continue training while symptomatic but usually with a deterioration in performance. In chronic cases, the patient experiences pain with any weight-bearing activity, including walking.

On physical examination, there is diffuse tenderness to palpation at the middle and distal thirds of the posteromedial tibia. This finding is important in distinguishing stress fractures, characterized by localized point tenderness from MTSS. Range of motion of the ankle typically does not reproduce the symptoms, although active plantar flexion may elicit pain. No neurologic or vascular abnormalities are present in patients with MTSS. A local injection of xylocaine into the affected soft tissue may decrease the pain along the tibia but is not specific at distinguishing MTSS from stress fractures.

Imaging

Plain films of the leg are usually normal. Occasionally, radiographs reveal mild cortical hypertrophy over the posteromedial tibia. This may be caused by bone remodeling due to repetitive stress on the overlying periosteum. Although MTSS is primarily a clinical diagnosis, nuclear imaging is the best tool for confirming the diagnosis. Bone scintigraphy with Tc-99 methylene diphosphonate is an excellent technique for distinguishing MTSS from stress fractures (60,69,70). In MTSS, the characteristic lesion involves increased longitudinal uptake along the periosteum of the posteromedial tibia (71). The injury involves a third of the length of the bone in the middle to distal sections of the tibia with increased uptake present only on the delayed images (phase III). Radionuclide images (phase I) and blood pool images (phase II) are normal. Both lateral and medial views of the leg are essential to localize the affected bone. In contrast to MTSS, the appearance of stress fractures on bone scans is characterized by focal intense uptake on all three phases.

The use of MRI as a diagnostic tool for MTSS remains experimental. In one report, Anderson et al. (72) performed MR images on 19 subjects with symptoms consistent with MTSS. They identified four MR patterns: normal appearance (37%), periosteal fluid only (26%), abnormal marrow signal intensity (26%), and stress fractures (11%). There was a strong correlation between chronicity of symptoms and a normal MR image. These findings raise questions concerning the pathophysiology of MTSS and whether a relationship exists between MTSS and stress fractures. The high cost and low yield of MRI in patients with suspected MTSS limit its utility.

Differential Diagnosis

The most common conditions that must be differentiated from MTSS are stress fractures of the tibia and fibula and chronic compartment syndromes (CCS) (59,61). Occasionally, two of these conditions may coexist in the same individual (55). Other conditions that must be included in the differential are tendinopathies, muscle strains, sciatica, nerve entrapment, arterial occlusion, fascial hernias, infections, tumors, and reflex sympathetic dystrophy.

Treatment

Rest is the mainstay of treatment for MTSS (47). Most patients can be treated successfully by abstinence from the offending activity for several days to 2 weeks. Andrish et al. (47) prospectively treated 97 subjects with MTSS with one of five different treatment regimes. Included in each treatment program was rest with variable adjuvants such as ice, aspirin, anti-inflammatories, heel-cord stretching exercises, and casting. The results demonstrated that no treatment combinations hastened the recovery faster than rest alone. Depending on the degree of pain, nonimpact exercises such as swimming or biking may be permitted (56).

Although unproven in clinical trials, several adjuvant treatments may still be beneficial. Whether these therapies truly affect the pathophysiology of MTSS or simply act as placebos is unknown. Because biopsies of affected tissue often demonstrate a periostitis, ice and nonsteroidals may limit the inflammatory response and decrease pain in the acute phase (53,60). Messier and Pittala (64) showed a trend toward less dorsiflexion in a group of patients with MTSS. Therefore, heel-cord stretching exercises are a reasonable addition to the treatment program.

As previously mentioned, excessive pronation and greater pronation velocity have been implicated in the development of MTSS (48,64,66). Hence, patients with pronation deformities should be evaluated for orthotic support (Fig. 49.10). Initially, the athlete's footwear should be assessed for overall fit, medial support, and cushioning ability. Running shoes with a narrow heel can decrease maximum pronation by providing hindfoot support (73). After the basics of a good running shoe are obtained, additional orthotic devices may be required. A medial heel wedge is recommended for athletes with a varus heel, whereas a medial post beneath the forefoot may be necessary for individuals with a varus foot.

In a retrospective study, orthotic shoe inserts were found to provide either a complete cure or improvement in 11 of 16 long distance runners with MTSS (74). Orthotic devices that are typically used for MTSS may be soft or semirigid. Soft orthotic devices are inexpensive and tend to be more comfortable. However, because the material loses its mechanical properties over 2 to 3 weeks, these devices should be limited to patients with mild deformities who require temporary relief. For patients requiring long-term orthoses, a semirigid device is more appropriate. Proper manufacturing of the orthosis is also a critical factor in determining the success of the device. Using high-speed filming, Smith et al. (75)

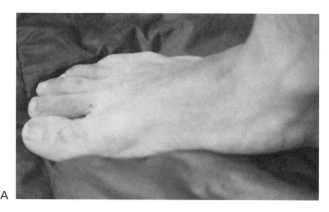
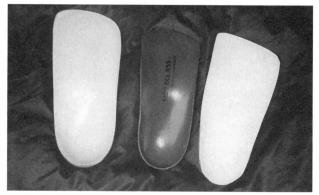

FIG. 49.10. Photograph of patient with flatfoot deformity **(A)** and orthotics that may be helpful in diminishing hyperpronation and the stress placed on the tibial insertion of the soleus in MTSS **(B)**.

found no statistical difference between soft and semi-rigid orthoses when measuring calcaneal eversion and maximum velocity of calcaneal eversion. However, this study was performed in new orthoses and did not take into account the rapid loss of strength of soft orthotic devices over a 2-week period.

Recurrence of symptoms in MTSS is not uncommon and usually occurs within the first few weeks after return to activities. Training errors, such as excessive mileage, infrequent rest periods, hard running surfaces, and poor footwear, are usually responsible. A gradual resumption of running over a 4- to 6-week period is recommended.

Surgical treatment is reserved for patients in whom a prolonged course of conservative therapy has failed. Candidates for operative therapy include patients who have persistent symptoms despite two to three well-supervised trials of rest. Often these subjects have been forced to abandon all physical activity. Before surgical intervention, it is critical to exclude other entities such as stress fractures or CCS.

Several authors have reported good results after fasciotomy of the periosteum along the entire posteromedial aspect of the tibia at the site producing pain (53,55,76). Detmer (55) performed the procedure on 18 patients (28 limbs) with MTSS using lidocaine and sedation in an outpatient setting. He proposed that the fasciotomy is effective because it detachs the fascia from the loosened painful periosteum. Patients with unilateral procedures resumed unassisted walking by the fifth day after surgery, whereas those with bilateral procedures required crutches for an additional 1 to 2 weeks. Rehabilitation included swimming and cycling by week 2 and running by week 3 postoperatively. At 3 months after surgery, 93% reported improvement in function, with 78% describing a complete cure. Holen et al. (76) reviewed 35 athletes who were treated for MTSS by fasciotomy along the entire length of the posteromedial tibial border through two short skin incisions. After a mean observation time of 16 months, most patients were satisfied.

Despite good subjective results, 22 patients had a lower activity level postoperatively.

Author's Preferred Method of Treatment

In the acute setting of a runner with pain in the distal half of the tibia, the treatment program is centered around rest. The training program and importance of rest are thoroughly discussed with the athlete and coach. Unless there is a high suspicion of a stress fracture based on clinical evaluation, plain films or nuclear studies are not mandatory during this phase. Although adjuvant therapies have not been proven to hasten recovery, they are important in stimulating the athlete's participation in the recovery process. Nonsteroidals are prescribed for 1 to 2 weeks to decrease pain and inflammation. Cryotherapy applied to the affected area two to three times per day also may diminish inflammation. Heel-cord stretching exercises are recommended in patients who lack full ankle dorsiflexion. Lower extremity alignment should be carefully analyzed. For patients with excessive foot pronation, a semirigid orthosis is recommended. During the healing period, aerobic conditioning can be maintained by switching to non–weight-bearing activities such as cycling and swimming.

After the symptoms have resolved, a graduated return to running is permitted over a 3- to 6-week period. The return to activities should be based on clinical resolution of symptoms, because scintigraphic lesions may remain positive for months after the symptoms have abated. During the first 2 weeks, running is permitted on soft level surfaces on an every other day basis. The intensity and mileage of running is restricted by at least 50%. If the athlete remains symptom free, the intensity may be increased to 75% during weeks 3 and 4. During weeks 5 and 6, a return to full activity, including sprinting and hurdling, can usually occur.

If the athlete's symptoms return, consideration is given to imaging studies or compartment monitoring to exclude other disease processes. The duration of the rest and rehabilitation periods should be increased with each recurrence. For the rare recalcitrant case that has failed at least three trials of conservative therapy, fasciotomy may be indicated.

COMPARTMENT SYNDROME

Compartment syndrome is a clinical condition resulting from prolonged elevation of tissue pressure within a closed fascial space (77,78). This elevated pressure can lead to diminished blood perfusion to the muscle and nerve within the compartment compromising tissue viability. Because of its tight fascial compartments, the lower leg is the most common site for compartment syndrome in the body. The anterior compartment is the most commonly affected compartment (79).

Pathogenesis

Compartment syndrome in athletes may occur in an acute (ACS) or chronic (CCS) form. The acute variety is a well-known entity, which is usually associated with tibial fractures and requires immediate fasciotomy. In athletes, ACS most frequently occurs after tibial fractures or muscle injury. Several case reports have described lateral compartment syndrome secondary to injury of the peroneal muscles (80–84). The mechanism typically involves an inversion injury to the ankle with a strain or tear of the peroneal muscle(s) resulting in compartmental hemorrhage. The diagnosis may initially be overlooked as an ankle sprain only to develop sufficient swelling 12 to 24 hours after the injury, resulting in a compartment syndrome. Another muscle that may rupture during sports participation leading to an ACS is the medial head of the gastrocnemius (85,86). In addition to indirect trauma to the leg muscles, compartment syndromes can also occur in contact sports in which blunt trauma to the muscle leads to hemorrhage and elevated compartment pressures.

In contrast to ACS, CCS or chronic exertional compartment syndrome involves intermittent compartment pressure elevation associated with exercise. The exact pathophysiology of CCS has yet to be elucidated. During exercise, the muscle bulk can increase up to 20% due to tissue perfusion. Intercompartmental pressures have been reported to increase up to 100 mm Hg during exercise (87). The combination of increased muscle size and elevated pressures in patients with noncompliant fascia may result in CCS symptoms. Alternatively, muscle herniation in patients with CCS may lead to vascular occlusion. Muscle herniae has been observed in approximately 30% to 50% of patients with CCS compared with 5% to 10% in control subjects (88,89).

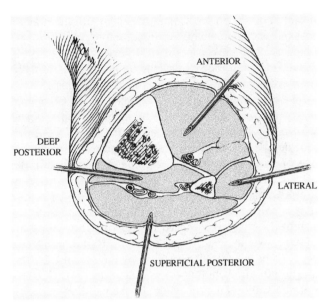

FIG. 49.11. Cross-section of tibia illustrates four major compartments and direction of needle insertion for testing each compartment.

Anatomy

The leg has been shown to contain at least four separate compartments: anterior, lateral, superficial, and deep posterior (Fig. 49.11) (90). Davey et al. (91) described a fifth compartment containing the tibialis posterior muscle, which is susceptible to its own compartment syndrome. Each of the four major compartments contains a sensory nerve that may be affected by elevated compartment pressures. The deep peroneal nerve lies within the anterior compartment, whereas the superficial peroneal nerve is located in the lateral compartment. The sural nerve runs through the superficial posterior compartment, and the posterior tibial nerve courses through the deep posterior compartment. Understanding the anatomy of each compartment is critical in diagnosis and treatment of this condition.

Clinical Evaluation

Early recognition of ACS is essential to prevent any permanent functional deficits. The classic presentation is pain out of proportion to the clinical situation (92). Patients present with severe pain and tense swollen compartment(s). Exacerbation of pain by passive stretching of the muscles in the affected compartment is the most sensitive clinical finding before the onset of ischemic dysfunction. The five P's (pain, pallor, paralysis, paresthesia, and pain) are late findings and indicate that ischemic injury has occurred. Fasciotomy at this stage yields suboptimal results. Of the five P's, paresthesias are usually the earliest symptom, occurring 1 to 2 hours after the onset of ischemia. Elevated pressures may be present despite normal pulses. Compartment syndrome may be masked in patients who are unconscious, on high-dose analgesics, or have a peripheral nerve block. In these patients, a high index of suspicion and tissue pressure measurements are critical for an early diagnosis.

The classic presentation of patients with CCS is pain in the leg that is brought on by exercise and relieved with rest. Symptoms are reproducible after an equivalent degree of exercise. Patients complain of paresthesias or dysesthesias from nerve compression within the affected compartment. On physical examination there are few characteristic findings. Patients with CCS may have a palpable muscle hernia, but this finding is inconsistent. Exercise is required to provoke the symptoms of pain, swelling, and/or paresthesias. Radiographs and bone scans are nondiagnostic in patients with CCS but are helpful in excluding other diagnoses (93). Ultrasonography allows measurement of the width of leg compartments at rest and during exercise but is less reliable than pressure measurements in diagnosing compartment syndrome (94). In one study, MRI was found to have delayed T1 recovery times postexercise in four of five patients with CCS (93). Nonetheless, the practical value of MRI is limited and unlikely to replace compartment pressure measurements.

Tissue pressure measurements are the gold standard for diagnosing compartment syndrome. Advances in technology have allowed easier and more precise techniques to measure compartment pressures. Early measurement devices used an infusion technique that allowed pressure readings over time (78). The disadvantages of this technique include the cumbersome and time-consuming setup of the device and the continuous infusion of saline into an already compromised compartment. The Wick and Slit catheters were designed to provide accurate interstitial fluid readings while minimizing tissue occlusion at the catheter tip (95,96). These devices transmit hydrostatic pressure from the catheter tip to a remote pressure transducer, thereby requiring precise positional control of the external transducer. Currently, the most commonly used monitor is the commercially available electronic Stryker STIC (solid-state transducer intercompartmental catheter) device (Fig. 49.12). This needle method allows multiple site recordings and repeated measurements with only minute injections of saline into the compartment (97). Hydrostatic column problems are eliminated by using a fiberoptic transducer-tipped catheter with a laterally positioned diaphragm. In the future, near-infrared spectroscopy and/or dynamic bone scans may prove to be useful noninvasive diagnostic tools for the detection of CCS (98,99).

The location of needle monitoring is important in obtaining accurate pressure readings. When ACS is suspected, tissue measurements should be evaluated in all four compartments. For closed tibial fractures, a gradi-

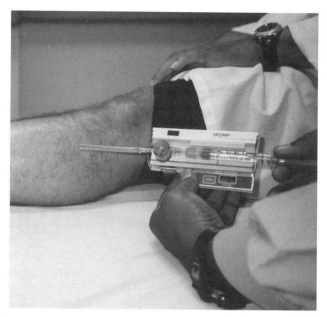

FIG. 49.12. Photograph of electronic STIC device used to measure compartment pressures.

ent may exist with highest pressures located within centimeters of the fracture site (100). Heckman et al. (100) recommended obtaining measurements at the level of the fracture and 5 cm proximal and distal to the injury. The highest pressure should be used in deciding whether a fasciotomy is necessary.

With a better understanding of the pathophysiology of compartment syndrome and the tolerance of muscle and nerve to ischemia, objective diagnostic criteria for ACS have been established. Normal resting compartment pressures range from 0 to 8 mm Hg. Levels greater than 30 to 40 mm Hg are associated with microcirculatory disturbances that can lead to muscle and nerve ischemia (101). Because compartment pressures depend on blood pressure, it is more accurate, especially in hypotensive trauma patients, to compare the difference between limb perfusion pressure and compartment pressure in determining whether surgical intervention is necessary (102,103). Compartment pressures within 20 mm Hg of diastolic pressure have been documented to significantly diminish tissue perfusion and are indicative of the need for fasciotomy (92).

In contrast to ACS, there is more controversy regarding the optimal diagnostic criteria for CCS. Although dynamic pressure recordings may be valuable in investigating the pathophysiology of CCS, they are not necessary for objective diagnosis of CCS. Because muscle contraction pressure requires standardization of muscle exertion between patients, it is more practical to emphasize muscle relaxation or rest pressure. In addition, muscle is normally perfused between muscle contractions during exercise (87). Therefore, static compartment pressures are the diagnostic modality of choice.

TABLE 49.3. *Indications for surgical decompression of CCS (Pedowitz)*

1. Preexercise compartment pressure >15 mm Hg
2. 1-min postexercise pressure >30 mm Hg
3. 5-min postexercise pressure >20 mm Hg

CCS, chronic compartment syndrome.

In patients suspected of having CCS, static compartment pressures are measured before exercise and at 1 and 5 minutes after exercise. The athletic activity should be of high intensity to reproduce the patient's symptoms. Most authors emphasize elevated postexercise pressures and a delay in return to preexercise values as important factors in diagnosing CCS. Because intramuscular pressure may be affected by joint angle, measurements should be performed with the knee and ankle in a standardized relaxed position for serial recordings (104). Although the diagnostic criteria for CCS vary between studies, the guidelines provided by Pedowitz et al. (89) are the most widely accepted. The authors proposed that any of the following compartment pressures are diagnostic of CCS of the leg: preexercise pressure more than 15 mm Hg, 1-minute postexercise pressure more than 30 mm Hg, or 5-minute postexercise pressure more than 20 mm Hg (Table 49.3).

Treatment

The treatment of ACS is emergent fasciotomy of the involved compartment(s). Muscles tolerate 4 hours of ischemia without any permanent damage. After 8 hours of ischemia, the damage is irreversible (105). Peripheral nerves develop neurapraxic changes after 4 hours of ischemia (106). Therefore, early diagnosis and prophylactic treatment of ACS by fasciotomy is essential in preventing permanent sequelae.

The double-incision fasciotomy is a safe and effective technique for decompressing all compartments of the leg (107). Wide skin incisions are necessary to completely decompress the compartments in ACS (108). An anterolateral longitudinal skin incision is performed midway between the tibial crest and the fibular shaft. A transverse incision through the fascia allows identification of the anterolateral intermuscular septum (109). Longitudinal fasciotomies are performed 1 to 2 cm anterior and 1 to 2 cm posterior to the septum, thereby decompressing the anterior and lateral compartments, respectively. The lateral compartment fasciotomy should avoid the superficial and anteriorly located superficial peroneal nerve. The superficial peroneal nerve exits the lateral compartment adjacent to the septum at the junction of the middle and distal thirds of the leg. When decompressing the distal aspect of the compartment, the fasciotome or scissors should be aimed poste-

riorly toward the lateral malleolus to avoid injury to the nerve.

The posteromedial incision allows decompression of the superficial and deep posterior compartments. The skin incision is placed 2 cm posterior to the posterior tibial margin. The skin edges are undermined, and the saphenous nerve and vein are retracted anteriorly. A transverse incision in the fascia is performed to allow visualization of the septum between the superficial and deep posterior compartments. The superficial compartment is decompressed first followed by the deep posterior compartment. Occasionally, the soleus origin must be detached from the tibia to decompress the deep compartment. The fascia over the tibialis posterior is divided to completely decompress the deep posterior muscles (91).

An alternative technique for decompressing all four compartments through one incision is the perifibular approach (78). A straight lateral incision is placed just posterior and parallel to the fibula from the level of the fibular head to the lateral malleolus. Proximally, the common peroneal nerve is exposed and protected. The posterior compartments are decompressed first followed by retraction of the anterior flap of the incision and decompression of the anterior and lateral compartments.

When the decompression is performed 6 to 8 hours after the onset of elevated pressure(s), debridement of necrotic tissue may be necessary to prevent infection. For ACS, all wounds are left open and managed with sterile dressings. Constrictive external dressings or a cast should be avoided because these devices may result in elevated intercompartmental pressures (110). Instead, a large nonrestrictive dressing should be applied. Once the swelling has sufficiently resolved, usually in 3 to 7 days, wound closure is performed (111). When the wound cannot be closed without undue tension, a skin-stretching device may be used to avoid the need for a split-thickness skin graft (112) (Fig. 49.13). With the skin-stretching device, the cosmetic appearance of the skin is maintained, donor morbidity is eliminated, and the in-hospital course is shortened.

Patients with CCS may opt for a trial of rest and activity modification. For those who return to their original activity level, the symptoms often recur. Therefore, operative decompression is frequently necessary for patients with CCS (88). In contrast to ACS, surgery for CCS involves small skin incisions and subcutaneous fasciotomies. In the presence of a fascial defect, the skin incision is placed directly over the muscle hernia (109). The fasciotomy is performed through the defect, being careful to protect the superficial peroneal nerve. Fascial defects should never be closed because of the risk of producing an ACS (88). Skin incisions are closed primarily at the completion of the operative procedure. Postoperatively, the patient begins

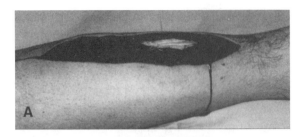

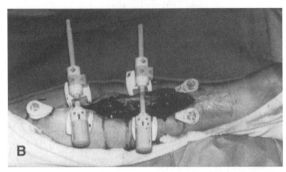

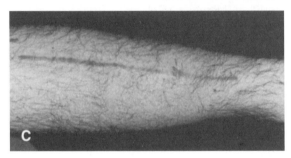

FIG. 49.13. Photograph of fasciotomy site in patient with tibia fracture **(A).** Skin stretching device **(B)** required 90 minutes to approximate skin edges for wound closure **(C).** (From Boden BP, Buinewicz BR. Management of traumatic cutaneous defects using a skin-stretching device. *Am J Orthop* 1995;24 [Suppl]:27–30, with permission.)

weight bearing as tolerated. During the first week, gentle stretching exercises are performed followed by strengthening exercises. By 2 to 3 weeks, the patent is usually sufficiently recovered to allow return to athletic activities.

Outcomes

In patients with ACS, the prognosis depends on the severity of the ischemia, time to decompression, and associated injuries. In addition to these factors, any patient who has undergone a fasciotomy may have diminished muscle strength in the affected compartment. In an animal study, Garfin et al. (113) documented a 15% loss of muscle strength without the constraining fascia. For CCS, good to excellent results have been reported in 60% to 95% of individuals undergoing decompression (88,89,114–116). The results of decompression of the deep posterior compart-

ment tend to be less favorable than decompression of the anterior compartment (114,115,117). This may be related to a delay in diagnosis, an incorrect diagnosis, difficulty measuring the deep posterior compartment pressure, or pitfalls associated with adequately decompressing the deep posterior compartment and the tibialis posterior muscle.

Author's Preferred Method of Treatment

Diagnosis of ACS is based on clinical signs and confirmed by compartment pressure measurements. The Stryker monitor is commercially available, reproducible, and easy to use. In patients with severe muscle injury, ACS may evolve over 1 to 3 days. These patients require hospital admission for observation and close monitoring. For normotensive patients, tissue pressures greater than 30 to 40 mm Hg indicate the need for fasciotomy. In patients who are hypotensive or hypertensive, fasciotomies should be performed when tissue pressures rise within 20 mm Hg of the diastolic pressure. The double-incision technique is effective at reaching all four major compartments. Meticulous dissection is required to adequately decompress the tibialis posterior muscle. If the wound cannot be closed without tension on a delayed basis, the skin-stretching device is a simple method to gain wound closure.

The most important factors in achieving a successful outcome in CCS is making the correct diagnosis and performing the surgery properly. The diagnostic guidelines proposed by Pedowitz et al. (89) are used to determine the need for surgery. Range of motion exercises should be performed as soon after the surgery as tolerated to prevent scar formation and stiffness from bleeding.

PROXIMAL TIBIOFIBULAR INSTABILITY

Instability of the proximal tibiofibular joint is an uncommon disorder. Disruption of this joint usually occurs as an isolated injury but may be associated with major limb trauma. Diagnosis requires a high index of suspicion, especially when a displaced tibial fracture is associated with an intact fibula. Instability of the proximal tibiofibular joint is classified into four different types. Acute injuries are treated with closed reduction and immobilization, whereas chronic injuries may require surgical intervention.

Pathoanatomy

The proximal tibiofibular articulation is a diarthrodial joint surrounded by a thickened capsule (118). In 10% of adults, the proximal tibiofibular joint communicates with the knee joint (119). Tibiofibular ligaments, which course superiorly and obliquely from the fibula to the tibia, stabilize the joint. The anterior tibiofibular ligaments are thicker and stronger than the posterior ligaments. These tibiofibular ligaments are reinforced by the biceps femoris tendon and the lateral (fibular) collateral ligament (LCL); both insert on the superior aspect of the fibula. The LCL and the biceps tendon are taut with knee extension and slack with knee flexion. The common peroneal nerve winds along the fibular neck coursing from posterior to anterior.

A bony sulcus on the tibia also provides some stability to the proximal fibula. Ogden (118) described two patterns of bony inclination at the proximal tibiofibular joint: horizontal and oblique. Although a continuum exists between horizontal and oblique, 20 degrees was chosen as a dividing point. Ogden proposed that the oblique inclination, greater than 20 degrees, is inherently less stable than the horizontal articulation.

During ankle motion the fibula undergoes vertical and rotatory displacements. The proximal fibula also undergoes slight anteroposterior movement with knee flexion and extension. Locking the position of the fibula to the tibia either by a syndesmotic screw or a bony synostosis (120) has been shown to affect ankle motion. The primary function of the proximal tibiofibular joint is to diminish torsional stresses at the ankle (121).

Clinical Evaluation

Common symptoms of a proximal tibiofibular injury include local pain, tenderness, and occasionally peroneal nerve involvement. At the time of injury the athlete experiences a "popping sensation" along the lateral aspect of the knee that may simulate a meniscal tear (122). The mechanism of injury is associated with direct or indirect trauma. The knee is typically in a flexed position, so that the LCL and biceps femoris tendon are relaxed.

On physical examination the fibular head is noted to be subluxated or dislocated. In addition to pain and a prominent fibular head, the biceps tendon appears as a tense band adjacent to the fibular head (123). Palpation of the fibular head elicits discomfort. Instability is detected by comparing a draw test of the proximal fibula with the unaffected contralateral side. After dislocation, patients often lack full extension of the knee. A careful neurologic evaluation should be performed to assess the status of the peroneal nerve. Physical examination of the knee, leg, and ankle are critical to exclude concomitant injuries.

Radiographs can be helpful in confirming the diagnosis. Multiple projections and comparison views of the contralateral extremity may be required to visualize the injury (124).

Radiographs of the leg in internal rotation will max-imize the distance between the lateral aspect of the tibia and the fibula.

Classification

The most commonly used classification system is that proposed by Ogden (125). Based on a review of 43 cases, he divided proximal tibiofibular instability injuries into four types (Fig. 49.14): subluxation (type 1), anterolateral dislocation (type 2), posteromedial dislocation (type 3), and superior dislocation (type 4). In his review, anterolateral dislocation was the most common type, accounting for 67.4%, followed by subluxations (23.3%), posteromedial dislocations (7%), and superior dislocations (2.3%). The injuries were further subdivided into acute or chronic.

Patients with subluxation have abnormal anteroposterior motion without frank dislocation (126). Bilaterality is common, although only one side may be symptomatic. The condition typically occurs in children who have hypermobility of their joints or in patients with an underlying pathologic condition such as muscular dystrophy or a connective tissue disorder. Subluxation may be the sequelae of a prior episode of proximal fibular dislocation.

Anterolateral dislocation of the proximal fibula is the most common type of dislocation as evidenced by Ogden's report and numerous case reports (121–123,125,127–131). The classic mechanism involves a fall on an inverted and plantar flexed foot with the knee flexed and the leg adducted (131). During inversion and plantar flexion of the foot, the anterolateral leg muscles contract, pulling the proximal fibula anteriorly. Flexion of the knee relaxes the stabilizing effect of the LCL and biceps tendon. The injuries frequently occur in soccer during a slide tackle or in baseball as the runner slides into a base. Lord and Coutts (132) reported the injury in parachutists during off-balanced landings. Because the injury occurs via an indirect mechanism, the skin is not contused. In addition to the usual symptoms, forceful ankle motion produces proximal pain due to the fibular motion (131).

Posteromedial dislocations are caused by direct high-energy trauma or by a twisting motion associated with a strong biceps femoris contraction. The fibular head shifts posteriorly behind the tibial plateau, making it less noticeable than the prominence associated with anterolateral dislocations. Concomitant injuries may include a peroneal nerve palsy and/or a lesion of the LCL.

Superior dislocations are extremely rare and usually associated with severe extremity trauma (133). These dislocations may accompany ankle injuries or displaced tibial shaft fractures with an intact fibula. Because of the high energy necessary to produce this lesion, neuro-

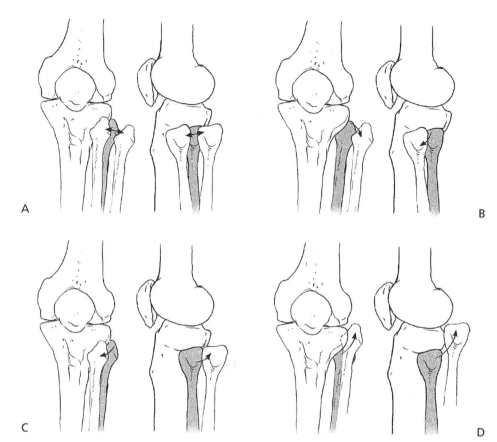

FIG. 49.14. Four types of tibiofibular instability as classified by Ogden: **A,** Type I, subluxation; **B,** type II, anterolateral dislocation; **C,** type III, posteromedial dislocation; **D,** type IV, superior dislocation.

vascular injuries and compartment syndromes can occur.

Treatment

After more serious injuries, such as tibia fractures or compartment syndromes, are addressed, attention should be turned to the proximal tibiofibular joint. Subluxation of the proximal fibula in children is often a self-limiting condition, which resolves with the onset of skeletal maturity (126). For persistent symptoms, a cylinder cast for 2 to 3 weeks is recommended. In acute dislocations, immediate closed reduction is the preferred treatment. The reduction can be attempted in the office, but if unsuccessful, sedation or general anesthesia in the operating room is required. The reduction maneuver involves flexion of the knee to 90 degrees and direct anterior or posterior pressure on the fibular head. There is disagreement as to the type and duration of immobilization. Some authors recommend an elastic bandage with crutches for comfort (131), whereas others advocate 3 weeks of immobilization (125).

For chronic instabilities, surgery is often required to relieve the symptoms. Arthrodesis of the superior tibiofibular joint has fallen out of favor because of resultant ankle symptoms due to the loss of fibular motion (125). Fusion of the proximal tibiofibular joint can be difficult to obtain with hardware failure and symptomatic nonunion. Several authors have reported good results after resection of the proximal fibula for chronic instability (121,131). In patients with chronic anterolateral instability, a more anatomic procedure has been described in which a strip of biceps femoris tendon and deep fascia of the anterior compartment of the leg is used to reconstruct the tibiofibular ligaments (134,135).

Return to activities depends on the type of injury and chronicity of symptoms. For acute dislocations that are immediately reduced, the recovery period takes approximately 6 weeks. The exception is posteromedial dislocations, where hamstring strengthening exercises should be avoided for 6 to 12 weeks. Rehabilitation after surgical correction of a chronic injury is more prolonged, often requiring 1 to 3 months of healing followed by an appropriate course of muscle strengthening.

Author's Preferred Method of Treatment

The most critical factor in treating proximal tibiofibular instabilities is making an early diagnosis. For acute injuries, closed reduction and immobilization for 2 to 3 weeks is recommended. Gentle range of motion exercises, two to three times per day, are permitted starting with the second week. This is followed by a 3-week course of strengthening exercises and gradual return to activities. In patients with a peroneal nerve palsy, a neurosurgical consult should be obtained to assist in determining whether the nerve needs to be explored and the timing of surgery. For patients with chronic instability, surgical correction is frequently required. Arthrodesis should be avoided because of the potential for ankle symptoms. Resection of the fibular head is a suboptimal procedure due to the loss of the LCL and biceps femoris tendon attachments. The ligament reconstruction procedure described by Giachino (134) appears to provide the most anatomic correction.

NERVE ENTRAPMENT

Peripheral nerve entrapment syndromes of the lower extremity are much less common than those of the upper extremity. In the leg, entrapment of the common peroneal nerve, the superficial peroneal nerve, and the sural nerve has been reported (136–139). The peroneal nerves are more commonly affected than the sural nerve.

Pathoanatomy

Common Peroneal Nerve

The common peroneal nerve is the lateral terminal branch of the sciatic nerve. The nerve passes between the biceps tendon and the lateral head of the gastrocnemius muscle to reach the posterior aspect of the fibular head. It then winds around the neck of the fibula between the two heads of the peroneus longus and divides into the deep and superficial peroneal nerves.

Several etiologic factors may be responsible for entrapment of the common peroneal nerve. Leach et al. (136) described eight athletes with peroneal nerve compression secondary to exercise. The authors proposed that the mechanism of injury involves contraction of the peroneal musculature when the foot is in a plantarflexed and inverted position. This places the nerve under stretch against a sharp fibrous edge at the peroneus longus origin. Other factors that may be responsible for peroneal nerve irritation include genu varum, posterolateral knee reconstructions, and mechanical pressure from proximal tibiofibular instability (140). An accessory ossicle (fabella) in the lateral head of the gastrocnemius or a ganglion cyst can also cause compression of the nerve.

Superficial Peroneal Nerve

The superficial peroneal nerve descends in the lateral compartment and innervates the peroneus brevis and longus muscles. The nerve pierces the deep fascia at the junction of the middle and distal thirds of the leg. After exiting the fascia, the nerve divides into the medial and intermediate dorsal cutaneous nerves to supply sensation to the dorsum of the foot except for the first web space.

The superficial peroneal nerve may be compressed proximally via one of the mechanisms described for the common peroneal nerve or distally as it exits the lateral compartment. Distal compression may be caused by a fascial hernia, fibula fracture, direct trauma, a space-occupying lesion, stretching of the nerve secondary to recurrent ankle sprains, or compression from high boots with tight laces (137,138).

Sural Nerve

The medial sural nerve courses between the heads of the gastrocnemius muscle proximally and just posterior to the peroneal tendons distally. At the ankle, it divides into two cutaneous nerves that supply sensation to the lateral heel and lateral border of the foot.

Entrapment neuropathy of the sural nerve is an extremely rare condition. Nerve compression may be caused by recurrent ankle sprains, calcaneal fractures, or space-occupying lesions such as a ganglion cyst or fibrous tissue around the ankle (139).

Clinical Evaluation

Patients with nerve entrapment present with pain at the site of compression. Sensory symptoms, such as paresthesias, dysesthesias, and hypesthesias, are often present. Motor weakness may occur in patients with common peroneal or deep peroneal involvement. Often, the patients complain of an exacerbation of symptoms during physical activity.

On physical examination, tenderness is elicited over the area of nerve entrapment. Neurologic deficits allow localization of the affected nerve. Neural irritability occurs with percussion of the nerve at the site of compression. For the superficial peroneal nerve, direct pressure at the site of entrapment while the patient actively plantarflexes and inverts the ankle often reproduces the symptoms. In addition, a fascial defect or muscle herniation may be palpable (141). Complete palpation of the affected area should be performed to exclude a soft tissue mass. An injection of local anesthetic into the region of nerve entrapment can temporarily alleviate the pain. Electrodiagnostic studies reveal prolonged conduction velocities or attenuated action potentials; however, a normal study does not rule out nerve entrapment (142). The differential diagnosis should include CCS and lumbar radiculopathies.

Treatment

Initial treatment of peripheral nerve entrapment syndromes consists of a trial of conservative therapy. For peroneal nerve entrapment syndromes with associated ankle instability, peroneal muscle strengthening exercises and an ankle brace may alleviate the symptoms. Compression via extrinsic factors such as tight shoes or taping should be avoided.

Patients who are unresponsive to conservative therapy are considered for operative decompression of the affected nerve. Complete fasciotomies and extensive neurolysis procedures are not necessary (143). Fascial defects should not be closed due to the risk of developing a compartment syndrome. Postoperatively, the patient is allowed to bear weight as tolerated. Return to full athletic activity is based on resolution of clinical symptoms and can usually be achieved by 3 weeks postsurgery.

POPLITEAL ARTERY ENTRAPMENT

Popliteal artery entrapment is a rare entity that has received more attention in the vascular literature than in the orthopedic literature. The syndrome is characterized by calf pain in young athletic individuals who may initially present to their orthopedic physician. The symptoms can mimic CCS of the posterior compartment. Accurate diagnosis depends on a high index of suspicion combined with angiography. Once diagnosed, most patients require surgical intervention.

Pathoanatomy and Classification

The etiology of popliteal artery entrapment has been attributed to various anatomic variations or congenital anomalies about the popliteal region (144–147). Although several classification systems have been proposed, the five types of entrapment described by a number of authors are the most widely accepted (145,148–150):

- Type I: Medial deviation of the popliteal artery around and deep to the medial head of the gastrocnemius (Fig. 49.15). Type I is the most common anomaly.
- Type II: Medial deviation of the popliteal artery around and deep to the medial head of the gastrocnemius. In Type II anomalies, the medial head of the gastrocnemius arises from a more lateral position on the medial femoral condyle.
- Type III: The popliteal artery is compressed by an accessory slip of muscle from a laterally positioned medial head of the gastrocnemius.
- Type IV: The popliteal artery is entrapped deep to the popliteus muscle or a fibrous band from the popliteus.

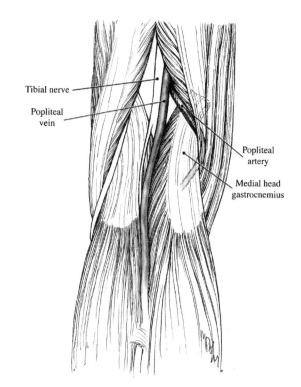

Tibial nerve

Popliteal vein

Popliteal artery

Medial head gastrocnemius

FIG. 49.15. Illustration of type I popliteal artery entrapment syndrome anomaly. Popliteal artery is displaced medially around and beneath the origin of the medial gastrocnemius.

- Type V: Any of the above variants in which the popliteal vein and artery are entrapped. This condition has been reported in 7.6% of cases (151).

Clinical Evaluation

The syndrome should be suspected in any young athlete with intermittent claudication pain in the calf (152). Most individuals with popliteal artery entrapment syndrome are young males under the age of 40 (151). Persky et al. (151) reported a 34% incidence of bilaterality. Patients complain of cramping in the calf and foot and occasional blanching, paresthesias, and numbness in the foot. The symptoms are typically associated with walking and relieved by rest. Interestingly, in patients with arterial compression without occluding thrombus, the calf pain may occur with walking but not with running (145,153,154).

Physical findings are limited in the early stages of this condition. Signs may include calf tenderness, diminished or absent pedal pulses, and knee warmth secondary to increased collateral circulation in the geniculate arteries. Provocation testing, such as exercise or knee hyperextension with active plantar flexion or passive dorsiflexion of the foot, may dampen pedal pulses. Knee extension and ankle dorsiflexion place the artery under stretch, whereas active plantar flexion causes the gastrocnemius to compress the popliteal artery. Evaluation of the venous system should also be performed. In contrast to CCS, intracompartmental pressure in patients with popliteal artery entrapment syndrome has been shown to diminish on exertion.

Imaging

Noninvasive duplex scanning may be helpful in identifying popliteal compression, especially with provocative testing (155). However, the definitive diagnosis is provided by arteriography. The most characteristic feature on the angiogram is medial deviation of the proximal popliteal artery (156). Other findings include segmental occlusion of the midpopliteal artery and poststenotic dilation (156). After obtaining neutral non-stressed views, stress arteriograms should be performed to elicit arterial compression.

Treatment

The risk of popliteal occlusion and lower extremity ischemic injury in young otherwise healthy individuals is high. Therefore, treatment should be operative correction by a vascular surgeon. When popliteal artery entrapment syndrome is diagnosed early and there is no arterial damage, transection of the compressing muscle or fascial band may be sufficient (146). If arterial damage is present, a vascular reconstructive procedure such as excision and reanastomosis or saphenous vein bypass grafting is necessary.

Outcomes

The best results are achieved when the syndrome is diagnosed early and treated by simple division of the constricting lesion. When arterial reconstruction is necessary, the recovery period is more prolonged. Duwelius et al. (144) measured ankle plantar flexion and dorsiflexion muscle strength 1 year after myotomy and arterial reconstruction in an athlete. They found no significant strength deficits in the affected leg compared with the contralateral extremity. Return to athletic participation depends on documentation of good blood flow in the extremity both at rest and with exercise.

TIBIOFIBULAR SYNOSTOSIS

Tibiofibular synostosis is an unusual cause of anterolateral leg pain that may mimic MTSS. The etiologies of tibiofibular synostosis are numerous but typically occur in athletes as a complication of ankle injuries. In athletically active individuals, the synostosis may restrict ankle motion, resulting in decreased performance. Conservative treatment is often successful, but in refractory cases surgical excision is necessary.

Pathoanatomy

The interosseous membrane is the primary bond between the tibia and fibula. The fibers of this membrane originate from the tibial periosteum and course distally and obliquely at an angle of approximately 15 to 20 degrees to insert on the fibula (157). Distally, the interosseous membrane is continuous with the interosseous ligament.

In addition to bearing one sixth of the weight supported by the leg, the fibula also has a dynamic stabilizing function at the ankle (157). During the midstance and preswing phases of the gait cycle, the fibula is pulled distally an average of 2.4 mm by the flexors of the foot (157). The effect of this movement is to enhance ankle stability and to increase tension in the interosseous membrane and tibiofibular ligaments. Restriction of this motion may lead to ankle and leg pain.

The causes of tibiofibular synostosis may be congenital or acquired (158,159). Congenital tibiofibular synostosis develops after intrauterine trauma or infection or as the result of developmental arrest after joint cavitation (158). Acquired synostosis may occur in association with leg length discrepancy, exostoses, tibia and/or fibular fractures, and posterolateral tibial bone grafting. In athletes, tibiofibular synostosis most commonly occurs after an ankle injury. The mechanism of injury either involves an external rotation or inversion force to the foot (157,160,161). These forces may result in tearing of the interosseous ligament and membrane with subsequent hemorrhage and ossification (160).

In addition to syndesmotic ankle sprains, synostoses have been reported to occur in association with stress fractures (159,162). The proposed mechanism is hemorrhage from a stress fracture that dissects along the interosseous membrane and ossifies over time (159). The ossification site is subject to fatiguing stresses as the muscles attempt to pull the fibula distally. This may lead to stress fractures of the ossifying mass, with further hemorrhage and bone formation.

Clinical Evaluation

Congenital tibiofibular synostosis may remain asymptomatic until the individual becomes athletically active (158). Once symptomatic, patients present with anterior leg pain over the synostosis during weight bearing and push-off. On physical examination, there is tenderness over the area of the synostosis. Dorsiflexion of the ankle may be limited due to the synostosis. The symptoms are often aggravated by physical activity. The diagnosis can usually be confirmed with radiographs (Fig. 49.16). In the early stages of synostosis, nuclear imaging may reveal a lesion that is not present on plain films.

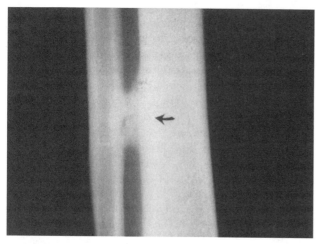

FIG. 49.16. Radiograph demonstrates a synostosis between the tibia and fibula at the junction of the middle and distal third of the leg. (From Henry JH, Andersen J, Cothren CC. Tibiofibular synostosis in professional basketball players. *Am J Sports Med* 1993;21:619–622, with permission.)

Treatment

Treatment recommendations in the literature vary. Some authors believe that a partial or complete synostosis is compatible with high-level performance (161,162). Nonoperative therapy consists of rest, nonsteroidals, evaluation for a custom-molded orthotic, and graduated return to activity once asymptomatic. In contrast, other authors report good clinical results and restoration of fibular biomechanics after surgical excision (157,159). After resecting the synostosis, meticulous hemostasis must be obtained to control hemorrhage and prevent recurrence. Waiting for the synostosis to mature before surgical excision and use of intraoperative bone wax are important factors in diminishing the risk of recurrence (159). Postoperatively, protected weight bearing with crutches is permitted for 1 month followed by a graduated return to athletic activities.

MEDIAL GASTROCNEMIUS INJURY

Injury to the medial gastrocnemius musculotendinous complex has often been referred to as tennis leg because of its frequency in tennis participants. The typical patient is a middle-aged recreational athlete who presents with a history of sharp pain in the posterior calf. The injury was once thought to be caused by rupture of the plantaris tendon. In a comprehensive review of the literature, Severance and Bassett (163) found no surgical or autopsy evidence supporting this hypothesis. It is now generally accepted that this injury involves the medial gastrocnemius.

Pathoanatomy

Several factors predispose the medial gastrocnemius muscle to injury as opposed to the other posterior calf muscles. In contrast to the slow-twitch soleus muscle, the gastrocnemius muscle fibers are fast twitch. Additionally, the gastrocnemius crosses two joints, making it vulnerable to injury during eccentric contractions when the muscle is being stretched (85). Although middle-aged patients present with an acute injury, there usually are preexisting chronic degenerative findings at the muscle–tendon unit.

Clinical Evaluation

Gastrocnemius injuries occur during explosive sprinting, jumping, or change of direction activities. There is usually simultaneous knee extension and ankle dorsiflexion, placing the muscle–tendon unit under stress. The patient experiences a sharp pain in the calf and often describes the sensation of being kicked.

Pain and tenderness are localized to the musculotendinous junction of the medial head of the gastrocnemius. Swelling and ecchymosis develop secondary to hematoma formation and may track distally to the ankle. Most patients are able to bear weight on the affected leg with pain. A thorough history and physical examination is usually sufficient to make a proper diagnosis. In addition to excluding other conditions, MRI can also help confirm the diagnosis by demonstrating a tear with surrounding hematoma (Fig. 49.17) (164).

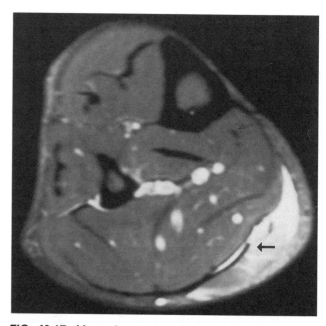

FIG. 49.17. Magnetic resonance imaging depicts injury to medial gastrocnemius. Notice swelling superficial to medial gastrocnemius muscle and retraction of tendon laterally (*arrow*).

The differential diagnosis should include thrombophlebitis, compartment syndrome, Achilles tendon rupture, Baker's cyst rupture, and neoplasm (85,165). Thrombophlebitis can be differentiated based on clinical findings and venography or Doppler studies if necessary. Rupture of the medial gastrocnemius has been reported in association with compartment syndromes (86). Symptoms such as pain out of proportion should alert the physician to a possible compartment syndrome. Pressure measurements may be required to exclude this diagnosis. Rupture of the Achilles tendon is distinguishable from a gastrocnemius injury based on clinical evaluation and a positive Thompson's test.

Treatment

Treatment of injuries to the medial head of the gastrocnemius is symptomatic. Although surgical intervention has been reported for this condition, good results have been documented with nonsurgical therapy (166). Early management consists of ice, elevation, compression with an Ace wrap, and crutches if weight bearing is painful. A heel lift helps relieve symptoms during the early symptomatic phase (167). Rehabilitation starts with early ankle and knee motion as tolerated. As the pain subsides, calf-strengthening exercises are initiated. For a complete muscle tear, full return to athletic participation can be expected in 3 to 12 weeks depending on the symptoms.

Author's Preferred Method of Treatment

The author prefers symptomatic nonsurgical management of gastrocnemius injuries. Initially, pain is alleviated through ice, elevation, compression, and nonsteroidals. Crutches may be necessary for several days after the injury followed by a heel lift once weight bearing can be tolerated. Rehabilitation consists of early stretching exercises followed by strengthening exercises and sports-specific activities. Return to full athletic participation is permitted when the patient is asymptomatic and has achieved close to 100% strength compared with the contralateral leg.

VENOUS THROMBOSIS

Effort-induced venous thrombosis is a well-documented condition affecting the axillary or subclavian veins of the upper extremity in throwing athletes (168). In the lower extremity, venous thrombosis is a rare entity in athletes (169). The condition may arise after trauma or strenuous exercise of the affected extremity (170,171). The symptoms include pain and swelling in the calf and/or thigh. Physical examination may demonstrate edema of the lower leg, popliteal or calf tenderness, and a positive Homan's sign. Pain is often present with the leg in a dependent position and diminished with elevation.

Venous Doppler studies or venography should be performed to confirm the diagnosis. In addition to effort thrombosis from running, other risk factors should be elicited: immobilization, oral contraceptives, tobacco use, malignancy, hemoglobinopathies, and prolonged bus or air transportation (169). The entity has also been reported in an athlete 2 weeks after a medial gastrocnemius muscle injury (172). The proposed mechanism was compression of the venous system from hematoma formation.

Treatment for venous thrombosis includes hospital admission, bedrest, and an internal medicine consultation. Anticoagulation is started with intravenous heparin and converted to oral warfarin. The possibility of a pulmonary embolus must be considered.

ACKNOWLEDGMENTS

Special thanks to Rachel I. Gafni, M.D., and Margaret Buda for their assistance in editing and preparing this chapter.

REFERENCES

1. Hulkko A, Orava S. Stress fractures in athletes. *Int J Sports Med* 1987;8:221–226.
2. Matheson GO, Clement DB, McKenzie DC, et al. Stress fractures in athletes: a study of 320 cases. *Am J Sports Med* 1987;15:46–58.
3. Bennell KL, Malcolm SA, Thomas SA, et al. The incidence and distribution of stress fractures in competitive track and field athletes. A twelve-month prospective study. *Am J Sports Med* 1996;24:211–217.
4. Carpintero P, Berral FJ, Baena P. Delayed diagnosis of fatigue fractures in the elderly. *Am J Sports Med* 1997;25:659–662.
5. Meyer SA, Saltzman CL, Albright JP. Stress fractures of the foot and leg. *Clin Sports Med* 1993;12:395–413.
6. McBryde AM. Stress fractures in athletes. *J Sports Med* 1976;3:212–217.
7. Stanitsk CL, McMaster JH, Scranton PE. On the nature of stress fractures. *Am J Sports Med* 1978;6:391–396.
8. Boden BP, Speer KP. Femoral stress fractures. *Clin Sports Med* 1997;16:307–317.
9. Barrow GW, Saha S. Menstrual irregularity and stress fractures in collegiate female distance runners. *Am J Sports Med* 1988;16:209–216.
10. Giladi M, Milgrom C, Simkin A, et al. Stress fractures and tibial bone width. A risk factor. *J Bone Joint Surg Br* 1987;69B:326–329.
11. Giladi M, Milgrom C, Simkim A, et al. Stress fractures. Identifiable risks. *Am J Sports Med* 1991;19:647–652.
12. Giladi M, Milgrom C, Stein M, et al. The low arch, a protective factor in stress fractures. A prospective study of 295 military recruits. *Orthop Rev* 1985;14:81–84.
13. Milgrom C, Giladi M, Simkin A, et al. An analysis of the biomechanical mechanism of tibial stress fractures among Israeli infantry recruits. *Clin Orthop* 1988;231:216–221.
14. Prather JL, Nusynowitz ML, Snowdy HA, et al. Scintigraphic findings in stress fractures. *J Bone Joint Surg Am* 1977;59A:869–874.
15. Wilcox JR Jr, Moniot AL, Green JP. Bone scanning in the evaluation of exercise-related stress injuries. *Radiology* 1977;123:699–703.
16. Zwas ST, Elkanovitch R, Frank G. Interpretation and classification of bone scintigraphic findings in stress fractures. *J Nucl Med* 1987;28:452–457.
17. Rupani HD, Holder LE, Espinola DA, et al. Three-phase radio-

nuclide bone imaging in sports medicine. *Radiology* 1985;156:187–196.

18. Rosen PR, Micheli LJ, Treves S. Early scintigraphic diagnosis of bone stress and fractures in athletic adolescents. *Pediatrics* 1982;70:11–15.

19. Chisin R, Milgrom C, Giladi M, et al. Clinical significance of nonfocal scintigraphic findings in suspected tibial stress fractures. *Clin Orthop* 1987;220:200–205.

20. Fredericson M, Bergman AG, Hoffman KL, et al. Tibial stress reaction in runners. Correlation of clinical symptoms and scintigraphy with a new magnetic resonance imaging grading system. *Am J Sports Med* 1995;23:472–481.

21. Arendt EA, Griffiths HJ. The use of MR imaging in the assessment and clinical mangement of stress reactions of bone in high-performance athletes. *Clin Sports Med* 1997;16:291–306.

22. Arendt EA, Griffiths HJ, Golloway HR, et al. The MR spectrum of stress injury to bone and its clinical relevance. *Am J Sports Med* (in press)

23. Milgrom C, Giladi M, Kashtan H, et al. A prospective study of the effect of a shock-absorbing orthotic device on the incidence of stress fractures in military recruits. *Foot Ankle* 1985;6:101–104.

24. Milgrom C, Burr DB, Boyd RD, et al. The effect of a viscoelastic orthotic on the incidence of tibial stress fractures in an animal model. *Foot Ankle* 1990;10:276–279.

25. Gardner LI, Dziados JE, Jones BH, et al. Prevention of lower extremity stress fractures: a controlled trial of a shock absorbent insole. *Am J Public Health* 1988;78:1563–1567.

26. Swenson EJ, DeHaven KE, Sebastianelli WJ. The effect of a pneumatic leg brace on return to play in athletes with tibial stress fractures. *Am J Sports Med* 1997;25:322–328.

27. Dickson T, Kichline P. Functional management of stress fractures in female athletes using a pneumatic leg brace. *Am J Sports Med* 1987;15:86–89.

28. Whitelaw GP, Wetzler MJ, Levy AS. A pneumatic leg brace for the treatment of tibial stress fractures. *Clin Orthop* 1991;270:301–305.

29. Green NE, Rogers RA, Lipscomb B. Nonunions of stress fractures of the tibia. *Am J Sports Med* 1985;13:171–176.

30. Blank S. Transverse tibial stress fractures. A special problem. *Am J Sports Med* 1987;15:597–602.

31. Chang PS, Harris RM. Intramedullary nailing for chronic tibial stress fractures. A review of five cases. *Am J Sports Med* 1996;24:688–692.

32. Rettig AC, Shelbourne KD, McCarroll JR, et al. The natural history and treatment of delayed union stress fractures of the anterior cortex of the tibia. *Am J Sports Med* 1988;16:250–255.

33. Shelbourne KD, Fisher DA, Rettig AC, et al. Stress fractures of the medial malleolus. *Am J Sports Med* 1988;16:60–63.

34. Reider B, Falroniero R, Yurkofsky J. Nonunion of a medial malleolus stress fracture. A case report. *Am J Sports Med* 1993;21:478–481.

35. Devas MB. Stress fractures of the tibia in athletes or "shin soreness." *J Bone Joint Surg Br* 1958;40B:227–239.

36. Devas MB, Sweetnam R. Stress fractures of the fibula. A review of fifty cases in athletes. *J Bone Joint Surg Br* 1956;38B:818–829.

37. Burrows HJ. Spontaneous fracture of the apparently normal fibula in its lower third. *Br J Surg* 1940;28:82–87.

38. Burrows JH. Fatigue fractures of the fibula. *J Bone Joint Surg Br* 1948;30:266–279.

39. Blair WF, Hanley SR. Stress fracture of the proximal fibula. *Am J Sports Med* 1980;8:212–213.

40. Strudwick WJ, Goodman SB. Proximal fibular stress fracture in an aerobic dancer. A case report. *Am J Sports Med* 1992;20:481–482.

41. Symeonides PP. High stress fractures of the fibula. *J Bone Joint Surg Br* 1980;62B:192–193.

42. Boden BP, Lohnes JH, Nunley JA, et al. Tibia and fibula fractures in soccer players. In review. Knee Surg Sports Traumatol Arthrosc 1999;7:262–266.

43. Teitz CC, Carter DR, Frankel VH. Problems associated with tibial fractures with intact fibulae. *J Bone Joint Surg Am* 1980;62A:770–776.

44. Slauterbeck JR, Shapiro MS, Liu S, et al. Traumatic fibular shaft fractures in athletes. *Am J Sports Med* 1995;23:751–754.

45. Garl TC, Alexander L, Ahlfeld SK, et al. Tibial fracture in a basketball player. Treatment dilemmas and complications. *Phys Sportsmed* 1997;25:41–53.

46. American Medical Association, Subcommittee on Classification of Sports Injuries. *Standard nomenclature of athletic injuries.* Chicago: American Medical Association, 1966:122–126.

47. Andrish JT, Bergfeld JA, Walheim JA. A prospective study on the management of shin splints. *J Bone Joint Surg Am* 1974;56A:1697–1700.

48. James SL, Bates BT, Osternig LR. Injuries to runners. *Am J Sports Med* 1978;6:40–50.

49. Watson AWS. Incidence and nature of sports injuries in Ireland. Analysis of four types of sport. *Am J Sports Med* 1993;21:137–143.

50. Wadley GH, Albright JP. Women's intercollegiate gymnastics. Injury patterns and "permanent" medical disability. *Am J Sports Med* 1993;21:314–320.

51. Puranen J. The medial tibial syndrome. Exercise ischemia in the medial fascial compartment of the leg. *J Bone Joint Surg Br* 1974;56B:712–715.

52. D'Ambrosia RD, Zelis RF, Chuinard RG, et al. Interstitial pressure measurements in the anterior and posterior compartments in athletes with shin splints. *Am J Sports Med* 1977;5:127–131.

53. Mubarak SJ, Gould RN, Lee YF, et al. The medial tibial stress syndrome. A cause of shin splints. *Am J Sports Med* 1982;10:201–205.

54. Holder LE. Bone scintigraphy in skeletal trauma. *Radiograph Clin North Am* 1993;31:739–781.

55. Detmer DE. Chronic shin splints. Classification and management of medial tibial stress syndrome. *Sports Med* 1986;3:436–446.

56. Detmer DE. Chronic leg pain. *Am J Sports Med* 1980;8:141–144.

57. Garth WP Jr, Miller ST. Evaluation of claw toe deformity, weakness of the foot intrinsics, and posteromedial shin pain. *Am J Sports Med* 1989;17:821–827.

58. Saxena A, O'Brien T, Bunce D. Anatomic dissection of the tibialis posterior muscle and its correlation to medial tibial stress syndrome. *J Foot Surg* 1990;29:105–108.

59. Slocum DB. The shin splint syndrome. Medical aspects and differential diagnosis. *Am J Surg* 1967;114:875–881.

60. Michael RH, Holder LE. The soleus syndrome. A cause of medial tibial stress (shin splints). *Am J Sports Med* 1985;13:87–94.

61. James T. Chronic lower leg pain in sport. *Austr Fam Phys* 1988;17:1041–1045.

62. Beck BR, Osternig LR. Medial tibial stress syndrome. The location of muscles in the leg in relation to symptoms. *J Bone Joint Surg Am* 1994;76A:1057–1061.

63. McKenzie DC, Clement DB, Taunton JE. Running shoes, orthotics, and injuries. *Sports Med* 1985;2:334–347.

64. Messier SP, Pittala KA. Etiologic factors associated with selected running injuries. *Med Sci Sports Exerc* 1988;20:501–505.

65. Sommer HM, Vallentyne SW. Effect of foot posture on the incidence of medial tibial stress syndrome. *Med Sci Sports Exerc* 1995;27:800–804.

66. Viitasalo JT, Kvist M. Some biomechanical aspects of the foot and ankle in athletes with and without shin splints. *Am J Sports Med* 1983;11:125–130.

67. Bates P. Shin splints—a literature review. *Br J Sports Med* 1985;19:132–137.

68. Clanton TO, Solcher BW. Chronic leg pain in the athlete. *Clin Sports Med* 1994;13:743–759.

69. Holder LE, Michael RH. The specific scintigraphic pattern of "shin splints in the lower leg": concise communication. *J Nucl Med* 1984;25:865–869.

70. Brill DR. Sports nuclear medicine. Bone imaging for lower extremity pain in athletes. *Clin Nucl Med* 1983;8:101–106.

71. Lieberman CM, Hemingway DL. Scintigraphy of shin splints. *Clin Nucl Med* 1980;5:31.

72. Anderson MW, Ugalde V, Batt M, et al. Shin splints: MR appearance in a preliminary study. *Radiology* 1997;204:177–180.

73. Ting A, King W, Yocum L, et al. Stress fractures of the tarsal navicular in long-distance runners. *Clin Sports Med* 1988;7:89–101.

74. Gross ML, Davlin LB, Evanski PM. Effectiveness of orthotic

shoe inserts in the long-distance runner. *Am J Sports Med* 1991;19:409–412.

75. Smith L, Clarke T, Hamill C, et al. The effects of soft and semi-rigid orthosis upon rearfoot movement in running. *Med Sci Sports Exerc* 1983;15:171.

76. Holen KJ, Engebretsen L, Grontvedt T, et al. Surgical treatment of medial tibial stress syndrome (shin splint) by fasciotomy of the superficial posterior compartment of the leg. *Scand J Med Sci Sports* 1995;5:40–43.

77. Rorabeck CH, Bourne R, Fowler P, et al. The role of tissue pressure measurement in diagnosing chronic anterior compartment syndrome. *Am J Sports Med* 1988;16:143–146.

78. Matsen FA, Winquist RA, Krugmire RB. Diagnosis and management of compartmental syndromes. *J Bone Joint Surg Am* 1980;62A:286–291.

79. Reneman RR. The anterior and lateral compartmental syndrome of the leg due to intensive use of muscles. *Clin Orthop* 1975; 113:69–80.

80. Arciero RA, Shishido NS, Parr TJ. Acute anterolateral compartment syndrome secondary to rupture of the peroneus longus muscle. *Am J Sports Med* 1984;12:366–367.

81. Davies JAK. Peroneal compartment syndrome secondary to rupture of the peroneus longus. A case report. *J Bone Joint Surg Am* 1979;61A:783–784.

82. Edwards PW. Peroneal compartment syndrome. Report of a case. *J Bone Joint Surg Br* 1969;51B:123–125.

83. Goodman MJ. Isolated lateral-compartment syndrome. Report of a case. *J Bone Joint Surg Am* 1980;62A:834.

84. Moyer RA, Boden BP, Marchetto PA, et al. Acute compartment syndrome of the lower extremity secondary to noncontact injury. *Foot Ankle* 1993;14:534–537.

85. Anouchi Y, Parker R, Seitz W. Posterior compartment syndrome of the calf resulting from misdiagnosis of a rupture of the medial head of the gastrocnemius. *J Trauma* 1987;27:678–680.

86. Straehley D, Jones WW. Acute compartment syndrome (anterior lateral and superficial posterior) following tear of the medial head of the gastrocnemius muscle. A case report. *Am J Sports Med* 1986;14:96–99.

87. Styf J, Korner L, Suurkula M. Intramuscular pressure and muscle blood flow during exercise in chronic compartment syndrome. *J Bone Joint Surg Br* 1987;69B:301–305.

88. Fronek J, Mubarak SJ, Hargens AR, et al. Management of chronic exertional anterior compartment syndrome of the lower extremity. *Clin Orthop* 1987;220:217–227.

89. Pedowitz RA, Hargens AR, Mubarak SJ, et al. Modified criteria for the objective diagnosis of chronic syndrome of the leg. *Am J Sports Med* 1990;18:35–40.

90. Matsen FA III. Compartmental syndrome. An unified concept. *Clin Orthop* 1975;113:8–14.

91. Davey J, Rorabeck C, Fowler P. The tibialis posterior muscle compartment. *Am J Sports Med* 1984;12:391–397.

92. Whitesides TE Jr, Heckman MM. Acute compartment syndrome. Update on diagnosis and treatment. *J Am Acad Orthop Surg* 1996;4:209–218.

93. Amendola A, Rorabeck CH, Vellett D, et al. The use of magnetic resonance imaging in exertional compartment syndromes. *Am J Sports Med* 1990;18:29–34.

94. Gershuni DH, Gosink BB, Hargens AR, et al. Ultrasound evaluation of the anterior musculofascial compartment of the leg following exercise. *Clin Orthop* 1982;167:185–190.

95. Mubarak SJ, Hargens AR, Owen CA, et al. The Wick catheter technique for measurement of intramuscular pressure. A new research and clinical tool. *J Bone Joint Surg Am* 1976;58A:1016–1020.

96. Rorabeck CH, Hardie PC, Logan J. Compartmental pressure measurement. An experimental investigation using the slit catheter. *J Trauma* 1981;21:446–449.

97. McDermott AGP, Marble AE, Yabsley RH, et al. Monitoring dynamic anterior compartment pressures during exercise. A new technique using the STIC catheter. *Am J Sports Med* 1982;10: 83–89.

98. Breit GA, Gross JH, Watenpaugh DE, et al. Near-infrared spectroscopy for monitoring of tissue oxygenation of exercising skeletal muscle in a chronic compartment syndrome model. *J Bone Joint Surg Am* 1997;79A:838–843.

99. Mohler LR, Styf JR, Pedowitz RA, et al. Intramuscular deoxygenation during exercise in patients who have chronic anterior compartment syndrome of the leg. *J Bone Joint Surg Am* 1997;79A:844–849.

100. Heckman MM, Whitesides TE Jr, Grewe SR, et al. Compartment pressure in association with closed tibial fractures. The relationship between tissue pressure, compartment, and the distance from the site of the fracture. *J Bone Joint Surg Am* 1994; 76A:1285–1292.

101. Mubarak SJ, Owen CA, Hargens AR et al. Acute compartment syndrome: Diagnosis and treatment with the aid of the Wick catheter. *J Bone Joint Surg Am* 1978;60A:1091–1095.

102. Heppenstall RB, Sapega AA, Scott R, et al. The compartment syndrome. An experimental and clinical study of muscular energy metabolism using phosphorus nuclear magnetic resonance spectroscopy. *Clin Orthop* 1988;226:138–155.

103. Heppenstall RB, Sapega AA, Izant T, et al. Compartment syndrome: a quantitative study of high-energy phosphorus compounds using 31P-magnetic resonance spectroscopy. *J Trauma* 1989;29:1113–1119.

104. Gershuni DH, Yaru NC, Hargens AR, et al. Ankle and knee position as a factor modifying intracompartmental pressure in the human leg. *J Bone Joint Surg Am* 1984;66A:1415–1420.

105. Whitesides T, Haney T, Morimoto K, et al. Tissue pressure measurements as a determinant for the need of fasciotomy. *Clin Orthop* 1975;113:43–51.

106. Whitesides TE Jr, Harada H, Morimoto K. Compartment syndromes and the role of fasciotomy, its parameters and techniques. *Instr Course Lect* 1977;26:179–196.

107. Mubarak SJ, Owen CA. Double-incision fasciotomy of the leg for decompression in compartment syndromes. *J Bone Joint Surg Am* 1977;59A:184–187.

108. Cohen MS, Garfin SR, Hargens AR, et al. Acute compartment syndrome. Effect of dermotomy on fascial decompression in the leg. *J Bone Joint Surg Br* 1991;73B:287–290.

109. Mubarak SJ. Surgical management of chronic compartment syndromes of the leg. *Op Techn Sports Med* 1995;3:259–266.

110. Garfin SR, Mubarak SJ, Evans KL, et al. Quantification of intracompartmental pressure and volume under plaster casts. *J Bone Joint Surg Am* 1981;63A:449–453.

111. Rorabeck CH. A practical approach to compartmental syndromes. Part III. *Instr Course Lect* 1983;32:102–113.

112. Boden BP, Buinewicz BR. Management of traumatic cutaneous defects by using a skin-stretching device. *Am J Orthop* 1995; 24[Suppl]Feb:27–30.

113. Garfin SR, Tipton CM, Mubarak SJ, et al. Role of fascia in maintenance of muscle tension and pressure. *J Appl Physiol* 1981;51:317–320.

114. Rorabeck CH, Fowler PJ, Nott L. The results of fasciotomy in the management of chronic exertional compartment syndrome. *Am J Sports Med* 1988;16:224–227.

115. Schepsis AA, Martini D, Corbett M. Surgical management of exertional compartment syndrome of the lower leg. Long-term followup. *Am J Sports Med* 1993;21:811–817.

116. Styf JR, Korner LM. Chronic anterior-compartment syndrome of the leg. Results of treatment by fasciotomy. *J Bone Joint Surg Am* 1986;68A:1338–1347.

117. Rorabeck CH, Bourne RB, Fowler PJ. The surgical treatment of exertional compartment syndrome in athletes. *J Bone Joint Surg Am* 1983;65A:1245–1251.

118. Ogden JA. The anatomy and function of the proximal tibiofibular joint. *Clin Orthop* 1974;101:186–191.

119. Resnick D, Newell JD, Guerra J, et al. Proximal tibiofibular joint: anatomic-pathologic-radiographic correlation. *AJR Am J Roentgenol* 1978;131:133–138.

120. Needleman RL, Skrade DA, Stiehl JB. Effect of the syndesmotic screw on ankle motion. *Foot Ankle* 1989;10:17–24.

121. Thomason P, Linson MA. Isolated dislocation of the proximal tibiofibular joint. *J Trauma* 1986;26:192–195.

122. Falkenberg P, Nygaard H. Isolated anterior dislocation of the proximal tibiofibular joint. *J Bone Joint Surg Br* 1983;65B: 310–311.

123. Andersen K. Dislocation of the superior tibiofibular joint. *Injury* 1985;16:494–498.

124. Veth R, Klasen H, Kingma L. Traumatic instability of the proximal tibiofibular joint. *Injury* 1981;13:159–164.

125. Ogden J. Subluxation and dislocation of the proximal tibiofibular joint. *J Bone Joint Surg Am* 1974;56A:145–154.

126. Ogden JA. Subluxation of the proximal tibiofibular joint. *Clin Orthop* 1974;101:192–197.

127. Christensen S. Dislocation of the upper end of the fibula. *Acta Orthop Scand* 1966;37:107–109.

128. Crothers OD, Johnson JTH. Isolated acute dislocation of the proximal tibiofibular joint. *J Bone Joint Surg Am* 1973;55A:181–183.

129. Harrison R, Hirdenach JCR. Dislocation of the upper end of the fibula. *J Bone Joint Surg Br* 1959;41B:114–120.

130. Sijbrandij S. Instability of the proximal tibio-fibular joint. *Acta Orthop Scand* 1978;49:621–626.

131. Turco VJ, Spinella AJ. Anterolateral dislocation of the head of the fibula in sports. *Am J Sports Med* 1985;13:209–215.

132. Lord CD, Coutts JW. A study of typical parachute injuries occurring in two hundred and fifty thousand jumps at the parachute school. *J Bone Joint Surg Am* 1944;26A:547–557.

133. Vigil AB, Barredo PM, Mortera SM. Traumatic luxation of the proximal tibiofibular joint, superior variety. A case report. *Acta Orthop Belg* 1983;49:479–482.

134. Giachino A. Recurrent dislocations of the proximal tibiofibular joint. *J Bone Joint Surg Am* 1986;68A:1104–1106.

135. Weinert CR, Raczka R. Recurrent dislocation of the superior tibiofibular joint. Surgical stabilization by ligament reconstruction. *J Bone Joint Surg Am* 1986;68A:126–128.

136. Leach RE, Purnell MB, Saito A. Peroneal nerve entrapment in runners. *Am J Sports Med* 1989;17:287–291.

137. Banerjee T, Koons DD. Superficial peroneal nerve entrapment. *J Neurosurg* 1981;55:991–992.

138. Kernohan J, Levack B, Wilson JN. Entrapment of the superficial peroneal nerve. Three case reports. *J Bone Joint Surg Br* 1985;67B:60–61.

139. Pringle RM, Protheroe K, Mukherjee SK. Entrapment neuropathy of the sural nerve. *J Bone Joint Surg Br* 1974;56B:465–468.

140. Moller BN, Kadin S. Entrapment of the common peroneal nerve. *Am J Sports Med* 1987;15:90–91.

141. McAuliffe TB, Fiddian NS, Browett JP. Entrapment neuropathy of the superficial peroneal nerve. A bilateral case. *J Bone Joint Surg Br* 1985;67B:62–63.

142. Sridhara CR, Izzo KL. Terminal sensory branches of the superficial peroneal nerve: an entrapment syndrome. *Arch Phys Med Rehabil* 1985;66:789–791.

143. Styf J. Entrapment of the superficial peroneal nerve. Diagnosis and results of decompression. *J Bone Joint Surg Br* 1989;71B:131–135.

144. Duwelius PJ, Kelbel JM, Jardon OM, et al. Popliteal artery entrapment in a high school athlete. A case report. *Am J Sports Med* 1987;15:371–373.

145. Love JW, Whelan TJ. Popliteal artery entrapment syndrome. *Am J Surg* 1965;109:620–624.

146. Rignault DP, Pailler JL, Lunel F. The "functional" popliteal entrapment syndrome. *Int Angio* 1985;4:341–343.

147. Taunton JE, Maxwell TM. Intermittent claudication in an athlete—popliteal artery entrapment: a case report. *Can J Appl Sports Sci* 1982;7:161–163.

148. Represa JAF, DeDiego JA, Molina LM, Popliteal artery entrapment syndrome. *J Cardiovasc Surg* 1986;27:426–430.

149. Delaney TA, Gonzalez LL. Occlusion of popliteal artery due to muscular entrapment. *Surgery* 1971;69:97–101.

150. Rich NM, Collins GJ Jr, McDonald PT, et al. Popliteal vascular entrapment. *Arch Surg* 1979;114:1377–1384.

151. Persky JM, Kempczinski RF, Fowl RJ. Entrapment of the popliteal artery. *Surg Gynecol Obstet* 1991;173:84–90.

152. Casscells SW, Fellows B, Axe MJ. Another young athlete with intermittent claudication. A case report. *Am J Sports Med* 1983;11:180–182.

153. Darling RC, Buckley CJ, Abbott WM, et al. Intermittent claudication in young athletes: popliteal artery entrapment syndrome. *J Trauma* 1974;14:543–552.

154. Lysens RJ, Renson LM, Ostyn MS, et al. Intermittent claudication in young athletes: popliteal artery entrapment syndrome. *Am J Sports Med* 1983;11:177–179.

155. diMarzo L, Cavallaro A, Sciacca V, et al. Diagnosis of popliteal artery entrapment syndrome: the role of duplex scanning. *J Vasc Surg* 1991;13:434–438.

156. McDonald PT, Easterbrook JA, Rich NM, et al. Popliteal artery entrapment syndrome. Clinical, noninvasive, and angiographic diagnosis. *Am J Surg* 1980;139:318–325.

157. Scranton PE, McMaster JH, Kelly E. Dynamic fibular function. A new concept. *Clin Orthop* 1976;118:76–81.

158. Gamble J. Proximal tibiofibular synostosis. *J Pediatr Orthop* 1984;4:243–245.

159. Flandry F, Sanders RA. Tibiofibular synostosis: an unusual cause of shin splint-like pain. *Am J Sports Med* 1987;15:280–284.

160. Fritschy D. An unusual ankle injury in top skiers. *Am J Sports Med* 1989;17:282–286.

161. Whiteside LA, Reynolds F, Ellsasser J. Tibio-fibular synostosis and recurrent ankle sprains in high performance athletes. *J Sports Med* 1978;6:204–208.

162. Henry JH, Andersen J, Cothren CC. Tibiofibular synostosis in professional basketball players. *Am J Sports Med* 1993;21:619–622.

163. Severance HW, Bassett FH. Rupture of the plantaris—does it exist? *J Bone Joint Surg Am* 1982;64A:1387–1388.

164. Menz MJ, Lucas GL. Magnetic resonance imaging of a rupture of the medial head of the gastrocnemius muscle. A case report. *J Bone Joint Surg Am* 1991;73A:1260–1261.

165. Robinson NA. Spontaneous rupture of the gastrocnemius muscle presenting as acute thrombophlebitis. *Am Surg* 1972;38:385–388.

166. Miller WA. Rupture of the musculotendinous junction of the medial head of the gastrocnemius muscle. *Am J Sports Med* 1977;5:191–193.

167. Froimson A. Tennis leg. *JAMA* 1969;209:415–416.

168. Wright RS, Lipscomb AB. Acute occlusion of the subclavian vein in an athlete: diagnosis, etiology and surgical management. *J Sports Med* 1974;2:343–348.

169. Harvey JS. Effort thrombosis in the lower extremity of a runner. *Am J Sports Med* 1978;6:400–402.

170. Gorard DA. Effort thrombosis in an American football player. *Br J Sports Med* 1990;24:15.

171. Zigun JR, Schneider SM. Effort thrombosis (Paget-Schroetter's syndrome) secondary to martial arts training. *Am J Sports Med* 1988;16:189–190.

172. Slawski DP. Case report: deep venous thrombosis complicating rupture of the medial head of the gastrocnemius muscle. *J Orthop Trauma* 1994;8:263–264.

Principles and Practice of Orthopaedic Sports Medicine,
edited by William E. Garrett, Jr., Kevin P. Speer, and Donald T. Kirkendall.
Lippincott Williams & Wilkins, Philadelphia © 2000.

CHAPTER 50

Athletic Injuries of the Midfoot and Hindfoot

Michael W. Bowman

The true incidence and severity of midfoot and hindfoot athletic injuries is vastly underestimated. The complex anatomy of the hindfoot and midfoot and the sophisticated biomechanics and function that takes place in this region are not easily understood, leading to both misdiagnosis and missed diagnosis. In our specialty orthopedic practice, which includes treatment of both recreational and professional athletes, a subtle but significant midfoot or hindfoot injury is often initially treated as a "foot or ankle sprain" and referred only when chronic disability results. Obviously, every possible athletic injury of the midfoot or hindfoot cannot be discussed in this chapter, but we review some of the more common and significant problems, concentrating on evaluation, differential diagnosis, and treatment. We first review the anatomy of the midfoot and forefoot as it applies to athletic injuries before discussing differential diagnoses and specific clinical problems.

MIDFOOT ANATOMY

Bony and Ligamentous Anatomy

The midfoot consists of 10 bones (Fig. 50.1). Together they form the slightly flexible but very stable longitudinal arch and transverse arch of the foot (Fig. 50.2). Eleven joints (5 tarsometatarsal joints, 3 naviculocuneiform joints, 2 intercuneiform joints, 1 naviculocuboid joint, and 1 cuneiform–cuboid joint) comprise the midfoot. The three cuneiforms and distal cuboid are wedge shaped in the coronal plane, creating a stable transverse arch. The base of the second metatarsal is inset 4 to 8 cm (1) more proximally than its neighbors, forming a "keystone" that contributes greatly to the stability of

the midfoot. Motion at each tarsometatarsal joint is limited to small ranges of dorsiflexion/plantar flexion (average 5 to 10 degrees) with slight abduction/adduction and slight pronation/supination allowed (2). The second tarsometatarsal joint is the most rigid, followed by the third tarsometatarsal joint (allowing 5 to 7 degrees dorsiflexion/plantar flexion). The fourth and fifth metatarsals articulate with the cuboid, allowing the most mobility (10 to 20 degrees of dorsiflexion/plantar flexion) and are known as the "mobile segment" of the midfoot (3). The first tarsometatarsal joint is usually very stable but may occasionally be hypermobile, allowing increased dorsiflexion in cases of flexible pes planus. Metatarsus primus varus may also be present as a normal variant. Together, enough midfoot motion is present to allow the metatarsals to adapt to irregular surfaces but provide a stable platform during push-off or jumping.

Very strong plantar intrinsic ligaments, the plantar tarsometatarsal ligaments and intermetatarsal ligaments, enhance midfoot stability (Fig. 50.3). No intermetatarsal ligament exists between the first and second metatarsal base; instead, a very strong Lisfranc's ligament runs from the lateral and plantar surface of the first (medial) cuneiform to the base of the second metatarsal. This ligament is only torn by high kinetic energy injuries of Lisfranc's joint that disrupts the second metatarsal base.

The dorsal tarsometatarsal and intermetatarsal ligaments are thin and more easily disrupted, which is evident in cases of Lisfranc's joint (tarsometatarsal) injuries. A significant twisting or axial force must be applied to disrupt the very strong plantar ligaments, as we will see.

The broad posterior tibial tendon insertion and peroneus longus sheath form a sling (Fig. 50.4) supporting the midfoot as well. Finally, the intrinsic muscles of the foot and the plantar fascia (windlass effect) support the arch of the midfoot (Fig. 50.5).

M. W. Bowman: Universiy of Pittsburgh, Pittsburgh, Pennsylvania 15260.

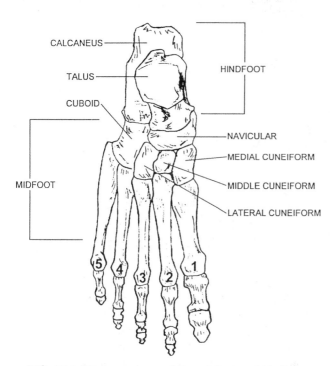

FIG. 50.1. Bony anatomy of the midfoot and hindfoot.

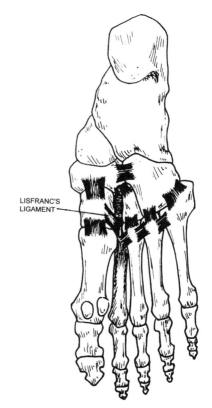

FIG. 50.3. Plantar view of the tarsometatarsal ligaments, including Lisfranc's ligament (labeled).

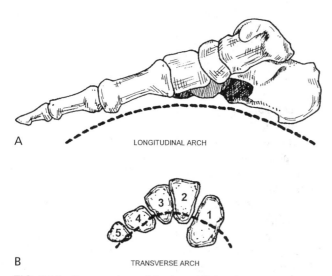

FIG. 50.2. Bony arches of the foot: (A) longitudinal arch and (B) transverse arch (proximal metatarsal level).

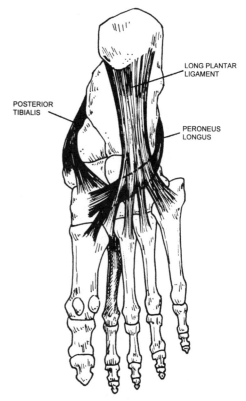

FIG. 50.4. Plantar view of the accessory structures supporting the plantar arch.

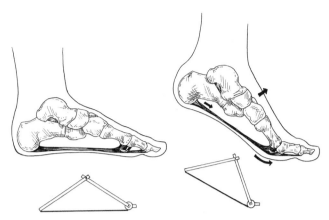

FIG. 50.5. The windlass effect of the plantar fascia. During the push-off phase of gait, metatarsophalangeal joint extension tightens the plantar fascia, elevating and supporting the arch. (Modified from Baxter, Pfeffer. *The foot and ankle in sport.* St. Louis: Mosby, 1995:197, with permission.)

Neurovascular Anatomy

The superficial peroneal nerve (the most variable nerve in the lower extremity) (Fig. 50.6) becomes cutaneous approximately 10.5 to 12 cm above the lateral malleolus (4–6) and courses distally across the midfoot from lateral to medial. As Kenzora (7) noted, the midfoot is a common area of iatrogenic injury and neuroma formation. The deep peroneal nerve runs in the anterior compartment underneath the extensor retinaculum (Fig. 50.7) and becomes superficial in the midfoot running across the first and second tarsometatarsal joints to supply sensation to the dorsal first/second web space and commonly a motor branch to the extensor digitorum brevis (8). It is commonly affected by spurs at the tarsometatarsal joint and may be injured during surgical approach (9).

The dorsalis pedis artery accompanies the deep pero-

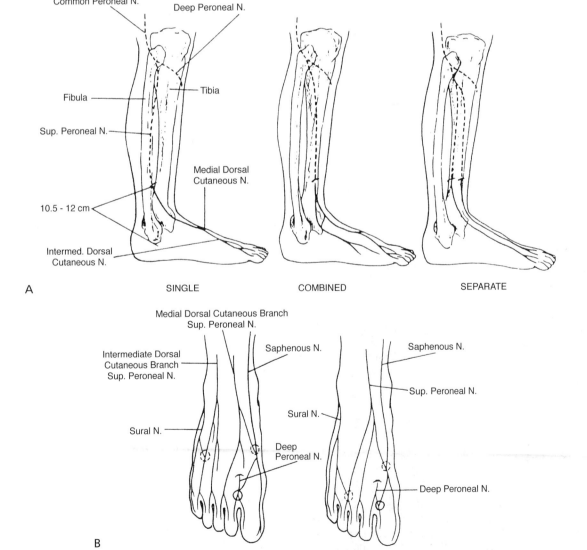

FIG. 50.6. Variations in the anatomy of the superficial peroneal nerve distribution: **(A)** lateral view and **(B)** dorsal view.

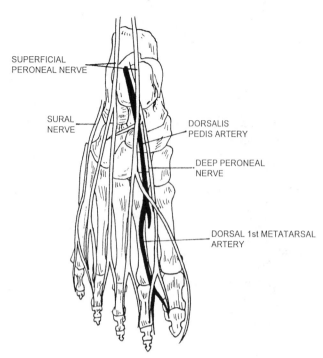

SUPERFICIAL
PERONEAL NERVE

SURAL
NERVE

DORSALIS
PEDIS ARTERY

DEEP PERONEAL
NERVE

DORSAL 1st METATARSAL
ARTERY

FIG. 50.7. Anatomy of the deep peroneal nerve.

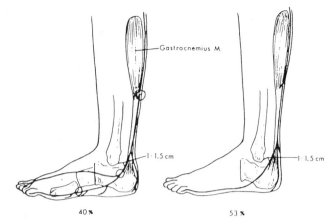

Gastrocnemius M.

1-1.5 cm

1-1.5 cm

40%

53%

FIG. 50.9. Variations in the anatomy of the sural nerve.

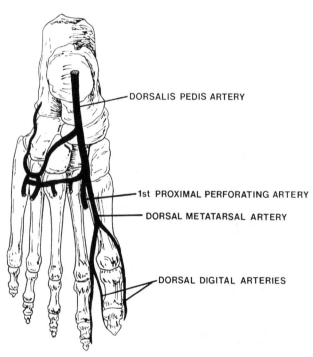

DORSALIS PEDIS ARTERY

1st PROXIMAL PERFORATING ARTERY

DORSAL METATARSAL ARTERY

DORSAL DIGITAL ARTERIES

FIG. 50.8. Dorsal arterial supply to the foot. The dorsalis pedis artery (a continuation of the anterior interosseous artery) is palpable over the navicular. The first proximal perforating artery may be injured by Lisfranc's joint injuries or first metatarsal osteotomy procedures.

neal nerve and a branch plunges plantarward between the first and second metatarsal base (Fig. 50.8). This artery may be injured by the initial midfoot injury, producing severe neurovascular compromise, or during surgery. Finally, the sural nerve (Fig. 50.9) is also very variable and may supply only the lateral side of the foot and fifth toe or the lateral half of the dorsum of the foot (10). It is frequently injured by surgical approach to the fourth and fifth tarsometatarsal joints, base of the fifth metatarsal, or lateral ankle.

HINDFOOT ANATOMY

Bony and Ligamentous Anatomy

As seen in Fig. 50.10, the spherical talonavicular joint and saddle-shaped calcaneocuboid joint have axes, which are aligned when the heel (calcaneus) is in eversion. This parallel alignment of the two joints comprising Chopart's joint allow increased midfoot motion (pronation and supination) and a more flexible midfoot that can provide shock absorption and adapt to a varied terrain (11–13). When the calcaneus inverts (such as in midstance or push-off), the axes of the talonavicular joint and the calcaneocuboid joint diverge, producing a stiffer more rigid midfoot platform for walking, running, or jumping.

A thick musculotendinous sling comprised of the plantar calcaneonavicular ligament ("spring ligament"), the thick plantar talonavicular capsule, and contributions from the posterior tibial tendon insertion provide stability at the talonavicular joint (Fig. 50.11). The Y-shaped bifurcate ligament (Fig. 50.12) (composed of the dorsal calcaneonavicular ligament and lateral calcaneocuboid ligament) supports the calcaneocuboid joint. As we see later, avulsion of the origin of the bifurcate ligament may result in a fracture of the anterior lateral process of the calcaneus.

The anatomy of the heel is rather specialized. The

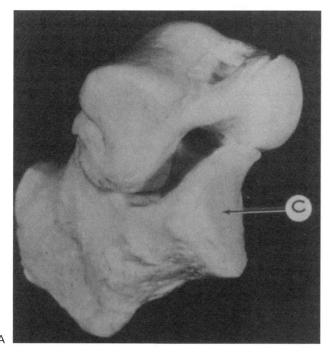

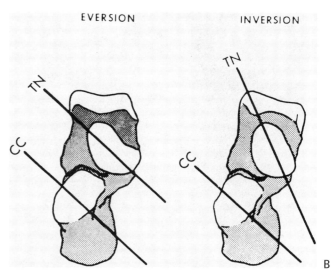

FIG. 50.10. A: Spherical talonavicular and saddle-shaped calcaneocuboid joints. (From Sarrafian SK. *Anatomy of the foot and ankle.* Philadelphia: J.B. Lippincott, 1983:392, with permission.) **B:** Effects of heel inversion and eversion upon alignment of the talonavicular (*TN*) and calcaneocuboid joints (*CC*). (From Mann RA. *Surgery of the foot and ankle,* 6th ed. Baltimore: Mosby, 1993:23, with permission.)

thick plantar aponeurosis (Fig. 50.13) runs from the interdigital spaces and plantar plates of the MTP joints along the arch deep to the subcutaneous tissue attaching to the medial calcaneal tubercle of the heel on its plantar surface. This calcaneal attachment runs along the "cap"

of the heel and becomes continuous with the insertion of the Achilles posteriorly (Fig. 50.14A). The posterior superior aspect of the heel is usually rounded but may occasionally be square, producing a Haglund's deformity. The Achilles tendon attaches to the calcaneus approximately 1 cm distal to the posterior superior edge of the calcaneus (14) and becomes continuous with the insertion of the plantar fascia distally. In the small space between the posterior superior border of the calcaneus and Achilles tendon, a small potential space exists known as the retrocalcaneal bursa (Fig. 50.14B) that is horseshoe shaped as noted by Frey et al. (15). Just superior to the posterior superior corner of the calcaneus and this bursa is a triangular-shaped collection of fatty tissue known as Kager's triangle that separates

FIG. 50.11. Superior view of the subtalar joint and the supporting structures of the talonavicular joint.

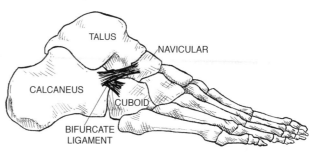

FIG. 50.12. Anatomy of the bifurcate ligament.

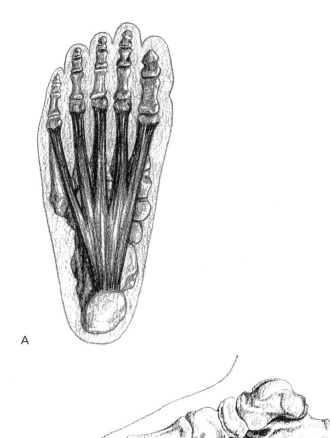

A

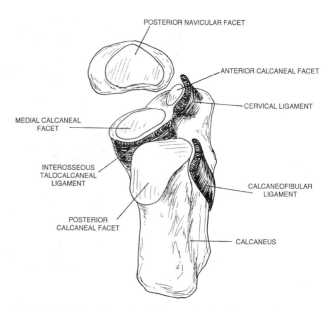

FIG. 50.15. Superior view of the subtalar joint displaying the ligamentous restraints.

FIG. 50.13. Plantar aponeurosis: **(A)** plantar view and **(B)** medial view.

the anterior surface of the Achilles tendon from the posterior ankle and the muscular and neurovascular structures.

As seen in Fig. 50.15, the subtalar joint is a complex joint consisting of a ball and socket-shaped anterior facet helping to support the talar head, a small medial facet, and large slightly curved posterior facet providing the main weight-bearing surface for the talus. Primary ligamentous support for the subtalar joint is extrinsic, provided by the calcaneofibular ligament. The cervical ligament and talocalcaneal interosseous ligament in order of importance provide the intrinsic stability of the

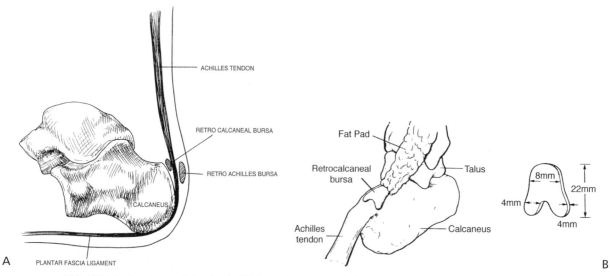

FIG. 50.14. Anatomy of the heel: **(A)** lateral view and **(B)** posterior view displaying the retrocalcaneal bursa. (From Frye C, Rosenberg Z, Shereff MJ, et al. *Foot Ankle* 1990;10:285–287, with permission.)

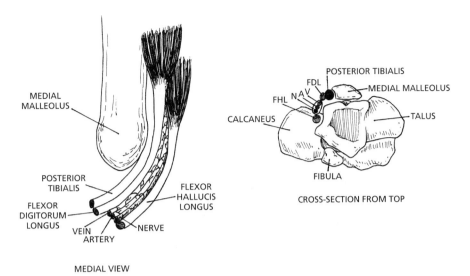

FIG. 50.16. Anatomic relationships of the posterior tibial nerve.

talocalcaneal joint. As noted by Inman (16), Manter (11), and others (13), this joint functions as a screw-shaped joint, permitting inversion and eversion and controlling the rigidity of the midfoot through the function of Chopart's joint.

Neurovascular Anatomy

The posterior tibial nerve is a direct continuation of the sciatic nerve running through the deep posterior compartment of the leg. In the lower one third of the leg (Fig. 50.16), the nerve lies between the flexor digitorum longus (anterior medially) and the flexor hallucis longus (posterior–lateral). The posterior tibial nerve is accompanied by the posterior tibial artery, which is anterior–medial to the nerve, and the venous plexus, which often has many branches wrapped around the nerve. The posterior tibial nerve courses behind the medial malleolus, tibialis posterior, and flexor digitorum longus under the flexor retinaculum, thus the mnemonic "Tom, Dick, and Harry." This area is commonly known as the tarsal tunnel. The posterior tibial nerve branches into a large medial plantar nerve anteriorly and a lateral plantar nerve posteriorly. Havel et al. (17) found that this branching occurs inside the tarsal tunnel in 93% of cadavers. The medial calcaneal nerve runs outside the tarsal tunnel in 45% of cases, supplying sensation to the medial heel and Achilles tendon area. It anastomoses with branches from the sural nerve (lateral calcaneal nerve), saphenous nerves, and superficial branches of the lateral plantar nerve. The medial plantar nerve (Fig. 50.17) runs through a fibroosseous tunnel plantarward of the posterior tibial tendon and just superficial to the intersection of the FDL and FHL at the thick fibrotic master knot of Henry. It then lies in the interval between the abductor hallucis and flexor digitorum brevis to sup-

ply the medial sole and plantar surface of the medial toes.

The lateral plantar nerve runs through a separate fibroosseous tunnel distal to the tarsal tunnel underneath the abductor hallucis fascia in the plane between the flexor digitorum brevis and quadratus plantae to lie in the interval between the flexor digitorum brevis and the intrinsic muscles to the little toe. It supplies sensation to the lateral plantar surface of the foot and the plantar surface of the lesser toes. A branch originating from either the posterior tibial nerve proper or as the first branch of the lateral plantar nerve, known as Baxter's nerve (18), also runs underneath the abductor fascia between the flexor digitorum brevis and quadratus plantae and courses transversely across the heel to the intrinsic muscles of the small toe, including the adductor digiti quinti. This nerve is also known as the nerve to the ADQ.

DIFFERENTIAL DIAGNOSES

Before discussing specific athletic injuries in detail, we list the differential diagnoses for midfoot and hindfoot injuries. Most midfoot or hindfoot injuries are accompanied by pain, usually swelling, and occasionally neurologic symptoms such as numbness or paresthesias.

Medial Midfoot Pain

Conditions that may cause symptoms of medial midfoot discomfort include

1. Medial Lisfranc's joint injury (ligamentous or fractures of the metatarsal base and/or cuneiform);
2. Chronic midfoot arthritis (chronic compression or sprain-type injuries producing arthritic changes,

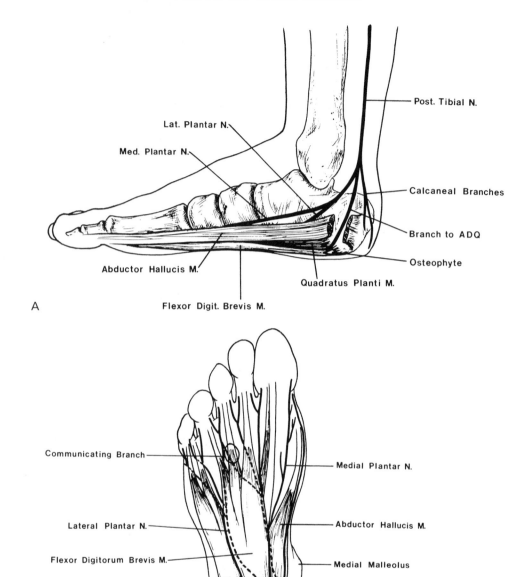

FIG. 50.17. Anatomy of the plantar nerves: (A) medial view and (B) plantar view.

spurs and avulsion fractures at the medial tarsometa-tarsal joints, naviculocuneiform joint);
3. Stress fracture of the first or second metatarsal (second metatarsal base fractures especially common in dancers);
4. Stress fracture of the navicular;
5. Posterior tibial tendinitis;
6. Painful accessory navicular due to posterior tibial tendinitis, "mass effect" from large accessory navicular rubbing against shoe, and painful synchondrosis between the accessory and main navicular;

7. FHL/FDL tendinitis at the master knot of Henry;
8. "Jogger's foot" (entrapment of the medial plantar nerve near the master knot of Henry).

Lateral Midfoot Pain

Conditions that may cause symptoms of lateral midfoot discomfort include

1. Avulsion fracture or Jones fracture at the base of the fifth metatarsal;

2. Stress fracture of the fourth or fifth metatarsal;
3. Lateral Lisfranc's joint injury (ligamentous or bony);
4. Stress fracture of the cuboid;
5. Painful os perineum/peroneus longus partial tear;
6. Peroneus brevis insertional tendinitis;
7. Sural nerve irritation at the base of the fifth metatarsal.

Anterior Midfoot Pain

Conditions that may cause symptoms of anterior midfoot discomfort include

1. Anterior tarsal syndrome (entrapment of the deep peroneal nerve);
2. Arthritic changes and spurring at the dorsal naviculo-cuneiform joint or tarsometatarsal joints;
3. Anterior tibial tendinitis;
4. Stress fracture of the lateral navicular.

Plantar Midfoot Pain

Conditions that may cause symptoms of plantar midfoot discomfort include

1. Lisfranc's injury (ligamentous/bony);
2. Plantar fasciitis;
3. Peroneus longus tendinitis;
4. FHL/FDL tendinitis;
5. Metatarsal stress fractures

Medial Hindfoot Pain

Conditions that may cause medial hindfoot discomfort include

1. Posterior tibial tendinitis/tenosynovitis;
2. Tarsal tunnel syndrome;
3. FDL/FHL tendinitis;
4. Talonavicular arthritis/sprain;
5. Calcaneal stress fracture;
6. Talar neck stress fracture;
7. Entrapment of the nerve to the ADQ;
8. Subtalar joint arthritis;
9. Tarsal coalition.

Lateral Hindfoot Pain

Conditions that may cause lateral hindfoot discomfort include

1. Peroneal tendinitis;
2. Subluxing peroneal tendons;
3. Entrapment of the peroneal tendons at the peroneal tubercle (calcaneus);
4. Avulsion fracture of the anterior lateral process of the calcaneus (bifurcate ligament);
5. Calcaneal stress fracture;

6. Lateral talar fracture;
7. Ankle or subtalar instability;
8. Subtalar joint arthritis;
9. Sinus tarsi syndrome;
10. Tarsal coalition;
11. Entrapment of the nerve to the ADQ.

Posterior Hindfoot Pain

Conditions that may cause posterior hindfoot discomfort include

1. Posterior impingement syndrome of the ankle;
2. Painful os trigonum;
3. Fracture, posterior talus;
4. Entrapment of flexor hallucis longus (trigger toe);
5. Distal Achilles insertional tendinitis, with or without spur;
6. Retrocalcaneal bursitis;
7. Painful Haglund's deformity;
8. Pump-bump (posterior lateral calcaneal exostosis).

Anterior Hindfoot Pain

Conditions that may cause anterior hindfoot discomfort include

1. Anterior talonavicular arthritis;
2. Anterior impingement syndrome, ankle;
3. Anterior tarsal syndrome (referred pain-motor branch from the deep peroneal nerve to extensor digitorum brevis).

STRATEGIES FOR DIAGNOSIS

As we might expect, the history of injury is very important to determine the nature of midfoot or hindfoot injury. The history may not be directly obtainable from the athlete because injuries occurring in the "heat of battle" are often not noticed or ignored until the end of competition. Injuries that occur in a "pile up" or at high speed are often difficult to recreate. Game films or training logs, if available, may often help to provide information about the mechanism/etiology of injury.

Physical examination, as we might expect, is the most valuable tool in narrowing the differential diagnosis to the specific injury. An immediate on-field or sideline examination often yields the most crucial information before swelling and discomfort set in. When you are not present, information provided by the training and/or coaching staff may also be helpful. Marked swelling, deformity, and ecchymosis produce suspicion of fracture or significant ligamentous injury, and standard high-quality x-rays should be obtained.

The standard anteroposterior (AP), lateral, and pronation oblique views provide a good initial x-ray evaluation of the midfoot. Supination oblique views may be necessary to demonstrate the medial navicular and presence of an accessory navicular. The AP and mortise (20-degree internal rotation) ankle view may be added for evaluation of the hindfoot. An oblique view of the heel may show an unusually large posterior lateral calcaneal exostosis or peroneal tubercle.

If fractures have been ruled out, specific joint by joint examination should be conducted with appropriate stress tests to rule out instability. If bony midfoot tenderness is present, despite normal x-rays, a computed tomography (CT) with coronal cuts and axial cuts along the axis of the metatarsals is very useful for determining Lisfranc's fracture dislocations, often showing missed tiny avulsion fractures at the base of the metatarsal/cuneiforms. Coronal and axial CT views of the ankle and hindfoot and occasional lateral reconstruction views are helpful in the evaluation of disorders of the hindfoot, especially the subtalar joint.

A triple-phase bone scan with magnified and coned views is often helpful for evaluation of arthritic changes, stress fractures, or occult fractures in patients with chronic discomfort of the midfoot or hindfoot. Magnetic resonance imaging (MRI) studies are frequently overdone in evaluation of midfoot or hindfoot injuries. Without good clinical correlation provided to the radiologist, they are also frequently over- and underinterpreted. The particular cuts obtained may not show the structures in question without properly consulting the radiologist beforehand. MRIs, however, are very useful in evaluating tendonopathies, early stress fractures, or stress reactions of bone, demonstrating the presence of joint effusion or showing avascular osteochondral lesions.

Selective joint injection with Xylocaine and/or cortisone is helpful in the evaluation of the midfoot and hindfoot where painful arthritis of a specific joint is suspected. Injection of a nerve proximal to its suspected source of entrapment with Xylocaine may also confirm entrapment neuropathy as the diagnosis.

ATHLETIC INJURIES OF THE MIDFOOT

Bony Lesions

Stress fractures in the lower extremity are common in athletes who run and jump, producing repetitive stresses on the bone (19). The incidence is higher in female athletes (20) due to initial lower bone mass, history of poor conditioning before athletic activity, and endocrine changes frequently seen in amenorrheic or oligomenorrheic athletes, especially runners. Frequent causes of stress fractures include training errors in which mileage or activity is increased too rapidly and equipment changes (such as shoes or foot orthoses) where weight-bearing forces are altered, resulting in a new and unaccustomed distribution of forces to the foot. Intrinsic

biomechanical problems, such as the athlete with extreme pes planus leading to over pronation or an athlete with a stiff varus foot producing excessive supination and weight on the lateral portion of the foot, may also lead to stress fractures.

Metatarsal Stress Fracture

Metatarsal stress fractures are the most common of lower extremity stress fractures, resulting in 55% of lower extremity stress fractures (21). Second metatarsal base fractures are very common (especially in dancers [22] or jumping athletes) due to the increased stability of the second metatarsal base that was mentioned previously and the fact that the second metatarsal is often the longest metatarsal, producing a long lever arm during push-off. Fifth metatarsal stress fractures are common in patients who excessively supinate or underpronate during gait.

Clinical Evaluation

Diagnosis of metatarsal stress fractures includes a history of pain and swelling, either specifically or diffusely in the midfoot. On examination, there should be swelling and point tenderness over the bone involved.

Imaging

Initial foot x-rays may be negative (Fig. 50.18A), show a radiolucent fracture line, or show cortical thickening and periosteal bony reaction. Serial x-rays, taken 3 weeks postinjury, or a triple-phase bone scan (Fig. 50.18B) are helpful in establishing the diagnosis. MRI, although much more expensive, is sometimes helpful in making the diagnosis of very early stress fractures.

Treatment

Treatment of metatarsal stress fractures consists of relative rest, limitation of weight bearing to tolerance, immobilization as needed for comfort, and cross-training to maintain cardiovascular status. I usually recommend vitamin D and calcium supplements for patients. Electromagnetic (23) or ultrasonic bone stimulator units (24,25) have also been used in acute and chronic cases with varying degrees of success.

Return to sports depends on diminution of swelling and absence of point bony tenderness followed by gradual return to weight bearing and progression to sports-related activities as tolerated. Rare cases of delayed union or nonunion may require drilling, bone grafting, and/or ORIF followed by immobilization and rehabilitation.

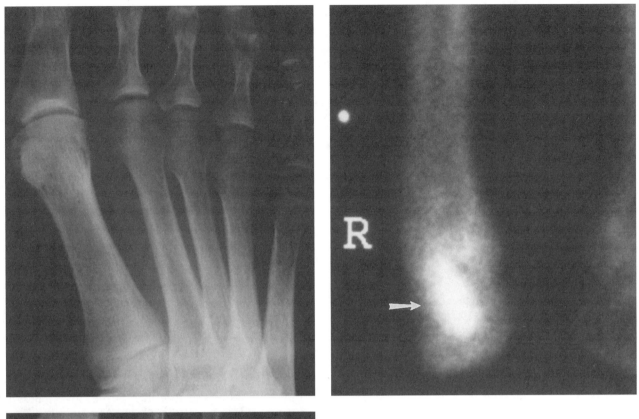

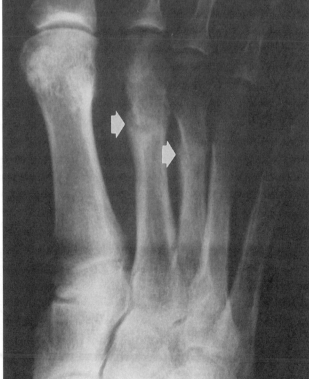

FIG. 50.18. Second and third metatarsal stress fractures in a 38-year-old speed walker: **(A)** initial anteroposterior radiograph (negative), **(B)** bone scan showing increased uptake at the proximal third and fourth metatarsals (*arrow*), and **(C)** final anteroposterior radiograph showing heel metatarsal stress fractures (*arrows*).

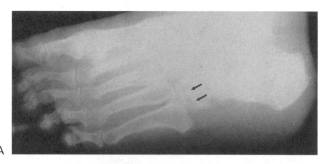
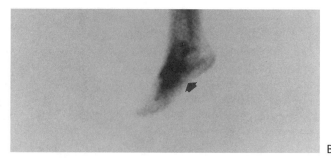

A

B

FIG. 50.19. Cuboid stress fractures of an 18-year-old runner: **(A)** oblique view showing increased radiodensity in the midbody of the cuboid (*black arrows*) and **(B)** lateral bone scan view showing increased uptake (*black arrows*) in the cuboid.

Cuboid Stress Fracture

Clinical Evaluation

Cuboid stress fractures, although less common with less than 1% of stress fractures (19,26), can present with lateral foot pain and swelling. Upon examination, the athlete is point tender over the cuboid, and it is sometimes difficult to differentiate between peroneus longus tendinitis, disorders of the os peroneum, calcaneocuboid arthritis, and a cuboid stress fracture.

Imaging

X-rays may show some increased radiodensity in the midcuboid (Fig. 50.19A). A bone scan (Fig. 50.19B) with magnified coned views may be positive and tomograms, CT, or MRI may show the stress fracture as well.

Treatment

The above-mentioned regimen of relative rest, limited weight bearing as tolerated, and cross-training with graduated activity as tolerated is also used to treat cuboid stress fractures.

Tarsal Navicular Stress Fracture

Stress fractures of the navicular are not uncommon but must be recognized and treated immediately due to their possible serious consequences (27–29). Because of the increased forces that the talar head places on the navicular and relative avascular midportion of the navicular (30), navicular stress fractures are prone to completely fracture, producing displacement or incongruity in the important talonavicular joint.

Clinical Evaluation

Athletes present with medial and anterior arch/ankle pain that is difficult to distinguish from posterior tibial or anterior tibial tendinitis, talonavicular arthritis, or a painful accessory navicular. Point tenderness over the medial or anterior lateral navicular should increase suspicion. Stress fractures of the navicular may occur medially near the posterior tibial tendon insertion or more commonly laterally and anterior near the midbody.

Imaging

Initial x-rays of the foot may be negative unless the fracture is displaced (Fig. 50.20). The standard pronation oblique foot view often yields the best view of the common lateral navicular fracture. The midbody fracture line runs anterior lateral to plantar medial. Scle-

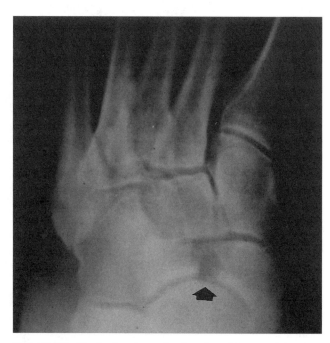

FIG. 50.20. Navicular stress fracture in a 22-year-old runner that progressed to complete fracture and separation. Anteroposterior radiograph showing complete midbody navicular fracture (*dark arrow*).

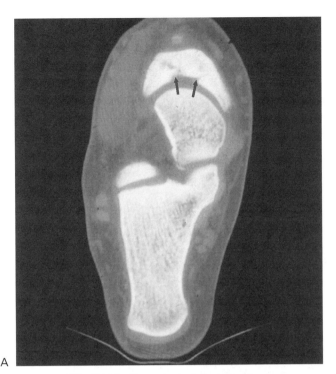
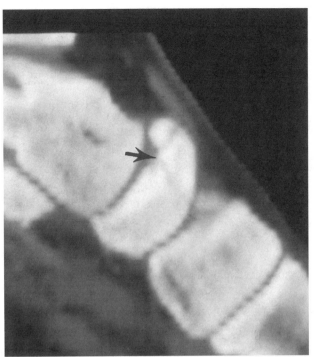

FIG. 50.21. Comminuted navicular fracture—computed tomography: **(A)** axial view of fracture (*arrows*) and **(B)** lateral reconstruction of fracture (*arrow*).

rosis around the fracture site or radiolucent lines may be present on cases that are more chronic. Cystic changes or displacement may occur in severe cases. Regular tomograms with AP and lateral views may be helpful in less obvious cases. CT (Fig. 50.21) is helpful, not only in determining the diagnosis but also in preoperative planning. A bone scan is useful as a screening tool in cases of chronic discomfort. MRI may also show the fracture (Fig. 50.22) but is an expensive screening tool.

Treatment

Nondisplaced navicular stress fractures should be treated aggressively with immobilization and non-

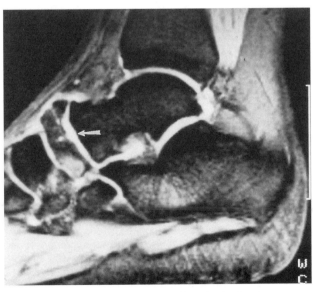
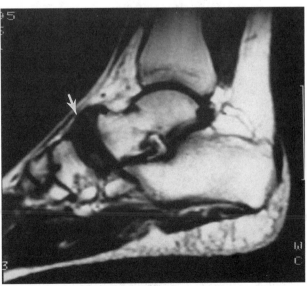

FIG. 50.22. Comminuted navicular fracture—magnetic resonance imaging: **(A)** stir scan showing fracture (*white arrow*) and **(B)** T1 scan showing decreased navicular vascularity (*white arrow*).

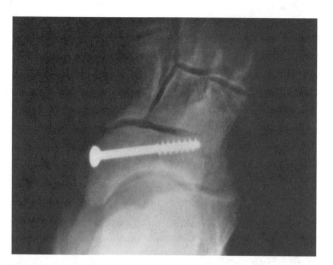

FIG. 50.23. Anteroposterior radiograph showing internal fixation and healing of navicular fracture in Figure 50.20.

weight bearing (31). Percutaneous screw fixation and compression is recommended for a minimally displaced fracture (Fig. 50.23). ORIF and bone grafting are indicated for displaced navicular fractures.

Postoperatively, the patient is immobilized and held in a non–weight-bearing status until the fracture is clinically and radiographically healed. Vitamin D and calcium supplements may be helpful. Electromagnetic or ultrasonic bone stimulator units are also often used because of the slowly healing nature of these fractures. Repeat tomograms or CT may be needed to definitively confirm healing.

After bony union, the athlete is begun on progressive weight-bearing exercises, a standard ankle rehabilitation program followed by gradual progression of running, jumping, and sports-related activities. Severe displaced navicular fractures may result in avascular

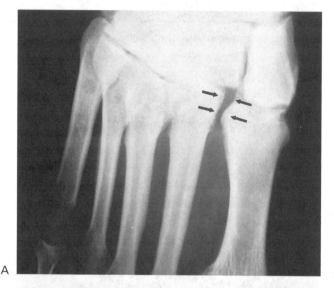

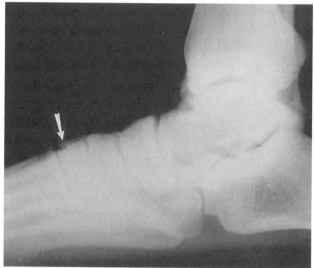

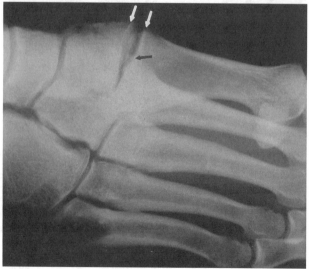

FIG. 50.24. Healed career ending Lisfranc's injury in a Hall of Fame linebacker: **(A)** anteroposterior radiograph showing residual separation (*dark arrows*) at the first–second metatarsal bases, **(B)** lateral view showing arthritic spurs (*white arrow*) at the tarsometatarsal joint, and **(C)** oblique view showing degenerative changes in the first tarsometatarsal joint (*white arrows*) and second tarsometatarsal joint (*dark arrow*).

necrosis of the navicular and/or talonavicular arthritis, resulting in the need for talonavicular fusion as a salvage procedure.

Lisfranc's Joint Injuries

Athletic injuries of Lisfranc's joint have been noted more frequently in recent literature (32). Heightened awareness of these chronic debilitating injuries has increased our ability to make the specific diagnosis, which was once simply labeled as a "foot sprain." A recent survey of the National Football League (NFL) shows that a significant number of Lisfranc's injuries occur each year, resulting in the inability to play for 6 to 10 weeks (33). Injuries range from the very subtle "midfoot sprain," which allows continuation of athletic play, to moderate or severe injuries causing persistent pain and swelling throughout the course of the season and affect the ability to compete. Severe injuries (Fig. 50.24) can result in the end of a Hall of Fame career.

There are several mechanisms of injury. An axial load to the midfoot (Fig. 50.25), common in pile-up situations, results in stretch of the relatively weak dorsal tarsometatarsal ligaments, fracture through the base of the second metatarsal, or a tear of Lisfranc's ligament and midfoot collapse. An alternative mechanism is a twisting injury to the midfoot, occurring when the forefoot is trapped by a large often 300-pound opponent (Fig. 50.26) and the rest of the foot and body are twisted away in an opposite direction. Landing injuries where a jumping athlete such as a volleyball player or basketball player comes down on a plantar flexed foot can also produce axial injuries (Fig. 50.27). Finally, injuries such as entrapment of the forefoot in bicycle toe clips or stirrups can result in a more traditional "equestrian-type injury."

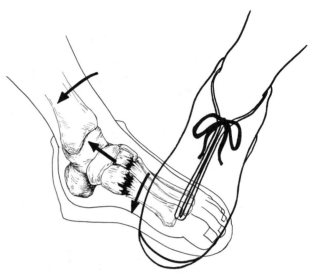

FIG. 50.26. Entrapment of the forefoot and twisting of the upper leg, producing a Lisfranc's joint injury.

Acute Lisfranc's joint injuries may be entirely ligamentous, producing dislocation of the midfoot. The dislocation will often spontaneously reduce, making initial x-rays negative. Multiple fractures also may occur through the base of the affected metatarsals and cuneiforms and/or cuboids. Permanent subluxation and deformity may also result. Hardcastle et al. (34), Quenu and Kuss (35), and others (36) have described the various patterns for fracture dislocation of Lisfranc's joint. Common patterns include lateral deviation of the forefoot (Fig. 50.28), medial displacement, and divergent displacement where the first ray and lateral forefoot are separated.

A chronic Lisfranc's dysfunction can occur in the pres-

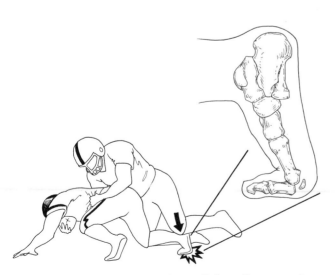

FIG. 50.25. Axial loading during a "pile up" can produce dorsal angulation at the Lisfranc's joint.

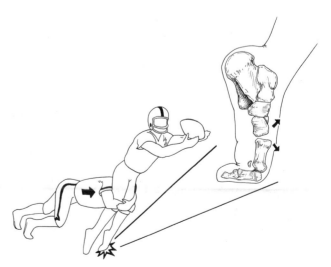

FIG. 50.27. "Landing" plantar flexion injury producing a Lisfranc's joint injury.

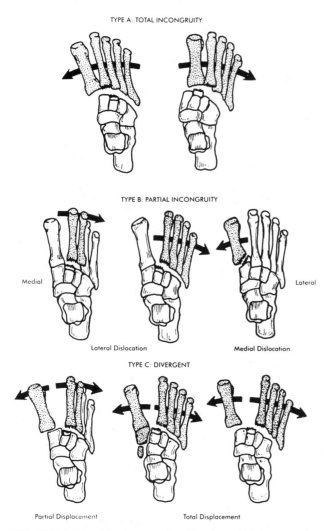

TYPE A: TOTAL INCONGRUITY

TYPE B: PARTIAL INCONGRUITY

Medial

Lateral

Lateral Dislocation

Medial Dislocation

TYPE C: DIVERGENT

Partial Displacement

Total Displacement

FIG. 50.28. The Hardcastle classification of Lisfranc's joint injuries. (From Baxter DE. *The foot and ankle in sport.* St. Louis: Mosby, 1995:110, with permission.)

ence of a severe pes planus deformity, caused by obesity or repeated trauma and producing midfoot collapse and arthritic changes, including spur formation.

Clinical Evaluation

Signs and symptoms range from pain and swelling only in a lesser sprain-type injury to severe swelling, ecchymosis, midfoot deformity, and neurovascular compromise in severe injuries. As noted previously in the anatomy section, the deep peroneal nerve and dorsalis pedis artery may be injured directly with this type of injury, producing neurovascular compromise. Sensation to the first web space may be altered or the dorsalis pedis pulse diminished.

Each of the five Lisfranc's joints and the naviculocuneiform joint and other cuneiform joints must be palpated to determine involvement. Stability of the joints

must be assessed by anterior/posterior manipulation performed by pushing upward and downward on the metatarsal head (Fig. 50.29).

Recognition of less-obvious Lisfranc's injuries may be more problematic. An axial load or twisting/forefoot trapping injury in an athlete may produce only a partial tear of the ligaments supporting the midfoot. As noted above, the thin dorsal ligaments are prone to injury first without necessarily tearing the stronger plantar ligaments and resulting in actual displacement or subluxation. The athlete may complain of swelling discomfort and continued pain in the midfoot with standing and push-off. This grade I or sprain-type injury can produce chronic discomfort and limited performance if not recognized early and treated appropriately. The metatarsal squeeze test (Fig. 50.30) will also produce discomfort at Lisfranc's joint after a grade I sprain or grade II injury. A Lisfranc's stress test, as suggested by Arntz et al. (37), may be performed.

Imaging

Regular x-rays (AP, lateral, and oblique) may be helpful but only if there is a persistent subluxation/dislocation or fracture of Lisfranc's joint. The subluxation or dislocation may spontaneously reduce, producing initial x-rays that are negative (Fig. 50.31). Be sure to look for widening in the gap between the first or medial cuneiform and the middle cuneiform. Widening of the intermetatarsal space (Fig. 50.31B) between the proximal base of the first and second metatarsals may be visible (38). Lateral dislocations may reveal only a medial border of the proximal fourth metatarsal that no longer lines up with the medial edge of the cuboid (Fig. 50.32).

In subtle Lisfranc's sprains (grade I to II), stress x-rays performed by stabilizing the heel and midfoot while manipulating the metatarsals may be helpful. CT with axial and coronal cuts will reveal fractures of the metatarsal bases and cuneiforms (Fig. 50.33) not seen on regular x-rays and aid in surgical planning. In chronic Lisfranc's injuries, a bone scan may be helpful to confirm posttraumatic degenerative changes.

Treatment

As mentioned above, the injured foot is assessed carefully to rule out fracture–dislocation. Stability is also assessed manually and, if needed, by stress x-rays. If fractures are present that are significantly displaced and/or intraarticular requiring reduction, open reduction internal fixation is usually performed as suggested by Hanson and others (39,40). One to three longitudinal anterior incisions allow full access to all five Lisfranc's joints, if necessary. Intervening soft tissue is removed; the fractures and joints are located and usually fixed securely

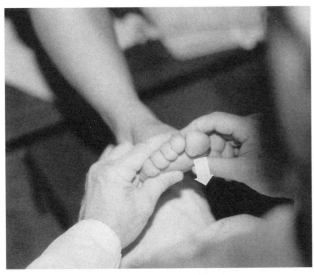
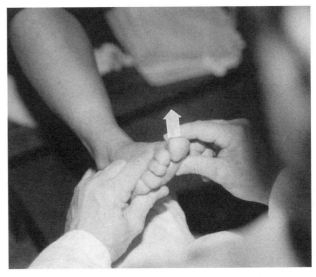

A

B

FIG. 50.29. Anterior–posterior stress test for laxity of the first tarsometatarsal joint: **(A)** downward pressure on the first metatarsal head shows no increased plantar flexion past the other metatarsal heads and **(B)** upward pressure on the first metatarsal head shows increased dorsal motion, suggesting slight tarsometatarsal laxity.

with screws (Fig. 50.34). My personal preference is 3.5-mm cannulated Synthes screws. It is important that the gap between the first ray and lateral midfoot (or gap between the medial and middle cuneiform) is reduced if present with transverse screws. Repair of the plantar ligaments or Lisfranc's ligament is usually not attempted.

Postoperatively, the patient may be placed in either a non–weight-bearing cast or, if the athlete is trustworthy, a molded bivalve AFO so immediate therapy can

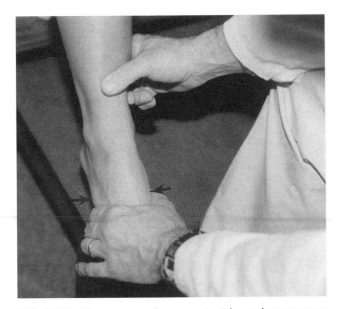

FIG. 50.30. The metatarsal squeeze test: inward pressure on the metatarsal necks may produce pain or abnormal motion.

be started for edema control and some gentle active range of motion. Progressive weight bearing is started after 6 to 8 weeks depending on residual pain, swelling, and discomfort. At 10 to 12 weeks, the screws can usually be removed on an outpatient basis. The athlete is then started on progressive loading programs, advancing from walking to jogging to agility exercises such as body slide, minitramp, and then on to sport-specific training.

Because there can be chronic residual midfoot discomfort, a molded semirigid foot orthosis and good shock-absorbing shoe with a light-weight carbon fiber insert to stiffen the shank may be used when the athlete returns to sports. Isolated tarsometatarsal joint fusions may be necessary in severe cases of tarsometatarsal arthritis to eliminate pain or instability.

In situations where no fracture exists but the midfoot is grossly unstable, as evidenced by manual testing or stress x-rays, the foot is immobilized and a short leg cast is applied for 6 to 8 weeks in the reduced position. Percutaneous Steinman pins or cannulated screws (my preference) are placed across the first, second, and fifth tarsometatarsal joints as needed to stabilize the midfoot. Stability and alignment are checked under fluoroscopy in the operating room. Inability to achieve anatomic alignment usually means soft tissue is interposed in the tarsometatarsal joint and open reduction is required. The above rehabilitation program is then instituted if the foot is stable and pain free upon removal from the cast.

Smaller insignificant avulsion-type fractures and situations where the foot is reasonably stable can be treated with a cast or AFO for 6 to 8 weeks, followed by the progressive rehabilitation program noted above. Again,

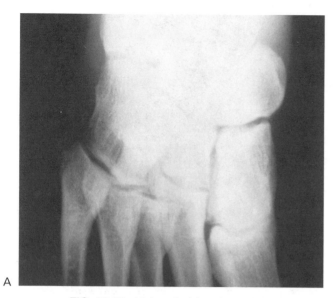

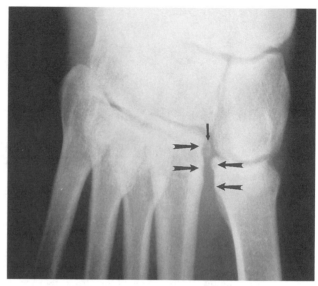

A

B

FIG. 50.31. Lisfranc's injury in an All Pro offensive lineman: **(A)** initial anteroposterior radiograph is negative and **(B)** anteroposterior radiograph at 2 weeks postinjury shows widening at the first–second metatarsal bases (*thick arrows*) and calcification, suggesting tear of Lisfranc's ligament (*thin arrow*).

progression of activities depends on assessment of stability and the level of pain and swelling with activities.

Finally in milder cases, such as a grade I or II sprain with no displacement or good stability, the patient may be treated with ice/edema control or compressive dressings to control swelling. Weight bearing is limited, depending on the amount of discomfort. This may range from no weight bearing with crutches, to partial weight bearing, to weight bearing with support. We will usually prescribe a semirigid foot orthosis to help support the arch with weight bearing. In some cases, a UCBL-type

orthosis may be used to provide better midfoot support. For these athletes, cross-training is initiated, such as water training with a swim vest or biking using heel weight bearing only on that side. The athlete's progress then depends on the amount of swelling and discomfort elicited with weight bearing. They can progress from

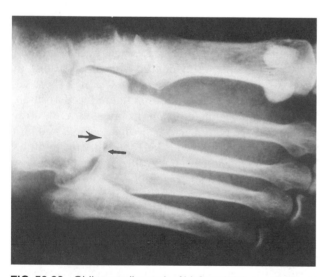

FIG. 50.32. Oblique radiograph of Lisfranc's injury with lateral subluxation. There is displacement between the medial edge of the cuboid (*thick arrow*) and the medial edge of the fourth metatarsal (*thin arrow*).

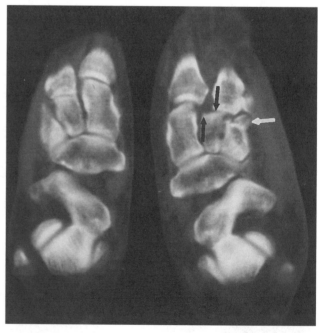

FIG. 50.33. Comminuted Lisfranc's fracture–dislocation. Anteroposterior computed tomogram view of the midfoot shows displacement of the second metatarsal base (*dark arrows*) and fractures of the lateral cuneiform (*white arrow*).

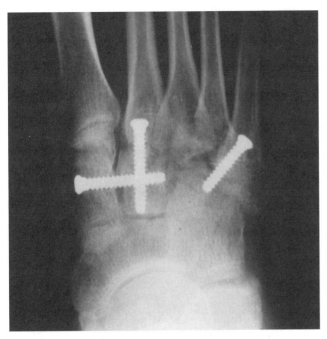

FIG. 50.34. Lisfranc's injury in a 24-year-old water skier. Anteroposterior radiograph showing internal fixation of the cuneiform diastasis and metatarsal subluxation.

pain-free weight bearing to running to minitramp, body slide, and then to figure-of-eight drills and sport-specific activities.

As with the above Lisfranc's injuries, these low-grade Lisfranc's sprains injuries can also be prone to some chronic foot discomfort and may require a semirigid foot orthosis for athletic activities.

In cases where chronic arthritis and pain exists secondary to a Lisfranc's fracture–dislocation, ice, nonsteroidal anti-inflammatory drugs, and selective cortisone injections may help, as well as orthoses. Isolated TMT fusions may be used to limit discomfort, swelling, and preserve function if conservative treatment fails (3). Fusion of the first, second, or third tarsometatarsal joint usually results in less functional problems because normal range of motion is limited. Fusion of the mobile segment (the fourth and fifth TMT joints) may lead to functional problems with running, jumping, and so forth and should be reserved as a salvage procedure.

Arthritis of the Midfoot

Athletes may suffer from arthritic changes, pain, and swelling in the midfoot joints, such as the tarsometatarsal joints or naviculocuneiform joints as a result of repeated or acute trauma. Repetitive sprain injury can cause capsular avulsion, bleeding, and formation of periarticular spurs. Repeated compression injuries secondary to weight (NFL linemen), pile-ups, and repetitive jumping can all produce degenerative changes in these joints (Fig. 50.35). Acute injuries (Lisfranc's fracture–dislocation) can also lead to chronic arthritic changes (even when treated properly).

Clinical Evaluation

The athlete may complain of dorsal or plantar midfoot pain and swelling at the affected joints. Palpation or anterior–posterior manipulation of the joint may produce pain. A painful spur may be present. The spur itself may cause painful impingement at the affected joint with weight bearing and may irritate adjacent structures such as the extensor tendons or the deep peroneal nerve, leading to extensor tendinitis or anterior tarsal syndrome, respectively. Selective injection with Xylocaine, with or without cortisone, is also an excellent diagnostic tool to help isolate the joints involved.

Imaging

Routine x-rays (AP, lateral, and two obliques) with metallic marker dots over the affected joints may show spur formation if present. CT or tomograms (AP and lateral views) may be helpful in evaluating the joint and assessing the degree or arthritic changes. Very often, the spurs occur only at the periphery of the joint and the remainder is normal. A magnified, coned, selective bone scan is helpful in isolating the affected joint in cases of chronic midfoot pain.

Treatment

Initial treatment for midfoot arthritis consists of anti-inflammatory medication, ice, and a semirigid foot orthosis or, in more severe cases, a UCBL-type device. Switching to a more shock-absorbing shoe may also be helpful. Light-weight carbon fiber inserts to stiffen the shoe may also help.

If spurs have formed at the affected joint and pro-

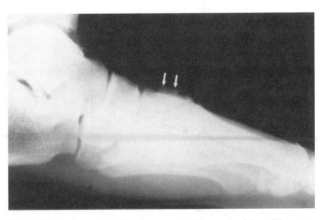

FIG. 50.35. Dorsal midfoot spurs (*white arrows*) in a 31-year-old 300-pound All Pro center.

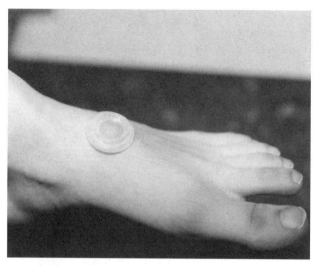

FIG. 50.36. Donut-shaped silicone for padding over a second tarsometatarsal spur.

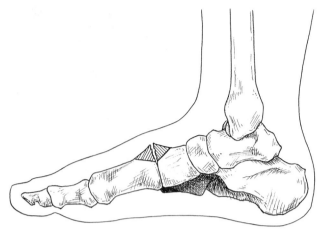

FIG. 50.38. "V"-shaped excision of tarsometatarsal spurs.

duced discomfort secondary to pressure from shoes, a donut-shaped pad or silicone-type pad (Fig. 50.36) may be helpful in reducing shoe pressure and friction. Alternative lacing techniques (41) (Fig. 50.37) may also be helpful in eliminating pressure of the shoe tongue on anterior spurs. Selective cortisone injections into the affected joints may be helpful for variable periods.

If the above-mentioned conservative treatments fail, surgery may be required. If only the periphery of the joint is involved with painful impingement of spurs, sur-

gical excision of the spurs in a V-shaped fashion (Fig. 50.38) may produce relief. If preoperative assessment shows that most of the joint is arthritic and involved, then isolated joint fusion may be required as a salvage procedure (3).

Painful Pes Planus

Flexible pes planus or a planovalgus foot configuration may be a normal congenital variation present in millions of athletes. A review of NFL players and other professional teams and many recreational athletes show that high-caliber athletic performance, even All Pro performance, is frequently possible, even with a severe flat foot deformity. No treatment is necessary if asymptomatic. We simply advise an athletic shoe with a good heel counter and good medial sole reinforcement and arch support to prevent excessive wear. Longitudinal studies have shown that treatment of young athletes with pes planus by insertion of orthotics or "cookies" does not lead to formation of an arch or guarantee prevention of future symptoms (42,43). Athletes who do present with severe excessive medial shoe wear or who are symptomatic with functional limitations require treatment.

Patients with excessive planovalgus configuration and pes planus may have medial and plantar arch pain, due to stretching of the plantar midfoot ligaments with arch collapse, posterior tibial tendinitis from repeated stretch, tarsal tunnel syndromes from stretch irritation of the tibial nerve, plantar fasciitis at the heel, lateral sinus tarsi pain due to severe valgus compression of the lateral subtalar joint, increased hallux valgus, and bunion discomfort with severe pronation of the first toe. An acute planovalgus deformity may also occasionally exist in athletes due to an acute plantar fascia tear, posterior tibial tendon tear, or Lisfranc's fracture–dislocation with midfoot subluxation. Acute severe tears

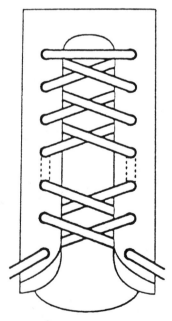

FIG. 50.37. Alternative lacing to avoid pressure on a dorsal spur. (From Frey C. *The foot and ankle in sport.* St. Louis: Mosby, 1995:359, with permission.)

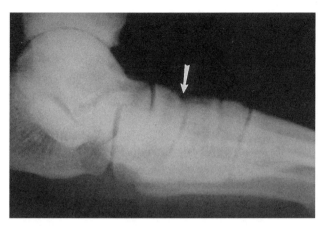

FIG. 50.39. Lateral radiograph showing pes planus and sagging at the naviculocuneiform joint (*white arrow*).

of the deltoid ligament may result in medial ankle instability and a severe valgus deformity as well.

Diagnosis

Diagnosis of painful pes planus is occasionally difficult because the deformity may also be associated with one of the above-mentioned specific problems. If other associated midfoot and hindfoot disorders have been ruled out, then painful pes planus may be the diagnosis of exclusion.

Physical examination will show a flattened arch and increased pronation. A posterior view will show increased heel valgus. Although no strict criteria exist to delineate pes planus, Harris-Beath print mats will show a widened arch print. As noted above, specific joint or tendon problems may be associated with or aggravated by pes planus. The physical examination will be positive for those specific problems as well.

Imaging

Lateral x-rays will show a sag (Fig. 50.39) at the tarsometatarsal, talonavicular, or naviculocuneiform joints.

An AP x-ray will frequently show increased pronation at the talonavicular as measured by Gould (44).

Treatment

For cases of chronic painful pes planus associated with other disorders as listed above, both the pes planus and specific problem may require treatment. Usually, a semirigid foot orthosis with a good arch support (Fig. 50.40) is selected as initial treatment. This is combined with a shoe that provides a good heel counter to hold the heel and a good medial sole support. In athletes with a severe flexible planovalgus deformity with marked heel valgus, a UCBL-type device may be required to help hold the heel out of valgus. If the subtalar joint is still flexible, controlling heel valgus and providing a semirigid support in the arch area with polyethylene or polypropylene usually will position the foot properly and still allow sufficient shock absorption of the foot for athletic endeavors. Simply attempting to build up the arch and push it upward is usually not successful and not tolerated by the athlete. Patients with severe painful chronic pes planus may not tolerate orthotic inserts but instead benefit from a medial wedge in the heel or sole of their shoe.

Surgical treatment for chronic painful flexible pes planus should be reserved as a last resort. Procedures include calcaneal osteotomy (45,46) to shift the heel inward or lengthen the lateral column (47), alone or combined with isolated talonavicular fusion (48), naviculocuneiform fusion (49), or first tarsometatarsal fusion (50). Calcaneal osteotomy can also be combined with posterior tibial tendon tightening or advancement and imbrication of the spring ligament (51). A salvage procedure is an isolated subtalar fusion or triple arthrodesis.

Treatment of acute pes planus due to midfoot fracture–dislocation consists of closed reduction or open reduction and immobilization. Limitation of weight bearing and immobilization are used in the case of a severe plantar fascia tear. Posterior tibial tendon repair and possible flexor digitorum longus graft (52) is used

A
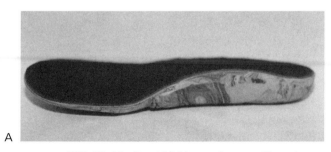
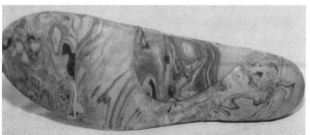
B

FIG. 50.40. Semirigid foot orthoses with arch support: **(A)** medial view and **(B)** plantar view. (Courtesy Foot Menders.)

for cases of acute posterior tibial tendon pathology that do not respond to conservative treatment.

Patients with chronic pes planus may participate in athletics as tolerated with conservative treatment. Patients requiring surgical treatment need protection for 6 to 10 weeks with a cast or molded AFO brace, followed by physical therapy for edema control, range of motion, and progressive resisted exercises and progressive weight bearing. Upon pain-free walking, progressive sports-related activities might be initiated. In cases of acute pes planus, weight bearing, progressive physical therapy, and progressive activities may be started after initial treatment and once pain-free weight bearing has been achieved.

PAINFUL ACCESSORY NAVICULAR/OS PERONEUM

Two accessory ossicles occur in the junction between midfoot and hindfoot that can produce pain in the hindfoot. The accessory navicular (prehallux) is present in 4% to 14% (53–55) of the population. It exists as either a pointed projection on the plantar medial aspect of the navicular or as a separate ossicle (43%) (56) imbedded within the posterior tibial tendon near its plantar insertion into the navicular.

The os peroneum is present as a fibrous or cartilaginous sesamoid, occasionally bony (20%) (57,58), inside the peroneus longus where it bends around the lateral corner of the cuboid to run across the plantar aspect of the foot in a fibroosseous tunnel toward its insertion on the plantar aspect of the first ray. As Sobel et al. (59) noted, there are several fibrous attachments from the base of the fifth metatarsal, cuboid and peroneus brevis, to the peroneus longus/os peroneum complex holding the peroneus longus and os peroneum in place.

Painful Accessory Navicular

A painful accessory navicular can cause medial arch and hindfoot pain in athletes, especially adolescent athletes. There are three main causes for pain from an accessory navicular. First is a mass effect due to the extra prominence rubbing on shoe wear. The athlete will typically give a history of discomfort with firmer or more tightly fitting shoe wear. Second, the athlete may experience posterior tibial tendinitis. The accessory navicular by its presence may alter the biomechanics of the posterior tibial tendon (56), resulting in posterior tibial tendinitis. In addition, a fair number of people with an accessory navicular may have pes planus as well. The third cause is painful synchondrosis, in which the cartilage connection between the accessory navicular and main navicular may break down from repeated overuse or an acute trauma, producing discomfort and swelling.

Clinical Evaluation

The athlete may have swelling and pain in the area of the accessory navicular. There may be direct pain over the accessory navicular secondary to friction and rubbing. A painful callus may also develop secondary to the mass effect. Posterior tibial tendon function may be weak upon resisted inversion or forced eversion. The posterior tibial tendon may be swollen as in tenosynovitis or simply tender to touch with tendinitis. Ballottment of the accessory navicular by manipulating the accessory navicular at the synchondrosis may produce discomfort. Injection with Xylocaine and cortisone in the synchondrosis, in this case, may relieve symptoms if only temporarily.

Imaging

An accessory navicular, when large, may be easily seen on the standard AP, lateral, and oblique films. In some cases, however, a supination oblique view (Fig. 50.41) may be required to clearly show the accessory navicular. In cases of chronic medial hindfoot pain, a bone scan may be positive in this area when ordered as a screening test. MRI may distinguish between increased fluid in the synchondrosis, swelling, and inflammation of the posterior tibial tendon at its distal insertion near the accessory navicular, a more proximal tenosynovitis, or posterior tibial tendon tear near the medial malleolus.

Treatment

For athletes suffering from the mass effect due to a prominent navicular, donut-shaped padding or a silicone gel-type pad (Fig. 50.42) may reduce friction and pressure on the accessory navicular mass. Nonsteroidal antiinflammatory medication and ice may also be helpful. Modification of shoe wear with a softer upper and wider shoe may also relieve pressure on the accessory navicular.

For athletes with posterior tibial tendinitis or a painful synchondrosis, ice and anti-inflammatory medication may help. Semirigid orthoses, relative rest, and crosstraining are used to reduce stress to the tendon and/or synchondrosis.

For cases of acute injury to the synchondrosis, casting for 4 to 6 weeks may help to return the athlete to a preinjury level of comfort and function. In cases of painful accessory navicular associated with a planovalgus or pes planus foot deformity, a semirigid orthosis or UCBL-type support may relieve pressure or may reduce force on the posterior tibial tendon and synchondrosis, relieving symptoms. Cortisone injection into the synchondrosis may be helpful as well.

Finally, if all above conservative measures have

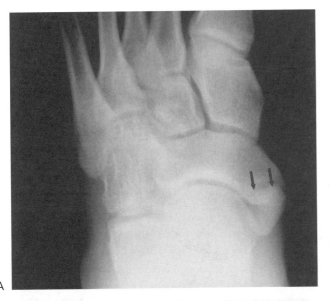

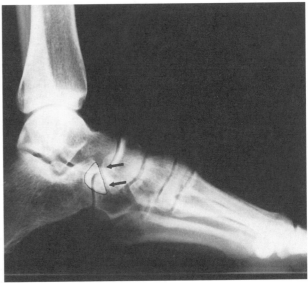

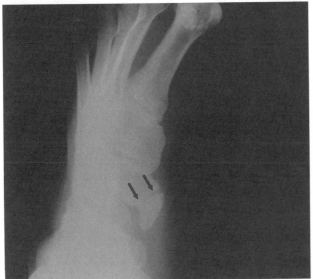

FIG. 50.41. Seventeen-year-old gymnast with a painful accessory navicular (*arrows*): **(A)** anteroposterior view, **(B)** lateral view, and **(C)** supination oblique view.

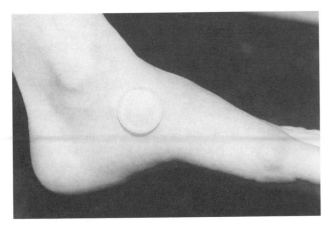

FIG. 50.42. Medial view—silicone gel pad for painful accessory navicular.

failed and the patient still exhibits significant soreness and limited function, excision of the accessory navicular and reconstruction of the posterior tibial tendon by securing the remainder of the posterior tibial insertion to the main body of the navicular with suture anchors (Figs. 50.43 and 50.44) may be helpful. Postoperatively, the patient is placed in a protective splint or cast, non-weight bearing, for 6 weeks. If the insertion of the posterior tibial tendon is still strong, gentle early active range of motion may be started to facilitate tendon gliding and prevent adhesions. After 6 weeks, progressive weight bearing is started along with resisted exercises. When motion is good and the strength of the posterior tibial tendon is 70% of the unaffected side, sport-specific activities are begun on a graduated basis. Athletes may still require semirigid orthotic support, especially those with pes planus.

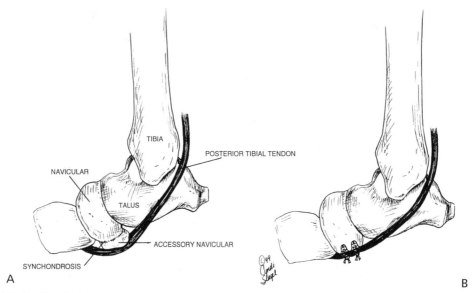

FIG. 50.43. Surgical treatment of a painful accessory navicular: **(A)** preoperative anatomy of painful accessory navicular and **(B)** postoperative excision of accessory navicular and fixation of the posterior tibial tendon to the navicular with suture anchors.

Painful Os Peroneum

Athletes may injure the os peroneum during an inversion sprain-type injury or by landing directly on the os peroneum when one player comes down upon another player's foot. Athletes with an old lateral ankle sprain and chronic lateral instability of the ankle also rely more heavily on the peroneals (the secondary stabilizer of the ankle). This can often produce degenerative tears in the peroneus brevis (60–65) and can lead to increased stress on the os peroneum. In situations like this, chronic attritional tears of the peroneus longus can result in an actual fracture of the os peroneum.

Clinical Evaluation

The patient may complain of "giving-way episodes." They also may complain of lateral foot pain or pain with attempted push-off due to lack of stabilization of the first ray. On examination, there may be tenderness along the peroneal sheath, pain with resisted peroneum longus function (resisted plantar flexion of the first metatarsal), resisted eversion, and forced supination of the foot and forced dorsiflexion of the first ray. There may also be swelling and point tenderness at the os peroneum.

Imaging

X-rays (AP, lateral, and oblique) may show migration or fracture of the os peroneum (Fig. 50.45). Occasionally in patients with chronic pain, serial x-rays may show documented widening of the os peroneum diastasis. In cases of chronic pain, a bone scan may or may not be positive in the area of the os peroneum and is to be differentiated from a cuboid stress fracture or basilar fifth metatarsal fracture. Tomograms or an MRI (66)

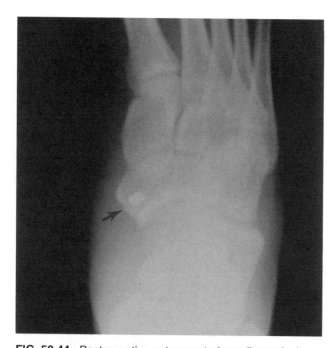

FIG. 50.44. Postoperative anteroposterior radiograph showing excision of accessory navicular and suture anchor fixation (*arrow*) of posterior tib tendon to the navicular.

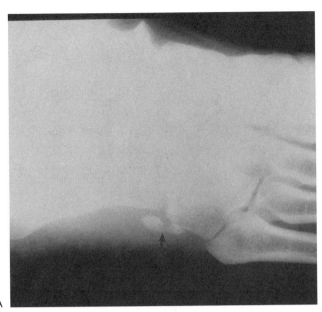

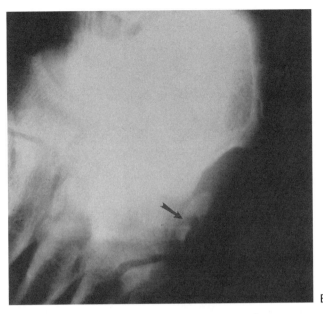

A   B

FIG. 50.45. Eighteen-year-old high school state tennis champion with fracture of the os peroneum and peroneus longus tear: **(A)** oblique foot radiographs showing diastasis of the os peroneum fracture (*arrow*) and **(B)** anteroposterior ankle radiograph clearly showing the diastasis (*arrow*).

may be helpful in evaluation of both the os peroneum and the peroneus longus (Fig. 50.46).

Treatment

In cases of acute os peroneal injury and nondisplaced fracture, cast immobilization may be indicated for 4 to

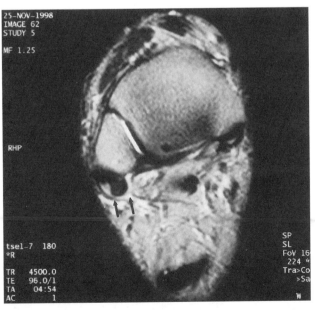

FIG. 50.46. Axial view just superior to the ankle showing fluid (*arrows*) around the peroneus longus.

6 weeks, until clinically and radiographically healed. For patients with chronic irritation of the os peroneum but no fracture, ice, anti-inflammatory medication, relative rest, and soft to semirigid molded orthoses with a good support underneath the first ray and pressure relief or a soft inlay underneath the os peroneum may be helpful in restoring function. Cortisone injection between the os peroneum and cuboid may be useful in cases of synovitis or mild degenerative changes but must be performed carefully to avoid the increased risk of peroneum longus rupture.

Surgery is indicated only when conservative treatment has failed. At the time of surgical exploration, if the peroneus longus is fairly intact but the os peroneum has been broken and is degenerative, excision of the os peroneum with tubular oversewing (67) of the peroneus longus is indicated. Postoperatively, early range of motion is begun with non-weight bearing for 4 to 6 weeks. Strengthening exercises and gradual progressive weight bearing is begun followed later by strengthening and sport-specific activities. In cases where the peroneum longus has ruptured and is not repairable, tenodesis (Fig. 50.47) to the peroneus brevis (68) may be indicated to provide additional lateral ankle support. If chronic instability of the lateral ankle exists, primary repair of the lateral ankle ligaments (69) (Brostrom-type repair) is indicated, and if needed the ruptured peroneus longus can be used for the graft augmentation. Any residual first ray instability may be assisted by a soft to semirigid orthotic with good support underneath the first ray and perhaps a first Morton's extension.

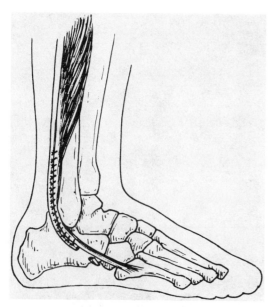

FIG. 50.47. Excision of the os peroneum and tenodesis of the peroneus longus to peroneus brevis.

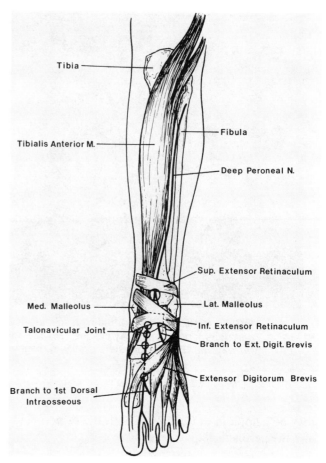

FIG. 50.48. Sites (*circles*) of possible entrapment of the deep peroneal nerve. (Modified from Baxter, Pfeffer. *The foot and ankle in sport.* St. Louis: Mosby, 1995:17, with permission.)

NEUROVASCULAR INJURIES OF THE MIDFOOT

Anterior tarsal syndrome, introduced by Kopel and Thompson (70) in 1963 and described by Marinachi (71) in the same year, describes compression of the deep peroneal nerve at the inferior edge of the extensor retinaculum. Although anterior tarsal syndrome receives less attention in the literature than tarsal tunnel syndrome, it is present more frequently than previously suspected. The diagnosis is often missed or delayed due to confusion with other conditions. Anterior tarsal syndrome has been seen in football players, basketball players, runners and athletes who wear tightly fitting shoes or boots (the ski boot syndrome) (72), cyclists, and equestrians as well. Wearing tight-fitting shoes, a common practice for sprinters or running backs and wide receivers in the NFL, may aggravate symptoms. Compression neuropathy of the deep peroneal nerve may also occur more distally in the midfoot (Fig. 50.48). Direct trauma to the deep peroneal nerve, which is in a superficial area, has been reported, such as in football players or basketball players having another player land directly on the dorsum of their instep.

Hypertrophic arthritic spurs (Fig. 50.49) over the talonavicular, naviculocuneiform, or tarsometatarsal joints and overlying bursitis (73,74) have been associated with compression of the nerve in the midfoot. These chronic spurs may result from repetitive compression injuries or capsular avulsion injuries due to repeated athletic trauma. Lisfranc's joint injuries with subluxation or dislocation can also produce entrapment or impingement on the deep peroneal nerve.

Clinical Evaluation

Athletes with anterior tarsal syndrome complain of dorsal foot pain, numbness, and hyperesthesia or paresthesia in the first web space. They may also complain of anterior lateral foot discomfort near the entrance of the

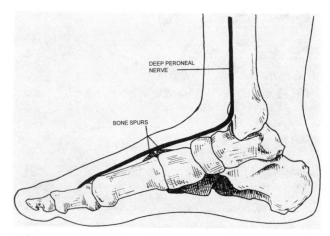

FIG. 50.49. Medial view: tarsometatarsal spurs producing irritation of the deep peroneal nerve.

sinus tarsi due to compression of the motor branch of the deep peroneal nerve to the extensor digitorum brevis. This is often confused with other conditions such as avulsion fracture of the anterior and lateral calcaneal process, sinus tarsi syndrome, or anterior lateral impingement ("the Duke lesion") of the ankle.

Swelling and tenderness may be noted along the course of the deep peroneal nerve from the anterior ankle where it exits underneath the superior retinaculum, across the dorsum of the navicular, and down to the dorsal first web space. Arthritic spurs, if present at the talonavicular joint or naviculocuneiform joint, may be palpated, producing discomfort. A boggy bursalike swelling or ganglion cyst may be present, entrapping the nerve. The deep peroneal nerve may be directly palpated and rolled back and forth over the bony prominence, cyst, or bursa, reproducing symptoms with either distal or retrograde paresthesias and numbness. A percussion test (Tinel's) may be acutely positive at the area of entrapment, at either the edge of the extensor retinaculum or the midfoot joints noted above, resulting in retrograde or antegrade paresthesias. Direct compression of the nerve (nerve compression test) may also reproduce symptoms.

In cases of entrapment of the motor branch to the extensor digitorum brevis, the patient may be noted to have weakness or atrophy of the extensor digitorum brevis in the area of the sinus tarsi. There may or may not be any direct tenderness there. However, pressure over the deep peroneal nerve proximally may produce referred pain to the sinus tarsi area. Injection of the deep peroneal nerve proximal to the area of compression should result in numbness over the deep peroneal distribution and resolution of symptoms.

Imaging

X-rays, including marker films with metal dots placed on the area of maximal tenderness, may show proximity of a midfoot joint with hypertrophic spurs secondary to arthritis or repeated trauma. Nerve conduction velocity studies may show increased distal sensory latency, but electromyograms may be normal due to entrapment of (75) the deep peroneal nerve below the motor branch to the EDB.

Treatment

Treatment of anterior tarsal syndrome begins with removal of any external compressive forces. Shoes should be inspected and properly sized, especially for athletes with a high arch cavovarus foot, and the appropriate width and depth must be provided. Alternative lacing techniques can reduce pressure on the specific area of the instep where compression occurs (Fig. 50.37). Pad-

ding techniques (Fig. 50.50) with either two pads parallel to the deep peroneal nerve or a donut-shaped pad over the area of compression and spurs may be helpful. Silicone-type pads that reduce friction and pressure may also be useful in the athletic shoe. Selective injections with Xylocaine and cortisone around the nerve are not only helpful diagnostically, but are also therapeutic in some early mild cases. Night splints (ankle/foot orthoses) may be helpful to avoid sleeping with the foot in the plantar flexed position. Nonsteroidal anti-inflammatory medication and ice may reduce inflammation around the nerve and adjacent joint. If conservative measures fail to provide relief within 3 months, repeat electrical studies may be performed.

If there is no improvement by clinical and diagnostic measurements and if symptoms continue to be functionally limiting, surgical exploration and neurolysis may be performed. In cases where the compression of the deep peroneal nerve is at the extensor retinaculum, the inferior arm of the retinaculum is totally released or lengthened in a Z-fashion.

If subluxation of a Lisfranc's joint exists, closed reduction and pinning of the joint may be required. If open reduction is necessary, the nerve should be explored and neurolysis performed as necessary. In the case of hypertrophic degenerative arthritis in the foot, the offending spurs are removed and a small portion of the joint resected in a V-shaped fashion (Fig. 50.38). If preoperative x-rays indicate that severe arthrosis of the joint exists, AP and lateral tomograms of the joint are

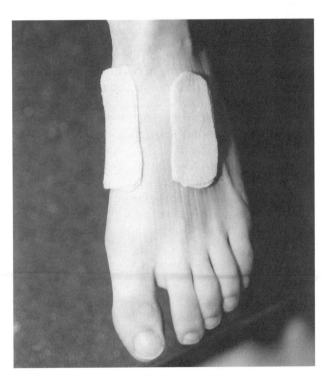

FIG. 50.50. Dorsal view: padding to reduce pressure on the deep peroneal nerve.

ordered preoperatively. If most of the joint is severely affected, a TMT or naviculocuneiform fusion may be performed to prevent reformation of the exostosis, synovitis, or joint subluxation and pain.

Postoperative management of neurolysis patients includes use of a soft nonconstrictive dressing and immediate active range of motion. Weight bearing is permitted, and patients are allowed active range of motion activities to promote nerve gliding and to reduce edema. After 2 weeks, when the wound is healed, patients begin a strengthening program and progressively return to sports activities.

COMPRESSION NEUROPATHY OF THE MEDIAL PLANTAR NERVE

"Jogger's Foot" or Distal Tarsal Tunnel Syndrome

As noted above, the medial plantar nerve exits the tarsal tunnel distally in a fibroosseous tunnel and courses plantar to the intersection of the FDL and FHL at the fibrotic master knot of Henry. In "jogger's foot," the medial plantar nerve may be compressed by osteophytes from the talonavicular joint or fibrosis at the master knot of Henry from repeated trauma such as running or jumping (76). Patients with a planovalgus foot deformity, especially those treated with a high rigid orthotic device, may become symptomatic. An accessory abductor hallucis (77) muscle and impingement at the "spring ligament" have also been noted as causing entrapment of the medial plantar nerve.

Clinical Evaluation

Athletes may present with pain, dysesthesia, and numbness over the medial plantar nerve distribution, including the medial sole of the foot and medial toes. However, they may complain of a deep, dull, aching medial plantar arch pain. Percussion and pressure tests may be positive over the medial plantar nerve near the navicular and the master knot of Henry. Forced pronation of the foot or pressure over the nerve with active flexion of the FHL and FDL may increase symptoms. Selective injection with Xylocaine and cortisone near the master knot of Henry or area of entrapment will differentiate this from tarsal tunnel syndrome.

Imaging

Routine foot x-rays may show talonavicular or plantar tarsometatarsal joint disease with spurring. A planovalgus foot may show severe sag of the midfoot joints on lateral x-ray (Fig. 50.39). Electrodiagnostic studies typically show only medial plantar nerve involvement if positive (78). Differential diagnosis is tarsal tunnel

syndrome, posterior tibial tendinitis, talonavicular disease, flexor hallucis longus tendinitis, and midfoot pain associated with midfoot sag and plantar ligament strain in severe planovalgus deformities.

Treatment

Conservative treatment includes nonsteroidal anti-inflammatory medication, ice, and contrast baths. Soft orthotic devices with medial heel posting or a UCBL for feet with a planovalgus configuration may be substituted. Soft silicone padding or donut padding around the master knot of Henry may be useful. Selective injection with Xylocaine and cortisone may be helpful in all cases.

Surgical treatment consists of neurolysis with release of the abductor hallucis deep fascia and neurolysis of the nerve near the master knot of Henry. In severe planovalgus deformity, a talonavicular fusion or triple arthrodesis may be needed. In cases with associated FHL/FDL tendinitis, the master knot of Henry is released.

BONY INJURIES OF THE HINDFOOT

Calcaneal Stress Fracture

Stress fractures of the calcaneus are not an uncommon source for heel pain and are usually seen in patients who perform repetitive jumping or running exercises. Female athletes who are amenorrheic or oligomenorrheic may be more slightly prone to this condition. Another common source is training errors where mileage or activity has been increased too much and too quickly. Worn out shoe wear with insufficient heel cushioning may also be a causative factor.

Clinical Evaluation

The athlete will usually complain of severe and diffuse heel pain that may be difficult for them to localize, but they may feel that the entire posterior heel hurts. A "pinch test" (Fig. 50.51), squeezing the medial and lateral portion of the midheel, may produce discomfort. There may be considerable swelling with this problem. Pain in this condition exists with direct weight-bearing pressure on the heel and push-off or lift-off.

Imaging

Lateral x-rays and Harris views may show linear or fluffy increased radiodensity, indicating bony healing (Fig. 50.52). The films, however, may be negative, and sometimes a bone scan (Fig. 50.53) may be necessary to confirm the diagnosis. Note that this appearance shows a more diffuse uptake and is different from the plantar

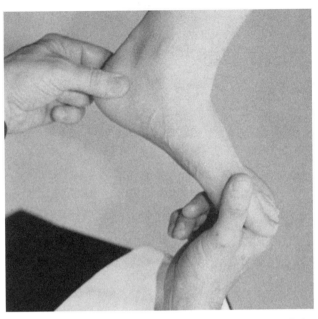

FIG. 50.51. Heel "pinch test": squeezing the sides of the posterior calcaneal tuberosity will cause pain in the calcaneal stress fracture.

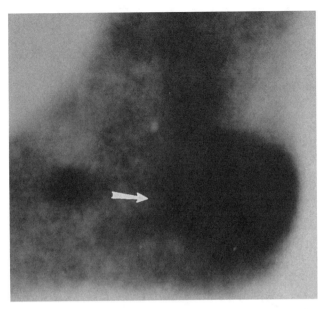

FIG. 50.53. Lateral bone scan, showing increased uptake across the posterior tuberosity of the calcaneus due to calcaneal stress fracture.

uptake seen with plantar fasciitis or the posterior uptake seen with distal Achilles tendinitis.

Treatment

Treatment usually consists of relative rest (modification of activities) consistent with the athlete's symptoms. This may range from reduction of mileage or activities, cross training, or even non-weight bearing with crutches.

Ice and anti-inflammatory medication are also helpful. Immobilization with an AFO, CAM walker, or cast may be necessary in severe cases until comfortable. Cardiovascular fitness and strength are maintained until the patient is pain free to palpation, swelling is limited, and they can comfortably bear weight. A gradual progression of activities from running to jumping to sport-specific activities is pursued with pain and swelling as guidelines. A cushioning heel cup, such as a viscoelastic

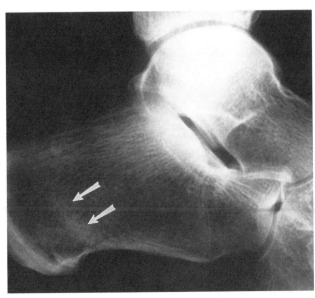

A

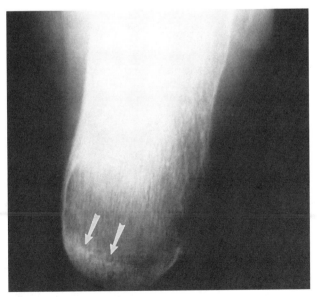

B

FIG. 50.52. Forty-two–year–old Masters runner with heel pain: (A) lateral radiograph shows increased radiodensity (*arrows*) due to stress fracture and (B) Harris axial view also showing radiodensity (*arrows*).

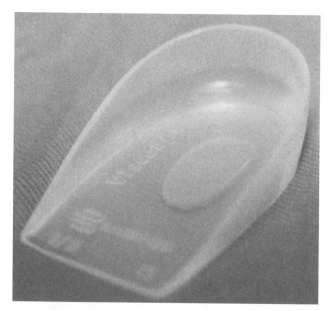

FIG. 50.54. Viscoelastic silicone heel cup.

heel cup (Fig. 50.54), may also be helpful in return to sports.

Fracture of the Anterior Lateral Process of the Calcaneus

Known as the "ankle sprain that does not heal," fracture of the anterior lateral process of the calcaneus produces discomfort and swelling on the lateral midfoot and is frequently missed upon initial examination. The usual two mechanisms of injury are a plantar flexion inversion injury similar to an ankle sprain or a dorsiflexion eversion injury (78). In the first scenario (Fig. 50.55A), the bifurcate ligament attached to this calcaneal process is stressed, pulling off a piece of the anterior calcaneal process and producing an avulsion-type fracture. Because of the continued forces of the bifurcate ligament on the fracture fragment, delayed union or nonunion of this fracture is common, producing chronic discomfort. In the second scenario, direct compression (Fig. 50.55B) on the anterior lateral calcaneal process leads to fracture.

Clinical Evaluation

As mentioned above, signs and symptoms consist of pain and swelling in the anterior lateral midfoot and tenderness to palpation at the tip of the anterior lateral process and over the sinus tarsi. Inversion and supination may produce discomfort by pulling on the fracture fragment.

Imaging

Routine x-rays (AP, lateral, and oblique views) may show the fracture. The oblique view is most helpful (Fig. 50.56). However, in some cases, especially chronic cases, x-rays may be equivocal. Tomograms with AP and lat-

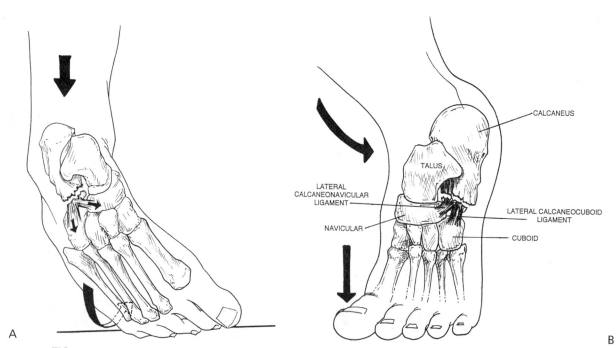

FIG. 50.55. A: Avulsion fracture of the anterior lateral process of the calcaneus by a plantar flexion inversion mechanism. **B:** Fracture of the anterior calcaneal process by dorsiflexion compression injury.

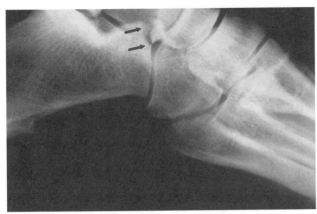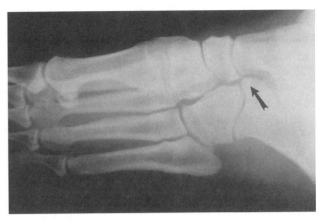

FIG. 50.56. Old fracture of the anterior lateral process in a 24-year-old aerobics instructor: **(A)** Lateral radiograph showing nonunion of the fracture (*arrows*) and **(B)** oblique radiograph (*arrow*).

eral views may be helpful. CT may also show this lesion, especially lateral reconstructions. For cases of chronic pain where a fracture or nonunion are suspected, a magnified, coned, down bone scan view is helpful as a screening tool.

Treatment

For acute cases, if the fracture is nondisplaced, a short leg cast is applied and a non–weight-bearing status maintained for 6 to 8 weeks or until x-rays confirm healing. After healing of the fracture and removal of the cast, progressive weight bearing is started, along with edema control and range of motion. The athlete progresses from pain-free walking to jogging and then to proprioceptive exercises and sport-specific activities.

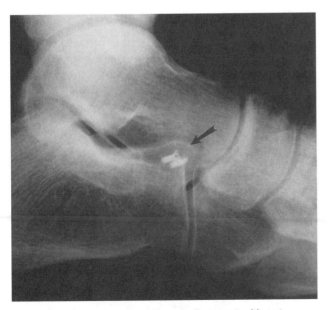

FIG. 50.57. Repair of the bifurcate ligament with suture anchors (*arrow*) after excision of the nonunion fragment.

If the fracture is displaced, it may be treated by open reduction internal fixation (when the piece big enough) or excision of the fragment and repair of the bifurcate ligament to the anterior lateral calcaneus with a suitable suture anchor (Fig. 50.57). The postoperative course is usually the same as mentioned above.

Occasionally, even when the fracture heals, the patient may develop some chronic arthritis at the dorsum of the calcaneocuboid joint as a result of irregularities at the fracture site. This condition may be determined by palpation of the calcaneocuboid joint, manipulation of that joint, or selective injection. A bone scan is usually helpful, and CT or tomograms are also helpful in assessing the degree of arthritic involvement in the joint.

If conservative treatment such as anti-inflammatory medication, selective injection, ice, and a molded support such as UCBL are not helpful, then operative treatment may be helpful. In this situation, an arthrotomy is made at the dorsum of the calcaneocuboid joint and the affected segment of the calcaneal process removed to decompress the joint. Usually, the segment of the affected joint is limited. Calcaneocuboid fusion is a last resort for severe arthritis of the calcaneocuboid joint, can produce severe functional problems for the athlete, and should be reserved as a salvage procedure.

Fracture of the Lateral Talar Process

Fracture of the lateral talar beak or lateral talar process is a frequently underdiagnosed problem. The athlete complains of lateral ankle discomfort and increased pain with activity, especially inversion/eversion type motions. The usual mechanism of injury is an inversion dorsiflexion sprain mechanism that is often combined with axial loading (78). This type of fracture may also be caused by an eversion loading injury ("snowboarders injury") (79). This fracture is relatively common, representing 24% of talar body fractures (80).

Clinical Evaluation

The diagnosis is made by the above history and swelling and tenderness at the lateral talar process. The athlete may also give a history of "giving-way" that is actually secondary to pain. Forced eversion/inversion may produce pain at the lateral talus. Because of its location, a fracture of the lateral talar process is easy to confuse with peroneal tendinitis.

Imaging

Routine ankle x-rays may show the fracture (Fig. 50.58); however, it is often easy to miss. A special AP view of the ankle with the foot in 30 degrees of plantar flexion and 45 degrees of internal rotation may show the fracture (81). CT is often the gold standard, showing the fracture and degree of displacement easily (Fig. 50.59).

Treatment

Acute nondisplaced cases are treated with immobilization in either an AFO or cast and limitation of weight bearing. Once the fracture is healed clinically and radiographically, progressive weight bearing and an ankle rehabilitation program is started. If the fragment is intraarticular and/or displaced, surgical treatment may be required, either excision of the fragment or open reduction internal fixation and bone grafting, if needed. In chronic nonunion cases, fragment excision or internal fixation may be required.

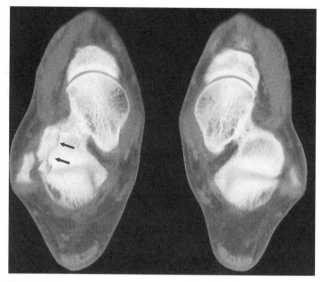

FIG. 50.59. Axial computed tomography of the patient in Figure 50.58. The minimally displaced lateral talar fracture is easily seen (*arrows*).

Painful Os Trigonum/Fracture of the Posterior Talus

The os trigonum ossicle is a normal variant present in 7% to 11% of the population (82–84) and often exists bilaterally. It exists at the junction of the ankle and subtalar joint and is a continuation of the posterior lateral talar process. The posterior talar process or "beak" is occasionally long (Stieda's process), extending posteriorly between the distal tibia and calcaneus and subject to injury. Of note, the flexor hallucis longus tendon sheath runs immediately adjacent to the os trigonum.

Acute plantar flexion injuries can produce injury to the synchondrosis between the posterior talus and os trigonum, causing swelling, or can produce a fracture of a long posterior talar beak. Either of these two injuries can produce posterior impingement syndrome, in which plantar flexion, especially with loading, produces posterior ankle pain (commonly seen in ballerinas and jumping athletes) (85), and flexor hallucis longus nodular tenovaginitis, leading to a "trigger toe" or rupture of the FHL.

Clinical Evaluation

In both cases, the athlete has pain in the posterior medial ankle and is tender to palpation at the posterior talar beak or os trigonum (Fig. 50.60). They may have tenderness with palpation of the posterior medial ankle during dorsiflexion/plantar flexion motion of the great toe, producing FHL motion. The posterior impingement test (Fig. 50.61) with forced plantar flexion of the foot may produce posterior discomfort. Extreme dorsiflexion may also produce discomfort in the posterior ankle as well.

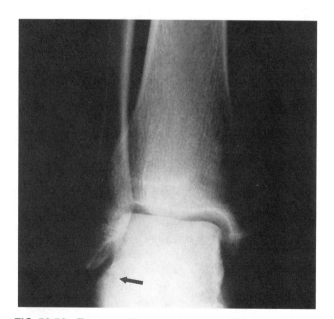

FIG. 50.58. Fracture of the lateral talus in a 21-year-old snowboarder. The anteroposterior radiograph of the ankle barely shows the fracture (*arrow*).

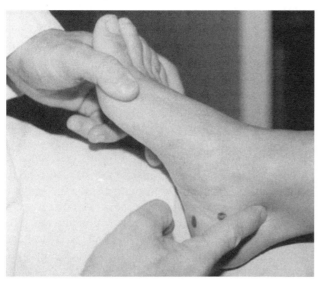

FIG. 50.60. Pressure on the posterior medial ankle may produce pain from a symptomatic os trigonum or fracture of the posterior process of the talus. This test may be accentuated by having the patient move the great toe up and down during palpation.

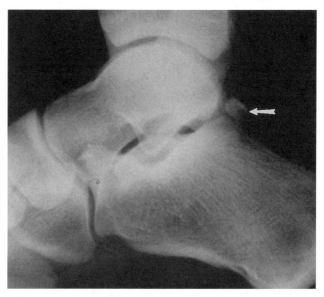

FIG. 50.62. Lateral radiograph showing a symptomatic os trigonum (*arrow*) in a 17-year-old cross-country runner.

Imaging

A lateral x-ray (Fig. 50.62) may show the presence of a large os trigonum or may show the presence of a fracture of the posterior talar beak. CT with axial and lateral reconstructions (Fig. 50.63) is also helpful in determining whether this is a fracture or an os trigonum. Tomograms have also been used. A bone scan will be positive in the posterior ankle joint but will not help determine the difference between a posterior talar fracture or symptomatic os trigonum.

Treatment

Fortunately, the treatment is the same for both conditions and is initially conservative. Nonsteroidal antiinflammatory medication and ice are used; training is modified to reduce jumping or hill running. For balleri-

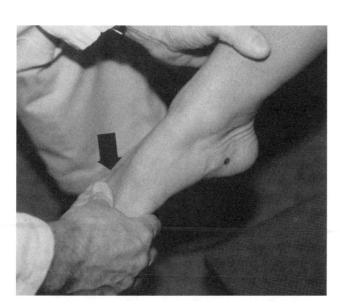

FIG. 50.61. The posterior impingement test to the ankle: forced plantar flexion will produce posterior ankle pain with a positive test.

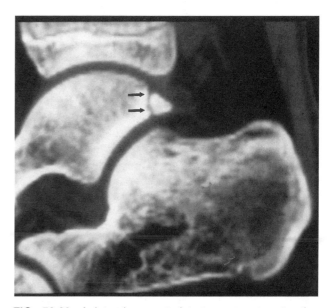

FIG. 50.63. A lateral computed tomogram reconstruction showing a posterior talar fracture (*arrows*) in a collegiate wide receiver.

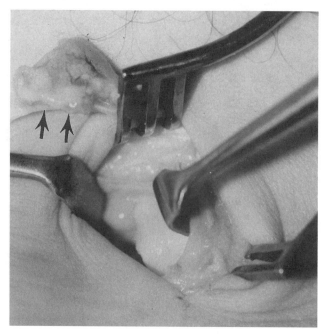

FIG. 50.64. Lateral view of surgical excision of a painful os trigonum (*arrows*). The peroneal tendons are retracted toward the toes (**right**).

nas, en pointe activities are restricted. If symptoms do not resolve, injection into the area of synchondrosis can be carefully performed approaching posterior to the neurovascular bundle. This may reduce pain at the synchondrosis and secondarily to the FHL (if FHL tendinitis is present). For acute posterior talar fractures that are nondisplaced, cast immobilization until healed may be helpful.

Surgery is required when conservative treatment fails and if there is a painful nonunion of a posterior talar fracture. Such treatment consists of excision of the os trigonum or posterior talar fracture fragment and FHL tenosynovectomy, if needed. A small longitudinal posterior lateral incision is used approaching from posterior to the peroneal tendons (Fig. 50.64). Postoperatively, the patient may start on immediate range of motion and progressive weight bearing as tolerated after approximately 2 weeks. Marumoto and Ferkel (86) introduced arthroscopic excision of the os trigonum. This is a new and exciting possibility, but results in other hands, when compared with the open approach, are still pending.

Subtalar Arthritis

Subtalar joint arthritis is another painful hindfoot condition occasionally affecting athletes. They complain of lateral or medial hindfoot pain with jumping, twisting, or planting activities. Causes for subtalar arthritic changes include trauma to the joint after inversion/eversion activities, an old fracture of the lateral talar process, or an old intraarticular calcaneus fracture. Another cause

is chronic instability of the subtalar joint. Athletes with flexible pes planus and severe heel valgus may experience lateral subtalar joint pain due to impingement of the lateral subtalar joint. Finally, adolescent or adult athletes with tarsal coalition may experience subtalar discomfort with increased activity due to stress upon an incomplete tarsal coalition.

Clinical Evaluation

Signs and symptoms are lateral (sinus tarsi) pain, tenderness, and occasionally medial subtalar joint discomfort, which may be confused with posterior tibial tendinitis. The athlete may have pain with inversion and eversion and limited subtalar motion. Pivoting activities and jumping or toe-raising activities may also cause discomfort because of the required subtalar inversion.

Imaging

X-rays (standard lateral and oblique views) may show arthritic changes (Fig. 50.65), especially in the posterior subtalar facet. CT (Fig. 50.66) is the gold standard for assessing subtalar changes. MRI, although more expensive, is helpful in showing increased fluid or synovitis in the subtalar joint. In cases of chronic pain, a bone scan (Fig. 50.67) may be helpful as a screening tool.

Treatment

Initial conservative treatment of subtalar arthritis includes anti-inflammatory medication, ice, and a UCBL-

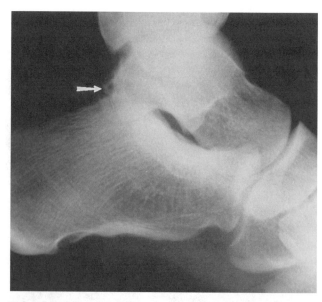

FIG. 50.65. Twenty-eight-year-old professional figure skater with posterior ankle pain. Lateral radiographs show sclerosis and degenerative changes in the posterior subtalar joint (*arrow*).

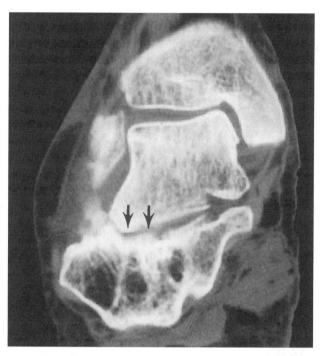

FIG. 50.66. Computed tomogram (coronal view) shows subtalar arthritis (*arrows*) in a patient with a healed calcaneus fracture.

type orthosis (Fig. 50.68) designed to limit motion but provide some flexibility. Cortisone injection may be helpful, although results have variable success.

Subtalar fusion (Fig. 50.69) is a last resort and may still allow the athlete to function well, particularly if the transverse tarsal joint (talonavicular and calcaneocuboid) is still normal with good mobility. The subtalar joint is fused in slight eversion to allow mobility of the midfoot. Postoperatively, the foot is immobilized in a cast or AFO with limited weight bearing for 6 to 10 weeks until the fusion is solid. Progressive weight bear-

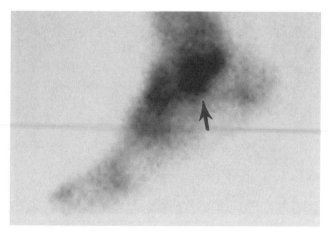

FIG. 50.67. Bone scan of the patient in Figure 50.66.

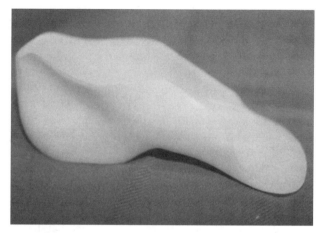

FIG. 50.68. A UCBL foot orthosis that supports and controls heel and subtalar motion.

ing and an ankle rehabilitation program are initiated, leading to return to sports.

Tarsal Coalition

A tarsal coalition is present in approximately 1% to 6% of the population (87,88) and bilateral in 50% to 60% of affected people. Coalitions may involve a single joint of the talocalcaneal, talonavicular, and calcaneonavicular complex or may involve more than one joint. The coalition is present to varying degrees, ranging from a fibrous connection, allowing some motion, to a partial bony coalition to a total bony fusion.

The athlete may complain of medial and lateral "ankle" discomfort, worse with increased weight-bearing, jumping, or pivoting activities and with varying terrain. They may have a high incidence of lateral ankle

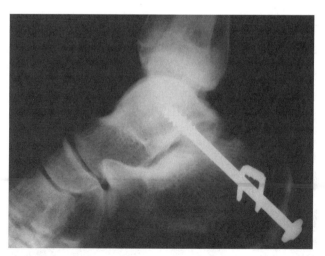

FIG. 50.69. Subtalar fusion in a young soccer player with a symptomatic tarsal coalition that did not respond to conservative management.

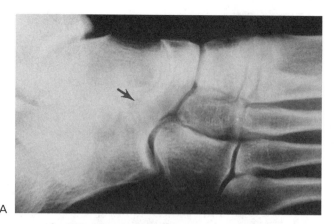

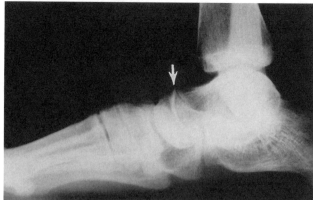

A

B

FIG. 50.70. Calcaneonavicular coalition: **(A)** oblique radiograph shows the bony connection (*arrow*) and **(B)** lateral radiograph shows dorsal talar beaking (*white arrow*).

"sprains" (89). This condition commonly presents in adolescent athletes and is also noted in young adults. Talocalcaneal coalitions with good residual transverse tarsal joint motion often present later.

Clinical Evaluation

On examination, there is frequently tenderness over the sinus tarsi or lateral subtalar joint. There may be pain medially over the subtalar joint as well. There is often decreased range of motion of the peritalar joints and pain with forceful inversion and eversion. A rigid flat foot with painful spastic peroneal tendons may be present in 10% (90). Selective injection in the subtalar joint with Xylocaine and cortisone may provide temporary relief, thus helping to establish the diagnosis.

Imaging

A standard oblique x-ray (Fig. 50.70) best shows a naviculocalcaneal coalition. A lateral x-ray view may show dorsal talar beaking, suggestive of a talocalcaneal coalition. A Harris axial view (Fig. 50.71), if properly oriented, may show a medial talocalcaneal fusion. The gold standard imaging study for tarsal coalition is the CT (91) (Fig. 50.72) with axial and coronal cuts, which not only shows an actual bony coalition, if present, but also varying degrees of arthritic changes in the remainder of the joint and adjacent joints. For chronic cases of hindfoot pain, a bone scan (92) may be helpful as a

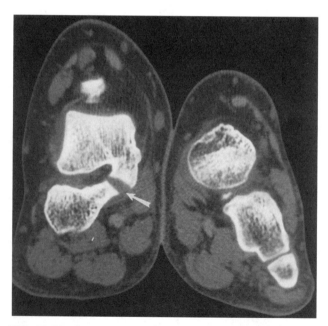

FIG. 50.71. Harris axial radiograph showing partial medial talocalcaneal coalition (*arrow*).

FIG. 50.72. Computed tomogram (coronal view) showing an incomplete talocalcaneal tarsal coalition (*arrow*).

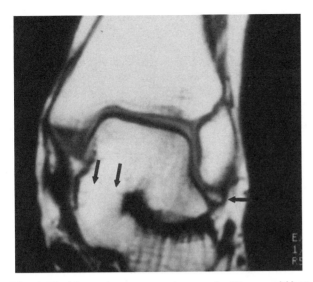

FIG. 50.73. Magnetic resonance image of a 19-year-old basketball player with lateral ankle pain. This coronal view shows a bony talocalcaneal coalition (*arrows*) and a small bony ossicle (*arrow*) at the tip of the fibula from multiple ankle sprains.

screening test. MRI (Fig. 50.73), although more expensive, is useful in cases where the suspected coalition is fibrous.

Treatment

Initial conservative treatment of tarsal coalition consists of nonsteroidal anti-inflammatory medication, ice, and limitation of weight bearing as needed. If pain is due to a recent traumatic event, rest in an AFO-type device or cast for 3 to 6 weeks may be helpful to return the athlete to his or her pain-free preinjury status. Localized injection with Xylocaine and cortisone may help to relieve irritation of the joint. A semirigid foot orthosis and supportive shoe with a good heel counter may help control hindfoot motion. A UCBL is also an excellent device to help control peritalar motion and reduce stress on the joint.

Surgical treatment may be necessary if conservative treatment fails to provide adequate relief and restore function. Resection of the bony coalition or fibrous coalition may be indicated in younger patients (Fig. 50.74) who have not developed arthritic changes and fibrosis of the surrounding structures. Resection is also indicated if the coalition affects less than 50% of the joint (93) and if imaging studies show that the rest of the affected joint is in good condition. Simple resection and interposition of fat grafts or muscle interposition (94–97) have proven effective in these cases. The athlete should be informed preoperatively that although pain relief may be gained, they might not realize increased motion in the affected joint.

Fusion of the affected joint may be necessary in older

athletes, where arthritic changes are already present (Fig. 50.69) or if more than 50% of the joint is affected by the coalition. After immobilization for 6 to 10 weeks and documented healing of the fusion, the patient may be started on a progressive weight-bearing program and ankle rehabilitation exercises. Patients with isolated talocalcaneal fusions do better if the remaining talonavicular and calcaneocuboid joints are mobile. A subtalar fusion is performed in slight eversion to allow maximum midfoot mobility.

HEEL PAIN

Heel pain is a common affliction affecting many athletes, with symptoms varying from mild to severely disabling. There are many different etiologies for heel pain, and an accurate diagnosis is critical to determine the proper treatment. Table 50.1 lists the various causes for heel pain (Fig. 50.75).

Insertional Plantar Fasciitis or Heel Pain Syndrome

One of the most common causes of heel pain in athletes is insertional plantar fasciitis, also known as heel pain syndrome (98), As noted in the section on anatomy, the plantar fascia is a dynamic stabilizer of the arch and undergoes tension during push-off and landing. Repetitive or acute traumatic stresses lead to microtears and occasional microfracture at the calcaneal attachment of the plantar fascia. In chronic insertional plantar fasciitis, metaplastic changes take place at the insertion as noted on biopsy or MRI. Athletes in sports that involve running and repetitive push-off or jumping are especially prone to this condition. Training errors such as swift increase in running mileage, improperly suited shoes,

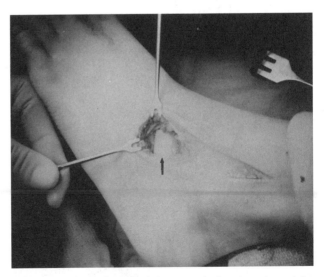

FIG. 50.74. Lateral surgical photograph showing a bony talocalcaneal bar (*arrow*) before excision.

TABLE 50.1. *Differential diagnosis of heel pain*

1. Heel pain syndrome (insertional plantar fasciitis)
2. Acute plantar fascial tear
3. Calcaneal stress fracture
4. Fat pad atrophy
5. Diffuse plantar fasciitis
6. Entrapment of Baxter's nerve (nerve to the ADQ)
7. Inflammatory heel pain (gout, rheumatoid arthritis; ankylosing spondylitis; systemic lupus erythematosus; Reiter's disease)

Posterior Heel Pain
8. Distal insertional Achilles tendinitis
9. Retrocalcaneal bursitis
10. Painful Haglund's deformity
11. Painful pump bump (posterior lateral calcaneal exostosis)
12. Retro Achilles bursitis

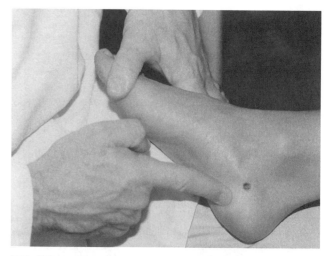

FIG. 50.76. Palpation of the insertion of the plantar fascia at the medial calcaneal tubercle.

lack of flexibility, and excessive hill training have been implicated, as well as biomechanical factors such as an overpronating planovalgus foot deformity or, at the opposite extreme, a rigid cavovarus foot.

Clinical Evaluation

The athlete complains of severe sharp pain in the plantar medial aspect of the heel, at the insertion of the plantar fascia on the medial calcaneal tubercle (Fig. 50.76). The pain may be sharp and localized, or pain may be more diffuse, extending distally across the plantar fascia. There is point tenderness, often at the medial calcaneal tubercle, and the athlete complains of pain in this area when pushing off or jumping and landing. In severe cases, swelling may also be noticed. Many athletes, consciously or unconsciously, compensate by supinating the foot to avoid push-off on the medial foot. Secondary lateral foot/ankle pain and anterior tibial or peroneal tendinitis may result from this supination posture.

Imaging

X-rays consisting of a lateral view of the foot and heel may or may not show a heel spur (Fig. 50.77). Heel

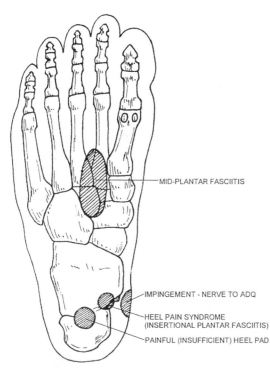

FIG. 50.75. Many causes for heel pain. (Modified from Baxter, Pfeffer. *The foot and ankle in sport.* St. Louis: Mosby, 1995:, with permission.)

Labels in figure:
MID-PLANTAR FASCIITIS
IMPINGEMENT - NERVE TO ADQ
HEEL PAIN SYNDROME (INSERTIONAL PLANTAR FASCIITIS)
PAINFUL (INSUFFICIENT) HEEL PAD

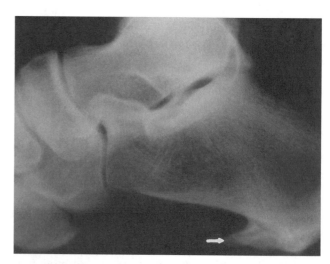

FIG. 50.77. Lateral radiograph of a patient with a large plantar calcaneal spur (*arrow*). This patient was seen for another unrelated foot problem and had no heel pain.

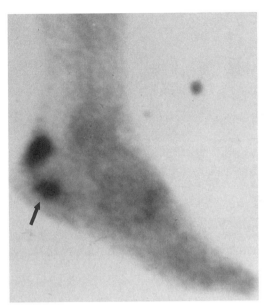

FIG. 50.78. Lateral bone scan of a patient with plantar fasciitis. Although both the Achilles insertion and plantar fascia insertion (*arrow*) show increased uptake, only the plantar fasciitis was symptomatic.

spurs, if present, have been noted in flexor brevis musculature and not the plantar fascia. Studies show that heel spurs are present in only 50% of patients with plantar fasciitis and that heel spurs may be seen in up to 15% of patients who are asymptomatic (99), thereby disproving the older notion of absolute cause and effect between the heel spur, if present, and plantar fasciitis.

A 45-degree medial oblique x-ray may show an ero-

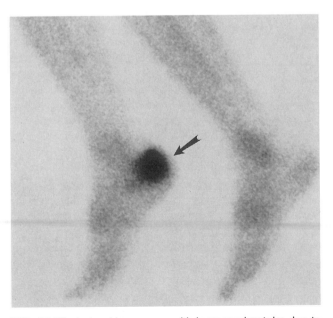

FIG. 50.79. Lateral bone scan with increased uptake due to calcaneal stress fracture (*arrow*).

sion or "saddle sign" (100) in the plantar surface of the spur (60%) and an increased soft tissue shadow, indicating edema. MRIs are expensive and should not be routinely ordered for the diagnosis of plantar fasciitis, although they may show edema, thickening, and inflammation at the insertion of the plantar fascia. A bone scan (Fig. 50.78) will often show increased uptake just at the plantar insertion of the fascia (101) and in chronic cases helps to distinguish it from a calcaneal stress fracture (Fig. 50.79).

Treatment

The treatment of insertional plantar fasciitis has been somewhat controversial. The National Heel Pain Study conducted by the American Orthopaedic Foot and Ankle Society and several other large studies (102–106) have suggested that the treatment of insertional plantar fasciitis is usually conservative. Although many different programs exist, there are several elements common to each. In our practice, we use a graduated protocol that is adaptable and customized to each patient/athlete.

First, any biomechanical or training causes for the plantar fasciitis must be determined. For a runner, training logs for reviewing their training habits may determine errors in training techniques that precipitated the heel pain. Mileage, in mild to moderate cases, may need to be reduced; hill training may need to be avoided to heal. In severe cases, running may need to be discontinued temporarily, and patients may need to be placed on cross-training activities such as biking, swim vest, and so forth. Athletes or patients who are grossly obese need to be reminded that complete pain relief may not be found until their weight is under control. Examination of the foot and gait or even running on a treadmill will reveal whether the patient has a pes planus and overpronating foot or, the opposite, rigid cavovarus foot. Inspection of the worn athletic shoes will reveal whether the patient is running in the proper shoe.

In addition to modified activity as noted above, antiinflammatory medication, ice, or contrast baths and massage of the affected area are started, either directly by hand massage or by rolling the foot over a tennis ball. Intrinsic stretching and strengthening exercises are performed with towel scrunches. Most importantly, plantar stretching exercises, Achilles stretching exercises, and hamstring stretching exercises are performed as needed. One of the most common findings in athletes is a very tight tendo-Achilles (especially the soleus). We have found that proper stretching is the key to recovery.

We also use physical therapy modalities such as phonophoresis or iontophoresis to the affected area. If athletes are still having discomfort and exhibit a tight Achilles with continued pain in the morning, a night

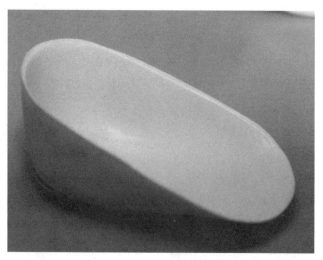

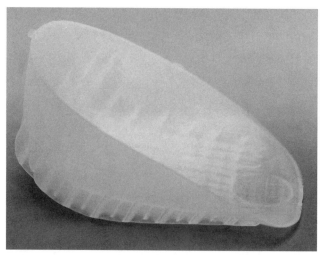

FIG. 50.80. Two commercially available heel cups.

dorsiflexion AFO (107) is added to promote Achilles stretching and plantar fascia stretching. During this period, most athletes, except for the most severe, will be able to train at some level.

For patients with a hyperpronating flexible pes planus, a soft semirigid custom foot orthosis is prescribed, and for patients with a high cavovarus foot, a soft molded orthosis is used. Note that there is much controversy over this particular area, with many people preferring prefabricated orthoses, arch supports, or heel cups (Fig. 50.80).

For patients who have not responded within a 3-

month period and have continued severe heel pain, a localized cortisone and Xylocaine injection is used with a plantar medial approach, arriving at the medial calcaneal tubercle. Note that repeated cortisone injections can cause withering or atrophy of the fat pad (108) and are strictly contraindicated. We usually reserve cortisone injections as a last resort before surgery. Casting for 3 to 6 weeks may also help at this stage (109).

Finally, for patients who have not responded to conservative measures within a 6-month period, a partial plantar fascia release, releasing the medial one third of the plantar fascia, may be performed (110–113). This

A

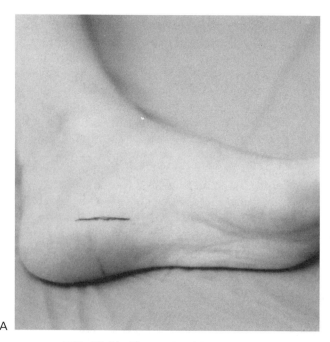

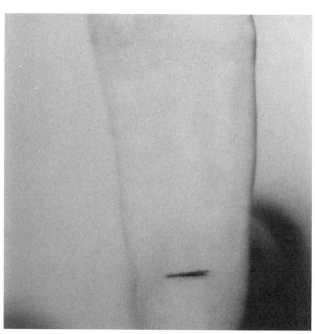

B

FIG. 50.81. Plantar fasciectomy surgical approaches: **(A)** medial Henry approach and **(B)** plantar transverse approach.

can be performed through either the standard medial Henry approach or a small transverse plantar approach (Fig. 50.81). Newer endoscopic plantar fasciectomy techniques (114,115) have been purported to promote early recovery, but there is no randomized prospective study that proves that these techniques are better. Indeed, there has been a higher reported incidence of complications (116) such as lateral arch pain, flattened arch, or lateral plantar nerve and artery injury noted (117). Once the patient has recovered, a set of maintenance exercises for Achilles and plantar fascia stretching is usually followed. General advice to athletes is that the longer their symptoms have been present, the longer it will require them to improve.

Acute Plantar Fascia Tear

Another variation of chronic plantar fasciitis is the acute plantar fascia tear (118) that is common in sports such as basketball or football where athletes may land or be pushed back on their foot with considerable weight.

Clinical Evaluation

The history is usually one of acute pain and swelling in the plantar surface of the foot, either in the midarch or near the insertion at the heel. There may be plantar ecchymosis, tenderness to touch, and the patient may notice a drop in arch height with cases of complete tear. Occasionally, a palpable defect can be felt in the plantar fascia as compared with the opposite side.

Imaging

X-rays of the heel and foot should be taken to rule out fracture but may be normal.

Treatment

Treatment depends on the severity of the symptoms. The athlete may be weight bearing as tolerated, ranging from modification of activities to non-weight bearing with crutches. Therapy should be directed around edema control and protection. In mild to moderate cases, the athlete may bear weight as tolerated with a CAM walker-type boot. In severe cases, cast immobilization may be required for 4 to 6 weeks until comfortable. Once the patient can comfortably bear weight, therapy is instituted to include mobilization, range of motion, strengthening exercises, and a gradual progression of weight-bearing activities. At this point, usually 4 to 6 weeks, a soft molded arch support may be helpful in reducing discomfort and improving function. Complete tears may result in loss of arch height (119–121), and lateral midfoot discomfort may be noted due to increased stress on the plantar midfoot ligaments from

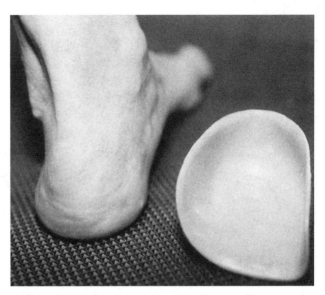

FIG. 50.82. Posterior view showing fat pad atrophy and heel pad flattening.

loss of the windlass mechanism. Again, soft or semirigid arch supports may help with this problem.

Fat Pad Insufficiency

Another cause for diffuse heel pain noted in older athletes is fat pad insufficiency. The fat pad atrophies with age and can produce diffuse heel pain due to inferior shock absorbing. This can also be seen in younger athletes where multiple cortisone injections have caused the fat pad to wither away (98). This tends to be a diagnosis of exclusion, and other causes must be ruled out, especially stress fracture. The tenderness is often diffuse, and having the athlete stand may show a flattening of the fat pad and widening of the subcutaneous tissue (Fig. 50.82).

Treatment

Treatment usually consists of ice, anti-inflammatory medication, and either a polyethylene or polypropylene heel cup (Fig. 50.80A) to hydrostatically contain the remaining fat pad and position it underneath the calcaneus or a viscoelastic-type heel cup, which provides increased cushioning and support. A good shock-absorbing shoe with increased shock absorption in the heel should also be selected.

Impingement of the Nerve to the ADQ

Another condition causing chronic plantar heel pain medially and laterally is impingement of the nerve to the ADQ (18,99,122,123) (Baxter's nerve). As mentioned in the first section, the nerve to the ADQ represents a

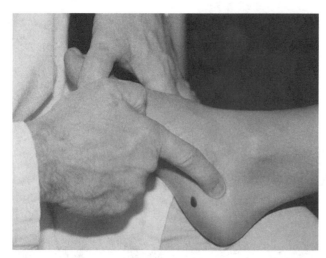

FIG. 50.83. Palpation of Baxter's nerve (nerve to the ADQ). Note that this is superior to the medial calcaneal tubercle of the plantar fascia insertion (*dot*).

branch of the posterior tibial nerve or first branch of the lateral plantar nerve that runs medially underneath the abductor hallucis fascia between the quadratus plantae and flexor brevis to reach the ADQ and intrinsic muscles of the little toe. It may be entrapped at the edge of the deep abductor hallucis fascia where it turns the corner. This produces a sharp burning heel pain, which may also feel electrical in nature.

Clinical Evaluation

There is tenderness to palpation medially over the nerve to the ADQ and especially where it turns (Fig. 50.83). Pressure there may produce medial heel pain or radiating pain to the lateral heel at its insertion on the ADQ. Electrical studies are occasionally helpful in showing increased latency to the nerve of the ADQ (123) or denervation but may frequently be normal or latencies may be unobtainable. Selective injection with Xylocaine and/or cortisone into the area of maximal tenderness may be not only diagnostic but therapeutic as well.

Conservative treatment is essentially the same for the treatment of insertional plantar fasciitis and as shown noted (124) should be pursued for 3 to 6 months before thinking of surgical treatment. Surgical treatment consists of decompression of the nerve to the ADQ (122). Baxter uses an oblique incision, set over the abductor fascia performed under local anesthesia with no tourniquet. My own preference is a curving posterior medial incision that is slightly more distal than the standard tarsal tunnel incision. I believe that this allows more exposure and also allows more complete release under direct vision. The inner or deep fascia of the abductor hallucis muscle is released and the nerve is decompressed past its turning point.

Postoperative weight bearing is limited for 2 weeks, but early range of motion exercises are started to promote nerve gliding, and progressive weight bearing is started between 2 and 6 weeks as comfort permits. Progressive activities are permitted as tolerated after 6 weeks.

Posterior Heel Pain

Posterior heel pain is also a common problem for athletes. Once again, there are multiple clinical entities that can produce this symptom, and accurate diagnosis is the key to proper treatment. The differential for posterior heel pain is seen in Table 50.1.

Distal Insertional Achilles Tendinitis

Distal insertional Achilles tendinitis is a common problem in jumping sports and may be produced by repetitive trauma, a direct blow, or insufficient stretching. Improper shoe wear with rubbing of the heel counter against the Achilles insertion can also be causative. Rarely, inflammatory causes such as Reiter's disease, lupus, gout, psoriasis, or rheumatoid arthritis can also produce distal Achilles tendinitis.

Clinical Evaluation

The patient will have tenderness and swelling at the distal insertion of the Achilles, and there is usually tenderness to direct posterior heel palpation (Fig. 50.84). Resisted plantar flexion, forced dorsiflexion, and tiptoe or jumping-type activities may reproduce discomfort.

Imaging

X-rays, lateral and oblique views of the heel, may be normal or may show some calcific spurs that are intra-

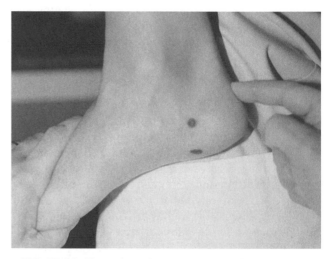

FIG. 50.84. Posterior palpation at the Achilles insertion.

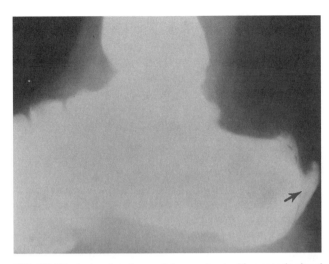

FIG. 50.85. Lateral radiograph in a patient with posterior heel pain. A large posterior calcific spur (*arrow*) resides within the Achilles insertion to the calcaneus.

tendinous at the insertion (Fig. 50.85), indicating a chronic inflammation. These spurs usually appear to be central within the insertion of the Achilles. MRI may show an area of inflammation or scarring at the insertion or slightly proximal (Fig. 50.90B). The swelling and spur (if present) may also produce a mass effect, rubbing against the shoe heel counter posteriorly.

Treatment

Treatment is initially conservative with anti-inflammatory medication, ice, contrast baths, phonophoresis or ultrasound, and an Achilles stretching program. Depending on the degree of symptoms, training may need to be modified with jumping or push-off activities lessened. In severe cases, weight bearing may need to be limited with crutches and immobilization in an AFO or cast (125). A donut-shaped or U-shaped pad (Fig. 50.86) or a silicone sleeve (Fig. 50.87) may be used posteriorly to avoid pressure and friction on the swollen area. A small quarter-inch to half-inch heel lift may be used in the shoe to decrease tension on the Achilles tendon during activities. Inspection of the athletic shoes should be made to see that there are no seams or ridges in the inner heel counter that can produce irritation and also to see that the heel lift will not bring the tender area into contact with such a seam or ridge.

In most cases, conservative treatment is effective; however, in chronic cases with considerable spur formation, surgical removal of the spur may be required. In the prone position, either a direct posterior approach, as advocated by Baxter and others, or a medial and lateral approach, as advocated by Jones (125), may be used. My personal preference is a single lateral longitudinal approach. Care must be taken to avoid significant

branches of the lateral calcaneal nerve (branch of the sural nerve) to avoid producing a painful neuroma. The sheath of the paratenon is split on the lateral side, and a curette is used under direct vision and fluoroscopy to gently remove the spur from within the tendon. If in removing the spur a significant amount of the Achilles becomes detached, the Achilles is reattached to the calcaneus with several bone anchors such as the Roc Anchor (Fig. 50.88).

The postoperative course depends on the patient and the degree of surgical trauma to the Achilles tendon. In cases where the spur and trauma to the Achilles is minimal, immediate range of motion is begun and weight bearing is tolerated in an AFO or CAM walker. Achilles strengthening is started at 2 to 6 weeks as tolerated. PREs and running activities are started at 6 weeks, and progression to jumping activities is allowed when the plantar flexion strength is 75% of the opposite side and dorsiflexion range of motion is normal. Return to sports (jumping activities) is permitted when isokinetic tests show strength equal to the other side and minitramp activities are nonpainful.

In cases with significant spurs and trauma to the Achilles requiring surgical reconstruction of the Achilles attachment with suture anchors, rehabilitation progresses at a slower pace. Trustworthy patients may start early range of motion of the ankle but remain non-weight bearing or touchdown gait in an AFO or CAM walker for 6 weeks, until the Achilles attachment is stronger. At 6 weeks, progressive resisted exercises and weight bearing as tolerated are initiated, following the rehabilitation program as discussed above. Less trustworthy patients or patients with severe Achilles pathology are

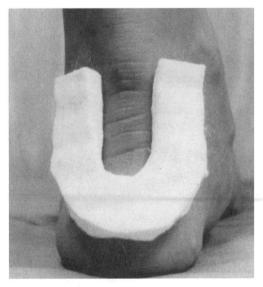

FIG. 50.86. Posterior U-shaped felt pad used to decrease pressure in an inflamed distal Achilles tendon.

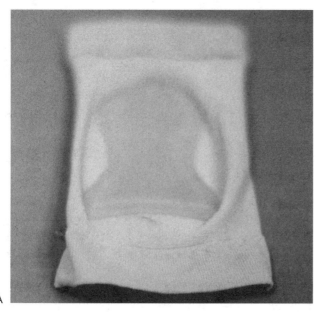

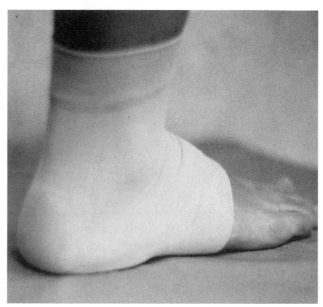

A   B

FIG. 50.87. Silicone pad and sleeve for posterior heel pain: **(A)** the silicone pad inside the sleeve and **(B)** lateral view of the sleeve applied.

placed in a short leg cast for 6 weeks, non-weight bearing, followed by the above program.

Haglund's Deformity

Another cause for posterior heel pain is prominence of the posterior superior calcaneus, known as Haglund's deformity. In between this prominence of the posterior

calcaneal tubercle and the distal Achilles tendon lies a potential space known as the retrocalcaneal bursa (Fig. 50.14) This U-shaped space becomes irritated and fluid filled, resulting in retrocalcaneal bursitis as it is trapped between the calcaneus and distal Achilles. This clinical entity is known as Haglund's syndrome (125).

Clinical Evaluation

Clinically, the athlete complains of posterior heel pain. The pinch test (Fig. 50.89) may be positive with tenderness to palpation medially and laterally just at the supe-

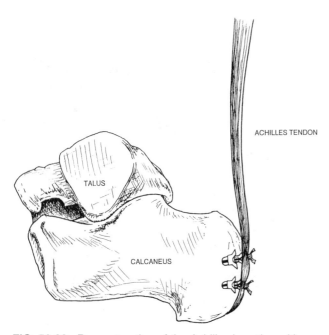

ACHILLES TENDON

TALUS

CALCANEUS

FIG. 50.88. Reconstruction of the Achilles insertion with suture anchors after excision of a large posterior calcaneal spur.

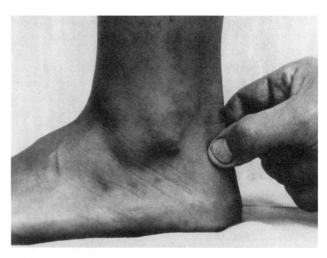

FIG. 50.89. "Pinch test" for Haglund's syndrome. This is superior and posterior to the pinch test for calcaneal stress fracture.

rior border of the posterior calcaneus. There may or may not be direct posterior tenderness.

Imaging

A lateral x-ray will show a squarish posterior–superior calcaneal prominence (Fig. 50.90A). There are several methods of determination for the presence of Haglund's deformity on x-rays such as Fowler's angle (126) or the parallel pitch angle (127). MRI (Fig. 50.90B) may show increased fluid in the retrocalcaneal bursa or increased

signal changes in the tendon adjacent to the "corner" of the Haglund's deformity, indicating irritation of the tendon by the prominence.

Treatment

Treatment includes anti-inflammatory medication, ice, Achilles stretching exercises, heel lift, and avoidance of a tightly fitting shoe with a sharp heel counter. Again, a U-shaped pad or a silicone-type heel sleeve may be helpful. If initial treatment fails, a single injection into

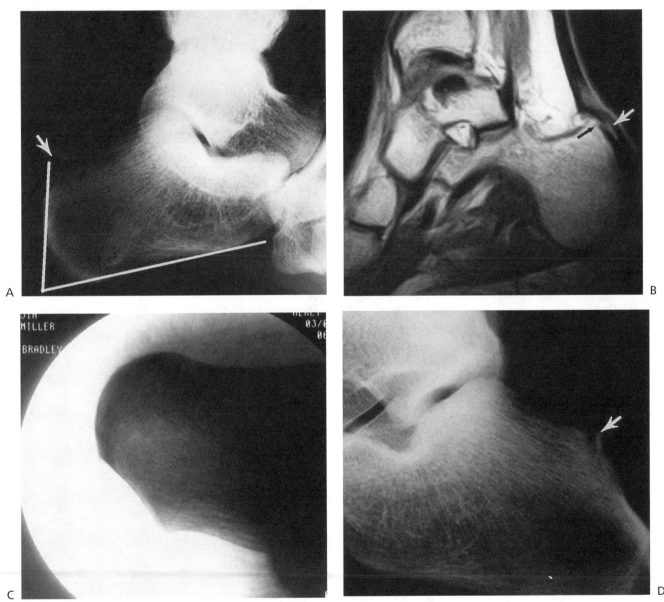

FIG. 50.90. A 24-year-old professional quarterback with chronic heel pain. **A:** Lateral radiograph—*arrow* shows Haglund's prominence. Fowler's angle is 80 degrees. **B:** Magnetic resonance image—lateral view shows inflammation of the Achilles tendon (*white arrow*) adjacent to the Haglund's prominence (*black arrow*). **C:** Intraoperative lateral fluoroscopic view showing excision of the Haglund's prominence. **D:** Lateral radiograph—6 months postoperatively, *white arrow* shows "cuff" of periosteal new bone formation.

the retrocalcaneal bursa with cortisone and Xylocaine may help. A word of caution: Injections must be in the retrocalcaneal bursa, not in the distal Achilles. A medial or lateral approach is used and the injection should flow smoothly. Attempts to overpressure the bursa or "completely fill up the space" may result in tendonopathy.

If conservative treatment fails, then surgical intervention may be considered. In the prone position, a small longitudinal lateral incision is made, and as noted above, care is taken to avoid major branches of the lateral calcaneal nerve. The Achilles tendon is gently pulled upward, the bursa resected, and an oscillating saw or osteotome is used to remove a portion of the posterior superior calcaneus, gently rounding the edges. A curette is used to carefully contour and smooth the opposite medial side of the calcaneus to avoid irritation of the Achilles insertion on that side. Fluoroscopy is used intraoperatively to assess the amount of calcaneus removal (Fig. 50.90C). In my experience, failure of surgical treatment is due to either lateral calcaneal neuroma or failure to remove enough bone. Note that in young athletes, the periosteal cuff can cause regrowth (Fig. 50.90D) of calcification, which in a few small cases may require removal. Treatment of the patient with Indocin in the postopertive phase may reduce this complication.

Retro-Achilles Bursitis

A retro-Achilles bursa is present as a potential space between the Achilles and subcutaneous skin posteriorly and may become traumatized due to increased pressure and friction from the shoe. This causes a retro-Achilles bursitis that is superficial, usually with direct tenderness posteriorly and a boggy feeling directly underneath the skin.

Treatment

Treatment is usually conservative, consisting of anti-inflammatory medication, ice, and protective padding. The shoe should also be inspected to make sure no seam or rough edge is producing aggravation. Aspiration may be used followed by compressive dressings. Rarely, when the condition does not resolve conservatively, excision of the bursa may be performed through a longitudinal medial or lateral incision.

Posterior Lateral Calcaneal Exostosis

The last condition producing posterior heel pain is the painful posterior lateral calcaneal exostosis or "pump bump." This bony prominence is posterior and lateral

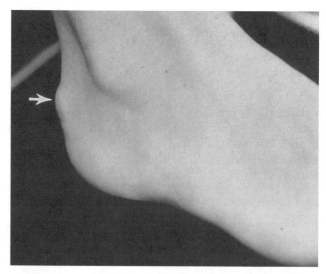

FIG. 50.91. Posterior lateral calcaneal exostosis or "pump bump" (*white arrow*).

to the Achilles insertion (Fig. 50.91) and produces discomfort often when rubbing against the heel counter. The bony prominence is a normal variation with overlying advantitial bursitis aggravated by shoe wear (98). Haglund's deformity may occur along with this painful prominence.

Clinical Evaluation

The pain, swelling, discomfort, and tenderness to palpation are posterior but lateral to the Achilles insertion as noted in Fig. 50.92.

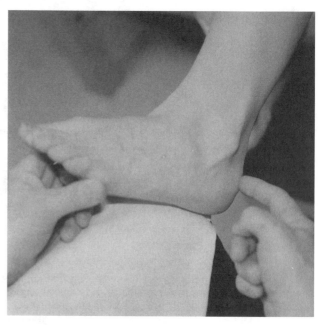

FIG. 50.92. Palpation of a posterior lateral "pump bump."

Imaging

An oblique heel x-ray may show the bony prominence.

Treatment

Treatment is also conservative consisting of ice, anti-inflammatory medication, and donut- or O-shaped padding. When conservative treatment fails, surgical intervention is used, consisting of excision of the bony prominence. A small longitudinal lateral incision is used. Progressively weight bearing and activities may be started approximately 2 weeks after surgery.

Inflammatory Heel Pain

As mentioned above, inflammatory conditions such as gout, rheumatoid arthritis, systemic lupus, psoriasis, ankylosing spondylitis, or Reiter's disease all can cause diffuse heel pain (128), especially at the Achilles tendon or plantar fascia insertions (an enthesopathy). The orthopedist should be cognizant of the possibility of these disorders as an etiology of heel pain and occasionally may be the first physician to make the diagnosis. Treatment is usually conservative with the appropriate anti-inflammatory medication and a soft silicone heel cup.

NEUROVASCULAR INJURIES OF THE HINDFOOT

Tarsal Tunnel Syndrome

Tarsal tunnel syndrome is perhaps the best known peripheral compression neuropathy of the lower extremities, with many articles and literature since its mention by Keck (129) and Lam (130). However, accounts of tarsal tunnel syndrome in athletes are few (73,131–136). Tarsal tunnel syndrome may be somewhat underreported in athletes because symptoms may be gradual and insidious in onset, such as the athlete who has numbness in the plantar aspect of his or her foot but no discomfort. The symptoms may also be confused with other conditions, such as posterior tibial tendinitis, painful pes planus, and medial ankle deltoid sprain in the case of the athlete who has posterior medial ankle discomfort.

Tarsal tunnel syndrome has been noted, not infrequently, in athletes with a severe pes planus and planovalgus deformity (133), resulting in undue tension on the medial and lateral plantar nerves. Jumping athletes who sustain a medial deltoid ligament tear of the ankle and resultant talar tilt may also become symptomatic. Posterior medial ankle synovitis and lesions such as posterior ankle ganglions or PVNS (75) can also lead to increased pressure on the contents on the tarsal tunnel. Posterior tibial tenosynovitis or flexor digitorum longus in running and jumping athletes can also produce tarsal tunnel syndrome.

Clinical Evaluation

Signs and symptoms include pain and tenderness at the tarsal tunnel; swelling and tenderness may also be present in the posterior tibial or FDL sheath. A percussion (Tinel's) may be positive over the tarsal tunnel, producing antegrade discomfort along the plantar nerve branches or retrograde discomfort up the tibial nerve. Sustained pressure over the tarsal tunnel (the nerve compression test) may also produce discomfort, dysesthesias, and/or numbness over the plantar distribution. Sensory mapping with the Semmes-Weinstein monofilament test may determine the degree of sensory loss, including loss of protective sensation in severe cases. Inflating a leg tourniquet above venous pressure proximal to the ankle may produce discomfort if varicosities are present (75). Forced pronation, together with pressure over the nerve, may increase symptoms. Claw toe deformities caused by intrinsic atrophy and associated weakness may be present late in severe cases.

Imaging

Routine x-rays are taken to rule out fracture, bony exostosis, or subtalar joint osteophytes, which could produce this condition. Earlier reports on the use of MRI in the evaluation of tarsal tunnel syndrome have been disappointing and not cost effective. However, recent reports by Erickson et al. (134) and Frey and Kerr (135) show that MRI is useful in evaluation of tarsal tunnel syndrome when space-occupying lesions are present. Zeiss et al. (136) recently suggested that MRI is useful in the evaluation of failed tarsal tunnel release.

Other Studies

Electrodiagnostic studies such as electromyogram and nerve conduction velocities have been helpful in evaluation (137–141), often demonstrating decreased conduction velocity, increased motor latency of the medial plantar nerve to the abductor hallucis muscle, increased motor latency of the lateral plantar nerve to the abductor digiti quinti, decreased sensory latency to the toes, decreased mixed nerve action potentials, and decreased motor evoked potentials. Goodgold et al. (142), Johnson and Ortiz (143), Kaplan and Kernahan (144), and Oh et al. (138,145) have worked toward a standardized electrical evaluation of tarsal tunnel syndrome. Decreased sensory action potential may be the most sensitive test (138) (90.5% positive but with a false-negative rate of 9.5%). It is important, however, to note that many series noted patients with obvious positive clinical findings and negative electric diagnostic studies (144,146,147).

Treatment

Initial treatment begins by determining any underlying condition that may cause tarsal tunnel syndrome and correcting that condition. Athletes with a severe flexible planovalgus foot may benefit from a semirigid foot orthosis or a UCBL-type orthosis to reduce heel valgus and tension on the tibial nerve. In some severe cases of pes planus such as we have seen in NFL linemen, a foot orthosis may not be tolerated, and instead a medial shoe wedge may help reduce tension and symptoms. In cases where an old ankle fracture or medial deltoid sprain has been involved, relative rest and an appropriate ankle rehabilitation program may be appropriate together with anti-inflammatory medication and ice as needed. For an athlete whose symptoms consist solely of numbness in the plantar aspect of the foot and where sensory mapping shows that protective sensation has not been lost, treatment is usually conservative. Cortisone injections along the nerve may help only in mild cases where the etiology of the nerve compression is local synovitis and are to be performed with great caution to avoid tendon rupture or direct interneural injection.

Severe cases of tarsal tunnel in athletes may warrant surgical decompression. The clinical criteria are marked discomfort, night pain, intrinsic muscle atrophy, loss of protective sensation, and failure to respond to conservative treatment. Cases where electrical diagnostic studies are positive with marked decreased nerve conduction velocity, increased motor and mixed nerve latencies, and intrinsic muscle denervation on electromyograms show a higher success rate than patients with clinical symptoms but negative electrical diagnostic tests (75).

Decompression of the tibial nerve and the medial and lateral plantar nerve branches is accomplished through a curving posterior medial incision approximately one fingerbreadth behind the medial malleolus. Authors have disagreed on the amount of decompression required (70,132,144). Any space-occupying lesions such as a giant cell tumor, ganglion cyst, or pigmented villonodular synovitis are removed, reducing pressure on the nerve. The venous plexus, which often wraps around the tibial nerve, may compress the nerve, especially when engorged by varicosities, and may be released on one side to decompress the nerve. This obviously must be undertaken under magnification.

A review of two large series reveals the rate of excellent results in tarsal tunnel surgery varies from 69% to 90% (149,150). Failure rates up to 25% have been reported (74,147). Causes for failure noted at the time of repeat surgery include cut nerve branches (especially medial calcaneal branches), inadequate decompression (especially distally and proximally), reformation of scar,

failure to release the venous plexus, incisional neuroma formation, and reflex sympathetic dystrophy. In our practice, decompression of the nerve, when required in athletes with a severe planovalgus foot deformity, must also be accompanied by orthotic or surgical treatment of the planovalgus deformity.

Exquisite homeostasis must be obtained at the time of surgery with a bipolar cautery and must be ensured by releasing the tourniquet before closing the wound. A compressive dressing is applied, and the athlete is non-weight bearing for 2 weeks while the wound heals. However, immediate range of motion is started to ensure nerve gliding and to reduce scarlike adhesions around the nerve. Progressive weight bearing as tolerated is begun during the 2- to 6-week postoperative period. At 6 weeks, resisted and strengthening exercises are started followed by a gradual return to sports-related activities. In several studies and in my own practice, the best results from tarsal tunnel surgery have been in those athletes where a specific constrictive band has been found compressing the nerve, specific compression by the venous plexus, or a space-occupying lesion such as giant cell tumor, ganglion cyst, PVNS, or subtalar joint spur.

CONCLUSION

Many athletic injuries can affect the multiple anatomic structures of the hindfoot and midfoot. Because of the complex anatomy, differential diagnosis is often difficult. Careful evaluation of the history (mechanism) of injury and a detailed physical examination based on anatomy will often help to narrow down the differential diagnosis. A healthy mix of suspicion is useful because many of these injuries tend to be subtle and often go undiagnosed for considerable periods of time. Also, as stated above, hindfoot and midfoot injuries can be chronically debilitating even when recognized promptly and treated aggressively.

REFERENCES

1. Sarrafian SK. *Anatomy of the foot and ankle descriptive, topographic, functional,* 2nd ed. Philadelphia: J.B. Lippincott, 1993:204.
2. Myerson M. The diagnosis and treatment of injuries to the Lisfranc's joint complex. *Orthop Clin North Am* 1989;20:655–664.
3. Bowman MW. Arthrodesis of the midfoot joints. *Techn Orthop* 1996;11:316–338.
4. Adkison DP, Bosse MJ, Gaccione DR, et al. Anatomical variations in the course of the superficial peroneal nerve. *J Bone Joint Surg Am* 1991;73A:112–114.
5. Herron M, Langkamer VG, Atkins RM. The anatomical variations of the distal course of the superficial peroneal nerve: recommendations to avoid injury during surgical procedures. *Foot* ;3:38–42.
6. Horwitz MT. Normal anatomy and variations of the peripheral nerves of the leg and foot: application IX. Operations for vascular disease: study of one hundred specimens. *Arch Surg* 1938;36:626–636.

7. Kenzora JE. Symptomatic incisional neuromas on the dorsum of the foot. *Foot Ankle* 1984;5:2.
8. Lambert EH. The accessory deep peroneal nerve: a common variation in innervation of extensor digitorum brevis. *Neurology* 1969;19:1169–1176.
9. Lawrence SJ, Botte MJ. The deep peroneal nerve in the foot and ankle: an anatomic study. *Foot Ankle* 1995;16:724–728.
10. Sarrafian SK. *Anatomy of the foot and ankle descriptive, topographic, functional,* 2nd ed. Philadelphia: J.B. Lippincott, 1993:356.
11. Manter JT. Movements of the subtalar and transverse tarsal joints. *Anat Rec* 1941;80:402.
12. Elftman M. The transverse tarsal joint and its control. *Clin Orthop* 1960;16:41.
13. Mann RA, Coughlin MJ. *Surgery of the foot and ankle,* 6th ed. Baltimore: Mosby, 1993:23–24.
14. Chao W. Achilles tendon insertion: an in vitro anatomic study. Presentation at 12th Annual AOFAS Summer Meeting, Hilton Head, SC, June 1996.
15. Frey C, Rosenberg Z, Shereff MJ, et al. The retrocalcaneal bursa: anatomy and bursography. *Foot Ankle* 1992;13:203–207.
16. Inman VT. *Inman's joints of the ankle,* 2nd ed. Baltimore: Williams & Wilkins, 1976.
17. Havel PE, Ebraheim NA, Clark SE, et al. Tibial branching in the tarsal tunnel. *Foot Ankle* 1988;9:117–119.
18. Baxter DE, Thigpen CM. Heel pain operative results. *Foot Ankle* 1984;5:16.
19. Matheson GE, et al. Stress fractures in athletes: a study of 320 cases. *Am J Sports Med* 1987;15:46–58.
20. Lloyd T. Women athletes with menstrual irregularities have increased musculoskeletal injuries. *Med Sci Sports Exerc* 1986;18:374.
21. Grana WA, Kalenak A. Clinical sports medicine. *Foot Ankle Sport* 1991;488.
22. O'Malley MJ, Hamilton WG, Munyak J, et al. Stress fractures at the base of the second metatarsal in ballet dancers. *Foot Ankle Int* 1996;2:89–94.
23. Rettig AC, Shelbourne KD, McCarroll JR, et al. The natural history and treatment of delayed union stress fractures of the anterior cortex of the tibia. *Am J Sports Med* 1988;16:250–255.
24. Jensen JE. Stress fracture in the world class athlete: a case study. *Med Sci Sports Exerc* 1997.
25. Heckman JD, Ryaby JP, McCabe J, et al. Acceleration of tibial fracture healing by non-invasive low-intensity pulsed ultrasound. *J Bone Joint Surg Am* 1994;76A:26–34.
26. Beaman DN, Roeser WM, Holmes JR, et al. Cuboid stress fractures: a report of two cases. *Foot Ankle* 1993;14:525–527.
27. Quirk R. Stress fractures of the navicular. *Foot Ankle Int* 1998;19:494–495.
28. Goergen TG, et al. Tarsal navicular stress fractures in runners. *AJR Am J Roentgenol* 1981;136:201.
29. Hunter L. Stress fractures of the tarsal navicular. *Am J Sports Med* 1981;9:217.
30. Torg JS, Pavlov H, Cooley LH, et al. Stress fractures of the tarsal navicular: a retrospective review of twenty-one cases. *J Bone Joint Surg Am* 1982;64:700–712.
31. Khan K, Fuller P, Brukner P, et al. Outcome of conservative and surgical management of navicular stress fractures in athletes. *Am J Sports Med* 1992;20:657–666.
32. Myerson MS. The diagnosis and treatment of injuries to the Lisfranc's joint complex. *Orthop Clin North Am* 1989;20:655–664.
33. Bradley JP. Personal communication.
34. Hardcastle PH, Reschauer R, Kutscha-Lissberg E, et al. Injuries to the tarsometatarsal joint. *J Bone Joint Surg Br* 1982;64B:349–356.
35. Quenu E, Kuss G. Etude sur les luxations du metatarse. *Rev Chir* 1909;39:231–336, 720–791, 1093–1094.
36. Myerson MS, Fischer RT, Burgess AR, et al. Fracture dislocations of the tarsometatarsal joints: end results correlated with pathology and treatment. *Foot Ankle* 1986;6:225.
37. Arntz T, Veith RG, Hansen ST. Fractures and fracture-dislocations of the tarsometatarsal joint. *J Bone Joint Dis* 1988;70A:173–181.
38. Shapiro MS, Wascher DC, Finerman GAM. Rupture of Lisfranc's ligament in athletes. *Am J Sports Med* 1994;22:687–691.
39. McClain EJ, Gruen GS, Hansen ST. Fracture-dislocation of the tarsometatarsal joint. Open reduction and internal fixation with screw fixation. In: Heckman JD, ed. *Perspective in orthopaedic surgery.* St. Louis, MO: Quality Medical Publishing, 1991:35–44.
40. Arntz CT, Hansen ST. Dislocations and fracture-dislocations of the tarsometatarsal joints. *Orthop Clin North Am* 1987;18:104–114.
41. Frey C. The shoe in sports. In: Baxter DE, ed. *The foot and ankle in sport.* St. Louis: Mosby, 1995:353–358.
42. Bordelon RL. Correction of hypermobile flatfoot in children by molded inserts. *Foot Ankle* 1980;1:143.
43. Wenger DR, Mauldin D, Speck G, et al. Corrective shoes and inserts as treatment for flexible flatfoot in infants and children. *J Bone Joint Surg Am* 1989;71A:800–810.
44. Gould N. Graphing the adult foot and ankle. *Foot Ankle* 1982;2:213–219.
45. Lord JP. Correction of extreme flatfoot: value of osteotomy of os calcis and inward displacement of posterior fragment (Gleich operation). *JAMA* 1923;81:1502.
46. Koutsogiannis E. Treatment of mobile flat foot by displacement osteotomy of the calcaneus. *J Bone Joint Surg Br* 1971;53:96.
47. Evans D. Calcaneo-valgus deformity. *J Bone Joint Surg Br* 1975;57:270–278.
48. Jacobs AM, Oloff LM. Surgical management of forefoot supinatus in flexible flatfoot deformity. *J Foot Surg* 1984;23:410–419.
49. Hoke M. An operation for the correction of extremely relaxed flatfeet. *J Bone Joint Surg* 1931;13:773.
50. Bordelon RL. Flatfoot in children and young adults. In: Mann RA, ed. *Surgery of the foot and ankle.* Vol. 2. St. Louis: Mosby, 1993.
51. Anderson AF, Fowler SB. Anterior calcaneal osteotomy for symptomatic juvenile pes planus. *Foot Ankle* 1984;4:274–283.
52. Porter DA, Baxter DE, Clanton TO, et al. Posterior tibial tendon tears in young competitive athletes: two case reports. *Foot Ankle Int* 1998;19:627–630.
53. Geist ES. The accessory scaphoid bone. *J Bone Joint Surg* 1925;7:570–574.
54. Harris RI, Beath T. *Army foot survey.* Vol. 1. Ottawa: National Research Council of Canada, 1947:52.
55. Grogan DP, Gasser SI, Ogden JA. The painful accessory navicular: a clinical and histopathological study. *Foot Ankle* 1989;10:164–169.
56. Kidner FC. The prehallux (accessory scaphoid) in its relation to flat foot. *J Bone Joint Surg* 1929;11:831–837.
57. Anatomical Society. Collective investigation: sesamoids in the gastrocnemius and peroneus longus. *J Anat Physiol* 1897;32:182.
58. Sarrafian SK. *Anatomy of the foot and ankle.* Philadelphia: J.B. Lippincott, 1983:87–88.
59. Sobel M, Pavlov H, Geppert MJ, et al. Painful os peroneum syndrome: a spectrum of conditions responsible for plantar lateral foot pain. *Foot Ankle* 1994;15:112–124.
60. Sammarco GJ, DiRaimondo CV. Chronic peroneus brevis tendon lesions. *Foot Ankle* 1989;9:163–170.
61. Sobel M, Levy ME, Bohne WHO. Longitudinal attrition of the peroneus brevis tendon in the fibular groove. *Foot Ankle* 1990;1:124–128.
62. Sobel M, Geppert MJ, Olson EJ, et al. The dynamics of peroneus brevis tendon splits: a proposed mechanism technique of diagnosis, and classification of injury. *Foot Ankle* 1992;13:413–422.
63. Clarke HD, Kiraoka HB, Ehman RL. Peroneal tendon injuries. *Foot Ankle* 1998;19:280–288.
64. Sobel M, Geppert MJ, Warren RF. Chronic ankle instability as a cause of peroneal tendon injury. *Clin Orthop* 1993;296:187–191.
65. Bonnin M, Tavernier T, Bouysset M. Split lesions of the peroneus brevis tendon in chronic ankle laxity. *Am J Sports Med* 1997;25:699–702.
66. Sobel M, Bohne WHO, Markisz JA. Cadaver correlation of peroneal tendon changes with magnetic resonance imaging. *Foot Ankle* 1991;11:384–388.
67. Peterson DA, Stinson W. Excision of the fractured os peroneum: a report on five patients and review of the literature. *Foot Ankle* 1992;13:277–281.

68. Sobel M, Mizel MS. Peroneal tendon injury. In: *Current practice in foot and ankle surgery.* Vol. 1. New York: McGraw-Hill, 1993.

69. Sobel M, Geppert MJ. Repair of concomitant lateral ankle ligament instability and peroneus brevis splits through a posteriorly modified Brostrom-Gould: technique tips. *Foot Ankle* 1992;13: 224–225.

70. Kopell HP, Thompson WAL. Peripheral entrapment neuropathies of the lower extremity. *N Engl J Med* 1960;262:56–60.

71. Marinacci AA. Neurological syndromes of the tarsal tunnels. *Bull L A Neurol Soc* 1968;33:90–100.

72. Lindenbaum BL. Ski boot compression syndrome. *Clin Orthop* 1979;140:19.

73. Schon LC, Baxter DE. Neuropathies of the foot and ankle in athletes. *Clin Sports Med* 1990;9:489–509.

74. Mann RA, Baxter DE. Diseases of the nerves. In: Mann RA, Coughlin MJ, eds. *Surgery of the foot and ankle,* 6th ed. St. Louis: Mosby, 1993:521–543.

75. Bowman MW. Compression neuropathies of the foot and ankle. In: *Current practice in foot and ankle surgery.* Vol. 2. New York: McGraw-Hill, 291–331.

76. Rask MR. Medial plantar neuropraxia (jogger's foot): report of three cases. *Clin Orthop* 1978;134:193.

77. Bhansali RM, Bhansali RR. Accessory abductor hallucis causing entrapment of the posterior tibial nerve. *J Bone Joint Surg Br* 1987;69B:479.

78. DeLee JC. Fractures and dislocations of the foot. In: Mann RA, ed. *Surgery of the foot and ankle.* Vol. 2. St. Louis: Mosby, 1993.

79. McCrory P, Bladin C. Fractures of the lateral process sof the talus: a clinical review. "Snowboarder's ankle." *Clin J Sport Med* 1996;6:124–128.

80. Shelton ML, Pedowitz WJ. Injuries to the talus and midfoot. In: Jahss MH, ed. *Disorders of the foot.* Vol. 2. Philadelphia: W.B. Saunders, 1982.

81. Mankey M. Fractures of the talus. *Foot Ankle* 1994;205–217.

82. Grant JCB. *A method of anatomy.* Baltimore: Williams & Wilkins, 1958.

83. McDougall A. The os trigonum. *J Bone Joint Surg Br* 1955;37: 257–265.

84. Bizarro AH. On sesamoid and supernumerary bones of the limbs. *J Anat* 1921;55:256–268.

85. Hamilton WG, Geppert MJ, Thompson FM. Pain in the posterior aspect of the ankle in dancers. *J Bone Joint Surg Am* 1996;78A: 1491–1500.

86. Marumoto JM, Ferkel RD. Arthroscopic excision of the os trigonum: a new technique with preliminary clinical results. *Foot Ankle* 1997;18:777–784.

87. Wray JB, Herndon CN. Hereditary transmission of congenital coalition of the calcaneus to the navicular. *J Bone Joint Surg Am* 1963;45A:365.

88. Stormont DM, Peterson HA. The relative incidence of tarsal coalition. *Clin Orthop* 1983;181:28.

89. Snyder RB, Lipscomb AB, Johnston RK. The relationship of tarsal coalitions to ankle sprains in athletes. *Am J Sports Med* 1981;9:313.

90. Elkus RA. Tarsal coalition in the young athlete. *Am J Sports Med* 1986;14:477.

91. Herzenberg JE, Goldner JL, Martinez S, et al. Computerized tomography of talocalcaneal tarsal coalition: a clinical and anatomic study. *Foot Ankle* 1986;6:273–288.

92. Mandell GA, et al. Detection of talocalcaneal coalitions by magnification bone scintigraphy. *J Nucl Med* 1990;31:1797.

93. Scranton PE Jr. Treatment of symptomatic talocalcaneal coalition. *J Bone Joint Surg Am* 1987;69A:533–539.

94. Gonzalez P, Kumar SJ. Calcaneonavicular coalition treated by resection and interposition of the extensor digitorum brevis muscle. *J Bone Joint Surg Am* 1990;72A:71–77.

95. Olney BW, Asher MA. Excision of symptomatic coalition of the middle facet of the talocalcaneal joint. *J Bone Joint Surg Am* 1987;69A:539–544.

96. Cowell HR. Tarsal coalition—review and update. *Instr Course Lect* 1982;31:264.

97. O'Neill DB, Micheli LJ. Tarsal coalition. A follow-up of adolescent athletes. *Am J Sports Med* 1989;17:544.

98. Dreeben S. Heel pain. *Orthopaedic knowledge update: foot and ankle.* Rosemont, IL: AAOS, 1994:179–182.

99. Tanz SS. Heel pain. *Clin Orthop* 1963;28:168–177.

100. Amis J, Jennings L, Graham D, et al. Painful heel syndrome: radiographic and treatment assessment. *Foot Ankle* 1988;9: 91–95.

101. Williams PL, Smibert JB, Cox R, et al. Imaging study the painful heel syndrome. *Foot Ankle* 1987;7:345–349.

102. Davis PF, Severud E, Baxter DE. Painful heel syndrome: results of nonoperative treatment. *Foot Ankle* 1994;15:531–535.

103. Wolgin M, Cook C, Graham C, Mauldin D. Conservative treatment of plantar heel pain: long-term follow-up. *Foot Ankle* 1994;15:97–102.

104. Graham CE. Painful heel syndrome: rationale of diagnosis and treatment. *Foot Ankle* 1983;3:261–267.

105. Martin RL, Irrgang JJ, Conti SF. Coutcome study of subjects with insertional plantar fasciitis. *Foot Ankle* 1998;19:803–811.

106. Lapidus PW, Guidotti FP. Painful heel: report of 323 patients with 364 painful heels. *Clin Orthop* 1965;39:178–186.

107. Wapner KL, Sharkey PF. The use of night splints for treatment of recalcitrant plantar fasciitis. *Foot Ankle* 1991;12:135–137.

108. Miller RA, Torres BA, McGuire M. Efficacy of first-time steroid injection for painful heel syndrome. *Foot Ankle* 1995;16:610–612.

109. Tisdel CL, Harper MC. Chronic plantar heel pain: treatment with a short leg walking cast. *Foot Ankle Int* 1996;17:41–42.

110. Snider MP, Clancy WG, McBeath AA. Plantar fascia release for chronic plantar fasciitis in runners. *Am J Sports Med* 1983;11: 215–219.

111. Leach RE, Seavey MS, Salter DK. Results of surgery in athletes with plantar fasciitis. *Foot Ankle* 1986;7:156–161.

112. Daly PJ, Kitaoka HB, Chao EYS. Plantar fasciotomy for intractable plantar fasciitis: clinical results and biomechanical evaluation. *Foot Ankle* 1992;13:188–195.

113. Anderson RB, Foster MD. Operative treatment of subcalcaneal pain. *Foot Ankle* 1989;9:317–323.

114. Page AE, O'Malley MJ, Cookl R. Endoscopic plantar fascia release: short-term clinical follow-up. The American Orthopaedic Foot and Ankle Society 14th Annual Summer Meeting, Boston, MA, July 24–26, 1998.

115. Shapiro SL. Endoscopic plantar fasciotomy for the treatment of intractable heel pain. The American Orthopaedic Foot and Ankle Society 14th Annual Summer Meeting, Boston, MA, July 24–26, 1998.

116. Laughlin R. Endoscopic plantar fascia release: an analysis of structures at risk. Paper presented at the annual meeting of the American Orthopaedic Foot and Ankle Society, Vail, CO, July 1995.

117. Gentile AT, Zizzo CJ, Dahukey A, et al. Traumatic pseudoaneurysm of the lateral plantar artery after endoscopic plantar fasciotomy. *Foot Ankle* 1997;18:821–822.

118. Leach R, Jones R, Silva T. Rupture of the plantar fascia in athletes. *J Bone Joint Surg Am* 1978;60A:537–539.

119. Kitaoka HB, Luo ZP, An KN. Mechanical behavior of the foot and ankle after plantar fascia release in the unstable foot. *Foot Ankle* 1997;18:8–15.

120. Thordarson DB, Kumar PJ, Hedman TP, et al. Effect of partial versus complete plantar fasciotomy on the windlass mechanism. *Foot Ankle* 1997;18:16–20.

121. Sharkey NA, Ferris L, Donahue SW. Biomechanical consequences of plantar fascial release or rupture during gait. Part 1. Disruptions in longitudinal arch conformation. *Foot Ankle* 1998;19:812–820.

122. Baxter DE, Pfeffer GB. Treatment of chronic heel pain by surgical release of the first branch of the lateral plantar nerve. *Clin Orthop* 1992;279:229–236.

123. Schon LC, Glennon TP, Baxter DE. Heel pain syndrome: electrodiagnostic support for nerve entrapment. *Foot Ankle* 1993;19:124–135.

124. Schon LC. Plantar fasciitis/heel pain. In: *Current practice in foot and ankle surgery.* Vol. 1. New York: McGraw-Hill, 254.

125. Jones DC. Posterior heel pain. In: *Current practice in foot and ankle surgery.* Vol. 2. New York: McGraw-Hill, 182.

126. Fowler A, Philip JF. Abnormality of the calcaneus as a cause of painful heel. *Br J Surg* 1945;32:494.

127. Pavlov H, Heneghan MA, Hersh A, et al. The Haglund syndrome: initial and differential diagnosis. *Diagn Radiol* 1982; 144:83–88.
128. Geppert MJ, Mizel MS. Management of heel pain in the inflammatory arthritides. *Clin Orthop* 1998;349:93–99.
129. Keck C. The tarsal tunnel syndrome. *J Bone Joint Surg* 1962; 44:180–182.
130. Lam SJS. Tarsal tunnel syndrome. *J Bone Joint Surg Br* 1967; 49:87–92.
131. Murphy PC, Baxter DE. Nerve entrapment of the foot and ankle in runners. *Clin Sports Med* 1985;4:753.
132. Baxter DE. *The foot and ankle in sport,* 1st ed. St. Louis, MO: Mosby, 1995.
133. Jackson DL, Haglund B. Tarsal tunnel syndrome in athletes: case reports and literature review. *Am Orthop Soc Sports Med* 1991;19:61–65.
134. Erickson SJ, Quinn SF, Kneeland JB, et al. MR imaging of the tarsal tunnel and related spaces: normal and abnormal findings with anatomic correlation. *AJR Am J Roentgenol* 1990;155: 323–328.
135. Frey C, Kerr R. Magnetic resonance imaging and the evaluation of tarsal tunnel syndrome. *Foot Ankle* 1993;14:159–164.
136. Zeiss J, Fenton P, Ebraheim N, et al. Magnetic resonance imaging for ineffectual tarsal tunnel surgical treatment. *Clin Orthop* 1991;264:264–266.
137. Schon LC, Baxter DE. Neuropathies of the foot and ankle in athletes. *Clin Sports Med* 1990;9:489–509.
138. Oh SJ, Savaria PK, Duba T, et al. Tarsal tunnel syndrome: electrophysiologic study. *Ann Neurol* 1979;5:327–330.
139. Johnson EW, Ortiz PR. Electrodiagnosis of tarsal tunnel syndrome. *Arch Phys Med Rehabil* 1966;47:776–780.
140. Kaplan JG. Modern electrodiagnostic studies. In: Jahss MH, ed. *Disorders of the foot and ankle: medical and surgical management,* 2nd ed. Philadelphia: W.B. Saunders, 1991:2026–2043.
141. Ballie DS, Keliklan AS. Tarsal tunnel syndrome: diagnosis, surgical technique, and functional outcome. *Foot Ankle Int* 1998;19: 65–71.
142. Goodgold J, Kopell HP, Spielholz NI. The tarsal tunnel syndrome: objective diagnostic criteria. *N Engl J Med* 1965;273: 742–745.
143. Johnson EW, Ortiz PR. Electrodiagnosis of tarsal tunnel syndrome. *Arch Phys Med Rehabil* 1966;47:776–780.
144. Kaplan PE, Kernahan WT. Tarsal tunnel syndrome: an electrodiagnostic and surgical correlation. *J Bone Joint Surg* 1981; 63:96–99.
145. Oh SJ, Arnold TW, Park KH, et al. Electrophysiological improvement following decompression surgery in tarsal tunnel syndrome. *Muscle Nerve* 1991;14:407–410.
146. Edwards WG, Lincoln R, Bassett FH, et al. The tarsal tunnel syndrome: diagnosis and treatment. *JAMA* 1969;207:716.
147. Linscheid RL, Burton RC, Fredericks EJ. Tarsal tunnel syndrome. *South Med J* 1970;63:1313–1323.
148. Baxter DE. *The foot and ankle in sport,* 1st ed. St. Louis, MO: Mosby, 1995.
149. Cimino WR. Tarsal tunnel syndrome: review of the literature. *Foot Ankle* 1990;11:47–52.
150. Radin EL. Tarsal tunnel syndrome. *Clin Orthop* 1983;161–167.

Principles and Practice of Orthopaedic Sports Medicine,
edited by William E. Garrett, Jr., Kevin P. Speer, and Donald T. Kirkendall.
Lippincott Williams & Wilkins, Philadelphia © 2000.

CHAPTER 51

Forefoot Injuries in the Athlete

James A. Nunley and Penny Lawlin

Injuries to the athlete's foot are not only common but can be devastating to an athletic career. Studies have cited anywhere from 55% to 90% of sporting injuries involve the hip, thigh, knee, leg, ankle, and foot (1). In a review of 16,754 athletic injuries, the foot accounted for 15.5% of all injuries (1) and overuse made up approximately 50% of all foot injuries. Studies looking at football players have found forefoot injuries to be the most commonly noted foot injury, ranking third behind injuries to the ankle and knee as the most common injury causing missed games and practices (2,3). Runners and dancers have a similar high propensity for disabling foot injury as well (4,5).

The athlete's foot is subjected to tremendous stresses. During walking, the magnitude of vertical force rarely exceeds 115% to 120% of body weight; however, during jogging and running, this force's magnitude increases to approximately 275% (5). Given the magnitude of these stresses during athletics and while performing activities of daily living, it is not surprising that foot injuries cause significant disability for the athlete.

In this chapter, the most frequently encountered injuries are reviewed. These include metatarsal fractures, both acute and stress; injury to the metatarsophalangeal (MTP) joint; sesamoid injuries; nerve dysfunction, hallux and lesser toe injuries; and common skin and nail conditions.

METATARSAL INJURIES

Metatarsal Stress Fractures

Stress fractures of all bones comprise as much as 10% of all sporting injuries (6). Stress fractures result from a characteristic response of bone, causing a complete

or partial fracture of the bone. Repeated subthreshold cyclical loading is the mechanism by which these injuries occur, thus their classification as overuse injuries.

On a cellular level, bone remodeling follows Wolff's law: any change in the stresses the bone encounters is followed by a change in its structure. With repeated rhythmic stressing, the resorptive phase of remodeling overwhelms the regenerative phase, and microfractures result. If the stress continues, these microfractures do not heal, instead propagating into fatigue or stress fractures. Healing only occurs when the regenerative phase is allowed to lay down enough new bone to support the stress it encounters.

The tibia is the most common site of stress fractures, followed by the metatarsals (6–9). Orava and Hulkko (7) divided these fractures further to show the third and second metatarsals to be the most common sites for stress fracture in the forefoot. Sullivan et al. (8) reviewed retrospectively their patient records of 51 runners and found a 16% incidence of stress fractures in the second and third metatarsal bones.

In transducer studies, bending strain and shear force were found to be highest under the second metatarsal head during running (10). Specifically, bending strain was estimated to be 6.9 times greater under the second metatarsal head compared with the first. This offers a biomechanical explanation for the higher incidence of stress fractures in the second metatarsal.

Several etiologic factors have been alluded to in the literature as predisposing to metatarsal stress fracture (11–23): congenital disorders of the first ray, a high longitudinal arch (cavus foot), female gender, excessive forefoot pronation, previous surgery to the first ray, footwear, and previous stress fracture.

Congenital disorders of the first ray include Morton foot and a short first metatarsal. A Morton foot combines a short first metatarsal and a longer second metatarsal with a hypermobile first ray. These anomalies in combination allow weight to shift from the first ray to the second or third metatarsal head, contributing to

J. A. Nunley: Department of Orthopaedic Surgery, Duke University Medical Center, Durham, North Carolina 27710.

P. Lawlin: Foot fellow, Duke University Medical Center, Durham, North Carolina 27710.

fatigue fractures. A short first metatarsal alone may also contribute, by again shifting weight to the second metatarsal, but Drez et al. (11) disputed this anomaly as an etiologic agent. When they reviewed radiographs of 65 patients with a metatarsal stress fracture and compared them with a control group, they found no difference between the first metatarsal length when the two groups were compared. This concurs with Harris and Beath (12), who showed no disability from a short metatarsal in their Canadian soldiers.

Weinfeld et al. (13) approached this issue and suggested that it is not the absolute metatarsal length that is the determining factor, but the function of the forefoot in the toe-off portion of the gait cycle. A short first metatarsal provides insufficient forefoot load sharing. When the hallux dorsiflexes in toe-off, the metatarsal head is depressed and the load beneath the first metatarsal increases regardless of its length. It is the hallux function that determines the load distribution in the forefoot. In hallux valgus, hallux rigidus, or after surgery on the first ray, the great toe has a diminished ability to bear weight and the adjacent metatarsals are subject to increased load, predisposing them to stress overload.

A low longitudinal arch, as in a flatfoot, has also been implicated in the etiology of metatarsal stress fractures (8,9,13–15). The cavus foot is more rigid and will not absorb much stress; instead, it transmits load to the tibia and femur. However, the flat foot absorbs much of the weight-bearing stress within the foot. Therefore, those with a lower longitudinal arch are predisposed to metatarsal fracture. Simpkin et al. (15) used an orthotic in their military recruits with low arches and found that their stress fracture rate was lower than those not wearing the orthotic.

Hyperpronation of the forefoot was suggested by Anderson (16) as a causative factor for stress fractures. He suggested that by pronating the forefoot, the load increases medially, especially to the distal first and second metatarsal heads. He thought that an element of hypermobility of the first ray was concurrently present, also shifting the load to the second metatarsal. This load shift was thought to cause an increase in stress fractures in this area.

Female gender as a risk factor is due to the osteopenia associated with secondary amenorrhea. Kadel et al. (17) reviewed their population of dancers and found 27 stress fractures in 17 dancers; 63% of these fractures occurred in the metatarsals. They found a relationship between these fractures and increased training time or menstrual irregularities. Specifically, their patients that danced more than 5 hours per day and had secondary amenorrhea of duration 6 months or more were at increased risk. They also added that those with loss of trabecular bone secondary to prolonged amenorrhea for greater than 6 months would not reverse the bone loss with estrogen replacement therapy alone. Another group found that the incidence of secondary amenorrhea was twice as common in dancers with stress fractures compared with uninjured dancers (18).

Previous corrective surgery to the first ray, which has been implicated in the etiology of metatarsal stress fracture, includes the Keller resection arthroplasty (19,20), Mayo excision arthroplasty (21), overcorrected McBride procedure (22), and fusion of the first MTP joint (16). The stress fractures were noted within a few months after surgery and were most likely due to an alteration of the relative lengths of the rays or to malalignment.

Frey (14) noted that an alteration of shoe wear can help to decrease the incidence of stress fracture. She suggested that the athletic shoes allow for better attenuation of the shock and better control of joint motion. Milgrom et al. (23) found in their military recruits that by changing their shoes from a standard military boot to a modified basketball shoe, they could significantly lower the incidence of metatarsal stress fractures.

Causes of stress fractures also include initiation of a new activity or a change in training. This change may be related to surface, distance, pace, or shoe wear, to list a few. These injuries are due to training error 60% to 75% of the time (6). In a series of 51 runners, these injuries occurred most often with training greater than 20 miles per week or on hard surfaces (8). Bilateral metatarsal stress fractures are more common in the novice runner who suddenly begins a training program (6).

McBryde (6) classified metatarsal stress injuries according to clinical and radiographic characteristics. Subclinical fractures do not exceed a threshold of recognizable pain and are generally an incidental finding on radiographs as cortical overgrowth. Subradiographic disease shows no radiographic findings but is symptomatic and is commonly diagnosed by a positive bone scan. Stress reaction of bone is an "ill-defined term describing bone pain related to remodeling" (6).

Clinically, the athlete with a stress fracture presents having insidious onset of pain in the forefoot. Upon questioning, the athlete may recount a recent change in training: more mileage, faster pace, more intense workouts, new shoes, or a new surface on which he or she is training. The pain is worse with activity; initially there is no effect on workouts, but progressively the pain worsens to the point where he or she cannot bear weight without noticing the pain. Generally, the pain has been present for a number of weeks before presentation to the physician.

On physical examination, there may be swelling along the dorsum of the foot. The site of the fracture is painful to palpation. It is important to differentiate pain from synovitis of the tarsometatarsal or MTP joints from metatarsal stress fracture pain. This is done through direct palpation along the shaft of the bone to elicit stress fracture pain and through passive range of motion

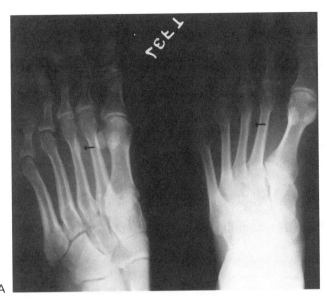 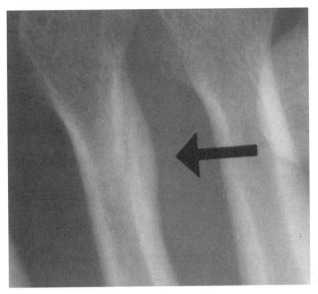

FIG. 51.1. Stress fracture of the metatarsal. **A:** Anteroposterior and oblique radiographs demonstrate periosteal new bone formation distally on the third metatarsal shaft (*arrows*). **B:** Endosteal thickening (*arrow*) may be seen on the enlarged view.

at the joint to elicit synovial irritation. Abnormalities in hindfoot alignment, rigidity of the foot, and forefoot alignment should also be noted.

Plain radiographs, including anteroposterior, lateral, and oblique views, reveal the fracture infrequently. When a fracture is identified, one may see periosteal new bone, endosteal thickening, or a radiolucent line (Fig. 51.1). If a radiolucent line is not seen, it is not unusual, because it does not become apparent until there is at least a 50% decrease in bone density (24). Other suggestive findings on plain radiographs include first metatarsal elevation above the plane of the second on lateral x-ray, indicating possible hypermobility of the first metatarsal. Additionally, slight hypertrophy of the second metatarsal medial cortex may be seen, insinuating chronic overload. If the fracture is not seen on initial radiographs, it may be seen on repeat radiographs taken after 3 weeks, when radiolucency at the fracture site due to fracture remodeling is present.

If clinical suspicion is high and no evidence of fracture is found on plain roentgenograms, bone scan should be obtained. Bone scans are more sensitive than plain radiographs for the detection of stress fractures but are less specific. The nuclear medicine studies may be positive within a few days of injury and may also show subclinical stress fractures elsewhere.

Stress fracture of the second metatarsal is most common (13,25,26), whereas the second, third, and fourth metatarsal stress fractures account for 90% of these injuries. First metatarsal stress fractures are rare. In nondancing athletes, the fractures occur in the diaphyseal portion of the bone; they occur proximally at the metadi-

aphyseal junction and may be associated with hyperpronation of the foot (16). Radiographic diagnosis is not always reliable, because one third of these fractures heal with intramedullary callus.

Activity modification with protected weight bearing in a wooden shoe for 4 to 8 weeks is the currently accepted treatment. A removable boot or walking short leg cast may be used for severe pain. Healing is assessed clinically by absence of pain on palpation and weight bearing and radiographically with appearance of callus. Surgery should be considered for delayed, nonunion, or malalignment. Surgery consists generally of open reduction with compression plating with or without bone graft.

Acute Metatarsal Fracture

Acute traumatic fractures of the metatarsals can occur in the distal shaft and neck. If a crushing mechanism was involved, compartment syndrome needs to be considered. In treating this fracture, it is helpful to know that transverse plane translation will not affect function unless painful synostosis with an adjacent metatarsal forms. However, plantar or dorsal angulation or shortening may be detrimental to the athlete because malalignment in these planes may cause a transfer of weight bearing to the other metatarsals or may interfere with comfort in shoe wear. Treatment of these injuries with satisfactory alignment is primarily supportive; however, as with all fractures, if alignment is poor, then open reduction and internal fixation may be needed.

METATARSOPHALANGEAL JOINT INJURIES

Metatarsophalangeal Joint Synovitis

Synovitis of the MTP joint is an often misdiagnosed condition. The athlete presents with a vague pain in the forefoot, which is exacerbated by walking, running, or any activity causing dorsiflexion of the MTP joint. The pain onset is insidious and gradually worsens with increasing activity. Synovitis of the MTP joint most commonly affects the second digit, with less frequent presentation involving the third digit or hallux. The cause is largely unknown, but some suggest forced dorsiflexion as a mechanism for injury (27). Synovitis of the MTP more commonly affects middle-aged athletes.

On examination, tenderness of the hallux MTP joint may be elicited by palpating the joint in the dorsoplantar plane. There is also pain with passive forced flexion of the digit. Swelling may be evident over the joint dorsally, and a spreading of the toes may be seen upon standing. Dorsal instability is assessed by performing an anterior drawer test (28) (Fig. 51.2). Deformities of the hallux should be noted, because hallux valgus may be seen in a significant number of patients with this malady in the second MTP joint (27).

Standing anteroposterior radiographs may reveal a widening of the joint space, the intermetatarsal space, degeneration of the joint, or spreading of the toes. Additionally, they allow assessment of hallux deformities. Any subluxation of the joint is important in determining treatment regimen. One may also rule out other abnormalities of the metatarsal head or proximal phalanx as a cause of similar presentation radiographically. These may include Freiberg's infraction, stress fracture of the metatarsal neck or head, or degenerative joint disease involving the MTP joint.

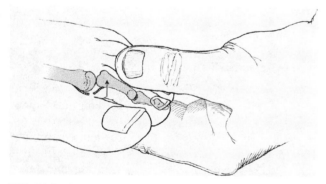

FIG. 51.2. Anterior drawer test. The metatarsal is stabilized with the examiner's nondominant hand while the dominant hand directs a dorsal force upon the toe to assess subluxability of the metatarsophalangeal (MTP) joint. Maintaining the index finger of the nondominant hand at the proximal border of the MTP allows the examiner to palpate directly the degree of joint motion. (Redrawn from Coughlin MJ. Second metatarsophalangeal joint instability in the athlete. *Foot Ankle* 1993;14(6):309–319, with permission.)

The natural history of long-standing synovitis of the MTP joint is eventual attrition of the capsule, plantar plate, and collateral ligaments. Chronic distention of the capsule, with the inflammatory response, are responsible for these changes (27–29). With loss of integrity of these stabilizing structures, joint subluxation and eventual dislocation may ensue. Dislocation will not occur until one or both of the collateral ligaments and the plantar plate are disrupted (30).

Initially, treatment of MTP synovitis is conservative, with activity modification to decrease the intensity of the workouts. Orthotics with shock-absorbing insoles may lessen the impact on the forefoot. Metatarsal pads placed just proximal to the involved joint's metatarsal head will decrease force on that joint. Taping to supinate the forefoot acts to decrease medial pressure. Active and passive exercises to strengthen the toe intrinsics and promote toe flexors and plantarflexion strengthening to help lift the metatarsal heads by flexing the toes against the weight-bearing surface of the floor will also decrease pressure on the MTP joint. Intraarticular injection of steroid is not suggested in the competitive, scholastic, or high-performance athlete, because the pain relief effected may cause the athlete to resume activities too quickly, which could further damage the capsule and ligaments. In recreational athletes, judicious use of intraarticular steroid, taking care to inject such that the needle does not injure the collateral ligaments, is effective. It should not be used before other modalities have been tried for a minimum of 6 weeks (27).

Surgical management is a consideration when conservative measures have failed. This includes open synovectomy, correction of deformity, and evaluation of the capsule, plantar plate, and collateral ligaments. Synovectomy should be complete. For mild hammertoe, MTP capsulotomy, extensor tenotomy, and arthrodesis of the PIP will give greater mechanical advantage to the long flexor tendon on the MTP joint by relieving the extensor as a deforming force and stabilizing the middle joint. For advanced hammertoe with dorsal dislocation of the MTP joint and medial angulation of the proximal phalanx, reduction of the joint with a Duvries plantar condylectomy of the metatarsal head can be performed. There is controversy as to whether to decompress the MTP joint by excising the proximal phalanx base or by excising part of the metatarsal head. Removing the proximal phalanx base is criticized because it removes a flexion force provided by the intrinsics on the MTP joint. However, with significant deformity, the intrinsics become a static deforming force, enhancing medial and/or dorsal angulation at the toe base. Removing the proximal phalanx base does not alter the weight-bearing capacity of the metatarsal head while removing the static deforming force. Excision of a portion of the plantar metatarsal head can reduce the joint but will alter the weight bearing of the remaining metatarsal.

Outcome of surgical treatment was evaluated for 42 patients followed a minimum of 6 months. Full relief was seen using the above guidelines for treatment with younger age, longer duration of symptoms, smaller hallux valgus angle, smaller angle of proximal phalanx elevation, greater medial or lateral angulation, greater relative length of the second metatarsal in relation to the first metatarsal, and fewer injections used in treatment (27).

Turf Toe

Artificial turf for playing surfaces first became popular in the late 1960s and early 1970s and was touted as a replacement for natural grass surfaces because it provided a more consistent surface—it maintained its firmness and an even grade. It also was found to allow water to drain through it. However, it has been found to become less compliant with age (3).

With the popularity of this playing surface came an increasing incidence of a condition now referred to as turf toe (31). The injury was not new, but the increased incidence corresponded with the increased popularity of synthetic turf. The term was coined in 1976 and refers to an injury to the hallux MTP joint resulting in pain and restriction of first MTP joint motion (32).

Anatomy

Important in the evaluation of this injury is an understanding of the first MTP joint anatomy (Fig. 51.3). The main stabilizing structures of this joint are capsuloligamentous. Minor stabilization is provided by the joint's bony interdigitation; the proximal phalanx has a shallow socket that articulates with the biconvex surface of the metatarsal head. Dynamic stabilizers include the surrounding musculotendinous structures: the short and long flexors and extensors, the abductor and adductor muscles, and the sesamoid complex that articulates with the metatarsal head plantarly.

The primary stabilizers of the first MTP joint are the capsule, collateral ligaments, and plantar plate. The collateral ligaments include both the MTP and metatarsosesamoid or suspensory ligaments. The MTP ligament takes origin from the lateral tubercle on the metatarsal head and fans out to insert on a wider area of the proximal phalanx base. The suspensory ligament originates on the lateral tubercle also but fans out more plantarly to insert on the sesamoids and plantar plate. The plantar plate is a thick fibrous structure that attaches firmly to the proximal phalanx base and loosely to the neck of the metatarsal via the capsule.

The architecture of the joint provides only minor stabilization. In the MTP, the instant centers of motion lie

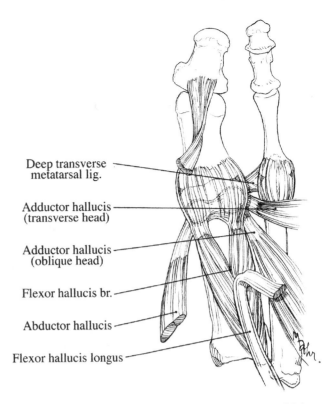

FIG. 51.3. Anatomy of the first metatarsophalangeal joint. The flexor hallucis longus tendon has been cut to visualize the relationship of the sesamoid complex. It lies between the sesamoids plantar to the intersesamoid ligament. [Redrawn from Rodeo SA, O'Brien S, Warren RF, et al. Turf-toe: an analysis of metatarsophalangeal joint sprains in professional football players. *Am J Sport Med* 1990;18:280–285, with permission (33).]

within the metatarsal head; motion occurs by a sliding action at the joint surface. This sliding action, when in full extension, changes to compression of the articular surfaces at the dorsal aspect of the metatarsal head and proximal phalanx. This effect provides for differential tension of the capsuloligamentous structures on changing toe position (14).

The dynamic stabilizers, including the short and long flexors and extensors, the abductor, and adductor, contribute to the stability by their incorporation within the capsuloligamentous complex. Medially, the abductor hallucis tendon inserts onto the medial sesamoid, continuing distally to insert onto the plantar and medial base of the proximal phalanx. Laterally, the adductor hallucis tendon inserts onto the fibular sesamoid and continues distally to insert onto the proximal phalanx base. The short flexors and extensors blend with the capsule at their insertions. The long flexor and extensors insert distally. Within the two heads of the flexor hallucis brevis tendon lay the medial and lateral sesamoids, which are connected to the plantar base of the proximal phalanx through the plantar plate.

Normal range of motion of the MTP joint is vital for continued function of the foot in gait. Range of motion is variable, but dorsiflexion usually is greater than plantarflexion. Passive plantarflexion may range from 3 to 43 degrees, whereas dorsiflexion ranges from 40 to 100 degrees (34). At least 60 degrees of dorsiflexion is necessary for barefoot walking on a level surface (35).

Etiology

One etiologic factor is related to the synthetic turf characteristics. Astroturf and grass were compared to determine parameters important in the performance of football maneuvers; stopping time, total impact duration, peak acceleration and deceleration, and average acceleration and deceleration were studied. When new, the artificial surface was comparative with grass; however, as the surface aged, the evaluation was repeated and was found to be worse in all parameters for the artificial turf that more closely resembled its asphalt base. The increased surface friction found in synthetic turf has been suggested to play a role in turf toe injuries (2). Firmness has also been implicated. However, the exact factor most responsible for this injury has yet to be elucidated (31–38).

Shoe wear used on these surfaces has changed from that used originally on grass and is also thought to contribute to the turf toe injury. The grass football shoe had seven cleats, which were attached to a metal sole plate; using these shoes on synthetic turf did not provide adequate traction, so athletes changed to a more flexible shoe that was multicleated, similar to a soccer shoe. This increase in shoe flexibility placed increased stress more directly onto the MTP joints, therefore opening a floodgate for injury.

Modifications to the turf shoe design have been suggested. Clanton et al. (2), while studying turf toe injury, evaluated shoe design; they compared football players who wore a flexible turf shoe with those using a modification providing a more stiff sole. Clanton et al. showed that the players wearing the stiff-soled shoe were less likely to sustain a turf toe injury.

Player position in football may also have an effect on the incidence of turf toe. Studies have suggested that positions such as offensive linemen, tight ends, and wide receivers have been found to have a higher incidence of turf toe (32,33). Rodeo et al. (33) found that 60% of offensive players had incurred this injury, whereas only 32% of defensive players exhibited evidence of turf toe; this, however, was not statistically significant but has been corroborated by another study (2). Thus, the etiologic agent still remains controversial.

Ankle and MTP joint range of motion has also brought debate. Authors have found that an increase in ankle dorsiflexion in the uninjured side of the injured athlete was higher when compared with the ankle mo-

tion of the unharmed athlete (33). Decreased MTP range of motion may also be related. Previous authors found no relation between MTP range of motion and turf toe injury. In their first evaluation of turf toe, Clanton et al. (2) cited restricted range of motion of the first MTP as a significant factor and advised protection of athletes having MTP extension of less than 60 degrees. Clanton and Ford (36) then followed this with an evaluation of players with which they followed these guidelines and found that the preseason range of motion carried no predictive value in determining who will sustain this injury.

Mechanism of Injury

The mechanism of injury has classically been thought to be hyperextension, although hyperflexion, valgus, and varus mechanisms have all been described (31–39). The mechanism may vary also by sport or position played.

Hyperextension is the most frequent mechanism cited. Typically, the foot is in dorsiflexion, with the forefoot fixed on the ground and the heel raised. Force is applied to the posterior aspect of the heel, driving the MTP joint into further dorsiflexion. An example is the football player involved in a pile up, laying prone on the field, with his foot outside the pile up. Another player will fall onto this foot, generating substantial force to dorsiflex forcefully the MTP joint and produce this injury (36). Given enough force, the joint capsule tears at its attachment to the metatarsal neck because this attachment is weaker than at the proximal phalanx. The dorsal articular surface of the metatarsal head simultaneously sustains a compression injury.

Hyperflexion has also been reported in the football population but is more often seen in professional beach volleyball players. In the latter, it has been termed "sand toe" (39). In this mechanism, the plantarflexed MTP is forced into an exaggerated position with resulting sprain of the dorsal capsule. The plantar portion of the metatarsal head is driven into the proximal phalanx. This can be seen in football when tackling a ball carrier from behind, when the knee is flexed, and another tackles the carrier from the front, forcing the body over the flexed knee and hyperplantarflexing the hallux (32). In volleyball, the injury is usually seen on landing after a running serve or spike (39).

Pure varus and valgus mechanisms are rare and are often associated with other injury mechanisms. A valgus mechanism may be seen in sudden acceleration, from the force of pushing off on the hallux. The varus mechanism has been reported in a basketball player (37) who externally rotated on a fixed forefoot. Surgical treatment was needed and allowed for examination of the pathology directly. The player was found to have avulsed both the transverse and oblique heads of the adductor hallucis muscle from their insertions distally.

Classification and Clinical Assessment

Classification of turf toe injury has been elucidated and is useful for the evaluation of these injuries. No studies have been completed to validate this system, but it allows a foundation in the assessment and treatment of these injuries. Radiographic examination is generally suggested to rule out capsular or ligamentous avulsions, to assess the sesamoid complex, or to evaluate for subluxation or frank dislocation of the MTP joint.

A grade 1 sprain incurs a stretch or minor tearing of the capsuloligamentous complex of the first MTP joint. Symptoms include localized plantar or medial tenderness, minimal swelling, and an absence of ecchymosis. There is minimal restriction in range of motion and weight bearing is possible. The athlete is able to participate with mild pain.

Grade 2 sprains show injury to the capsuloligamentous complex as a partial tear. Clinical presentation shows the tenderness to be more diffuse and intense. There is mild to moderate restriction on range of motion, and there is a mild limp on ambulation. The symptoms tend to worsen within the first day, and the athlete is unable to perform at a normal level.

In grade 3 sprains, there is a complete tear of the capsule, often with avulsion of the plantar plate from the metatarsal head/neck, and impaction of the proximal phalanx into the metatarsal head dorsally. There may be a concomitant fracture of a sesamoid or a separation of a bipartite sesamoid. Rarely, a tear of the sesamoid complex is distal to the sesamoids, resulting in a proximal migration of the complex. This may represent a dorsal dislocation of the MTP joint, which has spontaneously reduced. Clinically, there is severe pain and tenderness both plantarly and dorsally on the first MTP. Marked swelling and a large ecchymosis accompany severe restriction of the first MTP range of motion.

Treatment

Treatment for turf toe is largely conservative. Initial treatment will consist of rest, ice, compression if necessary, and elevation. Cryotherapy is continued for the first 48 hours. Thereafter, contrast whirlpool is recommended by some. This is followed by early joint mobilization. One regimen suggests removal of the initial compressive dressing at 3 days. At this evaluation, if swelling, tenderness, or significant pain persists, the dressing is reapplied. Taping has been used in the initial treatment. The purpose of the taping is to decrease swelling and to avoid extension of the MTP joint. Nonsteroidal anti-inflammatory medications may also be used; injection of cortisone and anesthetic agent is con-traindicated and can result in exacerbation of the original injury, leading to prolonged recovery.

The player is allowed to return to participation when near-normal or normal pain-free range of motion is achieved. The length of convalescence depends on the grade of injury. Typically, grade 1 injury requires only symptomatic treatment, with supportive taping or orthotics to decrease the shoe's flexibility through the forefoot. The player is allowed to continue participation as tolerated. In grade 2 injuries, a loss of playing time approximating 3 to 14 days is anticipated and return should include taping and a forefoot orthotic. Grade 3 injuries may require crutches for 2 to 3 days, and the loss of playing time ranges from 2 weeks to 6 months.

Operative treatment is rarely indicated; however, with chronic subluxation or repeated episodes of dislocation, soft tissue reconstruction may be necessary. Additionally, if painful symptoms continue despite appropriate conservative therapy, other additional injuries should be considered. These may include an intraarticular loose body, chondromalacia, or sesamoid pathology.

Outcome

Coker et al. (32) considered the turf toe injury more severe than frequent. They noted a significant number of patients treated conservatively with persistent pain with activities and decreased range of motion. They compared MTP joint injury to ankle sprains in their population of football players. During the 3 years of their evaluation, players sustained 74 ankle sprains and 18 toe injuries. They missed 152 practices for ankle sprains and 92 for toe injuries. Overall, they missed six games for ankle sprains and seven games for turf toe injury.

Clanton et al. (2) also followed patients to determine long-term disabilities. In 20 patients followed for a minimum of 5 years, they discovered a 50% incidence of persistent symptoms. They found an increased incidence of hallux valgus and early hallux rigidus in their population.

Others have also shown the injury to have a considerable morbidity (31–38). The injury is so disabling because large loads are necessarily transmitted to the forefoot in any standing, walking, or running activity (3). Push-off strength, necessary for sudden acceleration, is diminished. Additionally, the dorsiflexion necessary for push-off is often limited. The injury has become a source of considerable disability and playing time loss. Studies continue to look for new ways of decreasing morbidity and frequency of this injury.

First Metatarsophalangeal Dislocation

This injury lies on the continuum of first MTP joint injuries commonly referred to as turf toe. The mechanism of injury is hyperextension, and the dislocation is typically dorsal. Jahss (39) classified these dislocations according to the proposed anatomic structures disrupted (Fig. 51.4). Type I dislocation is one in which the sesamoid complex is not disrupted. Without this disruption, the dislocation may be irreducible by closed means. In these cases, the metatarsal head may be "button-holed" through the plantar capsule, with plantar plate interposed between the metatarsal head and base of the proximal phalanx. If medial subluxation is seen, the metatarsal head may be entrapped between the abductor hallucis and medial head of the flexor hallucis brevis. Similarly, if lateral subluxation is noted, the head may be caught between the lateral head of the flexor hallucis brevis and the adductor hallucis. Surgical management for this problem is controversial in that some prefer a dorsal and some prefer a plantar approach. Postoperatively, the patient is placed into a short leg walking cast, followed by a wooden shoe and vigorous physical therapy to restore motion.

Type II dislocations are divided into A and B subclassifications. IIA injuries have a disruption of the intersesamoid ligament without fracture of the sesamoid. The intersesamoid distance in increased on roentgenograms. IIB injuries have a concomitant fracture of the sesamoid. Both usually reduce by closed means. The

reduction maneuver includes longitudinal traction and manipulation to the reduced position by plantar-directed force on the proximal phalanx base. After reduction, the patient is placed in a short leg walking cast for 3 to 6 weeks.

Instability of Second Metatarsophalangeal Joint

This condition has been known for a long time. It was first noticed in those with hallux valgus, where continued pressure from the malaligned great toe over time destabilizes the second toe. This eventually caused subluxation or dislocation of the second toe (40). Others have studied this condition as a sequel to long-standing synovitis of the second MTP joint (28). In athletes, it may be seen with either of the above two situations or as the result of an acute injury.

The onset of pain is insidious and either isolated to the plantar second MTP or may be neuritic and radiatory in nature. Neuritic pain is generally caused from traction of the interdigital nerve lying beneath the transverse metatarsal ligament. On examination, the anterior drawer sign is positive for subluxation or dislocation of the joint. There may be dorsal, medial, or dorsomedial deviation of the second toe. Radiographic examination may show a long second metatarsal, with the average excess length of 9 mm. The joint also needs to be examined for congruency. Typically, patients with this disorder will have medial deviation of the second metatarsal head on the average of 2.8 degrees compared with the third metatarsal, which may average 8 degrees of lateral deviation (41,42).

Nonsurgical treatment should be attempted for those without deformity and with slight pain. For these patients, taping and or activity modification will relieve the symptoms. Surgical treatment should be reserved for those with deformity and pain not responding to conservative measures. Surgical management encompasses a dorsomedial capsular release, extensor tendon lengthening, lateral capsular reefing, and flexor digitorum longus transfer dorsally. If the problem is associated with a long second metatarsal, some advocate a shortening osteotomy of the second metatarsal concurrently.

Hallux Valgus

Hallux valgus is a deformity heavily studied in the general population. The deformity includes an abducted and pronated large toe, with callosities present on the medial aspect of the MTP joint. In addition, a "pinch callus" may be found at the level of the interphalangeal joint from pressure of this joint within the shoe. In athletes and the general population, shoe wear modification is the first line of therapy. However, in a persistently painful bunion or with decompensation of the

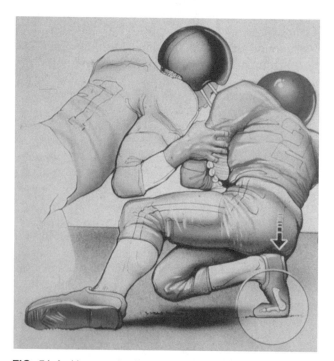

FIG. 51.4. Hyperextension as a mechanism of injury in turf toe. The foot is planted with the toes dorsiflexed. The tackle forces the foot into the ground, providing a hyperdorsiflexion injury to the hallux. [From Rodeo SA, O'Brien S, Warren RF, et al. Turf-toe: an analysis of metatarsophalangeal joint sprains in professional football players. *Am J Sport Med* 1990;18:280–285, with permission (33).]

deformity, surgery must be considered. Athletes present a special case for operative therapy due to the demands placed on this joint.

Some believe that in the athletic population, surgical correction of the deformity should be undertaken only with the understanding that future performance may not return to its preoperative level. In dancers, the deformity is exclusively treated nonoperatively with small modifications in the shoes (4). If they desire to have surgical intervention, the resultant stiffness is generally career ending. In sprinting, normal push-off strength is required to continue performing at an elite level; this strength is generally lost with surgical intervention for a bunion.

The natural history of a bunion deformity is that the joint may remain congruent, the pain tolerable with shoe modifications and conservative therapy. Alternatively, the joint may decompensate. If it decompensates, the deformity progresses relatively quickly; the pain increases, the joint becomes incongruous, and the first metatarsal no longer covers the lateral sesamoid. This progression often affects athletic performance. It is at this point that surgical intervention should be considered.

In mid and long distance runners, success has been reported with surgical correction in a small group of patients (43,44). In these athletes, a Chevron osteotomy was performed with minimal joint dissection, taking care to avoid any malalignment in the dorsoplantar plane. Both athletes returned to their preoperative performance level. Recommended also are the Chevron-Akin for a more severe deformity or a proximal metatarsal osteotomy for an increased intermetatarsal angle, with an uncovered lateral sesamoid. Important after any surgical intervention is an aggressive postoperative rehabilitation program for regaining range of motion at the MTP joint and push-off strength.

In general, arthroplasty procedures should be avoided in the athlete, because the implants do not hold up well against the rigors of the large forces generated at this joint. Other procedures to avoid include MTP fusion, the Lapidus procedure, and Keller arthroplasties. Both the fusion and the Lapidus procedure will provide a decreased range of motion of the MTP joint and therefore will decrease push-off strength. The Keller procedure eliminates the short flexor tendon, thus altering the mechanics of the joint and resulting in a decreased push-off as well.

In summary, hallux valgus deformities in the athlete provide a special problem in that high demands are placed on this joint. Range of motion of the joint and push-off strength are necessary for most sprinting sports. Although some believe that operating on a bunion deformity will certainly be career ending for most, some athletes in a given situation are candidates for corrective surgery.

Metatarsus Primus Varus

This is an underlying congenital defect, is familial in nature, and leads to secondary hallux valgus. It may present early in childhood. The deformity steadily increases. The natural history of this cause of hallux valgus is different from that described above in that its course is progressive. However, depending on the degree of deformity and the rapidity with which it is progressing, it may or may not be symptomatic. When hallux valgus develops later in life for a dancer, with or without metatarsus primus varus, no surgery should be undertaken until retirement.

Because of the young age at presentation, most athletes with symptomatic bunion from metatarsus primus varus are just starting their athletic career. Considerations for treatment include skeletal maturity of the patient and progression of the deformity. If the deformity has steadily progressed to a significant level or has been symptomatic, surgery should be offered; however, the operation is best timed if completed after skeletal maturity. Howse (45) recommended a Hohmann type of osteotomy, where the first metatarsal is osteotomized just proximal to the neck and the distal head and neck are moved laterally. A peg of bone fashioned on the lateral shaft impales the head and neck. This allows for correction of the valgus deformity while maintaining stability at the osteotomy site.

Metatarsalgia

Metatarsalgia is defined as pain located beneath the metatarsal heads on the plantar aspect of the foot. It is vague term and as such has a number of etiologies, including Freiberg's infraction and static deformities of the ankle. Ankle pathology is related to limitation of ankle dorsiflexion, most commonly from a contracted Achilles tendon or anterior ankle impingement; this equinus posture causes increased pressure on the metatarsals during stance leading to metatarsalgia.

Foot deformities predictably produce metatarsalgia in a given anatomic pattern. Cavus deformities will typically cause metatarsalgia under the first and fifth metatarsal heads. Pressure relief for these metatarsals is achieved by metatarsal padding placed just proximal to the prominent head. Flatfoot deformity will increase pressure on the middle metatarsal heads, which can be relieved by metatarsal pads, or an orthotic to provide arch support and pressure relief under the given metatarsal heads.

Freiberg's infraction is thought to be due to avascular necrosis of the metatarsal head. Young et al. (46) offered shearing of the articular cartilage as the primary process involved in this disease. It most commonly affects the second followed by the third metatarsal heads. Treatment early is protected weight bearing. Later in the course, flattening of the head occurs, and surgical debridement may be necessary. In treating the performance athlete with this disorder, one must avoid the imminent transfer metatarsalgia associated with excision of the metatarsal head or silastic replacement arthroplasty. The athlete should be counseled of the possibility that he or she may not return to the level of performance once achieved after treating this disorder.

INJURIES TO THE SESAMOIDS

Galen, in 180 AD, gave sesamoids their name, thinking that they resembled sesame seeds. They have been the source of frustration for many athletes suffering pain under their first metatarsal heads, where the differential diagnosis comprises a long list of disorders. Injuries to the sesamoid have accounted for 12% of all great toe injuries and 1.2% of all running injuries (44).

Anatomy and Function

Sesamoids may form from two or more centers of ossification. They usually ossify by age 11. Fusion failure of these ossification centers results in partite sesamoids. The tibial or medial sesamoid may be bipartite 10% to 19% of the time (47–49). Fibular or lateral sesamoids are rarely bipartite. In approximately 25% of those with a bipartite sesamoid, bilateral involvement is encountered. Congenital absence is rare. In further analyzing bipartite sesamoids, they were found to have asymmetric divisions 85% of the time.

The sesamoids are shaped convex plantarly and concave dorsally, the surface with which they articulated with the convex matatarsal condyles. They are suspended by the apparatus consisting of the MTP collateral ligaments and the sesamoid ligaments. They lie within the medial and lateral heads of the flexor hallucis brevis tendon. In normal stance, they lie just proximal to the first metatarsal head. In toe-off, with the first MTP joint in dorsiflexion, they move distally to lie just beneath the first metatarsal head. The adductor hallucis through its insertion onto the lateral sesamoid and proximal phalanx distally acts as a lateral stabilizer. The abductor hallucis acts similarly for medial stabilization.

Function of the MTP joint is dependent on the sesamoid complex. They increase the moment arm by which the flexor hallucis brevis acts upon the hallux, therefore providing a mechanical advantage in much the same fashion that the patella affects the extensor apparatus at the knee. Their incorporation into the plantar plate provides a static plantarflexion force at the MTP joint, also adding to the mechanical advantage afforded the flexor hallucis brevis. They act as shock absorbers to disperse forces acting on the head of the first metatarsal.

By means of their location and the position of the flexor hallucis longus tendon between them, they offer protection for that tendon as well (50).

Clinical Presentation

Sesamoid injury frequently presents as an insidious onset of plantar pain. The patient recounts having a several week history of pain, which may be poorly localized. The athlete's activities include more frequently running, racquet sports, basketball, volleyball, football, or soccer, among others. On examination, pain to palpation directly beneath the sesamoid and pain with passive extension of the hallux MTP is elicited. Active flexion of the MTP joint is weak. Hallux alignment may be affected by processes affecting the sesamoids and should be sought on examination. Swelling may be seen only in more advanced cases or with bursal inflammation. Erythema is uncommon in the absence of bursitis.

Radiographic evaluation should include standard anteroposterior and lateral examinations. Oblique examinations may allow visualization of each sesamoid. An additional view may be the tibial sesamoid view, which involves positioning the foot and ankle for a lateral radiograph, with the MTP joints extended 50 to 60 degrees and the beam angled 15 degrees cephalad, centered on the medial eminence of the first metatarsal. The axial sesamoid view, positions the patient prone, with the hallux resting on the cassette, which lay flat on the table. The hallux is dorsiflexed maximally and the beam is shot in the plane of the metatarsosesamoid joint.

Radiographic findings may include a diastasis of a partite sesamoid, an acute fracture, or changes in the bony architecture of the sesamoids (Fig. 51.5). In addition, increased intersesamoid distance may be seen. Using the axial view, the metatarsosesamoid joint can be evaluated for degeneration. Mottling or fragmentation of the sesamoid is found in osteochondral lesions and osteomyelitis of the sesamoid. If clinical suspicion is high but plain x-rays are negative, bone scan should be obtained, because stress fractures are often not visualized on plain radiographs.

Mechanism of Injury

Acute injury to the sesamoid complex is due to a hyperextension or combined hyperextension–abduction force to the hallux. Fracture has been produced experimentally by forced hyperextension and abduction of the great toe (51–59).

Pain may be caused by a number of processes involving the hallucal sesamoids: acute fracture, stress fracture, sesamoiditis, osteochondritis, osteomyelitis, bursitis, or a symptomatic separation of a partite sesamoid. With the exception of an acute fracture and osteomyeli-

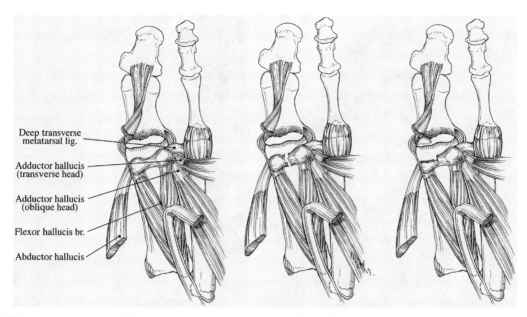

FIG. 51.5. Jahss classification for metatarsophalangeal joint dislocation. Type I dislocation dorsally without disruption of sesamoid complex. Type IIA dislocation dorsally with disruption of the intersesamoid ligament without sesamoid fracture. Type IIB dislocation dorsally with sesamoid fracture. [Redrawn from Jahss MH. Traumatic dislocations of the first metatarsophalangeal joint. *Foot Ankle* 1980;1:15–21, with permission (39).]

The labels on the figure read:
Deep transverse metatarsal lig.
Adductor hallucis (transverse head)
Adductor hallucis (oblique head)
Flexor hallucis br.
Abductor hallucis

tis, the remaining processes involve overuse injury. Because of their location and the first ray's relative weight bearing, the sesamoids are subject to large loads repeatedly. In his review of 26 sesamoid disorder patients, Scranton (54) found 14 cases involving long distance runners. In his patients, 8 had stress fractures, 3 had fractured through a partite sesamoid, 3 were found to have acute chondromalacia, 2 had an acute fracture, and 10 had anomalous sesamoids. He found that no matter what the cause of sesamoid injury, early motion was important. Limitation of dorsiflexion may result from adhesions forming in the retrocondylar space that tether the proximal phalanx.

Acute fracture has been described with dislocation of the first MTP joint. Additionally, direct trauma from landing after a fall may cause acute fracture. These are seen on radiographs and are initially treated conservatively with a weight-bearing cast with heel weight bearing for 6 weeks, after which the patient uses a metatarsal pad behind his or her first metatarsal head until approximately 3 months. If the fracture is displaced, some recommend excision of the fragment acutely (52), whereas others wait until an established nonunion is present, after which the symptomatic fragment is excised remotely (56). This aspect of treatment is the subject of debate presently.

Acute diastasis of a partite sesamoid misdiagnosed as turf toe was noted in four football players (58). In these athletes sustaining a hyperextension injury, they sustained a separation of their partite fragments with

symptoms of a fracture. The displacement occurred by proximal migration of the proximal fragment. The diagnosis was made by stress radiographs obtained with passive dorsiflexion of the toe, which showed the diastasis. The athletes were treated conservatively with protected weight bearing and dorsiflexion avoidance for 6 to 8 weeks. After nonunion occurred, the sesamoid was removed. They performed pathologic examination of the excised fragments and found granulation tissue without evidence of healing bone. They suggested early repair for those patients where activity requires rapid acceleration and deceleration.

Sesamoiditis, chondromalacia, and stress fractures of the sesamoid lie on a continuum of painful disorders affecting these bones. They are all caused to some extent by repeated loading cyclically to the sesamoids. Therefore, it is not difficult to understand the similarities in their diagnosis and treatment. Sesamoiditis is a diagnosis of exclusion in that the only positive findings are on physical examination, and stress fracture, chondromalacia, and osteochondritis need to be ruled out to use this diagnosis. Chondromalacia may be apparent on radiographic examination using the axial view to examine the metatarsosesamoid joint. However, often plain films are nondiagnostic, and bone scan may be obtained, which will show involvement of both the metatarsal head and sesamoid at their articulation (Fig. 51.6). Stress fractures may also be seen best on bone scan, because plain x-rays often are negative. The fracture will involve the sesamoid only in this case.

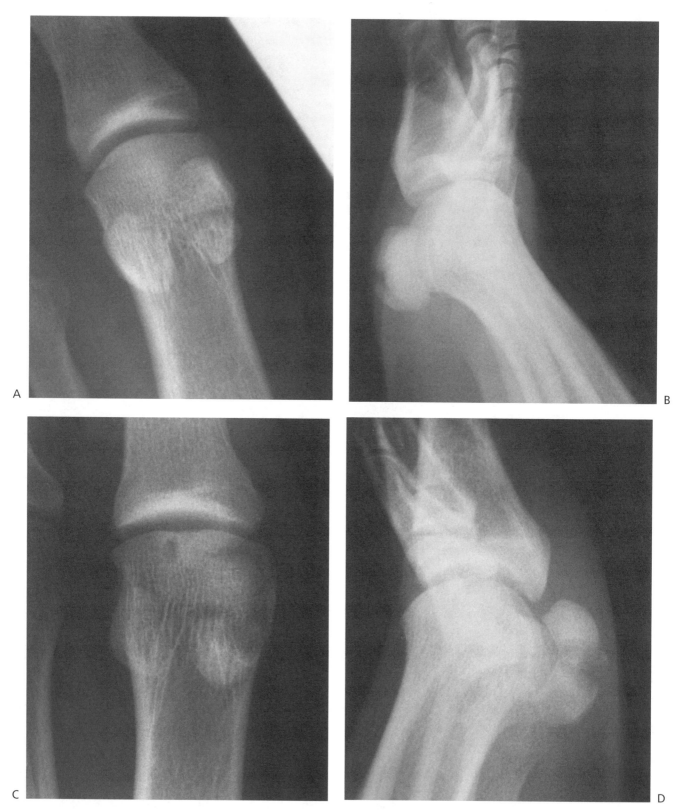

FIG. 51.6. Comparison of radiographic appearance of bipartite sesamoid (**A, B**), with sesamoid fracture (**C, D**). **A and B:** Bipartite medial sesamoid. Note the rounded smooth edges and mild asymmetry in fragment size and shape. The patient had no pain to palpation beneath the sesamoids. **C and D:** Sesamoid fracture. Note the irregular edges and almost symmetric split of the sesamoid. The patient presented with pain plantarly under the sesamoid, was tender to palpation, and had mild edema.

Treatment

Treatment of these disorders is through conservative management, with activity modification, molded shoe inserts, Morton's bar, nonsteroidal anti-inflammatory medications, and passive range of motion exercises (52,53,55). If this conservative therapy fails after a trial of 6 months (56), surgical management may be necessary.

Surgical treatment of sesamoid disorders is indicated infrequently. If sesamoiditis or stress fracture is related to a plantarflexed first metatarsal, dorsal closing wedge osteotomy may relieve pressure sufficiently to alleviate symptoms. Care must be taken to avoid overcorrection to avoid transfer metatarsalgia. If surgery is contemplated, one must remember that only those symptomatic portions of the sesamoid need be removed. The retention of a partial sesamoid will help maintain flexor tension and avoid establishing a cock-up, varus, or valgus hallux deformity. By the same token, once the sesamoid is removed, proper restoration of the flexor tension and plantar plate is vital to maintaining proper soft tissue balance surrounding this joint, therefore avoiding acquiring a hallux deformity. In general, excision of both sesamoids should not be taken lightly. If this is done, restoring soft tissue balance is not difficult, but weight bearing will no longer be cushioned, instead being transferred directly to the metatarsal head.

Removal of the sesamoid fragment may be undertaken for several reasons. For some, displaced fractures are an indication for removal. Those who advocate this indicate poor experience with healing of displaced fractures treated nonoperatively. Those who prefer conservative therapy may excise a continually symptomatic nonunion if this occurs. In sesamoiditis or osteochondritis resistant to conservative therapy for 6 months or longer, the general consensus is that the symptoms warrant excision. Additional indications for excision of a sesamoid include recurrent protracted sesamoid bursitis and osteomyelitis.

Postoperatively, the patient is placed in a well-padded splint. After 5 to 7 days, the splint is removed and a small dressing over the hallux and forefoot is put into place, and MTP active range of motion is begun. Manual passive range of motion and strengthening are started at 10 to 14 days postoperatively. Sports requiring rapid acceleration and deceleration may begin after 6 weeks.

Outcome

Migration of the hallux after resection of a sesamoid is a concern in operating on these disorders. This was first noticed after the original McBride procedure, which included excision of the fibular sesamoid. The toes drifted into varus 8% of the time in one study (56). After tibial sesamoidectomy, a 6.2-degree valgus drift

and a 2.2-degree increase in intermetatarsal angle was found (57). In an evaluation of 21 patients undergoing sesamoidectomy, varus or valgus drift was noticed in 10% of patients. The authors stressed the need to restore the tension on disrupted tissues after excision. The also found only 50% of the patients had complete relief of pain and were able to resume normal activities after sesamoidectomy (56).

Common in the literature reviewing operative treatment by sesamoidectomy is resultant disabilities. These included weakened plantarflexion of the hallux, necessary for forceful push-off. Restriction of MTP range of motion was also noted. A claw toe deformity was found in a few patients after this surgery, but some believe this result is technique dependent.

NERVE DISORDERS

Nerve disorders in the foot most commonly involve the deep and superficial peroneal and tibial nerves. Sites of compression or irritation differ by sporting activity, inherent deformities of the lower extremity, anomalous anatomy, and shoe wear. It is important in evaluating these disorders to rule out systemic problems or pathology in the more proximal peripheral or central nervous system before making the following diagnoses. The following discussion involves three of the most commonly seen nerve compression syndromes presenting with forefoot pain: interdigital neuroma, entrapment of the medial hallucal nerve, and anterior tarsal tunnel syndrome.

Interdigital Neuroma

Morton described this syndrome in 1876 when he recommended excision of the fourth metatarsal head as the treatment. We now know that this is not the best treatment option. It is a syndrome thought to be caused by perineural fibrosis surrounding the digital nerve at the level of the intermetatarsal ligament (60–67). Anatomically, the nerve is positioned just plantar to the intermetatarsal ligament.

The most frequently found cause is the common digital nerve becoming irritated by its adjacent ligament. However, trauma and space-occupying lesions may also cause the symptomatology complex. Trauma most often is from a fall or crush injury. Space-occupying lesions may consist of ganglion cysts, lipomas, synovitis of an adjacent joint, or bursitis to list a few. If a space-occupying lesion exists, malignancy should be ruled out.

The patient presents with neuritic pain radiating into the affected web space and toes, which may radiate proximally as well. It is most commonly seen in the third web space, followed by the second. Palpation between the metatarsal heads and compression mediolaterally on the foot at the level of the metatarsals will often recreate the pain. Decreased sensation in the web space and affected toes may be present. Increased activity or shoe wear compressing the metatarsal heads, such as women's high heels, will exacerbate the pain.

It is unusual, but not impossible, for more than one web space to be affected. The patient presenting with symptoms of the first or fourth web space affected should alert the examiner to rule out alternative processes involved. A diagnostic injection may be helpful in this situation. Injection of anesthetic with or without steroid will prove the diagnosis if pain is alleviated. Some caution against injection of steroid with an anesthetic for this condition in athletes (60–61). Those opposed to its use suggest that steroid causes fat pad atrophy with volar plate and collateral ligament degeneration. Others believe that injection of steroid and anesthetic may effect a cure approximately 50% of the time (29).

Treatment consists of starting with a wider shoe for the athlete to wear. Additionally, metatarsal pads and/or an arch support may also help to reduce pressure to the lateral metatarsal heads by preventing overpronation. When conservative measures fail, surgical excision of the nerve is the next line of therapy.

Controversial in surgical excision is whether a plantar or dorsal approach will be used and the importance of preservation of the intermetatarsal ligament (29,60–67). The choice of using a plantar incision is usually made for ease in identifying the nerve to resect, because it is located plantar to the intermetatarsal ligament. The downside of using plantar incisions is that they may form painful scars on which the patient walks. Dorsal incisions do not have the same problem, but dissection and visualization can be difficult. In the dorsal approach, some incise the intermetatarsal ligament, whereas others favor preserving the ligament. The attempt at preserving the ligament is thought to prevent instability of the MTP joint and allow a faster recovery. Three centimeters of nerve is suggested by one as the typical length of the resected nerve (29). Others recommend resecting to a level proximal to the metatarsal head and proceeding distally, taking care to lyse any and all communicating branches of the adjacent digital nerves (65). The proximal stump of the nerve should be stretched and cut, allowing it to retract into the forefoot fat pad proximal to the metatarsal heads.

With identification through injection of a single involved web space, 90% success with the above guidelines has been reported (29). However, the success in other studies report a 12 to 14% failure rate (67,68). After complete resection of the nerve, 32% of patients preserved their sensation in the operated web space (67). Additionally, of those not recorded as failures, 65% still complained of discomfort plantarly of a different character from their preoperative status. Overall, the results of both conservative and operative management

of this disorder are satisfactory in alleviating the symptomatology in most patients.

Medial Hallucal Nerve

The medial hallucal is a distal branch of the tibial nerve. The tibial nerve divides from 0 to 2 cm proximal to a line connecting medial malleolus to the calcaneal tuberosity. One to 2 cm distally, the lateral and medial plantar nerves enter the abductor hallucis through two separate fibroosseous tunnels. These tunnels are approximately 2 cm long. The medial hallucal branch takes off within or distal to its canal. Upon exiting the canal, it courses plantarly to provide sensation to the medial aspect of the large toe.

The nerve may become trapped within the canal, with hypertrophy of the abductor hallucis muscle, at its exit to the canal or as it courses medially by a prominent tibial sesamoid. It presents as pain under the medial aspect of the first MTP joint medially and is often mistaken for tibial sesamoiditis. It may be differentiated from this disorder by palpation of the nerve along its course.

Treatment is primarily conservative, with metatarsal pads behind sesamoids, nonsteroidal anti-inflammatory medications, and rest. If the pain persists, release at the nerve's egress from the abductor hallucis may be necessary. Additionally, if a hallux valgus deformity causing a prominent medial sesamoid and therefore a compression of the medial hallucal nerve at this level is present, surgical correction of this deformity may alleviate the compression.

Anterior Tarsal Tunnel Syndrome

The deep peroneal nerve may become entrapped, causing pain and/or numbness in the first web space. This branch of the common peroneal nerve travels between the extensor digitorum longus and extensor hallucis longus at the level approximately 3 to 5 cm proximal to the ankle. One centimeter proximal to the ankle, the nerve divides, giving off a lateral branch, which innervates the extensor digitorum brevis muscle. This division occurs beneath the oblique superior medial band of the inferior extensor retinaculum. A medial branch continues beside the dorsalis pedis artery underneath the oblique inferior medial band of the inferior extensor retinaculum. The nerve is generally compressed between the extensor retinaculum and ridges of the talonavicular joint. The nerve then continues distally between the extensor hallucis brevis and extensor hallucis longus tendons, providing sensation to the first web and adjacent borders of the first and second digits.

The compression may be caused by any space-occupying lesion on the dorsum of the foot in this area (e.g., talonavicular osteophyte, ganglion, lipoma, etc.).

Additionally, tying lace-up shoes too tightly may cause the compression.

Treatment includes anti-inflammatory medications, loosening up the lace-up shoes, or wearing shoes that will accommodate a more prominent dorsal arch. Surgical management includes decompression of the tunnel or removal of the space-occupying lesion.

FOREFOOT INJURIES IN DANCERS

Disorders of the forefoot in dancers present a constant challenge to the sport medicine physician. The patient performs specialized maneuvers, requiring positioning of their feet in unusual positions. These positions are held for extended periods of time over years of training. The combination of unusual positions for extended exposure periods cause a predicted set of conditions affecting their feet. This section is designed to review systematically some of the more commonly seen disorders seen in this specialized patient population.

Chronic Use Conditions

Bony Hypertrophy

Training to be a professional dancer begins well before skeletal maturity. Because of the redistribution of weight bearing experienced with altered foot positions, chronic changes occur in the forefoot. Wolff's law dictates that bone responds to altered stress patterns by remodeling accordingly. The dancer's metatarsal shafts are evidence of this process. Most commonly, the second metatarsal and lateral first metatarsal hypertrophy due to the transfer of load and increased stiffness of the second tarsometatarsal joint. This process is also seen more laterally in the third metatarsal. These hypertrophic changes are a normal response and should not be confused with stress fracture.

Stress Fracture

Metatarsal stress fractures are common injuries in the dancer. In this population, the metatarsal is the most frequent site of stress fracture. In contrast to running athletes, who sustain fractures distally in the metatarsal shafts, dancers tend to fracture proximally at the second metatarsal base (25,26,68). The fracture is located at the metadiaphyseal junction but may extend into the metatarsocuneiform joint. The fracture pattern is proximal lateral to distal medial.

Ballet dancers are susceptible to this type of fracture by dancing en pointe; the second metatarsal base is predisposed to fracture by its position while dancing en pointe, as well as its inherent stability. In the en pointe position, the metatarsals are hyperplantarflexed, with axial loads exceeding body weight repetitively applied primarily through the second ray. The second metatarsal base is locked into its position between the medial and lateral cuneiforms in a keystone configuration, providing a rigidly stable joint. Fractures occur in the metatarsals, carrying most of the load with the least mobility, the second followed by the third.

In their review of 54 female dancers, Kadel et al. (17) examined menstrual abnormalities, increased training time, and location of the stress fractures. They found 27 fractures in 17 dancers. In those who sustained fractures, a longer duration of amenorrhea could be found. They noted a loss of trabecular bone in those having amenorrhea of more than 6 months' duration. Estrogen replacement was not effective in decreasing the incidence of stress fractures in these dancers. Those dancers training more than 5 hours per day were more likely to sustain stress fracture. Stress fractures were found in the metatarsals 63% of the time, the tibia in 22%, and the spine 7%. This review provided a profile of at-risk athletes, which has been confirmed by subsequent studies (26,69).

Dancers present after insidious onset of forefoot pain exacerbated by dancing en pointe, performing a releve' maneuver, or after leaps. The average time from pain onset to presentation ranges from 2.5 to 5 weeks (26,69). It has only been seen in female dancers, because males dance in the demi pointe position.

Upon examination, the patient will have pain to palpation over the affected area. There may be swelling dorsally, with erythema. Stressing Lisfranc's joint may exacerbate the pain.

Routine radiographs are often insufficient for fracture visualization. In one series, plain radiographs were positive in only 37% of the patients. Oblique projections are helpful; however, the location at the base of the second metatarsal is difficult to assess because of bony overlap. To eliminate overlap at the second metatarsal base joints, O'Malley et al. (26) suggested obtaining a "dancer's view." This radiograph is obtained by positioning the patient's foot such that the dorsum is on the cassette, with the forefoot hyperplantarflexed, and aiming the beam for an anteroposterior view of the foot. If roentgenographic examination is negative and with high clinical suspicion, bone scan or magnetic resonance image may be obtained.

O'Malley et al. (26) studied the natural history and outcome of these stress fractures; this group reviewed the office records of 51 professional dancers in whom they found 64 fractures. Their average follow-up was 6.4 years, with a minimum of 1 year. They found a history of previous stress fracture in 19 and a delayed menarche in 61% of the dancers. The dancers were treated with a variety of methods, including activity modification by stopping all balletic activities, short leg walking cast, symptomatic treatment with a wooden shoe or sneaker, or resuming activity as tolerated. The time from injury to return to performance averaged 6.2 weeks. They saw eight refractures at an average of 4.3 years after the initial injury. At final follow-up, 14% complained of occasional stiffness or pain with dancing.

Stress fractures are common among dancing athletes. Like other athletes, the stress fractures result from repeated stress placed on the metatarsals. Dancers often continue to dance despite pain from stress fractures, until complete fracture ensues. When treated, stress fractures heal, with an average return to activities at approximately 6 to 8 weeks. Refracture is not common but may happen with repeated activity at a similar level.

Avascular Necrosis of the Metatarsal Head (Freiberg's Infraction)

Avascular necrosis is a devastating problem in dancers. This condition should be considered when the dancer complains of metatarsalgia of insidious onset. It usually occurs in the second or third metatarsal. Often, the dancer has ignored the pain, stiffness, and chronic swelling of the MTP joint for some time before presentation, such that when they present, there is end-stage disease. Treatment at this stage is primarily palliative, and the dancer should be counseled as to alternative careers.

Hamilton (68) provided staging for Freiberg's infraction; he described four types of involvement (Table 51.1). Type I involvement shows minimal deformity with little loss of motion. At this stage, the metatarsal head heals by creeping substitution. In type II disease, the head is misshapen but the articular surface remains intact. This usually provides limitation in dorsiflexion and may be treated with a "generous cheilectomy" to help restore motion. Type III involvement shows that the articular cartilage is loose within the joint. It has been peeled off the metatarsal head much like peeling an orange. Treatment is aimed at removing loose bodies and will generally require joint resection arthroplasty. At this stage, normal joint function cannot be expected to return, and the dancer should be encouraged to seek alternative means for a future career. Type IV refers to an involvement of multiple heads and may represent a form of epiphyseal dysplasia. It presents a difficult problem in that if one metatarsal head is resected or debrided the transfer to the other heads will lead to exacerbation of their problem. There is no satisfactory solution to this stage of problem for the dancer.

Alterations in Skin

Over time, the dancer's skin also undergoes changes to accommodate foot position, conform to shoe wear, and as a result of increased friction in those dancing in bare feet. One may see skin fissuring, calluses, and corns, with or without abscesses as a result of dancing stresses.

Fissures are usually seen in performers of modern dance. These artists usually do not wear shoes. Additionally, they may use rosin to enhance their stability on the floor. This increases the friction between their foot and the floor, allowing less slippage but also for translation of this energy to the soles of their feet. The MTP creases are at significant risk for fissuring. When fissuring occurs, it usually is not deep to the dermis, but upon breaching the dermis, the risk of infection and abscess formation is much increased. The treatment for superficial fissures is warm soaks, elevation, and antibiotic ointment. Until these heal, rosin use should be restricted and the dancer should wear shoes.

Calluses are formed at prominent points as the body's means of protection. Shaving of calluses should be avoided in dancers, as the calluses will recur and the dancer meanwhile will transfer this added stress to the bony prominence. Shoe wear may at times be adjusted to accommodate the prominences, after which the calluses may spontaneously resolve.

Corns are frequently seen in dancers' feet. The areas over the PIP joint and between the toes are at high risk. They are most often due to pressure from wearing the pointe shoe. Treatment is aimed at pressure relief for the skin through use of corn pads. When pain persists despite diligent efforts at padding, abscess should be suspected. Once abscess is documented, treatment con-

TABLE 51.1. *Treatment of Freiberg's infraction by type and deficit*

	Description	Deficit	Treatment
Type I	MT head heals by creeping substitution	Minimum deformity, minimum loss of motion	ROM
Type II	Articular surface intact, misshapen head	Limited DF	Cheilectomy, range of motion
Type III	Extensive MT head destroyed, articular surface loose in joint	Mechanical pain, severe ROM limitation	Resection arthroplasty, remove loose bodies
Type IV	Multiple heads involved	Any level	Difficult—counsel on career change

MT, metatarsae; DF, dorsiflexion; ROM, range of motion.
From Hamilton WG. Foot and ankle injuries in dancers. *Clin Sport Med* 1988;7:143–173, with permission (68).

sists of decompression and irrigation, with antibiotics. The dancer may return to training as tolerated after completion of 3 weeks of antibiotic therapy, with the addition of appropriate shoe padding.

Traumatic Aneurysm

Traumatic aneurysm of the dorsalis pedis arterial system is a rare condition in the dancing population. It is related to repetitive trauma to the balls of the feet and most commonly involves the common digital plantar artery. Dancers may present with symptoms consistent with a space-occupying lesion, which appears insidious. Clinically, they will have spreading of the metatarsal heads and widening of the web space. The dancer complains of a widened foot, changes in the way their shoes fit, or pain on demi pointe.

Treatment for this condition is through surgical excision through a dorsal incision, taking care to avoid and preserve adjacent structures. The nearby tendons and ligaments are usually not involved. Rehabilitation after such intervention includes immediate active and passive range of motion. Recovery can be expected to take up to 3 months.

Acute Conditions

Fracture of the Fifth Metatarsal

In ballet dancers, an acute fracture of the distal fifth metatarsal is the most frequently seen acute fracture (26). The mechanism of injury is with the foot positioned in demi pointe with plantarflexion of the ankle and weight bearing on the ball of the foot. The dancer rolls over the lateral border of the foot after losing balance. The mechanism is a twisting of the foot, producing a spiral oblique fracture that usually runs distal dorsal and lateral to proximal plantar and medial.

As with any metatarsal fracture, any significant displacement should be treated with reduction and fixation, with dorsal angulation avoided. That which constitutes significant displacement or angulation has not yet been agreed upon. Shereff (69) provided guidelines of displacement greater than 3 to 4 mm or angulation of greater than 10 degrees. These parameters have not yet been supported by any biomechanical or clinical studies.

A retrospective review of 35 dancers having sustained fractures of the distal fifth metatarsal shaft has been recently published (26). Average time from injury at follow-up was 6.5 years. Most fractures were treated without reduction in a walking cast, removable boot, or wrapped in an elastic bandage with a healing shoe. Of the remaining four, two required open reduction and two were reduced closed. All undergoing operation were held with Kirschner wire fixation. The authors found that the dancers could walk without pain at an

average of 6.1 weeks. On average, they returned to barre exercise at 11.6 weeks and to full performance at 19 weeks. Degree of displacement significantly impacted time away from dance, with dancers having a nondisplaced fracture returning at an average 7 weeks, those with minimally displaced fracture returning at 15.2 weeks, and those with a displaced fracture returning at 23 weeks. All the dancers in this review returned to professional performance without limitation.

Forefoot Deformities

Hallux Valgus

Hallux valgus deformity in the dancer presents a situation different from most other athletes. It may have a congenital component in metatarsus primus varus or may be acquired. When acquired, the deformity's etiology is related to the increased stress placed medially when pushing off in the demi pointe position. The repetitive loads on the medial ligametous support of the hallux MTP are increased with positions of extension, as seen in the demi pointe posture. Additionally, the pointe shoe is made with a generic shape that may be used with either shoe. In wearing such a shoe, the dancer increases the tension medially even with the toe in neutral.

Treatment for this deformity in dancing athletes is primarily nonoperative. Additional padding and alterations to the dancer's shoe toe box with anti-inflammatory medication are the treatments of choice. Only in progressive deformity or in disorders not responding to conservative management is surgery contemplated. When surgery is planned, the dancer needs to be aware that he or she may not return to dancing at an advanced level. The limitations in his or her ability are related to the loss of extension, which would not affect the nondancing population as severely. In addition, recovery can be expected to take up to 1 year.

Conditions Masquerading as Forefoot Problems

Hallux Saltans

Hallux saltans, or trigger toe, is a common problem in the dancing athlete. It represents the end stage of a spectrum of disorders of the flexor hallucis longus, starting as tenosynovitis and progressing to tendinosis. The lesion in this disorder is usually located in the ankle, where the flexor hallucis longus enters its tunnel as it passes beneath the sustentaculum tali; however, it has been described at the knot of Henry, the base of the first metatarsal, or as it passes between the sesamoids under the first metatarsal head (70). When the tendon sustains microtrauma, it becomes bulbous. This nodule will slide within the tendon sheath while continuing to enlarge until it eventually is unable to reenter the sheath after it has exited either proximally or distally. At this point, when the muscle contracts, the tendon does not slide, thus not allowing flexion of the hallux or pulling the toe into flexion. In the dancer, this lack of excursion proximally interferes with active flexion needed for the transition from demi pointe to pointe. If the nodule in the tendon pulls through the tunnel proximally, the tendon loses distal excursion—the toe will snap into flexion and the dancer is unable to hold the foot in pointe.

Sammarco and Cooper (70) reviewed 31 cases in 26 patients, both dancing and nondancing athletes. In the dancing population, they found the disorder to start with the insidious onset of pain posterior to the medial malleolus. In the remaining population, the onset was more sudden, and symptoms had been present for a much shorter duration than in the dancing population. The flexor hallucis longus was found to have torn in 71% of dancers and 30% of nondancers; triggering was found in 71% of dancers and only 23% of nondancers. Return to full activity was seen at 3 months in 14 of the 18 dancers and at 4 months in 12 of the 13 nondancers.

Tenosynovitis may be treated conservatively; however, triggering usually requires surgical release at the site of impingement to allow excursion of the tendon. Debridement of the tendon to the width of the normal tendon, repair of longitudinal tears, and excision of bony prominences, such as an os trigonum or a posterior talar process, should be performed at surgery.

Neurologic Conditions

Conditions affecting the nervous system proximal to the foot may occasionally present with complaints localized to the foot. Herniated nucleus pulposis should be ruled out with foot complaints, as the lower lumbar and sacral roots provide sensation to the foot. Tarsal tunnel syndrome may present with symptoms in the forefoot, including numbness and paresthesias beneath the metatarsal heads, medial foot, and hallux, or occasionally with clawing of the toes. The condition may be diagnosed with a positive tinel sign at the tarsal tunnel, but nerve conduction velocity measurements may be necessary for diagnosis. Treatment includes exploration of the nerve, with its branches and release of constricting bands.

The medial cutaneous branch of the deep peroneal nerve provides sensation to the first web space. The nerve may be irritated by the tight en pointe shoe or ballet shoe over the midfoot. Additionally, osteophytes over the midtarsal joints will irritate the nerve as it passes dorsally over the midfoot. Padding over the straps crossing the midfoot or resection of the offending osteophyte will relieve the pressure. This in combination with anti-inflammatory medication will usually alleviate the problem.

REFERENCES

1. Garrick JG, Requa RK. The epidemiology of foot and ankle injuries in sports. *Clin Sport Med* 1988;7:29–36.
2. Clanton TO, Butler JE, Eggert A. Injuries to the metatarsophalangeal joints in athletes. *Foot Ankle* 1986;7:162–176.
3. Sammarco GJ. Turf toe. *Instruct Course Lect* 1993;42:207–212.
4. Sammarco GJ, Miller EH. Forefoot conditions in dancers. *Foot Ankle* 1982;3:85–98.
5. Mann RA, Baxter DE, Lutter LD. Running symposium. *Foot Ankle* 1981;1:190–224.
6. McBryde AM Jr. Stress fractures in runners. *Clin Sport Med* 1985;4:737–751.
7. Orava S, Hulkko A. Delayed unions and nonunions of stress fractures in athletes. *Am J Sport Med* 1988;16:378–382.
8. Sullivan D, Warren RF, Pavlov H, et al. Stress fractures in 51 runners. *Clin Orthop* 1984;187:188–192.
9. Matheson GO, Clement DB, McKenzie DC, et al. Stress fractures in athletes. *Am J Sport Med* 1987;15:46–57.
10. Gross TS, Bunch RP. A mechanical model of metatarsal stress fracture during distance running. *Am J Sport Med* 1989;17:669–673.
11. Drez D Jr, Young JC, Johnston RD, et al. Metatarsal stress fractures. *Am J Sport Med* 1980;8:123–125.
12. Harris RI, Beath T. The short first metatarsal. *J Bone Joint Surg Am* 1949;31A:553–565.
13. Weinfeld SB, Haddad SL, Myerson MS. Metatarsal stress fractures. *Clin Sport Med* 1997;16:319–338.
14. Frey C. Footwear and stress fractures. *Clin Sport Med* 1997;16:249–257.
15. Simkin A, Leichter I, Giladi M, et al. Combined effect of foot arch structure and an orthotic device on stress fractures. *Foot Ankle* 1989;10:25–29.
16. Anderson EG. Fatigue fractures of the foot. *Injury* 1990;51:275–279.
17. Kadel NJ, Teitz CC, Kronmal RA. Stress fractures in ballet dancers. *Am J Sports Med* 1992;20:445–449.
18. Warren M, Brooks-Gunn J, Hamilton LH, et al. Scoliosis and fractures in young ballet dancers. *N Engl J Med* 1986;314:1348–1353.
19. Cleveland M, Winant EM. An end-result study of the Keller operation. *J Bone Joint Surg Am* 1950;32A:163–175.
20. Ford LT, Gilula LA. Stress fractures of the middle metatarsals following the Keller operation. *J Bone Joint Surg Am* 1977;59A:117–118.
21. Myerding HW, Pollock GA. March fractures. *Surg Gynecol Obstet* 1938;67:234–236.
22. Michetti ML. March fracture following a McBride bunionectomy. *J Am Podiatr Assoc* 1970;60:286–292.
23. Milgrom C, Giladi M, Kashtan H, et al. A prospective study of the effect of a shock absorbing orthotic device on the incidence of stress fractures in military recruits. *Foot Ankle* 1985;6:101–104.
24. Greaney RB, Gerber FH, Laughlin RL, et al. Distribution and natural history of stress fractures in U.S. Marine recruits. *Radiology* 1983;146:339–346.
25. Micheli L, Sohn R, Solomon R. Stress fracture of the second metatarsal involving Lisfranc's joint in ballet dancers. *J Bone Joint Surg Am* 1985;67A:1372–1375.
26. O'Malley MJ, Hamilton WG, Munyak J, et al. Stress fractures at the base of the second metatarsal in ballet dancers. *Foot Ankle* 1996;17:89–94.
27. Smith RW, Reischl SF. Metatarsophalangeal joint synovitis in athletes. *Clin Sport Med* 1988;7:75–88.
28. Mann RA, Mizel MA. Monoarticular nontraumatic synovitis of the metatarsophalangeal joint: a new diagnosis. *Foot Ankle* 1985;6:18–21.
29. Kay DB. Forefoot pain in the athlete. *Clin Sport Med* 1994;13:785–791.
30. Myerson M, Shereff M. Pathologic anatomy of claw and hammertoes. *J Bone Joint Surg Am* 1989;71A:45.
31. Bowers KD Jr, Martin RB. Turf-toe: a shoe related football injury. *Med Sci Sport Exerc* 1976;8:81–83.
32. Coker TP, Arnold JA, Weber DL. Traumatic lesions of the meta-

tarsophalangeal joint of the great toe in athletes. *Am J Sport Med* 1978;6:326–334.

33. Rodeo SA, O'Brien S, Warren RF, et al. Turf-toe: an analysis of metatarsophalangeal joint sprains in professional football players. *Am J Sport Med* 1990;18:280–285.

34. Joseph J. Range of movement of the great toe in men. *J Bone Joint Surg Br* 1954;36B:450–457.

35. Bojsen-Moller F, Lamoreaux L. Significance of free dorsiflexion of the toes in walking. *Acta Orthop Scand* 1979;50:471–479.

36. Clanton TO, Ford JJ. Turf toe injury. *Clin Sport Med* 1994; 13:731–741.

37. Mullis DL, Miller WE. A disabling sports injury of the great toe. *Foot Ankle* 1980;1:22–25.

38. Frey C, Andersen GD, Feder KS. Plantarflexion injury to the metatarsophalangeal joint ("sand toe"). *Foot Ankle* 1996;17:576–581.

39. Jahss MH. Traumatic dislocations of the first metatarsophalangeal joint. *Foot Ankle* 1980;1:15–21.

40. Branch HE. Pathologic dislocation of the second toe. *J Bone Joint Surg*;19:978–984.

41. Thompson FM, Hamilton WG. Problems of the second metatarsophalangeal joint. *Orthopedics* 1987;10:83–89.

42. Coughlin MJ. Second metatarsophalangeal joint instability in the athlete. *Foot Ankle* 1993;14:309–319.

43. Lillich JS, Baxter DE. Bunionectomies and related surgery in the elite female middle-distance and marathon runner. *Am J Sport Med* 1986;14:491–493.

44. McBryde AM Jr, Jackson DW, James CM. Injuries in runners and joggers. In: Schneider R, Kennedy JC, Plant ML, et al., eds. *Sports injuries.* Baltimore: Williams & Wilkins, 1985:395–416.

45. Howse J. Disorders of the great toe in dancers. *Clin Sport Med* 1983;2:499–505.

46. Young MC, Formasier VL, et al. Osteochondral disruption of the second metatarsal: a variant of Freiberg's infraction. *Foot Ankle* 1987;8:103–109.

47. Hubay CA. Sesamoid bones of the hands and feet. *AJR Am J Roentgenol* 1949;61:493–505.

48. Inge GAL, Ferguson AB. Surgery of the sesamoid bones of the great toe, an anatomical and clinical study with a report of 41 cases. *Arch Surg* 1933;27:466–489.

49. Powers JH. Traumatic and developmental abnormalities of the sesamoid bones of the great toe. *Am J Surg* 1934;23:315–321.

50. Burman MS, Lapidus PW. The functional disturbances caused by the inconstant bones and sesamoids of the foot. *Arch Surg* 1931;22:936–975.

51. Bizarro AH. The traumatology of the sesamoid structures. *Ann Surg* 1986;74:783–791.

52. Richardson EG. Injuries to the hallucal sesamoids in the athlete. *Foot Ankle* 1987;7:229–244.

53. Parra G. Stress fractures of the sesamoids of the foot. *Clin Orthop* 1960;18:218–285.

54. Scranton PE. Pathologic anatomic variations in the sesamoids. *Foot Ankle* 1981;1:321–326.

55. Coughlin MJ. Sesamoid pain: causes and surgical treatment. *Instruct Course Lect* 1990;39:23–35.

56. Mann RA, Coughlin MJ, Baxter D, et al. Sesamoidectomy of the great toe. Presented at the 15th Annual Meeting of the American Orthopaedic Foot and Ankle Society, Las Vegas, January 24, 1985.

57. Nayfa TM, Sorto LA Jr. The incidence of hallux abductus following tibial sesamoidectomy. *J Am Podiatry Assoc* 1982;72:617–620.

58. Rodeo SA, Warren RF, O'Brien SJ, et al. Diastasis of bipartite sesamoids of the first metatarsophalangeal joint. *Foot Ankle* 1993;14:425–434.

59. Baxter DE. Treatment of bunion deformity in the athlete. *Orthop Clin North Am* 1994;25:33–39.

60. Baxter DE. Functional nerve disorders in the athlete's foot, ankle, and leg. *Instruct Course Lect* 1993;42:185–194.

61. Murphy PC, Baxter DE. Nerve entrapment of the foot and ankle in runners. *Clin Sport Med* 1985;4:753.

62. Lillich JS, Baxter DE. Common forefoot problems in runners. *Foot Ankle* 1986;7:145–151.

63. Graham CE, Graham DM. Morton's neuroma: a microscopic evaluation. *Foot Ankle* 1984;5:150–161.

64. Lassman G. Morton's toe: clinical, light, and electron microscopic investigations in 133 cases. *Clin Orthop* 1979;142:73–92.

65. Mann RA, Baxter DE. *Surgery of the foot and ankle,* 6th ed. St. Louis: Mosby, 1993:544–554.

66. Mann RA, Reynolds JD. Interdigital neuroma: a critical clinical analysis. *Foot Ankle* 1983;3:238–244.

67. Bradley N, Miller WA, Evans JP. Plantar neuroma analysis of results following surgical excision in 145 patients. *South Med J* 1976;69:853–859.

68. Hamilton WG. Foot and ankle injuries in dancers. *Clin Sport Med* 1988;7:143–173.

69. Shereff MJ. Complex fractures of the metatarsals. *Orthopedics* 1990;13:875–882.

70. Sammarco GJ, Cooper PS. Flexor hallucis longus tendon injury in dancers and nondancers. *Foot Ankle* 1998;19:356–362.

Principles and Practice of Orthopaedic Sports Medicine,
edited by William E. Garrett, Jr., Kevin P. Speer, and Donald T. Kirkendall.
Lippincott Williams & Wilkins, Philadelphia © 2000.

CHAPTER 52

Toe Injuries and Related Conditions

Lamar L. Fleming

Forefoot injuries are often unrecognized by both the athlete and the clinician until the disorder becomes a disability. In this chapter we address painful greater and lesser toe conditions, including fracture, dislocation, hallux rigidus, and chronic lesser toe deformities. Related conditions include intractable plantar keratosis, interdigital neuromas, metatarsophalangeal synovitis, and hard and soft corns that contribute to metatarsalgia and toe pain. Hallux valgus and bunionette deformities are covered in separate sections.

Sporting injuries have been classified by Garrick and Requa (1) as generic or specific. Forefoot injuries can be considered specific relative to the more common ankle sprain. Certain sports promote identifiable patterns of injury based on unique physical demands during competition. Turf toe injury exemplifies a specific pattern of injury identified in a single sport. Bowers and Martin (2) observed this sprain injury pattern of the first metatarsophalangeal joint and related it to the combination of artificial turf and flexible cleated shoes used in football. The degree of disability resulting from the uncommon injury can represent a significant amount of missed competition compared with more common injuries such as an ankle sprain (3). Subsequent research characterizing the biomechanics of the injury has helped foster preventive measures and improve the health of the athlete (4–7).

In the absence of acute injury, the repetitive nature of athletic training contributes to cumulative musculoskeletal trauma. Proper equipment and athletic technique are important for the prevention of injury. Focus on education and prevention should be the goals for the clinician, along with returning the injured athlete to a preinjury level of performance.

The forefoot conditions outlined in this chapter primarily represent pain in one of three symptomatic locations: the metatarsophalangeal joint, over an exostosis or joint prominence, or between the toes. Many of these conditions are preventable with proper shoe wear and athletic technique. When an athlete becomes symptomatic, inspection of the athletic shoe wear is important. Understanding the individual sport is helpful for eliciting a proper history that can provide critical clinical information and help foster confidence in the physician–patient relationship. Conservative measures represent the primary form of treatment. Familiarity with various taping and splinting techniques will assist the athlete in the functional return to training and competition. When these efforts fail, appropriate operative treatment can be considered.

A number of acquired and congenital physiologic conditions of the lower extremity have been associated with forefoot pain. Factors extrinsic to the forefoot, including tendo-Achilles contracture, limb malalignment, and limb length discrepancy, can indirectly contribute to metatarsalgia (8). Intrinsic abnormalities are associated with dysfunction in the forefoot and include pes planus, pes cavus, hypermobile first ray, hallux valgus, and a long second ray Morton's toe (9).

In the absence of acute injury, chronic repetitive stress represents the primary mode of injury in the athlete. The variable expression of this chronic stress in the forefoot can range from painful callosities and toe deformities to stress fractures. The differential diagnosis for metatarsalgia includes sesamoiditis, nerve entrapment, joint capsulitis, and stress fracture.

Athletes represent a challenging population to treat. Psychological issues can make it difficult for the injured athlete to observe the prescribed rest and training restrictions. A proper diagnosis and well-coordinated treatment plan are important for recovery and preventing recurrent injury. Forthright discussion will help foster patient confidence and improve compliance. It

L. L. Fleming: Department of Orthopaedics, Emory University, Atlanta, Georgia 30322.

should be stressed that premature return to competition may prolong the recovery process.

FRACTURE OF THE TOES

In the general orthopedic population, toe fractures are the most common fractures in the forefoot and generally result from direct trauma (10–12). The proximal phalanx is involved more frequently than the middle or distal phalanges, with stubbing of the toe the most common cause of a phalanx fracture (11). Crush injuries can increase the risk of open fracture, particularly when the nail bed or a laceration is involved (13).

Great toe fractures are considered important with respect to diagnosis and treatment; anatomic reduction is essential (10). Malalignment and articular incongruity can cause significant disability in the great toe due to its structural and mechanical importance (14). Lesser toe fractures are considered functionally less significant with moderate deformity considered acceptable (11). Difficulty with shoe wear can be the likely result of a residual lesser toe deformity. Blodgett (11) observed the tendency of proximal phalanx fractures of the lesser toes to heal in a plantar angulated position, causing subsequent pain.

Soccer and kicking sports are associated with osteochondral fractures of the great toe that result from high valgus stresses (15). Joint sprains and dislocations can cause osteochondral fractures (16). Dancers, particularly ballet, subject the forefoot and toes to vertical loading forces that can typically result in diaphyseal phalanx fractures (14).

Stress fractures of the proximal phalanx of the great toe have been reported in the young mature athlete. Yokoe and Mannoji (17) described this condition using bone scans in symptomatic athletes, all with hallux valgus. These injuries were attributed to excessive training combined with the mechanical influence of the hallux valgus, producing increased strain on the medial side of the hallux. Shiraishi et al. (19) described epiphyseal fracture in the immature athlete characterized by a fragmentation pattern. Follow-up at maturity revealed no significant deformity or symptoms in this small series.

Clinical Evaluation

The evaluation of a painful toe includes a thorough history, physical examination, and inspection of the shoe wear. The onset of symptoms may help identify a chronic versus acute injury. Chronic toe injuries may result from impact of digits into the toe box of the shoe. The shoe may be small for the foot; this is commonly seen in soccer players. An individual may have a long second ray Morton's toe, contributing to direct impact of the phalanx into the shoe. The nail bed should be evaluated. A symptomatic subungual hematoma should be drained using a sterile hypodermic needle or heated paper clip (11,12). An abnormal-appearing nail bed may be indicative of an chronically traumatized toe. A recent history of trauma, including laceration, may introduce the possibility of an obvious or occult open fracture and risk of subsequent infection. Therefore, these injuries require more aggressive treatment (10).

Radiographic evaluation is useful in establishing the diagnosis of a phalanx fracture and assessing the joints for any associated dislocation. Standard radiographs, including anteroposterior (AP), lateral, and oblique views of the toes, can assist in identifying subtle fractures. Associated fracture patterns including comminution, displacement, periarticular involvement, and physeal involvement may influence subsequent treatment. Negative radiographic findings may represent a stress fracture, particularly in the great toe (19). Subtle fragmentation of the epiphysis may be indicative of a stress fracture in the immature athlete (18). Technetium bone scan has been used to diagnose stress fractures in the setting of normal radiographs.

Treatment

The primary treatment of phalanx fractures is conservative, with closed reduction successful in most cases (11). Rest, ice, immobilization, and anti-inflammatory medication are useful modalities. Adhesive taping is probably the most used form of stabilization. Shoe modification, using a postoperative-type shoe, can be helpful in relieving local pressure over the phalanx. Return to athletic activity is dictated by symptoms.

Operative treatment is indicated for displaced fractures involving the great toe, especially those with intraarticular involvement (10,11,20). Open fractures require immediate irrigation and appropriate antibiotic and tetanus prophylaxis (15). DeLee (20) advocated closed reduction of displaced fractures of the hallux, supplemented with Kirschner wire fixation: lesser toe fractures are treated primarily with closed reduction if needed, followed by adhesive taping to the adjacent toes. Hamilton (14) noted that posttraumatic deformity of the toes can undergo successful delayed reconstruction with resection arthroplasty procedures.

Rang (18) described operative treatment for displaced physeal fractures of the toes in the skeletally immature patient. Long-term sequelae include nail bed deformities, physeal growth arrest, and deformity. Chronic joint stiffness is associated with intraarticular injury patterns.

DISLOCATION OF THE TOES

Toe dislocations are the result of direct trauma. In the athlete, the mechanism most commonly results from sudden forced hyperextension. The first and fifth metatarsophalangeal joints are most commonly involved (22,23). Great toe metatarsophalangeal joint dislocations have been reported in football players (3,24). Artificial playing surfaces and the use of more flexible lightweight shoes have been associated with the increased incidence of sprains and dislocations observed in this sport (2,3). The metatarsophalangeal joints are involved more commonly than the interphalangeal joints. Simple dislocations respond to closed reduction. Complex dislocations require open reduction and are associated with bone fragment or soft tissue interposition preventing closed reduction (16,23–27).

Mechanism

Jahss (23) described the pathomechanics of first metatarsophalangeal joint dislocations and noted three patterns (Fig. 52.1). As with complex dislocations of the metacarpophalangeal joints in the hand, a type I dislocation involves rupture of the plantar (volar) plate from the base of metatarsal (metacarpal) neck. Dorsal dislocation of the intact sesamoid complex occurs. The dislocation is generally irreducible by closed means and requires open reduction. Type II dislocations occur with more forceful dorsiflexion; the intersesamoid ligament ruptures (IIA) or diastasis of the sesamoids (IIB) occurs. Closed reduction is effective in type II dislocations. Dislocation of the lesser metarsophalangeal joint also occurs by a forced dorsiflexion mechanism.

Clinical Evaluation

A thorough history and physical examination is performed, with attention to the neurovascular status of the dislocated toe. As with other dislocations, soft tissue integrity depends on a prompt diagnosis and anatomic reduction of the joint surfaces. Proper radiographic assessment includes standard AP, lateral, and oblique films of the foot. Identification of an avulsion fracture will likely require an open reduction.

Treatment

A closed reduction is performed by re-creating the original deforming dorsiflexion force. If this maneuver fails,

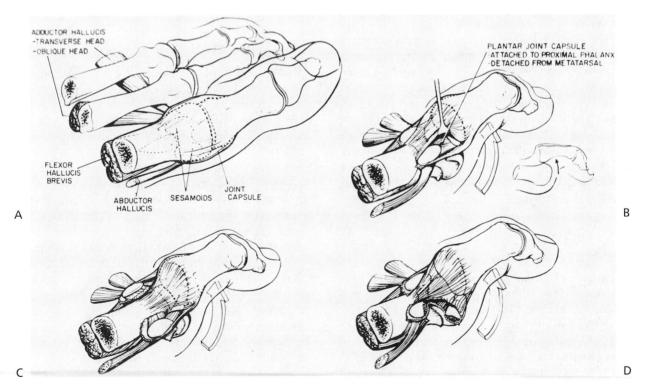

FIG. 52.1. A: The normal anatomic relationship of the first metatarsophalangeal joint and sesamoids. **B:** Type I dorsal dislocation of the joint with the intact sesamoid complex lying dorsal to the metatarsal head and neck. The metatarsal head is incarcerated through the volar capsule. This dislocation is usually irreducible with closed manipulation. **C:** Type IIA dorsal dislocation with a longitudinal tear of the intersesamoid ligament. This type is usually reducible using closed manipulation. **D:** Type IIB dorsal dislocation with fracture and incarceration of the sesamoid complex within the dorsal capsule. Open reduction is usually required. (From Jahss MH. Traumatic dislocations of the first metatarsophalangeal joint. *Foot Ankle* 1980;1:15–21, with permission.)

open reduction is typically done through a dorsal longitudinal incision for relocation of the interposed tissues. Treatment is based on the relative stability of the joint after reduction. A stable joint is maintained by an accommodative shoe and taping. Unstable joints require pinning to ensure reduction of the articular surfaces during the healing phase (28). Typically, fixation is maintained for 2 to 3 weeks after surgical treatment. Sequelae related to arthrofibrosis of the joint are common and usually asymptomatic. Reconstructive procedures for chronically symptomatic joints of the lesser toes include excisional arthroplasty or arthrodesis (28).

Chronic lesser toe dislocations observed in the athlete often cannot be reduced by closed means. Symptomatic open reduction alone may cause vascular impairment, and therefore a procedure such as DuVries arthroplasty or Keller arthroplasty can be used to reduce and correct the deformity (14). Stiffness can be problematic for certain athletes, including dancers, after such treatment.

TURF TOE

Bowers and Martin described turf toe in 1976 (2). This was in response to the notable increase in sprain injuries to the great toe observed in football players. Turf toe characteristically results from forced hyperextension of the first MP joint, causing a traumatic plantar capsuloligamentous sprain (29). The use of artificial playing surfaces and of flexible lightweight shoes to improve performance have been attributed to this specific injury pattern (2,4,30). Clanton and Ford (30) noted this injury ranking third to knee and ankle injuries in collegiate athletes and stressed the preventable nature of this disorder. Sprain injury to the first MP joint has also been observed in other sports, including soccer, basketball, volleyball, and dancing (14,31).

Mechanism

Four patterns of sprain injury to the first MP joint have been described (3). The most common is forced hyperextension of the first MP joint, described clinically as "turf toe." A fixed position of the forefoot, combined with axial loading over the hind portion of the foot, associated with tackling is a frequent scenario (Fig. 52.2) (2,3,30). Two additional mechanisms include varus and valgus deforming forces that can cause volar and collateral ligament disruption. Kicking sports in particular may contribute to the valgus pattern of strain injuries. Hyperflexion of the first MP joint has been observed in tennis, soccer, and volleyball and is an important variant to consider in the athlete with dorsal tenderness at the first MP joint with minimal plantar symptoms.

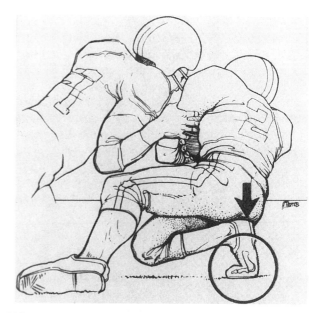

FIG. 52.2. A common mechanism for turf toe injury in the athlete. Forced hyperextension of the first metatarsophalangeal joint results from an axial load applied to the fixed dorsiflexed forefoot. The combination of artificial turf and the flexible cleated athletic shoe are important factors contributing to the injury. (From *Phys Sports Med* 17:132–147, with permission.)

CLASSIFICATION

Clanton and Ford (30) outlined a classification system for turf toe based on the clinical grading system used to characterize joint sprains. Grade I injuries are mild. The plantar tissues remain intact. Symptoms are minimal; there is minor swelling without ecchymosis. The athlete is able to bear weight and often continues to participate in competition after the acute injury. Athletes with acute grade I symptoms may act much like those with chronic turf toe disorder. Grade II injuries represent a partial tear of the capsular tissues. Symptoms are significant, with pain, ecchymosis, and restricted motion. The athlete is unable to perform at his or her usual level. In grade III injuries, there is a complete capsuloligamentous tear. There may have been an occult joint dislocation that spontaneously reduced. Symptoms are notable for pain, restricted motion, marked swelling, and ecchymosis. The athlete is unable to bear weight normally. Sesamoid fracture, diastasis, or periarticular fracture may be present.

Biomechanics

The function of the first MP joint is unique. It carries twice the mechanical load of to the lesser toes (9). It is important for the push-off strength required in athletic competition. Peak forces across this joint amount to 40% to 60% of the body weight (32). The forces increase to two to three times body weight with running or jogging and up to eight times with a running jump (33).

Anatomy

The plantar plate of the first MP joint is a thick fibrocartilaginous structure and serves as the primary stabilizer of the joint. It has a strong distal attachment to the proximal phalanx and a weaker proximal insertion to the metatarsal neck (34). Rupture of the volar plate is noted to occur more commonly at the proximal insertion, although it has been observed at variable locations.

The capsuloligamentous anatomy and relationship with the sesamoids is important in the understanding of the pathophysiology of turf toe (35). The medial and lateral sesamoids lie within the plantar plate and the respective flexor hallucis brevis tendons. The intermetatarsal ligament joins the sesamoids together and is a strong attachment of the lateral volar plate and capsule to the adjacent second metatarsal. The sesamoids serve to elevate the first metatarsal head and distribute a significant amount of force across the articulation. The blood supply of the medial sesamoid is unique. The medial plantar artery is the main vascular source, with a distal to proximal pattern of supply, which may predispose the sesamoids to injury, delayed healing, and nonunion (36). The incidence of bipartite sesamoid is approximately 30% and most commonly involves the medial sesamoid (35). Rodeo et al. (37) described sesamoid fracture with diastasis as the site of plantar tissue failure in the athlete (Fig. 52.3). The condition was associated with a bipartite medial sesamoid and is associated with progressive diastasis after turf toe injury.

Clinical Evaluation

The differential diagnosis of turf toe includes acute fracture, MP joint dislocation, stress fracture, osteochondral lesion, and flexor tendinitis. A thorough history and physical examination are performed. The ability of the athlete to recall the position of the foot at the time of injury may be helpful to the clinician. Pain localization and swelling can provide important clues to the degree of soft tissue injury. Tenderness over the sesamoids can help determine the likely pattern of injury. Depending on the degree of pain, stability of the joint should be assessed. Radiographic evaluation is generally based on symptomology; it is indicated for grades II and III sprain injuries and includes standard AP, lateral, and oblique films of the foot and an axial view of the sesamoids. Rodeo et al. (37) recommend obtaining dorsiflexion stress views in the athlete with a bipartite sesamoid and a grade III injury.

Treatment

Treatment of turf toe is primarily conservative. Rest, ice, compression, and elevation are important modalities in early treatment. An oral anti-inflammatory medication may be helpful. Restoration of range of motion is a major goal of treatment. The course of treatment is typically 4 to 6 weeks.

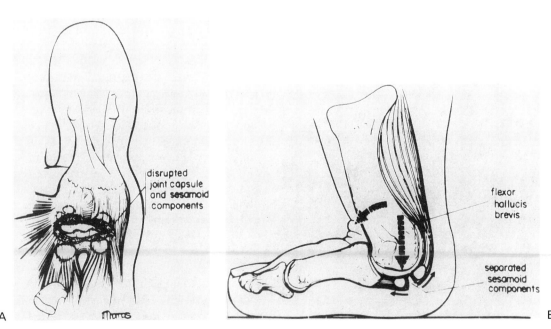

FIG. 52.3. A and B: Frontal and sagittal schematic views of turf toe injury to the first metatarsophalangeal joint with transverse fracture through sesamoids and volar capsular tissues. (From *Phys Sports Med* 17:132–147, with permission.)

Further supportive treatment includes taping and orthotic devices. Adhesive taping helps to stabilize the first MTP joint and may help to reduce the chance of reinjury during the functional phase of rehabilitation. A thin steel spring plate is typically used in the shoe to limit first MP joint movement. A custom-molded insole with a Morton's extension can be used if the more rigid insole is not tolerated (Fig. 52.4). Most athletes will recover within 4 to 6 weeks. Cast immobilization with the great toe in 10 degrees of plantar flexion for a period of up to 8 weeks should be considered if there is evidence of sesamoid fracture (10). Intraarticular cortisone injections are not indicated (29).

Operative treatment is considered in cases with persistent symptoms despite conservative care. Other surgi-cal indications include osteochondral fracture, proximal migration of sesamoids, and joint instability. Rodeo et al. (37) reported four cases of turf toe with progressive sesamoid diastasis. Surgical treatment included excision of the distal medial sesamoid and advancement of the remaining soft tissue sleeve to the remaining proximal fragment. Postoperative rehabilitation included 4 weeks of non-weight bearing, active plantar flexion at 4 weeks, and dorsiflexion allowed at 6 weeks. Return to sport occurred by 8 weeks postoperatively. They reported full recovery in their series with return to competitive athletics. Coker et al. (3) reported on a series of eight athletes with turf toe injuries, four of which underwent delayed surgical treatment. Findings at surgery included cartilaginous loose bodies, chondromalacia of the metatarsal head, capsular calcification, and medial sesamoid fracture. No specific conclusion could be drawn from this study with regard to surgical guidelines.

HALLUX RIGIDUS

Hallux rigidus presents a difficult clinical problem for the clinician and athlete. Sporting events that require jumping, cutting, and acceleration are dependent on dorsiflexion of the first MP joint and push-off from the hallux. Davies-Colley (38) described the disorder in 1887. Pain and reduced motion across the first MP joint are the most common symptoms. A dorsal bunion is typically the source of pain.

Clanton et al. (29) observed chronic first MP joint symptoms in a small group of athletes with previous turf toe injury. This suggests that turf toe and severe sprain injuries to the hallux may be an important predisposing factor in developing hallux rigidus; no present study has clearly defined this relationship.

The incidence of hallux rigidus is 2% in the general population, second only to hallux valgus (39). It is commonly observed in ages ranging from 30 to 60 years, although an adolescent subgroup is recognized. The etiology is multifactorial, with a number of conditions including osteochondritis dissecans, a long hallux, congenital squaring of the metatarsal head, metatarsus elevatus, shoe wear, and pes planus. Hallux rigidus is unilateral in approximately 70% of the general population, with a female predilection. The true incidence in the athlete is not known but is likely higher than in the general population.

Case Study

A 42-year-old male athlete presented with symptomatic hallux rigidus involving the right first MP joint. He described having to quit running and noted the tendency to walk on the outside of his foot. He also reported stiffness and anterior pain in his ipsilateral ankle. He had a significant history for participating in high school

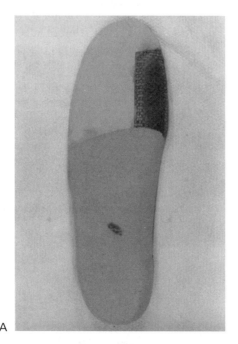

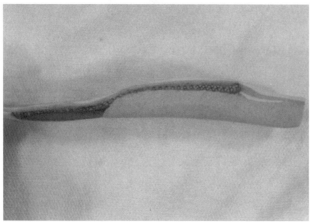

FIG. 52.4. A and B: Custom turf toe orthosis. A composite carbon fiber insert acts as a Morton's extension to dampen motion at the first metatarsophalangeal joint. It is inset into a full-length semirigid orthotic.

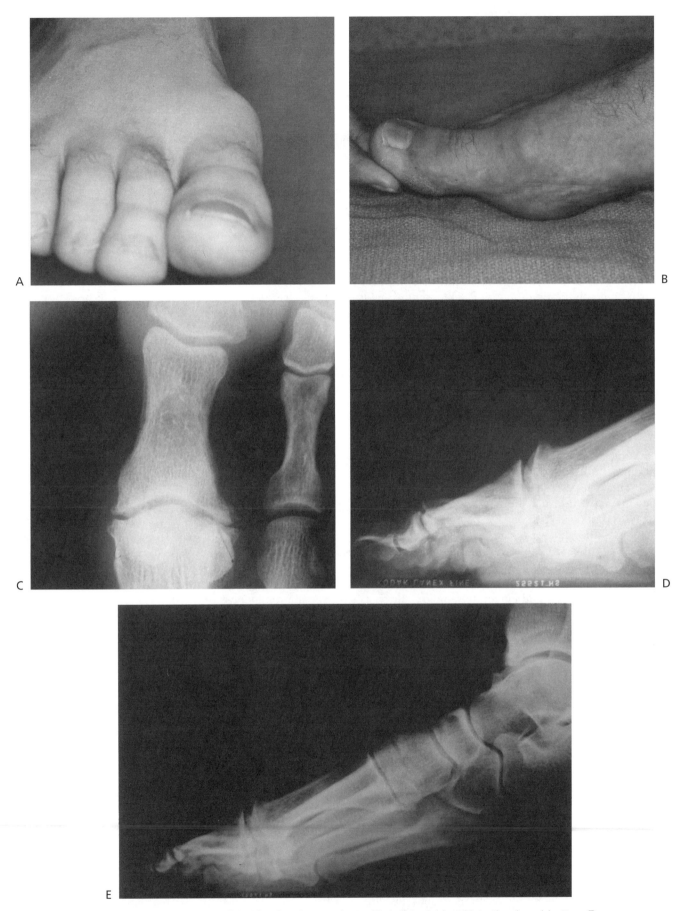

FIG. 52.5. A: Frontal view of the forefoot in a patient with hallux rigidus. Note the dorsal button. **B:** Lateral view of the medial forefoot with the maximal forced passive dorsiflexion of the first metatarsophalangeal joint demonstrated (<10 degrees). **C:** Weight-bearing anteroposterior radiograph of the first metatarsophalangeal joint shows squaring of the joint space with medial and lateral osteophytes. **D:** A lateral radiograph with magnification over the first MP joint demonstrates significant dorsal osteophytes involving the proximal phalanx and metatarsal head. **E:** A lateral radiograph of the foot. Note the anterior osteophytes involving both the distal tibia and talus at the ankle joint.

football as a lineman. During college he became an avid triathlete and marathon runner. He denied any specific injury to his forefoot during his athletic career. Before developing symptoms in his right foot, he had hallux rigidus of his left foot treated with a cheilectomy 5 years earlier. Examination of his right foot revealed a dorsal bunion over the first metatarsal head that was painful to palpation (Fig. 52.5A). Both active and passive dorsiflexion of the hallux revealed less than 10 degrees of motion and reproduced the patient's symptoms (Fig. 52.5B). Radiographic evaluation revealed significant osteophyte formation on both sides of the first MP joint that was appreciated on both the AP and lateral views (Fig. 52.5C, D, and E). The patient was managed conservatively with shoe modification, including a turf toe liner. The combination of anterior ankle impingement and hallux rigidus symptoms made it difficult to participate in any sport or exercise. Cheilectomy was subsequently performed at both the first MP and ankle joints. Postoperatively, he continues to be limited with respect to running but notes significant symptomatic and functional improvement.

Clinical Evaluation

The clinical examination commonly reveals a dorsal bunion deformity. Reduced motion of the first MP joint is present with pain elicited upon passive dorsiflexion. Synovitis and a dorsal callus may be present. Pain can also be reproduced with passive plantar flexion of the MP joint. Radiographic evaluation includes weight bearing AP, lateral, and oblique views of the foot. Hattrup and Johnson (40) described three grades of hallux rigidus based on the radiographic appearance. Grades I and II represent mild and moderate radiographic signs of arthritis and correlate well with positive outcome after cheilectomy. Grade III represents advanced arthritic changes, with notable joint space narrowing and significant osteophyte formation at both the proximal phalanx and metatarsal head. The differential diagnosis includes gout and underlying osteochondral injury, contributing to arthritis changes.

Treatment

Conservative treatment includes nonsteroidal antiinflammatory medication, a rigid insole, and consideration for corticosteroid injection. Shoe wear modification is important in relieving pressure over the dorsal bunion. A shoe with a wide and deep toe box with proper length is desirable. A stiff sole can help in reducing motion across the first MP joint; a turf toe liner or full length orthosis with a Morton's extension can be useful. Additional shoe modifications include installation of a metatarsal rocker bar. The athlete may encounter weakened push-off with the rigid insole.

Surgical management primarily incudes cheilectomy. First MP joint fusion is not tolerated well in the athlete and should not be considered. Similarly, implant arthroplasty and resection arthroplasty are not indicated procedures (41). Dorsal cheilectomy of 20% to 30% of the joint surface and exostosis is recommended, with debridement of medial and lateral osteophytes (42,43). Intraoperative motion of 60 to 70 degrees is desirable. For severe cases, the metatarsal cheilectomy can be combined with a dorsal closing wedge osteotomy as described by Moberg (43). The goal with this additional osteotomy is to allow clearance of the great toe during roll over in the stance. Mann and Clanton (41) reported the results of cheilectomy in 25 patients with improvement in average joint motion by 20 degrees. Most patients were satisfied at greater than 4 years after the surgical procedure.

DEFORMITIES OF THE TOES

Claw Toe

Clawing of the toes is characterized by dorsiflexion at the MP joints, with flexion at the interphalangeal joints of the toes. The deformity can be flexible or have a variable degree of rigidity. When all toes are involved, it may be associated with pes cavus, neurologic disorders of the foot, and systemic disorders including rheumatoid arthritis. Chronic regional disorders, including dependent edema, Sudeck's atrophy, and frostbite, can cause diffuse clawing of the toes. In the athlete the cause is usually idiopathic. Kelikian (45) described the disorder as an exaggerated form of hammertoe. The main functional difficulty with clawing of the toes is pain over the dorsal prominences of the deformity and metatarsalgia that results from focal pressure beneath the metatarsal heads.

The lesser toes stabilize the longitudinal arch during walking and maintain floor contact until the swing phase begins; fine adjustments in toe posture assist in balance control (46,47). An important dynamic relationship exists between the intrinsic and extrinsic muscle functioning to stabilize the toes (Fig. 52.6). Passive restraints at the MP joints include the joint capsule, collateral ligaments, plantar aponeurosis, and plantar plate. Mann and Hagy (47) studied muscle firing patterns in athletes and noted minimal intrinsic muscle activity compared with extrinsic plantar flexion tone in the running and jogging athlete. In the athlete, claw toes are more likely to occur without any associated deformity of the arch. Garth and Miller (48) theorized that medial tibial stress syndrome in the athlete resulted from primary foot intrinsic muscle weakness, resulting in compensatory extrinsic muscle substitution. This clinical entity observed in runners likely represents a similar form of dynamic muscle imbalance that contributes to clawing of the toes.

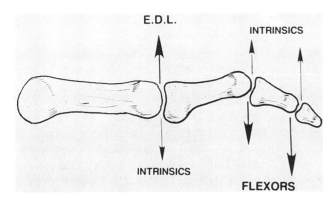

FIG. 52.6. The posture and function of the toes depends on both extrinsic and intrinsic muscle balance. An imbalance in this relationship due to intrinsic muscle weakness or the "cramming" effect of a shoe on the toes likely contributes to the common lessor toe deformities. (From Mann RA. *Surgery of the foot.* St. Louis: C.V. Mosby, 1986:148–170, with permission.)

Clinical Evaluation

Symptoms often result from dorsal corns, plantar calluses, and metatarsalgia. The deformity is characterized by MP joint extension, and PIP and DIP joint flexion; it can be fixed, semirigid, or flexible and usually involves all toes (48). Kelikian (45) described the push-up test to determine the flexibility of the claw deformity; passive correction is indicative of a flexible deformity (Fig. 52.7).

Treatment

Conservative treatment includes shaving the corns and calluses and use of metatarsal pads. The cavus foot is indicative of a more rigid arch. A custom semirigid full-length orthosis can help dissipate stresses in the fore-

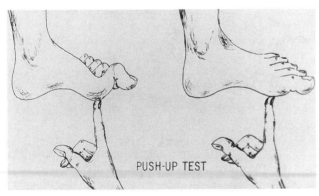

FIG. 52.7. The "push-up" test for determining the flexibility of claw toes is performed by placing dorsal pressure underneath the metatarsal heads of the foot. The claw toe deformity is considered flexible when the toes straighten and the clawing corrects. (From Kelikian H. *Hallux valgus: allied deformities of the forefoot and metatarsalgia.* Philadelphia: W.B. Saunders, 1965, with permission.)

foot. The shoes should have extra depth in the toe box to accommodate the claw toes.

Operative treatment of flexible claw toes include flexor to extension tendon transfer in the second through fourth toes (49,50). The fifth toe can be treated conservatively or with a flexor tenotomy. In the setting of flexible claw toes and a cavus foot, Kelikian (45) recommended correction of the cavus deformity with midfoot osteotomy, which spontaneously corrects the clawing deformity of the toes. Fixed deformities can be addressed with a PIP resection arthroplasty and pinning (46). If the joint is unreduced after the more distal correction, an MP joint capsulotomy and release is performed with an extensor tenotomy. Continued swelling and stiffness can be common residual symptoms after surgery and should be discussed with the patient before surgery.

Hammer Toe

Hammer toe is a common condition of the forefoot and is noticed by the athlete when symptoms develop secondary to a painful corn or plantar callus. The deformity is defined by flexion at the PIP joint, may be fixed or flexible, and may present with a variable degree of MP dorsiflexion that ranges from flexible to rigid (51). The distal interphalangeal joint typically remains flexible. It has been described as a swan's neck deformity of the toe. Pain often results from a dorsal corn over the PIP joint. The etiology is variable and is often attributed to shoe wear and restriction of the longer toes within the toe box of the shoe (45). Conservative treatment includes shoe wear modification. Symptomatic corns and calluses should be trimmed. Taping and pads can be helpful in relieving local pressure.

Flexible hammer toes that remain symptomatic despite appropriate conservative treatment can be effectively treated with a flexor–extensor tendon transfer (50). Operative treatment for rigid deformities include a PIP joint arthroplasty and a PIP joint fusion as described by Jones. Coughlin (46) reported favorable outcomes with surgical treatment of both flexible and rigid hammer toe deformities using these techniques. Significant relief pain is reported.

Rau and Manoli (52) reported a case of an acute hammer toe deformity in a kick boxer. The symptomatic toe was successfully treated with repair of the central extensor mechanism and lateral bands.

Mallet Toe

As with the hammer toe, mallet toe is a deformity resulting from shoe wear. The longer toes, particularly the second and third, are most commonly affected. The deformity is defined by flexion at the distal interphalangeal joint. A characteristic callous can form at the tip of the toe. Inflammatory processes, including psoriatic and rheumatoid arthritis, may cause the deformity.

As with the treatment of a hammer toe deformity, the mallet toe can be conservatively managed with pads to lessen impact at the tip of the toe. Shoe modification should also be considered to specifically accommodate the second and third toes.

Operative treatment for the flexible mallet toe includes release of the long flexor tendon. The rigid mallet deformity can be effectively treated through a dorsal approach with a resection arthroplasty of the distal portion of the middle phalanx and debridement of the articular surface of the distal phalanx; a flexor tenotomy can also be performed. Coughlin (53) reported a high satisfaction rate (86%) in 60 patients using this technique; fusion of the DIP joint occurred in 72% and a fibrous union in 28%.

Intractable Plantar Keratosis

A common source of metatarsalgia in the athlete is caused by a plantar callous. This buildup of keratinized epidermal tissue, better known as intractable plantar keratosis, identifies an area of increased plantar contact pressure in the forefoot.

Pain often brings the patient to the clinician for evaluation. Deformities associated with intractable plantar keratosis include metatarsal fracture malunion, hammer or claw toe, hallux valgus, bunionette, hypermobile first ray, and long second ray Morton's toe. These conditions disrupt the even distribution of contact pressures across the forefoot and metatarsal heads. Increased focal pressure beneath the symptomatic metatarsal head contributes to the formation of the reactive skin tissue in the form of a callous. Characteristically, the lesion is solitary and located beneath the symptomatic metatarsal head.

Clinical Evaluation

The patient's symptoms should be well characterized with respect to activity, shoe wear, and chronicity. The relationship with external factors, including changes in running or playing surfaces, new shoe wear, and recent competition, should be established. A Harris-Beath pressure mat can help localize the lesion visually and serves as a useful tool for educating the patient.

Radiographic evaluation includes weight-bearing AP, lateral, and oblique views of the foot. Hypertrophy of the second metatarsal can be evaluated and, if present, may be indicative of a hypermobile first ray or long second ray. The relative lengths of the metatarsal can also be evaluated.

Treatment

Conservative measures include shaving the lesion to reduce the plantar prominence. Metatarsal pads can help redistribute pressure to the metatarsal shaft and adjacent metatarsals. Orthotic devices can help provide long-term relief by allowing consistent pressure relief as the athlete's shoe wear changes. Attention to proper training techniques and increasing the variety of workouts can have a positive impact on the condition.

Surgical treatment is considered only when the conservative methods have been completely exhausted. Invasive methods to relieve metatarsalgia can cause transfer lesions to develop underneath the adjacent metatarsal heads. The ideal surgical procedure should relieve pressure beneath the symptomatic metatarsal head but not completely eliminate its ability to absorb stress and equalize the contact pressure across the forefoot. Malunion and nonunion are risks of performing complete metatarsal osteotomies without internal fixation. Mann and DuVries (54) advocated plantar condylectomy, which removes the plantar one fourth of the metatarsal head. Alternatively, distal oblique osteotomy (55) and proximal closing wedge metatarsal osteotomy (56) may be used to treat metatarsalgia resulting from intractable plantar keratosis. Athletic activity is generally allowed after clinical and radiographic healing is present.

Interdigital Neuromas

Morton (57) popularized the concept that paroxysmal pain resulting from irritation of the interdigital plantar nerve contributed to metatarsalgia. He described the third web space between the third and fourth metatarsal heads as a transition point between the medial (rigid) and lateral columns (mobile) of the foot that subjected the interdigital plantar nerve to chronic mechanical irritation (Fig. 52.8).

The athlete with an interdigital neuroma will typically complain of paroxysmal forefoot pain. The neuralgia can be accompanied by parasthesias into the web space and toes. Typically, the third web space is involved, followed by the second.

Clinical Examination

The lower extremities should be evaluated for any signs of radiculopathy, muscle atrophy, and weakness. Bilateral symptoms may suggest a proximal source of neuropathy symptoms. The MP joints should be evaluated for instability or synovitis, which are important in the differential diagnosis (58). Palpation of the painful interspace typically elicits symptoms. Mulder (59) described a diagnostic sign of neuroma that is elicited with compression of the adjacent metacarpal heads, producing a painful click. Diagnostic injection of an anesthetic agent into the suspected interdigital space can be useful in confirming the diagnosis (60,61).

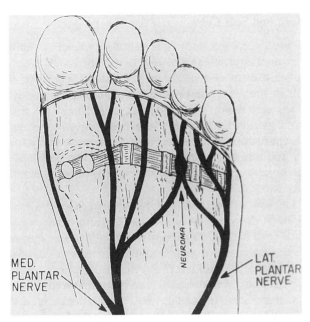

FIG. 52.8. The anatomy of the forefoot in the plane of the medial and lateral plantar nerves. The common digital nerve trunk in the third web pace is most commonly involved. It is bounded medially and laterally by metatarsal heads and superiorly by the intermetatarsal ligament. (From Kelikian H. *Hallux valgus: allied deformities of the forefoot and metatarsalgia.* Philadelphia: W.B. Saunders, 1965, with permission.)

(45). A long second ray has been associated with the disorder in athletes (65). Kelikian considered shoe wear and the impact of the long second ray in the toe box of the shoe as a causative factor, specifically in the hammertoe deformity observed in the second toe (45).

Metatarsophalangeal synovitis is observed commonly in the fifth decade of life (45,65,66). Hallux valgus was present in approximately 20% of cases in one series (62) and is consistent with the finding that abnormal contact pressures in the hallux is a causative factor in developing transfer stress to the adjacent metatarsals. The differential diagnosis includes interdigital neuroma, particularly with symptoms localizing to the second web space, and stress fracture of the metatarsal (45).

Clinical Evaluation

Diagnosis of MTP synovitis can be challenging for the clinician. Localizing the area of pain can be useful, with particular attention to the capsule of the suspected joint. The source of the interdigital pain can be difficult to diagnose. A history of paroxysmal pain and parasthesias involving the toes is indicative of a symptomatic neuroma and is helpful in differentiating this disorder from synovitis. An anterior drawer test will often elicit symptoms of pain and signs of instability (Fig. 52.9) (67).

Treatment

Conservative care includes shoe modification with a metatarsal pad and activity modification. Activity that exacerbates the pain should be discontinued on a trial basis. Corticosteroid injection may be considered (62).

Surgical treatment involves resection of the symptomatic common digital plantar nerve, typically done through a dorsal longitudinal incision. Transection of the deep transverse metatarsal ligament should be avoided (60). Circumferential compression of the forefoot is carried out for 6 weeks after surgery to allow healing of the deep transverse metatarsal ligament, and activity is increased according to symptoms (60). Mann and Reynolds (63) described a series of 56 patients with symptomatic interdigital neuromas occurring equally in both the second and third web space and reported improvement after excision in 80% of the cases.

Metatarsophalangeal Joint Synovitis

The second MP joint is prone to capsular disruption and instability (45,64–67). Pain, inflammation, and swelling characterize the disorder that primarily involves the second MP joint. This disorder is less frequently observed in the first and third MTP joints. Chronic symptoms can result in hammering, medial and sometimes lateral toe angulation, and subluxation of the involved MP joint

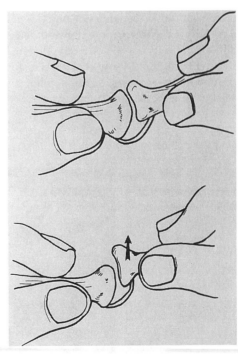

FIG. 52.9. The Thompson-Hamilton test for assessing metatarsophalangeal joint instability. The test is performed by stabilizing the metatarsal head and proximal phalanx of the toe. The thumb is used to apply dorsal pressure to the toe. Symptoms of pain are typically reproduced when instability is present. Laxity in the dorsal-plantar plane can be appreciated by the clinician. (From *Orthop Clin* 1989;20:535–551, with permission.)

Passive flexion at the symptomatic joint can cause significant pain. The clinical diagnosis can be difficult to make when normal toe alignment is present. Gradual deviation of the second toe in the medial and later the dorsal direction confirms the diagnosis of metatarsophalangeal synovitis. The possibility of an inflammatory arthritis should be considered. Diagnostic injection with a local anesthetic can be helpful in distinguishing interdigital neuroma from synovitis early in the disorder.

Routine weight-bearing AP, lateral, and oblique radiographs of the foot help to objectively evaluate the symptomatic joint. Symptoms present in the adolescent may be indicative of Freiberg infarction, which can be confirmed with radiographs.

Treatment

Conservative care involves taping the flexible toe in a neutral position (Fig. 52.10). Using the adjacent toe as a splint with adhesive taping can also be useful in alleviating symptoms (64,68). A well-positioned metatarsal pad promotes flexion at the MTP joint can serve to augment the effect of taping. When conservative measures, including activity modification, have been exhausted, surgical intervention is considered.

Open reduction at the metatarsophalangeal joint, with medial collateral ligament release and lateral ligament reconstruction, is recommended by Coughlin (64). In patients with a flexible hyperextension deformity of the MTP joint, extensor tendon lengthening and a Girdlestone-Taylor long flexor tendon transfer to the extensor tendon are performed. Progression to normal activity is begun 6 weeks postoperatively.

Hard and Soft Corns

A hard corn develops at a callous, typically over the proximal interphalangeal joint of the fifth toe. Soft corns develop most commonly on the lateral aspect of the fourth toe, over the proximal phalanx lateral condyle, at the metatarsophalangeal joint. Both conditions result from pressure caused by adjacent bony prominences. The hard corn forms in response to direct pressure from the toe box of the shoe, and the soft corn develops in response to pressure from the adjacent condyle of the fifth toe.

Clinical evaluation reveals hypertrophic epidermal tissue in the symptomatic areas. The appearance of the hard corn is characteristic of a typical callous. The soft corn may have a macerated appearance. Standard weight-bearing radiographs of the foot help to confirm the diagnosis and delineate the bony relationships.

Conservative treatment includes modification of the shoe wear. A ball and ring stretching device can help in relieving external pressure resulting from shoe wear. A shoe with adequate width and depth in the toe box recommended. A hard corn can be shaved with a scalpel. A doughnut-shaped pad can be placed over the hard corn to reduce local pressure. Padding placed in the web space is similarly used to reduce pressure over the soft corn.

Operative treatment for hard corns includes resection of the prominent lateral condyle at the PIP joint of the fifth toe (46). A lateral condylectomy of the proximal phalanx is recommended for surgical decompression of the soft corn (69). Care should be taken to repair the lateral collateral ligament to prevent joint subluxation. Return to athletic activity is indicated by clinical symptoms. Alternative approaches include partial proximal phalangectomy with syndactilization (45).

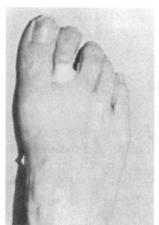 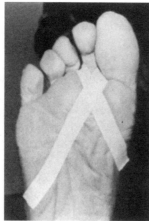

FIG. 52.10. Flexible deformity of the toe can be splinted using tape. The technique places a plantar directed force on the proximal phalanx to hold the toe in corrected position and allow healing. (From *Orthop Clin* 1989;20:535–551, with permission.)

REFERENCES

1. Garrick JG, Requa RK. The epidemiology of foot and ankle injuries in sports. *Clin Sports Med* 1988;7:29–36.
2. Bowers KD Jr, Martin RB. Turf-toe: a shoe-surface related football injury. *Med Sci Sports Exerc* 1976;8:81–83.
3. Coker TP, Arnold JA, Weber DL. Traumatic lesions of the metatarsophalangeal joint of the great toe in athletes. *Am J Sports Med* 1978;6:326–334.
4. Bonstingl RW, Morehouse CA, Niebel BW. Torques developed by different types of shoes on various playing surfaces. *Med Sci Sports* 1975;7:127–131.
5. Mueller FO, Blyth CS. North Carolina high school football injury study: equipment and prevention. *J Sports Med* 1974;2:1–10.
6. Nigg BM, Segesser B. The influence of playing surfaces on the locomotor system and on football and tennis injuries. *Sports Med* 1988;5:375–385.
7. Torg JS, Quedenfeld TC, Landau S. The shoe-surface interface and its relationship to football knee injuries. *J Sports Med* 1974;2:261–269.
8. Lillich JS, Baxter DE. Common forefoot problems in runners. *Foot Ankle* 1986;7:145–151.
9. Morton DJ. *The human foot. Its evolution, physiology and functional disorders.* New York: Columbia University Press, 1935.
10. Chapman MW. Fractures and fracture-dislocations of the ankle

and foot. In: Mann RA, ed. *DuVries' surgery of the foot,* 4th ed. St. Louis: Mosby-Year Book, 1978.

11. Blodgett WH. Injuries of the forefoot and toes. In: Jahss MH, ed. *Disorders of the foot.* Vol. 2. Philadelphia: W.B. Saunders, 1982.

12. Giannstras NJ, Sammarco GJ. Fractures and dislocations of the foot. In: Rockwood CA Jr, Green DP, eds. *Fractures.* Vol. 2. Philadelphia: J.B. Lippincott, 1975.

13. Guly HR. Fractures of the terminal phalanx presenting as paronychia. *Arch Emerg Med* 1993;10:301–305.

14. Hamilton WG. Foot and ankle injuries in dancers. In: Mann RA, Coughlin MJ, eds. *Surgery of the foot and ankle,* 6th ed. Vol. 2. St. Louis: Mosby, 1993:1245.

15. Jones P. Fatigue failure osteochondral fracture of the proximal phalanx of the great toe. *Am J Sports Med* 1987;15:616–618.

16. Fugate DS, Thompson JD, Christensen KP. An irreducible fracture-dislocation of a lesser toe: case report. *Foot Ankle* 1991; 11:317–318.

17. Yokoe K, Mannoji T. Stress fractures of the proximal phalanx of the great toe. A report of three cases. *Am J Sports Med* 1986;14:240–242.

18. Rang M. Foot. In: *Children's fractures,* 2nd ed. Philadelphia: J.B. Lippincott, 1983:215.

19. Shiraishi M, Mizuta H, Kubota K, et al. Stress fracture of the proximal phalanx of the great toe. *Foot Ankle* 1993;14:28–34.

20. DeLee JC. Fractures of the phalanges. In: Mann RA, Coughlin MJ, eds. *Surgery of the foot and ankle.* Vol. 2. Philadelphia: W.B. Saunders, 1982.

21. Noonan KJ, Saltzman CL, Dietz FR. Open physeal fractures of the distal phalanx of the great toe: a case report. *J Bone Joint Surg Am* 1994;76A:122–125.

22. Jahss MH. Chronic and recurrent dislocations of the fifth toe. *Foot Ankle* 1981;1:275–278.

23. Jahss MH. Traumatic dislocations of the first metatarsophalangeal joint. *Foot Ankle* 1980;1:15–21.

24. Wolfe J, Goodhart C. Irreducible dislocation of the great toe following a sports injury. A case report. *Am J Sports Med* 1989;17:695–696.

25. Eibel P. Dislocation of the interphalangeal joint of the big toe with interposition of a sesamoid bone. *J Bone Joint Surg Am* 1954;36A:880–882.

26. Katayama M, Murakami Y, Takahashi H. Irreducible dorsal dislocation of the toe. Report of thre cases. *J Bone Joint Surg Am* 1988;70A:769–770.

27. Lewis AG, DeLee JC. Type-I complex dislocation of the first metatarsophalangeal joint—reduction through a dorsal approach. A case report. *J Bone Joint Surg Am* 1984;66A:1120–1123.

28. Mann RA. *Surgery of the foot,* 5th ed. St. Louis: C.V. Mosby, 1986:1702.

29. Clanton TO, Butler JE, Eggert A. Injuries to the metatarsophalangeal joints in athletes. *Foot Ankle* 1986;7:162–176.

30. Clanton TO, Ford JJ. Turf toe injury. *Clin Sports Med* 1994;13:731–741.

31. Giannikas AC, Papachristou G, Papavasiliou N. Dorsal dislocation of the first metatarso-phalangeal joint. *J Bone Joint Surg Br* 1975;57B:384–386.

32. Sammarco GJ. Biomechanics of the foot. In: Frankel VH, Nordin M, eds. *Basic biomechanics of the skeletal system.* Philadelphia: Lea & Febiger, 1980:192–219.

33. Nigg BM. Biomechanical aspects of running. In: Nigg BM, ed. *Biomechanics of running shoes.* Champaign, IL: Human Kinetics, 1986:1–25.

34. Frey C, Anderson GD, Feder KS. Plantarflexion injury to the metatarsophalangeal joint ("sand toe"). *Foot Ankle Int* 1996;17:576–581.

35. Sarrafian SK. *Anatomy of the foot and ankle: descriptive, topographic, functional.* Philadelphia: J.B. Lippincott, 1993:91.

36. Chamberland PD, Smith JW, Fleming LL. The blood supply to the great toe sesamoids. *Foot Ankle* 1993;14:435–444.

37. Rodeo SA, Warren RF, O'Brien SJ, et al. Diastasis of bipartite sesamoids of the first metatarsophalangeal joint. *Foot Ankle* 1993;14:425–434.

38. Davies-Colley N. Contraction of the metatarsophalangeal joint of the great toe (hallux flexus). *BMJ* 1887;1:728.

39. Kile TA. Hallux rigidus. Athletic injuries of the foot and ankle: practical surgical strategies. AAOS Course Syllabus, April 11–13, 1997.

40. Hattrup SJ, Johnson KA. Subjective results of hallux rigidus following treatment with cheilectomy. *Clin Orthop* 1988;226: 182–191.

41. Mann RA, Clanton T. Hallux rigidus: treatment by cheilectomy. *J Bone Joint Surg Am* 1988;70A:400–406.

42. Mann RA, Coughlin MJ, DuVries HL. Hallux rigidus: a review of the literature and a method of treatment. *Clin Orthop* 1979;142:57–63.

43. Moberg E. A simple operation for hallux rigidus. *Clin Orthop* 1979;142:55–56.

44. Pfeffer GB. Cheilectomy. In: Johnson KA, ed. *The foot and ankle.* New York: Raven Press 1994.

45. Kelikian H. Deformities of the lesser toes. In: Kelikian H, ed. *Hallux valgus: allied deformities of the forefoot and metatarsalgia.* Philadelphia: W.B. Saunders, 1965.

46. Coughlin MJ. Lesser toe deformities. In: Mann RA, Coughlin MJ, eds. *Surgery of the foot and ankle,* 6th ed. St. Louis: C.V. Mosby, 1993.

47. Mann R, Hagy J. Function of the toes in walking, jogging and running. *Clin Orthop* 1979;142:24–29.

48. Garth WP Jr, Miller ST. Evaluation of claw toe deformity, weakness of the foot intrinsics, and posteromedial shin pain. *Am J Sports Med* 1989;17:821–827.

49. Barbari SG, Brevig K. Correction of claw toes by the Girdlestone-Taylor flexor-extensor transfer procedure. *Foot Ankle* 1984;5: 67–73.

50. Taylor RG. The treatment of claw toes by multiple transfers of flexor into extensor tendons. *J Bone Joint Surg Br* 1951;33B: 539–542.

51. Myerson MS, Shereff MJ. The pathological anatomy of claw and hammer toes. *J Bone Joint Surg Am* 1989;71A:45–49.

52. Rau FD, Manoli A 2nd. Traumatic boutonniere deformity as a cause of acute hammer toe: a case report. *Foot Ankle* 1991;11: 231–232.

53. Coughlin MJ. Operative repair of the mallet toe deformity. *Foot Ankle* 1995;16:109–116.

54. Mann RA, DuVries HL. Intractable plantar keratosis. *Orthop Clin North Am* 1973;4:67–73.

55. Pedowitz WJ. Distal oblique osteotomy for intractable plantar keratosis of the middle three metatarsals. *Foot Ankle* 1988;9:7–9.

56. Giannestras NJ. Shortening of the metatarsal shaft in the treatment of plantar keratosis. *J Bone Joint Surg Am* 1958;40A:61–71.

57. Morton TG. A peculiar and painful affection of the fourth metatarsophalangeal articulation. *Am J Med Sci* 1876;71:35–45.

58. Coughlin MJ. Soft tissue afflictions. In: Chapman M, ed. *Operative orthopaedics.* Philadelphia: J.B. Lippincott, 1988:1819.

59. Mulder JD. The causative mechanism in Morton's metatarsalgia. *J Bone Joint Surg Br* 1951;33B:94–95.

60. Coughlin MJ. Forefoot disorders. In: Baxter D, ed. *The foot and ankle in sport.* St. Louis: Mosby Year Book, 1995:231.

61. Greenfield J, Rea J Jr, Illfeld TW. Morton's interdigital neuroma: indications for treatment by local injections versus surgery. *Clin Orthop* 1984;185:142–144.

62. Rasmussen MR, Kitaoka HB, Patzer GI. Nonoperative treatment of plantar interdigital neuroma with a single corticosteroid injection. *Clin Orthop* 1996;326:188–193.

63. Mann RA, Reynolds JC. Interdigital neuroma—a critical clinical analysis. *Foot Ankle* 1983;3:238–243.

64. Coughlin MJ. Second metatarsophalangeal instability in the athlete. *Foot Ankle* 1993;14:309–319.

65. Goldner JL, Ward WG. Traumatic horizontal deviation of the second toe: mechanism of deformity, diagnosis and treatment. *Bull Hosp Jt Dis* 1987;47:123–125.

66. Mann RA, Mizel MS. Monarticular nontraumatic synovitis of the metatarsophalangeal joint: a new diagnosis? *Foot Ankle* 1985; 6:18–21.

67. Thompson FM, Hamilton WG. Problems of the second metatarsophalangeal joint. *Orthopaedics* 1987;10:83–89.

68. Smith RW, Reischl SF. Metatarsophalangeal joint synovitis in athletes. *Clin Sports Med* 1988;7:75–88.

69. Manwaring JGR. Corns, hammer-toes and bunions. *J Mich Med Soc* 1930;29:497–499.

Principles and Practice of Orthopaedic Sports Medicine,
edited by William E. Garrett, Jr., Kevin P. Speer, and Donald T. Kirkendall.
Lippincott Williams & Wilkins, Philadelphia © 2000.

CHAPTER 53

The Foot and Ankle Tendons

Roger A. Mann, Mark M. Casillas, and Michael J. Coughlin

ACHILLES TENDON

The gastrocnemius muscle originates from the medial and lateral femoral condyles and the popliteal surface of the femur (1). The soleus muscle originates from the posterior aspect of the upper third of the fibula, the soleal line on the tibia, and the fibrous arch between the tibia and fibula. The two muscles produce a common tendon, the Achilles tendon, which inserts into the inferior half of the posterior tuberosity of the calcaneus. The tendon measures 5 to 6 mm in thickness at the level of the ankle (2). Although the tendon does not have an accompanying synovial sheath, it is surrounded by a fibrous covering, paratenon, derived from the crural fascia. A synovial-lined bursa may be present anterior to the tendon, the retrocalcaneal bursa, or posterior to the tendon in a subcutaneous position, the retro-Achilles tendon bursa (3). Frey et al. (4) further delineated the anatomy of the retrocalcaneal bursa with bursography.

The gastrosoleus complex is a stance-phase muscle that acts primarily to decelerate the body as it passes over the foot. Eccentric contraction of the posterior calf muscles begins at 20% of the walking cycle, allowing controlled dorsiflexion of the ankle. This continues up to 40% of the walking cycle when plantar flexion of the ankle begins and the activity of the gastrosoleus complex becomes concentric. Curiously, although plantar flexion of the ankle continues until toe-off, the electrical activity of the gastrosoleus complex ceases at 50% of the walking cycle. It has been demonstrated that toe-off is a passive rather than an active event. In contrast, during steady

state running or acceleration (speed or direction change), toe-off is an active event (5).

The classification of Achilles tendon dysfunction is complicated by a bewildering number of terms that are applied inconsistently throughout the literature. In this section we address the most common types of Achilles tendon dysfunction using nomenclature based on anatomic and pathologic criteria: paratenonitis, tendinosis, partial or complete rupture, and retrocalcaneal inflammation. Paratenonitis is an inflammatory process limited to the paratenon without concomitant changes within the adjacent tendon. Tendinosis is an age-related degenerative process within the tendon substance that probably represents a precursor to partial or complete rupture. Retrocalcaneal inflammation is characterized by inflammation of the retrocalcaneal bursa that may or may not be associated with paratenonitis of the adjacent Achilles tendon.

Epidemiology

Dysfunction of the Achilles tendon is a common complaint among athletic individuals. One report followed 50 female gymnasts for a 1-year period; 8 of the 147 injuries were attributed to the Achilles tendon. One of these injuries had an acute onset, and seven had a gradual onset (6). The prevalence of Achilles paratenonitis varies among activities and reports. One report identified 109 cases (6.0%) among 1,650 runners that presented to a running clinic over a 2-year period (7). Among dance students, Achilles tendinitis or tendinosis accounted for 33 of the 352 injuries that occurred in an 8-month period among 185 dance students (8).

Mechanism of Injury and Pathoanatomy

Paratenonitis

Inflammation of the paratenon can typically be related to training errors or mechanical factors. Training errors

R. A. Mann: Foot and Ankle Fellowship, Oakland, California.

M. M. Casillas: Orthopaedic Surgeon, Orthopaedic Surgery Associates of San Antonio, San Antonio, Texas.

M. J. Coughlin: Staff Orthopaedic Surgeon, St. Alphonsus Regional Medical Center, Boise, Idaho.

include overuse, ineffective stretching, and ineffective warm-up period. Mechanical factors include excessive foot pronation, tight gastrosoleus motor unit, or faulty shoe wear. Impingement of the heel counter against the Achilles during plantarflexion may contribute to mechanical irritation of the surrounding soft tissues. Among 201 cases of surgically treated paratenonitis, each was found to have a thickened paratenon with fibrous adhesions extending to the tendon (9).

Tendinosis and Rupture

Intratendinous injuries, including tendinosis and rupture, are caused by intrinsic degeneration of the tendon substance, which tend to be age related (10). Åstrom and Rausing (10) performed histologic examination of tendon obtained from 163 patients with chronic Achilles tendinosis. They demonstrated abnormal fiber structure, focal hypercellularity, and vascular proliferation. Inflammatory cells were not present. Vascular studies have demonstrated an area of hypovascularity between 2 and 6 cm from the tendon insertion (11). This is the same region that is vulnerable to tendinosis and rupture. Arner and Lindholm (12) found three different mechanisms leading to rupture: push-off with the foot while extending the knee, sudden and unexpected dorsiflexion of the ankle, and violent dorsiflexion of the plantarflexed ankle.

Retrocalcaneal Inflammation

An enlarged or hyperconvex superior tuberosity of the calcaneus, Haglund's deformity, may predispose the Achilles tendon to injury just proximal to its insertion (13).

Clinical Evaluation

Patients with Achilles tendon dysfunction offer a history of pain along the course of the tendon. The type of pain, mode (acute vs. insidious) and date of onset of symptoms, type and level of athletic activity, type of shoe wear, and details regarding previous treatment are solicited. Physical examination of patients with Achilles tendon dysfunction includes gait analysis, a single heel rise test, and evaluation of the leg with the patient both standing and sitting.

The standing patient is examined from each side and from behind. Subtle swelling and defects in the contour of the Achilles tendon and surrounding tissues can be noted and compared with the well extremity. Calf atrophy may also be visualized or quantified with a tape measure.

The single heel rise test is performed with the patient facing a wall and standing approximately 12 inches from its base. The well leg is tested first by asking the patient to stand on the well leg with the symptomatic foot off the ground. The patient may use both hands to obtain stability against the wall. The patient then rises onto the toes of the well leg and slowly returns to the plantigrade position. The maneuver is repeated up to 10 times. The examiner notes the height of the heel rise and the degree of heel inversion. Next, the symptomatic leg is tested. A positive test includes pain over the course of the Achilles tendon, decrease in height, or inability to perform the heel rise.

Palpation of the entire posterior leg must be performed systematically. Proximal tenderness over the medial head of the gastrocnemius muscle suggests injury of that structure. Tenderness along the posterior medial border of the tibia suggests periostitis or stress fracture. Tenderness of the posterior calf musculature after exertion suggests compartment syndrome. Pain and swelling of the posterior–medial distal leg may be associated with an accessory soleus muscle (14). Tenderness of the posterior tuberosity of the calcaneus in the skeletally immature patient suggests Sever's disease (epiphysitis of the os calcis).

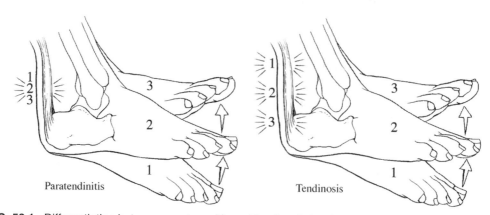

FIG. 53.1. Differentiation between paratenonitis and tendinosis by physical exam. As the foot is placed through a range of motion, the location of tenderne does not vary in the case of paratenonitis and does vary in the case of tendinosis.

Paratenonitis

Patients complain of pain over the Achilles tendon aggravated with activity. Examination reveals an antalgic gait; painful single heel rise; full strength of the gastrosoleus motor unit; and localized swelling, warmth, crepitus, and tenderness of the soft tissues surrounding the tendon. The location of tenderness does not change with the ankle in varying degrees of flexion (15) (Fig. 53.1).

Tendinosis

Achilles tendinosis is suggested by an antalgic gait; weakness when attempting to perform a single heel rise; decreased strength of the gastrosoleus motor unit; and localized or generalized thickening, warmth, and tenderness of the tendon. The location of tenderness changes with the ankle in varying degrees of flexion (Fig. 53.1). It is somewhat useful to consider patients with insertional tendinosis separately from those with more proximal tendon involvement.

Insertional tendon degeneration may be generalized or localized. Patients with localized degenerative changes are able to pinpoint the exact location of pain and tenderness on the Achilles insertion. The swelling is much less pronounce and typically confined to a small area. The patient is able to perform the single heel rise, although this may be painful. Patients with generalized degenerative changes demonstrate global swelling, warmth, and tenderness at the tendon insertion. These patients are unable to perform more than one or two single heel rises due to pain.

Rupture

Tendinosis may progress to rupture, either partial or complete. The patient complains of sudden pain in the calf or over the Achilles tendon, possibly associated with a pop or snap. The patient often notes a loss of power with active push-off or stair climbing. Squeezing the calf at midsubstance, the Thompson test (16), should produce plantarflexion of the foot. Failure of the midcalf squeeze to produce plantarflexion of the foot is considered a positive test and diagnostic for a complete rupture. Rupture of the Achilles tendon may produce a palpable defect; this defect may occur anywhere between the musculotendinous junction and the insertion.

Retrocalcaneal Inflammation

Tenderness and swelling just anterior to the Achilles tendon at the level of the superior tuberosity of the calcaneus is diagnostic for retrocalcaneal bursitis. Occasionally, the swollen bursa is palpable. This condition is typically not associated with degenerative changes at the adjacent Achilles tendon.

Imaging

Diagnostic imaging of the patient with symptoms related to the Achilles tendon begins with a weight-bearing plain radiographic lateral view of the foot. Intratendinous calcification is easily seen but not a common finding. Patients with localized insertional tendinosis may demonstrate calcification corresponding to the area of pain and tenderness. An enlarged or hyperconvex superior tuberosity of the calcaneus is noted. Magnetic resonance imaging (MRI) is the most useful diagnostic tool for imaging the Achilles tendon. The study may be of use in the treatment of patients with paratenonitis by delineating the extent of concomitant tendinosis. Tendinosis is confirmed by increased activity on T2 within the tendon itself; cystic changes, loss of a homogenous tendon signal, or loss of normal contours, such as localized thickening, are easily visualized. The ability to delineate the extent of disease within the tendon (staging) is our most common indication for obtaining this study. The presence of linear tears and incomplete or complete disruptions are also well demonstrated and differentiated by this modality. Computed tomography (CT) is useful in delineating the location of calcium deposits in patients with localized insertional tendinosis. This information would be useful only in preparation for surgical debridement.

Scintigraphy is used only to rule in stress fracture or tibial periostitis when these diagnoses are suggested by the clinical history and examination.

Frey et al. (4) suggested that bursography of the retrocalcaneal bursa may be used to differentiating retrocalcaneal bursitis from Achilles paratendinitis. The true utility of such an examination has not been demonstrated.

Economic Considerations

The clinical history and examination provide enough information for confident diagnosis of Achilles tendon dysfunction. MRI of the Achilles tendon is a staging study and should not be used as a screening test. CT and scintigraphy are not used for evaluation of the Achilles tendon.

Treatment of Injury

Paratenonitis and Tendinosis

Nonoperative

The initial treatment of acute pain related to paratenonitis or tendinosis is rest, ice application, and nonsteroidal anti-inflammatory medication (NSAID) therapy. Shoe modifications include lowering or softening the heel counter, adding a soft heel wedge, or the incorporation of an orthotic to resist excessive pronation. When symptoms fail to subside after 7 to 10 days of initial therapy or when symptoms are severe, the treatment must include enforced rest with a weight-bearing cast or removable cast boot.

Rehabilitation. Once the initial symptoms have subsided, stretching of the gastrosoleus motor unit must take precedent. Stretching is most effectively accomplished by standing 2 feet from a wall, balancing against the wall with both hands, separating both feet, and simultaneously internally rotating the feet 20 degrees. From this position the patient leans to the wall while maintaining the feet in a plantigrade position. The internal rotation of the feet is an important feature of this routine because it locks the transverse tarsal joint, thus preventing dorsiflexion through the midfoot. Training errors must be sought and corrected. A decrease in intensity or frequency of activity or cross-training may alleviate symptoms.

When to Refer. Patients with symptoms that fail to respond to a 6-week course of immobilization are referred to an orthopedic surgeon.

Surgical

Patients with Achilles paratenonitis that have failed an adequate course of conservative care and immobilization may require release of the thickened fibrous sheath (9,17). The tendon is also inspected and degenerative areas treated appropriately. Kvist and Kvist (9) reported 169 excellent, 25 good, and 7 poor results in a series of 201 cases of surgically treated for paratenonitis. Their approach differed from ours in that they began motion immediately after surgery. Rarely is this surgical intervention indicated because patients with this condition consistently respond to well-supervised nonoperative therapy.

Debridement of Achilles Paratenonitis. Under general anesthesia and tourniquet control, a longitudinal incision is made parallel to and 1.5 to 2 cm anterior to the medial border of the Achilles tendon. Sharp dissection is immediately directed to the Achilles tendon and the exposure of the tendon made between full-thickness flaps. The soft tissue must be managed with extreme caution because this area is predisposed to skin slough and wound breakdown. The paratenon is incised, and areas that appear to have inflammatory or degenerative changes are excised. The tendon is systematically inspected. Simple tears are directly repaired with a running 3-0 or 4-0 polydioxanone, PDS (Ethicon, Inc., Wayne, NJ), or nylon suture. If degenerative changes are significant, then reconstructive procedures such as those described below should be considered. No attempt is made to close the paratenon. The subcutaneous tissue is closed with absorbable suture and the skin closed with nylon or skin clips. A large

bulky dressing is placed with the foot and ankle in a neutral position. Plaster splints are added for immobilization.

After 10 days sutures are removed, weight bearing in a cast boot is allowed, and range of motion and strengthening with an elastic band is instituted. Immobilization is continued until complete resolution of the warmth and swelling adjacent to the tendon. Return to full activity is expected within 3 to 4 months.

Patients with Achilles tendinosis that have failed an adequate course of immobilization may require exploration of the degenerative tendon. If the area of degeneration is limited (less than 2 cm^2), then the plantaris tendon is weaved through the degenerative area. Using this technique the tendon is not compromised and the degenerative area is strengthened and a healing response stimulated by the local trauma. Eight of 10 patients we managed with a plantaris tendon weave had a successful result. If a large area of tendon is involved in the degenerative process, then a debridement of all compromised tendon is performed and a reconstructive procedure is performed. The reconstructive procedure combines transfer of the flexor hallucis longus tendon or the flexor digitorum longus tendon into the posterior superior calcaneus with advancement or turn-down of the Achilles tendon for a direct repair.

Reconstruction of Achilles Tendinosis with the Plantaris Tendon. Under general anesthesia and tourniquet control, a longitudinal incision is made parallel to and 1.5 to 2 cm anterior to the medial border of the Achilles tendon. Sharp dissection is immediately directed to the Achilles tendon and the exposure of the tendon made between full-thickness flaps. The soft tissue must be managed with extreme caution because it is predisposed to skin slough and wound breakdown. The paratenon is incised, and areas that appear to have inflammatory or degenerative changes are excised. The tendon is systematically inspected. If degenerative changes are significant, then reconstructive procedures such as those described below should be considered. If the degenerative changes within the tendon are limited, then a plantaris tendon weave is performed. The plantaris is located just adjacent to the medial aspect of the Achilles tendon. The tendon is harvested with the aid of a tendon stripper. A small incision is used for proximal exposure and release of the tendon. The distal insertion of the plantaris tendon is left intact. The tendon is woven through the degenerative section of Achilles tendon. This process is facilitated by passing a loop of 22-gauge wire through a large Mayo needle. The plantaris tendon is placed within the loop. As the needle is passed through the Achilles tendon, the wire and plantaris tendon follow. After the plantaris tendon has been passed through the degenerative section, it is secured to the Achilles tendon with a single nylon suture. No attempt is made to close the paratenon. The subcutaneous tissue is closed with absorbable suture and the skin closed with nylon or skin clips. A large bulky dressing is placed with the foot and ankle in a neutral position. Plaster splints are added for immobilization.

If the plantaris tendon is not present, a strip of the Achilles tendon may be harvested and woven through the Achilles as described above.

The sutures are removed at 10 days. The leg is maintained in a non–weight-bearing cast for 4 weeks followed by a removable cast boot for an additional 4 weeks. During the second 4 weeks, the patient is allowed to begin progressive weight bearing and to remove the cast for scheduled range of motion exercises of the foot and ankle. Once motion is reestablished, low resistance exercises with an elastic band are started. Localized areas of tendon swelling will not completely resolve but typically become pain free. The patient is allowed to resume unrestricted activity when local warmth and tenderness have completely resolved (3 to 6 months).

Debridement and Reconstruction of Achilles Tendinosis with the Flexor Hallucis Longus Tendon. Under general anesthesia and tourniquet control, a longitudinal incision is made parallel to and 1.5 to 2 cm anterior to the medial border of the Achilles tendon. Sharp dissection is immediately directed to the Achilles tendon and the exposure of the tendon made between full-thickness flaps. The soft tissue must be managed with extreme caution because this area is predisposed to skin slough and wound breakdown. The paratenon is incised, and areas that appear to have inflammatory or degenerative changes are excised. The tendon is systematically inspected. Degenerative areas are sharply excised. If the remaining tendon has been functionally compromised, then a reconstructive procedure should be performed.   The flexor hallucis longus tendon is harvested through a medial incision in which the abductor hallucis muscle is retracted in a plantar direction, allowing visualization of the plantar digital nerves and the flexor digitorum longus and the flexor hallucis longus tendons. While protecting the nerves, the flexor knot of Henry is released and the flexor hallucis longus tendon is released from all fascial connections that can be seen through the exposure. Next, the flexor hallucis longus tendon is tenodesed to the flexor digitorum longus tendon with no. 2 nonabsorbable suture. The tenodesis is placed as far distal as possible. The flexor hallucis longus tendon is divided just proximal to the tenodesis. The free end of the tendon is then pulled into the proximal exposure. A one-quarter–inch drill is used to make two drill holes through the superior tuberosity of the calcaneus. The holes, one through the medial surface and directed lateral and the second through the superior surface and directed inferior, are connected at their intersection. The distal end of the flexor hallucis longus tendon is secured with two no. 2 nonabsorbable suture. A suture

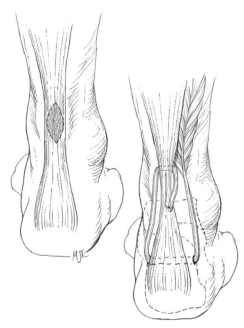

FIG. 53.2. Debridement and reconstruction of the Achilles tendon with the flexor hallucis longus tendon. The shaded area represents the area tendinosis and debridement.

passer is passed through the superior drill hole and out the medial drill hole. The sutures on the free end of the flexor hallucis longus are used to pull the tendon through the superior calcaneal tuberosity (Fig. 53.2). The foot is placed in a plantarflexed position, and the flexor hallucis longus tendon is then carefully placed under tension. The tension must approximate the tension of the contralateral Achilles tendon. The flexor hallucis longus is then sutured to itself with nonabsorbable suture. The reconstruction is further reinforced with the plantaris tendon if it is available. The tendon is weaved between the proximal and distal ends of the Achilles tendon. If the plantaris is not available, then the Achilles may be advanced onto itself by one of two methods: a turndown of the central one third of the tendon or by a V-Y advancement at the musculotendinous junction. The advanced section of the Achilles tendon is secured to the distal tendon with multiple interrupted no. 0 sutures. The subcutaneous tissue is closed with absorbable suture and the skin closed with nylon or skin clips. A large bulky dressing is placed with the foot and ankle in a plantarflexed position to reduce tension on the repair and the overlying skin. Plaster splints are added for immobilization.

The sutures are removed at 10 days. Depending on the condition of the skin, the foot is gradually brought to a neutral position between the second and fourth postoperative weeks. The leg is maintained in a non–weight-bearing cast for 4 weeks followed by a removable cast boot for 8 weeks. During the fifth week, the patient is allowed to begin range of motion exercises of the foot and ankle followed by low resistance exercises with an elastic band. Weight bearing is permitted after 12 weeks. The patient is allowed to resume unrestricted activity when local warmth and tenderness have completely resolved (6 to 9 months).

Ruptures

The ideal treatment of acute complete rupture of the Achilles tendon remains controversial. In a prospective randomized study conducted by Nistor (18), five ruptures occurred after nonsurgical treatment of 60 patients compared with two reruptures after surgical treatment of 45 patients. Nistor concluded that the results of both nonsurgical and surgical treatment appear to be uniformly good with only minor differences between the two groups. Nistor also reviewed 2,647 cases of surgically treated Achilles tendon rupture. The major complications included deep infection, 1%; fistulas, 3%; necrosis of skin or tendon or both, 2%; and rerupture, 2% (18). Inglis et al. (19) also reported that the rerupture rate for patients treated surgically is lower than for patients treated with cast immobilization; furthermore, the patients treated surgically were more satisfied with their results. It is our preference to treat patients with a primary surgical repair. These patients, in our experience, return to a higher level of performance earlier than patients treated with immobilization.

The treatment for chronic neglected rupture of the Achilles tendon is less controversial. Surgical repair or reconstruction is recommended for well-motivated and active individuals. If a secure reconstruction is not feasible with local tissue (Achilles tendon, plantaris tendon, V-Y advancement, or fascia turn down), then a tendon transfer can be added to the construct. The flexor hallucis longus (20), flexor digitorum longus (21), and peroneus brevis tendons (22) have each been used successfully. The addition of a functional motor unit may improve functional outcome. Reconstruction of chronic Achilles tendon rupture with the flexor hallucis longus tendon was successful in all seven patients treated by Wapner et al. (20). Similarly, Mann et al. (21) reported six excellent or good and one fair result after reconstruction of chronic rupture with the flexor digitorum longus tendon transfer.

Nonoperative

Patients with partial tears that do not compromise tendon function are treated with a non–weight-bearing gravity equinus cast for 4 weeks, followed by a weight-bearing cast for 4 to 8 weeks. Immobilization is discontinued when the tendon is nontender and the local warmth has subsided.

Patients with partial tears that compromise tendon function or complete tears are treated with either an equinus cast or operative repair, depending on the expectations and preference of the patient. Immobilization is discontinued when the tendon is nontender and the local warmth has subsided; the total amount of immobilization must be at least 8 weeks (23).

Rehabilitation. Once the initial symptoms have subsided, stretching of the gastrosoleus motor unit must take precedent. Stretching is most effectively accomplished by standing 2 feet from a wall, balancing against the wall with both hands, and simultaneously separating and internally rotating both feet. From this position the patient leans to the wall while maintaining the feet in a plantigrade position. The internal rotation of the feet is an important feature of this routine because it locks the transverse tarsal joint, thus preventing dorsiflexion through the midfoot. Training errors must be sought and corrected. A decrease in intensity or frequency of activity or cross-training may alleviate symptoms.

When to Refer. Patients with partial or complete and acute or chronic tears are referred to an orthopedic surgeon for supervision of the nonoperative treatment program.

Surgical

Primary Repair of Acute Achilles Tendon Rupture. Under general anesthesia and tourniquet control, a longitudinal incision is made parallel to and 1.5 to 2 cm anterior to the medial border of the Achilles tendon. Sharp dissection is immediately directed to the Achilles tendon and the exposure of the tendon made between full-thickness flaps. The soft tissue must be managed with extreme caution because this area is predisposed to skin slough and wound breakdown. The paratenon is incised, and areas that appear to have inflammatory or degenerative changes are excised. The tendon is systematically inspected, and blood clot from the rupture site is excised. The Achilles tendon is reapproximated and a primary repair performed (Fig. 53.3). A core suture, no. 3 nonabsorbable braided material, is used to reapproximate the tendon ends. Multiple peripheral sutures, no. 2-0 braided nonabsorbable, are used to complete the repair. If the plantaris is available, then it is woven through the repair site and secured with several no. 2-0 braided nonabsorbable sutures. If required, the Achilles may be advanced onto itself by one of two methods: a turn-down of the central one third of the tendon or a V-Y advancement at the musculotendinous junction. The advanced section of Achilles tendon is then secured to the distal tendon with multiple interrupted no. 0 sutures. No attempt is made to close the paratenon. The subcutaneous tissue is closed with absorbable suture and the skin closed with nylon or skin clips. A large bulky dressing is placed with the foot and ankle in plantarflexion in an attempt to remove tension

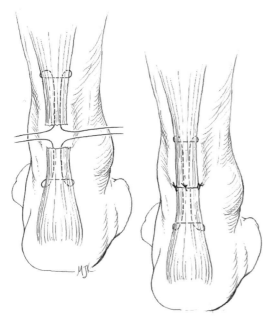

FIG. 53.3. Primary repair of acute Achilles tendon rupture with core suture.

from the repair and the overlying skin. Plaster splints are added for immobilization.

The skin sutures are removed at 10 days. A non–weight-bearing cast is used to gradually bring the ankle back to a neutral position during the initial postoperative month. A removable cast boot is placed at the fourth week, and the patient is allowed to begin range of motion exercises of the foot and ankle followed by low resistance exercises with an elastic band. Weight bearing is permitted after 8 weeks. The patient is allowed to resume unprotected weight bearing at 12 weeks and unrestricted activity when local warmth and tenderness have completely resolved (6 months).

An alternative rehabilitation program was proposed by Troop et al. (24) emphasizing early motion; passive and active motion started at an average of 10 and 23 days after surgery, respectively. Among 13 patients treated with open repair and early motion, 1 suffered a rerupture attributed to noncompliance with postoperative instructions.

Reconstruction of Chronic Neglected Achilles Tendon Rupture with the Flexor Hallucis Longus Tendon. Under general anesthesia and tourniquet control, a longitudinal incision is made parallel to and 1.5 to 2 cm anterior to the medial border of the Achilles tendon. Sharp dissection is immediately directed to the Achilles tendon and the exposure of the tendon made between full-thickness flaps. The soft tissue must be managed with extreme caution because this area is predisposed to skin slough and wound breakdown. The paratenon is incised, and areas that appear to have inflammatory or degenerative changes are excised. The tendon is sys-

tematically inspected. The tendon ends are debrided judiciously. The Achilles tendon is reapproximated and a primary repair performed if possible. A core suture, no. 3 nonabsorbable braided material, is used to reapproximate the tendon ends. Multiple peripheral sutures, no. 2-0 braided nonabsorbable, are used to complete the repair. If the plantaris is available, it is woven through the repair site and secured with several no. 2-0 braided nonabsorbable sutures. If required, the Achilles may be advanced onto itself by one of two methods: a turn-down of the central one third of the tendon or a V-Y advancement at the musculotendinous junction. The advanced section of Achilles tendon is then secured to the distal tendon with multiple interrupted no. 0 sutures.

If reconstruction is not possible with local tissue, the flexor hallucis longus is harvested and used to supplement the reconstruction. The flexor hallucis longus tendon is harvested through a medial incision in which the abductor hallucis muscle is retracted in a plantar direction, allowing visualization of the plantar digital nerves and the flexor digitorum longus and the flexor hallucis longus tendons. While protecting the nerves, the flexor knot of Henry is released and the flexor hallucis longus tendon is released from all fascial connections that can be seen through the exposure. Next, the flexor hallucis longus tendon is tenodesed to the flexor digitorum longus tendon with nonabsorbable suture. The tenodesis is placed as far distal as possible. The flexor hallucis longus tendon is divided just proximal to the tenodesis. The free end of the tendon is pulled into the proximal exposure. A one-quarter–inch drill is then used to make two drill holes through the superior tuberosity of the calcaneus. The holes, one through the medial surface and directed lateral and the second through the superior surface and directed inferior, are connected at their intersection. The distal end of flexor hallucis longus tendon is secured with two no. 2 nonabsorbable suture. A suture passer is passed through the superior drill hole and out the medial drill hole. The sutures on the free end of the flexor hallucis longus are used to pull the tendon through the superior calcaneal tuberosity (Fig. 53.4). The foot is placed in a plantar flexed position and the flexor hallucis longus tendon is carefully placed under tension. The tension must approximate the tension of the contralateral Achilles tendon. The flexor hallucis longus is sutured to itself with a no. 2 nonabsorbable suture. The free end of the tendon is weaved between the proximal and distal ends of the Achilles tendon. No attempt is made to close the paratenon. The subcutaneous tissue is closed with absorbable suture and the skin closed with nylon or skin clips. A large bulky dressing is placed with the foot and ankle in plantarflexion in an attempt to remove tension from the repair and the skin overlying the tendon. Plaster splints are added for immobilization.

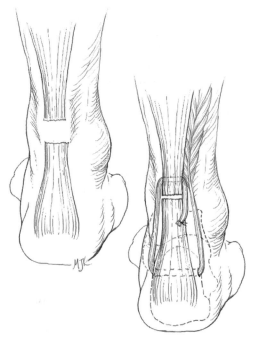

FIG. 53.4. Reconstruction of chronic neglected rupture of the Achilles tendon with the flexor hallucis longus tendon.

The skin sutures are removed at 10 days. A non–weight-bearing cast is used to gradually bring the ankle back to a neutral position during the initial postoperative month. A removable cast boot is placed at the fourth week, and the patient is allowed to begin range of motion exercises of the foot and ankle followed by low resistance exercises with an elastic band. Weight bearing is permitted after 8 weeks. The patient is allowed to resume unprotected weight bearing at 12 weeks and unrestricted activity when local warmth and tenderness have completely resolved (6 to 9 months).

Retrocalcaneal Inflammation

Nonoperative

The initial treatment of acute pain related to retrocalcaneal inflammation is rest, ice application, and NSAID therapy. Shoe modifications include lowering or softening the heel counter, adding a soft heel wedge. When symptoms fail to subside after 7 to 10 days of initial therapy or when symptoms are severe, the treatment must include enforced rest with a weight-bearing cast or removable cast boot.

Rehabilitation. Once the initial symptoms have subsided, stretching of the gastrosoleus motor unit must take precedent. Stretching is most effectively accomplished by standing 2 feet from a wall, balancing against the wall with both hands, separating both feet, and simultaneously internally rotating the feet 20 degrees.

From this position the patient leans to the wall while maintaining the feet in a plantigrade position. The internal rotation of the feet is an important feature of this routine because it locks the transverse tarsal joint, thus preventing dorsiflexion through the midfoot. Training errors must be sought and corrected. A decrease in intensity or frequency of activity or cross-training may alleviate symptoms.

When to Refer. Patients with symptoms that fail to respond to a 6-week course of immobilization are referred to an orthopedic surgeon.

Surgical

Patients with retrocalcaneal inflammation that have failed an adequate course of conservative management and immobilization may require debridement of the retrocalcaneal bursa and excision of the posterior superior aspect of the calcaneus. In one report, 4 of 14 patients managed with excision of the posterior superior calcaneus had unsatisfactory results; each patient was unable to return to the preinjury level of running (17). This procedure is designed to decompress the bursa and adjacent tendon. The tendon is also inspected and degenerative areas treated appropriately.

Excision of the Posterior Superior Calcaneus. Under general anesthesia and tourniquet control, a longitudinal incision is made parallel to and anterior to the medial border of the distal Achilles tendon and extended to the level of the Achilles tendon insertion. Sharp dissection is immediately directed to the Achilles tendon and the exposure of the tendon made between full-thickness flaps. The soft tissue must be managed with extreme caution because this area is predisposed to skin slough and wound breakdown. The paratenon is incised, and areas that appear to have inflammatory or degenerative changes are excised. The superior tuberosity of the calcaneus is exposed as the flaps are developed distally. The retrocalcaneal bursa is excised. The tendon is systematically inspected. If degenerative changes are significant, the reconstructive procedures such as those described above should be considered. The superior aspect of the calcaneus is exposed between the Achilles tendon insertion posteriorly and the posterior margin of the posterior facet of the subtalar joint anteriorly. The superior aspect of the calcaneus is resected with a wide osteotome. Care is taken to ensure that the Achilles insertion and posterior facet of the subtalar joint are not violated. The resection must provide complete decompression of the retrocalcaneal space. No attempt is made to close the paratenon. The subcutaneous tissue is closed with absorbable suture and the skin closed with nylon or skin clips. A large bulky dressing is placed with the foot and ankle in a neutral position. Plaster splints are added for immobilization.

Sutures are removed at 10 days. Weight bearing in a cast boot is allowed, range of motion and strengthening with an elastic band instituted, and immobilization continued until complete resolution of warmth and swelling adjacent to the tendon. Return to full activity is expected within 3 to 4 months.

FLEXOR HALLUCIS LONGUS TENDON

The flexor hallucis longus muscle originates from the inferior two thirds of the posterior fibula and the interosseous membrane; its tendon inserts at the base of the distal phalanx of the hallux (25). Activation of the flexor hallucis longus muscle produces plantar flexion of the hallux interphalangeal joint. The flexor hallucis longus muscle forms a tendon that courses distally between the medial and lateral posterior tubercles of the talus (the posterior talar grove) and crosses the inferior surface of the sustenaculum tali (26). The flexor hallucis longus tendon crosses deep to the flexor digitorum longus tendon at the knot of Henry. A tendinous slip from the lateral aspect of the flexor hallucis longus tendon inserts onto the flexor digitorum longus tendon (27). When a disruption occurs distal to this connection, proximal retraction of the tendon is limited. Furthermore, the connection may account for active flexion at the interphalangeal joint of the hallux when the flexor hallucis longus tendon is disrupted proximal to the tendinous connection. Two synovial-lined sheaths cover the flexor hallucis longus tendon in the foot and ankle. The proximal sheath begins 1 cm proximal to the ankle joint and ends just distal to knot of Henry. The second sheath begins at the level of the first metatarsal base and ends at the tendon insertion at the base of the distal phalanx (28).

Injury of the flexor hallucis longus tendon in the athletic individual can be grossly divided into overuse injuries (tenosynovitis, stenosing tenosynovitis, and partial longitudinal tears) and disruptions (closed and open).

Epidemiology

Tenosynovitis

Tenosynovitis of the flexor hallucis longus at the sustentaculum tali is most common among classical ballet dancers. The injury has also been described at the hallux were it was not related to ballet (29).

Stenosing Tenosynovitis

Tenosynovitis may progress to stenosing tenosynovitis with triggering phenomenon at the interphalangeal joint.

Partial Longitudinal Tears

Partial longitudinal tears of the flexor hallucis longus tendon have been reported infrequently. This injury may also lead to a triggering phenomenon at the interphalangeal joint. Injuries typically are related to athletic activity: cross-country skiing (30), classical ballet (31), dance (ballet, jazz, and tap) (30), and tennis (32).

Complete Closed Disruption

Complete closed disruption of the flexor hallucis longus tendon is a rare event. The injury does tend to occur in athletic individuals. Inokuchi and Usami (33) reported a single case of closed complete rupture of the flexor hallucis longus tendon and noted that a review of the literature revealed only six other cases. Six of the seven cases were directly related to athletic activity: one diving (34), one soccer (33), one walking (35), and three running (36–38).

Laceration

It is difficult to establish the incidence of flexor hallucis longus tendon laceration. In one report, the injury occurred in 13 of 46 cases of tendon injury about the foot and ankle (39).

Mechanism of Injury and Pathoanatomy

Tenosynovitis and Stenosing Tenosynovitis

Overuse injuries occur most commonly in the classic ballet dancer. The en pointe position is the most frequently implicated position. As the tendon passes beneath the sustenaculum tali, it is exposed to large stresses. The surrounding synovial sheath may become inflamed, which in turn places additional stress on the tendon. If the condition persists, it may lead to chronic changes, such as thickening of the sheath, partial longitudinal tears within the tendon, or nodular deformity of the tendon itself. Once this occurs, the tendon may become bound by a rigid structure resulting in triggering of the tendon. Structures capable of binding the tendon include the flexor tendon sheath behind the medial malleolus (40), the fibroosseous canal beneath the sustentaculum tali (41) (Fig. 53.5), and the sesamoid area of the hallux (29).

Hamilton (42) described a loss of hallux dorsiflexion when the ankle was placed in dorsiflexion, pseudohallux rigidus. This occurs when the flexor hallucis longus muscle is present on the distal tendon. As the hallux is dorsiflexed, the muscle is forced into the sheath beneath the sustentaculum talus.

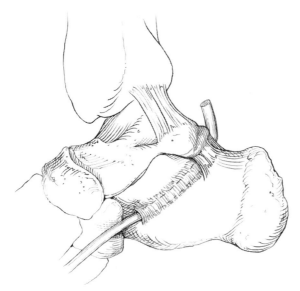

FIG. 53.5. Binding of the flexor hallucis longus tendon at the fibroosseous canal beneath the sustentaculum tali.

Partial Longitudinal Tear and Complete Closed Disruption

The onset of symptoms attributed to partial longitudinal tear may be acute or chronic; typically the onset is related to a specific injury (30,32). Closed disruption of the tendon has been described at a point 0.5 cm from the insertion (34), beneath the sustentaculum tali (35,36), just distal to the tendinous connection with the flexor digitorum longus tendon (37), beneath the metatarsal head (38), and at the posterior talar grove (33). The injury may occur with (33,36,38) or without (34,37) prodromal symptoms.

Laceration

Open disruption of the flexor hallucis longus tendon is associated with laceration to the plantar aspect of the foot. These injuries are typically the result of barefoot walking and are caused by sharp objects, usually broken glass.

Clinical Evaluation

Tenosynovitis and Stenosing Tenosynovitis

Evaluation of dancers with flexor hallucis longus tenosynovitis begins with careful questioning with regard to onset, localization of pain, current technique and practices, shoe wear, and response to previous treatment. Careful examination is required to localize the area of injury. Typically, crepitus, swelling, tenderness, warmth, and pain with motion of the hallux interphalangeal joint are localized behind the medial malleolus, behind the sustentaculum tali, or beneath the metatarsal

head. Pain and tenderness associated with flexor hallucis longus tenosynovitis must be differentiated from that caused by os trigonum (pain posterior lateral), Achilles paratenonitis (pain directly posterior), retrocalcaneal tenosynovitis (pain just anterior to Achilles tendon), peroneal tendon tenosynovitis (pain posterior lateral), and tarsal coalition (loss of subtalar motion). Advanced cases may feature triggering of the hallux interphalangeal joint due to stenosing tenosynovitis or partial longitudinal rupture. Hamilton (42) described a provocative maneuver used to demonstrate pseudo-hallux rigidus. The ankle is placed in full dorsiflexion as the hallux is tested for motion; pseudo-hallux rigidus is present when hallux dorsiflexion is limited.

Partial Longitudinal Tear and Complete Closed Disruption

The diagnosis of partial longitudinal rupture of the flexor digitorum longus tendon is difficult to make but must be suspected in the presence of localized pain and tenderness at the knot of Henry or posterior medial ankle. Pain with passive dorsiflexion of the hallux and weakness of interphalangeal joint flexion may be present. The diagnosis of complete closed disruption of the flexor digitorum longus tendon is made by demonstrating loss of active interphalangeal joint flexion. Prodromal symptoms and tenderness at the site of rupture are noted.

Laceration

When evaluating laceration of the tendon, the exact location of injury and the presence of residual hallux interphalangeal joint flexion, sensation of the plantar foot, and related injuries are noted.

Imaging

The initial imaging modality for patients with tenosynovitis is the weight-bearing anterior posterior and lateral radiograph of the ankle. The presence of an os trigonum, an enlarged posterior process of the talus, and degenerative changes of the ankle and subtalar joints are noted. Hamilton (42) recommended the addition of an en pointe (full plantar flexion) lateral radiograph to assess the significance of osteophyte impingement. For open lacerations, the radiographs may help identify radiopaque foreign bodies and bony injury. MRI may be useful in delineating the extent and location of tenosynovitis, tendinosis, rupture, or laceration. CT is indicated when tarsal coalition or os trigonum is suggested by clinical findings.

Pitfalls

MRI must be correlated with clinical findings to prevent interpretation of false positives.

Economic Considerations

Advanced imaging is used to confirm and stage the injury; it is not used for screening.

Treatment of Injury

Tenosynovitis

Nonoperative

Tenosynovitis is treated initially with modification of activity, stretching, ice therapy, and NSAID. More severe cases require enforced rest and immobilization with a weight-bearing cast or a cast boot.

Rehabilitation. Once the acute process has subsided, range of motion is maintained at the hallux interphalangeal and metatarsophalangeal joints.

When to Refer. Tenosynovitis almost always resolves with conservative measures. Patients are referred to an orthopedic surgeon after failure to respond to nonoperative management. Exploration and debridement of the tendon and tendon sheath may be considered for recalcitrant cases.

Stenosing Tenosynovitis at the Metatarsophalangeal Joint

Nonoperative

Stenosis at the metatarsophalangeal joint is treated initially with immobilization and NSAID. Once symptoms subside, range of motion of the toe is begun. Gould (29) reported on nine cases treated initially with distention of the tendon sheath with 1% lidocaine; three cases responded favorably, and the remaining required surgical tenolysis. Distention of the tendon sheath is performed with a 22-gauge needle inserted into the proximal aspect of the digital sheath. The lidocaine is forcible injected into the sheath in an attempt to rupture adhesions. If successful, active flexion of the hallux interphalangeal joint is restored. Repeated passive range of motion ensures complete release of adhesion.

Rehabilitation. Once the acute process has subsided, range of motion is maintained at the hallux interphalangeal and metatarsophalangeal joints.

When to Refer. Patients are referred to the orthopedic surgeon after failure to respond to nonoperative management.

Surgical

Patients that do not respond to conservative therapy require lysis of adhesions and release of the sheath be-neath the metatarsal head through a medial approach. Gould (29) used a more extensive exposure, the plantar full visualization approach.

Stenosing Tenosynovitis at the Fibroosseous Tunnel Beneath the Sustentaculum Tali

Nonoperative

Stenosis beneath the sustentaculum tali is treated initially with immobilization and NSAID. After the triggering and pain resolves, passive range of motion of the toe is instituted.

Rehabilitation. Once the acute process has subsided, range of motion is maintained at the hallux interphalangeal and metatarsophalangeal joints.

When to Refer. Patients are referred to the orthopedic surgeon after failure to respond to nonoperative management.

Surgical

Operative therapy in the professional dancer is considered only after the failure of a 4- to 6-month course of well-supervised nonoperative treatment. Surgical intervention is aimed at the release of the fibroosseous tunnel beneath the sustentaculum tali (41,42). In one report, release of the flexor hallucis longus at the fibroosseous tunnel beneath the talus in ballet dancers was effective and allowed 12 of 13 dancers to return to ballet as performers or students (41).

Release of the Fibroosseous Tunnel beneath the Sustentaculum. Typically, a general anesthetic is used for this procedure. The patient is placed in the supine position. Under tourniquet control, a curvilinear incision is made over the tarsal tunnel. The flexor retinaculum is exposed and then carefully divided. Great caution must be taken to avoid injuring the posterior tibial artery, vein, nerve, and their respective divisions. Once the neurovascular structures are isolated, they are carefully retracted anteriorly (41) or posteriorly (42). Motion of the hallux facilitates visualization of the flexor hallucis longus tendon within its sheath. The sheath is incised while using the hemostat to protect the underlying tendon. The tendon is followed as it passes beneath the sustenaculum tali. Stenosis is localized by moving the hallux. The fibroosseous tunnel is then carefully divided from proximal to distal until excursion of the tendon is unhindered. Synovium is sharply excised and tenolysis performed as required. The tendon is carefully inspected; partial longitudinal tears and nodules are debrided or repaired as required. The sheath is not closed. The subcutaneous tissue is closed with interrupted 4-0 absorbable suture and the skin closed with 4-0 nylon suture or skin clips. The foot and ankle are placed in a neutral position, covered with a comhpression dressing, and put into plaster splints for immobilization.

After a 10-day period of non-weight bearing, the patient returns for removal of skin sutures or clips. The foot is placed in a removable cast boot. The patient is instructed to begin weight bearing as tolerated and to remove the cast boot three times a day for active range of motion exercises. At the 3-week postoperative visit, a strengthening program is instituted and the patient is weaned out of the cast boot.

Partial Longitudinal Tear

Nonoperative

Patients with a partial longitudinal tear present with symptoms similar to tenosynovitis. Differentiating the presence of a partial longitudinal tear is difficult. The diagnosis is typically made at the time of surgical exploration. Nonoperative treatment for the symptom complex is identical to that of tenosynovitis.

Surgical

Repair of Partial Longitudinal Tear of the Flexor Hallucis Longus Tendon. When a tear is identified at the time of surgical exploration, it is repaired with a running polydioxanone, PDS (Ethicon, Inc.), or nylon suture. Knots are buried within the tendon to allow easy gliding. If the tear is related to chronic tenosynovitis, stenosis, or the tendinous connection between the flexor hallucis longus and flexor digitorum longus tendons, then these conditions must also be addressed at the time of surgery. The respective procedures and follow-up care are described above.

Subcutaneous and skin closure is performed. A bulky compression dressing is applied with plaster immobilization.

After a 10-day period of non-weight bearing, the patient returns for removal of skin sutures or clips. The foot is placed in a removable cast boot. The patient is instructed to begin weight bearing as tolerated and to remove the cast boot three times a day for active range of motion exercises. At the 8-week postoperative visit, a strengthening program is instituted and the patient is weaned out of the cast boot.

Complete Closed Disruption

Nonoperative

Complete closed disruption of the flexor hallucis longus tendon requires evaluation by an orthopedic surgeon. Emergent care includes immobilization of the foot and ankle in a non–weight-bearing splint.

Surgical

Repair or reconstruction of complete closed disruption of the flexor hallucis longus tendon in the athlete was performed in all five reported cases. The treatment consisted of fascia lata interposition graft (33), reinsertion of the tendon (34), primary repair (36,38), and primary repair followed by Z-lengthening of the tendon (37). Stiffness and loss of interphalangeal joint flexion are expected.

Laceration

Nonoperative

Laceration of the flexor hallucis longus tendon requires evaluation by an orthopedic surgeon. Emergent care includes tetanus prophylaxis and application of sterile dressing.

Surgical

Laceration of the flexor hallucis longus tendon requires careful clinical examination for appropriate surgical planning. Treatment options include routine wound care and primary skin closure alone or with primary repair of the tendon. The orthopedic literature does not clearly support either method (39,43). However, when an injury includes division of both heads of the flexor hallucis brevis and an irreparable division of the flexor hallucis longus tendon, then the distal part of the flexor hallucis longus tendon is sutured to the proximal flexor hallucis brevis muscle; this is done in an effort to prevent extension deformity of the hallux metatarsophalangeal joint (43).

We prefer primary repair of the flexor hallucis longus laceration, especially in the pediatric and athletic population. The patient must be informed that limited motion of the hallux is expected after primary repair. Adhesions at the site of primary repair produce effective tenodesis of the flexor hallucis longus tendon. This complication is difficult to prevent but does not seem to reduce functional outcome (43).

Primary Repair of Flexor Hallucis Longus Tendon Laceration. Perioperative prophylactic intravenous antibiotic, general anesthesia, and a thigh tourniquet are used. The wound is enlarged with proximal and distal extensions as required. Anatomy outside the zone of injury is identified. Systematic assessment of the flexor hallucis longus tendon, flexor digitorum brevis muscle and tendon, and local sensory nerves must be performed. The proximal end of the flexor hallucis longus tendon is retained by the interconnecting tendon, assuming that the laceration occurs distal to the interconnection. After meticulous debridement and irrigation of the wound, a primary tendon repair is performed.

Apposition is accomplished with a single core suture

of 2-0 nonabsorbable material. The peripheral edges are repaired with a smaller polydioxanone, PDS (Ethicon, Inc.), or nylon suture. The hallux interphalangeal joint is passively flexed and extended, and the excursion of the tendon at the repair site is observed. Any impediment to motion must be addressed. If the repair cannot be performed due to loss of tendon length, then a tenodesis to the flexor digitorum longus tendon is performed with both the proximal and distal ends of the flexor hallucis longus tendon. If the repair cannot be performed and both heads of the flexor hallucis brevis are not functional, then the distal end of the flexor hallucis longus tendon is sutured to the proximal flexor hallucis brevis muscle. If the repair cannot be performed due to retraction of the proximal tendon, tenodesis is performed or a secondary exposure is used and the tendon is located within its sheath at the ankle. After the tendon repair, divided digital nerves are released proximally and transplanted to a well-padded location such as a muscle belly. We do not perform primary repair of digital nerves in the foot. Surgical incisions are closed and the wound is loosely approximated to allow drainage. While maintaining the foot in slight plantarflexion, a bulky dressing is applied with plaster immobilization.

The wound is inspected postoperatively as mandated by surgical findings. At the first postoperative visit (within 10 days), the dressing is changed. The foot immobilization is gradually brought to neutral over the course of the next 2 to 3 weeks; when in a neutral position, a non–weight-bearing cast or a cast boot is placed. At 2 weeks, the sutures are removed and passive range of motion at the interphalangeal and metatarsophalangeal joints is instructed. The patient is instructed to begin weight bearing as tolerated at 6 weeks. At the 8-week postoperative visit, a strength-

ening program is instituted and the patient is weaned out of the cast boot.

PERONEUS BREVIS AND LONGUS TENDONS

The peroneus longus muscle originates from the lateral tibial condyle and the upper two thirds of the lateral surface of the fibula (44). The muscle forms a tendon that is retained by three tunnels (45). The first is the retromalleolar tunnel formed by the superior peroneal retinaculum (Fig. 53.6); this tunnel is shared with the anteriorly located peroneus brevis tendon. The second tunnel is formed by the inferior peroneal retinaculum; this tunnel receives the tendon after it has passed the malleolar tip and directs it anteriorly. The third tunnel is a fibrous tunnel that receives the tendon after it turns medially beneath the cuboid tubercle. At the cuboid tubercle a sesamoid, the os peroneum, is located within the substance of the tendon. The os peroneum has a reported incidence in anatomic and radiographic studies that varies from 5% to 26% (46). In a review of 1,000 radiographs, 143 os peroneum were noted and of these 27 were bipartite, 6 were tripartite, and 1 was multipartite (47). The peroneus longus tendon inserts at the base of the first metatarsal and lateral side of the medial cunieform.

The peroneus brevis muscle originates from the lower two thirds of the lateral surface of the fibula (48). The muscle forms a tendon that enters the retromalleolar tunnel between the fibular grove anteriorly and the peroneus longus tendon posteriorly. Beyond the tip of the fibula, the tendon turns anteriorly to enter a tunnel formed by the inferior peroneal retinaculum (49). The two peroneal tunnels are separated by fibrous tissue attached to the peroneal tubercle of the calcaneus. The

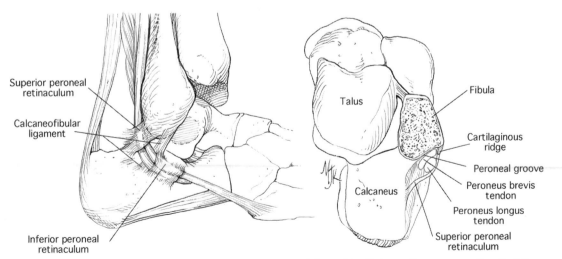

FIG. 53.6. Anatomic relationships at the lateral aspect of the ankle. Note on the cross-section that the peroneal groove is supplemented by a fibrocartilaginous ridge.

peroneus brevis inserts at the base of the fifth metatarsal.

The peroneal tendons share a common synovial sheath behind the malleolus (50). The sheath bifurcates above and below the malleolus. The peroneus brevis sheath ends 2 cm proximal to its insertion at the base of the fifth metatarsal. The peroneus longus tendon sheath ends at the cuboid tubercle; a second sheath covers the tendon until it reaches its insertion at the base of the first metatarsal.

Microvascular investigation has revealed that each peroneal tendon receives vascular supply through a posterior–lateral vincula (51). A zone of hypovascularity was not identified.

Both tendons pass behind the retromalleolar sulcus, a bony groove that is deepened by a fibrocartilaginous ridge (Fig. 53.6). Edwards (52) noted that the sulcus was very shallow in 82% of cases and not well formed in 18% of cases.

The superior peroneal retinaculum is the structure responsible for maintaining the peroneal tendons within the retromalleolar tunnel (53). Davis et al. (54) reported that the superior peroneal retinaculum consistently originated from the periosteum on the posterior–lateral ridge of the fibula. The retinaculum typically split into a superior and an inferior band. The superior band inserted into the anterior Achilles sheath or the posterior tuberosity of the calcaneus just inferior to the Achilles tendon insertion. The inferior band coursed parallel to and inserted just lateral to the calcaneofibular ligament. Numerous variations of the peroneal muscles and tendons have been described, including accessory muscles and variable or multiple insertions (55). Sobel et al. (56) reported the presence of a peroneus quartus in 21.7% of 124 cadaveric legs. The most common variation of the peroneus quartus took origin from the muscular portion of the peroneus brevis muscle in the lower third of the leg and inserted on the peroneal tubercle of the calcaneus. The tendon may be used in reconstruction of the superior peroneal retinaculum or the lateral ankle ligaments.

The relationship of the respective tendons to the axis of rotation of the ankle and subtalar joints illustrates their function as plantarflexors and evertors of the foot.

Injury of the peroneal tendons and their related structures in the athlete include tenosynovitis, traumatic subluxation and dislocation (acute and chronic), partial longitudinal rupture of the peroneus brevis, rupture, and fracture of the os peroneum.

Epidemiology

Tenosynovitis

The incidence of tenosynovitis of the peroneal tendons is difficult to establish. This is attributed to the use of inconsistent terminology throughout the orthopedic literature and the fact that early reports of tenosynovitis (57,58) are more appropriately discussed with tendon ruptures.

Traumatic Subluxation and Dislocation of the Peroneal Tendons

Anterior dislocation of the peroneal tendons is a well-recognized injury that unfortunately has the propensity to evade diagnosis. Lateral ankle sprains are often diagnosed exclusive of accompanying peroneal tendon dislocation. Failure to institute appropriate nonoperative treatment in a timely fashion may lead to the chronic condition. Clanton and Schon (59) reported that of the 265 reported cases of peroneal tendon dislocations, 97% occurred during athletic activity. Most of these cases were attributed to snow skiing (71%), followed by football (7%), running, soccer, and ice skating. In one report, 6,767 ski accidents resulted in 38 cases (0.6%) of peroneal tendon dislocation (60). Several reports have noted an interesting subgroup of patients that demonstrate subluxation of the peroneal tendons within the peroneal groove (61,62).

Partial Longitudinal Rupture of the Peroneus Brevis Tendon

Sobel et al. (63) reported splaying of the peroneus brevis tendon, partial thickness longitudinal split, or full-thickness longitudinal split of the peroneus brevis tendon in 14 of 124 cadaveric ankles (11%). Sammarco and DiRaimondo (64) reported that 11 of the 47 ankles undergoing ankle ligament reconstruction demonstrated longitudinal degenerative rents in the peroneus brevis tendon.

Rupture

Frank rupture of the peroneal tendons is a rare event. In one case, a 49-year-old man had experienced lateral foot pain for several months before rupturing the peroneus longus tendon during a 10-mile road race (65). In another case, a 20-year-old laborer sustained a peroneus longus tendon rupture subsequent to an inversion sprain of the foot that occurred during a soccer match (66). Two reported cases occurred in athletes (67,68).

Fracture of the Os Peroneum

Isolated fracture of the peroneus longus tendon is a rare event. Peterson and Stinson (46) noted that in contrast to peroneal tendon rupture, this injury occurs in a younger age group. They reported on five patients with an average age of 35 years. Two cases of the os peroneum fracture associated with concomitant rupture of the peroneus longus tendon have been reported (69,70).

Mechanism of Injury and Pathoanatomy

Tenosynovitis

Tenosynovitis of the peroneal tendons probably results from increased stress at the fibular tip where the direction of the tendons changes acutely. Plantarflexion-inversion injury (acute or chronic), subluxation (acute or chronic), or fracture of the fibula or calcaneus may account for the onset and persistence of this injury.

Traumatic Subluxation and Dislocation of the Peroneal Tendons

Most authors agree that the mechanism of injury is a sudden forceful passive dorsiflexion of the inverted foot with reflex contraction of the peroneal tendons and the foot plantarflexors (71–73). A forward fall while skiing is a common mechanism—the tip of the ski digs into the snow, producing dorsiflexion of the ankle. A shallow, flat, or convex peroneal groove may also contribute to the injury. The pathoanatomy of the injury is best illustrated by the classification of injury developed by Eckert and Davis (73) and subsequently modified by Oden (74) (Fig. 53.7). A type I injury is defined by an intact retinaculum that was elevated off its fibular

insertion; this allowed the peroneal tendons to translate out of the retrofibular tunnel and under the fibular periosteum. A type II injury is marked by an anterior tear of the retinaculum. A type III injury is an avulsion fracture of the retinaculum off the posterior fibular margin. A type IV injury is marked by a posterior tear of the retinaculum.

An alternative mechanism suggests that lateral ankle instability may lead to superior peroneal retinaculum incompetence (75). This mechanism is based on the fact that the inferior band (calcaneal band) of the superior peroneal retinaculum is parallel to the calcaneofibular ligament (54,75). Chronic adduction–inversion injury to the ankle associated with calcaneofibular ligament laxity may also attenuate the inferior band of the superior peroneal retinaculum.

For the subgroup of patients that demonstrate subluxation of the peroneal tendons within the peroneal grove, the reported mechanism of injury was either unknown (62) or repeat inversion injury to the ankle (61,62).

Partial Longitudinal Rupture of the Peroneus Brevis Tendon

Chronic subluxation of the peroneal tendons either clinical or subclinical is implicated as a major causative factor in the development of longitudinal tears of the peroneus brevis tendon (76,77). Laxity of the superior

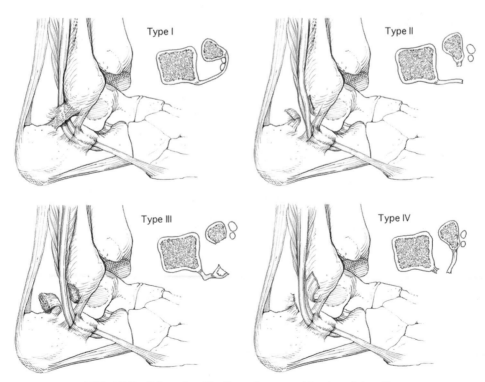

FIG. 53.7. Oden classification of peroneal tendon dislocation.

peroneal retinaculum allows subluxation of the peroneus brevis tendon over the posterior edge of the inferior fibula. The peroneus brevis tendon may be compressed by the peroneus longus tendon (76,77), the presence of peroneal musculature within the retromalleolar tunnel, or the presence of a peroneus quartus muscle (56).

Acute peroneal tendon longitudinal tear may also occur at the time of lateral ankle plantarflexion-inversion sprain. Among eight varsity athletes at Duke University, a tear of the peroneus brevis tendon (three patients) and peroneus longus tendon (five patients) occurred coincident with a plantarflexion-inversion ankle injury while participating in football, tennis, track, or cross-country running. Intraoperative findings failed to show evidence of concomitant peroneal tendon subluxation (78). In one series, 11 peroneus brevis tendon tears were noted among 47 patients undergoing lateral ankle ligament reconstruction (64).

Rupture

In one case report, the rupture of the peroneus longus tendon occurred during a 10-mile run; the patient had experienced pain for several months before the episode (65). A violent inversion of the foot on the leg was the mechanism for a complete rupture of the peroneus longus tendon (66).

Fracture of the Os Peroneum

In one series, all five fractures occurred with the foot in a position of inversion and plantarflexion (46).

Clinical Evaluation

Tenosynovitis

Patients present with pain of acute or chronic nature usually with a traumatic onset. Symptoms may localize to the retrofibular area, calcaneal tuberosity, cuboid groove, or the base of the fifth metatarsal. Examination reveals an antalgic gait; local swelling, tenderness, and warmth at the peroneal tendons; and painful passive inversion of the subtalar joint. Local anesthetic placed within the peroneal sheath may be used as a diagnostic aid.

Traumatic Subluxation and Dislocation of the Peroneal Tendons

Patients with acute anterior dislocation present with a history of pain behind the lateral malleolus after forceful passive dorsiflexion of the foot. The patient may recall sensing or hearing a snap or pop. The anteriorly dislocated tendons may have been identified by the patient

before reduction. For recurrent or chronic cases, the patient may note snapping or popping that occurs while walking or running. Examination reveals swelling and tenderness behind the lateral malleolus (60,71,73,79,80). If examined acutely, tenderness behind the lateral malleolus is noted, in contrast to an inversion ankle sprain that demonstrates tenderness in front of the lateral malleolus. Apprehension, subluxation, and possible dislocation is elicited by active dorsiflexion of the foot while the foot is held in a plantarflexed and everted position. The examination is carefully performed with several fingers gently palpating the peroneal tendons over the peroneal groove. Subluxation or frank dislocation of the tendon is palpable at the posterior–lateral margin of the lateral malleolus; comparison with the contralateral extremity is often helpful when attempting to differentiate physiologic from pathologic findings. Rarely, subluxation of the peroneal tendons occurs within the peroneal groove. The patient presents with the complaint of popping in the region of the peroneal tendons The popping is produced by the peroneus brevis tendon passing forcibly behind the peroneus longus tendon. The popping can be reproduced by the patient and the integrity of the superior peroneal retinaculum verified by inspection and palpation.

Partial Longitudinal Rupture of the Peroneus Brevis Tendon

Patients with partial longitudinal rupture of the peroneus brevis tendon present with a history of trauma to the ankle. Functionally, patients complain of subjective ankle instability on uneven terrain. Symptoms may include acute or chronic lateral ankle pain, retrofibular pain, lateral ankle swelling, lateral ankle instability, or popping.

Rupture

Patients presenting with a rupture of the peroneus longus tendon may offer a history of antecedent lateral ankle pain before experiencing a snap or a pop at the peroneal region. Difficulty walking, swelling, and tenderness over the peroneal tendons are noted on physical examination. Weakness of first ray plantarflexion may be present; however, this finding was not present in two reported cases (65,66).

Fracture of the Os Peroneum

Patients with fracture of the os peroneum present complaining of lateral foot pain, exacerbated by walking. The patients may report hearing a pop associated with the injury. Examination reveals local swelling and tenderness at the peroneus longus tendon where it crosses the cuboid. Pain at the os peroneum is reproduced with the single heel rise (81). Concomitant fracture of the fibula, rupture of the peroneus longus tendon, and injury to the brevis tendon or lateral ankle ligaments must be ruled out.

Imaging

Tenosynovitis

Plain radiographs are obtained as the initial imaging study. Concomitant ankle fracture is also ruled out. If lateral ankle instability is a significant complaint, stress views are obtained. MRI may be used to detect concomitant soft tissue injury such as partial longitudinal rupture of the peroneus brevis tendon or ankle ligament disruption.

Traumatic Subluxation and Dislocation of the Peroneal Tendons

Plain radiographs are obtained as the initial imaging study. Oden type III injuries may demonstrate a rim avulsion fracture of the lateral malleolus (Fig. 53.8). Concomitant ankle fracture is also ruled out. If lateral ankle instability is a significant complaint, stress views are obtained. CT may be used to define the anatomy of the peroneal groove. MRI may be used to detect peroneal tendon dislocation or concomitant soft tissue injury such a partial longitudinal rupture of the peroneus brevis tendon or ankle ligament disruption.

Partial Longitudinal Rupture of the Peroneus Brevis Tendon

Plain radiographs are obtained as the initial imaging study. Fracture of the ankle or os peroneum are ruled out. MRI is the modality of choice when evaluating chronic lateral ankle pain. Partial longitudinal tears are readily identified as linear areas of increased signal intensity within the peroneus brevis tendon. Peroneal tenography revealed peroneal tendon injury in eight pa-

tients all confirmed at surgery as longitudinal peroneal tendon tears (78).

Rupture

Plain radiographs taken in multiple projections and comparison views are used to identify a fractured os peroneum and to differentiate it from a multipartite os peroneum or a fractured cuboid. Repeat radiographs may demonstrate proximal migration of the os peroneum in the case of distal tendon rupture. MRI may also be used to identify the ruptured tendon, but the findings must be carefully correlated with the clinical presentation. In one case, MRI demonstrated increased signal uptake consistent with partial longitudinal tear, and subsequent surgical findings confirmed a complete intrasubstance rupture (65).

Fracture of the Os Peroneum

Plain radiographs taken in multiple projections and comparison views are used to identify a fractured os peroneum. As noted above, the occurrence of a bipartite or multipartite os peroneum is quite rare and strongly suggests the diagnosis of fracture when the clinical findings are in agreement. The presence of smooth sclerotic margins suggest a congenital bipartite or multipartite os peroneum (82). Scintigraphy may be used to distinguish a fracture from a congenital bipartite or multipartite os peroneum. MRI may be used to identify adjacent soft tissue injury and concomitant peroneus longus tendon rupture. Peterson and Stinson (46) successfully used ultrasound to confirm the integrity of the peroneus longus tendon surrounding a fractured os peroneum.

Treatment of Injury

Tenosynovitis

Nonoperative

The mainstay of treatment of peroneal tenosynovitis is rest, ice therapy, and NSAID. Shoe modifications may include a widened heel to increased lateral stability or a medial heel wedge to decompress calcaneal impingement. Recalcitrant cases require enforced rest with a weight-bearing cast or cast boot and continued therapy with NSAID.

Rehabilitation. Rehabilitation commences once the symptoms subside and emphasizes proprioception and strength training. Progressive return to full activity is expected. Surgical treatment of tenosynovitis is quite uncommon, especially when tenosynovitis occurs exclusive of peroneal subluxation and lateral ankle instability.

When to Refer. Persistent symptoms after 3 months of well-supervised nonoperative therapy suggests the possibility of a concomitant injury. Referral to an ortho-

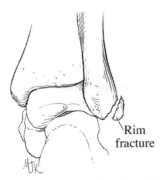

FIG. 53.8. Oden type III peroneal tendon dislocation with the characteristic rim fracture.

pedic surgeon is made for consideration of synovectomy and exploration.

Surgical

Synovectomy and exploration of the peroneal tendons is considered only after nonoperative therapy has been exhausted and the symptoms impair daily activity, including athletic activity. Proliferative synovium or reactive tissue is systematically and meticulously excised by sharp dissection. Careful inspection of the tendons and superior peroneal retinaculum are required to rule out concomitant tendon tears and subluxation.

Exploration of the Peroneal Tendons and Debridement of the Peroneal Sheaths. Typically, a general anesthetic is used for this procedure. The patient is placed in the supine position with a padded bump placed under the ipsilateral iliac crest. Under tourniquet control, a linear incision is made over the course of the peroneal tendons. The incision is centered over the symptomatic area. Care must be taken to avoid injury to the sural nerve and the anterior communicating branch when the exposure is made distal to the lateral malleolus. Once the nerves are isolated and protected, sharp dissection can be made to the tendon sheath. The sheath is sharply opened across the length of the surgical wound. Typically, an effusion will be noted within the tendon sheath and evidence of synovial proliferation and increased vascular activity. The synovium is sharply excised and tenolysis performed. Debridement of the sheath may require additional exposure. A 1-cm section of sheath and superior peroneal retinaculum is left intact at the lateral malleolus to function as a pulley and the remaining sheath is incised, inspected, and debrided as required. The tendons are carefully inspected. Partial longitudinal tears are debrided or repaired as discussed below. Evidence of tendinosis or rupture will require consideration for debridement of the tendon itself and possible reconstructive procedures. Decompression of calcaneal fibular impingement is performed when indicated. Assuming that the tendon itself appears healthy, the sheath is loosely closed with a running 3-0 nylon suture. The subcutaneous tissue is closed with interrupted 4-0 adsorbable suture and the skin closed with 4-0 nylon suture or skin clips. The foot and ankle are placed in a neutral position, covered with a compression dressing, and set in plaster splints for immobilization.

The patient is instructed to keep the foot elevated for the next 2 days. After a 10-day period of non-weight bearing, the patient returns for removal of skin sutures or clips. The foot is placed in a removable cast boot. The patient is instructed to begin weight bearing as tolerated and to remove the cast boot three times a day for active range of motion exercises. At the 3-week postoperative visit, a proprioceptive and strengthening program is instituted. Activities with the cast boot are gradually resumed, and finally the patient is weaned out of the cast boot.

Traumatic Subluxation and Dislocation of the Peroneal Tendons

Nonoperative

An initial acute dislocation deserves a trial of nonoperative intervention. A well-fitted short leg cast is placed with the foot in slight plantar flexion. A window is cut out of the cast directly over the peroneal tendons as they pass behind the peroneal groove. A felt pad is fitted over the tendons and the window is replaced. The amount of compression may be adjusted by the patient to maximize comfort. The patient remains non-weight bearing for 6 weeks. The cast is removed and integrity of the retinaculum is inspected. Casting may continue for another 4 weeks, at which time motion, strength, and proprioception must be emphasized. Stover and Bryan (72) reported excellent results for five of the seven patients treated with a non–weight-bearing cast.

Patients with recurrent or chronic dislocation are not likely to respond to nonoperative methods (71,79, 80,83–88).

Occasionally, popping caused by subluxation of the peroneal tendons within the peroneal sheath will be noted. The most reliable treatment for this entity is excision of abnormal peroneus brevis tendon and tenodesis of the peroneal tendons to each other.

Surgical

Once the patient develops a recurrent or chronic condition, then surgical intervention is the most reliable treatment option. The variety of surgical procedures is vast. In simplified terms, the procedures produce either a deepened peroneal groove, increase the competency of the superior peroneal retinaculum, or reroute the peroneal tendons. Procedures that deepen the peroneal groove may do so by physically deepening the groove (88) (Fig. 53.9) or by making the groove relatively deeper by placing a posterior bone block at the lateral margin of the groove (89,90) (Fig. 53.10). Procedures that increase the competency of the superior peroneal retinaculum include reattachment of the retinaculum to the posterior–lateral margin of the fibula with imbrication of redundant retinaculum (Fig. 53.11) or reconstruction of the retinaculum with peroneus brevis (79,91), peroneus quartus (92), Achilles (83), or plantaris (86) tendons. Rerouting procedures (93) require elevation of the calcaneofibular ligament and transposition of the peroneal tendons beneath the ligament followed by repair of the ligament.

For acute tears that have failed nonoperative treatment, we prefer to explore the injury and repair and

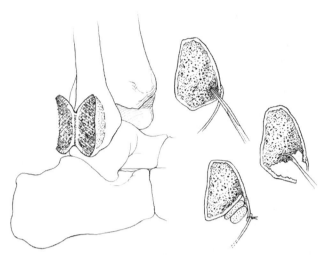

FIG. 53.9. Treatment of peroneal tendon dislocation with a groove-deepening procedure.

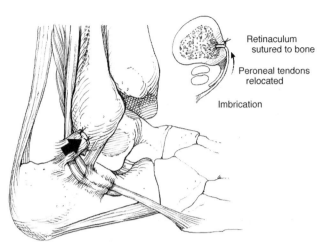

Retinaculum sutured to bone

Peroneal tendons relocated

Imbrication

FIG. 53.11. Treatment of peroneal tendon dislocation with repair and imbrication of the superior peroneal retinaculum.

imbricate the superior peroneal retinaculum as required. For chronic cases we perform a bone block procedure as described by DuVries (90). The use of a bone block provides effective containment of the tendons while preserving the smooth gliding surface of the peroneal groove.

Exploration, Repair, and Imbrication of the Superior Peroneal Retinaculum. Typically, a general anesthetic is used for this procedure. The patient is placed in the supine position with a padded bump placed under the ipsilateral iliac crest. Under tourniquet control, an "L"-shaped incision is made over the course of the peroneal tendons. Care must be taken to avoid injury to the sural nerve and its anterior communicating branch, which is found anterior to the lateral malleolus. Once the nerves are isolated and protected, sharp dissection is made to the tendon sheath. The superior peroneal retinaculum

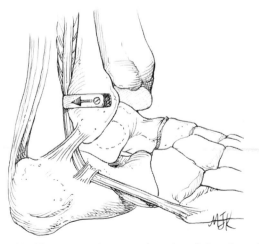

FIG. 53.10. Treatment of peroneal tendon dislocation with a sliding bone block.

is inspected and the type of injury noted. Further exposure of the peroneal tendons is accomplished by dividing the remaining retinaculum as required. If possible, a cuff of retinaculum is left on the fibula to facilitate repair and imbrication. Synovium is sharply excised and tenolysis performed. The tendons are carefully inspected. If present, a peroneus quartus is resected. If the peroneus brevis muscle extends to the peroneal groove, that section of muscle is excised. Partial longitudinal tears are debrided and repaired as discussed below.

For an Oden type I injury, the false space created by elevation of the fibular periosteum must be obliterated. Imbrication of the retinaculum and obliteration of this space is accomplished by securing the retinaculum to the fibula with nonabsorbable suture passed through drill holes in the posterior–lateral fibula. For Oden type II or IV injuries, the torn retinaculum is repaired and imbricated at the site of disruption. For Oden type III injuries, reduction and internal fixation is performed if the size of the fragment permits; otherwise, a repair and imbrication of the retinaculum through drill holes is performed.

For chronic cases that do not present sufficient retinaculum for repair, a bone block procedure is performed. A sagittal saw is used to cut a trapezoidal shaped graft at the lateral cortex of lateral malleolus. The graft must be wide enough to accommodate fixation with a small cancellous screw. The graft is translated posteriorly approximately 1 cm and fixation added. Tendon excursion and stability is verified before repaired and imbrication of the available retinaculum.

The subcutaneous tissue is closed with interrupted 4-0 absorbable suture and the skin closed with 4-0 nylon suture or skin clips. The foot and ankle are placed in a neutral position, covered with a compression dressing, and set with plaster splints for immobilization.

The patient is instructed to keep the foot elevated

for the next 2 days. After a 10-day period of non-weight bearing, the patient returns for removal of skin sutures or clips. The foot is placed in a removable cast boot, and the patient is instructed to remove the cast boot three times a day for active range of motion exercises. At the 6-week postoperative visit, the patient is allowed to begin weight bearing as tolerated and a proprioceptive and strengthening program is instituted. Activities with the cast boot are gradually resumed, and finally the patient is weaned out of the cast boot by 12 weeks postoperatively.

Partial Longitudinal Rupture of the Peroneus Brevis Tendon

The etiology of this lesion is related to laxity of the superior peroneal retinaculum and the subsequent subluxation of the peroneus brevis tendon over the posterior–lateral margin of the fibula. Furthermore, the tendon is compressed against the sharp posterior margin by the overlying peroneus longus tendon. Treatment must address both the tear and the recurrent subluxation.

Nonoperative

Most of these patients will present with lateral ankle pain. Treatment is initially symptomatic. If the diagnosis is made at the onset, the initial treatment addresses the concomitant peroneal tenosynovitis with rest, ice therapy, and NSAID. Recalcitrant cases require enforced rest with a weight-bearing cast or cast boot and continued therapy with NSAID. In the case of a competitive athlete, the ankle may be taped for symptomatic relief, allowing surgery to be performed at an elective date.

When to Refer. Typically, patients will present with persistent lateral ankle pain that is recalcitrant to nonoperative treatment. Referral to an orthopedic surgeon is made for consideration of exploration and treatment of the partial tear and incompetent superior peroneal retinaculum when indicated.

Surgical

Careful inspection of the superior peroneal retinaculum is required to rule out concomitant subluxation.

Repair of Partial Longitudinal Rupture of the Peroneus Brevis Tendon and Imbrication of the Superior Peroneal Retinaculum. Typically, a general anesthetic is used for this procedure. The patient is placed in the supine position with a padded bump placed under the ipsilateral iliac crest. Under tourniquet control, an L-shaped incision is made over the course of the peroneal tendons. Care must be taken to avoid injury to the sural nerve and the its anterior communicating branch, which

is found anterior to the lateral malleolus. Once the nerves are isolated and protected, sharp dissection can be made to the tendon sheath. The superior peroneal retinaculum is inspected. Laxity or frank incompetence is noted. The retinaculum is incised posterior to the lateral malleolus. A cuff of retinaculum is left on the fibula to facilitate repair and imbrication. The sheath is sharply opened across the length of the surgical wound. Typically, an effusion will be noted within the tendon sheath and evidence of synovial proliferation and increased vascular activity. The synovium is sharply excised and tenolysis performed. A 1-cm section of sheath and superior peroneal retinaculum is left intact inferior to the lateral malleolus to function as a pulley. The tendons are carefully inspected. If present, a peroneus quartus is resected. If the peroneus brevis muscle extends to the peroneal groove, that section of muscle is excised.

Partial longitudinal tears that appear degenerative due to fibrillation are debrided to normal-appearing tendon. If the remaining tendon is incompetent, then the degenerative section is excised and the proximal and distal ends of the peroneus brevis tendon are tenodesed to the adjacent peroneus longus tendon with multiple nonabsorbable sutures. If the remaining tendon appears to be competent, then the major tear is repaired with a running polydioxanone, PDS (Ethicon, Inc.), or nylon suture. The remaining tendon may be tubularized with a running suture. Subluxation of the peroneal tendons must be adequately addressed to prevent a recurrence. The sheath is loosely closed with a running 3-0 nylon suture. The subcutaneous tissue is closed with interrupted 4-0 absorbable suture and the skin closed with 4-0 nylon suture or skin clips. The foot and ankle are placed in a neutral position, covered with a compression dressing, and set in plaster splints for immobilization.

The patient is instructed to keep the foot elevated for the next 2 days. After a 10-day period of non-weight bearing, the patient returns for removal of skin sutures or clips. The foot is placed in a removable cast boot, and the patient is instructed to remove the cast boot three times a day for active range of motion exercises. At the 6-week postoperative visit, the patient is allowed to begin weight bearing as tolerated, and a proprioceptive and strengthening program is instituted. Activities with the cast boot are gradually resumed, and finally the patient is weaned out of the cast boot by 12 weeks postoperatively.

Rupture of the Peroneus Longus Tendon

Nonoperative

Complete intrasubstance rupture of a peroneal tendon requires surgical evaluation for consideration of primary repair or, in the case of delayed diagnosis, reconstruction. Emergent care includes immobilization with a well-padded splint, non-weight bearing, elevation of the extremity, and application of ice.

Surgical

A recent rupture of a peroneal tendon requires surgical exploration, synovectomy, debridement, and repair of partial tears and primary repair or reconstruction of the injured tendon. Among two cases of peroneus longus tendon rupture in an athletic individuals, one was treated with tendodesis to the adjacent peroneus brevis tendon (66) and the other by primary repair (65). Both outcomes appear to have been successful. When treating chronic cases, reconstruction of the tendon is recommended.

Repair or Reconstruction of Complete Rupture of a Peroneal Tenon. Typically, a general anesthetic is used for this procedure. The patient is placed in the supine position with a padded bump placed under the ipsilateral iliac crest. Under tourniquet control, a linear incision is made over the course of the peroneal tendons. The incision is centered over the rupture site. Care must be taken to avoid injury to the sural nerve and the anterior communicating branch when the exposure is made distal to the lateral malleolus. Once the nerves are isolated and protected, sharp dissection can be made to the tendon sheath. The sheath is sharply opened across the length of the surgical wound. Typically, an effusion will be noted. The synovium is sharply excised and tenolysis performed. Debridement of the sheath may require additional exposure. A 1-cm section of sheath and superior peroneal retinaculum is left intact at the lateral malleolus to function as a pulley. The remaining sheath is incised, inspected, and debrided as required. The tendons are carefully inspected. A complete rupture of a peroneal tendon is repaired primarily when possible.

Each end of the tendon is identified, excision of nonfunctional tendon performed. Apposition is accomplished with a single core suture of no. 0 nonabsorbable material. The peripheral edges are repaired with a smaller polydioxanone, PDS (Ethicon, Inc.), or nylon suture. When primary repair is not possible, reconstruction is most easily performed by tendodesis of the proximal and distal ends of the tendon to the adjacent peroneal tendon using a size 0 nonabsorbable material. When neither tendon is suitable for reconstruction, we recommend reconstruction with implantation of one of the peroneal tendons into the lateral calcaneus at the peroneal tubercle. This will provide active eversion to the hindfoot. The procedure requires preparation of a cancellous surface at the peroneal tubercle and fixation through bony tunnels made with the aid of a sharp towel clip. The tendon is prepared for transfer by exci-

sion of nonfunctional material, and one or two nonabsorbable sutures are passed through the tendon for secure fixation. The prepared tendon end is brought up to the cancellous surface of the peroneal tubercle; next, each group of sutures is passed through a single bony tunnel and tied to over a bony bridge. The peroneus tertius and quartus tendons may be harvested and used to reinforce the reconstruction. Decompression of calcaneal fibular impingement is performed when indicated. The sheath is loosely closed with a running 3-0 nylon suture. The subcutaneous tissue is closed with interrupted 4-0 absorbable suture and the skin closed with 4-0 nylon suture or skin clips. The foot and ankle are placed in an everted position, covered with a compression dressing, and set in plaster splints for immobilization.

The patient is instructed to keep the foot elevated for the next 2 days. After a 10-day period of non-weight bearing, the patient returns for removal of skin sutures or clips. The foot is placed in a removable cast boot, and the patient is instructed to remove the cast boot three times a day for active range of motion exercises. At the 6-week postoperative visit, the patient is allowed to begin weight bearing as tolerated, and a proprioceptive and strengthening program is instituted. Activities with the cast boot are gradually resumed, and finally the patient is weaned out of the cast boot by 12 weeks postoperatively.

Fracture of the Os Peroneum

Nonoperative

If fracture of the os peroneum is associated with a complete tear of the peroneus longus tendon, then referral should be made to an orthopedic surgeon for consideration of open reduction and internal fixation. The mainstay of treatment for an isolated fracture is enforced rest with a non–weight-bearing cast or cast boot. At 6 weeks, treatment may continue if examination and radiographs suggests progression to union.

Rehabilitation. Once the fracture becomes nontender and is radiographically united, a motion, strengthening, and proprioceptive rehabilitation may commence. Progressive return to full activity is expected.

When to Refer. Persistent symptoms after 3 months of well-supervised nonoperative therapy suggests the possibility of nonunion. Referral to an orthopedic surgeon is made for consideration of excision.

Surgical

Excision of the isolated fracture of the os peroneum is considered only if symptoms persist after an appropriate course of immobilization. When the tendon is intact, excision is probably the most predictable surgical procedure. Four of five patients treated with excision of a fractured os peroneum returned to their preinjury activity level (46). When a tendon rupture is associated with an os peroneum fracture, then open reduction and internal fixation of the fracture may be used to help restore continuity to the tendon.

Excision or Open Reduction and Internal Fixation of the Os Peroneum. Typically, a general anesthetic is used for this procedure. The patient is placed in the supine position with a padded bump placed under the ipsilateral iliac crest. Under tourniquet control, a linear incision is made parallel to and proximal to the course of the peroneus brevis. The incision is centered over the symptomatic area. Care must be taken to avoid injury to the sural nerve. The sheath is sharply opened across the length of the surgical wound. Typically, an effusion will be noted within the tendon sheath. The synovium is sharply excised and tenolysis performed. Debridement of the sheath may require additional exposure. If the tendon is not disrupted, the os peroneum is excised in a subperiosteal fashion. The remaining defect is then closed with a running polydioxanone, PDS (Ethicon, Inc.), or nylon suture. If the tendon is disrupted, primary repair is attempted with internal fixation of the fracture. The fracture is exposed, debrided, and reduced. Fixation is accomplished with large nonabsorbable suture passed through holes created with a sharp towel clip and through the tendon. The peripheral edges are repaired with a smaller polydioxanone, PDS (Ethicon, Inc.), or nylon suture. Excursion of the tendon is verified and the sheath loosely closed with a running 3-0 nylon suture. The subcutaneous tissue is closed with interrupted 4-0 absorbable suture and the skin closed with 4-0 nylon suture or skin clips. The foot and ankle are placed in an everted position, covered with a compression dressing, and immobilized with plaster splints.

The patient is instructed to keep the foot elevated for the next 2 days. After a 10-day period of non-weight bearing, the patient returns for removal of skin sutures or clips. The foot is placed in a removable cast boot, and the patient is instructed to remove the cast boot three times a day for active range of motion exercises. At the 6-week postoperative visit, the patient is allowed to begin weight bearing as tolerated, and a proprioceptive and strengthening program is instituted. Activities with the cast boot are gradually resumed, and finally the patient is weaned out of the cast boot by 12 weeks postoperatively. After open reduction and internal fixation, a non–weight-bearing cast is placed with the foot in a slightly everted position. At 6 weeks postoperatively, the patient is placed in a removable cast boot and instructed to begin weight bearing as tolerated. The cast boot is removed three times a day for active range of motion exercises. At 8 weeks postoperatively, a proprioceptive and strengthening program is instituted. Activities with the cast boot are gradually resumed, and

finally the patient is weaned out of the cast boot by 12 weeks postoperatively.

POSTERIOR TIBIAL TENDON

The posterior tibial muscle originates from the posterior surface of the proximal tibia, the proximal two thirds of the fibula, and the interosseous membrane (94). The muscle forms a tendon distally that passes behind the medial malleolus and subsequently divides into three distinct components (95). The largest component provides a direct insertion into the tuberosity of the navicular and the first cunieform. The remaining components provide insertions into the second and third cunieform; the cuboid; the peroneus longus tendon; the base of the second, third, fourth, and occasionally fifth metatarsals; and the sustentaculum tali. The tendon is surrounded by a synovial sheath beginning 6 cm proximal to the tip of the medial malleolus and ending near the tuberosity of the navicular (96). Frey et al. (97) demonstrated a zone of relative hypovascularity within the tendon behind and distal to the medial malleolus. The position of the posterior tibial tendon relative to the ankle and subtalar joint axes of rotation clearly illustrate its inversion and plantar flexion function (98) (Fig. 53.12). Because of the configuration of the subtalar and transverse tarsal joints, the longitudinal arch of the foot is stabilized by inversion of the heel. Between the foot flat and toe-off phase of the walking cycle (between 15% and 60% of the walking cycle), the posterior tibial muscle is active. Activation of the posterior tibial muscle and passive external rotation of the tibia produce inversion of the subtalar joint and subsequent stabilization of the longitudinal arch of the foot, thus providing a stable platform in preparation for toe-off (99).

This section reviews five conditions that affect the posterior tibial tendon in the athletic population: acute rupture, dislocation, acute tenosynovitis, chronic tenosynovitis, and chronic rupture.

Epidemiology

Acute Rupture

Acute rupture of the posterior tibial tendon, partial or complete, is uncommon among the young adult population. One case was reported in a 26-year-old man that occurred as he stepped up to a street car; the patient had no evidence of antecedent tenosynovitis (100). In four reported cases, the condition was attributed to a twisting ankle injury that occurred during volleyball (two cases), aerobics, or jogging (101).

Dislocation

Acute dislocation of the posterior tibial tendon is a rare event. In fact, Ballesteros et al. (102) found only 33

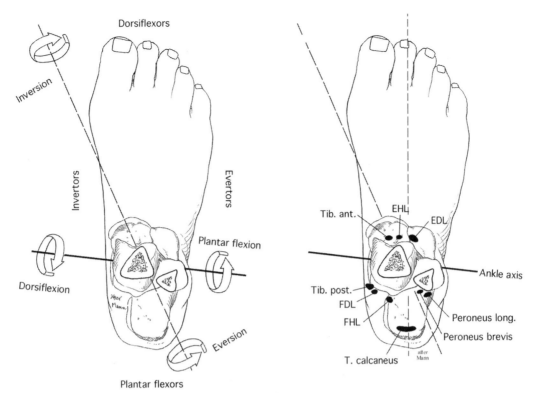

FIG. 53.12. Relationship of the tendons crossing the ankle relative to the axes of rotation for the ankle and subtalar joints.

reports in a review of the literature. The condition has occurred during running (103,104), gymnastics (105), and bullfighting (102).

Acute Tenosynovitis

More commonly, disorders of the posterior tibial tendon among athletes are due to acute tenosynovitis. In a review of 4,173 running injuries seen over a 4-year period, acute tenosynovitis accounted for 2.1% and 2.5% of all injuries among male and female patients, respectively (106). Another report identified 45 cases among 1,650 patients that presented to a runners clinic over a 2-year period (7). The incidence of this condition among runners has been calculated at 5% (107).

Chronic Tenosynovitis and Chronic Rupture

Chronic tenosynovitis and chronic rupture are related conditions that typically occur in older nonathletic adults. Woods and Leach (108) treated six athletic individuals with chronic rupture; they emphasized the importance of early recognition and treatment.

Mechanism of Injury and Pathoanatomy

Acute Rupture

Several variables probably contribute to tendon rupture, including age-related degenerative changes, a zone of hypovascularity (97), systemic disease, and traumatic or other mechanical factors. In one series of four acute ruptures, each occurring in an athletic individual, a twisting ankle injury was clearly associated with the onset of symptoms (101).

Dislocation

The mechanism for this rare injury is usually traumatic disruption of the flexor retinaculum caused by violent movement of the foot. One report (109) described a hypoplastic posterior tibial sulcus that contributed to the injury. Specific mechanisms include dorsiflexion and inversion of the foot caused by direct trauma (102,110), pronation–external rotation (104), or forced eversion–pronation and dorsiflexion of the foot (105,111).

Acute Tenosynovitis

Acute tenosynovitis is a painful syndrome caused by inflammation of the synovial sheath and the surrounding tissues. Most cases of acute tenosynovitis can be attributed to either overuse or the presence of a structural foot deformity such as an accessory navicular, excess heel valgus, or forefoot varus.

Chronic Tenosynovitis

Long-standing cases (more than 12 months) of tenosynovitis are arbitrarily termed chronic tenosynovitis and represent a painful syndrome typically associated tendon dysfunction due to degenerative changes within the substance of the tendon (tendinosis).

Chronic Rupture

Chronic rupture is an end stage of the dysfunctional tendon and commonly represents an elongated and nonfunctional tendon. Less commonly, this stage of the disease is caused by complete tear of the tendon.

Clinical Evaluation

Physical examination of the patient with posterior tibial tendon injury includes gait analysis, a single heel rise test, and evaluation of the foot with the patient both standing and sitting.

The single heel rise test is performed with the patient facing a wall and standing approximately 2 feet from the base. The well leg is tested first by asking the patient to stand on the well leg with the symptomatic foot off the ground. The patient may use both hands to obtain stability against the wall. The patient then rises onto the toes of the well leg and slowly returns to the plantigrade position. The maneuver is repeated up to 10 times. The examiner notes the height of the heel rise and the degree of heel inversion. Next, the symptomatic leg is tested. A positive test includes pain, weakness or absence of heel inversion, or decrease in height or inability to perform heel rise.

The standing patient is examined from behind. Knee alignment is assessed; excess genu valgum will place additional stress on the posterior tibial tendon. Heel valgus is noted and compared with the asymptomatic side. Swelling over the course of the posterior tibial tendon and forefoot adduction are also easily appreciated from this perspective. Manual motor testing is performed on all muscle groups of both lower extremities. The posterior tibial muscle is evaluated by instructing the patient to bring the foot from a position of plantarflexion and eversion to a position of plantarflexion and inversion. The patient is also asked to maintain a position of plantarflexion and inversion against resistance produced by the examiner.

The degree of fixed forefoot varus deformity is determined by examining the sitting patient; the hindfoot is held firmly by one of the examiner's hands and simultaneously the other hand is used to place a dorsiflexion force beneath the metatarsal heads. Care is taken to ensure the hand is raised in a plane parallel to the plantigrade position of the foot. The difference between the plantigrade position and the line drawn through the metatarsal heads defines the angle of fixed forefoot varus (normal, less than 7 degrees).

Acute Rupture

The patient with acute rupture of the posterior tibial tendon presents with a history of ankle injury with subsequent pain and inability to ambulate comfortably. A high degree of suspicion is required to make this diagnosis at the time of initial presentation. The presence of a concomitant ankle sprain or fracture may overshadow this condition. The physical examination demonstrates swelling and tenderness over the course of the posterior tibial tendon. Manual motor testing reveals the patient's inability to produce inversion of the plantarflexed foot. If the diagnosis is delayed, structural foot changes associated with chronic rupture may follow.

Dislocation

The patient with acute anterior dislocation of the posterior tibial tendon presents with a history of traumatic foot injury. The tendon may reduce spontaneously or remain anterior to the medial malleolus. Running and jumping are typically painful or not possible. The physical examination demonstrates swelling and tenderness over the retromalleolar area. The tendon is palpable anterior to the medial malleolus if it remains dislocated. Manual motor testing is painful and reveals profound weakness of the posterior tibial muscle.

Acute Tenosynovitis

Patients with tenosynovitis offer a history of pain along the course of the posterior tibial tendon, typically between the medial malleolus and the tendon's primary insertion at the navicular. For acute presentations, a change in athletic activity or shoe wear is solicited. Patients with tenosynovitis may have an antalgic gait. Normal heel inversion between 15% and 60% of the gait cycle is noted. The standing posture of the foot remains within normal limits. The single heel rise test is painful but otherwise normal. Manual motor testing of the posterior tibial muscle reveals either normal strength or loss of strength to varying degrees due to pain inhibition.

Chronic Tenosynovitis

Patients with long-standing tenosynovitis probably also have tendinosis or tendon degeneration. These patients also may have an antalgic gait. Loss of normal heel inversion between 15% and 60% of the gait cycle may also be detected. The foot may have flexible or fixed deformities such as heel valgus, flattening of the longitudinal arch, forefoot abduction, or forefoot varus. Manual motor testing of the posterior tibial muscle reveals loss of strength to varying degrees due to tendon failure.

Chronic Rupture

Patients with long-standing complete ruptures of the posterior tibial tendon demonstrate a loss of normal heel inversion between 15% and 60% of the gait cycle. The standing posture of the foot reveals heel valgus, flattening of the longitudinal arch, and forefoot abduction to varying degrees depending on the longevity of the dysfunction. Fixed heel valgus, forefoot varus, and contracture of the Achilles tendon also develop at the end stage. Manual motor testing of the posterior tibial muscle reveals little or no function.

Imaging

A weight-bearing plain radiographic series of the foot taken in the lateral and anterior posterior projections is the initial investigation. The presence of an enlarged or accessory navicular may predispose the patient to posterior tibial tendon injury. The alignment of the foot is noted with attention to midfoot breakdown on the lateral projection and forefoot abduction on the anterior posterior projection. A weight-bearing ankle series may reveal lateral tilt of the talus in the ankle mortise. Lateral tilt of the talus will contribute to hindfoot valgus and place chronic stress on the posterior tibial tendon. Lateral tilt may represent arthrosis of the talocrural joint; in such cases, a triple arthrodesis may lead to early and rapid progression of the talocrural arthrosis.

MRI is the preferred method for imaging the posterior tibial tendon. The method is useful for staging tendon disease and for preoperative planning when reconstruction is contemplated (112). The tendon is best demonstrated on the axial and sagittal images (113). The tendon is typically round to oval in shape with a homogenous low-signal throughout. Tenosynovitis is confirmed by increased water signal surrounding the tendon; the tendon itself remains well organized with no signal throughout its course. Tendinosis is confirmed by increased signal within the tendon. Pathologic findings consistent with tendinosis include loss of the homogenous low signal, a change to a fusiform or flattened shape, and the presence of partial linear tears. Dislocations and acute and chronic (114) disruptions are also well demonstrated. CT with high-definition soft tissue windows may be used to evaluate the posterior tibial tendon but is not the preferred imaging modality. CT and scintigraphy are used only to rule in tarsal coalition when this diagnosis is suggested by the clinical history and examination.

The use of real-time ultrasound in the evaluation of tendons about the foot and ankle has been advocated by several investigators (115,116). Reported advantages include widespread availability, low cost, lack of ionizing radiation, noninvasiveness, and ability to perform dynamic studies. The quality of information appears to be related to the experience of the person performing the examination. We have no experience with this modality.

Pitfalls

All routine radiographs must be weight-bearing studies to prevent underestimation of the deformity. When interpreting magnetic resonance images, Rosenberg et al. (113) noted that small amount of synovial fluid normally surrounds the tendon and should not be interpreted as a pathologic finding. They also noted that the tendon normally has a heterogeneous increased signal at its insertion into the navicular.

Economic Considerations

The clinical history and examination will provide enough information for diagnosis in most cases. MRI of the posterior tibial tenosynovitis remains a staging study and is not used as a screening test. CT and scintigraphy are not used for evaluation of the posterior tibial tendon.

Treatment of Injury

Acute Rupture

Nonoperative

Acute rupture of the posterior tibial tendon in the athletic individual must be repaired or reconstructed if the patients desires a return to a preinjury level of activity or performance.

Surgical

Treatment must restore the continuity of the posterior tibial tendon or replace its function with a transferred motor unit. Surgical exploration may reveal a secondary synovitis that requires debridement. An insertional tear may be reinserted into the navicular if the remaining tendon is free of degeneration and is long enough to accommodate the advancement. The use of suture anchors may allow the procedure to be done with a smaller amount of tendon, but we have no experience with this technique. A midsubstance rupture or a rupture through a degenerative tendon must be reconstructed with a transfer of the flexor digitorum longus tendon into the navicular tuberosity. Marcus et al. (101) reported excellent results in all four of their patients treated for acute rupture of the posterior tibial tendon. Three patients, despite functional improvements, failed to return to their preinjury activity level.

Exploration of the Ruptured Posterior Tibial Tendon and Reinsertion of the Tendon into the Navicular. Typically, a general anesthetic is used for this procedure. With the patient in the supine position and under tourniquet control, a linear incision is made over the course of the posterior tibial tendon from the posterior tip of the medial malleolus to the insertion of the posterior tibial tendon at the navicular, ending at the level of the medial cuneiform. Sharp dissection can be made to the tendon sheath. The sheath is sharply incised; using a hemostat to protect the underlying tendon, the sheath is opened across the length of the surgical wound. Proliferative synovium is sharply excised. The tendon itself is carefully inspected. Degenerative changes, represented by linear tears, tendon thickening, loss of tendon consistency, and change of color from white to yellow, are sharply resected. At this point a decision is made to reinsert the remaining tendon or reconstruct with a tendon transfer. For reinsertion of the tendon, enough length of healthy tendon must be present to allow passage of the tendon into the navicular. The deltoid and spring ligaments are inspected and repaired as necessary. A one-quarter–inch drill is then used to make a hole through the midportion of the navicular. The hole is started on the dorsum and directed out the plantar medial junction of the navicular. Once the drill is outside the plantar medial cortex of the navicular, a no. 15 scalpel is used to release soft tissue from the exit site. The distal end of the posterior tibial tendon is secured with two no. 2 nonabsorbable sutures; these sutures are weaved in a proximal direction to gain a substantial hold of the tendon. The sutures on the free end of the tendon are pulled through the navicular in a plantar to dorsal direction. The foot is placed in a plantarflexed and inverted position and the tendon is carefully advanced into the navicular. As the tendon is pulled through the navicular, the transfer is placed under maximum tension and the distal tendon is secured to the dorsal aspect of the navicular. Occasionally, the tendon may be split before passage into the navicular; in this case, one end of the tendon is passed through the navicular and then secured to the remaining end of the tendon. The posterior tibial tendon sheath is loosely closed with a running 3-0 nylon suture. The subcutaneous tissue is closed with interrupted 4-0 absorbable suture and the skin closed with 4-0 nylon suture or skin clips. The foot and ankle are placed in a plantarflexed and inverted position, covered with a compression dressing, and set in plaster splints for immobilization.

The patient is instructed to keep the foot elevated for the next 2 days. After a 10-day period of non–weight bearing, the patient returns for removal of skin sutures or clips. Non–weight bearing is continued in a plantarflexed and inverted cast. At the 6-week follow-up, the foot is placed in a plantigrade position and a removable cast boot is fitted. The patient is instructed to begin weight bearing as tolerated and to remove the cast boot three times a day for active range of motion exercises. At the 10-week postoperative visit, a strengthening program is instituted with an elastic band. Activities with the cast boot are gradually resumed, and finally the patient is weaned out of the cast boot.

Exploration of the Ruptured Posterior Tibial Tendon and Reconstruction with Transfer of the Flexor Digitorum Longus Tendon into the Navicular. Typically, a general anesthetic is used for this procedure. With the patient in the supine position and under tourniquet control, a linear incision is centered at the point of maximum tenderness. The incision is in line with the course of the posterior tibial tendon. The sheath is sharply incised; using a hemostat to protect the underlying tendon, the sheath is opened across the length of the surgical wound. Proliferative synovium is sharply excised. Debridement of the sheath may require additional proximal exposure. The skin incision is continued over the course of the tendon proximal to the medial malleolus. A 1-cm section of sheath and flexor retinaculum is left intact at the medial malleolus to function as a pulley, and the remaining sheath is incised, inspected, and debrided as required. The tendon itself is carefully inspected and the rupture well exposed. Degenerative changes, represented by linear tears, tendon thickening, loss of tendon consistency, and change of color from white to yellow, are sharply resected. The deltoid and spring ligaments are inspected and repaired as necessary. The flexor digitorum longus is harvested by extending the incision distally along the medial aspect of the first metatarsal. The fascia of the abductor hallucis muscle is released and the abductor hallucis muscle is retracted in a plantar direction, allowing visualization of the plantar digital nerves and the flexor digitorum longus and the flexor hallucis longus tendons. While protecting the nerves, the flexor knot of Henry is released and the flexor digitorum longus tendon is released from all fascial connections along its proximal course.

Next, the flexor digitorum longus tendon is tenodesed to the flexor hallucis longus tendon with nonabsorbable suture. The tenodesis is placed as far distal as possible. The flexor digitorum longus tendon is divided just proximal to the tenodesis. The free end of the tendon is pulled proximally into the middle section of the surgical wound. A one-quarter–inch drill is used to make a hole through the midportion of the navicular. The hole is started on the dorsum and directed out the plantar medial junction of the navicular. Once the drill is outside the plantar medial cortex of the navicular, a no. 15 scalpel is used to release soft tissue from the exit site. The distal end of the flexor digitorum longus is secured with two no. 2 nonabsorbable sutures. The sutures on the free end of the flexor digitorum longus tendon are pulled through the navicular in a plantar to dorsal direction. The sheath of the posterior tibial tendon is not used. The foot is placed in a plantarflexed and inverted position, and the flexor digitorum longus tendon is carefully advanced through the navicular. As the tendon is pulled through the navicular, the transfer is placed under maximum tension and the distal tendon is secured to the dorsal aspect of the navicular. At least three nonabsorbable sutures are placed through the tendon and into the tissue over the navicular. Excess tendon is sharply excised. The empty posterior tibial tendon sheath is loosely closed with a running 3-0 nylon suture. The subcutaneous tissue is closed with interrupted 4-0 absorbable suture and the skin closed with 4-0 nylon suture or skin clips. The foot and ankle are placed in a plantarflexed and inverted position, covered with a compression dressing, and set in plaster splints for immobilization.

The patient is instructed to keep the foot elevated for the next 2 days. After a 10-day period of non-weight bearing, the patient returns for removal of skin sutures or clips. Non-weight bearing is continued in a plantarflexed and inverted cast. At the 4-week follow-up, the foot is placed in a plantigrade position and a removable cast boot is fitted. The patient is instructed to begin weight bearing as tolerated and to remove the cast boot three times a day for active range of motion exercises. At the 8-week postoperative visit, a strengthening program is instituted with an elastic band. Activities with the cast boot are gradually resumed, and finally the patient is weaned out of the cast boot.

Dislocation

Nonoperative

Ouzounian and Meyerson (104) reported failure of nonoperative treatment for all seven of their patients with anterior dislocation of the posterior tibial tendon. Nonoperative treatment included cast or brace immobilization and physical therapy.

When to Refer. Patients with acute, persistent, or recurrent dislocation of the posterior tibial tendon are referred to an orthopedic surgeon.

Surgical

The literature suggests that the dislocation of the posterior tibial tendon anterior to the medial malleolus may be treated with the same principles used to manage peroneal tendon dislocation: The flexor retinaculum must be securely reduced and repaired or reconstructed and a flat flexor grove must be sufficiently deepened or supplemented by a bone block. Ballesteros et al. (102) described a modification of the Jones technique for reinforcement of the peroneal retinaculum. A medial flap of the Achilles tendon was mobilized keeping the insertion of the tendon at the calcaneal tuberosity intact. The flap was advanced into a drill hole just proximal to the medial malleolus. The treatment was successful in a competitive bullfighter. Ouzounian and Meyerson (104)

reported marked improvements in all seven patients each treated with a combination of several procedures, including retinaculum repair or reconstruction, tenodesis of the posterior tibial tendon to the flexor digitorum longus, or groove deepening. Six patients returned to a preinjury level of activity.

Acute Tenosynovitis

Nonoperative

Treatment of mild acute tenosynovitis begins with efforts aimed at the reduction of inflammation. A reduction or modification in athletic activity is the most sensible first step. NSAIDs are also judiciously administered and monitored. Treatment of moderate to severe acute tenosynovitis requires cessation of stressful activities. If the symptoms fail to respond within 4 weeks, then immobilization with a short leg walking cast or a removable cast boot is indicated.

When to Refer. All patients with acute tenosynovitis that fail to respond to a 4- to 6-week period of immobilization are referred to an orthopedic surgeon.

Surgical

Patients with acute tenosynovitis that have failed to respond to adequate conservative treatment require surgical exploration of the posterior tibial tendon and debridement of the posterior tibial tendon sheath (117). Proliferative synovium or reactive tissue should be systematically and meticulously excised by sharp dissection. Teasdall and Johnson (117) treated 19 patients with posterior tibial tendon dysfunction characterized by pain and swelling along the medial aspect of the ankle with synovectomy and debridement of the tendon sheath. Each patient had previously failed conservative therapy. At an average follow-up of 30 months, 14 patients reported complete relief, 3 patients reported the persistence of minor pain, 1 patient reported the persistence of moderate pain, and 1 patient reported the persistence of severe pain.

Exploration of the Posterior Tibial Tendon and Debridement of the Posterior Tibial Tendon Sheath. Typically, a general anesthetic is used for this procedure. With the patient in the supine position and under tourniquet control, a linear incision is made over the course of the posterior tibial tendon from the posterior tip of the medial malleolus to the insertion of the posterior tibial tendon at the navicular. Sharp dissection can be made to the tendon sheath. The sheath is incised, and while using the hemostat to protect the underlying tendon, the sheath is sharply opened across the length of the surgical wound. Typically, an effusion will be noted within the tendon sheath, as well as evidence of synovial proliferation and increased vascular activity. The synovium is sharply excised. Debridement of the sheath may require additional proximal exposure. The skin incision is continued over the course of the tendon proximal to the medial malleolus. A 1-cm section of sheath and flexor retinaculum is left intact at the medial malleolus to function as a pulley, and the remaining sheath is incised, inspected, and debrided as required. The tendon is carefully inspected. Partial longitudinal tears are debrided or repaired with a running 4-0 nylon suture. Evidence of tendinosis will require consideration for debridement of the tendon itself and a possible reconstructive procedure such as transfer of the flexor digitorum longus tendon to the navicular. Assuming that the tendon itself appears healthy, the sheath is loosely closed with a running 3-0 nylon suture. The subcutaneous tissue is closed with interrupted 4-0 absorbable suture and the skin closed with 4-0 nylon suture or skin clips. The foot and ankle are placed in a neutral position, covered with a compression dressing, and set in plaster splints for immobilization.

The patient is instructed to keep the foot elevated for the next 2 days. After a 10-day period of non-weight bearing, the patient returns for removal of skin sutures or clips. The foot is placed in a removable cast boot. The patient is instructed to begin weight bearing as tolerated and to remove the cast boot three times a day for active range of motion exercises. At the 4-week postoperative visit, a strengthening program is instituted with an elastic band. Activities with the cast boot are gradually resumed, and finally the patient is weaned out of the cast boot.

Chronic Tenosynovitis and Chronic Rupture

Nonoperative

Patients with chronic tenosynovitis or chronic rupture can be managed with an orthotic insert. The orthotic must incorporate a varus heel wedge (to reduce the tendency of the heel to assume a valgus position) and medial forefoot post (to compensate for forefoot varus).

When to Refer. Patients with chronic tenosynovitis or chronic ruptures that fail to improve with orthotic management are referred to an orthopedic surgeon. Referral for operative evaluation must be done in a timely manner because athletic performance is greatly inhibited by a nonfunctioning posterior tibial tendon and permanent structural changes will occur secondary to posterior tibial tendon dysfunction.

Surgical

Patients with chronic tenosynovitis that have not responded to an adequate course of conservative treatment or patients with chronic rupture and a flexible foot require debridement of the posterior tibial tendon sheath, excision of all degenerative tendon, and transfer of the flexor digitorum longus to the navicular.

Patients with chronic rupture and fixed subtalar valgus or fixed forefoot varus require subtalar, double, or triple arthrodesis. These reconstructive procedures are outside the scope of this chapter and in most cases preclude athletic competition.

Debridement of the Posterior Tibial Tendon and Reconstruction with Transfer of the Flexor Digitorum Longus Tendon into the Navicular. Typically, a general anesthetic is used for this procedure. With the patient in the supine position and under tourniquet control, a linear incision is made over the course of the posterior tibial tendon from the posterior tip of the medial malleolus to the insertion of the posterior tibial tendon at the navicular. Sharp dissection can be made to the tendon sheath. The sheath is sharply incised; using a hemostat to protect the underlying tendon, the sheath is opened across the length of the surgical wound. Typically, an effusion will be noted within the tendon sheath, as well as evidence of synovial proliferation and increased vascular activity. The synovium is sharply excised. Debridement of the sheath may require additional proximal exposure. The skin incision is continued over the course of the tendon proximal to the medial malleolus. A 1-cm section of sheath, and flexor retinaculum is left intact at the medial malleolus to function as a pulley and the remaining sheath is incised, inspected, and debrided as required. The tendon itself is then carefully inspected. Degenerative changes, represented by linear tears, tendon thickening, loss of tendon consistency, and change of color from white to yellow, are sharply resected. The deltoid and spring ligaments are inspected and imbricated or reconstructed as necessary. The flexor digitorum longus tendon is harvested by extending the incision distally along the medial aspect of the first metatarsal. The abductor hallucis muscle is retracted in a plantar direction, allowing visualization of the plantar digital nerves and the flexor digitorum longus and the flexor hallucis longus tendons. While protecting the nerves, the flexor knot of Henry is released and the flexor digitorum longus tendon is released from all fascial connections along its proximal course. Next, the flexor digitorum longus tendon is tenodesed to the flexor hallucis longus tendon with a nonabsorbable suture. The tenodesis is placed as far distal as possible. The flexor digitorum longus tendon is divided just proximal to the tenodesis. The free end of the tendon is pulled proximally into the middle section of the surgical wound. A one-quarter–inch drill is used to make a hole through the midportion of the navicular. The hole is started on the dorsum and directed out the plantar medial junction of the navicular. Once the drill is outside the plantar medial cortex of the navicular, a no. 15 scalpel is used to release soft tissue from the exit site. The distal end of the flexor digitorum longus is secured with two no.

2 nonabsorbable sutures. The sutures on the free end of the flexor digitorum longus tendon are pulled through the navicular in a plantar to dorsal direction. The sheath of the posterior tibial tendon is not used. The foot is placed in a plantarflexed and inverted position, and the flexor digitorum longus tendon is carefully advanced through the navicular. As the tendon is pulled through the navicular, the transfer is placed under maximum tension and the distal tendon is secured to the dorsal aspect of the navicular. At least three other nonabsorbable sutures are placed through the tendon and into the tissue over the navicular. Excess tendon is sharply excised. The empty posterior tibial tendon sheath is loosely closed with a running 3-0 nylon suture. The subcutaneous tissue is closed with interrupted 4-0 absorbable suture and the skin closed with 4-0 nylon suture or skin clips. The foot and ankle are placed in a plantarflexed and inverted position, covered with a compression dressing, and set in plaster splints for immobilization.

The patient is instructed to keep the foot elevated for the next 2 days. After a 10-day period of non-weight bearing, the patient returns for removal of skin sutures or clips. Non-weight bearing is continued in a plantarflexed and inverted cast. At the 4-week follow-up, the foot is placed in a plantigrade position and a removable cast boot is fitted. The patient is instructed to begin weight bearing as tolerated and to remove the cast boot three times a day for active range of motion exercises. At the 8-week postoperative visit, a strengthening program is instituted with an elastic band. Activities with the cast boot are gradually resumed, and finally the patient is weaned out of the cast boot.

TIBIALIS ANTERIOR, EXTENSOR HALLUCIS LONGUS, EXTENSOR DIGITORUM LONGUS, AND THE PERONEUS TERTIUS TENDONS

The muscles that originate within the anterior compartment of the leg include the tibialis anterior, extensor hallucis longus, extensor digitorum longus, and the peroneus tertius muscles. Each muscle forms a tendon that will pass anterior to the ankle joint, thus producing dorsiflexion of the foot. The tendons pass beneath the extensor retinaculum, a thickened section of the crural fascia. The retinaculum maintains the relationship of each tendon and prevents bowstringing. As the tendons pass across the ankle joint, they are surrounded by a synovial sheath, an individual sheath for the tibialis anterior tendon and the extensor hallucis longus tendon, and a common sheath for the extensor digitorum longus tendons (118). Proximal to the ankle joint, the anterior tibial artery and deep peroneal nerve are found between the tibialis anterior and extensor hallucis longus tendons. Distal to the ankle joint, the dorsalis pedis artery and deep peroneal nerve are found between the extensor hallucis longus and extensor digitorum longus tendons. Microvascular investigation of the tibialis anterior tendon demonstrated adequate blood supply to the entire tendon from proximal and distal ventral vinculae (119).

Injuries to the tendons in front of the ankle joint are uncommon. They typically occur in older less active persons but are reported in athletes of all ages. Injuries encountered in the athletic population include closed ruptures, lacerations, dislocations, and snapping.

Closed Rupture

Dooley et al. (120) noted that closed rupture of the tibialis anterior tendon tends to occur in patients between 60 and 70 years of age after relatively minor trauma. The subsequent functional deficit was mild, a mild to moderate foot drop, but was bothersome enough to three of the four patients in their series to warrant reconstruction. Ouzounian and Anderson (121) reported a series of 12 closed anterior tibial tendon ruptures. All seven of the surgically treated patients demonstrated improved function, and many returned to athletic activity. Based on their experience, they recommended bracing for elderly patients that present late with atraumatic ruptures and surgical repair or reconstruction for patients that present early with a traumatic ruptures.

Sim and DeWeerd reported a case of closed extensor hallucis longus tendon rupture in a 17-year-old snow skier. The proposed mechanism was constant dorsiflexion of the great toe produced by the patient trying to maintain the body's center of gravity behind the ski boot. The injury was treated successfully with primary repair, early range of motion, and 8 weeks of immobilization with the toe in hyperextension. A similar case of spontaneous extensor hallucis longus tendon rupture occurred in a 46-year-old hill walker. The disruption occurred at the level of the ankle and was successfully treated with a primary repair.

Laceration

The subcutaneous position of the tendons and neurovascular bundle at the anterior ankle predispose them to injury by direct trauma. Simonet and Sim described injury to the tibialis anterior tendon, extensor hallucis longus tendon, extensor digitorum longus tendon, dorsalis pedis artery, dorsalis pedis vein, or deep peroneal nerve by the blade of an ice skate. The injury occurred in five professional and collegiate hockey players; each skated with the tongue of the skate folded down, thus exposing the anterior ankle. Four patients treated with primary repair of the involved structures (tibialis anterior tendon, extensor hallucis longus tendon, and dorsalis pedis artery; extensor hallucis longus tendon and partial tibialis anterior tendon; tibialis anterior tendon;

extensor digitorum longus tendon, dorsalis pedis artery, and deep peroneal nerve) returned to professional hockey play. A single case of missed anterior tibialis tendon laceration in a college player was reconstructed 6 weeks after missed diagnosis. The reconstruction failed, and the patient was unable to return to the sport.

Griffiths reported a series of six open disruptions of the extensor hallucis longus tendon (ages 4 to 25). Five tendons were repaired primarily and one not repaired, each with a satisfactory result.

Traumatic disruption of the tibialis anterior in the athletic individual can be treated nonoperatively if the tendon ends remains well approximated. When displacement or retraction occurs, operative treatment is required. Repair can usually be accomplished with end to end or side to side repair. Occasionally, the proximal or distal tendon will require Z-lengthening before repair. Rarely, an interposition graft is required. Forst et al. reported the case of a 28-year-old female triathelete with a laceration of the tibialis anterior tendon caused by the bike chain guard. Primary repair failed due to infection. Reconstruction of the subsequent 9-cm defect was accomplished with a free peroneal brevis tendon graft from the ipsilateral leg. After scar revision, the woman returned to successful competition.

Dislocation

Akhtar and Levine reported a case of a 57-year-old man with dislocation of the extensor digitorum longus tendon after spontaneous rupture of the inferior retinaculum. The patient inverted the ankle while playing squash. Upon surgical inspection, the extensor retinaculum was ruptured and a fibrous band prevented reduction of the extensor digitorum longus tendon. After release of the band, the tendons spontaneously reduced and the retinaculum was repaired. The patient returned to full activity.

Snapping

Snapping of the tibialis anterior tendon near its insertion was reported in a 35-year-old scuba diver and swimmer. The pain began after a long dive with fins. The pain worsened, and a snapping of the tibialis anterior developed at the level of the navicular cuneiform joint. The symptoms failed to resolve with rest and NSAID. Operative findings revealed a ganglion cyst continuous with the navicular cuneiform joint. Complete recovery after excision was noted.

Authors' Preference

When surgical intervention is planned, the incision is in line with, but not over, the injured tendon in an effort to minimize adhesion with the overlying skin. Adhesion

between the repaired or reconstructed tendon and the extensor retinaculum are minimized by using techniques compatible with tendon surgery at the wrist or hand. Core sutures of nonreactive nonabsorbable material are buried within the tendon substance. The peripheral margin of the tendon ends are repaired with a smaller running suture made of nylon, polydioxanone, or PDS (Ethicon, Inc.).

REFERENCES

1. Hoppenfeld S, de Boer P. The tibia and fibula. In: *Surgical exposures in orthopaedics. The anatomic approach.* Philadelphia: J.B. Lippincott, 1984:462.
2. Sarrafian SK. Myology. In: *Anatomy of the foot and ankle,* 2nd ed. Philadelphia: J.B. Lippincott, 1993:279–281.
3. Sarrafian SK. Tendon sheaths and bursae. In: *Anatomy of the foot and ankle,* 2nd ed. Philadelphia: J.B. Lippincott, 1993:285–289.
4. Frey C, Rosenberg Z, Shereff M, et al. The retrocalcaneal bursa: anatomy and bursography. *Foot Ankle* 13:203–207.
5. Mann RA. Biomechanics of the foot and ankle. In: Mann RA, Coughlin MJ, eds. *Surgery of the foot and ankle.* 6th ed. 18–19.
6. Caine D, Cochrane B, Caine C, et al. An epidemiologic investigation of injuries affecting young competitive female gymnasts. *Am J Sports Med* 1989;17:811–820.
7. Clement DB, Taunton JE, Smart GW, et al. A survey of overuse running injuries. *Phys Sportsmed* 1981;9:47–58.
8. Rovere GD, Webb LX, Gristina AG, et al. Musculoskeletal injuries in theatrical dance students. *Am J Sports Med* 1983;11: 195–198.
9. Kvist H, Kvist M. The operative treatment of chronic calcaneal paratenonitis. *J Bone Joint Surg Br* 1980;62-B:353–357.
10. Åstrom M, Rausing A. Chronic Achilles tendinopathy. A survey of surgical and histologic findings. *Clin Orthop* 1995;316:151–164.
11. Lagergren C, Lindholm Å. Vascular distribution in the Achilles tendon. An angiographic and microangiographic study. *Acta Chir Scand* 1958;116:491–496.
12. Arner O, Lindholm Å. Subcutaneous rupture of the Achilles tendon. A study of 92 cases. *Acta Chir Scand* 1959; [Suppl]:239.
13. Bordelon RL. Heel pain. In: Mann RA, Coughlin MJ, eds. *Surgery of the foot and ankle,* 6th ed. 848.
14. Travis MT, Pitcher JD. Accessory soleus presenting as a posterior ankle mass: a case report and literature review. *Foot Ankle* 1995;16:651–654.
15. Williams JGP. Achilles tendon lesions in sport. *Sports Med* 1986;3:114–135.
16. Thompson TC. A test for rupture of the tendo Achilles. *Acta Orthop Scand* 1962;32:461.
17. Schepis AA, Leach RE. Surgical management of Achilles tendinitis. *Am J Sports Med* 1987;15:308–315.
18. Nistor L. Surgical and non-surgical treatment of Achilles tendon rupture. *J Bone Joint Surg Am* 1981;63-A:394–399.
19. Inglis AE, Scott WN, Sculco TP, et al. Rupture of the tendo achillis. An objective assessment of the surgical and non-surgical treatment. *J Bone Joint Surg Am* 1976;58-A:990–993.
20. Wapner KL, Pavlock GS, Hecht PJ, et al. Repair of chronic Achilles tendon rupture with flexor hallucis longus tendon transfer. *Foot Ankle* 1993;14:443–449.
21. Mann RA, Holmes GB, Seale KS, et al. Chronic rupture of the Achilles tendon: A new technique of repair. *J Bone Joint Surg Am* 1991;73-A:214–218.
22. Turco VJ, Spinella AJ. Achilles tendon ruptures—peroneus brevis transfer. *Foot Ankle* 1987;7:253–259.
23. Lea R, Smith L. Non-surgical treatment of tendo-achillis rupture. *J Bone Joint Surg Am* 1972;54-A:1398–1407.
24. Troop RL, Losse GM, Lane JG, et al. Early motion after repair of Achilles tendon ruptures. *Foot Ankle* 1995;16:705–709.
25. Hoppenfeld S, de Boer P. The tibia and fibula. In: *Surgical exposures in orthopaedics. The anatomic approach.* Philadelphia: J.B. Lippincott, 1984:462.

26. Sarrafian SK. Myology. In: *Anatomy of the foot and ankle*, 2nd ed. Philadelphia: J.B. Lippincott, 1993:235.
27. Sarrafian SK. Myology. In: *Anatomy of the foot and ankle*, 2nd ed. Philadelphia: J.B. Lippincott, 1993:240–242.
28. Sarrafian SK. Tendon sheaths and bursae. In: *Anatomy of the foot and ankle*, 2nd ed. Philadelphia: J.B. Lippincott, 1993:288.
29. Gould N. Stenosing tenosynovitis of the flexor hallucis longus tendon at the great toe. *Foot Ankle* 1981;2:46–48.
30. Boruta PM, Beauperthuy GD. Partial tear of the flexor hallucis longus at the Knot of Henry: Presentation of three cases. *Foot Ankle Int* 1997;18:243–246.
31. Sammarco J, Miller EH. Partial rupture of the flexor hallucis longus tendon in classical ballet dancers. *J Bone Joint Surg Am* 1979;61-A:149–150.
32. Trepman E, Mizel MS, Newberg AH. Partial rupture of the flexor hallucis longus tendon in a tennis player: a case report. *Foot Ankle Int* 1995;16:227–231.
33. Inokuchi S, Usami N. Closed complete rupture of the flexor hallucis longus tendon at the groove of the talus. *Foot Ankle Int* 1997;18:47–49.
34. Krackow KA. Acute, traumatic rupture of the flexor hallucis longus tendon: a case report. *Clin Orthop* 1980;150:261–262.
35. Thompson FM, Snow SW, Hershon SJ. Spontaneous atraumatic rupture of the flexor hallucis longus tendon under the sustentaculum tali: case report, review of the literature, and treatment options. *Foot Ankle* 1993;14:414–417.
36. Holt KW, Cross MJ. Isolated rupture of the flexor hallucis longus tendon: a case report. *Am J Sports Med* 1990;18:645–646.
37. Coghlan BA, Clark NM. Traumatic rupture of the flexor hallucis longus tendon in a marathon runner. *Am J Sports Med* 1993;21:617–618.
38. Romash MM. Closed rupture of the flexor hallucis longus tendon in a long distance runner: report of a case and review of the literature. *Foot Ankle Int* 1994;15:433–436.
39. Floyd DW, Heckman JD, Rockwood CA. Tendon lacerations in the foot. *Foot Ankle* 1983;4:8–14.
40. McCarroll JR, Ritter MA, Becker TE. Triggering of the great toe: a case report. *Clin Orthop* 1983;175:184–185.
41. Kolettis GJ, Micheli LJ, Klein JD. Release of the flexor hallucis longus tendon in ballet dancers. *J Bone Joint Surg Am* 1996;78-A:1386–1390.
42. Hamilton WG. Stenosing tenosynovitis of the flexor hallucis longus tendon and posterior impingement of the os trigonum in ballet dancers. *Foot Ankle* 1982;3:74–80.
43. Frenette JP, Jackson DW. Laceration of the flexor hallucis longus in the young athlete. *J Bone Joint Surg Am* 1977;59-A:673–676.
44. Hoppenfeld S, de Boer P. The tibia and fibula. In: *Surgical exposures in orthopaedics. The anatomic approach.* Philadelphia: J.B. Lippincott, 1984:465.
45. Sarrafian SK. Myology. In: *Anatomy of the foot and ankle*, 2nd ed. Philadelphia: J.B. Lippincott, 1993:227–229.
46. Peterson DA, Stinson W. Excision of the fractured os peroneum: a report of five patients and review of the literature. *Foot Ankle* 1992;13:277–281.
47. Burman M, Lapidius PW. The functional disturbances caused by inconstant bones and sesamoids of the foot. *Arch Surg* 1931;22:936–975.
48. Hoppenfeld S, de Boer P. The tibia and fibula. In: *Surgical exposures in orthopaedics. The anatomic approach.* Philadelphia: J.B. Lippincott, 1984:465.
49. Sarrafian SK. Myology. In: *Anatomy of the foot and ankle*, 2nd ed. Philadelphia: J.B. Lippincott, 1993:231.
50. Sarrafian SK. Tendon sheaths and bursae. In: *Anatomy of the foot and ankle*, 2nd ed. Philadelphia: J.B. Lippincott, 1993:284–285.
51. Sobel M, Geppert MJ, Hannafin JA, et al. Microvascular anatomy of the peroneal tendons. *Foot Ankle* 1992;13:469–472.
52. Edwards ME. The relationship of the peroneal tendons to the fibula, calcaneus, and cuboideum. *Am J Anat* 1928;42:213–253.
53. Purnell ML, Drummond DS, Engber WD, et al. Congenital dislocation of the peroneal tendons in the calcaneovalgus foot. *J Bone Joint Surg Br* 1983;65-B:316–319.
54. Davis WH, Sobel M, Deland J, et al. The superior peroneal retinaculum: an anatomical study. *Foot Ankle* 1994;15:271–275.
55. Sarrafian SK. Myology. In: *Anatomy of the foot and ankle*, 2nd ed. Philadelphia: J.B. Lippincott, 1993:231–235.
56. Sobel M, Levy ME, Bonhe WHO. Congenital variations of the peroneus quartus muscle: an anatomic study *Foot Ankle* 1990;11:81–90.
57. Webster FS. Peroneal tenosynovitis with pseudotumor. *J Bone Joint Surg Am* 1968;50-A:153–157.
58. Trevino S, Gould N, Korson R. Surgical treatment of stenosing tenosynovitis at the ankle. *Foot Ankle* 1981;2:37–45.
59. Clanton TO, Schon LC. Athletic injuries to the soft tissues of the foot and ankle. In: Mann RA, Coughlin MJ, eds. *Surgery of the foot and ankle*, 6th ed. 1167.
60. Escalas F, Figueras JM, Merino JA. Dislocation of the peroneal tendons. *J Bone Joint Surg Am* 1980;62-A:451–453.
61. McConkey JP, Favero KJ. Subluxation of the peroneal tendons within the peroneal tendon sheath: a case report. *Am J Sports Med* 1987;15:511–513.
62. Harper MC. Subluxation of the peroneal tendons within the peroneal groove: a report of two cases. *Foot Ankle* 1997;18:369–370.
63. Sobel M, Bonhe WHO, Levy ME. Longitudinal attrition of the peroneus brevis tendon in the fibular groove: an anatomic study. *Foot Ankle* 1990;11:124–128.
64. Sammarco GJ, DiRaimondo CV. Chronic peroneus brevis tendon lesions. *Foot Ankle* 1989;9:163–170.
65. Kilkelly FX, McHale KA. Acute rupture of the peroneal longus tendon in a runner: a case report and a review of the literature. *Foot Ankle* 1994;15:567–569.
66. Evans JD. Subcutaneus rupture of the tendon of the peroneus longus. Report of a case. *J Bone Joint Surg Br* 1966;48-B:507–509.
67. Tehranzadeh J, Stoll DA, Gabriele OM. Case report 271. Diagnosis: posterior migration of the os peroneum of the left foot, indicating a tear of the peroneal tendon. *Skeletal Radiol* 1984;12:44–47.
68. Konradsen L, Sommer H. Ankle instability caused by peroneal tendon rupture. A case report. *Acta Orthop Scand* 1989;60:723–724.
69. Mains DB, Sullivan RC. Fracture of the os peroneum. A case report. *J Bone Joint Surg Am* 55-A:1529–1530.
70. Peacock KC, Resnick EJ, Thoder JJ. Fracture of the os peroneum with rupture of the peroneus longus tendon. A case report and review of the literature. *Clin Orthop* 1986;202:223–226.
71. Murr S. Dislocation of the peroneal tendons with marginal fracture of the lateral malleolus. *J Bone Joint Surg Br* 1961;43-B:563–565.
72. Stover CN, Bryan DR. Traumatic dislocation of the peroneal tendons. *Am J Surg* 1962;103:180–186.
73. Eckert WR, Davis EA Jr. Acute rupture of the peroneal retinaculum. *J Bone Joint Surg Am* 1976;58-A:670–673.
74. Oden RF. Tendon injuries about the ankle resulting from skiing. *Clin Orthop* 1987;216:63–69.
75. Geppert MJ, Sobel M, Bohne WHO. Lateral ankle instability as a cause of superior peroneal retinacular laxity: an anatomic and biomechanical study of cadaveric feet. *Foot Ankle* 1993;14:330–334.
76. Sobel M, Geppert MJ, Olson EJ, et al. The dynamics of peroneus brevis tendon splits: a proposed mechanism, technique of diagnosis, and classification of injury. *Foot Ankle* 1992;13:413–422.
77. Brodsky JW, Krause JO. Peroneus brevis tendon tears: pathophysiology, surgical reconstruction, and clinical results.
78. Bassett FH, Speer KS. Longitudinal rupture of the peroneal tendon. *Am J Sports Med* 1993;21:354–357.
79. Arrowsmith SR, Fleming LL, Allman FL. Traumatic dislocation of the peroneal tendons. *Am J Sports Med* 1983;11:142–146.
80. McLennan JG. Treatment of acute and chronic luxations of the peroneal tendons. *Am J Sports Med* 1980;8:432–436.
81. Sobel M, Pavlov H, Gepper MJ, et al. Painful os peroneum syndrome: a spectrum of conditions responsible for plantar lateral foot pain. *Foot Ankle* 1994;15:112–124.
82. Truong DT, Dussault RG, Kaplan PA. Fracture of the os peroneum and rupture of the peroneus longus tendon as a complication of diabetic neuropathy. *Skeletal Radiol* 1995;24:626–628.
83. Jones E. Operative treatment of chronic dislocations of the peroneal tendons. *J Bone Joint Surg Am* 1932;14:574–576.

84. Martens MA, Noyez JF, Mulier JC. Recurrent dislocation of the peroneal tendons: results of rerouting the tendons under the calcaneofibular ligament. *Am J Sports Med* 1986;14:148–150.

85. Micheli LJ, Waters PM, Sanders DP. Sliding fibular graft repair for chronic dislocation of the peroneal tendons. *Am J Sports Med* 1989;17:68–71.

86. Miller JW. Dislocation of the peroneal tendons—a new operative procedure: a case report. *Am J Orthop* 1967;9:136–137.

87. Sarmiento A, Wolf M. Subluxation of the peroneal tendons: a case treated by rerouting the tendons under the calcaneofibular ligament. *J Bone Joint Surg Am* 1975;57-A:115–116.

88. Zoellner G, Clancy W Jr. Recurrent dislocation of the peroneal tendon. *J Bone Joint Surg Am* 1979;61-A:292–294.

89. Kelly RE. An operation for the chronic dislocation of the peroneal tendons. *Br J Surg* 1920;7:502–504.

90. DuVries HL. *Surgery of the foot.* St. Louis: Mosby-Year Book, 1965:256–257.

91. Stein RE. Reconstruction of the superior peroneal retinaculum using a portion of the peroneus brevis tendon: a case report. *J Bone Joint Surg Am* 1987;69-A:298–299.

92. Mick CA, Lynch F. Reconstruction of the peroneal retinaculum using the peroneus quartus. *J Bone Joint Surg Am* 1987;69-A:296–297.

93. Pozo JL, Jackson AM. A rerouting operation for dislocation of the peroneal tendons: operative technique and case report. *Foot Ankle* 1984;5:42–44.

94. Hoppenfeld S, de Boer P. The tibia and fibula. In: *Surgical exposures in orthopaedics. The anatomic approach.* Philadelphia: J.B. Lippincott, 1984:464.

95. Sarrafian SK. Myology. In: *Anatomy of the foot and ankle,* 2nd ed. Philadelphia: J.B. Lippincott, 1993:239–240.

96. Sarrafian SK. Tendon sheaths and bursae. In: *Anatomy of the foot and ankle,* 2nd ed. Philadelphia: J.B. Lippincott, 1993:285.

97. Frey C, Shereff M, Greenidge N. Vascularity of the posterior tibial tendon. *J Bone Joint Surg Am* 1990;72-A:884–888.

98. Mann RA. Biomechanics of the foot. In: *American Academy of Orthopaedic Surgeons atlas of orthotics,* 2nd ed. St. Louis: Mosby-Year Book, 1985:121.

99. Mann RA. Biomechanics of the foot and ankle. In: Mann RA, Coughlin MJ, eds. *Surgery of the foot and ankle,* 6th ed. 28–31.

100. Kettelkamp DB, Alexander HH. Spontaneous rupture of the posterior tibial tendon. *J Bone Joint Surg Am* 1969;51-A:759–764.

101. Marcus RE, Goodfellow DB, Pfister ME. The difficult diagnosis of posterior tibial tendon rupture in sports injuries. *Orthopaedics* 1995;18:715–721.

102. Ballesteros R, Chacon M, Cimarra A, et al. Traumatic dislocation of the tibialis posterior tendon: a new surgical procedure to obtain a strong reconstruction. *J Trauma* 1995;39:1198–2000.

103. Larsen E, Lauridsen F. Dislocation of the tibialis posterior tendon in two athletes. *Am J Sports Med* 1984;12:429–430.

104. Ouzounian TJ, Myerson MS. Dislocation of the posterior tibial tendon. *Foot Ankle* 1992;13:215–219.

105. Biedert R. Dislocation of the tibialis posterior tendon. *Am J Sports Med* 1992;20:775–776.

106. Macintyre JG, Taunton JE, Clement DB, et al. Running injuries: a clinical study of 4,173 cases. *Clin Sports Med* 1991;1:81–87.

107. Lynsholm J, Wilkander J. Injuries in runners. *Am J Sports Med* 1987;15:168–171.

108. Woods L, Leach RE. Posterior tibial tendon ruptures in athletic people. *Am J Sports Med* 1991;19:495–498.

109. Soler RR, Castany FJG, Ferret JR, et al. Traumatic dislocation of the tibialis posterior tendon at the ankle level. *Trauma* 1986;26:1049–1052.

110. Nava BE. Traumatic dislocation of the tibialis posterior tendon at the ankle: report of a case. *J Bone Joint Surg Br* 50-B:150–151.

111. Mittal RL, Jain NC. Traumatic dislocation of the tibialis posterior tendon. *Int Orthop* 1988;12:259–260.

112. Conti S, Michelson J, Jahss M. Clinical significance of magnetic resonance imaging in preoperative planning for reconstruction of posterior tibial tendon ruptures. *Foot Ankle* 1992;13:208–214.

113. Rosenberg ZS, Cheung Y, Jahss MH, et al. Rupture of posterior tibial tendon: CT and MR imaging with surgical correlation. *Radiology* 1988;169:229–235.

114. Alexander IJ, Johnson KA, Berquist TH. Magnetic resonance imaging in the diagnosis of disruption of the posterior tibial tendon. *Foot Ankle* 1987;8:144–147.

115. Miller SD, Holsbeeck MV, Boruta PM, et al. Ultrasound in the diagnosis of posterior tibial tendon pathology. *Foot Ankle Int* 1996;17:555–558.

116. Hsu T, Wang C, Wang T, et al. Ultrasonographic examination of the posterior tibial tendon. *Foot Ankle Int* 1997;18:34–38.

117. Teasdall RD, Johnson KA. Surgical treatment of stage I posterior tibial tendon dysfunction. *Foot Ankle Int* 1994;15:646–648.

118. Sarrafian SK. Tendon sheaths and bursae. In: *Anatomy of the foot and ankle,* 2nd ed. Philadelphia: J.B. Lippincott, 1993:283.

119. Geppert MJ, Sobel M, Hannafin JA. Microvasculature of the tibialis anterior tendon. *Foot Ankle* 1993;:261.

120. Dooley BJ, Kudelka P, Menelaus MB. Subcutaneous rupture of the tendon of the tibialis anterior. *J Bone Joint Surg Br* 62-B:471–472.

121. Ouzounian TJ, Anderson R. Anterior tibial tendon rupture. *Foot Ankle Int* 16:406–410.

Principles and Practice of Orthopaedic Sports Medicine,
edited by William E. Garrett, Jr., Kevin P. Speer, and Donald T. Kirkendall.
Lippincott Williams & Wilkins, Philadelphia © 2000.

CHAPTER 54

Concepts of Running Injuries

Stan James

EPIDEMIOLOGY

Distance running is a significant part of basic fitness programs for many people. The running boom began in the 1970s, particularly around 1972, after Frank Shorter's win in the marathon at Munich. Running virtually exploded in the 1970s, becoming a major form of fitness for millions of people throughout this country and Europe. In 1986, Jacobs and Berson (1) reported 30 million runners of all levels in the United States, with 10 million running regularly and roughly 1 million entering races. Its popularity stems from the fact that it requires only a pair of running shoes, appropriate clothing, and can be accomplished almost anywhere or at any time. There is also the additional reward of enhanced fitness, better health, cardiovascular benefits, and a better sense of well-being. Running injuries are frequent, but there is no doubt that the benefits far outweigh the disadvantages. At the start of the running boom, we knew very little about running injuries, their cause, and much less about their treatment. It soon became evident that with serious running (over 20 miles per week), the incidence of running injuries significantly increased. Van Mechelen (2) reported the incidence of running injuries from 24% to 77%, and when looking at data overall, it appears that the serious runner stands a chance of being injured somewhere between 37% and 56% of the time. Clement et al. (3) surveyed 1,650 runners, listing the 10 most frequently diagnosed conditions which accounted for about 69% of the total injuries, with most of the injuries being located from the knee distally.

James et al. (4) found that two thirds of running injuries were related to training errors, with excessive mileage accounting for 29% of the errors. In the group of 180 runners studied, the average mileage was 49 miles per week. Other significant factors involving injuries in this group were intense workouts, a rapid change in the training routine, and running on hills and hard surfaces. One of the goals of this study was to determine if there were any specific anatomic or biomechanical abnormalities associated with specific running injuries. No correlation was found in this study and to date any other study.

Through the years, we have also come to realize that certain people probably should not run long distances for aerobic fitness and would be better off in other sports or activities. Fortunately, with a recent change in attitudes toward fitness, people are much more willing to pursue other types of physical activity. Triathalons have attracted many people to the alternatives of swimming and cycling in addition to running, and there is an increased number of fitness centers where various types of exercise machines and aerobic-type indoor activities are offered. There seems little doubt that a broader-based fitness program (5) is more injury free than a fitness program that consists solely of distance running. No hard data support this premise, but empirically it does seem to be true and is an opinion shared by many coaches, athletes, fitness buffs, and physicians.

BIOMECHANICAL ABNORMALITIES ASSOCIATED WITH RUNNING INJURIES

A brief review of biomechanical function of the lower extremity is necessary but a subject that many orthopedists tend to shy away from due to its complexity. Nevertheless, much of the assessment of a running injury is based on biomechanical knowledge of how the lower extremity functions during running.

The stance phase or support phase is divided into an initial absorption phase and subsequently a generation phase. Most injuries occur during the stance or support phase of running. The function of the lower extremity during support phase is to absorb the impact of foot strike, support the body's weight, maintain forward mo-

S. James: Department of Exercise and Movement Science, University of Oregon, Eugene, Oregon 97401.

tion, and accelerate (propel) the body's center of gravity against internal and external resistance. The segmental articulation of the lower extremity, along with the mobile lumbar spine–pelvic unit, functions as a stable adjustable strut to ensure the body's center of gravity follows a smooth undulating path in the sagittal plane.

The support phase begins at the time the foot strikes the ground, most commonly on the lateral aspect of the heel, and terminates at toe-off at which point the limb passes into the recovery or swing phase. There is an initial relative shortening of the extremity during the absorption phase, with eccentric muscle activity until midsupport and then a relative lengthening during the generation phase before toe-off with concentric muscle contraction. Relative shortening is accomplished by a downward pelvic tilt, knee flexion, ankle dorsiflexion, and subtalar pronation. Relative lengthening is a function of upward pelvic tilt, posterior pelvic rotation, hip extension, knee extension, ankle plantar flexion, and resupination of the subtalar joint, creating a rigid lever of the foot for push-off during the generation phase.

The first absorption peak at foot strike can be five times body weight, whereas a second peak of ground reaction force occurs in the generation phase and can be up to seven times body weight. Running downhill may create shock at contact as high as 10 times body weight.

Scott and Winter (6) studied internal forces at chronic running injury sites, which included the Achilles tendon, lower leg, patellar tendon, patellofemoral joint, and plantar fascia. Peak loads were associated with midsupport and push-off when muscle activity was maximal, whereas the impact force of heel contact was determined to have no effect on the peak force seen at the chronic injury sites. Importantly, the peak tissue force occurred during the propulsive or generation phase and not during the absorption phase where much emphasis has been placed, particularly by shoe manufacturers in their attempt to modify the impact forces at foot strike with shoe design. Achilles tendon forces were 6 to 8 times the body weight, ankle bone-on-bone compressive forces 10 to 14 times body weight, lower leg compressive forces 10 to 14 times body weight, patellar tendon forces approximately 5 to 7 times body weight, and patellofemoral joint compressive forces 7 to 11 times body weight. Plantar fascial force was approximately one to three times body weight. These areas are chronic injury sites in runners, and it is not surprising when one considers the forces generated.

A great deal of attention has been given to pronation–supination through the subtarsal–midtarsal joint complex of the foot and its relationship to running injuries. A normal amount of pronation is absolutely essential during the support phase and coordinates with other events more proximally at the knee and hip. All these events must be synchronous for normal lower extremity function.

At foot strike, which in most runners is on the lateral aspect of the heel, there is initially a very rapid period of pronation that continues for approximately 70% of the weight-bearing phase with maximum pronation occurring at about 40% of the support phase, which is approximately when the center of gravity passes over the weight-bearing foot and also when transition from the absorption to generation phase is occurring. During this time, the midtarsal–subtalar joint complex is unlocked, allowing the foot to become more flexible to accommodate to the underlying surface. A certain amount of pronation is essential, but hyperpronation or compensatory pronation may be detrimental. Normally, after maximum pronation, the subtalar joint will gradually supinate and actually pass from pronation into supination at about 70% of the support phase, thus stabilizing the midtarsal–subtalar joint complex and creating a more rigid forefoot lever for push-off.

The problem arises with excessive or prolonged pronation during support phase, resulting in increased forces being applied to the supporting structures of the foot and leg by requiring additional effort of the intrinsic and extrinsic muscles in an attempt to stabilize the foot, normally accomplished by supination during the generation phase. The tibia obligatorily internally rotates with pronation and obligatorily externally rotates during supination. The degree of internal and external rotation, however, is not directly correlated with the amount of heel eversion during pronation and can vary considerably from runner to runner (7). Considerable individual difference for the movement is transferred from calcaneal eversion into tibial rotation. Nigg et al. (8) noted movement transfer between foot eversion (pronation) and tibial rotation to be small for subjects with low arches and higher for subjects with higher arches. They concluded that excessive pronation with substantial movement transfer of foot eversion into internal tibial rotation seemed to be a reasonable predictor for the development of overuse injuries, particularly involving the knee joint.

Excessive pronation of the foot or compensatory pronation is generally secondary to one or more of the following: tibia varum over 10 degrees, functional equinus with a tight tricep surae, subtalar varus, and forefoot supination (varus).

If internal tibia rotation is increased or prolonged with excessive pronation, which is secondary to one of the above anatomic malalignments of the foot or leg, it seems reasonable that more transverse rotation must be absorbed at the knee, which may account for the high incidence of knee injuries, particularly related to the extensor mechanism. Under these circumstances, normal tibial femoral rotation relationships and relationship of the patellofemoral joint is quite likely disturbed and may account for the much higher incidence of patellofemoral joint problems in runners (9).

Muscular function also influences the degree of pronation. The posterior tibialis muscle and tendon are ideally situated to resist pronation; however, Perry (10) explained how soleus muscle function is also associated with subtalar joint motion during the support phase of walking and running activities. The tibialis anterior, tibialis posterior, and soleus muscles are primary muscular restraints against subtalar eversion (pronation). The tibialis anterior is a primary muscle at initial heel contact, but once the forefoot comes into contact with the surface, the tibialis posterior replaces that of the tibialis anterior, and as the body weight moves forward at the ankle, the soleus begins to contract. The tibialis posterior has the longest inversion lever arm with the greatest mechanical advantage, but the soleus, even with a shorter lever arm, has twice the inversion torque on the calcaneus as that of the tibialis posterior due to its size and strength, thus overcoming the disadvantage of its shorter lever arm. This is quite likely associated with the development of medial tibial stress syndrome along the attachment of the soleus muscle. Even with maximum muscular participation, the ability of these muscles to meet the tremendous valgus torques (pronation) imposed upon the foot during the support phase dictates careful selection of the footwear and/or the use or orthotic devices to help control excessive eversion forces.

Nigg (11) emphasized that forces acting on the body during running have a magnitude, a point of application, and a direction, all of which much be considered in load analysis. He suggested that sports injuries are generally secondary to an overload of forces on a specific region of the body with the local forces or stresses exceeding the critical limit of the tissues involved. Overload can occur with a single force or event above that of the critical limits, resulting in an acute injury such as rupture of an Achilles tendon. In running, however, injury is more likely to occur secondary to cyclic forces occurring repetitively below the critical limit of the tissues involved, resulting in an accumulation of stress, particularly with continued abuse that eventuates in fatigue and injury secondary to repeated episodes of microtrauma. The tissues' inability to heal in the face of the continued abuse leads to a chronic inflammatory process (12). Nigg (11) suggested the most effective biomechanical strategies to reduce load and stresses on the locomotor system are as follows:

1. Movement: Changing the running style may alter abnormal forces, but from an empirical standpoint, it must be accomplished cautiously. Altering a runner's normal gait very dramatically can often lead to further problems.

2. Surface: Running on a softer surface as opposed to a harder surface or a smooth surface as opposed to a rough surface.

3. Shoe: Shoe structure can influence impact loading and foot motion and shoes can be modified or accommodated to the runner's needs.

4. Repetition: Diminishing the frequency of repetition or number of workouts such as reducing the mileage or frequency of workouts can help reduce the load and is often absolutely essential to avoid tissue overload. Continued abusive overload will lead to a chronic inflammatory processes that may virtually be impossible to ameliorate without cessation of running (12).

In summary, during the absorption phase the primary purpose is to decelerate kinetic energy with the joints placed in a position to maximize shock absorption under neuromuscular control. Deceleration occurs over a period of time with appropriate dissipation of the forces during the absorption phase (13). Running on rough on uneven surfaces may not allow the joints to be at their best position for shock absorption. For instance, if the knee joint is too straight during the absorption phase, more forces are applied to the bones and joints and to the elastic structure of the muscles and tendons, thus possible injury ensues. Also, the untrained athlete who is fatigued or who has contractures that prevent appropriate range of motion or proper positioning of joints may disrupt the timing of the kinetic system to correctly tension appropriate musculotendinous units. When they are not functioning at the appropriate time to allow stretch under tension, there is increased strain that can cause microinjury and subject other structures to greater stress because these forces are not being appropriately dissipated. Greater forces are generated during the generation phase than during the absorption phase and also during faster running. Usually tissues are subjected to the higher forces below the acute injury threshold, but repeated subthreshold forces over a long period of time without appropriate accommodation occurring in a physiologic fashion frequently leads to an injury.

CLINICAL EVALUATION

History

There are two very important elements to be considered in evaluating a runner's injuries. The first is to analyze the training program in detail. Approximately two thirds of runners' injuries relate to some mistake in the training program. This is discussed in more detail. Second, the entire lower extremity from pelvis distally to the foot should be examined, regardless of where the complaint is.

The subsequent discussion may seem a bit out of context in a sports medicine book, but understanding training principles is really the crux of the approach to treating runners' injuries. A weekly mileage of 20 to 25 miles separates the occasional runner from the more serious runner, with increased incidence of injury in the more serious runner. Without a knowledge of training techniques and the ability to determine what is appropriate or inappropriate, the physician is definitely handicapped. Runners usually recognize this fact. This along with a knowledge of the biomechanics of running is the cornerstone for successful treatment of runners' injuries. Guten's (14) *Running Injuries* and Noakes' (15) *Lore of Running* are two resources I personally highly recommend. Noakes text is perhaps the most comprehensive resource available, covering all aspects of running, including information on training and physiology and medical aspects of distance running.

Experienced runners are as likely to incur injuries as are the beginning runners. They all make basically the same training mistakes. The most common training errors are high mileage, high intensity, and any sudden change or rapid transition in the program. There is also a great tendency toward reinjury once an area has been injured. The body is an extremely adaptable mechanism, but it does demand time to accommodate the change in stress patterns and the time for accommodation differs for each individual and perhaps from time to time in the same individual. Continued abusive, repetitive, submaximal stress on the various tissues leads to tissue damage and chronic inflammation and is more difficult to treat than to simply alter the training program initially. To a lesser extent, shoes, surfaces, terrain, and anatomic factors also play a role in injury, but this is very difficult to quantify. Unfortunately, the same basic cause for an injury keeps cropping up repeatedly and frequently in the same individual who seems unaware of an obvious training mistake. It appears that most runners are fearful to deviate from the "accepted" training programs, which frequently consist of high mileage and high intensity. They avoid seeking an "optimal" training program. An optimal program is the least amount of training that will still maximize the runner's capabilities. This is a very difficult philosophy to sell, but the question a runner must ask is "Why go beyond this point and risk illness or injury?" A 10% increase in weekly mileage is about the maximum tolerated. It has been shown that the maximum training benefit for distance running lies somewhere between 80 to 90 km/wk (48 to 57 miles) (16). So the question has to be asked, "Why run more?" There appears to be a mind–body communication gap in runners. Unfortunately, regardless of how logical a training program may seem, the body will reject it if it is too stressful by creating an injury or illness. Basically, there are few "acts of God" relating to runners' injuries or illness with most being self-inflicted by simply exceeding the body's capacity to withstand physical and emotional stress.

Runners can maximally train their bodies for a given event at a mileage and intensity far below "the line" for which an injury or illness becomes a serious risk factor. Unfortunately, most people tend to train on or near the line with constant interruptions in the training program due to injury. How is an optimal level of training found? For the most part, it is an empirical process, but an astute coach can be extremely helpful. An individual may also refer to numerous books on distance training. In reality, everyone must seek out the ideal personal training program with an educated guess or trial and error. Errors are okay in training programs as long as they become learning experiences, not habitual recurrences.

Another approach is for a runner to review his or her training log. Often the runner will find a clue to the type of workout or sequence of workouts that produced an optimal performance. All or portions of it can be adapted as part of a program. Not everyone requires a structured program. Most individuals who are running recreationally can do with a general game plan, with the specifics of each day's training determined even the day of the workout. For the average runner or fitness buff, this may be a better approach. A competitive runner peaking for a specific event, however, will benefit from a customized more structured scheduled. Many runners who are running for general fitness and recreation will fair better with less structure and more flexibility. My advice to this individual is to ignore a predetermined time, distance, and intensity for workout and simply play off the body's feeling for a given day and tailor the workout accordingly. This philosophy does not appeal to a great number of individuals who prefer structure and unfortunately will often adhere to an inappropriate program regardless of the outcome. I know some very good coaches who present extremely rigid programs that may be highly successful for distance runners, providing they survive the training.

Some general guidelines for an appropriate training schedule, particularly for the runner who wants to maintain a reasonable high degree of fitness year after year but does not respond well to a continued structured program, is periodization in which there are alternate days, alternate weeks, and alternate months in which the training intensity and mileage varies. Intensity is not necessarily referring to a rapid pace. It can also refer to an extremely long run at a slower pace. Relatively hard or "quality" workouts should be interspersed with easier workouts. An easy day means not doing anything that will detract in the slightest from a planned quality day. Many runners seem to have a somewhat harder quality day and then a somewhat easier day, consequently never maximizing the effects from a good quality day or hard workout. Most runners do very well with two or perhaps three quality workouts over a 7- to 10-day period. As a general guideline, for most runners, one workout should have some element of quickness, another a moderate pace and distance, and a third with an overdistance run appropriate to the runner's event. However, these must be tailored to the runner's current conditioning. Workouts for speed and strength can vary from fartlek to formal interval workouts, depending on the runner's stage of training and conditioning. Hard workouts with very little change in intensity, duration, or distance day after day lead to staleness and frequently overuse injuries. Basically, a training program from 800 m through a marathon needs to develop high aerobic capacity by steady state training, develop lower body strength and flexibility with a hill phase of training, develop high anaerobic capacity with anaerobic training near the race schedule, and finally pursue a race prep phase in which speed and the ability to race are honed.

During training time, the runners should know what they are doing, how they are going to do it, and why they are doing it. Training and racing can be done at too fast or too slow a pace, and it is the responsibility of the coach to provide guidelines that help the athlete understand the correct sequence, quantity, and pace range. Runners often have a tendency to train too hard before they are in good shape and also to train too hard after they are in good shape. Resources are used during the challenge of a quality workout and are then replenished and improved upon during the recovery of the challenge, which is the basic theory of the hard/easy training regime. During recovery, there should be no challenge because it is during this period of time that adaption from the stress of the challenge takes place. Without adequate recovery, the adaption does not take place and the training effect is blunted. With too much challenge, the runner will actually regress and with too much recovery, there can be no progress. There has to be a proper balance between challenge and recovery so that the body will physiologically adapt and improve, which is the key to training. If the challenge to training is too severe, applied over too long a period time, or too many challenges are presented and recovery is insufficient, adaptation is soon replaced by boredom, fatigue, illness, and injury, accompanied by exhaustion and an overtrained state (Brown R, Training guide for the 800 through the marathon, unpublished data).

Runners who try to increase their training too quickly or challenge their bodies too severely in an attempt to concentrate on an aerobic response often find their program interrupted by a breakdown in the musculoskeletal system. I describe this as the theory of the "engine and the chassis," with the engine representing the cardiorespiratory system and the chasis the musculoskeletal system. The weak link is adaptation of the chasis causing a breakdown as the runner tries to train primarily the engine. It is not unusual for aerobic capacity to exceed musculoskeletal capacity, which often lags behind. An example is the situation typified by competitive cross-country skiers who finish the competitive season in early spring with superb aerobic fitness and then try to make a rapid transition to running for summer training and competition. Although their aerobic condition is excellent (the engine), the musculoskeletal system (the chassis) is not ready for the loads imposed by running. These individuals need to supplement their programs with alternative forms of aerobic exercise as running mileage is gradually and safely increased to an appropriate level.

There are several alternative forms of exercise that can benefit a runner by not only adding variety to the program to prevent staleness but also provide a safe mechanism for the runner who "needs the extra work" and also helps maintain conditioning during periods of injury. Moran and McGlynn (5) described cross-training for sports that are particularly adaptable. Numerous devices in fitness centers have low impact and can substitute for running. Perhaps the best form of alternative training, which seems to quite readily transfer to running and is also also an excellent mode for maintaining conditioning when the runner is unable to run, is running in water (17).

The runner should not ignore total body fitness. Frequently, runners have excellent lower extremity development and a poorly developed upper body. The core strength of the body comes from the trunk and pelvis. Resistance training should be a part of all runners' routine regime. This does not have to be heavy power lifting or body building but rather a well-designed circuit course that includes all muscle groups of the body, not only to enhance the efficiency of running but for injury prevention as well.

When taking a history from the runner, look for sudden changes in duration, frequency, or intensity of training based on the above principals. Include current complaints, history of past running injuries, running experience, training patterns, and running terrain. It is important to know where and when the pain occurs while running. For example, is it worse running uphill or downhill? Does it vary with the intensity of the run? At what phase of the running cycle does it occur? Walter et al. (18) in a study of 1,680 runners found that the risk of injuries was associated with increased running mileage and the history of previous injury. It apparently was not associated with other aspects of training such as pace, unusual running surface, hill running, or intense training. Injury rates were equal for all age and sex groups and were independent of years of running experience. Even though these factors do not appear to be directly associated in this study with injury, I have found them to be considerations in analyzing injury. This study also found runners with an injury the previous year had approximately a 50% higher risk for new injury during the follow-up period.

Keep in mind that many complaints are secondary to compensation for a previous injury that may not be the major area of complaint at the time of examination.

Physical Examination

The most important aspect of the physical examination is to include the entire lower extremity from pelvis to toes. This should include evaluation of extremity alignment in the frontal and transverse planes, extremity length from the anterior superior iliac spine to the medial malleolus, knee function, ankle dorsiflexion with the knee extended and flexed, configuration of the weight-bearing foot, leg heel alignment, heel forefoot alignment, assessment of subtalar joint motion, and assessment of footwear and shoe wear. Gross abnormalities are not always present on examination, nor should they necessarily be expected. Many anatomic factors and biomechanical factors that perhaps cause problems for runners are very subtle and would not cause any difficulty if not for the extreme repetitive stress that is applied to the lower extremity in distance running.

The level of the iliac wings will give some indication of whether or not there is a leg length discrepancy, but the mere fact that there is a discrepancy does not always indicate a problem. Generally, however, the short leg is considered to be at higher risk for stress-related injuries (19). In symptomatic runners, a discrepancy of more than 20 mm will perhaps require a shoe correction. No correction is indicated for a runner with a leg length discrepancy and no significant problems.

Patellar dynamics are particularly important and should be assessed with the patient walking and running and a thorough examination in the usual fashion. The presence of "squinting" patellae suggests rotational malalignment, particularly proximally, with an associated femoral neck anteversion and femoral torsion. A group of individuals that I have identified as having particular torsional problems in the lower extremity, often resulting in knee pain and making it extremely difficult for these people to distance run, is the group I refer to with "miserable malalignment." These individuals have femoral neck anteversion characterized by an increased internal rotation of the hip verses external rotation, a genu varum, squinting patellae, increased Q angles, perhaps a tibia varum, and stand fully pronated in a compensatory fashion. Their primary complaint is usually knee pain (20).

Ankle dorsiflexion should be assessed with the knee extended and flexed. A chronic gastrosoleus tightness is frequently found in runners (as are tight hamstrings), and with the foot in neutral position, dorsiflexion is limited to no more than neutral position or 0 degrees. A runner requires at least 10 degrees of ankle dorsiflexion during support phase or compensatory foot pronation will be required to provide adequate dorsiflexion through the subtalar–midtarsal joint complex. The overall alignment and configuration of both feet should be noted with the runner standing and walking.

The measurements of leg, heel, and heel forefoot alignment are extremely important. These measurements are based on three assumptions:

1. There is a position in which the foot will function efficiently with the least amount of stress being exerted on the joints, ligaments, and tendons.
2. With the weight-bearing foot, the foot should functionally be positioned such that the vertical axis of the heel is parallel to the longitudinal axis of the distal one third of the leg and the plane of the metatarsal heads is perpendicular to the vertical axis of the heel.
3. These relationships should exist at the subtalar joint in "neutral" position.

Clinically, the subtalar joint is placed in a neutral position by having the patient lie prone on the examination table with feet extended over the end of the table. The foot is grasped by the index finger and thumb at the fourth and fifth metatarsal heads and gently dorsiflexed until resistance is met. The foot is then moved through an arc of pronation and supination (eversion and inversion), and it is noted that through this arc of motion, there is a point at which the foot seems to fall off to one side or the other more easily. This "peak" is empirically the neutral position of the subtalar joint. The other index finger and thumb may be simultaneously placed on either side of the talar head, and as the foot is passed through its range of motion from inversion to eversion, the talar head will be felt to bulge medially with eversion and laterally with inversion. Position the foot such that the talar head does not seem to bulge to either side of the navicular. At this point the talus is congruently positioned in the navicular and the subtalar joint is assumed to be in its neutral position. Even though this is not an extremely precise clinical maneuver, it does seem to be adequate for the purposes intended.

To measure leg and heel alignment, place the runner prone on an examination table with the feet extended over the end of the table as previously described. A mark is placed over the midline of the calcaneus at the Achilles insertion site and another about 1 cm distally as close to the midline of the calcaneus as can be estimated. Two additional marks are placed over the midline of the distal one third of the leg to represent the longitudinal axis of the tibia. The measurement is carried out by placing the subtalar joint in its neutral position as previously described and then noting the alignment of the leg to the heel by the previously placed marks. The degree of angulation can be measured by a goniometer and most unweighted leg–heel alignment measurements will reveal the heel to be parallel to the distal one third of the leg or in 1 or 2 degrees of varus.

The forefoot heel alignment is then estimated by noting the relationship of the plane of the forefoot at the metatarsal head level in relation to the vertical axis of the heel. Normally, the plane of the forefoot at the metatarsal head level should be perpendicular to the vertical axis of the heel with the subtalar joint held in neutral position as previously described. If the plane is tilted such that the medial side of the foot rises above the neutral plane, the forefoot is supinated, and if the medial side of the foot drops below the neutral plane, the forefoot is said to be pronated. Most people have neutral alignment between heel and forefoot. The plane of the forefoot should be established in relation to the second, third, and fourth metatarsal heads rather than to all five metatarsal heads. Forefoot pronation is actually not very common and must be distinguished from a plantarflexed first ray. In this situation, the second, third, and fourth metatarsal heads are in the neutral plane in relation to the heel, but the first metatarsal is plantar flexed with the metatarsal head lying below the plane of the adjacent metatarsal heads. This condition is frequently associated with a cavus type of foot, which often demonstrates some reduction in range of motion of the midtarsal–subtalar joint complex as well. In some instances, the first ray may be hypermobile, shifting increased stress to the second and third metatarsal heads. This will often be evidenced by callous formation in this area.

The weight-bearing foot is described as cavus, neutral, or planus (pronated). The term pronated is current jargon used for planus but more correctly refers to motion about the subtalar joint (eversion, abduction, and dorsiflexion). Some pronation is normal for the weight-bearing foot, but excessive pronation is a compensatory motion usually secondary to the conditions discussed earlier. Keep in mind that an individual with a cavus or tendency toward a high arch foot may be standing fully pronated secondary to compensatory foot pronation. This is a difficult concept for many people to grasp, because they are associating pronation with pes planus.

Normal subtalar joint range in motion is 33 degrees plus or minus 7 degrees (4) with a ratio of inversion to eversion approximately 3:1. Normal subtalar joint motion should allow for approximately 8 degrees of eversion and 25 degrees of inversion. A disruption of this ratio is associated with compensatory pronation of the foot. When compensatory pronation is called upon, disruption in the lower extremity kinetic chain previously discussed can occur.

Examination of the training shoe can be very informative. A deformed shoe reflects adverse stresses upon the foot and may serve as a clue to a runner's problems. Individuals with compensatory foot pronation will often overrun the heel medially, and the more rigid cavus type foot perhaps with the heel in varus will overrun the outer side of the heel counter. Also pay attention to the integrity of the heel wedge and stiffness of the forefoot wedge along with outsole wear patterns.

RADIOGRAPHIC EXAMINATION

If radiographic examination of the involved areas is indicated, special views may be necessary in some instances. A runner seen for the first time with a very obvious soft tissue problem and no gross abnormalities noted clinically may not require an immediate radiographic examination. At the knee, routine radiographic examination includes at least four views: a weight-bearing anterior view, a lateral view at 45 degrees of flexion, a tangential view of the patella, and a notch view either with weight-bearing or a non–weight-bearing position. X-rays of the leg, ankle, and foot may also be used when appropriate, and in certain instances, ultrasonography, computer tomography (CT), and magnetic resonance imaging (MRI) may be of help. In most circumstances, the superior resolution of soft tissue, multiplanar capabilities, and lack of exposure to ionizing radiation makes the MRI the imaging modality of choice for evaluating disorders of soft tissues, particularly tendon structures. When abnormalities of associated osseus structures are of primary concern, the MRI may be inadequate and CT is a good alternative. Ultrasonography can also provide details about lesions, particularly in the Achilles tendon and patella tendon, but may have a limited application in smaller tendons.

CLINICAL CONDITIONS

In 1978, James et al. (4) found 71% of runners' injuries fit into six categories: knee pain 34%, posterior tibial syndrome (medial stress syndrome) 13%, Achilles tendonopathy 11%, plantar fasciitis 7%, and stress fractures 6%. The remaining 29% were miscellaneous problems. It is interesting that these percentages have remained reasonably constant through the years. In the group with knee problems, anterior knee pain accounted for approximately 25%, knee pain with no diagnosis 20%, iliotibial band syndrome 17%, parapatellar pain 15%, patellar tendinitis (tendonopathy) 7%, medial retanacular pain 6%, and miscellaneous 10%. By far, the patellofemoral joint and the iliotibial band syndrome accounted for most knee problems. The fact that the distribution of running injuries has remained so relatively constant through the years is somewhat puzzling. It either means that runners are making the same mistakes or that running at significant mileage makes injuries inevitable.

KNEE CONDITIONS

The knee is the most common site of problems in runners. Anterior knee pain is the most common knee complaint (20). In lay literature, this is often referred to as "runner's knee." Unfortunately, many professionals refer to it simply as "chondromalacia." Neither term is very specific or helpful. From a biomechanical standpoint, it is not difficult to see why this is the major area of injury. The extensor mechanism, including the patellar tendon, patella and quadriceps tendon, and retinaculae, are subjected to tremendous forces during both the absorption and generation or propulsion phase of running.

Patella Malalignment and Instability

Even minor maltracking problems for the patellofemoral joint can alter the pressure patterns in the patellofemoral joint with tremendous localized increased stress on the articular cartilage. The knee moments are created primarily by the quadriceps with the musculotendinous units being repetitively subjected to great forces during running, step after step, mile after mile, and day after day. As mentioned earlier, peak patellar tendon forces may reach 5 to 7 times body weight, with patellofemoral forces ranging from 7 to 11 times body weight. Anything that disrupts the normal function of the extensor mechanism during the act of running may cause an injury to the tissues and is generally characterized by rather diffuse pain, but often the runner can indicate that the patella as the major site of discomfort, although there are instances where the retinaculum also appears to be involved. There may be obvious tightness of the lateral retinaculum and the iliotibial band upon examination. If the condition is chronic, there may also be crepitus retropatellarly and tenderness along the lateral border of the patella indicative of possible degenerative changes in the lateral facet articular cartilage.

Patellar instability is also associated with anterior knee pain and may even be characterized by episodes of instability but rarely a true dislocation in runners. Patella subluxations, often associated with maltracking, alter the normal distribution of patellofemoral joint force, resulting in pain with or without articular cartilage damage. Some factors associated with instability are a relaxed medial retinaculum, a weak vastus medialis obliquus, increased Q angle, shallow sulcus, patella alta, genu valgum, femoral neck anteversion, and compensatory pronation (21).

Fortunately, conditions involving the patellofemoral joint will usually respond to a conservative program of closed-chain, concentric, and eccentric exercises for the quadriceps and hamstring muscles. Restoring muscle balance and endurance along with eliminating any muscle contractures, particularly of the hamstrings, are essential.

For the small group who might require surgical intervention for malalignment, an arthroscopic lateral retinacular release and perhaps a patellar chondroplasty, if indicated, is the option selected most often. A lateral release is compatible with return to running and is preferable to more extensive realignment procedures. The future of running depends largely on the degree of patellar chondrosis present. The surgeon and runner should be aware that some 8 to 12 weeks of rehabilitation will be required before returning to running after a retinacular release. Runners often anticipate a much quicker recovery because it does not seem to be a very complicated procedure. A more extensive surgical procedure involving proximal and distal extensor mechanism realignment must be done judiciously. In my experience, extensive realignment procedures have a very unpredictable result in terms of the ability to return to distance running. The simpler the procedure, the more likely are the prospects for return to running.

Quadriceps and Patellar Tendon Tendonopathy

Tendonopathy involving the quadriceps tendon and particularly the patellar tendon (ligament) are common conditions affecting the extensor mechanism, causing anterior knee pain. The patellar tendon insertion at the distal pole of the patella is the most common site of involvement. Microruptures may result in local areas of deep tendon degeneration or tendonosis and lead to structural deterioration with partial tissue failure but rarely with complete disruption.

Treatment of patellar tendonopathy is rather frustrating at times, but fortunately most can be solved conservatively with judicious application of concentric and eccentric exercises and modification of the running program. Orthotic inserts or shoe changes are all part of the treatment program as well. However, in my experience, once a demonstrable lesion is noted on MRI or ultrasonography, the chances of resolving it conservatively are quite slim in the face of continued running.

A conservative program should be pursued for at least 6 months before considering surgical exploration of the involved area, unless it has been present for quite some time and imaging studies reveal significant degenerative changes at the patellar tendon insertion site.

This is no place for an intratendinous steroid injection, however. Fortunately, the area involved is frequently quite small and can be surgically excised and the defect closed readily. If the attachment site is seriously involved with marked degeneration and localized disruption, it may require more extensive debridement, including freshening of the bony surface and reattaching of the tendon to the distal pole of patella (22,23). Return to running then takes 3 to 6 months, depending on the degree of involvement.

Pathologic Plica

A pathologic plica most commonly affects the medial parapatellar plica, which becomes fibrotic and rubs or snaps over the medial femoral condyle during flexion and extension. A large one may become impinged between the condyle and overlying medial patellar facet and can actually result in chondrosis of the involved areas. Occasionally, a plica may be in the suprapatellar area, causing pain deep to the quadriceps tendon, particularly with bent knee positions. On occasion I have found a plica laterally as well. The pathologic plica is a great mimic of numerous knee conditions and is often diagnosed by suspicion. It can also be overdiagnosed, resulting in misdiagnosis of other intraarticular conditions. A pathologic plica can be resolved easily arthroscopicaly, but if the involved band is not fibrotic, thickened, and avascular, it may well not be the source of pain. Other sources should be considered (24).

Iliotibial Band Friction Syndrome

Iliotibial band friction syndrome is the most common cause of lateral knee pain in the runner. Other conditions are a meniscal lesion, particularly common in older runners, and in some instances a popliteal tendon tenosynovitis that is rather rare but often associated with excessive downhill running. The runner will frequently have a genu varum or tibia varum along with heel varus and forefoot supination, resulting in compensatory pronation that can play a role with the initiation of iliotibial band friction syndrome (25). During the absorption phase when the knee is maximally flexed, the iliotibial band is pulled back across the prominence of the lateral femoral condyle. Simultaneously, particularly with a genu varum, there is an increase in varus moment at the knee due to the medial placed ground reaction force in relation to the knee. This requires an increased valgus moment by the iliotibial band laterally (13). The foot is in maximal pronation at this point in time with the tibia maximally internally rotated, thus advancing Gerdy's tubercle anteriorly and medially placing additional stress on the iliotibial band. Proximally, if there is abductor weakness and associated fatigue, the pelvis may sag to the contralateral side, again creating increased traction upon the distal portion of the iliotibial band. These factors cause increased force between the iliotibial band and the prominence of the lateral femoral condyle, resulting in an underlying synovitis between the iliotibial band and the lateral femoral condyle.

Conservative treatment is initiated with iliotibial band stretching and strengthening of the abductors of the hip. I have occasionally used a steroid injection once or twice with the injection being deep to the iliotibial band. This has been efficacious enough to warrant its use in the more acute cases as opposed to long-standing chronic cases.

Surgery is indicated for intractable cases. It is my feeling that arthroscopy should be initially carried out before release of the iliotibial band to rule out the possibility of a lateral meniscal lesion or other disorders such as a lateral pathologic plica. The procedure is simply to relax or release the iliotibial band with a cruciform incision and perhaps removing a small flap of fibrotic tissue over the prominence of the lateral femoral condyle. There also may be an involved bursa in the fibrotic tissue that is excised.

HINDFOOT PROBLEMS

The Achilles tendon is, indeed, the "Achilles heel" of the runner. Forces generated in the Achilles tendon during the running cycle are much greater than in walking, with forces ranging from six to eight times body weight. Achilles tendonopathy occurs not from the impact during the absorption phase, but from active muscle forces during the generation phase. Peak forces in the Achilles tendon are influenced by the shape of the midsole or thickness of the midsole that can affect the lever arm by reducing flexibility in the forefoot area of the shoe. Stresses can be minimized in the Achilles tendon if there is a straight line pull. It is important the heel counter, heel wedge, and outsole are correctly aligned and constructed and undue wear is not allowed. Proper shoes should have an adequate heel wedge, which is firm yet not too soft, and a well-formed supportive heel counter with a good fit, along with a flexible midsole. Intrinsic malalignment of the foot may also lead to Achilles tendonopathy with a rigid-type cavus foot or severe pes planus with compensatory pronation.

Posterior heel pain in runners is most commonly caused by Achilles tendonopathy (26) that includes injury to the muscular tendinous junction, peritendinitis, tendonosis, a combination of peritendinitis and tendonosis, retrocalcaneobursitis, and insertional tendonosis.

The most common area of involvement for Achilles tendonopathy is some 4 to 5 cm proximal to the insertion site in an area of diminished blood supply during propulsion. The blood supply alone is not the sole etiology. It is more likely due to microtrauma from repetitive forces at subthreshold level in an abusive fashion.

Proximal involvement at the musculotendinous junction usually responds quite readily to rest. The peritenon more distally may become adherent to the Achilles tendon itself. This is not truly a sheath but rather thin areolar tissue surrounding the Achilles tendon that can become inflamed and adherent. The Achilles tendon itself can be involved with various degrees of tendonosis ranging from a mucoid degeneration to a traumatic longitudinal tear and in some instances complete rupture (26).

The retrocalcaneal bursa is frequently involved, particularly with a rather prominent superior angle of the calcaneus applying excessive pressure to the bursa and overlying Achilles tendon near the insertion. Not uncommon is a cartilaginous ridge that develops in this area, applying even more pressure to the Achilles tendon and resulting in insertional tendonosis or Achilles tendon tendonosis near the insertion site. This ridge is not readily apparent on x-ray but seen frequently at surgery. Chronic recalcitrant cases may require a retrocalcaneal partial ostectomy to decompress the area. I highly recommend bilateral approaches to this area with a generous removal of bone from the superior angle of the calcaneus. In my experience, the cases that have required a second surgery have had insufficient removal of bone usually through a single incision.

The possibility of a calcaneal stress fracture causing posterior heel pain must also be considered, but it is not an extremely common finding in runners and can be readily diagnosed with a bone scan.

PLANTAR HEEL PAIN

Plantar heel pain is most commonly associated with a plantarfasciitis at the insertion of the medial band on the calcaneus. This has been referred to as "heel pain syndrome" (27) with actual plantar fasciitis occurring in the midportion of the plantar fascia. I have found this a very rare location for plantar fasciitis in runners. An additional source of plantar heel pain can be an insufficient heel pad. The heel pad is a very highly specialized structure of adipose tissue and fibrous septae that are ideally designed as a shock-absorbing mechanism. Any deficiency in this tissue imparts excessive forces to the calcaneus itself at heel strike and is more likely in an older runner.

Heel spurs are located within the substance of the flexor digitorium brevis and, if present, are a secondary phenomena due to some other abnormality of foot function. Removal of heel spurs in and of themselves will probably not solve the underlying problem.

Entrapment of the nerve to the abductor digitorium quinti (28), which passes deep to the insertion of the plantar fascia, is another source of heel pain. This is usually characterized by a burning type sensation and pain. An electromyogram may actually show some denervation of the abductor digitorium quintae. Conservative treatment of plantar fasciitis or plantar heel pain in my experience is best managed with a well-fabricated orthotic insert in the shoe. Surgical decompression is indicated if adequate conservative measures fail.

STRESS FRACTURES

Stress fractures account for approximately 5% of running injuries, with one third to one half occurring in the tibia. Menstrual irregularities and eating disorders are frequently associated with an increased incidence of stress fractures in women. The normal bone response to stress is osteoclastic removal of bone, whereas osteoblasts lay down new osteoid that mineralizes to form bone. Normally, this is a well-balanced mechanism in response to stress. Bone resists compression forces well but tolerates repetitive bending forces less well. Muscle forces reduce peak bending forces from 58% to 66% but not as well when they are fatigued (13). Appropriate training raises this fatigue limit, but it can be exceeded. Stress fractures occur when osteoclastic activity predominates due to excessive, submaximal, repetitive, bending moments. Stress fracture of the tibia, for instance, is caused by repetitive bending moments, not by axial forces during the support phase.

The diagnosis of stress fracture is largely one of suspicion from a history. Pain may have a gradual or a sudden onset and it may or may not be well localized, but persistent hip, thigh, or groin pain should raise suspicion. Tenderness may be localized over the area of the stress fracture, particularly in the tibia or metatarsals, which readily lend themselves to direct palpation. The runner may present with an antalgic gait to the involved side and hopping on the involved extremity will frequently elicit pain.

Fractures about the pelvis and sacrum are often diagnosed by suspicion and confirmed with a bone scan. In the pelvis, the most prominent site is the ischial pubic ramus and is more frequent in women than men. Physical findings are few, and the diagnosis is confirmed by bone scan. Femoral neck fractures often present as groin pain, and in some instances, the pain radiates down into the thigh. There may be an antalgic gait and some loss of range of motion with a positive hop test. Femoral neck stress fractures are critical and must be diagnosed promptly. This may require crutch-protected weight bearing, particularly if located on the superior portion of the femoral neck. Femoral stress fractures on the compression side of the femoral neck are unlikely to displace, but caution must be exercised. If there appears to be some widening of the fracture or if it is on the tension side of the femoral neck, the possibility of displacement must be seriously considered. Shin and Gillingham (29) recommended internal fixation in this situation.

Early diagnosis of stress fractures is confirmed by imaging studies. A triple-phase bone scan is quite sensitive and reveals early involvement. It is also quite inexpensive. A triple-phase bone scan can be used to track the progress with the delayed phase that increases for about 12 weeks and then slowly decreases for 3 to 8 months. The advantage of triple-phase bone scan is that it makes a diagnosis quite early, within perhaps 2 or 3 days after the onset of symptoms. It is readily available and relatively inexpensive. The MRI is very sensitive for stress fracture and reveals more detail of the bone involvement, and the progress of the stress fracture can also be tracked by MRI. One advantage of MRI is less exposure to ionizing radiation, but the disadvantage is expense and perhaps in some areas unavailability. Freidrickson et al. (30) report on the diagnosis of stress fractures with MRI, and when compared with radiographs and technetium bone scan, it was these authors' feeling that the MRI more precisely defined the anatomic location and the extent of the injury than did the other studies. Their conclusion was that MRI was more accurate in correlating the degree of bone involvement with clinical symptoms and allowed a more accurate recommendation for rehabilitation and return to running.

With the tibia being the primary site of stress fracture, the differential diagnosis of leg pain becomes essential (31). The differential diagnoses are tibial stress fracture, medial tibia stress syndrome, and chronic compartment syndrome. Stress fracture of the tibia is usually characterized by localized tenderness over a rather discreet area, and the triple-phase bone scan will reveal a round or focal area of intense labeling.

Medial tibia stress syndrome (32) reveals rather diffuse tenderness along the posterior medial tibia in line with the origin of the soleus muscle and/or posterior tibial muscle coincident to a periostitis. The triple-phase bone scan reveals a more linear involvement in the middle to distal one third of the posterior medial aspect of the tibia. Etiologically, medial tibial stress syndrome is likely related to stress at the origin of the soleus very commonly secondary to compensatory foot pronation where the soleus is one of the primary resistors for pronation along with the posterior tibial muscle. With compensatory pronation, these two muscles are used excessively in an attempt to stabilize the foot, particularly during the later portion of the support phase when the forefoot is not appropriately supinating.

Chronic compartment syndrome is characterized by pain in one or more of the four compartments of the leg; anterior, lateral, superficial posterior, or deep posterior (33). Clinically, there may be a tense palpable compartment and perhaps weakness and numbness of the foot during exercise or running. The triple-phase bone scan is negative, unless there happens to be an associated tibial stress fracture or medial tibial stress syndrome associated with the compartment syndrome. Compartment syndrome is confirmed by pressure studies, with resting pressure normally in the neighborhood of 10 mm Hg. The diagnosis of chronic compartment syndrome reveals a resting pressure of greater than 15 mm Hg and an immediate postexercise pressure greater than 30 mm Hg. A postexercise value at 5 minutes greater than 20 mm Hg and at 15 minutes greater than 15 mm Hg confirms the diagnosis. The exact pathophysiology of chronic compartment syndrome is not completely understood.

More distally in the foot, the most common area of stress fracture is the metatarsals, particularly the second and the third, and the tarsal navicular. A hypermobile short first metatarsal will cause a transfer of stress to the adjacent second and third metatarsals, frequently resulting in stress fracture, particularly with training excesses. During the propulsive phase, the maldistribution of forces across the forefoot can easily upset the normal balance of bone remodeling in the involved metatarsals subjected to excessive stress. Metatarsal stress fractures usually respond quite promptly to 4 to 6 weeks of nonimpact activity and perhaps orthotic inserts.

Although not as common, midfoot pain should at least raise suspicion of a stress fracture of the tarsal navicular. Routine x-rays are unhelpful for the most part. In the past, before CT and MRI, it required very careful positioning of the foot for tomographic demonstration of navicular stress fractures. Now with CT and MRI, it can be readily demonstrated, and a bone scan will also be helpful. Stress fractures of the navicular in a runner should be taken very seriously as with any athlete. The initial conservative treatment is a non–weight-bearing cast, and those that do not heal after an adequate period of time, surgical intervention may be necessary (34).

The treatment of stress fractures is generally no running from 3 to 8 weeks. The ischial pubic ramus fractures may take considerably longer. Recommended training is nonimpact, such as water running or aqua jogging or cross-training with biking, until the symptoms subside. The femoral neck fracture is one that demands extreme caution. Protected weight bearing until symptoms subside is necessary, and surgery for stabilization is indicated for compression side stress fractures involving 50% or more of the femoral neck and in most cases for tension side stress fractures (29).

The progress of stress fractures may be tracked by the delayed phase or triple-phase bone scan, particularly in runners whose training is critical to running schedules.

OSTEOARTHRITIS

A significant number of older master runners have been running for 25 to 30 years. The frequency of osteoarthritic conditions increases with age, but to date there is no evidence that running causes arthritis of the lower extremity joints (35). The relationship between running and osteoarthritis aside, once degenerative changes are established, the running program must be carefully customized and monitored. Runners often ask whether running will accelerate a known osteoarthritic condition and the answer is, yes it can. Generally, runners are unable to accept the advice to give up running, but they will frequently accept the advice to modify their program and to try to find one that is tolerated with minimal insult to the joint. It is often best to allow the runner to attempt to find an ideal program that can be tolerated, and then if they are unable to do so, it may be easier for them to decide to discontinue running rather than just being arbitrarily told they must stop.

Certainly, any program that causes pain and swelling in an involved joint is not being well tolerated. Low impact aerobic activities are possible alternatives to running, and these activities include ski machines, swimming, aerobic water exercises, biking, cross-country skiing, and race walking, all of which can be done in lieu of running or to supplement a limited amount of running. I have often advised patients to only run once or twice a week and derive the rest of their conditioning from nonimpact or very low impact activities. By reducing mileage, intensity, and duration, a runner can frequently find a level of running that is tolerated. Runners are cautioned that persistent pain and swelling are signs that the joint is not tolerating running well and they may have to discontinue it.

Minimal arthroscopic knee debridement to remove bothersome osteophytes, degenerative menisci, and loose bodies may help symptomatically but probably offer no long-term improvement. In my experience, extensive chondroplasty procedures or joint debridement procedures have not been effective in allowing a return to serious running. Running is not consistent with total joint arthroplasty.

PERSPECTIVES ON TREATING RUNNING INJURIES

Through the years I have established a treatment protocol (20) that is adaptable to virtually all runners' injuries regardless of location. In this chapter I have not discussed specific treatment for all the various injuries that runners can incur because most of these conditions are discussed in more detail elsewhere in the book.

I look upon this as a "toolbox" for the physician to pick and choose from and apply to the condition involved in an appropriate fashion. This is a rather generic approach to runners' injuries and may not appeal to many orthopedists who would prefer a "recipe" directed specifically at the injury, but I have found this not to be very effective in treating runners. Once the diagnosis is made, the treatment is not all that different from the same condition in other athletes, although there are some variations, as discussed.

The Training Program

At the risk of being redundant, the training program and application of training principals is of utmost importance in diagnosing a runner's injuries. Appropriate alterations in the training program in most cases will resolve the injuries in a conservative fashion. Total rest is the last piece of advice runners generally want to hear, but at times it does become necessary. Generally, a modification of the running program with reduced frequency, intensity, and duration is a more acceptable alternative. If the running program or training program

must be discontinued, then it can be supplemented by running in water with a flotation device as a excellent form of non–weight-bearing cross training. Wilber et al. (17) concluded that deep water running may serve as an effective training alternative to land-based running for the maintenance of aerobic fitness up to 6 weeks in trained endurance athletes. There are also other modes of low impact training, such as cross-country ski devices, steppers, biking, and rowing, all of which can benefit to supplement a modified program.

Shoe Modification

Running shoes generally come in one of the three following classifications: motion control, support, and cushion. Most running shoe manufacturers have shoes fitting into these three classifications. Unfortunately, shoe salesmen frequently do not understand this. A motion control shoe is for an individual who needs more control for compensatory pronation, and this is a board-lasted shoe with a straighter last and less flexibility. A support shoe is generally a combination-last in which there is partial board lasting and partial slip lasting that provides some support with more flexibility. The cushion shoes are for the runner with a more rigid type foot requiring more flexibility and cushion, and it is generally a slip-lasted shoe.

Shoes sometimes require modification, and an orthotist or shoe repair shop can modify running shoes for special problems such as leg length discrepancy where a thicker midsole and heel wedge are added to accommodate for the discrepancy. Changing the durometer or hardness of the midsole or heel wedge material and using a variable hardness heel wedge, which is softer on the lateral side and firmer on the inner side, can change foot mechanics by altering the rate of pronation and affect the duration of pronation. The heel wedge and midsole cushioning do very little to alter the ground reaction forces generated during the propulsive phase and are primarily effective during the short phase of impact. Much emphasis has been made by the shoe manufacturers on the cushioning effect or shock-absorbing effects on impact during running, but this is not as significant as the amount of ground reaction force during the propulsive phase. During the propulsive or generation phase, the midsole hardness probably has little effect on the forces being generated.

The temperature effect on midsole materials has not been seriously considered by the industry to date, and characteristics of midsole material can vary widely from cold to warm conditions. A cushion-type shoe in warm weather may not function as well in cold conditions with increased stiffness of the sole material. Likewise, a motion control shoe in extremely warm conditions may function more like a cushion-type shoe.

The fact that a shoe "looks okay" does not necessarily

mean that it is functioning as well as it did when it was new. Many running shoes begin to lose their effectiveness at approximately 300 miles and may require replacing even though the wear does not appear to be excessive. Needless to say, it is important to replace shoes that do begin to show excessive wear.

It is still difficult to prescribe a specific shoe for an individual based on foot type, although general guidelines do apply. Shoe selection is still largely empirical based on what fits and feels good along with what has worked in the past.

Muscle Reconditioning and Flexibility

The restoration of muscle strength, endurance, and balance of the entire lower extremity is essential after injury or surgery. An exercise program must be devised that duplicates the functions of the muscles as closely as possible and generally requires both concentric and eccentric exercises, preferably of the closed-chain variety. I have personally seen many situations where even after return to competition, a muscle group deficit has persisted because of a lack of specific reconditioning during rehabilitation.

Flexibility is important, but the literature does not support either the preventive aspect or rehabilitative aspect of stretching exercises. Empirically it does seem important, and that is an opinion commonly held among sports physicians, coaches, trainers, and athletes.

Taunton et al. (36) stressed the importance of appropriate rehabilitation directed at restoration of muscle strength and endurance. All muscle groups of the lower extremity from the hip distally must be considered in a rehabilitation program regardless of the site of injury. Particularly look for muscle deficiencies in the runner complaining that the lower extremity does not "feel right" or does "track right." These terms are nondescript and frustrating but are often secondary to muscular imbalance that the runner is incapable of clearly describing. The lower extremity functions as a synchronous unit, and any muscle imbalance or contractures can disrupt the normal kinetic sequence.

Orthotic Devices

Orthotic devices have been popular for runners since the running boom in the 1970s and have been used as a modality for treating a variety of running injuries (37). Data are still on the soft side for their efficacy (38), but empirically they have been effective, particularly for medial tibial stress syndrome, plantar fasciitis, and in some instances knee problems, particularly anterior knee pain.

The theory for an orthotic shoe device is that it can help control the subtalar–midtarsal joint motion, maintaining the subtalar joint at or near its neutral position with a more normal ratio of inversion to eversion. Orthotics will help to reduce compensatory pronation and its effect on obligatory tibial rotation. Depending on the materials with which they are fabricated, they may provide some functional shock absorption and more effective subtalar joint function.

Orthotics devices are classified as noncontrolling, partially controlling, or fully controlling. The noncontrolling or accommodating-type device provides more shock absorption with minimal control often required by the cavus type foot or the more rigid-type foot. A partially controlling device is for mild compensatory pronation and is generally fabricated from more resilient flexible materials. Fully controlling devices are for severe compensatory pronation and are more effective fabricated from less flexible materials. The disadvantage of an orthotic device is that it does add additional weight in the shoe, which can result in additional energy expenditure. The addition of weight to the runner's foot is the worse place that weight can be added.

Over the past few years, the market has been flooded with orthotic devices, and many are being prescribed indiscriminately and in some instances fabricated in a way that is not functional or useful. When prescribing an orthotic device, be certain that the instructions for taking appropriate molds or measurements are followed implicitly. An incorrect mold or measurement of the foot results in a poorly functioning orthotic device and is a waste of time and money.

Medications

Pain control and reduction of inflammation is the first step in treating runners' injuries and is accomplished largely with the use of nonsteroidal anti-inflammatory medication. Occasionally, diminishing doses of oral steroid can be helpful, particularly with acute soft tissue conditions such as an iliotibial band syndrome or Achilles peritendinitis. Narcotic analgesics should never be prescribed just to allow an individual to run. Steroid injections are sometimes indicated but certainly not directly into tendons.

The most frequent condition in which I have used a steroid injection is for acute iliotibial band syndrome. For acute Achilles peritendinitis accompanied by crepitus and swelling, a brisement is frequently beneficial. This is a technique used to lyse adhesions about the Achilles tendon with an injection of 10 mL of an analgesic agent. After skin preparation, the needle is introduced distal to the area of involvement at a very oblique angle so that the needle slides along the surface of the tendon and under the peritenon. When properly positioned, the fluid is forcefully injected and effectively performs a mechanical lysis of adhesions. This has been quite effective, particularly with an acute processes. One might consider adding a small amount of short-acting steroid to help reduce the immediate inflammatory response. The runner is instructed to discontinue running for 3 to 5 days after this procedure, but water activity is permitted.

Physical Therapy

Physical therapy modalities must be specifically directed for the condition involved, and again the entire lower extremity musculature should be included regardless of where the injury is located. Open-chain concentric rehabilitation exercises probably have little place in the rehabilitation of a runner's injury. Close-chain concentric and eccentric exercises are indicated, and a program should be designed to simulate the normal functions of the muscles as closely as possible and yet not aggravate the condition being treated. The therapist should seek out muscular imbalances and correct contractures. One tip for acute and chronic hamstring rehabilitation is to have the runner run uphill or upstairs. This is much better tolerated than running on the level, and it will allow the runner or even sprinter to return to training much earlier than running on the level.

Surgery

Most runners' injuries can be managed conservatively, but the program must be adequately supervised so that if it fails, the runner, the coach, and the physician will feel comfortable considering surgical treatment. Surgical indications in runners are really no different than those in any other athlete with a similar condition. Being conservative does not necessarily mean unusual or unwarranted delay but rather taking a methodical approach to the problem before surgery. It is important to point out to the runner that the condition could actually terminate his or her running despite well-indicated or well-performed surgery. In my experience, the most frequent surgery in runners has been for knee problems and Achilles tendonopathy.

In the knee, the most common conditions relate to the extensor mechanism, particularly maltracking problems, meniscal lesions, pathologic plica, patellar tendonopathy, or degenerative joint disease. The procedure should be explained in detail so the runner can make an informed decision and will not have unrealistic expectations of the result.

Rehabilitation

The surgeon must be director of postoperative rehabilitation with the athlete, trainer, physical therapist, and coach. The results of surgery may be negated by too rapid a return to running without adequate and careful rehabilitation. Similar problems can also occur after recovery from an injury even without surgery. My personal

TABLE 54.1. *Return to running protocol*

Week	Activity
1	Walk 1–2 miles, alternating 1 min fast and 1 min normal.
2	Walk 2–3 miles, alternating 1.5 min fast and 1.5 min normal. Also jog easy in lieu of fast walking.
3	Continue week 2 and if doing well, substitute (not add) a 10-min jog every other day in lieu of walk/jog.
4	Same as 3, but jog 15 min every other day in lieu of walk/jog.
5	Jog 15 min one day and 25 min the next.
6	Jog 20 min one day and 30 min the next.
7	Jog 20 min one day and 35 min the next.
8	Jog 20 min one day and 40 min the next.
9	Resume training at appropriate duration, intensity, and frequency.

rules of thumb for returning to running with missed training from whatever cause is as follows (39): for 1 week or less, resume an appropriate training program but monitor it very closely and correct training errors; for 1 to 2 weeks, reduce the training 25% for the first week of return and then resume an appropriate training program; for 2 to 3 weeks, reduce the training 50% for the first week of return, 25% the second week, and then resume training; and if 4 weeks or more, refer to the protocol in Table 54.1.

The emphasis is placed on a gradual return to running with guidelines rather than leaving it to the discretion of the runner. It is extremely important to emphasize to the runner that the purpose of this protocol is to condition the injured area and not aerobic conditioning, which can be maintained with cross-training activities if necessary. When following the protocol, the runner should run an easy comfortable pace, perhaps 7 to 10 minutes per mile, and the walk should be brisk. A rest day should be planned every 7 to 10 days. The runner should not be concerned about the mileage because this program is based on time rather than distance. The runner can hold at a given level or even drop back a level if conditions dictate. The program can be varied to meet individual needs. In some instances, runners can move faster and skip a week if they are progressing very well or levels can be shortened or lengthened depending on progress. The important point, however, is not to overtrain or attempt to return to running too fast without allowing proper conditioning of the injured area and its accommodation to the stress of running. General strengthening and flexibility exercises for the rest of the body should not be neglected during this period of time.

SUMMARY

Two thirds of running injuries are a result of improper training. The history must include a thorough analysis of the training program. Examination includes the entire lower extremity and not just the site of complaint. A basic understanding of appropriate training and the biomechanics of running are invaluable tools for the physician. Surgery is not frequently required, with most injuries responding to conservative treatment. A return to a running program must be carefully outlined after surgery or injury.

REFERENCES

1. Jacobs SJ, Berson BL. Injuries to runners: a study of entrants to a 10,000 meter race. *Am J Sports Med* 1986;14:151–155.
2. Van Mechelen W. Running injuries: a review of the epidemiological literature. *Sports Med* 1992;14:320–335.
3. Clement DB, Taunton JE, Smart GW, et al. A survey of overuse running injuries. *Phys Sports Med* 1981;9:47–58.
4. James SL, Bates BT, Osternig LR. Injuries to runners. *Am J Sports Med* 1978;6:40–50.
5. Moran GT, McGlynn GH. *Cross training for sports.* Champaign, IL: Human Kinetics, 1997.
6. Scott SH, Winter DA. Internal forces of chronic running injury sites. *Med Sci Sports Exerc* 1990;22:357–369.
7. Hinterman B, Nigg BM. Epidemiology of foot and ankle disorders. In: Nordin M, Andersson GBJ, Pope MH, eds. *Musculoskeletal disorders in the workplace: principles and practice.* St. Louis: Mosby, 1997:537–549.
8. Nigg BM, Cole GK, Nachbauer W. Effects of arch height of the foot and angular motion of the lower extremities in running. *J Biomech* 1993;26:909–916.
9. James SL, Jones DC. Biomechanical aspects of distance running injuries. In: Cavanagh PR, ed. *Biomechanics of distance running.* Champaign, IL: Human Kinetics, 1990:249–269.
10. Perry J. Anatomy and biomechanics of the hindfoot. *Clin Orthop* 1983;177:9–15.
11. Nigg BM. Biomechanics, load analysis and sports injuries in the lower extremities. *Sports Med* 1985;2:367–379.
12. Ledbetter WB. Aging effects upon the repair and healing of athletic injury. In: Gordon SL, Gonzalez-Mestre X, Garrett WE Jr, eds. *Sports and exercise in midlife.* Rosemont, IL: American Academy of Orthopaedic Surgeons, 1993.
13. Novachek TF, Trost JP, Schutte L. *Running and sprinting. Part 2. Injury mechanisms and training strategies* (Video/CDROM). St. Paul: Gillette Children's Hospital, 1996.
14. Guten GN. *Running injuries.* Philadelphia: W.B. Saunders, 1997.
15. Noakes T. *Lore of running,* 3rd ed. Champaign, IL: Leisure Press, 1991.
16. Wilmore JH, Costill JH. *Physiology of sport and exercise.* Champaign: Human Kinetics, 1994:152.
17. Wilber RL, Moffatt RJ, Scott BE, et al. Influence of water run training on the maintenance of aerobic performance. *Med Sci Sports Exerc* 1996;28:1056–1062.
18. Walter SD, Hart LE, McIntosh JM, et al. The Ontario cohort study of running-related injuries. *Arch Intern Med* 1989;149:2501–2504.
19. Baxter DE, Zingas C. The foot in running. *J Am Acad Orthop Surg* 1995;3:136–145.
20. James SL. Running injuries to the knee. *J Am Acad Orthop Surg* 1995;3:309–318.
21. Boden BP, Pearsall AW, Garrett WE, et al. Patellofemoral instability: evaluation of treatment. *J Am Acad Orthop Surg* 1997;5:47–57.
22. Blazina ME, Kerlan RK, Jobe FW, et al. Jumper's knee. *Orthop Clin North Am* 1973;4:665–678.
23. Fritschy D. Jumper's knee. *Oper Tech Sports Med* 1997;5:150–153.
24. Ewing JW. Plica: pathologic or not? *J Am Acad Orthop Surg* 1993;1:117–121.
25. Franco V, Cerullo E, Gianni E, et al. Iliotibial band friction syndrome. *Oper Tech Sports Med* 1997;5:153–156.
26. Benazzo F, Todesca A, Ceciliani L. Achilles tendon tendinitis and heel pain. *Oper Tech Sports Med* 1997;5:179–188.
27. Pfeffer GB. Plantar heel pain. In: Baxter DE, ed. *The foot and ankle in sports.* St. Louis: Mosby, 1995:195–206.
28. Baxter DE, ed. Functional nerve disorders. In: *The foot and ankle in sports.* St. Louis: Mosby, 1995:9–22.
29. Shin AY, Gillingham BL. Fatigue fractures of the femoral neck in athletes. *J Am Acad Orthop Surg* 1997;5:293–302.
30. Friedericson M, Bergman A, Hoffman KL, et al. Tibial stress reaction in runners. *Am J Sports Med* 1995;23:472–481.
31. Detmer DE. Chronic shin splints. Classification and management of medial tibial stress syndrome. *Sports Med* 1986;3:346–446.
32. Chambers HG. Medial tibial stress syndrome: evaluation and management. *Oper Tech Sports Med* 1995;3:274–277.
33. Mubarak SJ. Surgical management of chronic compartment syndrome. *Oper Tech Sports Med* 1993;3:259–266.
34. Torg JS, Pavlov H, Torg E. Overuse injuries in sport: the foot. *Clin Sports Med* 1987;6:291–320.
35. Paty JG Jr. Arthritis and running. In: Guten GN, ed. *Running injuries.* Philadelphia: W.B. Saunders, 1997:189–200.
36. Taunton JE, Clement DB, Smart GW, et al. Non-surgical management of overuse knee injuries in runners. *Can J Sports Med* 1987;12:11–18.
37. Gross ML, Napoli RC. Treatment of lower extremity injuries with orthotic shoe inserts. An overview. *Sports Med* 1993;15:66–70.
38. Jones DC, James SL. Foot orthoses. In: Baxter DE, ed. *The foot and ankle in sports.* St. Louis: Mosby, 1996:369–378.
39. James SL. Running injuries of the knee. In: Cannon D, ed. *AAOS Instructional Course Lectures.* Vol. 47. Rosemont, IL: American Academy of Orthopaedic Surgeons, 1997, 407–417.

Subject Index

Locators annotated with *f* indicate figures.
Locators annotated with *t* indicate tables.

A

A band, in sarcomeres, 4, 5*f*
Abdominal compartments
 anatomy of, 87–88
 compression syndrome of, 227
Abdominal hernias
 etiologies of, 218–219, 227
 referred hip pain from, 572, 572*t*
Abdominal wall injuries
 hernias, 218–219, 224, 227, 572*f*
 muscle strains, 218, 225
 nerve compression, 219–220, 220*f*
Abduction mechanisms, per joint. *See specific joint*
Abduction pillow, postoperative, for posterior shoulder capsulorrhaphy, 426, 426*f*
Abductor digit quinti (ADQ) muscle
 impingement of nerve to, 899, 933–934, 934*f*
 tendon insertions of, 898, 900*f*, 1020
Abductor pollicis longus (APL) tendon, DeQuervain's syndrome and, 283
ABN. *See* Acute brachial neuropathy
Abrasion arthroplasty
 for knee cartilage repair, 795, 802*f*, 855
 for patellofemoral arthritis, 737–739, 740*t*, 795
Abrasive wear, in articular cartilage, 789–791, 790*f*
Absorption phase, of running, 1011–1013
Acceleration, of arm. *See* Arm acceleration
Acceleration-deceleration injuries, intracranial, management of, 156–160, 158*t*
Accessory navicular, painful
 evaluation of, 914, 915*f*
 nonoperative treatment of, 914, 915*f*
 pathoanatomy of, 914
 surgical treatment of, 914–915, 916*f*
Acetaminophen, for knee degeneration, 852
Acetylcholine (ACh), in muscle contraction, 9, 10*f*
Achilles paratenonitis, 979–984
Achilles tendinitis
 distal insertional, 696, 934–936, 934*f*–936*f*
 from running, 1017, 1019–1020
Achilles tendinosis, 696, 979–984, 983*f*
Achilles tendon
 anatomy and physiology of, 23, 24*f*, 26, 26*f*, 979
 blood supply to, 30–31
 dysfunction of
  clinical evaluation of, 980–981, 980*f*
  epidemiology of, 979
  imaging studies of, 981
  injury mechanisms of, 979–980
  nonoperative treatment of, 981–982, 984, 986
  surgical treatment of, 982–987, 983*f*, 985*f*–986*f*
 functional considerations of, 32, 34–35
 as graft, for knee repair
  patellar tendon, 702, 704
  posterolateral, 683–684, 778, 814
 Haglund's deformity and, 936–938, 936*f*–937*f*, 980

 hindfoot insertions of, 897–898, 898*f*, 979
 immobilization devices for, 982–987
 inflammatory injuries of
  paratenonitis, 979–984
  retrocalcaneal, 980–981, 983, 986–987
  from running, 1017, 1019–1020
  tendinitis, 696, 934–936, 934*f*–936*f*
  tendinosis, 696, 979–984, 983*f*
 rehabilitation programs for, 982–984, 986–987
 retrocalcaneal bursa and, inflammatory injuries of, 980–981, 983, 986–987
 running force impact on, 1012–1013
  injuries from, 1017, 1019–1020
 shin splints and, 876
 tear injuries of
  clinical evaluation of, 981
  gastrocnemius injuries *versus,* 889
  magnetic resonance imaging of, 110
  mechanisms of, 980
  nonoperative treatment of, 984
  primary surgical repair of, 984–985, 985*f*
  reconstruction techniques for, 935–937, 936*f*, 985–986, 986*f*
Acquired immunodeficiency syndrome (AIDS), from allografts, 826
Acromioclavicular joint
 anatomy of, 337–339, 337*f*–338*f*, 369*f*
  inclination variations in, 511–512, 512*f*
  ligaments, 511–512, 512*f*
  muscle stabilizers, 512
 biomechanics of, 369–372, 369*f*–371*f*
  differential motions in, 512–513, 528
 clavicle fractures impact on, 535, 537–538
 dislocation injuries of
  active patient splinting with, 512, 512*f*, 516
  with brachial plexus injuries, 187–189, 191
  classifications of, 513–515, 514*f*–515*f*
  clavicle abnormalities with, 513, 514*f*, 516*f*–517*f*, 517, 519–521, 524
  clinical examination of, 516–517, 516*f*–517*f*
  ligament injuries with, 513–520, 514*f*–516*f*
  mechanisms of, 511, 513, 513*f*
  nonoperative treatment of, 521–522, 521*f*
  operative treatment of, 521–532
  radiographic studies of, 517–521, 518*f*–520*f*
  range of motion with, 371, 371*f*, 512–513, 516–517
  return to sport guidelines, 528–529, 532
  scapula abnormalities with, 500*f*, 501, 506, 516*f*–517*f*, 517, 520–521
  stability factors with, 514–517, 514*f*–517*f*
 range of motion of, 339, 370, 370*f*
  displacement impact on, 371, 371*f*, 512–513, 516–517
  post-screw fixation, 370–371, 512–513, 528
 rotator cuff injuries and, 480–483, 483*f*
 stability mechanisms of, 339, 512, 514–517
 surgical treatment of
  acromioclavicular fixation, 522*f*, 523, 525–528, 525*f*, 527*f*–528*f*
  acute injuries, 525–529, 525*f*–528*f*

 chronic injuries, 529–532, 529*f*–531*f*
 coracoclavicular cerclage, 522*f*–523*f*, 523
 coracoclavicular fixation, 522*f*, 523, 524*f*, 525–528, 527*f*, 530–531, 531*f*
 delayed, 515, 518, 521–522
 distal clavicle resection, 522*f*, 524, 529–531, 529*f*–531*f*
 dynamic muscle transfer, 524
 fixation procedures, 522*f*, 523, 523*f*–524*f*, 525–528, 525*f*–529*f*
 indications for, 521–522
 ligament reconstruction, 371–372, 522*f*–523*f*, 523–525, 529–531, 532*f*
 postoperative care with, 528–529, 531–532
Acromioclavicular ligaments
 anatomy of, 511–512, 512*f*
 injury mechanisms of, 513–515, 514*f*–515*f*, 520
 surgical reconstruction of, 371–372, 522*f*–523*f*, 523–525, 529–531, 532*f*
Acromionectomy, for rotator cuff impingement syndrome, 479–480
Acromion process
 in acromioclavicular fixation, 523
 elevation mechanisms of, 498–499, 519
 in glenoid labral tear repairs, 468, 472–475, 474*f*
 rotator cuff relationship to, 373, 373*f*, 374–375, 483*f*
  injury mechanisms with, 378–379, 378*f*–379*f*, 480, 480*f*
 in shoulder impingement, 332, 500*f*, 501
 types of, 332, 332*f*, 337, 373–374, 378
Acromioplasty
 anterior, for rotator cuff impingement syndrome, 479–480, 485–487, 492
  arthroscopic *versus* open, 485–486
 with glenoid labral tear repairs, 474–475
Actin
 in excitation-contraction coupling, 9–11, 10*f*–11*f*
 muscle regulation by, 4–6, 5*f*
Action potential, of peripheral nerves, in muscle contraction, 9, 10*f*
Active length-tension relationship, in muscle contractions, 10–11, 11*f*
Acute anterior spinal cord injury syndrome, 163, 166
Acute brachial neuropathy (ABN)
 clinical manifestations of, 184, 190–193
 prognosis for, 197–198
 treatment of, 196, 198–199
Acute compartment syndrome (ACS)
 clinical presentation of, 89–90
 diagnosis of, 91, 93
 injury mechanisms of, 604
 in lower leg, 879–882, 879*f*–880*f*, 881*t*, 882*f*
 pathophysiology of, 88–89
 of thigh, 604–606, 605*f*
 treatment of
  critical timing of, 605–606

Acute compartment syndrome (ACS) (*contd.*)
  decompressive techniques for, 89–95, 605, 605*f*
Acute low back pain, 203–205
ADAMs enzymes, articular cartilage degradation by, 62
Adductor brevis tendon, anatomy of, 584–585, 584*f*
Adductor canal syndrome, of thigh, 606
Adductor hallucis tendon, 897, 900*f*, 921
Adductor longus muscle
  anatomy of, 584–585, 584*f*
  strain injuries of
    classification of, 220, 593
    clinical presentation of, 220, 593
    epimysial release indications for, 227
    groin injuries from, 220–221, 220*f*, 228
      athletic pubalgia with, 223–224, 224*f*, 227, 227*f*
    hernias with, 218–219, 224, 226
    imaging studies of, 594
    mechanisms of, 593
    prognosis of, 221
    rehabilitation program for, 594
    return to sport guidelines, 221
    surgical repair of, 594
    tenotomy indications for, 221
    treatment per grade, 594
    treatment stages for, 220–221, 594
Adductor magnus muscle
  anatomy of, 583–585, 584*f*
  strain injuries of, 593
Adductor tubercle, injuries of, 595, 666
Adenosine triphosphatase enzyme
  in muscle contractions, 10, 10*f*
  muscle fiber typing with, 13–14, 15*f*, 16, 16*f*, 16*t*
Adhesion. *See* Cohesion
Adipose tissue
  estrogen conversion role of, 82
  magnetic resonance imaging intensity for, 100–101, 100*t*
Adolescents
  ankle injuries in, 992
  cervical spine injuries in, 161, 163–164
  elbow injuries in, 307
  hip injuries in, 571, 580–581, 581*f*, 596
  intracranial injuries in, 159
  knee injuries in, 615, 653, 666, 743
    tendon mechanisms, 687, 689, 698, 704–706
  lumbar spine injuries in, 204, 209–213
  pelvic apophyseal avulsion fractures in, 600–602
  shoulder injuries in, 401–402, 438, 465–466
  thigh muscle strain injuries in, 597
  toe injuries in, 976
ADQ. *See* Abductor digiti quinti muscle
AE. *See* Athletic exposure
Aerobic conditioning
  bone formation and, 83, 83*f*
  for hamstring strains, 591
  knee ligaments and, 670, 670*f*
  with leg injuries, 872, 878, 1015
  for lumbar spine injuries, 204–205, 207
  for runners, 872, 878, 1011, 1015, 1022
Aerobic metabolism, in tendon cells, 28–29
Afferent sensory neuron system, mechanoreceptors in, 31, 864
AFO. *See* Ankle-foot orthotics
Age factors
  of injuries. *See* Adolescents; Children
  of knee osteoarthritis, 62–63, 66, 845
Aggrecan, in articular cartilage, 54*t*, 55, 61–62
Aggrecanase, in articular cartilage, 62, 67
AIDS. *See* Acquired immunodeficiency syndrome
AIIS. *See* Anterior inferior iliac spine
Airway maintenance, for head and neck injuries, 154–155
AL. *See* Arcuate ligament
Alexander stress view, radiographic, for acromioclavicular dislocations, 519–520, 519*f*
Allen's test, for wrist injury evaluation, 274, 284–285

All-inside arthroscopic repair, of knee meniscus, 655, 655*f*–657*f*, 831
Allman classification, of clavicular injuries, 513–515, 535
Allografts
  autografts *versus*, 47, 235, 683–684, 829
  complications of, 826–827, 826*f*
  indications for. *See specific anatomy or injury*
  sterilization techniques for, 826
AMBRII syndrome, with Bankart lesion, 402
Ambulance, availability of, for head and neck injuries, 153–154
Amino acids. *See also* Proteins
  in muscle contractions, 11–12
Amnesia, from intracranial injuries, 157–158
AMZ. *See* Anteromedialization procedure
Anabolic steroids, risks of, 598
Anaerobic metabolism, in tendon cells, 28–29
Analgesics
  for acromioclavicular joint dislocations, 522
  nonsteroidal. *See* Nonsteroidal anti-inflammatory drugs
  post-knee repair, 755
  for runners' injuries, 1023
Analysis of variance (ANOVA)
  factorial, 133, 137
  repeated-measures, 133, 137
  in research studies, 133–134, 136–137, 144–145
Analytical models, of knee biomechanics, 639
Aneurysms
  compartment syndrome *versus*, 91–92
  of dorsalis pedis, in dancers, 961
  of thigh, 606–607
Angiofibroblastic hyperplasia, with elbow tendinosis, 290, 294, 300*f*, 303*f*
Angiography. *See* Arteriography
Anisotropic properties, of articular cartilage, 58, 58*f*, 60
Ankle
  anatomy of
    ligaments, 819–820, 823
    tendons, 979, 987, 991–992, 991*f*, 1000, 1007
  avulsion fractures of, 918, 922, 922*f*
  biomechanics of, 819–821, 883, 896–898, 897*f*, 927
  dome of, magnetic resonance imaging of, 110–111, 111*f*
  effusions of, 872, 998
  fractures of
    lateral process, 923–924, 924*f*
    posterior, 924–926, 925*f*–926*f*
  impingement syndromes of
    classification of, 821, 821*t*
    clinical evaluation of, 820, 924, 925*f*
    differential diagnosis of, 821, 821*t*, 919
    epidemiology of, 819
    expected outcomes of, 822, 822*f*
    imaging studies of, 820, 822–823
    injury mechanisms of, 111, 141, 142*f*, 819–820
    spectrum of, 819, 820*f*, 939–940
    tarsal, 899, 899*f*–900*f*, 939–940
    treatment of, 821–823, 822*f*
  injuries of
    associated leg injuries with, 872, 879, 883, 887
    fractures, 923–926, 924*f*–926*f*
    ligaments, 917, 917*f*, 939
    sprain, 819–823, 872, 879, 883, 887
  instability mechanisms of, 819–820, 820*f*, 822–823, 916–917
  ligaments of
    anatomy of, 819–820, 823
    injuries of, 110, 110*f*, 917, 939–940
  magnetic resonance imaging of
    for anterolateral impingement, 111, 141, 142*f*
    for ligamentous injury, 110, 110*f*
    for osteochondral injury, 110–112, 111*f*–112*f*
  pain mechanisms of, 819–820, 820*f*, 823, 920
  rehabilitation programs for, 820–822
  rotation of, posterior tibial tendon role in, 1000, 1001*f*
  sprains of
    chronic, 819–820
    epidemiology of, 819, 992

  impingement syndromes from, 819–823, 939–940
  mechanisms of, 819–820, 872, 879, 883, 887
  peroneus tendon mechanisms in, 992–998, 993*f*, 995*f*, 997*f*
  tendons of
    anatomy of, 979, 987, 991–992, 991*f*, 1000, 1007
    injuries of. *See specific tendon*
Ankle-foot orthotics (AFO), for foot injuries, 909, 921, 927, 929, 935
Ankylosing spondylitis, 215
ANOVA. *See* Analysis of variance
Antalgic gait
  with ankle tendon injuries, 994, 1002
  with patella pathology, 620, 621*f*
  from stress fractures, 1020
Anterior cruciate ligament (ACL), of knee
  anatomy of, 41, 626–627
  biomechanics of
    during exercise, 628–629
    force and strain measurements in, 625
    tensile property testing of, 40–41, 40*f*, 626
  counseling and education indications with, 748, 753–754, 866
  degenerative joint disease and, 848–850
  functional bracing of
    cautions with, 864–866
    design perspectives, 864–865
    goals for, 754, 863–864
    limitations of, 865–866
    mechanisms of, 864, 866
    objective testing of, 863–864, 866–867
    subjective reports of, 865–866
  physical examination of
    with injuries, 745–747, 746*f*
    pivot shift tests for, 614–617, 614*f*–616*f*
  reconstruction of
    with combined injuries, 44, 634, 744–745, 744*t*, 754–755, 780
    complications of, 756, 757*f*, 758, 758*t*
    expected outcomes of, 752–753
    fixation techniques for, 629, 632–633, 750
    goals of, 750
    graft complications of, 825–827, 826*f*
    grafts for, 44, 47–48, 48*f*, 626, 629–632, 750–751, 829
    historical perspectives of, 749–751
    patellar tendon graft advantages for, 630–632, 682, 750–751, 812
    range of motion perspectives of, 44–45, 45*f*, 627–628, 750–751, 758, 758*t*
    rehabilitation after, 755–756, 755*t*, 756*f*
    scar revision indications with, 757*f*, 758
    in skeletally immature athletes, 743, 748, 753–754
    strain considerations for, 625, 628–632
    tensile considerations with, 41–42, 626, 751, 755
    timing of, 750, 753
    tunnel complications with, 827–829, 827*f*–828*f*
    tunnel placement techniques for, 629–631, 751, 752*f*, 755, 815
  rehabilitation programs for
    active *versus* passive, 628–630, 749, 755
    knee positions for, 628–629, 748–749, 749*f*
    phases of, 748–749, 749*t*, 753, 755–756, 755*t*
    postoperative, 755–756, 755*t*, 756*f*
    preoperative, 753–754
    weight-bearing *versus* non–weight-bearing, 629, 749, 752, 865, 867
  stability braces for, 863–867
  stability role of, 626–628
  tear injuries of. *See also* Knee, multiligament injuries of
    clinical evaluation of, 745–747, 746*f*
    combined, 44, 634, 744–745, 744*t*, 754–755, 780
    epidemiology of, 743–744
    femoral intercondylar notch and, 744–745, 745*f*
    healing potential of, 43–44, 630, 632, 848

magnetic resonance imaging of, 102, 103f, 747–748, 748f
mechanisms of, 744–745, 744t, 745f
medial collateral ligament injuries with, 44, 634, 672–673, 744, 754
meniscus injuries with, 651, 653, 744–745, 744t, 747, 753–755
nonoperative treatment of, 748–749, 749f, 749t, 752. See also Anterior cruciate ligament, of knee, rehabilitation programs for
operative treatment of, 749–755, 752f. See also Anterior cruciate ligament, of knee, reconstruction of
posterior cruciate ligament injuries with, 763, 768, 771–772, 776–777, 780
radiographic studies of, 747
return to sport guidelines, 748–749, 749t, 752–753, 756, 865
in situ force measurement for, 45–47, 46f
tibia involvement with, 745, 745f, 747
treatment goals for, 750, 753
treatment outcomes for, 752–753
treatment phases for, 748–749, 753–758, 755t, 756f–757f, 758t
tensile strength of, 40–41, 40f
Anterior glenoid labrum, contact injuries of
arthroscopic treatment of, 446–449, 446f–450f
clinical evaluation of, 436, 438–442, 440f–441f
epidemiology of, 431–432
imaging analysis of, 442–445, 442f–444f
injury mechanisms of, 435–437
nonoperative treatment of, 445–446, 445f, 445t
postoperative rehabilitation for, 450
surgical treatment of, 446, 448
tack repair of, 447–450, 447f, 449f–450f
treatment algorithm for, 448–450, 449f–450f, 449t
Anterior inferior iliac spine (AIIS)
avulsion fractures of, 601, 601t
patella relationship to, 638, 702, 712
thigh relationship to, 585
Anterior interosseous syndrome, 548–549
Anteriorization procedure, of tibia tubercle
complications of, 834–835
for patellofemoral arthritis, 735–736, 736f, 739, 740t
Anterior shoulder instability
acute traumatic, 431, 445–449
clinical evaluation of, 402–404, 403f, 407
epidemiology of, 399
from glenoid labral injuries. See Anterior glenoid labrum
imaging analysis of, 404–406, 404f–405f
impingement with, 402, 406
injury mechanisms of, 401–402
labral injury mechanisms of
with contact sports, 431–454
with throwing motions, 343, 401–402, 407–409, 457–475
recurrence of, 402, 431–432, 435–436, 445–446, 445t
rehabilitation for, 406, 409
return to sport guidelines, 409
stability mechanisms, 399–401
treatment of, 406f, 407–409, 408f
Anterior slide test, for shoulder assessment, with labral tear injuries, 467
Anterior step-off, normal, posterior cruciate ligament injuries and, 769, 769f
Anterior superior iliac spine (ASIS)
avulsion injuries of, 217, 580, 601–602, 601t
thigh relationship to, 585
Anterior tarsal syndrome
evaluation of, 918–919
mechanisms of, 918–919, 918f, 958–959
nonoperative treatment of, 919, 919f
surgical treatment of, 919–920
Anterior tibial translation (ATT), functional bracing for, 863–867
Anterolateral corner compression syndrome, of ankle, 820–821
Anteromedialization (AMZ) procedure
for patellofemoral arthritis, 736–737, 739, 740t

for patellofemoral joint dislocations, 733–734, 733f
Anteversion, in glenohumeral instability, 501–502
Anthropomorphic factors
in knee osteoarthritis, 846, 851–852, 856
in leg injuries, 869, 876
Anticoagulation therapy, indications for, 810, 812, 889
Anti-inflammatory drugs. See Nonsteroidal anti-inflammatory drugs
APL. See Abductor pollicis longus tendon
Apley compression test, for knee injuries, 652, 652f, 850
Aponeurosis
of extensor carpi radialis brevis tendon, 299–302, 300f–301f
plantar, 897, 898f
of ulnar collateral ligament, 116, 116f, 244–245
Apophyses, avulsion injuries of
in iliac spine, 216–217, 580, 600–602, 601t
in knee, 689
Apprehension maneuver
in patellofemoral joint examination, 619–620, 620f, 712
for shoulder assessment, 403, 403f, 466–467, 483
Arches, of foot
bony, 893, 894f, 945, 1000
support for, 913f
Arcuate ligament (AL)
anatomy of, 676–677, 805–806
biomechanics of, 677, 766, 806–808
injuries of, 679–680, 683–685, 776–778
Arm acceleration
with golf swing, 393–394, 393f
with pitching
biomechanics of, 387f, 388, 459f–460f, 460, 552f, 554–555, 555f
pathologic, 557, 559f
with tennis, 392–393, 392f
Arm cocking
force couples with, 552, 554–555, 557
with pitching
biomechanics of, 459–460, 459f, 465, 552f, 559f
early, 387–388, 387f, 552–553, 552f–553f, 555–556
late, 387f–388f, 388, 552f–554f, 553–554, 556–567, 556f
pathologic, 555–558, 556f, 559f
scapula role in, 498, 501–503, 503t, 552–553, 553f
with tennis, 392, 392f, 498
Arm deceleration, with pitching, biomechanics of, 387f–388f, 388, 459f–460f, 460, 552f, 555
Arm kinematics
with golf swing, 393–394, 393f
with pitching. See Pitching
scapula role in, 498, 501–503, 503t, 552–553, 553f
with swimming, 391–392, 391f
with tennis, 392–393, 392f–393f, 498
with throwing, 387–388, 387f–388f
Arm position
glenohumeral joint stability per, 382, 384f, 386, 386f
shoulder injuries per, 418–421, 432
Arrow fixation. See Tack fixation
Arterial venous pressure gradient, in compartment syndrome, 88
Arteriography
for compartment syndromes, 91–92, 605
for knee injuries, 771, 810
for popliteal artery entrapment, 886–887
for thigh disorders, 606
for ulnar artery thrombosis, 285
Arterioles, of tendons, 31
Artery(ies)
axillary, injuries to, 185, 189, 191, 402
cerebral, injury impact on, 158–160
circumflex, of shoulder, 341, 342f, 343, 350, 352–355, 360
in compartment syndrome, 88, 91

dorsalis pedis, 895–896, 896f, 961, 1007
femoral, disorders of, 606
geniculate, 648–649, 765, 886
meningeal, epidural hematomas from, 158–159
popliteal
entrapment syndrome of, 886–887, 886f
knee injuries and, 765, 768, 808–809, 832
radial, wrist injuries and, 257, 274
subclavian, brachial plexus injuries and, 185, 189, 191
suprascapular, of shoulder, 353–355
tibial, 899, 899f, 1007
ulnar, wrist injuries and, 274, 285
Arthritis
degenerative. See Osteoarthritis
of elbow, 292–293, 321–323, 322f–323f
of hip region, 215
rheumatoid, 215, 292
from scaphoid fractures, 267, 269, 270f
of wrist, 274, 282
Arthrodesis
of calcaneocuboid joint, 923
forefoot indications for, 948
hindfoot indications for, 926–927, 927f, 929
knee indications for, 704
midfoot indications for, 911–913, 920
of subtalar joint, 926–927, 927f
of tibiofibular joint, 884
Arthrofibrosis
in articular cartilage, 58, 58f, 60, 62, 66
as bone-ligament-bone complex property, 39–41, 40f
post-graft reconstruction, 47–48, 48f
in knee
biomechanics of, 624, 626–627, 633
post-ligament repair, 758, 758f, 811–812, 829, 838
post-meniscal repair, 831
treatment of, 838–839
from toe injuries, 968
Arthrography
for elbow injuries, 311
for knee injuries, 691, 701
for rotator cuff injuries, 483–484
for wrist injuries, 277–278, 280
Arthrometer measurements, KT-100, of knee injuries, 749, 754, 763, 779, 866
Arthroplasty
for knee cartilage repair, 795, 802f, 855–858
for patellofemoral arthritis, 737–739, 740t, 795
for posterior shoulder dislocations, 422, 427
for toe deformities, 946, 953–954, 973
for toe injuries, 946, 966, 968, 972
Arthroscopy, diagnostic and therapeutic
for acromioclavicular joint dislocations, 525–526, 526f–527f
for ankle impingement syndromes, 820–822, 822f
for elbow injuries, 304, 313–315, 315f, 317, 321–325, 325f
for hindfoot injuries, 926
for hip injuries, 574–576, 574f, 576f, 579
for knee
articular cartilage indications, 792–793, 792f, 797, 800
compartment syndromes from, 90
degeneration, 854–855
indications for, 628, 635, 652–653, 828
ligament indications, 672–673, 744, 755, 758, 776, 780–781, 812
meniscus repair techniques, 653–656, 654f–657f, 831–832, 848
patellofemoral joint indications, 723–724, 724f, 726, 733
tendon indications, 695, 701
of quadriceps tendon ruptures, 599
for shoulder instability, 436, 445
anterior labral, 446–450, 446f–447f, 449f–450f
posterior labral, 416, 421, 423, 450–451, 451f
superior labral, 451–453, 453f, 470–474, 472f–474f

Arthroscopy, diagnostic and therapeutic (*contd.*)
 for wrist injuries, 277–278, 281
Articular cartilage
 biomechanics of, 57–58
  compression properties of, 59–60, 66, 793
  friction in, 60–61, 61*t*
  shear properties of, 58–59, 58*f*, 787, 788*f*,
   789
  swelling in, 60
  tension properties of, 58, 58*f*
 calcified-noncalcified junction in
  injury role of, 789–790
  structural properties of, 787–789, 789*f*
 cell structure of, 53, 54*t*, 56–57, 56*f*–57*f*
 chondrocytes in
  physiologic role of, 61–63, 66, 787, 794
  structural properties, 56–57, 56*f*–57*f*
 composition of, 53–56, 54*f*, 54*t*, 65
  age-related changes in, 57, 66
  collagen, 54–57, 56*f*, 61–62, 65–67, 787–789,
   789*f*
 degenerative changes in. *See also* Osteoarthritis
  pathoanatomy of, 62–67, 65*f*, 847, 849
  snapping hip syndrome from, 229, 574–576,
   574*f*, 576*f*
 function of, 53, 57–58, 789
 healing potential of, 63–64, 66, 791, 794
 hydrophilic property of, 53–55, 58*f*, 60, 65
 injuries to
  clinical evaluation of, 791
  functional changes with, 62–64, 790
  imaging studies of, 104–105, 105*f*–106*f*,
   791–793, 792*f*
  mechanisms of, 64, 789–791, 789*f*–790*f*
  open *versus* closed lesions, 792–793
  return to sport guidelines, 801
  treatment of, primary *versus* salvage, 793,
   800–801, 800*f*–802*f*
 laser chondroplasty of, 795–796, 795*f*–796*f*
  osteonecrosis from, 796, 832
 metabolism in, 61–63
  osteoarthritis impact on, 55–56, 66–67
 mineralization of, 54–55
 nutrition mechanisms, 54, 61
 organization of
  age-related changes in, 57, 66
  layers, 788–789, 789*f*
  matrix, 53, 56–57, 57*f*, 61–62, 66, 787–788,
   788*f*
  zonal, 56, 56*f*
 osteoarthritis and
  composition impact, 65–66
  etiologies of, 54–55, 62–64
  mechanics impact, 66
  metabolism impact, 55–56, 66–67
  morphology and histology impact, 64–65,
   65*f*
 Outerbridge classification of, in shoulder, 472
 permeability factors of, 53–56, 58, 58*f*, 60, 64,
  66
 regeneration of
  allografts for, 800–801, 800*f*–801*f*
  autogenous grafts for, 798–801, 799*f*–801*f*
  chondrocyte implants for, 67, 797–798,
   797*f*–798*f*, 856
  periosteal transplants for, 796–797, 796*f*–798*f*
  techniques for, 793, 796
  via growth factors, 67, 800
 rehabilitation exercises for, 793, 800–801
 repair of
  clinical modalities for, 67, 793–795
  intrinsic capabilities for, 63–64, 66, 791–794
  primary *versus* salvage, 800–801, 800*f*–802*f*
 softening of. *See* Chondromalacia
 stabilization and débridement of, 764*f*, 793–795,
  800
  failure mechanisms of, 801–802, 802*f*, 858
 swelling mechanisms of, 53–55, 59–60
 tensile properties of, 57–60, 58*f*
Articularis genus muscle, anatomy of, 585
Artificial turf
 grass *versus*, 950

toe sprain injuries from, 949, 968–970,
 968*f*–970*f*
ASIS. *See* Anterior superior iliac spine
Aspiration procedures, for olecranon bursitis,
 326
Aspirin
 for patellofemoral arthritis, 736
 for vascular compromise, with knee dislocations, 810
Athlete
 definition of, 224–225
 elite *versus* recreational, 273
Athletic exposure (AE), strain incidence per, 583,
 587, 593, 597
Athletic hernias, 218–219, 219*f*, 224, 227
Athletic pubalgia
 from adductor injuries, 223–225, 224*f*,
  228–230
 anatomy review, 223, 224*f*
 clinical presentations of, 225–226, 226*f*, 595
 definitions for, 224–225
 differential diagnosis of, 227–228, 595–596
 epidemiology of, 224–225
 imaging studies of, 225–227, 226*f*, 595
 injury mechanisms of, 223–224, 224*f*, 595
 physical therapy protocol for, 596, 596*t*
 specific syndromes of, 228–230
 surgical repair of, 226–227, 596
 treatment algorithms for, 227, 228*f*–229*f*
Atlantooccipital fusion, 175
Atlas fractures, 165–166, 177
ATPase. *See* Adenosine triphosphatase enzyme
ATT. *See* Anterior tibial translation
Attachments. *See* Insertions
Augmentation, for shoulder assessment, with labral contact injuries, 441–442
Autografts
 allografts *versus*, 47, 235, 683–684, 829
 indications for. *See specific anatomy or injury*
Avascular necrosis
 of femoral head
  blood supply occlusion and, 230
  laser-induced, 796, 832
  magnetic resonance imaging of, 112–113,
   113*f*
  from pelvic fractures, 216, 226
 of metatarsal head. *See* Freiberg's infraction
 of scaphoid bone, 116
Avulsion fractures
 of adductor tubercle, 595
 of ankle, 919, 922, 922*f*
 of foot, 909, 922, 922*f*
 of hand, 235, 236*f*, 237
 of iliac spine, 600–602, 601*t*
  apophyses, 216–217, 580, 600–602, 601*t*
 of ischial tuberosity, 217, 592
 of lumbar spine, 205
 of pelvis, 216–217
Avulsion injuries
 of distal interphalangeal joints, 249–250
 of flexor digitorum profundus tendon, 236,
  252–254, 253*f*–254*f*
 of knee, 666, 772, 772*f*, 774–775, 777, 812
 of nerve roots. *See* Neurotmesis
 of proximal interphalangeal joints, 247–248
 of triangular fibrocartilage complex, 274, 280,
  281*f*
Axial load injuries
 cervical
  mechanisms of, 159, 163, 165, 168, 168*f*, 170,
   174
  prevention strategies for, 172–174, 172*f*–173*f*,
   195
 of hands and wrists, 237, 247–248, 274
 of Lisfranc's joint, 907–908, 907*f*
 of toes, 968, 968*f*
Axial load test, for shoulder assessment, 403,
 403*f*, 420
 with labral injuries, 440, 440*t*, 466
Axial views, radiographic, of patellofemoral joint
 injuries, 718, 719*f*, 722*f*, 723

Axillary lateral view, radiographic. *See* West
 Point view
Axillary view, radiographic, of acromioclavicular
 joint injuries, 520–521
Axis fractures, 165–166, 177
Axonotmesis
 with brachial plexus injuries, 162, 183
 as nerve injury classification, 186, 543
Axons, injury mechanisms of, 179, 179*f*

B

Back. *See* Spine
Backboards, hitting against, injury risks with,
 295
Backhand strokes, with tennis, 392–393, 393*f*
Backpack palsy, 183–184, 189, 189*f*, 195, 197
Back swings, with golfing, 393–394, 393*f*
Baker's cyst, of knee, 620
Ballottement test, for lunotriquetral ligament injury, 279
Bankart lesion
 diagnostic techniques for, 468, 472
 repair techniques for
  anterior, 407–409, 408*f*, 448–450, 449*f*–450*f*
  posterior, 413–414, 423, 427
 shoulder instability with, 343, 401–402, 435,
  446, 446*f*
Basamania procedure, for clavicle fractures,
 537–538
Baseball. *See also* Pitching
 injuries from, 233, 249, 307, 883
Basketball, injuries from
 in foot and ankle, 819, 907, 918, 929*f*, 933, 968
 in knee, 691, 700, 721, 743
 in leg, 586, 597, 876
 in upper body, 233, 319
Bassett's ligament, in ankle sprains, 820
Bassini-type herniorrhaphy, for athletic pubalgia,
 596
Baxter's nerve, of hindfoot, impingement of, 899,
 933–934, 934*f*
Bayonet sign. *See* J sign
Beachchair position
 for acromioclavicular joint repair, 525, 525*f*
 for rotator cuff repairs, 490
Becker's muscular dystrophy, of thigh, 607
Bed rest, for lumbar spine injuries, 204, 207
Benign neglect, for acromioclavicular joint dislocations, 522
Bennett's fracture, of thumb, 239–240, 239*f*
Bennett's lesion, of shoulder labrum
 injury mechanisms of, 465–467, 468*f*
 treatment of, 473, 474*f*, 488–489
Bias, in research studies, 128, 130–132, 145–146
Biceps brachii muscle, anatomy of, 359–360
Biceps femoris tendon
 anatomy of, 583–584, 584*f*, 883
 strain injuries of, 585, 587
Biceps tendon
 anatomy of, 805
 biomechanics of, 806–808
 dislocations of, humerus and, 335, 343
 in glenohumeral joint stability, 385, 386*f*, 418
 glenoid rim origins of, 349–351, 350*f*, 359
 in knee repair, 682, 685, 813–814
 in rotator cuff biomechanics, 372, 372*f*–373*f*
 tear injuries of
  with elbow injuries, 309, 311
  with glenoid labrum tears, 457, 461, 470
  magnetic resonance imaging of, 108, 108*f*,
   114–115
Biceps tendon test. *See* O'Brien's test
Bicipital groove, shoulder anatomy of, 356, 359,
 373*f*
Bifurcate ligament, 896, 897*f*, 922
Biofeedback, for shoulder rehabilitation, 421
Biomechanics. *See also* Kinematics; *specific anatomy or sport*
 definition of, 624
Biopsy
 for heel pain, 929
 for thigh tumors, 607

Bipartite sesamoid, 969
Blatt procedure, for scapholunate injuries, 278, 278f
Blinding, in research sampling, 129–130, 132
Blocking splint, dorsal, for proximal interphalangeal joint ligament injuries, 247, 247f
Blocking techniques, football, for shoulder injury prevention, 437, 437f, 451
Blood pressure, compartmental. See Compartmental pressures
Blood supply
    anatomical. See Vascular anatomy; specific anatomy
    as wound healing prerequisite, 650
Blue line, in osteotendinous junction, 27
Blumensaat's line, in knee reconstructions, 827, 838
Body alignment. See also specific anatomy
    with golf swing, 563–564, 564f
    with pitching motion, 551–553, 552f, 559f
    pathologic, 555–557, 556f, 559f
    with running cycle, 1012–1013, 1016
Body weight
    as knee osteoarthritis factor, 846, 851–852, 856
    running kinematics and, 1012
Bone anchors, for Achilles tendon reconstruction, 935, 936f
Bone augmentation. See Bone blocks
Bone blocks
    for knee repair, 732, 777
        of ligaments, 683–685, 783–784
        osteochondral, 799, 799f
        patellar tendon, 703, 703f
    for peroneal tendon dislocations, 997, 997f
    for posterior shoulder dislocations, 414, 416, 422–423
    for posterior tibial tendon injuries, 1005
Bone cells
    functional morphology of, 78–79, 78f–79f
    proliferation rate with exercise, 80–83
    structure of, 76f–77f, 77
Bone cyst, aneurysmal, of femur, 607
Bone density, from mineralization, 78–83, 78f–79f
Bone formation
    estrogen and, 82–83, 83f
    exercise impact on, 79–83, 81f, 83f
    modulators of, 81–83, 83f
    process of, 77–79, 78f
Bone grafts
    autografts versus allografts, 47, 235
    for upper body injuries, 235, 422, 538
Bone growth plate
    hand, fractures of, 233, 236
    pelvic, avulsion fractures of, 216–217
Bone-ligament-bone complex, tensile properties of, 39–41, 40f
Bone marrow, composition of, 75, 77
Bone matrix
    composition of, 78–79
    mineralization of, 78–79, 78f–79f
Bone-patellar tendon-bone (PTB) grafts
    for anterior cruciate ligament reconstruction, 48, 626, 630, 632, 750–751
        quadruple hamstring graft versus, 47–48, 48f, 632, 829
    complications of, 825–826
    for patellar tendon reconstruction, 703
Bone plugs. See Bone blocks
Bones. See also specific bone
    adaptive response of
        endocrine factors, 81–82
        to high-intensity exercise, 80–81
        to low-intensity exercise, 80, 81f
        nutritional factors, 82–83, 83f
        parameters for, 79–80
        to space flight and weightlessness, 80
    blood supply of, 75, 76f, 77–78
    ion and fluid dynamics of, 77–79
    ligament relationship with, 27, 39
    mineralization of, 78–83, 78f–79f
    remodeling activity of, 77, 80, 81f

with exercise, 80–82
    with injuries. See specific anatomy or injury
    repair process of, 77–79
    structure of, 75–79
        cellular, 76f–79f, 77–78
        matrix, 78–79, 78f–79f
        osteons, 76f–77f, 77
        shapes, 75, 77–78
        tissue forms in, 76f–77f, 77, 79
    tendon attachments to, 21
Bone scans
    for Achilles tendon dysfunction, 981
    for articular cartilage injuries, 792
    for compartment syndromes, 92
    for foot injuries
        of forefoot, 947, 954–955
        of hindfoot, 902, 920, 926, 927f
        of midfoot, 902, 904–905, 914, 916
    for knee injuries, 735, 773, 780
    for leg injuries
        shin splints, 870, 870f, 870t, 875, 877
        stress fractures, 870, 870f, 870t, 1020–1021
    of lumbar spondylolisthesis, 211–212, 212f
    for pelvic evaluation, 216–217, 226
    for peroneus tendon injuries, 995
    for scaphoid fractures, 261, 263
    for thigh injuries, 603–604, 607
    for wrist injuries, 261, 263, 280
Bone spurs
    in hindfoot, 930–931, 930f, 935, 936f, 1020
    in midfoot, 911–912, 911f–912f, 918–919, 918f
Bone substitutes, for hand fracture grafting, 235
Bone-tendon-bone grafts, for knee repair, 683–684
Bone-tendon grafts, for knee repair, 683–684
Bone tissue
    cancellous (trabecular), 77
    cortical (compact), 76f, 77
        magnetic resonance imaging intensity for, 100–101, 100t
    lamellar (secondary), 76f–77f, 77, 79
    woven (primary), 77, 79
Boston brace, for lumbar spine injuries, 211
Boutonniere deformity, with hand injuries, 237, 251–252
Bowel-related disorders, 215
Boyd and Hawkin patellectomy, for patellofemoral arthritis, 738, 738f, 740t
Braces and bracing. See also Counterforce bracing; Splints and splinting
    for knee injuries
        with cartilage degeneration, 793, 854
        functional, for anterior cruciate ligaments, 754, 863–867
        hinged
            functional limitations of, 864–865
            for ligaments, 668, 671, 685, 749, 754
            patellofemoral joint, 729, 735
            tendon, 692–694, 699
        for leg stress fractures, 872–873
        for lumbar spine injuries, 205, 211
Brachial neuritis, 544
Brachial plexus
    anatomy of
        branch divisions of, 361, 361f, 544f
        cord divisions of, 361, 361f, 544f
        microstructure, 186
        nerve distributions, 184–185, 184f–185f, 544f
        root composition, 185–186, 185f–186f, 360–361, 544f
        trunk divisions of, 361, 361f, 544f
        upper arm distributions of, 360–361, 361f, 543, 544f
    clavicle relationship to, 330
    definition of, 161–183
    injuries of
        acute brachial neuropathy, 184, 190, 192, 196–198
        associated injuries with, 184, 189–193, 402

author's preferences regarding, 198–199
    burner syndrome, 187–188, 187f–188f, 192–197
    classification of, 186–187
    clinical evaluation of, 190–193, 192f
    compression mechanisms, 187–189, 188f–189f, 192, 195–197
    electrodiagnosis of, 193–194
    epidemiology of, 183–184
    imaging studies of, 116–117, 193–194, 193f
    mechanisms of, 161–163, 161f, 163f, 183–187, 186f, 189–190, 192
    muscle groups affected by, 187, 191, 195
    neurotmesis, 162, 183–186, 186f, 189–190, 192, 196–198
    prognosis for, 196–198
    rehabilitation for, 194–196, 195f
    return to sport guidelines, 196–199
    root avulsion, 189–190, 192, 196–197
    strength deficits with, 161–163, 191, 194–198
    surgical treatment of, 195–196
    treatment options for, 194–199, 195f
    with upper extremity injuries, 543–550, 544f
    postfixed, 185
    prefixed, 184
Brain herniation, 159
Brain resuscitation, 160
Brain swelling
    acute, 159–160
    delayed, 158, 160
Bristow procedure, in anterior shoulder dislocations, 407
Brostom lateral ligament reconstruction, of ankle, 821, 917
Buckle transducer, in knee biomechanics, 625
Buford complex, of glenohumeral capsule, 346, 351, 435, 435f, 469
Bulbocavernosus reflex, with cervical spine injuries, 164
Bumper model, of knee, 623
Bunion deformity. See Hallux valgus
Bunnel technique, for quadriceps tendon rupture repair, 599f, 600
Burner syndrome
    classifications of, 187
    clinical manifestations of, 187–188, 187f–188f, 192
    evaluation of, 190–195, 192f
    football etiologies, 183, 187f–188f
    mechanisms of, 161–163, 161f, 163f
    prognosis for, 196–197
    treatment of, 194–195, 195f, 198
Burns, compartment syndromes from, 89
Burr holes, for intracranial injuries, 159, 178
Bursa
    inflammation of. See Bursitis
    injuries to. See specific anatomy
Bursectomies, for snapping scapula, 506
Bursitis
    of hip, 112–113, 577–578
    of knee, 705, 721
    of olecranon, 325–326
    of pelvis and hip, 230
    septic versus non-septic, 325–326
Bursography, for Achilles tendon dysfunction, 981
Burst fractures, of cervical vertebrae, fusion indications for, 164, 167
Button fixation, for knee cruciate ligament reconstruction
    anterior, 47–48, 48f, 755
    posterior, 783–784, 814

C
Calcaneocuboid joint
    arthritis of, posttraumatic, 923
    arthrodesis indications for, 924
    saddle-shaped anatomy of, 896, 897f
    subtalar fusion and, 927
Calcaneocuboid ligament, lateral, 896, 897f

Calcaneofibular ligament
anatomy of, 898, 898f
decompression indications for, 996, 999
laxity of, ankle dislocations with, 992–993
sprain injuries of, 721, 819–820
Calcaneonavicular joint, coalition of, 927–929, 928f
Calcaneonavicular ligament
anatomy of, 896, 897f
pes planus and, 914, 920
repair indications of, 1004
Calcaneus. See also Hindfoot
anatomy of, 896–899, 897f–900f, 979, 991f
entrapment syndromes of, 1020
fractures of
anterior lateral process, 920–923, 922f–923f
avulsion, 918, 922, 922f
imaging studies of, 920–923, 921f–923f
stress, 920, 921f, 929–930, 931f
treatment of, 921–923, 922f–923f
Haglund's deformity and, 897, 936–938, 936f–937f
osteotomy indications for, 913, 986, 1020
pain syndromes of. See Heel pain
posterior lateral, exostosis of, 938–939, 938f
posterior superior, excision of, for Achilles dysfunction, 986–987
running injuries of, 1016, 1019–1020
Calcitonin, as bone formation stimulus, 82, 130
Calcium
in articular cartilage, 53, 54t, 55–56
bone formation and, 28, 79, 82
intracellular, spinal cord resuscitation and, 179, 179f
in muscle contraction, 5f, 6, 9–10, 10f, 28
Calcium phosphate crystals, in articular cartilage, 54t, 55
Calcium pyrophosphate deposition disease, knee meniscus tears with, 651
Calcium supplements, for foot injuries, 902, 906
Calf examination, with Achilles tendon dysfunction, 980–981
Calluses, in dancer's feet, 960–961
Calorie intake, bone formation and, 82–83
CAM walker, for hindfoot injuries, 921, 933, 935
Canals, in bone, 76f–77f, 77, 80
Capillaries
in compartment syndromes, 87–88, 88f
of tendons, 31
Capitate fractures, 271
Capitellum, in elbow injuries, 291, 308, 310–312, 319–321, 325f
Capsuloligamentous complex. See also specific joint or ligament
of metatarsophalangeal joint, 949, 949f, 951–952
of shoulder
anatomy of, 433–434, 433f–434f
posterior instability and, 417–418, 417f
Capsuloligamentous injuries, of wrist, 274–275
Capsulorrhaphies
for anterior shoulder dislocations, 408f, 409, 473
for glenoid labrum tears, radiofrequency technique for, 473–474, 473f–474f
for posterior shoulder dislocations
indications for, 415–416, 423, 427
posterior technique for, 423–426, 423f–426f
thermal-assisted technique for, 427, 473
Carcinoma. See also specific type
of thigh, 607
Cardiopulmonary resuscitation, for head and neck injuries, 153–154, 160
Carpal injuries. See Wrist
Carpal tunnel compression test, 285
Carpal tunnel syndrome, 284–285
Carpometacarpal (CMC) joints, fracture fixation procedures for, 238–239
Cartilage. See Articular cartilage
Cartilage oligomeric protein (COMP), in articular cartilage, 54t, 55, 66
Case-control studies, as research design, 124f, 128, 128f, 142

Case reports, as research design, 124, 124f
Case series, as research design, 124, 124f
Casts and cast boots
for Achilles tendon dysfunction, 982, 984–987
for flexor hallucis longus tendon injuries, 989–991
Casts and casts boots
for elbow tendinosis, 297
for forefoot injuries, 947, 961, 970
for hindfoot injuries, 921, 924, 933
for interphalangeal joint injuries, 251, 251f
for knee injuries, 692–693, 732, 758
for leg injuries, 877, 884
for midfoot injuries, 909, 915, 917
for peroneus tendon injuries, 996, 998, 1000
for posterior tibial tendon injuries, 1004–1007
for scaphoid fractures, 258–260, 260f, 263–267
for ulnar collateral ligament tears, 244–246, 245f
for wrist injuries, 280–281
Catch, in swimming stroke, 560, 560f
Cathepsins, articular cartilage degradation by, 62, 67
Catheter technique, for compartmental pressures, 880, 880f, 882
Caton index, of knee, 717, 718f
Cauda equina syndrome, from lumbar disk herniation, 206–207
Caudal central nucleus (CCN)
classifications per neurologic deficit, 170–171
recurrence rate of, 171, 172f
Cause-and-effect relationships, research designs for, 124, 124f, 127, 145
Cavus foot
with claw toe, 973
metatarsal injuries and, 945–946
CCS. See Chronic compartment syndrome
Cementing, in osteotendinous junction, 27
Censoring, in research studies, 139–140
Center of gravity, during running, 1012
Central pivot, in knee examination, 614–616, 614f
Central slip injuries, of proximal interphalangeal joints, 248, 250–252, 251f
Central tendency, in research studies, 135
Cerebral concussions
management of, 156–158
return to sport guidelines, 157–158, 158f
Cerebral edema, brain swelling versus, 159
Cervical collars, for head and neck injuries, 153–154, 163
Cervical spine
congenital conditions of, 175
functions of, 174
fusions of, 164–167, 178
injuries of
acute sprain syndrome, 160, 163
at-risk sports for, 172f–173f, 173–174
brachial plexus nerve roots, 161–163, 161f, 163f
in children, 161, 163–164
clinical presentations with, 161–165, 168
clinical stability considerations of, 165–166, 170, 177
emergency care of, 153–156, 155f
fractures and dislocations
of facet, 164, 166–167, 173, 176f, 177, 179
of lower region, 167, 168f, 177
management principles of, 164–165
of midcervical region, 166–167, 177
return to sport guidelines, 177–178
of upper region, 165–166, 177
immobilization devices for, 153–155, 155f, 162f, 163, 165
intervertebral disk herniations, 163–164, 169
with intracranial injuries, 160
ligament injuries with, 165–166, 176–177
osteoarthritis from, 163, 176, 188
prevention strategies for, 172–174, 172f–173
range of, 160–161
range of motion deficits with, 161–164, 168, 177–178
return to sport guidelines, 161, 163, 165, 174

congenital conditions and, 175
developmental conditions and, 175–177, 176f
traumatic conditions and, 177–178
spinal cord resuscitation with, 178–180
strength deficits with, 161–163
surgical treatment of, 164–167
lordosis of, from scapula fractures, 501, 503
reduction of, with fractures or dislocations, 164–165, 167, 180
stenosis of
brachial plexus injuries and, 188, 193
with cord neurapraxia, 168, 168f
magnetic resonance imaging of, 193
measurement methods for, 168–171, 169f, 171f–172f
return to contact activities with, 175–176
with transient quadriplegia, 168–170, 168f
Cervical sprain syndrome, acute, 160, 163
Cheilectomy
for Freiberg's infraction, 960, 960t
for hallux rigidus, 972
Chest examination, with clavicle fractures, 537
Chevron-Akin procedure, for toe deformities, 953
Children
acromioclavicular joint injuries in, 522
apophyseal avulsion fractures in, 600
cervical spine injuries in, 161, 163–164
clavicle fractures in, 535
elbow injuries in, 307, 319–321, 320f
hand fractures in, 233, 236, 239–240
hip dislocations in, 579
intracranial injuries in, 159
ischial tuberosity avulsion fractures in, 592
knee injuries in, 700–701, 743
tendon mechanisms, 687, 689, 698, 704–706
lumbar spine injuries in, 204, 209
thigh tumors in, 607
Chinese finger trap, 248
Chiropractic management, of lumbar spine injuries, 204
Chi-square test. See Pearson chi-square test
Chondral injuries. See Articular cartilage
Chondrocalcin, in articular cartilage, 54t, 55
Chondrocytes
in articular cartilage
healing role of, 791, 794
implants for repair, 67, 796–798, 797f–798f, 801, 856
osteoarthritis impact on, 64, 66
physiology of, 61–63, 787
structural properties, 56–57, 56f–57f
high-intensity exercise impact on, 81
in knee meniscus, 646, 650
in tendons, 27–28
transplants of, for knee cartilage regeneration, 67, 796–798, 856
Chondroitin sulfate
in articular cartilage, 55, 57, 787, 788f
in knee joint, 647, 852
in tendons, 25–26, 28
Chondromalacia
with elbow tendinosis, 291, 301f
knee injuries with, 689, 698, 705–706, 714, 1018
magnetic resonance imaging of, 104–105
Outerbridge classification of, 734
of patellofemoral joint, 636, 638, 734–735
of sesamoids, 954–955, 957
Chondroplasty
laser, of knee, 795–796, 795f–796f
of patella, 1018
Chondrosarcoma, of femur, 607
Chopart's joint, biomechanics of, 896, 899
Chronic compartment syndrome (CCS)
clinical presentation of, 90–91, 1021
diagnostic criteria for, 93–94
differential diagnosis of, 91–92, 877, 1021
exertional, of leg, 606, 879–882, 879f–880f, 881t, 882f, 1021
pathophysiology of, 88–89
recurrent, 95
treatment of, 95

Cinematography, for shoulder analysis, 387
Cineradiography, for wrist injuries, 276–277
Circumferential systems, in bone, 76f, 77
Clark compression test, for knee degeneration, 850
Clavicle
    acromioclavicular joint dislocations and abnormalities with, 513, 514f, 516f–517f, 517, 519–521, 524
        distal resection of, 522f, 524, 529–531, 529f–531f
    anatomy of, 329–330, 330f
    fractures of. See also Sternoclavicular joint
        brachial plexus injuries with, 189, 193, 195
        classification schemes for, 535–536, 536f
        clinical evaluation of, 536–537
        epidemiology of, 535
        imaging studies of, 537
        internal fixation of, 370–371, 537–538, 538f
        ligament attachments with, 535–536, 536f
        mechanisms of, 513, 530, 530f, 535–536, 536f
        reduction procedures for, 537–538, 538f
        return to sport guidelines, 537–538
        scapula dyskinesis with, 501, 506–507
        sling and swathe management of, 537–538
        treatment of, 537–538
        treatment outcomes with, 538
    functions of, 330, 367
    load displacement of, 368, 368f
    medial epiphyseal injuries of, 539–541, 539f
    muscle origins and insertions of, 330
    ossification process of, 329–330
    range of motion of, 369–371, 369f–370f
Clavicle collar, figure-of-eight, for scapula dyskinesis, 507, 507f
Claw toe, 939, 957, 972–973, 973f
Clinical relevance, of research studies, 143–145
Clinical series, as research design, 124–125, 124f
Closed chain exercises
    for knee rehabilitation, 629, 793, 801, 852
        with ligament injuries, 658, 658t, 685, 749, 754, 774
    for running injuries, 1024
    for scapular dyskinesis, 506–508, 507f
Closed head trauma. See Intracranial injuries
Closed reduction. See Reduction procedures
Clotting factor transfusions, for hemophiliacs, 606
Clunk test, for shoulder assessment, with labral tear injuries, 466–467, 467f, 471
CMC. See Carpometacarpal joints
Coccyx, ligament attachments to, 223, 224f
Cochran's rule, of statistical validity, 139
Cocking. See Arm cocking
Codivilla V-Y lengthening procedure. See V-Y lengthening technique
Coefficient of determination (r²), in research studies, 138
Coffee cup test, for elbow tendinosis, 292
Cofield translation testing, for shoulder instability, 420
Cohesion, in tendons, 23, 25, 32–33
Cohort study, as research design, 124f, 127–128, 140, 142
Collagenases, articular cartilage degradation by, 62
Collagen fiber
    of articular cartilage
        anatomy and physiology of, 53–57, 54t, 56f, 61–62, 787
        healing role of, 791, 794
        layered structure of, 788–789, 789f
        with osteoarthritis, 65–67
    in bone, 79
    in knee
        ligaments, 625–626, 667, 764–765
        meniscus, 645–647, 646f–647f
        tendons, 687–688, 690
    in ligaments, 39, 43, 625, 667
    mutations of, in articular cartilage, 54–55
    in tendons
        anatomy and physiology of, 23–24, 24f, 26–27
        biomechanical functions of, 32–33

degenerative factors of, 289, 291, 294
synthesis post-strain injuries, 586–587, 690
in tendon sheaths, 22–23, 22f
type I
    in bone, 79
    in knee, 646, 687
    in ligaments, 39, 43
    in rotator cuff, 353
    in tendons, 22–23, 25
type II
    in articular cartilage, 54, 54t, 57, 61–62, 67, 787
    in tendons, 27
type III
    in ligaments, 43
    in rotator cuff, 353
    in tendons, 22, 25
type V
    in articular cartilage, 54, 54t, 787
    in bone, 79
type VI, in articular cartilage, 54–55, 54t, 57, 66, 787
type VII, in bone, 79
type IX, in articular cartilage, 54, 54t, 66, 787
type X, in articular cartilage, 54–55, 54t, 66, 787
type XI, in articular cartilage, 54, 54t, 66, 787
type XII, in rotator cuff, 353
Collagen fibrils
    in bones, 76f, 77
    in tendons
        anatomy and physiology of, 23–24, 24f, 28
        biomechanical functions of, 32–33
        mineralized, 27
    in tendon sheaths, 22–23, 22f
Collagen scaffolds, for knee meniscus replacement, 649, 659
Collars
    for brachial plexus injuries, 162f, 163, 195, 195f
    figure-of-eight, for scapula dyskinesis, 507, 507f
    for head and neck injuries, 153–154, 163
Collateral ligaments. See specific anatomy or location
Collision injuries, cervical injuries from, 163, 177
Comatose athletes, emergency care of, with head and neck injuries, 159–160
COMP. See Cartilage oligomeric protein
Comparison groups, for research sampling, 132
Compartmental pressures
    criteria for compartment syndromes, 93–94
        of leg, 879–882, 881t, 1021
        of thigh, 605–606
    objective measurement techniques for, 92–93, 880, 880f
    volume relationship of, 87, 88f
Compartment syndromes
    acute. See Acute compartment syndrome
    in athletic pubalgia, 227
    chronic. See Chronic compartment syndrome
    clinical presentation of, 87, 89–91
    decompressive therapy for, 89–95. See also Fasciotomy; specific anatomy
    definition of, 87
    diagnostic criteria for, 93–94
    differential diagnosis of, 89, 91–92, 877
    exercise-induced, 89–91, 94, 604–605
    exertional, 89–91, 606, 879
    five P's of, 879–880
    with hand fractures, 234
    iatrogenic, 90
    locational aspects of, 87–88, 88f
    in lower extremities, 87–90, 88f, 835
        with knee injuries, 810, 835
        with leg injuries, 875, 877, 879–882, 1021
        with thigh injuries, 604–606
    magnetic resonance imaging of, 116–117
    medial tibial stress syndrome versus, 875, 877
    objective assessment of, 92–93
    pain assessment with, 90–91, 227–228
    pathophysiology of, 88–89
    treatment of, 94–95

in upper extremities, 87–88, 88f, 90–91
Compere's patellectomy, for patellofemoral arthritis, 738, 738f, 740t
Compression-flexion injuries
    to brachial plexus
        mechanisms of, 187–189, 188f–189f, 192
        treatment of, 195–196
    to cervical spine, 164, 168, 168f, 173, 173f
Compression fractures, of cervical vertebrae, 167, 168t
Compression injuries
    external
        articular cartilage response to, 58f, 59–60, 66
        bone response to, 80–81, 874
        calcaneal fractures and, 922, 922f
        compartment syndromes from, 89–90, 94
        magnetic resonance imaging for, 116–117
        of rotator cuff, 464–465, 471
    of nerves. See Nerve compression injuries
    of spinal cord. See Spinal cord
    of vessels. See Vascular compression injuries
Compression plates. See Plate fixation
Compression-rotation test, for shoulder assessment, with labral contact injuries, 442
Compression tests
    for knee degeneration, 850
    for knee meniscus tears, 652, 652f
    for patellofemoral joint, 712, 727, 850
Compression wrap, for knee tendon injuries, 697
Compressive loading. See Load
Computed tomography (CT)
    for Achilles tendon dysfunction, 981
    of clavicle fractures, 537
    for elbow injuries, 311
    for flexor hallucis longus tendon injuries, 988
    of foot and ankle, 111
        with hindfoot injuries, 902, 923–926, 927f, 928
        with midfoot injuries, 904, 908, 911
    for head and neck injuries, 155–156, 158–160, 167, 194
    for lumbar spine injuries, 205, 212, 212f
    for patellofemoral joint injuries, 719–721, 720f, 723
    for peroneus tendon injuries, 995
    for posterior tibial tendon dysfunction, 1003
    of running injuries, 1017
    of shoulder instability, 404, 421–422, 443, 444f
    single-photon emission. See Single-photon emission computed tomography
    of wrist and hand, 116, 281–282
        for scaphoid fractures, 258–259, 258f–259f, 261–263, 267
Computed tomography arthrography
    of elbow injuries, 311, 316f, 317, 321–322
    of knee instability, 104, 721
    of shoulder, 108–109
        with instability, 421, 443, 445, 467–468
Computed tomography myelography
    for brachial plexus injuries, 193
    for lumbar spondylolisthesis, 211
    for neck injuries, 161, 163
Computer simulations
    of injuries. See Injury modeling
    of joint motion, 49
Concavity/compression
    in glenohumeral joint, 498, 501, 508
    in rotator cuff, 353
Concentric muscle contractions
    force-velocity principle of, 12–13, 12f
    knee injuries from, 711
    pelvic apophyseal fractures from, 601–602
    in running cycle, 1012
Concussions. See Cerebral concussions
Condylectomy, Duvries plantar, of metatarsal head, 948–949
Confidence intervals, in research studies, 140–141, 143–144
Conformity, in knee, 614, 648
Confounding variables, in research studies, 125, 144

Congruence angle, of patellofemoral joint, 719, 719f
Connective tissue. See also specific type
  muscle matrix of, 3–4, 4f
Conoid ligaments
  in acromioclavicular joint
    anatomy of, 511–512, 512f
    injury mechanisms of, 514–515
  clavicle fractures and, 535–536, 536f
Consensus statements, as research design, 124f, 126
Contact sports. See also specific sport
  glenoid labrum injuries from, 431–454
Containment test, in patellofemoral joint examination, 620, 620f
Contingency tables, in research studies, 138–139, 141, 142f
Continuous passive motion machine (CPM), for knee rehabilitation, 755–756
Contractile filaments
  excitation-contraction coupling process in, 9–10, 10f
  mechanical properties of, 10–13, 11f–12f, 12t
  of muscle, 4–6, 5f, 17
Contractile proteins
  in excitation-contraction coupling, 9–10, 10f
  muscle hierarchy of, 4–5, 5f
  per muscle fiber types, 17
  regulatory role of, 5–6, 5f
Contractures
  with elbow injuries, 312, 321
  with interphalangeal injuries, 251–252, 254
  with knee injuries, 666, 693–694, 703, 735, 834
  running injuries and, 1018, 1024
Control groups, for research studies, 132–135, 144
Contusions
  intracranial, management of, 158–159
  of lumbar spine, fractures versus, 205
  of pelvis and hip, 230
  of quadriceps, 602–603
Cooper's ligament, for hernia repair, 227
Coordinate systems, for knee motion, 623, 625
Copper, in musculoskeletal metabolism, 28
Coracoacromial arch, rotator cuff and
  biomechanics of, 372–374, 373f
  injury mechanisms of, 378, 378f
Coracoacromial joint, ligaments of, 337–339, 337f–338f, 370f, 373f
Coracoacromial ligaments
  of acromioclavicular joint, stability role of, 337–339, 337f–338f, 370, 370f
  in glenohumeral joint stability, 382–383
  rotator cuff and
    biomechanics of, 374–375
    surgical repair procedures for, 486–487, 492
  surgical reconstruction of, 529–531, 532f
Coracobrachialis muscle, anatomy of, 356
Coracoclavicular joint, fixation procedures, for acromioclavicular joint dislocations, 522f, 523, 524f, 525–528, 527f, 530–531, 531f
Coracoclavicular ligaments
  in acromioclavicular joint
    anatomy of, 511–512, 512f
    injury mechanisms of, 513–515, 514f–515f, 520
    surgical reconstruction of, 371–372, 522f–523f, 523–525, 529–531, 532f
    cerclage procedure, for acromioclavicular joint repair, 522f–523f, 523
  clavicle fractures and, 535
Coracohumeral ligament
  in rotator cuff biomechanics, 372, 373f
  in thrower's shoulder pathology, 391, 391f
Coracoid process, of scapula
  acromioclavicular injuries and, 520, 520f, 525–528, 526f–528f, 530
  shoulder impingement role of, 331–332
Corner compression syndrome, anterolateral, 820–821
Corns, of feet, 960–961, 976
Coronary ligament, of knee meniscus, 645

Correlation analysis, in research studies, 137–138, 145
Correlation coefficient (r), in research studies, 125, 133, 137
Cortisol, bone formation and, 82
Cortisone injections
  for axillary nerve injuries, 546
  for elbow tendinosis, 294–295
  for foot injuries
    of hindfoot, 932, 938, 940
    of midfoot, 911–912, 914, 917, 919
  for hip pointers, 578
  for knee cartilage injuries, 793, 853
  for rotator cuff injuries, 489
Cost-benefit analysis, as research design, 124f, 126
Cost-effectiveness analysis, as research design, 124f, 126
Cost-identification studies, as research design, 124f, 126–127
Counterforce bracing, for elbow tendinosis, 296–298, 297f, 317, 550
Cowboy collar, for brachial plexus injuries, 162f, 163, 195, 195f
COX. See Cyclooxygenase enzyme
Cox's proportional hazards model, of survival curves, 141
CPM. See Continuous passive motion machine
Crank test, for shoulder assessment, with labral injuries, 441, 467
Creep
  articular cartilage and, 58–60
  definition of, 41–42, 42f
  of ligaments, 41–43, 42f, 48
  of tendons, 33, 687
Crepitus, in knee injuries, 619, 619f
  mechanisms of, 672, 714, 722, 735
Crimping, in ligaments, tensile strength and, 39
Critical closure theory, of compartment syndromes, 88
Critical zone, of rotator cuff, 354, 372, 377
Cronbach's alpha coefficient, in research studies, 133
Cross-body adduction view, radiographic, for acromioclavicular dislocations, 519, 519f
Cross-bridge cycling, in muscle contractions, 9–11, 10f–11f, 13, 17
Cross-sectional studies, as research design, 124f, 128–129
Cross-training, indications for. See specific anatomy or injury
Cruciate ligaments
  of femur-tibia complex, tensile property testing of, 40–41, 40f, 766–767
  of knee. See Anterior cruciate ligament; Posterior cruciate ligament
Cruciate linkage, as knee modeling approach, 624
Crush injuries, 94, 235, 239
Cryotherapy, 793, 951
CT. See Computed tomography
Cubital tunnel syndrome
  injury mechanisms, 284, 290–291, 547
  magnetic resonance imaging of, 114, 114f
  surgical repair of, 302–304, 303f, 547–548
Cuboid joint
  anatomy of, 893, 894f, 895–896, 897f
  stress fractures of, 904, 904f
Culture and sensitivity, of olecranon bursitis, 326
Cuneiform-cuboid joint
  anatomy of, 893, 894f
  injuries of, 904, 907, 911f
Current concepts, as research design, 124f, 126
Cutting exercises, for knee ligament injuries, 671, 864
Cycling, 284, 907, 918
Cyclooxygenase enzyme (COX), NSAIDs action on, 589, 853
Cyclops lesion, in knee reconstruction, 828–829
Cytokines
  in bone adaptation, 77–80, 82–83
  healing role of, 43, 63, 67, 690, 831

Cytoplasm, in tendon cells, 27, 29
Cytoskeleton, of muscle cell, 5–6

D
Dancers
  foot injuries in
    acute conditions, 961
    aneurysms, 961
    bony hypertrophy, 959
    chronic use conditions, 959–961, 960t
    with deformities, 961
    fractures, 961
    Freiberg's infraction, 960, 960f
    hindfoot, 924–926
    metatarsals, 946, 959–960
    midfoot, 907, 907f
    skin alterations, 960–961
    stress fractures, 959–960
    tendons, 979, 988
  hallux saltans in, 961–962
  neurologic conditions in, 962
Dancer's view, radiographic, for metatarsal fractures, 959
Data. See Research data
Dead arm syndrome, 481
Debridement
  arthroscopic. See Arthroscopy
  of elbow
    injury indications for, 321–323
    osteophyte indications for, 310, 312–315, 315f, 319, 326
  of foot and ankle injuries
    Achilles tendon inflammation, 982, 983f
    hallux saltans, 962
    peroneus tendon, 996, 999
    posterior tibial tendon, 1003, 1005–1007
    sprains, 822, 822f
  of hand injuries, 235, 247–248, 252
  of knee
    for articular cartilage injuries, 793–795, 794f, 800–801, 802f
    with ligament injuries, 782, 809, 828
    with meniscal repair, 832
    for osteoarthritis, 854–855, 1022
    with patellar repair, 835, 839
  of wrist ligament injuries, 278, 281
Deceleration, of arm. See Arm deceleration
Deceleration model, of thrower's shoulder, 388f, 389
Deceleration phase, of running, 1013
Decompressive therapy. See Fasciotomy; specific anatomy or pathology
Deep lateral ligament complex, of knee. See Posterolateral knee
Deep massage. See Massage therapy
Degenerative joint disease. See Osteoarthritis; specific joint
Degrees of freedom (DOF), of knee notion, with anterior cruciate ligament reconstructions, 44–45, 45f, 750–751
Deltoid ligament, of ankle, 939–940, 1004
Deltoid muscles
  in acromioclavicular joint injuries
    mechanisms of, 512–514, 514f
    surgical repair and, 526, 529–531
  anatomy of, 351–352, 351f, 546
  nerve injuries of, 546
  overhead throwing role of, 552–553, 553f, 555
  split guidelines for, with posterior shoulder capsulorrhaphy, 423–424, 424f, 426, 426f
  swimming stroke role of, 392, 560–562
Depolarization, of peripheral nerves, in muscle contraction, 9, 10f
DeQuervain's syndrome, of wrist, 282–283, 283f
Dermatan sulfate, 25, 647
Dermatomyositis, of thigh, 607
Dermotomy, for fasciotomy, 94–95
Descriptive research designs, 123–127, 124f, 135, 142
Desmin, in muscle contraction, 6
Diagnostic injections. See Nerve blocks
Diaphysis, of bone

adaptation to exercise, 80–82
composition of, 77–78, 77f
Diffuse axonal injury, clinical manifestations of, 156, 160
Digit injuries
of foot. See Toes
of hand. See Fingers
Dimple sign, with knee dislocations, 808, 810
DIP. See Distal interphalangeal joints
DISI. See Dorsal intercalated segmental instability
Diskectomy. See Vertebral diskectomy
Dislocations. See specific anatomy or injury
Distal interphalangeal joints (DIP)
fracture fixation procedures for, 235, 237
tendon injuries of
extensor, 249–250
flexor, 252–254, 253f–254f
tendon insertions of, 249, 253
toe deformities and, 973–974
Distal radial ulnar joint (DRUJ)
arthrography injections in, 277, 281
injuries of, 281–282
Distal tarsal tunnel syndrome, 920
Distributions, in statistical measurements, 136
Diving, injuries from, 174, 183, 462–463
DOF. See Degrees of freedom
Donor site morbidity, of autografts, 48
Doppler studies, for leg injuries, 889
Dorsal intercalated segmental instability (DISI), with wrist injuries, 275, 279
Dorsal rami, of spinal nerves, in brachial plexus, 184–186, 185f
Dose-responsive curve, of bone adaptation to exercise, 80–83, 83f
Downward phase, of golf swing, 564–565, 564f, 566f
Drawer tests
anterior versus posterior, 615, 745, 770
for knee injuries, 614–615, 628
of anterior cruciate ligament, 745, 746f, 747
with functional bracing, 865
of posterior cruciate ligament, 765–771, 779–780
grading method for, 769–770, 769f
postoperative, 778–779
for metatarsophalangeal injuries, 948, 948f, 952
quadriceps active, 770, 770f
Dreaded black line, of tibial stress fractures, 872, 872f
Dressings
compartment syndromes from, 89
for olecranon bursitis, 326
Drilling, as knee cartilage repair technique, 794–795, 855
Drop finger, injury mechanisms of, 249–250
Drug therapies. See specific class, drug, or pathology
DRUJ. See Distal radial ulnar joint
Duchenne muscular dystrophy, of thigh, 606–607
Duke lesion, of ankle, 919
Duplex scanning, noninvasive, for popliteal artery entrapment, 887
Duvries plantar condylectomy, of metatarsal head, 948–949
Dynamometers, for strength measurement, 191
Dystrophin, muscle content of, 6, 13

E
Eating disorders, 216, 869, 1020
Eccentric muscle contractions
ankle mechanisms of, 979
force-velocity principle of, 12f, 13, 35, 220
gastrocnemius injuries from, 888
knee injuries from, 691, 711
pelvic apophyseal fractures from, 601–602
strain injuries and, 586f, 590–591, 593, 597
Eccentric training, for muscle strain injuries, 586–587, 598
EC coupling. See Excitation-contraction coupling
Ecological studies, as research design, 124f, 125
ECRB. See Extensor carpi radialis brevis tendon
ECU. See Extensor carpi ulnaris tendon

EDC. See Extensor digitorum communis tendon
Efferent sensory neuron system, proprioception bracing and, 864
Effusions
of ankle, 872, 998
of knee, 714, 725, 745, 768
articular cartilage and, 791, 794
Elasticity
of articular cartilage, 58–60, 58f, 64
of bone, 77
of supraspinatus tendon, 375–376, 376f
in tendons, 22, 22f, 27, 32–34
Elastic tube exercises, for rotator cuff rehabilitation, 485, 485f–486f, 489
Elastin, 23, 647, 687
Elbow joint
blood supply of, 321
dislocations of, 307–308, 311–312
fractures of, 308
impingement syndromes of, 547–550, 547f–548f
with pitching, 555, 558–559, 559f
posterior, 308, 308f, 312–315, 313f–315f
injuries of
associated injuries with, 309, 312
clinical evaluation of, 308–310, 310f
epidemiology of, 307
lateral compression, 308–310, 308f
ligaments, 114–115, 114f–115f, 311–312, 315–319, 316f–318f
magnetic resonance imaging of, 113–115, 114f–115f, 311, 313, 319, 321
medial tension, 308–310, 308f, 312
nerve mechanisms of, 547–550, 547f–548f, 555, 558–559, 559f
posterior impaction, 308–310, 308f
radiography of, 293–294, 311–312, 311f
return to sport guidelines, 299, 312, 314, 318–324, 326
specific disorders, 311–326
tendons, 273–304
overuse injuries of
degenerative arthritis, 290–291, 322–323, 322f–323f
little league, 307, 319–320, 319f–320f
olecranon bursitis, 325–326
olecranon stress fractures, 308, 311, 323–324, 324f
osteochondritis dissecans, 114, 291–292, 320–322
posterior lateral instability, 324–325, 324f–325f
ulnar collateral ligament injuries, 308–310, 308f, 313–319, 316f–318f, 324–325
valgus extension overload, 308, 308f, 312–315, 313f–315f
reconstructive procedures for, 245–246, 312
grafts for, 317–318, 318f, 321, 325
swimming stroke role of, 562, 562f
tendinopathies of
associated syndromes with, 290–291, 298
clinical presentations of, 289, 291–292
conservative treatment of, 294–299, 296f–297f
epidemiology of, 289–290, 296
examination of, 291–292, 291f
injury mechanisms of, 273–288
pathoanatomy of, 290–291, 294
provocative tests for, 292–294
radiography of, 293–294
surgical treatment of, 294, 299–304, 300f–303f
Elbow pain, evaluation of, 291–294, 307–309, 311
nerve component of, 548–550
Electrical stimulation
for active tendon stress-strain curves, 34
for elbow tendinosis, 294–295
isometric, for postoperative muscle strengthening, 10, 10f
for knee rehabilitation, 669, 670f, 690, 694, 839
for leg stress fractures, 872
for lumbar spine injuries, 204
for shoulder rehabilitation, 421

Electrocautery, with knee arthroscopy, 724
Electrolytes
in articular cartilage, 53, 55
in bone, 77–79
Electromagnetic fields
in nuclear scanning, 100–101, 100t
safety of, 99–100
Electromagnetic stimulation, for stress fractures, 872, 902, 906
Electromyography (EMG)
axonotmesis impact on, 186
for brachial plexus injuries, 193–196
for carpal tunnel syndrome, 285
for compartment syndromes, 92
for elbow tendinosis, 293, 295
for foot injuries, 919, 939
for neck injuries, 161–163
for plantar heel pain, 1020
of running gait cycle, for strain risk analysis, 587
for shoulder analysis, 385, 387, 392, 394, 418
for thigh and groin pain, 587, 596
for upper extremity nerve injuries, 545, 547–549
Electronic STIC device, for compartmental pressures, 880, 880f, 882
Elmslie-Trillat realignment procedure, for patellofemoral joint dislocations, 732–734, 732f
Ely test, of knee, 705
Embolism, pulmonary, 889
Emergency management
of cervical spine injuries, 153–156, 155f, 160
of intracranial injuries, 153–156, 155f, 160
Endocrine system, bone remodeling and, 81–82
Endometriosis, 223
Endomysium, of muscle cell, 3–4, 4f
Endoneurium, of peripheral nerves, 186–187, 186f
Endoplasmic reticulum, rough, in tendon cells, 27, 29–30
Endotenon, of tendons, 22–23, 22f
blood supply to, 30–31
Endotracheal intubation, emergency, for head and neck injuries, 160
Endurance. See Muscle endurance
Endurance training, for runners, 1011, 1015, 1023
Energy. See Force; Kinetic energy; Load
Energy absorbed to failure
as bone-ligament-bone complex property, 39–40, 40f
in knee, 626, 858
Entrapment injuries. See also specific anatomy
of arteries. See Vascular compression injuries
of nerves. See Nerve compression injuries
Enzymes, articular cartilage degradation by, 62, 67
EPB. See Extensor pollicis brevis tendon
Epicondylitis, of elbow tendons. See Tennis elbow
Epidural hematoma, management of, 158–159
Epineurium, of peripheral nerves, 186–187, 186f
Epiphysis, of bone
growth influences on, 78, 80–82
injury mechanisms of, 580–581, 581f
Epiphysitis, with elbow injuries, 307, 310
Epitenon, of tendons, 22
EPL. See Extensor pollicis longus tendon
Equipment
for emergency care, of head and neck injuries, 153–156, 155f
improper racquet, injury risks from, 296
Erb's point, in brachial plexus injuries, 161, 161f, 185, 188, 191
Estrogen
adipose tissue conversion role, 82
bone formation and, 82–83, 83f
Ethylene oxide sterilization, of allografts, 826
Eversion
of ankle
biomechanics of, 819, 896, 897f, 926, 992
fractures with, 922–923, 922f
during running, 1012. See also Foot pronation
Evoked potentials, for brachial plexus injuries, 193–194

Ewing's sarcoma, of femur, 607
Examination under anesthesia. *See* Arthroscopy
Excitation-contraction coupling
  muscle contraction from, 9–11, 10*f*
  temporal summation and, 10, 10*f*
Exclusion criteria, for research sampling, 132
Excursion. *See also* Velocity
  in knee meniscus, 647, 647*f*
  in patellofemoral joint, 619, 619*f*
Exercise
  articular cartilage response to, 62–64
  bone adaptation to, 79–83, 81*f*, 83*f*
  compartment syndromes from, 89–91, 94,
    604–605
Exercise programs. *See* Rehabilitation programs
Exertional compartment syndromes
  chronic, of leg, 606, 879
  pathophysiology of, 89–91
Experimental research designs, 124*f*, 129–131, 144
Explanatory research designs, 124*f*, 127–131, 128*f*
Extension block pinning, for phalanx fractures,
    237–238
Extension-compression injuries, with cervical
    spine stenosis, 188
Extension exercises, for knee ligament injuries,
    669–670, 670*f*
Extension injuries. *See also* Hyperextension in-
    juries
  of phalanx, 237
Extension splinting
  for patellar entrapment syndrome, 839
  for ulnar nerve injuries, 547
Extensor carpi radialis brevis tendon (ECRB)
  aponeurosis of, 299–302, 300*f*–301*f*
  injury mechanisms of, 289–293
  resection and repair of, 300–302, 300*f*–302*f*
Extensor carpi ulnaris tendon (ECU), injuries of,
    279, 282, 284
Extensor digitorum brevis tendon, 895, 919
Extensor digitorum communis tendon (EDC), in-
    juries of, 252, 292
Extensor digitorum longus tendon, injuries of,
    1007–1008
Extensor hallucis longus tendon, injuries of,
    1007–1008
Extensor indicis proprius tendon, 284
Extensor pollicis brevis tendon (EPB), DeQuer-
    vain's syndrome and, 283
Extensor pollicis longus tendon (EPL), 283–284
Extensor tendon, of hand
  anatomy of, 248–249, 249*f*
  injuries of
    classification of, 249
    distal interphalangeal level, 249–250
    metacarpophalangeal level, 252
    proximal interphalangeal level, 250–252, 251*f*
External fixation. *See also* Immobilization and im-
    mobilization devices
  for hand fractures, 234–235, 234*f*
  for knee injuries, 704, 810
External rotation and retraction activities, for
    scapula dyskinesis, 508, 509*f*
External rotation model, maximal, of thrower's
    shoulder, 389–391, 389*f*–391*f*
External rotation recurvatum test, for knee liga-
    ment tears, 680, 771–772, 771*f*
Extraarticular fractures, of thumb, 239–240
Extrapolation, of research findings, 146
Extremity compartments
  anatomy of, 87–88, 88*f*
  compression syndromes of, 87–89, 88*t*, 90–91

F
Fabellofibular ligament (FFL)
  anatomy of, 676–677, 805–806
  biomechanics of, 677, 766, 806–808
  injuries of, 679–680, 683–685
Face mask
  at-risk playing with, in football, 172–174,
    172*f*–173*f*
  emergency removal of, for head and neck injur-
    ies, 153–154
Facet joints
  cervical dislocations of

  bilateral, 167, 173, 176*f*, 177
  unilateral, 164, 166–167, 173, 179
  lumbar injuries of, 203–204
Failure rates, as research design, 139–141, 140*f*
Fascicles. *See* Fiber bundles
Fasciotomy
  for compartment syndromes
    contraindications for, 94–95, 606
    emergent, 89–90
    incisions for, 94–95
    indications for, 94–95, 605
    lateral technique for, 605, 605*f*
    of lower leg, 879–882, 881*t*, 882*f*, 886
    prophylactic, 91, 93
    recovery patterns, 95
    of thigh, 605–606
  for medial tibial stress syndrome, 878–879
Fast glycolytic muscle fibers (FG), 14, 16–18, 16*t*,
    18*t*
Fast oxidative muscle fibers (FOG), 14, 16–18,
    16*t*, 18*t*
Fast spin echo pulse sequencing, for magnetic res-
    onance imaging, 101, 107, 405*f*
FATC. *See* Femur-anterior cruciate ligament-tibia
    complex
Fat grafts, for tarsal coalition, 929
Fatigue
  of ligaments, 42
  of muscles. *See* Muscle fatigue
  stress fractures from, 572, 574
Fat pad
  of heel, insufficiency of, 932–934, 933*f*
  of patellofemoral joint
    injuries of, 721–722
    physical examination of, 620, 620*f*
Fat pad syndrome, 721–722
FCU. *See* Flexor carpi ulnaris tendon
FDL. *See* Flexor digitorum longus tendon
FDP. *See* Flexor digitorum profundus tendon
FDS. *See* Flexor digitorum superficialis tendon
Female athletes
  injuries in, 572, 845, 946
  leg stress factors in, 869, 1020
Female athlete triad, 869, 1020
Femoral hernias, athletic pubalgia *versus*, 596
Femur. *See also* Thigh
  condyles of, running impact on, 1019
  epiphyseal injuries of, 580–581, 581*f*, 596
  fractures of, 216, 579, 604
    stress, 572–574, 573*f*, 603–604, 1020
  head of
    avascular necrosis of
      etiologies of, 216, 226, 230, 796
      magnetic resonance imaging of, 112–113,
        113*f*
    fractures of, 216, 579
  impingement syndrome of, 572, 572*t*, 594
  in knee injuries and reconstruction
    complications of, 827–829, 827*f*–830*f*,
      838–839
    distal varus osteotomies, 856–857
    intercondylar notch of, 682, 684–685, 755,
      758, 777
      anterior cruciate ligament tears and,
        744–745, 745*f*, 827–829, 828*f*–830*f*,
        838–839
      posterior cruciate ligament and, 763–764,
        764*f*, 769, 769*f*
      tunnel reconstruction procedures for,
        781–784, 783*f*–784*f*
  meniscus articulation with, 645, 646*f*
  neck of, stress fractures of, 572–574, 573*f*, 1020
  neoplasms of, 607
  patella articulations with, 637–639, 710–711,
    710*f*–711*f*, 719*f*. *See also* Patellofemoral
    joint
  tibia complex of, tensile property tesing of,
    40–41, 40*f*, 766–767
Femur-anterior cruciate ligament-tibia complex
    (FATC), 40–41, 40*f*
Femur-posterior cruciate ligament-tibia complex
    (FPTC), 766–767
FFL. *See* Fabellofibular ligament
FG. *See* Fast glycolytic muscle fibers

FHL. *See* Flexor hallucis longus
Fiber bundles, functional considerations of
  in ligaments, 39, 41
  in muscle, 3–4, 4*f*–5*f*
  in peripheral nerves, 186, 186*f*
  in tendon collagen, 22*f*, 23–26, 24*f*, 34
Fibrillation
  of articular cartilage, with osteoarthritis, 64, 65*f*,
    66
  of resting muscle, with brachial plexus injuries,
    194
Fibrin clot, in knee healing
  of articular cartilage, 791, 794, 800, 855
  meniscus injections of, 649–650, 657–658, 657*f*
Fibroblasts
  in healing process, 43, 646, 690
  of ligaments, 39, 43
  of tendons, 692
Fibrocartilage
  ligament insertions and, 39
  in osteotendinous junction, 26–27
Fibronectin
  in articular cartilage, 54*t*, 55, 57, 66
  in knee meniscus, 647, 650
  in tendons, 25, 28
Fibroosseous tunnel
  of forefoot, nerve entrapment in, 958
  of sustentaculum tali
    flexor hallucis longus tendon stenosing teno-
      synovitis of, 987, 988*f*, 989–990
    release technique for, 989–990
Fibrosarcoma, of thigh, 607
Fibrous dysplasia, of femur, 607
Fibrous histiocytoma, malignant, of thigh, 607
Fibrous sheaths. *See* Retinacula
Fibrous tissue, magnetic resonance imaging of,
    100–101, 100*t*, 116
Fibula
  fractures of
    incidence of, 874–875
    with knee dislocations, 809
    stress, 873–874, 873*f*–874*f*, 887
  head of. *See* Gerdy's tubercle
  instability mechanisms of, 882–885, 884*f*
  tendon insertions of, 991–992, 991*f*
  tibial articulation of. *See* Tibiofibular joint
Figure-4 position, for menisci examination, 617,
    618*f*
Finger extension test, for elbow tendinosis,
    292–293
Fingernails. *See* Nail bed injuries
Fingers
  fractures of. *See* Metacarpal fractures; Phalanx
    fractures
  injuries of. *See also* Thumb injuries
    collateral ligaments, 246–248, 247*f*
    extensor tendons, 248–252, 249*f*, 251*f*
    flexor tendons, 252–254, 253*f*–254*f*
  joints of. *See* Distal interphalangeal joints; Prox-
    imal interphalangeal joints
Finkelstein test, for DeQuervain's syndrome, 283
Fisher exact test, in research studies, 139
Fissures, skin, in dancer's feet, 960–961
Five P's, of compartment syndrome, 879–880
Fixation procedures. *See* Reduction procedures;
    specific device
  external. *See* External fixation
  internal. *See* Internal fixation
Flare response, with brachial plexus injuries, 192
Flat bones, structure of, 75
Flatfoot. *See* Foot pronation; Pes planus
Flexibility. *See also specific joint or test*
  in ligament stability tests. *See* Ligament cutting
    studies
  in patellofemoral joint evaluation, 715, 715*f*,
    735
  studies of. *See specific joint or test*
  as tendon function, 32
  in toe deformities, 973–974, 973*f*
Flexibility training
  for knee tendon injuries, 700
  of tendons, 692–697, 699, 701, 704–706
  for runners, 1011, 1015, 1023

Flexion injuries, of lower extremities. *See* Plantar-flexion injuries
Flexion rotation drawer test, for knee injuries, 746*f*, 747
Flexor carpi radialis tendon, 284, 554, 554*f*
Flexor carpi ulnaris tendon (FCU)
 overhead throwing role of, 554–555, 554*f*
 in tennis elbow, 290, 302–304
Flexor digitorum brevis tendon, 899, 900*f*, 990
Flexor digitorum longus tendon (FDL)
 in Achilles tendon reconstruction, 982, 984–985
 compression neuropathy and, 920, 939–940
 nerve relationships to, 899, 899*f*
 in posterior tibial tendon reinsertions, 1005–1007
 shin splints and, 876
 tear injuries of, 988, 991
 transfers, for metatarsophalangeal injuries, 952
Flexor digitorum profundus tendon (FDP)
 avulsion injuries of, 236, 252–254, 253*f*–254*f*
 miscellaneous injuries of, 250, 547
Flexor digitorum superficialis tendon (FDS)
 in interphalangeal injuries, 252–253
 overhead throwing role of, 554–555, 554*f*
Flexor hallucis brevis tendon
 injuries of, 990–991
 in metatarsophalangeal joint, 949, 949*f*
Flexor hallucis longus tendon (FHL)
 in Achilles tendon reconstruction, 982–986, 983*f*, 986*f*
 anatomy of, 949, 949*f*, 987
 compression neuropathy and, 920, 924–926
 immobilization devices for, 989–991
 injuries of
  epidemiology of, 961–962, 987
  evaluation of, 988–989
  mechanisms of, 987–988, 988*f*
  nonoperative treatment of, 989–990
  surgical treatment of, 989–991
 in metatarsophalangeal joint, 949, 949*f*
 nerve relationships to, 899, 899*f*
 rehabilitation programs for, 989–991
 stenosing tenosynovitis of, 987–990
  at fibroosseous tunnel beneath sustentaculum tali, 987, 988*f*, 989–990
  at metatarsophalangeal joint, 989
 tear injuries of
  complete closed, 987–988, 990
  lacerations, 987–988, 990–991
  partial longitudinal, 987–988, 990
 tenosynovitis of, 961, 987–989
FOG. *See* Fast oxidative muscle fibers
Follow-through motions
 with golf swing
  biomechanics of, 393–394, 393*f*, 564, 564*f*
  pathologic, 566, 566*f*
 with pitching
  biomechanics of, 387*f*–388*f*, 388, 459*f*, 460–461, 465, 552*f*, 555
  pathologic, 557, 559*f*
 with tennis, 392, 392*f*
Foot
 anatomy of. *See also specific anatomy or region*
  compartmental, 87
  tendons, 979, 987, 991–992, 991*f*, 1000, 1007
  angle measurements of, shin splints and, 876
 anterior. *See* Forefoot
 arches of, 893, 894*f*, 945, 1000
  support for, 913, 913*f*
 magnetic resonance imaging of
  ligamentous injury, 110, 110*f*
  osteochondral injury, 110–112, 111*f*–112*f*
 medial. *See* Midfoot
 posterior. *See* Hindfoot
 tendons of
  anatomy of, 979, 987, 991–992, 991*f*, 1000, 1007
  injuries of. *See specific tendon*
 weight-bearing alignment of, 1016–1017
Football
 ankle injuries from, 992, 994
 athletic pubalgia from, 223, 225

brachial plexus injuries from, 183, 187, 187*f*–188*f*
cervical spine injuries from, 167, 170, 172–174, 172*f*–173*f*
cervical spine stenosis from, 176–177, 176*f*
elbow injuries from, 326
foot injuries from
 forefoot, 950, 968–970, 968*f*–970*f*, 972
 hindfoot, 933, 937*f*, 940
 midfoot, 907, 907*f*–908*f*, 910*f*, 912, 918
 toes, 950, 968–970, 968*f*–970*f*, 972
hand fractures from, 233, 257
knee injuries from, 663, 671, 700, 743
muscle strains from, 585, 588, 597
shoulder injuries from, 431–454, 437*f*
wrist injuries from, 273
Foot pronation
 biomechanics of, 893, 896
 excessive
  congenital, 945–946
  during running, 1012–1013
 metatarsal injuries and, 945–946
 nerve compression with, 918–920
 orthotics for, 877, 878*f*
 shin splints and, 876–877
 with weight-bearing, 1016–1017
Foot strike, during running, 1011–1013
Foot supination
 biomechanics of, 893, 896
 during running, 1012–1013
Force. *See also* Load
 acromioclavicular joint response to, 513–515, 513*f*–515*f*
 foot injuries from, 907, 907*f*, 922–924, 922*f*, 925*f*, 945
 knee responses to, 625, 637–639
  with functional bracing, 793, 863–867
  injuries from, 679, 711, 711*f*, 767–768, 767*f*
  low-energy *versus* high-energy, 767, 808
  osteoarthritic, 847–849, 854, 856
  with reconstruction, *in situ* measurement of, 45–46, 46*f*
 leg injuries from, 869, 874–875, 887
 low-energy *versus* high-energy injuries, 767, 789–790, 808
 as muscle strain component, 586, 586*f*
 in running cycle, 1012–1013, 1016–1017
 shoulder responses to, 403, 403*f*, 420, 433–434
  as injury mechanism, 436–438, 437*f*, 461–465
 tendon buffer for, physiologic principles of, 23–25, 27, 32
 types of, 23, 27
Force couples, of shoulder, 374–375, 374*f*–375*f*, 499
 during cocking, 552, 554–555, 557
 during swimming, 560–561
Force-displacement curve, of knee, 615, 615*f*
Force-elongation curve, of tendons, 32–33
Force-generating axis, muscle arrangement per, 6–9, 7*f*–8*f*
Force production
 by muscle cell. *See* Muscle contractions
 in shoulder. *See also* Throwing motion
  positioning impact of, 418–419
  sequence of, 498, 499*f*
Force relaxation. *See* Stress relaxation
Force transmission
 by patellofemoral joint, 637–639
 by shoulder, 374–376, 374*f*–376*f*
 by tendons, 31–35
Force-velocity relationship, in muscle contractions, 12–13, 12*f*, 14*f*
Forearm
 compressive syndromes of, 87, 91
 strengthening exercises for, 298
Forefoot. *See also specific anatomy*
 deformities of
  hallux rigidus, 970, 971*f*, 972
  hallux valgus, 946, 951–953, 971*f*, 972
  mallet, 973–974
  metatarsus primus varus, 953
  Morton's, 945–946
 heel alignment measurements of, with running injuries, 1016–1017

impingement syndromes of
 anterior tarsal tunnel, 958–959
 interdigital neuroma, 957–958
 medical hallucal nerve, 958
 injuries of. *See also specific injury*
  bone scintigraphy, 947, 954–955
  in dancers, 907, 907*f*, 924–926, 946, 959–962, 960*t*, 979, 988
  imaging studies for, 947
  immobilization devices for, 947, 957, 961
  metatarsal, 945–947, 947*f*
  metatarsophalangeal, 948–954, 948*f*–949*f*, 952*f*
  nerves, 957–959
  padding devices for, 948, 958, 960–962
  radiography of, 947, 951–952, 954–955, 959
  return to sport guidelines, 947, 951, 961
  scope of, 945, 965, 1016–1017
  sesamoids, 954–957, 955*f*–956*f*
  shoe modifications for, 946, 950, 958–962
 rehabilitation programs for, 947–948, 951, 957, 961
Forehand strokes, with tennis, 392–393, 393*f*
Forward swings, with golfing, 393–394, 393*f*
Four-bar linkage, crossed, as knee modeling approach, 624, 633
Four-corner fusion, of carpal bones, for fractures, 269, 270*f*
FPTC. *See* Femur-posterior cruciate ligament-tibia complex
Fractures. *See also specific anatomy*
 bone healing process with, 77–80, 82–83
 compartment syndromes from, 89–90
Freiberg's infraction
 of metatarsophalangeal joints, 953–954
 of toes, 960, 976
 treatment of, by type and deficit, 960, 960*t*
Friction, articular cartilage response to, 60–61, 61*t*
Froment's sign, with wrist tendinopathies, 284
Frozen shoulder, 332
F statistic, in research studies, 137–138
Fulkerson realignment procedure, for patellofemoral joint
 arthritis, 736–737, 739, 740*t*
 dislocations, 733–734, 733*f*
Fulkerson relocation test, for patellofemoral joint instability, 713–714
Full flexion test, for knee meniscus tears, 652, 652*f*
Function, in knee physical examination, 613–616, 615*f*–616*f*, 620
Fusion procedures. *See* Arthrodesis
F-wave responses, with brachial plexus injuries, 194

G
Gadolinium, for magnetic resonance imaging, 116
GAGs. *See* Glycosaminoglycans
Gait analysis
 for Achilles tendon dysfunction, 979, 981
 for femoral epiphyseal injuries, 580
 with forefoot injuries, 946
 for heel pain, 931
 with hip fractures, 603
 in knee examination, 613–616, 615*f*–616*f*, 620, 621*f*
  with injuries, 669, 680, 838–839, 854
 of running
  abnormal biomechanics in, 1011–1013
  with injuries, 587, 876, 1020–1021
 with tibial tendon injuries, 1000, 1001*f*, 1002–1003
Gamekeeper's thumb, 116, 116*f*, 243
 bony, 238, 244
Gamma irradiation, of allografts, 826
Gardner-Wells tongs, for cervical spine reductions, 164
Gastrocnemius musculotendinous complex
 injuries of
  epidemiology of, 696
  evaluation of, 696–697, 889
  mechanisms of, 696, 888
  medial mechanisms, 888–889

Gastrocnemius musculotendinous complex
    (*contd.*)
    nonoperative treatment of, 697–698, 889
    operative treatment of, 697
    in knee repair, 683, 685, 777–778
Gastrosoleus complex, deceleration role of, 979
Gelatinase (MMP2), articular cartilage degrada-
    tion by, 62
Gender factors. *See* Female athletes
Generalization, of research findings, 146–147
Generation phase, of running, 1011–1013
Gene therapy, for knee healing, 667, 690
Genetics
    of osteoarthritis, 54–55, 847
    of spondylolisthesis, 209
Genitourinary system, pain etiologies of, 215, 572,
    572*t*
Gerdy's tubercle, 680, 805
    in knee repair, 682–684, 733, 813
Gilmore's groin. *See* Athletic pubalgia
Girdlestone-Taylor tendon transfer, for toe de-
    formities, 976
Glenohumeral capsule
    anatomy of, 343–344, 433–434, 433*f*–434*f*
    collagen layers of, 343–344, 344*f*
    functions of, 343, 345
    ligament functions in, 344–348, 345*f*, 347*f*–348*f*
    in shoulder dislocation stabilizations
        anterior, 408*f*, 409
        mini-shift procedures, 473–474, 473*f*–474*f*
        posterior, 415–416, 423–427, 423*f*–426*f*, 427
Glenohumeral index, 380–381, 381*f*
Glenohumeral joint. *See also* Shoulder
    abduction mechanisms of, 499
    anatomy of, 340–343, 341*f*–342*f*
        anterior *verus* posterior, 433–435, 433*f*–435*f*
        capsular, 344*f*–345*f*, 347*f*–348*f*, 433–434m
            343–348
        labral, 434–435, 434*f*–435*f*
        ligaments of, 343–348, 344*f*–345*f*, 347*f*–348*f*,
            382*f*, 433–434
        muscles of, 351*f*–353*f*, 352–356, 433
    articulation mechanisms of, 341, 341*f*, 343,
        380–381, 381*f*
    biomechanics of, 379, 380*t*, 386, 386*f*
        biceps tendon role in, 385, 386*f*
        dynamic mechanisms of, 384–386, 386*f*
        glenoid labrum in, 381–382, 381*f*
        glenoid version in, 380, 380*f*
        humeral version in, 379–380, 380*f*
        intraarticular pressure in, 382
        joint compression effect on, 384–385, 386*f*
        ligaments and capsule in, 382–385, 382*f*, 384*f*
        rotator cuff components of, 385
        scapular rotators in, 386
        surface area articulations in, 380–381, 381*f*
    blood supply of, 341, 342*f*, 343
    dislocations of
        with brachial plexus injuries, 187, 191, 546
        mechanisms of, 343–346, 345*f*
        posterior shoulder instability and, 416–417,
            417*f*, 420, 427
    inflexibility of, scapula dysfunction from, 500*f*,
        501
    instability of
        anterior. *See* Anterior shoulder instability
        classifications of, 431–433, 433*f*, 481
        from contact injuries, 431–454
        labral mechanisms of. *See* Glenoid labrum
        posterior. *See* Posterior shoulder instability
            with scapula dysfunction, 499, 500*f*, 501,
            505–509
        superior. *See* Superior glenoid labrum
            from throwing motions, 343, 401–402,
            407–409, 457–475
    microinstability mechanisms of, 344, 457–475
    overhead throwing role of, 552–555,
        553*f*–555*f*
    range of motion of, 341, 380–381, 380*t*, 381*f*,
        386, 386*f*
    rotator cuff and
        biomechanics of, 372–375, 373*f*, 375*f*

injury mechanisms, 479–481, 491, 491*f*
    scapula function in, 497–498, 499*f*
    stability of
        arm position impact on, 382, 384*f*, 386, 386*f*
        dynamic contributors to, 384–386, 386*f*, 401,
            433
        mechanisms of, 340, 343–348, 345*f*, 379, 380*t*,
            399–401
        static contributors to, 379–384, 380*f*–382*f*,
            380*t*, 384*f*, 400–401
        stretch receptors and, 385, 418
Glenohumeral ligaments. *See also specific lig-
    ament*
    anatomy of, 343–348, 344*f*–345*f*, 347*f*–348*f*,
        382*f*
    anterior *versus* posterior, 433–434, 433*f*–434*f*
    injuries of
        with contact sports, 433–438
        with throwing motions, 390–391, 457–465,
            458*f*, 462*f*
    joint stability role of, 382–384, 382*f*, 384*f*, 433
        in anterior shoulder, 400–401
        in posterior shoulder, 417–418, 417*f*–401
Glenohumeral muscle, in posterior shoulder stabil-
    ity, 418
Glenoid cavity
    in glenohumeral joint stability, 380, 380*f*
    humerus articulation index of, 380–381, 381*f*
    shoulder relationship with
        anatomy of, 332, 333*f*, 334
        in posterior instability, 416–417
Glenoid labrum
    anatomy of
        microanatomy, 457–458, 458*f*
        normal, 434–435, 434*f*–435*f*
        variations of normal, 435, 435*f*, 458
    anterior. *See* Anterior glenoid labrum
    biomechanics of, 381–382, 381*f*
    contact injuries of
        arthroscopic evaluation of, 436, 445
        classification of, 431–433, 432*f*
        clinical evaluation of, 438–442, 440*f*–441*f*
        epidemiology of, 431–433
        imaging analysis of, 442–445, 442*f*–444*f*
        joint biomechanics and, 433–435, 433*f*–435*f*
        pathoanatomy of, 435–438, 437*f*
        recurrence of, 432, 445–446, 445*t*
        rehabilitation for, 450–451, 453–454
        return to sport guidelines, 450–451
        treatment options for, 445–454, 445*f*–447*f*,
            449*f*–450*f*, 453*f*
    overhead throwing role of, 552, 553*f*
    posterior. *See* Posterior glenoid labrum
    superior. *See* Superior glenoid labrum
    tear injuries of
        arthroscopic treatment of, 470–473, 472*f*–474*f*
        Bankart lesions as, 343, 401–402, 407–409
        clinical evaluation of, 465–467, 465*t*,
            466*f*–467*f*
        debridement results for, 470–471, 473
        epidemiology of, 457
        imaging analysis of, 467–469, 468*f*–469*f*
        injury mechanisms of, 457–466, 458*f*–460*f*,
            462*f*–463*f*, 472, 472*f*
        nonoperative treatment of, 469–470
        rehabilitation of, 470, 474–475
Glenoid rim, of shoulder, biceps tendon origins
    from, 349–351, 350*f*
Glenoplasty, for posterior shoulder dislocations,
    414, 422
Glucocorticoids, bone formation and, 82
Glucosamine sulfate, for knee degeneration, 852
Glucosaminoglycan-like products, for knee degen-
    eration, 852
Gluteus maximus, iliotibial band relationship
    with, 585
α-Glycerophosphate dehydrogenase (α-GP)
    in articular cartilage, 54*t*, 55
    muscle fiber typing with, 14, 16*t*
Glycidic radicals, in tendon cell metabolism,
    28–29

Glycolytic activity, of muscle fibers, 14, 16–18,
    16*t*, 18*t*
Glycoproteins
    in articular cartilage, 54*t*, 55
    in knee meniscus, 645, 647
    in tendons, 25–28, 30
Glycosaminoglycans (GAGs)
    in articular cartilage, 55, 57, 61, 787–788, 788*f*
    in knee, 647, 687, 689
    low-intensity exercise impact on, 80
    in tendons, 25–28
Godfrey's sign. *See* Posterior sag sign
Golfer's elbow
    injury mechanisms of, 289–291, 293
    resection and repair of, 302–304, 303*f*
Golf swing
    impingement syndromes from, 289–291,
        302–304, 565–566, 566*f*
    phases of
        biomechanics of, 393, 393*f*, 563, 564*f*
        pathologic, 564–565, 565*f*–566*f*
    shoulder kinematics of, 393–394, 393*f*, 564
        pathologic, 564–566, 565*f*–566*f*
Golgi apparatus
    in articular cartilage cells, 61–62
    as mechanoreceptors, 31
    in tendon cells, 27, 29–30
Gonadal function, bone formation and, 82
Gortex grafts, for knee repair
    ligament failure with, 826–827, 826*f*–827*f*
    patellofemoral indications for, 835, 839
α-GP. *See* α-Glycerophosphate dehydrogenase
Gracilis muscle, anatomy of, 584–585, 584*f*
Gracilis syndrome, 229
Gracilis tendon graft
    for ligament reconstruction, 751, 828
    for tendon reconstruction, 693, 702, 702*f*, 704
    tensile strength of, 825
Gradient recalled echo sequencing (GRE), for
    magnetic resonance imaging, 101, 104–105
Grafts
    autografts *versus* allografts, 47, 235, 683–684,
        812–813
    bone. *See* Bone grafts
    ligament. *See* Ligament grafts
    meniscal, 658–659
    nerve. *See* Nerve grafts
    preconditioning of, impact on stress relaxation
        of, 42
    preservation techniques, 48
    for reconstruction. *See specific anatomy or
        injury*
Graft-tunnel motion, in knee reconstructions
    with anterior cruciate ligament, 47–48, 48*f*, 751,
        752*f*, 755, 815
    complications of, 827–829, 827*f*–828*f*
    with posterior cruciate ligament, 776, 778, 781–
        784, 782*f*–784*f*, 814
    posterolateral, 682, 684–685, 814–815
Gram stain, of olecranon bursitis, 326
Great toe
    deformities of. *See* Hallux rigidus; Hallux sal-
        tans; Hallux valgus; Toes
    injuries of, 966–967
Grip size, Nirschl technique for, 296, 296*f*
Groin muscles, strains of, 217–221, 220*f*, 593–595,
    596*t*
Groin pain
    bone etiologies of, 595
    chronic, 221, 226–227, 230
    clinical evaluation of, 225–226, 593
    imaging studies for
        magnetic resonance, 112, 113*f*, 221
        radiography, 587, 592, 594–595, 597, 599, 602,
            604
    injury mechanisms of, 223–224, 224*f*, 593
    medical etiologies of, 215, 595–596. *See also*
        Athletic pubalgia
    muscular etiologies of, 217–218, 220–221, 220*f*,
        593–595
    from nerve entrapment, 219, 220*f*
Grower's sign, 606–607

Growth factors
    for articular cartilage repair, 67, 800
    as bone formation stimulus, 78–79, 81–82
    for knee healing, 650, 690, 800
    for ligament healing, 44, 667
Growth plate injuries. *See* Bone growth plate
Guyon's canal, nerve compression in, tendinopathy from, 284
Gymnastics
    elbow injuries from, 307–308, 320–321
    foot and ankle injuries from, 915*f,* 979, 1001
    hand and wrist injuries from, 233, 273–274, 277–278, 285
    leg injuries from, 872, 872*f,* 875–876
    lumbar spine injuries from, 209
    muscle strains from, 586
Gynecologic disorders. *See* Menstrual disorders

H
Haglund's deformity, of hindfoot, 897, 936–938, 936*f*–937*f,* 980
Hall-effect strain transducer, in knee biomechanics, 625, 628, 867
Hallux rigidus
    case study of, 970, 971*f,* 972
    clinical evaluation of, 972
    incidence of, 951, 970
    metatarsal injuries and, 946
    metatarsophalangeal injuries and, 951
    treatment of, 972
Hallux saltans, 924–925, 961–962
Hallux valgus
    associated injuries with, 946, 951–952, 958, 975
    in dancers, 961
    of metatarsophalangeal joint, 952, 971*f,* 972
    surgical correction of, 952–953
Halo-brace immobilization, for cervical spine reductions, 164–165, 167
Hamate fractures, 271–272, 271*f*
Hamilton's staging, of Freiberg's infractions, 960, 960*t*
Hammer toe, 948, 973
Hamstrings. *See also specific muscle or tendon*
    as grafts, for knee repair
        for anterior cruciate ligament reconstruction, 47–48, 48*f,* 632, 751, 829
        complications of, 825
        posterolateral, 683, 777–778, 783, 784*f,* 815
    in hip injuries, growth-related, 580
    ischial tuberosity injuries and, 588, 592, 592*f*
    in knee injuries, 628, 631, 714*f,* 715, 735
    strain injuries of, 590–591, 591*f*
        acute treatment of, 589, 591, 591*f*
        chronic, 592
        classifications of, 588–589, 589*t*
        clinical evaluation of, 588, 588*f,* 696–697
        epidemiology of, 587, 696
        imaging studies of, 589, 589*f,* 592, 697
        mechanisms of, 587–588, 696
        nonoperative treatment of, 697
        prevention strategies for, 590
        rehabilitation program for, 587, 589–591, 591*f,* 697
        return to sport guidelines, 590–591, 591*f,* 697
        risk factors for, 587–588
        surgical repair of, 591–592, 592*f,* 697
        treatment per grade, 590–591, 591*f*
    thigh compartment anatomy of, 583–584, 584*f*
    in tibiofibular joint instability, 884–885
Hamstring syndrome, 228–229
Hand
    blood supply to, scaphoid fractures and, 257, 265
    fractures of
        bone grafting for, 235
        dislocation with, 233–239, 236*f,* 239*f*
        of distal phalanx, 235–236, 236*f*
        implant selection for, 234–235, 234*f*
        intraarticular considerations of, 233–235, 237–240, 239*f*
        mechanisms of, 233–234

    of metacarpals, 238–240, 239*f*
    of middle phalanx, 236–238
    of proximal phalanx, 238
    Salter-Harris classification of, 233, 236, 238, 240
    tendon injuries with, 236, 239, 239*f*
    treatment analysis for, 233–234
    injuries of
        of digits, 233–238, 246–254
        of ligaments, 238, 243–248
        return to sport guidelines, 233, 243–244, 247, 254
        of soft tissue, 233–235, 243–254, 273
        of tendons, 236, 239, 239*f,* 248–254, 253*f*–254*f*
        of thumb, 238–240, 243–246
    ligaments of, injuries of, 238, 243–248
    magnetic resonance imaging of, 115–116, 116*f*
    swimming stroke role of
        biomechanics of, 391–392, 391*f,* 559–561, 562*f*
        pathologic, 562–563, 562*f*
    tendons of
        anatomy and physiology of, 23, 248–249, 249*f*
        injuries of, 236, 239, 239*f,* 248–254, 253*f*–254*f*
Hand-held muscle testers, for strength measurement, 191
Hangman's fractures, 166
Hardcastle classification, of Lisfranc's joint injuries, 907–908, 908*f*
Harris-Beath print mats, for pes planus, 913
Harris view, radiographic, for talocalcaneal coalition, 928, 928*f*
Hauser realignment procedure, for patellofemoral joint dislocations, 639, 732–733, 732*f,* 834
Haversian systems, in bone, 76*f*
Hawkins impingement test, for shoulder injuries, 442, 482
Head injuries. *See* Intracranial injuries
Healing process (phases)
    of articular cartilage, 63, 67
    of bone, 77–80, 82–83
    of ligaments, 43
    of tendons, 290, 689–690
Heat therapy
    for lumbar spine injuries, 211
    for osteitis pubis, 595
Heel, pathoanatomy of. *See* Calcaneus
Heel counter
    Achilles tendon dysfunction and, 981–982
    hindfoot injuries and, 929, 934, 937–938
Heel cup
    for heel pain, 932–933, 933*f,* 939
    for hindfoot injuries, 921, 921*f*
Heel measurements, with running injuries, 1016
Heel pad, flattening of, 933, 933*f*
Heel pain
    acute plantar fascia tear, 933
    differential diagnosis of, 929, 930*f,* 930*t,* 934
    from fat pad atrophy, 932–934, 933*f*
    from impingement of nerve to the ADQ, 899, 933–934, 934*f*
    inflammatory, 939
    insertional plantar fasciitis, 929–933, 930*f*–932*f*
    magnetic resonance imaging of, 929, 931, 935, 937
    posterior
        differential diagnosis of, 930*t,* 934
        distal insertional Achilles tendinitis, 934–936, 934*f*–936*f*
        Haglund's deformity, 897, 936, 936*f*–937*f*
        posterior lateral calcaneal exostosis, 938–939, 938*f*
        retro-Achilles bursitis, 938
    postoperative rehabilitation for, 935–936, 939–940
    radiography of, 930–931, 933, 935, 937
    treatment of
        nonoperative, 635*f*–936*f,* 931–936, 938–939
        surgical, 932–936, 932*f,* 936*f*–937*f*

Heel pain syndrome, 929–933, 930*f*–932*f*
Heel pinch test
    for calcaneal fractures, 920, 921*f*
    for Haglund's deformity, 936–937, 936*f*
Heel rise test, single, for tendon dysfunction, 980, 1002
Heel slide exercises, for knee ligament injuries, 669, 669*f*
Heel spurs, 930–931, 930*f,* 1020
    Achilles tendinitis with, 935, 936*f*
Heel wedge
    for Achilles tendon dysfunction, 981–982
    for knee degeneration, 854
    for leg injuries, 877, 889
    for posterior tibial tendon injuries, 1006
    running injuries and, 1017, 1019, 1022
Helmets
    at-risk playing with, in football, 172–174, 172*f*–173*f*
    emergency removal of, for head and neck injuries, 153–155, 155*f*
Hemangioma, of thigh, 607
Hematomas
    acute subdural, 159
    epidural, 158–159
    intracerebral, 158
    with knee tendon ruptures, 692, 701
    magnetic resonance imaging of, 100–101, 100*t,* 116–117, 117*f*
    with quadriceps contusions, 602, 692
    subungual, 966
    with thigh muscle strains, 588, 588*f,* 592, 597
Hemiarthroplasty
    for patellofemoral arthritis, 737–739, 740*t*
    for posterior shoulder dislocations, 422, 427
Hemophiliacs, intramuscular bleeds of, 606
Hemorrhagic phase, of healing process, 43
Heparin sulfate, in tendons, 25, 28
Heparin therapy, for vascular compromise, 810, 889
Hepatitis viruses, graft transmission of, 826
Hernias
    athletic pubalgia *versus,* 595–596
    with compartment syndromes, 879
    repair results for, 224, 227
    from sports, 218–219, 219*f,* 227
Herniated nucleus pulposus (HNP)
    clinical presentations of, 205–206, 206*t*
    forefoot injuries *versus,* 962
    illustrative case of, 208–209, 208*f*
    imaging techniques for, 206–207, 208*f*
    natural history of, 206–207
    pathophysiology of, 205
    treatment of, 207–208
Herniation
    of brain, 159
    of spinal disks. *See* Vertebral disks
Herniography, contrast, 219, 219*f,* 221
Herniorrhaphy, Bassini-type, for athletic pubalgia, 596
High-intensity exercise, bone adaptation to, 80–81, 83*f*
Hiking, with backpacks, brachial plexus injuries from, 183–184, 189, 189*f,* 195
Hill-Sachs lesions, of humeral head
    imaging analysis of, 443, 443*f,* 468
    shoulder instability with, 343, 401, 413–414, 422, 427, 436
Hindfoot. *See also specific anatomy*
    anatomy of
        bones and ligaments, 894*f,* 896–899, 896*f*–898*f*
        neurovascular, 899, 899*f*–900*f*
    arthritis of
        posttraumatic, 923, 929
        subtalar joint, 926–927, 926*f*–927*f*
    biomechanics of, 896, 898*f*
    compression neuropathy of, 920
    deformities of, Haglund's, 897, 936, 936*f*–937*f*
    fractures of
        calcaneus, 920–923, 921*f*–923*f,* 929–930
        talus, 923–926, 924*f*–926*f*

Hindfoot. *See also specific anatomy (contd.)*
  impingement syndromes of, 924–926, 925f–926f
    of nerve to the ADQ, 899, 933–934, 934f
    tarsal tunnel, 939–940
  injuries of
    Achilles tendinopathy, 1019–1020
    arthrodesis indications for, 926–927, 927f, 929
    bone scans of, 902, 920, 926, 927f
    compression neuropathy of, 920, 939–940
    computed tomography of, 902, 923–926, 927f, 928
    cortisone injections for, 932, 938, 940
    diagnostic strategies for, 901–902
    differential diagnosis of, 899–901, 930
    fractures, 920–926, 929–930
    immobilization of, 921, 923–924, 932
    magnetic resonance imaging of, 902, 926–929, 931, 935, 937, 939
    nerve blocks for, 902, 928, 932, 938
    neurovascular, 939–940
    nonoperative treatment of, 921–927, 929, 940
    orthotics for, 921–927, 927f, 931–932, 937–938, 940
    padding devices for, 922, 935, 936f, 937–939
    radiography of, 902, 920–926, 928, 940
    return to sport guidelines, 921–922, 929, 933, 935–936, 940
    from running, 1019–1020
    shoe modifications for, 921–927, 927f, 931–932, 937–938, 940
    surgical treatment of, 923–924, 923f, 926–927, 926f–927f, 929, 930f, 939–940
    tarsal coalitions, 927–929, 928f–929f
  pain syndromes of, 901. *See also* Heel pain
    heel afflictions. *See* Heel pain
    os trigonum, 925–926, 925f–926f
    shin splints and, 876–877
    stability mechanisms of, 896–899, 897f–898f
    stress fractures of, calcaneal, 920, 921f, 929–930, 931f
Hip joint
  adduction pain syndromes of, 228–229
  apophyseal injuries of, 580
  forceful flexion of, muscle strains from, 218, 224–225, 224f
  fractures of
    etiologies of, 113, 572–574, 573f, 579
    pelvic fractures involvement of, 216–218
    rehabilitation for, 579–280
    treatment of, 573–574, 579
  hematoma of, 578–579
  infections of, 578
  injuries of
    acute conditions, 578–580
    athletic pubalgia *versus,* 596
    bursitis of, 112–113, 577–578
    contusion of, 578–579
    differential diagnosis of, 571–572, 572t
    dislocations of, 579–580
    epiphyseal, 580–581, 581f
    growth-related, 571, 580–581, 581f
    intraarticular pathology of, 229, 574–575, 574f
    magnetic resonance imaging of, 112–113, 113f
Hip joint
  mechanisms of, 571–578, 572t
  overuse injuries of
    bursitis, 577–578
    osteitis pubis. *See* Osteitis pubis
    snapping syndrome, 229, 574–576, 574f, 576f
    stress fractures, 113, 572–574, 573f
  referred pain in, differential diagnosis of, 571–572, 572t, 596
  rotation of
    with golf swing, 563–564, 564f
    with pitching motion, 551–552, 556, 559f
  running force impact on, 1012, 1016, 1019
  snapping syndrome of
    evaluation guidelines for, 575
    injury mechanisms of, 229, 574–575, 574f
    treatment of, 575–576, 576f
Hippocratic reduction technique, for anterior shoulder dislocations, 406, 406f

Hip pointer, 578–579
Histamine reflex test, for brachial plexus injuries, 192
Histiocytoma, malignant fibrous, of thigh, 607
Histochemistry, for muscle fiber typing, 13–16, 15f–16f, 16t
HIV. *See* Human immunodeficiency virus
HNP. *See* Herniated nucleus pulposus
Hockey
  athletic pubalgia from, 223, 225, 595
  brachial plexus injuries from, 183, 188
  glenoid labrum injuries from, 431–454
  knee injuries from, 663, 866
  leg tendon injuries from, 1007–1008
  muscle strains from, 586, 593
  wrist injuries from, 273
Hohmann osteotomy, of metatarsals, 953
Homan's sign, 91, 889
Homeostasis
  physiologic mechanisms of, 28, 41
  during surgery. *See specific anatomy, injury, or procedure*
Homogeneity, ligament tensile property and, 41
Hormonal imbalances, leg stress fractures from, 869, 871
Horner's syndrome, cervical nerve injuries with, 191–193, 197
Hueter-Volkman principle, of epiphyseal pressures, 80–81
Human immunodeficiency virus (HIV), graft transmission of, 812–813, 826
Humerus
  in glenohumeral joint stability, 379–380, 380f
  head of
    anatomy of, 334–335, 334f, 346–348, 346f
    compression fractures of. *See* Hill-Sachs lesions
    glenoid articulation index of, 380–381, 381f
    overhead throwing role of, 552, 553f, 554, 556
    in rotator cuff biomechanics, 372–375, 373f, 375f
    shoulder instability and, 401, 416–417, 417f, 420, 422, 427
  rotational osteotomy of, for posterior shoulder dislocations, 415, 422
  shoulder articulations with, 334–335, 334f. *See also* Glenohumeral joint
  swimming stroke role of, 392, 560–562, 562f
Humpback deformity, with scaphoid fractures, 263, 267
Hyaluronic acid, 28, 853
  in articular cartilage, 55–56, 61, 63
Hydrogen atom, in magnetic resonance imaging, 100
Hydrostatic factors, of compartment syndromes, 88–89
Hydroxyapatite crystals, in osteotendinous junction, 27
Hyperangulation model, of thrower's shoulder, 389, 389f
Hyperbaric oxygen, for compartment syndromes, 89
Hyperextension deformities, with hand injuries, 250
Hyperextension exercises, for knee rehabilitation, with anterior cruciate ligament repair, 748–749, 749f, 753, 755–756, 756f
Hyperextension injuries
  of cervical spine, 166, 168, 168f, 179
  of elbow, 292, 307–308, 311–312
  of interphalangeal joints, 246, 248–250
  of knee
    examination of, 616–617, 616f–617f, 620
    ligament mechanisms, 678–679, 765, 767–768, 768f, 808–809
  of lumbar spine, 203–204, 210
  of pelvic region, 223, 224f
  of toes, 950, 952, 954, 967–968, 968f
  of wrist, 233, 269, 273–278
Hyperflexion injuries
  of cervical spine, 168, 168f, 173, 173f, 179
  of distal interphalangeal joints, 249

of knee, 767–769, 767f
of quadriceps tendon, 598–600, 600f
of toes, 950, 968
of wrist, 279
Hyperpronation injuries, of metatarsals, 946
Hypothenar hammer syndrome, 285
Hypothesis testing
  error types in, 132–133, 144
  essential components of, 123, 132–133, 142
Hypoxia, in brain injuries, 178–179
Hysteresis
  of ligaments, 41–43, 42f
  of tendons, 33
H zone, of sarcomeres, 4, 5f

I

I band, in sarcomeres, 4, 5f, 11
Ice hockey. *See* Hockey
Ice therapy
  for Achilles tendon dysfunction, 981, 986
  for acromioclavicular joint dislocations, 522
  for adductor longus strains, 220
  for elbow injuries, 313
  for flexor hallucis longus tendon injuries, 989
  for foot injuries
    of hindfoot, 921, 925–929, 931, 935, 937, 939
    of midfoot, 911, 914, 917
  for hip injuries, 578, 580
  for knee ligament tears, 667, 667f
  for leg injuries, 877–878, 889
  for lumbar spine injuries, 204
  for peroneus tendon injuries, 995, 999
  for wrist pain, 278, 282, 285
IGHL. *See* Inferior glenohumeral ligament
IGHLC. *See* Inferior glenohumeral ligament complex
IKDC. *See* International Knee Documentation Committee
Iliac crest, grafts from
  for hand fractures, 235
  for scaphoid fractures, 260, 261f–262f, 266, 269
Iliac spine
  anterior inferior, 585, 601, 601t, 638, 702, 712
  anterior superior, 217, 580, 585, 601–602, 601t
  avulsion fractures of, 216–217, 580
Iliacus muscle, anatomy of, 585
Iliopsoas syndrome, 218, 229
Iliopsoas tendon, injuries of, 218, 580, 594–595
Iliotibial band (ITB)
  anatomy of, 585, 805–806
  friction syndrome of
    epidemiology of, 694–695
    evaluation of, 695
    nonoperative treatment of, 695–696, 1023–1024
    operative treatment of, 695
    pathoanatomy of, 229, 695
    from running, 1017, 1019, 1023–1024
  in knee injuries, 682, 685, 715, 723, 813
  tightness tests of, 715, 716f–717f
Iliotibial tract, anatomy of, 805–806
Immobilization and immobilization devices. *See also specific device*
  for Achilles tendon dysfunction, 982–987
  for acromioclavicular joint dislocations, 521f, 522
  articular cartilage changes with, 62–63
  bone adaptation to, 77, 80, 83, 83f
  compartment syndromes and, 89, 94–95, 605–606
  for elbow tendinosis, 297, 302
  for flexor hallucis longus tendon injuries, 989–991
  for foot injuries
    of forefoot, 947, 957, 961
    of hindfoot, 921, 923–924, 932
    of midfoot, 904, 906, 911, 913, 917, 920
    of toes, 966, 970
  for hand injuries
    fractures, 234–240, 234f
    soft tissue, 244–246, 245f, 250–252, 251f

for head and neck injuries
emergency care, 153–155, 155*f*
treatment indications, 162*f*, 163–164, 166–167
for knee injuries, 701, 810
ligaments, 666–667, 687–688, 725–726, 733, 748, 751
for leg injuries, 872–873, 877, 884
ligament tensile property and, 41, 666–667
for peroneus tendon injuries, 996, 998–1000
for posterior tibial tendon injuries, 1004–1007
for shoulder injuries, 406, 427, 450–451, 474
for wrist injuries
scaphoid fractures, 258–260, 260*f*, 263–267
soft tissue, 281–282, 284–285
Immunohistochemistry, muscle fiber typing with, 15*f*, 16
Impingement of nerve to the ADQ, 899, 933–934, 934*f*
Impingement syndromes. *See* Nerve compression injuries; *specific anatomy*
Implant devices, absorbable, for hand fractures, 234, 234*f*
Incidence, prevalence *versus,* 127, 129
Incidence study, as research design, 124*f*, 127–128
Incision and drainage, of olecranon bursitis, 326
Independence, of statistical measurements, 136
Infections
with hand fractures, 235, 247–248
post-Achilles tendon repair, 984
post-knee surgery, 756, 826, 832
with scaphoid fractures, 264
Inferior glenohumeral ligament (IGHL)
in anterior shoulder stability, 400–401, 409
functional anatomy of, 343, 345–348, 347*t*–348*t,* 382*f*
in throwing injuries, 390–391, 461
Inferior glenohumeral ligament complex (IGHLC)
in contact injuries, 433–436, 433*f*–434*f*
failure studies of, 435–436
functional anatomy of, 344, 347*f*–348*f,* 384*f*
humeral insertion bands of, 346–37, 346*f*
joint stability role of, 383–384, 384*f*
shoulder dislocations and, 401, 417–418, 417*f,* 420–421, 435–436
Inferior ramus, stress fractures of, 595
Inflammatory injuries. *See* *specific anatomy*
Inflammatory myopathy, of thigh, 606–607
Inflammatory phase, of healing process, 43, 63, 690
Infrapatellar contracture syndrome (IPCS)
etiologies of, 703, 834, 837–838
treatment of, 838–839
Infraspinatus muscle
anatomy of, 354
golf swing role of, 394, 564
nerve injuries of, 545
overhead throwing role of, 554, 554*f*
in rotator cuff biomechanics, 354, 372–373, 372*f*–373*f*
swimming stroke role of, 392, 561
Infusion technique, for compartmental pressures, 880
Inguinal hernias
athletic pubalgia *versus,* 595–596
mechanisms of, 218–219, 224
Inguinal pain. *See* Groin pain
Inguinal wall, repair procedures for, 219, 224, 227
Injuries. *See also specific anatomy or type*
from loading, 34–35. *See also* Load
multiple, treatment considerations for, 89
physical examination at time of, 613, 901
Injury modeling
for knee, 624–625
potential applications of, 49
Innominate bones, of pelvis, ligament attachments to, 223, 224*f*
Inorganic components
of bone, 78–80, 78*f*–79*f*
of tendons, 27–28
Insall-Salvati ratio, of knee, 703, 715, 717, 718*f,* 728

Insall's proximal realignment procedures, for patellofemoral joint dislocations, 729–730, 730*f,* 730*t*
Insertions
direct *versus* indirect, 39
of ligaments, 39, 47
of tendons, 21, 690
Inside-out arthroscopic repair, of knee meniscus, 653–654, 654*f,* 656, 831
Insoles, custom
for midfoot pathology, 913, 913*f,* 919
for toe injuries, 958, 970, 970*f,* 972
Instability cascade, of rotator cuff, 418
Instability mechanisms. *See* *specific anatomy or injury*
Insulin growth factors, for healing, 79, 82, 690, 800
Intercalary defects
with hand fractures, 234–235, 257
with scaphoid fractures, 267, 269
Intercompartmental pressures. *See* Compartmental pressures
Intercondylar notch impingement, femoral, with knee reconstructions, 827–829, 828*f*–830*f,* 838–839
Intercuneiform joints, anatomy of, 893, 894*f*
Interdigital neuromas
in forefoot, 957–958
of toes, 974–975, 975*f*
Intermetatarsal ligaments
anatomy of, 893, 894*f*
neuroma excisions and, 958
Internal fixation
of clavicle fractures, 370–371, 506, 537–538, 538*f*
for foot injuries
of hindfoot, 609, 902, 906*f,* 908–909, 911*f,* 919–920
of toes, 966, 968
for hand injuries
fractures, 233–240, 234*f,* 263–266, 269–272
ligament tears, 245–247
tendon lacerations, 250–253
for hip fractures, 573–574, 579, 581
of knee injuries
for anterior cruciate ligament repairs, 47, 48*f,* 629, 632–633, 750, 754–755
of ligaments, 682, 684–685
for posterior cruciate ligament repairs, 774–778, 775*f,* 781–784, 782*f*–784*f*
posterolateral, 682–683
of tendons, 692–694, 693*f,* 699
of leg fractures, stress, 873
for little league elbow, 319–320, 320*f*
for lumbar spondylytic defects, 211–212
for metatarsal fractures, 947, 961, 966, 1021
of os peroneum, 1000
for pelvic fractures, 216–217
of peroneus tendon injuries, 997–1000
of posterior tibial tendon injuries, 1003–1007
for scaphoid fractures, 258*f,* 260, 260*f,* 262*f,* 263–265, 265*f*
with dislocations, 267, 268*f*–269*f*
for scapula fractures, 506
for shoulder dislocations
anterior labral, 446–450, 446*f*–447*f,* 449*f*–450*f*
posterior labral, 450–451, 451*f*
superior labral, 451–453, 453*f,* 471
for wrist ligament injuries, 278
International Knee Documentation Committee (IKDC)
activity risks per, 749, 749*t*
knee examination criteria of, 614–616, 752
Interphalangeal joints
distal. *See* Distal interphalangeal joints
proximal. *See* Proximal interphalangeal joints
Interpretation, of research studies, 144–146
Interscalene block, for shoulder surgery, 490
Intersection syndrome, of wrist, 283
Intersesamoid ligament, 954, 955*f*
Interstitial systems, in bone, 76*f,* 77

Interval sports training, for shoulder rehabilitation, 475
Intervertebral disk injuries. *See* Vertebral disks
Intervertebral disk-space narrowing, with cervical spine injuries, 163–164, 188
Intraarticular disks, of shoulder joints
biomechanics of, 367, 367*f,* 369
dislocation repair consideration of, 526
Intraarticular pressure, in shoulder biomechanics, 382, 400
Intracerebral hematoma, 158
Intracompartmental pressures. *See* Compartmental pressures
Intracranial injuries
brain herniation with, 159
brain swelling, 158–160
in children, 159
diffuse
categories of, 156–159
return to sport guidelines, 157–158, 158*f*
focal brain syndromes, 158–159
immobilization devices for, 153–155, 155*f*
initial examination of, 156–157
management of, 160
emergency measures, 153–156, 155*f*
prevention strategies for, 172–174, 172*f*–173
primary mechanisms, 178
secondary mechanisms, 178
spinal cord resuscitation with, 178–180, 179*f*
Intracranial pressure, elevations of, with head injuries, 159–160
Intramedullary fixation
for hand fractures, 234, 234*f*
for knee injuries, 704
for lumbar spondylytic defects, 212
Intubation, of airway. *See* Endotracheal intubation
Inversion injuries, of ankle
biomechanics of, 819–821, 896, 897*f,* 926
fractures with, 922–923, 923*f*
leg injuries with, 879, 883
tendon injuries with, 992–994, 993*f*
Iontophoresis, 204, 721, 931
Ion transport
in bone, 77–79
enzymes for, in muscle contractions, 10, 10*f*
IPCS. *See* Infrapatellar contracture syndrome
Irrigation and debridement. *See* Debridement
Ischemia, occlusive
with compartment syndromes, 87–91, 88*f,* 881
with popliteal artery entrapment, 886–887
Ischial tuberosity
apophysitis of, 592–593
avulsion fractures of, 217, 592
hamstring strain injuries and, 588, 592, 592*f*
Isokinetic exercise, for muscle strain injuries, 589–591, 594, 598
Isokinetic testing, with thigh muscle strains, 590–591, 598
Isometric exercises, for scapular dyskinesis, 506–507
Isometric muscle contractions
active length-tension principle of, 10–12, 11*f*
electrical stimulation of, for muscle strengthening, 10, 10*f*
maximal voluntary, with pitching motion, 459–460
Isthmic spondylolisthesis
of lumbar spine, 209–213, 210*f,* 212*f*
treatment per grades of, 211–212
ITB. *See* Iliotibial band

J

Jersey finger, diagnosis and treatment of, 252–254, 253*f*–254*f*
Jogger's foot, 920
Joint motion
computer simulation of, 49
deficits in. *See* Range of motion deficits
degrees of freedom with, for knee reconstruction, 44–45, 45*f,* 48*f*

Joint stability
  cartilage degeneration and, 62–63
  mechanisms of. *See specific joint*
J sign, with patellofemoral joint injuries, 712, 727, 850
Jumper's knee. *See* Patellar tendinitis

K

Kager's triangle, of hindfoot, 897–898, 898*f*
Kaplan-Meier survival curve, in research studies, 140
Kappa coefficient, in research studies, 133
Keinbach's disease, of lunate bone, 270
Keller arthroplasty, for toe deformities, 946, 953
Kellgren-Lawrence scale, of knee osteoarthritis, 845
Kendall tau test, in research studies, 137, 139
Kennedy classification, of multiligament injuries of knee, 808
Kenny Howard shoulder harness, modified, for acromioclavicular joint dislocations, 521*f*, 522
Keratan sulfate
  in articular cartilage, 55, 57, 787, 788*f*
  in knee meniscus, 647
Ketorolac, post-knee repair, 755
Kicking, injuries from, 588, 966, 968
Kidney stones, 215
Kinematics
  with knee reconstructions, robotic measurement of, 45–46, 46*f*, 627–628
  of running gait cycle, 1011–1013
  of shoulder, with throwing, 418–419, 498, 499*f*
  of tendons, 32
Kinetic energy chain
  from arm cocking, 552, 554–555
  of overhead throwing
    scapula abnormalities impact on, 502–503, 503*t*
    scapula sequencing of, 418–419, 498, 499*f*
    with running, 1013, 1017
  of scapula function, 418–419, 498, 499*f*, 502–503
    rehabilitation exercises for, 506–509, 507*f*–509*f*
Kirschner wire fixation
  for hand injuries
    fractures, 234–240, 234*f*
    tendon lacerations, 250–251
  for toe fractures, 966
  for ulnar collateral ligament tears, 245–246
  for wrist ligament injuries, 278, 278*f*
Klippel-Feil anomaly, of spine, 175
Knee joint
  ACL-deficient. *See* Anterior cruciate ligament
  anatomy of
    articular cartilage, 54*f*, 62–64, 787–789, 788*f*–789*f*
    articulations, 623, 637–639, 645, 646*f*
    bursae, 721*f*
    ligaments, 39, 41, 626–627, 636–637, 645, 646*f*, 663–664, 664*f*
    menisci, 645–649, 646*f*–648*f*
    patellofemoral joint, 636, 709–711, 710*f*
    posterolateral, 675–679, 763–765, 764*f*–765*f*
    tendons, 687
  arthrodesis indications for, 704
  arthroplasty of. *See* Knee, reconstruction of
  biomechanics of
    ligaments, 625–634, 765–767, 806–808
    meniscal, 634–636, 647–648
    patellofemoral joint, 636–639, 711, 711*f*
    principles of, 624–625
    stiffness approach to, 624, 626–627, 633
    tensile property testing of, 40–41, 40*f*, 624–625, 807–808
  bumper model of, 623
  bursitis of, 705, 721
  chondral lesions of
    clinical evaluation of, 791, 849–850
    imaging studies of, 791–793, 792*f*
    mechanisms of, 789–791, 789*f*–790*f*
    treatment of, 793–801, 800*f*–801*f*, 854–855

degenerative disease of
  abrasion arthroplasty for, 795, 802*f*, 855
  anatomy-specific, 636, 638, 687, 689, 734–740
  arthroscopic interventions for, 854–855
  articular cartilage damage, 849
  clinical evaluation of, 849–850, 857
  cystic, 617, 618*f*
  drilling repair of, 794–795, 855
  epidemiology of, 845–847
  grading schemes for, 64–65, 845, 851, 855
  imaging studies for, 850–851
  with ligament injury, 766, 776
  mechanical factors, 847–849, 851–852, 854
  microfracture repair of, 794–795, 800, 855
  nonoperative treatment of, 851–853
  Outerbridge classification of, 472, 855
  patellar, 636, 638, 734–740
  pathoanatomy of, 62–67, 65*f*, 617, 618*f*, 636, 732, 847–849
  post-meniscal repair, 830, 832
  repair techniques for, osteotomies as, 856–858
  transplant regeneration for, 796–797, 796*f*–798*f*, 856
dislocations of. *See* Knee, multiligament injuries of
effusions of, 714, 725, 745, 768
  articular cartilage and, 791, 794
force displacement of, 615, 615*f*, 624–626
force transmission by, 637–639
hyperextension tests of, 616–617, 616*f*–617*f*
injuries of
  chondral, 787–804. *See also* Articular cartilage
  cruciate. *See* Anterior cruciate ligament; Posterior cruciate ligament
  decision-making with, 621–622
  hyperextension, 616–617, 616*f*–617*f*, 620, 678–679
  iliotibial band in, 682, 685, 715, 723
  immobilization devices for, 666–667, 687–688, 701, 725–726, 733
  ligaments
    combined, 44, 634, 679, 681, 805–817. *See also* Knee, multiligament injuries of
    isolated. *See specific ligament*
  low-energy *versus* high-energy, 767, 789–790, 808
  magnetic resonance imaging of, 102–105, 102*f*–106*f*, 675
  mechanisms of, 229, 598, 666
  medial and posteromedial, 663–674
  meniscal. *See* Meniscus
  muscle-tendon units in, 679, 688–689, 696, 705
  patella. *See* Patellofemoral joint
  posterolateral, 675–685
  return to sport guidelines
    with ligaments, 667–668, 671–672
    with tendons, 694–695, 697, 699–701, 704, 706
  from running, 1017–1019
  tendons, 687–708
instability of
  ligament mechanisms, 39–40, 40*f*, 42, 47–48, 626–634
  meniscus mechanisms of, 635–636
  patellofemoral joint mechanisms, 638–639
  tests for, 614*f*–620*f*, 615–616
ligaments of. *See also specific ligament*
  anatomy of, 39, 41, 625–626, 645, 663–664, 664*f*
  biomechanics of, 624–634, 765–767
  combined injuries of. *See* Knee, multiligament injuries of
  failure factors of, 39–40, 40*f*, 42, 47–48, 626, 743
  functional tests of, 614–616, 614*f*–616*f*
  grafts for, 47–48, 48*f*, 629–633, 682–685, 750–751
  immaturity injuries of, 743, 748, 753–754

reconstruction complications with, 825–830, 826*f*–830*f*
load displacement of, 624–626
  by cruciate ligaments, 626–633
  by medial and lateral collateral ligaments, 633–634
load impact in, on tendons, 687–688, 700
magnetic resonance imaging of, 621
  chondral and osteochondral injuries, 104–105, 105*f*–106*f*
  ligamentous injuries, 102, 103*f*–104*f*, 104, 598
  meniscal injuries, 102, 102*f*–103*f*, 617, 652
meniscus of. *See* Meniscus
modeling approaches for, 624, 638
multiligament injuries of. *See also specific ligaments*
  anatomical perspectives, 805–806
  with anterior cruciate, 744–745, 744*t*, 754–755, 780
  biomechanical perspectives, 806–808
  bony injuries with, 809–811
  classification of, 808
  definition of, 805
  emergency care of, 809
  evaluation of, 809–811
  incidence of, 808
  instability measurements for, 807–808, 811
  mechanisms of, 44, 634, 808
  with medial collateral, 663, 672–673, 744, 754, 766, 771–772, 776–778
  nerve injuries with, 809–811
  operative repair of
    anterior cruciate reconstruction, 815
    approach for, 813
    grafts for, 812–813
    indications for, 807, 809, 811–812
    lateral side techniques, 813–814
    medial side techniques, 814
    posterior cruciate reconstruction, 814–815
    ten-step order for, 815, 815*f*
    timing of, 809, 812
  with posterior cruciate, 763, 771–772, 771*f*, 774, 776–778, 780
  posterolateral mechanisms, 675, 679, 681, 685, 771–772, 771*f*
  preoperative evaluation of, 812
  reduction maneuvers for, 809–810
  rehabilitation of, 815
  vascular injuries with, 809–810, 812
osteotomies of
  degenerative indications for, 856–857
  distal varus, 857
  proximal tibial, 857
patellar extension of. *See* Patellofemoral joint
PCL-deficient. *See* Posterior cruciate ligament
physical examination of. *See also specific anatomy*
  central pivot tests for, 614–616, 614*f*
  conduct of, 613–614
  imaging studies for, 617, 621
  philosophy of, 613, 621–622
  secondary restraint comparisons in, 616–620, 616*f*–620*f*
range of motion of
  degrees of freedom of, 44–45, 45*f*, 623
  with exercise, 628–629
  meniscus function in, 647–648
  tests of, 615–616, 615*f*–616*f*
reconstruction of
  grafts for, 630–633, 672, 682–685, 701–704
  kinematic measurements of, 45–46, 46*f*, 627–628
  ligament component. *See specific ligament*
  for osteoarthritis, 795, 802*f*, 855–858
  patellar tendon, 701–706, 702*f*–703*f*
  patellofemoral component, 638–639
  rehabilitation programs for, 667–672, 668*f*–670*f*, 668*t*
    of articular cartilage, 793, 800–801
    ligament injuries, 628–630, 638, 673, 815. *See also specific ligament*
    meniscus repair, 657–658, 658*t*

patellofemoral injuries, 721, 723–724, 728–729, 731, 733, 735–736
tendon injuries, 692–697, 699, 701, 704–706
rotation mechanisms of
    with anterior cruciate ligament reconstructions, 44–45, 45f
    ligament role in, 623, 625–634, 647, 765–767
    with multiligament reconstructions, 807–808
    with posterior cruciate ligament reconstructions, 763–767, 764f, 769–775, 769f
    tests for, 615–617
stability of
    ligament role in, 625–626, 765–767
        cruciates, 626–633, 763–766
        medial and lateral collateral, 633–634, 766
    meniscus role in, 635–636, 647–648
    patellofemoral joint role in, 638–639
    posterolateral mechanisms, 805–808. See also Posterolateral knee
    posteromedial mechanisms, 806–807. See also Posteromedial knee
surgical complications of
    with ligament reconstruction, 825–830, 826f–830f
    with meniscal procedures, 830–833
    patellar entrapment as, 829, 833, 837–839, 838f
    with patellofemoral procedures, 833–837, 836f–837f
tendons of. See also specific tendon
    age-related changes in, 687, 689, 700
    anatomy of, 687
    healing processes of, 689–691
    immaturity injuries of, 689, 705–706
    injuries of, 691–705
    injury mechanisms of, 688–689
    mechanical load effect on, 687–688
    metabolic disorders affecting, 688
    rehabilitation programs for, 692–697, 699, 701, 704–706
total replacement of, indications for, 795, 802f, 855–858
translation mechanisms of, 623, 647
    with anterior cruciate ligament reconstructions, 44–45, 45f
    ligament role in, 625–634, 763, 765–766
    with multiligament reconstructions, 807–808
    with posterior cruciate ligament reconstructions, 765–766
    tests for, 615–616
transplantation techniques for, 796–797, 796f–798f, 856
treatment decisions for, conceptual perspectives of, 621–622
Knick deformation, of collagen fibrils, 33
Knot of Henry, in foot injuries, 899, 920, 961
    of tendons, 983, 985, 987–988
Krackow technique, for knee ligament repairs, 673
KT-100 measurement. See Arthrometer measurements
K-wires. See Kirschner wire fixation
Kyphosis. See Spine

L

Labrum
    of glenoid. See Glenoid labrum
    of hip, magnetic resonance imaging of, 113
    of shoulder. See also Glenoid labrum
        anatomy of, 348–351, 349f–350f
        magnetic resonance imaging of, 108–110, 109f
        stability significance of, 108
Lacerations, of hand tendons
    extensor considerations, 248–252, 249f, 251f
    flexor considerations, 248, 252–254, 253f–254f
Lachman test
    for knee stability, 614–615, 624, 628, 696, 850, 865
        with ligament injuries, 680, 745–746, 746f
    for shoulder assessment, with labral tear injuries, 466, 466f

Lacing alternatives, for foot injuries, 912, 912f, 919, 959
Lactate dehydrogenase (LDH), in tendon cell metabolism, 28–29
Lacunae, in bone, 76f–77f, 77
Laminectomy, posterior cervical, indications for, 164
Laminin, in tendons, 25, 28
Lapidus procedure, for toe deformities, 953
Laser chondroplasty, for knee repair, 795–796, 795f–796f
Laser-induced osteonecrosis, post-knee repair, 796, 832
Laser stimulation therapy, for knee tendon injuries, 690
Lateral collateral ligament (LCL), of elbow, injuries of, 311, 324–325, 324f
Lateral collateral ligament (LCL), of knee
    anatomy of, 676, 805–806
    biomechanics of, 676, 766, 806–808
    injuries of
        magnetic resonance imaging of, 102
        mechanisms of, 679–680, 771
        surgical repair of, 682, 684, 776–778, 813
        physical examination of, 616–617, 616f–617f, 680
        stability role of, 627, 633–634, 676, 883
Lateral patellar pressure syndrome
    clinical evaluation of, 722–723, 722f
    natural history of, 722, 737
    rehabilitation programs for, 723–724
    treatment of
        nonoperative, 723
        operative, 723–724, 724f, 737, 739, 740t
Lateral patellofemoral angle, measurement of, 718, 719f, 735
Lateral scapular slide. See Scapular slide
Lateral slide test, of scapular strength, 504–505, 504f, 505t, 508–509
Latissimus dorsi muscle
    anatomy of, 359
    golf swing role of, 394, 564
    overhead throwing role of, 553–555, 553f, 557
    swimming stroke role of, 560–561
Laxity tests. See Ligament laxity tests
LDH. See Lactate dehydrogenase
Leg. See also Thigh
    anatomy of
        compartmental, 87, 879, 879f
        nerve supply, 879, 879f, 1007
        tendons, 979, 987, 991–992, 991f, 1000, 1007
    ankle injuries impact on, 872, 879, 883, 887
    compartment syndromes of
        clinical evaluation of, 879–881, 880f, 881t
        fasciotomy indications for, 879–880, 881t, 882, 886
        fasciotomy techniques for, 881–882, 882f
        pathogenesis, 89, 91, 94, 879
        pressure measurements with, 880–882, 880f, 881t
        in thigh, 604–606, 605f
    entrapment syndromes of
        nerves, 885–886
        popliteal artery, 886–887, 886f
    fractures of
        associated injuries with, 869, 875
        incidence of, 874–875
        stress, 871–874, 871f–874f, 887, 1020
    medial gastrocnemius injury of, 888–889, 888f
    return to sport guidelines, 872–874, 882, 887–889
    running injuries in, 869, 871, 873, 875–876, 886, 889, 1016
    shin splints of. See Medial tibial stress syndrome
    stress fractures of
        clinical evaluation of, 869–870
        epidemiology of, 869
        fibular distal, 873–874, 873f–874f, 887
        fibular proximal, 874
        imaging studies of, 870–871, 870f, 870t–871t
        medial malleolus, 872–873, 873f

pathogenesis of, 869, 887
return to sport guidelines, 872–874
    from running, 1020–1021
    tibial anterior cortex, 872, 872f
    tibial shaft, 871–872, 871f
    treatment of, 871
tendons of. See also specific anatomy or tendon
    anatomy of, 979, 987, 991–992, 991f, 1000, 1007
    anterior injuries of, 1007–1008
    posterior injuries of. See Achilles tendon; Posterior tibial tendon
    surgery preferences for, 1008
tibiofibular injuries of
    proximal instability of, 882–885, 884f
    synostosis, 887–888, 888f
venous thrombosis of, 76, 91, 758, 889
Legg Calve Perthes disease, 230
Length-tension relationship, of muscle contractions, 10–13, 11f, 12t, 14f
Levator scapulae muscle
    anatomy of, 357
    golf swing role of, 564
    overhead throwing role of, 552–553, 553f
Lidocaine injection. See Nerve blocks
Life-table methods, in research studies, 140
Lift-off test, for rotator cuff injuries, 482, 482f
Ligament cutting studies
    of glenohumeral ligaments, 382–385
    of knee ligaments, 624–625, 627, 633, 678, 765, 807
Ligament grafts
    for acromioclavicular joint repair, 523–525, 530–531, 531f
    in knee
        complications of, 825–829, 826f–830f
        techniques for. See specific ligament
    for quadriceps tendon rupture repair, 600
Ligament laxity tests
    for ankle instability, 820, 823
    for knee instability, 616–617, 626–627, 776, 780
        with multiligament injuries, 807–808, 811
        with reconstruction, 629–633, 749, 781
    for shoulder instability, 420–421, 466
    volar plates and, 250, 257
Ligament of Humphrey (anterior meniscofemoral ligament), 645, 764f, 765
Ligament of Wrisberg (posterior meniscofemoral ligament), 645, 767
Ligaments. See also specific joint or ligament
    anatomy of, 39, 41
    collagen organization in, 39, 43
    failure of
        factors of, 39–40, 40f, 42, 626
        post-reconstruction, 47–48, 858
    fatigue of, stress relaxation impact on, 42
    function of, 39
    grafts for
        autografts versus allografts, 44, 47–48
        tensile considerations for, 41–42
    healing of
        enhancement of, 44, 667
        potential of, 43–44, 48–49
        scarring with, 757f, 758, 820
    injuries of
        combined versus isolated, 44
        immobilization impact on, 666–667
    reconstruction of, future directions of, 48–49
    remodeling activity of, 667
    sprain processes of, 820
    strain theories for, 40f, 41–43
    tensile properties of
        bone-ligament-bone complex, 39–41, 40f
        homeostasis, 41, 41f
        homogeneity, 41
        parameters for, 39–40, 40f
        strain rate effect, 41
        viscoelasticity and, 41–43, 42f
Lipids, in articular cartilage, 54t, 55
Lipomas, of thigh, 607
Liposarcoma, of thigh, 607

Lisfranc's joint, injuries of
  clinical evaluation of, 908, 909f
  degenerative changes with, 908, 911
  dislocations with, 907–908, 910f–911f, 920
  Hardcastle classification of, 907–909, 908f
  mechanisms of, 906f–907f, 907–908
  nonoperative treatment of, 908–911
  operative treatment of, 908–909, 911f
Lisfranc's ligament
  anatomy of, 893, 894f
  in joint injuries, 907, 909, 910f
Lisfranc's stress test
  for forefoot injuries, 959
  for midfoot injuries, 908, 909f
Lister's tubercle, in wrist injury mechanisms, 261, 283–284
Literature review, critical evaluation of, 121–122, 122f
Lithotripsy, for elbow tendinosis, 295
Little league elbow, 307, 319–320, 319f–320f
Load
  articular cartilage response to, 54–55, 57–64, 58f, 61t, 66
    with injury mechanisms, 789–791, 789f–790f
  axial. See Axial load
  bone response to, 77, 80–81
  exercise applications of. See Strength training
  foot injuries from, 923–924, 923f, 945, 955, 959
  head and neck responses to, 159, 163, 165, 168, 168f, 170–174, 173f
  hip injuries from, 572, 574, 578
  injuries from, 34–35. See also specific anatomy or injury
  knee responses to
    with functional bracing, 793, 863–867
    ligament mechanisms, 624–628, 632–634, 766–767
    meniscus mechanisms, 634–636, 647–648
    osteoarthritic, 847–849, 852, 854, 856
    patellofemoral joint mechanisms
    tendon mechanisms, 687–689, 700
  leg responses to
    shin splints as, 875
    stress fractures as, 869, 874, 887
  ligament response to, 39–43, 40f–42f
    post-graft reconstruction, 47–48, 48f
    in thumb articulations, 244
  muscle response to, 3, 12, 12f
  oppositional. See Shear load
  pelvic injuries from, 216–217
  in running cycle, 1012–1013, 1016–1017
  shoulder responses to, 357, 359, 367, 372–373, 403, 403f, 420, 433–435
  spinal injuries from
    cervical. See Axial load injuries
    lumbar, 209
  as stretching. See Tensile load
  tendon response to, 25, 31–35, 33f, 34–35
  tibiofemoral joint response to, 623–624, 627, 634–635
  toe responses to, 968–969, 968f
  valgus versus varus. See Valgus loading; Varus loading
Load and shift test. See Axial load test
Load-elongation curve
  of knee, 625–626
  of ligaments, 39–40, 40f, 42, 42f
Loading-unloading curve, cyclic
  of bone, 80
  of ligaments, 42, 42f
Load sensors, implantable telemeterized, for patellofemoral joint, 639
Load-transmission, as menisci function, 634–636
Load transmission, by knee meniscus, 634–635, 648
Local anesthetic blocks. See Nerve blocks
Locked posterior dislocation (LPD), of shoulder
  injury mechanisms of, 413–415, 419
  treatment of, 422–427
Log rank test, in research studies, 141
Log rolling procedure, 154
Long bones
  circulatory system of, 78
  growth processes of, 80–82

clavicle variation of, 329–330
structure of, 75, 77
Longitudinal muscles, physiologic principles of, 6–7, 7f
Lordosis. See Spine
Low back pain. See Acute low back pain
Lower extremities
  compartment syndromes in, 87–89, 88f, 90, 835
  injuries of. See specific anatomy
  muscle architecture of, 7–8, 8f
Low-intensity exercise, bone adaptation to, 80, 81f, 83f
LPD. See Locked posterior dislocation
LT. See Lunotriquetral ligament
Lubrication, for tendons, 22–23
Lumbar spine
  fusions of, spondylolisthesis indications for, 212
  injuries of
    acute pain syndrome, 203–205
    fractures and dislocations of, acute, 205
    herniated disks, 205–209, 206f, 208f
    imaging techniques for, 204, 206–207, 208f, 210–211, 212f
    referred hip pain from, 571–572, 572t
    return to sport guidelines, 203–207
    soft tissue, 203, 205, 208
    spondylolisthesis, 209–213, 210f, 212f
    spondylolysis, 209–213, 212f
    treatment considerations, 203–205, 207, 211–212
  lordosis of
    with pitching, 557, 559f
    from scapula fractures, 503
Lumbosacral corset, 205
Lunate fractures, 269–270
Lunotriquetral ligament (LT), injuries of, 274, 279–280, 279f–280f
Lymphocytes, in healing process, 43
Lymphoma, malignant, of femur, 607
Lysosomes, in tendon cells, 27, 29
Lytic pars defect, spondylolisthesis from, 209–212

M

Magnetic resonance arthroscopy
  of elbow, 114, 114f, 311
  of knee, 104–105
  of shoulder, 105–106, 108–110, 109f, 421, 468
Magnetic resonance imaging (MRI)
  of ankle, 110–112, 110f–112f, 141, 142f
    impingement syndromes, 821, 821t, 823
  for anterior shoulder instability, 404–406, 405f
  for brachial plexus injuries, 193–194
  of burner syndrome, 187–188
  for compartment syndromes, 89, 92
  of elbow, 113–115, 114f–115f
    for injury evaluation, 311, 313, 319, 321
  of foot, 110–112, 110f–112f
    for hindfoot injuries, 902, 926, 929, 931, 935, 937, 939
    for midfoot injuries, 902, 904–905, 914, 916
  of hand, 115–116, 116f
  for head injuries, 155–156, 159–160
  of heel pain, 929–931, 935, 937
  of hip, 112–113, 113f
    for injury evaluation, 573–575, 573f
  impact in sports medicine, 99
  of knee, 102–105, 102f–106f, 720
    for injury evaluation, 617, 621, 652, 792, 851
    for ligament injuries, 666, 681, 747–748, 748f
    for tendon injuries, 692, 695, 697, 699–701
  for leg injuries
    miscellaneous, 877, 888, 888f
    stress fractures, 870, 870f, 871t, 1020–1021
  for lumbar spine injuries, 204, 206
  of muscle injuries, 113f, 116–117, 117f, 594
    hamstring strains, 587, 589, 589f–590f, 592
    quadriceps, 597, 599–600
  for neck injuries, 155–156, 161, 163
  of pelvis, 112–113, 113f, 216
    for groin pain, 225–227, 226f, 595
  physics of, 100–102, 100t

pulse sequencing options for, 101–102
  for rotator cuff injuries, 484, 484f
  of running injuries, 1017
  safety of, 99–100
  of scaphoid fractures, 116, 261, 263
  of shoulder, 105–110, 107f–109f
    for anterior instability, 404–406, 405f
    for labral injuries, 443–445, 444f, 467–468, 469f
    for posterior instability, 421
  signal intensity of tissues, 100–101, 100t
  of stress fractures. See Stress fractures
  of tendon injuries, 116–117, 117f
    Achilles dysfunction, 981
    flexor hallucis longus, 988–989
    peroneus tendon, 995
    posterior tibial tendon, 1003
  terminology of, 100–102
  for thigh injuries, 587, 589, 594, 597–604
  of ulnar collateral ligament, 116, 116f, 317, 317f
  of wrist, 115–116, 116f
    for injury evaluation, 277, 280–281, 281f
Magnuson-Stack procedure, in anterior shoulder dislocations, 407
Magnuson-type debridement, for knee degeneration, 855
Major histocompatibility complex (MHC), muscle fiber typing with, 15f, 16
Malleolus ligaments, in ankle sprains, 819–820
Mallet finger, 249–250
Mallet fractures, of distal phalanx, 235, 236f, 249
Mallet toe, 973–974
Manganese, in musculoskeletal metabolism, 28
Mankin grading scheme, for osteoarthritis, 65
Mann-Whitney U test, in research studies, 139
Manual motor testing. See Strength deficits
Maquet anteriorization procedure, for patellofemoral arthritis, 735–736, 736f, 739, 740t
  complications of, 834–835
Martin-Grueber anastomosis, median nerve pathology with, 549
Masking, in research sampling, 129–130, 132
Mass, in shoulder function, 502–503, 503t
Massage therapy
  for athletic pubalgia, 223
  for knee tendon injuries, 695, 699
  for lumbar spine injuries, 204
Mathematical models, of knee biomechanics, 624, 638
Matrix molecules
  adhesive, 28
  in articular cartilage, 54–55, 54t, 66
  in knee meniscus, 645–647
  in tendons, 25–28, 30, 690
Maximal voluntary isometric contraction (MVIC), with pitching motion, 459–460
Maximum oxygen capacity, bone formation and, 83, 83f
Mayfield spiral injury, of lunotriquetral ligament, 279, 279f
M band, in sarcomeres, 5, 5f, 11
McBride arthroplasty, for forefoot injuries, 946, 957
McBryde classification, of metatarsal stress fractures, 946
MCL. See Medial collateral ligament
McMurray test, for knee injuries, 651f, 652, 850
McVay procedure, for hernia repair, 227
Mean, in research studies, 135
Mechanical loading. See Load
Mechanoreceptors, role of, 31, 334, 350
Medial collateral ligament (MCL), of elbow
  injuries of
    magnetic resonance imaging of, 114, 114f
    mechanisms of, 289, 291–293, 291f
    resection and repair of, 302–304, 303f, 814
    overhead throwing role of, 554, 554f, 559f
Medial collateral ligament (MCL), of knee
  anatomy of, 39, 663–664, 664f
  physical examination of, 616–617, 616f–617f
  rehabilitation programs for
    expected outcome of, 671–672
    with nonoperative treatment, 667–672, 668f–669f, 668t

phase III of, 667, 668t, 670–671
phase II of, 667, 668t, 670, 670f
phase I of, 667–671, 668f–669f, 668t
postoperative, 673
stability role of, 41, 626, 633–634, 806
superficial, 663, 664f, 673
tear injuries of
classification of, 665–666, 671–672
clinical evaluation of, 664–666, 664f–665f
combined, 663. See also Knee, multiligament
injuries of
combined, with anterior cruciate ligament, 44,
634, 672–673, 744, 754
combined, with posterior cruciate ligament,
766, 768, 771–772, 776–778, 780
healing potential of, 43–44, 633–634
imaging studies of, 102, 103f, 666
immobilization impact on repair of, 41
mechanisms of, 663–664, 664f, 768
nonoperative treatment of, 666–672,
667f–670f, 668t
operative treatment of, 671–673, 780
return to sport guidelines, 667–668, 671–672
Medialization procedures, for patellofemoral joint
with arthritis, 736–737, 739, 740t
with dislocations, 733–734, 733f
Medial malleolus, stress fractures of, 872–873,
873f
Medial retinacular complex, knee injuries of, magnetic resonance imaging of, 102, 104, 104f
Medial tibial stress syndrome (MTSS)
biomechanics of, 876, 1013
chronic, 876–879
clinical evaluation, 876–877
compartment syndrome versus, 875, 877
differential diagnosis of, 875, 877, 887, 1021
epidemiology of, 875
imaging studies of, 870, 870f, 870t, 875, 877
pathoanatomy of, 875–876, 876f
pathogenesis of, 875, 972, 1021
treatment of
conservative, 877–879, 878f
fasciotomy indications, 878–879
Median, in research studies, 135
Mediastinum, compression of, with sternoclavicular dislocations, 539–540
Medical team, emergency care responsibilities of,
153–156, 155f
Membrane components
of muscle contraction, 6, 10, 10f
per muscle fiber types, 18
Meniscectomy
arthroscopic, indications for, 652, 848
biomechanical impact of, 634–636, 648
complete
functional impact of, 634–636
indications for, 652, 658
complications of, 832–833, 848
lateral, 635–636
medial, 635
partial
functional impact of, 635–636, 648
indications for, 652–653, 658
rehabilitation program for, 657–658, 658t
Meniscofemoral ligaments, knee articulations of,
645, 764f–765f, 765, 767
Meniscoid lesions, in ankle sprains, 819–820
Meniscus, of knee
anatomy of
gross, 645, 646f
ultrastructure, 645–647, 646f–647f
vascular, 648–649, 648f
arthroscopic repair of
all-inside technique, 655, 655f–657f, 831
indications for, 635, 652
inside-out technique, 653–654, 654f, 656, 831
outside-in technique, 654–655, 654f
tack fixation technique, 655, 657f
T-fix system for, 655, 656f
biomechanics of, 634–636
collagen fiber in, 645–647, 646f–647f
degenerative changes in, 63, 617, 618f, 790, 848
post-repair, 830, 832–833
discoid, vulnerability of, 651

functions of
anatomical basis of, 646–647, 647f
load transmission as, 634–636, 648
stability as, 635–636, 647–648
as graft, for ligament repair, 658–659, 777–778
healing processes of, 649–650, 649f, 658–659
fibrin clot injections for, 649–650, 657–658,
657f
vascularity factor in, 649–650, 653, 657,
830–831
physical examination of, 614, 617–619, 618t
repair of. See also Meniscectomy
arthroscopic, 635, 652–656, 654f–657f, 658,
831
complications of, 658, 790, 830–833
excision versus, 652–653
open, 652–653, 658
rehabilitation program for, 657–658, 658t, 833
suture considerations for, 653, 656–657
vascular versus avascular, 649–650, 653, 657
synovial fringe of, 648–650, 648f
tear injuries of
with anterior cruciate ligament tears, 651,
653, 744–745, 744t, 747, 753–755
classification of, 650f, 651, 744
clinical evaluation of, 651–652, 651f–652f
epidemiology of, 650
magnetic resonance imaging of, 102,
102f–103f, 617, 652
mechanisms of, 650–651, 653
treatment of, 635, 652–658, 654f–657f
treatment options for, 635, 652
vascular classifications of, 649, 657
transplantation of, 658–659, 831, 833
Menstrual disorders
athletic pubalgia and, 215, 225
lower extremity injuries and, 869, 920, 946, 959,
1020
Merchant's axial view, of patellofemoral joint,
718, 719f, 725, 728, 735
Mesenchymal syndrome, 291
Mesotenon, of tendons, 22, 30
Meta-analysis, as research design, 124f, 126, 130
Metabolic disorders
in knee pathology, 688, 847
leg stress fractures from, 869, 871
Metabolism
in articular cartilage, 61–63
per muscle fiber types, 17–18, 18t
in tendon cells, 28–29, 29f
Metacarpal fractures, implant selection for,
233–235, 234f
Metacarpophalangeal joint (MP)
dislocations of, 248
injury mechanisms of. See also Fingers
extensor tendon, 252
flexor tendon, 253–254, 254f
ligament, 244, 245f, 246, 248
stability importance of, 238, 243–244, 249, 251
Metalloproteinases (MMPs), articular cartilage
degradation by, 62, 66, 855
Metastatic disease, of femur, 607
Metatarsalgia, 953–954
Metatarsals
bony hypertrophy of, 959
dance injuries in. See Dancers
deformities of, primus varus, 953
dislocations of, 966–968, 967f
fractures of
acute, 947, 961, 966, 1021
stress, 902, 903f, 945–947, 947f, 959, 966
head of, avascular necrosis of. See Freiberg's infraction
osteotomy indications for, 952–954, 974
stress fractures of
classification of, 946
evaluation of, 946–947, 947f
mechanisms of, 902, 903f, 945–947, 947f, 959,
966
risk factors for, 945–946, 959–960
treatment of, 947
Metatarsal squeeze test, for Lisfranc's joint injuries, 908, 909f

Metatarsophalangeal joint (MP, MTP). See also
Toes
anatomy of, 949–950, 949f, 969, 969f
biomechanics of, 949–950, 954, 968–969
deformities of
bunion, 971f, 972
cavus, 945–946, 953, 973
claw, 972–973, 973f
corns, 976
hallux rigidus, 970, 971f, 972
hallux valgus, 946, 951–953, 971f, 972
hammer, 973
intractable plantar keratosis, 974
joint synovitis, 948–949, 949f, 975–976,
975f–976f
mallet, 973–974
metatarsus primus varus, 953
dislocations of, 966–968, 967f
classifications of, 952, 954, 955f
of first joint, 951–952, 952f
sesamoid complex and, 951–952, 954, 955f
first joint
dislocations of, 951–952, 952f
functional anatomy of, 949–950, 949f
flexor hallucis longus tendon stenosing tenosynovitis of, 961–962, 989–990
infractions of, 953–954, 960, 960t
injuries of
dislocations, 951–952, 966–968
infractions, 953–954, 960, 960t
sprains, 968–970, 968f–970f
turf toe, 949–950, 968–970
instability of
second joint, 952
tests for, 975–976, 975f
interdigital neuromas of, 957–958, 974–975,
975f
metatarsal fractures and, 946
metatarsalgia syndrome of, 953–954
osteotomy indications for, 953
range of motion of, 949–950, 954
sprain injuries of, 968–970, 968f–970f
stability mechanisms of, 949
synovitis of
clinical evaluation of, 948, 948f, 975–976,
975f
incidence of, 975
nonoperative treatment of, 948, 976
surgical treatment of, 948–949, 949f, 976, 976f
Metatarsophalangeal ligament, 949, 949f, 954
Metatarsosesamoid ligament, 949, 949f
Methylprednisolone
for knee degeneration, 853–854
for spinal cord injuries, 156, 165, 180
MGHL. See Middle glenohumeral ligament
MHC. See Major histocompatibility complex
Microcapillary infusion technique, for compartmental pressures, 92–93
Microfracture
as forefoot injury, 945
as knee cartilage repair technique, 794–795,
800, 855
Microinstability injuries, of shoulder, 344,
457–475
Microtrauma, repetitive. See Overuse injuries
Microvascular occlusion, compartment syndromes
from, 87–89, 88f
Middle glenohumeral ligament (MGHL)
in anterior shoulder stability, 400–401
in contact injuries, 433–434, 433f–434f
functional anatomy of, 345–347, 347f–348f,
382f, 383
in posterior shoulder stability, 417–418, 417f
in throwing injuries, 390–391
Midfoot. See also specific anatomy
anatomy of
bones and ligaments, 893, 894f–895f
neurovascular, 895–896, 896f
arthritis of, 911–912, 911f–912f, 919
arthrodesis indications for, 909, 912
bony arches of, 893, 894f, 1000
support for, 913, 913f
compression neuropathy of, 920
deformities of

Midfoot. *See also specific anatomy (contd.)*
  cavus, 945–946, 953, 973
  flat. *See* Pes planus
  fractures
    avulsion, 909
    dislocations with, 907–909, 908f, 910f–911f, 913
    stress, 903–906, 903f–906f
  in gait cycle. *See* Foot pronation; Foot supination
  impingement syndromes of, 907, 907f, 911, 918–920, 918f–919f
  injuries of
    bone scans of, 902, 904, 908, 916
    computed tomography of, 905–906, 908, 911
    cortisone injections for, 911, 914, 917, 919
    diagnostic strategies for, 901–902
    differential diagnosis of, 899–901
    fractures and dislocations of, 902–909, 903f–906f, 908f, 910f–911f, 913
    immobilization of, 904, 906, 911, 913, 917, 920
    internal fixation, 902, 906, 906f, 909, 912f
    of Lisfranc's joint, 906f–911f, 907–911
    magnetic resonance imaging of, 902, 904–905, 914, 916
    nerve blocks for, 902, 911, 914, 919–920
    neurovascular, 902, 911, 918–920, 918f–919f
    nonoperative treatment for, 902, 904, 910–914, 917, 919
    operative treatment for, 902, 906, 908–909, 912–913, 915, 917, 919
    orthotics for, 909–911, 913–915, 913f, 917, 919
    padding devices for, 912–913, 912f–913f, 915f, 919, 919f
    physical therapy for, 903, 909–912, 914–915, 917
    radiography of, 902, 904–905, 908, 911–914, 916
    return to sport guidelines, 92, 906, 914, 917, 920
    shoe modifications for, 911–914, 912f–913f, 915f, 917, 919, 919f
  neurovascular injuries of, 918–920, 918f–919f
  osteotomy indications for, 973
  pain syndromes in, 899–901
    accessory navicular, 914–917, 915f–918f
    os peroneum, 916–917, 917f–918f
    pes planus, 912–914, 913f
  range of motion of, 893, 894f
  rehabilitation programs for, 902, 909–912, 914–915, 917, 919
  stability mechanisms of, 893, 894f
  stress fractures of
    cuboid, 904, 904f
    mechanisms of, 902
    metatarsals, 902, 903f
    tarsal navicular, 904–907, 904f–906f, 1021
Mineralization, of bone, 78–79, 78f–79f
  exercise impact on, 80–83
Minerals, for musculoskeletal metabolism, 28
Mitochondria, in tendon cells, 29–30
MMPs. *See* Metalloproteinases
MO. *See* Myositis ossificans
Mobility deficits. *See also* Gait analysis
  with lumbar spine injuries, 203–204
Mobilization, as ligament injury treatment, 41, 43
Mode, in research studies, 135
Moire topographic analysis, of scapular position, 505
Monocytic cells, in healing process, 43
Morton foot, metatarsal fractures and, 945–946
Morton's bar, for sesamoid injuries, 957
Morton's extension insole, for toe injuries, 917, 970, 970f, 972
Mosaicoplasty, in joint reconstructions, 321, 798
Motor evoked potentials, for brachial plexus injuries, 193–194
Motor ganglia, of spinal nerves, in brachial plexus, 185–186, 185f, 191
MP. *See* Metacarpophalangeal joint; Metatarsophalangeal joint

MRI. *See* Magnetic resonance imaging
MTJ. *See* Myotendinous junction
MTP. *See* Metatarsophalangeal joint
MTSS. *See* Medial tibial stress syndrome
Multipennate muscles, physiologic principles of, 7, 7f
Muscle contractions
  actin regulation of, 4–6, 5f
  concentric, 12–13, 12f
  contractile protein hierarchy for, 4–5, 5f
  cytoskeleton proteins for, 5–6
  eccentric, 12f, 13, 35
  fused, 10
  isometric. *See* Isometric muscle contractions
  length-tension relationships of, 4–5, 5f, 7, 10–13, 11f, 14f
  mechanical properties of, 3, 7–8, 8f–9f, 13
    active length-tension relationship, 10–11, 11f
    architecture impact on, 13, 14f
    force-velocity relationship, 12–13, 12f, 14f
    passive length-tension relationship, 11–12, 11f, 12t
  membrane activation of, 6, 10, 10f
  myosin role in, 4–5
  neural activation of, 9–10, 10f
  physiologic cross-sectional area impact on, 7–8, 8f–9f, 13
  temporal summation of, 10, 10f
  tendon relationship with, 32, 34
  tetanic, 10–11, 10f–11f
  velocity-force relationships of, 3, 7–8, 8f–9f, 12–13, 12f, 14f
Muscle endurance, 17, 1023
Muscle fatigue
  physiologic principles of, 9, 17
  as strain injury component, 586, 588, 590, 597
Muscle fiber bundles
  functional anatomy of, 3–4, 4f–5f
  strain gage analysis of, in knee, 624–625, 628–630, 633
Muscle fibers
  cell structure of, 3–6, 4f–5f
  compartment syndrome impact on, 87, 88f
  fast, 5, 7, 13–14, 16–17
  macroscopic arrangement of, 6–9, 7f–9f
  slow, 5, 7, 13–14, 17
  tendon relationship with, 32, 34
  types of
    histochemical, 13–16, 15f, 16t
    morphologic properties of, 17–18, 18t
    physiologic properties of, 16–17
    size relationship with, 16, 16f
Muscle fiber typing
  by ATPase histochemistry, 13–14, 15f, 16, 16t
  by combined histochemistry, 13–14, 15f, 16t
  fiber size relationship with, 16, 16f
  by immunohistochemistry, 15f, 16
Muscle hypertension syndrome, compartment syndrome versus, 94
Muscle hypertrophy, 3, 116, 420
Muscle infarction, in thigh, 606
Muscle length
  contraction relationship with, 3, 7–8, 8f–9f, 10–13, 11f, 14f
  term definitions for, 11–12, 12t
Muscle mass, tension relationship to, 7
Muscle relaxation, physiologic principles of, 10, 10f
Muscles. *See also specific muscle or tendon*
  of abdominal wall, 218
  atrophy of, magnetic resonance imaging of, 116
  brachial plexus injuries impact on, 161–163, 187, 191, 194–196
  of hip, adduction, 218, 224–225, 224f, 228–229
  lumbar spine injuries impact on, 203–204, 206, 206t
  magnetic resonance imaging intensity for, 100–101, 100t
  of pelvis, 223, 224f, 226
  physiologic types of, 6–7, 7f, 13, 16–17
  rupture injuries of
    compartment syndromes from, 89–90

magnetic resonance imaging, 113f, 116–117, 117f
  skeletal. *See* Skeletal muscle
Muscle spasms
  abdominal adductor, 218–219
  with lumbar spine injuries, 203–204
Muscle strain injuries. *See also specific muscle*
  of abdominal wall, 218
  of groin muscles, 593–596, 596t
  of hamstrings, 587–593, 588f–592f, 589t
  hematomas with, 588, 588f, 592, 597
  imaging studies of, 587
  of lower back, 203
  muscle-tendon units in, 24, 24f, 33–34
    of knee, 679, 688–689, 696
    of thigh, 586, 586f, 593
  pathophysiology of, 586–587, 586f
  of quadriceps, 596–603, 599f–600f, 601t
  RICE treatment for, 587, 589, 591, 594–595, 597
  risk factors for, 585–587
  of thigh adductors, 593–596, 596t
  treatment strategies for, 587
Muscle-tendon units
  anatomy and physiology of, 25–27, 25f–26f
  biomechanical functions of, 31, 33
  stress-strain curve of, 24, 24f, 33–34, 33f
    in knee injuries, 679, 688–689, 696, 705
    in thigh injuries, 586, 586f, 593
Muscle tension
  active length relationship of, 10–11, 11f
  passive length relationship of, 11–12, 12t
  physiologic principles of, 4–5, 5f, 7, 17
  tendon response to, 32
Muscle transfers
  for acromioclavicular joint repair, 524
  for long thoracic nerve injuries, 544
  for tarsal coalition, 929
Muscle viability tests, with compartment syndromes, 94
Muscular dystrophies, 6, 606–607
Musculotendinous junction. *See* Myotendinous junction
MVIC. *See* Maximal voluntary isometric contraction
Myelography, for brachial plexus injuries, 193
Myofibrils
  anatomy and physiology of, 4, 5f
  mechanical properties of, 10–13, 11f–12f, 12t
Myopathies, inflammatory, of thigh, 606–607
Myosin
  in excitation-contraction coupling, 9–11, 10f–11f
  as muscle motor, 4–5
Myositis ossificans (MO), 230, 603
Myotendinous junction (MTJ)
  anatomy and physiology of, 21, 25–26, 25f–26f
  blood supply to, 30–31
  functional considerations of, 26, 32, 34
  strains of
    in abdominal wall, 218
    in groin, 220, 223, 230

N
Nail bed injuries, with phalanx injuries, 235–236, 966
National Athletic Association, helmet removal guidelines of, 155, 155f
Natural remedies, for knee degeneration, 852
Navicular injuries. *See* Tarsal navicular
Naviculocapitate syndrome, 271–272
Naviculocuboid joint, anatomy of, 893, 894f
Naviculocuneiform joints
  anatomy of, 893, 894f
  injuries of, 908, 918, 920
Neck injuries. *See* Cervical spine
Neck rolls, for brachial plexus injuries, 195
Needle electrode examination, for neck injuries, 162
Neer classification, of clavicle fractures, 535–536, 536f

Neer impingement test, for shoulder injuries, 442, 482, 563, 563f
Neer's stages, of rotator cuff impingement, 479–480, 480t
Neoepitopes, of proteoglycans, in articular cartilage, 66–67
Neoplasms. *See also* specific tumor
  benign, of lower extremity, 607, 620
  malignant, of thigh, 607
Nerve(s)
  action potential of, 9, 10f
  axillary
    injury mechanisms of, 402, 545–546
    shoulder distributions of, 330, 344, 352, 361, 545–546
  Baxter's, impingement of, 899, 933–934, 934f
  in bone, 76f, 77
  brachial plexus. *See* Brachial plexus
  calcaneal, 899, 899f, 935
  cluneal, 572, 572t
  cranial
    injury mechanisms of, 543–544
    shoulder distributions of, 357–359
  digital, neuromas of, 957–958, 974–975, 975f
  femoral cutaneous
    entrapment syndrome of, 572, 572t, 594
    thigh distribution of, 583, 584f, 585, 592
  foot distribution of
    hindfoot, 899, 899f–900f, 1020
    midfoot, 895–896, 895f–896f, 919
  groin distribution of, 219, 220f
  hallucal, medial, 958
  injuries to. *See also* Brachial plexus; *specific anatomy, injury or nerve*
    classifications of, 186–187, 543
    compression. *See* Nerve compression injuries
    electrodiagnosis of, 193–194
    imaging studies of, 116–117, 583, 592
    recovery potential of, 543, 546, 549
    referred hip pain with, 572, 572t
    scapula dysfunction from, 500f, 501, 505
    with upper extremity injuries, 543–550, 545f–548f
  knee distribution of, 682, 765
  leg distribution of, lower, 879, 885–886, 1007
  long thoracic, 357, 501, 505, 544, 544f
  median, 548–549, 548f
  microstructure of, 186, 186f
  muscle contraction role of, 9–10, 10f
  musculocutaneous, 524, 546–547
  neuromas of, digital, 957–958, 974–975, 975f
  obturator, 584–585, 585f, 596
  peroneal
    common, 885, 895, 896f, 958
    deep, 879, 895–896, 895f–896f
      entrapment syndromes of, 918–920, 919f–920f, 958–959, 962
      laceration injuries of, 1007–1008
    knee injuries and, 682, 765, 771, 809, 811, 833
    leg injuries and, 879, 881, 883, 885
    superficial, 879, 881, 885, 896, 896f
  plantar, 899, 900f
    compression neuropathy of, 920, 939–940
    digital, neuroma of, 974–975, 975f
    posterior articular, 765
    posterior interosseous (PIN), 285, 291–293, 297, 549–550
  radial
    tunnel syndrome of, 285, 291–293, 297, 549–550
    wrist injuries and, 283–285, 299
  rami divisions of, 184–185, 185f
  saphenous, 831–833, 899
  sciatic, 583–585, 584f, 592, 592f, 899
    pain syndrome of, 205–208, 206t, 228–229, 620
  spinal accessory, 357, 501, 505, 543–544, 544f
  suprascapular, 524, 544–545, 545f
  sural
    foot distributions of, 895f–896f, 896, 899
    leg injuries and, 879, 885

  surgical consideration of, 935, 997–998
  in tendons, 31
  tibial
    injury mechanisms of, 809, 879, 939–940, 958
    posterior, 899, 899f
  ulnar
    elbow injuries and
      caution with surgical repair of, 317–319
      conservative treatment of, 547
      decompression surgery for, 302–304, 303f, 547–548
      injury mechanisms of, 290–291, 297, 308–310, 547, 547f
    wrist tendinopathy and, 284
Nerve blocks, diagnostic and therapeutic
  for elbow tendinosis, 294
  for forefoot injuries, 958
  for glenohumeral joint, 334
  for hand fracture reduction, 237
  for hindfoot injuries, 902, 928, 932, 938
  for leg entrapment syndromes, 885
  for midfoot injuries, 902, 911, 914, 919
  for obturator nerve entrapment, 596
  for scaphoid fracture reduction, 264
  for snapping hip syndrome, 575
  for ulnar artery thrombosis, 285
Nerve compression injuries. *See also* specific anatomy, nerve, or sport
  brachial plexus mechanisms of, 183–184, 188, 192, 195–198
  with burner syndrome, 188
  with carpal tunnel syndrome, 285
  with elbow tendinosis, 291–294
  in foot
    forefoot, 957–959
    midfoot, 918, 918f–919f, 920
  in groin, 219–220, 220f
  in heel, 899, 924–926, 925f–926f, 933, 934f, 939–940
  with knee dislocations, 809–811
  in lower leg, 879–881
  with lumbar spine injuries, 204–207, 210
  of rotator cuff, 378–379, 379f
  shoulder mechanisms of, 331–332, 402, 406, 419, 442, 461–465
  with upper extremity injuries, 543–550
  in wrist, 284–285
Nerve conduction evaluation
  for brachial plexus injuries, 193–194
  for carpal tunnel syndrome, 285
  for midfoot injuries, 919
  for suprascapular nerve injuries, 545
Nerve endings
  classifications of, 31
  in scar tissue, 290
Nerve grafts, upper extremity indications for, 544
Nerve roots, injuries to
  avulsions. *See* Neurotmesis
  in brachial plexus. *See* Brachial plexus
  with cervical fractures, 164–165
  impingement. *See* Nerve compression injuries
Neurapraxia
  with brachial plexus injuries, 161–163, 183, 194
  with cervical spinal stenosis, 168, 168f
    measurement methods for, 168–171, 169f, 171f–172f
  as nerve injury classification, 186, 543
Neurological assessment
  with elbow injuries, 291–294, 309–310, 310f, 312
  with head and neck injuries, 154–156, 161–164, 167
  recovery correlations, 179–180
  with wrist injuries, 274, 276, 276f, 279, 283–285
Neurologic deficits, with lumbar spine injuries, 204–207, 206t
Neurolysis, for midfoot entrapment syndromes, 919–920
Neuromas
  heel pain and, 935
  interdigital

  in forefoot, 957–958
  of toes, 974–975, 975f
Neuromuscular junctions, muscle contraction role of, 9, 10f
Neurotmesis
  with brachial plexus injuries
    imaging techniques for, 193–194
    mechanisms of, 162, 183–186, 186f, 189–190, 192
    treatment options for, 196–198
  as nerve injury classification, 186–187, 194, 543
Neurovascular examinations
  with clavicle fractures, 536–537, 540
  for compartment syndromes, 89–92
  with knee injuries, 747, 758, 771, 808–811
Neurovascular injuries
  of hindfoot, 939–940
  of midfoot, 902, 911, 918–920, 918f–919f
Nirschl technique
  for racquet grip size determination, 296, 296f
  for tennis elbow repair
    lateral tendon, 300–302, 300f–302f
    medial tendon, 302–304, 303f
Nonsteroidal anti-inflammatory drugs (NSAIDs)
  for Achilles tendon dysfunction, 981, 986
  action mechanism of, 589, 852–853
  for elbow injuries, 294, 313, 326, 548–550
  for flexor hallucis longus tendon injuries, 989
  for foot injuries
    of hindfoot, 920, 925–926, 929, 931, 933, 935, 939
    of midfoot, 914, 917, 919
  for hip injuries, 578, 580
  for knee injuries, 736, 793, 839
    degenerative, 852–854
    tendons, 690, 692–697, 699, 701, 704–706
  for leg injuries, 877–878, 889
  for lumbar spine injuries, 204, 207, 211
  for muscle strains, 220, 587, 589, 591, 594–595, 598
  for osteitis pubis, 218, 595
  for peroneus tendon injuries, 995, 998
  for runners' injuries, 1023
  side effects of, 852–853
  for wrist injuries, 278–279, 281–282, 285
Non-weight-bearing exercises. *See* Open chain exercises
Nucleus pulposus, herniations of, in lumbar spine, 205–208, 206t, 208f
Nutrition
  for articular cartilage, 54, 61
  bone remodeling and, 82–83, 83f
  stress fractures and, 572, 869, 871
  for tendons, 22

O

Ober's test, for iliotibial band tightness, with patellofemoral joint injuries, 695, 715, 716f–717f
Obesity, as knee osteoarthritis factor, 846, 851–852
O'Brien's test, for shoulder assessment, with labral contact injuries, 442
Observational research designs, 124f, 127–129, 128f
Obturator externus muscle, anatomy of, 584–585, 584f
Occupational exposure, as knee osteoarthritis factor, 846
OCD. *See* Osteochondritis dissecans
Odds ratio, in research studies, 128, 142
Oden's classification, of peroneal tendon dislocations, 993, 993f, 995, 995f, 997
Odontoid
  congenital anomalies of, 175
  fractures of, 165–166, 177
Ogden's classification, of tibiofibular instability, 883–884, 884f
Olecranon
  bursitis of, 325–326
  in elbow injuries
    stress fractures of, 308, 311, 323–324, 324f

Olecranon (*contd.*)
  tendinosis and, 292–293, 304
  treatment considerations of, 310, 312–315, 315*f*
Open chain exercises
  for knee rehabilitation, 629, 685, 773–774, 793
  for running injuries, 1024
  for scapular dyskinesis, 508–509, 508*f*–509*f*
Open reduction. *See* Reduction procedures
Opponens splint, short, for ulnar collateral ligament tears, 244, 245*f*
Optical mapping technique, for knee strain, 625
Origin, of tendons, 21
Orthotics. *See also specific device*
  for foot positioning
    with hindfoot injuries, 921–927, 927*f*, 931–932, 937–938, 940
    with midfoot injuries, 909–911, 913–915, 913*f*, 917, 919
  non-foot indications for, 712, 811
  for knee degeneration, 811, 854
  for leg stress fracture prevention, 871
  for posterior tibial tendon injuries, 1006
  for runners, 1023
  for shin splints, 877, 878*f*
  for toe deformities, 973–974
  for toe injuries, 970, 970*f*, 972
Osgood-Schlatter disease
  hip injuries with, 580
  knee tendon injuries with, 689, 698, 705–706
Osmotic factors, colloid, of compartment syndromes, 88–89
Osmotic pressure gradients, in articular cartilage, 53–55, 60
Os peroneum
  fracture of
    epidemiology of, 992–993
    evaluation of, 994–995
    mechanisms of, 994
    nonoperative treatment of, 999
    surgical treatment of, 999–1000
  pain syndrome of
    clinical evaluation of, 916, 994–995
    imaging studies of, 916–917, 916*f*–917*f*
    pathoanatomy of, 914, 916
    treatment of, 918, 918*f*
Osseofascial compartment
  pressure elevations in. *See* Compartment syndromes
  pressure-volume relationship in, 87, 88*f*
  measurement techniques for, 92–93
Osteitis pubis
  evaluation and treatment of, 576–577, 595
  gracilis syndrome with, 229
  injury mechanisms of, 576–577, 595
  pain syndrome with, 112, 217–218, 220, 226, 577
  range of motion of, 217
  rectal muscle disruption with, 223–227, 224*f*, 226*f*
Osteoarthritis
  as age-related degeneration, 62–64, 66, 822, 845, 1021
  biomarkers of, 66
  cartilage changes with, 55–56, 64–67, 65*f*
  clinical presentations of, 64
  genetic etiologies of, 54–55, 847
  grading schemes for, 64–65, 845, 851
  mechanisms of. *See specific anatomy or injury*
  primary *versus* secondary, 846
  in runners, 1021–1022
Osteoblasts, functional morphology of, 78–79, 78*f*–79*f*, 82
Osteochondral fragments
  of ankle, magnetic resonance imaging of, 111, 821
  of knee, removal of, 726
Osteochondral grafts, for knee cartilage, 796, 798–801, 799*f*–801*f*, 856
Osteochondritis dissecans (OCD)
  with elbow injuries
    evaluation of, 114, 317, 320–321
    pathoanatomy of, 291–292, 320–321

    treatment of, 321–322
    magnetic resonance imaging of
      of ankle, 110–111, 111*f*
      of elbow, 114, 317
      of knee, 105, 106*f*
    osteochondrosis *versus*, 320
Osteochondroma, of femur, 607
Osteochondrosis, of elbow, 320
Osteoclasts
  function of, 78, 79*f*, 80, 82
  in leg stress fractures, 869, 1020
Osteocytes, function of, 77–80, 77*f*–79*f*
Osteoid osteoma, of femur, 607
Osteonecrosis
  with carpal fractures, 263, 267, 269–270
  with hip fractures, 574
  laser-induced, post-knee repair, 796, 832
Osteopenia, hip stress fractures from, 572
Osteophytes
  in dancer's feet, 962
  with elbow injuries, 307–308, 313
    olecranon repair indications with, 310, 312–315, 315*f*, 319, 326
    tendinosis, 292–293, 304
  knee degeneration and, 845, 847, 850–851
Osteoporosis, 869
Osteosarcoma, of femur, 607
Osteotendinous junction (OTJ), anatomy and physiology of, 21, 26–27, 26*f*, 31–32
Os trigonum, painful
  evaluation of, 924–925, 925*f*, 988
  pathoanatomy of, 924
  treatment of, 925–926, 926*f*
Outerbridge classification
  of articular cartilage, 472, 855
  of chondromalacia, 734
Outliers, in research studies, 138
Outside-in arthroscopic repair, of knee meniscus, 654–655, 654*f*
Overhead athlete. *See also* Throwing motion; *specific sport*
  dominant extremity range of motion of, 420
  injury concepts for, 551, 559*f*, 562*f*, 566–567, 566*f*
  operative intervention impact on, 422
  scapula role in, 497–498, 499*f*
    biomechanics of, 499–501, 500*f*
  shoulder instability in
    anterior, 402
    biomechanics of, 389–391, 389*f*–391*f*
    from labral injuries, 438, 457–475
    posterior, 413, 418, 420, 422
    sternoclavicular subluxation with, 539
Overuse injuries. *See also* Training errors
  of ankle tendons, 979–980, 987
  with distance running, 871, 875–878, 1011, 1022
  of elbow, 289–291, 294, 312–326
  of hip, 572–578, 573*f*–574*f*, 576*f*
  of knee, 614, 689, 695–696, 701, 712
    patellar tendon, 598, 698–700
  of leg, 871, 875–878
  of lumbar spine, 205–209
  of pelvis, 215–217, 224*f*
  risk factors for, 289–290
  of shoulder
    biomechanics of, 377, 402, 413, 418
    golf sprain *versus* strain, 565
    labrum, 461, 463, 474
    scapula, 501
  of thigh adductor tendons, 594
Oxidative activity, of muscle fibers, 13–14, 15*f*–16*f*, 16–18, 16*t*, 18*t*
Oxygen, for emergency care, of head and neck injuries, 153–154

P

Pacinian corpuscles, as mechanoreceptors, 385, 418
Pads and padding devices
  for forefoot injuries, 948, 958, 960–962
  for hindfoot injuries, 922, 935, 936*f*, 937–939

  for midfoot injuries, 912–913, 912*f*–913*f*, 915*f*, 919, 919*f*
  for shoulders, 154–155, 188, 195
Paget's disease, injuries with, 607, 688
Pain control. *See* Analgesics; *specific drug*
Pain receptors, musculoskeletal, 31
Pain syndromes. *See specific anatomy or injury*
Pairwise comparisons, in research studies, 137
Palmar lip fractures, 237–238
Palmar plate arthroplasty, with phalanx fractures, 237–238
Palmar pole fractures, with carpal fractures, 257, 259*f*, 260, 263, 264*f*, 265, 269, 271
Palmer classification, of triangular fibrocartilage complex injury, 280–282, 280*f*
Pancoast tumor, brachial plexus injuries and, 191, 193
Paratenon, of tendons, 22, 30–31
Paratenonitis, of Achilles tendon, 979–984
Paresthesias
  with carpal tunnel syndrome, 285
  with cervical spine injuries, 161–164, 168
  with compartment syndromes, 879–880
Par interarticularis defect. *See* Spondylolysis
Parsonage-Turner syndrome, 544
Passive length-tension relationship, in muscle contractions, 11–12, 11*f*, 12*t*
Patella. *See* Patellofemoral joint
Patella alta, 698, 706, 726, 728, 851
Patella baja, 691, 834–835, 836*f*, 851
Patella glide
  with injuries, 383, 712–713, 839
  tests for, 619–620, 620*f*, 713, 713*f*
Patella infera, 838–839
Patellar entrapment syndrome (PES)
  post-knee repair, 703, 829, 833, 837–839
  primary *versus* secondary, 838
  stages of, 838, 838*f*
  treatment of, 839
Patellar ligament, anatomy of, 709, 710*f*
Patellar plica, from running, 1018–1019
Patellar pressure syndrome. *See* Lateral patellar pressure syndrome
Patellar prosthesis, for degenerative arthritis, 737, 737*f*
Patellar resurfacing, for patellofemoral arthritis, 737–739, 740*t*
Patellar tendinitis
  epidemiology of, 698, 700
  evaluation of, 698–699, 714–715, 714*f*
  injury mechanisms of, 598, 638, 689, 698, 705, 721
  treatment of
    nonoperative, 699, 721–722
    operative, 699–700, 722
    results and complications of, 700
Patellar tendon
  anatomy of, 709, 710*f*
  avulsion fractures of, 705
  as graft, for knee repair, 700
    of anterior cruciate ligament, 630–632, 682, 750–751, 812
    of posterior cruciate ligament, 776, 778, 781–782, 784, 784*f*
    posterolateral, 683–684
  healing processes of, 689–690
  reconstruction techniques for, 701–704, 702*f*–703*f*
  rehabilitation programs for, 701, 704
  running force impact on, 1012, 1016–1018
  rupture injuries of
    acute *versus* chronic, 702–704, 703*f*
    epidemiology of, 700
    evaluation of, 701
    grafts for, 701–704
    mechanisms of, 598, 688–689, 698, 700–701
    nonoperative treatment of, 701
    operative treatment of, 701–704, 702*f*–703*f*
    from overuse, 598, 698–700
    partial *versus* complete, 701
    results and complications of, 704–705

Patellar tracking. *See* Patellofemoral tracking
Patella tilt, with injuries, 712–713, 838–839
  chronic pressure syndrome from, 722–724, 722*f*, 724*f*
  radiographic measurement of, 715, 718–720, 719*f*–720*f*
Patella-trochlea joint, biomechanics of, 636–638
Patellectomy, for patellofemoral arthritis, 737–739, 738*f*, 740*t*
Patellofemoral joint
  acute dislocations of
    etiology of, 724
    evaluation of, 725, 725*f*
    outcomes of, 726, 726*t*–727*t*
    treatment of, 725–727
  alignment of
    complications of, 833–835, 836*f*
    measurements of, 718–721, 719*f*–720*f*
    treatment considerations of, 638–639, 704, 712, 726, 729–740
  anatomy of, 636, 709–710, 710*f*
    articulation models of, 637–639, 710–711, 710*f*
  arthritis of
    arthroplasty for, 737–739, 740*t*, 795
    chondromalacia classifications, 734–735
    degenerative, 636, 638, 732, 734–740, 834, 850–851
    evaluation of, 734–735
    nonoperative treatment of, 735–736
    operative treatment of, 736–740, 736*f*–738*f*, 740*t*
    treatment outcomes for, 739–740, 740*t*
  arthroscopy indications for, 723–724, 724*f*, 726, 733
  biomechanics of
    abnormal tracking in, 638, 694, 699
    contact area, 636–638, 710–711, 710*f*
    force transmission, 637–639, 711, 711*f*
  chondromalacia of, 636, 638, 734–735
  compression tests for, 712, 727, 850
  dislocations of
    acute, 724–727, 725*f*, 726*t*–727*t*
    with knee ligament tears, 666
    radiographic measurement of, 715, 718–721, 719*f*–720*f*
    recurrent, 727–734, 728*f*, 730*f*–733*f*, 730*t*
  impingement syndromes of. *See* Patellar entrapment syndrome
  injuries of
    articular cartilage mechanisms, 791, 793
    clinical evaluation of, 711–715, 712*f*–715*f*
    computed tomography of, 719–721, 720*f*, 723
    dislocations of, 666, 724–734, 725*f*, 726*t*–727*t*, 728*f*, 730*f*–733*f*, 730*t*
    magnetic resonance imaging of, 102, 104, 104*f*, 720
    mechanisms of, 636, 711–712, 711*f*, 768
    patellar tracking with, 712, 721–723, 726, 729
    radiographic evaluation of, 715–719, 718*f*–719*f*, 725, 728, 735
    soft tissue, 639, 714, 714*f*, 721–722, 721*f*, 731–734, 731*f*–733*f*
    with tendon ruptures, 691–692, 704
    vastus medialis obliquus muscle in, 712, 714, 723–724, 726, 729, 730*f*, 732, 735
  instability mechanisms of, 711–715, 724–734, 726*t*–727*t*
    from running, 1017–1018
  lateral pressure syndrome of, 722–724, 722*f*–724*f*, 737, 739, 740*t*
  malalignment, from running, 1017–1018
  measurements of
    articular surface ratios, 838
    congruence angle, 719, 719*f*
    for knee degeneration, 850–851
    lateral angel, 718–719, 719*f*
    lateral patellofemoral angle, 718, 719*f*, 735
    Q angle, 638, 702, 712, 724, 727, 735
    sulcus angle, 718–719, 719*f*, 724, 735
  pain syndromes of, 637–638, 723, 734–735
    with knee reconstruction, 828–829, 833

  palpation of, 714–715, 714*f*, 721
  post-repair procedures, 833–837, 836*f*–837*f*
  physical examination of, 619–620, 619*f*–620*f*
    with injuries, 711–715, 712*f*–715*f*, 721
  quadriceps role in, 636–638, 709, 711*f*
    with injuries, 712, 715, 715*f*
  reaction forces of, 636–639, 711, 711*f*
  realignment procedures for
    anterior techniques, 735–736, 736*f*, 739, 740*t*
    complications of, 833–835, 836*f*
    distal techniques, 731–734, 731*f*–733*f*
    proximal techniques, 729–731, 730*f*, 730*t*
  recurrent dislocations of
    distal realignment procedures for, 731–734, 731*f*–733*f*
    evaluation of, 727–728, 728*f*
    incidence of, 727
    proximal realignment procedures for, 729–731, 730*f*, 730*t*
    treatment of, 728–729
  rehabilitation programs for, 638, 721–724, 728–729, 731, 733, 735–736
  running force impact on, 1012–1013, 1016, 1018
  salvage procedures for
    anteromedialization, 733–734, 733*f*, 736–737, 739, 740*t*
    complications of, 834–835, 839
    Maquet anteriorization, 735–736, 736*f*, 739, 740*t*
  soft tissue injuries. *See also* Patellar tendinitis
    mechanisms of, 714, 714*f*, 721–722, 721*f*
    reconstruction of, 639, 731–734, 731*f*–733*f*, 740*t*. *See also* Patellar tendon
  stability mechanisms of, 709–711, 710*f*
  surgical complications of
    hemarthrosis, 835
    with lateral release, 833–834
    nonunion, 837, 837*f*
    pain syndromes as, 833–839, 836*f*–838*f*
    patella baja, 834–835, 836*f*
    with realignments, 834–835
    with salvage procedures, 834–835
Patellofemoral joint reaction (PFJR), force dynamics of, 636–638, 711, 711*f*
Patellofemoral ligament, medial, anatomy of, 709, 710*f*
Patellofemoral pain syndrome
  with injuries, 637–638, 712, 723, 734–735
  with knee reconstruction, 828–829, 833
  post-repair procedures, 833–839, 836*f*–838*f*
Patellofemoral tracking
  biomechanics of, 638, 1018
  with patellofemoral joint injuries, 712, 721–723, 726, 729, 735
  with tendon injuries, 694, 699, 701
PCL. *See* Posterior cruciate ligament
Pearson chi-square test, in research studies, 128, 138–140
Pectineus muscle, anatomy of, 585
Pectoralis major muscle
  anatomy of, 358
  golf swing role of, 394
  overhead throwing role of, 553–555, 553*f*
  swimming stroke role of, 392, 560
Pectoralis minor muscle, 358, 544
Pediatric injuries. *See* Children
Pedorthotics, for knee degeneration, 854
Pelligrini-Stieda sign, with knee ligament tears, 666
Pelvic floor repair, for athletic pubalgia, 226–227, 596
Pelvic inflammatory disease, 215
Pelvis
  anatomy of, 223, 224*f*
    compartmental, 87–88
    ligaments, 223, 224*f*, 229
    muscles of, 220, 223, 224*f*, 226
  fractures of
    avulsion, 216–217, 226, 600–602, 601*t*
    simple, 229
    stress, 216, 229, 1020
  injuries of

  adductor, 220–224, 220*f*, 224*f*, 227–229, 227*f*
  osteitis pubis, 112, 217–218, 220, 226, 229
  overuse, 215–217, 224*f*, 229
  soft tissue, 230
  magnetic resonance imaging of, 112–113, 113*f*, 216
  ossification centers of, 600–601
  pain etiologies of, 215, 572, 572*t*
  rotation of, with golf swing, 563–565, 564*f*, 566*f*
  running force impact on, 220, 1012, 1016, 1019
Pennate muscles, physiologic principles of, 6–7, 7*f*, 13
Pentose phosphate shunt, in tendon cells, 28–29
Percussion test. *See* Tinel's sign
Perichondral transplants, for knee cartilage regeneration, 796, 856
Perineurium, of peripheral nerves, 186–187, 186*f*
Periosteum, of bone
  anatomy of, 76, 76*f*, 78
  biopsies of, for tibial inflammation, 875
  stripping of, impact on healing, 78
  transplants of, for knee cartilage regeneration, 796–797, 796*f*–798*f*
Peritendinitis, in lower extremities, 689, 696, 698
Peritendinous sheaths, of tendons, 21
Permeability factors, of compartment syndromes, 88–89
Peroneal groove, deepening of, for dislocation repairs, 996–998, 997*f*
Peroneal retinaculum, superior
  anatomy of, 991–992, 991*f*
  incompetence mechanisms of, 992–994, 996, 998
  repair and imbrication of, for tendon injuries, 996–999, 997*f*, 1005
Peroneus brevis tendon
  in Achilles tendon reconstruction, 984
  anatomy of, 991–992, 991*f*
  in os peroneum, 916, 917*f*
  partial longitudinal rupture of, 992–995
  tenosynovitis of, 992–996
  traumatic subluxation of, 992–998, 993*f*, 995*f*, 997*f*
Peroneus longus tendon
  anatomy of, 893, 894*f*, 991, 991*f*
  isolated fracture of, 992–995, 999–1000
  in os peroneum, 917, 917*f*
  painful syndrome of. *See* Os peroneum
  rupture of, 992, 994–995, 998–999
  tenosynovitis of, 992–996
  traumatic subluxation of, 992–998, 993*f*, 995*f*, 997*f*
Peroneus muscle/tendons
  anatomy of, 991–992, 991*f*, 994
  function of, 992
  immobilization devices for, 996, 998–1000
  injuries of
    clinical evaluation of, 994–995
    epidemiology of, 992–993
    imaging studies of, 995, 995*f*
    mechanisms of, 993–994, 993*f*
    nonoperative treatment of, 995–996, 998–999
    surgical treatment of, 996–1000, 997*f*
  isolated fracture of, 992–995, 999–1000
  rehabilitation programs for, 995–996, 998–1000
  rupture of, 992–995, 998–999
  tenosynovitis of, 992–996
  traumatic subluxation and dislocation of
    pathoanatomy of, 992–996, 993*f*, 995*f*
    surgical repair of, 996–998, 997*f*
  variations of, 992
Peroneus tertius tendon, injuries to, 1007–1008
Perthes disease, 596
PES. *See* Patellar entrapment syndrome
Pes anserinus, 584–585, 806
Pes planus
  forefoot injuries with, 946, 953
  of midfoot
    associated injuries with, 912–913, 920, 927, 939

Pes planus (*contd.*)
    clinical presentations of, 912–913
    imaging studies of, 913, 913*f*
    nerve compression with, 920, 939
    treatment of, 914, 914*f*, 932, 932*f*, 940
PEVK region, of sarcomeres, 11–12
PFJR. *See* Patellofemoral joint reaction
PFL. *See* Popliteofibular ligament
Phagocytosis, 30, 43
Phalanx fractures
    of fingers
        bone grafting for, 235
        distal, 235–236, 236*f*
        implant selection for, 234–235, 234*f*
        ligament injuries with, 238
        middle, 236–238
        proximal, 238
        stability classification of, 237
        treatment of, 233–234
    of toes, 966
Phalen's test, for carpal tunnel syndrome, 285
Phonophoresis, for heel pain, 931, 935
Phosphate, in bone mineralization, 79
Phospholipids, in articular cartilage, 54*t*, 55
Phosphorylation. *See* Oxidative activity
Physical examinations
    focused. *See* specific anatomy or injury
    at time of injury, value of, 613, 901
Physical therapy. *See also* Rehabilitation pro-
        grams; *specific modality*
    for acute brachial neuropathy, 196
    for adductor longus strains, 220–221
    for ankle sprains, 821, 822*f*
    for athletic pubalgia, 596, 596*t*
    for compartment syndromes, 605–606
    for elbow tendinosis, 294
    for flexor hallucis longus tendon injuries,
        989–991
    for foot injuries
        heel pain, 931–936, 935*f*, 938–939
        of hindfoot, 920–921, 923–927, 929, 940
        of midfoot, 903, 909–912, 914–915, 917
        of toes, 966–967, 969–970, 972
    for hip injuries, 578–579
    for knee injuries
        of ligaments, 628–630, 658
            anterior cruciate, 748–749, 749*f*, 755–756,
                755*t*, 756*f*
            posterior cruciate, 773–775
            posterolateral, 667, 667*f*, 685, 780
        meniscus repair, 657–658, 658*t*
        patellofemoral joint, 721, 723–724, 728–729,
            731, 733, 735–736
        of tendons, 690, 692–697, 699–701, 704–706
    for leg injuries, shin splints, 877–879
    for lumbar spine injuries, 204, 207, 211
    for muscle strains, 587, 589–590, 594, 598
    for peroneus tendon injuries, 995–996,
        998–1000
    for quadriceps injuries, 598, 600–603
    for running injuries, 1024
    for shoulder rehabilitation, 421, 426–427,
        474–475
Physiologic cross-sectional area (PCSA)
    of lower limb muscles, 7–8, 8*f*
    as muscle force parameter, 7, 13, 17
    of upper limb muscles, 8–9, 9*f*
Physis, of bone. *See* Diaphysis
Pie throwing, by pitchers, 556, 559*f*
Pigmented villonodular synovitis (PVNS), tarsal
        tunnel syndrome and, 939–940
PIN. *See* Nerve(s), posterior interosseous
Pincer mechanism, in cervical cord compression,
        168–169, 168*f*
Pinched nerve syndrome. *See* Burner syndrome;
        Nerve compression injuries
Pinch test. *See* Heel pinch test
Pin fixation
    for hand fractures, 234–236, 234*f*, 238–239
    for hip injuries, 573–574, 581
    of midfoot injuries, 908–909, 911*f*

for patellar tendon repair, 702
for wrist injuries
    ligamentous, 278, 280
    for scaphoid fractures, 267, 268*f*
Pinocytosis, in tendon cells, 30
Piriformis syndrome, 228–229
Pisiform fractures, 270–271
Pitching, overhand
    acceleration in
        biomechanics of, 388, 459*f*–460*f*, 460, 552*f*,
            554–555, 555*f*
        pathologic, 557
    arm cocking in
        biomechanics of, 459–460, 459*f*, 552*f*
            early, 387–388, 387*f*, 552–553, 552*f*–553F
            late, 388, 388*f*, 552*f*–554*f*, 553–554
        pathologic
            early, 555–556
            late, 556–557, 556*f*
    deceleration in, biomechanics of, 388, 388*f*, 460,
        460*f*, 552*f*, 555
    elbow injuries from, 558–559, 559*f*
    follow-through in
        biomechanics of, 388, 388*f*, 459*f*, 460–461,
            552*f*, 555
        pathologic, 557
    impingement syndromes in, 461–465, 463*f*, 468,
        557–559, 559*f*, 566*f*
    off-season maintenance programs for, 469–470
    phases of
        biomechanics of, 387, 387*f*–388*f*, 458, 459*f*,
            552*f*
        pathologic, 551, 558–559, 559*f*, 566–567, 566*f*
    shoulder injuries from
        anatomical mechanisms, 557, 559*f*
        anterior dislocations as, 402
        deceleration mechanisms, 558, 558*f*
        glenoid labral tears as, 461–465, 462*f*–463*f*
        as instability continuum, 558, 559*f*
    shoulder kinematics for, 387–388, 387*f*–388*f*
    stride with, 387–388, 387*f*, 458–459, 459*f*
    wind-up in
        biomechanics of, 387, 458, 459*f*, 551–552, 552*f*
        pathologic, 555
Pivoting exercises, for knee ligament injuries, 671
Pivot shift test
    for elbow injuries, 310, 310*f*, 325
    in knee examination, 614–616, 616*f*
        with ligament injuries, 672, 746–747, 772
Planovalgus deformity, of foot. *See* Pes planus
Plantar aponeurosis, anatomy of, 897, 898*f*
Plantar fascia
    acute tear of, 933
    inflammation of. *See* Plantar fasciitis
    release of, for heel pain, 933
    running force impact on, 1012, 1020
    windlass effect of, in gait cycle, 893, 895*f*
Plantar fasciitis, insertional
    acute tears with, 933
    clinical evaluation of, 930, 930*f*
    imaging studies of, 930–931, 930*f*–931*f*
    injury mechanisms of, 929–930
    treatment of
        nonoperative, 931–932, 932*f*
        surgical, 932–933, 932*f*
Plantar-flexion injuries
    of ankle, 819–820, 993–994, 993*f*
    of forefoot, 961
    of hindfoot, 922, 922*f*, 924, 925*f*
    of midfoot, 907, 907*f*
Plantaris tendon
    in Achilles tendon reconstruction, 982–983
    rupture of, 888
Plantar keratosis, intractable, of toes, 974
Plantar ligaments. *See also specific ligament*
    of hindfoot
        anatomy of, 896, 897*f*–898*f*
        Lisfranc's joint injuries and, 907, 909
    of midfoot, 893, 894*f*
Plantar plate
    dislocation injuries of, 967, 967*f*

in metatarsophalangeal joint, function of, 949,
    949*f*
sesamoid resections and, 957
Plastic deformation. *See* Creep
Plate fixation
    for acromioclavicular joint dislocations, 523
    for clavicle fractures, 538, 538*f*
    for hand fractures, 234–239, 234*f*
    for knee repair, 682
    for patellar tendon repair, 704
Platelet-derived growth factors, for knee healing,
    650, 690
Plica, pathologic patellar, from running,
    1018–1019
Plyometrics, for shoulder rehabilitation, 475, 508,
    508*f*
Polyester tape fixation, for anterior cruciate liga-
    ment reconstruction, 47, 48*f*
Polymyositis, of thigh, 607
Pool therapy, for lumbar spine injuries, 204
Popliteal artery entrapment syndrome
    classification of, 886, 886*f*
    clinical evaluation of, 92, 886–887, 886*f*
    treatment of, 887
Popliteofibular ligament (PFL)
    anatomy of, 677–678, 805–806
    biomechanics of, 675–678, 806–807
    evolution of knowledge of, 675–676
    injuries of, 679, 682–684
Popliteus tendon
    anatomy of, 676, 805–806
    biomechanics of, 766, 806–808
    healing processes of, 689–690
    injuries of
        epidemiology of, 696
        evaluation of, 696–697
        mechanisms of, 696
        nonoperative treatment of, 697–698
        surgical repair of, 682–683, 685, 697
Postconcussion syndrome, 157–158
Posterior cruciate ligament (PCL), of knee
    anatomy of, 41, 626–627
        gross, 763–765, 764*f*
        meniscofemoral ligaments in, 765, 765*f*
        neurovascular supply of, 765
    biomechanics of, 765–767
    chronic insufficiency of, 778–781
    degenerative disease of, 766, 776
    physical examination of
        drawer tests for, 765–771, 769*f*, 778–780
        pivot shift tests for, 614–617, 614*f*–616*f*, 680,
            772
    reconstruction of, 632–633
        for acute injuries, 776–778
        avulsion fractures of tibial insertion, 774–775,
            774*f*–775*f*
        for chronic insufficiency, 778–779
        for combined injuries, 776–778, 780
        graft complications of, 825–827, 826*f*
        for isolated injuries, 776
        tunnel placement techniques for, 776, 778,
            781–784, 782*f*–784*f*, 814
    rehabilitation for
        for isolated injuries, 775–776
        nonoperative, 773–774, 779–780
        phases of, 774
        postoperative, 779
        weight-bearing *versus* non-weight-bearing,
            774, 779
    stability role of, 627–628, 632–633, 763–765,
        764*f*
    tear injuries of
        acute, 776–778
        chronic insufficiency, 778–781
        clinical evaluation of, 768–772, 779–780
        combined. *See also* Knee, multiligament injur-
            ies of
            evaluation of, 771–772, 771*f*, 774
            operative treatment of, 776–778, 780
        epidemiology of, 763
        isolated, 768–770, 769*f*–770*f*, 775–776

magnetic resonance imaging of, 102, 103*f*, 772–773, 773*f*
mechanisms of, 767–768, 767*f*–768*f*
nonoperative treatment of, 773–776
operative treatment of, 774–779. *See also* Posterior cruciate ligament, of knee, reconstruction of
pathoanatomy of, 765–767
return to sport guidelines, 779
tibial insertion avulsions, 772, 772*f*, 774–775
treatment outcomes of, 774, 776, 779
tensile strength of, 766–767
Posterior glenoid labrum, contact injuries of
arthroscopic treatment of, 450–451, 451*f*
clinical evaluation of, 438–442, 440*f*–441*f*
epidemiology of, 432
imaging analysis of, 442–445, 442*f*–444*f*
injury mechanisms of, 437–438, 437*f*
nonoperative treatment of, 450–451
pathoanatomy of, 436
Posterior interosseous neuropathy, 549
Posterior oblique ligament (POL), of knee, 617, 617*f*, 806
Posterior sag sign, in posterior cruciate ligament injuries, 769
Posterior shoulder instability
acute dislocations from, 413, 422, 427
biomechanics of, 416–418, 417*f*
classifications of, 413, 419, 422
evaluation of, 419–421
from glenoid labral injuries. *See* Posterior glenoid labrum
incidence of, 416
labral injury mechanisms of
with contact sports, 431–454
with throwing motions, 343, 401–402, 407–409
as locked posterior dislocations
injury mechanisms of, 413–415, 419
treatment of, 422–427
pathoanatomy of, 413, 416–418
psychological disorders and, 419, 427
as recurrent posterior subluxations
injury mechanisms of, 413–416, 418–419
treatment of, 421–427
rehabilitation of
as initial treatment, 421–422, 427
postoperative, 426–427
return to sport guidelines, 422, 427
treatment of
capsulorrhaphy indications, 415–416, 423
posterior technique for, 423–426, 423*f*–426*f*
thermal-assisted technique for, 427
expected outcomes of, 422, 427
literature review of, 413–416
nonoperative, 421–422
operative indications, 421–423
Posterior superior glenoid impingement, as rotator cuff injury, 481
Posterior tests, in research studies, 137
Posterior tibial tendon
anatomy of, 893, 894*f*, 896, 897*f*, 1000, 1001*f*
degenerative changes in, 1001–1004
dislocation of, 1000–1002, 1005
function of, 1000
immobilization devices for, 1004–1007
magnetic resonance imaging of, 110, 110*f*, 1003
in nerve impingement syndromes, 914–915, 916*f*, 939
reconstruction procedures for, reinsertion into navicular, 1003–1004
with transfer of flexor digitorum longus tendon, 1004–1007
rehabilitation programs for, 1004–1007
tear injuries of
acute, 1000–1005
chronic, 1001–1003, 1006–1007
epidemiology of, 1000–1001
evaluation of, 1002–1003
mechanisms of, 1000–1002
nonoperative treatment of, 1003, 1005–1006
surgical repair of, 1003–1007

tendinitis of, 914–915
tenosynovitis of
acute, 1001–1002, 1005–1006
chronic, 1001–1002, 1006–1007
surgical repair of, 1005–1007
Posterolateral knee. *See also specific anatomical component*
anatomy of
complex components of, 675–679, 766, 805
layers, 805–806
variability in, 806
biomechanics of, 675–676, 678, 766, 806–808
evolution of knowledge of, 675–676
grafts for, 682–685
injuries of
acute *versus* chronic, 679–680
combined, 675, 679, 685, 771–772, 771*f*. *See also* Knee, multiligament injuries of
evaluation of, 679–681
mechanisms of, 678–679, 766, 771
nonoperative treatment of, 681, 685
operative treatment of, 681, 685, 780
fixation procedures, 681–683
graft reconstructions, 682–685
reconstruction of, 682–685, 776–778, 780
stability of, 676, 678–680
Posteromedial knee
anatomy of, 663–664, 664*f*, 806
biomechanics of, 806–808
injuries of
evaluation of, 664–666, 664*f*–665*f*
mechanisms of, 663–664, 664*f*
nonoperative treatment of, 666–672, 667*f*
operative treatment of, 672–673
rehabilitation program for, 666–673, 668*f*–670*f*, 668*t*
Postganglionic injuries, in brachial plexus, 184*f*–186*f*, 185–186, 192
Posture, scapula and, 503, 506–507, 506*f*–507*f*
Posturing, with intracranial injuries, 158, 160
Potassium, in articular cartilage, 53, 55
Power analysis, for research sampling, 132–133
Predictive values, of research studies, 138, 141
Preganglionic injuries, in brachial plexus, 184*f*–186*f*, 185–186, 192
Pregnancy, 215
Pressure-volume relationship, in osseofascial compartments, 87, 88*f*
measurement techniques for, 92–93
Prevalence, incidence *versus,* 127, 129
Prevalence studies, as research design, 128–129
PRICEMM principles, for elbow tendinosis, 294
Primary reports, as research designs, 124–125, 124*f*
Proliferative phase, of healing process, 43, 690
Pronation, of foot. *See* Foot pronation
Pronator syndrome, 293, 548
Pronator teres, overhead throwing role of, 554
Prone hang exercises, for knee ligament injuries, 669, 669*f*
Proprioception
in glenohumeral joint stability, 385
knee mechanisms of, 648, 864
Proprioceptive training
for ankle injuries, 821, 923, 996, 998–1000
for anterior cruciate ligament injuries, 864
for scapula dyskinesis, 508, 508*f*
Prostatitis, athletic pubalgia *versus,* 596
Proteinases, articular cartilage degradation by, 62, 67
Protein intake, bone formation and, 82–83
Proteins
in articular cartilage, 54*t*, 55–56
matrix. *See* Matrix molecules
in muscle contraction, 4–6, 5*f*, 9, 11–12
Proteoglycans
in articular cartilage, 54*t*, 55–57, 56*f*–57*f*, 61, 787–788, 788*f*
with osteoarthritis, 66–67
definition of, 55
in knee, 645, 647, 687
in tendons, 23, 25, 27–28, 30

Protons, in magnetic resonance imaging, 100–101, 100*t*
Provocative pain tests
for elbow tendinosis, 292–293
for flexor hallucis longus tenosynovitis, 988
for popliteal artery entrapment, 886–887
Provocative scaphoid shift test, for scapholunate injury, 276, 276*f*
Proximal interphalangeal joints (PIP)
collateral ligaments of, immobilization treatment for, 246–247, 247*f*
corns over, 960–961
dislocation injuries of, 246–247
dorsal, 247
metacarpophalangeal, 248
volar, 247–249
fracture considerations of, 233, 236–238
tendon injuries of
extensor, 250–252, 251*f*
flexor, 252–254, 253*f*–254*f*
tendon insertions of, 249, 253
toe deformities and, 973, 976
Pseudoaneurysms, 606
Psoas muscle, anatomy of, 585
Psychological disorders, posterior shoulder instability and, 419, 427
PTB. *See* Bone-patellar tendon-bone grafts
Pubalgia. *See* Athletic pubalgia
Pubic rami, stress fractures of, 572–574
Pubic symphysitis. *See* Osteitis pubis
Pull-through, in swimming stroke
early
biomechanics of, 391, 559–560, 560*f*
pathologic, 561, 562*f*
late, biomechanics of, 391, 560–561, 560*f*
mid, pathologic, 561–562, 562*f*, 564*f*
Pulmonary embolism, 889
Pulses, with compartment syndromes, differential assessment of, 87, 88*f*, 90–91, 880
Pulse sequencing, for magnetic resonance imaging, 101–102
Pump bump, of ankle, 938–939, 938*f*
Push-up test, for claw toe flexibility, 973, 973*f*
Putti-Platt procedure
in anterior shoulder dislocations, 407
reverse of, for posterior shoulder dislocations, 413, 415, 422–423
P value
in research studies, 121, 123, 128, 137–139
in significance testing, 142–145
PVNS. *See* Pigmented villonodular synovitis

Q

Q angle, of patellofemoral joint, 638, 702, 712, 724, 727, 735
Quadriceps. *See also specific muscle or tendon*
anatomy of, 709, 710*f*
contusions injuries of, 602–603
as graft
for patellar tendon repair, 703–704, 703*f*
for posterior cruciate ligament, 783
iliac apophysis avulsion fractures and, 600–602, 601*t*
injuries of
contusions, 602–603
epidemiology of, 596–597
return to sport guidelines, 598, 600, 602–603
ruptures, 598–600, 599*f*–600*f*
strains, 597–598
myositis ossificans of, 603
patellofemoral joint and
injury applications of, 712, 715, 715*f*, 723, 728–729, 735
kinematics of, 637–638, 709, 711*f*
in patellofemoral joint kinematics, 636–638, 709, 711, 711*f*
running impact on, 1018
rupture injuries of
bilateral, 598–599, 691
chronic, 694
clinical evaluation of, 599, 691
diagnostic studies for, 599–600, 691–692

Quadriceps. *See also specific muscle or tendon* (*contd.*)
    epidemiology of, 691
    mechanisms of, 598–599, 688, 691
    nonoperative treatment of, 692
    outcomes and complications of, 694
    partial, 598
    rehabilitation of, 693–694
    risk factors for, 598–599
    surgical repair of, 599f–600f, 600, 692–694, 693f
    strength training for, with knee repairs
        of anterior cruciate ligament, 748–749, 754–756
        of posterior cruciate ligament, 773–774, 776, 780
    thigh compartment anatomy of, 585, 585f, 596–597
Quadriceps active drawer test, for posterior cruciate ligament, 770, 770f
Quadrilateral space, in shoulder anatomy, 355–356, 360, 360f, 362, 546
Quadriplegia
    permanent
        from head and neck injuries, 167, 170
        from spearing with helmets, 172–174, 172f–173f
    transient
        with cervical spinal stenosis, 168–170, 168f
        from head and neck injuries, 163, 166
Quasi linear viscoelastic theory, for ligaments, 42–43

R
R. *See* Correlation coefficient
R². *See* Coefficient of determination
Racquet sports. *See also* Tennis
    miscellaneous injuries from, 183, 189, 225, 289
    proper equipment for, 296
    wrist injuries from, 271, 273, 280, 282–283
Radial bone, head fractures of, with elbow injuries, 291, 312
Radial collateral ligament, ulnar, 246, 324–325, 324f
Radial extrusion test, for menisci examination, 617, 618f
Radial tunnel syndrome, 285, 291–293, 297, 549–550
Radiculopathy. *See* Nerve compression injuries
Radiocarpal joint, arthrography injections in, 277, 281
Radiofrequency capsulorrhaphies, for glenoid labrum tears, 473–474, 473f–474f
Radiofrequency fields
    in nuclear scanning, 100–101
    safety of, 99–100
Radiography
    for acromioclavicular joint injuries, 517–521, 518f–520f
    of ankle impingement syndromes, 820–823, 821t, 822f
    for brachial plexus injuries, 193–194, 193f
    of clavicle fractures, 537
    of elbow injuries, 293–294, 311–312, 311f
    for flexor hallucis longus tendon injuries, 988
    for foot injuries
        of forefoot, 947, 951–952, 954–955, 959
        of hindfoot, 902, 920–926, 928, 940
        of midfoot, 902, 904–905, 908, 911–914, 916
        of toes, 966–967, 969, 974
    for hand injuries
        fractures, 233, 235, 237, 239
        soft tissue, 243–244, 246–247, 249
    for head and neck injuries
        diagnostic indications for, 161, 163–167
        emergency indications, 155–156
        flexion-extension indications, 164–167, 176f, 177
    for hip injuries, 575, 577, 579–581, 581f
    for knee injuries, 621, 791, 850–851
        ligaments, 666, 680–681, 747, 772
        patellofemoral joint, 715–719, 718f–719f, 725, 728, 735
        tendons, 691, 695, 697, 699, 701

    for leg injuries, 870, 871t, 1017
    for lumbar spine injuries, 204–205, 210–211, 210f
    of myositis ossificans, 603
    for pelvic apophyseal avulsion fractures, 601–602
    for peroneus tendon injuries, 995
    for posterior tibial tendon dysfunction, 1003
    for rotator cuff injuries, 483, 483f
    of scaphoid fractures, 258, 259f–260f, 261, 263, 264f–265f, 267
    for shoulder instability
        anterior *versus* posterior, 404, 404f, 421
        from labral injuries, 442–443, 442f–443f, 468, 468f, 471
    for sports hernias, 219, 219f
    for thigh injuries, 587, 589, 594, 597–604
    for wrist injuries, 275f, 276–277, 279–282, 280f–281f
Rami, of spinal nerves, in brachial plexus, 184–185, 185f
Randomized clinical trials (RCT), as research design, 124f, 129–130, 132, 140
Range, in research studies, 135
Range of motion deficits
    with adductor longus strains, 220–221
    with brachial plexus injuries, 191
    with cervical spine injuries, 161–164, 168, 177–178
    with counterforce bracing, 296–298, 297f
    with hand injuries, 244, 246–248, 250, 252
    with knee injuries, 628–630, 837–839, 838f. *See also specific injury*
    with lumbar spine injuries, 204
    with scaphoid fractures, 261, 267, 269, 270f
    with shoulder instability, 420, 427, 439
Range of motion mechanisms. *See specific joint*
Range of motion therapy
    for elbow injuries, 312, 317, 321–322
    for hand injuries, 244, 246–248, 250, 253–254
    for knee injuries, 668, 668f, 673
        active *versus* passive, 628–630, 839
    for scaphoid fractures, 266–267
    for shoulder injuries, 450–451, 453–454, 470, 474–475
RARE pulse sequencing, for magnetic resonance imaging, 101, 107
RCT. *See* Randomized clinical trials
Realignment procedures. *See* Reduction procedures; *specific anatomy or injury*
Reconstructive procedures. *See specific anatomy*
Recovery phase
    of running, 1012–1013
    of swimming stroke
        biomechanics of, 391, 560f, 561
        pathologic, 562, 562f
Rectal exam, indications for, 215
Rectus muscle
    disruption from pubis, 223–227, 224f, 226f
    injuries of, 585, 597
Recurrent posterior subluxations (RPS), of shoulder
    mechanisms of, 413–416, 418–419, 421
    treatment of, 421–427
Recurvatum test, external rotation, for knee ligament tears, 680, 771–772, 771f
Red-red tears, of knee meniscus, 649, 653
Reduction procedures. *See also* Internal fixation
    for carpal fractures, 263–266, 269–272
    for clavicle fractures, 537–538, 538f
    for elbow dislocations, 312
    for femoral neck fractures, 216
    for foot injuries, 902–903, 905–906, 906f, 919, 924
    for hand injuries
        fractures, 234–240, 263, 269
        soft tissue, 247–248
    for hip dislocations, 579
    with instrumentation, for lumbar spondylytic defects, 212
    for knee dislocations, 809–810
    for leg injuries, 873, 873f, 884
    for little league elbow, 319–320, 320f
    for os peroneum, 1000

    for shoulder dislocations
        anterior, 406, 406f, 445, 445f
        posterior, 421–423, 427
    for sternoclavicular dislocations, 540–541
    for toe injuries, 966–968, 976
    for wrist injuries
        scaphoid fractures, 263–266, 269–272
        soft tissue, 278, 278f, 282
Red-white tears, of knee meniscus, 649
Reflection pulleys, for tendons, 21
Reflex arcs, in glenohumeral joint stability, 385
Reflex deficits
    with brachial plexus injuries, 191–192
    with spine injuries, 164, 206, 206t
Reflex sympathetic dystrophy, post-knee repair, 832, 838
Regression analysis, in research studies, 137–138
Rehabilitation programs. *See also* Physical therapy
    for brachial plexus injuries, 194–196
    for foot injuries
        of forefoot, 947–948, 951, 957, 961
        heel pain, 635f–936f, 931–941
        of midfoot, 902, 909–912, 914–915, 917, 919
        of toes, 969–970, 976
    for hand injuries
        fractures, 233, 236
        soft tissue, 243–244, 252–253
    for hip injuries, 578–579
    for knee injuries, 667–672, 668f–670f, 668t
        articular cartilage, 793, 800–801
        ligaments, 628–630, 638, 673, 815. *See also specific ligament*
        meniscus repair, 657–658, 658t
        patellofemoral joint, 721, 723–724, 728–729, 731, 733, 735–736
        tendons, 692–697, 699–701, 704–706
    for leg injuries, 872–874, 877–879, 882
    for lumbar spine injuries, 204, 207, 211
    for muscle/tendon injuries
        Achilles dysfunction, 982–984, 986–987
        adductor longus, 220–221
        flexor hallucis longus, 989–991
        gastrocnemius complex, 697–698, 889
        hamstrings, 587, 589–591, 591f
        peroneus, 995–996, 998–1000
        posterior tibial, 1004–1007
        quadriceps, 598, 600–603
        thigh adductors, 594
        wrist, 282, 284
    for pelvic apophyseal avulsion fractures, 601–602, 601t
    for rotator cuff, 450–451, 470, 475, 485, 489, 493
    for running injuries, 1018, 1021, 1023–1024
    for shoulder injuries
        anterior dislocations, 406, 409
        from glenoid labrum contact injuries, 450–451, 453–454
        from glenoid labrum tear injuries, 470, 474–475
        posterior dislocations, 421–422, 426–427
    for tennis elbow, 289–290, 294, 297–299
    for tibiofibular joint, 883–884
    for wrist injuries, 266–267, 278, 281–282, 284
Reiter's syndrome, 215
Relative lengthening, in running cycle, 1012
Relative risk, research determination of, 127, 129, 142
Relative shortening, in running cycle, 1012
Reliability, of statistical measurements, 133
Relocation tests
    for patellofemoral joint instability, 713–714
    for shoulder stability assessment, 403–404, 403f
        with labral contact injuries, 441, 441f
        with labral tear injuries, 466–467
Remodeling activity
    of bone, 77, 80, 81f
        foot injuries and, 945, 959
    of ligaments, 667
    of tendons, 587, 690–691
Remodeling phase, of healing process, 43, 690
Repair and regeneration
    biological. *See* Homeostasis
    techniques for. *See specific anatomy or injury*

Repetitive microtrauma. *See* Overuse injuries
Repetitive motion injuries
    of elbow, 289–290, 294, 307
    of hip joint, 572
    of knee, 229
    of toes, 965
    of wrist, 273–274, 280, 283–284
Rescue breathing, for head and neck injuries, 154
Research data
    analysis methods for, 142–146
    types of, 135–136, 135*f*
Research designs
    appropriate selection of, 123, 124*f*
    descriptive category, 123–127, 124*f*
    experimental, 124*f*, 129–131
    explanatory category, 124*f*, 127–131, 128*f*
    observational, 124*f*, 127–129, 128*f*
    primary reports, 124–125, 124*f*
    synthetic evaluations, 124*f*, 125–127
Research objectives, identification importance of,
        122–123
Research studies
    application of findings, 146–147
    background information presentation for,
        133–135
    bias in, 128, 130–132, 145–146
    critical evaluation of, 121–122, 122*f*
    data analysis methods for, 142–146
    designs for, 123–131, 124*f*, 128*f*
    interpretation of results, 144–146
    question and objective identification for,
        122–123
    sample selection for, 131–133
    statistical tests for
        appropriateness of selection of, 135–142,
            135*f*, 140*f*, 142*f*
        evaluation parameters for, 123, 125, 133–134
Resistance training
    for rotator cuff rehabilitation, 485, 485*f*–486*f*
    for runners, 1015
    for shoulder rehabilitation, 475
Response rate, in research studies, 134
Rest, as treatment strategy. *See* Overuse injuries
Resting winging, with scapular dyskinesis, 503,
        503*f*, 544
Retinacula
    of leg tendons, 1007
        peroneus. *See* Peroneal retinaculum
    for tendon gliding, 21–22
Retinacula, of knee
    anatomy of, 709, 710*f*
    inferior release of, indications for, 919
    injury mechanisms of, 714–715
        lateral pressure syndrome as, 722–724,
            722*f*–724*f*, 737, 739, 740*t*
        lateral *versus* medial, 709, 710*f*, 712, 713*f*
        medial, 724–725
    lateral release of
        complications of, 833–834
        indications for, 723, 726, 729, 731, 733, 737,
            839, 1018
        techniques for, 723–724, 724*f*, 737, 739, 740*t*
Retraction/protraction function, of scapula
    abnormal, 501–502, 502*f*
    normal, 498, 500*f*, 501
Retro-Achilles bursitis, 938
Retrocalcaneal bursa
    Achilles tendon relationship to, 979
    Haglund's syndrome of, 936–937, 937*f*, 980
    of hindfoot, 897, 898*f*
    inflammatory injuries to, 979–981, 986–987
Retrocalcaneal inflammation, of Achilles tendon
    clinical evaluation of, 981
    injury mechanisms of, 979–980
    treatment of, 986–987
Retroversion, in glenohumeral instability,
        379–380, 380*f*
Return to sport guidelines
    for acromioclavicular joint injuries, 528–529,
        532
    for adductor longus strains, 221
    for ankle impingement syndromes, 822, 822*f*

for brachial plexus injuries, 196–199
for cerebral concussions, 157–158, 158*f*
for cervical spine injuries, 161, 163, 165,
        174–178
for clavicle fractures, 537–538
for elbow injuries, 299, 312, 314, 318–324, 326
for foot injuries
    of forefoot, 947, 951, 961
    of hindfoot, 921–922, 929, 933, 935–936, 940
    of midfoot, 92, 906, 914, 917, 920
    of toes, 965–966, 970
for groin pain, 225
for hamstring strains, 590–591, 591*f*, 697
for hand injuries, 233, 243–244, 247, 254
for knee injuries
    anterior cruciate ligament, 748–749, 749*t*,
        752–753, 756, 865
    chondral lesions, 801
    medial collateral ligament, 667–668, 671–672
    posterior cruciate ligament, 774, 779
    tendons, 694–695, 697, 699–701, 704, 706
for leg injuries
    miscellaneous, 882, 887–889
    stress fractures, 872–874
    of tibiofibular joint, 883–885, 887
for quadriceps injuries, 598, 600, 602–603
for running injuries, 1018, 1024, 1024*t*
for shoulder instability, 409, 422, 427, 450, –451,
        475
for spine injuries, 178, 203–207
for sternoclavicular dislocations, 540–541
for wrist fractures, 263–264, 266–267, 273
Reverse pivot shift test, for posterior cruciate liga-
        ment injuries, 772
Review articles, as research design, 124*f*, 126
Rhabdomyosarcoma, of thigh, 607
Rhomboid muscles
    anatomy of, 357
    golf swing role of, 564
    overhead throwing role of, 552–553, 553*f*
    in scapula function, 499
    swimming stroke role of, 392, 560–561
RICE (rest, ice, compression, and elevation)
    for muscle contusions, 602
    for muscle strains, 587, 589, 591, 594–595, 597
Risk factors, research determination of, 127, 129,
        142
RNA, messenger, articular cartilage matrix synthe-
        sis by, 61–62
Robotic/universal force-moment sensor (UFS sys-
        tem), for knee reconstructions, 45–46, 46*f*,
        807
Rockwood classification, of acromioclavicular
        joint dislocations, 513–515, 514*f*–515*f*
Rolando's fracture, of thumb, 239
Rotation mechanisms
    of injuries. *See* specific anatomy or injury
        per joint. *See* specific joint
    with sport activities. *See* specific sport
Rotation tests, for knee injuries, 627–634, 680,
        850
Rotator cable. *See* Rotator cuff-joint capsule
        complex
Rotator cuff
    acromion process relationship to, 373, 373*f*,
        374–375
        injury mechanisms with, 378–379, 378*f*–379*f*,
            480, 480*f*, 483*f*
    anatomy of, 352–353, 352*f*–353*f*
        microstructure, 372–373, 373*f*
        muscles of, 353–355, 372, 372*f*
        tendons, 23, 372–373, 373*f*
    biomechanics of, 372–379
        biceps tendon role in, 372, 372*f*–373*f*
        conceptual models of, 374–375, 374*f*–375*f*
        coracoacromial arch role in, 372–374, 373*f*
        force responses in, 374–376, 375*f*–376*f*
        infraspinatus muscle role in, 354, 372–373,
            372*f*–373*f*
        subscapularis muscle role in, 354–355,
            372–373, 372*f*–373*f*
        supraspinatus muscle role in, 353–354,
            372–375, 372*f*–373*f*, 375*f*–376*f*

teres minor muscle role in, 355, 372–373,
        372*f*–373*f*
    blood supply of, 353–354, 372
    collagen types in, 353, 373
    critical zone of, 354, 372, 377
    glenohumeral joint involvement, 385, 479–481,
        491, 491*f*
    impingement of
        anatomical description of, 331–332
        with brachial plexus injuries, 192
        Neer's stages of, 480, 480*t*
        outlet syndrome, 479–480, 480*f*, 480*t*
        posterior superior glenoid, 481
        secondary, 479–481
        surgical treatment of, 485–487, 489
    inflammatory mechanisms of, 376–377, 376*f*
    overhead throwing role of, 553–554
    reconstruction results of, 375, 379
    rehabilitation programs for, 450–451, 470, 475,
        485, 489, 493
    repair options for
        nonoperative, 484–485, 486*f*, 489
        operative, 375, 379, 479, 485–493
    surgical treatment options for
        acromioplasty indications, 479–480, 485–487,
            492
        anatomical markings for, 490, 490*f*
        arthroscopic, 485–483
        basic operating room setup for, 490–491
        for Bennett's lesion, 488–489
        bursa considerations, 479, 481, 491–493, 492*f*
        coracoacromial ligaments, 486–487, 492
        debridement only, 487
        decompressive, 486–487, 489
        for full-thickness tears, 487–488, 490
        glenohumeral arthroscopy, 491, 491*f*
        historical perspective of, 479
        for impingement, 485–487, 489
        for isolated subscapularis tendon ruptures,
            488
        mini-open, 487–488, 492–493, 493*f*
        open, 485–488, 493
        for partial-thickness tears, 487, 489–490
    tear injuries of
        acromion process and, 378–379, 378*f*–379*f*,
            480, 480*f*, 483*f*
        bursa involvement, 479, 481, 491–493, 492*f*
        clinical evaluation of, 481–483, 482*f*, 489
        epidemiology of, 479
        etiology of, 377–379, 479–481
        histopathology of, 376–377, 376*f*–377*f*
        imaging techniques for, 483–484, 483*f*–484*f*
        magnetic resonance imaging of, 105–107,
            107*f*–108*f*, 484, 484*f*
        mechanisms of, 372–375, 378–379, 378*f*
        microtrauma mechanisms, 413, 418–419, 421,
            481
        nerve compression, 378–379, 379*f*
        pathoanatomy of, 376–377, 376*f*–377*f*,
            480–481, 480*f*, 480*t*
        scapula dyskinesis with, 502, 506–509
        SLAP lesions and, 432–433, 432*f*, 436,
            438–439, 442
        with tennis elbow, 298
        with throwing, 464–465, 467
        treatment of, 484–493
        vascular involvement, 481
    tendinitis of, 376–377
    training modification programs for, 484–485
Rotator cuff-joint capsule complex, biomechanics
        of, 372–373, 372*f*–373*f*, 375
Rotator interval, anatomy of, 353, 353*f*, 355–356
Roux-Elmsli-Trillat procedure, for patellofemoral
        joint realignment, 638–639
Roux-Goldthwait realignment procedure, for pa-
        tellofemoral joint dislocations, 731–732,
        731*f*, 734, 834
RPS. *See* Recurrent posterior subluxations
Ruffini corpuscles, as mechanoreceptors, 31, 385,
        418
Rugby, injuries from, 586, 597, 663
Runner's knee, 689, 698, 705–706, 714, 1018

Running
  aerobic conditioning for, 872, 878, 1011, 1015,
    1022
  gait phases of, 1011–1013
  injuries from
    in ankle, 992, 994, 1000–1001
    biomechanics of, 1011–1013
    clinical presentations of, 889, 1017
    epidemiology of, 1011
    evaluation of, 1013–1017
    in foot, 1019–1020
      forefoot, 954, 979
        midfoot and hindfoot, 904f, 918, 920, 921f,
          923, 925f
    in knee, 691, 694–695, 1017–1019
    in leg, 869, 871, 873, 875–876, 886, 889
    muscle strains, 587
    orthotics for, 871, 877, 878f, 1023
    osteoarthritis, 1021–1022
    rehabilitation programs for, 1018, 1021,
      1023–1024
    return to sport guidelines, 872–874, 1018,
      1024, 1024t
    stress fractures, 1020–1021
    surgery indications for, 1018–1020, 1024
    treatment of, 1022–1024
  load reduction strategies for, 1013
  medial tibial stress syndrome from, 875–876,
    1021
  progressive program of, for knee ligament injur-
    ies, 671
  stress fractures from
    in femur, 603–604
    in hindfoot, 920, 921f
    in hip joint, 572, 1020
    in leg bones, 869, 871, 873, 1020–1021
  total body fitness for, 872, 878, 1011, 1015,
    1022–1023
  training principles for, 1013–1016, 1022
Rupture injuries
  of ligaments. See specific joint or ligament
  of tendons
    biomechanics of, 33–35
    per joint. See specific joint or tendon
R × C table, in research studies, 138–139

S
Sacroiliac disorders, 229, 572, 572t
Sacrum
  ligament attachments to, 223, 224f
  stress fractures of, 1020
Salter-Harris classification, of hand fractures, 233,
  236, 238, 240
Sample selection, for research studies, 131–133,
  139
Sand toe, 950, 968
Sarcomeres
  anatomy and physiology of, 4–5, 5f
  in muscle contractions, 9–12, 10f–11f
Sarcoplasmic reticulum (SR), in muscle contraction, 6, 9, 10f, 18, 18t
Sartorius muscle, anatomy of, 585
Scaffolds. See Collagen scaffolds
Scaphoid bone
  anatomy of, 257
  excision of, for fracture complications, 269, 270f
  fractures of
    acute treatment of, 263–266, 264f–265f
    clinical evaluation of, 260–261
    complexities and dislocations, 267, 268f–269f
    computed tomography of, 258–259,
      258f–259f, 261–263, 267
    displacement with, 258–260, 258f,
      260f–262f, 263, 264f–265f
    grafts for, 260, 261f–262f, 266–267, 269
    immobilization of, 258–260, 260f, 263–267
    magnetic resonance imaging of, 116, 261, 263
    mechanisms of, 257
    morphology of, 257–260, 258f–260f
    radiography of, 258, 259f–260f, 261, 263,
      264f–265f, 267
    rehabilitation of, 266–267

  treatment classifications, 257–260
  treatment results, 259f, 260, 261f–262f,
    263–264, 267, 269, 270f
  impingement, chronic manifestations of, 277
Scaphoid impaction syndrome, 278–279
Scapholunate ligament (SL)
  arthroscopy applications for, 277–278
  Blatt reconstructive procedure for, 278, 278f
  injuries of
    evaluation of, 275–277, 276f
    mechanisms of, 274–275, 275f
    treatment of, 277–278, 278f
Scapula
  abnormalities, with acromioclavicular joint dislo-
    cations, 500f, 501, 506, 516f–517f, 517,
    520–521
  acromion elevation by
    abnormal, 332, 500f, 501–502
    normal, 498–499, 505
  anatomy of, 330–334, 331f–333f, 497
  biomechanics of, 499, 500f, 501
  dyskinesis of
    diagonal patterns of, 508, 508f
    measurements of, 503–505, 504f–505f, 505t
    mechanisms of, 501–503, 502f, 503t, 506, 544
    rehabilitation considerations in, 506–509,
      506f–509f
    resting winging with, 503, 503f, 544
    rotator cuff involvement with, 502, 506–509
    treatment considerations for, 505–506
  evaluation guidelines for, 503–505, 503f–504f,
    505t
  fractures of, 501, 506
  impingement syndrome of, 500f, 501–502,
    505–506, 544
  muscle origins and insertions of
    as stabilizers, 331–332, 331f, 386, 499, 501
    strength measurements of, 503–505
    in throwing motions, 498
    treatment options for, 505–506
  ossification process of, 331–332
  overhead throwing role of
    biomechanics of, 497–498, 499f, 501–503,
      503t, 552–553, 553f
    pathologic, 556–557, 556f
  physiology of, 499–501, 500f
  posture relationship to, 503, 506–507, 506f–507f
  retraction/protraction function of
    abnormal, 501–502, 502f
    normal, 498, 500f, 501, 505
  shoulder functions of
    with injuries, 501–503, 502f, 503t
    stability, 380, 380f, 497–498
    throwing, 497–498, 499f
  snapping, 340, 503, 506
  swimming stroke role of, 392, 560–561
  translation mechanisms of, 499
Scapular assistance test, 503
Scapular slide, lateral
  biomechanics of, 501–503, 502f, 503t
  measurements of, 504–505, 504f, 508–509
Scapulothoracic joint
  anatomy of, 339–340, 356–358
  bursitis of, 503, 506
  dissociation versus dislocation of, 340
  dyskinesis of
    measurements of, 503–505, 504f–505f, 505t
    mechanisms of, 501–503, 502f, 503t
    rehabilitation considerations in, 506–509,
      506f–509f
  range of motion of, 339–340
Scar tissue
  in ligament healing, 820
  of knee, 757f, 758, 812, 828
  nerve endings in, 290
Sciatica
  acute, from herniated nucleus pulposus,
    205–208, 206t
  knee pain and, 620
  with piriformis syndrome, 228–229
Scintigraphy. See Bone scans; specific anatomy
Screw fixation

  for acromioclavicular joint dislocations, 522f,
    523, 525–528, 525f–528f
  range of motion and, 370–371, 512–513, 528
  for clavicle fractures, 538
  for femoral neck fractures, 216
  for hand fractures, 234–239, 234f
  for knee injuries
    ligament repairs, 632, 673, 750
    patellar repair, 703, 703f, 835
    posterolateral, 682, 814–815
  for lumbar spondylytic defects, 211–212
  of midfoot injuries, 906, 906f, 909, 911f
  for scaphoid fractures, 260, 260f, 262f, 263–265,
    264f–265f, 268f, 269
  for shoulder injuries, 447, 447f, 452, 471
Scrotal exam, indications for, 219
Scuderi's proximal realignment procedures, for patellofemoral joint dislocations, 730t, 731
Scuderi technique, for quadriceps tendon rupture
  repair, 599f, 600, 693–694
SD. See Standard deviation
SDH. See Succinate dehydrogenase
SE. See Standard error
Second impact syndrome, 158, 160
Segond fracture, with knee ligament tears, 666,
  747
SEM. See Standard error of the mean
Semimembranosus muscle, anatomy of, 583–584,
  584f, 806
Semitendinosus muscle, anatomy of, 583–584,
  584f
Semitendinosus tendon grafts
  for ligament reconstruction, 675, 751, 777, 783,
    828
  for tendon reconstruction, 693, 702, 702f, 704
  tensile strength of, 825
Semmes Weinstein monofilament test, 274, 939
Sensitivity, in research studies, 141
Sensory deficits
  with brachial plexus injuries, 191
  with lumbar spine injuries, 206, 206t
Sensory evoked potentials
  for brachial plexus injuries, 193–194
  for wrist injuries, 274
Sensory ganglia, of spinal nerves, in brachial
  plexus, 185–186, 185f, 191
Sensory mapping. See Semmes Weinstein monofilament test
Serratus anterior muscle
  anatomy of, 357
  golf swing role of, 564
  nerve injuries of, 544
  overhead throwing role of, 552–553, 553f,
    556–557
  in shoulder pathology, 501–502, 505
  strength assessment of, 503
  swimming stroke role of, 392, 560–562
Serving activities. See also Overhead athlete
  scapula role in, 497–498, 499f
    biomechanics of, 499–501, 500f
Sesamoid complex
  metatarsophalangeal dislocations and, 951–952,
    954, 955f
Sesamoidectomy, 957
Sesamoiditis, 954–955, 957–958
Sesamoid ligaments
  anatomy of, 949, 949f, 954, 955f
  painful accessory syndrome of. See Os per-
    oneum
  toe injuries and, 949f, 967–970, 967f, 969f
Sesamoids
  anatomy of, 954
  bipartite, 954, 956f, 969
  bursitis of, 954
  chondromalacia of, 954–955
  diastasis of, with toe injuries, 969–970, 969f
  fractures of, 954–955, 956f, 957
  injuries of
    evaluation of, 954–955, 955f–966f
    mechanisms of, 954–955, 958
    treatment and outcome of, 957
  osteochondritis of, 954, 957

osteomyelitis of, 954–955, 957
Sex steroids, bone formation and, 82
Sexually transmitted diseases, 215
SFA (Societ Franaise Arthroscopie) score, for os-
teoarthritis, 65
SGHL. *See* Superior glenohumeral ligament
Sharpey's fibers, in tendons, 26, 39
Shear load
  articular cartilage response to, 58–59, 58*f*, 64,
    787, 788*f*, 789
    injury mechanisms with, 789–791, 789*f*–790*f*,
      793
  cervical spine injuries from, 166
  as knee injury mechanism, 627, 633, 687, 847
  as scapula injury mechanism, 502
  tendon buffer for, 27
Shear test, for lunotriquetral ligament injury, 279
Shelf sign, with patellar entrapment syndrome,
  838, 838*f*
Shell bilateral post design, for knee braces,
  864–865
Shift test, for shoulder assessment, 403, 403*f*
Shin guards, leg fractures and, 874, 874*f*
Shin splints. *See* Medial tibial stress syndrome
Shoe inserts. *See also* Heel wedge; Insoles
  for knee cartilage injuries, 793
Shoes
  Achilles tendon dysfunction and, modifications
    for, 981
  forefoot injuries and
    in dancers, 960–962
    modifications of, 946, 950, 958–959
  hindfoot injuries and, modifications of,
    921–927, 927*f*, 931–932, 937–938, 940
  midfoot injuries and
    lacing alternatives for, 912, 912*f*, 919
    modifications of, 911–914, 912*f*–913*f*, 915*f*,
      917, 919, 919*f*
  for running, 1013, 1017, 1019
    modifications of, 1022–1023
  toe deformities and, 972–975, 973*f*
  toe injuries and, 950, 966, 970, 970*f*, 972
Short bones, structure of, 75
Short lateral ligament (SLL), of knee
  anatomy of, 676–677, 805–806
  biomechanics of, 677, 806–808
  injuries of, 679–680, 683–685
Short tau inversion recovery (STIR), for magnetic
  resonance imaging, 101, 112, 116
Shoulder girdle, atrophy of, with rotator cuff injuries, 481, 482*f*
Shoulder grinding factor, 462
Shoulder instability, return to sport guidelines,
  409, 422, 427, 450, –451, 475
Shoulder joint. *See also* Glenohumeral joint
  abduction of
    mechanisms of, 346–348, 347*f*–348*f*, 351–352,
      359
    per joint. *See specific joint*
  acute brachial neuropathy of, 184, 190. *See also*
    Brachial plexus
  anatomy of
    bones, 329–335, 330*f*–334*f*
    bursae, 361–362, 362*f*
    joints, 329, 335–343, 336*f*–338*f*, 341*f*–342*f*
    labrum, 348–351, 349*f*–350*f*
    ligaments, 343–348, 344*f*–345*f*, 347*f*–348*f*
    muscles, 351–360, 351*f*–353*f*, 360*f*
    nerve supply, 330, 344, 352, 354–361, 361*f*
    normal, 433–435, 433*f*–435*f*, 457–458, 458*f*
    spaces, 355–356, 360, 360*f*, 362–363
    vascular, 330, 339, 341, 342*f*, 343, 350,
      352–358, 360
  biomechanics of, 367
    acromioclavicular joint, 369–372, 369*f*–371*f*
    coracoacromial arch, 373–374, 373*f*
    force resistance per position, 418–421, 432
    glenohumeral joint, 379–386, 380*f*–382*f*, 380*t*,
      384*f*, 386*f*
    rotator cuff, 372–379, 372*f*–379*f*
    sternoclavicular joint, 367–369, 368*f*–369*f*
  bone anatomy of, 329

clavicle, 329–330, 330*f*
  humerus, 334–335, 334*f*
  scapula, 330–334, 331*f*–333*f*
bursae
  anatomy of, 361–362, 362*f*
  rotator cuff tears and, 479–481, 491–492, 492*f*
electromyography analysis of, 385, 387, 392, 394
force couples of, 374–375, 374*f*–375*f*
imaging techniques for, 381
impingement syndromes in
  arthroscopic findings of, 471–472
  from golfing, 289–291, 302–304, 565–566,
    566*f*
  with instability, 402, 406, 419, 442
  mechanisms of, 192, 277, 331–332, 543–547
  scapula involvement with, 500*f*, 501
  from swimming, 563, 563*f*, 566*f*
  from throwing, 461–465, 463*f*, 468, 557–559,
    559*f*, 566*f*
injuries of
  capsular. *See* Glenohumeral capsule
  force as mechanism of, 436–438, 437*f*,
    461–465
  from golfing, 564–566, 565*f*–566*f*
  joint-related. *See* Glenohumeral joint; Gleno-
    humeral ligaments
  labral. *See* Glenoid labrum
  from pitching. *See* Pitching
  scapula role in, 501–503, 502*f*, 503*t*
instability and dislocations of
  anterior mechanisms. *See* Anterior shoulder
    instability
  microinstability, 344, 457–475
  in overhead athletes, 389–391, 389*f*–391*f*,
    402, 413, 418
  posterior mechanisms. *See* Posterior shoulder
    instability
  rotator cuff mechanisms of. *See* Rotator cuff
  superior mechanisms. *See* Superior glenoid
    labrum
  with throwing motions, 389–391, 389*f*–391*f*,
    402
joint anatomy of, 329
  acromioclavicular, 337–339, 337*f*–338*f*
  capsule and glenohumeral ligaments,
    343–348, 344*f*–345*f*, 347*f*–348*f*
  glenohumeral, 340–343, 341*f*–342*f*
  scapulothoracic, 339–340
  sternoclavicular, 335–337, 336*f*
kinematics of
  with golf swing, 393–394, 393*f*
  with swimming, 391–392, 391*f*
  with tennis, 392–393, 392*f*–393*f*
  with throwing, 387–391, 387*f*–391*f*
labrum of
  anatomy of, 348–351, 349*f*–350*f*
  injuries to. *See* Glenoid labrum
  magnetic resonance imaging of, 108–110,
    109*f*
  stability significance of, 108
ligaments
  anatomy of, 343–348, 344*f*–345*f*, 347*f*–348*f*,
    368*f*–370*f*
  biomechanical functions of, 367–388
  sport kinematics of, 387–394
magnetic resonance imaging of
  instability, 107–110, 107*f*, 109*f*
  rotator cuff tears, 105–107, 107*f*–108*f*
muscle anatomy of, 351
  glenohumeral group, 351*f*–353*f*, 352–356
  multiple joint group, 358–360, 360*f*
  scapulothoracic group, 356–358
nerve supply to, 344, 352, 354–359
  brachial plexus as, 184–185, 184*f*–185*f*, 330,
    360–361, 361*f*
  injury mechanisms of, 543–547, 545*f*
range of motion of
  mechanisms of, 329–330, 336–340, 351–360
  per joint. *See specific joint*
rotation of
  mechanisms of, 346–348, 347*f*–348*f*, 354–357,
    359
  per joint. *See specific joint*
space anatomy of, 355–356, 360, 360*f*, 362–363

stability of
  anterior mechanisms, 399–401
  evolution of, 329–330
  mechanisms of, 107–110, 345, 347–348, 350,
    353–354, 359
  per joint. *See specific joint*
stereophotogrammetry of, 378*f*, 379, 381
translation mechanisms of
  anatomical basis of, 355–356, 433–434
  biomechanical principles of, 371, 371*f*,
    374–375, 381, 383–385
  with dislocations, 401, 418–420
  grading per glenoid fossa, 440–441, 440*f*
  with labral contact injuries, 440–442,
    440*f*–441*f*
Shoulder pads
  for burner syndrome prevention, 188, 195
  emergency removal of, for head and neck injur-
    ies, 154–155
Significance testing
  clinical importance *versus,* 143–145
  statistical, 123, 141–144
Sinding-Larsen-Johansson disease, knee tendon injuries with, 705–706
Single-integral finite strain theory, for ligaments,
  42–43
Single-photon emission computed tomography
  (SPECT)
  for compartment syndromes, 89
  for lumbar spondylolisthesis, 211–212, 212*f*
Sinusoidal wave pattern. *See* Crimping
Sinus tarsi syndrome, 919
Skeletal muscle
  anatomy and physiology of
    architecture of, 6–9, 13, 17
    cell structure of, 3–6
    neural activation of, 9–10, 10*f*
  mechanical properties of, 3, 7–8, 8*f*–9*f*, 13
    active length-tension relationship, 10–11,
      11*f*
    force-velocity relationship, 12–13, 12*f*, 14*f*
    passive length-tension relationship, 11–12,
      11*f*, 12*t*
  types of
    histochemical, 13–16, 15*f*–16*f*, 16*t*
    morphologic properties of, 17–18, 18*t*
    physiologic properties of, 16–17
Skeletal muscle architecture
  impact on mechanical properties, 13, 14*f*
  of lower limb, 7–8, 8*f*
  physiologic principles of, 6–7, 17
  types of, 6–7, 7*f*
  of upper limb, 8–9, 9*f*
Skeletal muscle cell
  connective tissue matrix of, 3–4, 4*f*
  contractile protein hierarchy of, 4–5, 5*f*
  diameter and length of, 3
  force production by, 3, 4*f*–5*f*, 5–6. *See also* Mus-
    cle contractions
Skeletal traction
  brachial plexus injury from, 162–163
  for cervical fractures and dislocations, 164,
    166–167
  for hand injuries, 238, 248, 251*f*
  for patellar tendon repair, 702
Ski boot syndrome, 918–920, 918*f*–919*f*
Skiing
  foot and ankle injuries from, 918–920,
    918*f*–919*f*, 992–993
  knee injuries from, 743–744
Skillful neglect. *See* Benign neglect
Skin disorders
  in dancer's feet, 960–961
  of thigh, 607
Skin grafts, for leg fasciotomies, 881
SL. *See* Scapholunate ligament
SLAP lesions, of glenoid labrum
  arthroscopic treatment of, 451–453, 453*f*,
    470–471
  classification of, 432–433, 432*f*, 463–464, 472*f*
  contact injury mechanisms of, 436, 438–439

SLAP lesions, of glenoid labrum (contd.)
  tear injury mechanisms of, 463–464
  tests for, 442
Sling immobilization, for dislocations
  of acromioclavicular joint, 521f, 522, 528,
    531–532
  of shoulder dislocations, 406, 409, 450–451
  of sternoclavicular joint, 537–538, 540–541
Slip injuries
  of capital femoral epiphysis, 596
  in lumbar spine. See Spondylolysis
  of proximal interphalangeal joints, 248,
    250–252, 251f
SLL. See Short lateral ligament
Slow oxidative muscle fibers (SO), 14, 16–18, 16t,
    18t
Snakebites, compartment syndromes from, 89,
    94–95
Snapping hip syndrome, 229, 574–576, 574f, 576f
Snapping scapula, 340, 503, 506
Snapping tibialis anterior tendon, 1008
Snyder classification of superior labrum injuries.
    See SLAP lesions
SO. See Slow oxidative muscle fibers
Soccer
  ankle injuries from, 820, 987, 992
  athletic pubalgia from, 223, 225
  knee injuries from, 691, 700, 743
  leg injuries from, 874, 883
  thigh muscle strains from, 585–588, 593, 597
  toe injuries from, 966, 968
Sodium, in articular cartilage, 53, 55
Soft tissue decompression, for rotator cuff injur-
    ies, 487
Soft tissue fixation, of anterior cruciate ligament
    grafts, 47–48, 48f, 750–751, 752f
Soft tissue injuries
  with cervical spine injuries, 164–165
  compartment syndromes from, 89, 94–95
  of hand
    with fractures, 233–235
    ligaments, 238, 243–248
    tendons, 236, 239, 239f, 248–254
  knee cartilage changes with, 63
  of lumbar spine, 203, 205, 208
  of patellofemoral joint, 714, 714f, 721–722,
    721f. See also Patellar tendinitis
  of pelvis and hip, 230
  of wrists
    ligaments, 274–282, 275f–276f, 278f–281f
    tendons, 279, 282–285, 283f
Soft tissue reconstruction
  for patellofemoral dislocations, 731–734,
    731f–733f
  for shoulder dislocations
    nerve injuries and, 544
    posterior, 415, 422–423
Soft tissue tumors, 607, 620
Soleus bridge, in medial tibial stress syndrome,
    876, 876f, 1013
Soleus muscles, running force impact on, 1013
Soleus syndrome. See Medial tibial stress syn-
    drome
Space flight, bone adaptation to, 80
Spear tackler's spine, 176–177, 176f
  cervical spine injuries from, 172–174, 172f–173f,
    197
Specificity, in research studies, 141
SPECT. See Single-photon emission computed to-
    mography
Spectroscopy, for compartment syndromes, 94
Speed test, for shoulder assessment, with labral
    tear injuries, 466
Spina bifida occulta, 175
Spinal canal
  mean diameter of, 170, 171f
  measurement methods for, with cervical steno-
    sis, 168–171, 169f, 171f–172f
  vertebral body ratio to, 168–169, 169f, 175
Spinal column injuries. See specific spinal region

Spinal cord
  compression of. See also Nerve compression in-
    juries
    canal relationship to, 168–171
    with cervical fractures or dislocations, 156,
      164–165, 168, 168f
    helmet spearing and, 173–173, 173f
  injuries of
    acute anterior syndrome, 163, 166
    with cervical fractures or dislocations
      lower region, 167–168, 168f, 177
      management principles for, 164–165
      midcervical region, 166–167, 177
      upper region, 165–166
    methylprednisolone guidelines for, 156, 165,
      180
    neurologic recovery from, 178–180, 179f
    paralysis from. See Quadriplegia
    pincer mechanism of, 168–169, 168f
    prevention strategies for, 172–174, 172f–173
    steroid indications for, 156, 164–165
    resuscitation of, 164, 178–180, 179f
Spinal shock, from cervical spine injuries, 164,
    178–180, 179f
Spine
  alignment of, scapular dyskinesis and, 501, 503,
    506, 506f–507f
  evaluation of, with scapula assessment,
    503–505, 504f–505f, 505t
  fusions of. See specific spinal region
  kyphosis of, from scapula fractures, 501, 506,
    506f
  lordosis of
    with pitching, 557, 559f
    from scapula fractures, 501, 503
  stabilization of, 207
  stenosis of. See Cervical spine
Spine boards, for emergency care, of head and
    neck injuries, 153–154, 155f
Spin echo pulse sequencing, for magnetic reso-
    nance imaging, 101
Spin-lattice relaxation, in magnetic resonance im-
    aging, 100
Spinoglenoid ligament, nerve injuries and, 545
Spin-spin relaxation, in magnetic resonance im-
    aging, 100
Splints and splinting
  for Achilles tendon dysfunction, 982–983, 985
  available options for, 250
  for elbow tendinosis
    as counterforce bracing, 296–298, 297f, 317
    postoperative, 302, 302f, 319–320, 325–326
  figure-of-eight
    for clavicle fractures, 537–538
    for scapula dyskinesis, 507, 507f
  for flexor hallucis longus tendon injuries, 990
  for foot injuries, 909, 911, 913–915, 914f, 919,
    957
  for hand fractures, 235–238
  hip-knee-foot, post-hamstring repair, 592
  for interphalangeal joint injuries, 247, 247f,
    250–254, 254f
  for peroneus tendon injuries, 999–1000
  for posterior tibial tendon injuries, 1006–1007
  for scaphoid fractures, 266–267
  for ulnar collateral ligament tears, 244, 245f
  for upper extremity nerve injuries, 547,
    549–550
  for wrists
    for hyperextension injury prevention,
      278–279
    injury stabilization, 280–281, 284–285
Spondyloarthropathies, pelvic pain from, 215
Spondylolisthesis
  classification of, 209
  of lumbar spine
    etiology of, 209
    illustrative case of, 212–213, 212f
    natural history of, 209–210
    radiologic evaluation of, 210–211, 210f
    treatment of, 211–212, 212f

Spondylolysis, of lumbar spine, 209–213, 212f
Sports
  compartment syndromes during, 89–91, 94
  hernias from, 218–219, 219f
  injuries from. See specific anatomy, injury, or
    sport
  loads from. See Force; Load
Sprains
  of ankle, 819–823, 872, 879, 883, 887
    impingement syndromes from, 819–823,
      939–940
  cervical syndrome from, 160, 163
  of shoulder, 565
  of toes, 949, 968–970, 968f–970f
  of wrist, 261, 273–274
Spring ligament. See Calcaneonavicular ligament
Sprinting, injuries from, 580, 585, 590, 601
Spurling's maneuver, for cervical neck injuries,
    162, 192, 192f
Spurs. See Bone spurs; Heel spurs
Squatting
  ankle arthrosis from, 821
  jumping from, leg fractures with, 874
  patellofemoral joint function with, 636–638, 725
SR. See Sarcoplasmic reticulum
Stability mechanisms. See specific anatomy or
    injury
Stair climbing
  for anterior cruciate ligament rehabilitation, 749
  patellofemoral joint function with, 637, 725
Stance phase, of running, 1011–1013
Standard deviation (SD), in research studies, 133,
    135
Standard error (SE), in research studies, 135–136
Standard error of the mean (SEM), in research
    studies, 133, 136
Staple fixation
  for shoulder injuries, 446–447
  for tibial avulsion fractures, 774–775, 775f
Starling equation, of capillary fluid dynamics, 88
Static deformity, in wrists, 275, 278–280
Statistical analysis, types of, 142–146
Statistical practices, critical evaluation of
  application of findings, 146–147
  background information presentation, 133–135
  data analysis methods, 142–144
  interpretation of results, 144–146
  key questions for, 121–122, 122f
  sample selection, 131–133
  study design appropriateness, 123–131, 124f,
    128f
  study question and objective identification,
    122–123
Statistical tests and techniques
  appropriate selection of, 135
  of confidence, 140–141, 143–144
  of correlation, 125, 133, 137, 145
  diagnostic value of, 141–142, 142f
  independence of, 136
  for multiple comparisons, 137
  nonparametric, 136, 138–139
  parametric, 136–138
  predictive, 138, 141
  of regression, 137–138
  reliability of, 133
  of significance, 123, 141–145
  for small samples, 139
  summarization methods for, 133–134
  survival analysis as, 139–141, 140f
  validity of, 134, 139
  of variance, 133–137, 145
Statistics
  descriptive, 135, 142
  inferential, 135, 146
Stener lesion, 116, 244, 246
Step-off, normal anterior, posterior cruciate liga-
    ment injuries and, 769, 769f
Step-up exercises, for knee ligaments, 670, 670f
Stereophotogrammetry, for shoulder analysis,
    378f, 379, 381
Sterilization techniques, for allografts, 826
Sternoclavicular joint

anatomy of, 335–337, 336f, 368f
biomechanics of, 367–369, 368f–369f
dislocation injuries of
  with brachial plexus injuries, 187, 191
  classification of, 539
  epidemiology of, 538
  evaluation of, 539–540, 539f–540f
  mechanisms of, 337, 539, 539f
  nonoperative treatment of, 540–541
  operative treatment of, 369, 540
  return to sport guidelines, 540–541
  treatment outcomes for, 369, 540–541
range of motion of, 336–337, 369, 369f
stability mechanisms of, 336, 367–368, 368f
Steroids, injections and oral. See also specific type
  for acute brachial neuropathy, 196
  anabolic, risks of, 598
  for ankle sprains, 821, 822f
  for elbow injuries, 294–295, 326
  for forefoot injuries, cautions with, 948, 951, 958
  for knee injuries, 695–698, 705, 721–722, 839, 853
    knee tendon injuries from, 688, 691, 700, 1018
  for lumbar spine injuries, 207
  for muscle strains, 594
  for runners' injuries, 1023–1024
  for spinal cord injuries, 156, 164, 180
  for wrist ligament injuries, 281–282, 284–285
Stieda's process, of ankle, fracture of, 924–926, 925f–926f
Stiffness. See Arthrofibrosis
Stinger syndrome. See Burner syndrome
STIR. See Short tau inversion recovery
Stool, hemoccult analysis of, 215
Strain energy density, of ligaments, 40, 40f
Strain gage analysis
  of glenohumeral ligaments, 382–384, 391, 435–436
  of knee, 625–626
    anterior cruciate ligament, 627–629
    with functional bracing, 866–867
    muscle bundle comparisons, 624–625, 628–630, 633
Strain injuries
  of knee, 625
  of ligaments, 40f, 41–43
  of muscles. See Muscle strain injuries
  of musculotendinous junction, 26, 34, 218, 220, 223, 230
  of scapula, 502
  of shoulder, 565
  of tendons, 594–595
Strength deficits
  with acute cervical sprains, 163
  with lower extremity injuries
    of nerves, 885–886
    of popliteal artery, 886–887
  with tibial tendon dysfunction, 1002–1003
  with upper extremity nerve injuries, 545, 547
    brachial plexus mechanisms, 161–163, 191, 194–198
Strength testing, 191, 754
Strength training
  for adductor longus strains, 221
  for ankle sprains, 821, 822f
  for brachial plexus rehabilitation, 195–196
  closed chain. See Closed chain exercises
  for forearm, 298–299, 321–322
  for hamstring strains, 590–591, 591f
  for knee injuries
    of anterior cruciate ligament, 748–749, 754–756
    of articular cartilage, 793, 801, 852
    meniscus repairs and, 657–658, 658t
    of patellofemoral joint, 723–724, 728, 735
    of posterior cruciate ligament, 773–774, 776, 780
    of tendons, 697, 699, 701, 706
  for knee ligaments, 670, 670f
  muscle response to, 3
  open chain. See Open chain exercises

patellofemoral joint response to, 636
  for pelvic mobility, 217–218
  for rotator cuff rehabilitation, 485, 485f–486f
  for runners, 1011, 1023
  for shoulder instability, 409, 450–451, 453, 470, 475
  for tibiofibular joint instability, 884–885
  for ulnar collateral ligament tears, 244–245, 317
Stress
  as healing stimulus, 587, 667
  in ligaments, 40, 40f, 667
  in patellofemoral joint, 636–639
Stress fractures
  compartment syndrome versus, 91–92
  of cuboid joint, 904, 904f
  of femur, 113, 572–574, 573f, 603–604, 1020
  of forefoot, 959–960, 966
    metatarsals, 902, 903f, 945–947, 947f, 959, 966
    tarsal navicular, 903, 905, 905f–907f, 1021
  of hindfoot, 920, 921f, 929–930, 931f
  of hip, 113, 572–574, 573f, 603–604, 1020
  of inferior ramus, 595
  of leg bones, 869–874, 870f, 870t–871t, 887, 1020–1021
    fibula, 873–874, 873f–874f, 887
    medial malleolus, 872–873, 873f
    tibia, 870–872, 871f–872f, 871t, 1021
  magnetic resonance imaging of
    in elbow, 311, 324
    in foot and ankle, 111, 112f, 1021
    in hip, 113, 573, 573f
    in leg, 1020–1021
  of midfoot, 902–906, 903f–906f
  of olecranon, 308, 311, 323–324, 324f
  of pelvis, 216, 229, 1020
  from running
    bone-specifc, 869–874, 870f–874f, 870t–871t, 887
    mechanisms of, 869–871, 1020–1021
Stress relaxation
  articular cartilage and, 58–60, 66
  cyclic. See Creep
  definition of, 41, 42f
  of ligaments, 41–43, 42f
  of tendons, 33
Stress-strain curve
  of ligaments, 40, 40f
  of tendons, 24, 24f, 33–34, 33f
Stress testing
  of elbow injuries, 310, 310f, 312
  for midfoot injuries, 908, 909f
  for posterior shoulder instability, 420
Stress views, radiographic
  for acromioclavicular dislocations, 518–520, 519f
  for ankle impingement syndrome, 821–822, 822f
  for knee ligament injuries, 747, 772
Stretchers, for emergency care, of head and neck injuries, 153–154
Stretch force, as muscle strain component, 586, 586f
Stretching exercises
  for Achilles tendon dysfunction, 982–984
  for elbow injuries, 313, 322, 324
  for flexor hallucis longus tendon injuries, 989
  for hamstring strains, 590
  for heel injuries, 931, 935
  importance of, 42
  for knee injuries, 657, 721, 729
  for lumbar spine injuries, 204, 207
  for pelvic mobility, 217–218
  for rotator cuff rehabilitation, 485
  for scapular dyskinesis, 506
  for shin splints, 877–878
  for shoulder throwing functions, 470, 475
Stretch receptors, in glenohumeral joint stability, 385, 418
Stride, with pitching, 387–388, 387f, 458–459, 459f
Stroke techniques. See Swimming; Tennis

Stromelysin (MMP3), articular cartilage degradation by, 62
Stryker monitor, for compartment pressures, 880, 880f, 882
Stryker Notch view, radiographic
  of acromioclavicular joint injuries, 520, 520f
  for shoulder instability, 442–443, 443f, 468, 468f, 471
Study groups, in research, 131–135
Subacromial bursa, anatomy of, 361–362
Subchondral bone, articular cartilage injuries and, 55, 63–64, 67
Subclavius muscle, anatomy of, 358
Subdural hematomas, acute, 159
Subfascicles, in tendon collagen, 22f, 23–24
Sublabral foramen, as common variant, 350–351
Subluxations. See specific anatomy
Subscapularis bursa, anatomy of, 361–362, 362f
Subscapularis muscle
  anatomy of, 354–355
  in anterior shoulder stabilizations, 408f, 409
  golf swing role of, 394, 564
  overhead throwing role of, 553–555, 553f, 557
  in rotator cuff biomechanics, 354–355, 372–373, 372f–373f
  swimming stroke role of, 392, 561–562
Subscapularis tendon, isolated rupture of, 488, 488f
Subtalar joint
  anatomy of, 898–899, 898f
  arthritis of, 926–927, 926f–927f
  arthrodesis indications for, 927–929, 929f
  ossicle variation of. See Os trigonum
  rotation of, posterior tibial tendon role in, 1000, 1001f
Subtalar-midtarsal joint complex, running force impact on, 1012–1013
  alignment measurements with, 1016–1017
Succinate dehydrogenase (SDH), muscle fiber typing with, 13–14, 15f, 16t
Sulcus angle, of patellofemoral joint, 718–719, 719f, 724, 735
Sulcus sign, of shoulder instability, 403, 420, 440–441, 466
Superficial zone protein, in articular cartilage, 54t, 55
Superior glenohumeral ligament (SGHL)
  in contact injuries, 433–434, 433f–434f
  functional anatomy of, 344–346, 382–383, 382f
  in shoulder stability
    anterior, 400–401
    posterior, 417–418, 417f, 420
  in throwing injuries, 390–391, 461
Superior glenoid labrum
  contact injuries of
    arthroscopic treatment of, 451–454, 453f
    classification of, 432–433, 432f
    clinical evaluation of, 438–442, 440f–441f
    epidemiology of, 432–433
    imaging analysis of, 442–445, 442f–444f
    injury mechanisms of, 436, 438
    nonoperative treatment of, 451, 453–454
  tear injuries of
    arthroscopic treatment of, 470–473, 472f–474f
    mechanisms of, 463–464
Superior shoulder instability, from glenoid labral injuries. See Superior glenoid labrum
Superior sulcus tumor, brachial plexus injuries and, 191, 193
Supination, of foot. See Foot supination
Support phase, of running, 1011–1013
Supraspinatus muscle
  anatomy of, 353–354
  biomechanics of, 375–376, 376f
    rotator cuff and, 353–354, 372–375, 372f–373f, 375f
  overhead throwing role of, 552–555, 553f
  swimming stroke role of, 392, 560–561
Supraspinatus tendon
  critical zone of, 354, 372, 377
  rotator cuff relationship with

Supraspinatus tendon (*contd.*)
  biomechanics of, 373–374, 373*f*
  injury mechanisms of, 378–379, 378*f*
Surgical hardware, magnetic resonance imaging interaction with, 99–100
Survival analysis, as research design, 139–141, 140*f*
Suspensory ligaments, of forefoot, 949, 949*f*
Sustentaculum tali
  fibroosseous tunnel release of, 989–990
  stenosing tenosynovitis of, 987, 988*f*, 989–990
Suture fixation
  in Achilles tendon repair, 982–986, 983*f*, 985*f*
  for acromioclavicular joint dislocations, 523, 523*f*–524*f*, 529*f*
  for clavicle fractures, 538
  of flexor hallucis longus tendon injuries, 990–991
  for hindfoot injuries, 923, 923*f*
  for knee repair
    of ligaments, 682, 684–685
    of posterior cruciate ligaments, 774–775, 775*f*, 777
    of tendons, 692–694, 693*f*, 699, 701–704, 702*f*
  for peroneus tendon injuries, 997–1000
  of posterior tibial tendon injuries, 1004–1007
  for quadriceps tendon rupture repair, 600, 600*f*
  for rotator cuff tears, 493
  for shoulder dislocations, with labral injuries, 447–448, 447*f*, 452, 471, 473, 473*f*
  for tibial avulsion fractures, 774–775, 775*f*, 777
Swan-neck deformity, with hand injuries, 237, 250
Sweet spot, in racquet sports, 295–296
Swimming, freestyle
  athletic pubalgia from, 225
  elbow injuries and, 319, 324
  impingement syndrome from, 563, 563*f*, 566*f*
  shoulder kinematics of, 391–392, 391*f*, 560
    pathologic, 109*f*, 562–563, 562*f*–563*f*
  stroke phases of
    biomechanics of, 391, 391*f*, 559, 560*f*, 562*f*
    early pull-through, 391, 559–560, 560*f*
    late pull-through, 391, 560–561, 560*f*
    pathologic, 561–563, 562*f*–563*f*
    recovery, 391, 560*f*, 561
  thoracic outlet syndrome from, 189
Swing phase, of running, 1012–1013
Syndesmotic sprains, of ankle, 819
Synovial abrasion, for knee meniscus healing, 650, 657
Synovial fluid
  articular cartilage relationship with, 61, 66–67
  in knee, 764–765, 853–854
  ligament cell proliferation and, 43
Synovial fringe
  of knee meniscus, 648*f*, 649–650, 657
  of tendons, 30–31
Synovial sheaths, of tendons, 21–22
  vascular, 30–31
Synovitis, of metatarsophalangeal joints, 975–976, 975*f*–976*f*
Synthetic evaluations, as research design, 124*f*, 125–127

T

Tack fixation, bioabsorbable
  for knee meniscus repairs, 655, 657*f*
  for shoulder dislocations
    anterior labral, 447–451, 447*f*, 449*f*–450*f*
    superior labral, 451–453, 453*f*, 471
Takeaway phase, of golf swing
  biomechanics of, 563–564, 564*f*
  pathologic, 565, 566*f*
Talocalcaneal joint
  anatomy of, 895–899, 897*f*–898*f*
  coalition of, 927–929, 928*f*–929*f*
Talofibular ligaments, of ankle, sprain injuries of, 819–821
Talonavicular capsule, anatomy of, 896, 897*f*
Talonavicular joints
  anatomy of, 896, 897*f*
  arthrodesis indications for, 920, 929

coalition of, 927–929
  subtalar fusion and, 927
Talotibial exostosis, 821
Talus. *See* Ankle
Tangential views, of patellofemoral joint, 718, 719*f*
Tanner staging, for anterior cruciate ligament repair, 754
Taping techniques
  for forefoot injuries, 948, 951–952
  patellar, 729, 735
  for phalanx fractures, 237–238, 246–248, 966
  for proximal interphalangeal joint ligament injuries, 246–248
  for toe injuries, 966, 970, 976, 976*f*
Tarsal coalition, in hindfoot
  evaluation of, 928–929
  imaging studies of, 928–929, 928*f*–929*f*, 988
  treatment of, 929, 930*f*
Tarsal navicular joints
  accessory, painful syndrome of, 914–915, 914*f*–915*f*
  accessory ossicles in, 914
  os peroneum of, painful, 914, 917–918, 917*f*–918*f*
  stress fractures of, 903, 905, 905*f*–907*f*, 1021
  tibial tendon reinsertion procedures for, 1003–1004
Tarsal tunnel syndrome
  anterior. *See* Anterior tarsal syndrome
  distal, 920–921
  of forefoot, 958–959, 962
  of hindfoot, 899, 899*f*–900*f*, 939–940
Tarsometatarsal joints (TMT)
  anatomy of, 893, 894*f*
  arthrodesis indications for, 911, 914, 920
  in Lisfranc's joint injuries, 907, 908*f*–911*f*, 909
Tarsometatarsal ligaments
  anatomy of, 893, 894*f*
  of hindfoot, Lisfranc's joint injuries and, 908–909, 909*f*–910*f*
Team physician
  emergency care responsibilities of, 153–154
  physical examinations by, at time of injury, 613, 901
Teardrop fractures, of cervical vertebrae, 167, 168*f*
Tear injuries. *See specific joint, ligament, or tendon*
Telos machine, for anterior cruciate ligament evaluation, 747
Temporal summation, principles of, 10, 10*f*
Tenascin
  in articular cartilage, 54*t*, 55, 66
  in tendons, 25, 26*f*
Tenderness and temperature, in knee injuries, 614, 619–620, 619*f*, 666, 696, 705
  patellofemoral, 705, 714–715, 721
Tendinitis
  of Achilles tendon, 696, 934–936, 934*f*–936*f*
  of knee. *See* Patellar tendinitis
  of posterior tibial tendon, 914–915
  of rotator cuff, 376–377
  tendinosis *versus*, 290, 689
Tendinosis
  of Achilles tendon, 696, 980–984
  of elbow. *See* Tennis elbow
  of foot, 961–962
  of knee, 689, 698
  pathophysiology of, 289–291
  tendinitis *versus*, 290, 689
Tendoblasts, function of, 23, 28–30, 29*f*
Tendocytes, function of, 23, 28–30, 29*f*
Tendon-bone junction, in knee injuries, 689–690, 692, 700
Tendon bursae, 21
Tendon cells
  metabolism role of, 23, 29–30, 29*f*
  morphology of, 24*f*, 28–29, 29*f*
Tendon grafts
  for knee repair, 630–633, 672

of anterior cruciate ligament, 47–48, 48*f*, 626, 629–632, 750–751
  of posterior cruciate ligament, 776–778, 781–784, 784*f*
  posterolateral, 682–685, 814–815
  of tendons, 701–702
  for peroneus tendon repairs, 996–999, 997*f*
  for ulnar collateral ligament repair, 317–318, 318*f*, 325
Tendon plates, muscle fiber attachments to, 3–4, 4*f*
Tendons. *See also specific muscle or tendon*
  anatomy and physiology of
    cellular, 23, 28–30, 29*f*
    elastic fibers, 22, 22*f*, 27
    extracellular ground substance, 28
    fiber orientation, three-dimensional, 23–25, 24*f*, 34
    inorganic components, 27–28
    internal architecture, 23–25, 24*f*
    macroscopic structure, 21
    myotendinous junction, 21, 25–26, 25*f*–26*f*
    nerve distribution, 31
    osteotendinous junction, 21, 26–27, 26*f*
    surrounding structures, 21–23, 22*f*
    vascular, 30–31, 290
  biomechanics of, 32–33, 33*f*
  collagen organization in, 22–25, 22*f*, 24*f*, 27
  degeneration of. *See* Tendinosis
  functions of, 31–32
  healing processes in
    enhancement of, 690–691
    intrasynovial *versus* extrasynovial, 689–690
    physiological, 688–690
  injuries of, magnetic resonance imaging of, 116–117, 117*f*, 277, 280–281, 281*f*
  insertion mechanisms of, 21, 690
  ruptures of
    biomechanics of, 33
    per tensile force, 34–35
  stress-strain curve of, 24, 24*f*, 33–34, 33*f*
  tensile strength of, 31–32, 34–35
Tendon sheaths
  anatomy and physiology of, 21–22, 30
  two-layer, 22–23, 22*f*
Tendon transfers
  for Achilles tendon repair, 982–986, 983*f*, 985*f*–986*f*
  with posterior tibial tendon reinsertions, 1005–1007
  for toe deformities, 976
Tendon zone, of osteotendinous junction, 26
Tennis
  elbow injuries from. *See* Tennis elbow
  foot injuries from, 917*f*, 994
  knee injuries from, 721
  leg injuries from, 888–889, 888*f*
  serve
    kinetic energy sources for, 418–419, 498, 499*f*
    scapula role in, 497–499, 499*f*
  stroke, shoulder kinematics of, 392–393, 392*f*–393*f*
Tennis elbow
  conservative treatment of, 294–299, 296*f*–297*f*, 550
  epidemiology of, 289–290, 296
  lateral
    injury mechanisms of, 289–293
    resection and repair of, 300–302, 300*f*–302*f*
  maximum tenderness point of, 291–292, 291*f*
  medial
    injury mechanisms of, 289–291, 293
    resection and repair of, 302–304, 303*f*
  pathoanatomy of, 289–291
  posterior
    injury mechanisms of, 290, 293
    resection and repair of, 304
  provocative tests for, 292–294
  radiography of, 293–294
  return to sport guidelines, 299
  sport mechanics impact on, 295–296
  surgical treatment of

general principles of, 299
lateral procedures, 300–302, 300f–302f
medial procedures, 302–304, 303f
posterior procedures, 304
treatment principles, 294, 299, 550
Tennis leg, 888–889, 888f
Tenodesis, for posterior shoulder dislocations, 414
Tenosynovitis
with elbow injuries, 299, 301f, 314
of flexor hallucis longus tendon, 961–962, 987–990
of peroneus tendons, 992–996
of posterior tibial tendon, 1001–1002, 1005–1007
of wrist extensors, 282, 284
Tensile load
as bone-ligament-bone complex property, 39–41, 40f
post-graft reconstruction, 47–48
knee response to, 40–41, 40f, 625–626
tendon injuries in, 688–689
Tensile strength
of articular cartilage, 57–60, 58f, 62–63, 66
of bone, 79–81, 83
of ligaments, 39–43, 40f–42f. See also specific ligament
of tendons, 31–32, 34–35. See also specific tendon
Tension
in muscles. See Muscle tension
tissue response to. See Tensile strength
Teres major muscle, anatomy of, 356
Teres minor muscle
anatomy of, 355
overhead throwing role of, 554–555, 554f
in rotator cuff biomechanics, 355, 372–373, 372f–373f
swimming stroke role of, 392, 560
Terosis, 82
Terry Thomas sign, for scapholunate injury, 275, 275f
Testicular exam, indications for, 219
Tetanic muscle contractions, 10–11, 10f–11f
Tetanus prophylaxis, 990
TFCC. See Triangular fibrocartilage complex
T-fix repair system, for knee meniscus tears, 655, 656f
Therapeutic injections. See Nerve blocks; Steroids
Thermal-assisted capsulorrhaphies. See Radiofrequency capsulorrhaphies
Thigh. See also Leg
adductor canal syndrome of, 606
adductor functions of
anatomy of, 583–585, 584f
muscle strains and, 593–596, 596t
anatomy of
iliotibial band, 585
muscle compartments, 87, 583–585, 584f–585f
nerve distributions, 583–585, 584f–585f
vascular, 230, 584–585, 584f–585f
compartment anatomy of, 87, 583–585
anterior, 583, 585, 585f, 596–597
medial, 583–585, 584f
posterior, 583–584, 584f
compartment syndromes of
acute, 604–606, 605f
chronic exertional, 606
extensor functions of
anatomy of, 583, 585, 585f
fracture injuries of, 600–604
muscle strains and, 596–598, 599f–600f, 601t
rupture mechanisms of, 598–600, 599f–600f
flexor functions of
anatomy of, 583–584, 584f
muscle strains and, 587–593, 588f–592f, 589t
hemophiliac pseudotumors of, 606
injuries of
femur fractures, 603–604
incidence of, 583
radiography for, 587, 589, 594, 597–604
strains, 587–594, 596–603
miscellaneous muscle disorders of, 606–607

muscle strains of
adductors, 593–596, 596t
hamstrings, 587–593, 588f–592f, 589t
quadriceps, 596–603, 599f–600f, 601t
vascular injuries of, 606
Thigh wraps, injury indications for, 603
Thompson test, for Achilles tendon dysfunction, 981
Thoracic outlet syndrome, neurogenic
clinical manifestations of, 189, 192–193
treatment of, 195–197
Thoracic wall, scapula retraction and protraction along, 498, 500f, 501–502
Thromboses
arterial, 285, 606
deep venous, 76, 91, 758, 889
with knee injuries, 76, 758, 810, 812
treatment of, 889
Thrombospondin
in articular cartilage, 54t, 55, 62
in knee meniscus, 647
in tendons, 28
Thrower's exostosis, 465–467, 468f, 473, 474f
Thrower's shoulder
deceleration model of, 388f, 389
glenoid labrum and, 457, 461–465, 462f–463f
hyperangulation in, 389, 389f
maximal external rotation model of, 389–391, 389f–391f
mechanisms of, 388f–391f, 389–391, 402, 406, 418–419
rotator cuff and, 464–465, 467
treatment of, 469–475, 472f–474f
Thrower's Ten Program, for rehabilitation, 475
Throwing motion. See also Pitching
impingement syndromes from, 461–465, 463f, 468, 557–559, 559f, 566f. See also Elbow joint; Shoulder joint
injuries from. See also specific injuries
in elbow, 308, 308f
rehabilitation exercises for, 406, 409, 470, 474–475
in shoulder. See Thrower's shoulder
instability mechanisms with, 389–391, 389f–390f, 402, 413, 418
off-season maintenance programs for, 469–470
overhead. See Overhead athlete
phases of, 307–308, 387, 387f, 458, 459f
scapula role in, 497–498, 499f
shoulder kinematics of, 387–388, 387f–388f
Thumb injuries
fracture mechanisms, 238–240
of ligaments, 243
radial collateral, 243, 246
ulnar collateral, 238, 243–246, 245f
Thumb spica cast
for scaphoid fractures, 263, 265–266
for ulnar collateral ligament tears, 244–245, 245f
Thumb spica splints, for scaphoid fractures, 266–267
Tibia
fractures of
avulsion, 666, 705, 772, 774–775, 777, 809, 812
incidence of, 874–875
plateau, with knee dislocations, 809
spine classifications, 747
stress, 870–872, 871f–872f, 871t, 1021
functional bracing of, with anterior cruciate ligament injuries, 863–867
instability mechanisms of, 882–885, 884f
knee injuries and. See also Maquet anteriorization procedure; Tunnel fixation
anterior cruciate ligament tears, 745, 745f, 747, 863–867
complications with, 827, 827f, 829, 829f–830f
ligament rotation and translation with, 627–634, 680–681, 754, 769–775, 769f
osteotomy indications for, 680–682, 733, 835, 837, 856–857
posterior cruciate ligament and

avulsion fractures of insertions of, 772, 772f, 774–775, 774f–775f, 812
injury evaluations and, 769–770, 769f
tunnel reconstruction procedures for, 781–784, 782f, 784f
meniscus articulation with, 645, 646f
muscles of, running force impact on, 1013
osteotomies of
complications of, 835, 837, 837f
for degeneration, 856–857
ligament indications for, 680–682, 733, 733f
rotation and translation of
functional bracing for, 863–867
with knee injuries, 627–634, 680–681, 754
posterior cruciate ligament role in, 763–767, 764f
running impact on, 1012–1013, 1016
stress fractures of
anterior cortex, 872, 872f
imaging grading system for, 870–871, 871t, 1021
shaft, 871–872, 871f
stress syndrome of. See Medial tibial stress syndrome
in tensile property testing, 40–41, 40f
tubercle of
patellofemoral considerations of, 638, 702, 712, 732–733, 732f–733f, 834
anteriorization for arthritis, 735–736, 736f, 739, 740t
prominence in adolescents, 705–706
Tibial external rotation test, for knee ligament tears, 627–634, 680
Tibial tendon, injuries of
anterior, 1007–1008
gait analysis with, 1000, 1001f, 1002–1003
in painful accessory navicular, 914–915, 916f
posterior. See Posterior tibial tendon
Tibiofemoral joint
degenerative arthritis of, 735
functional bracing of, 864
in knee biomechanics, 623–624, 627, 634–635
Tibiofibular joint
distal, syndesmosis of, 819–820, 883
instability of, proximal
classification of, 883–884, 884f
clinical evaluation of, 883
pathoanatomy of, 882–883
return to sport guidelines, 883–885, 887
treatment of, 884–885
proximal
anatomy of, 678
instability of, 882–885, 884f
in knee repair, 681–682
posterolateral knee stability role of, 678–679
rehabilitation program for, 883–884
superior, arthrodesis of, 884
synostosis of, 887–888, 888f
Tibiofibular ligaments, stability role of, 882–883, 887
Tibiofibular syndesmosis, distal
ankle motion and, 883
sprain injuries of, 819–820
Tibiofibular synostosis
acquired versus congenital, 887
clinical evaluation of, 887, 888f
treatment of, 888
Tinel's sign
with brachial plexus injuries, 191
with elbow injuries, 291, 316, 547
with foot injuries, 919, 939, 962
with wrist tendinopathies, 284–285
Tissue. See also specific type
magnetic resonance imaging of
pulse sequencing and, 101–102
signal intensity for, 100–101, 100t
Tissue engineering, for articular cartilage repair, 67
Tissue necrosis, from compartment syndromes, 88–90, 604–606
Titin, in muscle contraction, 6, 11–12

TMT. *See* Tarsometatarsal joints
Toe-off event
    biomechanics of, 979, 1000
    metatarsal injuries and, 946
Toe region, of ligament load-elongation curve,
        39–40, 40f
Toes. *See also specific bones or joints*
    deformities of
        bunion, 971f, 972
        claw, 972–973, 973f
        corns, 976
        hammer, 973
        intractable plantar keratosis, 974
        joint synovitis, 975–976, 975f–976f
        mallet, 973–974
        nonoperative treatment of, 973–976, 976f
        operative treatment of, 973–976
        shoe modifications for, 972–975, 973f
    dislocations of
        classification of, 967, 967f
        clinical evaluation of, 967
        mechanisms of, 966–967
        treatment of, 967–968
    fractures of, 966, 1021
    hallux rigidus of, 970–972, 971f
    injuries of
        dislocations, 966–968, 967f
        fractures, 966, 1021
        mechanisms of, 965–966
        nonoperative treatment of, 966–967, 969–970,
            972
        operative treatment of, 966, 968, 970, 972
        orthotics for, 970, 970f
        radiography for, 966–967, 969, 974
        return to sport guidelines, 965–966, 970
        shoe modifications for, 966, 970, 970f, 972
        sprains, 968–970, 968f–970f
        taping indications for, 966, 970, 976, 976f
    interdigital neuromas of, 957–958, 974–975,
        975f
    ligaments of, stability role of, 967
    osteotomy indications for, 972
    reconstruction techniques for, 966, 968
    rehabilitation programs for, 970, 976
    tendons of, tensile strength of, 34
Tomograms
    for carpal fractures, 261, 269–271
    of elbow, 311, 321
Tourniquet applications, compartment syndromes
        from, 90
Trace elements, importance of, 28, 82–83
Track and field, injuries from, 585, 588, 597, 994
Traction
    diagnostic, for shoulder instability, 403, 403f
    therapeutic. *See* Skeletal traction; *specific device*
Traction/countertraction closed reduction maneu-
        ver, for shoulder dislocations, 406, 406f,
        445, 445f
Traction injuries
    to brachial plexus, 162–163, 183–184, 187
    to tibia, 875
Trainers, emergency care responsibilities of,
        153–154
Training errors. *See also* Overuse injuries
    elbow injury risks from, 290, 295–296
    foot injuries from
        in forefoot, 945–946, 955
        in midfoot and hindfoot, 902, 903f–905f, 920,
            929, 931
        of tendons, 979–980
    leg injuries from, 871, 875–878
    running injuries from, 1011, 1013–1016
Training programs
    modification of. *See specific injury or sport*
    progressive, bone adaptation with, 83, 83f
    transitions in, injury risks during, 290
Transducer studies
    of knee biomechanics, 625, 628, 867
    of metatarsal injuries, 945
Transforming growth factors, for knee healing,
        690, 800
Translation movements. *See specific joint*

Transportation team, responsibilities of, for head
        and neck injuries, 153–154
Transscaphoid perilunate fracture-dislocation, 267,
        268f
Transverse tubular system (T system), of muscle
        contraction, 6, 9, 10f, 18, 18t
Trapezium fractures, 271
Trapezius muscle
    in acromioclavicular joint injuries, 512–514,
        514f, 517
        in surgical repair procedures, 526, 529–531
    anatomy of, 356–357
    golf swing role of, 564
    overhead throwing role of, 552–553, 553f
    in shoulder pathology, 501–502, 505–506, 544
    swimming stroke role of, 392, 560–561
Trapezoid ligaments
    in acromioclavicular joint
        anatomy of, 511–512, 512f
        injury mechanisms of, 514–515, 515f, 524
    clavicle fractures and, 535–536, 536f
Treadmill studies, on bone remodeling, 80–81,
        81f
Trephines, for vascular access channels, 657
Trial-and-error technique, for knee reconstruc-
        tion, 681, 684–685
Triangular fibrocartilage complex (TFCC), of
        wrist
    function of, 274–275
    injuries of
        degenerative classification, 280–282
        differential diagnosis of, 274, 277, 281
        distal radial ulnar joint instability with,
            281–282
        mechanisms of, 279–280, 282
        traumatic classification, 280–281, 280f
        treatment of, 281–282
Triangular space, in shoulder anatomy, 355–356,
        360, 360f, 362–363
Triceps brachii muscle
    anatomy of, 360
    tendinosis of, 290, 293, 304
Trigger toe, 924, 961–962
Triquetrohamate impaction syndrome, 282
Triquetrum fractures, 270
Tropomyosin, in muscle contraction, 5f, 6
Troponin, in muscle contraction, 5f, 6, 9
Trunk
    evaluation of, with scapula assessment,
        503–505, 504f–505f, 505t
    rotation of
        with golf swing, 564–565, 564f, 566f
        with pitching motion, 551–553, 552f, 559f
        pathologic, 555–557, 556f, 559f
T sign, of ulnar collateral ligament tears,
        316f–317f, 317
T system. *See* Transverse tubular system
t tests, in research studies, 136, 139, 143
TUBS syndrome, with Bankart lesion, 402
Tubular bones, structure of, 75
Tumors. *See* Neoplasms; *specific type*
Tunnel fixation, for knee reconstructions
    with anterior cruciate ligament, 629–631, 751,
        752f, 755, 815
    complications of, 827–829, 827f–828f
    with posterior cruciate ligament, 776, 778, 814
    posterolateral, 682, 684–685, 814–815
Turf toe
    biomechanics of, 968–969
    classification of, 951, 968
    clinical evaluation of, 951, 969
    etiology of, 950
    incidence of, 949, 968
    injury mechanism of, 950–951, 952f, 968, 968f
    metatarsophalangeal anatomy and, 949–950,
        949f
    outcomes of, 951
    pathoanatomy of, 969, 969f
    treatment of, 951, 969–970, 970f

U

UCBL-type orthotics
    for hindfoot injuries, 920, 923, 926–927, 927f,
        940

for midfoot injuries, 910–911, 913–914
UCL. *See* Ulnar collateral ligament
UFS system. *See* Robotic/universal force-moment
        sensor
Ulna
    deviation of, for scaphoid fracture imaging, 261,
        263
    distal resection of, for wrist ligament injuries,
        281–282
    fractures of, tennis elbow *versus,* 292
    injuries of, dorsal *versus* volar, 282
Ulnar collateral ligament (UCL)
    aponeurosis of, 116, 116f, 244–245
    bundle anatomy of, 315–316, 316f
    insertions of, 243–244
    overhead throwing role of, 554–556, 554f
    reconstructive procedures for, 245–246, 312, 325
        with grafts, 317–318, 318f, 325
    tear injuries of
        with bony fragments, 245–246
        examination guidelines for, 244, 310–311, 316
        imaging of, 116, 116f, 316–317, 316f–317f
        immobilization treatment of, 244–246, 245f
        mechanisms of
            with elbow injuries, 308–310, 308f,
                313–319, 316f–318f, 324–325
            with hand injuries, 238, 243–244
        nerve injuries with, 547–548
        from pitching, 557–559
        posterior lateral elbow instability with,
            324–325, 324f–325f
        prognosis for, 245–246
        surgical treatment of, 245–246, 312, 317–319,
            318f
Ultrasonography
    diagnostic
        of compartment syndromes, 91
        of knee tendon injuries, 691–692, 697, 699
        of muscle strains, thigh adductors, 594
        of running injuries, 1017
    therapeutic
        for knee tendon injuries, 690, 695, 699
        for lumbar spine injuries, 204
        for midfoot stress fractures, 902, 906
Unconscious athletes, emergency care of, with
        head and neck injuries, 153–160, 155f
Unipennate muscles, physiologic principles of, 7,
        7f
Upper extremities. *See also specific anatomy*
    compartment syndromes in, 87–88, 88f, 90–91
    injuries of. *See also specific anatomy*
        nerve mechanisms, 183–199, 543–550
        soft tissue, 243–254 , 273–285
        tendinopathies, 289–304
    muscle architecture of, 8–9, 9f
    nerves distributions in, 184–185, 184f–185f, 543
    nerves injuries in
        brachial plexus mechanisms, 183–199, 543,
            544f
        with elbow pathology, 547–550, 547f–548f
        with shoulder pathology, 543–547, 545f
Urinary tract infections, 215

V

Valgus extension overload test, for elbow injuries,
        310, 312
Valgus loading
    elbow injuries from
        mechanics of, 308, 308f, 312–313
        with pitching, 555, 558–559
        treatment of, 313–315, 313f–315f
    in knee
        hyperextension and, 616–617
        ligament mechanisms of, 626–627, 629, 633,
            807
            anterior cruciate, 744
            medial collateral, 663, 671–672
            posterior cruciate, 766, 772
        meniscus mechanisms of, 635–636
        osteotomy indications with, 856–857
        patellofemoral joint and, 712
    in toe injuries, 950, 968

Valgus stress test, for knee ligament tears,
665–666, 672
Validity, of research findings, 134, 146
Variance formulas, for research studies, 133–137,
145
Varus loading
in knee
hyperextension and, 616–617, 620, 678–679
ligament mechanisms of, 627, 629, 633, 680,
807
anterior cruciate, 744
posterior cruciate, 766, 771
meniscus mechanisms of, 635–636
osteotomy indications with, 856–857
in toe injuries, 950–951, 968
Varus rotation test, for knee injuries, 680, 850
Vascular access channels, for knee meniscus healing, 657
Vascular anatomy. See also Artery(ies); Vein(s)
of Achilles tendon, 30–31
of articular cartilage, 63, 67
of bone, 75, 76f, 77–78
of glenohumeral joint, 341, 342f, 343
of hand, 257, 265
of ligaments, disruption with injuries, 43–44
of lower leg, 1007
of meniscus, 648–650, 648f
of posterior cruciate ligament, 765
of rotator cuff, 353–354, 372
of shoulder, 330, 339, 341, 342f, 343, 350,
352–354, 357–358, 360
of tendons, 30–31, 290
of thigh, 230, 584–585, 584f–585f, 606
Vascular compression injuries
with clavicle fractures, 537
of popliteal vessels, 92, 810, 886–887, 886f
with knee injuries, 765, 768, 808–809, 832
Vastus intermedius muscle, injuries of, 585, 597
Vastus lateralis oblique muscle (VLO)
anatomy of, 585, 709, 710f, 806
in patellofemoral joint injuries, 729–730, 730f,
732
Vastus medialis oblique muscle (VMO)
anatomy of, 585, 709, 710f
in patellofemoral joint injuries, 712, 714,
723–724, 726, 729, 730f, 732, 735
strain injuries of, 596–597
Vater-Pacini corpuscles, as mechanoreceptors, 31
Vein(s)
of hindfoot, 899, 899f
popliteal, knee injuries and, 810
Vein grafts, for ulnar artery thrombosis, 285
Velocity
force relationship with, 12–13, 12f, 14f
muscle fiber length and, 3, 7–8, 8f–9f, 13, 14f
muscle fiber type and, 17
shin splints and, 876
in shoulder function, 498, 499f, 502–503, 503t
weather impact on, 295
Venography, indications for, 91, 889
Venous pressure, in compartment syndrome, 88
Ventral rami, of spinal nerves, in brachial plexus,
184–186, 185f
Vertebrae, injuries of. See Facet joints; specific spinal region
Vertebral body
forward displacement of. See Spondylolisthesis
fracture locations on, 205
spinal canal ratio to, 168–169, 169f, 175
Vertebral diskectomy
anterior cervical, indications for, 164, 166
lumbar, macro- versus micro-, 208
Vertebral disks
herniations of
from cervical injuries, 163–164, 169, 178
from lumbar injuries, 205–209, 206t, 208f, 962
injuries of
acute versus chronic, 163–164, 178
return to sport guidelines, 178
space narrowing of, with cervical spine injuries,
163–164, 188
Viral disease, graft transmission of, 812–813, 826
Viscoelasticity
of articular cartilage, 55–56, 58–60

of knee meniscus, 647–648
of ligaments, 41–43, 42f
of tendons, 33
Viscoplasticity, of ligament grafts, 48
VISI. See Volar intercollated segment instability
Vitamin D supplements, for foot injuries, 902,
906
Vitamins
bone formation and, 82–83
supplement indications for, 902, 906
VLO. See Vastus lateralis oblique muscle
VMO. See Vastus medialis oblique muscle
Volar flexion template, for central slip rehabilitation, 252
Volar intercollated segment instability (VISI),
with wrist injuries, 279–280
Volar ligaments, of toes, injuries of, 967–969,
967f, 969f
Volar plate
laxity risks for, 250, 257
of proximal interphalangeal joints
injury mechanisms of, 244, 247–249
ligament insertions of, 244, 246, 249
splinting options for, 250
Volkmann canals, in bone, 76f, 77
Volkmann's ischemic contractures, 87
Volleyball
foot injuries from, 907, 1000
hand fractures from, 233
knee injuries from, 691, 698
toe injuries from, 950, 968
V-Y lengthening technique
for Achilles tendon repair, 983–985, 983f
for knee tendon repair, 600, 693–694

W
Wad of Henry, mobile, elbow tendinosis and, 291
Waist-to-hip ratio, as knee osteoarthritis factor,
846
Wallerian degeneration, with nerve injuries, in
brachial plexus, 186
Wall slide exercises, for knee ligament injuries,
669, 669f
Warm-up exercises, importance of, 42, 289–290
Warping, of articular cartilage, 60
Warren technique, for knee reconstruction, 681,
684–685
Wartenberg's sign, with wrist tendinopathies,
284–285
Water, magnetic resonance imaging intensity for,
100–101, 100t
Water content, of articular cartilage, 53–55, 54t,
65
Water exercises. See Pool therapy
Watson test, for scapholunate injury, 276, 276f
Weaver-Dunn procedure, for clavicle fractures,
538
Weight-bearing
exercises for. See Closed chain exercises
foot alignment with, 1016–1017
knee osteoarthritis and, 846, 854, 856
Weighted image principles, of magnetic resonance
imaging, 100–101, 100t
Weighted kappa, in research studies, 133
Weightlessness, bone adaptation to, 80, 83, 83f
Weight lifting
compartment syndromes from, 90
lumbar spine injuries and, 205
quadriceps tendon ruptures from, 598–599
as shoulder instability rehabilitation, 409
wrist injuries from, 266, 273, 282, 285
Weight training. See Strength training
West Point view, radiographic, for shoulder instability, 421, 442, 442f, 468
Wheal formation, with brachial plexus injuries,
192
White-white tears, of knee meniscus, 649–650,
657
Wilcoxon two-sample test, in research studies, 139
Williams flexion exercises, for lumbar spine injuries, 207

Windlass effect, of plantar fascia, in gait cycle,
893, 895f
Wind-up motions
with pitching
biomechanics of, 387, 387f, 458, 459f,
551–552, 552f
pathologic, 555, 559f
with tennis, 392, 392f
Wire fixation
for hand injuries
fractures, 234–240, 234f
tendon lacerations, 250–251
for patellofemoral joint, 702, 735–736, 736f,
739, 740t
for toe fractures, 966
Wolff's law, of bone remodeling, 75, 80–81, 945,
959
Workmen's compensation claims
for groin pain, 225
for lumbar spine injuries, 203–207
Wound healing
phases of. See Healing process
prerequisites for, 650
Wrestling, injuries from, 183, 233, 431–454
Wright's maneuver, for brachial plexus injuries,
192
Wrist
anatomy of, 257, 274
four-corner fusion of, for fracture complications, 269, 270f
fractures
displacement with, 258–260, 258f, 260f–262f,
263, 264f–265f, 269–272
epidemiology of, 257
fixation of, 258f, 260, 260f, 262f, 263–265,
265f, 267, 268f–269f
imaging of, 116, 258–259, 261–263, 267,
269–271
immobilization of, 258–260, 260f, 263–267,
271–272
ligament and tendon injuries with, 267,
268f–269f, 269–271
miscellaneous bones, 269–272, 271f
ganglions of, 277
injuries of
capsuloligamentous, 274–275
case-control study on, 128, 128f
epidemiology of, 273–274
evaluation of, 274
imaging techniques for, 275f, 276–277,
279–282, 280f–281f
ligaments, 275–282, 275f–276f, 278f–281f
with fractures, 267, 268f–269f, 269–270
soft tissue, 274–282, 275f–276f, 278f–281f
magnetic resonance imaging of, 115–116,
116f
return to sport guidelines, 263–264, 266–267,
273
scaphoid bone, 257–269
of soft tissue, 273–285
tendons, 279, 282–285, 283f
instability mechanisms of, 275, 279
sprains of, diagnostic cautions with, 261,
273–274
tendinopathies of
carpal tunnel syndromes, 284–285
DeQuervain's, 282–283, 283f
extensor, 279, 283–284
flexor, 284
second compartment, 283
vascular disorders of, 285
Wrist pain
chronic, 273–274
radial-sided, 274
from scaphoid impaction syndrome, 278–279
from scapholunate injury, 274–278,
275f–276f, 278f
ulnar-sided, 274–275
from carpal tunnel syndrome, 284–285
from DeQuervain's syndrome, 282–283, 283f
from distal radial ulnar joint injury, 280–282,
280f–281f

Wrist pain (*contd.*)
  from extensor carpi ulnaris subluxation, 282
  from lunotriquetral ligament injury, 274,
    279–280, 279*f*–280*f*
  from tendinopathy, 282–284
  from triquetrohamate impaction syndrome,
    282

X
Xylocaine injection. *See* Nerve blocks

Y
Yates continuity correction, for small research
  studies, 139
Yergason test, for shoulder assessment, with labral tear injuries, 466
Young's modulus measure, of articular cartilage,
  60, 690

Z
Zanca view, radiographic

for acromioclavicular dislocations, 518,
  518*f*
for rotator cuff injuries, 483, 483*f*
Z band, in sarcomeres, 4–6, 5*f*, 11, 18, 18*t*
Zinc, importance of, 28, 82–83
Z-plasty lengthening technique, for tendon
  repair
  in ankle, 990, 1008
  in foot, 919
  in knee, 693–694, 704